PEDIATRIC
Pharmacotherapy

Second Edition

PEDIATRIC
Pharmacotherapy

Second Edition

Editors

Sandra Benavides, Pharm.D., FCCP, FPPA
Pharmacy Clinical Specialist
Salah Foundation Children's Hospital
Broward Health Medical Center
Fort Lauderdale, Florida

Milap C. Nahata, Pharm.D., M.S., FCCP, FAPhA, FASHP, FPPA
Director, Institute of Therapeutic Innovations and Outcomes
Professor Emeritus of Pharmacy, Pediatrics and Internal Medicine
Colleges of Pharmacy and Medicine
Department of Pharmacy Practice and Science
The Ohio State University College of Pharmacy
Columbus, Ohio

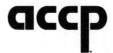

American College of Clinical Pharmacy
Lenexa, Kansas

Senior Director, Professional Development and Member Services: Nancy M. Perrin, M.A., CAE
Director of International Programs & Associate Director of Professional Development: Wafa Y. Dahdal, Pharm.D.
Managing Editor: Peter Burns
Cover Design: Dane Anderson; Layout: Steven M. Brooker
Senior Medical Editor: Kimma J. Sheldon-Old, Ph.D., M.A.
Copy Editor: Deanna Laing, ELS

For order information or questions, contact:
American College of Clinical Pharmacy
13000 West 87th Street Parkway, Suite 100
Lenexa, Kansas 66215
(913) 492-3311
(913) 492-0088 (Fax)
accp@accp.com

Printed in the United States of America
ISBN (print): 978-1-952291-03-6
ISBN (eBook): 978-1-952291-04-3
Library of Congress Control Number: 2020939196

Dedication

To Josh, Joshua, and Jude: You have given me the strength, encouragement, and purpose to live my life as it is meant to be lived, and for that I am forever grateful.

S. Benavides

I dedicate this work to my students and fellows, patients and caregivers, colleagues and collaborators, mentors and friends, and family in the United States and India for their inspiration, affection, and support.

M. Nahata

CONTENTS

CONTRIBUTORS

Susan M. Abdel-Rahman, Pharm.D.
Marion Merrell Dow/Missouri Chair in
*   Pediatric Clinical Pharmacology*
Chief, Section of Therapeutic Innovation,
*   Children's Mercy Hospital Kansas City*
Director, Health Care Innovation, Children's
*   Mercy Research Institute*
Professor of Pediatrics, University of
*   Missouri-Kansas City School of Medicine*
Department of Pediatrics
Kansas City, Missouri

Nicole M. Arwood, Pharm.D., BCPPS
Clinical Pharmacist—Hematology/Oncology
Department of Pharmacy
Ann & Robert H. Lurie Children's Hospital
*   of Chicago*
Chicago, Illinois

Alberto Augsten, Pharm.D., M.S., BCPP,
    DABAT
Pharmacy Clinical Manager
Long-Acting Therapy Clinic (LAT) Manager
PGY2 Psychiatric Pharmacy Residency
*   Director*
Board-Certified Clinical Toxicologist
Department of Pharmacy
Memorial Healthcare System
Hollywood, Florida

Sandra Benavides, Pharm.D., FCCP, FPPA
Pharmacy Clinical Specialist
Salah Foundation Children's Hospital
Broward Health Medical Center
Fort Lauderdale, Florida

Kim W. Benner, Pharm.D., FASHP, FPPA,
    BCPS
Professor of Pharmacy Practice
Department of Pharmacy Practice
Samford University McWhorter School of
*   Pharmacy*
Homewood, Alabama

M. Brooke Bernhardt, Pharm.D., M.S.,
    BCOP, BCPPS
Assistant Professor
Department of Pediatrics, Section of
*   Hematology/Oncology*
Baylor College of Medicine
Houston, Texas

Varsha Bhatt-Mehta, Pharm.D., M.S.
    (CRDSA), FCCP
Clinical Professor, Clinical Pharmacy
Clinical Professor, Pediatrics and
*   Communicable Diseases*
Department of Clinical Pharmacy, College of
*   Pharmacy*
Pediatrics and Communicable Diseases,
*   Michigan Medicine*
University of Michigan
Ann Arbor, Michigan

Sasigarn A. Bowden, M.D.
Professor of Pediatrics
Department of Pediatrics
The Ohio State University/Nationwide
*   Children's Hospital*
Columbus, Ohio

Jacob T. Brown, Pharm.D., M.S.
Assistant Professor
Pharmacy Practice and Pharmaceutical
*   Sciences*
University of Minnesota, College of
*   Pharmacy*
Duluth, Minnesota

Joshua Caballero, Pharm.D., FCCP, BCPP
Professor and Chair
Department of Clinical and Administrative
*   Sciences*
Larkin University, College of Pharmacy
Miami, Florida

Andria Farhat Church, Pharm.D., BCPS,
    BCPP
Assistant Professor of Pharmacy Practice
Department of Pharmacy Practice
Palm Beach Atlantic University—Lloyd L.
*   Gregory School of Pharmacy*
West Palm Beach, Florida

Michelle Condren, Pharm.D., FPPA,
    BCPPS, CDE, AE-C
Professor and Vice Chair for Research
Department of Pediatrics
University of Oklahoma School of
*   Community Medicine*
Tulsa, Oklahoma

Christina L. Cox, Pharm.D., BCPS, BCPPS
Clinical Associate Professor
Clinical Pharmacy and Outcomes Sciences
University of South Carolina College of
*   Pharmacy*
Columbia, South Carolina

Catherine M. Crill, Pharm.D., FCCP,
    BCNSP
Director, Office of Experiential Learning
*   and International Programs, College of*
*   Pharmacy*
Associate Professor, Departments of Clinical
*   Pharmacy & Translational Science and*
*   Pediatrics*
The University of Tennessee Health Science
*   Center*
Memphis, Tennessee

Rustin D. Crutchley, Pharm.D., AAHIVP
Clinical Associate Professor
Department of Pharmacotherapy
Washington State University, College of
*   Pharmacy and Pharmaceutical Sciences*
Yakima, Washington

Alix A. Dabb, Pharm.D.
Clinical Pharmacy Specialist, Oncology
*   Clinical Decision Support*
Department of Pharmacy
The Johns Hopkins Hospital
Baltimore, Maryland

Jean Dinh, Pharm.D., Ph.D.
Research Faculty
Clinical Pharmacology, Toxicology, and
*   Therapeutic Innovation*
Children's Mercy Hospital
Kansas City, Missouri

Kimberly Le Dinh, Pharm.D.
Clinical Pharmacy Specialist
Department of Pharmacy
Texas Children's Hospital
Houston, Texas

Duchess Domingo, Pharm.D.
Pediatric Pharmacist
Department of Pharmacy
Golisano Children's Hospital of Southwest
*   Florida*
Fort Myers, Florida

Elizabeth Farrington, Pharm.D., FCCP,
    FCCM, FPPA, BCPS, BCNSP
Clinical Pharmacist—Pediatrics
Department of Pharmacy
New Hanover Regional Medical Center,
*   Betty H. Cameron Women's and*
*   Children's Hospital*
Wilmington, North Carolina

Adinoyi O. Garba, Pharm.D., BCPS
Clinical Assistant Professor
Department of Pharmacy Practice
D'Youville School of Pharmacy
Buffalo, New York

Brooke L. Gildon, Pharm.D., BCPS, BCPPS
Associate Professor
Southwestern Oklahoma State University
*   College of Pharmacy*
Department of Pharmacy Practice
Weatherford, Oklahoma

Heather L. Girand, Pharm.D., BCPPS
Professor
Department of Pharmacy Practice
Ferris State University College of Pharmacy
Kalamazoo, Michigan

Mark R. Haase, Pharm.D., FCCP, BCPS
Associate Professor
Department of Pharmacy Practice
Texas Tech University Health Sciences Center
*   Jerry H. Hodge School of Pharmacy*
Amarillo, Texas

Tracy M. Hagemann, Pharm.D., FCCP, FPPA
Professor and Associate Dean
Department of Clinical Pharmacy and Translational Science
University of Tennessee, College of Pharmacy
Nashville, Tennessee

Rohan K. Henry, M.D., M.S.
Attending Physician
Nationwide Children's Hospital
Section of Endocrinology & Diabetes
Assistant Professor of Pediatrics
The Ohio State University College of Medicine
Columbus, Ohio

Cherry W. Jackson, Pharm.D., FCCP, FASHP, BCPP
Professor of Pharmacy
Auburn University
Clinical Professor, Psychiatry and Behavioral Neurobiology
University of Alabama, Birmingham
Birmingham, Alabama

Peter N. Johnson, Pharm.D., FPPA, FCCM, BCPS, BCPPS
Professor of Pharmacy Practice
President's Associate Presidential Professor
The University of Oklahoma College of Pharmacy
Clinical Pharmacy Specialist—Pediatric Critical Care
The Children's Hospital at OU Medical Center
Oklahoma City, Oklahoma

Tiffany Kessler, Pharm.D., BCPS
Associate Professor
Department of Pharmacy Practice
Southwestern Oklahoma State University
Weatherford, Oklahoma

Kristin C. Klein, Pharm.D., FPPA, BCPPS
Clinical Professor and Clinical Pharmacist Specialist
College of Pharmacy and Department of Pharmacy
University of Michigan and Michigan Medicine
Ann Arbor, Michigan

Tiffany-Jade M. Kreys, Pharm.D., BCPP
Assistant Dean of Student Affairs & Admissions
Assistant Professor
Clinical & Administrative Science Department
California Northstate University
Elk Grove, California

Robert J. Kuhn, Pharm.D., FCCP, FPPA, FASHP
Professor of Pharmacy Practice and Science
Pharmacy Practice and Science and Pediatrics
University of Kentucky College of Pharmacy
Lexington, Kentucky

Weng Man Lam, Pharm.D., M.S., BCPS, BCPPS
Pediatric Critical Care Clinical Pharmacist Specialist
Department of Pharmacy
Children's Memorial Hermann Hospital
Houston, Texas

Stacie J. Lampkin, Pharm.D., BCACP, BCPPS, AE-C
Associate Professor/Clinical Pediatric Ambulatory Care Pharmacist
Department of Pharmacy Practice
D'Youville School of Pharmacy
Buffalo, New York

Jennifer Le, Pharm.D., MAS, FCCP, FIDSA, FCSHP, BCPS-AQ ID
Professor of Clinical Pharmacy
Skaggs School of Pharmacy and Pharmaceutical Sciences
University of California San Diego
La Jolla, California

Teresa V. Lewis, Pharm.D., BCPS
Associate Professor
The University of Oklahoma Health Sciences Center
College of Pharmacy
Oklahoma City, Oklahoma

Lisa Lubsch, Pharm.D., FPPA, BCPPS, AE-C
Clinical Professor and Pediatric Pharmacist
Department of Pharmacy Practice
Southern Illinois University Edwardsville School of Pharmacy and Cardinal Glennon Children's Hospital
St. Louis, Missouri

Shirin Madzhidova, Pharm.D.
Assistant Professor—Pediatrics
Department of Pharmacy Practice
Philadelphia College of Osteopathic Medicine Georgia
Suwanee, Georgia

Kalen Manasco, Pharm.D., FCCP, FPPA, BCPS
Clinical Professor/Clinical Specialist
Department of Pharmacotherapy and Translational Research
University of Florida College of Pharmacy and UF Health Shands
Gainesville, Florida

Jamie L. Miller, Pharm.D., FPPA, BCPS, BCPPS
Professor
Department of Pharmacy: Clinical and Administrative Sciences
PGY1 Pharmacy Residency Program Director
University of Oklahoma College of Pharmacy
Oklahoma City, Oklahoma

Amy C. Min, Pharm.D., BCACP, AAHIVP
Clinical Assistant Professor
Department of Pharmacy Practice
Temple University School of Pharmacy
Philadelphia, Pennsylvania

Brady S. Moffett, Pharm.D., MPH, MBA
Assistant Director, Pharmacy
Department of Pharmacy
Texas Children's Hospital
Assistant Professor, Pediatrics
Department of Pediatrics
Baylor College of Medicine
Houston, Texas

Milap C. Nahata, Pharm.D., M.S., FCCP, FAPhA, FASHP, FPPA
Director, Institute of Therapeutic Innovations and Outcomes
Professor Emeritus of Pharmacy, Pediatrics and Internal Medicine
Colleges of Pharmacy and Medicine
Department of Pharmacy Practice and Science
The Ohio State University College of Pharmacy
Columbus, Ohio

Stephanie D. Natale, Pharm.D.
Pharmacist
Rady Children's Hospital
San Diego, California

Johanna L. Norman, Pharm.D., BCPPS
Critical Care Clinical Pharmacist
Le Bonheur Children's Hospital
Memphis, Tennessee

Vinita B. Pai, Pharm.D., M.S.
Associate Professor of Clinical Pharmacy and Advanced Patient Care Pharmacist
Department of Pharmacy Practice and Sciences/Pharmacy
The Ohio State University/Nationwide Children's Hospital
Columbus, Ohio

Hanna Phan, Pharm.D., FCCP, FPPA
Associate Professor and Assistant Department Head
Department of Pharmacy Practice & Science
The University of Arizona, College of Pharmacy
Associate Professor
Department of Pediatrics
The University of Arizona, College of Medicine
Tucson, Arizona

Stephanie V. Phan, Pharm.D., BCPP
Clinical Pharmacist Researcher
Pharmacy and Quality Measurement Division
Health Services Advisory Group
Tampa, Florida

Amy L. Potts, Pharm.D., BCPPS
Program Director, Quality/Safety &
Education
Monroe Carell Jr. Children's Hospital at
Vanderbilt
Department of Pharmacy
Franklin, Tennessee

David E. Procaccini, Pharm.D., MPH,
BCPS, CACP
Clinical Pharmacy Practitioner, Pediatric
Intensive Care & Cardiology/Heart
Transplant
Department of Pharmacy
The Johns Hopkins Hospital
Baltimore, Maryland

Jose A. Rey, Pharm.D., M.S., BCPP
Professor
Department of Pharmacy Practice
Nova Southeastern University
Davie, Florida

Juan Carlos Rodriguez, Pharm.D., BCPPS
Clinical Manager
Department of Pharmacy
Joe DiMaggio Children's Hospital
Hollywood, Florida

Anita Siu, Pharm.D., BCPPS
Clinical Professor
Department of Pharmacy Practice and
Administration
Rutgers, The State University of New Jersey/
Ernest Mario School of Pharmacy
Piscataway, New Jersey
Neonatal/Pediatric Pharmacotherapy
Specialist
Department of Pharmacy and Pediatrics
Jersey Shore University Medical Center/
K. Hovnanian Children's Hospital
Neptune, New Jersey

Joanie Spiro Stevens, Pharm.D., BCPS,
BCPPS
Pharmacy Clinical Manager
PGY2 Pediatric Residency Program Director
Pharmacy Department
Joe DiMaggio Children's Hospital
Hollywood, Florida

Jeremy Stultz, Pharm.D., BCPPS
Assistant Professor
Clinical Pharmacy and Translational Science
University of Tennessee Health Science
Center College of Pharmacy
Antimicrobial Stewardship Pharmacist
Department of Pharmacy
Le Bonheur Children's Hospital
Memphis, Tennessee

Christopher A. Thomas, Pharm.D., MBA,
BCPPS
Manager of Clinical Pharmacy Services
Department of Pharmacy Services
Phoenix Children's Hospital
Phoenix, Arizona

M. Tuan Tran, Pharm.D., BCPS
Infectious Disease Pharmacist
Department of Pharmacy Services
CHOC Children's Hospital
Orange, California

Heidi Trinkman, Pharm.D.
Clinical Pharmacy Specialist, Pediatric
Hematology/Oncology and Stem-Cell
Transplantation
Department of Pharmacy
Cook Children's Medical Center
Fort Worth, Texas

Jose Valdes, Pharm.D., BCPP
Medical Science Liaison
U.S. Clinical Development & Medical Affairs
Novartis Pharmaceuticals Corporation
Windermere, Florida

Jeffrey L. Wagner, Pharm.D., MPH, BCPS
Assistant Vice President
Pharmacy, Respiratory Care, and ECMO
Services
Texas Children's Hospital
Houston, Texas

Mary A. Worthington, Pharm.D., FPPA,
BCPPS, BCPS
Professor
Department of Pharmacy Practice
Samford University
Birmingham, Alabama

Tara E. Wright, Pharm.D., BCOP, BCPPS
Pediatric Hematology/Oncology Clinical
Pharmacist
Department of Pharmacy
Seattle Children's Hospital
Seattle, Washington

Reviewers

Titilola Afolabi, Pharm.D., BCPS, BCPPS
Assistant Professor
Department of Pharmacy Practice
Midwestern University—Glendale, College of Pharmacy
Glendale, Arizona

Danielle M. Alm, Pharm.D., BCPS, BCPPS
Assistant Professor of Clinical Pharmacy
Department of Pharmacy Practice & Pharmacy Administration
Philadelphia College of Pharmacy at University of the Sciences
Philadelphia, Pennsylvania
Pediatric Clinical Pharmacy Specialist— Pediatrics
Department of Pharmacy
Children's Regional Hospital at Cooper University Health Care
Camden, New Jersey

Joni Beck, Pharm.D., BC-ADM, CDE
Clinical Professor and Clinical Programs Director
OUHSC College of Medicine
Pediatric Diabetes & Endocrinology
Oklahoma City, Oklahoma

M. Brooke Bernhardt, Pharm.D., M.S., BCOP, BCPPS
Assistant Professor
Department of Pediatrics, Section of Hematology/Oncology
Baylor College of Medicine
Houston, Texas

Brookie M. Best, Pharm.D., MAS
Associate Dean for Pharmacy Education
Professor of Clinical Pharmacy and Pediatrics
Skaggs School of Pharmacy and Pharmaceutical Sciences
Pediatrics Department, School of Medicine— Rady Children's Hospital San Diego
University of California, San Diego
La Jolla, California

Allison B. Blackmer, Pharm.D., FCCP, BCPS, BCPPS
Associate Professor of Pharmacy
Department of Clinical Pharmacy
University of Colorado Skaggs School of Pharmacy and Pharmaceutical Sciences
Clinical Pharmacy Specialist
Special Care Clinic
Children's Hospital Colorado
Aurora, Colorado

Gabriella Blyumin, Pharm.D., BCPPS
Clinical Pharmacy Specialist—Pediatric Intensive Care
Department of Pharmacy
Nicklaus Children's Hospital
Miami, Florida

Kelly S. Bobo, Pharm.D., MBA, BCPS, BCPPS
Clinical Pharmacy Manager
Department of Pharmacy
Le Bonheur Children's Hospital
Memphis, Tennessee

Laura R. Bobolts, Pharm.D., BCOP
Senior Vice President, Pharmacy
Oncology Analytics, Inc.
Coconut Creek, Florida

Brian K. Brown, Pharm.D., BCPS, BCPPS
CVICU/Cardiac Transplant Clinical Pharmacist
Department of Pharmacy
Johns Hopkins All Children's Hospital
St. Petersburg, Florida

Joshua Caballero, Pharm.D., FCCP, BCPP
Professor and Chair
Department of Clinical and Administrative Sciences
Larkin University, College of Pharmacy
Miami, Florida

Andrea Calvert, Pharm.D.
Clinical Pharmacy Specialist—Neurology
Department of Pharmacy
Children's Hospital Colorado
Aurora, Colorado

Roxane Carr, Pharm.D., BCPS
Clinical Coordinator
Department of Pharmacy
Children's & Women's Health Centre of BC
Assistant Professor, Part-time
Faculty of Pharmaceutical Sciences
University of British Columbia
Vancouver, British Columbia, Canada

Rachel B. Carroll, Pharm.D., BCPPS
Clinical Pharmacy Specialist, Pediatric Hematology, Oncology, Bone Marrow Transplant
Department of Pharmacy
Children's Healthcare of Atlanta
Atlanta, Georgia

Benjamin Chavez, Pharm.D., BCPP, BCACP
Director of Behavioral Health Pharmacy Services
Salud Family Health Center
Ft. Lupton, Colorado

Allison M. Chung, Pharm.D., FCCP, BCPPS
Associate Professor
Department of Pharmacy Practice
Auburn University, Harrison School of Pharmacy
Adjunct Associate Professor
Department of Pediatrics
University of South Alabama, School of Medicine
Mobile, Alabama

Abigail Clark, Pharm.D., BCOP
Medical Science Liaison
Department of Medical Affairs
Clovis Oncology
Indianapolis, Indiana

Christina L. Cox, Pharm.D., BCPS, BCPPS
Clinical Associate Professor
Clinical Pharmacy and Outcomes Sciences
University of South Carolina College of Pharmacy
Columbia, South Carolina

Julianna Crain, Pharm.D., BCPPS, AE-C
Pediatric Critical Care Pharmacy Clinical Specialist
Department of Pharmacy
Joe DiMaggio Children's Hospital
Hollywood, Florida

Jessica Forster, Pharm.D., BCPS, BCPPS
Pediatric Pharmacist
Department of Pharmacy Services
UC Davis Children's Hospital
Sacramento, California

Elizabeth A.S. Goswami, Pharm.D., BCPS, BCPPS
Clinical Pharmacy Specialist
Department of Pharmacy
The Johns Hopkins Hospital
Baltimore, Maryland

Sean G. Green, Pharm.D., BCOP
Pediatric Clinical Pharmacy Specialist, Hematology/Oncology
Department of Pharmacy
Lucile Packard Children's Hospital, Stanford University
Stanford, California

Brent Hall, Pharm.D., BCPPS
Senior Pharmacist, Pediatrics
Department of Pharmacy
UC Davis Health
Sacramento, California

Robin N. Hieber, Pharm.D., BCPP
Clinical Pharmacy Specialist, Mental Health
VISN 23 Clinical Resource Hub
Veterans Affairs
Antioch, Illinois

David S. Hoff, Pharm.D., FCCP, FPPA, BCPPS
Clinical Leader
Pharmacy Department
Children's Hospitals and Clinics of Minnesota
Minneapolis, Minnesota

Naomi House, Pharm.D., BCPP
Clinical Pharmacy Practitioner, Psychiatry
Department of Pharmacy
Wolfson Children's Hospital
Jacksonville, Florida

Bethany W. Ibach, Pharm.D., BCPPS
Assistant Professor
Department of Pharmacy Practice
Texas Tech University Health Sciences Center
Jerry H. Hodge School of Pharmacy
Abilene, Texas

Todd A. Kociancic, Pharm.D., BCPPS
Clinical Pharmacist
Department of Pharmacy Services
Phoenix Children's Hospital
Phoenix, Arizona

Karen Kovey, Pharm.D., BCPS, BCPPS
Pediatric Clinical Specialist
Department of Pharmacy
Mission Children's Hospital
Asheville, North Carolina

Kristen Lamberjack, Pharm.D., BCACP, AAHIVP
Advanced Patient Care Pharmacist
Nationwide Children's Hospital
Columbus, Ohio

Allison Lardieri, Pharm.D., BCPPS
Safety Evaluator
Division of Pharmacovigilance
U.S. Food and Drug Administration
Silver Spring, Maryland

Joseph M. LaRochelle, Pharm.D., FCCP, BCPPS
Coleman Endowed Professor of Pharmacy Practice and Vice Chair
Division of Clinical and Administrative Sciences
Xavier University of Louisiana College of Pharmacy
Clinical Professor
Louisiana State University Health Sciences Center School of Medicine
New Orleans, Louisiana

Bernard R. Lee, Pharm.D., BCPS, BCPPS
Clinical Pharmacist
Department of Pharmacy
Mease Countryside Hospital—BayCare Health
Safety Harbor, Florida

Alex Lopilato, Pharm.D., BCPPS
Pediatric Cardiology Pharmacy Specialist, Residency Program Director
Children's Pharmacy
AdventHealth for Children
Orlando, Florida

Jenana Maker, Pharm.D., BCPS
Professor
Department of Pharmacy Practice
University of the Pacific School of Pharmacy
Stockton, California
Staff Pharmacist
Pharmacy Department
University of California Davis Medical Center
Sacramento, California

Kelly L. Matson, Pharm.D., B.S., BCPPS
Clinical Professor
Department of Pharmacy Practice
University of Rhode Island
Kingston, Rhode Island

Chephra McKee, Pharm.D., BCPPS
Assistant Professor
Department of Pharmacy Practice
Texas Tech University Health Sciences Center
Jerry H. Hodge School of Pharmacy
Abilene, Texas

Jamie L. Miller, Pharm.D., FPPA, BCPS, BCPPS
Professor
Department of Pharmacy: Clinical and Administrative Sciences
PGY1 Pharmacy Residency Program Director
University of Oklahoma College of Pharmacy
Oklahoma City, Oklahoma

Jill A. Morgan, Pharm.D., BCPS, BCPPS
Professor and Chair
Department of Pharmacy Practice and Science
University of Maryland School of Pharmacy
Baltimore, Maryland

Jennifer L. Morris, Pharm.D., BCPS, BCPPS
Assistant Director of Clinical Services—Specialty Pharmacy
Clinical Pharmacy Specialist—Dialysis
Department of Pharmacy
Texas Children's Hospital
Houston, Texas

Allison L. Mruk, Pharm.D., BCPPS
Clinical Pharmacy Specialist—Critical Care
Department of Pharmacy Services
Phoenix Children's Hospital
Phoenix, Arizona

Michael D. Nailor, Pharm.D., BCPS
Clinical Specialist—Infectious Diseases
Department of Pharmacy Services
St. Joseph's Hospital and Medical Center
Phoenix, Arizona

Sarah D. Newman, Pharm.D., BCPS, BCPPS
Clinical Hospital Pharmacist—Pediatric Emergency Medicine
Department of Pharmacy Services
Holtz Children's Hospital—Jackson Health System
Miami, Florida

Catherine E. O'Brien, Pharm.D.
Associate Professor of Pharmacy Practice
Department of Pharmacy Practice
University of Arkansas for Medical Sciences College of Pharmacy
Little Rock, Arkansas

Kirsten H. Ohler, Pharm.D., BCPS, BCPPS
Clinical Associate Professor
Clinical Pharmacist Specialist, Pediatrics/NICU
Program Director, PGY1 Pharmacy Residency
Department of Pharmacy Practice
University of Illinois at Chicago
University of Illinois Hospital & Health Sciences System
Chicago, Illinois

Karisma Patel, Pharm.D., BCPPS, BCIDP
Clinical Specialist Pharmacist, Pediatric Infectious Diseases
Department of Pharmacy
Children's Health
Dallas, Texas

Rebecca S. Pettit, Pharm.D., B.A., BCPS, BCPPS
Pediatric Pulmonary Ambulatory Specialist
Department of Pharmacy
Riley Hospital for Children at IU Health
Indianapolis, Indiana

Denise I. Pinal, Pharm.D., BCPPS
Clinical Assistant Professor
Department of Pharmacy Practice and Clinical Sciences
University of Texas at El Paso School of Pharmacy
El Paso, Texas

Renee F. Robinson, Pharm.D., MPH, MSPharm
Associate Professor
Department of Pharmacy Practice and Administration
University of Alaska/Idaho State University College of Pharmacy
Anchorage, Alaska

Cheryl L. Sargel, Pharm.D., BCCCP
Advanced Patient Care Pharmacist
Department of Pharmacy
Nationwide Children's Hospital
Columbus, Ohio

Anita Siu, Pharm.D., BCPPS
Clinical Professor
Department of Pharmacy Practice and Administration
Rutgers, The State University of New Jersey/Ernest Mario School of Pharmacy
Piscataway, New Jersey
Neonatal/Pediatric Pharmacotherapy Specialist
Department of Pharmacy and Pediatrics
Jersey Shore University Medical Center/K. Hovnanian Children's Hospital
Neptune, New Jersey

Kimberly Tallian, Pharm.D., APh, BCPP
Advanced Practice Pharmacist—Neuropsychiatry
Department of Pharmacy
Scripps Mercy Hospital, San Diego
San Diego, California

Marla C. Tanski, Pharm.D., MPH, BCPPS
Clinical Pharmacy Manager
Department of Pharmacy
Johns Hopkins All Children's Hospital
St. Petersburg, Florida

Mary Temple-Cooper, Pharm.D., M.S., B.S.,
  BCPS
Clinical Manager
Department of Pharmacy
Hillcrest Hospital—Cleveland Clinic
Mayfield Heights, Ohio

Jena Valdes, Pharm.D., BCPPS
Inpatient Pharmacy Manager
Department of Pharmacy
Johns Hopkins All Children's Hospital
St. Petersburg, Florida

DISCLOSURE OF POTENTIAL CONFLICTS OF INTEREST

Consultancies: Susan M. Abdel-Rahman (Missouri HealthNet; American Regent; Becton-Dickinson; WHO); Alberto Augsten (Janssen); Sandra Benavides (Handtevy; Alkermes [spouse or significant other]); Kim W. Benner (Alabama Pharmacy Association; Alabama Society of Health-System Pharmacists; Pediatric Pharmacy Association [PPA]); Varsha Bhatt-Mehta (LexiComp; Precision Xtract; Rxescue); Allison B. Blackmer (American Society for Parenteral and Enteral Nutrition [ASPEN]; American College of Clinical Pharmacy [ACCP]; Colorado Department of Health Care Policy & Financing; American Association of Colleges of Pharmacy [AACP]; PPA); Kelly S. Bobo (Board of Pharmacy Specialties [BPS]; Cumberland Pharmaceuticals); Joshua Caballero (American Society of Health-System Pharmacists [ASHP]; Alkermes); Andrea Calvert (LexiComp); Benjamin Chavez (BPS; College of Psychiatric and Neurologic Pharmacists [CPNP]); Allison M. Chung (ACCP; Ozanam Charitable Pharmacy; MobilCare); Andria Farhat Church (CPNP); Michelle Condren (LexiComp); Alix A. Dabb (NCUN); Tracy M. Hagemann (LexiComp; Dispensary of Hope; Cumberland Emerging Technologies Life Sciences Center); David S. Hoff (Midwest Inquiry); Cherry W. Jackson (ACCP; CPNP; ASHP); Peter N. Johnson (ASHP); Tiffany Kessler (Oklahoma Society of Health-System Pharmacists); Kristin C. Klein (PPA); Robert J. Kuhn (Cystic Fibrosis Foundation [CFF]); Kristen Lamberjack (Oscar); Stacie J. Lampkin (New York State Department of Health); Jennifer Le (Antimicrobial Drugs Advisory Committee, FDA; Agency for Healthcare Research and Quality, Healthcare Patient Safety and Quality Improvement Research; NIH, Special Emphasis Panel/Scientific Review Group, Respiratory Sciences—Small Business Study Section); Kelly L. Matson (Rhode Island Department of Health; East Greenwich Substance Misuse Task Force; PPA; AACP Pediatric Pharmacy SIG); Jamie L. Miller (ASHP); Jill A. Morgan (Church & Dwight; NFID Summit on Vitamin A in Measles Management; ASHP); Milap C. Nahata (Global Alliance for TB Drug Development); Rebecca S. Pettit (Gilead Sciences; Vertex Pharmaceuticals); Hanna Phan (Wolters Kluwer); Amy L. Potts (Institute for Safe Medication Practices; ASHP; LexiComp); Anita Siu (BPS); Heidi Trinkman (LexiComp); Jeffrey L. Wagner (Omniceutical); Mary A. Worthington (PPA)

Stock Ownership: Allison M. Chung (MobilCare [spouse or significant other]); Abigail Clark (Clovis Oncology); Catherine E. O'Brien (Radius Health [spouse or significant other]); Jose Valdes (Novartis)

Royalties: Sandra Benavides (ASHP [self and spouse or significant other]); Jean Dinh (ReveraGen BioPharma); Tracy M. Hagemann (ASHP); Jennifer Le (ACCP); Vinita B. Pai (Harvey Whitney Books); Hanna Phan (ASHP); David E. Procaccini (Silvergate/Azurity)

Grants: Susan M. Abdel-Rahman (Nabriva; NIH-NICHD; Merck Sharp & Dohme); M. Brooke Bernhardt (Celgene); Allison B. Blackmer (Department of Clinical Pharmacy Faculty Grant Program; NIH; Clinical and Operational Effectiveness and Patient Safety Small Grants Program; FDA; ASPEN); Jacob T. Brown (Whiteside Institute for Clinical Research); Roxane Carr (Canadian Society of Hospital Pharmacists); Allison M. Chung (Auburn University, Biggio Center); Christina L. Cox (University of South Carolina School of Medicine); Tracy M. Hagemann (Merck; GlaxoSmithKline); Cherry W. Jackson (Auburn University); Peter N. Johnson (University of Oklahoma [OU] College of Pharmacy; OU College of Medicine—Department of Pediatrics [Section of Critical Care]); Jamie L. Miller (OU College of Pharmacy); Jill A. Morgan (CERSI/FDA); Jennifer L. Morris (National Institute of Allergy and Infectious Diseases [NIAID]); Rebecca S. Pettit (Theravance); Hanna Phan (CFF; NHLBI/NIH); David E. Procaccini (Grifols Pharmaceuticals/Medical Affairs); Anita Siu (Catalant); Jeremy Stultz (NIAID; Fresenius Kabi AG)

Honoraria: Susan M. Abdel-Rahman (Abbott Nutrition Health Institute); Alberto Augsten (Janssen; Alkermes); Kim W. Benner (Jefferson County Pharmaceutical Association); Laura R. Bobolts (*Pharmacy Times* Continuing Education); Christina L. Cox (ACCP); Sean G. Green (Stanford University/Jazz Pharmaceuticals); Cherry W. Jackson (ACCP; Mississippi Pharmacists Association and Mississippi Society of Health-System Pharmacists; Auburn University); Joseph M. LaRochelle (ACCP); Lisa Lubsch (PTCS; NACFC); Kelly L. Matson (Association of Regulatory Boards of Optometry; American Pharmacists Association); Chephra McKee (Texas Society of Health-System Pharmacists); Jose A. Rey (Otsuka America; Janssen; Alkermes); Cheryl L. Sargel (Chicagoland Critical Care Conference); Jeremy Stultz (PPA Meeting Presentations); Heidi Trinkman (Jazz Pharmaceuticals; BTG/Boston Scientific)

Other: M. Brooke Bernhardt (Children's Oncology Group, continuing education committee chair); Jeremy Stultz (pending grant submissions could total 5%–20% salary release that would go to institution, University of Tennessee Health Science Center); Jose Valdes ("During the time this manuscript was initiated, Jose Valdes worked at Nova Southeastern University, College of Pharmacy. Prior to publication of the manuscript [06/2020], he started employment as a Medical Science Liaison at Novartis Pharmaceuticals Corporation.")

Nothing to disclose: Titilola Afolabi; Danielle M. Alm; Nicole M. Arwood; Joni Beck; Brookie M. Best; Gabriella Blyumin; Sasigarn A. Bowden; Brian K. Brown; Rachel B. Carroll; Julianna Crain; Catherine M. Crill; Rustin D. Crutchley; Kimberly Le Dinh; Duchess Domingo; Elizabeth Farrington; Jessica Forster; Adinoyi O. Garba; Brooke L.

Gildon; Heather L. Girand; Elizabeth A.S. Goswami; Mark R. Haase; Brent Hall; Rohan K. Henry; Robin N. Hieber; Naomi House; Bethany W. Ibach; Todd A. Kociancic; Karen Kovey; Tiffany-Jade M. Kreys; Weng Man Lam; Allison Lardieri; Bernard R. Lee; Teresa V. Lewis; Alex Lopilato; Shirin Madzhidova; Jenana Maker; Kalen Manasco; Amy C. Min; Brady S. Moffett; Allison L. Mruk; Michael D. Nailor; Stephanie D. Natale; Sarah D. Newman; Johanna L. Norman; Kirsten H. Ohler; Karisma Patel; Stephanie V. Phan; Denise I. Pinal; Renee F. Robinson; Juan Carlos Rodriguez; Joanie Spiro Stevens; Kimberly Tallian; Marla C. Tanski; Mary Temple-Cooper; Christopher A. Thomas; M. Tuan Tran; Jena Valdes; Tara Wright

PREFACE

Optimal use of pharmacotherapy in pediatric patients continues to advance as a result of increased research of childhood diseases and treatments, approval of new medications, and availability of clinical guidelines. However, many challenges still exist in selecting optimal drug therapy for individual pediatric patients. Because the pediatric population is distinct from the adult population, drugs must often be used differently in pediatric patients. The uniqueness of neonates, infants, children, and adolescents goes beyond the physical and developmental distinctions. Consequently, drugs behave differently in this population. Medications may not be absorbed, distributed, metabolized, or eliminated the same as in adults, and the pharmacokinetics of medications may vary across the age continuum from birth to adolescence. Furthermore, medications may have altered pharmacodynamics in children compared with adults, causing increased or decreased efficacy or safety, about which much is still unknown. Adding to the complexity of optimal use of pharmacotherapy in pediatric patients are the unique health conditions that affect children, which may not yet be fully understood.

Each day, pediatric clinicians face challenges in selecting the appropriate pharmacotherapy for children and adolescents. Yet until the past decade, there was no resource to guide aspiring pediatric pharmacists in selecting the best pharmacotherapeutic approach. Since publication of the first edition of *Pediatric Pharmacotherapy* in 2013, several other resources have been developed for pediatric pharmacists at varying degrees of practice. However, to be most helpful to pharmacy students, residents, and practitioners caring for pediatric patients, the second edition of *Pediatric Pharmacotherapy* remains uniquely focused on common illnesses and pharmacotherapies. Written, reviewed, and edited by experienced clinicians and educators, this book presents an overview of disease pathophysiology, clinical features of disease, clear goals for therapy, and insightful treatment considerations specific to pediatric patients on the basis of the primary literature, the clinical guidelines, and extensive clinical experience. Contributors to the book offer essential knowledge in each topic, together with a detailed description of pharmacotherapeutic options. As educators and clinicians, they understand the need for a concise, easy-to-understand, yet thorough resource that will allow readers to serve their patients most effectively.

The second edition includes new chapters on acute kidney injury, oncologic emergencies, and adrenal insufficiency. Each of these clinical conditions has specific areas in which pharmacists can positively affect patient care. Also new to the second edition are patient-specific cases in all disease-specific chapters, developed to help readers apply the information presented in each chapter. Cases highlight common pediatric disorders or diseases that may be encountered in clinical care in an ambulatory, community, or acute setting, and guide readers through the Pharmacists' Patient Care Process to develop and implement appropriate pharmacotherapeutic care plans.

The vision for the second edition remains the same as for the first: to create a resource to help students, residents, and practitioners learn about the unique intricacies of pediatric patients and pediatric pharmacotherapies. For students using this textbook in a pediatric elective or advanced pharmacy practice experience, we hope it will spark their interest in pursuing practice in this dynamic and rewarding specialty. For PGY1 residents gaining experience in a pediatric rotation, we hope it will be their initial point of reference to understand an approach to treating patients. For those early in their careers, or those occasionally caring for pediatric patients in any setting, we hope it will inspire them to learn more about medication use in children. In the second edition, our overarching intent continues to be to empower readers to positively affect the care of the pediatric population.

Sandra Benavides
Milap C. Nahata

ACKNOWLEDGMENTS

We, the editors of the second edition of *Pediatric Pharmacotherapy*, would like to express our appreciation for the time and work invested by its dedicated authors, particularly for their diligence to the revisions that came from the reviewers, editors, and medical editor. We also appreciate the time given by each expert who reviewed the chapters to ensure the authors had presented the most current and relevant issues. We know the time devoted to these tasks usually took authors and reviewers away from other activities, responsibilities, and family, and we are grateful for their sacrifices.

Moreover, the second edition would not have been possible without the many ACCP staff members who contributed. We appreciate your dedication to the book.

With its mission to "improve human health by extending the frontiers of clinical pharmacy," ACCP has been instrumental in promoting clinical pharmacy through research, practice, and education. Throughout the creation of the book, we stayed true to ACCP's vision to produce a text that would teach pharmacy students, residents, and practitioners about the uniqueness of pharmacotherapy in pediatric patients. We are grateful to ACCP for its ongoing and enthusiastic support of this project.

Finally, we thank all the practitioners who care for children on a daily basis and those who contribute to the literature through original research, review articles, and case reports. Without these clinical experiences and publications, our vision for this book would never have been accomplished.

5-ASA	5-Aminosalicylate		ASPEN	American Society of Parenteral and Enteral Nutrition
5-HIAA	5-Hydroxyindoleacetic acid		AST	Aspartate aminotransferase
6-MP	6-Mercaptopurine		AT	Angiotensin
25-OH-D	25-Hydroxyvitamin D		ATN	Acute tubular necrosis
AACAP	American Academy of Child and Adolescent Psychiatry		ATRA	All–trans-retinoic acid
AAN	American Academy of Neurology		AUC	Area under the curve
AAP	American Academy of Pediatrics		AUC/MIC	Area under the curve/minimum inhibitory concentration
ABC	ATP-binding cassette		AUC_{0-24}	24-Hour area under the curve
ABC-I	Aberrant Behavior Checklist—Irritability subscale		AV	Atrioventricular
ABPM	Ambulatory blood pressure measurement		AVNRT	Atrioventricular nodal reentrant tachycardia
ABR	Annual bleeding rate		AVRT	Atrioventricular reentrant tachycardia
ABRS	Acute bacterial rhinosinusitis		B	Bolus dose
AC	Activated charcoal		BBB	Blood-brain barrier
ACE	Angiotensin-converting enzyme		BCMA	Barcode medication administration
ACEI	Angiotensin-converting enzyme inhibitor		BDD	B-domain deleted
ACIP	Advisory Committee on Immunization Practices		BED	Binge eating disorder
ACS	Acute chest syndrome		BFM	Berlin-Frankfurt-Munster
ACT	Activated clotting time		BG	Blood glucose
ACTH	Adrenocorticotrophic hormone		BI	Bullous impetigo
ADA	American Diabetes Association		BID	Twice daily
ADE	Adverse drug event		β-Blocker	β-Adrenergic receptor blocker
ADH	Antidiuretic hormone		BMD	Bone mineral density
ADHD	Attention-deficit/hyperactivity disorder		BMI	Body mass index
ADHD-SRS	ADHD Symptoms Rating Scale		BN	Bulimia nervosa
ADME	Absorption, distribution, metabolism, and elimination		BP	Blood pressure
ADR	Adverse drug reaction		BPCA	Best Pharmaceuticals for Children Act
AgRP	Agouti-related peptide		BPD	Bipolar disorder
AHA	American Heart Association		BPD	Bronchopulmonary dysplasia
AI	Adrenal insufficiency		BPI	Bipolar I disorder
AIDS	Acquired immunodeficiency syndrome		BPII	Bipolar II disorder
AIEOP	Associazione Italiana Ematologia Oncologia Pediatrica		BPO	Benzoyl peroxide
AIN	Acute interstitial nephritis		BRUE	Brief resolved unexplained event
AKI	Acute kidney injury		BSA	Body surface area
AKIN	Acute Kidney Injury Network		BT	Blalock-Taussig (shunt)
ALK	Alkaline phosphatase		BU	Bethesda unit
ALL	Acute lymphoblastic leukemia		BUN	Blood urea nitrogen
α-MSH	α-Melanocyte stimulating hormone		C	Continuous infusion; conventional hemodialysis
ALT	Alanine aminotransferase		Ca	Calcium
AML	Acute myelogenous leukemia, acute myeloid leukemia		CaCC	Calcium activated chloride channel
AMPK	AMP-activated protein kinase		CAH	Congenital adrenal hyperplasia
AN	Anorexia nervosa		cAMP	Cyclic adenosine 3',5'-monophosphate
ANC	Absolute neutrophil count		CA-MRSA	Community-acquired methicillin-resistant *Staphylococcus aureus*
Anti-Xa	Antifactor Xa		CANMAT	Canadian Network for Mood and Anxiety Treatments
AO	Aorta		CAP	Community-acquired pneumonia
AOM	Acute otitis media		CARS	Childhood Autism Rating Scale
AOP	Apnea of prematurity		cART	Combination antiretroviral therapy
AOX	Aldehyde oxidases		CART	Cocaine- and amphetamine-related transcript
aPCC	Activated prothrombin complex concentrate		CAVH	Continuous arteriovenous hemofiltration
APL	Acute promyelocytic leukemia		CAVHD	Continuous arteriovenous hemodialysis
aPTT	Activated partial thromboplastin time		CAVHDF	Continuous arteriovenous hemodiafiltration
AR	Allergic rhinitis		CBC	Complete blood count
ARB	Angiotensin receptor blocker		CBE	Chloride bicarbonate exchanger
ARC	Arcuate nucleus		CBF	Core-binding factor
ARDS	Acute respiratory distress syndrome		CBT	Cognitive behavioral therapy
ARI, Ari	Aripiprazole		CBT-E	Enhanced cognitive behavioral therapy
ARIA	Allergic Rhinitis and its Impact on Asthma		CBZ	Carbamazepine
ART	Antiretroviral therapy		CC	Clindamycin
ARV	Antiretroviral		CCB	Calcium channel blocker
ASD	Antiseizure drug		CCG	Children's Cancer Group
ASD	Atrial septal defect		CCR5	C-C chemokine receptor type 5
ASD	Autism spectrum disorder		CD	Celiac disease; Crohn disease
ASHP	American Society of Health-System Pharmacists		CDC	Centers for Disease Control and Prevention
			CDI	*Clostridioides difficile* infection
			CDRS	Children's Depression Rating Scale

CDRS-R	Child Depression Rating Scale-Revised
CDSS	Clinical decision support system
CEBPA	CCAAT/enhancer binding protein alpha
CES	Carboxylesterases
CF	Cystic fibrosis
CFCS	Child Facial Coding System
CFF	Cystic Fibrosis Foundation
CFRD	Cystic fibrosis-related diabetes
CFTR	Cystic fibrosis-transmembrane conductance regulator
CFU	Colony-forming unit
CGI-I	Clinical Global Impression Scale-Improvement Scale
CGM	Continuous glucose monitoring
CGRP	Calcitonin gene-related peptide
CHAMP study	Childhood and Adolescent Migraine Prevention study
CHF	Congestive heart failure
CHr	Reticulocyte hemoglobin content
CI	Continuous intravenous infusion
CINV	Chemotherapy-induced nausea and vomiting
cJET	Congenital junctional ectopic tachycardia
CKD	Chronic kidney disease
C/L	Communication/language impairments
Cl, Cl⁻	Chloride
CLD	Chronic lung disease
CMP	Comprehensive metabolic panel
CMV	Cytomegalovirus
CNI	Calcineurin inhibitor
CNS	Central nervous system
CO	Cardiac output
CO₂	Carbon dioxide
COBI	Cobicistat
CP	Cerebral palsy
CPAP	Continuous positive airway pressure
CPOE	Computerized prescriber order entry
C-R	Concentration response
CR	Complete remission; controlled release
CrCl	Creatinine clearance
CRES	CAR T cell–related encephalopathy syndrome
CRF	Corticotropin-releasing factor
CRH	Corticotropin-releasing hormone
CRP	C-reactive protein
CRRT	Continuous renal replacement therapy
CRS	Cytokine release syndrome
CRS-R	Conners Rating Scales-Revised
CRTZ	Chemoreceptor trigger zone
CSF	Cerebrospinal fluid
CSII	Continuous subcutaneous insulin infusion
CT	Computed tomography
CVP	Central venous pressure
CVVH	Continuous venovenous hemofiltration
CVVHD	Continuous venovenous hemodialysis
CVVHDF	Continuous venovenous hemodiafiltration
CXCR4	C-X-C motif chemokine receptor type 4
CYP	Cytochrome P450
CYP3A4	Cytochrome P450 3A4 isoenzyme
D/M	Dual/mixed
DA₂	Dopamine receptor
DBP	Diastolic blood pressure
DBPC	Double-blind, placebo-controlled
DCOG	Dutch Childhood Oncology Group
DEA	Drug Enforcement Agency
DEET	*N,N*-diethyl-*m*-toluamide
DEXA	Dual-energy x-ray absorptiometry
DFE	Dietary folate equivalent
DHE	Dihydroergotamine
DHHS	U.S. Department of Health and Human Services
DIOS	Distal intestinal obstruction syndrome
DKA	Diabetic ketoacidosis
DM	Diabetes mellitus
DMSA	Dimercaptosuccinic acid
DOPA	Dopamine
DPI	Dry powder inhaler
DRESS	Drug reaction with eosinophilia and systemic symptoms
DRP	Digoxin reduction product
DSM-5	*Diagnostic and Statistical Manual of Mental Disorders, Fifth Edition*
DSM-IV	*Diagnostic and Statistical Manual of Mental Disorders, Fourth Edition*
DSM-IV-TR	*Diagnostic and Statistical Manual of Mental Disorders, Fourth Edition, Text Revision*
DT	Diphtheria and tetanus toxoids
DTaP	Diphtheria, tetanus, and acellular pertussis
D-test	Double-disk diffusion
DVT	Deep venous thrombosis
DXA	Dual-energy x-ray absorptiometry
E	Erythromycin
EC	Enteric coated
ECF	Extracellular fluid
ECG	Electrocardiogram; electrocardiographic
eCrCl	Estimated creatinine clearance
ECT	Electroconvulsive therapy
ED	Emergency department
EEG	Electroencephalographic
EFAD	Essential fatty acid deficiency
EFS	Event-free survival
EHEC	Enterohemorrhagic *Escherichia coli*
EHL	Extended half-life
EIA	Enzyme immunoassay
EIB	Exercise-induced bronchospasm
EKG	Electrocardiogram
ELBW	Extremely low birth weight
ELISA	Enzyme-linked immunosorbent assay
EN	Enteral nutrition
ENaC	Epithelial sodium channel
EORTC-CLG	European Organization for the Research and Treatment of Cancer-Children Leukemia Group
EPS	Extrapyramidal symptoms
ER	Extended release
ESH	European Society of Hypertension
ESPGHAN	European Society for Pediatric Gastroenterology, Hepatology, and Nutrition
ESR	Erythrocyte sedimentation rate
ESRD	End-stage renal disease
ET	Endotracheal tube
ETEC	Enterotoxigenic *Escherichia coli*
ETP	Early T cell precursor
FabAV	Crotalidae polyvalent immune Fab antivenom
FAT	Focal atrial tachycardia
FBT	Family-based therapy
Fc	Crystallizable fragment
FDA	U.S. Food and Drug Administration
FDAMA	Food and Drug Administration Modernization Act
FDASIA	Food and Drug Administration Safety and Innovation Act
FDC	Fixed-dose combination
FEIBA	Factor eight inhibitor bypass activity
FEV₁	Forced expiratory volume in 1 second
FGA	First-generation antihistamine; first-generation antipsychotic
FIO₂	Fraction of inspired oxygen
FIX	Factor IX
FLACC	Face Legs Activity Cry Consolability Scale
FLT3	FMS-like tyrosine kinase-3
FLT3-/ITD	FMS-like tyrosine kinase 3 internal tandem duplication
FMEA	Failure mode effects analysis
FODMAPs	Fermentable oligosaccharides, disaccharides, monosaccharides, and polyols
FP	Fusion Protein
FR-SSNS	Frequently relapsing steroid-sensitive nephrotic syndrome
FRNS	Frequently relapsing nephrotic syndrome

FSGS	Focal segmental glomerulosclerosis		IBS-D	Diarrhea-predominant IBS
FVIII	Factor VIII		IBS-M	Mixed IBS
FVC	Forced vital capacity		IBW	Ideal body weight
FWD	Free water deficit		IC	Impetigo contagiosa
G6PD	Glucose-6-phosphate dehydrogenase		ICF	International Classification of Functioning, Disability and Health; intracellular fluid
GA	Gestational age		ICH	Intracranial hemorrhage
GABA	γ-Aminobutyric acid		ICHD-3	*International Classification of Headache Disorders, 3rd edition*
Gal	Galactosidase			
GAS	Group A β-hemolytic *Streptococcus*		ICN	Intensive care nursery
GATA	GATA-binding protein		ICP	Intracranial pressure
GATA1	GATA-binding protein 1 (globin transcription factor 1 or *GATA1* gene)		ICS	Inhaled corticosteroids
			ICU	Intensive care unit
GATLA	Argentine Group for the Treatment of Acute Leukemia		IDA	Iron-deficiency anemia
			IDMS	Isotope dilution mass spectrometry
GBS	Guillain-Barré syndrome		IDSA	Infectious Diseases Society of America
G-CSF	Granulocyte colony-stimulating factor		Ig	Immunoglobulin
GER	Gastroesophageal reflux		IgA	Immunoglobulin A
GERD	Gastroesophageal reflux disease		IgE	Immunoglobulin E
GFD	Gluten-free diet		IgG	Immunoglobulin G
GFR	Glomerular filtration rate		IgM	Immunoglobulin M
GHB	γ-Hydroxybutyrate		IH	Infantile hemangioma
GI	Gastrointestinal		IIV	Inactivated influenza vaccine
GLP-1	Glucagon-like peptide 1		IL	Interleukin
GMFCS	Gross Motor Function Classification System		ILAE	International League Against Epilepsy
GST	Glutathione S-transferase		ILE	Intravenous lipid emulsion
GVHD	Graft-versus-host disease		IM	Intramuscular; intramuscularly
H$_1$	Histamine-1		INCS	Intranasal corticosteroid
H$_2$	Histamine-2		IND	Investigational new drug
H$_2$RA	Histamine-2 receptor antagonist		iNO	Inhaled nitric oxide
HbA	Normal adult hemoglobin		INR	International normalized ratio
HbC	Hemoglobin C		INSTI	Integrase strand transfer inhibitor
HbF	Fetal hemoglobin		IO	Intraosseous infusion
HBIG	Hepatitis B immunoglobulin		IOM	Institute of Medicine
HbS	Sickle hemoglobin		IPV	Inactivated polio vaccine
HbS βthal	Sickle cellβ-thalassemia		IR	Immediate release; intermediate risk
HbSC	Compound heterozygous hemoglobin (sickle hemoglobin and hemoglobin C)		ISBD	International Society for Bipolar Disorders
			ISMP	Institute for Safe Medication Practices
HbSS	Homozygous form of sickle cell disease		ITI	Immune tolerance induction
HBV	Hepatitis B vaccine; hepatitis B virus		IV	Intravenous; intravenously
HCO$_3$	Serum bicarbonate		IVC	Inferior vena cava
Hct	Hematocrit		IVIG	Intravenous immunoglobulin
HCV	Hepatitis C virus		JET	Junctional ectopic tachycardia
HD	Hemodialysis; high-dose		JNC VIII	Eighth Report of the Joint National Committee on Prevention, Detection, Evaluation, and Treatment of High Blood Pressure
HDL-C	HDL cholesterol			
HEENT	Head, eyes, ears, nose, and throat			
HFA	Hydrofluoroalkane		K	Potassium
HFMD	Hand, foot, and mouth disease		KD	Kawasaki disease; ketogenic diet
Hgb	Hemoglobin		KDIGO	Kidney Disease Improving Global Outcomes
HHS	U.S. Department of Health and Human Services		KDOQI	Kidney Disease Outcomes Quality Initiative
HHV	Human herpes virus		K-SADS	Kiddie Schedule for Affective Disorders and Schizophrenia
Hib	*Haemophilus influenzae* type b			
HINE	Hammersmith Infant Neurological Examination		LA	Left atria; long acting
HIT	Heparin-induced thrombocytopenia		LABA	Long-acting β-agonist
HIV	Human immunodeficiency virus		LAGB	Laparoscopic adjustable gastric band
HLA	Human leukocyte antigen		LAIV	Live attenuated influenza vaccine
HLHS	Hypoplastic left heart syndrome		LAME	Leucémie Aiguë Myéloblastique Enfant
HPA	Hypothalamic–pituitary–adrenal		LCOS	Low cardiac output syndrome
HPD	High permeability dialysis		LD	Lethal dose
HPV	Human papillomavirus		LDH	Lactate dehydrogenase
HR	Heart rate; high risk		LDL-C	Low-density lipoprotein cholesterol
HS	At bedtime		LE	Leukocyte esterase
HSCT	Hematopoietic stem-cell transplantation		LES	Lower esophageal sphincter
HSTCL	Hepatosplenic T-cell lymphoma		LET	Lidocaine, epinephrine, and tetracaine
HSV	Herpes simplex virus		LFT	Liver function test
Ht	Height		LGA	Large for gestational age
HTN	Hypertension		LGS	Lennox-Gastaut syndrome
HUS	Hemolytic uremic syndrome		Li	Lithium
I&D	Incision and drainage		LOCF	Last observation carried forward
IBD	Inflammatory bowel disease		LP	Lumbar puncture
IBS	Irritable bowel syndrome		LQTS	Long QT syndrome
IBS-C	Constipation-predominant IBS			

LR	Low risk	**NICE**	National Institute for Health and Care Excellence
LRTI	Lower respiratory tract infection	**NICU**	Neonatal intensive care unit
LSD	Lysergic acid diethylamide	**NIDA**	National Institute on Drug Abuse
LTB4	Leukotriene B4	**NIPS**	Neonatal Infant Pain Scale
LTRA	Leukotriene receptor antagonist	**NMDA**	*N*-methyl-D-aspartate
LV	Left ventricle	**NNRTI**	Nonnucleoside reverse transcriptase inhibitor
LVES	Left ventricular end systolic	**NOPHO**	Nordic Society of Pediatric Haematology and Oncology
MAC	*Mycobacterium avium* complex	**NP-Y**	Neuropeptide Y
MAO	Monoamine oxidase	**NR**	No recommendations; not recommended
MAOIs	Monoamine oxidase inhibitors	**NRDS**	Neonatal respiratory distress syndrome
MAP	Mean arterial pressure	**NRS**	Numeric Rating Scale
Max	Maximum	**NRTI**	Nucleoside reverse transcriptase inhibitor
MCD	Minimal change disease	**NS**	Normal saline
M-CHAT-R/F	Modified Checklist for Autism in Toddlers–Revised with Follow-Up	**NSAID**	Nonsteroidal anti-inflammatory drug
MCH	Mean corpuscular hemoglobin	**NSDUH**	National Survey on Drug Use and Health
MCHC	Mean corpuscular hemoglobin concentration	**NTS**	Nontyphoidal *Salmonella*; nucleus tractus solitarius
MCT	Medium chain triglyceride	**OAT**	Organic anion transporter
MCV	Mean corpuscular volume; meningococcal conjugate vaccine	**OATP**	Organic-anion-transporting polypeptide
MDAC	Multiple-dose activated charcoal	**OC**	Orbital cellulitis
MDD	Major depressive disorder; maximum daily dose	**OCS**	Oral corticosteroids
MDI	Metered dose inhaler	**OCT**	Organic cation transporter
MDMA	Methylenedioxymethamphetamine	**ODT**	Oral disintegrating tablet
MDPV	Methylenedioxypyrovalerone	**OI**	Opportunistic infection; osteogenesis imperfecta
MDR	Multidrug resistance	**OLZ**	Olanzapine
MenB	Meningococcal serogroup B	**OM**	Otitis media
MIC	Minimum inhibitory concentration	**OROS**	Osmotic-release oral system
MLL	Mixed lineage leukemia	**ORS**	Oral rehydration solution
MMF	Mycophenolate mofetil	**ORT**	Oral rehydration therapy
MMR	Measles, mumps, and rubella	**OS**	Overall survival
MMRV	Measles, mumps, rubella, and varicella	**OXC**	Oxcarbazepine
MOH	Medication overuse headache	**P**	Plasma derived
MRC	Metabolic research council	**PA**	*Pseudomonas aeruginosa*
MRD	Minimal residual disease	**PA**	Pulmonary artery
MRI	Magnetic resonance imaging	**Pao$_2$**	Alveolar oxygen partial pressure
mRNA	Messenger RNA	**PBD**	Pediatric bipolar disorder
MRP	Multidrug resistance protein	**PC**	Periorbital cellulitis
MRSA	Methicillin-resistant *Staphylococcus aureus*	**PCA**	Patient-controlled analgesia
MSD	Maximum single dose	**PCC**	Prothrombin complex concentrate
MSSA	Methicillin-sensitive *Staphylococcus aureus*	**PCDAI**	Pediatric Crohn Disease Activity Index
MSSA	Methicillin-susceptible *Staphylococcus aureus*	**Pco$_2$**	Partial pressure of carbon dioxide
MTCT	Mother-to-child-transmission	**PCP**	Phencyclidine; *Pneumocystis jirovecii* pneumonia
MTF	Monitoring the Future	**PCR**	Polymerase chain reaction
MU	Million units	**PCV**	Pneumococcal conjugated vaccine
MUP	Medication use process	**PD**	Peritoneal dialysis; pharmacodynamics
N/A	Not applicable; not available	**PDA**	Patent ductus arteriosus
Na, Na$^+$	Sodium	**PDD**	Pervasive developmental disorder
NaCl	Sodium chloride	**PDD-NOS**	Pervasive developmental disorder–not otherwise specified
NAPA	*N*-acetyl procainamide	**PDE**	Phosphodiesterase
NaPO$_4$	Sodium phosphate	**PE**	Pulmonary embolism
NAPQI	*N*-acetyl-*p*-benzoquinonimine	**PedMIDAS**	Pediatric Migraine Disability Assessment Score
NAS	Intranasal	**PedsQL**	Pediatric Quality of Life
NASPGHAN	North American Society for Pediatric Gastroenterology, Hepatology, and Nutrition	**PEF**	Peak expiratory flow
NCA	Nurse-controlled analgesia	**PEG**	Polyethylene glycol
NCC MERP	National Coordinating Council for Medication Error Reporting and Prevention	**PEGylation**	Modification of the factor molecule to include polyethylene glycol
NCCPC-PV	Non-communicating Child's Pain Checklist-Postoperative Version	**PERT**	Pancreatic enzyme replacement therapy
NCHS	National Center for Health Statistics	**PFO**	Patent foramen ovale
NCI	National Cancer Institute	**PG**	Plasma glucose
ND	No data	**PGE**	Prostaglandin
NEC	Necrotizing enterocolitis	**P-gp**	P-glycoprotein
Neuro	Neurologic	**Ph**	Philadelphia chromosome
NF	Necrotizing fasciitis	**PHIS**	Pediatric Health Information System
NFCS	Neonatal Facial Coding System	**PHQ-9**	Patient Health Questionnaire-9 Item
NG	Nasogastric (tube)	**PHTN**	Pulmonary hypertension
NGAL	Neutrophil gelatinase-associated lipocalin	**PI**	Protease inhibitor
NHL	Non-Hodgkin lymphoma	**PICU**	Pediatric intensive care unit
NHLBI	National Heart, Lung, and Blood Institute	**PINDA**	National Program for Antineoplastic Drugs for Children
		PIPP	Premature Infant Pain Profile

PIVKA-II	Proteins induced by vitamin K absence
pJET	Postoperative junctional ectopic tachycardia
PJRT	Permanent junctional reciprocating tachycardia
PK	Pharmacokinetics
PLE	Protein-losing enteropathy
Plt	Platelet
PN	Parenteral nutrition
PNALD	Parenteral nutrition–associated liver disease
PO	Oral, orally
Po_2	Partial pressure of oxygen
PO_4	Phosphate
POG	Pediatric Oncology Group
POMC	Pro-opiomelanocortin
PPA	Pediatric Pharmacy Association
PPAR-γ	Peroxisome proliferator-activated receptor gamma
PPD	Purified protein derivative
PPI	Proton pump inhibitor
PPLLSG	Polish Pediatric Leukemia/Lymphoma Study Group
ppm	Parts per million
PPSV23	23-Valent pneumococcal polysaccharide vaccine
PR	Rectal
PREA	Pediatric Research Equity Act
pRIFLE	Pediatric risk, injury, failure, loss, end stage renal disease
PRSP	Penicillin-resistant *Streptococcus pneumoniae*
PT	Prothrombin time
PTH	Parathyroid hormone
Pts	Patients
PUCAI	Pediatric UC activity index
PVL	Panton-Valentine leukocidin
PVR	Pulmonary vascular resistance
Q	Every
QAM	Every morning
QD	Daily
QHS	Every night
QID	Four times daily
QOD	Every other day
QPM	Every evening
QUE	Quetiapine
RA	Receptor agonist; right atria
RAAS	Renin–angiotensin–aldosterone system
RADT	Rapid antigen detection test
RBC	Red blood cell
RCD	Refractory celiac disease
RCT	Randomized controlled trial
RDA	Recommended daily allowance
RDS	Respiratory distress syndrome
RDW	Red cell distribution width
REMS	Risk evaluation and mitigation strategy
rFIX	Recombinant factor IX
rFVIIa	Recombinant activated factor VII
rFVIII	Recombinant factor VIII
RIFLE	Risk, injury, failure, loss, end stage renal disease
Ris	Risperidone
RISP	Risperidone
RNA	Ribonucleic acid
RR	Respiratory rate
RRT	Renal replacement therapy
RSV	Respiratory syncytial virus
RT	Room temperature
RV	Right ventricle; rotavirus
RYGB	Roux-en-Y gastric bypass
SABA	Short-acting β-agonist
SBP	Systolic blood pressure
SC	Single chain; subcutaneous; subcutaneously
SCD	Sickle cell disease
SCID	Severe combined immunodeficiency
SCr	Serum creatinine
SCT	Sickle cell trait
SDNS	Steroid-dependent nephrotic syndrome
SE	Status epilepticus
SFD	Solute fluid deficit
SGA	Second-generation antihistamine; second-generation antipsychotic; small for gestational age
SHARE	Support, Help, and Resources for Epilepsy
SHL	Standard half-life
SIADH	Syndrome of inappropriate antidiuretic hormone secretion
SIB	Self-injurious behavior
SJS	Stevens-Johnson syndrome
SLC	Solute carrier transporter
SMBG	Self-monitoring of blood glucose
SMZ	Sulfamethoxazole
SNAP-IV	Swanson, Nolan, and Pelham-IV questionnaire
SNP	Sodium nitroprusside
SNRI	Serotonin norepinephrine reuptake inhibitor
SNS	Sympathetic nervous system
SOI	Syrup of ipecac
SPA	Suprapubic aspiration
SR	Sustained release
S/RB	Stereotype/repetitive behaviors
SRNS	Steroid-resistant nephrotic syndrome
SSNRI	Selective serotonin and norepinephrine reuptake inhibitor
SSNS	Steroid-sensitive nephrotic syndrome
SSRI	Selective serotonin reuptake inhibitor
SSSS	Staphylococcal scalded skin syndrome
SSTI	Skin and soft tissue infection
STAR*D	Sequenced Treatment Alternatives to Relieve Depression
STAT	Immediately
SUD	Substance use disorder
SULT	Sulfotransferase
SVC	Superior vena cava
SVR	Systemic vascular resistance
SVT	Supraventricular tachyarrhythmia
T1DM	Type 1 diabetes
TAF	Tenofovir alafenamide
TBW	Total body water
TC	Total cholesterol
TCA	Tricyclic antidepressant
TCMAP	Texas Children's Medication Algorithm Project
Tco_2	Total carbon dioxide
Td	Tetanus and diphtheria
Tdap	Tetanus, diphtheria, and acellular pertussis
TDF	Tenofovir disoproxil fumarate
TDM	Therapeutic drug monitoring
TdP	Torsades de pointes
TEN	Toxic epidermal necrolysis
TFD	Total fluid deficit
TG	Triglycerides
TGA	Transposition of the great arteries
TID	Three times daily
TIW	Three times/week
TJC	The Joint Commission
TKI	Tyrosine kinase inhibitor
TLESR	Transient lower esophageal sphincter relaxation
TLS	Tumor lysis syndrome
Tmax	Maximum temperature
TMD	Transient myeloproliferative disorder
TMP	Trimethoprim
TMP/SMX, TMP/SMZ	Trimethoprim/sulfamethoxazole
TNA	Total nutrient admixture
TNF	Tumor necrosis factor
TNFα	Tumor necrosis factor alpha
TOF	Tetralogy of Fallot
TORDIA	Treatment of SSRI-Resistant Depression in Adolescent trial
TPMT	Thiopurine S-methyltransferase
TPN	Total parenteral nutrition
TSAT	Transferrin saturation

TSH	Thyroid-stimulating hormone
TTG	Tissue transglutaminase
UC	Ulcerative colitis
UFH	Unfractionated heparin
UGT	UDP-glucuronosyltransferase
UGT1	UDP glucuronosyltransferase 1 family
UK MRC	United Kingdom Medical Research Council
ULN	Upper limit of normal
uNGAL	Urine neutrophil gelatinase-associated lipocalin
UNICEF	United Nations Children's Fund
uPCR	Urine protein to creatinine ratio
URTI	Upper respiratory tract infection
US	Ultrasonography
USDA	U.S. Department of Agriculture
USP	United States Pharmacopeia
UTI	Urinary tract infection
VAERS	Vaccine Adverse Event Reporting System
VAL	Valproate
VAR	Varicella
VAERS	FDA Vaccine Adverse Event Reporting System
VARS	Vanderbilt ADHD Rating Scale
VCUG	Voiding cystourethrography
V$_d$	Volume of distribution
VF	Ventricular fibrillation
VHC	Valved holding chamber
VILI	Ventilator induced lung injury
VLBW	Very low birth weight
VMH	Ventromedial nucleus
VO$_2$	Oxygen uptake
VSD	Ventricular septal defect
VT	Ventricular tachycardia
VUR	Vesicoureteral reflux
VWF	von Willebrand factor
VZV	Varicella zoster virus
WBC	White blood cell
WBI	Whole bowel irrigation
WHO	World Health Organization
WPW	Wolff-Parkinson-White (syndrome)
Wt	Weight
XR	Extended release
YMRS	Young Mania Rating Scale
YRBS	Youth Risk Behavior Survey
ZIP	Ziprasidone

PEDIATRIC
Pharmacotherapy

Second Edition

Section I

General Principles

CHAPTER 1

Introduction to Pediatrics

Hanna Phan, Pharm.D., FCCP, FPPA; and
Milap C. Nahata, Pharm.D., M.S., FCCP, FAPhA, FASHP, FPPA

LEARNING OBJECTIVES

1. Define the different age groups and corresponding developmental milestones in pediatric patients.

2. Describe differences in vital signs and laboratory normal values based on age.

3. Describe fundamental differences between pediatric and adult patients regarding drug therapy, including availability of treatment options, clinical data, and administration challenges.

4. Define off-label medication use and its implications in pediatric drug therapy.

5. Apply general pharmacotherapeutic concepts and pediatric-specific factors toward providing care and education to patients and families.

ABBREVIATIONS IN THIS CHAPTER

AAP	American Academy of Pediatrics
BMI	Body mass index
CDC	Centers for Disease Control and Prevention
FDAMA	Food and Drug Administration Modernization Act
GFR	Glomerular filtration rate
PD	Pharmacodynamics
PK	Pharmacokinetics
WHO	World Health Organization

THE ROLE OF A PEDIATRIC PHARMACIST

Pediatric patients are not simply "smaller adults"—they are their own population with a need for specialized patient care.[1] Pediatric pharmacy practice focuses on the provision of safe and effective drug therapy in infants, children, and adolescents. As such, the American Society of Health-System Pharmacists recognizes the specialized nature of pediatric pharmacy practice through its statement regarding pediatric pharmaceutical services and its accreditation of postgraduate residency training programs in pediatric pharmacy practice.[2-4] The Pediatric Pharmacy Association offers therapeutic position statements and guidance on pediatric pharmacy practice including the role of pediatric pharmacists in personalized medicine and clinical pharmacogenomics.[5,6] The American College of Clinical Pharmacy also supports pediatric pharmacy practice through the Pediatric Practice Research Network and contributions such as the opinion paper about pediatric pharmacy education and training.[7] Similarly, other

professional organizations support the role of pharmacists in pediatric patient care. The American Academy of Pediatrics (AAP) acknowledges the importance of interdisciplinary teams in pediatric patient care. In fact, the AAP recommends that prescribers use pharmacist consultation, when available, including the integration of clinical pharmacists in patient care rounds and activities that involve reviewing medication use procedures and orders.[8] Other professional organizations, American College of Clinical Pharmacy and Pediatric Pharmacy Association, also collaborated in support of the pediatric pharmacist's role in patient care through a joint opinion paper regarding recommendations for meeting the needs of pediatric patients.[9] In 2015, the Board of Pharmacy Specialties administered the first round of Pediatric Pharmacy Certification examination for pharmacists to become Board Certified Pediatric Pharmacy Specialists.[10] The need for pediatric pharmacists persists with more than 60 postgraduate year two Pediatric Pharmacy programs compared with more than 200 pediatric medical residencies in the United States.[9,11,12] In addition, with the expansion of health systems by adding pediatric towers or hospitals across the United States, the scarcity is likely to continue of pediatric-trained pharmacists available to ensure safe and effective medication use in infants, children, and adolescents.

Drug selection and use, monitoring of effectiveness and toxicity, prevention of medication errors, patient and caregiver education, and contributions to knowledge through research are among the responsibilities of pharmacists when caring for pediatric patients.[13] Pharmacists who care for pediatric patients should possess knowledge regarding acute and chronic disease states and drug therapy as well as the skills to apply this knowledge to practice. Pediatric practice includes a wide range of patient ages, with conditions varying from lower respiratory tract infection to trauma. Examples of chronic disease states that affect pediatric patients include type 1 diabetes mellitus, asthma, or congenital heart disease. This introductory chapter provides a broad discussion of pediatric drug therapy considerations, and subsequent chapters further discuss specific pediatric illnesses and treatment strategies for these patients.

CLASSIFICATION OF PEDIATRIC PATIENTS

Pediatric patients are a specialized patient population. Classification is often age-dependent, expressed in days, weeks, months, or years. Common age terms in pediatrics are neonates, infants, children, and adolescents (Table 1). Some government agencies combine adolescents with young adults, who are up to 24 years of age.[1,14-16] Additional classifications are based on other factors such as birth weight and gestational age (Table 1). An appreciation of the classification of pediatric patients is important in guiding medication selection

Table 1. Pediatric Age Classification and Definitions[1,14-16]

Common Age Classification	
Neonate	Age ≤ 28 days
Infant	Age 29 days to < 12 mo
Child	Age > 12 mo to 12 yr
Adolescent	Age 13–17 yr (some use definition up to 21 yr)
Neonatal Terminology	
Gestational Age (GA)	Age from date of mother's first day of last menstrual period to date of birth
Full Term	Born at ≥ 37 wks' gestation
Premature	Born at < 37 wks' gestation
Chronological (Postnatal) Age	Age from birth to present, measured in days, wk, mo, or yr
Corrected (Adjusted) Age	May be used to describe age of a premature child ≤ 3 yr: **Corrected age equation**: Chronological age in mo – [(40 – GA at birth in wk) × 1 mo ÷ 4 wk]
Neonatal Weight Classification	
Low Birth Weight	Premature infant with birth weight between 1500 and 2500 g
Very Low Birth Weight	Premature infant with birth weight 1000 g to < 1500 g
Extremely Low Birth Weight	Premature infant with birth weight < 1000 g
Small for Gestational Age (SGA)	Birth weight < 10th percentile among neonates of the same GA
Large for Gestational Age (LGA)	Birth weight > 90th percentile among neonates of the same GA

because some medications are contraindicated for patients of certain ages. Medication dosing can also be affected by such classifications because dosing may depend on organ function development, which progresses with age, such as for the kidney or liver. For example, neonates and infants lack the ability to effectively metabolize alcohol by alcohol dehydrogenase whereas adults have this ability. For this reason, elixir formulations should be avoided whenever possible in neonates and infants.[16,17]

DISTINCTNESS OF PEDIATRIC PHARMACOTHERAPY

Pediatric patients are distinct from their adult counterparts because of their differences with respect to pharmacokinetics and pharmacodynamics (PK/PD), psychosocial influences on drug therapy selection, and treatment options. Developmental changes in PK/PD affect drug therapy selection and dosage requirements in the pediatric age continuum, from birth to 18 years (Pediatric Pharmacokinetics chapter). Pediatric clinicians must also consider factors that affect patients' and/or caregiver's hesitance for medication administration. These factors include health and cultural beliefs, socioeconomic status, and psychosocial differences among patient age groups (e.g., child vs. adolescent). Pediatric patients also require special consideration regarding selection of drug formulations. For example, because children younger than 6 years are generally unable to swallow solid dosage forms, oral liquids are preferred for this age group.

Off-label medication use occurs often because of the limited availability of U.S. Food and Drug Administration (FDA) label-approved indications for the pediatric patient population. Such practices are noted by the AAP as especially important and complex for those patients age younger than 2 years and those with chronic and/or rare diseases.[18] Among pediatric patients with prescriptions, almost 40% were prescribed to one or more off-label medications; among these, many (56.4%) were used for an unapproved indication.[19] Other studies have shown 67% to 96% of outpatient prescriptions and about 79% of inpatient admissions involve off-label medication use in the United States.[20,21] With limited evidence-based data (e.g., randomized controlled trials) available for many needed medications, the selection and dosing of pediatric drugs are a considerable obstacle for health care professionals. Pharmacists who specialize in pediatrics are an important and integral part of the patient care team, both in the outpatient and inpatient care settings, because they are equipped with skills to evaluate drug information and possess specialized knowledge about developmental PK/PD.[7]

EPIDEMIOLOGY OF THE PEDIATRIC POPULATION IN THE UNITED STATES

The pediatric population accounts for almost 25% of the U.S. population.[22] Patients younger than 17 years face various chronic conditions, with asthma in more than 10 million and attention deficit-hyperactivity disorder in almost 5 million in the United States.[22] More than 13% of children (10 million) in the United States take a prescription medication chronically for at least 3 months during a year.[23,24] Also in the United States, around 11.2 million children have special health care needs. This subpopulation of pediatric patients, termed *children and youth with special health care needs* by the Association of Maternal Child Health Programs, include children who have chronic conditions, medically complex health issues, and/or behavioral or emotional conditions.[25] Given the variety of conditions that require potentially off-label and complex therapy regimens, pediatric pharmacists can play a key role in ensuring safe and effective use of these medications.

Infants, children, and adolescents are a considerable proportion of the patients in a variety of health care settings, including community pharmacies, ambulatory clinics, emergency departments, and hospitals. With more than 210 visits per 100 people per year in the ambulatory care setting among patients from birth to age 17 years, pediatric patients expend a considerable amount of outpatient resources.[24] Overall within this group, hospitalization rates of pediatric patients younger than 17 years were lower than for older patients, but still considerable, with approximately 5.8 million hospital stays versus an estimated 8.9 million hospital stays by patients age 18 to 44 years in 2012.[26,27] In addition, more than 23 million emergency department visits occurred among pediatric patients younger than 15 years, which is comparable to the 20 to 35 million visits among adults age 25 to 74 years in 2013. Based on a survey of more than 2,800 pediatric caregivers from 1998 to 2007, about 56% of children in the United States used at least one medication in a given week, with 20% being prescription medications.[28] These data emphasize a continued need for pediatric-specific care, especially drug therapy.

GROWTH AND DEVELOPMENT

Infants and children are often monitored for growth and development. Markers of physical growth include weight, length or height, head circumference, weight-for-length, and body mass index (BMI). These markers are age- and sex-dependent; therefore, the use of correct tools for measuring pertinent variables based on these factors is important for proper nutritional status and assessment of the physical growth of pediatric patients. For infants and children younger than 2 years, the World Health Organization (WHO) growth charts are recommended to assess these variables (Figure 1). The WHO growth charts reflect growth based on the standard for infant feeding, represented by infants who were predominantly breastfed for a duration of at least 4 months and continued through 12 months of age. The Centers for Disease Control and Prevention (CDC) growth charts are recommended when assessing children 2 years and older (Figure 2).[29] Growth charts provide a graphic representation of a child's growth with respect to the general pediatric population among six countries, including the United States. To use these charts, a patient's data (e.g., age and BMI) should be plotted on each axis, finding the cross-coordinate between the two variables. This point should correlate with a percentile (e.g., 10th percentile).[29] Nutritional status is often assessed on the basis of growth percentiles, such as BMI (Parenteral and Enteral Nutrition and Pediatric Obesity chapters). Also noteworthy is the gradual development of organ function, such as in the kidney and liver, and drug distribution space, such as total body water, affecting the PK/PD of drugs administered to the patients (Pediatric Pharmacokinetics chapter).

Motor development milestones involve the ability to perform an activity such as sitting up straight or taking first steps. Motor skills can be divided into two classifications. *Gross motor skills* are often considered large movements; smaller movements often associated with appendages or mouths are considered *fine motor skills*. Both skill types are monitored closely, especially during the first 2 years of life. Examples of gross motor skills include holding the head steady while upright, sitting upright on one's own, beginning to walk, beginning to run, and beginning to jump at ages 3, 6, 12, 18, and 24 months, respectively. Fine motor skills also develop in tandem with grasping toys, transferring objects from hand to hand, grasping with fingers, stacking building blocks, and the ability to hold eating utensils, assessed for the same time intervals as for gross motor skills.[30-32] These markers of normal physical development from birth to young adulthood can affect medication administration. For example, the ability to grasp and hold objects is needed in manipulating and self-administering dosage forms such as metered dose inhalers.

The *Piaget stages* are often used to describe cognitive development and include *sensorimotor, preoperational, concrete operations*, and *formal operations*. These stages span the ages from birth to 18 years and indicate the progression of comprehending language and knowledge (Communicating with Children, Adolescents, and Their Caregivers chapter).[33] Cognitive development is important for medication administration and for education about medications and techniques. Comprehension of language and knowledge can affect one's understanding of medication administration instructions and the importance of treatment. A poor understanding of why and how to take medications can affect medication adherence and patient outcomes. Assessments of growth, motor, and cognitive developmental milestones are recommended during each pediatric preventive care visit, also known as *a well-child visit*, to detect developmental delay as early as possible.[34]

Pediatric patients should be seen by their primary care provider (e.g., pediatrician) on a regular schedule to monitor for developmental milestones and provide preventive care, including routine childhood immunizations. These appointments are known as *well-check visits* and occur more often early in life (i.e., every 1 to 2 months in infancy) and then annually. Pediatric pharmacists can also play a role in the provision of this care in the ambulatory care setting. These well-check visits not only ensure close monitoring for motor and social and development, early diagnosis of childhood conditions, and minimize vaccine-preventable disease, but also provide the opportunity for caregivers to raise any concerns they may have and to engage in their child's health.[34]

DIFFERENCES IN PEDIATRIC PATIENT DATA—VITAL SIGNS, LABORATORY VALUES, AND CALCULATIONS

Assessment of vital signs, as in adult medicine, is imperative in the evaluation of pediatric patients. Changes in vital signs can be indicative of effectiveness and safety in drug therapy. For example, respiratory rate and heart rate can be used

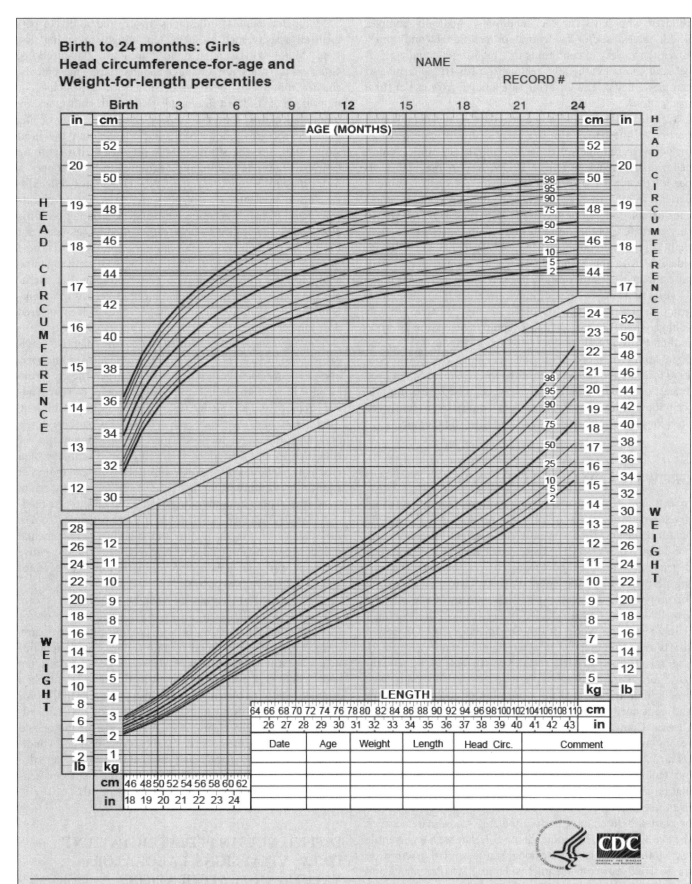

Figure 1. Example of World Health Organization (WHO) growth chart: Girls (age 0–24 months), head circumference-for-age and weight-for-length percentiles.[29]

Reprinted from World Health Organization Growth Standards (www.who.int/childgrowth/en), published by the Centers for Disease Control and Prevention, November 1, 2009.

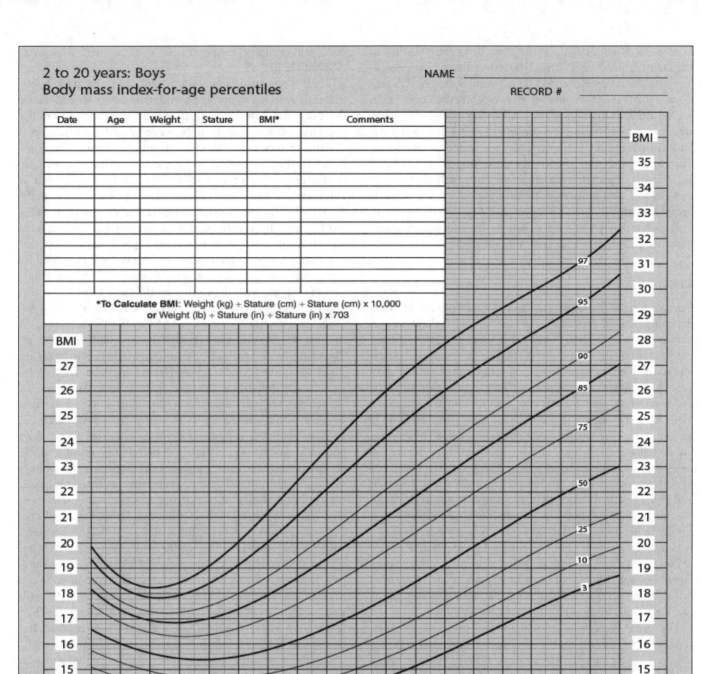

2 to 20 years: Boys
Body mass index-for-age percentiles

NAME _____

RECORD # _____

Date	Age	Weight	Stature	BMI*	Comments

*To Calculate BMI: Weight (kg) ÷ Stature (cm) ÷ Stature (cm) x 10,000
or Weight (lb) ÷ Stature (in) ÷ Stature (in) x 703

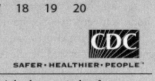

Figure 2. Example of Centers for Disease Control and Prevention (CDC) growth chart: Boys (age 2–20 years), body mass index-for-age percentiles, 2000.[29]

BMI = body mass index.

Reprinted from Centers for Disease Control Growth Charts (www.cdc.gov/growthcharts) developed by the National Center for Health Statistics in collaboration with the National Center for Chronic Disease Prevention and Health Promotion, May 30, 2000 (modified October 16, 2000).

as markers of efficacy and adverse reactions from the use of albuterol, respectively. Normal values for heart rate, respiratory rate, blood pressure, and body temperature are different from adult values because of physiologic differences. Pain scores are also an important marker for assessing a pediatric patient and should be considered "vital" in their care. Pain is perceived by patients of all ages, including newborns. Therefore, pain assessment should be part of the routine assessments of pediatric patients. Laboratory values of infants and children also differ from those of their adult counterparts because of physiologic differences, and they should be evaluated appropriately. Different equations are also used to assess pediatric patient data (e.g., creatinine clearance).

VITAL SIGNS

Normal ranges for heart rate and respiratory rate are age-dependent. Blood pressure ranges are not only reliant on age, but also on sex and height percentile (Pediatric Hypertension chapter). It is important to be familiar with normal ranges and individualized patient data to optimize the monitoring of patient outcomes on drug therapy. Reference ranges for heart and respiratory rates can vary by resource and are not necessarily evidence based.[35] In general, for patients from birth up to age 3 months, the normal heart rate is between 85 beats/minute and 205 beats/minute, and the heart rate range decreases to a range of 100–190 beats/minute at 2 years. The heart rate of children ranges from 80–140 beats/minute at 2 to 10 years, and among patients older than 10 years is closer to the heart rate range of adults at 60–100 beats/minute. Respiratory rate is similar to heart rate in its downward trend with increasing age, with ranges of 30–60 breaths/minute for infants, 24–40 for children up to 3 years, and 22–34 for children age 3 to 5 years. For school-age children up to about 12 years of age, respiratory rate is between 18–30 breaths/minute; around adolescence, the rate approaches adult values at 12–16 breaths/minute.[36]

The AAP guidelines provide blood pressure reference ranges for assessment on the basis of age, sex, and height for children 1 year or older. In general, systolic blood pressure at the 50th percentile can range from 80–98 mm Hg, 91–106 mm Hg, and 99–122 mm Hg, and diastolic pressure can range from 34–56 mm Hg, 53–63 mm Hg, and 59–70 mm Hg at age ranges 1 to 5, 6 to 11, and 12 to 17 years, respectively. For specific ranges based on height percentile, sex, and age, one should refer to the Report on Diagnosis, Evaluation, and Treatment of High Blood Pressure in Children and Adolescents.[37] Overall, *heart and respiratory rates decrease with age*, and *blood pressure increases with age.*

Body temperature can be determined via the rectal, oral, axillary, and tympanic route. Rectal temperature measurement is recommended by the AAP for children younger than 4 years. For older children, oral measurement can be used. Axillary measurement can be used for patients as young as 3 months, although it is thought to be less accurate than oral and rectal measurements. Tympanic measurement is considered potentially less accurate because of cerumen accumulation.[38,39] Some institutions use temporal artery thermometry, which is most accurate in patients older than 3 months.[40] In general, the difference in body temperature between rectal, oral, and axillary temperatures, from highest to lowest, is about 1°F (0.6°C).

Fever is a normal physiologic response involving the hypothalamic reaction to pyrogens, and its presence should not be the cause for immediate drug therapy in otherwise healthy pediatric patients unless it is accompanied by discomfort. Patients at increased risk of severe infection should be evaluated further. In general, with a mean normal temperature considered a reading of 98.6°F (37°C), a low-grade fever is considered a body temperature ranging from 100°F–102°F (37.8°C–39°C). A high fever, temperature greater than 104°F (40°C), may have greater risk of heat-related adverse outcomes. Antipyretics such as acetaminophen may be given for body temperatures greater than 101°F (38.3°C), measured by any route, if the patient presents with discomfort.[41] The definition of *fever* can vary depending on the route of measurement and patient age. For example, a rectal temperature of 100.4°F (38°C) in a neonate is considered a fever. In infants up to age 3 months, the fever threshold is higher, up to 100.7°F (38.2°C).[42] The vital signs for premature and term infants or neonates are discussed in the Introduction to Neonatology chapter.

It is also important to assess pain in pediatric patients. Difficulties in pain assessment are most common among patients with a limited ability to have direct communication, such as neonates, infants, and young children. Some older pediatric patients (e.g., critically ill individuals) may be unable to verbally express pain symptoms. In these cases, indicators of pain include physiologic markers, such as increased respiratory and/or heart rate and oxygen desaturations, as well as changes in behavior (e.g., grimacing or high-pitched crying). Standardized assessment scales such as the Neonatal Infant Pain Scale (NIPS) and the Face, Legs, Activity, Cry, Consolability (FLACC) scale use these physiologic or behavioral indicators for neonates or infants and children up to age 4 years, respectively.[43,44] The Wong-Baker FACES scale, with graphic facial expressions, is often used in children older than 4 years.[45] A visual analog scale, or a numeric pain scale, can be used in older children (e.g., age 10 years) who can verbalize and comprehend number values. Additional information regarding the assessment and treatment of pain can be found in the Pain Management chapter.

LABORATORY VALUES

Normal laboratory values in infants and children can differ from those seen in adults. Physiologic differences account for variation in normal ranges by age and are noted throughout the book in reference to the disease states discussed. With the advances in software technology, laboratories now often report abnormal values with adjacent normal ranges based on the age of pediatric patients. Standard pediatric handbooks or references such as *The Harriet Lane Handbook* or the *Pediatric & Neonatal Dosage Handbook* also serve as resources for normal laboratory values for pediatric patients.[46,47]

CALCULATIONS

In addition to differences in normal vital signs and laboratory value ranges, calculations used to assess pediatric patients

Table 2. Common Equations Used for Data Calculations in Pediatric Patients[48–50,53-57,73]

Calculation	Equation
Body surface area (BSA)[a]	BSA (m^2) = square root [(height × weight) ÷ 3600]
Body mass index (BMI)[a]	BMI = weight ÷ height ÷ height × 10,000
Ideal body weight (IBW)[a]	IBW (kg) = [(height)^2 × 1.65] ÷ 1000
Creatinine clearance (CrCl) or estimated glomerular filtration rate (GFR)	**Original Schwartz Equation** CrCl (mL/minute/1.73 m^2) = [k × L] ÷ SCr k = proportionality constant L = length in centimeters SCr = serum creatinine in mg/dL Premature infant age ≤ 1 yr: k = 0.33 Term infant age ≤ 1 yr: k = 0.45 Child (male or female) or adolescent female: k = 0.45 Adolescent male: k = 0.7 **Bedside Schwartz Equation (Modified Schwartz Equation)** for patients age 1–18 years CrCl = [0.413 × height (in cm)]/SCr (in mg/dL)
Estimation of pediatric dosing when limited pediatric-dosing data are available	Approximate pediatric dose = adult dose × [BSA (in m^2) ÷ 1.73 m^2]

[a]With height in centimeters, weight in kilograms.

differ from those used for adult patients. Body surface area, BMI, and ideal body weight calculations are sometimes used in the dosing of certain medications and in assessing nutritional status (Table 2).[48-50] Creatinine clearance is used to assess a patient's renal function and is applied in dosing when renal dysfunction is present or when the patient is taking a potentially nephrotoxic drug. The Cockcroft-Gault and Jeliffe equations have been studied and validated in healthy adult populations but should not be applied when evaluating pediatric patients.[51,52] The Schwartz equation is used to calculate estimated creatinine clearance in pediatric patients, including low-birth-weight infants and patients up to age 21 years.[53,54] Although use of the Schwartz equation is a common approach to estimating glomerular filtration rate (GFR) in pediatric patients, this equation has limitations. For example, the Schwartz equation can potentially overestimate GFR, especially in moderate to severe renal insufficiency, because serum creatinine is a crude marker of GFR.[54,55] Thus, alternative methods based on additional factors such as cystatin C or blood urea nitrogen have been proposed to estimate GFR in children with renal insufficiency such as chronic kidney disease.[56,57] Most of the equations listed in Table 2 apply to infants, children, and adolescents; however, application of these equations is limited in the neonatal population. Assessment methods for neonates and premature infants can be found in the Introduction to Neonatology chapter.

CHALLENGES OF MEDICATION ADHERENCE

Adherence, defined as "the extent to which a person's behavior – taking medication, following a diet, and/or executing lifestyle changes, corresponds with agreed recommendations from a health care provider," is a challenge for all patient populations, and pediatric patients are no exception to this continued health care issue.[58] Although chronic illnesses, such as cystic fibrosis and diabetes mellitus, are often associated with a high potential for poor adherence, short antibiotic treatment courses for conditions such as acute otitis media are also worth investigating.[59] Consequences of nonadherence include delayed or absent clinical improvement, worsening of illness, and unnecessary therapy modifications that can lead to adverse clinical outcomes. Medication adherence is often difficult to document in ambulatory care practice environments. Approaches to measuring medication adherence include self-report, clinician's impression, dose count (e.g., pills or inhaler counter), refill verification, electronic dose monitoring services, and monitoring of serum drug concentrations when appropriate.[60,61] Devices such as electronic monitors have been used in research settings. However, these are not commonplace in clinic settings and are cost-prohibitive for routine use at this time.[62,63]

Nonadherence, often defined as adhering to a prescribed therapy less than 80% of the time, is multifaceted in nature. It is seen in all age groups, from infancy to adolescence. Reasons for poor adherence include incorrect timing because of forgetting to administer a dose, conflict with caregiver's and/or patient's personal beliefs, socioeconomic limitations, adverse drug effects, and unpleasant or inconvenient medication formulation or schedules, as well as psychological factors, such as peer acceptance among adolescents. In general, children younger than 5 years have greater medication adherence to the treatment of chronic illnesses, in most cases because of caregiver responsibility and action in administering necessary medication.[61] However, it should not be assumed that all caregivers adhere to prescribed treatment regimens. A reason for poor adherence in this subpopulation is apprehension regarding medication adverse effects. An example is nonadherence to inhaled corticosteroid therapy for asthma because of the fear of growth suppression. Other reasons for nonadherence in this younger population can include the caregiver's inability and unavailability to administer the drugs in a timely manner.[61]

Inappropriate measurements of a medication dose can also affect medication adherence. For example, if a caregiver uses a measuring device to administer a liquid medication that results in larger doses (e.g., a large kitchen spoon), adverse drug effects as well as early therapy discontinuation may ensue. Conversely, if caregivers use a device that provides a smaller amount of medication (e.g., a small dining teaspoon), subtherapeutic dosing and poor patient outcomes with respect to efficacy may ensue. Thus, caregivers should be provided with and educated about proper measuring devices such as oral syringes. Some caregivers may also miss doses because of resistance from the child. As a child grows older and enters early adolescence, responsibility for medication administration shifts from the caregiver to the child or adolescent. Approaches to improve medication adherence should address the transition from childhood to adolescence, which involves factors such as peer pressure, perceived invisibility, and potential for oppositional or rebellious behavior.[64]

Different approaches have been suggested to improve medication adherence. Behavioral and educational approaches such as motivational interviewing have received the most emphasis in studies regarding chronic diseases such as pediatric asthma and diabetes mellitus.[65,66] Caregiver education regarding medications should be reinforced at several points of health care visits because it is important to enhance the caregiver's understanding of the importance and benefit of completing treatment and the risk of adverse effects. Ease of administration, including palatable dosage forms and the need for less frequent dosing, can help caregivers keep to a treatment schedule. Poor palatability of medication, specifically liquid medications, can negatively affect medication adherence. Despite the lack of extensive research data, clinician and parental experiences have shown the importance of palatability as a target to improve adherence for oral medications.[61,63] The use of a reward system and positive reinforcement may aid in decreasing resistance by young children during treatment periods. Empowering older children and adolescents positively with knowledge about their disease may improve self-management of drug therapy and medication adherence.[64]

OFF-LABEL MEDICATION USE IN PEDIATRIC PATIENTS

Off-label medication use is defined as the use of a medication outside its FDA label-approved indications, which include the *age group in which a medication is used*, the *disease or illness it treats*, and the *route of administration*. Currently, more than 75% of the drugs approved for use in adults lack dosing, efficacy, and safety data pertaining to pediatric patients.[21] Off-label use is legal and well accepted as long as the use is based on appropriate clinical judgment. However, limitations to off-label medication use exist, including the potential for

denied insurance provider coverage of the medication. Other limitations to off-label medication use are possible medical liability because of serious adverse effects, limited experience for treatment of a condition or specific age group (e.g., neonates), and limited available formulations for use in young populations. Thus, a strong need remains for additional clinical trials to determine the appropriateness of selecting and dosing medications in the pediatric population.

Regulatory changes have been made to decrease the off-label use of drugs in the pediatric population. The Pediatric Rule, issued in 1994, permitted manufacturers to label drugs for pediatric use on the basis of extrapolated efficacy data and additional PK/PD data specific to the pediatric population when disease and therapy response were considered similar to those of their adult counterparts.[67] Unfortunately, this permission resulted in only a few well-conducted studies regarding infants and children because of the difficulties involved in predicting dose-response from adult data. The Food and Drug Administration Modernization Act (FDAMA) followed in 1997, offering a financial incentive of extended market exclusivity for 6 months for performing pediatric studies.[68] Because of the FDAMA, additional drugs were assigned pediatric labeling. However, efficacy data were still lacking. In 2002, an incentive-based Best Pharmaceuticals for Children Act was implemented, extending the FDAMA including the provision from the 1997 FDAMA offering an additional 6 months of patent exclusivity for on-patent drugs being tested for pediatric use, thereby encouraging industry to conduct pediatric studies for branded products labeled only for adults.[69] The Pediatric Research Equity Act (PREA) of 2003 also provided potential requirements for the pediatric assessment of drug applications submitted to the FDA for approval in adults.[67] This assessment includes the potential use and evaluation of risk versus benefit in pediatric patients. The FDA pediatric decision tree, a process whereby agents are evaluated for pediatric study regarding PK/PD, efficacy, and safety, is shown in Figure 3.[70] For rare diseases with an occurrence of 200,000 people or fewer in the United States, such as inborn errors of metabolism, the Orphan Drug Act provides support in the development of needed treatment.[71]

The 2002 Best Pharmaceuticals for Children Act has been effective primarily for the blockbuster drugs to receive 6-month patent exclusivity. Thus, the concern remains when extrapolating adult data to treat pediatric patients for many branded products with a limited market and for generic drugs with no incentives. Extrapolation is challenging because this approach is not always accurate when determining safe and effective pediatric dosing. A wide range of evidence in pediatric drug therapy through the identification of well-designed, appropriate biomedical literature is needed to provide optimal, evidence-based care to the pediatric population. The use of available guidelines, such as those commissioned by the National Asthma Education and Prevention Program and National Heart, Lung and Blood Institute for asthma,[72] is recommended, although their individualized application to specific patients is necessary in pediatric patient care.

Because of limited pediatric-specific guidelines for much of drug therapy, use of primary literature is crucial in providing evidence-based care to infants, children, and adolescents.

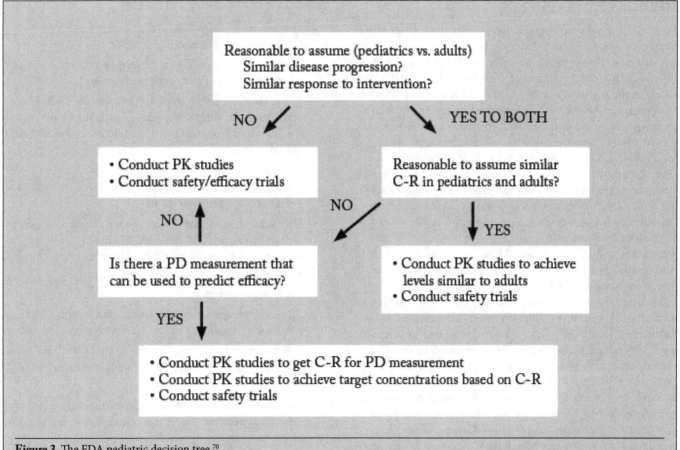

Figure 3. The FDA pediatric decision tree.[70]

C-R = concentration response; PD = pharmacodynamic; PK = pharmacokinetic.

Reprinted from U.S. Food and Drug Administration: Guidance for Industry: Exposure–Response Relationships—Study Design, Data Analysis, and Regulatory Applications. Available at www.fda.gov/downloads/Drugs/GuidanceComplianceRegulatoryInformation/Guidances/ucm072109.pdf. Accessed April 24, 2018.

Although randomized, placebo-controlled trials are considered the "gold standard" of primary literature, much of the available literature consists of retrospective cohort studies of the pediatric population. Careful evaluation of these data should guide the applicability of the results in clinical practice. Evaluation of literature includes appropriateness of study design, generalizability to the population under study, and appreciation for statistical and clinical significance of findings. Furthermore, the use of case reports and case series can provide some data regarding unknown effects of newer drug therapy. However, given the small patient populations in these reports, clinicians should assess the appropriateness of applying them to their own patients.

Another dilemma for many drug therapy options is that adult dosing often involves a standard dose for most of the population regardless of age and weight (e.g., omeprazole 20 mg orally daily), whereas pediatric dosing is often weight-dependent (e.g., omeprazole 1 mg/kg orally daily). Pediatric dosages may also be based on age (e.g., neonate vs. child). Rounding of doses is an issue not often seen in the care of adults. In pediatric patients, doses of wide-therapeutic index medications (e.g., antibiotics) can be rounded for ease of measurement. Some institutions round doses by 10% to 20%, depending on the risks associated with a given medication.

In the past, approaches to dosing included different rules to estimate dosing when pediatric-specific data were not available. However, these equations differentiated a child from an adult using a ratio of one factor of difference such as *age in months* (*Fried's Rule*) or *age in years* (*Young's Rule*) or *weight in pounds* (*Clark's Rule*). This approach oversimplifies the known complex differences between the pediatric and adult populations. As a result, these approaches can over- or underestimate dosing in pediatric patients. Thus, these methods are no longer recommended for estimating off-label dosing in pediatric patients. If there is no alternative therapy—or if limited or no pediatric data exist for dosing, but evidence supports the safety of the drug in pediatric patients—some clinicians may elect to dose on the basis of the body surface area ratio if the child is in the normal range for height and weight for age (Table 1).[73] Of note, however, this method is not a well-studied approach to off-label medication dosing, and caution should be used when considering this option. A potential exists for unaccounted differences in PK/PD between pediatric and adult patients when using this dose-estimating approach, resulting in differences in efficacy and safety. Thus, clinical judgment should be applied when considering off-label medication use and dosing in instances of limited pediatric data.

MEDICATION SAFETY

Medication errors are preventable events that result from human or system flaws.[8] Pediatric patients are at increased risk of medication errors, with an error rate of 15% of pediatric medication orders compared with 5% of adult medication orders in the acute care setting.[8] Prescribing and transcription errors account for many of the medication errors—50% of all errors—in neonatal and pediatric intensive care units in the United States. Because pediatric doses are often calculated (e.g., milligram per kilogram), the risk of calculation error is high. Accuracy and consistency in the units of measurement used are important in preventing calculation and prescribing errors. Decimal errors, such as trailing zeros (e.g., 5.0 mg) and missing leading zeros (e.g., .5 mg), also result in 10-fold or greater errors. As with any patient, the *five rights of patient medication administration* should be reviewed every time to help ensure medication safety: *right patient, right drug, right dose, right route,* and *right time.*

Medication safety is also compromised with errors in medication preparation, dilution, and dose measurement.[74] Calculation inaccuracies can lead to prescribed dose errors, especially when medications are compounded into intravenous solutions or oral suspensions. One should also be cautious of potential dispensing errors when the incorrect strength of a medication is selected. Calculation errors can be reduced through computer physician order entry, which can provide automated medication-dosing calculators and mandatory prescription order fields.[75] The use of an alert-based decision support system can potentially prevent several errors; however, it also has the potential to cause "alert fatigue" because of too many unnecessary alerts, which can lead a clinician to bypass warnings for incorrect medication orders. Barcode technology has also helped reduce the incorrect selection and administration of medications.[76] Medication administration error rates have also decreased with the use of technologies such as smart pumps for parenteral medications in daily care.[77] Despite technological advances, however, a potential for human or system error remains during the process of preparing, dispensing, and administering medications. Thus, medication error prevention is a multifaceted task involving the active participation of the health care team as well as the patient and caregiver. Communication between all parties and continued efforts to improve medication use practice are essential in the provision of safe patient care (Medication Safety chapter).

FUNDAMENTALS OF PEDIATRIC PATIENT CARE

Application of pediatric-specific knowledge and clinical skills is vital to the successful care of infants, children, and adolescents. Within each subpopulation, it is imperative to recognize differences because of patient-specific factors (e.g., age, disease, culture) and adapt approaches to suit each individual to provide optimal patient care. The following "checklists" are clinical pearls to keep in mind when caring for patients within each age subpopulation in pediatrics.

INFANTS AND YOUNG CHILDREN

- For neonates and premature infants, please refer to the Introduction to Neonatology chapter.

- Educate the caregiver about the purpose, effectiveness, and potential adverse effects of the medication.

- For children younger than 3 years, review birth history and history of illness, including hospitalizations; review medical record for assessment of cognitive and motor skills development.

- Note body weight, height, and head circumference (for infants), and assess growth percentiles (e.g., by using the WHO or CDC growth chart).

- For infants, evaluate weight-based dosing regularly, especially for medications used in chronic illnesses that require dose adjustments with growth (e.g., weight gain).

- Use an up-to-date weight available to verify appropriate doses (e.g., mg/kg).

- Elixir formulations should be avoided because of alcohol content, especially in neonates and young infants, or when chronic use or larger volumes are indicated.

- Minimize use of dosage forms with preservatives (e.g., benzyl alcohol) in neonates.

- Be aware of the palatability of medications—if an oral liquid formulation tastes bad, investigate whether an alternative exists in a solid dosage form that is safe to administer as either a crushed tablet or an opened capsule, mixing the contents into a palatable delivery method. An example of a poor-tasting oral solution is clindamycin; if a dose fits a capsule size, some clinicians elect opening the capsule in soft food (e.g., applesauce) versus administering the liquid oral formulation.

  ○ Approaches to help alleviate unpalatable medications can include use of food items to help mask the unpleasant aftertaste of some medications. Always ask about any food or medication allergies before suggesting items. For bitter or salty tasting medications, chocolate may serve to mask the taste (e.g., use of chocolate syrup with doses). For those medications with a metallic taste, fruit flavors (e.g., strawberry syrup) may help mask unpleasant taste. Other possible approaches to offset unpleasant taste is to offer a cold treat (e.g., sorbet) before and after a dose. The cold may help numb papillae of the tongue and minimize medication aftertaste.

  ○ Many pharmacies also offer patients and caregivers the option of services to add flavoring agents to liquid dosage formulations. Considerations when using flavor agents are dosage form stability with the addition as well flavor compatibility to best mask unpleasant taste.

- Do not crush or modify extended- or sustained-release solid dosage forms.

- Use appropriate measuring devices (e.g., oral syringe) with oral liquid formulations.

- Be aware of potential medication contraindications because of age (e.g., ceftriaxone use in premature neonates because of potential to displace bilirubin from albumin and increase the risk of kernicterus).
- Often, children around age 6 years can swallow a tablet or capsule, but this ability should not be assumed for all children. Ask the patient and caregiver whether liquid or solid dosage forms are preferred.

OLDER CHILDREN AND ADOLESCENTS

- Use an up-to-date weight available to verify appropriate doses (e.g., mg/kg).
- Maximum doses are often adult doses; however, verify such dosing using a pediatric dosing reference. A common body weight at which adult dosing is applied is when a child reaches 40 kg.[78]
- Educate patients and caregivers about the purpose, effectiveness, and potential adverse effects of the medication.
- Consider issues that are more mature or adult in nature affecting health including alcohol, tobacco, illicit drug use, sexual activity, and psychosocial concerns.
- Adolescence is often considered a "nadir" of medication adherence; thus, education and age-appropriate approaches to improve adherence should be initiated.
- Be aware of the need for increasing independence, including medication administration.
- Involve the patient as an active participant in overall care.

OVERALL DRUG THERAPY ASSESSMENT

The following are examples of general items that should be considered and assessed as part of selecting, using, and monitoring drug therapy for all pediatric patients[2,3,5,7]:

- Use correct age, weight (in kilograms), and height.
- Consider social factors such as patient or caregiver health beliefs and culture.
- Correctly use units of measurement such as dose (e.g., milligram vs. gram) and body weight (e.g., kilogram vs. pound).
- Calculate and verify doses by body weight (e.g., actual, ideal, adjusted) as appropriate.
- Evaluate current conditions and determine optimal drug therapy for such conditions.
- Consider comorbidities.
- Evaluate appropriateness of current drug therapy including complementary and alternative medications, supplements, and over-the-counter drugs.
- Assess medication adherence.
- Be careful about inappropriate abbreviations and notations such as trailing zeros (e.g., 1.0 mg) and missing leading zeros (e.g., .1 mg).
- Evaluate for potential adverse drug effects (i.e., ask open-ended questions of patients and caregivers).

- Evaluate for drug-drug and drug-food interactions.
- Round doses to measurable amounts. Dose rounding by 10% to the closest measurable dose is common practice. Dose rounding should be avoided in medications with a narrow therapeutic index (e.g., digoxin).
- Develop a monitoring plan for drug therapy with identification and assessment of the values for efficacy or safety.
- Reconcile medications and dosage regimens at each patient encounter.
- Provide patient and caregiver education. Not a one-time activity, education should be reinforced at several points of care (e.g., hospital, clinic, pharmacy)—*Repetition is beneficial!*

PATIENT AND CAREGIVER EDUCATION

Patient and caregiver education is fundamental to the care of pediatric patients. Drug therapy can be daunting to some caregivers, especially to new parents or caregivers of patients with a new disease diagnosis. Clinicians should be considerate of their approach when communicating with patients and caregivers including health literacy, culture or beliefs, socioeconomic status, and family structure/dynamic. Information that patients and caregivers should be privy to includes:

- Reasons for medication use
- Expected therapy outcomes
- Dose measurement (with appropriate device)
- Medication storage
- Potential adverse drug effects
- Therapy duration
- If therapy is chronic and requires laboratory monitoring, then discuss what these tests are, why they are used for monitoring efficacy or safety, and how often monitoring is performed.

Education should be specific regarding the type of drug therapy a patient is using. For example, specialized information is needed when discussing aerosolized or nebulized medication and use of a nebulizer device. An important educational point in this case is administration technique in the use of a metered dose inhaler with or without a spacer. Other medication administration techniques that patient and caregivers may not be as familiar with are the proper administration of otic drops, ophthalmic drops or ointments, and nasal sprays. Additional information is provided in the Communicating with Children, Adolescents, and Their Caregivers chapter. Patient and caregiver education should be provided in all patient care settings in both inpatient and outpatient environments. Reinforcement of essential points is critical in optimizing medication adherence and safety. Transitions of care should include clear communication between inpatient and outpatient clinic and/or community pharmacy settings. This bridge of care involving health care providers as well as patients and their families is necessary in providing optimal patient care. Pharmacists can bridge the gaps by encouraging patients and their families to ask questions and by providing information about current medications. For example, pharmacists can provide means for patients and their families to maintain medication lists (written or electronic), thereby empowering them to participate in their health care.

THE PRESENT AND FUTURE OF PEDIATRIC PHARMACY PRACTICE

Pediatric patients are seen in all health care settings, including community pharmacies, ambulatory clinics, community hospitals, and large academic, tertiary institutions. A fundamental understanding of the needs of this special population is essential for the provision of patient care by pharmacists. Although pharmacists in the community setting often lack specialty training in pediatric practice, all pharmacy practitioners should have an appreciation of general concepts in pediatrics, such as approaches to dosing (e.g., milligram per kilogram), pharmacokinetics, and drug administration needs, as well as the ability to identify potential drug-related problems (e.g., contraindicated medications for certain age groups). Examples of available resources can be found as part of various pharmacy professional organizations, such as the American College of Clinical Pharmacy, Pediatric Pharmacy Association, and American Society of Health-System Pharmacists.[79-81]

Pediatric pharmacy practice is a growing specialty area of pharmacy practice, serving future generations of patients with a mission focused on patient advocacy and provision of safe and effective drug therapy through professional responsibility, education, and research. This area of practice will continue to grow with its expansions in the professional pharmacy school curriculum, including specialty pediatrics tracks for doctor of pharmacy degrees, as well as continued education and training in pediatric postgraduate residencies and fellowships. Practice opportunities in pediatric pharmacy have expanded beyond the pharmacy counter, with an increasing number of pharmacists working as part of interdisciplinary teams in the care of infants, children, and adolescents, from intensive care units to specialist clinics such as cystic fibrosis centers nationwide. Opportunities exist to advance pediatric practice for present and future generations of pharmacists, including expanding the role of pharmacists in areas such as pediatric immunizations, chronic care management, and continuity of care between inpatient and outpatient care. Pharmacists must also initiate and participate in pediatric pharmacotherapy research to advance health care and the profession. Examples of pharmacist-driven innovations include increasing the understanding of approaches to drug therapy management, discovering new therapeutic approaches, and developing behavioral interventions to optimize medication adherence. This partnership of advanced practice and scholarship is what the pharmacy profession must promote to make contributions to the body of knowledge in pediatrics and provide quality patient care.

ADDITIONAL GENERAL PEDIATRIC RESOURCES

Additional information regarding pediatric patient care, including medication dosing, extemporaneous compounding, and an overview of general pediatric diseases, can be found in various resources from the Internet to print books (Box 1).[46,47,78-87] With the growth in information technology, many drug-dosing references are also available by smartphone or tablet computers. Clinicians caring for pediatric patients should have access to at least one reference regarding pediatric-specific dosing and one reference on general pediatric disease pathophysiology and treatment options.

Box 1. Examples of General Pediatric Resources[79-88]

Websites

American Academy of Pediatrics (AAP)—www.aap.org

Pediatric Pharmacy Association (PPA)—
www.ppag.org

References

*Hughes HK, Kaul LK. The Harriet Lane Handbook, 21st ed. Philadelphia: Elsevier Mosby, 2018.

*Buck ML, Hendrick AE. Pediatric Medication Education Text, 5th ed. Lenexa, KS: American College of Clinical Pharmacy, 2009.

*Kliegman RM, St. Geme J. Nelson Textbook of Pediatrics, 21st ed. Philadelphia: Saunders, 2019.

*Taketomo CK, Pediatric & Neonatal Dosage Handbook, 26th ed. Hudson, OH: Lexi-Comp, 2019 [also available as online database version].

*Nahata MC, Pai VB. Pediatric Drug Formulations, 7th ed. Cincinnati: Harvey Whitney, 2019.

Phelps SJ, Hagemann TM, Lee KR, et al. Pediatric Injectable Drugs: The Teddy Bear Book, 11th ed. Bethesda, MD: American Society of Health-System Pharmacists, 2018.

*Available in print and electronically.

REFERENCES

1. Kearns GL, Abdel-Rahman SM, Alander SW, et al. Developmental pharmacology-drug disposition, action, therapy in infants and children. N Engl J Med 2003;349:1157-67.

2. Pediatric Pharmacy Administration Group Committee on Pediatric Pharmacy Practice. Pediatric pharmacy practice guidelines. Am J Hosp Pharm 1991;48:2475-7.

3. American Society of Hospital Pharmacists. ASHP guidelines for providing pediatric pharmaceutical services in organized health care systems. Am J Hosp Pharm 1994;51:1690-6.

4. American Society of Health-System Pharmacists and Pediatric Pharmacy Advocacy Group. Educational Outcomes, Goals, and Objectives for Postgraduate Year Two (PGY2) Pharmacy Residencies in Pediatrics. Available at https://www.ashp.org/-/media/assets/professional-development/residencies/docs/pgy2-newly-approved-pediatric-pharmacy-2016.ashx-?la=en&hash=E3AA8593C06B82F81A85B6294B3D7DFA760E35BC. Accessed May 20, 2019.

5. Pediatric Pharmacy Association. Practice Statements and Guidelines. Available at https://www.ppag.org/index.cfm?pg=PositionStatements. Accessed November 10, 2019.

6. Kennedy MJ, Phan H, Benavides S, et al. Pediatric Pharmacy Advocacy Group, position statement: the role of the pediatric pharmacist in personalized medicine and clinical pharmacogenomics for children. J Pediatr Pharmacol Ther 2011;16:118-122.

7. Aucoin RG, Buck ML, Dupuis LL, et al. Pediatric pharmacotherapeutic education: current status and recommendations to fill the growing need. Pharmacotherapy 2005;25:1277-82.

8. American Academy of Pediatrics Committee on Drugs; American Academy of Pediatrics Committee on Hospital Care. Prevention of medication errors in the pediatric inpatient setting. Pediatrics 2003;112:431-6.

9. Bhatt-Mehta V, Buck ML, Chung AM, et al. Recommendations for meeting the pediatric patient's need for a clinical pharmacist: a joint opinion of the Pediatrics Practice and Research Network of the American College of Clinical Pharmacy and the Pediatric Pharmacy Advocacy Group. Pharmacotherapy 2013;33:243-251.

10. Board of Pharmacy Specialties (BPS). Pediatric Pharmacy. Washington DC: Board of Pharmacy Specialties. Available at www.bpsweb.org/bps-specialties/pediatric-pharmacy/. Accessed May 20, 2019.

11. Association of American Medical Colleges. Electronic Residency Application Service, 2018 Participating Specialties and Programs. Available at https://services.aamc.org/eras/erasstats/par/index.cfm. Accessed April 23, 2018.

12. American Society of Health-System Pharmacists (ASHP). Online Residency Directory. Available at https://accred.ashp.org/aps/pages/directory/residencyprogramsearch.aspx. Accessed April 23, 2018.

13. Phan H, Pai VB, Nahata MC. Pediatrics. In: Chisholm-Burns MA, Schwinghammer TL, Wells BG, et al., eds. Pharmacotherapy: Principles and Practice, 4th ed. New York: McGraw-Hill, 2016;19-29.

14. American Academy of Pediatrics, Committee on Fetus and Newborn. Age terminology during the perinatal period. Pediatrics 2004;114:1362-4.

15. U.S. Department of Health and Human Services, Food and Drug Administration, Center for Drug Evaluation and Research (CDER), and Center for Biologics and Evaluation and Research (CBER). Guidance for Industry, E11 Clinical Investigation of Medicinal Products in the Pediatric Population. December 2000. Available at www.fda.gov/downloads/drugs/guidancecomplianceregulatoryinformation/guidances/ucm073143.pdf. Accessed April 24, 2018.

16. Mulye TP, Park MJ, Nelson CD, et al. Trends in adolescent and young adult health in the United States. J Adolesc Health 2009;45:8-24.

17. Strolin Benedetti M, Baltes EL. Drug metabolism and disposition in children. Fundam Clin Pharmacol 2003;17:281-99.

18. Committee on Drugs. Off-label use of drugs in children. Pediatrics. 2014;133:563-67.

19. Palmaro A, Bissuel R, Renaud N, et al. Off-label prescribing in pediatric outpatients. Pediatrics. 2015:135:49-58.

20. Bazzano AT, Mangione-Smith R, Schonlau M, et al. Off-label prescribing to children in the United States outpatient setting. Acad Pediatr 2009;9:81-8.

21. Shah SS, Hall M, Goodman DM, et al. Off-label drug use in hospitalized children. Arch Pediatr Adolesc Med 2007;161:282-90.

22. U.S. Census Bureau. National Population by Characteristics: 2010-2017. Available at www.census.gov/data/tables/time-series/demo/popest/2010s-national-detail.html. Accessed May 20, 2019.

23. Bloom B, Jones LI, Freeman G. Summary Health Statistics for U.S. children: National Health Interview Survey, 2012. National Center for Health Statistics. Vital Health Stat 2013;10(258). Available at www.cdc.gov/nchs/data/series/sr_10/sr10_258.pdf. Accessed April 24, 2018.

24. Rui P, Okeyode T. National Ambulatory Medical Care Survey: 2015 State and National Summary Tables. Available at www.cdc.gov/nchs/ahcd/ahcd_products.htm. Accessed April 23, 2018.

25. Association of Maternal & Child Health Programs. Children & Youth With Special Health Care Needs. Available at www.amchp.org/programsandtopics/CYSHCN/Pages/default.aspx. Accessed April 24, 2018.

26. Witt WP (Truven Health Analytics), Weiss AJ (Truven Health Analytics), Elixhauser A (AHRQ). Overview of hospital stays for children in the United States, 2012. Rockville, MD: Agency for Healthcare Research and Quality. December 2014. HCUP Statistical Brief #187. Available at www.hcup-us.ahrq.gov/reports/statbriefs/sb187-Hospital-Stays-Children-2012.jsp. Accessed April 24, 2018.

27. Rui P, Kang K, Albert M. National Hospital Ambulatory Medical Care Survey: 2013 Emergency Department Summary Tables. Available at www.cdc.gov/nchs/data/ahcd/nhamcs_emergency/2013_ed_web_tables.pdf. Accessed April 24, 2018.

28. Vernacchio L, Kelly JP, Kaufman DW, et al. Medication use among children <12 years of age in the United States: Results from the Slone Survey. Pediatrics 2009;124:446-54.

29. Centers for Disease Control and World Health Organization. Growth charts. Available at www.cdc.gov/growthcharts. Accessed April 24, 2018.

30. Feigelman S. The first year. In: Kliegman RM, Stanton BF, St. Geme JW, et al. eds. Nelson Textbook of Pediatrics. Philadelphia: Saunders Elsevier, 2016:62-5.e1.

31. Feigelman S. The second year. In: Kliegman RM, Behrman RE, Jenson HB, et al. eds. Nelson Textbook of Pediatrics. Philadelphia: Saunders Elsevier, 2016:70-6.e1.

32. Council on Children with Disabilities; Section on Developmental Behavioral Pediatrics; Bright Futures Steering Committee; Medical Home Initiatives for Children With Special Needs Project Advisory Committee. Identifying infants and young children with developmental disorders in the medical home: an algorithm for developmental surveillance and screening. Pediatrics 2006;118:405-20.

33. Piaget J, Inhelder B. The psychology of the child. New York: Basic Books, 1969.

34. Committee on Practice and Ambulatory Medicine and Bright Futures Periodicity Schedule Workgroup. American Academy of Pediatrics. 2016 Recommendations for Preventive Pediatric Health Care. Pediatrics 2016;137:26-27.

35. Fleming S, Thompson M, Stevens R, et al. Normal ranges of heart rate and respiratory rate in children from birth to 18 years of age: a systematic review of observational studies. Lancet 2011;377:1011-8.

---

36. American Heart Association. Pediatric Advanced Life Support Provider Manual. Dallas: American Heart Association, 2006.

37. National High Blood Pressure Education Program Working Group on High Blood Pressure in Children and Adolescents. The fourth report on the diagnosis, evaluation, and treatment of high blood pressure in children and adolescents. Pediatrics 2004;114 (2 suppl 4th report):555-76.

38. American Academy of Pediatrics. (2007). Parenting Corner Q&A: What's the Best Way to Take a Child's Temperature? Available at www.healthychildren.org/English/health-issues/conditions/fever/pages/How-to-Take-a-Childs-Temperature.aspx. Accessed April 24, 2018.

39. Doezema D, Lunt M, Tandberg D. Cerumen occlusion lowers infrared tympanic membrane temperature measurement. Acad Emerg Med 1995;2:17-9.

40. Greenes DS, Fleisher GR. Accuracy of a noninvasive temporal artery thermometer for use in infants. Arch Pediatr Adolesc Med 2001;155:376-81.

41. Sullivan JE, Farrar HC. Section on Clinical Pharmacology and Therapeutics and Committee on Drugs. Clinical report—fever and antipyretic use in children. Pediatrics 2011;127:580-7.

42. Baraff LJ, Bass JW, Fleisher GR, et al. Practice guideline for the management of infants and children 0 to 36 months of age with fever without source. Agency for Health Care Policy and Research. Ann Emerg Med 1993;22:1198-210.

43. Lawrence J, Alcock D, McGrath P, et al. The development of a tool to assess neonatal pain. Neonatal Netw 1993;12:59-66.

44. Merkel SI, Voepel-Lewis T, Shayevitz JR, et al. The FLACC: a behavioral scale for scoring postoperative pain in young children. Pediatr Nurs 1997;3:293-7.

45. Hockenberry MJ, Wilson D, Winkelstein ML. Wong's Essentials of Pediatric Nursing, 7th ed. St. Louis: Mosby, 2005:1259.

46. Arcara K, Tschudy M. The Harriet Lane Handbook, 20th ed. Philadelphia: Elsevier Mosby, 2015.

47. Taketomo CK, Hodding JH, Kraus DM. Pediatric & Neonatal Dosage Handbook, 23rd ed. Hudson, OH: Lexi-Comp, 2016 [also available as online database version].

48. Mosteller RD. Simplified calculation of body surface area. N Engl J Med 1987;317:1098.

49. Mei Z, Grummer-Strawn LM, Pietrobelli A, et al. Validity of body mass index compared with other body-composition screening indexes for the assessment of body fatness in children and adolescents. Am J Clin Nutr 2002;75:978-85.

50. Traub SL, Kichen L. Estimating ideal body mass in children. Am J Hosp Pharm 1983;40:107-10.

51. Cockroft DW, Gault MH. Prediction of creatinine clearance from serum creatinine. Nephron 1976;16:31-41.

52. Jeliffe RW. Creatinine clearance: bedside estimate. Ann Intern Med 1973;79:604-5.

53. Schwartz GJ, Brion LP, Spitzer A. The use of plasma creatinine concentration for estimating glomerular filtration rate in infants, children, and adolescents. Pediatr Clin North Am 1987;34:571-90.

54. Staples A, LeBlond R, Watkins S, et al. Validation of the revised Schwartz estimating equation in a predominantly non-CKD population. Pediatr Nephrol 2010;25:2321-6.

55. Seikaly MG, Browne R, Bajaj G, et al. Limitations to body length/serum creatinine ratio as an estimate of glomerular filtration in children. Pediatr Nephrol 1996;10:709-11.

56. Filler G, Lepage N. Should the Schwartz formula for estimation of GFR be replaced by cystatin C formula? Pediatr Nephrol 2003;18:981-5.

57. Schwartz GJ, Muñoz A, Schneider MF, et al. New equations to estimate GFR in children with CKD. J Am Soc Nephrol 2009;20:629-37.

58. Sabate E. Adherence to long-term therapies: evidence for action. World Health Organization. 2003. Available at http://www.who.int/chp/knowledge/publications/adherence_full_report.pdf?ua=1. Accessed May 20, 2019.

59. Osterberg L, Blaschke T. Adherence to medication. N Engl J Med 2005;353:487-97.

60. Matsui DM. Drug compliance in pediatrics clinical and research issues. Pediatr Clin North Am 1997;44:1-14.

61. Matsui D. Current issues in pediatric medication adherence. Pediatr Drugs 2007;9:283-8.

62. De Bleser L, De Geest S, Vincke B, et al. How to test electronic adherence monitoring devices for use in daily life: a conceptual framework. Comput Inform Nurs 2011;29:489-95.

63. Winnick S, Lucas DO, Hartman AL, et al. How do you improve compliance? Pediatrics 2005;115:e718-24.

64. Ou HT, Feldman SR, Balkrishnan R. Understanding and improving treatment adherence in pediatric patients. Semin Cutan Med Surg 2010;29:137-40.

65. McQuaid EL, Kopel SJ, Klein RB, et al. Medication adherence in pediatric asthma: reasoning, responsibility, and behavior. J Pediatr Psychol 2003;28:323-33.

66. Bond GG, Aiken LS, Somerville SC. The health belief model and adolescents with insulin-dependent diabetes mellitus. Health Psychol 1992;11:190-8.

67. Pediatric Research Equity Act. Public Law 108-155. Available at https://www.fda.gov/drugs/development-resources/pediatric-research-equity-act-prea. Accessed May 20, 2019.

68. Food and Drug Administration Modernization Act of 1997 (FDAMA). Enacted 21 November 1997. Available at https://www.fda.gov/regulatory-information/food-and-drug-administration-modernization-act-fdama-1997/fda-backgrounder-fdama. Accessed May 20, 2019.

69. Best Pharmaceuticals for Children Act. Public Law 107-109. Available at https://www.fda.gov/science-research/pediatrics/best-pharmaceuticals-children-act-and-pediatric-research-equity-act. Accessed April 24, 2018.

70. U.S. Food and Drug Administration: Guidance for Industry: Exposure-Response Relationships—Study Design, Data Analysis, and Regulatory Applications. Available at www.fda.gov/downloads/Drugs/GuidanceComplianceRegulatoryInformation/Guidances/ucm072109.pdf. Accessed April 24, 2018.

71. Orphan Drug Act. Available at www.fda.gov/ForIndustry/DevelopingProductsforRareDiseasesConditions/Howtoapplyfor OrphanProductDesignation/ucm364750.htm. Accessed April 24, 2018.

72. National Asthma Education and Prevention Program National Heart, Lung and Blood Institute. Expert Panel Report 3: Guidelines for the Diagnosis and Management of Asthma. Washington, DC: U.S. Department of Health and Human Services, 2007.

73. Shirkey HC. Drug dosage for infants and children. JAMA 1965; 193:443-6.

74. Rinke ML, Bundy DG, Velasquez CA, et al. Interventions to reduce pediatric medication errors: a systematic review. Pediatrics 2014;134:338-360.

75. Potts AL, Barr FE, Gregory DF, et al. Computerized physician order entry and medication errors in a pediatric critical care unit. Pediatrics 2004;113:59-63.

76. Poon EG, Keohane CA, Yoon CS, et al. Effect of bar-code technology on the safety of medication administration. N Engl J Med 2010;362:1698-707.

77. Larsen GY, Parker HB, Cash J, et al. Standard drug concentrations and smart-pump technology reduce continuous-medication-infusion errors in pediatric patients. Pediatrics 2005; 116:e21-5.

78. Matson KL, Horton ER, Capino AC; Advocacy Committee for the Pediatric Pharmacy Advocacy Group. Medication dosage in overweight and obese children. J Pediatr Pharmacol Ther 2017;22:81-3.

79. Pediatric Pharmacy Association (PPA) Position Statements and Guidelines. Available at https://www.ppag.org/index.cfm?pg=PositionStatements. Accessed November 10, 2019.

80. American Society of Health-System Pharmacists (ASHP) Resource Centers, Pediatrics. Available at https://www.ashp.org/pharmacy-practice/resource-centers/pediatrics. Accessed April 23, 2018.

81. American College of Clinical Pharmacy Practice and Research Networks. Available at www.accp.com/about/prns.aspx. Accessed April 23, 2018.

82. American Academy of Pediatrics (AAP) [homepage on the Internet]. Available at www.aap.org/. Accessed April 23, 2018.

83. Pediatric Pharmacy Association (PPA) [homepage on the Internet]. Available at www.ppag.org/. Accessed April 23, 2018.

84. Nahata MC, Pai VB. Pediatric Drug Formulations, 7th ed. Cincinnati: Harvey Whitney, 2019.

85. Kliegman RM, St. Geme J. Nelson Textbook of Pediatrics, 21st ed. Philadelphia: Saunders, 2019.

86. Phelps SJ, Hagemann TM, Lee KR, et al. Pediatric Injectable Drugs: The Teddy Bear Book, 11th ed. Bethesda, MD: American Society of Health-System Pharmacists, 2018.

87. Buck ML, Hendrick AE. Pediatric Medication Education Text, 5th ed. Lenexa, KS: American College of Clinical Pharmacy, 2009.

88. Hughes HK, Kaul LK. The Harriet Lane Handbook, 21st ed. Philadelphia: Elsevier Mosby, 2018.

CHAPTER 2

Introduction to Neonatology

Varsha Bhatt-Mehta, Pharm.D.,
M.S. (CRDSA), FCCP

LEARNING OBJECTIVES

1. Define the human neonate on the basis of gestational and postnatal age.

2. Understand the physiologic development for neonates of varying gestational ages that differentiates them from older infants and children, and understand neonate drug dosing and disposition.

3. Describe the most common disease states associated with premature and full-term neonates.

4. List the challenges of drug administration in the neonate, including dosage forms and methods of administration.

ABBREVIATIONS IN THIS CHAPTER

ADME	Absorption, distribution, metabolism, and elimination
CDC	Centers for Disease Control and Prevention
DBP	Diastolic blood pressure
ELBW	Extremely low birth weight
HBIG	Hepatitis B immunoglobulin
HBV	Hepatitis B vaccine
ICN	Intensive care nursery
MAP	Mean arterial pressure
NEC	Necrotizing enterocolitis
NRDS	Neonatal respiratory distress syndrome
PDA	Patent ductus arteriosus
SBP	Systolic blood pressure
VLBW	Very low birth weight

EVOLUTION OF THE SCIENCE OF NEONATAL–PERINATAL MEDICINE

HISTORICAL PERSPECTIVE

In 1960, Alexander Schaffer coined the term neonatology.[1] This term refers to the art and science of diagnosis and treatment of the diseases in the newborn infant. The science of neonatology is quite young, yet it has carved a niche of its own. The term perinatal defines the time between the obstetric and neonatal periods. Perinatologists specialize in maternofetal medicine. They take care of pregnant women who are at high risk of pregnancy-related complications. In large academic centers, the perinatal obstetricians and neonatologists work side by side in perinatal centers, giving rise to the specialty of neonatal–perinatal medicine. The first neonatal intensive care nurseries (ICNs) were formed around the early 1900s. Mainly reserved for the premature infant, these ICNs provided "warmth, rest, diet, quiet, sanitation, space"—to use Florence Nightingale's words[1]—and other amenities that prevail today in the modern high-tech ICN and were essential to the growth and survival of the premature neonate.

CONNECTION BETWEEN NEONATAL CARE SETTINGS: INTENSIVE CARE NURSERY, NEWBORN NURSERY, AND HOME CARE

Neonatology bridges obstetrics with pediatrics. Since ancient times, care for pregnant women has relied on midwives, grandmothers, and other experienced female elders. This approach worked well for uncomplicated pregnancies, but crises were common in complicated pregnancies, accounting for a significant number of maternal deaths. Specialty care was not provided to the neonate, resulting in high neonatal mortality, especially of premature neonates or those with congenital malformations. Today, the successful care of premature neonates requires a team of health care providers including obstetricians, perinatologists, and neonatologists.

ETHICAL DILEMMAS OF NEONATAL PRACTICE

The practice of neonatal–perinatal medicine is full of ethical dilemmas, including neonates with congenital malformations, extreme prematurity, and respiratory depression at birth. The lives of these neonates can be prolonged by modern technology and certain medications such as those that support blood pressure or sedative and analgesic agents to allow certain technologies such as mechanical ventilation to be more effective and provide life support for prolonged durations. However, the long-term neurologic outcome of such births is uncertain. Neonatologists face the ethical dilemma of how much life support to offer and for how long. In some cases, there may be a difference of opinion between the neonatologist and the family. Specialized ethics committees are required in such situations to determine the futility of the situation. While ethical discussions are ongoing, all health care professionals involved in the care of such patients must provide their full support to the treating physicians, who are ultimately responsible for the neonate's outcome.

EPIDEMIOLOGY

Neonatal deaths may be subdivided into *early neonatal deaths*, occurring during the first 7 days of life, and *late neonatal deaths*, occurring after the seventh day but before 28 completed days of life. *Perinatal mortality* (early neonatal death), defined as the number of stillbirths and deaths in the first week of life per 1000 live births, is a useful additional indicator of maternal and newborn health care and a main component of perinatal mortality reports. During the neonatal–perinatal period, the mother and fetus grow at a fast rate. At birth, the fetus is required to make an abrupt transition from the protective environment of the uterus to the extrauterine environment. This transition requires the baby to undergo significant physiologic stress. Thus, the highest number of neonatal deaths occurs in the first 24 hours of life. *Neonatal mortality rate*, defined by the World Health Organization as the number of deaths during the first 28 completed days of life per 1000 live births in a given year or period, is highest during the first month of life.

Globally, the mortality rate for children younger than age 5 years has decreased by 58%, from an estimated rate of 93 deaths per 1000 live births in 1990 to 39 deaths per 1000 live births in 2017. During the same period, 47% of all deaths for children younger than 5 years were newborn infants, an increase from 40% in 1990. Neonates who die within the first 28 days of birth have conditions and diseases associated with lack of quality care at birth or skilled care and treatment immediately after birth and in the first days of life. Preterm birth, intrapartum-related complications (birth asphyxia or lack of breathing at birth), infections, and birth defects cause most neonatal deaths in this age group (Figure 1). Reducing neonatal mortality is increasingly important because the proportion of deaths for children younger than 5 years that occur during the neonatal period is increasing, despite a decline in the overall mortality for this age group (Figure 2). The health interventions needed to address the major causes of neonatal deaths generally differ from those needed to address other deaths for children younger than 5 years.[2,3]

Preterm birth is an important perinatal health problem across the globe. Every year, an estimated 15 million neonates are born preterm (before 37 completed weeks of gestation), and this number is rising. Preterm birth complications are the leading cause of death among children younger than 5 years, responsible for around 1 million deaths in 2015. Of these deaths, 75% could be prevented with current, cost-effective interventions.

More than 60% of preterm births occur in Africa and South Asia, but preterm birth is truly a global problem. In the lower-income countries, on average, 12% of neonates are born too early compared with 9% in higher-income countries. Within countries, poorer families are at higher risk. The difference in survival of premature neonates depending on where they are born is dramatic. For example, more than 90% of extremely preterm neonates (less than 28 weeks) born in low-income countries die within the first few days of life, yet less than 10% of extremely preterm neonates die in high-income countries.[4-6]

The most recent data on infant mortality in the United States are from the National Center for Health Statistics, a branch of the Centers for Disease Control and Prevention (CDC). The total infant mortality rate declined from 6.75 infant deaths per 1000 births in 2007 to 6.07 in 2011, but since then did not change significantly through 2016 (5.87 infant deaths) (Figure 3). Infant mortality in the United States is highest among non-Hispanic black mothers (Figure 4). These

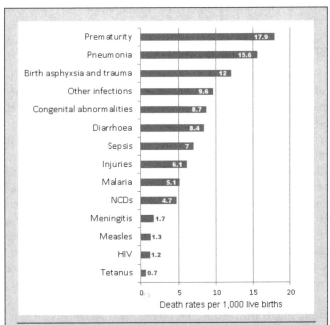

Figure 1. Global causes of death in 2016 among children younger than 5 years.

Neonatal deaths were 46% of deaths in this population.

Reprinted with permission from WHO-MCEE methods and data sources for child cause of death 2000- 2016. Global Health Estimates Technical Paper WHO/HMM/IER/GHE/2018.1 Available at https://www.who.int/maternal_child_adolescent/data/causes-death-children/en/. Accessed October 21, 2019.

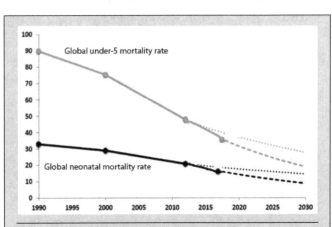

Figure 2. Global mortality rates in 2017 of children younger than age 5 years.

-------- = projected mortality rate;

········ = projected mortality rate to achieve the United Nation's Sustainable Development Goal (SDG) target that states all countries should aim to reduce neonatal mortality to at least as low as 12 deaths per 1000 live births and under-5 mortality to at least as low as 25 deaths per 1000 live births by 2030.

Reprinted with permission from WHO-MCEE methods and data sources for child cause of death 2000- 2016. Global Health Estimates Technical Paper WHO/HMM/IER/GHE/2018.1 Available at https://www.who.int/maternal_child_adolescent/data/causes-death-children/en/. Accessed October 21, 2019.

data were recently published in the National Vital Statistics Report of the National Center for Health Statistics branch of the CDC. Infants at younger gestational age have a large impact on U.S. mortality rates because of their higher risk of death. Figure 5 presents the distribution of live births and infant deaths by gestational age in the United States in 2007; infants younger than 34 weeks' gestation account for less than 5% of all infant births but greater than 50% of infant deaths.

HOW DOES THE NEONATAL POPULATION DIFFER FROM OTHER PEDIATRIC POPULATIONS?

DEFINING THE HUMAN NEONATE

Gestation is defined as the period between conception and birth. In humans, full gestation occurs during 37–40 weeks. Infants born before 37 weeks or 259 days of gestation are defined as *preterm* (or *premature*) *neonates*. The neonatal period commences at birth and ends at 28 completed days after birth. A *neonate* is defined as a newborn infant during the first 28 days of life after full gestation. After 28 days, the neonate is referred to as an *infant*.

Premature neonates may be further divided into subgroups by either gestational age or birth weight. Defining premature neonates by gestation is complicated because in many situations the weight and gestational age of the fetus may not correspond because growth retardation has occurred in utero from several different causes, for example, small-for-gestational-age infants who are small because of undernourishment in utero.

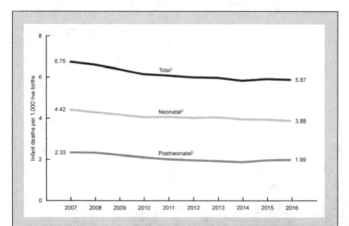

Figure 3. Total infant, neonatal, and postneonatal mortality rates in the United States from 2007–2016.[a]

[a]2013 Data are from the linked Birth/Infant Death datasets.

[1]Significant decreasing trend for 2007–2011 (p<0.05); stable trend for 2011–2016.

[2]Significant decreasing trend for 2007–2016 (p<0.05).

[3]Significant decreasing trend for 2007–2014 (p<0.05); stable trend for 2014–2016.

Information from the National Vital Statistics Report, National Center for Health Statistics (NCHS), Centers for Disease Control and Prevention (CDC). Infant Mortality by Age at Death in the United States, 2016. NCHS Data Brief No. 326, November 2018. Available at www.cdc.gov/nchs/products/databriefs/db326.htm. Accessed March 23, 2019.

Similarly, large-for-gestational-age infants weigh much more than anticipated at a given gestation.

The term *low birth weight* defines all infants born with a birth weight less than 2500 g. The term *very low birth weight* (VLBW) refers to infants weighing less than 1500 g, whereas the term *extremely low birth weight* (ELBW) refers to infants weighing less than 1000 g at birth. The care of VLBW and ELBW infants constitutes an important part of all ICNs and is a significant portion of the cost of care.[4] Another term more commonly used in the past 5 years is *late preterm infant*. This term signifies infants born between 34 and 37 weeks' gestation, although some controversy surrounds the lower end of gestational age.

Despite these dilemmas, for consistency of care among health care providers in everyday practice, some general definitions are necessary to describe the premature neonates' age after birth. The most commonly used descriptions include *postnatal age*, which refers to the actual chronologic age of the infant after birth, and *corrected gestational age*, *postmenstrual age*, and *postconceptional age*, which all refer to the same period, expressed differently—the sum of gestational age and postnatal age.

MULTIPLE GESTATIONS

The incidence of multiple gestations has increased during the past 2 decades, especially in some affluent countries, because of the increased number of pregnancies in older women as well as the increased use of fertility enhancement therapies. The number of births from twin gestations was about 25 per 1000 live births in the mid-1990s, whereas the number of births from higher-order multiple gestations was around 1.3 per 1000 live births.[6] Fetuses of a multifetal pregnancy are more likely to be born prematurely. Such pregnancies are also more likely to be complicated by pregnancy-induced hypertension, premature onset of labor, and antenatal and postpartum hemorrhages, among other complications.

DEVELOPMENTAL DIFFERENCES: ORGAN ONTOGENY AND FUNCTION

The development and function of organs in an infant are a matter of gestational age and postnatal age. In a full-term neonate, the organs in the body are mature for age at the time of birth. In a premature neonate, birth has occurred before the internal organs of the body are fully developed. However, compared with infants and children, both premature and full-term neonates are still considered to have immature organ function.

The ontogeny of organs affects the absorption, distribution, metabolism, and excretion (ADME) of drugs.[7] Developmental changes in surface area of the skin, gastrointestinal tract, and other mucosal surfaces such as the rectum and oral cavity can affect the rate and extent of drug absorption significantly in the neonatal period. Changes in body composition occur with increasing age. About 70% to 80% of a neonate's body weight is water. This composition affects the distribution of drugs significantly, resulting in larger volumes of distribution for water-soluble drugs in neonates compared with infants, older children, and adolescents. Conversely, lipid-soluble drugs do not distribute extensively in water, so lower doses may be needed. The plasma-binding proteins such as albumin and α-1-acid glycoprotein are present in lower concentrations, especially in premature neonates, resulting in much higher plasma concentrations of free or pharmacologically active drugs that are highly protein bound.

Hepatic metabolism of drugs is also limited and varies according to gestational age, especially in the premature neonate. Phase I oxidative metabolism and phase II reactions such as glucuronidation are slow in the premature neonate and later mature around age 6 months.

The functional and anatomic maturation of the kidneys is a dynamic process in the neonate, beginning around 9 weeks' gestation and continuing well into early childhood. The glomerular filtration rate increases rapidly in the first 2 weeks of life in the term neonate. In the premature neonate, this maturation is slower, thus affecting the clearance of compounds exclusively eliminated by the kidney. Dosage adjustments for drugs eliminated extensively by the renal route are essential when renal function is compromised because of age, underlying illness, or both. The Introduction to Pediatrics chapter and the Pediatric Pharmacokinetics chapter discuss drug dosage for this population in more detail.

FUNDAMENTALS IN NEONATE CARE

MATERNAL OBSTETRIC, LABOR, AND DELIVERY HISTORY

A mother may be exposed to many prescribed and unprescribed substances during the course of pregnancy as well as during labor and delivery that may adversely affect the neonate. In caring for the neonate, a detailed history of drug or other substance exposure in utero is critical because such substances may transfer to the fetus through the placenta and affect the initial treatment of the neonate.

In utero, the fetus relies on the placenta (the fetus is connected to the placenta by the umbilical cord) almost completely for nutritional, respiratory, and excretory functions. The placenta grows in parallel with the fetus. During pregnancy, substances may cross the placenta by the following processes: *simple diffusion*; *facilitated diffusion*, also called *gradient-dependent diffusion*; *active transport*, requiring specific transporters that use energy to transfer substances, mostly for lipid-insoluble substances; *receptor-mediated endocytosis*; and other mechanisms.

Most drugs travel across the placenta by active transport or passive diffusion. Exposure of the mother to anesthetic or analgesic agents, tocolytic agents, nicotine, cocaine, or other substances of abuse can have adverse effects on the neonate. Knowledge of such history before the delivery of the neonate can help the health care provider be prepared for successful resuscitation of the neonate.

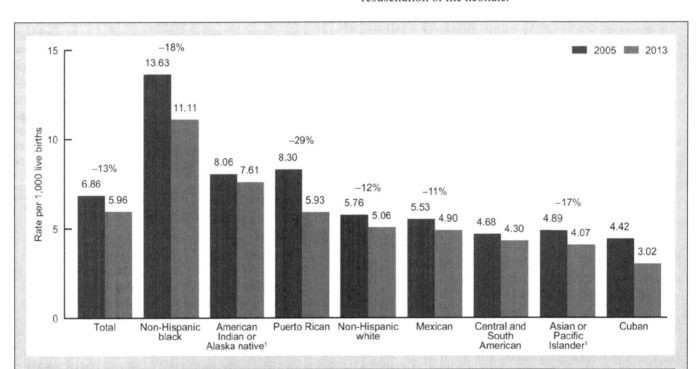

Figure 4. Infant, neonatal, and postneonatal mortality rates by race and Hispanic origin of mothers in the United States from 2005 and 2013.

[1]Includes persons of Hispanic and Non-Hispanic origin.

Neonatal is less than 28 days and postneonatal is 28 days to under 1 year.

Reprinted from Mathews TJ, MacDorman, MF, Thoma, ME, Division of Vital Statistics. Infant Mortality Statistics From the 2013 Period Linked Birth/Infant Death Data Set. National Vital Statistics Report 2015 August; 64:9. Available at https://www.cdc.gov/nchs/data/nvsr/nvsr64/nvsr64_09.pdf. Accessed March 6, 2019.

NEONATE-SPECIFIC CONSIDERATIONS

NEONATAL RESUSCITATION

The transition from fetal to extrauterine life is a complex process that requires understanding of in utero physiology and potential complications that may occur during the process of labor and delivery. Most full-term and low-birth-weight newborn infants transition from intrauterine to extrauterine life with little or no assistance. They are vigorous and cry at birth, breathing easily afterward. Other neonates may require varying degrees of resuscitation for restoring cardiopulmonary function to allow adjustment to extrauterine life.

NORMAL PHYSIOLOGIC EVENTS AT BIRTH

In utero, the fetal lungs are filled with fluid, providing an area of high resistance. The oxygenation of the blood occurs in the placenta. This circulation is maintained by two main patent fetal shunts—the foramen ovale and ductus arteriosus. These shunts provide connections to the right atrium and aorta, respectively, shunting the blood away from the pulmonary circulation. Relatively little blood reaches the lungs because of high pulmonary vascular resistance.

Clamping of umbilical vessels removes the low-resistance placental circulation and raises the systemic blood pressure. The pulmonary vascular resistance decreases with lung expansion and increased oxygenation, resulting in increased pulmonary blood flow (Figure 6). As a result, the pulmonary

venous return and the left atrial pressure increase. In full-term neonates, this process results in closure of the two fetal shunts, thus creating normal systemic circulation. This transition takes about 24–48 hours. Anatomic closure follows in about 8–10 days, causing permanent closure of the shunts.

ABNORMAL PHYSIOLOGIC EVENTS AT BIRTH

If the lungs fail to expand after birth and spontaneous respiration is not established, the result is residual lung fluid, hypoxemia and acidosis, and hypercapnia caused by inefficient breathing and pulmonary vasoconstriction, leading to reduced pulmonary blood flow. The systemic vascular resistance does not increase. The fetal shunts remain open and continue to shunt blood. The direction of the shunting is dependent on the resistance present in the lungs and the systemic circulation. In such situations, complications arise, leading to the use of mechanical ventilation to support respiratory function and blood pressure medications to support the systemic blood pressure.

An abnormal physiologic transition sometimes requires significant resuscitative measures in the neonate, including cardiopulmonary resuscitation with bag-mask ventilation, chest compressions, and use of medications such as epinephrine when indicated. The course of events that follows abnormal physiologic transition at birth can result in different types of complications in the premature and full-term infant. Some of these complications are discussed briefly later in this chapter.

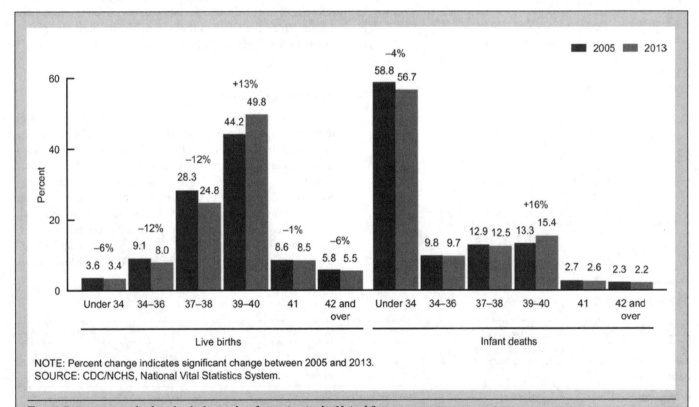

NOTE: Percent change indicates significant change between 2005 and 2013.
SOURCE: CDC/NCHS, National Vital Statistics System.

Figure 5. Percentage of infant deaths by weeks of gestation in the United States.

Reprinted from Mathews TJ, MacDorman, MF, Thoma, ME, Division of Vital Statistics. Infant Mortality Statistics From the 2013 Period Linked Birth/Infant Death Data Set. National Vital Statistics Report 2015 August; 64:9. Available at www.cdc.gov/nchs/data/nvsr64/nvsr64_09.pdf. Accessed March 6, 2019.

INITIAL STABILIZATION AND ASSESSMENT

When a neonate is born, the first step in the stabilization process is thermoregulation. Newborn infants have immature thermoregulatory systems and lack adequate body fat. The large surface area-to-body mass ratio is susceptible to cold stress. Both of these factors predispose the neonate to hypothermia. This predisposition is especially important in a term or preterm neonate who is hypoxic at birth. Hypoxia blunts the normal response to cold and can make the neonate hypothermic. Hypo- and hyperthermia both can lead to adverse neurologic consequences, so it is essential to gain control of body temperature as soon as possible. To prevent excessive heat loss from the body caused by external environmental factors, the neonate must be received in a warm blanket after birth and dried immediately. The full-term neonate acquires the ability to maintain adequate body temperature soon after birth. In some cases, however, the neonate may need to be placed under a radiant warmer for 24–48 hours to maintain normal body temperature. Premature infants are initially placed under radiant warmers and then transitioned to thermoregulated incubators as soon as possible after stabilization. They stay in the controlled-temperature environment until they have acquired an adequate surface area-to-body mass ratio, typically around 2000 g of body weight.

APGAR SCORES

Initial assessment of a newborn infant during the resuscitative phase includes assessment of appearance and vital signs, APGAR scores (Table 1), gestational age assessment, and measurement of weight, length, and head circumference, as well as a complete physical examination to identify any congenital anomalies.[8] The neonate's initial weight, length, and head circumference are plotted on the day of birth, and the growth thereafter is followed through 36 months of life to determine whether the infant has normal progression. The Introduction to Pediatrics chapter provides examples of growth charts. Separate charts exist for premature neonates beginning at 22 weeks' gestation. These charts allow a growth comparison, first with the fetus as early as 22 weeks and then with the term infant to 10 weeks' corrected gestational age.[9] There are separate charts for male and female infants. Growth charts are available from the CDC in their Vital Health Statistics series, available at www.cdc.gov/nchs/data/nvsr/nvsr64/nvsr64_09.pdf.[10]

GESTATIONAL AGE ASSESSMENT

The best estimate of gestational age is antenatal ultrasonography. If the infant's gestational age is uncertain, it can be determined to within around 2 weeks using a standardized scoring system such as the Ballard scoring method.[11] The New Ballard Score is a set of procedures developed by the physician Jeanne L. Ballard to determine gestational age through the neuromuscular and physical assessment of a newborn infant, including the extremely premature newborn infant. The method uses score sheets for neuromuscular and physical maturity and assigns scores for each. The gestational age is derived from these scores.

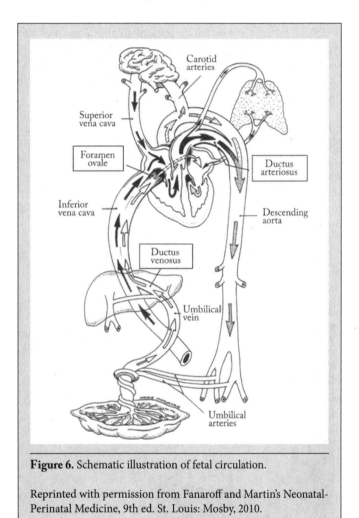

Figure 6. Schematic illustration of fetal circulation.

Reprinted with permission from Fanaroff and Martin's Neonatal-Perinatal Medicine, 9th ed. St. Louis: Mosby, 2010.

Table 1. APGAR Scoring System[8]

Sign	Score[a]		
	0	1	2
Heart rate	Absent	< 100 beats/minute	> 100 beats/minute
Respiratory effort	Absent	Slow, irregular	Good, crying
Muscle tone	Flaccid	Some flexion of extremities	Active motion
Reflex irritability	No response	Grimace	Vigorous cry
Color	Pale	Cyanotic	Completely (whole body) pink

[a]In practice, patients are scored at 1 and 5 minutes of life. Maximum score = 10; minimum score = 0.

CARING FOR THE FULL-TERM NEONATE

A standard nursery can provide routine care for healthy, full-term newborn infants born at 37 weeks' or more gestation. Neonates born at 35 weeks' gestation weighing at least 2000 g and otherwise healthy may also be cared for in a standard nursery. Close monitoring for respiratory distress, poor color, diaphoresis, jitteriness, or abnormal tone should occur for the first 6–12 hours of life.

FEEDINGS

Full-term healthy neonates should be offered feeding by mouth. Breast milk is the preferred nutrition for a newborn infant. Breastfeeding is initiated shortly after birth once the neonate shows signs of hunger. However, at times, breast milk must be avoided because of maternal intake of prescription drugs that may cross into breast milk and adversely affect the neonate. If breast milk is unavailable or if the mother chooses not to breastfeed, an iron-fortified cow milk–based infant formula should be used. Most term infants will take 15–30 mL every 3–4 hours in the first 1–3 days of life and about 75–90 mL by day 5 of life.

PREVENTION OF HEMORRHAGIC DISEASE: VITAMIN K

The American Academy of Pediatrics recommends that every neonate receive a single intramuscular dose of 0.5–1 mg of vitamin K (phytonadione) within 1 hour of birth to prevent vitamin K–dependent hemorrhagic disease of the newborn. This neonatal condition is caused by vitamin K deficiency that is the combined result of a lack of unbound maternal vitamin K, inability of vitamin K to cross the placental wall, immaturity of the fetal liver, and lack of vitamin K–producing bacteria in the infant colon. Clinically, the condition may arise abruptly in the early postpartum period with spontaneous nasogastric or intracranial hemorrhage. The condition affects up to 1 in 1000 neonates and carries a 5% to 30% mortality rate if untreated. The condition may be more common in breastfed infants and is more severe and of earlier onset in infants of mothers receiving anticonvulsants. Breastfed infants are at higher risk of developing hemorrhagic disease because of low concentrations of vitamin K in breast milk together with colonization of bacteria in the gut that are unable to produce vitamin K.

PROPHYLAXIS FOR OPHTHALMIC INFECTIONS

All newborn infants should receive an application of a 1- or 2-cm ribbon of sterile erythromycin (0.5%) eye ointment immediately following birth for prophylaxis against gonococcal ophthalmia neonatorum and chlamydia eye infection, ensuring that the treatment reaches all parts of the conjunctival sac. This treatment is recommended by American Academy of Pediatrics for all newborn infants, including those born by cesarean delivery.

NEONATE SCREENING

Each state has developed guidelines for screening the newborn infant. This preventive public health strategy is used for early identification of treatable disorders that significantly affect health and development. The disorders screened vary from state to state depending on the prevalence of the disorders in each state. Some of the more commonly screened disorders may include disorders of amino acid metabolism; fatty acid oxidation disorders; organic acid disorders; endocrine disorders, such as congenital hypothyroidism and congenital adrenal hypoplasia; hemoglobinopathies, such as β-thalassemia; cystic fibrosis; galactosemia; and biotinidase deficiencies. Screening for these disorders has had a significant impact on the morbidity and mortality from metabolic disorders.

PHYSIOLOGIC NEONATAL JAUNDICE

Neonatal physiologic jaundice (also referred to as *indirect hyperbilirubinemia*) is a condition in which the level of unconjugated bilirubin is increased because of the neonate's inability to rapidly clear it from the body. This condition can occur in both premature and full-term infants. Jaundice is usually seen first in the face and then progresses to the trunk and extremities. Because high bilirubin levels stain the skin and eye sclera yellow, parents or caregivers are often the first to recognize the condition and bring the yellow staining to the attention of the health care providers. Two-thirds of all neonates will appear jaundiced during the first few days of life. In most cases in which the neonate is feeding well, this condition will resolve itself without intervention. Breastfed full-term neonates have higher bilirubin levels than formula-fed infants. Frequent breastfeeding every 2–3 hours helps resolve this problem.

When feeding cannot be established well in the first few days of life—which is most often the case in premature neonates, but can also occur in full-term neonates—hyperbilirubinemia may become a pathologic issue needing intervention. If intervention is needed, the American Academy of Pediatrics guidelines for evaluation and treatment of jaundice should be followed.[12] Untreated indirect hyperbilirubinemia can have severe neurologic consequences. Acute bilirubin encephalopathy can cause lethargy, hypotonia, and poor sucking reflexes. In advanced stages, irreversible neurologic damage can occur and may sometimes lead to coma and death if left untreated for a prolonged time.

IMMUNIZATIONS

All neonates (premature, low birth weight, and full term) born to mothers who are positive for hepatitis B surface antigen must routinely receive hepatitis B immunoglobulin (HBIG) (0.5 mL intramuscularly) and hepatitis B vaccine (HBV) (0.5 mL intramuscularly) within 12 hours of life. This administration prevents or significantly reduces the vertical transmission of the disease in infants born to mothers with a positive test for hepatitis B surface antigen. If HBV cannot be administered to a full-term infant together with or soon after HBIG, then HBV should be administered within the first

7 days of life. For premature infants or sick low-birth-weight infants in whom the vaccine cannot be given within the prescribed period with HBIG, it must be given within the first month of life or at the earliest opportunity when the infant is clinically able to tolerate the vaccine. All infants born to hepatitis B surface antigen–positive mothers should receive additional HBV at 1, 2–3, and 6–7 months of chronologic age for four doses total. Full-term neonates born to hepatitis B surface antigen–negative mothers should receive the vaccine by 2 months of age. For preterm infants weighing less than 2 kg born to hepatitis B surface active antigen–negative mothers, the optimal time to initiate the first dose of HBV is at 30 days' chronologic age if medically stable or at hospital discharge if stabilization occurs before 30 days of age.[13] The Pediatric Vaccines chapter discusses this topic in greater detail.

FULL-TERM SICK NEONATES

Many full-term neonates are at risk of developing perinatally acquired infections. Neonatal sepsis in full-term newborn infants is rare, but it can be potentially life threatening. Risk factors for acquiring such infections include prolonged rupture of fetal membranes, maternal chorioamnionitis, maternal colonization with group B *Streptococcus*, prematurity, and maternal urinary tract infection. Thus, the most common organisms found in the perinatal period include group B *Streptococcus* and *Escherichia coli*. These sick full-term neonates require cardiorespiratory support and intensive nursing care. Such neonates are admitted to the ICN, where they are assessed for sepsis. Other common diseases found in these infants that may require ICN admission and close observation include transient tachypnea of the newborn period, meconium aspiration syndrome, neonatal seizure, neonatal hypoxic-ischemic encephalopathy, acute hypoglycemia in infants of diabetic mothers, and congenital surgical or cardiac conditions.

These neonates are cared for in the ICN until the underlying illness has resolved or been surgically treated and the infant is fully recovered, able to maintain temperature without assistance, and able to breathe without assistance, in addition to having well-established nutrition to meet nutritional needs for growth and development.

SELECT COMMON DISEASES OF THE FULL-TERM NEONATE

INFANTS OF DIABETIC MOTHERS

Diabetes mellitus is a common medical complication of pregnancy, affecting 2%–3% of all pregnancies. Infants of diabetic mothers are generally macrosomic, meaning large for gestational age. They are at risk of developing cardiomegaly, hyperbilirubinemia, respiratory distress, and polycythemia, and they may have congenital malformations. Good control of maternal glucose concentrations during pregnancy is important for the well-being of the fetus. Because of the increased glucose demand by the growing fetus, the plasma glucose concentrations in normal and diabetic pregnancies are lower than in the immediate postpartum period. For women who develop gestational diabetes, as well as for those who were

diabetic before becoming pregnant, maintaining tight glucose control and glucose concentrations near normal values for adults is essential.

In the immediate postnatal period, these infants may develop acute hypoglycemia: blood glucose less than 35 mg/dL in full-term infants and less than 25 mg/dL in premature infants. Low glucose concentrations may cause lethargy, hypotonia, seizures, poor feeding, apnea, or jitters. Metabolic derangements such as hypocalcemia and hypomagnesemia are also common.

Fluids and electrolytes are the mainstay of treatment. Acute hypoglycemia should be treated with an initial bolus dose of glucose 10% (2–5 mL/kg), and early, frequent oral feeding should be instituted. Intravenous continuous glucose infusion, with electrolytes if needed, should be initiated to deliver an initial glucose load of 7–8 mg/kg/minute or higher in some cases, depending on the severity of hypoglycemia. This dose can be weaned gradually as oral feedings are established. Frequent blood glucose concentration checks are needed until a stable oral nutritional regimen is established that maintains blood glucose in the normal range (40–60 mg/dL).

MECONIUM ASPIRATION

Meconium is the earliest stools of an infant. It is composed of materials ingested while the infant is in the uterus and consists of intestinal epithelial cells, lanugo, mucus, amniotic fluid, bile, and water. Meconium is almost sterile, viscous, and sticky like tar, with no odor. It should be completely passed by the end of the first few days of life, with the stools progressing toward yellow (digested milk). The presence of meconium in the amniotic fluid suggests an in utero asphyxia episode. Aspiration of this meconium can lead to significant morbidity and mortality if left untreated. The passage and aspiration of meconium are not seen in neonates younger than 34 weeks' gestation. At delivery, if the amniotic fluid is meconium stained, then aggressive suctioning of the meconium at the perineum is indicated. After the neonate is delivered, the oropharynx should be suctioned below the vocal cords to ensure that the meconium is not aspirated into the lungs. Meconium aspiration can lead to chemical pneumonitis and respiratory distress, with severe cases requiring mechanical ventilator support. Supportive measures may include the use of vasopressors for maintaining blood pressure, intravenous fluids, and sedatives and analgesics to keep the neonate adherent with mechanical ventilation. In severe cases, pulmonary hypertension may develop. Inhaled nitric oxide is often used as a pulmonary vasodilator in such cases.

CARING FOR THE PREMATURE NEONATE

Premature neonates are born at younger than 37 weeks' gestation. Shorter pregnancies carry greater risks of mortality and morbidity. The earliest gestational age at which the infant has at least a 50% chance of survival is generally believed to be 24 weeks, although rare exceptions exist. Surviving premature neonates are at risk of short- and long-term complications, including the following: *gastrointestinal*, such as necrotizing enterocolitis (NEC); *respiratory*, such as respiratory distress syndrome and chronic lung disease; *neurologic*, such as apnea of prematurity, hypoxic-ischemic encephalopathy, intraventricular hemorrhage, retinopathy of prematurity, cerebral palsy, and developmental delay; *cardiovascular*, such as patent ductus arteriosus (PDA); and *hematologic*, such as pathologic jaundice. In addition, premature neonates are at higher risk of infectious complications, such as sepsis and pneumonia.

In developed countries, all premature neonates are cared for in ICNs. Modern ICNs allow continuous cardiorespiratory monitoring, administration of intravenous fluids and nutrition, mechanical ventilator support, and administration of a variety of intravenous medications. However, premature infants cared for in an ICN are also at greater risk of nosocomial infections, which contribute to the morbidity and mortality of these patients.

VITAL SIGN AND LABORATORY ASSESSMENT

Temperature. It is unusual for neonates to develop fever except in response to environmental factors. Rectal temperature is less likely to be affected by environmental changes unless the changes are prolonged; therefore, rectal temperature is a better measure than skin temperature. A sustained rectal temperature of more than 100.4°F (38°C) requires further evaluation of the neonate for infectious or neurologic issues. Premature neonates often become hypothermic in response to environmental temperature fluctuations. Prolonged hypothermia also requires further evaluation.

Respiratory and heart rate. The respiratory rate in a full-term neonate is measured by counting chest movements for a full minute. The normal rate in a full-term healthy neonate is 30–60 inspirations per minute. Premature neonates may have respiratory rates at the upper end of the normal range.

The heart rate in healthy full-term neonates is generally 110–160 beats/minute. Premature neonates have resting heart rates at the upper end of the normal range. Heart rate may vary significantly in sick full-term and premature neonates. *Tachycardia*, defined as a heart rate persistently greater than 160 beats/minute, warrants further investigation. In preterm infants, a heart rate persistently less than 90 beats/minute constitutes *bradycardia* that requires further investigation.

Blood pressure. Blood pressure varies widely at different gestational ages. At least three separate measurements are needed before diagnosing hypertension in a neonate. The range of normal blood pressures in the neonate depends on the method of measurement (invasive vs. noninvasive measurements) as well as gestational age. In general, the mean arterial pressures provide a better estimate of blood pressure than systolic or diastolic blood pressure alone because it considers both the systolic and diastolic blood pressure. The calculation of mean arterial pressure is as follows:

$$MAP = [(2 \times DBP) + (SBP)]/3$$

The average systolic, diastolic, and mean blood pressure during the first 12 hours of life in normal newborn infants grouped according to birth weight have been described.[14] Sick newborn infants may experience significant blood pressure fluctuations and may deviate substantially from the normal blood pressures shown in this reference.

Hypotension is more common in critically ill infants. The treatment threshold for hypotension varies significantly depending on whether the hypotension is compromising systemic perfusion, which is measured by clinical indicators such as capillary refill, skin color, and urine output. Therefore, the perfusion status of an individual infant is a far better determinant of the significance of hypotension.

Laboratory values. There are no neonate-specific reference ranges of laboratory values for commonly used tests such as blood chemistries, hematology tests, or liver function tests. These values in neonates are generally compared with those in older children or adults. The serum creatinine in the first 48 hours of life is not a reliable indicator of kidney function in the neonate because it often reflects the mother's serum creatinine. In the full-term infant, the values reflect true renal function in about 48 hours after feedings or intravenous hydration is established.

The reference ranges used also do not differ for pre- and full-term neonates. However, ELBW infants pose a particular challenge in maintaining a normal electrolyte balance because of their inability to conserve sodium and bicarbonate, given their immature kidney function. These infants often have metabolic acidosis and hypernatremia during the first few days of life. In premature infants, it is difficult to predict when renal function will become normal because renal dysfunction may be a consequence of prematurity as well as underlying illness. In the neonatal period, it is often more useful to follow trends in laboratory values rather than single values to assess the fluid and electrolyte status and organ function.

SELECT COMMON DISEASES AND COMPLICATIONS OF THE PREMATURE NEONATE

APNEA OF PREMATURITY

Premature neonates have an immature respiratory pattern because of an underdeveloped brain stem. Periodic breathing (short recurring pauses in respiration lasting 5–10 seconds) is common in prematurity and considered the normal respiratory pattern at that age. A respiratory pause that is prolonged (more than 20 seconds) with complete cessation of breathing or one that is associated with cyanosis and/or bradycardia is defined as *apnea of prematurity*. The problem increases in severity and frequency with decreasing gestational age. The causes of apnea with or without bradycardia and desaturation may be multifactorial and may include the following: thermal instability; metabolic disorders, such as electrolyte abnormalities and hypoglycemia; central nervous system disorders, such as intraventricular hemorrhage, seizures, and encephalopathies; infection; decreased oxygen delivery to the brain secondary to PDA, hypotension, or shock; or airway obstruction from an ill-positioned neck or a mechanical obstruction of the oropharynx, all of which should be ruled out when apneic episodes begin. Once other causes are ruled out, then the diagnosis of true idiopathic apnea of prematurity is confirmed.

Treatment includes nonpharmacologic and pharmacologic measures. Nonpharmacologic measures include tactile stimulation, increasing fraction of inspired oxygen, and use of respiratory support such as continuous positive airway pressure or mechanical ventilation.

Pharmacologic measures primarily include the use of methylxanthines (caffeine and theophylline), which theoretically increase the sensitivity of the chemoreceptors in the brain to carbon dioxide, although this mechanism has not been proven in the human neonate.[15] Apnea of prematurity is generally resolved at greater than 34 weeks' corrected gestational age. At this time, all neonates should be challenged to breathe without the help of methylxanthines, and treatment should be weaned, preferably before discharge.[16] Further details about apnea of prematurity management are available in the Apnea of Prematurity chapter.

NECROTIZING ENTEROCOLITIS

Necrotizing enterocolitis is among the most common gastrointestinal problems in the premature neonate. It is characterized by partial- or full-thickness intestinal ischemia. Although the terminal ileum is usually involved, NEC can occur in any part of the intestine. The exact cause of NEC is unknown, but factors leading to intestinal ischemia are implicated. Reperfusion injury after acute ischemia to the intestines has been proposed as a mechanism for injury. The most commonly known risk factors include prematurity, formula feeding (especially hyperosmolar formulas), neonatal stress, infection, and surgery in the newborn period. Feeding precedes NEC symptomatology in most NEC cases. It is unclear whether the volume or rate of feeding plays a major role in the pathogenesis of NEC. Overall, NEC appears to be a multifactorial disorder that requires a delicate balance between intestinal perfusion, intestinal flora, and type of enteral nutrition.

The clinical features of NEC are nonspecific. Temperature instability, lethargy, feeding intolerance, and abdominal distension are generally the first signs of NEC. Blood may be present in the stools. Apnea, bilious vomiting, and signs of shock may develop with advanced disease possibly caused by infection from enteric bacteria. An abdominal radiograph in NEC is characteristic with pneumatosis intestinalis (free air in the peritoneum) and portal venous gas in advanced disease.

Treatment includes bowel rest, nasogastric suction, intravenous fluids (including parenteral nutrition), and broad-spectrum antibiotics for about 2 weeks. Medications to support blood pressure may be necessary. Intestinal perforation warrants surgical intervention. Occasionally, portions of the intestine may become necrosed and require surgical removal. These infants have permanent short bowel. Long-term complications of NEC include the formation of strictures in the affected part of the intestine and difficulty with feeding, especially in short bowel syndrome, and prolonged need for parenteral nutrition, which can lead to intestinal failure associated liver disease.[17]

NEONATAL RESPIRATORY DISTRESS SYNDROME

Neonatal respiratory distress syndrome (NRDS) is a condition produced by surfactant deficiency in the lungs. It is present to some extent in all premature infants born younger than 34 weeks' gestation. The extent of deficiency is inversely proportional to gestational age. The surfactant is a substance consisting of phospholipids and proteins naturally produced by the body. Its function is to produce surface tension at the interface of the alveoli and the air in the lungs and to keep the alveoli open so that adequate gas exchange may occur. Neonatal respiratory distress syndrome is most common in VLBW and ELBW infants, although it does occur in low-birth-weight infants. The ELBW infants are intubated for mechanical ventilator support within minutes of birth. These infants may not exhibit the typical clinical course of NRDS.

Early signs and symptoms of surfactant deficiency include difficulty in initiating normal respirations, expiratory grunting, sternal and intercostal retractions, nasal flaring, cyanosis on room air, and tachypnea. Chest radiography shows a reticulogranular, ground-glass pattern with air bronchograms, which is characteristic of NRDS. Physiologically, there is reduced lung compliance, ventilation perfusion mismatch caused by decreased alveolar ventilation resulting in hypoxemia, and hypercarbia with metabolic acidosis, if the hypoxemia is severe.

Treatment of NRDS consists primarily of surfactant replacement therapy and mechanical ventilator support. Premature infants may be administered surfactant as soon as the diagnosis of NRDS is confirmed by radiologic examination and intubation has been performed. In ELBW infants, it may be beneficial to administer prophylactic surfactant as soon as possible after intubation. Surfactant administration results in improved lung compliance with improved oxygenation and lower requirements for the fraction of inspired oxygen. Improved compliance allows effective ventilation at lower peak inspiratory pressures, thus reducing the potential for lung injury. Complications of surfactant treatment, such as oxygen desaturation and bradycardia, are common secondary to airway occlusion during surfactant administration. A rapid change in lung compliance may result in hyperventilation and overdistension, potentially increasing the risk of pneumothorax.

Several surfactant products are commercially available. These products and other options for treating neonatal respiratory distress syndrome are described in detail in the Neonatal Respiratory Distress Syndrome and Bronchopulmonary Dysplasia chapter.[18]

PATENT DUCTUS ARTERIOSUS

Patent ductus arteriosus is an essential shunt in utero (Figure 6). Once the fetus is delivered, successful transition from fetal to neonatal circulation is essential and occurs naturally in full-term neonates. When such transitions are incomplete or delayed, PDA results. The incidence of PDA is inversely related to gestational age. An untreated, symptomatic PDA can result in significant morbidity and mortality. Congestive heart failure and hypoperfusion of the brain (increased potential for intraventricular hemorrhage), kidneys (acute tubular necrosis), and intestine (potential for NEC) secondary to PDA can cause increased morbidity.

Clinical diagnosis of a PDA is made when a systolic murmur is detected together with a hyperdynamic precordium, bounding palmer pulses, increased pulse pressure, and signs of congestive heart failure, including tachypnea, tachycardia, edema, and hepatomegaly. Occasionally, refractory hypotension or pulmonary hemorrhage is also seen. Chest radiography reveals pulmonary edema and an enlarged heart. Definitive diagnosis is made by an echocardiogram that shows a PDA with a left-to-right shunt detected by Doppler studies.

Treatment of PDA is warranted in neonates who are symptomatic from it. Management of PDA falls into three categories: medical, pharmacologic, and surgical. Medical management includes use of fluid restriction and diuretics to manage congestive heart failure and to allow the PDA time to close physiologically. This approach is sometimes successful, with some PDAs closing permanently, whereas others close transiently and reopen, requiring a more definitive intervention. Fluid restriction may severely restrict the caloric intake of the neonate regardless of the mode of nutrition. Electrolyte abnormalities and the need for higher mechanical ventilator settings are common with this approach.

Pharmacologic management includes the use of drugs that cause ductal closure. The ductus arteriosus is sensitive to prostaglandins. While in utero, its patency is maintained by the high levels of circulating prostaglandins produced by the placenta. The arterial oxygen concentration, which is low in utero, also plays a role in keeping the ductus open. Once the neonate is separated from the placenta, prostaglandin concentrations are decreased and oxygenation is established, increasing oxygen concentrations in the blood. Both of these factors aid in ductal closure. Although this process occurs as part of normal adaptation in the full-term infant, in premature neonates the circulating prostaglandin levels remain high after birth, allowing the ductus to remain open in the postnatal period.

Nonsteroidal inflammatory agents are useful in the treatment of PDA by inhibiting prostaglandin production. Both intravenous ibuprofen and indomethacin are effective in ductal closure. Intravenous ibuprofen has some advantages over indomethacin such as reduced adverse effect on renal function compared with the severe oliguria often seen with intravenous indomethacin.[19] Surgical ligation is indicated when pharmacologic treatment has failed or when it is contraindicated. Further information is provided in the Congenital Heart Disease chapter.

OTHER COMMON CONDITIONS IN FULL-TERM AND PREMATURE NEONATES

NEONATAL SEPSIS

Around 1–5 of 1000 newborn infants are afflicted with sepsis. The incidence increases to 40–50 in 1000 in infants weighing less than 2500 g, with further increase as birth weight decreases.[20,21] Neonatal sepsis at any stage carries significant morbidity and mortality. Surviving infants may sustain significant neurodevelopmental sequelae.

The pathogens responsible during early sepsis (younger than 5 days of life) are those vertically transmitted at birth. Group B Streptococcus and coliforms (E. coli) are the most common organisms colonizing the birth canal. Clinical signs and symptoms of neonatal sepsis are nonspecific and may include temperature instability, hypotension, frequent oxygen desaturations, apnea, increased work of breathing, and poor weight gain. Early sepsis is suspected in infants of mothers with chorioamnionitis, ill infants of mothers with unknown group B streptococcal status, prematurity when there is no obvious explanation for premature delivery, and prolonged rupture of membranes (generally 18–24 hours before birth). Empiric treatment is provided with ampicillin for treatment of group B Streptococcus and gentamicin or cefotaxime for treatment of coliform bacteria.

Late-onset infections are generally those that occur after the first 5 days of life. The most common pathogens suspected in late-onset sepsis may be community acquired (Streptococcus pneumoniae, Haemophilus influenzae, or late-onset group B streptococcal infections) or hospital ICN acquired (coagulase-negative and coagulase-positive staphylococci, E. coli, Enterococcus spp., and Klebsiella spp.). Clinical signs and symptoms of late-onset sepsis are also nonspecific and may include manifestations such as lethargy, poor feeding, apnea, jaundice, cyanosis, hypotension, metabolic acidosis, and respiratory distress. Common risk factors include the following: prolonged instrumentation, such as the presence of indwelling central or peripheral catheters for intravenous access; endotracheal tubes for mechanical ventilation; repetitive or prolonged courses of antibiotics; and other nosocomial risk factors such as human handling of ELBW infants.

Prompt diagnosis of early- and late-onset infections and initiation of early empiric treatment until microbiologic results are returned are essential. Once the microbiologic results are known, then therapy can be tailored on the basis of institution-specific susceptibility results. Doses and duration of selected antibiotic regimens should consider efficacy, toxicity, organ function, pharmacokinetic information about the agent, appropriate coverage of suspected organisms, and the site of infection.

SEIZURE DISORDERS

In pre- and full-term infants, seizures can be caused by a wide variety of underlying conditions. Repetitive seizures are associated with increased morbidity and mortality and require prompt treatment. Neonatal seizures are relatively common and rarely idiopathic. In most cases, they are of consequence if there is an underlying cause that should be sought and treated. Neonatal seizures are clinically distinct from those in older infants and children. Seizures in neonates are generally more difficult to diagnose clinically and may require electroencephalogram monitoring. Neonatal jitteriness is sometimes confused with seizures. The two entities can be distinguished by the effectiveness of applying mild pressure to the body, which will stop jitteriness but not seizures. More than 50% of neonatal seizures occur on the first day of life.[22] Risk factors include the following: hypoxic–ischemic encephalopathy; electrolyte abnormalities; hyperbilirubinemia; inborn errors of metabolism; drug toxicity, including in utero exposure immediately before delivery, which should be suspected if seizures occur within a few hours of birth; drug withdrawal; and idiopathic neonatal seizures. Seizures in neonates can be subtle, focal, or generalized.

Diagnosis is made on the basis of the results obtained in a complete workup for metabolic derangements, labor and delivery history, toxicology screening to identify in utero drug exposure, and imaging studies of the brain, including a video electroencephalogram if warranted. Treatment of neonatal seizures involves treating the underlying cause, if one is identified, as well as the seizures themselves. Etiology-specific therapy is critical because it may prevent further brain injury. This point is particularly true for the seizures associated with some metabolic disorders (e.g., hypoglycemia, hypocalcemia, and hypomagnesemia) and with central nervous system or systemic infections. Furthermore, neonatal seizures may not be effectively controlled with antiepileptic drugs unless their underlying cause is treated. Pharmacologic management of the seizures themselves is aimed at halting seizure activity. Intravenous phenobarbital and phenytoin are used as first-line agents.[23] Benzodiazepines may be used for immediate control of status epilepticus. Appropriate monitoring of plasma concentrations of drugs as well as adverse effects is essential. Other supportive measures such as vasopressors for hemodynamic support and mechanical ventilation for respiratory support may be necessary.

CONSIDERATIONS FOR MEDICATION ADMINISTRATION IN THE NEONATE

Neonates in the ICN pose specific challenges to the system for prescribing, dispensing, administering, and monitoring medications, primarily because of the lack of available well-researched data on how to use medications effectively in this population.[24] Issues of drug administration in the neonate can be categorized into three groups: ADME, choice of administration route, and dosage preparation and drug compatibility. Physiologic differences between children and adults are well recognized. In pre- and full-term neonates, these differences are enhanced a step further—in fact, the physiologic differences between pre- and full-term neonates are significant enough to warrant dosing modifications. Nevertheless, little is known about the ADME of many drugs used in this population. Clinicians must often use their own knowledge of the physiologic basis of drug effectiveness and the dosage form at hand to determine a safe and effective dose and route of drug administration in a neonate. (The Pediatric Pharmacokinetics chapter addresses this point in more detail.) The second issue is safe drug administration. Although many different administration routes are possible for many drugs, in neonates, the use of these formulations is limited because of insufficient absorption of the active compound by oral, rectal, or intramuscular routes. Most drugs in critically ill neonates are administered intravenously.

INTRAVENOUS ACCESS AND MEDICATION ADMINISTRATION

Intravenous drug administration requires the infant to have an intravenous catheter placed for drug administration.[25,26] The catheter may be placed in a large vein (central venous catheter) or in a small peripheral vein. The insertion site has implications in drug administration because drugs with a high osmolar load may cause vein irritation if administered by the peripheral vein route. Decisions regarding drug concentrations and acceptable osmolarities must be made with knowledge regarding catheter placement. Most intravenous drugs used in neonates will require further dilution before administration to measure accurately. The dispensing pharmacists must provide a chemically stable, appropriately diluted solution that may be safely administered without the risk of vein irritation and fluid overload in the infant, who may have fluid restrictions merely because of their body size.

Intravenous access is often very limited in neonates. Once the drug is received at the bedside, a determination must be made about its compatibility with other solutions running through the intravenous catheter. Incompatibilities can result in precipitation of the drug in the catheter, and infused precipitate can act as a nidus for clot formation in the vein, leading to compromised blood flow. Smart pumps are routinely used in ICNs for drug administration. Although these infusion pumps are designed for safe drug administration, errors in pump setting can lead to medication administration errors. A streamlined medication use process from prescribing to drug administration is necessary for the safe and effective administration of medications in the ICN.[27]

DRUG DOSING IN NEONATES

Drug dosing in neonates is generally based on weight. Factors such as organ maturation may also be considered. Thus, neonatal dosing recommendations may be given on the basis of weight as well as postnatal age or postconceptional age. The ADME of a drug may vary depending on gestational age and/or postnatal age. Few dosing guidelines are available for commonly used drugs in the neonate. Neonatal pharmacy practitioners must be aware of the current literature and use their knowledge of pharmacokinetics and pharmacodynamics to determine a safe dose. Neonates will lose about 10% of their body weight in the first week of life. Thus, it is appropriate to use birth weight as dosing weight during this time. Once the neonate has regained birth weight, subsequent dosing may be based on actual weight. However, this approach may not always be possible in critically ill neonates who may have increased total body weight because of water retention and body edema. In such cases, an estimate of dry weight corresponding to the infant's gestational and postnatal age may be obtained from standardized growth charts available from sources such as the CDC.

FUTURE OF NEONATAL PHARMACY PRACTICE

Neonatal pharmacy practice requires skilled personnel with a clear understanding of the impact of the ontogeny of organ function on the ADME and the pathogenesis of neonatal disease states. Appropriately experienced and trained neonatal clinical pharmacy practitioners are vital to the safe and effective treatment of diseases in a very special subpopulation at high risk of adverse events. Despite advances in diagnostic technology and newer technologically advanced methods of drug preparation and administration, this population remains vulnerable to medication errors. Drug dosing in neonates continues to remain a challenge after more than 50 years of the inception of this science, and it continues to test the knowledge and skills of the neonatal practitioner, who must make clinical judgments on the basis of knowledge of the disease states, pharmaceutical dosage forms, and existing drug dosage information in older populations. Pediatric health care professionals outside the pharmacy profession now recognize the need for such skills.[28] Neonatal clinical pharmacy practitioners of the future will require advanced training and experience in domains such as epidemiology, pathophysiology, and pharmacotherapeutics of neonatal diseases, as well as in-depth knowledge of pharmacokinetics, pharmacodynamics, and pharmacogenomics. They will also need to understand the impact of interplay of these processes on drug disposition and issues in neonatal medication safety, as well as gain expertise in neonatal translational research, to contribute to the current gaps in knowledge of neonatal pharmacotherapeutics. Neonatal pharmacy practitioners will need to become more integrated in the care of the neonate in the future, keeping pace with and working hand in hand with the neonatologists and perinatologists as essential members of an interprofessional team to sustain and further advance the improvement in outcomes made in neonatal care in the past decade by reducing practice variations in neonatal pharmacy practice.[29]

CONCLUSIONS

Neonatal-perinatal medicine and neonatal pharmacotherapeutics have progressed significantly since the inception of these sciences in the 20th century. Challenges of the 21st century are highlighted in hope that the advances in understanding of neonatal disease states at the molecular level will allow more targeted drug therapy and advances in neonatal pharmacotherapeutics.

REFERENCES

1. Schaffer AJ. Diseases of the Newborn. Philadelphia: Saunders, 1960:1.
2. United Nations, Department of Economic and Social Affairs: Population Division. Levels and Trends in Child Mortality Report 2018 [monograph on the Internet]. Available at https://www.who.int/maternal_child_adolescent/data/causes-death-children/en/. Accessed October 21, 2019.
3. United Nations Inter-agency Group for Child Mortality Estimation (UN IGME). Levels & Trends in Child Mortality: Report 2018, Estimates developed by the United Nations Inter-agency Group for Child Mortality Estimation. United Nations Children's Fund. New York, 2018.
4. Beck S, Wojdyla D, Say L, et al. The worldwide incidence of preterm birth: a systematic review of maternal mortality and morbidity. Bull World Health Organ 2010;88:31-8.
5. Blencowe H, Cousens S, Oestergaard M, et al. National, regional and worldwide estimates of preterm birth [estimates from 2010]. Lancet 2012;379:2162-72.
6. World Health Organization [homepage on the Internet]. Preterm Birth [fact sheet]. Available at https://www.who.int/news-room/fact-sheets/detail/preterm-birth. Accessed March 7, 2019.
7. Kearns GL, Abdel-Rahman SM, Alander SW, et al. Developmental pharmacology—drug disposition, action, and therapy in infants and children. N Engl J Med 2003;349:1157–67.
8. Apgar V. A proposal for a new method of evaluation of the newborn infant. Curr Res Anesth Analg 1953;32:260-7.
9. Fenton TR. A new growth chart for preterm babies: Babson and Bend's chart updated with recent data and a new format. BMC Pediatr 2003;3:13.
10. Centers for Disease Control and Prevention (CDC). 2000 CDC Growth Charts for the United States: Methods and Development. Vital Health Statistics [series]. 2002 May:11;246. Available at www.cdc.gov/nchs/data/series/sr_11/sr11_246.pdf. Accessed March 23, 2019.
11. Ballard JL, Khoury JC, Wedig K, et al. New Ballard score, expanded to include extremely premature infants. J Pediatr 1991;119:417-23.
12. American Academy of Pediatrics, Subcommittee on Hyperbilirubinemia. Management of hyperbilirubinemia in the newborn infant 35 or more weeks of gestation. Pediatrics 2004;114:297-316.
13. Sarri TN. Immunization of preterm and low birth weight infants. Pediatrics 2003;112:193-8.
14. Versmold HT, Kitterman JA, Phibbs RH, et al. Aortic blood pressure during the first 12 hours of life in infants with birth weight 610–4220 grams. Pediatrics 1981;67:611.
15. Erenberg A, Leff RD, Haack DG, et al.; Caffeine Citrate Study Group. Caffeine citrate for the treatment of apnea of prematurity: a double-blind, placebo-controlled study. Pharmacotherapy 2000;20:644-52.
16. Henderson-Smart DJ, Steer PA. Caffeine versus theophylline for apnea in preterm infants. Cochrane Database Syst Rev 2010;1:CD000273.
17. Hartman GE, Boyjian MJ, Choi SS, et al. General Surgery: Necrotizing Enterocolitis. Neonatology: Pathophysiology and Management of the Newborn, 5th ed. Philadelphia: Lippincott Williams & Wilkins, 1999.
18. Wirbelauer J, Speer CP. The role of surfactant treatment in preterm infants and term newborns with acute respiratory distress syndrome. J Perinatol 2009;29:S18-S22.
19. Thomas RL, Parker GC, Overmeire BV, et al. A meta-analysis of ibuprofen vs indomethacin for closure of patent ductus arteriosus. Eur J Pediatr 2005;164:135-40.
20. Faix RG. Infectious emergencies. In: Donn SM, Faix RG, eds. Neonatal Emergencies. Mount Kisco, NY: Futura Publications, 1991:209-30.
21. Feigin RD, Adcock LM, Miller DJ. Postnatal bacterial infections. In: Fanaroff AA, Martin RJ, eds. Neonatal-Perinatal Medicine. Diseases of the Fetus and Infant. St. Louis: Mosby, 1992:619-61.
22. Volpe JJ. Neonatal seizures. Current concepts and revised classification. Pediatrics 1989;84:422-8.
23. Painter MJ, Scher MS, Stein AD, et al. Phenobarbital compared with phenytoin for the treatment of neonatal seizures. N Engl J Med 1999;341:485-9.
24. Conroy S, McIntyre J, Choonara I. Unlicensed and off label drug use in neonates. Arch Dis Child Fetal Neonatal Ed 1999;80:F142-4.
25. Donn SM. Vascular access. In: Donn SM, ed. Michigan Manual of Neonatal Intensive Care, 3rd ed. Philadelphia: Hanley and Belfus, 2003:46-9.
26. Workman E. Percutaneous intravenous catheters. In: Donn SM, ed. Michigan Manual of Neonatal Intensive Care, 3rd ed. Philadelphia: Hanley and Belfus, 2003:50-2.
27. Kunac DL, Reith DM. Identification of priorities for medication safety in neonatal intensive care. Drug Saf 2005;28:251-61.
28. American Academy of Pediatrics. Committee on Fetus and Newborn. Levels of neonatal care. Pediatrics 2004;114:1341-7.
29. Horbar JD, Edwards EM, Greenberg T, et al. Variation in performance of neonatal intensive care units in the United States. JAMA Pediatr 2016;4396.

CHAPTER 3

Pediatric Pharmacokinetics

Jean Dinh, Pharm.D., Ph.D.;
Jacob T. Brown, Pharm.D., M.S.; and
Susan M. Abdel-Rahman, Pharm.D.

LEARNING OBJECTIVES

1. Review the impact of ontogeny on drug disposition in children.

2. Understand the physiologic basis for recommended doses in children.

ABBREVIATIONS IN THIS CHAPTER

ABC	ATP-binding cassette
AOX	Aldehyde oxidases
AUC	Area under the curve
CES	Carboxylesterases
CYP	Cytochrome P450
DRP	Digoxin reduction product
FDA	U.S. Food and Drug Administration
GFR	Glomerular filtration rate
GST	Glutathione *S*-transferase
IDSA	Infectious Diseases Society of America
mRNA	Messenger RNA
MRP	Multidrug resistance protein
MRSA	Methicillin-resistant *Staphylococcus aureus*
OAT	Organic anion transporter
P-gp	P-glycoprotein
SLC	Solute carrier transporter
SULT	Sulfotransferase
UGT	UDP-glucuronosyltransferase
V_d	Volume of distribution

INTRODUCTION

The safe and effective use of medications is guided by an understanding of the relationship between dose, exposure, and response. For special populations, including children, much of this knowledge is nonexistent.[1] Despite regulatory initiatives designed to increase the conduct of clinical trials that would enhance our knowledge of pediatric pharmacokinetics, the number of sponsored drug trials conducted in children remains limited.[2-5] As a result, the drug label tends to offer few data that can be used to guide pediatric pharmacotherapy.[6]

Fortunately, many of the factors that influence dose-exposure relationships are understandable and predictable from recognized patterns of developmental physiology.[7] However, the impact of some physiologic processes on drug disposition is not readily apparent, despite well characterized ontogeny (i.e., developmental trajectories of physiological and biochemical processes), because of limited data that correlate physiology and disposition (i.e., relatively few drugs are susceptible to the biologic process in question). The physiologic factors that drive the disposition of other drugs are not yet defined, and, for these drugs, the impact of development will remain unappreciated without the conduct of pediatric pharmacokinetic studies.[7]

The sections that follow discuss pediatric drug disposition in the context of existing knowledge on developmental anatomy and physiology. The impact of disease and other chronic conditions on the disposition of drugs in children is left to other chapters in this textbook. Where human data are lacking, data on the ontogeny of drug disposition pathways in animals are introduced. Attention is drawn to the areas of pediatric pharmacokinetics in which the impact of growth and development remains unknown.

ABSORPTION

Absorption describes the process by which a drug passes from an extravascular compartment into systemic circulation. The pharmacokinetic term used to describe the rate and extent to which a drug is absorbed is *bioavailability*. This parameter measures the relative amount of a drug entering into systemic circulation when administered from an extravascular site compared with the amount entering circulation from a reference formulation. The term *absolute bioavailability* describes when the reference formulation is given by intravascular administration, given that intravascular drugs have by definition a bioavailability equal to 1. When the reference formulation is administered by an extravascular route, the term *relative bioavailability* is used.

The amount of drug in systemic circulation is often measured by either: (1) determining the maximum concentration, or (2) determining the area under the curve (AUC) by measuring drug concentration as a function of time in either serum or plasma. Drugs administered by any extravascular route (e.g., oral, sublingual, buccal, intramuscular, percutaneous, rectal) encounter physical, chemical, and mechanical barriers to absorption, irrespective of a patient's age. For a drug to be absorbed, it must first be dissolved in biological fluid, and then cross at least one phospholipid membrane layer. In addition, drugs may be substrates for transporters, which are proteins that can either increase or decrease absorption. These proteins are also subject to ontogenic and genetic variability, which can cause interindividual differences in this pharmacokinetic variable. Thus, factors that affect both the solubility and permeability of the drug are highly influential in absorption. Of importance, the fundamental mechanisms by which drugs overcome these barriers do not change with age, but the rate and extent to which these processes occur are altered because of normal growth and development.

ENTERAL ADMINISTRATION

Oral administration is the most common route for drug delivery. Although several chemical and physical factors influence the bioavailability of drugs administered by mouth, one of the most overlooked barriers to oral drug administration resides with the ability to move the drug past the oropharynx. Children will reject medications on the basis of color, taste, texture, and temperature, rendering even the most potent of medicines useless. Taste and smell both play a significant role in the acceptability of oral medications, and clear ontogenic patterns are attributed to gustatory and olfactory development. The ability to perceive sweet tastes appears to be present at birth, with evidence to suggest that the perception of sweet can be detected in utero (e.g., increased fetal swallowing is observed when sweetened solutions are injected into the amniotic sac).[8] The ability to detect bitter, salty, and sour flavors appears to develop by age 2 years, whereas the response to trigeminal stimuli (e.g., texture, temperature, piquancy) develops within the first 1–2 years of life. Of interest, a child's willingness to accept certain flavors is influenced by the mother's diet during breastfeeding and the variability of flavors to which the infant is exposed during the first years of life.[9] Of note, the affective response to odor does not fully mature until about age 5–7 years.[8] Consequently, the common formulation strategy of trying to mask an aversive taste with a pleasant odor may not be effective in younger children.[6]

Beyond the oropharynx, several ontogenic processes can influence the bioavailability of orally administered drugs. Children experience a period of relative achlorhydria shortly after birth, despite increased concentrations of circulating gastrin.[10-12] This failure to produce adult levels of gastric acid is believed to result from a decrease in receptor responsiveness to gastrin, leading to a higher gastric pH early in life. Discussions of pH are inevitably accompanied by a reference to the Henderson-Hasselbalch equation and the ionized/unionized ratio; however, the stomach is not the primary absorptive site for most orally administered drugs. As such, the consequence of increased pH in the young infant is less applicable to the degree of ionization and more relevant to

the chemical stability of the drug being administered. For example, many of the β-lactam and macrolide antibiotics are acid labile, and in adults, a significant fraction of the delivered dose can be broken down before entering the intestine (if an acid-resistant formulation is not used). In contrast, these same drugs are relatively protected in the stomach of a young infant. As a result, more intact drug will reach the intestine and be available for absorption. Figure 1 illustrates the impact of gastric pH on the absorption profile of penicillin administered at comparable weight-based doses to neonates, infants (2 weeks – 2 years), and children (2 – 13 years). As predicted, given our knowledge of developmental gastric physiology, pre- and full-term neonates achieve concentrations five to six times higher compared with concentrations observed in infants and children.[13]

For drugs formulated in lipid-based vehicles or lipophilic drugs that require solubilization by bile acids, maturation of biliary function can play a key role in absorption. Postprandial sampling of two major bile salts in the circulation of newborns and young infants reveals that their concentrations exceed those observed in adults; however, the corresponding concentrations within the intestinal lumen are lower through the first 6 months of life. This finding is likely the result of immature bile salt transport into the biliary canaliculi.[14,15] As a result, the extent of fat absorption is lowest early in the neonatal period.[16-18] The clinical relevance of this finding can be illustrated by pharmacokinetic studies of the antipicornaviral agent pleconaril, which is formulated in a vehicle of medium-chain triglycerides. Dose escalation in adults shows a proportional increase in total body exposure, whereas a 50% increase in dose delivered to neonates (gestational age greater than or equal to 32 weeks and postnatal age between 0 – 32 days) produces no change in either the plasma maximum concentration or AUC.[19,20] The capacity-limited absorption observed in the pleconaril studies and in similar studies of a lipid-based chloramphenicol formulation supports the assertion that knowledge of developmental physiology can guide our understanding of age-dependent changes in dose-exposure relationships.[21] Of note, both intrinsic (i.e., physiology) and extrinsic (i.e., formulation) factors were involved in determining the disposition profiles of these anti-infectives such that the magnitude of their combined influence might not have been predicted without carefully constructed and executed pharmacokinetic studies.

Irrespective of a drug's physiochemical properties, the rate of gastric emptying influences the rate at which the drug is presented to the primary absorptive site (i.e., the small intestine). Gastric-emptying rates increase dramatically during the first week of life; however, several other factors influence this rate of drug absorption in the newborn period, including prematurity, gastroesophageal reflux, respiratory disease, congenital heart disease, and the caloric density of feeds.[22] By extension, intestinal motility also controls the rate at which medications are distributed along the primary absorptive site. The frequency and amplitude of intestinal contractions are reduced in the newborn and young infant, contributing to irregular peristaltic activity shortly after birth.[23] Although highly variable, most children usually attain adult motility patterns by age 6–8 months.[24] The impact of altered motility

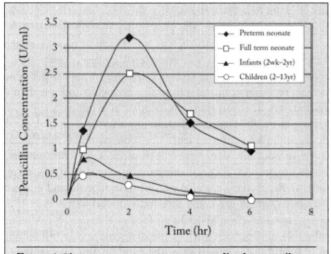

Figure 1. Plasma concentration vs. time profiles for penicillin in neonates, infants, and children after oral administration of a single 10,000-units/lb dose.

on drug absorption will depend, in large part, on the disintegration and dissolution characteristics of the drug molecule and the formulation in which it is administered.

The combined effect of both reduced gastric emptying and poorly coordinated intestinal contractility is well illustrated by the pharmacokinetic profiles for cisapride. The time to achieve maximal plasma concentrations averages 5.0 hours in infants 28–36 weeks' postconception, 4.3 hours in infants 36–42 weeks' postconception, and 2.2 hours in infants 42–54 weeks' postconception compared with 1.8 hours in adults.[25] Even when pharmacologic intervention is used to enhance gastric emptying and intestinal motility, the maximal attainable absorption rate is limited by age. Neonates younger than 30 days and infants older than 30 days respond to the prokinetic metoclopramide with an increase in the absorption rate of a concomitantly administered sugar (Figure 2).[24]

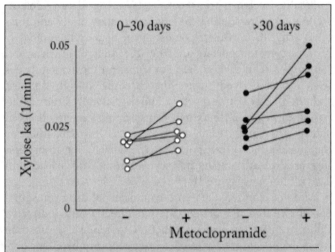

Figure 2. Absorption rate constant of xylose in neonates (younger than 30 days) and young infants (older than 30 days) with and without concurrently administered metoclopramide. Adapted with permission from Heimann G. Enteral absorption and bioavailability in children in relation to age. Eur J Clin Pharmacol 1980;18:43-50.

However, neonates do not attain the same absolute absorption rate as observed in young infants, suggesting that other developmental factors restrict absorption in the young infant. This difference has led many pediatric clinicians to attribute reduced absorption rates in young infants to diminished intestinal surface area; yet, considered in the context of an infant's primary function (i.e., to assimilate nutrients and grow), a reduction in intestinal surface area would seem counterintuitive.[26,27] In fact, a careful examination of anatomic and anthropometric data reveals that intestinal villi mature by 20 weeks of gestation and that overall intestinal length, as a percentage of adult values, exceeds other measures including total body length, body weight, and body surface area (Figure 3).[26] These data refute the assertion of decreased intestinal surface area, leaving no clear explanation for delayed absorption in the young infant. We hypothesize that differences in absorption rate are partially attributed to differences in splanchnic blood flow. Preprandial blood flow velocity increases by 30% to 40% during the first few weeks of life, which may influence the concentration gradient across the intestinal mucosa.[28-30]

The intestinal lining of the gastrointestinal tract is also an active site of drug biotransformation, affecting the amount of active drug that moves into systemic circulation. Both phase I and phase II enzymes (described in greater detail in the Metabolism section of this chapter) are found at varying levels along the gastrointestinal tract. Unfortunately, few studies have examined intestinal enzyme expression as a function of age. Early work examined the activity of several intestinal enzymes from biopsies taken at the duodenojejunal flexure. Among these enzymes were epoxide hydrolase, glutathione peroxidase, and aryl hydrocarbon hydroxylase, now referred to as cytochrome P450 (CYP) 1A1 (CYP1A1). Of the three enzymes examined, only CYP1A1 appeared to show some level of developmental dependence, with activity increasing with increasing age.[31] For orally administered medications that are inactivated by CYP1A1, reduced presystemic clearance in younger children would be expected. Since this initial study, other CYPs have been reported to be expressed in the intestine, and ontogeny data are accumulating, including the following: CYP1B1, CYP2C, CYP2D6, CYP2E1, CYP2J2, CYP2S1, CYP2W1, and CYP3A5.[32]

The duodenal expression and activity of CYP3A has been the most investigated of the CYPs. Neither protein nor activity was detected to any appreciable extent in the fetus; however, a steady increase in both expression and activity was observed from the neonatal period through early adolescence.[33,34] In contrast, a study noted the opposite effect, wherein protein content appeared stable in pediatric samples, and messenger RNA (mRNA) expression decreased with age in duodenal tissue; however, it should be noted that this relationship was not statistically significant.[35] Although most investigations involving

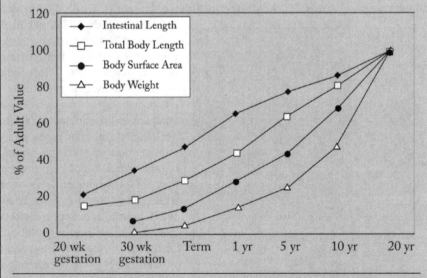

Figure 3. Intestinal length, total body length, body surface area, and body weight with age as a percentage of adult values.

CYP2J2 are regarding the role that this enzyme plays in arachidonic acid oxidation, this enzyme has significant substrate overlap with CYP3A and may play a bigger role in presystemic clearance than previously thought.[35,36] Expression of CYP2J2 has been detected in fetal tissue, and levels appear to be higher in pediatric tissue compared with adults; thus, contribution of this enzyme may have a bigger impact in younger patients.[32] The CYP2C enzymes are also detectable in intestinal fetal tissue; however, their abundance relative to adults has yet to be determined. For drugs metabolized by CYP3A and/or CYP2J2, the impact of ontogeny appears to be variable and drug specific. As a whole, the impact of ontogeny on expression of the remaining phase I drug metabolizing enzymes in the intestine requires further investigation.

Phase II conjugation in the intestine may result in increased biotransformation of substrates. The following phase II enzyme families have been reported to be found in the gastrointestinal tract: glutathione S-transferases (GSTs), UDP-glucuronosyltransferases (UGTs), and sulfotransferases (SULTs). Busulfan, an alkyl sulfonate used in the treatment of cancer, is a substrate of GSTA1-1.[37] The ontogeny of this enzyme's activity can be extrapolated from studies evaluating the conjugation rate of the drug. The glutathione-conjugating capacity of distal duodenal biopsies on busulfan appears to be highest in children younger than 5 years compared with children older than 8 years and early adolescents.[38] Of note, the age-dependent activity observed in vitro parallels the changes in the apparent oral clearance of busulfan in vivo, implying that younger children (i.e., less than 8 years of age) may require higher doses of drugs for which the primary route of clearance is by glutathione conjugation. Other phase II enzymes that are expressed along the intestinal tract display levels comparable with or in excess of those found in the liver; however, no attempts have been made to examine the influence of ontogeny on their expression and/or activity.[39]

Although relevant to only a few drugs, we would be remiss not to mention the role of normal intestinal flora on the inactivation (by metabolism) and reactivation (by deconjugation) of orally administered medications. Anaerobic intestinal bacteria that predominate in the intestines of adults mediate digoxin inactivation to digoxin reduction products (DRPs). Recovery of DRPs in the urine of patients receiving digoxin increases steadily from birth through adulthood, with the biggest increase occurring near the time of weaning. This increase in urinary DRPs coincides with an increase in DRP-positive cultures that can be recovered from the stool.[40] Of importance, the predominant bacterial organisms observed in the intestinal tract differ substantially within and between pediatric populations, depending on age and the constitution of feeds.[41] In addition, the composition and diversity of microbiota is also affected by mode of delivery (cesarean or vaginal delivery), particularly in infants from birth to age 3 months, adding yet another level of complexity during this early period of life. These differences typically disappear at about age 6 months.[42] As such, predicting the impact of age on the activity of intestinal microflora is unrealistic.

Finally, intestinal transporters play a considerable role in facilitating or restricting the uptake of many orally administered drugs. Unfortunately, most of the data on the ontogeny of intestinal transporters are from the study of nutrient and ion uptake in animal models. For some transporter substrates (e.g., lactose-derived sugars that use the apically situated sodium-glucose cotransporter 1 and basolaterally situated glucose transporter 2), maximal translocation can be observed shortly after birth.[43] For others, such as iron (absorbed by the divalent metal transporter 1), the capacity for absorption increases linearly during infancy, attaining adult capacity in early childhood (Figure 4).[44,45]

Although limited, data on the ontogeny of drug transporters in children are being acquired directly and indirectly. Efflux transporters, which function to remove a substrate from a cell, can greatly impact drug exposure by either preventing (when localized on the apical membrane) or promoting (when localized on the basolateral membrane) drug entering systemic circulation. The most studied efflux transporters belong to the ATP-binding cassette (ABC) superfamily of proteins. The most widely studied of these proteins include the following: P-glycoprotein (P-gp), encoded by the *ABCB1* gene; breast cancer resistance protein, encoded by *ABCG2*; multidrug resistance protein 1 (MRP1), encoded by *ABCB1*; and MRP2, encoded by *ABCB2*. Ontogeny investigations of these transporters involve evaluating expression by either mRNA or protein levels as a function of age. These analyses are conducted in either post-mortem human tissue or in animal models. Studies examining the expression of P-gp suggest that this transporter is present within the intestine as early as age 1 month and appears stabilized by 12 weeks of gestation, albeit with wide interindividual variability.[46,47] The expression of breast cancer resistance protein is detected and appears to be constant in tissues that range

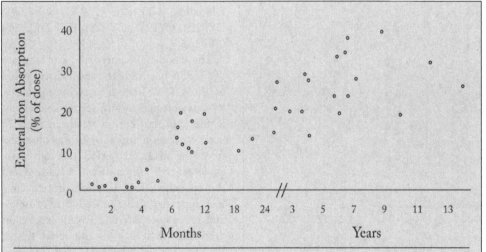

Figure 4. Enteral iron absorption as a percentage of the dose administered. Adapted with permission from Gladtke E, Rind H. Iron therapy during childhood. Ger Med Mon 1966;11:438–42.

in age from 5.5 to 28 weeks. The expression of MRP1 is lower in tissues evaluated from neonatal donors; however, the pattern and level of expression progress to those of adult by 7 weeks of gestation. The expression of MRP2, similarly to P-gp, appears to be constant in neonatal tissue throughout adulthood. The extent of expression of MRP2 is highly variable in the population.[47]

The second major family of transporters that contribute to drug absorption are the solute carrier (SLC) transporters. Particularly for drug molecules that are charged at physiological pH, these transporters are the means to cell entry. Most data for SLC transporter ontogeny are for organic anion transporter (OAT) P2B1 (encoded by *SLCO2B1*). This protein appears to be highly expressed in neonates, and then decreases as a child develops and matures.[47]

Other studies allow us to acquire this information indirectly through the use of probe substrates that can report on the activity of a transporter. Pharmacokinetic investigations of the histamine-2 receptor blocker nizatidine reveal very little of an age effect when the drug's terminal elimination rate constant is examined. By contrast, apparent oral clearance shows appreciable age-dependent changes, providing support for the developmentally dependent expression of one or more transporters for which the drug may be a substrate.[48] Of note, dietary constituents and phytochemicals can alter the activity of several intestinal transporters, including those found in apple juice.[49] Thus, the potential for drug–nutrient interactions will depend largely on the age-dependent level of expression for the transporters in question.

EXTRA-ENTERAL ADMINISTRATION

Although used less commonly as a means of drug delivery, extra-enteral formulations also encounter developmental barriers that influence the rate and extent to which the drugs they contain enter the body. Rectal administration is an efficient means of drug delivery and is often used in children for whom oral administration is not an option or has proven difficult. However, both formulation and developmental physiology must be considered when using the rectal route. The number of *high-amplitude pulsatile contractions* (defined as an amplitude of 80 mm Hg or greater, lasting at least 10 seconds, and propagating at least 30 cm) of the lower gastrointestinal tract is more common in infants than in older children and adults.[50] Although the impact on drug absorption from rectal solutions or fast-melt suppositories may not be significantly affected, suppositories that deliver their contents over hours will very likely be expelled before liberating the entire drug dose.

The impact of altered lower gastrointestinal motility on drug absorption is illustrated by the age-related differences observed in erythromycin concentrations between neonates and children. When administered intravenously, the differences in AUC between neonates, infants, and children are negligible. However, when equivalent weight-based doses are delivered by suppository, bioavailability is markedly lower in neonates (28%) than in infants (36%) and children (54%).[51] Similarly, acetaminophen delivered rectally at comparable weight-based doses reveals reduced absorption in full-term neonates compared with children and adults. However,

preterm neonates show enhanced absorption, likely the result of differences in both motility and metabolism.[52-54]

Percutaneous drug application is rarely exploited for systemic drug delivery in pediatrics. This mode of drug delivery can be particularly advantageous in situations for which continuous drug delivery is needed and/or when adherence may be of concern. Transdermal delivery has been used in children mostly in the areas of psychiatry (e.g., clonidine, methylphenidate, dexamphetamine) or pain control (e.g., paracetamol and fentanyl).[55-58] Nonetheless, topical drug administration in children can be accompanied by significant systemic exposure. Children demonstrate a markedly larger surface area per unit of mass than do adults (Figure 3), a greater degree of hydration to their skin (as measured by capacitance, conductance, and transepidermal water loss), and higher rates of perfusion, all of which contribute to enhanced drug permeability.[59,60] In addition, premature infants show a thinner stratum corneum than do older children and adults, further facilitating the enhanced translocation of drugs. Although the epidermal and dermal layers can be thinner in full-term newborns and young infants, the primary percutaneous barrier constituted by the uppermost layers of the skin are fully mature in the full-term newborn and even in the preterm newborn by 2 weeks of life.[61] All of these findings, in concert, contribute to an increased risk of systemic toxicity—and, in some cases, death—in infants and children after topical exposure to a variety of chemicals ranging from the therapeutically active (e.g., antihistamines, steroids, silver sulfadiazine) to the seemingly inert (i.e., talcum powder, laundry detergent).[62,63]

Subcutaneous drug delivery is administration directly to the fatty layer of tissue beneath the skin (i.e., the hypodermis).[64] Although currently used to a limited extent in children, this mode of drug delivery is expected to be used more often given the increasing number of biologic pharmacotherapies being introduced into the market. Similar to percutaneous delivery, this route of administration can be advantageous when a sustained release is desired, such as with biological protein-based therapy (i.e., insulin, growth hormone, or monoclonal antibodies).[64,65] Studies evaluating insulin pharmacokinetics and pharmacodynamics showed high inter- and intra-individual variability in both absorption and response.[64,66] This example highlights a major issue pertinent to all subcutaneously administered drugs, which is the substantial variability in absorption that may explain some variability in response.[67] However, the major sources for the variability have not been fully elucidated. Drugs administered by this route reach systemic circulation through uptake by either blood vessels or lymphatic capillaries. Uptake is size dependent, with smaller molecules (less than 10 nm) typically being reabsorbed by blood capillaries. Larger molecules (about 10–100 nM) are typically reabsorbed by the lymphatic system.[68] The hypodermis is poorly perfused with blood and lymph capillaries, making absorption into systemic circulation slow from the drug depot. Therefore, some factors that are likely to affect subcutaneous pharmacotherapy absorption in pediatrics include the following: the variable composition of the hypodermis as a function of body site, age, and gender; and the ontogeny of blood and lymph capillaries in the organization in the hypodermis.[64,66,69]

Intramuscular absorption is the final extra-enteral route of drug delivery reviewed here. It is often suggested that absorption after intramuscular administration is erratic in children. For many drugs, however, intramuscular injection can be a very efficient route of drug delivery. Apart from the variability contributed by formulation, capillary density is one of the primary intrinsic drivers of drug absorption when medications are administered by intramuscular injection. Partly because of an increase in metabolic demand, young infants show a 25% increase in skeletal muscle capillary density compared with children in their early adolescence and a 56% increase compared with adults.[70] This increase in capillary density results in greater intramuscular bioavailability for many drugs, including the aminoglycoside and β-lactam antibiotics (Figure 5).[71,72]

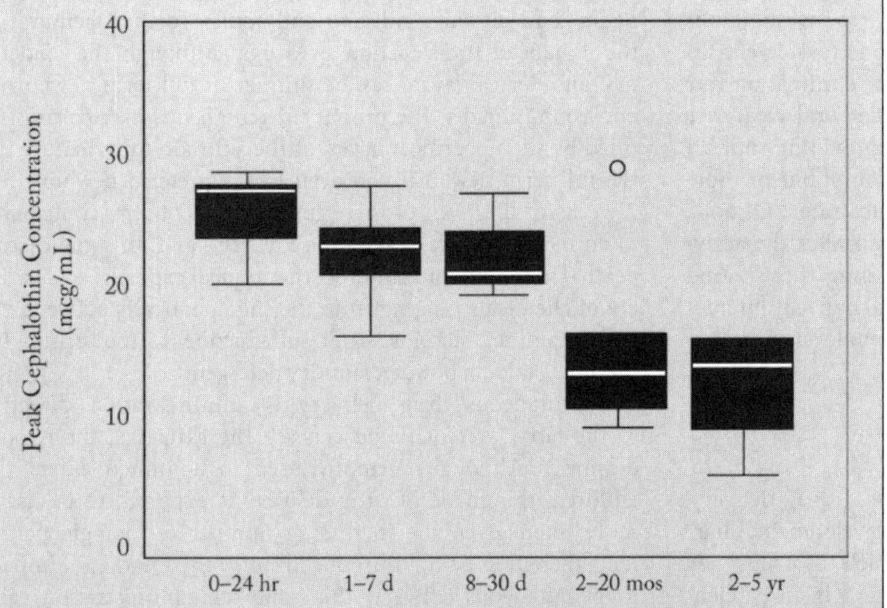

Figure 5. Maximal cephalothin plasma concentrations observed in neonates, infants, and young children after intramuscular administration of a 12.5-mg/kg injection.

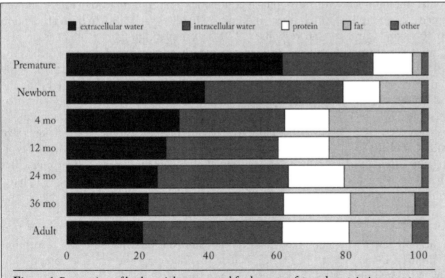

Figure 6. Proportion of body weight accounted for by water, fat, and protein in neonates, infants, young children, and adults.

DISTRIBUTION

Distribution describes the process by which the drug moves from systemic circulation, sometimes considered the "central" compartment, into interstitial and intracellular fluids. The ability of a drug to do so depends on the following: (1) the water-to-fat composition of the various tissues into which a drug can move and be soluble; (2) perfusion into those tissues; (3) the fraction of drug unbound in circulation; and (4) the ability of drug to translocate phospholipid membranes. The pharmacokinetic term used to describe this process is *volume of distribution* (V_d), which reflects the size of a compartment necessary to account for the total amount of drug administered, presuming that the drug is present throughout the body at the same concentration as observed in the plasma. Therefore, between two drugs in which equal amounts are given, the drug with lower plasma concentration would actually exhibit a larger V_d. Of importance, this theoretical "compartment" does not always correspond to a true physiologic space, and it can be difficult to discern into which tissues a drug distributes without quantitative tissue studies. As a result, the impact of development on drug distribution is not apparent for all drugs; however, this knowledge is available for some drugs that share selected physiochemical characteristics.

At birth, humans exhibit larger fractions of total body water than at any other point in their life. Around 80% of a pre- or full-term neonate's body weight is composed of water, a fraction that gradually decreases throughout the first 4 months of life (Figure 6).[73] Even the fat stores in these youngest infants consist of a higher proportion of water and a lower proportion of lipid compared with the fat of mature adults. Consequently, hydrophilic drugs that restrict their distribution to body water stores show larger apparent distribution volumes and lower plasma concentrations in neonates and young infants.

The clinical impact of expanded body water stores is well illustrated by several classes of antibiotics. The aminoglycosides distribute into a V_d that approximates extracellular fluid. Given their higher extracellular fluid stores, young children experience considerably lower peak gentamicin concentrations after the administration of equivalent weight-based doses. Compared with infants, young children have peak concentrations that are almost 33% greater and almost 50% greater in older children.[74] When their reduced renal clearance is accounted for in the selection of a dosing interval, infants will eventually achieve gentamicin concentrations comparable to those observed in adults. However, the delay can have deleterious clinical consequences for this concentration-dependent drug.[75,76] Attaining high peak plasma concentrations early in therapy affords rapid bacterial killing while minimizing the risk of adaptive resistance.[77,78]

Linezolid, an oxazolidinone antibiotic, provides a similar example for drugs that distribute into a volume approximating total body water. Based on age-dependent changes in total body water stores, linezolid displays higher V_d values in the neonatal population (0.83 ± 0.18 L/kg) and correspondingly lower maximal plasma concentrations (12.5 ± 3.5 mg/L) after a comparable weight-based dose compared with children (0.71 ± 0.18 L/kg, 17.0 ± 5.2 mg/L) and adults (0.63 ± 0.13 L/kg, 19.7 ± 4.9 mg/L). When coupled with the more rapid rate of clearance observed in infants, the clinical implications for this time-dependent antibiotic become apparent. If linezolid were administered with the same weight-adjusted dose and dosing frequency across all age groups, infants would be predicted to spend just 20% to 35% of the dosing interval above the minimum inhibitory concentration for susceptible organisms. By comparison, it is predicted that children and adults would spend 35% to 70% and 70% to 100%, respectively, of the dosing interval above the minimum inhibitory concentration.[79]

In contrast to body water stores, body fat stores are limited in the premature and newborn infant. Considerable increases in body fat stores are seen between 24 and 36 months of life, when the percentage of body fat approaches that of adult values (Figure 6). Although this observation may seem to suggest that highly lipophilic drugs will exhibit smaller distribution volumes in infants and young children, these drugs, in fact, associate with lipids and other cellular components such that marked distinctions in V_d with age are not as readily apparent.

Another factor that influences drug distribution is the amount of free drug available to translocate from the circulation into peripheral tissue sites. The free fraction of drug is determined, in part, by the binding affinity of the drug for circulating proteins, the concentration of circulating proteins, and the presence of endogenous circulating ligands that have the ability to displace drugs from their protein binding sites (e.g., bilirubin, free fatty acids).[80-82] Several physiologic differences in the neonate and young infant predispose them to increases in the free fraction of drugs, among which are the reduction in circulating plasma proteins (e.g., albumin, α-1-acid glycoprotein).[83] In addition, a proportion of the circulating albumin in newborns is constituted by fetal albumin, for which many drugs appear to have a lower binding affinity. Consequently, neonates and young infants (typically younger than 6 months) experience higher unbound fractions of drugs than do older children and adults.

Thiopental, a short-acting barbiturate used primarily for sedation, binds mainly to albumin. Because neonates display higher circulating bilirubin levels and lower albumin stores, they experience a lower percentage of protein binding of thiopental (73.2%) compared with adults (84.4%), resulting in higher free fractions.[84] Sufentanil, a derivative of the opioid analgesic fentanyl, offers a similar example of drugs bound to α-1-acid glycoprotein. Because of reductions in this glycoprotein, the free fraction of sufentanil is significantly increased in neonatal (19.5%) and infant (11.5%) populations compared with children (8.1%) and adults (7.8%).[85]

The clinical impact of developmental differences in protein binding depends in large part on the drug under consideration. For a drug like phenytoin, with its high degree of protein binding and narrow therapeutic index, small changes in protein binding can result in dramatic increases in the drug's free fraction and a corresponding increase in the risk of toxicity. A reduction from 99% protein binding (1% free) to 98% protein binding (2% free) effectively doubles the free fraction of the drug. By contrast, a reduction in ampicillin binding from 22% in adults to 10% in neonates results in a modest (15%) increase in free fraction and a negligible alteration in risk profile.[86]

Finally, growing attention has been paid to the many transport proteins that facilitate the vectorial transport of endogenous compounds (e.g., steroids, peptides, nucleotides, electrolytes) as well as a wide range of xenobiotics within the body. The normal biologic substrates of these transporters support somatic development and maintain homeostasis in the growing child. Within different tissues, they are used to different extents at different times throughout development. As such, adaptive mechanisms likely contribute to variability in the tissue-specific expression, quantitative expression, affinity, and turnover rate of transporter proteins during human maturation. Unfortunately, only scant data describe a change in the tissue-specific expression of transport proteins with age. A single study examining P-gp expression in postmortem brain tissue from neonates born between 23 and 42 weeks' gestation suggests that by late gestation, the pattern of P-gp localization is similar to that of adults; however, the quantitative abundance is significantly reduced.[87] By contrast, animal studies have suggested that changes in blood flow and pore density account for differences in central nervous system drug penetration with age; however, the relevance of these findings to humans is unclear. The contribution of transport proteins to distribution in humans is difficult (if not impossible) to assess at this time because of the current limitations in the inability to measure drug at target organs.

METABOLISM

The human liver is responsible for an array of synthetic, metabolic, and homeostatic functions in addition to its prominent role in the removal of toxins and other foreign substrates from the blood. The pharmacokinetic term used to describe the rate of metabolism is *clearance*, defined as the volume of biological fluid that is cleared of drug (or drug metabolites) per unit time. Although hepatic detoxification pathways likely arose to deal with endogenous ligands and exogenous chemicals or toxins found in nature (e.g., phytochemicals), these pathways serve a dual role as major routes of clearance for an array of medications to which children are exposed. Those classified as phase I enzymes covalently modify drugs (by oxidation, reduction, hydrolysis) to increase their polarity, whereas phase II enzymes act to conjugate endogenously synthesized polar functional groups to the parent drug or any of its phase I metabolites. Of note, several phase I and phase II enzymes are located in tissues other than the liver (e.g., kidney, lung, adipose, intestine, skin); however, these extrahepatic sites (with the exception of the intestine) are of limited quantitative importance, and the discussion that follows will be restricted to the liver.

In the context of interindividual variation in drug metabolism, a review of the literature reveals that far more emphasis is placed on genetic polymorphisms than ontogeny. Scientific investigations that followed the tragedy of chloramphenicol and the "gray baby syndrome" were among the first to reveal the contribution of development to drug biotransformation, and respectable efforts have been made to describe the ontogeny of various hepatic drug metabolism pathways.[88] However, most publications focus on the consequence of sequence variations on enzyme activity. Given that genetically encoded variations in the structure or function of drug-metabolizing enzymes remain constant with age, we will not spend time reviewing their significance. However, we would be remiss not to point out the potential relevance (or lack thereof) of polymorphisms in the context of ontogeny. Sequence variations that encode for an enzyme with low or no function have no bearing on the disposition of a substrate if the developmental signal to "turn on" and express the protein has yet to be received. Thus, the following ontogenic profiles described inform more than simply age-dependent changes in the rate and extent of drug biotransformation; they inform whether and to what extent the potential for drug–drug, drug–food, drug–environment, and drug–gene interactions may be experienced.

PHASE I METABOLISM

The primary drug-metabolizing enzymes responsible for carrying out phase I reactions are the CYPs. As oxidative enzymes, the classical chemical reaction catalyzed by CYPs involves insertion of a single atom of oxygen (from molecular oxygen $-O_2$) between a carbon–hydrogen bond. It should be noted that this reaction is not the only one that CYPs are capable of catalyzing. The relative contribution of CYPs to medication therapy are the CYP3A family, followed closely by CYP2D6, the CYP2C family, CYP2E1, and finally CYP1A2. A strategy to increase drug metabolic stability used by drug companies in recent years is to purposefully design drugs that do not have a high affinity for CYP enzymes. The result of this approach is that other mechanisms of clearance become more prominent, particularly with newer drugs. The major phase I enzymes involved in non-CYP metabolism are aldehyde oxidases (AOXs) and carboxylesterases (CES; CES1 and CES2 being the most relevant in humans).[89] The ontogeny and genetic variability of these enzymes may become increasingly important as more drugs are designed to minimize CYP metabolism. The AOXs oxidize both aliphatic and aromatic aldehydes to the corresponding carboxylic acids, hydroxylate heteroaromatic rings, and can reduce amino- and sulfo-groups.[90] The CES enzymes are hydrolytic enzymes and insert a molecule of water to cleave ester, thioester, and amide bonds.[91]

It is important to note that CYP3A4 is estimated to be involved in the metabolism of more than 50% of available medications, including benzodiazepines, calcium channel blockers, and statins. Humans experience a CYP3A isoform switch shortly after birth, transitioning from the expression of CYP3A7 (responsible for the 16α-hydroxylation of dehydroepiandrosterone) to CYP3A4 (responsible for the 17β-hydroxylation of testosterone). Levels of CYP3A4 increase steadily throughout infancy, maturing to adult levels by age 1 year.[92,93] Consistent with this observation, the clearance of sildenafil, a phosphodiesterase inhibitor metabolized primarily by CYP3A4, rapidly increases within the first 10 days of life, correlating with an increase in the expression of CYP3A4.[94] Similarly, the terminal half-life of cisapride, a prokinetic agent also primarily metabolized by CYP3A4, is significantly longer in preterm infants younger than 36 weeks' gestational age (11.7 hours) compared with term infants older than 36 weeks' gestational age (7.7 hours), infants older than 42 weeks (4.8 hours), and adults (4.1 hours).[25,95]

The CYP2D6 enzyme is estimated to contribute to the metabolism of 25% of the drugs on the market, including β-blockers, antidepressants, and antipsychotics. The CYP2D6 enzyme is highly polymorphic, with significant interindividual differences observed within and between populations. A study examining CYP2D6 activity from birth through year 1 of life revealed that activity comparable with that of adults can be detected by age 2 weeks and confirmed that the impact of inheritance on interindividual CYP2D6 variability is of greater significance than development.[96] In fact, CYP2D6 genetic polymorphisms and the associated variability in enzymatic activity is the primary reason that the U.S. Food and Drug Administration (FDA) has issued warnings regarding the use of codeine in children younger than 12 years. Codeine is a prodrug that is metabolized by CYP2D6 to the active metabolite morphine. Children who are faster metabolizers may experience increased adverse effects because of increased exposure to the active metabolite.[97]

Distinct developmental profiles are seen between the two primary isoforms of the CYP2C family. In vitro quantitation of immunoreactive protein from hepatic tissue reveals that CYP2C9 expression appears to be rather invariant with postnatal age, whereas the expression of CYP2C19 appears to increase during the first 6 months of life.[98] Of interest, clinical pharmacokinetic data suggest that the terminal half-life of phenytoin (a primary substrate for CYP2C9) decreases from an average of 20 hours at birth to 8 hours by 2 weeks of life.[99,100] By contrast, the proton pump inhibitor omeprazole (a substrate for CYP2C19) shows higher rates of clearance in young infants and correspondingly faster half-lives normalizing during the first 5 years of life.[101-105] Both examples highlight the challenge that can arise when attempting to predict in vivo disposition on the basis of in vitro protein or transcript expression data.

The CYP2E1 enzyme is involved in the metabolism of various anesthetics, including enflurane, halothane, and isoflurane. Transcript, protein, and activity levels are all negligible during prenatal life, with a gradual increase in expression and activity observed throughout childhood. Levels with 80% of adult values are attained after the first year of life.[106,107]

The CYP1A2 enzyme metabolizes various substrates, including theophylline, caffeine, clozapine, haloperidol, and duloxetine. Activity levels of CYP1A2 are absent throughout fetal development and extremely low in the neonatal population (4% to 5% of adult levels). A steady increase is observed thereafter, with infants age 1–3 months showing 10% to 15% of adult levels, infants 3–12 months exhibiting 20% to 25% of adult activity, and children 1–9 years displaying 50% to 55% of the activity of an adult.[108] Of note, dietary factors can also influence the rate of CYP1A2 metabolism. Examining changes in the disposition of caffeine with age reveals that breastfed infants are slower to decrease their caffeine half-life compared with infants who are formula fed.[109,110]

Of the carboxylesterases, CES1 is predominantly expressed in the liver and is responsible for the hydrolysis of several commonly used medications, including methylphenidate, oseltamivir, and clopidogrel, whereas CES2 is predominantly expressed in the intestine and hydrolyze medications such as valacyclovir, tenofovir, and irinotecan.[111] Recently, microsomal and cytosolic protein expression of CES1 and CES2 in children from 1 day of life to age 18 years in 165 children has been described. For both enzymes, infants younger than 3 weeks showed significantly decreased protein expression, suggesting their rate of hydrolysis may be reduced in CES1 and CES2 substrates. Similar age-dependent increases in both CES1 and CES2 protein have been described.[112,113]

The relevance of AOX to exogenous substrate metabolism is still being established; as such only a small amount of data is available on ontogeny of this family of enzymes in humans. Development of AOX activity was characterized in a cohort of 101 Japanese neonates and children to age 10 years by measuring urinary ratio of pyridine to N(1)-methylnicotinamide, an AOX substrate. Neonates appeared to have about 10% to 15% the activity of an adult, but a linear increase by age 1 year reached the level of adult activity. Of note was the substantial variability (4-fold) in the cohort. An immunoblot assay to measure protein expression of AOX in set of 16 human livers, age 13 days to 45 years, noted a similar pattern of protein expression.[114,115]

PHASE II METABOLISM

Phase II reactions entail the conjugation of drug molecules with endogenously synthesized functional groups (e.g., glucuronic acid, glutathione, glycine, sulfate). These reactions further increase the polarity of intermediate metabolites, making the compound more water-soluble and thereby enhancing its excretion. Several major gene families have been identified that are involved in phase II reactions, including N-acetyltransferases, UGTs, GSTs, and SULTs. Analogous to the CYP families, these gene families also have individual isoforms displaying their own ontogenic profile.

The UGTs are among the most well-characterized phase II gene families. Metabolism of acetaminophen, ibuprofen, and warfarin, among other medications, involves UGT1A1. Activity of UGT1A1 is absent in fetal liver, followed by the immediate acquisition of activity shortly after birth and reaching adult levels between 3 and 6 months of life.[116] By contrast, UGT1A9 (substrates include ethinyl estradiol, ibuprofen, and acetaminophen) transcript expression is about 44% of adult values by age 6 months and is still only 64% by age 2 years.[117] In combination with the UGTs1A, UGT2B7 is responsible for the glucuronidation of morphine. Pharmacokinetic data from which morphine clearance is derived suggest that clearance (and, by extension, UGT2B7 activity) is lowest in premature neonates, increasing exponentially during the first year of life to activity levels that exceed those of adults.[118]

The SULTs play a role in steroid hormone biosynthesis, catecholamine metabolism, and thyroid hormone homeostasis. SULT1A1 is present in the fetal liver, and its expression appears consistent from birth through adolescence. By contrast, SULT2A1 activity levels increase substantially within the first 3 months of life and achieve activity comparable to that of adults after age 3 months.[119] Finally, both GSTA1 and GSTA2 are present in the prenatal liver; however, adult values are not achieved until age 1–2 years.[120]

Despite the wide array of developmental profiles observed for the phase I and phase II drug-metabolizing enzymes, neonates and young infants are not always disadvantaged in terms of clearing xenobiotics. The element of redundancy built into human detoxification pathways means that many drugs undergo biotransformation by multiple enzymes. For some drugs, compensatory mechanisms ensure that the overall clearance rate does not change with age. For other drugs, the contribution of minor pathways, although important, may be less efficient, resulting in delayed drug clearance until maturation of the primary pathway occurs. Acetaminophen offers a great example of the latter scenario. The major routes of metabolism are UGT1A6 and SULT1A1. Sulfate conjugates account for most acetaminophen metabolites recovered in newborns, with a shift in ratio observed with increasing age (Figure 7).[121] However, infants still exhibit longer overall half-lives than do young children and adolescents.[122] Ultimately, the impact of ontogenic changes in drug metabolism on drug disposition and action will depend on the nature of the chemical moiety (active drug vs. prodrug), its therapeutic index, and the number of pathways for which the drug serves as a substrate.

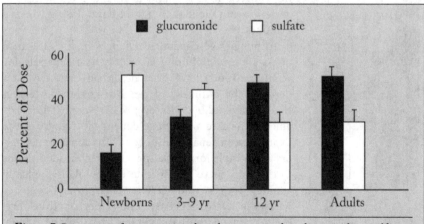

Figure 7. Percentage of an acetaminophen dose recovered as glucuronide or sulfate conjugates in newborns, children, and adults.

ELIMINATION

Although the body uses many organs to facilitate the removal of xenobiotics and endobiotics, the kidneys remain a major organ of elimination for many drugs and/or their metabolites. Both active and passive processes work in concert to clear endogenous and foreign substrates while maintaining normal fluid and electrolyte homeostasis. Of note, the kidney serves as a prototypic organ for which the completion of organogenesis does not signal structural and functional maturation of the organ. Nephrogenesis is complete by 36 weeks' gestation, yet maturation continues through childhood, as reflected by changes in the anatomic dimensions of the organ. Macroscopically, kidney length more than doubles from birth to age 12 years. Kidney weight exhibits a comparable linear increase during this same time. Microscopically, the diameter of the average glomerulus in a newborn is about one-third that of an adult, and the average proximal tubule is about one-tenth the length of that in an adult.[123] The radius of the small pores in the glomerulus increases by more than 25% during the first 3 months of life (from 19.6 to 25 Å), whereas the ratio of large pores to small pores shifts in favor of the former. Neonates also experience an increase in vascular resistance and reduced renal blood flow, with fractional cardiac output to the kidney increasing almost 4-fold during the first year of life.[124]

Because of these and other changes, renal function in children differs quantitatively from that of adults, with both passive and active processes showing clear developmental profiles (Figure 8). Glomerular filtration rate (GFR) increases abruptly after birth, more than doubling in the first 2 weeks of life and increasing uninterrupted until growth is complete. However, when examined with respect to body surface area, adult filtration capacity is achieved in the first 1–2 years of life.[124,125] Of note, GFR is significantly decreased in the premature newborn, and postnatal acquisition of functional filtration capacity follows a different trajectory in these children (Figure 9).[126] Analogous to GFR, concentrating capacity in newborns is significantly diminished at birth, increasing from less than 600 mOsm/kg of water to greater than 900 mOsm/kg of water during the first month of life and ultimately to 1200 mOsm/kg of water when growth is complete.[126]

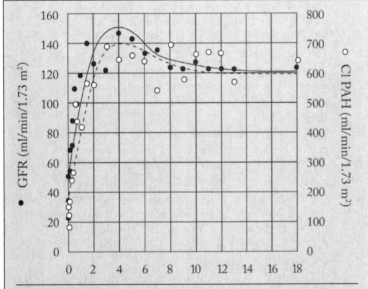

Figure 8. Changes in glomerular filtration (solid circles, solid line) rate and para-aminohippurate clearance (open circles, dashed line) as a function of age.

Based on these observations, gestational and postmenstrual age, in addition to comorbid disease processes and coadministered drugs, should be considered when determining age-appropriate pediatric dosage regimens. In young children with decreased renal function, clearance is significantly reduced and the corresponding half-life significantly prolonged, necessitating longer dosing intervals. For example, the half-life of fluconazole in premature infants (88 hours) is considerably longer than in their full-term counterparts (19.5–25 hours). Consequently, fluconazole is dosed as follows: in infants younger than 29 weeks of gestation and younger than age 14 days, dosing is every 72 hours; in infants younger than 29 weeks of gestation and older than age 14 days or infants 30–36 weeks of gestation and younger than age 14 days, dosing is every 48 hours; and in infants 30–36 weeks of gestation and older than age 14 days, dosing is every 24 hours.[127]

Although age-dependent changes in the clearance of para-aminohippurate (a prototypical substrate for renal transport) have been described, very few data describe the ontogeny of renal drug transporters in the human kidney. However, clear support is available for the assertion of age-dependent changes in the expression of renal transporters. The renal transporters responsible for regulating sodium chloride balance in the body serve to illustrate this point. The apically situated Na^+/H^+ and Cl^-/OH^- transporters, together with the Na^+/K^+-ATPase and chloride transporters located on the basolateral surface of the tubule, all show diminished activity in fetal and young animals.[128-132] Animal studies suggest that there is little

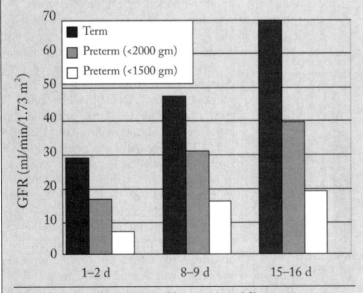

Figure 9. Postnatal acquisition of functional renal filtration capacity as a function of gestational age.

evidence to implicate the presence of specific transporter isoforms in the young or a difference in the affinity of these transporters for their respective substrates with age. Rather, differences in activity appear to be related to the existence of these transporters in lower abundance along the entire length of the nephron in young animals compared with adult animals.[128-130]

Although these renal sodium chloride transporters are not directly involved in drug transport, a substantial number of other proteins situated on both the basolateral and apical surfaces of the tubule take on the task of facilitating diffusion or actively transporting drugs in the kidney.[132-134] Table 1 highlights the predominant renal transporters that have been characterized to date and offers select examples of drugs that depend on these transporters for their elimination.[128] The transporters in the kidney, which have been the most extensively studied, are the following: P-gp, breast cancer resistance protein, OAT, OAT3, and multidrug and toxin extrusion proteins. It should be noted that at the time of writing, drug transporters are a relatively new field of study. As such,

ontogeny data on drug transporters in the kidney are limited to data on P-gp. Expression of this protein was detected as early as 11 weeks of gestation.[47] Because of the limited ontogeny data in humans, their known ontogenic profiles in rats (OAT, organic cation transporter) and mice (MRP) are illustrated in Figure 10.[135-139] For reference, the analogous developmental stages between selected animal species and humans are detailed in Table 2.[140]

An additional, often overlooked route of drug elimination is biliary excretion. Immaturity in the expression of transporters responsible for the translocation of drugs and their metabolites across the biliary canaliculus restricts the biliary clearance of drugs during the first few weeks of life.[141] To compensate, the fractional urinary excretion of many drugs that otherwise rely on biliary transport is increased in the neonate. Around 70% of a ceftriaxone dose is recovered in the urine of neonates compared with children and adults (40% to 60%).[142] Similarly, the amount of cefoperazone recovered in the urine of preterm newborns (55%) is substantially greater than that of full-term neonates (18%).[143] Although

Table 1. Clinically Relevant Renal Drug Transporters

Common Name	Gene	Substrates	Inhibitors
SLC21A3	OATP-A	Chlorambucil, fexofenadine, ouabain, rocuronium	Dexamethasone, erythromycin, lovastatin, naloxone, naltrindole, quinidine, verapamil
SLC21A9	OATP-B	Benzylpenicillin	
SLC21A11	OATP-D	Benzylpenicillin	
SLC21A12	OATP-E	Benzylpenicillin	
OCT1	SLC22A1	Acyclovir, ganciclovir	Acebutalol, amantadine, cimetidine, clonidine, disopyramide, midazolam, procainamide, prazosin, quinine, quinidine, vecuronium, verapamil
OCT2	SLC22A2	Amantadine, memantine	Desipramine, procainamide, quinine
OCT3	SLC22A3	Cimetidine	Clonidine, desipramine, imipramine, prazosin, procainamide
OCTN1	SLC22A4	Quinidine, verapamil	Cephaloridine, cimetidine, procainamide, quinine
OCTN2	SLC22A5	Pyrilamine, quinidine, valproate, verapamil	Cephalosporins, cimetidine, clonidine, desipramine, procainamide, pyrilamine, quinine
OAT1	SLC22A6	Methotrexate, acyclovir	ß-Lactam antibiotics, NSAIDs, diuretics
OAT2	SLC22A7	Zidovudine	ß-Lactam antibiotics, NSAIDs, diuretics
OAT3	SLC22A8	Zidovudine, cimetidine, methotrexate, salicylate	ß-Lactam antibiotics, diuretics, NSAIDs, quinidine
OAT4	SLC22A11	Azathioprine, cimetidine, methotrexate	ß-Lactam antibiotics, diuretics, NSAIDs
MRP1	ABCC1	Etoposide, methotrexate	Indomethacin, sulfinpyrazone
MRP2	ABCC2	Furosemide, indomethacin, methotrexate, vinblastine	Cyclosporin
MRP3	ABCC3	Methotrexate	
MRP4	ABCC4	Adefovir, azidothymidine, methotrexate	Sildenafil
MRP5	ABCC5	Adefovir, mercaptopurine	Sildenafil

ABC = ATP (adenosine triphosphate) binding cassette; MRP = multidrug resistance protein; NSAIDs = nonsteroidal anti-inflammatory drugs; OAT = organic anion transporter; OATP = organic-anion-transporting polypeptide; OCT = organic cation transporter; SLC = solute carrier.

Table 2. Analogous Developmental Stages Between Humans and Selected Animal Species

Developmental Stage	Age			
	Human	**Rat**	**Dog**	**Pig**
Neonate	Birth–1 mo	Birth–1 wk	Birth–3 wk	Birth–2 wk
Infant	1 mo–2 yr	1–3 wk	3–6 wk	2–4 wk
Child	2–12 yr	3–9 wk	6 wk–5 mo	4 wk–4 mo
Adolescent	12–16 yr	9–13 wk	5–9 mo	4–7 mo
Adult	> 16 yr	> 13 wk	> 9 mo	> 7 mo

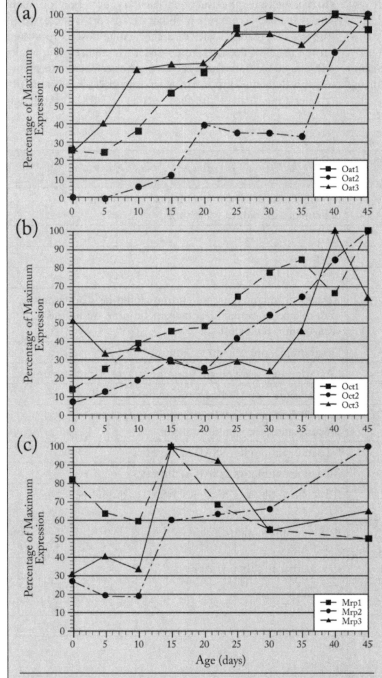

Figure 10. Average transcript expression levels of selected (a) organic anion transporter (OAT), (b) organic cation transporter (OCT), and (c) multidrug resistance protein (MRP) genes in male and female rodent kidneys.

compensatory clearance pathways exist, the overall rate of clearance for drugs eliminated through the bile will be reduced in neonates. Both P-gp and MRP2 ontogeny have been investigated to some extent in bile canaliculi. Both proteins were detected in the wall of the bile canaliculi in fetuses as early as 14 weeks by immunohistochemistry and mRNA levels. In the fetus and neonate, P-gp mRNA levels are around 20- to 30-fold lower than adult. Rapid increase occurs soon after birth, and in infants between 1–12 months the mRNA levels were only 5-fold lower than that of adults. Of interest, protein expression and mRNA levels in P-gp do not correlate because no difference has been observed in P-gp protein expression in livers ranging in age from 1 month to 12 years. In addition, another data set evaluated P-gp expression in liver samples and found no age dependence in P-gp in livers from age 7–70 years. For MRP2, mRNA levels were also initially low in fetal tissue and also increased with age. Unlike P-gp, the difference in mRNA levels between adult and fetal and infant tissue (age 1–12 months) was much more dramatic (200-fold lower in fetal tissue vs. 100-fold in young infants). Protein expression levels of MRP2 exhibited age dependence to the age of 7 years, at which point these levels stabilized and were similar to adult level.[47] For drugs in which biliary excretion plays a significant role, and are also substrates of P-gp and/or MRP2, dosing in children may need to be adjusted to account for reduced biliary excretion capacity.

PEDIATRIC DOSING BASED ON SCALING, MODELING, AND SIMULATION

The effect of ontogeny poses a challenge to dosing medications in the pediatric population because of the many physiological processes that change as a child develops. Adding to this complexity is the fact that organs mature at different rates and different proteins have variable expression patterns as a child develops. To accurately describe drug pharmacokinetics in a pediatric population, clinical studies must be conducted in children. However, children have been historically excluded in drug trials for many reasons, including, but not limited to, the following: ethics of involving minors in studies; safety concerns for the child; the amount of blood needed to conduct a pharmacokinetic study; and additional costs to drug companies. Unfortunately, the result of this lack of data means that in practice as much as 50% to 75% of medications being given to children are being dosed off-label.[144] While carefully conducted pediatric trials are now being encouraged, another way to obtain these data are through modeling and simulation. The typical approach is *allometric scaling*, which is adjusting an average dose that is appropriate for an adult to that of a child based on either weight, age, or body surface area, and may also include a scaling factor (typically 0.75). This scaling factor takes into account that changes in total bodyweight and organ weight/function are not typically linear.[144] Allometric scaling can be a suitable option for dose selection when used for older children because it factors in differences in organ size between adults and children. However, this method is inadequate in younger children where the ontogeny of drug metabolizing enzymes and transporters can be a critical factor to variability in drug pharmacokinetics.[145] In addition, this method is unable to take into account comorbidities and the effect these physiological changes have on individual pharmacokinetics. An area of current concern is that allometric scaling would be insufficient for dosing in the obese pediatric population. Childhood obesity is a concern particularly in the United States, but is of increasing relevance in other parts of the world. This condition has the potential to affect V_d and clearance, which cannot be captured by estimations of organ size alone.[146-148] Because both distribution and clearance are affected, it is highly likely that drug pharmacodynamics will be altered as well. The extent to which pharmacokinetics and pharmacodynamics is affected by obesity is most likely drug dependent.

Another way to individualize dosing in pediatrics is through modeling and simulation. Population pharmacokinetic models typically describe compartmental pharmacokinetics from a dataset that includes a large number of individuals. Often the data are scavenged and scattered, versus the intense data collection from a small number of individuals as is traditional in drug development. These models also can take into account multiple different patient covariates and evaluate the impact of each variable on a population basis.[149] Physiologically based pharmacokinetic models are computational algorithms that predict drug concentration based on prior knowledge of drug absorption, distribution, metabolism, and excretion as well as data on physiological characteristics in different populations (e.g., organ size, blood flow). When the pharmacokinetic data are from previous in vivo clinical studies, the model is considered *top-down*. Population pharmacokinetic models are considered a type of top-down model. Conversely, when the model incorporates pharmacokinetic data generated using in vitro systems, such as hepatic cell lines or subcellular fractions of organ cells, the model is considered *bottom-up*. Some models will incorporate both types of data and are occasionally referred to as *middle-out*, a model for which an example of successful implementation is valganciclovir.[150] The authors of the study were successfully able to extend an already developed valganciclovir population pharmacokinetic model for adults into neonates using in vitro generated data on kidney transporters. Their suggestions on dosing were incorporated into the FDA drug label.[150] Indeed, more drug labels are now including results from physiologically based pharmacokinetic studies as evidence for dosing recommendations for pediatric populations.[151] Although these physiologically based models offer a link between adult and pediatric pharmacokinetics, it must be noted that this approach is but one aspect of pharmacology and dosing. There is still a need to understand and describe pediatric pharmacodynamics and clinical outcomes of a drug. This area of research is one that is currently of major interest in pediatric clinical pharmacology.

CONCLUSIONS

To provide optimal care for any special population, clinicians require knowledge of how physiology and pathology intersect to affect the disposition and action of drugs. Children represent a "special population" in whom processes involved in normal growth and development overlay the processes that govern disease presentation and progression. Consequently, a fundamental working knowledge of developmental biology is essential for any clinician who chooses to care for children. This knowledge enables the pediatric care provider to make rational recommendations for drug regimen selection when data are limited in the product label to guide pediatric dosing.

It should be recognized that gaps in our knowledge will be present as long as there are drugs for which the sum total of all disposition processes have yet to be elucidated as well as known disposition pathways for which the impact of ontogeny has yet to be characterized. In these settings, data generated from carefully constructed clinical pharmacokinetic studies, including scaling, modeling, and simulation, can be used to expand our knowledge of developmental biology. The thoughtful clinician transitioning into pediatric practice should, over the course of a career, seek to accumulate and assemble both types of knowledge to construct the framework for optimal pediatric pharmacotherapy.

Patient Case | OSTEOMYELITIS IN A YOUNG CHILD

A 5-year-old boy is brought to the emergency department with leg pain and fever. The patient displays a limp when walking, and recently his parents and caregivers have had to carry him even short distances. He lives at home in urban Missouri with mother, father, and two older sisters. His family notes that he has not recently traveled or experienced trauma; however, his history is significant for recurrent methicillin-resistant *Staphylococcus aureus* (MRSA) skin infections.

Vital signs: Tmax: 38.5°C (101.3°F), Wt 16 kg, Ht 43 inches

Laboratory findings:

CRP 17.7 mg/L

Erythrocyte sedimentation rate 103 mm/hr

Creatinine phosphokinase 108 U/L

SCr 0.5 mg/dL

WBC 13.5×10^3 cells/mm^3

Neutrophil predominance 80%

Pain Score: 8/10

Magnetic resonance imaging and bone scan: positive for osteomyelitis in the right fibula.

The infectious disease team notes that their immediate suspicion is osteomyelitis caused by MRSA. They decide that drainage and debridement followed by antibiotic therapy are needed for this patient. They follow the Infectious Diseases Society of America (IDSA) guidelines for treatment of MRSA recommending vancomycin 15 mg/kg/dose intravenously every 6 hours.

After surgery and 1 week of vancomycin therapy, the patient remains febrile and still reports pain of 8/10 in the right leg. Culture of a surgical sample confirms MRSA and is sensitive to vancomycin and daptomycin. The team decides to change therapy to daptomycin 8 mg/kg/day intravenously based on the IDSA guidelines. However, this dose is in excess of the recommended adult dose.

1. Based on the differences between children and adults with respect to renal elimination, and the fact that around 80% of daptomycin is cleared by the kidney, why is the recommended dose of daptomycin for this child higher than would be administered to an adult?

Renal function, as measured by glomerular filtration rate (GFR) and para-aminohippurate clearance, displays a rapid linear increase shortly after birth and reaches a maximum around age 4 years (Figure 8). Then, by about age 12 years, the GFR and para-aminohippurate clearance decrease and become comparable with that for adults. Supporting this point is the fact that the renal clearance of daptomycin in younger children is observed to be higher than that of an adult.[152] When dosing daptomycin, the pharmacodynamic target is an area under the curve (AUC)/minimum inhibitory concentration. Because an increased clearance would result in a lower AUC, the increased dose recommendation is made to achieve an AUC that is comparable with that for adults.

2. As a substrate of P-glycoprotein (P-gp), what pharmacokinetic features are of most concern for daptomycin? How does the ontogeny of P-gp affect these pharmacokinetic variables?

The P-gp protein expression and messenger RNA (mRNA) data in the bile canaliculi are conflicting. However, based on the data for both overall, full P-gp activity has most likely been reached in a child who is age 5 years; in younger children (less than age 1 year), lower expression levels from mRNA are anticipated. Therefore, the impact of ontogeny of P-gp is not likely to factor greatly for this child. In addition, because the primary route of clearance is renal (as mentioned previously), any loss of biliary excretion because of age is unlikely to affect overall clearance in this child.

REFERENCES

1. Committee on Drugs. Guidelines for the ethical conduct of studies to evaluate drugs in pediatric populations. Pediatrics 1995;95:286-94.
2. Best Pharmaceuticals for Children Act. Public Law 107–109, 4 January 2002. Available at www.gpo.gov/fdsys/pkg/PLAW-107publ109/content-detail.html. Accessed August 19, 2018.
3. Pediatric Research Equity Act. Public Law 108–155, 3 December 2003. Available at www.congress.gov/108/plaws/publ155/PLAW-108publ155.pdf. Accessed August 19, 2018.
4. U.S. Food and Drug Administration. Food and Drug Administration Modernization Act of 1997 (FDAMA). Enacted 21 November 1997. Available at www.fda.gov/regulatory information/lawsenforcedbyfda/significantamendmentstothe fdcact/fdama/default.htm. Accessed August 19, 2018.
5. Benjamin DK, Smith PB, Murphy MD, et al. Peer-reviewed publication of clinical trials completed for pediatric exclusivity. JAMA 2006;296:1266-73.
6. Abdel-Rahman SM, Wells T, Reed M, et al. Considerations in the rational design and conduct of pediatric clinical pharmacology trials: avoiding the problems and pitfalls. Clin Pharmacol Ther 2007;81:483-94.
7. Abdel-Rahman SM, Kauffman RE. The integration of pharmacokinetics and pharmacodynamics: understanding dose-response. Annu Rev Pharmacol Toxicol 2004;44:111-36.
8. Lawless H. Sensory development in children: research in taste and olfaction. J Am Diet Assoc 1985;85:577-85.
9. Menella JA. Ontogeny of taste preferences: basic biology and implications for health. Am J Clin Nutr 2014; 99:704S-11S.
10. Agunod M, Yamaguchi N, Lopez R, et al. Correlative study of hydrochloric acid, pepsin, and intrinsic factor secretion in newborns and infants. Am J Dig Dis 1969;14:400-14.
11. Moazam F, Kirby WJ, Rodgers BM, et al. Physiology of serum gastrin production in neonates and infants. Ann Surg 1984; 199:389-92.

12. Rodgers BM, Dix PM, Talbert JL, et al. Fasting and postprandial serum gastrin in normal human neonates. J Pediatr Surg 1978;13:13-6.
13. Huang NN, High RH. Comparison of serum levels following the administration of oral and parenteral preparations of penicillin to infants and children of various age groups. J Pediatr 1953;42:657-8.
14. Poley JR, Dower JC, Owen CA, et al. Bile acids in infants and children. J Lab Clin Med 1964;63:838-46.
15. Suchy FJ, Balistreri WF, Heubi JE, et al. Physiologic cholestasis: elevation of the primary serum bile acid concentrations in normal infants. Gastroenterology 1981;80:1037-41.
16. Filer LJ, Mattson FH, Fomon SJ. Triglyceride configuration and fat absorption by the human infant. J Nutr 1969;99:293-8.
17. Lee PC, Borysewicz R, Struve M, et al. Development of lipolytic activity in gastric aspirates from premature infants. J Pediatr Gastroenterol Nutr 1993;17:291-7.
18. Hamosh M, Bitman J, Liao TH, et al. Gastric lipolysis and fat absorption in preterm infants: effect of medium-chain triglyceride or long-chain triglyceride-containing formulas. Pediatrics 1989;83:86-92.
19. Abdel-Rahman SM, Kearns GK. Single oral dose escalation pharmacokinetics of pleconaril (VP 63843) capsules in adults. J Clin Pharmacol 1999;39:613-8.
20. Kearns GL, Bradley JS, Jacobs RF, et al. Single-dose pharmacokinetics of a pleconaril in neonates. Pediatr Infect Dis J 2000;19:833-9.
21. Shankaran S, Kauffman RE. Use of chloramphenicol palmitate in neonates. J Pediatr 1984;105:113-6.
22. Gupta M, Brans YW. Gastric retention in neonates. Pediatrics 1978;62:26-9.
23. Berseth CL. Gestational evolution of small intestine motility in preterm and term infants. J Pediatr 1989;115:646-51.
24. Heimann G. Enteral absorption and bioavailability in children in relation to age. Eur J Clin Pharmacol 1980;18:43-50.
25. Kearns GL, Robinson PK, Wilson JT, et al. Cisapride disposition in neonates and infants: in vivo reflection of cytochrome P450 3A4 ontogeny. Clin Pharmacol Ther 2003;74:312-25.
26. Weaver LT, Austin S, Cole TJ. Small intestinal length: a factor essential for gut adaptation. Gut 1991;32:1321-3.
27. Helander HF, Fandriks L. Surface area of the digestive tract—revisited. Scand J Gastroenterol 2014;49:681-9.
28. Yanowitz TD, Yao AC, Pettigrew KD, et al. Postnatal hemodynamic changes in very-low-birthweight infants. J Appl Physiol 1999;87:370-80.
29. Martinussen M, Brubakk AM, Vik T, et al. Mesenteric blood flow velocity and its relation to transitional circulatory adaptation in appropriate for gestational age preterm infants. Pediatr Res 1996;39:275-80.
30. Martinussen M, Brubakk AM, Linker DT, et al. Mesenteric blood flow velocity and its relation to circulatory adaptation during the first week of life in healthy term infants. Pediatr Res 1994;36:334-9.
31. Stahlberg MR, Hietanen E, Maki M. Mucosal biotransformation rates in the small intestine of children. Gut 1988;29:1058-63.
32. Xie F, Ding X, Zhang QY. An update on the role of intestinal cytochrome P450 enzymes in drug disposition. Acta Pharmacuetica Sinica B 2016;6:374-83.
33. Johnson TN, Tanner MS, Taylor CJ, et al. Enterocytic CYP3A4 in a paediatric population: developmental changes and the effect of coeliac disease and cystic fibrosis. Br J Clin Pharmacol 2001;51:451-60.
34. Betts S, Bjorkhem-Bergman L, Rane A, et al. Expression of CYP3A4 and CYP3A7 in human foetal tissues and its correlation with nuclear receptors. Basic and Clin Pharm and Toxicol 2015;117:261-6.
35. Chen YT, Trzoss L, Yang D, et al. Ontogenic expression of human carboxylesterase-2 and cytochrome P450 3A4 in liver and duodenum: postnatal surge and organ dependent regulation. Toxicology 2015;330:55-61.
36. Lee CA, Neul D, Clouser-Roche A, et al. Identification of novel substrates for human cytochrome P450 2J2. Drug Metab Dispos 2010;38:347-56.
37. Gibbs JP, Yang JS, Slattery JT. Comparison of human liver and small intestinal glutathione S-transferase-catalyzed busulfan conjugation in vitro. Drug Metab Dispo 1998;23:52-5.
38. Gibbs JP, Liacouras CA, Baldassano RN, et al. Up-regulation of glutathione S-transferase activity in enterocytes of young children. Drug Metab Dispos 1999;27:1466-9.
39. Tukey RH, Strassburg CP. Genetic multiplicity of the human UDP-glucuronosyltransferases and regulation in the gastrointestinal tract. Mol Pharmacol 2001;59:405-14.
40. Linday L, Dobkin JF, Wang TC, et al. Digoxin inactivation by the gut flora in infancy and childhood. Pediatrics 1987;79:544-8.
41. Orrhage K, Nord CE. Factors controlling the bacterial colonization of the intestine in breastfed infants. Acta Paediatr Suppl 1999;88:47-57.
42. Rutayisire E, Huang K, Liu Y, et al. The mode of delivery affects the diversity and colonization pattern of the gut microbiota during the first year of infants' life: a systematic review. BMC Gastroenterol 2016;16:86.
43. Pacha J. Development of intestinal transport function in mammals. Physiol Rev 2000;80:1633-67.
44. Garrick MD. Human iron transporters. Genes Nutr 2011;6:45-54.
45. Gladtke E, Rind H. Iron therapy during childhood. Ger Med Mon 1966;11:438-42.
46. Fakhoury M, Litalien C, Medard Y, et al. Localization and mRNA expression of CYP3A and P-glycoprotein in human duodenum as a function of age. Drug Metab Dispos 2005;33:1603-7.
47. Brouwer KLR, Aleksunes, LM, Brandys B, et al., on behalf of the Pediatric Transporter Working Group. Human ontogeny of drug transporters: review and recommendations of the Pediatric Transporter Working Group. Clin Pharmacol Ther 2015;98:266-87.
48. Abdel-Rahman SM, Johnson F, Connor J, et al. Developmental pharmacokinetics and pharmacodynamics of nizatidine. J Pediatr Gastroenterol Nutr 2004;38:442-51.
49. Abdel-Rahman SM, Johnson FK, Gauthier-Dubois G, et al. The bioequivalence of nizatidine (Axid) in two extemporaneously and one commercially prepared oral liquid formulations compared with capsule. J Clin Pharmacol 2003;43:148-53.
50. Di Lorenzo C, Flores A, Hyman P. Age-related changes in colon motility. J Pediatr 1995;127:593-6.
51. Strachunsky LS, Nazarov AD, Firsov AA, et al. Age dependence of erythromycin rectal bioavailability in children. Eur J Drug Metab Pharmacokinet 1991;3:321-3.
52. Beck DH, Schenk MR, Hagemann K, et al. The pharmacokinetics and analgesic efficacy of larger dose rectal acetaminophen in adults: a double-blinded randomized study. Anesth Analg 2000;90:431-6.
53. Coulthard KP, Nielson HW, Schroder M, et al. Relative bioavailability and plasma paracetamol profiles of Panadol suppositories in children. J Paediatr Child Health 1998;34:425-31.
54. van Lingen RA, Deinum JT, Quak JME, et al. Pharmacokinetics and metabolism of rectally administered paracetamol in preterm neonates. Arch Dis Child Fetal Neonatal Ed 1999;80:59-63.
55. Isaac M, Holvey C. Transdermal patches: the emerging mode of drug delivery system in psychiatry. Ther Adv Pyschopharmacol 2012;2:255-63.
56. Sintov AC, Krymberk I, Gavrilov V, et al. Transdermal delivery of paracetamol for paediatric use: effects of vehicle formulations on the percutaneous penetration. J Pharm Pharmacol 2003;55:911-9.
57. Collins JJ, Dunkel IJ, Gupta SK, et al. Transdermal fentanyl children with cancer pain: feasibility, tolerability, and pharmacokinetic correlates. J Pediatrics 1999;134:319-23.

58. Zernikow B, Michel E, Anderson B. Transdermal fentanyl in childhood and adolescence: a comprehensive literature review. J Pain 207;8:187-207.

59. Okah FA, Wickett RR, Pickens WL, et al. Surface electrical capacitance as a noninvasive bedside measure of epidermal barrier maturation in the newborn infant. Pediatrics 1995;96:688-92.

60. Fluhr JW, Pfisterer S, Gloor M. Direct comparison of skin physiology in children and adults with bioengineering methods. Pediatr Dermatol 2000;17:436-9.

61. Rutter N. Percutaneous drug absorption in the newborn: hazards and uses. Clin Perinatol 1987;14:911-30.

62. West DP, Worobec S, Solomon LM. Pharmacology and toxicology of infant skin. J Invest Dermatol 1981;76:147-50.

63. Parekh D, Miller MA, Borys D, et al. Transdermal patch medication delivery systems and pediatric poisonings, 2002–2006. Clin Pediatrics 2008;47:659-63.

64. Richter WF, Bhansali SG, Morris ME. Mechanistic determinants of biotherapeutics absorption following SC administration. AAPS J 2012;14:559-70.

65. Kim H, Park H, Lee SJ. Effective method for drug injection into subcutaneous tissue. Sci Rep 2017;7:9613.

66. Heinemann L. Variability of insulin absorption and insulin action. Diabetes Technol Ther 2002;4:673-82.

67. Kagan L. Pharmacokinetic modeling of subcutaneous absorption of therapeutic proteins. Drug Metab Dispos 2014;42:1890-1905.

68. Swartz MA. The physiology of the lymphatic system. Adv Drug Deliv Rev 2001;50:3-20.

69. Leung A, Balaji S, Keswani SG. Biology and function of fetal and pediatric skin. Facial Plast Surg Clin North Am 2013;21:1-6.

70. Carry MR, Ringel SP, Starcevich JM. Distribution of capillaries in normal and diseased human skeletal muscle. Muscle Nerve 1986;9:445-54.

71. Kafetzis DA, Sinaniotis CA, Papadatos CJ, et al. Pharmacokinetics of amikacin in infants and pre-school children. Acta Paediatr Scand 1979;68:419-22.

72. Sheng KT, Huang NN, Promadhattavedi V. Serum concentrations of cephalothin in infants and children and placental transmission of the antibiotic. Antimicrob Agents Chemother 1964;10:200-6.

73. Friis-Hansen B. Water distribution in the foetus and newborn infant. Acta Paediatr Scand 1983;305:7-11.

74. Siber GR, Echeverria P, Smith AL, et al. Pharmacokinetics of gentamicin in children and adults. J Infect Dis 1975;132:637-51.

75. Moore RD, Smith CR, Lietman PS. The association of aminoglycoside plasma levels with mortality in patients with gram-negative bacteremia. J Infect Dis 1984;149:443-8.

76. Noone P, Parsons TMS, Pattison JR, et al. Experience in monitoring gentamicin therapy during treatment of serious gram negative sepsis. BMJ 1974;1:477-81.

77. Gerber AU, Craig WA. Aminoglycoside-selected subpopulations of *Pseudomonas aeruginosa*. J Lab Clin Med 1982;100:671-81.

78. Blaser J, Stone BB, Groner MC, et al. Comparative study with enoxacin and netilmicin in a pharmacodynamic model to determine importance of ratio of antibiotic peak concentration to MIC for bactericidal activity and emergence of resistance. Antimicrob Agents Chemother 1987;31:1054-60.

79. Kearns G, Abdel-Rahman S, Blumer J, et al. Single dose pharmacokinetics of linezolid in infants and children. Pediatr Infect Dis J 2000;19:1178-84.

80. Fredholm BB, Rane A, Persson B. Diphenylhydantoin binding to proteins in plasma and its dependence on free fatty acid and bilirubin concentration in dogs and newborn infants. Pediatr Res 1975;9:26-30.

81. Windorfer A, Kuenzer W, Urbanek R. The influence of age on the activity of acetylsalicylic acid-esterase and protein-salicylate binding. Eur J Clin Pharmacol 1974;7:227-31.

82. Nau H, Luck W, Kuhnz W. Decreased serum protein binding of diazepam and its major metabolite in the neonate during the first postnatal week relate to increased free fatty acid levels. Br J Clin Pharmacol 1984;17:92-8.

83. Kanakoudi F, Drossou V, Tzimousli V, et al. Serum concentrations of 10 acute-phase proteins in healthy term and preterm infants from birth to age 6 months. Clin Chem 1995;41:605-8.

84. Kingston H, Kendrick A, Sommer K, et al. Binding of thiopental in neonatal serum. Anesthesiology 1990;72:428-31.

85. Mestelman C, Benhamou D, Barre J, et al. Effects of age on plasma protein binding of sufentanil. Anesthesiology 1990;72:470-3.

86. Ehrenbo M, Agurell S, Jalling B, et al. Age differences in drug binding by plasma proteins: studies on human foetuses, neonates and adults. Eur J Clin Pharmacol 1971;3:189-93.

87. Tsai C, Ahdab-Barmada M, Daood MJ, et al. P-glycoprotein expression in the developing human central nervous system: cellular and tissue localization. Pediatr Res 2001;47:436A.

88. Young WS III, Lietman PS. Chloramphenicol glucuronyl transferase: assay, ontogeny and inducibility. J Pharmacol Exp Ther 1978;204:203-11.

89. Argikar UA, Potter PM, Hutzler JM, et al. Challenges and opportunities with non-CYP enzyme aldehyde oxidase, carboxyesterase, and glucuronosyltransferase: focus on reaction phenotyping and prediction of human clearance. AAPS J 2016;18:1391-405.

90. Terao M, Romao MJ, Leimkuhler S, et al. Structure and function of mammalian aldehyde oxidases. Arch Toxicol 2016;90:753-80.

91. Ross MK, Borazjani A. Enzymatic activity of human carboxylesterase. Curr Prot Toxicol 2007;33:4.24.1-4.24.14.

92. Stevens JC, Hines RN, Chungang GU, et al. Developmental expression of the major human hepatic CYP3A enzymes. J Pharmacol Exp Ther 2003;307:573-82.

93. LaCroix D, Sonnier M, Moncion A, et al. Expression of CYP3A in the human liver: evidence that the shift between CYP3A7 and CYP3A4 occurs immediately after birth. Eur J Biochem 1997;247:625-34.

94. Mukherjee A, Dombi T, Wittke B, et al. Population pharmacokinetics of sildenafil in term neonates: evidence of rapid maturation of metabolic clearance in the early postnatal period. Clin Pharmacol Ther 2009;85:56-63.

95. Maya MT, Domingos CR, Guerreiro MT, et al. Comparative bioavailability of two immediate release tablets of cisapride in healthy volunteers. Eur J Drug Metab Pharmacokinet 1998;23:377-81.

96. Blake MJ, Gaedigk A, Pearce RE, et al. Ontogeny of dextromethorphan O- and N-demethylation in the first year of life. Clin Pharmacol Ther 2007;81:510-6.

97. U.S. Food and Drug Administration. Codeine and Tramadol Can Cause Breathing Problems for Children. FDA Consumer Health Information, 20 April 2017. Available at www.fda.gov/ForConsumers/ConsumerUpdates/ucm315497.htm. Accessed August 19, 2018.

98. Koukouritaki SB, Manro JR, Marsh SA, et al. Developmental expression of human hepatic CYP2C9 and CYP2C19. J Pharmacol Exp Ther 2004;308:965-74.

99. Bourgeois BF, Dodson WE. Phenytoin elimination in newborns. Neurology 1983;33:173-8.

100. Whelan HT, Hendeles L, Haberkern CM, et al. High intravenous phenytoin dosage requirement in a newborn infant. Neurology 1983;33:106-8.

101. Faure C, Michaud L, Shaghaghi EK, et al. Intravenous omeprazole in children: pharmacokinetics and effect on 24-hour intragastric pH. J Pediatr Gastroenterol Nutr 2001;33:144-8.

102. Jacqz-Aigrain E, Bellaich M, Faure C, et al. Pharmacokinetics of intravenous omeprazole in children. Eur J Clin Pharmacol 1994;47:181-5.

103. Vinayek R, Amantea MA, Maton PN, et al. Pharmacokinetics of oral and intravenous omeprazole in patients with the Zollinger-Ellison syndrome. Gastroenterology 1991;101:138-47.

104. Marier JF, Dubuc MC, Drouin E, et al. Pharmacokinetics of omeprazole in healthy adults and in children with gastroesophageal reflux disease. Ther Drug Monit 2004;26:3-8.

105. Andersson T, Hassall E, Lundborg P, et al. Pharmacokinetics of orally administered omeprazole in children. Am Coll Gastroenterol 2000;95:3101-6.

106. Vieira I, Sonnier M, Cresteil T. Developmental expression of CYP2E1 in the human liver: hypermethylation control of gene expression during the neonatal period. Eur J Biochem 1996;238:476-83.

107. Flockhart DA. Drug Interactions: Flockhart Table. Indiana University School of Medicine (2019). Available at https://drug-interactions.medicine.iu.edu/MainTable.aspx. Accessed September 30, 2019.

108. Sonnier M, Cresteil T. Delayed ontogenesis of CYP1A2 in the human liver. Eur J Biochem 1998;251:893-8.

109. Le Guennec JC, Billon B. Delay in caffeine elimination in breast-fed infants. Pediatrics 1987;79:264-8.

110. Blake MJ, Abdel-Rahman SM, Pearce RE, et al. Effect of diet on the development of drug metabolism by cytochrome P-450 enzymes in healthy infants. Pediatr Res 2006;60:717-23.

111. Laizure SC, Herring V, Hu Z, et al. The role of human carboxylesterases in drug metabolism: have we overlooked their importance? Pharmacotherapy 2013;33:210-22.

112. Hines RN, Simpson PM, McCarver DG. Age-dependent human hepatic carboxylesterase 1 (CES1) and carboxylesterase 2 (CES2) postnatal ontogeny. Drug Metab Dispos 2016;44:959-66.

113. Boberg M, Vrana M, Mehrotra A, et al. Age-dependent absolute abundance of hepatic carboxylesterases (CES1 and CES2) by LC-MS/MS proteomics: application to PBPK modeling of oseltamivir in vivo pharmacokinetics in infants. Drug Metab Dispo 2017;45:216-23.

114. Tamaya Y, Miyake K, Sugihara K, et al. Developmental changes of aldehyde oxidase activity in young Japanese children. Clin Pharmacol Ther 2007;81:567-72.

115. Tayama Y, Sugihara K, Sanoh S, et al. Developmental changes of aldehyde oxidase activity and protein expression in human liver cytosol. Drug Metab Pharmacokinet 2012;27:543-7.

116. de Wildt SN, Kearns GL, Leeder JS, et al. Glucuronidation in humans. Pharmacogenetic and developmental aspects. Clin Pharmacokinet 1999;36:439-52.

117. Strassburg CP, Strassburg A, Kneip S, et al. Developmental aspects of human hepatic drug glucuronidation in young children and adults. Gut 2002;50:259-65.

118. Scott CS, Riggs KW, Ling EW, et al. Morphine pharmacokinetics and pain assessment in premature newborns. J Pediatr 1999;135:423-9.

119. Duanmu Z, Weckle A, Koukouritaki SB, et al. Developmental expression of aryl, estrogen, and hydroxysteroid sulfotransferases in pre- and postnatal human liver. J Pharmacol Exp Ther 2006;316:1310-7.

120. Strange RC, Davis BA, Faulder CG, et al. The human glutathione S-transferases: developmental aspects of the GST1, GST2, and GST3 loci. Biochem Genet 1985;23:1011-28.

121. Miller RP, Roberts RJ, Fischer LJ. Acetaminophen elimination kinetics in neonates, children, and adults. Clin Pharmacol Ther 1976;19:284-94.

122. Allegaert K, Van der Marel CD, Debeer A, et al. Pharmacokinetics of a single dose intravenous propacetamol in neonates: effect of gestational age. Arch Dis Child Fetal Neonatal Educ 2004;89:25-8.

123. McCrory WM. Embryonic development and prenatal maturation of the kidney. In: Edelmann CM, ed. Pediatric Kidney Disease. Boston: Little, Brown and Company, 1978:3-25.

124. Spitzer A. Renal physiology and functional development. In: Edelmann CM, ed. Pediatric Kidney Disease. Boston: Little, Brown and Company, 1978:25-128.

125. Schwartz GJ, Feld LG, Langford DJ. A simple estimate of glomerular filtration rate in full-term infants during the first year of life. J Pediatr 1984;104:849-54.

126. John TR, Moore WM, Jeffries JE, eds. Children Are Different: Developmental Physiology, 2nd ed. Columbus, OH: Ross Laboratories, 1978.

127. Saxen H, Hoppu K, Pohjavuori M. Pharmacokinetics of fluconazole in very low birth weight infants during the first two weeks of life. Clin Pharmacol Ther 1993;54:269-77.

128. Shah M, Quigley R, Baum M. Maturation of proximal straight tubule NaCl transport: role of thyroid hormone. Am J Physiol Renal Physiol 2000;278:596-602.

129. Guillery EN, Karniski LP, Mathews MS, et al. Maturation of proximal tubule Na+/H+ antiporter activity in sheep during transition from fetus to newborn. Am J Physiol 1994;267:537-45.

130. Petershack JA, Nagaraja SC, Guillery EN. Role of glucocorticoids in the maturation of renal cortical Na+-K+-ATPase during fetal life in sheep. Am J Physiol 1999;276:1825-32.

131. Shah M, Quigley R, Baum M. Neonatal rabbit proximal tubule basolateral membrane Na+/H+ antiporter and Cl-/base exchange. Am J Physiol 1999;276:1792-7.

132. Lee W, Kim RB. Transporters and renal drug elimination. Annu Rev Pharmacol Toxicol 2004;44:137-66.

133. Tsuji A. Transporter mediated drug interactions. Drug Metabol Pharmacokinet 2002;17:253-74.

134. Wright SH, Dantzler WH. Molecular and cellular physiology of renal organic cation and anion transport. Physiol Rev 2003; 84:987-1049.

135. Buist SC, Cherrington NJ, Choudhuri S, et al. Gender-specific and developmental influences on the expression of rat organic anion transporters. J Pharmacol Exp Ther 2002;301:145-51.

136. Slitt AL, Cherrington NJ, Hartley DP, et al. Tissue distribution and renal developmental changes in rat organic cation transporter mRNA levels. Drug Metab Dispos 2002;30:212-9.

137. Alnouti Y, Petrick J, Klaassen C. Tissue distribution and ontogeny of organic cation transporters in mice. Drug Metab Dispos 2006;34:477-82.

138. Rosati A, Maniori S, Decorti G, et al. Physiological regulation of P-glycoprotein, MRP1, MRP2 and cytochrome P450 3A2 during rat ontogeny. Dev Growth Differ 2003;45:377-87.

139. Maher JM, Slitt AL, Cherrington NJ, et al. Tissue distribution and hepatic and renal ontogeny of the multidrug resistance-associated protein (MRP) family in mice. Drug Metab Dispos 2005;33:947-55.

140. Gad SC. Regulatory requirements for INDs/FIH (first in human) studies. In: Gad SC, ed. Preclinical Development Handbook: ADME and Biopharmaceutical Properties. Hoboken, NJ: John Wiley & Sons, 2008:1267-303.

141. Rollins DE, Klaassen CD. Biliary excretion of drugs in man. Clin Pharmacokinet 1979;4:368-79.

142. Hayton WL, Stoeckel K. Age-associated changes in ceftriaxone pharmacokinetics. Clin Pharmacokinet 1986;11:76-86.

143. Rosenfeld WN, Evans HE, Batheja R, et al. Pharmacokinetics of cefoperazone in full-term and premature neonates. Antimicrob Agents Chemother 1983;23:866-9.

144. Samant TS, Mangel N, Lukacova V, et al. Quantitative clinical pharmacology for size and age scaling in pediatric drug development: a systematic review. J Clin Pharmacol 2015;55:1207-17.

145. Sage DP, Kulczar C, Roth W, et al. Persistent pharmacokinetic challenges to pediatric drug development. Front Genet 2014;5:218.

146. Kendrick JG, Carr RR, Ensom MHH. Pediatric obesity: pharmacokinetics and implications for drug dosing. Clin Ther 2015; 37:1897-923.

147. Harskamp-van Ginkel MW, Hill KD, Becker KC, et al., Best Pharmaceuticals for Children Act—Pediatric Trials Network Administrative Core Committee. Drug dosing and pharmacokinetics in children with obesity: a systematic review. JAMA Pediatr 2015;169:678-85.

148. Rowe S, Siegel D, Benjamin DK Jr., Best Pharmaceuticals for Children Act—Pediatric Trials Network Administrative Core Committee. Gaps in drug dosing in obese children: a systematic review of commonly prescribed acute care medications. Clin Ther 2015;37:1924-32.

149. Sheiner LB, Ludden TM. Population Pharmacokinetics/ Dynamics. Ann Rev Pharmacol Toxicol 1992;32:185-209.

150. Jorga K, Chavanne C, Frey N, et al. Bottom-up meets top-down: complementary physiologically based pharmacokinetic and population pharmacokinetic modeling for regulatory approval of a dosing algorithm of valganciclovir in very young children. Clin Pharmcol Ther 2016;100:761-9.

151. Maharaj AR, Edginton AN. Physiologically base pharmacokinetic modeling and simulation in pediatric drug development. CPT Pharmacometrics Syst Pharmacol 2014;3:e148.

152. Bradley JS, Benziger D, Bokesch P, et al. Single-dose pharmacokinetics of daptomycin in pediatric patients 3–24 months of age. Pediatr Infect Dis J 2014;33:936-9.

CHAPTER 4

Drug Formulations

*Vinita B. Pai, Pharm.D., M.S.; and
Milap C. Nahata, Pharm.D., M.S., FCCP, FAPhA,
FASHP, FPPA*

LEARNING OBJECTIVES

1. Describe the legislative actions undertaken by the U.S. Congress to encourage the pharmaceutical industry to conduct drug trials supporting pediatric labeling of their drugs and develop pediatric formulations.

2. Recognize the need for extemporaneous formulations in infants and children.

3. List the most common extemporaneously compounded oral liquid formulations.

4. Describe the different extemporaneous options available for providing a suitable dosage form for a child.

5. Explain the methods involved in compounding an extemporaneous formulation and the factors that affect its use in clinical practice.

ABBREVIATIONS IN THIS CHAPTER

ASHP	American Society of Health-System Pharmacists
BPCA	Best Pharmaceuticals for Children Act
FDA	U.S. Food and Drug Administration
FDAMA	Food and Drug Administration Modernization Act
FDASIA	Food and Drug Administration Safety and Innovation Act
PREA	Pediatric Research Equity Act
USP	United States Pharmacopeia

INTRODUCTION

An estimated 73.6 million children, from age birth to 18 years, resided in the United States in 2015. Of these children, 19.9 million were 5 years or younger.[1] In December 2010, the *Wall Street Journal* reported that according to one of the largest U.S. pharmacy benefits providers, Medco Health Solutions, around 25% of children and 30% of adolescents between ages 10 and 19 years were taking a medication for a chronic condition in 2009.[2] Almost 7% of these children and adolescents were taking two or more drugs for long-term therapy. The total number of prescriptions or refills dispensed to children and adolescents were as follows (from most to least): asthma drugs 45,388,000; attention-deficit/hyperactivity disorder drugs 24,357,000; antidepressants 9,614,000; antipsychotics 6,546,000; antihypertensives 5,224,000; sleep aids

307,000; oral hypoglycemic drugs 424,000; and statins 94,000. Many of these drugs, however, are not labeled for use in the 0- to 9-year-old age group and thus are not available in suitable dosage forms.

Research and development of most pharmaceuticals are focused on providing safe and efficacious drugs for adults. Initial efficacy and safety trials for most drugs often exclude infants, children, and pregnant women. Drugs routinely used in pediatric patients may not have U.S. Food and Drug Administration (FDA)–approved pediatric labeling. Without these trials, information regarding the effective dose per patient weight (milligram per kilogram per dose), the frequency of dosing, and the adverse effects of a drug in the pediatric population may come from pilot observations, from case reports or series, and by trial-and-error methods. Drugs without pediatric labeling are often unavailable in dosage forms suitable to administer to children. For example, tacrolimus is used as an immunosuppressive agent in adult and pediatric solid-organ and peripheral stem cell transplants. However, it is available only as a capsule. A liquid formulation has to be extemporaneously compounded for use in infants and children.

In 1997, the Food and Drug Administration Modernization Act (FDAMA) was signed into law (Public Law 105-115).[3] According to Section 111, pharmaceutical companies with a drug already on the market or submitting a new drug application to the FDA were offered an additional 6 months of patent protection (exclusivity to market that drug) in exchange for conducting requested trials in children. The goal was to encourage the pharmaceutical industry to conduct trials supporting the pediatric labeling of their drugs and develop a pediatric formulation for their product. In 2002, the FDAMA was reauthorized as the Best Pharmaceuticals for Children Act (BPCA); in 2007, this act was signed into law.[4,5] Under this law, the FDA would accept, on a case-by-case basis, pediatric labeling directions for preparing an extemporaneous pediatric formulation as an alternative to a stable commercial formulation. The BCPA also encouraged companies to conduct studies in neonates.

In 1998, the FDA mandated an assessment of new drugs, new indications, new dosing regimens, new active ingredients, and new dosage forms for pediatric patients, which was formalized as the Pediatric Research Equity Act (PREA) in 2003. The Food and Drug Administration Safety and Innovation Act (FDASIA) was signed into law in 2012 and permanently renewed and strengthened the BPCA and PREA. FDASIA requires submission of a pediatric study plan by the manufacturer subject to PREA, even if the new drug application is intended for adults. This gives greater authority to the FDA to ensure that the sponsor meets PREA requirements to conduct pediatric studies as planned or to seek an extension or deferral for failing to comply. FDASIA also requires inclusion of a staff member with expertise in neonatology on the

Pediatric Review Committee.[6] It is encouraging that the FDA has approved 680 labeling changes for children and that more than 230 drugs have been granted pediatric exclusivity under BPCA.[7] However, these changes have come at a high cost in certain instances. The average wholesale acquisition price of commercially manufactured liquid dosage forms of enalapril and lisinopril may cost 21 and 775 times the generically available solid dosage forms, respectively. The availability of these products precludes pharmacies from extemporaneously compounding the formulations for the same drug. A one-month supply of an extemporaneously prepared drug costing less than $20 may have a wholesale acquisition cost of $1000 or more for a commercially marketed liquid of certain medications.[8]

NEED FOR EXTEMPORANEOUS FORMULATIONS

A pharmacist may need to compound an oral extemporaneous formulation for pediatric and adult patients who are unable to swallow solid dosage forms or who are receiving their medication through a nasogastric tube or gastrostomy tube. In addition, most children younger than 6 years, even when given specific training, are unable to swallow a solid dosage form such as a tablet or capsule.[9,10] Most pediatric drug doses are based on body weight (milligram per kilogram per dose) or body surface area (milligram per square meter per dose). Such individualized doses cannot be easily administered and titrated using the available solid dosage forms, which contain a fixed amount of drug. For drugs requiring drug concentration monitoring (e.g., tacrolimus), dose adjustments to achieve safe and effective blood concentrations may result in doses that are not commercially available. In addition, the presence of an inactive ingredient or a high concentration of the inactive ingredient in a commercially available liquid dosage form may prevent the use of a particular drug in premature or full-term neonates (e.g., Dexamethasone Intensol containing 30% alcohol). Toxicity may not be observed after a single dose of this medication; however, toxicity because of the long-term administration and additive effects of certain excipients cannot be ignored. Stability of the drug in the oral extemporaneous formulation and ability to accurately administer a dose should be ensured before use in patients.

Pharmacists also compound parenteral drugs extemporaneously. Parenteral drugs are supplied in a commercially available ready-to-use concentration, a concentrated solution requiring further dilution, or a dry, lyophilized powder for reconstitution. Some intravenous drugs (e.g., phenobarbital, morphine, furosemide, fentanyl) may be too concentrated for accurate measurement of the small doses (volumes) needed for treatment of neonates and infants. These doses may require further dilution before intravenous administration. For example, furosemide is available as a 10-mg/mL solution for injection. A neonate weighing 0.7 kg would require a dose of 0.7 mg intravenously or 0.07 mL, which cannot be accurately measured with the commercial formulation. Under these circumstances, the intravenous drug requires further dilution with a suitable diluent to prevent errors in measuring the amount. The drug stability and sterility of this parenteral extemporaneous formulation must be documented before its use in patients.

MOST COMMONLY PREPARED PEDIATRIC EXTEMPORANEOUS FORMULATIONS

Information regarding the most commonly compounded extemporaneous formulations for children in the United States is available through surveys published in the literature. A 1998–1999 survey of 57 small and large hospitals caring for pediatric patients identified the five most commonly compounded formulations as follows: spironolactone, captopril, ursodiol, metronidazole, and allopurinol.[11] Oral, nasogastric, and gastric were the most common routes of administration of these medications. The same survey also identified 103 drug formulations prescribed by pediatricians that had no compounding and/or stability information.

In 2009, another survey was conducted to determine the scope and frequency of use of extemporaneous liquid formulations in children's hospitals.[12] The five most commonly compounded formulations in 20 pediatric U.S. hospitals identified by this survey were lansoprazole, spironolactone, captopril, sildenafil, and ursodiol. This survey identified a total of 231 drugs or drug combinations that were compounded into liquid formulations for 28% of all inpatient admissions during a 12-month period.

OPTIONS FOR PROVIDING EXTEMPORANEOUS FORMULATIONS

Pharmacists who often compound extemporaneous formulations will need informational resources providing formulation recipe, compounding method, storage conditions, and stability data. The most common and immediate resource is the United States Pharmacopeia (USP).[13] It contains official monographs of compounded preparations that include valid stability data to establish a *beyond-use date* or *expiration date* (i.e., the date beyond which a compounded preparation is not to be used, which is determined from the date of preparation). Compounding information supported by stability studies and beyond-use dates may be available in the package insert of drugs such as losartan, benazepril, lisinopril, and rifampin. This information usually is included in the package inserts of brand-name products because the manufacturer most often has a pediatric labeling for the drug.

Tertiary publications such as the *Pediatric & Neonatal Dosage Handbook*, which was designed as a dosing reference for neonates, infants, and children, and *NeoFax*, which is a reference specific for the dosing and administration of drugs in neonates, contain necessary information regarding the extemporaneous compounding of a drug formulation.[14,15] *Pediatric Drug Formulations* and *Extemporaneous Formulations for Pediatric, Geriatric, and Special Needs Patients* are two tertiary publications that compile information regarding formulation recipes, methods of compounding, storage conditions, and stability data.[16,17] Primary peer-reviewed publications regarding specific formulations can be obtained by conducting a literature search through PubMed using search terms such as "extemporaneous drug formulations," "extemporaneous compounding," and "extemporaneous preparations children," combined with the name of the drug being researched.

Another resource for locating information about the compounding of extemporaneous formulations is the Investigator's Brochures or reports, but these documents are usually not easily available or accessible because of their confidential or proprietary nature. Before using the compounding information from the Investigator's Brochures or pharmaceutical industry–generated reports, pharmacists should ascertain that the formulation stated in the brochure is not being investigated for its stability, bioavailability, or bioequivalence through ongoing clinical trials. If such trials are under way, the formulation cannot be dispensed for routine patient care until trial results indicate successful achievement of the study goals. Manufacturers of the solid dosage forms can be contacted to obtain information regarding any preclinical testing of extemporaneous formulations. However, when a drug does not have pediatric labeling, the potential for legal liabilities may prevent manufacturers from providing information about formulations used in preclinical studies.

When compounding and stability information for an oral commercially manufactured product is unavailable, some pediatric hospital pharmacies may compound it as a suspension or solution. The liquid preparation is usually packaged in a tight, light-resistant container (amber plastic bottle) and stored at controlled temperatures to observe for signs of physical changes. For water-containing formulations prepared from solid ingredients, the USP-recommended beyond-use date is no later than 14 days for liquid preparations when stored at cold temperatures between 35.6°F (2°C) and 46.4°F (8°C).[18] The USP recommendations should be used with caution, especially because the stability of a drug in liquid depends on several physicochemical properties such as pH and oxidation-reduction reactions. For example, captopril (0.75 mg/mL) in cherry syrup is only stable for 2 days at room temperature or when refrigerated, and it is stable for 10 days or less in a 1:1 mixture of Ora-Sweet and Ora-Plus or Ora-Sweet SF and Ora-Plus, depending on the storage temperature. Thus, without the stability data, labeling these captopril formulations with a beyond-use date of 14 days according to the USP would be inappropriate.[19]

Under these circumstances, preparing powder papers or using dosage forms intended for adults with or without alterations seems to be a logical option. The procedure for preparing powder papers includes crushing the tablets or opening the capsules, uniformly redistributing the contents with inactive ingredients such as lactose to achieve the required dilution, weighing out each powder paper, and then folding it. This preparation is time-consuming and labor-intensive. In addition, the contents of the powder paper will still have to be reconstituted into a liquid before administration. Solid dosage forms without an extemporaneous formulation can also be administered by splitting or crushing a tablet and opening a capsule and administering the content with food. These modifications may result in a compromise in the physicochemical stability of the drug, an altered rate of drug absorption, and improper dosing because of the inaccurate splitting of tablets or spillage during reconstitution or mixing with a large amount of food that is not completely ingested by the patient. For a solid dosage form with a water-soluble active ingredient, crushing the tablet or mixing the contents of a capsule

with a specified amount of water and drawing up the exact amount for a dose can be done. However, this process can be time-consuming and has the potential for calculation errors. Alternatively, the injectable solution of the same drug can be administered orally, provided both formulations contain the same salt form with similar bioavailability. However, the cost of the injectable solution can be a limitation to using this method.

METHODS OF PREPARING DIFFERENT EXTEMPORANEOUS FORMULATIONS

The most commonly compounded extemporaneous formulation for children involves making a liquid formulation from a solid dosage form, which could be formulated as a solution or a suspension. For a more comprehensive review of preparing extemporaneous formulations, the clinician is referred to the American Society of Health-System Pharmacists (ASHP) website at www.ashp.org and other valuable resources.[20,21] The ASHP website provides guidelines that address areas of extemporaneous compounding through the following two documents: *ASHP Technical Assistance Bulletin on Compounding Nonsterile Products in Pharmacies,*[22] and *ASHP Guidelines on Quality Assurance for Pharmacy-Prepared Sterile Products.*[23]

A suspension is the most commonly compounded oral formulation because most drugs (active ingredients) are not completely water soluble. Even if the active ingredient is completely water soluble, the inactive ingredients (excipients) may not be soluble. A suspending agent that can uniformly suspend the active and inactive ingredients after shaking is necessary to accurately withdraw a dose and should be used in the compounding recipe. Adding a suspending agent to a formulation with soluble active but insoluble inactive ingredients allows a more pharmaceutically elegant preparation. Without a suspending agent, the insoluble ingredients will settle rapidly. This settling may result in the caregiver's inaccurate assumption that he or she is unable to withdraw a uniform dose from the preparation. Preparation of an extemporaneous liquid dosage form from tablets involves crushing and triturating them in a mortar into a fine powder, whereas capsule contents are emptied into a mortar and mixed well. The powder is then levigated into a smooth paste using small portions of the selected vehicle, which usually consists of a combination of a suspending agent and a sweetening agent. The uniform paste is mixed with the rest of the vehicle in geometric proportions with constant mixing until the desired volume is almost achieved. The mixture is then transferred to a measuring device (graduated cylinder), and the selected vehicle is added to make up the required volume according to the recipe. The preparation should then be transferred to an appropriate container, such as an amber bottle, and labeled with a beyond-use date under storage conditions, as indicated in the stability studies. Prescription bottles should not be used as measuring devices because the graduation marked on these bottles is inaccurate.

Ingredients (raw materials) used in compounding extemporaneous formulations should always be of USP or equivalent grade. Carboxymethylcellulose and methylcellulose are common suspending agents. A carboxymethylcellulose sodium suspension is easier to compound, but it has a pH of about 10, which can affect drug solubility, stability, and absorption. The preparation of a methylcellulose suspension is difficult and time-consuming because it requires four hours to remove entrapped air bubbles. However, the advantage of using a methylcellulose 1%/simple syrup suspension (1:1) is that it is an inert, nonreactive, and pH-neutral (pH 6.8) vehicle. Most pharmacists in the United States prefer to use commercially available ready-to-use vehicles. A vehicle can be easily prepared by combining Ora-Plus (Paddock Laboratories, Minneapolis, MN), a carboxymethylcellulose-containing suspending agent, with Ora-Sweet (Paddock Laboratories) syrup, in a 1:1 volume. Ora-Sweet SF (Paddock Laboratories), a sugar-free syrup vehicle, can be used instead of Ora-Sweet. All three have an acidic pH, which should be considered in compounding suspensions when drug stability data are unavailable for the preparation. Ora-Blend and Ora-Blend SF, marketed by the same manufacturer, are sweetened (with sugar or sugar free) suspending agents, eliminating the need to prepare a 1:1 mixture of Ora-Plus with Ora-Sweet or Ora-Plus with Ora-Sweet SF. Other available vehicles include SyrSpend SF, SyrSpend SF Alka, SyrSpend SF Cherry, SyrSpend SF Alka Cherry, SyrSpend SF Grape, and SyrSpend SF Alka Grape (Gallipot, St. Paul, MN).

Certain characteristics of an oral liquid dosage form such as taste, odor, palatability, texture, color, and sweetness may enhance a patient's acceptance of the medication therapy. Children usually prefer a sweet taste with fruity flavors. Choice of flavoring agents may also depend on the characteristic taste of the drug itself because certain flavoring agents mask certain tastes well. Cocoa-flavored vehicles may mask bitter-tasting drugs, whereas fruit or citrus flavors may mix well with sour or acidic-tasting drugs, and salty drugs can be made more palatable if masked by raspberry- or orange-flavored vehicles. Formulations can be made to taste sweet using vehicles such as simple syrup USP or Ora-Blend. Flavored vehicles such as SyrSpend SF Cherry or SyrSpend SF Grape can also be used. Adding a flavoring agent to an extemporaneous formulation when it was not used in the original formulation could alter the stability and concentration of the medication. If additional flavoring is needed, the agent can be added to each dose immediately before administration of the dose. Adding coloring agents may make the formulation esthetically more appealing. However, the stability of the formulation may be affected by the presence of these chemical coloring agents because most of the dyes are affected by the formulation pH, presence of oxidizing or reducing substances, or exposure to light. Thus, many institutions do not add coloring agents to extemporaneous formulations.

FACTORS THAT AFFECT THE USE OF EXTEMPORANEOUS FORMULATIONS IN CLINICAL PRACTICE

STABILITY

A stable extemporaneous formulation is one that retains the characteristics and properties it possessed at the time of preparation throughout its storage and use, termed *shelf life*.

An extemporaneous formulation should be physically, chemically, microbiologically, therapeutically, and toxicologically stable during its shelf life. Stability is affected by temperature, radiation, light, humidity, particle size, pH, water and other solvents, container properties, and other chemicals that may be present in the formulation. All compounded preparations require a beyond-use date labeling. Several factors determine this beyond-use date. The expiration date for a commercially manufactured product cannot be directly extrapolated to assign a beyond-use date for a nonsterile preparation compounded from it.

Physical stability includes the lack of change in color, odor, taste, texture, and consistency of the preparation. This stability can be tested by storing the compounded formulation at various commonly used storage conditions (temperatures and containers) and periodically (e.g., at weeks 0, 1, 2, 4, 8, and 12) testing for components of physical stability. The most common storage temperatures for medications include room temperature (68°F–77°F [20°C–25°C]), refrigerated temperature (35.6°F–46.4°F [2°C–8°C]), and freezer temperature (-77°F to -68°F [-25°C to -20°C]). Storage containers generally consist of amber plastic prescription bottles unless specified in the stability studies.

Chemical stability of drugs in an extemporaneous formulation (both sterile and nonsterile) involves the measurement of the active ingredient(s) to ensure its potency during storage and use. During storage, no more than a 10% change in the active ingredient concentration should occur. Pharmacists should consult and apply specific and general stability documentation and literature when available. Testing for chemical stability involves the use of certain analytic methods. The analytic method should be accurate, efficient, specific, reproducible, and stability-indicating. No single method can be used to test all drugs. Many analytic tests are not available in the pharmacy or health care facility; thus, they may need to be outsourced to contract laboratories. A contract laboratory chosen for conducting analytic tests should follow USP General Chapter standards using official methods and techniques for testing. The chemical stability of the active ingredient(s) is usually reported as a percentage of the initial concentration. In general, formulations with storage conditions and beyond-use dates, which preserve the potency of the active ingredient(s) within 90% to 110% of the initial concentration, should be used; however, the USP monograph for the specific drug should be consulted for acceptable variance for each active ingredient being evaluated.

Most pharmacies involved in dispensing extemporaneous formulations lack the resources to undertake such chemical stability studies. Instead, they may have to rely on books, peer-reviewed publications, or a commercially available or institution-specific computer database with recipes for extemporaneous formulation recipes. A search of the literature for stability data on an extemporaneous formulation may reveal several studies using different compounding agents, storage conditions, and duration of stability for the same drug. All stability data must be carefully interpreted with respect to the particular compounded formulation. Ease and convenience of compounding, duration of stability of the formulation, easy availability of the compounding ingredients, and cost are factors to consider in choosing a particular recipe as your institution's primary formulation for a compounded product. Formulations with limited demand and a shorter duration of stability should not be prepared in large amounts to avoid waste of unused medications.

Because most extemporaneous liquid preparations are aqueous, they are at risk of contamination with microorganisms that can multiply during storage. These microbes may include molds, yeasts, and bacteria. The susceptible preparations should be protected using preservatives. An effective preservative should be nontoxic; inhibit the growth of microorganisms likely to contaminate the preparation; be sufficiently water soluble to achieve the necessary concentration; be in an ionized form to penetrate the microorganism; be nonirritating and nonsensitizing; have adequate stability; be compatible with all the other ingredients of the formulation; and be nonreactive with the container and closure used to dispense the formulation. The most commonly used preservatives include derivatives of benzoic acid such as sodium benzoate and methylparaben and derivatives of sorbic acids such as potassium sorbate. An example is Ora-Plus, which contains both potassium sorbate and methylparaben. If the alcohol content in alcoholic and hydroalcoholic extemporaneous formulations is sufficient to prevent microbial growth, then these formulations may not need additional chemical preservatives. However, a high alcohol content may preclude the use of these products in certain pediatric patients, especially premature neonates and newborns. Necessary caution must be used while compounding so that the pH is not altered and that the preservative is not diluted to less than its effective concentration.

STERILITY

Sterility testing is required for compounded parenteral products. All hospitals are required to comply with the USP Revised General Chapter <797> Pharmaceutical Compounding—Sterile Preparations Guidelines, which set practice standards to ensure that compounded sterile preparations are of high quality and prevent harm or fatality to patients caused by microbial contamination, excessive bacterial endotoxins, and errors caused by the presence or absence of labeled ingredients or presence in inaccurate amounts.[24] Most pharmacies involved with the compounding of sterile preparations have undertaken major renovations to their "Clean Rooms" while also actively training and evaluating their personnel in aseptic manipulation skills. The guidelines assign compounded sterile preparations three risk levels on the basis of their probability of microbial contamination and physical and chemical contamination. These risk levels (low, medium, and high) refer to the quality of the compounded sterile preparation immediately after the final aseptic manipulation or immediately after the final sterilization. These guidelines offer pre-administration exposure duration and temperature limits (beyond-use date and storage temperature) in the absence of direct testing results or appropriate information sources that justify different limits. The USP Revised General Chapter <797> Pharmaceutical Compounding—Sterile Preparations Guidelines provide

a more comprehensive review of sterility requirements for extemporaneously compounded parenteral formulations.[24]

EFFICACY AND SAFETY OF EXTEMPORANEOUS FORMULATIONS

The ultimate goal of preparing an extemporaneous formulation is to make it effective and safe in patients. Care must be taken to maximize safety; for example, a sustained-release tablet should not be crushed when preparing a liquid formulation, and a preservative such as benzyl alcohol should be avoided in a formulation intended for a neonate. Propylene glycol, ethanol, and sorbitol are examples of other excipients that have been associated with adverse effects in pediatric patients and should be avoided in pediatric formulations. Ideally, extemporaneous formulations should be studied in patients to establish their efficacy and safety. However, such studies are generally cost-prohibitive because of lack of funding for the performance of clinical studies. Efficacy and safety data of an extemporaneous formulation obtained in adult studies may not be reproducible in a pediatric population because of specific characteristics of the formulation. Omeprazole, a proton pump inhibitor, is often administered by a nasogastric tube for stress ulcer prophylaxis in critically ill mechanically ventilated patients. An extemporaneous suspension of omeprazole in sodium bicarbonate is formulated to prevent degradation of the drug granules by the gastric acid. This suspension has been effective in preventing clinically significant upper gastrointestinal bleeding in critically ill adults, and it effectively maintained excellent control of the gastric pH.[25,26] In a study of mechanically ventilated critically ill pediatric patients, administration of the same extemporaneous suspension did not produce the expected gastric acid suppression, despite the use of recommended standard doses.[27] The inadequate amount/volume of bicarbonate in the smaller pediatric dose to protect omeprazole degradation from the acid in the child's stomach was hypothesized to cause this difference in bioavailability and efficacy.

A concern about the use of many extemporaneous formulations is lack of bioavailability, efficacy, and safety data in pediatric patients. However, the use of these formulations should be guided by justified need, application of principles discussed in this chapter, and documentation of stability data, which are increasingly available and shared within the professional community. Despite the lack of specific efficacy and safety studies, extemporaneous formulations should be prepared using general principles already discussed in this chapter. Each formulation should be made specifically based on available data. For example, variations in the use of drug and excipients, method of preparation, and storage conditions can compromise stability as well as the expected efficacy and safety of the formulation. Patients receiving extemporaneous formulations should be monitored to ensure they achieve the expected clinical benefit and experience no harmful effects. Clinical experience should be shared through presentations at national meetings, discussions on websites, and publications in peer-reviewed journals. With the exception of nonsterile or contaminated products, safety concerns have seldom been reported with the use of extemporaneous formulations.

Although no specific agency or group receives reports of adverse events associated with extemporaneous formulations, such occurrences should be reported to the FDA and be widely shared with health care professionals through accessible publications.

One of the efforts made towards ensuring safety of intravenous and oral liquid medications is the Standardize 4 Safety Initiative started by ASHP.[28] This initiative is coordinating a national and interprofessional endeavor in standardizing drug concentrations to reduce errors, especially during transitions of care. Proposed standard concentrations for pediatric intravenous continuous infusion dosage units have been posted by ASHP. Similarly, it would be important to standardize concentrations of extemporaneously compounded oral formulations to ensure safe medication use.

COST

Reimbursement for the preparation and dispensing of extemporaneous formulations can be difficult, especially for community pharmacies, based on the patient's insurance carrier. Insurance authorization is often required, and the process can be time-consuming. For each extemporaneous formulation, the total cost includes the cost of the active ingredient(s), other ingredients needed to compound the formulation such as vehicles, and the pharmacist's compounding time. Reimbursement may not cover all the costs, especially if expensive ingredients such as injectables are needed. Thus, pharmacists preparing extemporaneous formulations should inquire with insurance carriers to determine how they will be reimbursed. Specialty pharmacies involved in compounding various extemporaneous formulations do not usually accept health insurance and will directly bill the patient for the total cost of the extemporaneous formulations.

CONCLUSIONS AND FUTURE PERSPECTIVES ON DEVELOPMENT OF PEDIATRIC DRUG FORMULATIONS

The need for extemporaneous formulations will continue to exist both for new drugs under patent protection and for generic drugs. Pharmacists play an essential role in the preparation of stable, effective, and safe formulations for pediatric patients of all age groups. However, the challenge of finding adequate information and financial resources for conducting stability and sterility as well as efficacy and safety studies with all extemporaneously prepared formulations of new and generic drugs is likely to continue. The use of these preparations should be monitored for efficacy and safety in patients, and these data should be shared through presentations at national meetings and publications in journals and books. Finally, funding agencies should provide resources to conduct studies with extemporaneous formulations to make important drugs accessible to infants and children.

Patient Case — DRUG FORMULATIONS

A 36-day-old male infant weighing 4 kg who has severe combined immunodeficiency disorder undergoes hematopoietic stem cell transplantation. In preparation for the patient's discharge, the caregiver brings the following prescriptions to the pharmacy: fluconazole 24 mg by mouth daily; trimethoprim/sulfamethoxazole 10 mg by mouth twice daily on Saturday and Sunday; and tacrolimus 0.35 mg by mouth twice daily.

1. Which of the prescriptions can be filled with commercially available formulations? Calculate the dose in mL for each drug based on the available strength.

The infant would be unable to swallow any medications dispensed as solid dosage forms. In addition to verifying that the patient is receiving accurate doses using either milligram per kilogram per dose or milligram per kilogram per day, the pharmacist must ascertain if all of these medications are available in a liquid dosage form.

The following medications are available in liquid dosage form:

(1) **Fluconazole 24 mg by mouth daily**: Fluconazole is available as powder for reconstitution into a suspension. It is available in two strengths, 10 mg/mL and 40 mg/mL. Most pharmacies may carry only one concentration. Using 40 mg/mL allows for administering smaller volumes compared with the 10 mg/mL. If the 40 mg/mL suspension is dispensed, then the patient's dose will be 0.6 mL. If 10 mg/mL suspension is dispensed, then the patient's dose will be 2.4 mL.

(2) **Trimethoprim/sulfamethoxazole 10 mg orally twice daily on Saturday and Sunday**: This combination antibiotic is available as sulfamethoxazole 200 mg and trimethoprim 40 mg per 5 mL as a suspension. The dose is always based on the trimethoprim component. The infant's dose is 10 mg of trimethoprim or 1.25 mL orally twice daily Saturday and Sunday.

(3) **Tacrolimus 0.35 mg by mouth twice daily**: Tacrolimus is available only as 0.5 mg, 1 mg, and 5 mg capsules; therefore, administering the prescribed dose of 0.35 mg is impossible using the available dosage form and strengths. The prescription could only be filled if tacrolimus were compounded to a liquid formulation of a suitable strength.

2. What information resources are needed to fill the tacrolimus prescription?

To prepare a formulation that is appropriate, it is necessary to research information regarding formulation recipe, compounding method, storage conditions, and stability for tacrolimus. The most common and immediate resource to find this information is the USP. This resource contains official monographs of compounded preparations that include valid stability data to establish a beyond-use or expiration date. A recipe for a liquid suspension of tacrolimus together with the compounding method, storage conditions, and expiration date is available in USP 39-NF 34. If this information is currently unavailable in USP, then tertiary publications such as the *Pediatric & Neonatal Dosage Handbook*, *NeoFax*, *Pediatric Drug Formulations* and *Extemporaneous Formulations for Pediatric, Geriatric, and Special Needs Patients* could be used. In addition, an extemporaneous formulation should be researched in primary literature through online databases such as PubMed. This approach allows the pharmacist to locate any additional studies published after the last updates to the tertiary references. However, not all pharmacies have access to such databases or individual publications. A last resource is the Investigator's Brochures or reports; however, this information is confidential or proprietary in nature and not easily available.

3. How is the tacrolimus suspension prepared for this infant?

Tacrolimus capsules to obtain	50 mg of tacrolimus
1:1 proportion of Oral-Plus and Syrup NF quantity sufficient	100 mL

The recipe for a liquid formulation of tacrolimus in available in USP 39-NF 34. The recipe provides the pharmacist a list of ingredients, quantities, and compounding instructions to prepare a liquid formulation of a certain concentration (milligram per milliliter). The quantity of each ingredient is calculated based on the total amount to be prepared. The exact number of tacrolimus capsules are opened and emptied in a suitable mortar. Preparation of the extemporaneous formulation will be performed based on the pharmacy's standard operating procedure for handling hazardous drugs. This approach is to prevent personnel from being exposed to aerosolized tacrolimus powder while opening the capsules and mixing the ingredients. Ora-Plus and Syrup NF are mixed in equal quantities to form the vehicle. The vehicle is added in small portions to the mortar, and then triturated into a smooth paste. The vehicle is added in volumetric proportions and mixed well until the liquid is pourable. The contents of the mortar are transferred to a graduated cylinder. The mortar is rinsed with small quantities of the vehicle and added to the bottle to bring to final volume. The contents of the bottle should be mixed well.

4. How should the prescription be labeled?

Among other elements that the State Board of Pharmacy requires to appear on a label, the following information should be included for this prescription:

Concentration of the product: 0.5 mg/mL

Storage conditions: Protect from light, store at controlled room temperature

Administration instructions: Shake well before use

Do not use beyond: This date is no more than 90 days after the date on which the medication was compounded.

5. What patient education information specific to this formulation would be appropriate?

The caregiver should be educated about the storage conditions for this preparation, which are storage at room temperature but away from areas of too much heat or humidity. In addition, the caregiver should be educated on the importance of shaking the bottle well so that the contents are uniformly mixed before drawing a dose, using appropriately sized oral syringes, and the volume of the liquid to be administered by drawing their attention to the markings on the syringe for the accurate measurement of the dose.

REFERENCES

1. U.S. Census Bureau. Annual Estimates of the Resident Population for Selected Age Groups by Sex for the United States, States, Counties, and Puerto Rico Commonwealth and Municipios: April 1, 2010 to July 1, 2015. Available at https://factfinder.census.gov/faces/tableservices/jsf/pages/productview.xhtml?pid=PEP_2015_PEPAGESEX&prodType=table. Accessed March 12, 2019.

2. Mathews AW. So young and so many pills: more than 25% of kids and teens in the U.S. take prescriptions on a regular basis. Wall Street Journal. December 28, 2010. Available at www.wsj.com/articles/SB10001424052970203731004576046073896475588. Accessed March 12, 2019.

3. U.S. Food and Drug Administration. Food and Drug Administration Modernization Act of 1997. Available at www.fda.gov/regulatoryinformation/lawsenforcedbyfda/significantamendmentstothefdcact/fdama/default.htm. Accessed March 12, 2019.

4. U.S. Food and Drug Administration. Best Pharmaceuticals for Children Act, January 2, 2002. Available at https://bpca.nichd.nih.gov/Pages/default.aspx. Accessed March 12, 2019.

5. U.S. Food and Drug Administration. Food and Drug Administration Amendments Act (FDAAA) of 2007. Available at www.fda.gov/regulatoryinformation/lawsenforcedbyfda/significantamendmentstothefdcact/foodanddrugadministrationamendmentsactof2007/default.htm. Accessed March 26, 2019.

6. Pediatric Provision in the Food and Drug Administration Safety and Innovation Act (FDASIA). Available at www.fda.gov/RegulatoryInformation/LawsEnforcedbyFDA/SignificantAmendmentstotheFDCAct/FDASIA/ucm311038.htm. Accessed March 12, 2019.

7. PREA and BPCA: Spurring Pediatric Drug Development. Available at https://www.phrma.org/fact-sheet/prea-and-bpca-spurring-pediatric-drug-development. Accessed March 12, 2019.

8. Probst LA, Welch TR. Pediatric drug formulations—unintended consequences of legislation. New Engl J Med 2017;376:795-6.

9. Michele TM, Knorr B, Vadas EB, et al. Safety of chewable tablets for children. J Asthma 2002;39:391-403.

10. Czyzewski DI, Runyan RD, Lopez MA, et al. Teaching and maintaining pill swallowing in HIV-infected children. AIDS Reader 2000;10:88–95.

11. Pai V, Nahata MC. Need for extemporaneous formulations in pediatric patients. J Pediatr Pharmacol Ther 2001;6:107–19.

12. Lugo R, Cash J, Trimby R, et al. A survey of children's hospitals on the use of extemporaneous liquid formulations in the inpatient setting. J Pediatr Pharmacol Ther 2009;14:156.

13. United States Pharmacopoeia–National Formulary [USP 39 NF 34]. Official monographs USP. Rockville, MD: United States Pharmacopeial Convention, Inc., 2016.

14. Taketomo CK, Hodding JH, Kraus DM, eds. Pediatric & Neonatal Dosage Handbook 2015–2016. Hudson, OH: Lexi-Comp, 2016.

15. Neofax 2017. Micromedex Solutions. Columbus, OH: Truven Health Analytics, 2017.

16. Nahata MC, Pai VB. Pediatric Drug Formulations. 7th ed. Cincinnati, OH: Harvey Whitney Books Co., 2019.

17. Jew RK, Soo-Hoo W, Erush SC, eds. Extemporaneous Formulations for Pediatric, Geriatric, and Special Needs Patients. Bethesda, MD: American Society of Health-System Pharmacists, 2016.

18. United States Pharmacopoeia-National Formulary [USP 39 NF 34]. <795>Pharmaceutical Compounding—Non-sterile Preparations. Rockville, MD: United States Pharmacopeial Convention, Inc., 2016.

19. Allen LV Jr, Erickson MA III. Stability of baclofen, captopril, diltiazem hydrochloride, dipyridamole, and flecainide acetate in extemporaneously compounded oral liquids. Am J Health Syst Pharm 1996;53:2179–84.

20. American Society of Health-System Pharmacists. ASHP Policy Positions: Drug Distribution and Control. Available at https://www.ashp.org/pharmacy-practice/policy-positions-and-guidelines/browse-by-topic/drug-distribution-and-control. Accessed March 12, 2019.

21. Allen LV Jr, ed. The Art, Science, and Technology of Pharmaceutical Compounding. Washington, DC: American Pharmacists Association, 2008.

22. American Society of Health-System Pharmacists. ASHP Technical Assistance Bulletin on Compounding Nonsterile Products in Pharmacies. Available at www.ashp.org/pharmacy-practice/policy-positions-and-guidelines/browse-by-topic/drug-distribution-and-control. Accessed March 12, 2019.

23. American Society of Health-System Pharmacists. ASHP Guidelines on Quality Assurance for Pharmacy-Prepared Sterile Products. Available at www.ashpmedia.org/softchalk/softchalkleadsurveyorresourcelink/1%20PrepGdlQualAssurSterile.pdf. Accessed March 12, 2019.

24. United States Pharmacopoeia-National Formulary [USP 39 NF 34]. <797>Pharmaceutical Compounding—Sterile Preparations. Rockville, MD: United States Pharmacopeial Convention, Inc., 2016.

25. Phillips JO, Metzler MH, Palmieri TL, et al. A prospective study of the simplified omeprazole suspension for the prophylaxis of stress-related mucosal damage. Crit Care Med 1996;24:1793–800.

26. Lasky MR, Metzler MH, Phillips JO. A prospective study of omeprazole suspension to prevent clinically significant gastrointestinal bleeding from stress ulcers in mechanically ventilated trauma patients. J Trauma 1998;44:527–33.

27. Haizlip JA, Lugo RA, Cash JJ, et al. Failure of nasogastric omeprazole suspension in pediatric intensive care patients. Pediatr Crit Care Med 2005;6:182–7.

28. American Society of Health-System Pharmacists. Standardize 4 Safety Initiative. Available at www.ashp.org/pharmacy-practice/standardize-4-safety-initiative. Accessed March 12, 2019.

CHAPTER 5

Communicating with Children, Adolescents, and Their Caregivers

Michelle Condren, Pharm.D., FPPA, BCPPS, CDE, AE-C

LEARNING OBJECTIVES

1. Describe Piaget's four stages of cognitive development.

2. Develop patient education for children related to their developmental stage.

3. List eight tips for developing rapport with children of all ages.

4. State the potential advantages of engaging children in medication education.

5. Provide examples of pediatric-specific patient education that are not included in standard medication information handouts.

INTRODUCTION

Verbal and written communications are essential components of health care that help ensure adherence to therapy, patient safety, improved outcomes, and patient satisfaction. Health care providers are trained in communication techniques for adult patients, but many providers state that they do not have as much experience in communicating health information to children.[1] Although many principles of communicating with adults also apply to children, communicating with children requires a different approach that considers the child's developmental level as well as the child–caregiver interaction. Because children often depend on an adult caregiver to assist with medication administration, the practitioner should provide caregivers with education that is specific to the child to increase the caregivers' confidence in the treatment. If the health care provider shows interest, takes the time to answer questions and address concerns, and involves the child in the communication, parents and caregivers are more likely to be satisfied with the care received and to adhere to the prescribed treatment.[1,2]

It is as important for pharmacists to talk with children about their medications as it is to talk with their parents. However, community pharmacists report that they talk with children about their medications only 20%–30% of the time.[2,3] Medication education for children can occur in many settings, including community pharmacies, hospitals, clinics, group education visits, schools, and health fairs. This chapter will review the benefits associated with communicating with children about medications as well as techniques for delivering age-appropriate information and gaining rapport with this specific patient population. In addition, this chapter will provide tips for educating parents and caregivers about the medications for their children.

COMMUNICATION TO DECREASE ERRORS AND IMPROVE ADHERENCE

Once the medication leaves the pharmacy, it is the caregiver's and child's responsibility to ensure appropriate dosing and administration. As evidenced by previous studies, medical visits, and calls to poison control centers, many unintentional overdoses occur each year because of improper measurement and accidental ingestion. Difficulty measuring the proper dose can result from low health literacy or a simple misunderstanding of the directions. Studies have shown that without intervention, only 50% of caregivers give an accurate dose of liquid medications to the children in their care.[4] This rate of accuracy can be increased to 95% by using a 1- to 3-minute intervention of demonstrating how to use a dosing device, having the caregiver demonstrate use of the device, and providing pictogram-based information handouts.[4] This study also concluded that the additional education resulted in an improved adherence rate of 62%–91%.[4]

In another study, parents were asked to measure 1 teaspoon or 5 mL of acetaminophen by a dosing cup, dropper, dosing spoon, and oral syringe.[5] When a dosing cup was used, most doses measured resulted in an overdose. This study also concluded that dosing errors with cups and dosing spoons were more common in parents with lower health literacy. Clinicians must be aware of the challenges that caregivers face in administering medications and be proactive in providing information and appropriate dosing devices as well as ensuring caregivers' understanding of the medication and its administration.

COMMUNICATION PRINCIPLES FOR CHILDREN AND ADOLESCENTS

Children can generally begin providing and receiving information during health care visits at age 3 years, with an even greater level of involvement starting at age 7 years.[6] However, many children have become accustomed to being silent observers during health care visits and may develop disinterest in or resentment toward their health care. The United States Pharmacopeia has developed a position statement outlining the principles for teaching children and adolescents about medications.[7] Included in these principles are that children want to know about medications, so health care providers should communicate directly with them about both what they want to know and what they need to know. In addition, providers can encourage children to ask questions about medications. A good approach is to always end an encounter with a child by asking a question such as, "What questions do you have for me about your medicine?"

Communications with children can be for the goal of obtaining information from the child, expressing empathy with the child, relaying information to the child, or confirming the child's understanding. Each of these points requires the use of age-specific techniques that provide age-appropriate information and establish rapport, as discussed in the following sections.

COGNITIVE DEVELOPMENTAL STAGES

When communicating with children, health care providers should ensure that the message is delivered at a level that the child can understand. Identifying a child's developmental stage can help narrow the scope of information to be communicated and improve efficiency and effectiveness. One of the methods used to help identify a child's developmental stage is Piaget's classification of cognitive development. The four stages of cognitive development are *sensory motor*, *preoperational*, *concrete operational*, and *formal operational*. Table 1 describes Piaget's developmental stages and how to apply them to those receiving medication education.[8,9] When applying any system for staging a child's developmental level, it is important to recognize that the stages are estimates and that

Table 1. Piaget's Cognitive Developmental Stages and How They Affect Medication Education[8,9]

Age Range (yr)	Stage	Features	Medication Counseling
Birth–2	Sensory motor	Do not see the connection between self and external objects	Learning about medications is not possible
2–7	Preoperational	Can consider only a single aspect of a situation Can consider only the "here and now" Have no concept of cause and effect Have difficulty conceptualizing time Do not understand the connection between an action and their health Can use symbols or pictures to represent objects	Hands-on activities are the most effective Include the taste of medication in the education Example of information to provide: "This medication will keep you from getting sick. You will take it when you wake up in the morning and before you go to sleep at night. Your mom or dad or the grown-up who is taking care of you will help you take the medication."
7–11	Concrete operational	Can focus on many aspects of a situation Can think about concrete events but have difficulty with hypothetical situations Can distinguish between self and effects of the outside world Can best understand concrete or observable situations Can understand that diseases are preventable Can see things from different points of view	Give them time to ask questions, and explain concepts to them Discuss the adverse effects of medications that should be reported to an adult Example information to provide: "This medication will go into your lungs and make it easier for you to run and play. You will take it when you wake up and before you go to bed. If you do not take it two times a day, it will not work. You need to brush your teeth after using the medication. Work with your mom and dad or the grown-up who is taking care of you to make sure you take the medication right and remember to take the medication."
≥ 12	Formal operational	Capable of hypothetical thought and logical reasoning Can understand how illness occurs and how it is affected by their actions Begin to understand they can have control of their health	Typically able to receive a message at the same level as an adult Keep in mind they may be more embarrassed by certain topics Example information to provide: "This medication works in your lungs to decrease mucus and swelling so that you can breathe better and have less cough. Because you are breathing things into your lungs every day that cause the problem, this medication works only if used every day, twice a day. It is important to keep using this medication even when you start feeling better because the asthma will still be there. Work with your parents or adults who care for you to help make this part of your everyday routine."

they vary among patients. As children are exposed to situations and experiences, they may more quickly enter a new developmental stage than other children who have not had the same experiences.[6] In addition, traditional methods of staging development do not apply to children with learning disabilities or disease states that impair development (e.g., autism spectrum disorders). Health care providers should assess each child individually for the level of development, and then educate the child at that level.

DEVELOPING RAPPORT

Many children and adolescents are hesitant to talk to adults they do not know. Therefore, the first step for the health care communicator is to try to gain the child's trust and express an interest in the child as an individual. General tips recommended to adults communicating with children of all ages include the following: (1) sit at the child's eye level; (2) begin by discussing a topic that is of interest to the child; (3) avoid commenting on characteristics about which the child may be self-conscious (e.g., hair color, height, shyness); (4) use a normal tone of voice; (5) do not "talk down" to the child; (6) maintain a calm demeanor; (7) pay attention to the child; and (8) listen actively.[8] Additional items are summarized in Box 1. Finally, the clinician should always consider differences in culture that may affect a person's likelihood of maintaining eye contact and interest in self-care.

INFANTS

The importance of gaining patient rapport starts in infancy. Although medication education cannot be delivered to infants, interacting with an infant's parents or caregivers will be much easier if the infant is at ease. Health care providers should not lean over an infant's face or take the infant out of the caregiver's arms if the infant is anxious about leaving the

---

Box 1. General Tips for Communicating with Children and Adolescents[7,8,10,11]

Sit at or below their eye level

Begin by discussing a topic of interest to the child or adolescent

Remain calm and nonjudgmental

Be aware of their body language and then respond, if needed

Speak in a normal tone of voice

Allow them to express concerns and ask questions

Give them ample time to respond to questions

Give them your full attention

Listen attentively and repeat to ensure you understand them

Allow them to participate in decision-making about their medications

---

caregiver. In addition, adults should not force playing with an infant. An infant who is interested in playing will reach out or make sounds, whereas a distressed infant will likely become more anxious if the adult tries to play. It is often difficult to communicate with parents or caregivers when their infant is irritable; thus, giving them time to comfort their infant will be beneficial.

TODDLERS AND PRESCHOOLERS

At age 1–5 years, children are developing new skills and do not yet understand the importance of health care visits and listening to others. They often have difficulty communicating because they are learning new words and learning how to formulate sentences. Therefore, when obtaining information from children, the health care provider should show patience to give the child time to think about what to say and communicate a sentence. When the child becomes distracted or disruptive, clinicians can provide a playful distraction, such as an opportunity to draw or play with a toy, which will help redirect the child to a new activity. Because children do not have a good concept of time, the provider should avoid asking the child for a prolonged recall of information. Instead, the goal is to deliver information in simple terms, with brevity and honesty.

SCHOOL-AGE CHILDREN

For school-age children, it is easier to obtain information using open-ended questions and allowing them to explain how they perceive a situation. They will begin to provide a more accurate recall of symptoms and activities, and they will often give a more accurate account of their current symptoms than their parents or caregivers. Because they have a better understanding of cause and effect by this age, they will have a greater need to know information and to have a chance to express their concerns and questions. School-age children can begin contributing to the decision-making process about their treatment plan. If they state that they do not like a medication, then the health care provider can offer alternatives for the child to choose and educate the child on how the alternatives differ. Children at this age respond well to visual displays of disease states and medications and enjoy interacting with adults by way of games and challenges.

ADOLESCENTS

Adolescents are the least likely to trust that adults have their best interest in mind and may be unwilling to provide a great deal of information. The health care provider can begin the conversation by asking about a topic that may be of interest to the adolescent patient, rather than starting with the provider's own agenda. If adolescents feel that their viewpoint is not being considered or understood, they are likely to withdraw or even become angry. Before rapport is established, many adolescents will not maintain eye contact, but it will improve as their trust increases.

The adolescent should be the primary person giving information during an encounter, and then the parents/caregivers

---

should be asked to confirm or add information. Adolescents should learn to advocate for their own health care and learn to communicate their needs. Adolescents often provide information that may alarm or shock the provider. It is important to remain calm and nonjudgmental in these circumstances. When developing a treatment plan, the best approach is to include adolescents in the decision-making process and affirm that their questions and concerns have been addressed.

The health care provider should also give adolescents an opportunity to talk with the provider privately. If planning to ask the adolescent patient about contraception, sexual health, or alcohol, drug, or tobacco use, then the provider should try to speak with the adolescent in private rather than in a parent's presence. This approach will allow the adolescent patient more comfort to speak freely and will communicate that the provider respects their privacy and perspective. Common situations that require privacy and sensitivity when communicating with adolescents include counseling on the proper use of contraception, on drug interactions that may increase the risk of unintended pregnancy while using oral contraception, and on interactions between alcohol and medications. Adolescents may be unwilling to talk about these issues in a first encounter, but they will likely become more open after the clinician has developed trust in follow-up encounters. Parents and caregivers may resist this approach, but the health care provider should emphasize that adolescents need to learn to communicate directly with the provider and begin to take responsibility for their medical care.

ADDITIONAL COMMUNICATION CONSIDERATIONS FOR CHILDREN AND ADOLESCENTS

The technique and skill required for obtaining information differs from that required to deliver information. When obtaining information, open-ended questions are preferable. However, the questions must be specific and often need to be followed up with more straightforward, closed-ended questions. With closed-ended questions, children and adolescents may give responses that they think will please the provider.[10] The clinician may need to let them know it is acceptable to be honest. An example of a statement to help encourage truth in recalling medication adherence is: "A lot of people have trouble remembering to take their medicine; do you find it hard to remember to take your medicine?" The provider can then follow with additional open-ended questions to obtain further details.

Children often refer to a medication by appearance or color, and sometimes what they use the medication for, rather than by the name of the drug. When interviewing the patient, if the child does not know the name of the medication, the health care provider can ask if the child can describe what it looks like. Then the provider can emphasize the importance of knowing the medication name and can assess patient recall at future visits. When providing medication information to children, it is important to select the most salient points and deliver them using the principles discussed in the previous

sections. Essential components of medication education for children include the following:

1. Why do I need this medicine?
2. How does the medicine taste?
3. When do I take the medicine?
4. How will it make me feel better?
5. How long will I take it?
6. What are the adverse effects?

Other important points to emphasize include informing children to tell an adult if they take too much medication or if they see someone else taking their medication, in addition to encouraging the child to tell an adult if they have any new feelings or adverse effects while taking the medication.

When a child or adolescent is asked to demonstrate a skill such as inhaler technique, smaller children may be fearful, embarrassed, or shy. For children who are fearful or anxious, the clinician may give them the spacer to play with before trying to demonstrate the technique so that they can learn that it is not a harmful object. For those who seem embarrassed, it is important to ensure as much privacy as possible and to consider demonstrating the technique before asking them to do so. In addition, the health care provider can give children and adolescents choices, but only when a choice truly exists. For example, it is not effective to ask "Would you like to show me how you use your inhaler?" if the intention is to have patients demonstrate the technique, even if their answer is "No." The provider will lose rapport by proceeding with having them demonstrate the technique after they have responded that they are not interested. A more appropriate statement might be, "I need to watch you use your inhaler so I can make sure it is working; would you like to show me now or after when we talk about your medicines?" Effective techniques to assist children with medication adherence are patient-specific. Asking children and adolescents what they believe will help them remember to take their medications is helpful because no single approach works for everyone. Potential methods to assist in remembering include posting dosing calendars with or without medication pictures on them, providing cell phone reminders or alarms, placing the medications in an area of high visibility, using pill boxes, and using phone-based applications. Two examples of phone-based applications include MyMedSchedule (https://secure.medactionplan.com/mymed schedule/) and Medisafe (https://www.medisafeapp.com/).

COMMUNICATING WITH PARENTS AND CAREGIVERS

Studies show that parental and caregiver satisfaction with medical care is determined by the practitioner's interpersonal skills. If they feel they were not treated with respect or that their fears were not addressed, then they will be dissatisfied and less likely to follow through with medical advice.[11] In interviews of parents during physician visits, 88% wanted to be addressed by their names rather than as "mom" or "dad."[12] The practitioner is encouraged to ask parents how they prefer to be addressed. There is a fine balance between including the child in the encounter and ensuring that the parents feel included as well. It is helpful for providers to let parents know that they plan to ask the child questions and to provide them with information before starting. Box 2 summarizes items to consider when talking with parents or caregivers.

Written information dispensed with prescriptions is not phrased with a child in mind and can be frightening and confusing to parents or caregivers. Many fear giving their children any medications; thus, reading this information may cause them not to give the medication. An example is the use of fluoroquinolones in children. The American Academy of Pediatrics recommends fluoroquinolones in children if no other alternatives exist for treatment of infection. However, many patient information handouts state that these medications should not be used in children because of the lack of a U.S. Food and Drug Administration label-approved indication and because of safety concerns. Parents or caregivers who see this information may be resistant to giving the medication to their child unless they are educated on the data that exist and informed that no alternative exists.

In addition, written information should be at the sixth-grade reading level to ensure understanding by those with low health literacy. Most materials are estimated to be written at a 10th- or 11th-grade reading level.[13] Methods of assessing readability include the Flesch-Kincaid formula (http://www.readabilityformulas.com/flesch-grade-level-readability-formula.php) and the McLaughlin Simple Measure of Gobbledygook (https://www.readabilityformulas.com/smog-readability-formula.php). The United States Pharmacopoeia has developed a guide to assist in developing and evaluating educational materials.[14] This guide includes not only readability, but also the balance of words and pictures and the appropriateness of content for the child's age. Parent-friendly medication information handouts are available that are more specific to children and are easier to read.[15] These handouts are available in English or Spanish. Lexi-Comp online also provides pediatric-specific patient education handouts in 18 different languages. If these resources are unavailable, the clinician can point out differences that may be relevant to the child compared with the information provided on the medication handout from the pharmacy. Examples are provided in Box 3.

In addition, parents or caregivers may need assistance in determining how the information in a warning label applies to their child. For example, the statement "Do not operate heavy machinery while taking this medicine" has a different meaning for a child. In this case, the health care provider should counsel them that their child should avoid tall playground equipment and should be careful riding a bicycle or any motorized toys while taking that medication.

It is important to determine who will be giving children their medication. Medication is often given at school or by a grandparent, or it may be given at another house if the parents do not live together. If the person accompanying the child to the visit is not the only one to administer the medication, the adult who is present at the visit should be educated on the importance of providing all information to anyone who will be responsible for giving the child's medication. Too often, children are held responsible for transporting medications between homes and remembering to take them, placing them at risk of not receiving the medication consistently. Providing adequate information to the school ensures the safe and appropriate administration of the medication in that setting.

Another important component of the health care encounter is to verify the identity of the person with the child. Another relative, a babysitter, or a stepparent may be with the child. In some cases, the health care provider may need to contact the parents if they are not at the visit to ensure they have the information needed to safely use their child's medication. This practice will also help avoid uncomfortable moments that occur when the adult's identity is assumed.

CONCLUSIONS

Because children and adolescents are important consumers of health care, they should receive the information they need to use medications safely and effectively. Pharmacists play an important role in communicating with children, adolescents, and their parents and caregivers. The techniques discussed in this chapter will help facilitate the pharmacist's effectiveness and efficiency in communicating with this special patient population. With practice, communicating with children and adolescents will become a rewarding experience and will positively affect the health and safety of these vulnerable patients.

Box 2. General Tips for Communicating with Parents and Caregivers[7,8,10,11]

Inform them you will be talking with their child or adolescent

Learn their names, and use their names during communication

Provide guidance on how much their child should be involved in self-administering medication

Encourage them to provide their child with some autonomy, when appropriate

Allow them to express concerns and ask questions

Respond respectfully about any misconceptions or fears they may express

---

Box 3. Information Needed to Supplement Medication Information Handouts

How to measure the dose

How to administer the medication

How the adverse effects may manifest in a child

How the warning labels apply to a child

Reassurance that the medication may be used for an indication other than those listed

---

A 6-year-old boy is admitted to the hospital for an asthma exacerbation. His medical history is significant for asthma and allergic rhinitis. The family reports good adherence to medications overall but states that the boy has needed albuterol about 4 days a week for the past month. His home medications are fluticasone hydrofluoroalkane 110 mcg 1 puff with spacer twice daily, cetirizine 10 mg 1 tablet by mouth once daily, and albuterol hydrofluoroalkane 2 puffs before exercise and every 4 hours as needed.

In preparation for hospital discharge, he will be changed to fluticasone/salmeterol 45/21 mcg 2 puffs with spacer twice daily and prednisolone 2 mg/kg/day for 3 days. The pharmacist is asked to provide patient and family education regarding the patient's new medications.

1. Given that this patient is 6 years old, which developmental stage most likely describes this patient?

A normally developing 6-year-old would be in the preoperational stage, according to Piaget's classification.

2. When talking with this 6-year-old patient, what principles are important to remember related to the type of educational message the pharmacist should deliver?

Children in the preoperational stage should receive very straightforward information about their medications. At this age, they generally do not understand cause and effect. For example, the boy will not be able to understand that taking medications regularly will prevent another hospital visit. This concept is important for the family to understand, but education specific to the child should be limited to demonstrating inhaler technique, showing pictures to demonstrate what asthma is, explaining that his parents or caregivers will be giving him the medication every day, and outlining basic symptoms he should report to an adult. All other educational points should be directed toward the parents.

3. State the general communication techniques that will help build rapport with this 6-year-old patient.

To help children feel more comfortable talking with the pharmacist, it is best to be at their eye level rather than above in a position of authority. Children often wear something that indicates their interests, and talking with them about their interest opens the communication and helps them to start talking and feel more comfortable. Giving them ample time to answer questions is important because children take longer to process their thoughts than adults. Moreover, children should always be given an opportunity to ask questions. The health care provider's tone of voice should be the same as if talking to another adult.

REFERENCES

1. Nilaward W, Mason H, Newton G. Community pharmacist-child medication communication: magnitude, influences, and content. J Am Pharm Assoc 2005;4:354-62.
2. Ranelli P, Bartsch K, London K. Pharmacists' perceptions of children and families as medicine consumers. Psychol Health 2000;15:829-40.
3. Pradel F, Obeidat N, Tsoukleris M. Factors affecting pharmacists' pediatric asthma counseling. J Am Pharm Assoc 2007;47:737-46.
4. Yin H, Dreyer B, vanSchaick L, et al. Randomized controlled trial of a pictogram-based intervention to reduce liquid medication dosing errors and improve adherence among caregivers of young children. Arch Pediatr Adolesc Med 2008;162:814-22.
5. Yin H, Mendelsohn A, Wolf M, et al. Parents' medication administration errors: role of dosing instruments and health literacy. Arch Pediatr Adolesc Med 2010;164:181-6.
6. Borzekowski D. Considering children and health literacy: a theoretical approach. Pediatrics 2009;124:S282-8.
7. Bush P, Ozias J, Walson P, et al. Ten guiding principles for teaching children and adolescents about medicines. Clin Ther 1999;21:1280-4.
8. Deering C, Cody D. Communicating with children and adolescents. Am J Nurs 2002;102:34-41.
9. Hameen-Anttila K, Bush P. Healthy children's perceptions of medicines: a review. Res Soc Admin Pharm 2008;4:98-114.
10. Krahenbuhl S, Blades M. The effect of interviewing techniques on young children's responses to questions. Child Care Health Dev 2006;32:321-31.
11. Levetown M, American Academy of Pediatrics Committee on Bioethics. Communicating with children and families: from everyday interactions to skill in conveying distressing information. Pediatrics 2008;121:e1441-60.
12. Amer A, Fischer H. "Don't call me 'mom'": how parents want to be greeted by their pediatrician. Clin Pediatr 2009;48:720-2.
13. Wallace L, Keenum A, DeVoe J. Evaluation of consumer medical information and oral liquid measuring devices accompanying pediatric prescriptions. Acad Pediatr 2010;10:224-7.
14. Bush PJ. Guide to Developing and Evaluating Medicine Education Programs for Children and Adolescents. Kent, OH: American School Health Association, 1998.
15. Buck M, Hendrick A. Pediatric Medication Education Text, 5th ed. Lenexa, KS: American College of Clinical Pharmacy, 2009.

Section II

Medication Safety

CHAPTER 6

Medication Safety
Amy L. Potts, Pharm.D., BCPPS

LEARNING OBJECTIVES

1. Provide a background for the basis of medication safety as a national public health initiative.

2. Explain differences in medication safety specific to pediatric patients that make them more vulnerable to adverse drug events.

3. Describe specific preventive strategies for medication errors and important considerations for pediatric patients.

4. Describe the role of automation and technology in medication safety with considerations for pediatric patients.

ABBREVIATIONS IN THIS CHAPTER

ADE	Adverse drug event
BCMA	Barcode medication administration
CPOE	Computerized prescriber order entry
FDA	U.S. Food and Drug Administration
IOM	Institute of Medicine
ISMP	Institute for Safe Medication Practices
MUP	Medication Use Process
TJC	The Joint Commission

INTRODUCTION

Medical errors are common, and costly, and they may result in significant harm or injury.[1] In 1999, the Institute of Medicine (IOM) published its initial report *To Err Is Human*, which served as the catalyst for health care reform and patient safety. The IOM estimated that 44,000–98,000 people experience a medical error annually, making medical errors the eighth leading cause of death, with a multibillion-dollar price tag. These alarming statistics provided the necessary leverage to make creating a safer health care system part of the national agenda and a public health concern.[1] In 2001, the IOM released a follow-up report titled *Crossing the Quality Chasm*, which provided the blueprint for health care redesign with a focus on health care technology.[2]

Progress has been made to improve patient safety overall; however, complete reform of health care has not been achieved.[2] The 2007 progress report from the IOM, *Preventing Medication Errors: Quality Chasm Series*, served as a more comprehensive analysis of quality and safety and provided the framework to advance the health care industry to a higher standard.[3] The IOM summarized several recommendations

as part of this health care improvement plan, including patient-focused care, medication management standards, implementation of technology, and improved communication among health care providers. The IOM also recommended more funding for medication safety research and additional oversight by regulatory organizations to provide incentives for institutions that have implemented best practices in the safe use of medications. Pharmacy-specific recommendations included monitoring of medication adverse events, patient education and discharge teaching, medication reconciliation, use of electronic prescribing, minimizing alerts from clinical decision support tools, and surveillance of patients at risk of adverse events.

Medications are estimated to harm at least 1.5 million people annually.[3] Pediatric patients are at highest risk because of several differences characteristic of this patient population. This chapter provides the foundation for a basic understanding of medication safety and a summary of key preventive strategies, with a focus on pediatric-specific considerations.

DEFINITIONS

The National Coordinating Council for Medication Error Reporting and Prevention defines a *medication error* as follows:

> any preventable event that may cause or lead to inappropriate medication use or patient harm, [while]... the drug is in the control of the health care professional, patient, or consumer. Such events may be related to professional practice, health care products, procedures, and medication use systems including prescribing; order communication; product labeling, packaging, and nomenclature; compounding; dispensing; distribution; administration; education; monitoring; and use.[4]

The National Coordinating Council for Medication Error Reporting and Prevention categorizes medication errors on the basis of severity, as shown in Figure 1.[5] Medication errors may or may not result in harm to the patient. An *adverse drug event* (ADE) occurs as a result of harm caused by the use of a drug. Potential ADEs are events that could result in harm but did not harm the patient. Not all ADEs are the result of a medication error, but all medication errors have the potential to result in an ADE.[6] When a medication error is intercepted before the medication is administered to the patient, it is referred to as a *near miss*. This type of error can provide an opportunity for systems to be reviewed for error-prone steps, allowing institutions to be proactive instead of reactive to errors. Specific medication error types and common causes for medication errors are summarized in Table 1 and Box 1.

Adverse drug reactions are defined as unintended, undesired, or excessive responses to therapy that are typically

---

unpreventable and may be associated with a medication dosed normally over time or with a single dose. Adverse effects of a medication are not adverse drug reactions. Adverse effects are expected and based on known drug properties, versus adverse drug reactions, which are the unexpected harmful effects of a drug when used appropriately. Pharmacists are responsible for monitoring and reporting adverse drug reactions as part of an organized medication safety program.[6-8]

INCIDENCE/PREVALENCE

In 1984, the Harvard Medical Practice Study estimated 3.7% of hospitalized adult patients experience an adverse event related to medication therapy. Of these events, about 70% were preventable, and 30% of patients experienced significant morbidity and mortality as a result.[9-11] The Adverse Drug Event Prevention Study further described medication errors and ADEs.[12] This study found that medication-related ADEs occurred commonly in adults at a rate of 6.5 per 100 patient admissions, and most were preventable. In addition, a systems analysis of ADEs found that the most common system defects included a lack of communication and readily accessible drug and patient information in a timely manner.[12,13] In a later study, the incidence of medication errors in hospitalized adults was 5.3 per 100 medication orders, with most errors being preventable and occurring at the point of ordering.[14,15]

Adverse drug events occur more often in pediatric patients than in adults.[16-18] In 2001, the incidence of medication errors in pediatric patients was 5.7 per 100 medication orders. In addition, these researchers classified medication errors as *actual errors* or *potential errors*. Most (79%) potential ADEs in children occurred at the stage of ordering, primarily involving dosing errors. The most common drug classes included intravenous anti-infectives, electrolytes and fluids, and analgesics and sedatives.[16] Subsequently, a Sentinel Event Alert aimed at preventing pediatric medication errors was issued by The Joint Commission (TJC): The most common types of errors in children were dosing error (37.5%), omission error (19.9%), wrong drug (13.7%), and prescribing error (9.4%). The most common causes included performance deficit (43%), knowledge deficit (29.9%), procedure/protocol not followed (20.7%), and miscommunication (16.8%).[17]

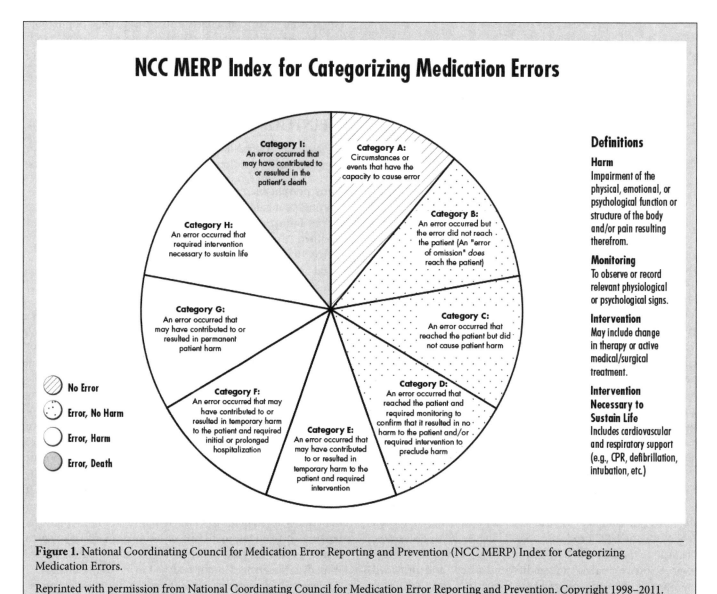

Figure 1. National Coordinating Council for Medication Error Reporting and Prevention (NCC MERP) Index for Categorizing Medication Errors.

Reprinted with permission from National Coordinating Council for Medication Error Reporting and Prevention. Copyright 1998–2011.

VULNERABILITY OF PEDIATRIC PATIENTS

Caring for pediatric patients can be operationally complex and requires specialized clinical decision-making skills. Limited drug information is available for pediatric patients, who often require off-label use of medications approved by U.S. Food and Drug Administration (FDA) and extrapolation of safety and efficacy data from the adult literature. In using this approach, clinicians must be aware of important considerations for developmental growth and maturation in this patient population that need to be carefully evaluated.

Pediatric care can also present challenges to the standard medication use process (MUP). Commercially available drug formulations are often unsuitable for pediatric patients and are not readily available from manufacturers.[19] As a result, manipulation of both oral and injectable commercial products is often required. As described in following text, developmental differences and required deviations from readily available preparations make infants and children more susceptible to medication errors and related injuries.[16,19,20]

DEVELOPMENTAL DIFFERENCES

Pediatric patients can be further classified into groups based on developmental stages as follows: *neonates* (*term neonates* and *preterm neonates*), *infants*, *toddlers*, *children* and *adolescents*. During each developmental stage, a pediatric patient

Table 1. Types of Medication Errors[7]

Type[a]	Definition
Prescribing error	Incorrect drug selection (based on indications, contraindications, known allergies, existing drug therapy, and other factors), dose, dosage form, quantity, route, concentration, rate of administration, or instructions for use of a drug product ordered or authorized by physician (or other legitimate prescriber), illegible prescriptions, or medication orders that lead to errors that reach the patient
Omission error[b]	Failure to administer an ordered dose to a patient before the next scheduled dose, if any
Wrong time error	Administration of medication outside a predefined time interval from its scheduled administration time (this interval should be established by each individual health care facility)
Unauthorized drug error[c]	Administration to the patient of medication not authorized by a legitimate prescriber for the patient
Improper dose error[d]	Administration to the patient of a dose that is greater or less than the amount ordered by the prescriber or administration of duplicate doses to the patient (i.e., one or more dosage units in addition to those that were ordered)
Wrong dosage-form error[e]	Administration of a drug product in a different dosage form than ordered by the prescriber
Wrong drug-preparation error[f]	Drug product incorrectly formulated or manipulated before administration
Wrong administration-technique error[g]	Inappropriate procedure or improper technique in the administration of a drug
Deteriorated drug error[h]	Administration of a drug that has expired or for which the physical or chemical dosage-form integrity has been compromised
Monitoring error	Failure to review a prescribed regimen for appropriateness and detection of problems, or failure to use appropriate clinical and laboratory data for adequate assessment of patient response to prescribed therapy
Compliance error	Inappropriate patient behavior regarding adherence to a prescribed medication regimen
Other medication error	Any medication error that does not fall into one of the above predefined categories

[a]These categories may not be mutually exclusive because of the multidisciplinary and multifactorial nature of medication errors.
[b]Omission error assumes no prescribing error. Excluded from this type of error are (1) a patient's refusal to take the medication, and (2) a decision not to administer the dose because of recognized contraindications. If an explanation for the omission is apparent (e.g., patient was away from nursing unit for tests or medication was unavailable), then that reason is documented in the appropriate records.
[c]Unauthorized drug error includes, for example, wrong drug, a dose given to the wrong patient, unordered drugs, and doses given outside a stated set of clinical guidelines or protocols.
[d]Improper dose error exclusions are (1) allowable deviations based on preset ranges established by individual health care organizations in consideration of measuring devices routinely provided to those who administer drugs to patients (e.g., not administering a dose based on a patient's measured temperature or blood glucose concentration) or other factors such as conversion of doses expressed in the apothecary system to the metric system, and (2) topical dosage forms for which medication orders are not expressed quantitatively.
[e]Wrong dosage-form error exclusions are accepted protocols (established by the Pharmacy & Therapeutics Committee or its equivalent) that authorize pharmacists to dispense alternative dosage forms for patients with special needs (e.g., liquid formulations for patients with nasogastric tubes or those who have difficulty swallowing), as allowed by state regulations.
[f]Wrong drug-preparation error includes, for example, incorrect dilution or reconstitution, the mixing of drugs that are physically incompatible, and inadequate product packaging.
[g]Wrong administration-technique error includes doses administered (1) by the wrong route (different from the route prescribed), (2) by the correct route but at the wrong site (e.g., left eye instead of right eye), and (3) at the wrong rate of administration.
[h]Deteriorated drug error includes, for example, administration of expired drugs and improperly stored drugs.

Reprinted with permission from American Society of Health-System Pharmacists. Copyright 1993.

has variable pharmacokinetic and pharmacodynamic parameters. Dramatic changes in drug absorption, distribution, metabolism, and elimination occur during the first year of life. These changes pose challenges for health care providers in optimizing the effectiveness of drug therapies and minimizing adverse effects. Neonates grow rapidly during their first months of life, doubling their birth weight by 3 to 4 months. This degree of rapid growth can necessitate frequent dose adjustments. Dosing is individualized based on age, weight, or body surface area, requiring individualized dosing calculations. In addition, infants, young children, and older children with developmental delays are unable to verbally communicate possible ADEs to caregivers, making it difficult to detect when an ADE has occurred. Because of these differences, pediatric patients are less likely to avoid harm or injury when errors do occur.[16]

LACK OF COMMERCIALLY AVAILABLE DOSAGE FORMS

The lack of available dosage forms suitable for infants and children proves challenging for pharmacies that service children. Age-appropriate drug formulations are essential to the care of smaller infants and children. Manipulation of commercial products can lead to changes in bioavailability, stability, and sterility, increasing the risk of harm.[19,20]

ORAL EXTEMPORANEOUS PREPARATIONS

Oral dosage formulations for infants and children are not readily accessible. In addition, the liquid preparations that are available by the manufacturer are often unpalatable. Extemporaneous liquid formulations are needed to make drugs accessible for pediatric patients. Pharmacies can prepare oral liquid dosage forms from tablets, capsules, or powder with supporting evidence of appropriate stability and mixing instructions based on specific drug properties. This specialized compounding, which can be time intensive, is not performed in all pharmacies and can be burdensome on families and caregivers. In addition, it is not uncommon for parents or caregivers to be asked to open and empty capsules to sprinkle the contents onto food. Caregivers may also be asked to crush tablets, dilute the tablet contents in water, and give an aliquot of this preparation to their child. This process has significant risk and potential for error, especially in families with limited education or language barriers. This risk and potential for error emphasizes the importance of discharge teaching and targeted education for patients and caregivers. Also noteworthy in the outpatient setting is that the measuring of oral liquid preparations is inconsistent. For example, some caregivers use oral syringes, cups, dosing spoons, or teaspoons for medication delivery, which results in variability of medication administration. It is important to consider this type of error and to ensure adequate understanding when providing patient and caregiver education. Community pharmacists play a large role in educating patients and caregivers about medications and their appropriate administration and use.

INTRAVENOUS STOCK DILUTIONS

For injectable medications, a dilution of a commercial product through sterile compounding may be required for pediatric patients, especially neonates. Dilutions are typically necessary for doses measuring less than 0.1 mL to improve accuracy during medication dispensing and administration. For example, furosemide is a common diuretic used in pediatric patients. The recommended dose of furosemide is 1 mg/kg/dose. If the patient weighs less than 1 kg, the patient's dose will be too small to measure using the standard concentration 10 mg/mL available from the manufacturer. As a result, the drug must be diluted to 1 mg/mL. The dilution process requires careful calculation and manipulation, both of which have a potential for error. In addition, when a stock dilution is made to prepare many patient-specific doses simultaneously, an error in the dilution process may affect many patients or an entire patient care unit.

MULTIPLE CONCENTRATIONS

The use of several concentrations for both oral and intravenous preparations can be confusing. Many drugs are available commercially in significantly different concentrations to meet the requirements of very small infants as well as older children and adults. In fact, some medications are labeled as "infant" or "pediatric" drugs, such as gentamicin, naloxone, and sodium bicarbonate. As a result, potential harm or injury can occur when the wrong concentration is used inadvertently. The use of standardized concentrations when feasible is highly recommended to avoid error that may result in 10-fold differences.[21,22]

Similarly, for drugs that are available in multiple concentrations, dosing errors may also occur when doses are expressed in units of volume only. For example, if the prescriber writes a prescription for 1 teaspoon (5 mL) of amoxicillin, then it is unclear which commercially available concentration is to be dispensed—125 mg/5 mL, 250 mg/5 mL, or 400 mg/5 mL. If the prescriber writes a prescription for 250 mg (5 mL) of amoxicillin, then it is clear that the

---

Box 1. Common Causes of Medication Errors

Ambiguous strength designation on labels or in packaging
Drug product nomenclature (look-alike or sound-alike names, use of lettered or numbered prefixes and suffixes in drug names)
Equipment failure or malfunction
Illegible handwriting
Improper transcription
Inaccurate dosage calculation
Inadequately trained personnel
Inappropriate abbreviations used in prescribing
Labeling errors
Medication unavailable

Reprinted with permission from American Society of Health-System Pharmacists. Copyright 1993.

250-mg/5-mL concentration should be used. Methadone has two oral liquid concentrations available 1 mg/mL and 10 mg/m. Dosing by volume for methadone may result in a 10-fold overdose if the prescriber does not adequately clarify the concentration to be dispensed. A 10-fold error with high-risk agents such as opioids or digoxin may result in significant injury or death. *It is recommended that doses always be expressed in milligrams and milliliters*—not just milliliters.

PREVENTIVE STRATEGIES FOR MEDICATION ERROR

Patient safety is a top priority for all health care providers and several organizations have position statements, guidance toward improved safety, and best practice recommendations regarding error prevention strategies. These organizations include but are not limited to organizations such as Institute for Safe Medication Practices (ISMP), Agency for Healthcare Research and Quality, FDA, American Society of Health-System Pharmacists, and the Pediatric Pharmacy Association. In addition, TJC has adopted medication management standards to which hospitals are held accountable for patient safety.

The ISMP has established its role as a leader in medication safety education and preventive strategies. This organization has provided the framework for developing medication safety programs and has published several tools to help practitioners implement these strategies.[2,23-25] The regular distribution of ISMP safety newsletters encourages the reporting of error-prone practice patterns and actual medication errors using a collaborative approach.

As an international nonprofit professional pharmacy association, Pediatric Pharmacy Association is dedicated to promoting safe and effective medication use in children through communication, research, education, and advocacy. In 2001, Pediatric Pharmacy Association, in collaboration with ISMP and American Academy of Pediatrics, published guidelines for the prevention of medication errors in pediatric patients.[26] This collaborative identified medication safety strategies and recommendations specific to pediatric patients, highlighting challenges in this vulnerable population. These recommendations were endorsed by the American Society of Health-System Pharmacists in support of established standards for pediatric pharmacy practice, most recently updated in 2017, to establish minimum requirements for hospitals that care for infants and children.[7,27,28]

In summary, many organizations endorse the preventive strategies for medication safety promoted by the IOM, which include support for a culture of safety, training, and education; medication management standard and best practices; patient-centered care; and the judicious use of technology. In the next section, these principles will be discussed as they pertain to pediatric pharmacy practice.

CULTURE OF SAFETY

A critical step in medication error prevention is establishing a culture of safety within the organization, focusing on systems—versus individuals—to improve safety. A transparent quality improvement strategy encourages ADE reporting and allows frontline staff to offer recommendations for improving processes to enhance safety, optimize resources, reduce costs, or provide better workflow and efficiency. It is vital that the organization support nonpunitive actions when errors occur or are reported as part of its culture. At some institutions, the staff still receives corrective action and disciplinary consequences when errors are recognized or reported. Although practitioners should be held accountable, organizations should concentrate on system failures versus individual performance. Errors are seldom the result of practitioner negligence, and the blaming of individuals must be restrained. A high priority for each organization should be to establish best practices within the MUP to support its employees and minimize risk.

The MUP consists of several steps including *prescribing, transcribing, dispensing, administration, monitoring,* and *documenting.* Figure 2 provides a summary of each step in more detail.[29] The likelihood of error increases with each step in a process, especially when humans are involved. *Human error,* known as an *active failure,* occurs because of a single failure point within a system. An example of an active failure is nonadherence to policy or procedure. However, most errors occur as a result of several failures within a system, which are termed *latent failures.* Latent failures differ from active failures because they lie dormant within the system and are often undetected until an error occurs. These failures are considered the weaknesses or gaps of the system. Tools used to evaluate risk or determine why an error occurred include *failure mode effects analysis* (FMEA) and *root cause analysis.* Failure mode effects analysis is often performed prospectively to determine latent failures and may be used as a gap analysis for complex systems or processes within a system before an event occurs. Root cause analysis is typically completed retrospectively to determine the cause and effect of an actual error because of an event that occurred.[30-32] As described in following text in more detail, system failures in training or education, standardization, communication, complexity, and limited technology may also increase the risk of medication errors.

EDUCATION AND TRAINING

Caring for infants and children requires a basic foundation of education and clinical skill that should be more accessible in pharmacy schools. Pediatrics should be a required therapeutics course in the curriculum of schools of pharmacy. Most often, pediatric therapeutics is offered as an abbreviated course with minimal content, or it may only be offered as an elective course. Some pharmacy students are never exposed before graduation to the challenges and differences of pediatrics and medication therapy.[33-35]

Residency training is often necessary to gain the foundational knowledge base and clinical decision-making skills to apply to pediatric pharmacy practice. The development and expansion of residency programs in any organization can help promote pharmacy services that are more focused on pediatric patients. There are fewer pediatric pharmacy residency programs compared with more generalized pharmacy practice residency programs and other specialties. Some institutions provide only 1 year of training as either pediatric pharmacy practice or a higher-level specialty residency. Some institutions offer both a pharmacy practice and specialty residency program in pediatrics. This approach provides a more comprehensive pharmacy practice and specialized residency training experience, with additional exposure in a particular subspecialty (e.g., neonatal intensive care unit, critical care, oncology) after pharmacists complete 2 years of residency training in an exclusively pediatric environment.

Board certification in pediatric pharmacotherapy has been established by the Board of Pharmaceutical Specialties. This most specialized and clinically significant accomplishment is aimed to set a standard for highly skilled pediatric practitioners following the same strategy as for other recognized specialties.[36]

Health care systems and organizations should develop age-based training and education programs that promote basic competencies required for pediatric pharmacy practice. Providing essential age-specific training to practitioners in areas such as developmental pharmacology, common drugs and disease states, medication safety, and pediatric-specific considerations establishes a basic foundation for practitioners who care for infants and children.[28]

MEDICATION MANAGEMENT STANDARDS AND BEST PRACTICES

Medication management standards have been established by TJC that provide a basic framework for medication error prevention.[37,38] These standards, in conjunction with the national patient safety goals, provide guidance in drug ordering, administering, storage, and dispensing to optimize the MUP. Box 2 summarizes a checklist for organizations as a tool for evaluating medication management in the pediatric population.[17]

A formulary management system provides a framework to establish safe and cost-effective medication use. Pharmacists must play a large role in formulary selection, procurement, management of drug shortages, and medication use evaluation. A standard approach to drug request and review for formulary consideration should be established, including, at a minimum, important efficacy and cost data, any potential safety implications, and similar formulary medications that can be removed.[39,40]

Several tools have been developed to aid in standardizing medication use. The ISMP serves as a resource for clinical practice and as a liaison to manufacturers in recommending improved drug delivery systems and relabeling or renaming a *look-alike/sound-alike* drug. These recommendations include a standardized drug nomenclature (i.e., *tallman lettering*), problem-prone abbreviations, and confusing drug names (i.e., look-alike/sound-alike drug names), and, most recently, standardized concentrations for neonates.[41-44] In addition to these tools, other medication error prevention strategies to promote safety should be established. These strategies might include a process for medications that look or sound alike to be stored separately to prevent confusion.

The ISMP has also identified an extensive list of high-alert medications including anticoagulants, narcotics, insulin, neuromuscular-blocking agents, intravenous digoxin, dialysis solutions, and total parenteral nutrition. These drugs are more commonly associated with significant harm if used in error. Strategies recommended to improve safety with these agents

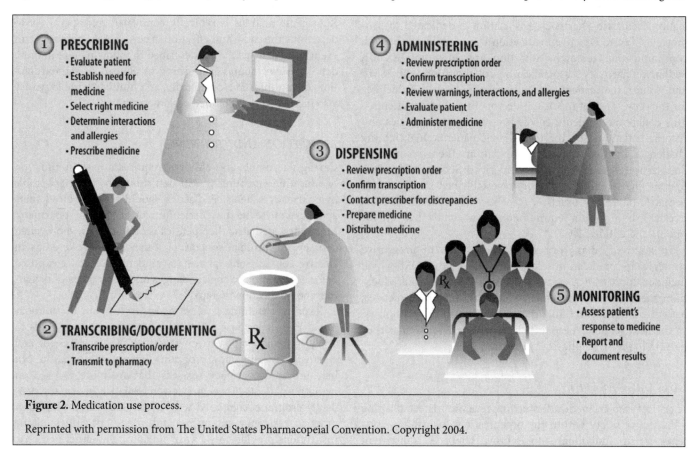

Figure 2. Medication use process.

Reprinted with permission from The United States Pharmacopeial Convention. Copyright 2004.

include limiting access, making use of auxiliary labels and alerts, making independent double checks, and using standardization throughout the MUP.[45]

Box 2. Evaluation Checklist for Medication Management in Pediatric Populations

Note: The following checklist is not meant to be comprehensive. Organizations may use it as a model, adding items based on recommendations from government agencies or professional associations.

Protocols for drug evaluation, selection, storage, and administration are standardized for the pediatric population.

Concentrations and dose strengths of high-risk medications are limited and standardized.

When adult medications are used off-label for children, the drugs are prepared and dispensed in patient-specific "unit doses" or "unit-of-use" containers.

A pharmacist reviews and verifies all pediatric medication orders (except in emergency situations).

A pharmacist with expertise in pediatric medications is on-call at all times.

Up-to-date references for pediatric medications are readily available in all areas where pediatric patients may be treated.

All pediatric patients are weighed at the time of admission.

Weight is always recorded in kilograms.

No high-risk drug is dispensed to a pediatric patient unless the patient has been weighed (except in emergency situations).

Medication orders/prescriptions are standardized, and the guidelines for inclusion of all necessary information are enforced.

If a computerized physician order entry system is used, the system has been adapted to pediatric populations and provides alerts, for example, if necessary information is missing or a dose adjustment is required.

Adult and pediatric doses or medications are stored separately, and products that have been repackaged for pediatric use are clearly labeled as such.

Barcoding technology (if applicable) has been adapted to pediatric codes, such as small-volume, patient-specific dose labels.

All staff members who may be involved in the care of children receive specialty training, including medication risks and double checks to reduce those risks.

Staff members who educate parents and other caregivers about patients' medications include all necessary information such as information about adverse effects and administration method.

Reprinted with permission from Joint Commission on Accreditation of Health Care Organizations. Copyright 2007.

In addition, emphasized by TJC is the use of standardized concentrations and patient-specific medication dispensing in the most ready-to-administer form. These best practices are challenging for pediatric institutions where medication orders are complex with limited standard doses, and manipulation of drug formulations are often required to meet the needs of the pediatric patient. When the volume of doses dispensed for adults are compared with the volume of pediatric workload, the additional steps in the dispensing process, including time, are often unaccounted for as part of the workload data. In addition, appropriate weight-based dosing must be verified for all inpatient and outpatient orders. These additional steps in the dispensing process should be considered when allocating resources, although they are difficult to quantify.

PATIENT- AND FAMILY-CENTERED CARE

Patient- and family-centered care provides a comprehensive approach to medical management by incorporating all members of the health care team in deciding treatment strategies, with a focus on patients and their families/caregivers. Clinical pharmacists have emerged as providers in comprehensive drug management to patients and providers by optimizing medication therapy, monitoring for effectiveness and adverse effects, and promoting health, wellness, and disease prevention. Studies have shown that clinical pharmacy services improve patient outcomes and reduce cost.[16,46,47] Establishing safe medication practices has also become the primary role of pharmacists, and ownership of continuous quality improvement efforts and measurement of medication safety are mainstays of current practice.

Unit-based or decentralized clinical pharmacists establish a model for more comprehensive and patient and family-focused care. This approach has shown reductions in medication errors in both adult and pediatric patients through the provision of more accessible drug information, patient education, and medication reconciliation, together with other clinical pharmacy services.[16,46,47]

Most recently, the American Society of Health-System Pharmacists Pharmacy Practice Model Initiative provided a summary of recommendations to advance pharmacy practice to meet the needs of changing health care systems. As part of this initiative, key stakeholders and leaders in pharmacy collectively provided a blueprint for establishing pharmacists as having a direct patient care role. As drug therapy experts, pharmacists must leverage technology and clinical skills to optimize patient care and improve safety, focusing on drug therapy management.[48]

JUDICIOUS USE OF TECHNOLOGY

Implementation of technology provides a safer environment for patients through standardization of the MUP. This standardization includes the use of computerized prescriber order entry (CPOE) with clinical decision support systems, electronic medical records, pharmacy systems, automated dispensing cabinets, smart infusion pumps, barcode medication administration (BCMA) and pharmacy workflow managers (e.g., DoseEdge; Baxter Healthcare Corp., Round Lake, IL).

The ISMP offers self-assessment tools and guidelines to help organizations implement new modes of technology and evaluate existing systems for areas of improvement compared with best practices and national standards. However, many of the advances in commercial technology are marketed to adult patients; therefore, caution and careful consideration must be used when implementing them in the pediatric setting. A recent publication by the Agency for Healthcare Research and Quality provides an expert consensus on core functionality necessary in pediatric electronic health records and serves as an essential resource for technology components targeted to the MUP specific to pediatric patients.[49]

In the following section, each of these tools and their impact on medication safety will be summarized, with pediatric considerations highlighted.

COMPUTERIZED PRESCRIBER ORDER ENTRY

Computerized prescriber order entry is a key technology to reduce medication errors and has been endorsed by several leading patient safety organizations since the initial IOM reports were published. Although increasingly more common within the health care community, the implementation of CPOE remains a challenge. When implemented correctly, CPOE requires a reasonable timeline, resources, and capital funding, which are often barriers to progress.[50]

Studies in adults support CPOE as an important tool in medication error prevention.[51,52] Overall, CPOE provides more legible and complete medication orders with limited use of abbreviations. However, in pediatrics, data are limited and sometimes conflicting.[42-60] One study found that medication prescribing errors and rule violations were almost eliminated and that potential ADEs were reduced 41% in critically ill pediatric patients.[55] In critically ill neonates, CPOE implementation has shown improved safety and reductions in medication prescribing errors.[56] Box 3 summarizes factors associated with an "ideal" CPOE system.[26] Some data suggest that CPOE implementation can result in increased mortality.[58] However, subsequent studies did not show similar results.[59,60] Some studies have reported increases in mortality rates after CPOE implementation and correlate short implementation timelines with difficulty accessing critical medications because of poorly customized applications.[61]

A strategic timeline for implementation with focused design of clinical decision support systems (CDSS) is essential for improved medication prescribing benefits. Forced functions also allow a more streamlined approach to medication ordering, assisting in drug selection and dosing in accordance with best practices. For example, a drug that is only provided as an oral dosage form should not be orderable as an injection.[50] The use of basic drug–drug interactions, drug–allergy interactions, and duplicate therapy warnings provides warnings to the end user during order entry, but this approach must be clinically justifiable to avoid excessive alerting. Advanced CDSS provides additional guidance to the prescriber beyond what typically if offered with the commercial software license. This level of customization is often needed for pediatric patients, especially neonates for whom dosing is often based on weight and gestational age with regard to the pharmacodynamic complexities that make this population at highest risk of medication errors. Examples include specific corrected age- or weight-based dosing recommendations and rounding logic; dosing calculators; order set development and standardized ordering pages for error-prone medications (e.g., continuous infusions, total parenteral nutrition, patient-controlled anesthesia, anticoagulation); patient-specific code dosing sheets; pharmacy and therapeutics initiatives; drug shortage alerts; FDA warnings and safety alerts; and customized dosing advisors.

Alert fatigue from too many unnecessary alerts can be problematic. Alerts displayed to the prescriber should be carefully reviewed, monitored, and minimized to those requiring specific action or considered significant. Minimizing alerts through periodic review and customization will result in more meaningful alerts that are actionable to the targeted audience.[62] In summary, CPOE with clinical decision support targets the most error-prone step of this process and reduces medication prescribing errors. Of importance, success is often related to a well-executed implementation plan and the feasibility of customization from the commercial software. Customization is essential to success in pediatrics, and pediatric-specific resources will need to be allocated for long-term development and maintenance.

PHARMACY SYSTEMS

Ideally, the pharmacy verification system interfaces with the CPOE system, which eliminates the need to transcribe medication orders and supports a "paperless" process. For

---

Box 3. Functionality Associated With an "Ideal" Computerized Prescriber Order Entry System[26]

Prescriber order entry for verification by nurse and pharmacist

Computer-generated medication administration records

Current medication list that is readily accessible

Two-way interface between pharmacy and other electronic documentation tools

Access to archived patient information

Age- and weight-based dosing recommendations

Allergies and weight required and forced-upon order entry

Access to vital patient information at the point of order entry

Clinical decision support that provides appropriate patient-specific drug information, such as the following: dose checks, allergy alerts, renal function, drug interactions and contraindications, laboratory warnings

Provide forced functions by limiting inappropriate options for order entry based on the drug that is ordered

Reprinted with permission from Pediatric Pharmacy Advocacy Group. Copyright 2001.

order verification, it is important for the pharmacy system to require minimal manipulation of medication orders. For pediatric patients, most orders that are verified require frequent manipulation, which sometimes results in miscellaneous orders or other workarounds to accommodate the specific needs of these patients. This process introduces risk and often takes time away from other clinical pharmacy services and responsibilities. Pharmacy workflow managers (e.g., DoseEdge) help to standardize dispensing practices to improve efficiency and safety. These systems offer barcode scanning technology to verify accurate medication selection, and some systems offer picture-taking capability to allow for remote order verification.

Pediatric dosage forms are most commonly dispensed as patient-specific medication from the pharmacy, but some medications can be stored in an automated dispensing cabinet in standard doses to provide quicker access for common non-high risk medications (i.e., amoxicillin, famotidine and ondansetron). Automatic dispensing cabinets help standardize the dispensing process at the unit level, providing quicker access to select medications. Consequently, however, the storage of look-alike/sound-alike and high-alert medications may introduce risk, so consistent use of medication error prevention strategies should be established. Medications approved for override need to be monitored and approved through a formal process. Patient profiling and scanning on restock are both important aspects for the use of an automated dispensing cabinet that should not be overlooked because these actions provide additional safety within the process.

BARCODE MEDICATION ADMINISTRATION

Medication administration errors are difficult to intercept and have the most potential for harm. Barcode medication administration is recommended as a tool to improve medication safety during drug delivery. This tool provides emphasis on the five patient rights as follows: *right patient, right drug, right dose,* and *right route,* at the *right time.* A recent survey found that around 30% of hospitals nationwide have implemented BCMA, a significant improvement from less than 10% in 2005.[62,63]

The benefits of BCMA on medication errors have not been well established in adult or pediatric patients.[64] Recent studies have shown reductions in medication errors of between 27.3% and 87% with BCMA use, but a significant return on investment has been difficult to quantify.[65] It is important to understand specific barriers and other obstacles in nursing workflow because these often create workaround or frustration with the system. Some researchers have studied the use of BCMA in several hospitals, identifying 15 workarounds by nursing. Also reported were 31 causes of these workarounds to BCMA, including the following: unreadable barcode labels, missing or unreadable armbands, malfunctioning scanners, medications without barcodes, failing batteries, uncertain wireless connectivity, and emergencies.[66]

For pediatric patients, specific limitations of the system and other considerations need to be evaluated before implementation. For example, it is difficult to scan the armband of a swaddled neonate requiring temperature regulation in an incubator bed. In addition, barcoding from the manufacturer, which is the concept for the accuracy of these systems, is tailored specifically to adult dosage forms. Many of the pediatric formulations are not conveniently available from the manufacturer; therefore, each institution must establish its process for patient-specific barcodes and be able to provide the resources to maintain this process.

SMART INFUSION PUMPS

Smart pump technology provides a safety net for appropriate medication administration of intermittent and continuous infusions. Guidelines published by ISMP are available to guide institutions through critical points of a successful implementation of smart pump technology.[67] Pharmacists play an essential role in drug library development, which provides the "guardrails" for safe drug delivery. These parameters are based on published drug dosing recommendations and established clinical practices within the institution. Most companies offer electronic data collection to allow periodic review for continuous quality improvement. This data review provides a summary of drug use and clinical practice patterns. The number of overrides of the guardrails can be monitored, which helps identify questionable practices or the need to adjust the library to avoid unnecessary alerts. More importantly, the drug library can be customized to meet the needs of the institution and promotes the use of standardized concentrations. Pediatric settings often require more than one standard concentration to meet the needs of the large variability in size within the pediatric population. This requirement demands a larger and more customized drug library compared with that in adult settings. This demand should be considered upon initial implementation, and resource allocation should be evaluated for the development and maintenance of subsequent updates.

MEASURING MEDICATION SAFETY

Measuring medication safety should be systematic and demonstrate the impact on outcomes associated with process improvement strategies. Benchmarking medication safety is more than just defining error rates and comparing internally and externally. Determining what to measure can be challenging but should follow a standardized approach for selecting outcomes and appropriate data collection. Without required outcomes or measures established by quality organizations, institutions are left to monitor ADEs and establish their own goals as a part of internal medication safety programs. Most often, institutions will collaborate together to establish more meaningful benchmarking and medication safety goals with the primary goal to improve patient safety.[68]

Voluntary reporting is another way to identify potential failures within the MUP and make suggestions for improvement. However, voluntary reporting significantly underestimates the occurrence of medication errors and ADEs. Fewer than 5% of ADEs are actually reported through this process, and near misses are seldom included.[68-70] Near-miss data help identify error-prone steps in a process before an event occurs. Occurrence reports should never be discouraged or used as a means to quantify medication error rates. Internal reporting should be rewarded as part of a nonpunitive, just culture with the goal of increasing voluntary reporting. Occurrence reporting, when used in conjunction with other methods, is helpful in identifying vulnerability and risk within the MUP as part of a medication safety program.

Adverse drug event surveillance tools, pharmacovigilance, and direct observation are more reliable in capturing ADEs.[70-75] The use of known "triggers" to identify ADEs is effective and provides a way to prioritize patients on the basis of risk. These tools help provide more accurate and timely data in determining whether patients have experienced an ADE. Through a validated methodology and retrospective chart review, these events help determine system failures and opportunities for improvement. Unfortunately, this process is time-consuming and costly, and it still accounts for a small percentage of actual ADEs. An electronic "trigger tool" can provide real-time aggregate data by surveillance of all patients against the triggers without timely and costly chart review. The ADE surveillance provides additional utility to the framework of medication safety programs when used in collaboration with occurrence reporting and external reporting systems.

Markers of performance, core measures, patient outcome data, regulatory and compliance standards, continuous quality data from technology (such as alerts and overrides), and medication events can also be considered part of a medication safety program. For institutions that have implemented the use of technology, compliance with these systems and possible workarounds that need to be addressed may be considered.[61,68]

CONCLUSIONS

Medication errors occur commonly, and most are preventable, with pediatric patients at highest risk. Infants and children offer challenges and developmental differences that make this population more vulnerable. Their needs require additional steps in the MUP and complex clinical decision-making skills. Leadership support to promote a culture of safety and a systems approach to medication errors is necessary in developing successful medication safety programs. Additional training and education in the area of pediatrics will provide the necessary foundation of knowledge. For pharmacists, this training and education include age-based competencies or additional didactic and residency training in basic pediatric pharmacy practice. Pharmacists trained in pediatric pharmacy practice are essential for appropriate patient care of both outpatients and inpatients. Community pharmacists collaborate with other health care professionals to ensure the correct medication use for pediatric patients. Clinical pharmacists providing clinical services in an inpatient setting should be available at the unit level to the multidisciplinary team in support of patient and family-centered care. Technology provides a standardized approach for error-prone steps in the MUP such as ordering and medication administration. When used judiciously, technology has the potential to enhance patient safety. Because most systems are developed for adult patients, additional resources must be allocated to customize and maintain technology systems to meet the needs of pediatric patients. Noncompliance and workarounds to the use of this technology should be evaluated to avoid unintended consequences and address vulnerabilities within the system. In addition, alerts and warnings should be kept to a minimum to avoid alert fatigue. Pharmacists play a key role in medication error prevention. Careful attention to the needs and vulnerability of pediatric patients should be a focus for patient safety standards and goals of national and regulatory agencies to provide children's hospitals the resources and governance needed to create a safer culture and environment.

Patient Case — UNDERSTANDING MEDICATION SAFETY RISKS AND STRATEGIES TO IMPROVE THE MEDICATION USE PROCESS

A 6-year-old, 20-kg girl presents to the emergency department for complex cardiac management, failure to thrive with a lack of adequate oral intake, and potential gastrostomy tube placement. Medical history is complicated, with prematurity, congenital heart disease, diabetes, and gastroesophageal reflux disease.

Current medications:	
Hydrochlorothiazide 25 mg orally daily	Insulin glargine 15 units subcutaneous at bedtime
Enalapril 10 mg orally daily	Baclofen 5 mg orally every 8 hours
Omeprazole 20 mg orally daily	Oxcarbazepine 300 mg orally every 12 hours
	Acetaminophen 325 mg orally every 4-6 hours as needed for pain

1. Why are pediatric patients at a higher risk of medication errors?

Different and changing pharmacokinetic parameters; complex calculations; lack of available dosage forms; need for more accurate measuring and drug delivery; lack of published data.

Many factors place pediatric patients at increased risk of medication errors, including the following: (1) Different and changing pharmacokinetic parameters between patients at various ages and stages of maturational development; (2) need for calculation of individualized doses based on the patient's age, weight (mg/kg), body surface area (mg/m²), and clinical condition; (3) lack of available dosage forms and concentrations appropriate for administration to neonates, infants, and children; often dosage formulations are extemporaneously compounded and lack stability, compatibility, or bioavailability data; (4) need for precise dose measurement and appropriate drug delivery systems; and (5) lack of published information or FDA label approval regarding dosing, pharmacokinetics, safety, efficacy, and clinical use of drugs in the pediatric population.

2. Which of this patient's medications is defined as "high alert" based on the Institute for Safe Medication Practices (ISMP) high alert medication list for acute care settings?

Insulin glargine.

Insulin is the only medication on this patient's medication list that poses highest risk of harm if used in error based on the ISMP high alert medication list for acute care settings.

3. How is a "high alert" medication defined according to the ISMP?

Poses a heightened risk of patient harm when used in error; requires special safeguards to prevent error; results in safety events reported through internal or external reporting systems.

High-alert medications are drugs that bear a heightened risk of causing significant patient harm when they are used in error. Although mistakes may or may not be more common with these drugs, the consequences of an error are clearly more devastating to patients. Acute care settings have been asked to establish a list of high-alert medications to determine which medications require special safeguards to reduce the risk of errors. This safeguarding may include strategies such as standardizing the ordering, storage, preparation, and administration of these products; improving access to information about these drugs; limiting access to high-alert medications; using auxiliary labels and automated alerts; and using redundancies such as automated or independent double checks when necessary.

4. What safety strategies can be put in place to help minimize risk with high-alert medications?

Standardization; limiting access; independent double checks; increased awareness and education; designating high-alert storage and labeling.

For this patient and insulin specifically, storage of insulin may be limited to the pharmacy only and double check the type of insulin, concentration, and amount/dose being dispensed to reduce risk because this medication is classified as high alert. Consider adding "high alert" labeling to notify others to be more cautious with this medication.

Several safety strategies can be considered overall to help reduce risk with high alert medication, including strategies such as standardizing the ordering, storage, preparation, and administration of these products; improving access to information about these drugs; limiting access to high-alert medications; using auxiliary labels and automated alerts; and using redundancies such as automated or independent double checks when necessary.

5. The patient has undergone a gastrostomy tube insertion, and you are the pharmacist dispensing to the patient's family/caregiver on discharge. What are important patient counseling considerations regarding the baclofen oral suspension?

Dispensing errors are more common with compounded oral medications because of a lack of standard concentrations; always include the milligram and the milliliter dose on the medication label instructions to help avoid confusion; educate the family/caregiver to use metric unit dosing cups or syringes.

The lack of standardization locally and nationally with oral compounded medications leads to inconsistencies and increases the risk of error. Although efforts have been made in some states, such as Michigan, a national standard is still lacking. In an effort to avoid confusion with varied concentrations, it is important for pharmacists to include both the milligram dose and the milliliter amount on the patient label. Lastly, education on the use of metric-only delivery devices such as a syringe or dosing cup should be emphasized. Adverse drug events have been associated with dosing errors and variability because caregivers may use standard kitchen teaspoons for convenience instead of using the correct measuring tools.

REFERENCES

1. Institute of Medicine, Kohn LT, Corrigan JM, Donaldson MS, eds. To Err Is Human: Building a Safer Health System. Washington, DC: National Academy Press, 2000.
2. Institute of Medicine. Crossing the Quality Chasm: A New Health System for the 21st Century. Washington, DC: National Academy Press, 2001.
3. Institute of Medicine, Committee on Identifying and Preventing Medication Errors, Board on Health Care Services. Preventing Medication Errors. Washington, DC: National Academies Press, 2007. Available at www.nap.edu/read/11623/chapter/1. Accessed May 23, 2019.
4. National Coordinating Council for Medication Error Reporting and Prevention. About Medication Errors. Available at www.nccmerp.org/about-medication-errors. Accessed May 17, 2018.
5. National Coordinating Council for Medication Error Reporting and Prevention Medication Error Index. NCC MERP Index for Categorizing Medication Errors. Available at http://nccmerp.org/sites/default/files/indexBW2001-06-12.pdf. Accessed May 17, 2018.
6. Nebeker JR, Barach P, Samore MH. Clarifying adverse drug events: a clinician's guide to terminology, documentation, and reporting. Ann Intern Med 2004;140:795-801.
7. American Society of Hospital Pharmacists. ASHP guidelines on preventing medication errors in hospitals. Am J Hosp Pharm 1993;50:305-14.
8. American Society of Health-System Pharmacists. ASHP Guidelines on Adverse Drug Reaction Monitoring and Reporting. Available at https://www.ashp.org/-/media/assets/policy-guidelines/docs/guidelines/adverse-drug-reaction-monitoring-reporting.ashx. Accessed May 17, 2018.
9. Brennan TA, Leape LL, Laird N, et al. Incidence of adverse events and negligence in hospitalized patients: results from the Harvard Medical Practice Study I. N Engl J Med 1991;324:370-6.
10. Leape LL, Lawthers AG, Brennan TA, et al. Preventing medical injury. Qual Rev Bull 1993;19:144-9.
11. Leape LL, Brennan TA, Laird NM, et al. The nature of adverse events in hospitalized patients: results from the Harvard Medical Practice Study II. N Engl J Med 1991;324:377-84.
12. Bates DW, Cullen D, Laird N, et al., for the ADE Prevention Study Group. Incidence of adverse drug events and potential adverse drug events: implications for prevention. JAMA 1995;274:29-34.
13. Bates DW, Leape LL, Petrycki S. Incidence and preventability of adverse drug events in hospitalized adults. J Gen Intern Med 1993;8:289-94.
14. Bates DW, Boyle DL, Vander Vliet MB, et al. Relationship between medication errors and adverse drug events. J Gen Intern Med 1995;10:199-205.
15. Leape LL, Bates DW, Cullen DJ, et al., for the ADE Prevention Study Group. Systems analysis of adverse drug events. JAMA 1995;274:35-43.
16. Kaushal R, Bates DW, Landrigan C, et al. Medication errors and adverse drug events in pediatric inpatients. JAMA 2001;285:2114-20.
17. The Joint Commission. Sentinel Event Alert, Issue 39: Preventing Pediatric Medication Errors. Available at www.jointcommission.org/sentinel_event_alert_issue_39_preventing_pediatric_medication_errors/. Accessed May 1, 2018.
18. Kunac DL, Kennedy J, Austin N, et al. Incidence, preventability, and impact of adverse drug events (ADEs) and potential ADEs in hospitalized children in New Zealand: a prospective observational cohort study. Paediatr Drugs 2009;11:153-60.
19. Ivanovska V, Rademaker C, van Dijk L, et al. Pediatric drug formulations: a review of challenges and progress. Pediatrics 2014;143:361-72.
20. Nahata MC, Pai VB. Pediatric Drug Formulations, 6th ed. Harvey Whitney Books Co., Cincinnati, 2014.
21. University of Michigan College of Pharmacy. State-Wide Initiative to Standardize the Compounding of Oral Liquids in Pediatrics. Available at www.mipedscompounds.org. Accessed September 30, 2019.
22. Institute for Safe Medication Practices. Standard Concentrations of Neonatal Drug Infusions. Available at www.ismp.org/Tools/PediatricConcentrations.pdf. Accessed September 30, 2019.
23. Institute for Safe Medication Practices. Pathways for Medication Safety—leading a Strategic Planning Effort. Available at www.ismp.org/resources/strategic-planning. Accessed May 1, 2018.
24. Institute for Safe Medication Practices. Looking Collectively at Risk. Pathways for Medication Safety Tool #2. Chicago, IL: American Hospital Association, 2003.
25. Institute for Safe Medication Practices. Assessing Bedside Bar-Coding Readiness. Available at http://forms.ismp.org/selfassessments/PathwaySection3.pdf. Accessed May 1, 2018.
26. Levine SR, Cohen MR, Blanchard NR, et al. Guidelines for preventing medication errors in pediatrics. J Pediatr Pharmacol Ther 2001;6:427-43.
27. American Society of Hospital Pharmacists. ASHP guidelines for providing pediatric pharmaceutical services in organized health care systems. Am J Hosp Pharm 1994;51:1690-2.
28. American Society of Health-System Pharmacists. ASHP-PPAG guidelines for providing pediatric pharmaceutical services in organized health care systems. Am J Health-Syst Pharm 2018;75:e136-50
29. U.S. Pharmacopeia. The Standard. Rockville, MD: U.S. Pharmacopeia, 2019.
30. Cohen MR. One hospital's method of applying failure mode and effects analysis. In: Cohen MR, ed. Medication Errors. Washington, DC: American Pharmaceutical Association, 1999:561-4.
31. Cohen MR, Senders J, Davis NM. Failure mode and effects analysis: a novel approach to avoiding dangerous medication errors and accidents. Hosp Pharm 1994;29:319-30.
32. Institute of Medicine. Failure Mode Effects Analysis Tool. Available at www.ihi.org/resources/Pages/Tools/FailureModesandEffectsAnalysisTool.aspx. Accessed May 1, 2018.
33. Aucoin RG, Buck ML, Dupuis LL, et al. Pediatric pharmacotherapeutic education: current status and recommendations to fill the growing need. Pharmacotherapy 2005;25:1277-82.
34. Low JK, Baldwin JN. Pediatric pharmacy education for U.S. entry-level doctor of pharmacy programs. Am J Pharm Educ 1999;63:323-7.
35. Bahal-O'Mara N, Nahata MC. Teaching paediatric pharmacotherapy at colleges of pharmacy in the United States and Canada. J Clin Pharm Ther 1994;19:3-6.
36. Bhatt-Mehta V, Buck ML, Chung AM, et al. Recommendations for meeting the pediatric patient's need for a clinical pharmacist: a joint opinion of the Pediatrics Practice and Research Network of the American College of Clinical Pharmacy and the Pediatric Pharmacy Advocacy Group [PRN Opinion Paper]. Pharmacotherapy 2013;33:243-251.
37. Joint Commission on Accreditation of Healthcare Organizations. 2002 Hospital Accreditation Standards. Oakbrook Terrace, IL: Joint Commission on Accreditation of Healthcare Organizations, 2002:51-61, 101, 111-5, 148, 161-74, 345.
38. The Joint Commission. 2018 National Patient Safety Goals. Available at www.jointcommission.org/standards_information/npsgs.aspx. Accessed May 17, 2018.
39. American Society of Health-System Pharmacists. ASHP Guidelines on Medication-Use Evaluation. Available at www.ashp.org/-/media/assets/policy-guidelines/docs/guidelines/medication-use-evaluation.ashx. Accessed May 1, 2018.
40. American Society of Health-System Pharmacists. ASHP Guidelines on the Pharmacy and Therapeutics Committee and the Formulary System. Available at https://www.ashp.org/-/

media/assets/policy-guidelines/docs/guidelines/gdl-pharmacy-therapeutics-committee-formulary-system.ashx. Accessed May 1, 2018.

41. Institute for Safe Medication Practices. Look-alike drug names with recommended tall man letters. Available at www.ismp.org/recommendations/tall-man-letters-list. Accessed May 23, 2019.

42. Institute for Safe Medication Practices. List of error-prone abbreviations. Available at www.ismp.org/recommendations/error-prone-abbreviations-list. Accessed May 23, 2019.

43. Institute for Safe Medication Practices. List of confused drug names. Available www.ismp.org/recommendations/confused-drug-names-list. Accessed May 23, 2019.

44. Institute for Safe Medication Practices. List of standard concentrations of neonatal drug infusions. Available at www.ismp.org/recommendations/standard-concentrations-neonatal-drug-infusions. Accessed May 23, 2018.

45. Institute for Safe Medication Practices. List of high-alert medications. Available at www.ismp.org/recommendations/high-alert-medications-acute-list. Accessed May 23, 2019.

46. Folli HL, Poole RL, Benitz WE, et al. Medication error prevention by clinical pharmacists in two children's hospitals. Pediatrics 1987;79:718-22.

47. Wang JK, Herzog NS, Kaushal R, et al. Prevention of pediatric medication errors by hospital pharmacists and the potential benefit of computerized physician order entry. Pediatrics 2007;119:e77-85.

48. The consensus of the Pharmacy Practice Model Summit. Am J Health-Syst Pharm. 2011;68:1148-52.

49. Dufendach KR, Eichenberger JA, McPheeters ML, et al. Core functionality in pediatric electronic health records. Rockville, MD: Agency for Healthcare Research and Quality, Technical Brief No. 20; April 2015. Available at www.ncbi.nlm.nih.gov/books/NBK293626/. Accessed May 28, 2019.

50. ASHP guidelines on pharmacy planning for implementation of computerized provider-order-entry systems in hospitals and health systems. Am J Health Syst Pharm 2011;68:e9-e31.

51. Bates DW, Cullen DJ, Laird N, et al. Incidence of adverse drug events and potential adverse drug events. Implications for prevention. ADE Prevention Study Group. JAMA 1995;274:29-34.

52. Koppel R, Metlay JP, Cohen A, et al. Role of computerized physician order entry systems in facilitating medication errors. JAMA 2005;293:1197-203.

53. Walsh KE, Landrigan CP, Adams WG, et al. Effect of computer order entry on prevention of serious medication errors in hospitalized children. Pediatrics 2008;121:e421-7.

54. Van Rosse F, Maat B, Rademaker CM, et al. The effect of computerized physician order entry on medication prescription errors and clinical outcome in pediatric and intensive care: a systemic review. Pediatrics 2009;123:1184-90.

55. Potts AL, Barr FE, Gregory DF, et al. Computerized physician order entry and medication errors in a pediatric critical care unit. Pediatrics 2004;113:59-63.

56. Cordero L, Kuehn L, Kumar RR, et al. Impact of computerized physician order entry on clinical practice in a newborn intensive care unit. J Perinatol 2004;24:88-93.

57. Walsh KE, Landrigan CP, Adams WG, et al. Effect of computer order entry on prevention of serious medication errors in hospitalized children. Pediatrics 2008;121:e421-7.

58. Han YY, Carcillo JA, Venkataraman ST, et al. Unexpected increased mortality after implementation of a commercially sold computerized physician order entry system. Pediatrics 2005;116:1506-12.

59. Longhurst CA, Parast L, Sandborg CI, et al. Decrease in hospital-wide mortality rate after implementation of a commercially sold computerized physician order entry system. Pediatrics 2010;126:14-21.

60. Keene A, Ashton L, Shure D, et al. Mortality before and after initiation of a computerized physician order entry system in a critically ill pediatric population. Pediatr Crit Care Med 2007; 8:268-71.

61. Van Rosse F, Maat B, Rademaker CM, et al. The effect of computerized physician order entry on medication prescribing errors and clinical outcome in pediatric and intensive care: a systematic review. Pediatrics 2009;123:1184-90.

62. Stultz JS, Nahata MC. Computerized clinical decision support for medication prescribing and utilization in pediatrics. J Am Med Inform Assoc 2012;19:942-53.

63. Pedersen CA, Schneider PJ, Scheckelhoff DJ. ASHP national survey of pharmacy practice in hospital settings: monitoring and patient education—2009. Am J Health Syst Pharm 2010;67:542-58.

64. Pedersen CA, Schneider PJ, Scheckelhoff DJ. ASHP national survey of pharmacy practice in hospital settings: dispensing and administration—2011. Am J Health Syst Pharm 2012;69:768-85.

65. Sakowski J, Newman JM, Dozier K. Severity of medication administration errors detected by a bar-code medication administration system. Am J Health Syst Pharm 2008;65:1661-6.

66. Miller DF, Fortier CR, Garrison KL. Bar code medication administration technology: characterization of high-alert medication triggers and clinician workarounds. Ann Pharmacother 2011;45:162-8.

67. Koppel R, Wetterneck T, Telles JL, et al. Workarounds to barcode medication administration systems: their occurrences, causes, and threats to patient safety. J Am Med Inform Assoc 2008;15:408-23.

68. Institute for Safe Medication Practices. Proceedings from the ISMP Summit on the use of smart infusion pumps: guidelines for safe implementation and use. Available at www.ismp.org/guidelines/safe-implementation-and-use-smart-pumps. Accessed September 30, 2019.

69. Cohen MR. Managing Medication Risks Through a Culture of Safety. In: Cohen MR, ed. Medication Errors. Washington, DC: American Pharmaceutical Association, 1999:643-49.

70. Agency for Healthcare Research and Quality. Pediatric Toolkit for Using the AHRQ Quality Indicators. Available at www.ahrq.gov/professionals/systems/hospital/qitoolkit/pediatrictoolkit.html. Accessed September 30, 2019.

71. Takata GS, Mason W, Taketomo C, et al. Development, testing, and findings of a pediatric-focused trigger tool to identify medication-related harm in US children's hospitals. Pediatrics 2008;121:e27-e395.

72. Fabiano V, Mameli C, Zuccotti GV. Adverse drug reactions in newborns, infants and toddlers: pediatric pharmacovigilance between present and future. Expert Opin Drug Saf 2012;11:95-105.

73. Kilbridge PM, Noirot LA, Reichley RM, et al. Computerized surveillance for adverse drug events in a pediatric hospital. J Am Med Inform Assoc 2009;16:607-12.

74. Ferranti J, Horvath MM, Cozart H, et al. Reevaluating the safety profile of pediatrics: a comparison of computerized adverse drug event surveillance and voluntary reporting in the pediatric environment. Pediatrics 2008;121:e1201-7.

75. Stockwell DC, Kane-Gill SL. Developing a patient safety surveillance system to identify adverse events in the intensive care unit. Crit Care Med 2010;38(6 suppl):S117-25.

CHAPTER 7

Pediatric Toxicology

Mark R. Haase, Pharm.D., FCCP, BCPS

LEARNING OBJECTIVES

1. Describe the methods of poisoning data collection and how they affect poisoning prevention and therapy efforts.

2. Determine the incidence of pediatric poisonings in the United States based on the National Poison Data System Annual Report.

3. Evaluate the poisoned child.

4. Assess the efficacy of gastric decontamination methods.

5. Manage select pediatric poisonings.

ABBREVIATIONS IN THIS CHAPTER

AC	Activated charcoal
FabAV	Crotalidae polyvalent immune Fab antivenom
MDAC	Multiple-dose activated charcoal
NAPQI	*N*-acetyl-*p*-benzoquinonimine
SOI	Syrup of ipecac
WBI	Whole bowel irrigation

INTRODUCTION

Despite increased educational efforts, childhood poisonings remain a common occurrence, although not a common cause of morbidity and mortality in this population.[1] Each year, more than 2 million toxic exposures are reported, with more than half of these exposures occurring in children younger than 6 years. Medical management of poisoned children is similar to that for adults; however, important differences must be considered. This chapter will introduce the reader to the reporting system used to document epidemiologic trends in toxic exposure incidence and management, the evaluation of the poisoned child, decontamination principles, and the management of selected poisonings.

EPIDEMIOLOGY

NATIONAL POISON DATA SYSTEM

The National Poison Data System is the only comprehensive resource in the United States for poisoning surveillance. It is owned and managed by the American Association of Poison Control Centers, and since 1983 the organization has used these data to publish an annual report.[2] The current database holds data on more than 68 million reported toxic exposures. Poison centers serve all 50 states and several U.S. territories and are typically staffed by pharmacists and nurses. Pharmacists fill many roles at poison centers, including, but not limited to, poison information specialist and director of the poison center. Poison specialists are available 24 hours/day and can be reached through the national poison hotline at (800) 222-1222. Poison centers provide data to the National Poison Data System from incoming calls by an online reporting system that allows real-time surveillance of poisoning data. In 2017, poison centers received over 2.1 million calls for human exposures. In 1983, more than 250,000 human exposures were reported, although for the past 20 years, the number has been more than 2 million per year.[2] Of note, the database contains information from reported exposures only; many more exposures occur that are unreported, including those that cause serious injuries or fatalities.[3] In addition, some clinicians manage poisonings without consulting a poison center, and therapeutic errors that result in toxicity may not be reported.[1,2] Nevertheless, these data are very important because they can help inform policy decisions in many areas. A wealth of information for health care professionals and the lay public regarding epidemiology, prevention, and management of poisonings is available at websites provided by the American Association of Poison Control Centers and the Centers for Disease Control and Prevention (www.aapcc.org and www.cdc.gov/HomeandRecreationalSafety/Poisoning/index.html).

EPIDEMIOLOGIC TRENDS

Historically, children younger than 6 years have accounted for about 50% of all reported exposures. In 2017, children younger than 3, 6, and 20 years accounted for 34%, 45%, and 60% of reported toxic exposures, respectively.[2] Despite these high percentages, children account for only a small minority of fatalities, with less than 1% occurring in children younger than 6 years in 2017 when the toxin contributed in some way to death.[2]

The type of poisons most often encountered by children has remained much the same for many years. Analgesics, cosmetics, and household cleaning substances are consistently the most common toxins encountered overall. In addition, foreign bodies, topical preparations, vitamins, antihistamines, cough and cold preparations, pesticides, and plants are often ingested.[2]

EVALUATION OF THE POISONED CHILD

For many reasons, an infant, toddler, or young child will ingest or be exposed to substances to which an older child or adolescent will not be exposed. As children age, they become more mobile, allowing them to satisfy their natural curiosity and investigate their surroundings that they could not explore before. They can mimic adult activities such as taking medicine. They may mistake pharmaceuticals such as ferrous sulfate for candy or household cleaning products for flavored drinks. Fortunately, in children, most exposures are without intent to harm, and most result in minimal, if any, adverse outcomes.[2] However, any time a child presents with an altered level of consciousness, metabolic disturbance, neurologic dysfunction, or cardiac or pulmonary distress, it is important to include toxic exposure as part of the differential diagnosis.[4] In many ways, the evaluation of a poisoned child is similar to that of an adolescent (or an adult), but there are some important differences in supportive care, history, and evaluation.

SUPPORTIVE CARE

Supportive care, always a key component in managing toxic exposures, begins with airway stabilization and should follow Pediatric Advanced Life Support guidelines.[5] Some substances, such as tricyclic antidepressants, can cause rapid loss of consciousness and result in the need for rapid sequence intubation for airway protection, ventilation, and oxygenation. In addition, early antidote administration may be necessary, such as naloxone in opioid ingestions. Table 1 lists antidotes to selected poisonings. A more complete listing of available antidotes has been provided in other resources.[6]

HISTORY AND PHYSICAL EXAMINATION

A thorough history of ingestion in small children is usually easier to obtain than in adolescents. In general, caregivers provide as much detail as possible, including ingested volume estimates, tablet counts, containers of the substance in question, and a complete review of toxic substances in the vicinity of the child when the exposure occurred. The toxin involved and the time of ingestion are easiest to ascertain, whereas the amount ingested is typically more difficult to determine. These factors are important because they significantly affect the decision to implement decontamination strategies.[7] It is important to inquire about other places that the child may have been because roughly 15% of toxic ingestions in children occur outside the home.[1] A thorough history in an adolescent patient can be more difficult because the ingestion is more likely intentional or the result of substance abuse, and these patients may not be as forthcoming. Any information obtained from the patient about the ingestion must be taken in context of the clinical condition of the patient.[1] Other important contrasts between children and adolescents or adults are as follows: children more often present within a few hours of ingestion; multiple toxins are more likely involved in adolescent or adult exposures; in children, the toxin is more likely nontoxic; and children ingest a smaller amount in most instances.[1] Although children more often encounter nontoxic substances or ingest an amount that results in minimal harm, there are several toxins or drugs that may cause serious harm or death in very small amounts (Table 2).[1,8]

The physical examination centers on mental status and vital signs, including pulse; respiratory rate, quality, and effort; blood pressure; temperature; skin tone and color; hydration status; peripheral pulses; and perfusion.[9] A neurologic examination should be performed, including an evaluation of pupil size and reactivity. Many signs and symptoms of toxic exposures manifest in clusters called *toxidromes* (Table 3). Specific toxins, identified from the history or presentation, may allow the caregiver to narrow the physical examination to focus on expected or possible complications of the poisoning.

LABORATORY EVALUATIONS

Laboratory evaluations should be directed by the history and physical examination, although most patients presenting with suspected poisoning should have serum chemistries

Table 1. Antidotes for Selected Poisonings or Toxicities[6,9]

Antidote	Poisoning or Toxicity
Atropine/Pralidoxime	Organophosphates/Carbamates
Dantrolene	Malignant hyperthermia caused by the disease process such as neuroleptic malignant syndrome or heat stroke, or caused by drug toxicity such as from monoamine oxidase inhibitors or baclofen withdrawal
Deferoxamine	Iron
Digoxin antibody fragments (Fab)	Digoxin
Flumazenil	Benzodiazepines
Edetate calcium disodium (EDTA)/dimercaprol (British Anti-Lewisite [BAL])/succimer (dimercaptosuccinic acid)	Lead
Methylene blue	Methemoglobinemia
Protamine	Heparin
Sodium and amyl nitrite/sodium thiosulfate	Cyanide
Sodium bicarbonate	Salicylates, tricyclic antidepressants
Vitamin K	Warfarin

and acid–base status assessed. If the history indicates the possibility of alcohol ingestion, serum osmolality may be useful. Ingestions of cardiovascular agents such as β-adrenergic blockers or calcium channel blockers warrant an electrocardiogram.[4] A chemistry allows a calculation of the anion gap ([Na-{Cl + HCO_3}]; normal value 4–12 mEq/L). An elevated gap may indicate poisoning. A common mnemonic device to identify potentially causative mechanisms of an elevated anion gap is MUDPILES ([M] methanol; [U] uremia; [D] diabetic ketoacidosis; [P] propylene glycol; [I] isoniazid, iron, infection; [L] lactic acidosis; [E] ethylene glycol, ethanol; [S] salicylates).[9] Serum concentrations of acetaminophen—and, to a lesser extent, salicylates, ethanol, or iron—should be strongly considered because acetaminophen is so widely available in many products, and symptoms may not occur until several hours after ingestion. Other specific serum concentrations are generally not required and should be dictated by the specific ingestion.[4]

DECONTAMINATION

Although gastric decontamination offers the only therapy available other than supportive care for many orally ingested poisons, few data suggest any effect on outcomes. Reasons for this lack of evidence include significant interpatient variability (even in similar ingestions) and that most ingestions result in only minor to moderate adverse effects. Very large trials would be required to detect differences in outcome, a requirement that is especially true in children.[10] The lack of evidence of efficacy has resulted in significant decreases in the use of gastric decontamination. In 1985, syrup of ipecac (SOI) or activated charcoal (AC) was given in almost 20% of child exposures, whereas in 2017, less than 1% of children received these agents.[2] This trend has also been influenced by statements from the American Academy of Pediatrics and the American Academy of Clinical Toxicology.[11,12] The American Academy of Pediatrics statement, which is a summary of the evidence

Table 2. Substances That May Result in Severe Toxicity in Children with Small Exposure[1,8]

Substance	Potentially Significant Exposure in Children	Definitive Management or Antidote Beyond Supportive Care and Decontamination
Antihistamines	Diphenhydramine 10–15 mg/kg	Benzodiazepines for seizures or delirium Sodium bicarbonate for arrhythmias
Benzocaine	¼ teaspoon of 7.5% gel in infants ½ teaspoon in older children	Methylene blue for methemoglobinemia
β-Adrenergic antagonists	Propranolol > 4 mg/kg (40-mg tablet in 10-kg infant)	Pressor support Glucagon, insulin, glucose for cardiovascular support
Calcium channel blockers	Diltiazem > 1 mg/kg	Calcium Pressor support Glucagon, insulin, dextrose for cardiovascular support
Camphor	5 mL of camphorated oil (1 g of camphor)	Airway management Seizure management
Clonidine	0.1 mg Chewing clonidine patch	Pressor support Arrhythmia management Seizure management Naloxone
Diphenoxylate/ atropine	> 0.5–2 tablets	Naloxone
Methyl salicylate	> 150 mg/kg Several salicylate sources 1 mL of oil of wintergreen = 1400 mg of acetyl-salicylic acid	Dextrose and electrolytes Forced diuresis/alkalinization Seizure and cerebral edema management

Opioids	Hydrocodone 2.5 mg reported lethal
	  in infants (1 teaspoon of hydrocodone/
	  acetaminophen solution)
		Naloxone
		Pressor support
		Seizure management

Sulfonylureas	Chlorpropamide 250 mg Glipizide 5 mg Glyburide 2.5 mg	Intravenous dextrose Glucagon

Tricyclic antidepressants	10–20 mg/kg considered potentially lethal
	  in infants and young children
		Sodium bicarbonate, lidocaine, phenytoin,
		  or magnesium for arrhythmias
		Seizure management

Adapted with permission from McGraw-Hill. Hines EQ, Fine JS. 31: Pediatric principles. In: Nelson LS, Howland M, Lewin NA, et al., eds. Goldfrank's Toxicologic Emergencies, 11e. New York, NY: McGraw-Hill; 2019. Available at http://accessemergencymedicine.mhmedical.com/content.aspx?bookid=2569&-Sectionid=210270170. Accessed June 20, 2019.

for managing poisoning in the home, suggests that SOI not be used routinely in the home and that insufficient evidence exists to recommend use of AC in the home. The American Academy of Clinical Toxicology statement notes that SOI use at home or in the emergency department should be avoided; in fact, it may now be unavailable in most places, and manufacturing in the United States has stopped. The statement also notes that AC should generally be reserved for affected toxins within 1 hour of exposure. Table 4 summarizes gastric decontamination methods, and a brief discussion of each is provided in sections that follow. A review of decontamination techniques has been provided in other resources.[12-16]

SYRUP OF IPECAC

Syrup of ipecac is no longer recommended for use in poisoned patients, in either children or adults.[13] There are reports of gastric returns when SOI is administered, but these returns are variable and do not alter outcome.[17-20] An analysis of poison exposure data in children found that the use of SOI had no impact on either emergency department referral or outcomes.[21] In addition, although the administration of SOI has proved to be safe, rare serious adverse events can occur and the potential for abuse exists, which can lead to myopathy, cardiomyopathy, and death with chronic use.[22,23] Because of this lack of impact on clinical outcomes and because in many cases toxin ingestion by children results in no to minimal harm, SOI is no longer recommended for routine use.[11,13]

GASTRIC LAVAGE

Because of a lack of evidence of effectiveness and a relatively high complication rate, routine use of gastric lavage is not recommended.[14] A review of data available since the publication of the consensus statement in 2004 by the American Academy of Clinical Toxicology and the European Association of Poison Centres and Clinical Toxicologists has not altered that recommendation.[14] In addition, gastric lavage poses serious risks, including delaying definitive antidote administration, aspiration, mechanical injury, hyponatremia, hypothermia, and death.[24] In the rare instance that a risk-benefit analysis predicts potential benefit to gastric lavage, it is recommended that this procedure be performed within 1 hour of ingestion and only by properly trained caregivers.[14] However, clear gastric returns do not exclude a significant ingestion or guarantee that all toxin has been removed. In addition, the possibility remains that a significant amount of drug is still available in the stomach several hours after ingestion, although lavage appears variably effective at best in these situations.[25,26]

ACTIVATED CHARCOAL

Activated charcoal (AC) is produced when substances high in carbon content (e.g., wood, peat) are heated and then treated with steam or carbon dioxide.[12] This process results in a high surface area that allows the adsorption of other substances. Activated charcoal remains the method of gastric decontamination most often used.[2] Current recommendations call for considering the use of AC within 1 hour in patients with a potentially toxic ingestion.[12] Data available since the 2005 consensus statement by the American Academy of Clinical Toxicology and the European Association of Poison Centres and Clinical Toxicologists have supported this recommendation, suggesting that AC provides minimal if any benefit in poisoned patients and has decreased efficacy 1–2 hours after

Table 3. Toxic Syndromes

Group	Vital Signs				Mental Status	Pupil Size	Peristalsis	Diaphoresis	Other
	BP	HR	RR	T					
Anticholinergics	– /↑	↑	±	↑	Delirium	↑	↓	↓	Dry mucus membranes, flush, urinary retention
Cholinergics	±	±	– /↑	–	Normal to depressed	±	↑	↑	Salivation, lacrimation, urination, diarrhea, bronchorrhea, fasciculations, paralysis
Ethanol/sedative hypnotics	↓	↓	↓	– /↓	Depressed, agitated	±	↓	–	Hyporeflexia, ataxia
Opioids	↓	↓	↓	↓	Depressed	↓	↓	–	Hyporeflexia
Serotonin toxicity	↑	↑	– /↑	– /↑	Normal to agitated delirium	= /↑	↑	↑	Clonus, tremor, seizures
Sympathomimetics	↑	↑	↑	↑	Agitated	↑	– /↑	↑	Tremor, seizures
Withdrawal from ethanol/sedative hypnotics	↑	↑	↑	↑	Agitated, disoriented, hallucinations	↑	↑	↑	Tremor, seizures
Withdrawal from opioids	↑	↑	–	–	Normal, anxious	↑	↑	↑	Vomiting, rhinorrhea, piloerection, diarrhea, yawning

BP = blood pressure; HR = heart rate; RR = respiratory rate; T = temperature; ↑= increases; ↓ = decreases; ± = variable; – = change unlikely.
Reprinted with permission from McGraw-Hill. Nelson LS, Howland M, Lewin NA, et al. 3: Initial Evaluation of the Patient: Vital Signs and Toxic Syndromes. In: Nelson LS, Howland M, Lewin NA, et al., eds. Goldfrank's Toxicologic Emergencies, 11e. New York, NY: McGraw-Hill; 2019. Available at http://accesspharmacy.mhmedical.com/content.aspx?bookid=2569&Sectionid=210267208. Accessed June 20, 2019.

ingestion.[27-30] However, other data suggest AC can be effective in preventing sequelae and hastening the elimination of toxin, even when given later than 1 hour after ingestion.[31-33]

Administration of AC to children in the home has been investigated in an effort to increase efficacy by earlier administration. Safe administration appears feasible for parents and caregivers, but inconsistent; considering the risk of too-common and inappropriate use, home administration is not recommended.[11,34,35]

An AC/drug ratio of 10:1 is recommended. However, in most poisonings, the exact amount of drug ingested is unknown. Thus, it is suggested that adults receive 50–100 g (providing adsorption of around 5–10 g of drug) and that children receive 0.5–1 g/kg; note that these recommendations

are based more on tolerance and more could be needed in large overdoses.[10] If the 10:1 ratio is unlikely to be achieved with a maximally tolerated single dose, multidose AC or other decontamination methods should be considered. Activated charcoal is a relatively safe intervention. Vomiting is the most likely complication in children, and vomiting before administration and nasogastric tube placement appears to increase the risk.[36] Complications that are more serious, such as aspiration or bowel perforation, are much less common.[12,37]

Multiple-dose activated charcoal (MDAC) is defined as the administration of more than two sequential doses.[38] Multiple doses provide benefit by preventing prolonged absorption or enterohepatic recirculation (termed *gastric dialysis*).[39,40] Drugs are present in the gastrointestinal tract not only because

Table 4. Gastric Decontamination Methods[12-15,24,36,37]

Method	Mechanism	Indications	Contraindications	Adverse Effects	Comments
Syrup of ipecac	Alkaloids emetine and cephaline activate vomiting center in CRTZ and act directly in small intestine; vomiting usually occurs within 20 minutes	Not recommended for use; can be considered in potentially toxic ingestions presenting within 1 hour in alert patient; clinical benefit has not been demonstrated	Caustic, hydrocarbon, battery, and sharp ingestions; ingestions expected to cause altered level of consciousness; significant prior vomiting; nontoxic ingestion	Persistent vomiting, sedation, vagal bradycardia, delay of definitive therapy, esophageal tear, pneumomediastinum (rare); relatively safe when used appropriately	May be most useful in large ingestions when/where AC not effective; early administration can result in significant returns, so availability in remote areas may be prudent; alternative cause should be suspected for vomiting > 2 hours after dose; use requires expectation of normal state of consciousness at least 1 hour after use; because of very limited clinical utility, reported use has decreased from 15% of exposures in 1985 to less than 0.01% of exposures in 2014; availability limited; U.S. production halted
Gastric lavage	Gastric intubation with 22- to 28-Fr orogastric tube; patient placed in left lateral decubitus position; 10–15 mL of warm saline/kg administered and removed	Life-threatening ingestions presenting within 1 hour; risk-benefit assessment recommended (e.g., iron tablet ingestion; anti-cholinergic or other agents that may slow gut motility, or agents that may form bezoars, like aspirin)	Hydrocarbon, caustic ingestions, unprotected airway, patient at risk of hemorrhage or perforation, head trauma, uncooperative patient (relative)	Airway or esophageal injury, hypoxia, electrolyte and core temperature disturbances	Saline should be used in children to prevent electrolyte disturbances; process is physically and emotionally traumatic in children; airway protection is imperative because children often vomit during tube placement; tube size in small children is prohibitive, contributing to decline in use of this method; in rare cases lavage is deemed useful should only be performed by properly trained caregivers
Activated charcoal	Reversible adsorption, possibly by hydrogen/ ionic binding, van der Waals forces; high surface area maximizes adsorption	Potentially toxic ingestions when administered within 1 hour (e.g., acetaminophen, aspirin, and most ingestions not in contraindication list)	Caustic, alcohol, metal, hydrocarbon ingestions; ileus, gastric, or intestinal perforation	Vomiting (from AC or NG tube placement) more common if coadministered with sorbitol; aspiration; bowel injury rare but severe	Unpalatable because of thick, gritty texture; if not premixed, combine with water or cola in a 1:8 ratio, disguise preparation, or administer by NG tube; airway must be protected; sorbitol should only be given with initial dose, if at all
Whole bowel irrigation	Polyethylene glycol and electrolyte solution flushes gastrointestinal tract	Very large ingestions when poor outcome is likely; SR or EC product poisonings, iron, potassium, or lithium, particularly in those presenting > 2 hours after ingestion; ingestions when AC is ineffective; removal of drug packets from gastrointestinal tract	Ileus, gastrointestinal hemorrhage, perforation, obstruction, uncontrolled vomiting, diarrhea with volume depletion or hemodynamic instability	Vomiting, bloating, cramping; colonic perforation, esophageal tears, aspiration rare	Balanced solution prevents electrolyte imbalances; continue until effluent clear or no opacities on radiograph if present before therapy; may be useful in select poisonings but clinical benefit unproven

AC = activated charcoal; CRTZ = chemoreceptor trigger zone; EC = enteric coated; Fr = French; NG = nasogastric; SR = sustained release.
Reprinted with permission from Haase MR. Poisoning and envenomation. In: Richardson M, Chant C, Chessman KH, et al., eds. Pharmacotherapy Self-Assessment Program, seventh ed. Pediatrics. Lenexa, KS: American College of Clinical Pharmacy, 2010:53.

of ingestion but also because of diffusion from the circulation back into the lumen of the gut. Drug concentrations in the circulation decline as metabolism and elimination occur, limiting the amount of drug that can diffuse back into the gut lumen. Administration of AC causes enhanced elimination of drug from the gut through adsorption and elimination in the stool. This process results in a "sink," described by an increased drug gradient between the circulation and the gut lumen, allowing more drug to diffuse into the gut lumen where it can be adsorbed by AC and eliminated. Repeated administration of AC enhances this process of gastric dialysis of certain drugs.

Clinical outcome data are scant to support the use of MDAC. However, there may be benefit in treating poisoning from agents to which children are exposed, including phenobarbital, carbamazepine, theophylline, amitriptyline, digoxin, and phenytoin.[38] Publications since the 1999 American Academy of Clinical Toxicology position statement have shown mixed efficacy.[27,28,32,41,42] However, in large overdoses when protein binding is exceeded, enterohepatic recirculation occurs, or absorption or first-pass metabolism is slowed, MDAC may be clinically useful.[10] If MDAC is used, then a standard loading dose should be given, followed by 0.5 g/kg every 4–6 hours for up to 24 hours or until the patient's condition has improved or drug serum concentrations are no longer in the toxic range.[38,43]

An important consideration is the potential for AC to adsorb not only the ingested poison, but also other agents used in managing the poisoning. For example, AC causes a statistically significant decrease in the absorption of acetylcysteine when administered concurrently. Clinically, this effect does not appear to be significant. However, the interaction can be minimized by separating the administration of the two agents by 1–2 hours or using the intravenous acetylcysteine preparation.[44]

WHOLE BOWEL IRRIGATION

Whole bowel irrigation (WBI) is performed using a polyethylene glycol and electrolyte solution to essentially flush out the gastrointestinal tract. This preparation prevents electrolyte abnormalities associated with older cathartics such as sodium phosphate.[45] Use should be considered in patients who have overdosed sustained-release or enteric-coated drugs, ingested iron or other metals, or acted as carriers of illicit drug packages. Some investigations have used WBI in overdoses when it would not be considered clinically (e.g., acetaminophen), and use of WBI could potentially decrease the adsorptive capacity of AC.[10,46]

The solution can be given orally, but in children, administration by nasogastric tube is often easier. Small children should receive 0.5 L/hour, whereas older children and adolescents should receive 1.5–2 L/hour. The older patient should sit on a toilet, whereas diapers are required in small children and infants. Administration for up to 4–6 hours may be necessary to achieve a clear effluent.[45] Several products are available for WBI, including GoLYTELY (Braintree Laboratories, Inc., Braintree, MA), NuLYTELY (Braintree Laboratories), and CoLyte (Meda Pharmaceuticals, Somerset, NJ), and these

may be flavored for palatability. However, MiraLAX (Bayer HealthCare, Whippany, NJ), commonly used for managing constipation in children, should not be used for WBI because it contains no electrolytes, increasing the risk of electrolyte abnormalities.[45]

REVIEW OF MANAGEMENT OF SELECT POISONINGS

A review of the management of multiple toxic exposures is beyond the scope of this chapter. However, poisonings occur that have several aspects of management specific to the pediatric population, although perhaps not the most common statistically. Analgesics, particularly acetaminophen, are quite commonly ingested by children, and the toxic dose differs from that of adults on a kilogram basis. Antidote therapy for toxic alcohol exposure has changed in recent years, and additional pediatric data have guided the management of these exposures in children. Management of snakebites in children is similar to that in adults, but many issues need to be considered when administering antivenin to children. Care of children who have ingested or been exposed to these three toxins is discussed in the following paragraphs.

ACETAMINOPHEN

When dosed therapeutically, acetaminophen has a very good safety profile in children.[47-49] Acetaminophen is also widely available in many dosage forms and drug combinations. Therefore, it is not surprising that in 2017, almost 25,000 toxic exposures to acetaminophen alone occurred in children younger than 6 years; this does not include acetaminophen combination products.[2] Overall, acetaminophen combination products and acetaminophen alone were the sixth and seventh most common toxins associated with death, respectively, involved in almost 15% of all poisoning fatalities combined. Outcomes in children are generally good.[2] However, acetaminophen is the most commonly identified cause of acute liver failure in children.[50]

After absorption, around 90% of an acetaminophen dose is glucuronidated and sulfated. These metabolites, and a small percentage of unchanged drug, are eliminated in the urine. The rest is metabolized by the cytochrome P450 system to a toxic metabolite, N-acetyl-p-benzoquinonimine (NAPQI). This metabolite is rapidly toxic to liver cells, but natural stores of glutathione conjugate it, and this complex is eliminated in the urine. In an overdose, glutathione stores become depleted, NAPQI is no longer detoxified, and direct liver damage results.[44] In untreated patients, acetaminophen toxicity typically progresses through the following four stages. In *stage 1*, after ingestion, gastrointestinal symptoms such as nausea and vomiting predominate, although patients may be asymptomatic. No liver damage has occurred yet. *Stage 2* may occur as early as 12 hours in large overdoses, but typically by 24–36 hours after ingestion, there is evidence of *acetaminophen-induced hepatotoxicity*, defined as aspartate aminotransferase concentrations greater than 1000 IU/L. *In stage 3*, maximal liver damage occurs, 3–4 days after ingestion. Patients may experience fulminant hepatic failure, encephalopathy, coma, and hemorrhage. Alanine aminotransferase and aspartate aminotransferase may exceed 10,000 IU/L, and elevations in prothrombin time and international normalized ratio are possible. Kidney damage can occur with or without the presence of liver toxicity, but it more often occurs shortly afterward. The incidence of kidney injury is unclear and is thought to be a rare event; however, it has been reported to be as high as 8.9%.[44,51,52] Death occurs in 3–5 days because of multiple organ failure. *Survival to stage 4* should result in recovery of liver function, with laboratory values returning to normal within 1 month.[44] Of note, although published data suggest a wide variation in outcomes, risk of fulminant or fatal hepatotoxicity is significant in patients with acetaminophen poisoning who do not receive treatment. However, even without treatment, fatality rates likely do not exceed 20%.[53]

The decision to initiate therapy for acetaminophen poisoning is dictated by the amount ingested. Acute ingestions of 7.5–15 g in adults or 150 mg/kg in children have conventionally been considered toxic. However, a recent publication in patients 12 years or older attempting to link reported dose to antidote requirement suggested that exposure to less than 10 g results in a 10% chance or less of treatment need.[54] In children, no data support this 150 mg/kg exposure limit, and it is unlikely that significant liver toxicity would occur with doses less than 200 mg/kg.[55-57] With the recent U.S. Food and Drug Administration (FDA) labeling of intravenous acetaminophen in the United States, 10-fold dosing errors have become a concern. Toxicity has been reported in children with intravenous acetaminophen in doses well under 200 mg/kg.[58-60] However, in most cases, exposure to intravenous acetaminophen should result in no more risk than an oral exposure, and management of a potentially toxic dose should be similar to the approach to an oral ingestion.[61] Still, some advocate for initiation of treatment after a dose of 60 mg/kg or more of the intravenous product.[44,58] Even though acetaminophen is absorbed relatively quickly and an effective antidote exists, gastric decontamination can be considered if the patient presents early after ingestion. Gastric lavage and SOI are typically not indicated. Activated charcoal can be given within 1–2 hours after ingestion and may help keep serum concentrations below the treatment line of the Rumack-Matthew nomogram.[44] The Rumack-Matthew nomogram (Figure 1) permits a single acetaminophen concentration obtained at least 4 hours after ingestion to be used to assess the risk of hepatotoxicity.[44] The treatment line, at 25% below the dotted line in Figure 1, is used to justify antidote therapy. If the serum concentration is on or above the treatment line between 4 and 24 hours, therapy is initiated. Of note, the Rumack-Matthew nomogram is validated only for use in single, acute, oral ingestions. The toxicity risk of the extended-release acetaminophen product can be reliably assessed because peak acetaminophen concentrations occur in a time frame similar to that of immediate-release products. However, if the initial serum concentration is below the treatment line, it is prudent to repeat a measurement at about 8 hours after ingestion to confirm risk assessment because a small percentage of patients may cross above the treatment line.

Antidote therapy is provided with acetylcysteine. It can prevent hepatotoxicity by providing a substrate for glutathione production and binding NAPQI directly, and it can decrease present hepatotoxicity by free radical scavenging and antioxidant effects.[62] Acetylcysteine may be administered orally or intravenously. Some authors have suggested that the oral route be used in patients presenting within 8–10 hours of ingestion and that intravenous acetylcysteine be administered when presenting 10 hours or more after ingestion,[63] whereas others have suggested that the opposite approach is true.[64,65] However, in most cases, it appears efficacy should be equivalent, particularly when given within 8 hours.[59,64] One apparent advantage to intravenous administration is the 21-hour infusion time (150 mg/kg over 1 hour; then 50 mg/kg over 4 hours; then 100 mg/kg over 16 hours) compared with the 72-hour oral regimen (140 mg/kg for the first dose; then 70 mg/kg every 4 hours for 17 doses). This opportunity for decreased length of hospital stay offsets the higher cost of the intravenous acetylcysteine product. However, several authors have found that shorter courses of the oral product may be as effective as the traditional 72-hour regimen.[66-68] Use of these shorter regimens would make the oral route more cost-effective. The cases for which the intravenous formulation likely should be favored are in patients who already have liver failure, patients with intractable vomiting, and pregnant patients.[44]

Both formulations have proved to be safe in acetaminophen overdose. The most common adverse events with oral administration are nausea, vomiting, and diarrhea, whereas anaphylactoid reactions (rarely serious) are more common with the intravenous preparation.[62,65,69] An additional consideration with standard dilution of the intravenous product is the potential for excess free water administration, resulting in hyponatremia and seizures. In younger patients, more concentrated solutions should be administered.[62,70] For example, in adults, the three infusions are given in volumes of 200 mL, 500 mL, and 1000 mL, respectively, resulting in concentrations ranging from about 40 mg/mL to less than 5 mg/mL. To prevent the development of hyponatremia in children, the product should be diluted to a concentration of 40 mg/mL for all three phases.

ETHYLENE GLYCOL AND METHANOL

Ethylene glycol and methanol pose serious risks to children because they can be found in the home in several different products, and very small amounts can be deadly in small children.[71,72] Ethylene glycol is the primary ingredient in engine coolant, and the sweet taste increases the likelihood of significant ingestion in unsuspecting children and pets. Methanol can be found in solvents, antifreeze, fuels, and photocopying fluid, but it is most often encountered in windshield washer fluid.[73,74] In 2017, there were 5583 single exposures to ethylene glycol (about 9% of cases were in children younger than 6 years), and almost 1200 (15% in children younger than 6 years) single exposures to methanol products were reported. There were 16 fatalities from exposures to these alcohols overall, but none in children.[2]

Aside from central nervous system depression, ethylene glycol and methanol are not in themselves responsible for the toxic effects. In the first several hours after exposure,

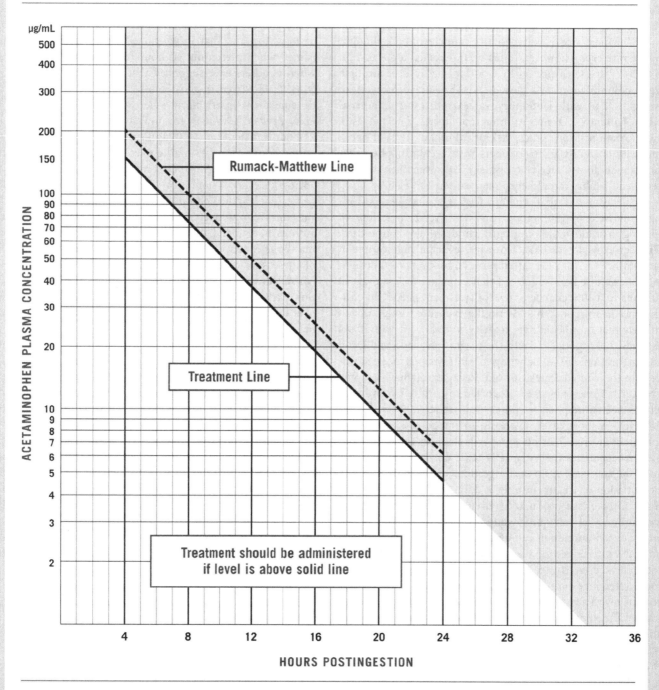

Figure 1. Rumack-Matthew nomogram.

Reprinted with permission from McGraw-Hill. Hendrickson RG, McKeown NJ. 33. Acetaminophen. In: Nelson LS, Howland M, Lewin NA, et al., eds. Goldfrank's Toxicologic Emergencies, 11e. New York, NY: McGraw-Hill; 2019. Available at http://accesspharmacy.mhmedical.com/content.aspx?bookid=2569&Sectionid=210270383. Accessed June 20, 2019.

patients with ethylene glycol ingestions may present with decreased mental status, ataxia, slurred speech, and, in larger ingestions, coma. During this time, ethylene glycol is metabolized by alcohol dehydrogenase to glycoaldehyde and then by aldehyde dehydrogenase to glycolic acid (most responsible for metabolic acidosis), which is further metabolized to glyoxylic acid and oxalic acid.[73,74] In the 12–24 hours after ingestion, these metabolites result in cardiopulmonary compromise such as respiratory distress, tachycardia, congestive heart failure, and cardiovascular collapse. From 1–3 days after ingestion, nephrotoxicity predominates because of calcium precipitation of oxalic acid in renal tubules. Significant hypocalcemia leading to tetany or changes in electrocardiogram may occur as well.[72-74] Methanol is metabolized by alcohol dehydrogenase to formaldehyde and then by aldehyde dehydrogenase to formic acid, which is most responsible for metabolic acidosis.[73] Symptoms in the first 12–24 hours after ingestion include depressed mental status and tachypnea. The accumulation of formic acid can result in hallmark visual disturbances such as blurriness (termed *snow field vision*) and blindness, which can be permanent.[75] Other signs and symptoms can include gastrointestinal distress, headache, shock, and seizures.[72-74]

Initial management includes supportive care and efforts to resolve metabolic acidosis. Laboratory evaluation should include serum chemistries, lactate, and ionized calcium. Serum ethylene glycol or methanol concentrations should be obtained if available, although at many institutions, this measurement must be sent to a reference laboratory, limiting clinical utility; although controversial, serum concentrations of ethylene glycol and methanol above 25 mg/dL are considered toxic. Anion gap and osmolar gap calculations can be completed to assist in diagnosing exposures. However, a normal gap does not rule out clinically significant poisoning.[73]

Gastric decontamination is, in most cases, not recommended in toxic alcohol ingestions. Syrup of ipecac is not indicated because of central nervous system depression, and AC does not effectively adsorb alcohols.[43] It may be useful to insert a nasogastric tube to aspirate stomach contents in intubated patients in some cases, particularly in large ingestions for which absorption may be delayed.[73] Other potentially helpful supportive measures include administering folic acid in methanol poisoning and giving pyridoxine and thiamine in ethylene glycol poisoning to enhance the elimination of toxic metabolites.[72-74,76-78] Folic acid or folinic acid can be given intravenously at 1 mg/kg (maximal dose 50 mg) every 4–6 hours for 24 hours or until methanol and formic acid have been eliminated. Pyridoxine and thiamine can be given intravenously in doses of 100 mg/day until ethylene glycol is eliminated. Data regarding the efficacy of these adjunctive therapies are limited, but the risk–benefit ratio is sufficiently low that they should be administered in all patients.

Definitive therapy is aimed at preventing the metabolism of ethylene glycol or methanol to its more toxic metabolites. Historically, the only available option has been ethanol, which has an affinity for alcohol dehydrogenase several times that of ethylene glycol and methanol.[79] This characteristic prevents the accumulation of toxic metabolites and allows renal and pulmonary elimination of the parent alcohols. Ethanol has been used safely in children, and it can be given intravenously or orally, with the goal of maintaining serum concentrations of 100–150 mg/dL. This concentration can typically be achieved by administering an intravenous loading dose of 8 mL/kg of 10% ethanol over 1 hour, followed by an infusion of 0.8 mL/kg/hour. Serum ethanol concentrations will need to be obtained often because of the variability in patient pharmacokinetics.[79] However, use of ethanol has several disadvantages. Administration of intravenous ethanol requires a central venous catheter because of the high osmolarity. Ethanol can contribute to central nervous system and respiratory depression, and it may cause hypothermia, hypoglycemia, and hyponatremia, necessitating intensive care monitoring.[79,80] In addition, repeated serum ethanol concentrations are required because metabolic rates vary significantly, and although ethanol can be used safely in children, the potential for significant adverse reactions exists.[74,81] If used, ethanol should be continued until ethylene glycol or methanol concentrations are less than 25 mg/dL.

Fomepizole (4-methylpyrazole) was made available for use in the United States in 1997. It is a competitive alcohol dehydrogenase inhibitor with an affinity several thousand times that of ethanol for alcohol dehydrogenase.[71,82] Fomepizole is effective in the management of both ethylene glycol and methanol ingestions.[80,81,83,84] Several advantages of fomepizole over ethanol are as follows: no alteration in level of consciousness; no effect on blood glucose or electrolytes; no requirement of central venous access; and no requirement for intensive care if the patient is stable. Perhaps of more importance, fomepizole appears to be associated with fewer errors during administration.[85] Patients should receive a loading dose of 15 mg/kg, followed by 10 mg/kg every 12 hours for four doses, and then 15 mg/kg every 12 hours until serum ethylene glycol or methanol concentrations are less than 25 mg/dL.[82] A course of fomepizole costs about 4 times that of a course of ethanol. However, the lack of need for intensive care monitoring likely makes fomepizole more cost-effective than ethanol, and this drug has become first-line therapy in toxic alcohol ingestions.[71,80,86,87] The need for hemodialysis as a treatment modality has decreased significantly since fomepizole became available. However, hemodialysis still may be necessary in patients with severe acidosis, end-organ toxicity, serum concentrations of ethylene glycol or methanol above 50 mg/dL, large ingestions, or late presentation, in whom significant metabolite buildup has occurred and inhibition of alcohol dehydrogenase would be ineffective.[72,73]

CROTALINE ENVENOMATIONS

Crotaline snakes (Viperidae, subfamily Crotalinae) include the rattlesnake, copperhead, and cottonmouth. These snakes are also referred to as *pit vipers* because they have a heat-sensing pit posterior to the nostrils. Additional features that distinguish the Crotaline snakes from nonvenomous North American snakes include a triangle-shaped head, visible fangs, and elliptical pupils.[88,89] It is estimated that 8000 snakebites occur annually in the United States.[88] In 2017, 4075 envenomations caused by crotaline snakes were reported.[2]

Crotaline venom contains a large number of substances, including enzymes, peptides, amino acids, metallic ions, lipids, and carbohydrates. These components are present in varying quantities and potencies, depending on the age and nutritional status of the snake, geographic region, season, and climate. Once injected, venom is absorbed through lymphatic and venous drainage. The venom then results in local tissue damage, including capillary endothelial destruction, leading to leakage of plasma and red blood cells into tissues, causing significant edema, erythema, and ecchymosis.[89,90] After local tissue destruction, hematologic toxicity is the most prominent effect of venom and includes coagulopathy, hemolysis, and thrombocytopenia.[88,91] Prothrombin times may be extremely high, even early after a bite, and platelet counts may be very low. Although local and hematologic effects predominate, respiratory, cardiovascular, and neurologic effects may manifest as well. Symptom severity caused by envenomation is related to the amount of venom injected, which depends on fang penetration, the amount of time the snake is allowed to bite, and the length of time since the snake last expended venom. About one-fourth of bites are "dry," meaning no venom is released by the snake.[89,90] The severity of the envenomation can be assessed by one of several scoring systems.[92,93] In general, scoring is as follows: (1) with minimal envenomation, there is local pain and swelling only, with no systemic manifestations; (2) with moderate envenomation, there is local tissue involvement in addition to non–life-threatening systemic signs and symptoms with possible coagulation abnormalities, but no evidence of bleeding; (3) with severe envenomation, there is local tissue damage in addition to altered mental status, hypotension, tachycardia, and coagulation abnormalities with severe bleeding or possible severe bleeding.[71,91]

After envenomation, symptoms usually occur within several minutes, if not immediately. Patient presentation includes fear, anxiety, intense pain (more than would be expected from the size of the wound), weakness, and dizziness. Those with more severe envenomations can present with altered mental status, tachycardia, visual disturbances, and a metallic taste.[89] Prehospital supportive care involves first moving the victim away from the snake and then transporting the victim to a health care facility as soon as possible. It is not recommended to search for or to try to capture or kill the snake. Instead, the focus should be on calming the patient and keeping him or her warm, and the affected limb should be immobilized and positioned below heart level. Tight-fitting clothing and jewelry such as wedding bands should be removed. Application of ice or tourniquets, incision or excision of the wound, or use of suction devices is highly discouraged.[89,90] Emergency department management involves first ensuring airway, breathing, and circulation. A detailed history of the event, as well as any comorbid conditions and allergy history, should be obtained. A detailed physical examination should be performed, and the initial laboratory evaluation should include a complete blood cell count, platelet count, coagulation studies, serum electrolytes, and urinalysis.[89,90]

Definitive therapy for crotaline envenomation was formerly provided with antivenin (Crotalidae) polyvalent, an equine-derived whole immune globulin antibody formulation.

This preparation, in use since the 1950s, has proved to be effective and significantly reduced mortality caused by Crotalidae envenomations. However, 25%–50% of patients receiving antivenin (Crotalidae) polyvalent had an acute reaction, including vomiting, rash, dyspnea, cyanosis, and anaphylaxis, and the rate of serum sickness ranged from almost 20% to more than 80% of patients.[94] Antivenin (Crotalidae) polyvalent is no longer manufactured.

In 2000, Crotalidae polyvalent immune Fab antivenom (FabAV) was approved for use. This product is indicated for treating the victims of envenomation by North American crotaline snakes. It is a monovalent ovine Fab derived by inoculating sheep with the venom of the western diamondback, eastern diamondback, Mojave rattlesnake, or cottonmouth rattlesnake, although case reports suggest efficacy against several other types of snake as well.[94-98] The final product is a lyophilized mixture of antibodies from all four antivenins.[99] Crotalidae polyvalent immune Fab antivenom binds venom that has reached the intravascular space, and the complex is eliminated renally. The Fab fragments are small enough to reach interstitial spaces, preventing further tissue damage.[88]

The severity of the envenomation determines the FabAV dose. Of note, dosing is not based on the size of the child. This antivenom works by neutralizing a specific amount of venom; thus, the dosing recommendations apply to both children and adults. From 4 to 6 vials, each containing up to 1 g of total protein, should be administered over 1 hour in 250 mL of normal saline. If the venom has been neutralized (no progression of local tissue damage; normalization of systemic signs and symptoms and coagulation disturbances), a maintenance regimen of 2 vials every 6 hours for up to 18 hours should be administered. If, after 1 hour, control of the envenomation is not achieved, an additional dose of 4–6 vials should be administered; this regimen should be repeated until signs and symptoms have ceased to progress. Ideally, administration should occur within 4–6 hours of the bite.[99]

Although a relatively small amount of literature describes the use of FabAV in children, it is proven to be effective in managing pediatric snakebite victims.[100-104] Most patients achieve initial control with the first dose. Still, delayed complications, including recurrent coagulopathy, have been reported in children despite initial therapeutic success.[105,106] Follow-up within 1 week after discharge seems prudent. This antivenom appears to be well tolerated in children. Overall, adverse events are less common with FabAV than with antivenin (Crotalidae) polyvalent because only about 10% to 20% of patients experience acute and delayed reactions.[94] However, later data in children and adults suggest adverse event rates appear to be lower.[107,108] The infusion rate may contribute to adverse events, necessitating dose titration. It is recommended that the initial infusion be given at 25 mL/hour for the first 10 minutes. This rate may be increased as tolerated up to 250 mL/hour, although the infusion should be given over at least 1 hour.[92,99] Pretreatment with diphenhydramine may be considered, and epinephrine, albuterol, and corticosteroids should be available during an acute reaction.

An additional administration concern in children is volume overload, particularly in infants or in large envenomations requiring several doses of FabAV. Although there are no published reports of volume overload occurring, caution should be taken in children with pulmonary, cardiac, or renal conditions. Some institutions provide the initial 4- to 6-vial dose in 2-vial increments in 100 mL of normal saline, which may guard against potential volume overload in small children.[92] Such incremental dosing may also prevent waste if it is determined that the entire dose is not necessary. This approach is important because acquisition costs can exceed $2000 per vial or gram. Time to reconstitute vials must be considered as well. The package insert recommends diluting vials in 10 mL of sterile water for injection before final preparation. This can take several minutes; thus, early notification of the pharmacy department is important in providing rapid administration. Some data suggest that diluting each vial in 25 mL of sterile water for injection and then hand-mixing will result in significant decreases in reconstitution times.[109]

In October 2018, a new equine immune Fab (Crotalidae Immune F(ab')₂ (Equine) – Anavip; Rare Disease Therapeutics, Inc., Franklin, TN) was made available for the treatment of rattlesnake envenomation in adults and children.[110] There are several differences between the two products, including: ovine versus equine source; purification process in manufacturing; venom used in production obtained from snakes in different geographical regions; and, it appears most importantly, molecular weight and pharmacokinetics, especially elimination half-life.[111] The equine product appears to be more effective at preventing recurrent coagulopathy that can often require readmission and further treatment with antivenom several days after the initial treatment of the bite. It will likely require some time to determine if this advantage will result in more effective treatment of crotalidae envenomations in various geographical regions.

MANAGEMENT OF OTHER COMMON PEDIATRIC EXPOSURES

As noted, most pediatric toxic exposures result in minimal to no effects. Many calls to the poison center involve exposures to essentially harmless substances, such as cosmetics, toothpaste, and crayons (although it is of note that colognes and perfumes contain significant amounts of ethanol and can result in significant toxicity). Other common exposures like household cleaners, foreign bodies (batteries), and cough and cold preparations, although usually not serious, can result in significant toxicity. A discussion of these exposures is provided in the following section.

HOUSEHOLD CLEANER AND CAUSTIC EXPOSURE

In 2017, household cleaning substances were the second most commonly reported exposure in children younger than 6 years; in fact, these substances are the second most commonly reported exposure overall.[2] Yet the number of children younger than 6 years requiring emergency department management of injuries from household product exposure has decreased significantly.[112] Examples of household cleaner products encountered include bleaches, detergents, and soaps. Examples of caustics include acids and alkalis found in products such as toilet, drain, and oven cleaners.

In most pediatric exposures to these substances, there is no intent to self-harm, so ingestion or exposure quantities are likely to be limited, minimizing the risk of an adverse outcome. However, even with small to moderate exposure, symptoms may be observed. Ingestion of detergents and soaps may result in drooling, nausea, vomiting, gastric pain, and respiratory distress, if aspirated. Some products, if sufficiently alkaline, may result in esophageal injury, whereas strong acids are more likely to cause gastric injury.[113] Bleach exposure presents similarly, although the risk of esophageal injury is low with household-strength preparations (usually 3% sodium hypochlorite). Medical management in most children involves supportive care. Fluids may be offered to the asymptomatic or mildly symptomatic child, and observation is typically sufficient.[114] Vomiting should not be induced.[115,116] Neutralization—offering acidic beverages in alkaline ingestions and alkaline beverages in acidic ingestions—should not be performed. After large ingestions or ingestions of highly concentrated substances, endoscopy, surgical, and further medical and pharmacological intervention such as corticosteroids, proton pump inhibitors, or antibiotics may be necessary.[116-118]

FOREIGN BODY INGESTION

Foreign body ingestion can include coins, toys, disc batteries, and ornaments. Unless the object is composed of a significantly toxic agent (e.g., lead) or is aspirated, management usually consists of observation, although manual removal may be necessary in esophageal impaction. However, disc batteries, because of their composition, present further risk. In 2017, more than 3400 disc battery exposures were reported.[2] Most batteries are obtained by children from products such as games, hearing aids, watches, calculators, and remote controls.[119]

In most cases of battery ingestion, the disc passes the esophagus into the stomach. From there, it usually passes through the intestinal tract within 1–2 weeks and results in no symptoms. However, the battery may become lodged in the esophagus and result in serious and life-threatening complications such as burns, perforations, and fistulae.[120-122] This damage is caused by alkaline electrolyte leakage from the battery, pressure necrosis, and external current generation when the battery comes in contact with tissue.[119,122,123] Signs and symptoms include vomiting, diarrhea, abdominal pain, fever, refusal to eat or drink, and dysphagia.[121] When impaction occurs, the battery should be removed immediately. Of note, in addition to the esophagus, one may encounter children with batteries lodged in the nose, ears, or other body cavities, and it is important in these cases to remove the battery as soon as possible as well. The larger the battery, the more likely impaction will occur. Battery diameter can range from just more than 5 mm–25 mm, and children ingesting batteries of 20 mm in diameter or more are more likely to develop significant complications.[119] In addition to the national poison hotline, a national battery ingestion hotline available at (800) 498-8666 exists to provide guidance in managing an ingestion. The following website at the National Capital Poison Center provides further information: www.poison.org/battery.

COUGH AND COLD PREPARATIONS

Little, if any, evidence supports the use of cough and cold preparations in children for the management of cold symptoms.[124,125] In fact, evidence exists that these preparations are associated with fatalities and apparent life-threatening events.[126-128] Pseudoephedrine is most commonly associated with fatalities. In most instances of death reported in these publications, the drug was given at home and at higher-than-recommended doses. Often, the child was given several drugs with similar ingredients, the dose measurement was inaccurate, an adult formulation was used, or the child was given doses by multiple caregivers.

In 2007, an FDA Advisory Panel recommended that these drugs be avoided in children younger than 6 years, although the FDA still recommends that they be avoided in children younger than 2 years. However, partly because of this recommendation, manufacturers have voluntarily withdrawn cough and cold products intended for children younger than 2 years, and the Consumer Healthcare Products Association has updated labels to state that use should be avoided in children younger than 4 years. Since that time, evidence shows that use of over-the-counter cough and cold products and reports of adverse events and toxicity from use in young children has decreased.[129-132]

Management of toxicity from these products is primarily supportive, as discussed previously in this chapter. Gastric decontamination, primarily AC, can be used if the patient presents early and the airway is protected. Symptomatic therapy may be necessary, including the management of hypertension (e.g., labetalol, nicardipine, clonidine, nitroprusside), arrhythmias (e.g., lidocaine, amiodarone, procainamide), and seizures (e.g., benzodiazepines, phenytoin, levetiracetam).

CAREGIVER ROLE IN POISON PREVENTION

Whereas most toxic exposures in children are not serious, a few steps taken by parents and caregivers can help prevent serious or fatal outcomes from poisonings. Many poison centers publish guides on their websites; for example, the Texas Poison Center Network provides *A Parent's Guide to Poison Prevention*.[133] Information for caregivers may include: lists of medications or substances that are common in the home that can be very dangerous to young children; poison prevention tips; and the Poison Help phone number at (800) 222-1222.

CONCLUSIONS

Although most toxic exposures occur in the pediatric population, serious or fatal outcomes are quite rare. The American Association of Poison Control Centers and the National Poison Data System provide health care professionals with information that can shape public health and educational efforts. Any pharmacist or health care professional involved in the care of children should be familiar with this resource.

Medical management of the poisoned child can be similar to that of an adult patient in many respects. However, obtaining an accurate history, particularly the amount ingested, can be difficult, making physical and laboratory examination and patient presentation key to effective management. Knowledge of and familiarity with available resources, especially the poison control center, will help clinicians of any experience level provide the best care for pediatric patients who have been poisoned.

Patient Case — ACETAMINOPHEN OVERDOSE

A 3-year-old, 15-kg boy who was found to have eaten two full 24-count bottles of 80-mg chewable acetaminophen tablets (given to him by his 4-year old sister who obliged him when he asked for candy) is brought to the emergency department. His parents found him finishing the last of the tablets about 2 hours before presentation. The child has been previously healthy and is on no chronic medications.

On physical examination, the patient is a cooperative child who appears healthy and in no apparent distress; other examination findings are within normal limits. Vital signs are blood pressure 96/54 mmHg, heart rate 104 beats/minute, respiratory rate 18 breaths/minute, and Tmax 98.6°F (37°C).

1. What are the key components of the initial evaluation of this child?

A thorough history provided by child's parents is of utmost importance. Given that the sister gave the child the acetaminophen, it is crucial to ascertain whether any other medications or substances could have been ingested. Fortunately, in cases such as this, parents are typically very thorough and cooperative in their investigation and contribution to the history of the event. In this case, it is clear that an acetaminophen ingestion occurred, and no other substances were ingested.

The physical assessment is important as well. In this case, there are no outward signs of toxicity—vital signs are normal, and

the physical examination findings, including fluid status, skin color and tone, pulses, and neurological status, are also normal. If the toxin is unknown, then a clinician could make use of the classic presentations of certain toxins (*toxidromes*) to aid in identifying the ingested substance. Table 3 provides examples of toxidromes.

Laboratory analysis is important in determining the extent of an exposure or ingestion. The history of the ingestion can provide direction for specific laboratory studies to be ordered, although it is usual practice to at least obtain a serum chemistry. Of course, if concentrations of a suspected toxin can be readily measured, this assessment should be done at the appropriate time.

2. What methods of decontamination should be attempted, if any, in this child?

Gastric decontamination should be used sparingly because there is little evidence that these procedures improve outcomes in poisoned patients. The decision to perform gastric decontamination will depend primarily on the substance ingested (including the amount and likelihood of a severe or life-threatening course) and the time elapsed from ingestion to presentation at health care facility. In this case, syrup of ipecac is not indicated; in fact, it is no longer recommended in poisoned patients. Neither is gastric lavage indicated for this patient because it is not effective and it carries serious risks. Although whole bowel irrigation is theoretically useful, it would unlikely be of clinical benefit in an acetaminophen overdose. Activated charcoal could be considered because the patient was evaluated within 1–2 hours, and absorption of acetaminophen could be lessened. If activated charcoal were used, a reasonable dose would be 15 g given one time orally or by nasogastric tube. However, because this case is a single ingestion of acetaminophen presenting very early, the most impactful intervention will be administration of the antidote.

3. A serum acetaminophen concentration is obtained 4 hours after ingestion is 223 mcg/mL. How should the child be managed?

In any ingestion, airway, breathing, and circulation must be assessed. Baseline serum chemistry including liver transaminases, complete blood count, and coagulation studies should be obtained. Given that the child ingested just more than 250 mg/kg, it can likely be assumed that a 4-hour concentration is in the toxic range. Therefore, the antidote, acetylcysteine, would be initiated before the first acetaminophen concentration being drawn.

For this patient, the concentration is found to be above the treatment line, so acetylcysteine should and will be administered. Because the child presented early, oral and intravenous administration should be equally effective. The intravenous regimen may be preferred because it would be complete in less than 24 hours, whereas the traditional oral regimen schedule is 72 hours, which prolongs admission time. Even though oral acetylcysteine is less expensive than the intravenous form, the 3-day course and hospital stay would eliminate that cost advantage. However, shorter oral treatment regimens are effective, even being given only until the acetaminophen concentration is undetectable, and no coagulation or liver transaminase abnormalities have been noted. Thus, an abbreviated oral regimen could be used in this case, and the patient discharged in a similar time frame as if the intravenous regimen were given, avoiding hospitalization costs. If the intravenous regimen were chosen, it is important to make sure the dilution is the same 40 mg/mL for all three phases of dosing.

4. What supportive care measures and follow-up evaluations should be performed?

Supportive care measures in overdose are often not specific to a particular toxin and may apply to many patients. In this case, supportive care includes maintaining adequate hydration, in part by managing nausea or vomiting; typically, this management is all that is necessary, especially if the antidote is administered within 8 hours of ingestion. Beyond that approach, managing hepatic or kidney injury—should these effects occur—is paramount. Blood glucose monitoring or vitamin K administration may be useful in a patient with liver damage, and, if severe, blood product administration may be necessary to reverse coagulopathy.

Continued monitoring depends in part on the acetaminophen and initial hepatic transaminase concentrations. If the initial aspartate transaminase concentration is normal, then re-evaluation after completion of the antidote is recommended. If this concentration is elevated, then coagulation studies and kidney function should be assessed and repeated at least every 24 hours. In practice, a complete metabolic panel (including hepatic transaminase, albumin, alkaline phosphatase, and bilirubin), together with coagulation studies, is often obtained with initial laboratory studies. Acetaminophen concentrations are usually obtained until it is no longer detectable.

REFERENCES

1. Hines EQ, Fine JS. 31: Pediatric Principles. In: Nelson LS, Howland M, Lewin NA, et al., eds. Goldfrank's Toxicologic Emergencies, 11e. New York, NY: McGraw-Hill, 2019. Available at http://accesspharmacy.mhmedical.com/content.aspx?bookid=2569&Sectionid=210270170. Accessed June 20, 2019.
2. Gummin DD, Mowry JB, Spyker DA, et al. 2017 Annual Report of the American Association of Poison Control Centers' National Poison Data System (NPDS): 35th annual report. Clin Toxicol 2018;56:1213-415.
3. Linakis JG, Frederick KA. Poisoning deaths not reported to the regional poison control center. Ann Emerg Med 1993;22:1822-8.
4. Hanhan UA. The poisoned child in the pediatric intensive care unit. Pediatr Clin North Am 2008;55:669-86.
5. de Caen AR, Berg MD, Chameides L, et al. Part 12: Pediatric advanced life support—2015 American Heart Association Guidelines update for cardiopulmonary resuscitation and emergency cardiovascular care. Circulation 2015;132(Suppl 2):S526-42.
6. Nelson LS, Howland M, Lewin NA, et al. 4: Principles of Managing the Acutely Poisoned or Overdosed Patient. In: Nelson LS, Howland M, Lewin NA, et al., eds. Goldfrank's Toxicologic Emergencies, 11e. New York, NY: McGraw-Hill, 2019. Available at https://accesspharmacy.mhmedical.com/content.aspx?bookid=2569&Sectionid=210267250. Accessed June 20, 2019.
7. Frithsen IL, Simpson WM. Recognition and management of acute medication poisoning. Am Fam Physician 2010;81:316-23.
8. Micromedex Solutions [homepage on the Internet]. Ann Arbor, MI: Truven Health Analytics, Inc. Available at www.micromedexsolutions.com. Accessed June 14, 2018.
9. Nares MA, Cantwell GP, Weisman RS. Poisoning. In: Rogers' Textbook of Pediatric Intensive Care, 5th ed. Philadelphia: Wolters Kluwer, 2016:476-98.
10. Hoegberg LG. 5: Techniques Used to Prevent Gastrointestinal Absorption. In: Nelson LS, Howland M, Lewin NA, et al., eds. Goldfrank's Toxicologic Emergencies, 11e. New York, NY:

McGraw-Hill; 2019. Available at http://accesspharmacy.mh medical.com/content.aspx?bookid=2569&Sectionid=210267333. Accessed June 20, 2019.

11. American Academy of Pediatrics Committee on Injury, Violence, and Poison Prevention. Policy Statement: poison treatment in the home. Pediatrics 2003;112:1182-5.

12. American Academy of Clinical Toxicology and European Association of Poisons Centres and Clinical Toxicologists. Position paper: single dose activated charcoal. Clin Toxicol 2005; 43:61-87.

13. Hojer J, Troutman WG, Ederman A, et al. Position paper update: ipecac syrup for gastrointestinal decontamination. Clin Toxicol 2013;51:134-9.

14. Benson BE, Hoppu K, Troutman WG, et al. Position paper update: gastric lavage for gastrointestinal decontamination. Clin Toxicol 2013;51:140-6.

15. Thanacoody R, Caravati EM, Troutman WG, et al. Poison paper update: whole bowel irrigation for gastrointestinal decontamination of overdose patients. Clin Toxicol 2015;53:5-12.

16. Barrueto F, Gattu R, Mazer-Amirshahi M. Updates in the general approach to the pediatric poisoned patient. Pediatr Clin N Am 2013;60:1203-20.

17. Neuvonen P, Olkkola K. Activated charcoal and syrup of ipecac in the prevention of cimetidine and pindolol absorption in man after administration of metoclopramide as an antiemetic. J Toxicol Clin Toxicol 1984;22:103-14.

18. Neuvonen P, Vartiainen M, Tokola O. Comparison of activated charcoal and ipecac syrup in prevention of drug absorption. Eur J Clin Pharmacol 1983;24:557-62.

19. Saetta JP, Quinton DN. Residual gastric content after gastric lavage and ipecacuanha induced emesis in self-poisoned patients: an endoscopic study. J R Soc Med 1991;84:35-8.

20. Garrison J, Shepherd G, Huddleston WL, et al. Evaluation of the time frame for home ipecac syrup use when not kept in the home. J Toxicol Clin Toxicol 2003;41:217-21.

21. Bond GR. Home syrup of ipecac use does not reduce emergency department use or improve outcome. Pediatrics 2003; 112:1061-4.

22. Palmer E, Guay A. Reversible myopathy secondary to abuse of ipecac in patients with major eating disorders. N Engl J Med 1985;313:1457-9.

23. Schiff RJ, Wurzel CL, Brunson SC, et al. Death due to chronic syrup of ipecac use in a patient with bulimia. Pediatrics 1986; 78:412-6.

24. Eddleston M, Haggalla S, Sudarshan RK, et al. The hazards of gastric lavage for intestinal self-poisoning in a resource poor location. Clin Toxicol 2007;45:126-42.

25. Kimura Y, Kamada Y, Kimura S. A patient with numerous tablets remaining in the stomach even 5 hours after ingestion. Am J Emerg Med 2008;26:118.e1-e2.

26. Djogovic D, Hudson D, Jacka M. Gastric bezoar following venlafaxine overdose [letter]. Clin Toxicol 2007;45:735.

27. Eddleston M, Juszczak E, Buckley NA, et al. Multiple-dose activated charcoal in acute self-poisoning: a randomized controlled trial. Lancet 2008;371:579-87.

28. Lurie Y, Bentur Y, Levy Y, et al. Limited efficacy of gastrointestinal decontamination in severe slow-release carbamazepine overdose. Ann Pharmacother 2007;41:1539-43.

29. Cooper GM, Le Couteur DG, Richardson D, et al. A randomized clinical trial of activated charcoal for the routine management of oral drug overdose. QJM 2005;98:655-60.

30. Mullins M, Froelke BR, Regina-Paz Rivera M. Effect of delayed activated charcoal on acetaminophen concentration after simulated overdose of oxycodone and acetaminophen. Clin Toxicol 2009;47:112-5.

31. Spiller HA, Winter ML, Klein-Schwartz W, et al. Efficacy of activated charcoal administered more than four hours after acetaminophen overdose. J Emerg Med 2006;30:1-5.

32. Brahmi N, Kouraichi N, Thabet H, et al. Influence of activated charcoal on the pharmacokinetics and the clinical features of carbamazepine poisoning. Am J Emerg Med 2006;24:440-3.

33. Wang X, Mondal S, Wang J, et al. Effect of activated charcoal on apixaban pharmacokinetics in healthy volunteers. Am J Cardiovasc Drugs 2014;14:147-54.

34. Spiller HA, Rodgers GC. Evaluation of administration of activated charcoal in the home. Pediatrics 2001;108:e100.

35. Bond GR. Activated charcoal in the home: helpful and important or simply a distraction? Pediatrics 2002;109:145–6.

36. Osterhoudt KC, Durbin D, Alpern ER, et al. Risk factors for emesis after therapeutic use of activated charcoal in acutely poisoned children. Pediatrics 2004;113:806-10.

37. Green JP, McCauley W. Bowel perforation after single-dose activated charcoal. CJEM 2006;8:358-60.

38. American Academy of Clinical Toxicology and European Association of Poisons Centres and Clinical Toxicologists. Position statement and practice guidelines on the use of multi-dose activated charcoal in the treatment of acute poisoning. Clin Toxicol 1999;37:731-51.

39. Berg MJ, Berlinger WG, Goldberg MJ, et al. Acceleration of the body clearance of phenobarbital by oral activated charcoal. N Engl J Med 1982;307:642-4.

40. Levy G. Gastrointestinal clearance of drugs with activated charcoal. N Engl J Med 1982;307:676-8.

41. de Silva HA, Fonseka MMD, Pathmeswaran A, et al. Multiple-dose activated charcoal for treatment of yellow oleander poisoning: a single-blind, randomized, placebo-controlled trial. Lancet 2003;361:1935-8.

42. Skinner CG, Chang AS, Matthews AR, et al. Randomized controlled study on the use of multiple-dose activated charcoal in patients with supratherapeutic phenytoin levels. Clin Toxicol 2012;50:764-69.

43. Smith SW, Howland M. A1: Activated Charcoal. In: Nelson LS, Howland M, Lewin NA, et al., eds. Goldfrank's Toxicologic Emergencies, 11e. New York, NY: McGraw-Hill; 2019. Available at http://accesspharmacy.mhmedical.com/content.aspx?bookid= 2569&Sectionid=210266863. Accessed June 20, 2019.

44. Hendrickson RG, McKeown NJ. 33: Acetaminophen. In: Nelson LS, Howland M, Lewin NA, et al., eds. Goldfrank's Toxicologic Emergencies, 11e. New York, NY: McGraw-Hill; 2019. Available at http://accesspharmacy.mhmedical.com/content.aspx?bookid= 2569&Sectionid=210270383. Accessed June 20, 2019.

45. Smith SW, Howland M. A2: Whole Bowel Irrigation and Other Intestinal Evacuants. In: Nelson LS, Howland M, Lewin NA, et al., eds. Goldfrank's Toxicologic Emergencies, 11e. New York, NY: McGraw-Hill; 2019. Available at http://accesspharmacy.mh medical.com/content.aspx?bookid=2569&Sectionid=210266921. Accessed June 20, 2019.

46. Lapatto-Reiniluoto O, Kivisto KT, Neuvonen PJ. Activated charcoal alone and followed by whole-bowel irrigation in preventing the absorption of sustained-release drugs. Clin Pharmacol Ther 2001;70:255-60.

47. Lavonas EJ, Reynolds KM, Dart RC. Therapeutic acetaminophen is not associated with liver injury in children: a systematic review. Pediatrics 2010;126:e1430-e1444.

48. Shaoul R, Novikov J, Maor I, et al. Silent acetaminophen-induced hepatotoxicity in febrile children: does this entity exist? Acta Paediatr 2004;93:618-22.

49. Kozer E, Greenberg R, Zimmerman DR, et al. Repeated supratherapeutic doses of paracetamol in children—a literature review and suggested clinical approach. Acta Paediatr 2006;95:1165-71.

50. Squires RH, Shneider BL, Bucuvalas J, et al. Acute liver failure in children: the first 348 patients in the pediatric acute liver failure study group. J Pediatr 2006;148:652-8.

51. Waring WS, Jamie H, Leggett GE. Delayed onset of acute renal failure after significant paracetamol overdose: a case series. Human Exp Toxicol 2010;29:63-8.

52. Ozkaya O, Genc G, Bek K, et al. A case of acetaminophen (paracetamol) causing renal failure without liver damage in a child and review of literature. Ren Fail 2010;32:1125-7.

53. Chun LJ, Tong MJ, Busuttil RW, et al. Acetaminophen hepatotoxicity and acute liver failure. J Clin Gastroenterol 2009;43:342-9.

54. Dufful SB, Isbister GK. Predicting the requirement for N-acetylcysteine in paracetamol poisoning from reported dose. Clin Toxicol 2013;51:772-6.

55. Tenenbein M. Acetaminophen: the 150 mg/kg myth. J Toxicol Clin Toxicol 2004;42:145-8.

56. Bond GR. Reduced toxicity of acetaminophen in children: it's the liver. J Toxicol Clin Toxicol 2004;42:149-52.

57. Cook MD, Clark RF. Acetaminophen toxicity [letter]. Pediatr Emerg Care 2005;21:703-4.

58. Beringer RM, Thompson JP, Parry S, et al. Intravenous paracetamol overdose: two case reports and a change to national treatment guidelines. Arch Dis Child 2011;96:307-8.

59. Gray T, Hoffman RS, Bateman DN. Intravenous paracetamol—an international perspective of toxicity. Clin Toxicol 2011;49:150-2.

60. Berling I, Anscombe M, Isbister GK. Intravenous paracetamol toxicity in a malnourished child. Clin Toxicol 2012;50:74-6.

61. Dart RC, Rumack BH. Intravenous acetaminophen in the United States: iatrogenic dosing errors. Pediatrics 2012;129:349-53.

62. Hendrickson RG, Howland M. A3: N-Acetylcysteine. In: Nelson LS, Howland M, Lewin NA, et al., eds. Goldfrank's Toxicologic Emergencies, 11e. New York, NY: McGraw-Hill; 2019. Available at http://accesspharmacy.mhmedical.com/content.aspx?bookid=2569&Sectionid=210261914. Accessed June 20, 2019.

63. Kanter MZ. Comparison of oral and i.v. acetylcysteine in the treatment of acetaminophen poisoning. Am J Health Syst Pharm 2006;63:1821-7.

64. Yarema MC, Johnson DW, Berlin RJ, et al. Comparison of the 20-hour intravenous and 72-hour oral acetylcysteine protocols for the treatment of acute acetaminophen poisoning. Ann Emerg Med 2009;54:606-14.

65. Whyte AJ, Kehrl T, Brooks DE, et al. Safety and effectiveness of acetadote for acetaminophen toxicity. J Emerg Med 2010;39:607-11.

66. Betten DP, Cantrell FL, Thomas SC, et al. A prospective evaluation of shortened course oral N-acetylcysteine for the treatment of acute acetaminophen poisoning. Ann Emerg Med 2007;50:272-9.

67. James LP, Wells E, Beard RH, et al. Predictors of outcome after acetaminophen poisoning in children and adolescents. J Pediatr 2002;140:522-6.

68. Woo OF, Mueller PD, Olson KR, et al. Shorter duration of oral N-acetylcysteine therapy for acute acetaminophen overdose. Ann Emerg Med 2000;35:363-8.

69. Heard K. A multicenter comparison of the safety of oral versus intravenous acetylcysteine for treatment of acetaminophen overdose. Clin Toxicol 2010;48:424-30.

70. Marzullo L. An update of N-acetylcysteine treatment for acute acetaminophen toxicity in children. Curr Opin Pediatr 2005;17:239-45.

71. White ML, Liebelt EL. Update on antidotes for pediatric poisoning. Pediatr Emerg Care 2006;22:740-6.

72. Henry K, Harris CR. Deadly ingestions. Pediatr Clin North Am 2006;53:293-315.

73. Wiener SW. 106: Toxic Alcohols. In: Nelson LS, Howland M, Lewin NA, et al., eds. Goldfrank's Toxicologic Emergencies, 11e. New York, NY: McGraw-Hill; 2019. Available at http://accesspharmacy.mhmedical.com/content.aspx?bookid=2569&Sectionid=210275462. Accessed June 20, 2019.

74. Michael JB, Sztajnkrycer MD. Deadly poisons: nine common agents that kill at low doses. Emerg Med Clin North Am 2004;22:1019-50.

75. Sanaei-Zadeh H, Zamani N, Shadnia S. Outcomes of visual disturbances after methanol poisoning. Clin Toxicol 2011;49:102-7.

76. Smith SW, Howland M. A12: Folates: Leucovorin (Folinic Acid) and Folic Acid. In: Nelson LS, Howland M, Lewin NA, et al., eds. Goldfrank's Toxicologic Emergencies, 11e. New York, NY: McGraw-Hill; 2019. Available at http://accesspharmacy.mhmedical.com/content.aspx?bookid=2569&Sectionid=210262439. Accessed June 20, 2019.

77. Howland M. A15: Pyridoxine. In: Nelson LS, Howland M, Lewin NA, et al., eds. Goldfrank's Toxicologic Emergencies, 11e. New York, NY: McGraw-Hill; 2019. Available at http://accesspharmacy.mhmedical.com/content.aspx?bookid=2569&Sectionid=210262584. Accessed June 20, 2019.

78. Hoffman RS. A27: Thiamine Hydrochloride. In: Nelson LS, Howland M, Lewin NA, et al., eds. Goldfrank's Toxicologic Emergencies, 11e. New York, NY: McGraw-Hill; 2019. Available at http://accesspharmacy.mhmedical.com/content.aspx?bookid=2569&Sectionid=210263242. Accessed June 20, 2019.

79. Howland M. A34: Ethanol. In: Nelson LS, Howland M, Lewin NA, et al., eds. Goldfrank's Toxicologic Emergencies, 11e. New York, NY: McGraw-Hill; 2019. Available at http://accesspharmacy.mhmedical.com/content.aspx?bookid=2569&Sectionid=210263617. Accessed June 20, 2019.

80. De Brabander N, Wojciechowski M, De Decker K, et al. Fomepizole as a therapeutic strategy in paediatric methanol poisoning. A case report and review of the literature. Eur J Pediatr 2005;164:158-61.

81. Brent J. Fomepizole for the treatment of pediatric ethylene and diethylene glycol, butoxyethanol, and methanol poisoning. Clin Toxicol 2010;28:401-6.

82. Howland M. A33: Fomepizole. In: Nelson LS, Howland M, Lewin NA, et al., eds. Goldfrank's Toxicologic Emergencies, 11e. New York, NY: McGraw-Hill; 2019. Available at http://accesspharmacy.mhmedical.com/content.aspx?bookid=2569&Sectionid=210263559. Accessed June 20, 2019.

83. Brent J, McMartin K, Phillips S, et al. Fomepizole for the treatment of ethylene glycol poisoning. N Engl J Med 1999;340:832-8.

84. Brent J. Fomepizole for ethylene glycol and methanol poisoning. N Engl J Med 2009;60:2216-23.

85. Lepik KJ, Sobolev BG, Levy AR, et al. Medication errors associated with the use of ethanol and fomepizole as antidotes for methanol and ethylene glycol poisoning. Clin Toxicol 2011;49:391-401.

86. Barceloux DG, Krenzelok EP, Olson K, et al. American Academy of Clinical Toxicology practice guidelines on the treatment of ethylene glycol poisoning. J Toxicol Clin Toxicol 1999;37:537-60.

87. Barceloux DG, Bond GR, Krenzelok EP, et al. American Academy of Clinical Toxicology practice guidelines on the treatment of methanol poisoning. J Toxicol Clin Toxicol 2002;40:415-46.

88. Goto CS, Feng SY. Crotalidae polyvalent immune Fab for the treatment of pediatric crotaline envenomation. Pediatr Emerg Care 2009;25:273-9.

89. Ruha A, Pizon AF. 119: Native (US) Venomous Snakes and Lizards. In: Nelson LS, Howland M, Lewin NA, et al., eds. Goldfrank's Toxicologic Emergencies, 11e. New York, NY: McGraw-Hill; 2019. Available at http://accesspharmacy.mhmedical.com/content.aspx?bookid=2569&Sectionid=210277153. Accessed June 20, 2019.

90. Gold BS, Barish RA, Dart RC. North American snake envenomation: diagnosis, treatment, and management. Emerg Med Clin North Am 2004;22:423-43.

91. Schmidt JM. Antivenom therapy for snakebites in children: is there evidence? Curr Opin Pediatr 2005;17:234-8.

92. Weant KA, Johnson PN, Bowers RC, et al. Evidence-based, multidisciplinary approach to the development of a crotalidae polyvalent antivenin (CroFab) protocol at a university hospital. Ann Pharmacother 2010;44:447-55.

93. Sotelo N. Review of treatment and complications in 79 children with rattlesnake bite. Clin Pediatr 2008;47:483-9.

94. Gold BS, Dart RC, Barish RA. Bites of venomous snakes. N Engl J Med 2002;347:347-56.

95. Bush SP, Green SM, Moynihan JA, et al. Crotalidae polyvalent immune Fab (ovine) antivenom is efficacious for envenomations by Southern Pacific rattlesnakes (Crotalus helleri). Ann Emerg Med 2002;40:619-24.

96. Schier JG, Wiener SW, Touger M, et al. Efficacy of Crotalidae polyvalent antivenin for the treatment of hognosed viper (Porthidium nasutum) envenomation. Ann Emerg Med 2003;41:391-5.

97. Lavonas EJ, Gerardo CJ, O'Malley G, et al. Initial experience with Crotalidae polyvalent immune Fab (ovine) antivenom in the treatment of copperhead snake bite. Ann Emerg Med 2004; 43:200-6.

98. Trinh HH, Hack JB. Use of CroFab antivenin in the management of a very young pediatric copperhead envenomation. J Emerg Med 2005;29:159-62.

99. CroFab [package insert]. West Conshohocken, PA: BTG International Inc., 2018.

100. Dart RC, Seifert SA, Carroll L, et al. Affinity-purified, mixed monospecific crotalid antivenom ovine Fab for the treatment of crotalid venom poisoning. Ann Emerg Med 1997;30:33-9.

101. Dart RC, Seifert SA, Boyer LV, et al. A randomized multicenter trial of crotaline polyvalent immune Fab (ovine) antivenom for the treatment for crotaline snakebite in the United States. Arch Intern Med 2001;161:2030-6.

102. Pizon AF, Riley BD, LoVecchio F, et al. Safety and efficacy of Crotalidae polyvalent immune Fab in pediatric Crotaline envenomations. Acad Emerg Med 2007;14:373-6.

103. Corneille MG, Larson S, Stewart RM, et al. A large single-center experience with treatment of patients with crotalid envenomations: outcomes with and evolution of antivenin therapy. Am J Surg 2006;192:848-52.

104. Farrar HC, Grayham T, Bolden B, et al. The use and tolerability of crotalidae polyvalent immune FAB (ovine) in pediatric envenomations. Clin Pediatr 2012;51:945-9.

105. Miller AD, Young MC, DeMott MC, et al. Recurrent coagulopathy and thrombocytopenia in children treated with Crotalidae polyvalent immune Fab; a case series. Pediatr Emerg Care 2010; 26:576-82.

106. Ruha AM, Curry SC, Albrecht C, et al. Late hematologic toxicity following treatment of rattlesnake envenomation with Crotalidae polyvalent immune Fab antivenom. Toxicon 2011;57:53-9.

107. Johnson PN, McGoodwin L, Banner W Jr. Utilisation of Crotalidae polyvalent immune Fab (ovine) for Viperidae envenomations in children. Emerg Med J 2008;25:793-8.

108. Schaeffer TH, Khatri V, Reifler LM, et al. Incidence of immediate hypersensitivity reaction and serum sickness following administration of crotalidae polyvalent immune Fab antivenom: a meta-analysis. Acad Emerg Med 2012;19:121-31.

109. Quan AN, Quan D, Curry SC. Improving Crotalidae polyvalent immune Fab reconstitution times. Am J Emerg Med 2010; 28:593-5.

110. Anavip [package insert]. Franklin, TN: Rare Disease Therapeutics, Inc., 2018.

111. Bush SP, Ruha A, Seifert SA, et al. Comparison of F(ab')$_2$ versus Fab antivenom for pit viper envenomation: a prospective, blinded, multicenter, randomized clinical trial. Clin Toxicol 2015;53:37-45.

112. McKenzie LB, Ahir N, Stolz U, et al. Household cleaning product-related injuries treated in US emergency departments in 1990-2006. Pediatrics 2010;126:509-16.

113. Kay M, Wyllie R. Caustic ingestions in children. Curr Opin Pediatr 2009;21:651-4.

114. Meyer S, Eddleston M, Bailey B, et al. Unintentional household poisoning in children. Klin Padiatr 2007;219:254-70.

115. Betalli P, Rossi A, Bini M, et al. Update on management of caustic and foreign body ingestion in children. Diagn Ther Endosc 2009:Article ID 969868.

116. Shub MD. Therapy of caustic ingestion: new treatment considerations. Curr Opin Pediatr 2015;27:609-13.

117. Dogan Y, Erkan T, Cokugras FC, et al. Caustic gastroesophageal lesions in childhood: an analysis of 473 cases. Clin Pediatr 2006;45:435-8.

118. Usta M, Erkan T, Cokugras FC, et al. High doses of methylprednisolone in the management of caustic esophageal burns. Pediatrics 2014;133:e1518-24.

119. Litovitz T, Whitaker N, Clark L. Preventing battery ingestions: an analysis of 8648 cases. Pediatrics 2010;125:1178-83.

120. Kimball SJ, Park AH, Rollins MD, et al. A review of esophageal disc battery ingestions and a protocol for management. Arch Otolaryngol Head Neck Surg 2010;136:866-71.

121. Marom T, Goldfarb A, Russo E, et al. Battery ingestion in children. Int J Pediatr Otorhinolaryngol 2010;74:849-54.

122. Wurzel DF, Masters IB, Choo KL, et al. A case for early bronchoscopic airway assessment after battery disc ingestion. Pediatr Pulmonol 2014;49:E72-4.

123. Samad L, Ali M, Ramzi H. Button battery ingestion: hazards of esophageal impaction. J Pediatr Surg 1999;34:1527-31.

124. Bell EA, Tunkel DE. Over-the-counter cough and cold medications in children: are they helpful? Otolaryngol Head Neck Surg 2010;142:647-50.

125. Goldman RD. Treating cough and cold: guidance for caregivers of children and youth. Paediatr Child Health 2011;16:564-6.

126. Pitetti RD, Whitman E, Zaylor A. Accidental and nonaccidental poisonings as a cause of apparent life-threatening events in infants. Pediatrics 2008;122:e359-62.

127. Wingert WE, Mundy LA, Collins GL, et al. Possible role of pseudoephedrine and other over-the-counter cold medications in the deaths of very young children. J Forensic Sci 2007;52:487-90.

128. Dart RC, Paul IM, Bond GR, et al. Pediatric fatalities associated with over-the-counter (nonprescription) cough and cold medications. Ann Emerg Med 2009;53:411-7.

129. Hampton LM, Nguyen DB, Edwards JR, et al. Cough and cold medication adverse events after market withdrawal and labeling revision. Pediatrics 2013;132:1047-64.

130. Mazer-Amirshahi M, Rasooly I, Brooks G, et al. The impact of pediatric labeling changes on prescribing patterns of cough and cold medications. J Pediatr 2014;165:1024-8.

131. O'Donnell K, Mansbach JM, LoVecchio F, et al. Use of cough and cold medications in severe bronchiolitis before and after a health advisory warning against their use. J Pediatr 2015;167:196-8.

132. Mazer-Amirshahi M, Reid N, van den Anker J, et al. Effect of cough and cold medication restriction and label changes on pediatric ingestions reported to United States poison centers. J Pediatr 2013;163:1372-6.

133. Texas Poison Center Network. A Parent's Guide to Poison Prevention. Available at https://www.poisoncontrol.org/a-parents-guide-to-poison-prevention/. Accessed June 20, 2019.

Section III

Cardiovascular Disorders

CHAPTER 8

Congenital Heart Disease

Brady S. Moffett, Pharm.D., MPH, MBA; and
David E. Procaccini, Pharm.D., MPH, BCPS, CACP

LEARNING OBJECTIVES

1. Review the basic anatomy and pathophysiology of common congenital heart defects.

2. Select and appropriately monitor pharmacotherapy for a patient with a congenital heart defect.

3. Describe the pathophysiology, diagnosis, and pharmacotherapy for treatment of low cardiac output syndrome.

ABBREVIATIONS IN THIS CHAPTER

ACEI	Angiotensin-converting enzyme inhibitor
ASD	Atrial septal defect
BT	Blalock-Taussig (shunt)
HLHS	Hypoplastic left heart syndrome
LA	Left atria
LCOS	Low cardiac output syndrome
LV	Left ventricle
NSAID	Nonsteroidal anti-inflammatory drug
PA	Pulmonary artery
PDA	Patent ductus arteriosus
PFO	Patent foramen ovale
PGE	Prostaglandin
PLE	Protein-losing enteropathy
PVR	Pulmonary vascular resistance
RA	Right atria
RV	Right ventricle
SVR	Systemic vascular resistance
TGA	Transposition of the great arteries
TOF	Tetralogy of Fallot
VSD	Ventricular septal defect

INTRODUCTION

Congenital heart disease is the most common birth defect and occurs in about 8 of every 1000 live births.[1,2] Since the first report of a congenital heart defect in 1945, tremendous strides have occurred in the diagnosis, repair, and management of congenital heart disease.[3,4]

Application of pharmacotherapy in pediatric patients with congenital heart disease can be complex, and data for efficacy of many therapies are limited.[5-8] Many patients with congenital heart disease have several cardiac defects, involvement of other organ systems (e.g., asplenia and intestinal malrotation in patients with heterotaxy syndrome), or genetic mutations (e.g., Trisomy 21 with complete atrioventricular canal) that can complicate pharmacotherapy.[1,2] Moreover, strategies for managing congenital heart disease are often subject to institutional bias. For example, institutions vary in their use of corticosteroids in the cardiopulmonary bypass circuit, recombinant factor VIIa to control postoperative bleeding, or peritoneal dialysis as a strategy for removing fluid and inflammatory mediators in postoperative patients, all of which could potentially affect pharmacotherapy.[9-12]

A complete understanding of pathophysiology, hemodynamics, and pediatric clinical pharmacology is necessary to appropriately apply pharmacotherapy in a patient with congenital heart disease. This chapter aims to summarize the pathophysiology and pharmacotherapy for common congenital heart defects in pediatric patients. This discussion includes the epidemiology of congenital heart defects, clinical presentation, diagnosis, course and prognosis of the disease, and surgical or interventional procedures associated with the various defects. Each defect presented is evaluated as if a patient were presenting with an isolated lesion. It is important to note that many congenital heart defects occur in combination with other comorbidities.

The pharmacotherapy for each congenital heart defect will be summarized with respect to the preoperative (or surgically unrepaired) period, the immediate postoperative period, and the long-term (or chronic) management of surgically repaired congenital heart disease. Table 1 and Table 2 summarize the surgical management, common complications, and basic pharmacotherapy for each of the lesions.[13] Because a large portion of the pharmacotherapy for congenital heart disease is in the immediate postoperative period, the etiology, diagnosis, and treatment of postoperative low cardiac output syndrome (LCOS) will be addressed.

A brief overview of fetal versus neonatal circulation is included, but the focus of the chapter will be congenital heart disease in the neonate and infant. This chapter will only focus on the pathophysiology and pharmacotherapy related directly to congenital heart defects and will not cover areas such as postoperative pain and sedation management, or infectious disease prophylaxis. In addition, the normal circulation and structure of the heart will not be presented, and the reader is encouraged to understand the anatomy and physiology of the normal heart before engaging with the material in this chapter.

LOW CARDIAC OUTPUT SYNDROME

Encountered primarily after surgical repair of congenital heart disease, *low cardiac output syndrome* is often defined as the inability of the heart to deliver sufficient oxygenated blood to the end organs and tissues.[14-16] The primary etiology

Table 1. Common Congenital Heart Defects and Surgical Repairs

Defect	Lesion Description	Surgical or Interventional Repair
Patent ductus arteriosus	Communication between PA and aorta	Ductus ligation Coil or device insertion (interventional)
Atrial septal defect	Communication between right and left atria by a hole in the atrial septum	Patch repair of defect[a] Device insertion (interventional)
Ventricular septal defect	Communication between right and left ventricle by a hole in the ventricular septum	Patch repair of defect[a] Device insertion (interventional)
Tetralogy of Fallot	PA stenosis, ventricular septal defect, overriding aorta, right ventricular hypertrophy	Ventricular septal defect closure and repair of PA stenosis[a]
Transposition of the great arteries	Switched locations of the PA and aorta, resulting in 2 separate circulations	Arterial switch operation[a]
Coarctation of the aorta	Narrowing of the aorta; categorized as preductal or postductal	End-to-end anastomosis surgery (if coarctation does not involve carotid arteries) Patch repair surgery[a] (if coarctation involves carotid arteries)
Hypoplastic left heart syndrome	Absence of left ventricle and aortic narrowing (atresia) First stage of HLHS palliation	1) Norwood procedure[a] (first stage of HLHS palliation): Combination of PA and aorta to form a "neo-aorta," BT shunt, atrial septectomy) OR Sano modification[a] OR hybrid procedure 2) Bidirectional Glenn (second stage of HLHS palliation): Takedown of BT shunt, anastomosis of superior vena cava to PA[a] 3) Fontan (third stage of HLHS palliation): Attachment of inferior vena cava to PA by an extracardiac conduit[a] (with or without fenestration)

[a]Requires cardiopulmonary bypass to perform surgical procedure.
BT = Blalock-Taussig; HLHS = hypoplastic left heart syndrome; PA = pulmonary artery; SVC = superior vena cava.

Table 2. Significant Sequelae of Congenital Heart Disease Before and After Surgical Intervention

Defect	Preoperative	Immediate Postoperative	Long Term
Patent ductus arteriosus	CHF, PHTN	None	None
Atrial septal defect	CHF, PHTN	HTN	None
Ventricular septal defect	CHF, PHTN	Systolic HTN, arrhythmias	None
Tetralogy of Fallot	CHF, hypercyanotic episodes, chronic cyanosis, clubbing	LCOS, PHTN, HTN, ventricular tachycardia, thrombus formation	Ventricular tachycardia, exercise intolerance
Transposition of the great arteries	Cardiogenic shock, cyanosis	LCOS, coronary vasospasm	None (arterial switch)
Coarctation of the aorta	Cardiogenic shock (neonates), CHF, left ventricular enlargement	LCOS (particularly in neonates), HTN	HTN, re-coarctation
Hypoplastic left heart syndrome	Cardiogenic shock, cyanosis	LCOS, arrhythmias, PHTN, cyanosis	Sudden death, low weight gain, poor feeding
Bidirectional Glenn	Sudden death, low weight gain, poor feeding	LCOS, arrhythmias, PHTN	CHF, cerebral swelling, headache
Fontan	CHF, cerebral swelling, headache	LCOS, arrhythmias, PHTN, chylous effusions, thrombus formation	Arrhythmias, effusions, protein-losing enteropathy, thrombi, plastic bronchitis

CHF = congestive heart failure; HTN = hypertension; LCOS = low cardiac output syndrome; PHTN = pulmonary hypertension.

of LCOS is myocardial "stunning," which occurs after cardiac surgery, together with elevated circulating levels of interleukins and other inflammatory mediators. The use of cardiopulmonary bypass is often implicated in LCOS, as is aortic cross clamping during surgery (resulting in myocardial ischemia), myocardial tissue incision, and the use of cardioplegia solutions.[14,17] Studies have shown a decline in cardiac output, an increase in pulmonary vascular resistance (PVR), and an increase in systemic vascular resistance (SVR) occurring 6–18 hours after cardiac surgery, particularly in neonates that have undergone cardiopulmonary bypass during surgery.[15,16,18]

Low cardiac output syndrome is diagnosed based on an aggregation of symptoms. Subjectively, patients may appear gray or dusky, versus pink, with a sluggish capillary refill time (greater than 3 seconds). Additional signs of poor systemic perfusion include reduction in peripheral temperatures compared with their core body temperature, decreased urine output, and elevated serum lactate levels from poorly perfused tissues undergoing anaerobic metabolism.[15,16,19] Subsequently, if unmanaged, accumulation of lactate can lead to an elevated anion-gap acidosis.

The role of pharmacotherapy in the postoperative patient with congenital heart disease is to prevent or minimize LCOS. Considering the classic equation for cardiac output (cardiac output = stroke volume × heart rate) (Figure 1), the prevention or minimization of LCOS is primarily achieved by manipulation of stroke volume. Thus, the primary goals include: (1) optimizing preload, (2) reducing afterload, and (3) augmenting contractility. These methods will be discussed throughout this chapter, and a summary of medications used in the immediate postoperative period is provided in Table 3 and Table 4.

PRELOAD

Optimizing preload is essential for maintaining maximal cardiac output. If preload is too high, patients will experience venous congestion and edema; however, if preload is too low, cardiac output is diminished. Monitoring of preload is based on the patient's physical examination (e.g., hepatomegaly, pulmonary edema), or by direct monitoring of right atrial pressure by assessing central venous pressure.[13] Appropriate preload can be titrated using crystalloid or colloid solutions administered as continuous infusions or intermittent boluses.[20] Preload reduction usually occurs with diuresis. Loop and thiazide diuretics are commonly used as the pharmacologic agent of choice for fluid removal in a cardiac patient.[21-23] Furosemide may be administered as an intermittent or continuous infusion, and continuous infusions have shown benefit in maintaining diuresis while limiting drug exposure.[24,25] Bumetanide and torsemide have also been used but have less published experience.[26,27] Thiazide diuretics may be used synergistically with loop diuretics because they inhibit sodium and chloride reabsorption distally from the ascending loop of Henle. Thiazides may be preferred in patients with concomitant chronic lung disease, or in patients who require long-term use based on their ability to reabsorb calcium and mitigate bone fractures.[28,29] Spironolactone can also be used, particularly when patients require increased doses of loop diuretics to achieve adequate urine output.[30] Potassium supplementation may be necessary in patients receiving high doses of diuretics.[31] Hypochloremic metabolic alkalosis is an adverse event associated with high doses and long-term therapy with loop diuretics. The use of acetazolamide and/or chloride supplementation may be necessary in some patients to reverse the alkalosis.[13,32]

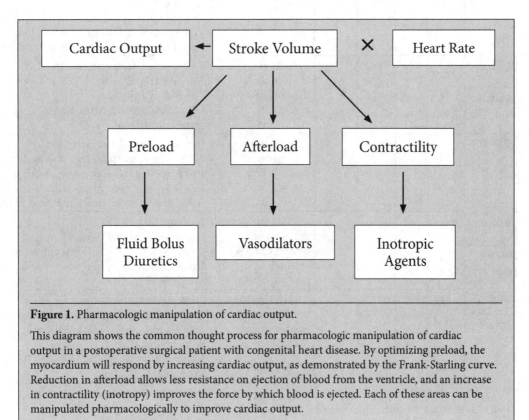

Figure 1. Pharmacologic manipulation of cardiac output.

This diagram shows the common thought process for pharmacologic manipulation of cardiac output in a postoperative surgical patient with congenital heart disease. By optimizing preload, the myocardium will respond by increasing cardiac output, as demonstrated by the Frank-Starling curve. Reduction in afterload allows less resistance on ejection of blood from the ventricle, and an increase in contractility (inotropy) improves the force by which blood is ejected. Each of these areas can be manipulated pharmacologically to improve cardiac output.

AFTERLOAD

Reduction in afterload is primarily accomplished by medications that dilate the systemic vasculature. Dobutamine, fenoldopam, milrinone, nitroprusside, nicardipine, and nesiritide are examples of continuous-infusion agents that promote systemic vascular dilation. Milrinone has the largest amount of supportive literature associated with pediatric postoperative cardiac surgical patients, including pharmacokinetic data.[17,33-37] Patients should be monitored for potential adverse events including arrhythmias (dobutamine, milrinone), thrombocytopenia (milrinone), cyanide/thiocyanate toxicity with high doses (greater than 2 mcg/kg/minute) and longer duration (greater than 48 hours) of nitroprusside, and hypotension (all agents).[17,33-46] Nesiritide has preload reducing effects in light of lack of response to diuretics, as well as vasodilatory effects. Nesiritide however has been noted to be associated with acute kidney injury; thus it is not recommended as first-line therapy in patients with decompensated heart failure, and should only be considered when other treatment modalities to lower central venous pressure have been exhausted.[47-57] The vasodilatory effects of fenoldopam tend to be less potent than those of other agents, but may be useful in increasing urine output in patients receiving high doses of diuretics.[58,59] Angiotensin-converting enzyme inhibitors (ACEIs) (e.g., captopril, enalapril) have also been used as oral afterload-reducing agents.[7,60-65] Enalaprilat provides an intravenous form of ACEI that may be used in patients who are unable to take oral medication. In particular, hypotension, acute kidney injury, and hyperkalemia have been observed when using ACEIs in patients with congenital heart disease.[13,65-69]

Table 3. Common Continuous Adrenergic Vasoactive Infusions in Congenital Heart Disease

Drug	Dose (mcg/kg/min)	Adrenergic and Dopaminergic Activity[a]				Titration (mcg/kg/min)[b]	Cautions/Comments
		α_1	β_1	β_2	DOPA		
Dobutamine	2–20	+	+++	+	0	1–2 every 10 min until desired effect is reached	• Increases CO • Higher doses can cause tachyarrhythmias and changes in BP leading to myocardial ischemia
	Max 30						
Dopamine	< 5	0	++	+	++++	1–5 every ≥ 5 min	• Initial dose based on clinical indication and patient status • < 5 mcg/kg/min = renal, coronary, mesenteric, and cerebral arterial vasodilation and natriuretic response • 5–10 mcg/kg/min = increased contractility/CO • > 10 mcg/kg/min = increased contractility/CO and vasoconstriction/increase in SVR • If > 20 mcg/kg/min needed, a more direct-acting vasoactive agent should be added (i.e., epinephrine, norepinephrine) • Can induce arrhythmias • Prolonged infusions can deplete endogenous norepinephrine resulting in a loss of vasopressor response
	5–10	++	+++	+	++	1–10 every ≥ 5 min	
	> 10	++++	+++	0	+		
Epinephrine	0.01–1	++	+++	++	0	0.01–0.1 every ≥ 1 min until desired effect is reached	• Low doses increase contractility and CO • Escalating doses increase SVR and BP • Can induce arrhythmias • (+) Inotropic/chronotropic effects can induce myocardial ischemia
	Max 2						
Isoproterenol	0.05–2	0	0	++++	++++	0.05–0.1 every ≥ 10 min until desired effect is reached	• Increases CO and decreases SVR • Affinity for β_2 receptors leads to vasodilation • Has a prominent chronotropic effect • Use in hypotensive patients is limited to situations in which hypotension results from bradycardia
Norepinephrine	0.05–1	++++	++	0	0	0.01–0.1 every ≥ 2 min until desired effect is reached	• Increases SVR and BP • Decreases renal perfusion • Can induce tachyarrhythmias and myocardial ischemia • Extravasation can produce ischemic necrosis and sloughing
	Max 2						
Phenylephrine	0.04–2	++++	0	0	0	0.05–0.3 every ≥ 5 min until desired effect is reached	• Decreases renal perfusion • Pure α-adrenergic agonist with minimal cardiac activity • Rapid increase in systolic and diastolic BP can cause reflex bradycardia • Extravasation can produce ischemic necrosis and sloughing
	Max 4						

[a]Adrenergic and dopaminergic activity range: 0 (no activity) to ++++ (most activity).
[b]Titrations may vary based on clinical indication and patient status.
BP = blood pressure; CO = cardiac output; CVP = central venous pressure; DOPA = dopamine; SVR = systemic vascular resistance.

Table 4. Common Continuous Non-Adrenergic Vasoactive and Vasodilator Agents

Drug	Dose	Mechanism/Clinical Effects	Titration[a]	Cautions/Comments
Esmolol	Loading: 100–500 mcg/kg infused over 1 min Initial: 50–100 mcg/kg/min Range: 50–250 mcg/kg/min Max: 1000 mcg/kg/min	• Competitively blocks β1 stimulation with little effect on β2 receptors • (-) Chronotropic effect/decrease in HR • Lusiotropy	• 50–100 mcg/kg/min every ≥ 10 min until desired effect is reached • Smaller titrations may be warranted in asthma/reactive airway disease	• Bradycardia, hypotension, peripheral ischemia • Phlebitis, necrosis after extravasation • Diaphoresis • Caution when discontinuing infusions to prevent rebound hypertension
Fenoldopam	Initial: 0.05 mcg/kg/min Range: 0.05–0.8 mcg/kg/min	• DOPA-1 receptor agonist • Peripheral vasodilation • Enhanced renal perfusion and urine output	0.02–0.05 mcg/kg/min every ≥ 20 min until desired effect is reached	• Headache, flushing • Hypotension, bradycardia • ST-T abnormalities on ECG
Labetalol	Loading: 0.2–1 mg/kg (max 20 mg) Initial: 0.25–1.2 mg/kg/hr Max: 3 mg/kg/hr Max adult dose: 10 mg/minute	• Non-selective β-blockade of both β1 and β2 receptors; also antagonizes α1 receptors • (-) Chronotropic effect/decrease in HR	• 0.1 mg/kg/hr every ≥ 15 min until desired effect is reached • Smaller titrations may be warranted in asthma/reactive airway disease	• Hypotension, AV conduction abnormalities, bradycardia • Drowsiness, fatigue, dizziness • Bronchoconstriction ○ Caution in asthma/reactive airway disease ○ Discontinue with occurrence • Dose adjustments may be needed in hepatic dysfunction
Milrinone	Loading: 50–100 mcg/kg Initial: 0.5–1 mcg/kg/min Range: 0.25–1 mcg/kg/min Max: 1.5 mcg/kg/min	• Non-catecholamine, PDE-3 inhibitor • Positive inotropic effects/increase in CO • Reduction in SVR/afterload • Lusiotropy	0.125–0.25 mcg/kg/min every ≥ 30 min until desired effect is reached	• Arrhythmias • Duration of effects for about 6 hr in normal renal function • Lower doses may provide response in renal failure • Long-term use associated with thrombocytopenia
Nesiritide	Loading: 1 mcg/kg Range: 0.01–0.03 mcg/kg/min	• B-type natriuretic peptide • Natruresis and diuresis • Vasodilation/reduction in SVR	0.005 mcg/kg/min every ≥ 3 hr until desired effect is reached	• Headache, flushing • Hypotension • Acute kidney injury • Not recommended as first-line therapy for decompensated heart failure; consider only when alternative treatment modalities to lower CVP have failed
Nicardipine	Initial: 0.5–1 mcg/kg/min Range: 0.5–5 mcg/kg/min Max: 7 mcg/kg/min Max adult dose: 250 mcg/min	• Causes relaxation of vascular smooth muscle and coronary vasodilation	0.2–0.3 mcg/kg/min every ≥ 15 min until desired effect is reached	• Hypotension, flushing, vasodilation, palpitation, tachycardia, peripheral edema, angina • Headache, dizziness • Constipation • Titrate with caution in cardiac, renal, or hepatic dysfunction • Caution in pheochromocytoma and portal hypertension

(continued)

Table 4. Common Continuous Non-Adrenergic Vasoactive and Vasodilator Agents (*continued*)

Drug	Dose	Mechanism/Clinical Effects	Titration[a]	Cautions/Comments
Nitroglycerin	Initial: 0.25–0.5 mcg/kg/min Range: 0.25–3 mcg/kg/min Max: 5 mcg/kg/min Max adult dose: 400 mcg/min	• Converted to nitric oxide in vascular smooth muscle leading to vasodilation of venous and arterial smooth muscle ○ Venous effect greater than arterial	0.5–1 mcg/kg/min every ≥ 3 min until desired effect is reached	• Patients who do not respond hemodynamically with doses of ~200 mcg/minute should be considered nonresponders[130] • Administer with nitro-tubing and nitro-clave • Headache, flushing, hypotension, pallor, reflex tachycardia • With abrupt withdrawal: severe hypotension, bradycardia, acute coronary vascular insufficiency • Contraindicated in patients with glaucoma, severe anemia, increased ICP, hypotension, uncontrolled hypokalemia, pericardial tamponade, constrictive pericarditis • Use with extreme caution with PDE-5 inhibitors
Nitroprusside	Initial: 0.25–0.5 mcg/kg/min Range: 0.25–3 mcg/kg/min Max: 10 mcg/kg/min Max adult dose: 400 mcg/min	• Induces release of nitric oxide leading to vasodilation of venous and arterial smooth muscle	0.5–1 mcg/kg/min every ≥ 5 min until desired effect is reached	• Product should be protected from light, even during administration • Headache, flushing, hypotension, pallor, reflex tachycardia • With abrupt withdrawal: severe hypotension, bradycardia, acute coronary vascular insufficiency • Contraindicated in severe anemia, increased ICP, hypotension, uncontrolled hypokalemia, pericardial tamponade, constrictive pericarditis • Metabolized to cyanide in the bloodstream, then to thiocyanate in the liver, which is then renally eliminated • Use with PDE-5 inhibitors increases the risk of systemic and cerebral vasodilation and hypotension; use with extreme caution
Prostaglandin E$_1$	Initial: 0.05–0.1 mcg/kg/min • Once therapeutic response is achieved, reduce to lowest effective maintenance dose Range 0.01–0.4 mcg/kg/min	• Direct vasodilation to vascular smooth muscle	0.03–0.1 mcg/kg/min every ≥ 20 min Therapeutic response indicated by: • Increase in systemic BP and pH in those with restricted systemic blood flow and acidosis • Increase in oxygenation (pO$_2$) in those with restricted pulmonary blood flow	• Flushing • Hypotension, bradycardia • Thrombocytopenia (with prolonged infusion) • Apnea most common in patients < 2 kg and with doses > 0.015 mcg/kg/min
Vasopressin (Pressor Effect)	Initial: 0.05 milliunits/kg/min Range: 0.05–2 milliunits/kg/min	• Vasoconstriction/increase in SVR and BP	0.05–0.5 milliunits/kg/min every ≥ 30 min until desired effect is reached	• Vasoconstriction • Hypervolemia • Hyponatremia

[a]Titrations may vary based on clinical indication and patient status.

AV = atrioventricular; BP = blood pressure; CO = cardiac output; CVP = central venous pressure; DOPA = dopamine; ECG = electrocardiogram; HR = heart rate; ICP = intracranial pressure; PDE = phosphodiesterase; SVR = systemic vascular resistance.

Although this section has focused on systemic cardiac output, many patients also require pharmacologic manipulation of the pulmonary vasculature to improve cardiac output to the lungs. Agents such as oxygen, nitric oxide, bosentan, sildenafil, epoprostenol, treprostinil, and iloprost have been used to augment cardiac output to the pulmonary vascular bed.[70-82]

INOTROPY

Increased contractility (inotropy) in the immediate postoperative period can be achieved with a wide variety of continuous-infusion medications, such as dobutamine, dopamine, epinephrine, norepinephrine, and milrinone. Catecholamines, such as epinephrine and norepinephrine, should be used in lower doses to improve contractility and minimize peripheral vasoconstriction and increased afterload. Dopamine may be used as an inotropic agent, but reports have associated its use with an increase in postoperative arrhythmias.[83,84] Dobutamine can be used as an inotropic agent with the beneficial effect of reduced afterload from peripheral vasodilation, but arrhythmias have also been noted with its use.[38-40]

Catecholamine refractory shock, a condition in which increasing doses of catecholamines do not induce changes in vasculature tone or inotropy, can occur in patients who have undergone congenital heart disease surgery. Vasopressin is an agent that can be considered in patients with catecholamine refractory shock. Vasopressin is a potent vasoconstrictor that, when used at very low doses, has profound effects on the periphery and the coronary arteries when traditional catecholamines cease being effective.[85-90] Catecholamine refractory shock also coincides with adrenal insufficiency, which is more prominent in patients with previous cardiac surgeries.[91] Bolus administration or continuous infusion of hydrocortisone for 5 days postoperatively improves catecholamine responsiveness and hemodynamic variables without suppression of the hypothalamic-pituitary-adrenal access.[92]

A comprehensive understanding of the pharmacology and physiologic effects of medications used for the prevention and treatment of LCOS is necessary to make informed decisions/recommendations. Optimal postoperative management requires use of nonpharmacologic and pharmacologic modalities. Nonpharmacologic options, such as peritoneal dialysis, ventilator strategies, or mechanical support, are often used.[11,12,14] Pharmacotherapy should be applied in a selective manner that incorporates not only the patient's cardiac pathophysiology, but also other comorbidities that are present (Figure 2).

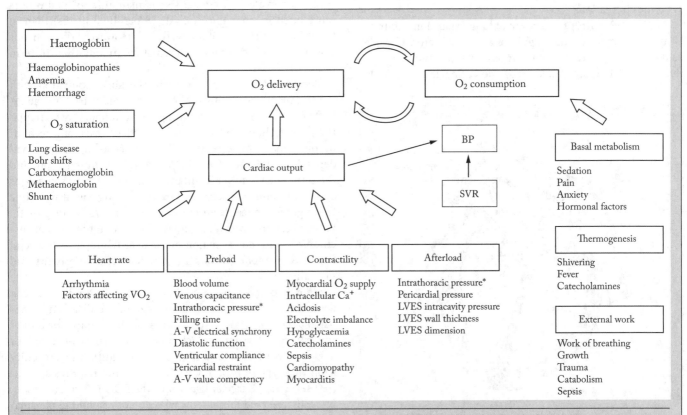

Figure 2. Monitoring of cardiac output.

This diagram shows the complicated assessment and treatment of postoperative low cardiac output syndrome for a patient who has undergone surgical repair of a congenital heart defect. The goal of treating low cardiac output syndrome is to improve the delivery of oxygen to end organs, adequately providing tissues with oxygen as needed according to demand. Pharmacologic manipulation of cardiac output focuses on optimizing preload, increasing contractility, and decreasing afterload.

* Common intensive care scenarios augmenting intrathoracic pressure include mechanical ventilation, pneumothorax, and pleural/pericardial fluid collections.

A-V (AV) = atrioventricular; BP = blood pressure; LVES = left ventricular end systolic; SVR = systemic vascular resistance; VO$_2$ = oxygen uptake.

Reprinted with permission from: Tibby SM, Murdoch IA. Monitoring cardiac function in intensive care. Arch Dis Child 2003;88:46-52.

FETAL VS. NEONATAL CIRCULATION

The primary difference between fetal circulation and neonatal circulation, as it pertains to congenital heart disease, is the oxygenation of blood by the placenta instead of the lungs. Fetal pulmonary vasculature is typically constricted, allowing only a small amount of blood to the lungs and resulting in high right-sided pressures. The lungs are bypassed in utero by three shunts: (1) the *ductus venosus*, which connects the inferior vena cava to the intra-hepatic portion of the umbilical vein; (2) the *ductus arteriosus*, which connects the pulmonary artery (PA) to the aorta; and (3) the *foramen ovale*, which is a communication through the atrial septum connecting the left atria (LA) and right atria (RA). Oxygenated blood is delivered to the heart from the placenta and travels through the right atrium. About 66% of the blood empties into the right ventricle (RV) and is pumped through the PA, where it then shunts across the patent ductus arteriosus (PDA) to the aorta. Because of a high PVR, only about 10% of this blood traveling through the fetal PA will actually pass through the pulmonary vasculature. The remaining blood in the RA is shunted from the right atrium to the left atrium (a right to left shunt) across the patent foramen ovale (PFO), emptied into the left ventricle (LV), and is then pumped to the aorta and into the systemic circulation.[93]

At birth, PVR drops as a result of lung expansion and inhalation of oxygen, a potent pulmonary vasodilator. The placenta is no longer responsible for oxygenation, and when it is removed, SVR increases, thereby increasing left ventricular

and left atrial pressure. This increase in pressure, together with increased blood return from the lungs to the left atrium, causes the PFO to close. Closure of the ductus venosus occurs after the termination of umbilical blood flow, which decreases pressure in the inferior vena cava and right atrium. The concentration of prostaglandin E$_2$ (PGE$_2$), a potent vasodilator, drops, and the ductus arteriosus begins to close within the first 12 hours, with complete closure occurring in about 96 hours. When these shunts have completely closed, the heart is considered to have mature circulation.[93]

CONGENITAL HEART DISEASE

PATENT DUCTUS ARTERIOSUS

The ductus arteriosus connects the PA and the aorta, which is necessary to bypass the pulmonary vasculature in utero. The ductus arteriosus should completely close about 96 hours after birth, secondary to a reduction in endogenous PGE$_2$ synthesis and concentration (Figure 3).[5,6,93] A PDA that does not close spontaneously, which accounts for around 10% of all congenital heart disease, occurs as an isolated defect without other congenital heart disease in as many as 90% of cases. A PDA is twice as prevalent in female versus male infants, and occurs more often in premature infants (8 per 1000 births) than in term infants (1 per 5000 births).[1,2] However, spontaneous closure is more common in premature infants than in term infants.[94-97]

Because of higher pressures in the aorta compared with the PA, blood ejected from the LV with shunt back to the PA (left to right shunting) resulting in pulmonary overcirculation, congestion, and eventual left-sided heart failure and/or pulmonary hypertension. The degree of symptoms will depend on the size of the PDA, the age at presentation, and the ratio of SVR to PVR. Infants with a PDA may show signs and symptoms of heart failure, including sweating while feeding, tachypnea, feeding intolerance, and/or poor growth. Patients can be given a diagnosis of a PDA on the basis of auscultation, with confirmation by echocardiography. Closure of the PDA is important to minimize long-term morbidity and mortality.[94,96]

Choice of therapy modality is multifactorial and can depend on the age of the patient, size of the PDA, and other patient-related factors. Nonpharmacologic therapy for a PDA consists of interventional closure by insertion of a coil or device into the ductus arteriosus. Morbidity and mortality from this type of procedure is very low, but requires specialized services.[98] Surgical ligation of the PDA is also an option, typically reserved for patients who do not respond to pharmacologic therapy, who have a very large PDA, or when coinciding with other heart defects.

Before closure of a PDA, pharmacotherapy is focused on reducing pulmonary congestion, heart failure, and pulmonary overcirculation. Restriction of fluids and use of diuretics is common practice.[94] However, the use of loop diuretics, such as furosemide, should be approached with caution as they have been noted to increase PGE synthesis, thus potentially impairing closure of the PDA.[99-101] Primary pharmacologic therapy for closure of a PDA consists of the nonsteroidal

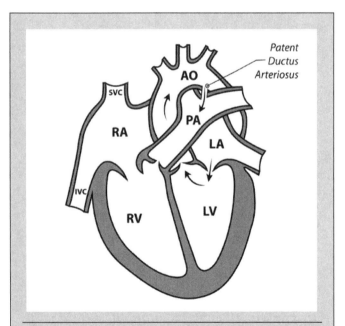

Figure 3. Patent ductus arteriosus.

This diagram shows the anatomic description of a PDA and the movement of blood flow in a patient with a PDA. The arrows represent blood shunting from the higher-pressure (left) side to the lower-pressure pulmonary arterial (right) side, resulting in pulmonary overcirculation and congestion.

AO = aorta; IVC = inferior vena cava; LA = left atria; LV = left ventricle; PA = pulmonary artery; PDA = patent ductus arteriosus; RA = right atria; RV = right ventricle; SVC = superior vena cava.

anti-inflammatory drugs (NSAIDs) indomethacin (0.2 mg/kg/dose intravenously initially, with subsequent doses based on post-natal age) or ibuprofen (10 mg/kg/dose intravenously initially, followed by 5 mg/kg/dose intravenously at 24 and 48 hours).[66] By administering these agents, circulating concentrations of PGEs are decreased, thus promoting constriction and closure of the PDA. Intravenous indomethacin has traditionally been the agent of choice for pharmacologic closure of a PDA, and is given in escalating doses during a 72-hour period. A lack of clinically significant differences between intravenous ibuprofen and intravenous indomethacin for closure of a PDA in a term infant have been reported, although ibuprofen may have fewer adverse events in preterm neonates, such as lower serum creatinine values and higher urine output.[101] The preferential agent for PDA closure varies among institutions. Adverse events associated with indomethacin and ibuprofen therapy include necrotizing enter colitis, bleeding (including intracranial hemorrhage), and acute kidney injury. Acetaminophen has also been used for PDA closure, primarily in extremely low-birth-weight and preterm neonates, and appears to be a promising alternative to NSAIDs with possible fewer adverse effects. Acetaminophen may therefore be considered for patients without clinical need for surgical repair and with contraindications to NSAID therapy.[102,103] After closure of an isolated PDA, long-term survival is excellent, and a normal life span is expected.

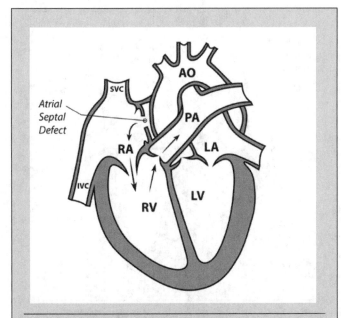

Figure 4. Atrial septal defect.

This diagram shows the anatomic description of an ASD and the movement of blood flow in a patient with an ASD. The arrows represent blood shunting from the higher-pressure (left) side to the lower-pressure pulmonary arterial (right) side, resulting in pulmonary overcirculation, congestion, and potential right atrial enlargement.

AO = aorta; ASD = atrial septal defect; IVC = inferior vena cava; LA = left atria; LV = left ventricle; PA = pulmonary artery; RA = right atria; RV = right ventricle; SVC = superior vena cava.

ATRIAL SEPTAL DEFECT

An atrial septal defect (ASD) is a communication between the RA and LA through the atrial septum (Figure 4). About 10% of all congenital heart defects are ASDs, and ASDs occur twice as often in female versus male infants.[1,2] Most ASDs occur in the middle of the septum (ostium secundum ASD), but others can occur close to the atrioventricular valves (ostium premium ASD) or close to the superior vena cava (sinus venosus ASD). In a common ASD, oxygenated blood is shunted from LA into the RA (left to right shunt), resulting in pulmonary overcirculation and congestion, right atrial enlargement, and, potentially, right-sided heart failure. Right atrial enlargement, caused by volume overload from the left to right shunt, can result in atrial arrhythmias, particularly in older children and adults. In cases associated with concomitant pulmonary arterial stenosis or increased PVR, however, blood may actually shunt deoxygenated blood from the RA to the LA (right to left shunt), resulting in cyanosis.[13] Most patients with an ASD will (initially) remain asymptomatic, and some ASDs close spontaneously; the degree of symptomatology is often related to the size of the ASD.[104] Large ASDs may have significant shunting and should undergo surgical or interventional closure in the cardiac catheterization laboratory. Interventional closure carries less morbidity than surgical closure, but it can only be performed in select patients. Overall mortality for surgical or interventional closure is very low, and patients can be expected to have a normal life span after their procedure.[105,106]

Preoperative pharmacotherapy is limited in patients with ASDs associated with significant shunting because closure of the ASD is the curative course. Relief of symptoms including pulmonary congestion can be achieved with diuretics. Surgical closure of an ASD may require pharmacologic therapy to treat postoperative hypertension, which is not often observed after device closure. Nicardipine or nitroprusside are commonly used for treatment of hypertension in the immediate postoperative period.[107-110] If needed, β-Blockers and ACEIs are viable options for continuations of therapy thereafter, and also mitigate progression to heart failure.[110-112] Anticoagulation after surgical or interventional closure of an ASD is often indicated until endothelialization of the surgical patch or device has occurred. Typically, low-dose aspirin (1–5 mg/kg/day; maximum 81 mg/day) is used for 3–6 months after closure despite limited data on the efficacy of this practice. Patients without comorbidities can be expected to live a normal life span.

VENTRICULAR SEPTAL DEFECT

A ventricular septal defect (VSD) is a communication between the LV and RV, which may occur anywhere along the septum (Figure 5). As the most common congenital heart defect, VSDs are about 20% to 30% of all congenital heart defects.[1,2] Typically, oxygenated blood is shunted from the LV to RV (left to right shunt; a "restrictive" VSD), resulting in pulmonary overcirculation, congestion, right-sided heart failure, and, possibly, pulmonary hypertension.[13] Like with an ASD, the degree (and direction) of shunting and symptomology depends on the size of the VSD and the ratio of PVR and SVR. Patients with very small VSDs may be asymptomatic; otherwise symptoms may include dyspnea, poor feeding, failure to thrive, or signs and symptoms of heart failure. However, VSDs may be large enough ("nonrestrictive") to allow shunting of deoxygenated blood from the RV to LV (right to left shunt), resulting in cyanosis.[13] Right to left shunting and cyanosis can also occur in patients with VSD, with concomitant pulmonary arterial stenosis or increased PVR. Patients with a VSD are at increased risk of developing bacterial endocarditis, regardless of VSD size. Diagnosis of a VSD can be made by auscultation, and echocardiography is often used to confirm the diagnosis and determine the size and shunting direction of the VSD.[93]

Up to 25% of patients with a VSD have spontaneous closure during childhood, and small VSDs are more likely to spontaneously close than a large VSD.[113] Clinically significant VSDs that do not spontaneously close require surgical or catheter-directed closer, both of which are associated with very low rates of mortality. Surgical intervention should take place in neonates and infants with significant clinical presentation (i.e., failure to thrive) and signs and symptoms of heart failure. In addition, children with pulmonary hypertension, regardless of the size of VSD, should undergo surgical or interventional closure.

The goal of preoperative pharmacotherapy in patients with a VSD is to minimize pulmonary congestion, prevent heart failure, and maintain growth. Various agents have been used to reduce afterload and minimize congestion. Hydralazine was initially the agent of choice, but recently, furosemide (or other diuretics), digoxin, and ACEIs have been used.[63,65,114-118] Caution is warranted when using ACEIs because of the risk of acute kidney injury, particularly in very young patients with a VSD.[63,66,68] Immediate postoperative management consists of maintaining cardiac output and management of postoperative hypertension. Patients may still be hypertensive after discharge and should be followed until blood pressure has normalized. Unlike ASD, low-dose aspirin is not generally indicated as higher ventricular (vs. atrial) pressures decrease the propensity for cardiac hemostasis. However, low-dose aspirin for 3–6 months after a surgical procedure may be considered for patients with lower ventricular performance or with additional risk factors for venous thromboembolism. Patients without comorbidities can be expected to live a normal life span.

TETRALOGY OF FALLOT

The anatomic description of tetralogy of Fallot (TOF) consists of four components: pulmonary stenosis, aorta overriding the ventricular septum, right ventricular hypertrophy, and VSD (Figure 6).[5,6,93] Tetralogy of Fallot accounts for about 10% of all congenital heart defects, and it is the most common

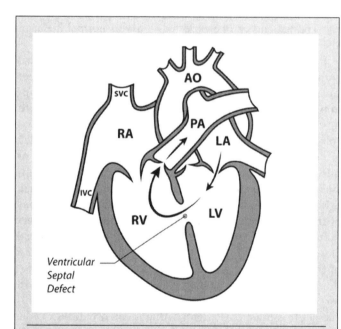

Figure 5. Ventricular septal defect.

This diagram shows the anatomic description of a VSD and the movement of blood flow in a patient with a VSD. The arrows represent blood shunting from the higher-pressure (left) side to the lower-pressure pulmonary arterial (right) side, resulting in pulmonary overcirculation, congestion, and heart failure. Left ventricular enlargement can also occur, secondary to increased blood return from the lungs to the LA and LV, resulting in systolic dysfunction and heart failure.

AO = aorta; IVC = inferior vena cava; LA = left atria; LV = left ventricle; PA = pulmonary artery; RA = right atria; RV = right ventricle; SVC = superior vena cava; VSD = ventricular septal defect.

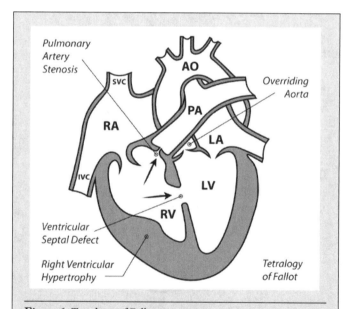

Figure 6. Tetralogy of Fallot.

This diagram shows the four components of tetralogy of Fallot: pulmonary artery stenosis, right ventricular hypertrophy, aorta overriding the ventricular septum, and ventricular septal defect. Patients experience hypercyanotic episodes ("Tet spells") when pulmonary vascular resistance is elevated, and unoxygenated blood is shunted from right to left and to the systemic circulation.

AO = aorta; IVC = inferior vena cava; LA = left atria; LV = left ventricle; PA = pulmonary artery; RA = right atria; RV = right ventricle; SVC = superior vena cava.

cyanotic heart defect in patients younger than 1 year.[1,2] The degree and frequency of shunting, as well as symptomology, is based on the severity of the pulmonary stenosis. Patients with mild pulmonary stenosis have more prominent left to right shunting across the VSD, leading to heart failure. These patients are often referred to as a *pink tet*. In patients with moderate to severe pulmonary stenosis, blood flow is more limited to the pulmonary vasculature, and right to left shunting of blood is more prominent, resulting in cyanosis, otherwise known as a *blue tet*. Most patients will present within the first year of life, and signs and symptoms can include decreased growth or poor feeding, dyspnea on exertion, or decreased tolerance to physical activity. Older patients will also show signs of clubbing from chronic cyanosis.

When PVR is acutely greater than the pressure in the LV, the right to left shunting of deoxygenated blood ensues, resulting in acute cyanosis, which is termed a *hypercyanotic episode*, or *Tet spell*. Hypercyanotic spells often occur when patients are ill or agitated or when they have been unable to inhale enough oxygen to maintain pulmonary vasodilation (e.g., crying). These are medical emergencies, and interventions are urgently required to shunt blood from left to right and into the pulmonary vasculature.[119,120] Patients

at risk of having a Tet spell are often placed on propranolol, which minimizes the spasm of the infundibulum below the PA and relaxes the RV and right ventricular outflow tract.[121,122] Treatment of a Tet spell focuses on elevating SVR and decreasing PVR. Older patients may have a characteristic movement known as *squatting* in response to a Tet spell, also referred to as the *knee-to-chest maneuver*.[65,118] By bringing the knees to the chest, SVR is increased, left ventricular pressure is increased, and blood is shunted from left to right. Pharmacologic interventions include oxygen (decreases PVR), morphine (decreases PVR), fluids (increases right ventricular filling and pulmonary blood flow), β-blockers, and intravenous phenylephrine (increases afterload).

Preoperative management consists of minimizing right to left shunting and preventing heart failure. Surgical intervention is the curative approach for TOF. The VSD is closed in such a way that the aorta then originates only from the LV. To relieve the PA stenosis, infundibular masses can be resected, the PA can be augmented with a patch, or the PA can be completely replaced with synthetic valved conduit. Preliminary use of a Blalock-Taussig (BT) shunt, which connects the aorta to the PA, bypassing the stenotic region of the PA, is sometimes considered for patients who maintain adequate oxygen saturations while unrepaired; these patients generally then undergo a full repair between ages 3–6 months. This approach, however, is now uncommon unless the patient has specific morbidities that do not allow an immediate complete repair.[13]

Immediate postoperative management consists of maintaining cardiac output, treating postoperative hypertension, and ensuring adequate pulmonary blood flow. Inhaled nitric oxide has been used to improve pulmonary blood flow after surgical correction.[123] Alternatively, inhaled epoprostenol has also been used to reduce PVR postoperatively.[124] Patients are often given low-dose aspirin for 3–6 months after placement of foreign material, such as a PA patch, or patients may take aspirin indefinitely if a pulmonary valve has been placed.[125] Long-term management of surgically corrected TOF focuses on prevention and treatment of heart failure and treatment of right ventricular dysfunction. Sustained postoperative arrhythmias have also been reported, with older age and presence of valvular regurgitation being primary risk factors.[126] Treatments may include surgical resection, cryoablation, an implantable cardioverter-defibrillator, and anti-arrhythmic agents. The choice of antiarrhythmic agent is dependent on the specific arrhythmia and will not be discussed in this chapter. The long-term survival for patients with surgically corrected TOF is good (estimated at 86% at older than 30 years), but it is still less than that for patients without congenital heart disease.[1,127]

TRANSPOSITION OF THE GREAT ARTERIES

Transposition of the great arteries (TGA) is a defect in which the PA arises from the LV, and the aorta arises from the RV (Figure 7). This defect accounts for about 7% of all congenital heart defects, and it is most often diagnosed prenatally by echocardiography or in infancy.[1,2] In utero, the communication between the PA and aorta by the PDA and PFO allow

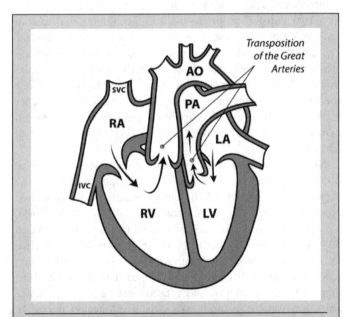

Figure 7. Transposition of the great arteries.

This diagram shows the anatomy of TGA, in which the aorta (AO) arises from the right ventricle (RV), and the pulmonary artery (PA) arises from the left ventricle (LV). In utero, the PDA would connect the AO and PA. After birth, once the PDA begins to constrict, two separate circulations form in the patient with TGA: (1) unoxygenated blood travels from the IVC/SVC → RA → RV → AO → systemic circulation without going to the pulmonary vasculature; and (2) oxygenated blood travels from the pulmonary veins → LA → LV → PA → lungs without going to the systemic circulation. In summary, oxygenated blood never reaches the end organs, and unoxygenated blood is continually cycled through the systemic circulation.

IVC = inferior vena cava; LA = left atria; PDA = patent ductus arteriosus; RA = right atria; SVC = superior vena cava; TGA = transposition of the great arteries.

for delivery of oxygenated blood to the systemic circulation. In TGA, closure of the PDA and PFO after birth results in reversed pulmonary and systemic circulations, with delivery of deoxygenated blood to the systemic circulation. Patients may or may not have a septal defect in conjunction with TGA. The lack of oxygenated blood delivery to end organs will result in profound acidosis and shock. Patients without a prenatal diagnosis often present in shock about 24–72 hours after birth, when the PDA begins to close. Echocardiography after birth can definitively diagnose TGA.

Surgical correction by the arterial switch procedure is the standard for patients with TGA. Prior to repair, the left ventricle is pumping blood to the pulmonary vasculature, which has a lower pressure than that of systemic vasculature. In order to preserve left ventricular function needed to deliver blood to the higher pressure of the systemic vasculature, surgical repair should ideally occur within the first 2 weeks of life.[13,93] The arterial switch procedure consists of keeping the roots of both the PA and the aorta in the original location, but removing the remainder of each vessel and anastomosing each to the opposite root. In addition, the coronary arteries are removed from aortic root in the RV and reattached to the PA root in the LV. Before the arterial switch procedure, the Mustard procedure, which consists of a complex series of intracardiac baffles to shunt blood to the appropriate vessels, was a common surgical approach. Patients with TGA in combination with pulmonary

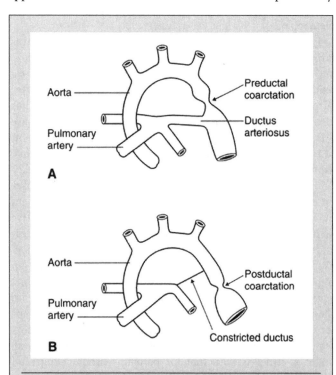

Figure 8. Coarctation of the aorta.

These diagrams show two versions of coarctation of the aorta. A coarctation can occur before the ductus arteriosus (A) or after the ductus arteriosus (B). In addition, the preductal coarctations can occur further up the aortic arch and involve the carotid or subclavian arteries.

Reprinted with permission from: Lilly L. Pathophysiology of Heart Disease, 2nd ed. Baltimore: Lippincott Williams & Wilkins, 1998.

stenosis may still undergo the Mustard procedure to avoid placing the stenotic PA in the aortic position.[128]

Preoperative pharmacotherapy of TGA consists of maintaining the PDA to ensure that oxygenated blood flows from the PA to the aorta. This goal is accomplished by using a PGE E1 (PGE$_1$) infusion to maintain ductal patency.[129] Immediate postoperative pharmacotherapy should manage LCOS. Patients may also be placed on a prophylactic nitroglycerin infusion, as a coronary vasodilator, to prevent coronary vasospasm after their surgical manipulation (although unlikely to exceed adult dosing of nitroglycerin, the total flat dose should always be determined to avoid potential adverse effects; Table 4).[130] Long-term pharmacotherapy is minimal because patients should have normal circulation, and long-term survival for patients after the arterial switch procedure is good, cited at about 85%.[131,132]

COARCTATION OF THE AORTA

A patient with coarctation of the aorta has a narrowing of the aorta, which restricts blood flow to the systemic circulation (Figure 8). Aortic coarctations are often associated with other congenital heart defects and account for about 6% of all congenital heart defects. Coarctations are also typically divided into two categories: preductal and postductal.[1,2] *Preductal coarctation* occurs most often in a fetus with another cardiac anomaly that restricts blood flow to the aorta and is associated with aortic arch hypoplasia. *Postductal coarctation* occurs as an isolated lesion most often after birth and is most likely the result of ductal tissue in the aorta that constricts after birth.[13,93] Both forms of coarctation can result in decreased cardiac output and left ventricular hypertrophy because of aortic obstruction.

Neonatal patients with preductal coarctation can exhibit differential cyanosis (differing oxygen saturations on the upper and lower parts of the body) because of deoxygenated blood shunting from the PA through the PDA to the aorta. Coarctations can also cause differential blood pressures based on the location of the coarctation in relation to the ductus; for example, if the ductus is after the subclavian arteries, then blood pressure will be higher in the arms than in the legs. Some patients with mild coarctation may never experience any symptomatology and may grow and develop normally. Mild coarctations can present with tachypnea, hepatomegaly, dyspnea, and tachycardia. Neonates with severe coarctation will present in shock with profound acidosis, caused by lack of blood flow to end organs, and they may develop heart failure.[13,93] Collateral arteries may develop spontaneously in some patients to accommodate for the lack of blood flow through the aorta, and these collateral arteries can erode through the ribcage.[13,93] A coarctation may sometimes be diagnosed in older patients who experience dyspnea on exertion or syncope, however this approach to diagnosis is less common. Echocardiography or magnetic resonance imaging can be used to confirm the diagnosis.[13,93]

Surgical correction is necessary to eliminate the coarctation. Two surgical methods are commonly used: end-to-end anastomosis or patch repair. The *end-to-end anastomosis* does not routinely involve cardiopulmonary bypass and can occur when the coarctation does not involve the carotid arteries. During this procedure, both ends of the coarctation are clamped, the narrowed section is dissected, and the aorta is then sutured together. The *patch repair technique* involves cardiopulmonary bypass, with dissection of the coarctation followed by repair of the aorta with a prosthetic patch. Operative mortality is reported at less than 2%, but it can be higher in neonates presenting in shock or with ventricular dysfunction.[13]

Preoperative pharmacotherapy is aimed at maintaining cardiac output in the presence of an obstruction. For preductal coarctations, PGE_1 may be used to maintain the PDA and deliver systemic blood flow postductus.[130] Managing heart failure and decreasing afterload are also strategies for maintaining cardiac output before surgical intervention. In the immediate postoperative period, many patients experience hypertension after coarctation repair, which is imperative to treat to avoid rupturing aortic sutures.[130] The etiology of this hypertension is not completely understood; however, it may involve enhanced sympathetic activity to compensate for the previously elevated SVR before surgical repair and/or high-circulating levels of catecholamines after repair. Based on these proposed mechanisms, afterload-reducing agents (e.g., nicardipine, nitroprusside) are generally preferred; however, β-blockers (e.g., esmolol, labetalol) may also be considered if contraindications to afterload-reducing agents ensue; nitroprusside should be avoided or used with caution in patients with hepatic and/or renal dysfunction because of the increased risk of cyanide/thiocyanate toxicity.[45,133-140] Long-term management of hypertension is often necessary for up to 6 months after the surgical procedure. In general, ACE-inhibitors are preferred in patients without presence or risk factors for renal dysfunction. β-Blockers (e.g., propranolol, atenolol) may also be considered; however, there are fewer data on the use of these agents for this indication, specifically in neonates and infants. Patients should be followed routinely because of a potential for re-coarctation. The long-term survival rate for patients with coarctation repair is excellent.

HYPOPLASTIC LEFT HEART SYNDROME

Patients with hypoplastic left heart syndrome (HLHS) have a small to nonexistent LV and narrow (or atretic) aorta (Figure 9). Patients are unable to survive with HLHS without surgical treatment because of insufficient blood flow from the LV through the aorta, to the systemic circulation. Only about 1% of all congenital heart defects are HLHS; however, the syndrome requires the largest amount of resources for repair compared with other congenital cardiac defects.[1,2]

Hypoplastic left heart syndrome is not compatible to life; however, because of intracardiac shunting as a fetus, infants may not be given a diagnosis until they present postnatally in shock as the PDA begins to close. This condition was uniformly fatal before the early 1980s, when Dr. William Norwood introduced the three-stage approach to surgical repair of HLHS.[141] Immediately after birth, PGE_1 is used to maintain the PDA and deliver systemic blood flow postductus. In addition, before initial surgical intervention, patients may require a balloon atrial septostomy to create an ASD if the PFO has closed or if it is too small. The ASD is necessary

for survival because it allows shunting of oxygenated blood from the LA to the RA. This right to left shunting allows for the mixing of oxygenated and deoxygenated blood in the RA, which would then be ejected from the RV to the systemic circulation by the PDA, until the first surgical procedure can be performed. The first stage of the surgical palliation occurs within the first few days of life and includes the following procedures: (1) combining the aorta and PAs into one "neo-aorta" (also called the *Damus-Kaye-Stansel procedure*); (2) creating a large ASD, and (3) placing one of two aortopulmonary shunts: *a BT shunt*, which is a subclavian to PA connection, or a *Sano shunt*, which is an RV to PA shunt.[142] Sano shunts may have a potential advantage because they maintain higher diastolic pressure, thus avoiding diastolic runoff and presumably providing better coronary perfusion. Long-term outcomes between the two shunts remain inconclusive.[143] These interventions allow oxygenated blood from the lungs to flow from the pulmonary veins to the LA, across the septum to the RA—where it mixes with deoxygenated blood from the inferior vena cava/superior vena cava—to the RV. Blood then flows through the neo-aorta and then either to the lungs (by the BT shunt or Sano shunt) or the systemic circulation by the aorta. Hybrid procedures have been performed that involve stenting the PDA open to supply blood flow to the aorta from the PA, together with banding of the branch PAs, which restricts pulmonary blood flow and prevents overcirculation.[144-146] Because of complete mixing of oxygenated and deoxygenated blood at the atrial level, oxygen saturations after the Norwood procedure and other associated procedures should be at about 75% to 85%. This percentage represents an equal amount of blood flow to the pulmonary and systemic circulations (a Qp/Qs ratio of 1:1).[13]

Preoperative pharmacotherapy for HLHS before the Norwood procedure consists of maintaining the PDA to ensure blood flow through the aorta to the systemic circulation with PGE_1 administration, as well as managing the signs and symptoms of heart failure.[147,148] Infusions of PGE_1 are titrated to the lowest possible dose that will maintain ductal patency and minimize adverse events, such as hypotension or apnea. In the immediate postoperative period, treatment of LCOS and balancing of systemic and pulmonary blood flow are the goals of cardiovascular pharmacotherapy. Patients are often anticoagulated with a low-dose heparin infusion (6–10 units/kg/hour) until they are able to receive enteral medications; then low-dose aspirin (1–5 mg/kg/day) is used as an antiplatelet agent for the prevention of BT shunt thrombosis.[149] The ideal long-term or interstage management strategy for patients after a single ventricle palliation remains unclear.[150,151] However, use of digoxin after the Norwood procedure is performed has been associated with significantly reduced interstage mortality.[152] Sudden death during the interstage period can occur, and an exact etiology for this phenomenon is unknown.[153] In addition, the lack of inter-stage weight gain has been noted for patients after single ventricle palliation, which has been thought to contribute to mortality.[154-156] Pharmacotherapy has elicited few improvements in this area, with recent publications showing the ineffectiveness of ACEIs and other medications in improving interstage weight gain.[7] Current best practice appears to be close monitoring of weight

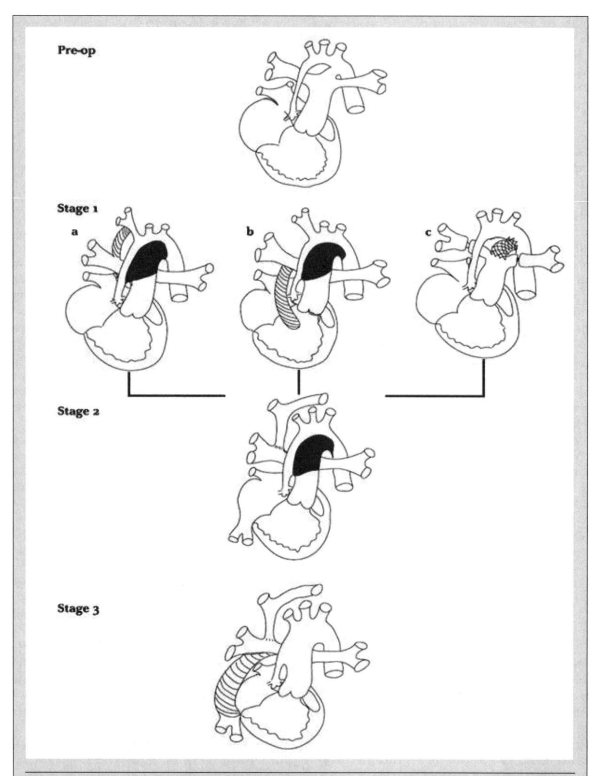

Figure 9. Hypoplastic left heart syndrome and three-stage surgery.

This diagram represents the anatomy of unrepaired hypoplastic left heart syndrome (HLHS). Note the aortic atresia and small left ventricle. Stage 1 represents three options for the initial palliation of HLHS: (a) the classic Norwood procedure combines the aorta and pulmonary artery (also known as the *Damus-Kaye-Stansel procedure*), creation of an atrial septal defect, and placement of a Blalock-Taussig (BT) shunt; (b) the Sano procedure replaces the BT shunt with a right ventricle to pulmonary artery conduit; and (c) a hybrid procedure involves stenting of the ductus arteriosus and banding of the branch pulmonary arteries. Stage 2 is the bidirectional Glenn procedure, in which the Blalock-Taussig shunt or right ventricle to pulmonary artery conduit is taken down, and the superior vena cava is attached to the pulmonary artery. Stage 3 is the Fontan procedure, in which an extracardiac conduit is used to attach the inferior vena cava to the pulmonary artery, subsequently dividing pulmonary and systemic circulations.

Reprinted with permission from: Stumper O. Hypoplastic left heart syndrome. Heart 2010;96:231-6.

and frequent follow-up before the second-stage procedure, the bidirectional Glenn procedure.[154-156]

The bidirectional Glenn procedure occurs at 4–6 months of life. The goal of the procedure is to remove the BT shunt or Sano shunt from the earlier Norwood procedure, and then attach the superior vena cava to the PA.[157] This approach delivers a greater amount of blood flow to the pulmonary vascular bed, and oxygen saturations generally increase to about 80% to 85%.[13]

Little information exists for the pharmacotherapeutic management of the patient after the bidirectional Glenn procedure. Immediate postoperative management consists of maintaining cardiac output and preventing thrombus with a low-dose heparin infusion (6–10 units/kg/hour). Anecdotally, a nitroglycerin infusion has been used to help maintain the patency of the superior vena cava to PA anastomosis. The increase in pulmonary blood flow can result in pulmonary congestion, for which diuretic therapy may be warranted. Patients who have undergone bidirectional Glenn and have elevated PVR may experience headaches caused by poor cerebral venous drainage through the super vena cava into the PA. This symptom can be treated with NSAIDs, acetaminophen, or diuretics to decrease pulmonary congestions, or an alternative is to use modalities that reduce PVR.[158,159] Long-term pharmacotherapy in patients after the bidirectional Glenn is directed toward the prevention of heart failure.

The Fontan procedure is the final stage of palliation, which consists of attaching the inferior vena cava, through a conduit, to the PA.[160] This procedure occurs at about age 3 years and completely separates the pulmonary and systemic circulations. The separated circulations should allow oxygen saturations to return to normal (95% to 100%) with the single RV pumping oxygenated blood to the systemic circulation. A small fenestration is usually created between the conduit and the right atrium to relieve pressure in the conduit if the PVR becomes too high, and to avoid hepatic congestion.[13] The fenestration is most often used in the immediate postoperative period when PVR is higher after cardiopulmonary bypass and during mechanical ventilation.

Immediate postoperative management of the patient after the Fontan procedure is focused on maintaining cardiac output and preventing LCOS. Patients are at risk of developing pleural or chylous effusions after the Fontan procedure. Protocolized management which includes postoperative diuretics, ACEI, fluid restriction, low-fat diets, and use of low-flow nasal cannula have been used and have been shown to mitigate chylous effusions and time to chest-tube removal.[161] The use of octreotide after the Fontan procedure has also been used with variable efficacy.[162-164] Protein-losing enteropathy (PLE) can also occur in postoperative Fontan patients. Treatment options of PLE include use of subcutaneous heparin injections based on its proposed anti-inflammatory effects, albumin replacement, and use of enteral budesonide.[165-167] Additional literature exists on the use of octreotide for PLE; however, the response is quite variable and often unsuccessful.[168]

One of the most controversial areas in pharmacotherapy for the Fontan patient is anticoagulation. Because of the physiology and hemodynamics of the Fontan circuit, the RA can become enlarged, with patients potentially developing atrial arrhythmias (i.e., atrial fibrillation, atrial flutter), thus increasing the propensity for thrombus formation. Previous, smaller population studies have evaluated the risks and benefits of aspirin anticoagulation compared with warfarin anticoagulation in the Fontan patient without arrhythmias, finding that bleeding risk is increased with warfarin, but thrombus formation is increased with aspirin use.[169-173] More recently, a 10-year analysis comparing thrombus and bleeding outcomes in 475 patients concluded no difference in the hazard rates of late thromboembolic events between aspirin and warfarin beyond the first year after the extracardiac conduit Fontan procedure.[174] Patients post-operative from the Fontan procedure also have significant variability in response to warfarin and an increased risk of bleeding, both of which are associated with a prolonged hospital admission.[175] Although there is no consensus on optimal anticoagulation strategies, for Fontan patients without contraindications aspirin alone may be considered postoperatively; warfarin should be considered for patients with additional risk factors for thromboembolism, including arrhythmias and hypercoagulable states.[126,176]

Long-term pharmacotherapeutic management of the Fontan patient includes the prevention and management of heart failure. There is currently no consensus on the optimal management or prevention of heart failure in a patient with a single RV, and practice varies widely.[5] In addition, heart failure in Fontan patients is primarily caused by right ventricular overload, which is comparatively different than in other adult populations. Enalapril and sildenafil have been studied in Fontan patients, but neither improved symptoms or exercise tolerance.[177-180] β-Blockers may show some benefit in Fontan patients with heart failure, but large trials have not been performed.[181,182] Further research in this area is warranted to improve long-term outcomes.

Because the Fontan procedure is the terminal operation in the staged repair of HLHS, patients can develop several complications throughout their lifetime. Many patients undergo revisions of their original Fontan circuit because of decreased exercise tolerance or increasing cyanosis. Life expectancy and quality of life have improved with time. As surgical and medical management continues to improve, patients will live longer, and health care providers will require specialized training and knowledge to appropriately care for patients with a single ventricle.

FUTURE DIRECTIONS

As surgical and medical management of congenital heart disease in children improves, patients are surviving into adulthood. The population of adult patients with congenital heart disease is growing by 5% per year, representing well over 1 million patients in the United States alone.[183-185] Management of the adult patient with congenital heart disease is an area that requires clinicians to have specialized knowledge in both pediatric and adult cardiovascular diseases. Morbidity can be high in this patient subset, and currently few centers have developed to care for this patient population.[186,187] The specific cardiac pathophysiologies and comorbidities in this patient population make application of pharmacotherapy challenging and ripe for research and evaluation.[188] In addition, the neurologic complications that can be associated with cardiopulmonary bypass, chronic cyanosis, and low-flow states are undergoing evaluation. It is well known that patients with congenital heart disease can have lower levels of cognitive function, and future directions include research to eliminate this morbidity.[189-193]

CONCLUSIONS

The pharmacotherapeutic management of patients with congenital heart disease is complex and plagued by a lack of data compared with that for adult patients with cardiac pathophysiology. A comprehensive understanding of pathophysiology, hemodynamics, and pediatric pharmacology is necessary to optimize outcomes for this challenging patient population.

Patient Case | MANAGEMENT OF POSTOPERATIVE HYPERTENSION AFTER COARCTECTOMY

A 4-month-old girl is referred to pediatric cardiology after a well child check at a pediatrician. The patient had mild hepatomegaly at the pediatrician office visit, and four extremity blood pressures showed elevated blood pressures in the right and left upper extremities. The cardiologist subsequently performed an echocardiogram, which showed a coarctation of the aorta occurring after the subclavian arteries. The patient underwent end-to-end anastomosis surgical repair by left thoracotomy. She has now been admitted to the intensive care unit for postoperative management of hypertension.

On examination in the immediate postoperative period (day 0), the patient is intubated and sedated, and she has two thoracostomy tubes with minimal drainage. She appears warm and well perfused and in no acute distress.

Medications: Fentanyl 1 mcg/kg/hour intravenously, pantoprazole 1 mg/kg/dose every 24 hours, and cefazolin 25 mg/kg/day intravenously every 8 hours; fluids are 5% dextrose with 0.45% sodium chloride at 50% of maintenance values

Physical examination: BP 145/96 mm Hg (arterial line), HR 120 beats per minute, brisk capillary refill (2–3 seconds), urine output 1.5 ml/kg/hour, Wt 10 kg

Laboratory findings:

SCr	0.4 mg/dL
Serum lactate	0.9 mg/dL
Na	139 mEq/L
K	3.7 mEq/L
HCO$_3$	26 mEq/L
Cl	101 mEq/L
ALT	37 U/L
AST	25 U/L
INR	1.2

1. What hypertensive agent do you recommend in the immediate postoperative period, as well as for long-term management if necessary?

An intravenous infusion of nicardipine or nitroprusside would be most appropriate in the immediate postoperative period because the patient would likely be unable to take enteral medications, and antihypertensive medications would need to be titrated sooner to maintain blood pressure at this time—specifically to mitigate the risk of suture rupture, as well as of postoperative bleeding and thoracostomy tube output. Esmolol could also be considered; however, without the presence of renal dysfunction, afterload-reducing agents are generally used first. Milrinone would not be an appropriate choice for antihypertensive effects because its primary use is to improve cardiac output through increased inotropy and vasodilation. In addition, this patient did not require cardiopulmonary bypass and does not have low cardiac output syndrome, as evidenced by the low lactate, adequate capillary refill, and normal urine output. For long-term management, once the blood pressure is normalized, transitioning to enalapril when the patient is able to take enteral medications would be preferred given the patient is without renal dysfunction. Enalapril is also commercially available as a solution and has data for use in neonates and infants. Atenolol would

not be a superior choice compared with enalapril in this scenario. Additionally, there are limited data for the use of atenolol in infants, and it also requires extemporaneous compounding.

2. What dosage regimen (dose, route, duration) and monitoring guidelines would you recommend for nitroprusside before the transition to enalapril for this patient?

A nitroprusside intravenous continuous infusion could be initiated at 0.5 mcg/kg/min and titrated every 5 minutes or more until goal blood pressures are reached. Serum lactate and other markers of perfusion (i.e., capillary refill, urine output, peripheral vs. core temperature) would be useful to ensure that the patient continues to deliver oxygen to end organs through the low cardiac output state, which occurs 6–18 hours after surgery. Cyanide and thiocyanate concentrations would not be necessary in this patient because of a very low risk of toxicity in the presence of normal renal and hepatic functions. However, if the patient were to develop signs or symptoms of cyanide/thiocyanate toxicity and/or to develop renal dysfunction, in conjunction with higher nitroprusside doses (generally more than 2 mcg/kg/min) and/or longer duration of therapy (more than 48 hours), then monitoring of cyanide/thiocyanate concentrations may be warranted. In addition, an elevated anion gap, lactate, and methemoglobin levels would ensue and should be monitored if a patient were symptomatic (i.e., lethargic, cyanotic) and/or cyanide/thiocyanate values were unavailable. Serum creatinine and electrolyte values should also be routinely monitored before and after initiation of enalapril because of the increased propensity of the drug to result in acute kidney injury and alterations in serum potassium.

REFERENCES

1. Mitchell SC, Korones SB, Berendes HW. Congenital heart disease in 56,109 births. Incidence and natural history. Circulation 1971;43:323-32.
2. Hoffman JI, Kaplan S. The incidence of congenital heart disease. J Am Coll Cardiol 2002;39:1890-900.
3. Blalock A, Taussig HB. Landmark article May 19, 1945: The surgical treatment of malformations of the heart in which there is pulmonary stenosis or pulmonary atresia. By Alfred Blalock and Helen B. Taussig. JAMA 1984;251:2123-8.
4. Gersony WM. Major advances in pediatric cardiology in the 20th century: II. Therapeutics. J Pediatr 2001;139:328-33.
5. Anderson PA, Breitbart RE, McCrindle BW, et al. The Fontan patient: inconsistencies in medication therapy across seven pediatric heart network centers. Pediatr Cardiol 2010;31:1219-28.
6. Pasquali SK, Hall M, Slonim AD, et al. Off-label use of cardiovascular medications in children hospitalized with congenital and acquired heart disease. Circ Cardiovasc Qual Outcomes 2008; 1:74-83.
7. Hsu DT, Zak V, Mahony L, et al. Enalapril in infants with single ventricle: results of a multicenter randomized trial. Circulation 2010;122:333-40.
8. Shaddy RE, Boucek MM, Hsu DT, et al. Carvedilol for children and adolescents with heart failure: a randomized controlled trial. JAMA 2007;298:1171-9.
9. Pasquali SK, Hall M, Li JS, et al. Corticosteroids and outcome in children undergoing congenital heart surgery: analysis of the Pediatric Health Information Systems database. Circulation 2010;122:2123-30.
10. Agarwal HS, Bennett JE, Churchwell KB, et al. Recombinant factor seven therapy for postoperative bleeding in neonatal and pediatric cardiac surgery. Ann Thorac Surg 2007;84:161-8.
11. Hanson J, Loftness S, Clarke D, et al. Peritoneal dialysis following open heart surgery in children. Pediatr Cardiol 1989;10:125-8.
12. Weng KP, Hsieh KS, Huang SH, et al. Peritoneal dialysis in treatment of postoperative heart failure after cardiac surgery in infants. Acta Paediatr Taiwan 2004;45:81-4.
13. Chang AC, Hanley FL, Wernovsky G, et al. Pediatric Cardiac Intensive Care. Baltimore: Lippincott Williams & Wilkins, 1998.
14. Shekerdemian L. Perioperative manipulation of the circulation in children with congenital heart disease. Heart 2009;95:1286-96.
15. Auler JO Jr, Barreto AC, Gimenez SC, et al. Pediatric cardiac postoperative care. Rev Hosp Clin Fac Med Sao Paulo 2002;57:115-23.
16. Cuadrado AR. Management of postoperative low cardiac output syndrome. Crit Care Nurs Q 2002;25:63-71.
17. Hoffman TM, Wernovsky G, Atz AM, et al. Efficacy and safety of milrinone in preventing low cardiac output syndrome in infants and children after corrective surgery for congenital heart disease. Circulation 2003;107:996-1002.
18. Wernovsky G, Wypij D, Jonas RA, et al. Postoperative course and hemodynamic profile after the arterial switch operation in neonates and infants. A comparison of low-flow cardiopulmonary bypass and circulatory arrest. Circulation 1995;92:2226-35.
19. Rocha TS, Silveira AS, Botta AM, et al. Serum lactate as mortality and morbidity marker in infants after Jatene's operation. Rev Bras Cir Cardiovasc 2010;25:350-8.
20. Schroth M, Plank C, Meissner U, et al. Hypertonic-hyperoncotic solutions improve cardiac function in children after open-heart surgery. Pediatrics 2006;118:e76-e84.
21. Chemtob S, Kaplan BS, Sherbotie JR, et al. Pharmacology of diuretics in the newborn. Pediatr Clin North Am 1989;36:1231-50.
22. Prandota J. Clinical pharmacology of furosemide in children: a supplement. Am J Ther 2001;8:275-89.
23. van der Vorst MM, Kist JE, van der Heijden AJ, et al. Diuretics in pediatrics: current knowledge and future prospects. Paediatr Drugs 2006;8:245-64.
24. van der Vorst MM, Ruys-Dudok van Heel I, Kist-van Holthe JE, et al. Continuous intravenous furosemide in haemodynamically unstable children after cardiac surgery. Intensive Care Med 2001;27:711-5.
25. van der Vorst MM, den HJ, Wildschut E, et al. An exploratory study with an adaptive continuous intravenous furosemide regimen in neonates treated with extracorporeal membrane oxygenation. Crit Care 2007;11:R111.
26. Senzaki H, Kamiyama M, Masutani S, et al. Efficacy and safety of torasemide in children with heart failure. Arch Dis Child 2008;93:768-71.
27. Marshall JD, Wells TG, Letzig L, et al. Pharmacokinetics and pharmacodynamics of bumetanide in critically ill pediatric patients. J Clin Pharmacol 1998;38:994-1002.
28. Brion LP, Primhak RA, Ambrosio-Perez I. Diuretics acting on the distal renal tubule for preterm infants with (or developing) chronic lung disease. Cochrane Database Syst Rev 2000; 3:CD001817.
29. García-Nieto V, Monge-Zamorano M, González-García M, et al. Effect of thiazides on bone mineral density in children with idiopathic hypercalciuria. Pediatr Nephrol 2012;27:261-8.
30. Buck ML. Clinical experience with spironolactone in pediatrics. Ann Pharmacother 2005;39:823-8.
31. Moffett BS, McDade E, Rossano JW, et al. Enteral potassium supplementation in a pediatric cardiac intensive care unit: evaluation of a practice change. Pediatr Crit Care Med 2011;12:552-4.
32. Moffett BS, Moffett TI, Dickerson HA. Acetazolamide therapy for hypochloremic metabolic alkalosis in pediatric patients with heart disease. Am J Ther 2007;14:331-5.
33. Bailey JM, Miller BE, Lu W, et al. The pharmacokinetics of milrinone in pediatric patients after cardiac surgery. Anesthesiology 1999;90:1012-8.
34. Bailey JM, Hoffman TM, Wessel DL, et al. A population pharmacokinetic analysis of milrinone in pediatric patients after cardiac surgery. J Pharmacokinet Pharmacodyn 2004;31:43-59.
35. Chang AC, Atz AM, Wernovsky G, et al. Milrinone: systemic and pulmonary hemodynamic effects in neonates after cardiac surgery. Crit Care Med 1995;23:1907-14.
36. Duggal B, Pratap U, Slavik Z, et al. Milrinone and low cardiac output following cardiac surgery in infants: is there a direct myocardial effect? Pediatr Cardiol 2005;26:642-5.
37. Ramamoorthy C, Anderson GD, Williams GD, et al. Pharmacokinetics and side effects of milrinone in infants and children after open heart surgery. Anesth Analg 1998;86:283-9.
38. Berg RA, Donnerstein RL, Padbury JF. Dobutamine infusions in stable, critically ill children: pharmacokinetics and hemodynamic actions. Crit Care Med 1993;21:678-86.
39. Bohn DJ, Poirier CS, Edmonds JF, et al. Hemodynamic effects of dobutamine after cardiopulmonary bypass in children. Crit Care Med 1980;8:367-71.

40. Habib DM, Padbury JF, Anas NG, et al. Dobutamine pharmacokinetics and pharmacodynamics in pediatric intensive care patients. Crit Care Med 1992;20:601-8.

41. Beekman RH, Rocchini AP, Dick M, et al. Vasodilator therapy in children: acute and chronic effects in children with left ventricular dysfunction or mitral regurgitation. Pediatrics 1984;73:43-51.

42. Moffett BS, Price JF. Evaluation of sodium nitroprusside toxicity in pediatric cardiac surgical patients. Ann Pharmacother 2008;42:1600-4.

43. Przybylo HJ, Stevenson GW, Schanbacher P, et al. Sodium nitroprusside metabolism in children during hypothermic cardiopulmonary bypass. Anesth Analg 1995;81:952-6.

44. Flynn JT, Mottes TA, Brophy PD, et al. Intravenous nicardipine for treatment of severe hypertension in children. J Pediatr 2001;139:38-43.

45. Nakagawa TA, Sartori SC, Morris A, et al. Intravenous nicardipine for treatment of postcoarctectomy hypertension in children. Pediatr Cardiol 2004;25:26-30.

46. Thomas CA, Moffett BS, Wagner JL, et al. Safety and efficacy of intravenous labetalol for hypertensive crisis in infants and small children. Pediatr Crit Care Med 2011;12:28-32.

47. Behera SK, Zuccaro JC, Wetzel GT, et al. Nesiritide improves hemodynamics in children with dilated cardiomyopathy: a pilot study. Pediatr Cardiol 2009;30:26-34.

48. Feingold B, Law YM. Nesiritide use in pediatric patients with congestive heart failure. J Heart Lung Transplant 2004;23:1455-9.

49. Jefferies JL, Denfield SW, Price JF, et al. A prospective evaluation of nesiritide in the treatment of pediatric heart failure. Pediatr Cardiol 2006;27:402-7.

50. Jefferies JL, Price JF, Denfield SW, et al. Safety and efficacy of nesiritide in pediatric heart failure. J Card Fail 2007;13:541-8.

51. Mahle WT, Cuadrado AR, Kirshbom PM, et al. Nesiritide in infants and children with congestive heart failure. Pediatr Crit Care Med 2005;6:543-6.

52. Marshall J, Berkenbosch JW, Russo P, et al. Preliminary experience with nesiritide in the pediatric population. J Intensive Care Med 2004;19:164-70.

53. Moffett BS, Jefferies JL, Price JF, et al. Administration of a large nesiritide bolus dose in a pediatric patient: case report and review of nesiritide use in pediatrics. Pharmacotherapy 2006; 26:277-80.

54. Price JF, Mott AR, Dickerson HA, et al. Worsening renal function in children hospitalized with decompensated heart failure: evidence for a pediatric cardiorenal syndrome? Pediatr Crit Care Med 2008;9:279-84.

55. Ryan A, Rosen DA, Tobias JD. Preliminary experience with nesiritide in pediatric patients less than 12 months of age. J Intensive Care Med 2008;23:321-8.

56. Simsic JM, Scheurer M, Tobias JD, et al. Perioperative effects and safety of nesiritide following cardiac surgery in children. J Intensive Care Med 2006;21:22-6.

57. Kirk R, Dipchand AI, Rosenthal DN, et al. The International Society for Heart and Lung Transplantation Guidelines for the management of pediatric heart failure: Executive summary [corrected]. J Heart Lung Transplant 2014;33:888-909.

58. Moffett BS, Orellana R. Use of fenoldopam to increase urine output in a patient with renal insufficiency secondary to septic shock: a case report. Pediatr Crit Care Med 2006;7:600-2.

59. Moffett BS, Mott AR, Nelson DP, et al. Renal effects of fenoldopam in critically ill pediatric patients: a retrospective review. Pediatr Crit Care Med 2008;9:403-6.

60. Dutertre JP, Billaud EM, Autret E, et al. Inhibition of angiotensin converting enzyme with enalapril maleate in infants with congestive heart failure. Br J Clin Pharmacol 1993;35:528-30.

61. Dyadyk AI, Bagriy AE, Lebed IA, et al. ACE inhibitors captopril and enalapril induce regression of left ventricular hypertrophy in hypertensive patients with chronic renal failure. Nephrol Dial Transplant 1997;12:945-51.

62. Leversha AM, Wilson NJ, Clarkson PM, et al. Efficacy and dosage of enalapril in congenital and acquired heart disease. Arch Dis Child 1994;70:35-9.

63. Momma K. ACE inhibitors in pediatric patients with heart failure. Paediatr Drugs 2006;8:55-69.

64. Thompson LD, McElhinney DB, Culbertson CB, et al. Perioperative administration of angiotensin converting enzyme inhibitors decreases the severity and duration of pleural effusions following bidirectional cavopulmonary anastomosis. Cardiol Young 2001;11:195-200.

65. Webster MW, Neutze JM, Calder AL. Acute hemodynamic effects of converting enzyme inhibition in children with intracardiac shunts. Pediatr Cardiol 1992;13:129-35.

66. Dutta S, Narang A. Enalapril-induced acute renal failure in a newborn infant. Pediatr Nephrol 2003;18:570-2.

67. Moffett BS, Goldstein SL, Adusei M, et al. Risk factors for postoperative acute kidney injury in pediatric cardiac surgery patients receiving angiotensin-converting enzyme inhibitors. Pediatr Crit Care Med 2011;12:555-9.

68. Tan LH, Du LZ, Carr MR, et al. Captopril induced reversible acute renal failure in a premature neonate with double outlet right ventricle and congestive heart failure. World J Pediatr 2011;7:89-91.

69. Taketomo C, Hodding J, Kraus D. Pediatric Dosage Handbook. Hudson, OH: Lexi-Comp, 2011.

70. Allman KG, Young JD, Carapiet D, et al. Effects of oxygen and nitric oxide in oxygen on pulmonary arterial pressures of children with congenital cardiac defects. Pediatr Cardiol 1996;17:246-50.

71. Bizzarro M, Gross I. Inhaled nitric oxide for the postoperative management of pulmonary hypertension in infants and children with congenital heart disease. Cochrane Database Syst Rev 2005;4:CD005055.

72. Carroll CL, Backer CL, Mavroudis C, et al. Inhaled prostacyclin following surgical repair of congenital heart disease—a pilot study. J Card Surg 2005;20:436-9.

73. Daftari B, Alejos JC, Perens G. Initial experience with sildenafil, bosentan, and nitric oxide for pediatric cardiomyopathy patients with elevated pulmonary vascular resistance before and after orthotopic heart transplantation. J Transplant 2010;2010:656984.

74. Day RW, Hawkins JA, McGough EC, et al. Randomized controlled study of inhaled nitric oxide after operation for congenital heart disease. Ann Thorac Surg 2000;69:1907-12.

75. Hermon M, Golej J, Burda G, et al. Intravenous prostacyclin mitigates inhaled nitric oxide rebound effect: a case control study. Artif Organs 1999;23:975-8.

76. Huddleston AJ, Knoderer CA, Morris JL, et al. Sildenafil for the treatment of pulmonary hypertension in pediatric patients. Pediatr Cardiol 2009;30:871-82.

77. Kovacikova L, Zahorec M, Nosal M. Sildenafil as a pulmonary vasodilator after repair of congenital heart disease. Bratisl Lek Listy 2007;108:453-4.

78. Limsuwan A, Wanitkul S, Khosithset A, et al. Aerosolized iloprost for postoperative pulmonary hypertensive crisis in children with congenital heart disease. Int J Cardiol 2008;129:333-8.

79. Nemoto S, Umehara E, Ikeda T, et al. Oral sildenafil ameliorates impaired pulmonary circulation early after bidirectional cavopulmonary shunt. Ann Thorac Surg 2007;83:e11-e13.

80. Schulze-Neick I, Hartenstein P, Li J, et al. Intravenous sildenafil is a potent pulmonary vasodilator in children with congenital heart disease. Circulation 2003;108:II167-73.

81. Uhm JY, Jhang WK, Park JJ, et al. Postoperative use of oral sildenafil in pediatric patients with congenital heart disease. Pediatr Cardiol 2010;31:515-20.

82. Kovach J, Ibsen L, Womack M, et al. Treatment of refractory pulmonary arterial hypertension with inhaled epoprostenol in an infant with congenital heart disease. Congenit Heart Dis 2007;2:194-8.

83. Hoffman TM, Bush DM, Wernovsky G, et al. Postoperative junctional ectopic tachycardia in children: incidence, risk factors, and treatment. Ann Thorac Surg 2002;74:1607-11.

84. Padbury JF, Agata Y, Baylen BG, et al. Pharmacokinetics of dopamine in critically ill newborn infants. J Pediatr 1990;117:472-6.

85. Burton GL, Kaufman J, Goot BH, et al. The use of arginine vasopressin in neonates following the Norwood procedure. Cardiol Young 2011;21:536-44.

86. Jerath N, Frndova H, McCrindle BW, et al. Clinical impact of vasopressin infusion on hemodynamics, liver and renal function in pediatric patients. Intensive Care Med 2008;34:1274-80.

87. Lechner E, Dickerson HA, Fraser CD Jr, et al. Vasodilatory shock after surgery for aortic valve endocarditis: use of low-dose vasopressin. Pediatr Cardiol 2004;25:558-61.

88. Mastropietro CW, Clark JA, Delius RE, et al. Arginine vasopressin to manage hypoxemic infants after stage I palliation of single ventricle lesions. Pediatr Crit Care Med 2008;9:506-10.

89. Masutani S, Senzaki H, Ishido H, et al. Vasopressin in the treatment of vasodilatory shock in children. Pediatr Int 2005;47:132-6.

90. Rosenzweig EB, Starc TJ, Chen JM, et al. Intravenous arginine-vasopressin in children with vasodilatory shock after cardiac surgery. Circulation 1999;100:II182-6.

91. Bangalore H, Checchia PA, Ocampo EC, et al. Cortisol response in children after second cardiopulmonary bypass. Pediatr Cardiol 2019;40:47-52.

92. Suominen PK, Dickerson HA, Moffett BS, et al. Hemodynamic effects of rescue protocol hydrocortisone in neonates with low cardiac output syndrome after cardiac surgery. Pediatr Crit Care Med 2005;6:655-9.

93. Lilly L. Pathophysiology of Heart Disease, 2nd ed. Baltimore: Lippincott Williams & Wilkins, 1998.

94. Archer N. Patent ductus arteriosus in the newborn. Arch Dis Child 1993;69:529-32.

95. Hammerman C, Kaplan M. Patent ductus arteriousus in the premature neonate: current concepts in pharmacological management. Paediatr Drugs 1999;1:81-92.

96. Hamrick SE, Hansmann G. Patent ductus arteriosus of the preterm infant. Pediatrics 2010;125:1020-30.

97. Laughon MM, Simmons MA, Bose CL. Patency of the ductus arteriosus in the premature infant: is it pathologic? Should it be treated? Curr Opin Pediatr 2004;16:146-51.

98. Moore JW, Levi DS, Moore SD, et al. Interventional treatment of patent ductus arteriosus in 2004. Catheter Cardiovasc Interv 2005;64:91-101.

99. Lee BS, Byun SY, Chung ML, et al. Effect of furosemide on ductal closure and renal function in indomethacin-treated preterm infants during the early neonatal period. Neonatology 2010;98:191-9.

100. Brion LP, Campbell DE. Furosemide for symptomatic patent ductus arteriosus in indomethacin-treated infants. Cochrane Database Syst Rev 2000;2:CD001148.

101. Thomas RL, Parker GC, Van OB, et al. A meta-analysis of ibuprofen versus indomethacin for closure of patent ductus arteriosus. Eur J Pediatr 2005;164:135-40.

102. Luecke CM, Liviskie CJ, Zeller BN, et al. Acetaminophen for patent ductus arteriosus in extremely low-birth-weight neonates. J Pediatr Pharmacol Ther 2017;22:461-6.

103. Ohlsson A, Shah PS. Paracetamol (acetaminophen) for patent ductus arteriosus in preterm or low-birth-weight infants. Cochrane Database Syst Rev 2015;3:CD010061.

104. Cockerham JT, Martin TC, Gutierrez FR, et al. Spontaneous closure of secundum atrial septal defect in infants and young children. Am J Cardiol 1983;52:1267-71.

105. Murphy JG, Gersh BJ, McGoon MD, et al. Long-term outcome after surgical repair of isolated atrial septal defect. Follow-up at 27 to 32 years. N Engl J Med 1990;323:1645-50.

106. Pastorek JS, Allen HD, Davis JT. Current outcomes of surgical closure of secundum atrial septal defect. Am J Cardiol 1994;74:75-7.

107. Tobias JD. Nicardipine to control mean arterial pressure after cardiothoracic surgery in infants and children. American Journal of Therapeutics 2001; 8:3-6.

108. Flynn JT, Mottes TA, Brophy PD, et al. Intravenous nicardipine for treatment of severe hypertension in children. J of Pediatrics 2000;139:38-43.

109. Harer MW, Kent AL. Neonatal hypertension: an educational review. Pediatr Nephrol 2018 Jul 5.

110. Rad EM and Assadi F. Management of hypertension in children with cardiovascular disease and heart failure. Int J Prev Med 2014; 5:S10-6.

111. Alabed S, Sabouni A, Al Dakhoul S, et al. Beta-blockers for congestive heart failure in children. Cochrane Database Syst Rev 2016;1:CD007037.

112. Prijic S, Buchhorn R, Kosutic J, et al. Beta-blockers (carvedilol) in children with systemic ventricle systolic dysfunction—systematic review and meta-analysis. Rev Recent Clin Trials 2014;9:68-75.

113. Miyake T, Shinohara T, Inoue T, et al. Spontaneous closure of muscular trabecular ventricular septal defect: comparison of defect positions. Acta Paediatr 2011;100:e158-62.

114. Beekman RH, Rocchini AP, Rosenthal A. Hemodynamic effects of hydralazine in infants with a large ventricular septal defect. Circulation 1982;65:523-8.

115. Nakazawa M, Takao A, Shimizu T, et al. Afterload reduction treatment for large ventricular septal defects. Dependence of haemodynamic effects of hydralazine on pretreatment systemic blood flow. Br Heart J 1983;49:461-5.

116. Nakazawa M, Takao A, Chon Y, et al. Significance of systemic vascular resistance in determining the hemodynamic effects of hydralazine on large ventricular septal defects. Circulation 1983;68:420-4.

117. Vazquez-Antona CA, Simon RS, Rijlaarsdam M, et al. [Oral enalapril in patients with symptomatic ventricular septal defects] [in Spanish]. Arch Inst Cardiol Mex 1996;66:496-504.

118. Sluysmans T, Styns-Cailteux M, Tremouroux-Wattiez M, et al. Intravenous enalaprilat and oral enalapril in congestive heart failure secondary to ventricular septal defect in infancy. Am J Cardiol 1992;70:959-62.

119. Apitz C, Webb GD, Redington AN. Tetralogy of Fallot. Lancet 2009;374:1462-71.

120. Armstrong BE. Congenital cardiovascular disease and cardiac surgery in childhood. Part 1. Cyanotic congenital heart defects. Curr Opin Cardiol 1995;10:58-67.

121. Graham EM, Bandisode VM, Bradley SM, et al. Effect of preoperative use of propranolol on postoperative outcome in patients with tetralogy of Fallot. Am J Cardiol 2008;101:693-5.

122. Garson A Jr, Gillette PC, McNamara DG. Propranolol: the preferred palliation for tetralogy of Fallot. Am J Cardiol 1981;47:1098-104.

123. Booker PD, Prosser DP, Franks R, et al. Nitric oxide in the treatment of acute right ventricular failure after surgical correction of tetralogy of Fallot. J Cardiothorac Vasc Anesth 1996;10:973-4.

124. Brown AT, Gillespie JV, Miquel-Verges F, et al. Inhaled epoprostenol therapy for pulmonary hypertension: Improves oxygenation index more consistently in neonates than in older children. Pulm Circ 2012;2:61-6.

125. Monagle P, Chalmers E, Chan A, et al. Antithrombotic therapy in neonates and children: American College of Chest Physicians Evidence-Based Clinical Practice Guidelines (8th Edition). Chest 2008;133:887S-968S.

126. Gatzoulis MA, Balaji S, Webber SA, et al. Risk factors for arrhythmia and sudden cardiac death late after repair of tetralogy of Fallot: a multicentre study. Lancet 2000;356:975-81.

127. Page GG. Tetralogy of Fallot. Heart Lung 1986;15:390-401.

128. Carrel T, Pfammatter JP. Complete transposition of the great arteries: surgical concepts for patients with systemic right ventricular failure following intraatrial repair. Thorac Cardiovasc Surg 2000;48:224-7.

129. Johnson BA, Ades A. Delivery room and early postnatal management of neonates who have prenatally diagnosed congenital heart disease. Clin Perinatol 2005;32:921-46, ix.

130. Coons JC, McGraw M, Murali S. Pharmacotherapy for acute heart failure syndromes. Am J Health Syst Pharm 2011;68:21-5.

131. Jonas RA. Advances in surgical care of infants and children with congenital heart disease. Curr Opin Pediatr 1995;7:572-9.

132. Gorler H, Ono M, Thies A, et al. Long-term morbidity and quality of life after surgical repair of transposition of the great arteries: atrial versus arterial switch operation. Interact Cardiovasc Thorac Surg 2011;12:569-74.

133. Bojar RM, Weiner B, Cleveland RJ. Intravenous labetalol for the control of hypertension following repair of coarctation of the aorta. Clin Cardiol 1988;11:639-41.

134. Gidding SS, Rocchini AP, Beekman R, et al. Therapeutic effect of propranolol on paradoxical hypertension after repair of coarctation of the aorta. N Engl J Med 1985;312:1224-8.

135. Moltzer E, Mattace Raso FU, Karamermer Y, et al. Comparison of candesartan versus metoprolol for treatment of systemic hypertension after repaired aortic coarctation. Am J Cardiol 2010;105:217-22.

136. Rouine-Rapp K, Mello DM, Hanley FL, et al. Effect of enalaprilat on postoperative hypertension after surgical repair of coarctation of the aorta. Pediatr Crit Care Med 2003;4:327-32.

137. Sealy WC. Paradoxical hypertension after repair of coarctation of the aorta: a review of its causes. Ann Thorac Surg 1990;50:323-9.

138. Tabbutt S, Nicolson SC, Adamson PC, et al. The safety, efficacy, and pharmacokinetics of esmolol for blood pressure control immediately after repair of coarctation of the aorta in infants and children: a multicenter, double-blind, randomized trial. J Thorac Cardiovasc Surg 2008;136:321-8.

139. Wiest DB, Garner SS, Uber WE, et al. Esmolol for the management of pediatric hypertension after cardiac operations. J Thorac Cardiovasc Surg 1998;115:890-7.

140. Will RJ, Walker OM, Traugott RC, et al. Sodium nitroprusside and propranolol therapy for management of postcoarctectomy hypertension. J Thorac Cardiovasc Surg 1978;75:722-4.

141. Norwood WI, Lang P, Hansen DD. Physiologic repair of aortic atresia-hypoplastic left heart syndrome. N Engl J Med 1983;308:23-6.

142. Sano S, Ishino K, Kawada M, et al. Right ventricle-pulmonary artery shunt in first-stage palliation of hypoplastic left heart syndrome. J Thorac Cardiovasc Surg 2003;126:504-9.

143. Rosenthal DN. Single ventricle reconstruction trial: a work in progress. Circulation 2014;129:2000-1.

144. Bockeria L, Alekyan B, Berishvili D, et al. A modified hybrid stage I procedure for treatment of hypoplastic left heart syndrome: an original surgical approach. Interact Cardiovasc Thorac Surg 2010;11:142-5.

145. Michelfelder E, Polzin W, Hirsch R. Hypoplastic left heart syndrome with intact atrial septum: utilization of a hybrid catheterization facility for cesarean section delivery and prompt neonatal intervention. Catheter Cardiovasc Interv 2008;72:983-7.

146. Galantowicz M, Cheatham JP, Phillips A, et al. Hybrid approach for hypoplastic left heart syndrome: intermediate results after the learning curve. Ann Thorac Surg 2008;85:2063-70.

147. Reddy SC, Saxena A. Prostaglandin E1: first stage palliation in neonates with congenital cardiac defects. Indian J Pediatr 1998;65:211-6.

148. Talosi G, Katona M, Racz K, et al. Prostaglandin E1 treatment in patent ductus arteriosus dependent congenital heart defects. J Perinat Med 2004;32:368-74.

149. Li JS, Yow E, Berezny KY, et al. Clinical outcomes of palliative surgery including a systemic-to-pulmonary artery shunt in infants with cyanotic congenital heart disease: does aspirin make a difference? Circulation 2007;116:293-7.

150. Baker-Smith CM, Neish SR, Klitzner TS, et al. Variation in postoperative care following stage I palliation for single-ventricle patients: a report from the Joint Council on Congenital Heart Disease National Quality Improvement Collaborative. Congenit Heart Dis 2011;6:116-27.

151. Schidlow DN, Anderson JB, Klitzner TS, et al. Variation in interstage outpatient care after the Norwood procedure: a report from the Joint Council on Congenital Heart Disease National Quality Improvement Collaborative. Congenit Heart Dis 2011;6:98-107.

152. Oster ME, Kelleman M, McCracken C, et al. Association of digoxin with interstage mortality: results from the Pediatric Heart Network Single Ventricle Reconstruction Trial Public Use Dataset. J Am Heart Assoc 2016;5:e002566.

153. Hehir DA, Dominguez TE, Ballweg JA, et al. Risk factors for interstage death after stage 1 reconstruction of hypoplastic left heart syndrome and variants. J Thorac Cardiovasc Surg 2008;136:94-9, 99e1-3.

154. Ghanayem NS, Hoffman GM, Mussatto KA, et al. Perioperative monitoring in high-risk infants after stage 1 palliation of univentricular congenital heart disease. J Thorac Cardiovasc Surg 2010;140:857-63.

155. Ghanayem NS, Hoffman GM, Mussatto KA, et al. Home surveillance program prevents interstage mortality after the Norwood procedure. J Thorac Cardiovasc Surg 2003;126:1367-77.

156. Jaquiss RD, Ghanayem NS, Hoffman GM, et al. Early cavopulmonary anastomosis in very young infants after the Norwood procedure: impact on oxygenation, resource utilization, and mortality. J Thorac Cardiovasc Surg 2004;127:982-9

157. Bridges ND, Jonas RA, Mayer JE, et al. Bidirectional cavopulmonary anastomosis as interim palliation for high-risk Fontan candidates. Early results. Circulation 1990;82:IV170-6.

158. Ahmad W, Miteff F, Collins N. Headache in a patient with complex congenital heart disease: diagnostic and therapeutic considerations. Heart Lung Circ 2015;24:e184-7.

159. Martínez-Quintana E, Rodríguez-González F. Complications after a bidirectional cavopulmonary anastomosis with accessory sources of pulmonary blood flow. Int J Angiol 2016;25:e51-3.

160. Fontan F, Baudet E. Surgical repair of tricuspid atresia. Thorax 1971;26:240-8.

161. Pike NA, Okuhara CA, Toyama J, et al. Reduced pleural drainage, length of stay, and readmissions using a modified Fontan management protocol. J Thorac Cardiovasc Surg 2015;150:481-7.

162. Kocyildirim E, Yorukoglu Y, Ekici E, et al. High-dose octreotide treatment for persistent pleural effusion after the extracardiac Fontan procedure. Anadolu Kardiyol Derg 2008;8:75-6.

163. Chan SY, Lau W, Wong WH, et al. Chylothorax in children after congenital heart surgery. Ann Thorac Surg 2006;82:1650-6.

164. Chan EH, Russell JL, Williams WG, et al. Postoperative chylothorax after cardiothoracic surgery in children. Ann Thorac Surg 2005;80:1864-70.

165. Ryerson L, Goldberg C, Rosenthal A, et al. Usefulness of heparin therapy in protein-losing enteropathy associated with single ventricle palliation. Am J Cardiol 2008;101:248-51.

166. Schumacher KR, Cools M, Goldstein BH, et al. Oral budesonide treatment for protein-losing enteropathy in Fontan-palliated patients. Pediatr Cardiol 2011;32:966-71.

167. Thacker D, Patel A, Dodds K, et al. Use of oral budesonide in the management of protein-losing enteropathy after the Fontan operation. Ann Thorac Surg 2010;89:837-42.

168. John AS, Phillips SD, Driscoll DJ, et al. The use of octreotide to successfully treat protein-losing enteropathy following the Fontan operation. Congenit Heart Dis 2011;6:653-6.

169. Barker PC, Nowak C, King K, et al. Risk factors for cerebrovascular events following Fontan palliation in patients with a functional single ventricle. Am J Cardiol 2005;96:587-91.

170. Cheung YF, Chay GW, Chiu CS, et al. Long-term anticoagulation therapy and thromboembolic complications after the Fontan procedure. Int J Cardiol 2005;102:509-13.

171. Jacobs ML, Pourmoghadam KK, Geary EM, et al. Fontan's operation: is aspirin enough? Is coumadin too much? Ann Thorac Surg 2002;73:64-8.

172. John JB, Cron SG, Kung GC, et al. Intracardiac thrombi in pediatric patients: presentation profiles and clinical outcomes. Pediatr Cardiol 2007;28:213-20.

173. Mahnke CB, Boyle GJ, Janosky JE, et al. Anticoagulation and incidence of late cerebrovascular accidents following the Fontan procedure. Pediatr Cardiol 2005;26:56-61.

174. Iyengar AJ, Winlaw DS, Galati JC, et al., Australia and New Zealand Fontan Registry. No difference between aspirin and warfarin after extracardiac Fontan in a propensity score analysis of 475 patients. Eur J Cardiothorac Surg 2016;50:980-7.

175. Crone E, Saliba N, George S, et al. Commencement of warfarin therapy in children following the Fontan procedure. Thromb Res 2013;131:304-7.

176. Monagle P, Cochrane A, McCrindle B, et al. Thromboembolic complications after Fontan procedures—the role of prophylactic anticoagulation. J Thorac Cardiovasc Surg 1998;115:493-8.

177. Giardini A, Balducci A, Specchia S, et al. Effect of sildenafil on haemodynamic response to exercise and exercise capacity in Fontan patients. Eur Heart J 2008;29:1681-7.

178. Goldberg DJ, French B, McBride MG, et al. Impact of oral sildenafil on exercise performance in children and young adults after the Fontan operation: a randomized, double-blind, placebo-controlled, crossover trial. Circulation 2011;123:1185-93.

179. Kouatli AA, Garcia JA, Zellers TM, et al. Enalapril does not enhance exercise capacity in patients after Fontan procedure. Circulation 1997;96:1507-12.

180. Reinhardt Z, Uzun O, Bhole V, et al. Sildenafil in the management of the failing Fontan circulation. Cardiol Young 2010;20:522-5.

181. Ishibashi N, Park IS, Takahashi Y, et al. Effectiveness of carvedilol for congestive heart failure that developed long after modified Fontan operation. Pediatr Cardiol 2006;27:473-5.

182. Ishibashi N, Park IS, Waragai T, et al. Effect of carvedilol on heart failure in patients with a functionally univentricular heart. Circ J 2011;75:1394-9.

183. Brickner ME, Hillis LD, Lange RA. Congenital heart disease in adults. First of two parts. N Engl J Med 2000;342:256-63.

184. Brickner ME, Hillis LD, Lange RA. Congenital heart disease in adults. Second of two parts. N Engl J Med 2000;342:334-42.

185. Moodie DS. Adult congenital heart disease. Curr Opin Cardiol 1995;10:92-8.

186. Rodriguez FH III, Moodie DS, Parekh DR, et al. Outcomes of hospitalization in adults in the United States with atrial septal defect, ventricular septal defect, and atrioventricular septal defect. Am J Cardiol 2011;108:290-3.

187. Schoormans D, Sprangers MA, Pieper PG, et al. The perspective of patients with congenital heart disease: does health care meet their needs? Congenit Heart Dis 2011;6:219-27.

188. Webb GD. Challenges in the care of adult patients with congenital heart defects. Heart 2003;89:465-9.

189. Bellinger DC, Jonas RA, Rappaport LA, et al. Developmental and neurologic status of children after heart surgery with hypothermic circulatory arrest or low-flow cardiopulmonary bypass. N Engl J Med 1995;332:549-55.

190. Newburger JW, Jonas RA, Wernovsky G, et al. A comparison of the perioperative neurologic effects of hypothermic circulatory arrest versus low-flow cardiopulmonary bypass in infant heart surgery. N Engl J Med 1993;329:1057-64.

191. Shillingford AJ, Wernovsky G. Academic performance and behavioral difficulties after neonatal and infant heart surgery. Pediatr Clin North Am 2004;51:1625-39, ix.

192. Wernovsky G, Shillingford AJ, Gaynor JW. Central nervous system outcomes in children with complex congenital heart disease. Curr Opin Cardiol 2005;20:94-9.

193. McKenzie ED, Andropoulos DB, DiBardino D, et al. Congenital heart surgery 2005: the brain: it's the heart of the matter. Am J Surg 2005;190:289-94.

CHAPTER 9

Pediatric Arrhythmias

Brady S. Moffett, Pharm.D., MPH, MBA

LEARNING OBJECTIVES

1. Describe the epidemiology and pathophysiology of common pediatric arrhythmias.

2. Recommend first-line and alternative pharmacologic options for the acute and chronic treatment of common pediatric arrhythmias.

3. Identify monitoring variables for therapeutic efficacy and toxicity for pharmacotherapy of common pediatric arrhythmias.

ABBREVIATIONS IN THIS CHAPTER

AV	Atrioventricular
AVNRT	Atrioventricular nodal reentrant tachycardia
AVRT	Atrioventricular reentrant tachycardia
cJET	Congenital junctional ectopic tachycardia
ECG	Electrocardiogram; electrocardiographic
FAT	Focal atrial tachycardia
JET	Junctional ectopic tachycardia
LQTS	Long QT syndrome
NAPA	*N*-acetyl procainamide
pJET	Postoperative junctional ectopic tachycardia
PJRT	Permanent junctional reciprocating tachycardia
TdP	Torsades de pointes
VF	Ventricular fibrillation
VT	Ventricular tachycardia
WPW	Wolff-Parkinson-White (syndrome)

INTRODUCTION

This chapter will focus on arrhythmias common to the pediatric population, divided into three major subsections: supraventricular tachyarrhythmias, ventricular tachyarrhythmias, and bradyarrhythmias. The goal of this chapter is to review pharmacotherapy management strategies for the most common arrhythmias seen by a pediatric clinical pharmacist. However, because there are exceptions to the strategies presented, particularly for those practicing in large, tertiary referral centers, the reader will be given references for further investigation of uncommon arrhythmias.

Some assumptions were made when writing this chapter. Because this textbook focuses on the pediatric age group, only aspects of arrhythmia pathophysiology, medical care, or pharmacotherapy that are specific to the pediatric population will be discussed. Because of space limitations and the availability of other excellent resources, basic cardiovascular anatomy and physiology (including an in-depth discussion of the mechanism of cardiac conduction) will not be covered in this chapter. Similarly, a basic understanding of electrocardiographic (ECG) interpretation will be assumed. If readers would like an update on these aspects of cardiovascular anatomy and physiology, they are directed to other sources.[1,2]

As shown throughout this chapter, many different agents can be used to treat similar arrhythmias, and single agents can be used in a wide variety of indications. The basic pharmacology of each class will be reviewed, and salient points will be addressed regarding each of the antiarrhythmic agents discussed in the chapter that may affect decision making when initiating pharmacotherapy. Specifically, this section will focus on dosing, drug concentration monitoring, dosage forms, and adverse events. Dosing information for pediatric patients is summarized in Table 1. For other information regarding antiarrhythmic drug properties, such as pharmacokinetic factors, the reader is urged to consult a comprehensive drug reference.[3]

NORMAL CARDIAC CONDUCTION

The cardiac conduction system consists of the sinoatrial node, the atrioventricular (AV) node, the bundle of His with the left and right bundle branches, and the Purkinje fibers. In a normal heart, electrical impulses are generated in the sinoatrial node and are transmitted through the atria to the AV node, then to bundle of His, and then left and right bundle branches to the Purkinje fibers, which finally stimulates myocardial contraction.

The basis of electrical conduction begins with the shifting of ions into and out of cells, thus generating a change in polarization, known as the *action potential*. The action potential involves four phases, with specific ions involved in each phase (Figure 1). Developmentally, changes in ion transport channels appear to occur with age, leading to increased expression of potassium and calcium channels with older age.[4] In addition, the electrophysiological characteristics of the AV node have been noted to change in pediatric patients as they age.[5] However, the impact of this change on the pharmacotherapy for pediatric arrhythmias is currently unknown.

SUPRAVENTRICULAR TACHYARRHYTHMIAS

Supraventricular tachyarrhythmias are the most common arrhythmia in childhood, occurring in about one in every 250 children. A higher prevalence has been reported in patients

Table 1. Summary of Antiarrhythmic Medication Dosing in Pediatric Patients[5]

Drug	Dosage	Pharmacotherapy Notes
Class Ia (Na⁺ Channel Blockade—Moderate)		
Quinidine sulfate	Oral: 30 mg/kg/day or 900 mg/m²/day given in 5 daily doses; range 15–60 mg/kg/day in 4–5 divided doses IV: 2–10 mg/kg/dose every 3–6 hr as needed	Two forms available: sulfate and gluconate; drug concentration monitoring typically not performed; IV not routinely recommended
Procainamide	IV loading dose: 3–6 mg/kg/dose; max 100 mg/dose; may be repeated to total max of 15 mg/kg IV continuous infusion: 20–80 mcg/kg/min	Procainamide and *N*-acetyl procainamide concentrations used to guide therapy
Disopyramide	Oral, by patient age: < 1 yr: 10–30 mg/kg/day in 4 divided doses 1–4 yr: 10–20 mg/kg/day in 4 divided doses 4–12 yr: 10–15 mg/kg/day in 4 divided doses 12–18 yr: 6–15 mg/kg/day in 4 divided doses	Drug concentration monitoring typically not performed
Class Ib (Na⁺ Channel Blockade—Mild)		
Lidocaine	IV bolus: 1 mg/kg/dose IV continuous infusion: 20–50 mcg/kg/min	Drug concentration monitoring useful for guiding therapy
Mexiletine	Oral: 1.4–5 mg/kg/dose every 8 hr	—
Class Ic (Na⁺ Channel Blockade—Strong)		
Flecainide	Oral: Starting dose: 1–3 mg/kg/day or 50–100 mg/m²/day divided 3 times/day Max: 8 mg/kg/day or 200 mg/m²/day Average effective dose: 4 mg/kg/day or 140 mg/m²/day	Drug concentration monitoring useful for guiding therapy
Propafenone	Oral: 200–300 mg/m²/day divided 3–4 times/day Max: 600 mg/m²/day divided 3–4 times/day	Drug concentration monitoring typically not performed
Class II (β-Blockade)		
Propranolol	Oral: Neonates: 0.25 mg/kg/dose every 6 hr; max: 5 mg/kg/day Oral: Infants and children: 0.5–1 mg/kg day in divided doses every 6–8 hr Usual dose: 2–4 mg/kg/day; max: 60 mg/day	—
Esmolol	IV bolus: 100–500 mcg/kg/dose over 1 min IV continuous infusion: 300–1000 mcg/kg/min	—
Atenolol	Oral: 0.5–1 mg/kg/day given 1–2 times/day; max: 2 mg/kg/day or 100 mg/day	—
Metoprolol	Oral: Age 1–17 yr: 1–2 mg/kg/day given twice daily Max: 6 mg/kg/day or 200 mg/day	Extended-release tablets given once daily
Nadolol	Oral: 0.5–1 mg/kg/day given daily Max: 2.5 mg/kg/day	—
Class III (K⁺ Channel Blockade)		
Sotalol	Oral: Age ≤ 2 yr: 30 mg/m²/dose every 8 hr adjusted per age nomogram OR 2 mg/kg/day divided every 8 hr OR 80–200 mg/m²/day divided every 8 hr Oral: Age > 2 yr: 80–200 mg/m²/dose divided every 8 hr	Institutional practices vary for dosing sotalol; ECG monitoring is important for QT-interval prolongation
Amiodarone	IV bolus: 5 mg/kg/dose up to 15 mg/kg; max dose varies based on indication IV continuous infusion: 10–20 mg/kg/day or 5–15 mcg/kg/min Oral: 10–20 mg/kg/day or 600–800 mg m²/day 1–2 times/day	Initial dosing may be loaded for 1–2 wk because of long half-life; reduction to most effective dose can occur after loading

(continued)

Table 1. Summary of Antiarrhythmic Medication Dosing in Pediatric Patients[5] *(continued)*

Drug	Dosage	Pharmacotherapy Notes
Class IV (Ca++ Channel Blockade)		
Verapamil	IV: Age 1–15 yr: 0.1–0.3 mg/kg/dose; max: 5 mg/dose Oral: 4–8 mg/kg/day in 3 divided doses OR Age 1–5 yr: 40–80 mg every 8 hr Age > 5 yr: 80 mg every 6–8 hr	IV use not recommended for age < 1 yr because of the risk of cardiovascular collapse
Diltiazem	Oral: Children: 1.5–2 mg/kg/day in 3–4 divided doses Max: 8 mg/kg/day	Extended-release formulations can be given once daily
Digoxin	Oral and IV: *Loading and maintenance doses are not summarized here because they vary considerably based on age* Oral: *Historically, oral maintenance doses range is 5–10 mcg/kg/ day divided 1–2 times/day*	Drug concentration monitoring usually useful only in assessment of toxicity
Adenosine	IV: 0.1 mg/kg/dose; subsequent doses 0.2 mg/kg/dose, up to 0.3 mg/kg/dose	Administer by rapid push with rapid flush through IV access closest to heart

ECG = electrocardiogram; IV = intravenous; max = maximum.

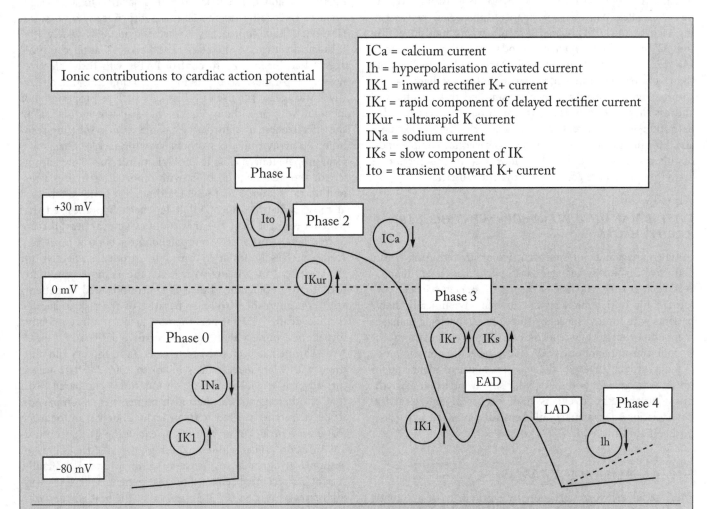

Figure 1. Action potential of the Purkinje fibers and the associated ion shifts. Phase 0 consists of Na+ influx into the cell, resulting in a positive charge. At phase 1, K+ effluxes from the cell, followed by Ca++ ions. In phase 2, K+ ions efflux from the cell. Phase 3 includes more K+ efflux from the cell, to decrease the action potential threshold. Phase 4 spontaneous depolarization occurs only in pacemaker cells. Early afterdepolarizations (EAD) and late afterdepolarizations (LAD) represent "extra" depolarizations that can occur in patients with prolonged phase 2 and phase 3 (K+ channel) repolarizations, potentially resulting in arrhythmias.

Reprinted with permission from Chakrabarti A, Stuart AG. Understanding cardiac arrhythmias. Arch Dis Child 2005;90:1086-90.

who have undergone cardiac surgery or have congenital heart disease.[6] However, most patients with supraventricular tachyarrhythmias have structurally normal hearts, and patients are commonly given a diagnosis on a routine office visit.[7] Most supraventricular tachyarrhythmias are paroxysmal (lasting 30 seconds or less), but they can be incessant, resulting in significant hemodynamic compromise and heart failure in as little as 24–48 hours.[8] Patients can become symptomatic, exhibiting signs of heart failure such as poor feeding, sweating, and tachypnea in infants and fatigue, tachypnea, and peripheral edema in older patients.[8] Although overall mortality from supraventricular arrhythmias is low, rapid diagnosis and appropriate treatment are essential to minimize patient morbidity.[9]

Overall, supraventricular tachyarrhythmias have been traditionally defined as an abnormally rapid heart rhythm originating above the bundle of His.[10] Within this broad heading are many different pathophysiologic mechanisms of arrhythmias, including those with focal atrial tachycardias (FATs); reentrant mechanisms mediated by an accessory pathway outside the AV node (Wolff-Parkinson-White syndrome [WPW] and concealed pathways, permanent junctional reciprocating tachycardia [PJRT]); and a reentrant mechanism within the AV node (atrioventricular nodal reentrant tachycardia [AVNRT]), or junctional ectopic tachycardia (JET). More than 90% of the supraventricular arrhythmias diagnosed in children have a reentrant mechanism, and this chapter will address these arrhythmias in the most detail.[11] Typically, the definition of supraventricular tachyarrhythmias excludes atrial fibrillation and atrial flutter; however, for completeness in this discussion, both will be addressed in this section as arrhythmias that are generated above the ventricles.

INITIAL MANAGEMENT OF SUPRAVENTRICULAR ARRHYTHMIAS

Initial management of supraventricular arrhythmias, before definitive diagnosis, has standard approaches. Vagal maneuvers, such as ice to the face or carotid massage, have been performed for initial management in hemodynamically stable patients with limited success.[12] Initial pharmacologic management often consists of adenosine as a diagnostic and therapeutic tool, causing temporary AV block, depending on the mode of tachycardia.[13,14] Despite the widespread use of adenosine for initial management and therapy for supraventricular arrhythmias, proarrhythmic effects have occurred, and electrical defibrillation equipment should be readily available when adenosine is administered.[15]

FOCAL ATRIAL TACHYCARDIAS

Focal atrial tachycardias, consisting primarily of automatic atrial ectopic tachycardias, account for 4% to 14% of all supraventricular arrhythmias in children and are typically refractory to pharmacologic management.[16,17] Although most forms of supraventricular tachyarrhythmias are reentrant in nature, FATs consist of a site within the myocardium that exhibits pacemaker cell characteristics, generating action potentials from areas other than the sinoatrial or AV node. Various other forms of FATs can occur, including micro-reentrant atrial tachycardia, chaotic atrial tachycardia, or multifocal atrial tachycardia.[11,18] Patients who have undergone cardiac surgery are often the most likely patient subset for FATs, although some FATs are caused by other disease states or are idiopathic.[16] Patients with FATs will present with an elevated heart rate, typically greater than 200 beats/minute for infants and children. The ECG findings for FATs can be difficult to identify, particularly in patients with heart failure or in neonates.[19] Electrocardiographic readings will show an elevated heart rate with normal QRS and an extended R-P interval, although it may be difficult to see P waves in this type of tachycardia.[16,19] The clinical course of FATs can vary depending on age.[16,20,21] Ventricular dysfunction and heart failure can ensue if FATs are not corrected in a timely manner.[22] Catheter ablation may be necessary as a nonpharmacologic intervention for incessant FATs refractory to medical therapy.[23]

The goals of pharmacotherapy for FATs are to decrease the automaticity of the ectopic focus, potentially decrease the conduction velocity of the impulse through the Purkinje fibers, and slow the ventricular rate. Pharmacologic management of FATs, after diagnosis, is based primarily on case-series data, and approaches to treatment vary widely.[16,20,21] Historically, digoxin and class Ia and class IV antiarrhythmic agents have been used to control FATs, with little effectiveness.[16,23,24] β-Blockers are the most common first-line antiarrhythmic agent. The use of β-blockers such as propranolol or atenolol, with or without digoxin, has had varying results on the effectiveness of control, with some reports showing resolution of arrhythmia, but others showing lack of effect.[16,24,25] Oral propafenone, a class Ic antiarrhythmic, has shown promise for the treatment of FATs, with reported arrhythmia resolution rates from 33% to 89%, although it is not often used at most pediatric centers.[26-29] It has been hypothesized that patients younger than 1 year without structural heart disease have a better response to propafenone for control of FATs.[30] Another class Ic antiarrhythmic, flecainide, is effective for the treatment of patients with FATs and is more commonly used than propafenone, but it is contraindicated in patients with congenital heart disease because of the risk of sudden cardiac death.[31,32] Pharmacotherapy is often more effective in patients younger than 3 years versus older than 3 years.[21] Amiodarone has been used to treat FATs in infants and children, with high success rates of up to 100%.[16,33,34] However, the adverse effect profile of amiodarone, compared with that of other agents, can be much higher.[34] In a comparison study of infants treated with procainamide or amiodarone for supraventricular arrhythmias (excluding JET), continuous-infusion procainamide had a higher incidence of control without any greater incidence of adverse effects.[35] Finally, sotalol has recently been used to treat patients with FATs with high rates of success.[36-38] It appears that the best efficacy with sotalol occurs in younger patients who receive higher doses.[30] The combination of flecainide and sotalol has been used to treat FATs and other arrhythmias with high success rates in patients who have been refractory to single-agent therapy.[39] Nevertheless, despite advances in antiarrhythmic therapy, β-blockers remain the most common first-line agent for the treatment of FATs.

ATRIOVENTRICULAR NODAL REENTRANT TACHYCARDIA

Of the two primary reentrant mechanisms, AVNRT is more common in older children, seldom occurring before age 2 years.[11,40,41] To have a reentrant rhythm, two separate pathways capable of conducting an action potential must be present. The pathophysiology of AVNRT consists of these two pathways within the AV node (termed *dual AV nodal physiology*), a slow pathway and a fast pathway, allowing a reentrant circuit (Figure 2).[42] In typical AVNRT, an ectopic beat must conduct down the slow pathway and then turn around and go back up the fast pathway to set up a circuit of rapid tachycardia.[43] Most patients have typical AVNRT as just described, with a few patients having atypical AVNRT consisting of conduction down the fast pathway and up the slow pathway.[42,44-47] Patients with AVNRT generally present with a rapid heart rate and, occasionally, chest pain, shortness of breath, and light-headedness. Those in prolonged tachycardia can present with signs and symptoms of heart failure. Neonates and infants will present with poor feeding, sweating while feeding, cough, cyanosis, and pallor with a marked decrease in activity.[48] Typically, patients with AVNRT will present with a rapid heart rate and narrow QRS on ECG, with a P wave occurring immediately after the QRS (termed *short RP tachycardia*); however, often a few characteristics differentiate AVNRT from other supraventricular tachyarrhythmias.[49,50] Ablation of the slow pathway is often performed in the cardiac catheterization laboratory, with initial success rates greater than 95% in experienced centers and recurrence rates after ablation of less than 10%.[45,47,51]

The goal of pharmacotherapy is to block the reentrant cycle within the AV node. Using antiarrhythmic medications to increase the refractory period, decrease automaticity, and/or decrease conduction velocity, the cycle can be broken. Initial management consists of vagal maneuvers and adenosine. The pharmacotherapy for AVNRT is highly varied, and many modalities have been used. Medications that decrease AV nodal conduction (digoxin, β-blockers, verapamil) are typically initiated as first-line oral agents and have a high rate of efficacy.[46,52] Propranolol is usually the first-line choice for a β-blocker in infants.[53] Atenolol and nadolol have also been used in the treatment of AVNRT in older children.[54] The percentage of breakthrough AVNRT in patients receiving β-blockers is significant (about 30%), even if tachycardia is initially well controlled.[41] Flecainide and propafenone have also been used for arrhythmias recalcitrant to initial therapies. Of the class Ic agents, flecainide has the largest experience in the treatment of refractory AVNRT, with up to 100% resolution of arrhythmias in one report and 81% success in another report.[31,55] However, flecainide is contraindicated in

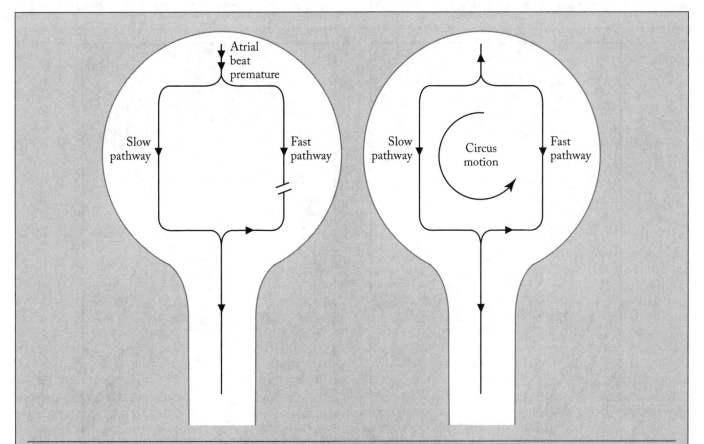

Figure 2. Atrioventricular nodal reentrant tachycardia (AVNRT). This figure shows the dual pathways that can occur in an atrioventricular node. The fast pathway typically conducts before the slow pathway and is refractory when the slow pathway reaches it, thus causing the slow pathway conduction to stop. However, a premature atrial beat may cause extra conduction down the slow pathway, which then conducts retrograde up the fast pathway, resulting in a reentrant circuit, sometimes referred to as circus motion.

Reprinted with permission from Esberger D, Jones S, Morris F. ABC of clinical electrocardiography. Junctional tachycardias. BMJ 2002;324:662-5.

the presence of congenital heart disease.[31,55] Few data exist for the use of amiodarone in AVNRT, potentially because of the high rates of resolution with other antiarrhythmic agents. Amiodarone appears to be a suitable last-line agent for arrhythmias refractory to all other agents on the basis of reports of effectiveness when treating other arrhythmias.[56,57] Similarly, sotalol has few data describing its use in AVNRT, although initial data are favorable as treatment of refractory AVNRT.[58,59]

In conclusion, the greatest body of evidence suggests that first-line therapy for AVNRT is a β-blocker or digoxin. Recent data have suggested that propranolol or digoxin have similar outcomes.[60,61] In general, medical therapy is used in very young patients who may be at higher risk of complications during a catheter-based ablation procedure. Recalcitrant arrhythmias should be treated with flecainide, sotalol, or amiodarone.

ACCESSORY PATHWAY–MEDIATED REENTRANT TACHYCARDIAS

The second mechanism for reentrant arrhythmia uses an accessory pathway as an essential component of the tachycardia circuit. These are known as *atrioventricular reentrant tachycardias* (AVRTs) and are composed of two major subsets: WPW syndrome and concealed accessory pathways including PJRT.

To have an accessory pathway–mediated tachycardia, four components are necessary: the atrium, the AV node, the ventricle, and the accessory pathway. Most commonly, an ectopic beat travels down the AV node and activates the ventricle, resulting in retrograde conduction up the accessory pathway to the atrium and back down the AV node (termed *orthodromic tachycardia*) (Figure 3). Although many accessory tracts have been identified, the most common is the Kent bundle, a residual fiber along the AV valve annulus, allowing electrical conduction between the atrium and the ventricle. Accessory pathway–mediated tachycardias can be distinguished by the direction of the impulse through the accessory tract during tachycardia: *antidromic* (from the atria to the ventricles) or *orthodromic* (from the ventricles to the atria).[62] Evidence of an accessory pathway can sometimes be seen on the surface ECG, with findings of a short PR interval, a slurred QRS upstroke (delta wave), and a wide QRS complex, and is considered the classic definition of the WPW pattern of ventricular preexcitation.[62] Wolff-Parkinson-White syndrome is diagnosed by the presence of pre-excitation on an ECG and evidence of a supraventricular tachycardia. Accessory pathways with only retrograde conduction cannot be seen on a surface ECG and are termed *concealed accessory pathways*, which can still create a circuit for AVRT.[62]

Orthodromic tachycardia, the most common form of AVRT, usually appears as a narrow QRS tachycardia and is

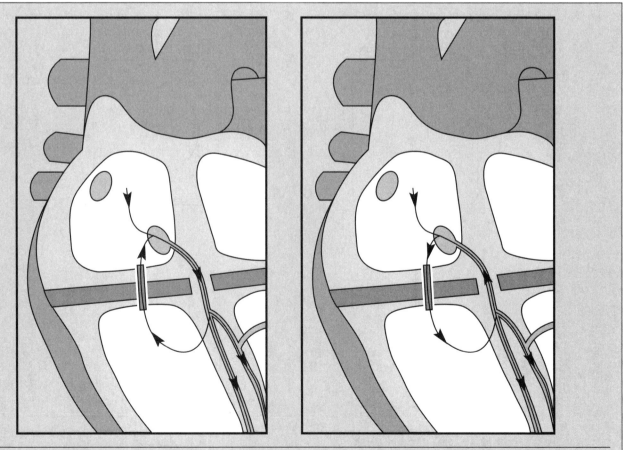

Figure 3. Accessory pathway reentrant arrhythmias. This diagram represents orthodromic (left) and antidromic (right) reentrant tachycardia through a Kent bundle. The reentrant circuit is started when an ectopic beat conducts through the atrioventricular node.

Reprinted with permission from Esberger D, Jones S, Morris F. ABC of clinical electrocardiography. Junctional tachycardias. BMJ 2002;324:662-5.

often difficult to distinguish from AVNRT on ECG.[62] This difficulty is because the ventricles are depolarized by the normal conduction system, and the accessory tract is conducting retrograde in tachycardia. Antidromic AVRT occurs less often, is marked by ventricular pre-excitation, and is more often a wide QRS complex because of more rapid ventricular activation through the accessory pathway.[62]

Most patients with supraventricular tachycardia who present at younger than 1 year will have some form of accessory pathway–mediated tachycardia. More than 90% will spontaneously resolve by age 1 year.[7] However, a recurrence rate of about 30% has been reported after initial resolution.[63] An increased incidence of supraventricular arrhythmias occurs in infancy and then again later in childhood, with a final peak in adolescence.[63] The long-term prognosis for patients with WPW is excellent for those with structurally normal hearts, in the absence of other comorbidities.[9,43] However, asymptomatic pediatric patients with WPW left untreated have about a 55% chance of becoming symptomatic by age 40 years.[64] Evaluation of all patients with WPW is necessary to prevent long-term morbidity, including risk of atrial fibrillation and risk of developing cardiomyopathy.

Initial treatment of AVRT is similar to treatment of other supraventricular arrhythmias—vagal maneuvers and adenosine. Long-term management of AVRT often includes ablation of the accessory tract, which has proven to be very successful and is considered the standard of care by many.[43,65-70] The goals of pharmacotherapy are to break the reentrant cycle by decreasing the automaticity of the pacemaker cells, decreasing the conduction velocity, and/or increasing the refractory period. As previously described, adenosine is often used as initial pharmacologic therapy before a definitive diagnosis.

Digoxin was a mainstay of treatment in patients with AVRT and WPW for decades, and some practitioners still use it.[71-74] Digoxin can decrease the refractory period of the accessory pathway in WPW, and it can increase the signal transmission from the atria to the ventricles, potentially resulting in rapid ventricular conduction in patients with atrial fibrillation.[75] However, some consider these effects primarily a risk to patients younger than 1 year because accessory pathway refractory periods are much shorter in children than in adults.[73] Even though digoxin has been used effectively in pediatric patients with WPW and supraventricular tachycardia, other agents have shown similar efficacy without the risk of ventricular arrhythmias.[7]

As with digoxin, verapamil use has been discouraged in the treatment of AVRT because it also decreases the refractory period of accessory pathways and can result in rapidly conducted ventricular arrhythmias.[7,76-79] Verapamil, particularly the intravenous formulation, is contraindicated in neonates and infants because of the risk of cardiovascular collapse.

β-Blockers are most often considered the first-line agent for patients with AVRT.[7,58] Propranolol, atenolol, and nadolol have all been used with high efficacy and low adverse event profiles in pediatric patients.[7,53,54,80-82] In patients with a need for intravenous medication, such as postoperative patients, intravenous esmolol has been used to treat supraventricular arrhythmias.[83-89]

Traditionally, the use of class Ia agents (quinidine or, more commonly, procainamide) is a next step in patients who do not experience control with β-blockade.[7,8,41] The intravenous form has been used in infants and neonates, but with few data on efficacy for refractory AVRT.[74,90,91,92]

A substantial body of literature is associated with the use of class Ic agents in patients with WPW. Propafenone was initially a drug of choice for patients whose previous therapies had failed.[27-29,93,94] Now, oral flecainide represents an effective option for patients with supraventricular arrhythmias and WPW because of the large body of experience with the agent.[31,39,55,95-102] Clinicians, however, are hesitant to use flecainide in patients with structural heart disease (i.e., congenital heart disease) because of the increased mortality risk identified in adult and pediatric data.[103-105]

The class III agents are often reserved for the treatment of refractory AVRT, but they can be very effective. Amiodarone has been used with high rates of success (60% to 100% complete resolution), but it has also been reported to have a high incidence of adverse events, including hypotension, QT prolongation, and proarrhythmia.[34,88,106-108] Sotalol has also been used for refractory WPW with good success, but the published experience to date has been much smaller than that for other agents.[37,38,59,109-111] In addition, the concerns with sotalol are the risk of ventricular proarrhythmia, caused by QT-interval prolongation and development of torsades de pointes (TdP), and hypotension.

In summary, oral β-blockers are the typical first-line agents for the treatment of supraventricular arrhythmias in patients with WPW. Patients with refractory arrhythmias may benefit from the addition of a second agent before progressing therapy to a class III agent. Depending on the patient's age, ability to take oral medications, and underlying pathophysiology, intravenous procainamide or oral flecainide is a reasonable next step. Finally, before multi-agent therapy, oral or intravenous amiodarone or sotalol may be used.

PERMANENT JUNCTIONAL RECIPROCATING TACHYCARDIA

Although a large portion of supraventricular arrhythmias are caused by reentrant mechanisms, PJRT as a subset is relatively rare. Permanent junctional reciprocating tachycardia differs from the other reentrant tachycardias because it is characterized by an accessory pathway that exhibits only slow decremental retrograde conduction from the ventricles to the atria.[62] This conduction results in an ECG pattern of long RP tachycardia with inverted P waves in the inferior leads. Permanent junctional reciprocating tachycardia is often incessant and, if left untreated, can result in cardiomyopathy and heart failure.[62,112,113] Although PJRT can spontaneously resolve, it has a high degree of morbidity resulting from the incessant tachycardia, which often forces practitioners to treat it.[112-114] Depending on the refractory nature of the tachycardia and the patient's age and ventricular function, use of ablation is often considered the standard of care for older children with PJRT, and it is rarely used in infants.[112,113]

Pharmacotherapy for PJRT consists of case reports or case series because of the relative infrequency of the arrhythmia.

Drugs used have included propranolol, flecainide, propafenone, sotalol, and amiodarone.[27,31,59,107,114] β-Blockers alone are often ineffective. Propafenone has been used with limited success.[26,27] Early experience with treatment of PJRT showed success with flecainide, in which six of seven patients were successfully treated.[31] Amiodarone was also used early with limited success (about 50% resolution).[107] Multidrug therapy has also been used to treat PJRT, using flecainide and propranolol, flecainide and sotalol, or amiodarone and propranolol.[114] The largest study of PJRT reported that most patients (79%) did not respond to first-line therapy and that as many as nine different pharmacotherapeutic strategies had to be tried before control was gained. The highest rate of complete or partial effectiveness (84% to 94%) occurred with either amiodarone or verapamil (alone or in combination with digoxin).[112]

Permanent junctional reciprocating tachycardia is a difficult arrhythmia to treat with antiarrhythmic medications, and few data are available to guide therapy. β-Blockers remain first-line therapy. However, escalation of therapy to class I, class III, class IV, or multidrug regimens is likely.

ATRIAL FLUTTER, ATRIAL FIBRILLATION, AND INTRA-ATRIAL REENTRANT TACHYCARDIA

The last three supraventricular arrhythmias are addressed together because of their shared characteristics and relative infrequency in the pediatric population. These arrhythmias are often considered "macro-reentrant" tachycardias because the entire atrium often consists of one large reentrant circuit.[6,115-118] Atrial flutter and atrial fibrillation are rare in neonates, infants, and children and are often found in patients with concomitant heart disease and in patients who have undergone surgical correction of congenital heart disease.[6,115-120] Presentation of atrial flutter in neonates typically occurs within the first 48 hours of life.[118] Atrial flutter appears as a "saw-tooth" pattern on ECG, whereas atrial fibrillation is described as "irregularly irregular" with no discernable pattern.[121] Intra-atrial reentrant tachycardia has also been termed *scar flutter* because it is seen in patients with a history of heart surgery. Direct current cardioversion is often used to convert patients to normal sinus rhythm (with anticoagulation possibly indicated before cardioversion).[6,115-118] First-line therapy for intra-atrial reentrant tachycardia is pharmacologic, but patients often require catheter ablation, placement of an implantable pacemaker or cardioverter–defibrillator, or surgery.[122] The use of transesophageal pacing for conversion of atrial flutter and atrial fibrillation in neonates and infants has shown success, but direct current cardioversion remains the mainstay of therapy.[120] However, for older children, the presence of atrial fibrillation or intra-atrial reentrant tachycardia, particularly in conjunction with congenital heart disease, is often treated with pharmacotherapy before cardioversion or in conjunction with cardioversion, depending on a patient's hemodynamic state.[123]

Many agents have been used in the treatment of atrial flutter. Atrial flutter in neonates may not require pharmacotherapy because rates of spontaneous conversion or use of cardioversion can resolve the arrhythmia with a low incidence of recurrence.[115,118,124-126] Neonates with atrial flutter

have historically been treated with digoxin, despite the low rates of success (less than 50%), and most clinicians would not treat a patient for longer than 1 year after diagnosis if there were no signs of recurrence.[115,118,124,126] β-Blockers, including propranolol, have often been used as a first-line agent for the treatment of neonatal atrial flutter after cardioversion.[125,127,128] Other agents such as amiodarone, procainamide, quinidine, and sotalol have also been used for the treatment of neonatal atrial flutter.[38,115,129-133] Treatment of atrial flutter in older infants and children has shown efficacy with the use of propafenone but poor results with the use of flecainide.[27,31,32,94] Amiodarone may be the most effective agent for the treatment of atrial flutter in infants and children, showing a 94% resolution rate.[123] Sotalol has also been used, however, with lower rates of conversion than with amiodarone.[110,130] Overall treatment recommendations for neonates with atrial flutter include a β-blocker as a first-line therapy, but progression to other agents may be necessary for intractable arrhythmias. Infants and older children with atrial flutter may benefit from amiodarone, but the adverse events that can be associated with it must be weighed against the benefit gained.

Atrial fibrillation pharmacotherapy has primarily been extrapolated from adult data because atrial fibrillation is extremely rare in children but common in adults. Digoxin has been used to slow ventricular response in atrial fibrillation with the addition of procainamide or quinidine if therapy initially fails.[119,134,135] Often, progression of pharmacotherapy to sotalol or amiodarone becomes necessary.[111,130] Currently, the data for treatment of atrial fibrillation are sparse and likely subject to institutional bias; thus, treatment decisions should be considered on a case-by-case basis.

JUNCTIONAL ECTOPIC TACHYCARDIA

Although JET is a rare supraventricular arrhythmia, the mortality and morbidity associated with JET can be as high as 35% to 40%.[6,22,136-147] Junctional ectopic tachycardia is most often associated with postoperative cardiac surgical patients and patients with myocarditis.[6,22,136-144] The ECG pattern of JET can have a wide or narrow QRS complex depending on the presence of underlying bundle branch block. It classically has a QRS morphology similar to that of sinus rhythm for that particular patient.[22] Early recognition and treatment of JET is important because the tachycardia can result in profound decreases in cardiac output and lead to cardiovascular collapse, particularly in the postoperative patient.[148] Patients with JET will often present in severe heart failure.[149] Junctional ectopic tachycardia can be particularly difficult to treat because the tachycardia-associated decrease in cardiac output can result in increased adrenergic tone, which can subsequently further increase the junctional rate.[22] Nonpharmacologic interventions for the treatment of postoperative JET (pJET) include cooling of the patient to reduce automaticity, sedation, decrease in environmental stimuli, reduction in inotropic agents, overdrive pacing, or His bundle ablation.[22,143-145,148,149] Congenital JET (cJET) typically is not as life threatening as pJET, but unlike pJET, which can resolve in 48–72 hours, cJET often requires chronic treatment.[22,137,140,144] In addition, 50% of patients with cJET have a family history of JET.[22]

For pJET, intravenous amiodarone should be considered a first-line agent after nonpharmacologic intervention.[34,150-154] Other agents such as digoxin or propafenone have been previously used with much lower success rates.[94,155] Before cardiac surgery, the supplementation of magnesium and use of propranolol are both proven to decrease the incidence of pJET.[151,156] The treatment of cJET with amiodarone has also shown good results, whereas the use of a β-blocker with or without digoxin has been fairly unsuccessful.[144] Oral propafenone has shown variable results in treating cJET, yet it can still be considered an agent for initial therapy.[28,157,158] Finally, sotalol has also been used for the treatment of cJET in some patients.[109,139] The most effective agent for the treatment of pJET or cJET at this time appears to be amiodarone.

VENTRICULAR TACHYARRHYTHMIAS

Ventricular tachycardia (VT) and ventricular fibrillation (VF) are of great concern, particularly because of their association with sudden cardiac death in children and adolescents. This section will focus on VT and the subsequent potential progression to VF in pediatric patients.

VT AND FIBRILLATION

The etiologies of VT in pediatric patients are varied, and they differ considerably from typical adult etiologies. Patients with congenital heart disease, particularly patients with tetralogy of Fallot, have been noted to have a higher incidence of VT than the general pediatric population.[159] In addition, patients with cardiomyopathies, such as hypertrophic cardiomyopathy or left ventricular noncompaction syndrome, are at a very high risk of sudden death because of VT leading to VF.[160] Other etiologies of VT include surgery for congenital heart disease, genetic disorders (Brugada syndrome, long QT syndrome [LQTS]), catecholamine-sensitive polymorphic tachycardia, arrhythmogenic right ventricular dysplasia, myocarditis, and electrolyte disturbances.[6,161,162] Many drugs have been implicated in the development of VT, primarily caused by QT-interval prolongation and TdP, which will be addressed in a separate section of this chapter. Despite the many identified pathologies for VT, the etiology is often idiopathic. The incidence of spontaneous VT has been reported to be as high as 3% in patients with no preexisting cardiac disease.[163,164]

Pediatric patients with VT can present with chest pain, syncope with exertion, or cardiac arrest.[165] Ventricular tachycardia is defined as three or more consecutive beats originating in the ventricles, and it appears as a wide QRS complex tachycardia on ECG.[165,166] Long-term prognosis of pediatric patients with VT is variable and dependent on many factors. These include the etiology of VT, severity of cardiovascular compromise with VT, and patient comorbidities.[167]

Treatment of patients with VT requires that their hemodynamic status be considered before therapy initiation. According to Pediatric Advanced Life Support guidelines, patients with hemodynamic compromise caused by VT/VF are emergently treated.[168] For in-depth summaries of acute pharmacologic management of VT/VF, the algorithms in the Pediatric Advanced Life Support guidelines should be consulted.[168]

Patients with chronic episodes of hemodynamically stable VT are managed differently, with the focus on prevention of VT/VF by medical or pharmacologic interventions. First-line therapy for chronic management of nonsustained VT in pediatric patients is often β-blockers, but this approach has been extrapolated from adult data.[169] Atenolol, metoprolol, or nadolol have been used for treatment of VT and LQTS in children, whereas propranolol has been used in infants.[170,171] Mexiletine has also been used for the treatment of ventricular arrhythmias in pediatric patients with congenital heart disease.[117,172] Pharmacotherapy for the prevention of VT/VF often depends on the underlying substrate for VT; therefore, first-line therapies should be chosen on the basis of patient-specific pathophysiology. Primary therapies that have been evaluated include β-blockers or amiodarone.[167] Disopyramide can also be considered for patients with VT and hypertrophic obstructive cardiomyopathy as an adjunct to β-blockers.[173]

TORSADES DE POINTES

Torsades de pointes is a form of polymorphic VT that is associated with a prolonged QT interval, which was previously discussed. Torsades de pointes occurs because of prolongation of the QT interval, which can occur with various disease states, including congenital LQTS, drug-induced long QT, and other forms of acquired long QT.[174] Patients with a QT interval on ECG of 450 milliseconds or greater if they are male or 460 milliseconds if female are considered to have prolonged QT interval and therefore are at risk of TdP or other ventricular arrhythmias.[175] These numbers, however, are not absolute, and a patient's entire clinical scenario should be evaluated when determining QT-interval prolongation. Electrocardiographic findings for TdP are reflective of its name: the peaks of the QRS complexes appear to "twist"—thus, the term in French, *torsades de pointes*, or *twisting of the points*.[166] Many medications have been implicated in causing TdP, with prolongation of the QT interval as the most common reason for the removal of medications from the market in the United States.[176] Table 2 shows select medications that cause QT-interval prolongation and that may be used in pediatric patients.

Management strategies are two-fold: prevention of TdP and treatment of patients with TdP. Prevention of TdP focuses on the management of congenital LQTS, maintenance of electrolyte homeostasis, and minimization of exposure to medications that can potentially prolong the QT interval. It is beyond the scope of this chapter to summarize all the information associated with congenital LQTS because the various mutations often dictate pharmacotherapy.[177,178] In general, β-blocker therapy is indicated as first-line pharmacologic therapy in patients with high-risk LQTS mutations. If the mutations for LQTS affect sodium channels, mexiletine and flecainide have shown some initial benefit in adult patients.[179] Patients may occasionally require a pacemaker or an implantable cardioverter–defibrillator. Acute management of TdP requires the use of intravenous magnesium sulfate for treatment (25–50 mg/kg/dose) and subsequent removal of any medications that may be prolonging the QT interval.[180,181]

BRADYARRHYTHMIAS

Two primary forms of bradyarrhythmias are most commonly seen in pediatric patients: sinus bradycardia and AV nodal block.

SINUS BRADYCARDIA

Sinus bradycardia is defined as a heart rate less than the lower limit of normal values, and it can occur in a wide variety of patient subsets, from preterm infants to well-trained athletes.[182-189] Rarely is sinus bradycardia a cause for medical treatment unless hemodynamic instability occurs, such as in cardiogenic shock or if the patient has notable symptoms related to bradycardia. Patient presentation for bradycardia can vary on the basis of age and can include poor feeding and lack of weight gain (in neonates and infants), fatigue, exercise intolerance, and, in severe bradycardia, cardiogenic shock or seizures.[187] Sinus node dysfunction, or "sick sinus syndrome," is a common cause of sinus bradycardia. Etiologies of sinus node dysfunction include medications, excessive vagal tone, electrolyte imbalances, elevated intracranial pressure,

Table 2. Select Medications Responsible for QT Prolongation That May Be Used in Pediatric Patients[a,218]

Class and Notes	Medications
Class I (Highest Risk) • Prolongs the QT interval • May put patients at risk of proarrhythmia, including TdP	Amiodarone Chlorpromazine Clarithromycin Disopyramide Erythromycin Haloperidol Methadone Pentamidine Procainamide Quinidine Sotalol
Class II (Moderate Risk) • Some reports suggest QT-interval prolongation and possible induction of proarrhythmia, but insufficient evidence for causing TdP • Patients may be at risk of TdP if class 2 agents are used with other risk factors for development of TdP	Amantadine Azithromycin Chloral hydrate Dolasetron Escitalopram Flecainide Foscarnet Fosphenytoin Granisetron Levofloxacin Nicardipine Octreotide Ondansetron Quetiapine Risperidone Tacrolimus Venlafaxine Voriconazole
Class III (Low Risk) • Weak evidence for development of TdP • Unlikely to cause arrhythmia when used in normal doses in patients without other risk factors	Amitriptyline Ciprofloxacin Citalopram Diphenhydramine Fluconazole Fluoxetine Imipramine Itraconazole Paroxetine Ritonavir Sertraline Trazodone Trimethoprim/sulfamethoxazole

[a]Medications and classifications are constantly modified according to the most recent literature. The CredibleMeds website at www.crediblemeds.org provides complete listings and classifications of medications.
TdP = torsades de pointes.

and congenital heart disease (particularly after repair of a congenital heart lesion).[185] A genetic component to sinus node dysfunction has been identified that is associated with LQTSs.[190,191] Cardiac pacing is an option because pharmacotherapy for sinus bradycardia is not currently indicated. Limitation or removal of agents that can cause sinus bradycardia, or correction of preexisting patient pathophysiologies that can lead to bradycardia, is warranted.[185]

AV NODAL BLOCK

Atrioventricular nodal block, defined as a delay in signal conduction from the atria to the ventricles, primarily involves the AV node and/or the bundles of His.[185] Atrioventricular block is classified according to the degree of PR-interval prolongation and the association of P waves with QRS complexes. First-degree AV block, or PR-interval prolongation in adults, is defined as a PR interval greater than 0.2 milliseconds while maintaining a 1:1 atria-to-ventricle conduction ratio. Second- and third-degree (or complete) AV block are characterized by increasing the degree of AV dissociation.[185] Complete AV block has no associated conduction between atria and ventricles, and it is characterized by an atrial rate that is higher than the ventricular rate.[185]

Primary modalities for treatment of higher-grade or symptomatic AV block include pacemaker insertion and correction of the underlying pathophysiology that is leading to AV block.[192] Removal of offending agents, such as medications, is indicated for the treatment of AV block. Pharmacotherapy is rarely beneficial as primary treatment.

ANTIARRHYTHMIC AGENT SELECTION

Antiarrhythmic medications affect ion transport in myocardial cells. Three primary modes of electrical signal transduction and generation are affected as follows: (1) *automaticity*—the rate of action potential generation; (2) *conduction velocity*—the speed of action potential movement through the myocardium; and (3) *refractory period*—the time to repolarize. All antiarrhythmic medications are classified by Vaughan-Williams categories based on their primary mechanism of action as shown in Table 1. The dosing and monitoring of these agents is often individualized on the basis of the arrhythmia being treated and other patient comorbidities.[5] In addition, the effect of each of these medications on electrophysiologic and hemodynamic factors has been summarized. Each of these drugs will be evaluated in depth regarding their effect on various arrhythmias in the following sections (Table 3).

Table 3. Common Pediatric Arrhythmias and Suggested Pharmacologic Interventions

Arrhythmia	First Line	Alternative	Comments
AVRT, AVNRT	IV: Adenosine PO: Propranolol, Digoxin	IV: Esmolol, Procainamide, Sotalol, Amiodarone PO: Flecainide, Sotalol, Amiodarone	IV route should be reserved for patients with poor perfusion or unable to take PO
Focal atrial tachycardias	IV: Esmolol PO: Propranolol, Digoxin	IV: Procainamide, Sotalol, Amiodarone PO: Flecainide, Sotalol, Amiodarone	
Wolff-Parkinson-White syndrome	IV: Esmolol PO: Propranolol	IV: Sotalol, Amiodarone PO: Sotalol, Amiodarone	Digoxin should be avoided in this syndrome
Atrial fibrillation	IV: Esmolol PO: Propranolol, Atenolol	IV: Sotalol, Amiodarone PO: Sotalol, Amiodarone	Cardioversion is first line before pharmacologic therapy
Atrial flutter	IV: Esmolol PO: Propranolol, Atenolol	IV: Sotalol, Amiodarone PO: Sotalol, Amiodarone	Cardioversion is first line before pharmacologic therapy
Intra-atrial re-entrant tachycardia	IV: Esmolol PO: Propranolol, Atenolol, Digoxin	IV: Sotalol, Amiodarone PO: Sotalol, Amiodarone	
Junctional ectopic tachycardia (post-operative)	IV: Amiodarone	IV: Digoxin, multidrug therapy	Cooling and neuromuscular blockade should also be used
Ventricular tachycardia	IV: Amiodarone PO: Metoprolol, Atenolol, Nadolol		Defibrillation may also be indicated for poor perfusion
Ventricular fibrillation	IV: Amiodarone PO: Metoprolol, Atenolol, Nadolol		Defibrillation may also be indicated for poor perfusion
Torsades des pointes	IV: Magnesium		Removal of medications that prolong the QT interval

AVNRT = atrioventricular nodal reentrant tachycardia; AVRT = Atrioventricular reentrant tachycardia; IV = intravenous; PO = by mouth.

CLASS IA

The class Ia agents block sodium channel uptake in the fast sodium channels. In relation to other class I agents, the blockade would be considered moderate, and the resultant effects of a decrease in automaticity, an increase in refractory period, and a decrease in conduction velocity would also be considered moderate. The QT interval can be moderately prolonged, with little to no effect on QRS duration or PR interval. Left ventricular dysfunction and hypotension with therapy have been noted.[30,58]

QUINIDINE

Quinidine has been used to treat children with rare arrhythmias, such as the Brugada.[193] Pharmacokinetic studies highlighting doses with quinidine have been performed.[194] Clearance of quinidine is inversely proportional with age in pediatric patients; therefore, younger patients may require higher doses.[195] A trough serum concentration of 2–7 mcg/mL is considered therapeutic for the treatment of arrhythmias.[5]

However, quinidine is not used often because of the high rate of adverse events, proarrhythmia (i.e., TdP), central nervous system toxicity, and hypotension with the intravenous form.[196] Quinidine is available in two different forms (gluconate and sulfate), with dosing differences between them, and requires special attention to minimize medication errors. Careful consideration should occur before the use of quinidine regarding the risk-benefit ratio. A formulation for an extemporaneous preparation of a suspension is available.[197]

PROCAINAMIDE

Because of the paucity of data for the dosing of procainamide in neonates, infants, and children, dosing and monitoring strategies have been primarily extrapolated from adult literature. Intravenous dosing consists of a loading dose followed by a continuous infusion of 20–80 mcg/kg/minute, with doses to achieve therapeutic concentrations on the lower end for neonates and preterm neonates, likely because of decreased clearance.[92,198] Patients with renal dysfunction or receiving renal replacement therapy have reduced clearance of procainamide and metabolites and require dosage adjustments.[92]

Monitoring of drug concentrations is indicated for intravenous procainamide. Concentrations of procainamide and its active metabolite, N-acetyl procainamide (NAPA), are drawn after an intravenous bolus and every 12 hours during continuous-infusion therapy.[5] Goal concentrations have been reported at 4–10 mcg/mL for procainamide, but they can vary depending on institutional practices.[5] Procainamide therapy is usually not titrated to NAPA concentrations, but these concentrations are useful to determine whether the patient is a "fast acetylator" (a NAPA/procainamide ratio of 1:1 or greater) and will therefore need higher doses.[92]

The most common adverse events associated with procainamide are hypotension, primarily with continuous-infusion administration, and proarrhythmia, such as heart block. Recent reports have documented that procainamide is associated with fewer adverse events than amiodarone, with similar efficacy in certain situations.[35]

DISOPYRAMIDE

Minimal data are available for disopyramide use in pediatric patients because newer agents are more effective at controlling arrhythmias or have fewer adverse events.[173] Disopyramide dosing should be adjusted in patients with renal dysfunction.[5] Serum concentrations of disopyramide can be measured, although there is no correlation with drug efficacy in pediatric patients.[5] Adverse events with therapy include proarrhythmia.[5] A formulation for an extemporaneous preparation of a suspension is available.[5]

CLASS IB

Medications in class Ib are considered to have the least potent sodium channel blockade, affecting the fast sodium channels in the phase 0 upstroke of the action potential. Class Ib agents decrease both automaticity and conduction velocity and increase the refractory period, but all effects are to a lesser extent compared with the other class I antiarrhythmics. Class Ib medications have little effect on the QRS duration, PR interval, QT interval, or left ventricular function.

LIDOCAINE

Lidocaine can be given as an intravenous bolus or as continuous infusion for acute ventricular arrhythmias.[5] Pharmacokinetic factors have been described in pediatric patients with congenital heart disease.[199] Serum lidocaine concentrations can be monitored at steady state to prevent toxicity, with goal ranges reported from 1.5–5 mcg/mL.[5] Hypotension, central nervous system toxicity, and proarrhythmia are the adverse events reported on bolus intravenous injection or continuous intravenous infusion.[5]

MEXILETINE

Few data are available for the use of mexiletine in pediatric patients for treating ventricular arrhythmias and certain types of LQTS.[172,200] Mexiletine is structurally similar to lidocaine, but orally active. Serum mexiletine concentrations can be monitored as trough concentrations to minimize toxicity.[5] Potential adverse events include proarrhythmia and ataxia.[5] A formulation for an extemporaneous preparation of a suspension is available.[200]

CLASS IC

The phase 0 upstroke involving sodium ion channel blockade is blocked to the greatest degree by class Ic agents. Similarly, decreases in automaticity and conduction velocity and increases in refractory period are the most pronounced of all the class I agents. The PR interval, QT interval, and QRS duration are all prolonged.

FLECAINIDE

Dosing is controversial regarding whether dosing per kilogram or by body surface area should be used to achieve therapeutic concentrations.[5,31,55] Flecainide interacts with milk;

therefore, concentrations can be lower (or doses will need to be higher) in patients who are breastfeeding or receiving milk and concentrations may change when the patient's diet changes if not immediately given around a feed.[5,55] Sex, race, and cytochrome P450 2D6 enzyme expression affect flecainide disposition.[201-203] Flecainide is contraindicated in patients with congenital heart disease because of reports of increased mortality.[103]

Flecainide concentrations can be monitored when initiating therapy and on a regular basis thereafter. Therapeutic range for treatment of arrhythmia is 0.2–1 mcg/mL drawn as a trough, but the use of flecainide concentration monitoring on patient outcomes is unknown.[5] Concentrations may not need to be measured if using low doses because the effectiveness of therapy can be monitored by QRS widening. In-hospital initiation of flecainide is usually required.

Adverse events are relatively uncommon, primarily consisting of neurologic changes and proarrhythmia (less than 1%), and they are rare when concentrations are within therapeutic ranges.[5,55] A formulation for an extemporaneous preparation of a flecainide suspension is available.[5]

PROPAFENONE

Propafenone dosing is controversial regarding whether milligram-per-kilogram dosing or body surface area should be used.[5,27,91] Patients who received the lower range of dosing had decreased effectiveness when undergoing treatment of WPW compared with patients who received higher doses (300–380 mg/m^2/day).[58] Serum concentration monitoring is not typically used for propafenone because concentrations do not correlate well with ECG findings.[204] A formulation for an extemporaneous preparation of a suspension is available.[205]

CLASS II

The β-blockers make up the class II agents and exhibit their actions primarily on the pacemaker cell action potentials by limiting catecholamine stimulation. These effects primarily result in decreased automaticity, and they subsequently increase the effective refractory period of the Purkinje fibers. Use of β-blockers can acutely decrease left ventricular function and will prolong the PR interval. There is usually no effect on the QT interval or QRS duration. Caution should be used when a β-blocker is administered in a patient with reactive airway disease, in particular propranolol, which is nonselective by nature (β1 and β2).[5]

PROPRANOLOL

Standard dosing regimens for propranolol have been established, and most centers commonly use a maximum of 4 mg/kg/day.[5,8] Drug concentration monitoring for propranolol is not currently indicated. Reported adverse events with propranolol include hypotension, bradycardia, and hypoglycemia. Propranolol is currently available in two different concentrations of a commercially available solution: 4 mg/mL and 8 mg/mL for enteral use.[5] Intravenous propranolol is also available, but with limited experience.[5]

ESMOLOL

Esmolol can be used as a continuous infusion for treatment of supraventricular arrhythmias or ventricular arrhythmias.[5] Pharmacokinetic and dosing studies have been performed in children, and esmolol is often used when a quick onset and short half-life of β-receptor blockade are beneficial.[83,206] Adverse events are similar to those of other β-blockers and consist of bradycardia and hypotension.[5]

ATENOLOL

Atenolol has been used for arrhythmias in children, but with less experience than other β-blockers such as propranolol.[54,170] Pharmacokinetic and pharmacodynamic studies have been performed with atenolol in children, and drug concentration monitoring is not currently indicated.[54,82,207] Common adverse events associated with atenolol include bradycardia and hypotension.[5] There is a formulation for an extemporaneous preparation of an atenolol suspension.[5]

METOPROLOL

Metoprolol has not typically been used for the treatment or prevention of arrhythmias in pediatric patients; thus, few data are available to guide therapy.[171,208] Metoprolol is more cardiospecific in its β-blockade than other β-blockers and may have a lower incidence of bronchospasm.[5] Care should be taken that patients receive the correct formulation of tablet: metoprolol tartrate or metoprolol succinate (extended release). A formulation for an extemporaneous preparation of a suspension is available.[209]

NADOLOL

Pharmacokinetic studies have been performed for nadolol in children, and the authors of the study warn of using nadolol in children younger than 2 years because of wide variations in pharmacokinetic factors.[210] Common adverse events for nadolol include bradycardia and hypotension.[5] No formulation for a suspension is currently available.

CLASS III

The class III agents exhibit their antiarrhythmic effects primarily through potassium channel blockade, extending phase 4 of the action potential and increasing the refractory period. However, agents in this class often have several mechanisms of action. Sotalol has nonselective β-blockade effects in addition to potassium channel-blocking effects. Amiodarone has sodium channel-blocking effects, β-blocking effects, and calcium channel-blocking effects. Electrocardiographic findings in patients receiving class III antiarrhythmics include prolonged PR and QT intervals and increased QRS duration. The prolongation of the QT intervals places patients at risk of TdP.

SOTALOL

Sotalol dosing for neonates, infants, and children has been controversial. Currently three dosing methods have been suggested for patients younger than 2 years.[5] A dosing nomogram for patients younger than 2 years has been proposed, with reductions in dose for younger patients on the basis of body surface area.[5] Other pharmacokinetic studies have been performed showing that lower doses of sotalol are effective in patients younger than 2 years but that sotalol should be dosed on a milligram-per-kilogram basis.[211,212] Recent data have supported dosing on body surface area, with no reduction in dose for age or renal function, and show good outcomes.[213] Younger patients may be more tolerant of higher doses of sotalol than older patients.[30] The ideal method for dosing sotalol in this age subset is unclear. Monitoring of ECG for QT-interval prolongation is necessary when initiating or titrating therapy.

Primary adverse events associated with sotalol are arrhythmia related. Bradycardia and TdP can occur with sotalol use, and female patients are more likely to have TdP with sotalol compared with male patients.[5,196] Maintenance of electrolyte homeostasis (i.e., potassium and magnesium) is important for preventing TdP, and frequent ECG monitoring is indicated. In-hospital initiation of sotalol is usually required.

Sotalol is available as a tablet, and there is a formulation for an extemporaneous preparation of a suspension.[5] Intravenous sotalol has recently become available; however, no pediatric experience is available to date with intravenous sotalol.

AMIODARONE

Amiodarone can be dosed either on body surface area or per body weight for continuous-infusion or chronic therapy.[5] In the acute setting, body weight dosing is primarily used for intravenous bolus.[5] Amiodarone serum concentrations can be drawn, but few data are available to interpret concentrations or their effect on antiarrhythmic efficacy.[214,215]

Many adverse events are associated with amiodarone therapy. Pulmonary fibrosis, thyroid toxicity, corneal deposits, hepatotoxicity, decreased growth, developmental delay, dermatologic hypersensitivity, and proarrhythmia (i.e., TdP) have all been reported with amiodarone therapy, and a baseline evaluation for potentially affected organ system function is warranted.[216-218] Hypotension is a common adverse event after the intravenous administration of amiodarone.[219-221] Some centers may precede an infusion of amiodarone with an infusion of calcium to prevent hypotension. Drug interactions with amiodarone are also significant because it affects cytochrome P450 enzymes and P-glycoprotein drug transport mechanisms.[5]

Although an intravenous formulation of amiodarone is available, it is only compatible with a 5% dextrose solution.[5] In addition, amiodarone intravenous solutions must be given through tubing that does not have bis(2-ethylhexyl)phthalate in the formulation because a solubility component of intravenous amiodarone (Polysorbate 80) has been noted to leach this phthalate from the tubing, potentially causing sterility in male patients.[5] A formulation for an extemporaneous preparation of a suspension is available.[222] Hypotension can occur, particularly with intravenous amiodarone. Because amiodarone is highly lipid soluble, special care must be taken when preparing a suspension.

CLASS IV

The class IV agents include the nondihydropyridine calcium channel blockers (i.e., verapamil and diltiazem). In contrast to dihydropyridine calcium channel blockers (i.e., nifedipine), the class IV agents more specifically act on the myocardium and on the pacemaker cell action potential by blocking slow L-type calcium channels. Calcium channel blockade decreases phase 4 depolarization by increasing the refractory period of the pacemaker cell and decreasing conduction velocity in the AV node. Electrocardiographic findings include an increased PR interval. These agents can decrease left ventricular function and cause hypotension; they are not recommended for children younger than 1 year.

VERAPAMIL

Dosing for treatment or prevention of arrhythmias is not well established in pediatric patients, with limited pharmacokinetic studies performed to date.[223,224] In general, the use of verapamil in patients younger than 1 year is discouraged, despite some reports of successful use.[225-227] Intravenous verapamil therapy for the treatment of arrhythmias in neonates and infants is discouraged because of cases of proarrhythmia, including AV block and cardiovascular collapse after administration.[76,69,228] Different strategies to avoid the cardiovascular adverse effects have been tried, including administering intravenous calcium with verapamil and using slow infusion rates.[229]

Verapamil is available in different extended-release formulations. Therefore, attention to dosage forms is important to minimize errors. A formulation for an extemporaneous preparation of a suspension is available.[209]

DILTIAZEM

Few data are available for the use of diltiazem to treat or prevent arrhythmias in pediatric patients.[230] Proarrhythmic effects, including AV block and hypotension, are two primary concerns for adverse events.[5] Diltiazem is available as immediate- and extended-release formulations, and a formulation for an extemporaneous preparation of a suspension is available.[231]

DIGOXIN

Digoxin acts by blocking the sodium/potassium ATPase pump in the myocardium, which results in decreased conduction velocity (by decreasing the rate of transmission through the AV node) and increased refractory period. Sinus bradycardia and AV block can occur, particularly when serum digoxin concentrations are elevated.

Digoxin use in pediatric patients for the treatment of arrhythmias has a large body of literature because it has historically been first-line therapy for many types of arrhythmias.[30,58] Pharmacokinetic studies of children have been performed to delineate dosing.[232] Digoxin toxicity can occur in patients with renal dysfunction, electrolyte imbalances, or drug interactions.[233] Serum digoxin concentrations are not indicated for routine therapy because concentrations do not correlate with efficacy, but they may be useful in the assessment of digoxin toxicity.[234] In addition, neonates may have false-positive results for elevated digoxin concentrations because of digoxin-like interacting substances in the blood.[235] Digoxin toxicity manifests as bradycardia (including AV block), nausea and vomiting, and visual disturbances.[232] Digoxin-immune Fab is used to treat symptomatic digoxin toxicity.[233] Digoxin should be avoided in patients with WPW because of the risk of ventricular arrhythmias. Precautions should be taken when administering digoxin because dosing is in micrograms, and errors have occurred when using a commercially available digoxin solution.[236]

ADENOSINE

Adenosine is an endogenous nucleoside that directly affects potassium currents, which depresses AV nodal function. The ECG often shows no conduction after the administration of adenosine (in reentrant arrhythmias), or depressed nodal activity, which lasts a few seconds.

Published experience with adenosine in pediatric patients is extensive.[14,237-242] Patients may require several doses of adenosine to achieve the desired effect. Adenosine, which has a short half-life (6–10 seconds), should be administered as a rapid intravenous push, followed by a rapid flush, through intravenous access that is closest to the heart, to ensure adequate delivery of the drug to the myocardium before metabolism.[5]

Despite extensive experience with adenosine, adverse effects have been noted, including the generation of wide complex tachyarrhythmias.[15] Caution should be used when using adenosine in patients with asthma because bronchospasm can occur. Only experienced personnel should administer adenosine in a setting where life-support equipment is available.

CONCLUSIONS

The pharmacotherapy for pediatric arrhythmias can be complex and highly variable. A comprehensive knowledge of arrhythmia pathophysiology and antiarrhythmic pharmacology and an understanding of the impact of pediatric growth and development on these conditions are essential to ensure optimal outcomes. Future efforts to refine the pharmacotherapy for pediatric arrhythmias are warranted to minimize morbidity and maximize efficacy.

Patient Case NEONATAL SUPRAVENTRICULAR TACHYCARDIA

A 3-week-old, 4.2-kg, term male infant is admitted to the emergency department (ED) after a well child check-up at the pediatrician office. The patient was referred to the ED because of a heart rate of about 280 beats per minute. On arrival to the ED, he appears pale with cool extremities.

> **Medical history:** No pertinent medical history before this event
>
> **Medications:** No current medications
>
> **Physical examination:** Patient appears dusky and cool, but in no
>
> acute distress; HR 294 beats/minute on electrocardiogram; mildly sluggish capillary refill of 3 seconds
>
> **Electrocardiogram:** Narrow complex tachycardia
>
> A cardiology consultation is sought, and a diagnosis of supraventricular tachycardia is made.

1. What is the first choice for treatment of supraventricular tachycardia in this patient?

Intravenous adenosine 0.4 mg (0.1 mg/kg/dose) would be the best choice for initial pharmacotherapy for this patient. Because the patient appears to have compromised perfusion (i.e., pale appearance, cool extremities, sluggish capillary refill), the use of a rapidly acting medication is indicated versus an enteral medication with a slower onset. Ice to the face or other vagal maneuvers typically have limited success. Esmolol could potentially be an option if the supraventricular tachycardia does not resolve after several doses of adenosine and the patient requires management in an intensive care unit.

Case (continued). The arrhythmia is terminated after two doses of adenosine in the ED; the patient is in sinus rhythm and regains acceptable cardiac output. The cardiology service recommends discharge from the ED with antiarrhythmic therapy and follow-up within the next week.

2. What pharmacotherapy would you recommend?

Oral propranolol 4 mg (1 mg/kg/dose) every 6 hours or digoxin 20 mcg (5 mcg/kg/dose) orally every 12 hours would be acceptable answers for this patient scenario. Both are commercially available solutions, and the data for treatment of infant supraventricular tachycardia have shown no differences in efficacy. Propranolol must be administered more often than digoxin, but digoxin has a greater risk of toxicity, and overdoses with digoxin have been reported. Amiodarone would not be an acceptable first choice because of the many associated toxicities and the difficulty in preparation of a suspension. Sotalol, although available commercially as a suspension, should be reserved for patients for whom initial therapy with propranolol or digoxin has failed. After initiation of pharmacotherapy, the patient should have resolution of the arrhythmia with no breakthrough seen on electrocardiography or 24-hour Holter monitoring.

REFERENCES

1. Lilly L. Pathophysiology of Heart Disease, 6th ed. Baltimore: Lippincott Williams & Wilkins, 2015.

2. Sanoski CA, Bauman JL. The arrhythmias. In: DiPiro JT, Talbert RL, Yee GC, et al., eds. Pharmacotherapy: A Pathophysiologic Approach, 10th ed. New York: McGraw-Hill, 2016.

3. Taketomo C, Hodding J, Kraus D. Pediatric & Neonatal Dosage Handbook, 19th ed. Hudson, OH: Lexi-Comp, 2012.

4. Wetzel GT, Klitzner TS. Developmental cardiac electrophysiology recent advances in cellular physiology. Cardiovasc Res 1996;31: E52-60.

5. Cohen MI, Wieand TS, Rhodes LA, et al. Electrophysiologic properties of the atrioventricular node in pediatric patients. J Am Coll Cardiol 1997;29:403-7.

6. Hoffman TM, Wernovsky G, Wieand TS, et al. The incidence of arrhythmias in a pediatric cardiac intensive care unit. Pediatr Cardiol 2002;23:598-604.

7. Deal BJ, Keane JF, Gillette PC, et al. Wolff-Parkinson-White syndrome and supraventricular tachycardia during infancy: management and follow-up. J Am Coll Cardiol 1985;5:130-5.

8. Garson A Jr, Gillette PC, McNamara DG. Supraventricular tachycardia in children: clinical features, response to treatment, and long-term follow-up in 217 patients. J Pediatr 1981;98:875-82.

9. Salerno JC, Garrison MM, Larison C, et al. Case fatality in children with supraventricular tachycardia in the United States. Pacing Clin Electrophysiol 2011;34:832-6.

10. Josephson ME, Wellens HJ. Differential diagnosis of supraventricular tachycardia. Cardiol Clin 1990;8:411-42.

11. Ko JK, Deal BJ, Strasburger JF, et al. Supraventricular tachycardia mechanisms and their age distribution in pediatric patients. Am J Cardiol 1992;69:1028-32.

12. Sreeram N, Wren C. Supraventricular tachycardia in infants: response to initial treatment. Arch Dis Child 1990;65:127-9.

13. Cetta F, Porter CB. Diagnostic use of adenosine in two pediatric patients. Pediatr Emerg Care 1995;11:100-2.

14. Ralston MA, Knilans TK, Hannon DW, et al. Use of adenosine for diagnosis and treatment of tachyarrhythmias in pediatric patients. J Pediatr 1994;124:139-43.

15. Kipel G, Rossi AF, Steinberg LG, et al. Malignant wide complex tachycardia after adenosine administration to a postoperative pediatric patient with congenital heart disease. Pediatr Cardiol 1995;16:36-7.

16. Mehta AV, Sanchez GR, Sacks EJ, et al. Ectopic automatic atrial tachycardia in children: clinical characteristics, management and follow-up. J Am Coll Cardiol 1988;11:379-85.

17. Naheed ZJ, Strasburger JF, Benson DW Jr, et al. Natural history and management strategies of automatic atrial tachycardia in children. Am J Cardiol 1995;75:405-7.

18. Salim MA, Case CL, Gillette PC. Chaotic atrial tachycardia in children. Am Heart J 1995;129:831-3.

19. Stambach D, Bermet V, Bauersfeld U. Clinical recognition and treatment of atrial ectopic tachycardia in newborns. Swiss Med Wkly 2007;137:402-6.

20. Bauersfeld U, Gow RM, Hamilton RM, et al. Treatment of atrial ectopic tachycardia in infants < 6 months old. Am Heart J 1995;129:1145-8.

21. Salerno JC, Kertesz NJ, Friedman RA, et al. Clinical course of atrial ectopic tachycardia is age-dependent: results and treatment in children < 3 or > or =3 years of age. J Am Coll Cardiol 2004;43:438-44.

22. Case CL, Gillette PC. Automatic atrial and junctional tachycardias in the pediatric patient: strategies for diagnosis and management. Pacing Clin Electrophysiol 1993;16:1323-35.

23. Kugler JD, Danford DA, Deal BJ, et al. Radiofrequency catheter ablation for tachyarrhythmias in children and adolescents. The Pediatric Electrophysiology Society. N Engl J Med 1994; 330:1481-7.

24. Dhala AA, Case CL, Gillette PC. Evolving treatment strategies for managing atrial ectopic tachycardia in children. Am J Cardiol 1994;74:283-6.

25. Gillette PC, Garson A Jr. Electrophysiologic and pharmacologic characteristics of automatic ectopic atrial tachycardia. Circulation 1977;56:571-5.

26. Beaufort-Krol GC, Bink-Boelkens MT. Oral propafenone as treatment for incessant supraventricular and ventricular tachycardia in children. Am J Cardiol 1993;72:1213-4.

27. Guccione P, Drago F, Di Donato RM, et al. Oral propafenone therapy for children with arrhythmias: efficacy and adverse effects in midterm follow-up. Am Heart J 1991;122:1022-7.

28. Janousek J, Paul T, Reimer A, Kallfelz HC. Usefulness of propafenone for supraventricular arrhythmias in infants and children. Am J Cardiol 1993;72:294-300.

29. Janousek J, Paul T. Safety of oral propafenone in the treatment of arrhythmias in infants and children (European retrospective multicenter study). Working Group on Pediatric Arrhythmias and Electrophysiology of the Association of European Pediatric Cardiologists. Am J Cardiol 1998;81:1121-4.

30. Luedtke SA, Kuhn RJ, McCaffrey FM. Pharmacologic management of supraventricular tachycardias in children. Part 2. Atrial flutter, atrial fibrillation, and junctional and atrial ectopic tachycardia. Ann Pharmacother 1997;31:1347-59.

31. Perry JC, McQuinn RL, Smith RT Jr, et al. Flecainide acetate for resistant arrhythmias in the young: efficacy and pharmacokinetics. J Am Coll Cardiol 1989;14:185-91.

32. Zeigler V, Gillette PC, Ross BA, et al. Flecainide for supraventricular and ventricular arrhythmias in children and young adults. Am J Cardiol 1988;62:818-20.

33. Figa FH, Gow RM, Hamilton RM, et al. Clinical efficacy and safety of intravenous amiodarone in infants and children. Am J Cardiol 1994;74:573-7.

34. Perry JC, Fenrich AL, Hulse JE, et al. Pediatric use of intravenous amiodarone: efficacy and safety in critically ill patients from a multicenter protocol. J Am Coll Cardiol 1996;27:1246-50.

35. Chang PM, Silka MJ, Moromisato DY, et al. Amiodarone versus procainamide for the acute treatment of recurrent supraventricular tachycardia in pediatric patients. Circ Arrhythm Electrophysiol 2010;3:134-40.

36. Colloridi V, Perri C, Ventriglia F, et al. Oral sotalol in pediatric atrial ectopic tachycardia. Am Heart J 1992;123:254-6.

37. Tanel RE, Walsh EP, Lulu JA, et al. Sotalol for refractory arrhythmias in pediatric and young adult patients: initial efficacy and long-term outcome. Am Heart J 1995;130:791-7.

38. Tipple M, Sandor G. Efficacy and safety of oral sotalol in early infancy. Pacing Clin Electrophysiol 1991;14:2062-5.

39. Price JF, Kertesz NJ, Snyder CS, et al. Flecainide and sotalol: a new combination therapy for refractory supraventricular tachycardia in children <1 year of age. J Am Coll Cardiol 2002;39:517-20.

40. Tanel RE, Walsh EP, Triedman JK, et al. Five-year experience with radiofrequency catheter ablation: implications for management of arrhythmias in pediatric and young adult patients. J Pediatr 1997;131:878-87.

41. Weindling SN, Saul JP, Walsh EP. Efficacy and risks of medical therapy for supraventricular tachycardia in neonates and infants. Am Heart J 1996;131:66-72.

42. Van Hare GF, Chiesa NA, Campbell RM, et al. Atrioventricular nodal reentrant tachycardia in children: effect of slow pathway ablation on fast pathway function. J Cardiovasc Electrophysiol 2002;13:203-9.

43. Salerno JC, Seslar SP. Supraventricular tachycardia. Arch Pediatr Adolesc Med 2009;163:268-74.

44. Anand RG, Rosenthal GL, Van Hare GF, et al. Is the mechanism of supraventricular tachycardia in pediatrics influenced by age, gender or ethnicity? Congenit Heart Dis 2009;4:464-8.

45. Drago F, Russo MS, Silvetti MS, et al. Cryoablation of typical atrioventricular nodal reentrant tachycardia in children: six years' experience and follow-up in a single center. Pacing Clin Electrophysiol 2010;33:475-81.

46. Gross GJ, Epstein MR, Walsh EP, et al. Characteristics, management, and midterm outcome in infants with atrioventricular nodal reentry tachycardia. Am J Cardiol 1998;82:956-60.

47. Topilski I, Rogowski O, Glick A, et al. Radiofrequency ablation of atrioventricular nodal reentry tachycardia: a 14 year experience with 901 patients at the Tel Aviv Sourasky Medical Center. Isr Med Assoc J 2006;8:455-9.

48. Gilljam T, Jaeggi E, Gow RM. Neonatal supraventricular tachycardia: outcomes over a 27-year period at a single institution. Acta Paediatr 2008;97:1035-9.

49. Jaeggi ET, Gilljam T, Bauersfeld U, et al. Electrocardiographic differentiation of typical atrioventricular node reentrant tachycardia from atrioventricular reciprocating tachycardia mediated by concealed accessory pathway in children. Am J Cardiol 2003;91:1084-9.

50. Tipple MA. Usefulness of the electrocardiogram in diagnosing mechanisms of tachycardia. Pediatr Cardiol 2000;21:516-21.

51. Van Hare GF, Javitz H, Carmelli D, et al. Prospective assessment after pediatric cardiac ablation: recurrence at 1 year after initially successful ablation of supraventricular tachycardia. Heart Rhythm 2004;1:188-96.

52. Bouhouch R, El Houari T, Fellat I, et al. Pharmacological therapy in children with nodal reentry tachycardia: when, how and how long to treat the affected patients. Curr Pharm Des 2008;14:766-9.

53. Pickoff AS, Zies L, Ferrer PL, et al. High-dose propranolol therapy in the management of supraventricular tachycardia. J Pediatr 1979;94:144-6.

54. Mehta AV, Subrahmanyam AB, Anand R. Long-term efficacy and safety of atenolol for supraventricular tachycardia in children. Pediatr Cardiol 1996;17:231-6.

55. Perry JC, Garson A Jr. Flecainide acetate for treatment of tachyarrhythmias in children: review of world literature on efficacy, safety, and dosing. Am Heart J 1992;124:1614-21.

56. Bouillon T, Schiffmann H, Bartmus D, et al. Amiodarone in a newborn with ventricular tachycardia and an intracardiac tumor: adjusting the dose according to an individualized dosing regimen. Pediatr Cardiol 1996;17:112-4.

57. Burri S, Hug MI, Bauersfeld U. Efficacy and safety of intravenous amiodarone for incessant tachycardias in infants. Eur J Pediatr 2003;162:880-4.

58. Luedtke SA, Kuhn RJ, McCaffrey FM. Pharmacologic management of supraventricular tachycardias in children. Part 1. Wolff-Parkinson-White and atrioventricular nodal reentry. Ann Pharmacother 1997;31:1227-43.

59. Pfammatter JP, Paul T, Lehmann C, et al. Efficacy and proarrhythmia of oral sotalol in pediatric patients. J Am Coll Cardiol 1995;26:1002-7.

60. Moffett BS, Lupo PJ, delaUz CM, et. al. Efficacy of digoxin in comparison with propranolol for treatment of infant supraventricular tachycardia: analysis of a large, national database. Cardiol Young 2015;25:1080-5.

61. Sanatani S, Potts JE, Reed JH, et. al. The study of antiarrhythmic medications in infancy (SAMIS): a multicenter, randomized controlled trial comparing the efficacy and safety of digoxin versus propranolol for prophylaxis of supraventricular tachycardia in infants. Circ Arrhythm Electrophysiol 2012;5:984-91.

62. Perry JC, Garson A Jr. Supraventricular tachycardia due to Wolff-Parkinson-White syndrome in children: early disappearance and late recurrence. J Am Coll Cardiol 1990;16:1215-20.

63. Munger TM, Packer DL, Hammill SC, et al. A population study of the natural history of Wolff-Parkinson-White syndrome in Olmsted County, Minnesota, 1953-1989. Circulation 1993;87:866-73.

64. Brugada J, Closas R, Ordonez A, et al. Radiofrequency catheter ablation of an incessant supraventricular tachycardia in a premature neonate. Pacing Clin Electrophysiol 2002;25:866-8.

65. Case CL, Gillette PC, Oslizlok PC, et al. Radiofrequency catheter ablation of incessant, medically resistant supraventricular tachycardia in infants and small children. J Am Coll Cardiol 1992;20:1405-10.

66. Case CL, Gillette PC. Indications for catheter ablation in infants and small children with reentrant supraventricular tachycardia. J Am Coll Cardiol 1996;27:1551-2.

67. Chiu SN, Lu CW, Chang CW, et al. Radiofrequency catheter ablation of supraventricular tachycardia in infants and toddlers. Circ J 2009;73:1717-21.

68. De Santis A, Fazio G, Silvetti MS, et al. Transcatheter ablation of supraventricular tachycardias in pediatric patients. Curr Pharm Des 2008;14:788-93.

69. Erickson CC, Walsh EP, Triedman JK, et al. Efficacy and safety of radiofrequency ablation in infants and young children < 18 months of age. Am J Cardiol 1994;74:944-7.

70. Mantakas ME, McCue CM, Miller WW. Natural history of Wolff-Parkinson-White syndrome discovered in infancy. Am J Cardiol 1978;41:1097-103.

71. Giardina AC, Ehlers KH, Engle MA. Wolff-Parkinson-White syndrome in infants and children. A long-term follow-up study. Br Heart J 1972;34:839-46.

72. Byrum CJ, Wahl RA, Behrendt DM, et al. Ventricular fibrillation associated with use of digitalis in a newborn infant with Wolff-Parkinson-White syndrome. J Pediatr 1982;101:400-3.

73. Wong KK, Potts JE, Etheridge SP, et al. Medications used to manage supraventricular tachycardia in the infant: a North American survey. Pediatr Cardiol 2006;27:199-203.

74. Gillette PC, Garson A Jr, Kugler JD. Wolff-Parkinson-White syndrome in children: electrophysiologic and pharmacologic characteristics. Circulation 1979;60:1487-95.

75. Epstein ML, Kiel EA, Victorica BE. Cardiac decompensation following verapamil therapy in infants with supraventricular tachycardia. Pediatrics 1985;75:737-40.

76. Kirk CR, Gibbs JL, Thomas R, et al. Cardiovascular collapse after verapamil in supraventricular tachycardia. Arch Dis Child 1987;62:1265-6.

77. Gulamhusein S, Ko P, Klein GJ. Ventricular fibrillation following verapamil in the Wolff-Parkinson-White syndrome. Am Heart J 1983;106:145-7.

78. Gulamhusein S, Ko P, Carruthers SG, et al. Acceleration of the ventricular response during atrial fibrillation in the Wolff-Parkinson-White syndrome after verapamil. Circulation 1982;65:348-54.

79. Gillette P, Garson A Jr, Eterovic E, et al. Oral propranolol treatment in infants and children. J Pediatr 1978;92:141-4.

80. Mehta AV, Chidambaram B. Efficacy and safety of intravenous and oral nadolol for supraventricular tachycardia in children. J Am Coll Cardiol 1992;19:630-5.

81. Trippel DL, Gillette PC. Atenolol in children with supraventricular tachycardia. Am J Cardiol 1989;64:233-6.

82. Adamson PC, Rhodes LA, Saul JP, et al. The pharmacokinetics of esmolol in pediatric subjects with supraventricular arrhythmias. Pediatr Cardiol 2006;27:420-7.

83. Cuneo BF, Zales VR, Blahunka PC, et al. Pharmacodynamics and pharmacokinetics of esmolol, a short-acting beta-blocking agent, in children. Pediatr Cardiol 1994;15:296-301.

84. Das G, Tschida V, Gray R, et al. Efficacy of esmolol in the treatment and transfer of patients with supraventricular tachyarrhythmias to alternate oral antiarrhythmic agents. J Clin Pharmacol 1988;28:746-50.

85. Gray RJ, Bateman TM, Czer LS, et al. Esmolol: a new ultrashort-acting beta-adrenergic blocking agent for rapid control of heart rate in postoperative supraventricular tachyarrhythmias. J Am Coll Cardiol 1985;5:1451-6.

86. Ko WJ, Chu SH. A new dosing regimen for esmolol to treat supraventricular tachyarrhythmia in Chinese patients. J Am Coll Cardiol 1994;23:302-6.

87. Trippel DL, Wiest DB, Gillette PC. Cardiovascular and antiarrhythmic effects of esmolol in children. J Pediatr 1991;119:142-7.

88. Wiest DB, Trippel DL, Gillette PC, et al. Pharmacokinetics of esmolol in children. Clin Pharmacol Ther 1991;49:618-23.

89. Shahar E, Barzilay Z, Frand M, et al. Amiodarone in control of sustained tachyarrhythmias in children with Wolff-Parkinson-White syndrome. Pediatrics 1983;72:813-6.

90. Bryson SM, Leson CL, Irwin DB, et al. Therapeutic monitoring and pharmacokinetic evaluation of procainamide in neonates. DICP 1991;25:68-71.

91. Moffett BS, Cannon BC, Friedman RA, et al. Therapeutic levels of intravenous procainamide in neonates: a retrospective assessment. Pharmacotherapy 2006;26:1687-93.

92. Heusch A, Kramer HH, Krogmann ON, et al. Clinical experience with propafenone for cardiac arrhythmias in the young. Eur Heart J 1994;15:1050-6.

93. Vignati G, Mauri L, Figini A. The use of propafenone in the treatment of tachyarrhythmias in children. Eur Heart J 1993; 14:546-50.

94. Fenrich AL Jr, Perry JC, Friedman RA. Flecainide and amiodarone: combined therapy for refractory tachyarrhythmias in infancy. J Am Coll Cardiol 1995;25:1195-8.

95. Ferlini M, Colli AM, Bonanomi C, et al. Flecainide as first-line treatment for supraventricular tachycardia in newborns. J Cardiovasc Med (Hagerstown) 2009;10:372-5.

96. Musto B, D'Onofrio A, Cavallaro C, et al. Electrophysiologic effects and clinical efficacy of flecainide in children with recurrent paroxysmal supraventricular tachycardia. Am J Cardiol 1988;62:229-33.

97. Musto B, Cavallaro C, Musto A, et al. Flecainide single oral dose for management of paroxysmal supraventricular tachycardia in children and young adults. Am Heart J 1992;124:110-5.

98. Nunez F, Ruiz-Granell R, Martinez-Costa C, et al. Safety and efficacy of flecainide in the treatment of symptomatic children with Wolff-Parkinson-White syndrome. Pediatr Cardiol 2010; 31:1162-5.

99. Till JA, Shinebourne EA, Rowland E, et al. Paediatric use of flecainide in supraventricular tachycardia: clinical efficacy and pharmacokinetics. Br Heart J 1989;62:133-9.

100. Wren C, Campbell RW. The response of paediatric arrhythmias to intravenous and oral flecainide. Br Heart J 1987;57:171-5.

101. Zeigler V, Gillette PC, Hammill B, et al. Flecainide for supraventricular tachycardia in children. Am J Cardiol 1988;62:41D-43D.

102. Fish FA, Gillette PC, Benson DW Jr. Proarrhythmia, cardiac arrest and death in young patients receiving encainide and flecainide. The Pediatric Electrophysiology Group. J Am Coll Cardiol 1991;18:356-65.

103. Ruskin JN. The cardiac arrhythmia suppression trial (CAST). N Engl J Med 1989;321:386-8.

104. Echt DS, Liebson PR, Mitchell LB, et al. Mortality and morbidity in patients receiving encainide, flecainide, or placebo. The Cardiac Arrhythmia Suppression Trial. N Engl J Med 1991;324:781-8.

105. Celiker A, Ceviz N, Ozme S. Effectiveness and safety of intravenous amiodarone in drug-resistant tachyarrhythmias of children. Acta Paediatr Jpn 1998;40:567-72.

106. Coumel P, Fidelle J. Amiodarone in the treatment of cardiac arrhythmias in children: one hundred thirty-five cases. Am Heart J 1980;100:1063-9.

107. Soult JA, Munoz M, Lopez JD, et al. Efficacy and safety of intravenous amiodarone for short-term treatment of paroxysmal supraventricular tachycardia in children. Pediatr Cardiol 1995; 16:16-9.

108. Celiker A, Ayabakan C, Ozer S, et al. Sotalol in treatment of pediatric cardiac arrhythmias. Pediatr Int 2001;43:624-30.

109. Maragnes P, Tipple M, Fournier A. Effectiveness of oral sotalol for treatment of pediatric arrhythmias. Am J Cardiol 1992;69:751-4.

110. Miyazaki A, Ohuchi H, Kurosaki K, et al. Efficacy and safety of sotalol for refractory tachyarrhythmias in congenital heart disease. Circ J 2008;72:1998-2003.

111. Vaksmann G, D'Hoinne C, Lucet V, et al. Permanent junctional reciprocating tachycardia in children: a multicentre study on clinical profile and outcome. Heart 2006;92:101-4.

112. Lindinger A, Heisel A, von Bernuth G, et al. Permanent junctional re-entry tachycardia. A multicentre long-term follow-up study in infants, children and young adults. Eur Heart J 1998;19:936-42.

113. Drago F, Silvetti MS, Mazza A, et al. Permanent junctional reciprocating tachycardia in infants and children: effectiveness of medical and non-medical treatment. Ital Heart J 2001;2:456-61.

114. Dunnigan A, Benson W Jr, Benditt DG. Atrial flutter in infancy: diagnosis, clinical features, and treatment. Pediatrics 1985; 75:725-9.

115. Herzberg GZ, Rossi AF. Atrial flutter in a pediatric patient in the immediate period after the Fontan procedure: control with oral propafenone. Pacing Clin Electrophysiol 1997;20:3002-3.

116. Kertesz NJ, Towbin JA, Clunie S, et al. Long-term follow-up of arrhythmias in pediatric orthotopic heart transplant recipients: incidence and correlation with rejection. J Heart Lung Transplant 2003;22:889-93.

117. Texter KM, Kertesz NJ, Friedman RA, Fenrich AL Jr. Atrial flutter in infants. J Am Coll Cardiol 2006;48:1040-6.

118. Radford DJ, Izukawa T. Atrial fibrillation in children. Pediatrics 1977;59:250-6.

119. Rhodes LA, Walsh EP, Saul JP. Conversion of atrial flutter in pediatric patients by transesophageal atrial pacing: a safe, effective, minimally invasive procedure. Am Heart J 1995;130:323-7.

120. Saoudi N, Cosio F, Waldo A, et al. A classification of atrial flutter and regular atrial tachycardia according to electrophysiological mechanisms and anatomical bases; a Statement from a Joint Expert Group from The Working Group of Arrhythmias of the European Society of Cardiology and the North American Society of Pacing and Electrophysiology. Eur Heart J 2001;22:1162-82.

121. Kannankeril PJ, Fish FA. Management of intra-atrial reentrant tachycardia. Curr Opin Cardiol 2005;20:89-93.

122. Garson A Jr, Gillette PC, McVey P, et al. Amiodarone treatment of critical arrhythmias in children and young adults. J Am Coll Cardiol 1984;4:749-55.

123. Casey FA, McCrindle BW, Hamilton RM, et al. Neonatal atrial flutter: significant early morbidity and excellent long-term prognosis. Am Heart J 1997;133:302-6.

124. Martin TC, Hernandez A. Atrial flutter in infancy. J Pediatr 1982;100:239-42.

125. Mendelsohn A, Dick M, Serwer GA. Natural history of isolated atrial flutter in infancy. J Pediatr 1991;119:386-91.

126. Fazio G, Visconti C, D'Angelo L, et al. Pharmacological therapy in children with atrial fibrillation and atrial flutter. Curr Pharm Des 2008;14:770-5.

127. Garson A Jr, Bink-Boelkens M, Hesslein PS, et al. Atrial flutter in the young: a collaborative study of 380 cases. J Am Coll Cardiol 1985;6:871-8.

128. Dilber E, Mutlu M, Dilber B, et al. Intravenous amiodarone used alone or in combination with digoxin for life-threatening supraventricular tachyarrhythmia in neonates and small infants. Pediatr Emerg Care 2010;26:82-4.

129. Beaufort-Krol GC, Bink-Boelkens MT. Sotalol for atrial tachycardias after surgery for congenital heart disease. Pacing Clin Electrophysiol 1997;20:2125-9.

130. Beaufort-Krol GC, Bink-Boelkens MT. Effectiveness of sotalol for atrial flutter in children after surgery for congenital heart disease. Am J Cardiol 1997;79:92-4.

131. Knirsch W, Kretschmar O, Vogel M, et al. Successful treatment of atrial flutter with amiodarone in a premature neonate. Case report and literature review. Adv Neonatal Care 2007;7:113-21.

132. Rowland TW, Mathew R, Chameides L, et al. Idiopathic atrial flutter in infancy: a review of eight cases. Pediatrics 1978; 61:52-6.

133. Moller JH, Davachi F, Anderson RC. Atrial flutter in infancy. J Pediatr 1969;75:643-51.

134. Zaldivar N, Gelband H, Tamer D, et al. Atrial fibrillation in infancy. J Pediatr 1973;83:821-2.

135. Andreasen JB, Johnsen SP, Ravn HB. Junctional ectopic tachycardia after surgery for congenital heart disease in children. Intensive Care Med 2008;34:895-902.

136. Batra AS, Chun DS, Johnson TR, et al. A prospective analysis of the incidence and risk factors associated with junctional ectopic tachycardia following surgery for congenital heart disease. Pediatr Cardiol 2006;27:51-5.

137. Braunstein PW Jr, Sade RM, Gillette PC. Life-threatening postoperative junctional ectopic tachycardia. Ann Thorac Surg 1992;53:726-8.

138. Cilliers AM, du Plessis JP, Clur SA, et al. Junctional ectopic tachycardia in six paediatric patients. Heart 1997;78:413-5.

139. Grosse-Wortmann L, Kreitz S, Grabitz RG, et al. Prevalence of and risk factors for perioperative arrhythmias in neonates and children after cardiopulmonary bypass: continuous Holter monitoring before and for three days after surgery. J Cardiothorac Surg 2010;5:85.

140. Hoffman TM, Bush DM, Wernovsky G, et al. Postoperative junctional ectopic tachycardia in children: incidence, risk factors, and treatment. Ann Thorac Surg 2002;74:1607-11.

141. Maiers JA, Ebenroth ES. Junctional ectopic tachycardia following complete heart block associated with viral myocarditis. Pediatr Cardiol 2006;27:367-8.

142. Mildh L, Hiippala A, Rautiainen P, et al. Junctional ectopic tachycardia after surgery for congenital heart disease: incidence, risk factors and outcome. Eur J Cardiothorac Surg 2011;39:75-80.

143. Villain E, Vetter VL, Garcia JM, et al. Evolving concepts in the management of congenital junctional ectopic tachycardia. A multicenter study. Circulation 1990;81:1544-9.

144. Gillette PC, Garson A Jr, Hesslein PS, et al. Successful surgical treatment of atrial, junctional, and ventricular tachycardia unassociated with accessory connections in infants and children. Am Heart J 1981;102:984-91.

145. Gillette PC, Garson A Jr, Porter CJ, et al. Junctional automatic ectopic tachycardia: new proposed treatment by transcatheter His bundle ablation. Am Heart J 1983;106:619-23.

146. Gillette PC. Evolving concepts in the management of congenital junctional ectopic tachycardia. Circulation 1990;81:1713-4.

147. Darst JR, Kaufman J. Case report: an infant with congenital junctional ectopic tachycardia requiring extracorporeal mechanical oxygenation. Curr Opin Pediatr 2007;19:597-600.

148. Sarubbi B, Musto B, Ducceschi V, et al. Congenital junctional ectopic tachycardia in children and adolescents: a 20 year experience based study. Heart 2002;88:188-90.

149. Emmel M, Sreeram N, Brockmeier K. Catheter ablation of junctional ectopic tachycardia in children, with preservation of atrioventricular conduction. Z Kardiol 2005;94:280-6.

150. Kelly BP, Gajarski RJ, Ohye RG, et al. Intravenous induction of therapeutic hypothermia in the management of junctional ectopic tachycardia: a pilot study. Pediatr Cardiol 2010;31:11-7.

151. Raja P, Hawker RE, Chaikitpinyo A, et al. Amiodarone management of junctional ectopic tachycardia after cardiac surgery in children. Br Heart J 1994;72:261-5.

152. Plumpton K, Justo R, Haas N. Amiodarone for post-operative junctional ectopic tachycardia. Cardiol Young 2005;15:13-8.

153. Kovacikova L, Hakacova N, Dobos D, et al. Amiodarone as a first-line therapy for postoperative junctional ectopic tachycardia. Ann Thorac Surg 2009;88:616-22.

154. Grant JW, Serwer GA, Armstrong BE, et al. Junctional tachycardia in infants and children after open heart surgery for congenital heart disease. Am J Cardiol 1987;59:1216-8.

155. Mahmoud AB, Tantawy AE, Kouatli AA, et al. Propranolol: a new indication for an old drug in preventing postoperative junctional ectopic tachycardia after surgical repair of tetralogy of Fallot. Interact Cardiovasc Thorac Surg 2008;7:184-7.

156. Lucet V, Do ND, Fidelle J, et al. [Anti-arrhythmia efficacy of propafenone in children. Apropos of 30 cases.] Arch Mal Coeur Vaiss 1987;80:1385-93.

157. Reimer A, Paul T, Kallfelz HC. Efficacy and safety of intravenous and oral propafenone in pediatric cardiac dysrhythmias. Am J Cardiol 1991;68:741-4.

158. Deanfield JE, McKenna WJ, Presbitero P, et al. Ventricular arrhythmia in unrepaired and repaired tetralogy of Fallot. Relation to age, timing of repair, and haemodynamic status. Br Heart J 1984; 52:77-81.

159. McKenna WJ, Deanfield JE. Hypertrophic cardio-myopathy: an important cause of sudden death. Arch Dis Child 1984;59:971-5.

160. Denjoy I, Lupoglazoff JM, Guicheney P, et al. Arrhythmic sudden death in children. Arch Cardiovasc Dis 2008;101:121-5.

161. Kuhl U, Schultheiss HP. Myocarditis in children. Heart Fail Clin 2010;6:483-4ix.

162. Roggen A, Pavlovic M, Pfammatter JP. Frequency of spontaneous ventricular tachycardia in a pediatric population. Am J Cardiol 2008;101:852-4.

163. Dickinson DF, Scott O. Ambulatory electrocardiographic monitoring in 100 healthy teenage boys. Br Heart J 1984;51:179-83.

164. Doniger SJ, Sharieff GQ. Pediatric dysrhythmias. Pediatr Clin North Am 2006;53:85-105, vi.

165. Passman R, Kadish A. Polymorphic ventricular tachycardia, long Q-T syndrome, and torsades de pointes. Med Clin North Am 2001; 85:321-41.

166. Alexander ME, Berul CI. Ventricular arrhythmias: when to worry. Pediatr Cardiol 2000;21:532-41.

167. de Caen AR, Maconochie IK, Aickin R, et. al. Part 6: Pediatric Basic Life Support and Pediatric Advanced Life Support: 2015 International Consensus on Cardiopulmonary Resuscitation and Emergency Cardiovascular Care Science With Treatment Recommendations. Circulation 2015 Oct 20;132:S177-203.

168. Priori SG, Blomström-Lundqvist C, Mazzanti A, et. al. Task Force for the Management of Patients with Ventricular Arrhythmias and the Prevention of Sudden Cardiac Death of the European Society of Cardiology (ESC). Europace 2015;17:1601-87.

169. Trippel DL, Gillette PC. Atenolol in children with ventricular arrhythmias. Am Heart J 1990;119:1312-6.

170. Das SN, Kiran U, Saxena N. Perioperative management of long QT syndrome in a child with congenital heart disease. Acta Anaesthesiol Scand 2002;46:221-3.

171. Moak JP, Smith RT, Garson A Jr. Mexiletine: an effective antiarrhythmic drug for treatment of ventricular arrhythmias in congenital heart disease. J Am Coll Cardiol 1987;10:824-9.

172. Ostman-Smith I. Hypertrophic cardiomyopathy in childhood and adolescence - strategies to prevent sudden death. Fundam Clin Pharmacol 2010;24:637-52.

173. Garson A Jr, Dick M, Fournier A, et al. The long QT syndrome in children. An international study of 287 patients. Circulation 1993;87:1866-72.

174. Villain E, Levy M, Kachaner J, et al. Prolonged QT interval in neonates: benign, transient, or prolonged risk of sudden death. Am Heart J 1992;124:194-7.

175. Roden DM. Drug-induced prolongation of the QT interval. N Engl J Med 2004;350:1013-22.

176. Chiang CE, Roden DM. The long QT syndromes: genetic basis and clinical implications. J Am Coll Cardiol 2000;36:1-12.

177. Berger S, Dhala A, Friedberg DZ. Sudden cardiac death in infants, children, and adolescents. Pediatr Clin North Am 1999; 46:221-34.

178. Benhorin J, Taub R, Goldmit M, et al. Effects of flecainide in patients with new SCN5A mutation: mutation-specific therapy for long-QT syndrome? Circulation 2000;101:1698-706.

179. Hoshino K, Ogawa K, Hishitani T, et al. Successful uses of magnesium sulfate for torsades de pointes in children with long QT syndrome. Pediatr Int 2006;48:112-7.

180. Sasse M, Paul T, Bergmann P, et al. Sotalol associated torsades de pointes tachycardia in a 15-month-old child: successful therapy with magnesium aspartate. Pacing Clin Electrophysiol 1998;21:1164-6.

181. Richards JM, Alexander JR, Shinebourne EA, et al. Sequential 22-hour profiles of breathing patterns and heart rate in 110 full-term infants during their first 6 months of life. Pediatrics 1984; 74:763-77.

182. Southall DP, Johnston F, Shinebourne EA, et al. 24-hour electro-cardiographic study of heart rate and rhythm patterns in population of healthy children. Br Heart J 1981;45:281-91.

183. Montague TJ, Taylor PG, Stockton R, et al. The spectrum of cardiac rate and rhythm in normal newborns. Pediatr Cardiol 1982;2:33-8.

184. Mangrum JM, DiMarco JP. The evaluation and management of bradycardia. N Engl J Med 2000;342:703-9.

185. Rein AJ, Simcha A, Ludomirsky A, et al. Symptomatic sinus bradycardia in infants with structurally normal hearts. J Pediatr 1985;107:724-7.

186. Yabek SM, Jarmakani JM. Sinus node dysfunction in children, adolescents, and young adults. Pediatrics 1978;61:593-8.

187. Guilleminault C, Coons S. Apnea and bradycardia during feeding in infants weighing greater than 2000 gm. J Pediatr 1984; 104:932-5.

188. Hiss RG, Lamb LE, Allen MF. Electrocardiographic findings in 67,375 asymptomatic subjects. X. Normal values. Am J Cardiol 1960;6:200-31.

189. Bricker JT, Garson A Jr, Gillette PC. A family history of seizures associated with sudden cardiac deaths. Am J Dis Child 1984; 138:866-8.

190. Mehta AV, Chidambaram B, Garrett A. Familial symptomatic sinus bradycardia: autosomal dominant inheritance. Pediatr Cardiol 1995;16:231-4.

191. Epstein AE, DiMarco JP, Ellenbogen KA, et al. ACC/AHA/HRS 2008 Guidelines for Device-Based Therapy of Cardiac Rhythm Abnormalities: a report of the American College of Cardiology/ American Heart Association Task Force on Practice Guidelines (Writing Committee to Revise the ACC/AHA/NASPE 2002 Guideline Update for Implantation of Cardiac Pacemakers and Antiarrhythmia Devices): developed in collaboration with the American Association for Thoracic Surgery and Society of Thoracic Surgeons. Circulation 2008;117:e350-e408.

192. Probst V, Denjoy I, Meregalli PG, et al. Clinical aspects and prognosis of Brugada syndrome in children. Circulation 2007; 115:2042-8.

193. Burckart GJ, Marin-Garcia J. Quinidine dosage in children using population estimates. Pediatr Cardiol 1986;6:269-73.

194. Szefler SJ, Pieroni DR, Gingell RL, et al. Rapid elimination of quinidine in pediatric patients. Pediatrics 1982;70:370-5.

195. Ali KM. Collateral effects of antiarrhythmics in pediatric age. Curr Pharm Des 2008;14:782-7.

196. Allen LV Jr, Erickson MA. Stability of bethanechol chloride, pyrazinamide, quinidine sulfate, rifampin, and tetracycline hydrochloride in extemporaneously compounded oral liquids. Am J Health Syst Pharm 1998;55:1804-9.

197. Singh S, Gelband H, Mehta AV, et al. Procainamide elimination kinetics in pediatric patients. Clin Pharmacol Ther 1982; 32:607-11.

198. Burrows FA, Lerman J, LeDez KM, et al. Pharmacokinetics of lidocaine in children with congenital heart disease. Can J Anaesth 1991;38:196-200.

199. Holt DW, Walsh AC, Curry PV, et al. Paediatric use of mexiletine and disopyramide. Br Med J 1979;2:1476-7.

200. Nahata MC, Morosco RS, Hipple TF. Stability of mexiletine in two extemporaneous liquid formulations stored under refrigeration and at room temperature. J Am Pharm Assoc (Wash) 2000;40:257-9.

201. Doki K, Homma M, Kuga K, et al. Effect of CYP2D6 genotype on flecainide pharmacokinetics in Japanese patients with supraventricular tachyarrhythmia. Eur J Clin Pharmacol 2006;62:919-26.

202. Doki K, Homma M, Kuga K, et al. Gender-associated differences in pharmacokinetics and anti-arrhythmic effects of flecainide in Japanese patients with supraventricular tachyarrhythmia. Eur J Clin Pharmacol 2007;63:951-7.

203. Ito S, Gow R, Verjee Z, et al. Intravenous and oral propafenone for treatment of tachycardia in infants and children: pharmacokinetics and clinical response. J Clin Pharmacol 1998;38:496-501.

204. Juarez OH, Flores PC, Ramirez MB, et al. Extemporaneous suspension of propafenone: attending lack of pediatric formulations in Mexico. Pediatr Cardiol 2008;29:1077-81.

205. Abrams J, Allen J, Allin D, et al. Efficacy and safety of esmolol vs propranolol in the treatment of supraventricular tachyarrhythmias: a multicenter double-blind clinical trial. Am Heart J 1985;110:913-22.

206. Buck ML, Wiest D, Gillette PC, et al. Pharmacokinetics and pharmacodynamics of atenolol in children. Clin Pharmacol Ther 1989;46:629-33.

207. Hepner SI, Davoli E. Successful treatment of supraventricular tachycardia with metoprolol, a cardioselective beta blocker. Clin Pediatr (Phila) 1983;22:522-3.

208. Allen LV Jr, Erickson MA III. Stability of labetalol hydrochloride, metoprolol tartrate, verapamil hydrochloride, and spironolactone with hydrochlorothiazide in extemporaneously compounded oral liquids. Am J Health Syst Pharm 1996;53:2304-9.

209. Mehta AV, Chidambaram B, Rice PJ. Pharmacokinetics of nadolol in children with supraventricular tachycardia. J Clin Pharmacol 1992;32:1023-7.

210. Saul JP, Ross B, Schaffer MS, et al. Pharmacokinetics and pharmacodynamics of sotalol in a pediatric population with supraventricular and ventricular tachyarrhythmia. Clin Pharmacol Ther 2001;69:145-57.

211. Shi J, Ludden TM, Melikian AP, et al. Population pharmacokinetics and pharmacodynamics of sotalol in pediatric patients with supraventricular or ventricular tachyarrhythmia. J Pharmacokinet Pharmacodyn 2001;28:555-75.

212. Knudson J, Cannon BC, Kim JJ, et al. High-dose sotalol is safe and effective in neonates and infants with refractory supraventricular tachyarrhythmias. Pediatr Cardiol 2011;32:896-903.

213. Maling T. Amiodarone therapeutic plasma concentration monitoring. Is it practical? Clin Pharmacokinet 1988;14:321-4.

214. Kannan R, Yabek SM, Garson A Jr, et al. Amiodarone efficacy in a young population: relationship to serum amiodarone and desethylamiodarone levels. Am Heart J 1987;114:283-7.

215. Anastasiou-Nana MI, Anderson JL, Nanas JN, et al. High incidence of clinical and subclinical toxicity associated with amiodarone treatment of refractory tachyarrhythmias. Can J Cardiol 1986;2:138-45.

216. Ardura J, Hermoso F, Bermejo J. Effect on growth of children with cardiac dysrhythmias treated with amiodarone. Pediatr Cardiol 1988;9:33-6.

217. Bowers PN, Fields J, Schwartz D, et al. Amiodarone induced pulmonary fibrosis in infancy. Pacing Clin Electrophysiol 1998;21:1665-7.

218. Costigan DC, Holland FJ, Daneman D, et al. Amiodarone therapy effects on childhood thyroid function. Pediatrics 1986;77:703-8.

219. Haas NA, Camphausen CK. Acute hemodynamic effects of intravenous amiodarone treatment in pediatric patients with cardiac surgery. Clin Res Cardiol 2008;97:801-10.

220. Ng GY, Hampson Evans DC, Murdoch LJ. Cardiovascular collapse after amiodarone administration in neonatal supraventricular tachycardia. Eur J Emerg Med 2003;10:323-5.

221. Nahata MC. Stability of amiodarone in an oral suspension stored under refrigeration and at room temperature. Ann Pharmacother 1997;31:851-2.

222. Sapire DW, O'Riordan AC, Black IF. Safety and efficacy of short- and long-term verapamil therapy in children with tachycardia. Am J Cardiol 1981;48:1091-7.

223. de Vonderweid U, Benettoni A, Piovan D, et al. Use of oral verapamil in long-term treatment of neonatal, paroxysmal supraventricular tachycardia. A pharmacokinetic study. Int J Cardiol 1984;6:581-6.

224. Casta A, Wolf WJ, Richardson CJ, et al. Successful management of atrial flutter in a newborn with verapamil. Clin Cardiol 1985;8:597-8.

225. Chan KY, Yip WC, Ng MP, et al. Efficacy of verapamil in the conversion of supraventricular tachycardia in Singapore children. Ann Acad Med Singapore 1987;16:334-6.

226. Lie KI, Duren DR, Cats VM, et al. Long-term efficacy of verapamil in the treatment of paroxysmal supraventricular tachycardias. Am Heart J 1983;105:688.

227. Garland JS, Berens RJ, Losek JD, et al. An infant fatality following verapamil therapy for supraventricular tachycardia: cardiovascular collapse following intravenous verapamil. Pediatr Emerg Care 1985;1:198-200.

228. Haft JI, Habbab MA. Treatment of atrial arrhythmias. Effectiveness of verapamil when preceded by calcium infusion. Arch Intern Med 1986;146:1085-9.

229. Pass RH, Liberman L, Al-Fayaddh M, et al. Continuous intravenous diltiazem infusion for short-term ventricular rate control in children. Am J Cardiol 2000;86:559-62, A9.

230. Allen LV Jr, Erickson MA III. Stability of baclofen, captopril, diltiazem hydrochloride, dipyridamole, and flecainide acetate in extemporaneously compounded oral liquids. Am J Health Syst Pharm 1996;53:2179-84.

231. Bendayan R, McKenzie MW. Digoxin pharmacokinetics and dosage requirements in pediatric patients. Clin Pharm 1983; 2:224-35.

232. Wells TG, Young RA, Kearns GL. Age-related differences in digoxin toxicity and its treatment. Drug Saf 1992;7:135-51.

233. Park MK. Use of digoxin in infants and children, with specific emphasis on dosage. J Pediatr 1986;108:871-7.

234. Bertrand JM, Langhendries JP, Gras A, et. al. Digoxin-like immunoreactive substance in serum of preterm and full-term neonates. Eur J Pediatr 1987;146:145-6.

235. Alexander DC, Bundy DG, Shore AD, et al. Cardiovascular medication errors in children. Pediatrics 2009;124:324-32.

236. Clarke B, Till J, Rowland E, et al. Rapid and safe termination of supraventricular tachycardia in children by adenosine. Lancet 1987;1:299-301.

237. De Wolf D, Rondia G, Verhaaren H, et al. Adenosine triphosphate treatment for supraventricular tachycardia in infants. Eur J Pediatr 1994;153:668-71.

238. Losek JD, Endom E, Dietrich A, et al. Adenosine and pediatric supraventricular tachycardia in the emergency department: multicenter study and review. Ann Emerg Med 1999;33:185-91.

239. Overholt ED, Rheuban KS, Gutgesell HP, et al. Usefulness of adenosine for arrhythmias in infants and children. Am J Cardiol 1988;61:336-40.

240. Paul T, Pfammatter JP. Adenosine: an effective and safe antiarrhythmic drug in pediatrics. Pediatr Cardiol 1997;18:118-26.

241. Till J, Shinebourne EA, Rigby ML, et al. Efficacy and safety of adenosine in the treatment of supraventricular tachycardia in infants and children. Br Heart J 1989;62:204-11.

242. Celiker A, Tokel K, Cil E, et al. Adenosine induced torsades de pointes in a child with congenital long QT syndrome. Pacing Clin Electrophysiol 1994;17:1814-7.

CHAPTER 10

Pediatric Hypertension

Christopher A. Thomas, Pharm.D., MBA, BCPPS

LEARNING OBJECTIVES

1. Outline the history, incidence, and epidemiology of pediatric hypertension.

2. Review the pathophysiology, including neurohormonal and humoral pathways, of pediatric hypertension.

3. Describe the clinical presentation, criteria for diagnosis, blood pressure measurement methodology, and approach to management of pediatric hypertension and hypertensive crisis.

4. Explain the pharmacology and pediatric implications for each drug class used in the treatment of pediatric hypertension and hypertensive crisis.

ABBREVIATIONS IN THIS CHAPTER

AAP	American Academy of Pediatrics
ABPM	Ambulatory blood pressure measurement
ACE	Angiotensin-converting enzyme
AHA	American Heart Association
ARB	Angiotensin receptor blocker
AT	Angiotensin
β-Blocker	β-Adrenergic receptor blocker
BP	Blood pressure
CCB	Calcium channel blocker
ESH	European Society of Hypertension
JNC VIII	Eighth Report of the Joint National Committee on Prevention, Detection, Evaluation, and Treatment of High Blood Pressure
RAAS	Renin–angiotensin–aldosterone system
SNP	Sodium nitroprusside
SVR	Systemic vascular resistance

INTRODUCTION

Ancient works have referred to *hypertension* as "hard pulse disease," but modern medicine most simply defines it as the persistence of elevated arterial blood pressure (BP).[1] Although the adverse effects of hypertension have been known in adult arenas since 2600 BC, pediatric medicine was late to recognize or even consider childhood hypertension as an illness without suggestive signs and symptoms until the late 1960s.[1-4] Not until this period were the first reference BP ranges developed for children. Established pediatric BP norms were unavailable until this era because normal values for pediatric hypertension were typically borrowed from adult literature because of a lower incidence of hypertension in pediatric patients and a lack of knowledge regarding its adverse effects in this patient population. Although the incidence of pediatric hypertension is relatively low, its damaging effects may be experienced throughout all pediatric age groups. With the initial contributions of the investigators of the Muscatine and Bogalusa Heart Studies, which began in 1971 and 1972, respectively, interest and research in pediatric hypertension and cardiovascular disease began to gain momentum.[5,6] These studies helped pave the way for hypertension research in children and established the importance of evaluating pediatric BP on the basis of age, sex, and height. In the past 45 years, however, much research has focused on the identification, definition, treatment, and now prevention of hypertension in the pediatric patient.[7]

Research leading to a subsequent increase in pediatric hypertension literature has afforded clinicians more evidence-based resources to manage this disease state.[7] In contrast to the available adult literature, the amount of quality pediatric data are limited. Also unlike existing adult data, robust clinical trials evaluating the treatment of pediatric hypertension are scant. Many studies suggest that pediatric hypertension "tracks" into adulthood; however, data showing that the treatment of pediatric hypertension reduces or prevents this tracking phenomenon are nonexistent.[8-12] There are data, however, to support that the adoption of a healthy lifestyle may halt the hypertension tracking phenomenon from adolescence to adulthood.[13] The most recent evidence-based guidelines to aid pediatric clinicians in the management of hypertension were produced by the American Academy of Pediatrics (AAP) in 2017 and the European Society of Hypertension (ESH) in 2009.[14,15] Suggested updates to the 2009 ESH guidelines have been published in 2014 to include ambulatory BP measurement (ABPM) guidelines[16] This chapter will review pertinent aspects of these guidelines, including pathologic mechanisms and pharmacotherapy in addition to relevant recently published clinical literature regarding the treatment of pediatric hypertension and hypertensive crisis.

EPIDEMIOLOGY

The incidence of hypertension in children and adolescents is about 1%–5% of the healthy pediatric population.[17] Other investigations, however, estimate the incidence to be as high as 11%.[18] Although the rate of pediatric hypertension is rising, it is relatively low compared with a 33% incidence of hypertension in adults in 2014.[19] With evidence suggesting that children and adolescents with high BP are more likely to be hypertensive adults, diagnostic screening, preventive measures, and pharmacologic treatment of hypertension in children with the goal of minimizing potential long-term deleterious effects have been deemed of great importance by many expert clinicians.[8-12,14]

PATHOPHYSIOLOGY

Cardiovascular function is regulated by a complex cascade of neurohormonal mechanisms that influence hemodynamics. Neural mechanisms include sympathetic tone, the baroreflex system, and cardiopulmonary reflex. Humoral regulation occurs through the renin–angiotensin–aldosterone system (RAAS), endothelial vasoactive factors, glucocorticoids, arginine vasopressin, and natriuretic peptides.[20-24] Although many pathways exist, not one has proved to be the sole cause of primary pediatric hypertension. For this reason, many pharmacologic agents have been developed to address potential underlying imbalances in hemodynamic regulation mechanisms.

NEURAL REGULATION

The central nervous system plays an essential role in the regulation of BP by allocating autonomic tone to various areas of the cardiovascular system through receptors that detect pressure changes in the vasculature and changes in the chemical composition of the blood. These α- and β-receptors reside on the pre- and postsynaptic surfaces of sympathetic terminals and regulate norepinephrine release.[21,22,25] Stimulation of central α_2-receptors inhibits the release of norepinephrine, whereas activation of central β-receptors has the opposite effect.[21,22,25] The response seen on arterioles and venules as a result of peripheral α_1-receptor activation is vasoconstriction.[21,22] β_1-Receptors are very densely dispersed within the heart, and β_2-receptors are abundant within the lungs as well as the arterioles and venules. β_1-Activation produces an increase in heart rate and contractility, and β_2-activation causes vasodilation.[21,22]

The negative feedback mechanism regulating sympathetic tone and ultimately short-term BP control is called the *baroreflex system*.[22] Receptors designed to detect changes in arterial BP are mainly located in the aorta and carotid arteries.[21,22] Other baroreceptors are located in the afferent arterioles of the kidneys, but their main role is involved in renin release.[23] Increased baroreceptor activity occurs because of an acute intravascular pressure elevation that results in decreased heart rate and contractility in addition to peripheral vasodilation.[21,22] This effect is illustrated by the use of carotid massage to treat supraventricular tachycardia. By manually palpating the carotid artery, this nonpharmacologic intervention attempts to increase vagal tone by mimicking increased arterial pressure. An acute BP decrease has the opposite baroreceptor effect, causing vasoconstriction and an increase in heart rate and contractile force because of decreased baroreceptor activity. As children age, their physiologic normal BP increases with increasing body size.[20] Baroreceptors subsequently adjust to changing BP norms as children mature to help maintain safe hemodynamic control.[20]

HUMORAL REGULATION

Together with neural regulation, many humoral mechanisms contribute to the maintenance of cardiovascular function and homeostasis. Alterations in any or all of these mechanisms may lead to the pathologic development of hemodynamic abnormalities.

The RAAS is primarily regulated by the kidney's effect on electrolyte and fluid balance, sympathetic tone, vascular smooth muscle tone, and BP. In humans, angiotensin-converting enzyme (ACE) activity leads to increased production of angiotensin (AT) II, decreased bradykinin concentrations, sympathetic norepinephrine release, and aldosterone release. Inhibition of this pathway by ACE inhibitors such as captopril causes vasodilation, decreased afterload, increased cardiac output, and mild diuresis.[23,24,26] In the first months of life, it is crucial to consider the differences existing in the RAAS. Plasma renin activity and subsequent AT II concentrations in newborns and infants are very high.[26] This difference may cause significant hypotension in neonates if caution is not observed in dose initiation and titration of ACE inhibitors.

Other pharmacologic RAAS targets for antihypertensive effects in pediatric patients include AT-receptors.[27] The pediatric AT_1-receptor regulates the function of the cardiovascular system, but the AT_2-receptor has no important role in cardiovascular homeostasis.[27] Because the activation of AT_1-receptors produces direct arterial vasoconstriction, increased sympathetic tone, and aldosterone release, angiotensin receptor blockers (ARBs) are also used in children to combat hypertension.

ASSESSMENT

Together with a thorough knowledge of the physiologic mechanisms behind hemodynamic homeostasis in children, it is important to understand how to assess BP in pediatric patients. In this section, the differences between primary and secondary hypertension will be reviewed, with appropriate pediatric BP measurement techniques; diagnostic criteria for pediatric hypertension; and normal physiologic BP ranges in infants, children, and adolescents.

MEASUREMENT OF BP

The AAP 2017 Clinical Practice Guideline for Screening and Management of High Blood Pressure in Children and Adolescents (AAP Guidelines) recommended a methodology for measuring BP in children, as listed in Box 1.[14] These guidelines urge clinicians to begin routine BP measurements at age 3 years because of the difficulty measuring BP in younger children. Neonates, infants, and toddlers can certainly develop hypertension, so care should be taken to routinely evaluate BP in children younger than 3 years if they have certain comorbid diseases as defined in the AAP Guidelines.[14] Examples include neonatal complications requiring intensive care, congenital heart disease, and kidney disease.[14] For all pediatric patients, special consideration should be focused on investigating the presence of preexisting circumstances that may cause BP elevation at measurement. For example, an infant who is crying during measurement may have a falsely elevated BP compared with BP at rest. To aid the clinician in recognizing the pharmacologic causes of hypertension, a brief list highlighting common childhood and adolescent prescriptions, over-the-counter drugs, food, and supplements that can elevate BP are listed in Table 1.[28-30]

Routine BP assessment in pediatric patients can be measured by auscultation or oscillometric devices if validated in pediatric patients.[14] Auscultation should be performed by placing the stethoscope over the brachial artery (proximal and medial to the antecubital fossa) and just below the bottom edge of the BP cuff.[31,32] For pediatric patients, special attention should be placed on selecting the appropriate cuff size.[31,32] The American Heart Association (AHA) recommends selecting a cuff with a bladder that will cover 80% to 100% of the patient's arm circumference.[31,32] Children with large arms are recommended to use small, standard, or large adult cuffs and, if necessary, a thigh cuff.[32] The importance of using the appropriate-size cuff when measuring pediatric BP is paramount because using an incorrect size may provide false readings.[32] Smaller cuffs tend to yield falsely high measurements, whereas larger cuffs underestimate BP.[33,34] It is recommended that infants and neonates (or patients with faint Korotkoff sounds) have an indirect BP measurement with an ultrasonic flow detector.[35]

Box 1. Methodology for Pediatric Blood Pressure Measurement[14,15]

- Measure BP annually in patients age > 3 years, or at every health care visit if obese, receiving medications that increase BP, have kidney disease, diabetes, or a history of aortic arch obstruction/coarctation
- Oscillometric monitoring devices may be used if validated in pediatrics
- Auscultation monitoring is preferred to confirm elevated oscillometric readings
- Choose appropriate cuff size
- Avoid stimulants (drugs or food) before measurement
- Rest quietly in a seated position for at least 3–5 minutes before measurement
- Use right arm, seated position, back supported, feet resting on floor (supine position for infants)
- High BP should be remeasured and confirmed by ambulatory BP measurement for a duration of 1 year or more or with stage 1 hypertension for three clinic visits to diagnose hypertension

BP = blood pressure.

DIAGNOSIS

The AAP Guidelines define normal and abnormal pediatric BP values in percentiles with reference to age, sex, and height.[14] The Eighth Report of the Joint National Committee on Prevention, Detection, Evaluation, and Treatment of High Blood Pressure (JNC VIII) simply defines hypertension in adults younger than 60 years as 140/90 mm Hg or greater and 150/90 mm Hg for those age 60 or older.[36] The JNC VIII adult definitions of hypertension are based on known risk factors for cardiovascular disease.[36] The strategy of using static systolic BP and diastolic BP measurements, as used for adults, is inappropriate in children for two reasons. First, pediatric evidence is lacking to link hypertension to increased risk of cardiovascular disease, outside of surrogate markers such as carotid intima-media thickness and left ventricular mass. Second, because normal BP values change as children grow, clinicians must rely on data that compare pediatric BP values with those of their pediatric peers.[14,37] Population-based

Table 1. Substance-Induced Hypertension[28-30]

Prescription and Over-the-Counter Medications	Drugs of Abuse	Food	Environmental Exposure	Drug Withdrawal
Amphetamines	Alcohol	Black licorice	Cadmium	Benzodiazepines
Cyclosporine	Anabolic steroids	Calcium	Lead	β-Blockers
Decongestants	Caffeine	Sodium	Mercury	Clonidine
Darbepoetin alfa	Cocaine			Opioids
Epoetin alfa	Ecstasy			
Ergot alkaloids	Ephedrine			
Glucocorticoids	Nicotine			
Ketamine				
Levothyroxine				
Lithium				
Metoclopramide				
Nonsteroidal anti-inflammatory agents				
Oral contraceptive agents				
Phenylephrine				
Pseudoephedrine				
Scopolamine				
Tacrolimus				
Tricyclic antidepressants				

normal BP values (represented in percentiles) for children age 1–13 years are grouped by age, sex, and height, and have been published previously in the AAP Guidelines.[14] The definition of hypertension in adolescents age 13 years more closely mimics the methodology of standard BP breakpoints that JNC VIII uses for the definition of high BP in adults.[14] These pediatric guidelines should be reviewed by any clinician involved in the diagnosis, evaluation, and treatment of childhood hypertension.[14] Classification of pediatric hypertension based on percentiles for age, gender, and height as well as the standard cutoff ranges for adolescents age 13 years and older is shown in Table 2. The BP range that meets the classification for stage 1 hypertension in patients age 1–13 years, for example, is greater than or equal to the 95th percentile for age, gender, and height up to less than the 95th percentile plus 12 mm Hg, or 130/80–139/89 mm Hg (whichever is lower).[14]

The ESH embraces similar principles regarding BP norms based on patient demographics; however, it is important to note that the normal values listed by the AAP Guidelines are slightly lower than the ESH values across each demographic category.[14,15] Thus, it is recommended that U.S. clinicians follow the BP values in the AAP Guidelines when diagnosing and treating hypertension, whereas European clinicians should follow the ESH report. Guidelines for normal BP values in newborns and infants can be found in the Report of the Second Task Force on Blood Pressure Control in Children.[14,33] Definitions of varying severities of hypertension in children based on percentiles for age, sex, and height as well as adolescents age 13 years and older are listed in Table 2.[14] Whereas some have criticized the current BP tables provided by the AAP Guidelines as too complex, others have aimed to simplify the thresholds for the identification of hypertension

Table 2. Classification of Hypertension in Children and Adolescents, with Measurement Frequency and Therapy Recommendations

Classification	Age 1–13 years: SBP or DBP (mm Hg) Percentile[a]	Age ≥ 13 years (mm Hg)	Measurement Frequency	Therapeutic Lifestyle Changes	Pharmacologic Therapy
Normal	< 90th	< 120/< 80	Annually	Encourage healthy diet, sleep, and physical activity	Not indicated
Elevated	90th to < 95th or if BP > 120/80 to < 95th percentile[b]	120/< 80 to 129/< 80	• Recheck in 6 months by auscultation with upper and lower extremity measurement • If 6-month recheck is elevated, then repeat a third measurement in 6 months using ABPM	Weight-management counseling if overweight; introduce physical activity and diet management[c]	None unless compelling indications such as chronic kidney disease, diabetes mellitus, heart failure, or left ventricular hypertrophy exist
Stage 1	> 95th to < 95th + 12 mm Hg or 130/80 to 139/89[b]	130/80 to 139/89	• Recheck in 1–2 weeks or sooner if the patient is symptomatic by auscultation with upper and lower extremity measurement • If 1-2 week recheck is elevated, then repeat a third measurement in 3 months using ABPM; if persistently elevated on two additional occasions, then evaluate or refer to source of care within 1 month	Weight-management counseling if overweight; introduce physical activity and diet management[c]	Initiate therapy based on clinical indications or other compelling indications exist (as shown above)
Stage 2	> 95th percentile + 12 mm Hg or ≥ 140/90[b]	≥ 140/90	• Perform measurement via auscultation with upper and lower extremity measurement • Evaluate or refer to source of care within 1 week or immediately if the patient is symptomatic; initiate ABPM	Weight-management counseling if overweight; introduce physical activity and diet management[c]	Initiate therapy[d]

[a]For sex, age, and height measured on at least three separate occasions; if systolic and diastolic categories are different, categorize by the higher value.
[b]Whichever value is lower.
[c]Parents and children trying to modify the eating plan to the Dietary Approaches to Stop Hypertension Study eating plan could benefit from consultation with a registered or licensed nutritionist to begin the plan.
[d]More than one drug may be required.
ABPM = ambulatory blood pressure monitoring; BP = blood pressure; DBP = diastolic blood pressure; SBP = systolic blood pressure.

in children.[38-41] The tables in the AAP Guidelines, however, remain the gold standard for pediatric thresholds for the diagnosis of hypertension in childhood.

AMBULATORY BLOOD PRESSURE MEASUREMENT

Ambulatory BP measurement recently gained acceptance in the essential diagnosis and treatment of hypertension in pediatric patients.[14,15] It is most simply defined as the repeated measurement of BP in the outpatient setting while the patient is participating in normal daily living activities, including sleep.[42] Pediatric patients may have dramatically different BP readings in a physician's office compared with BP readings in everyday ambulatory settings. Such patients meet the defining criteria for *white-coat hypertension*. However, pediatric patients who are normotensive in the office and hypertensive outside are considered to have *masked hypertension*. Techniques such as ABPM may reveal the presence of either diagnosis.[14,19] According to the AAP Guidelines as well as the ESH and AHA, ABPM is effective in detecting white-coat hypertension, masked hypertension, and differences in nocturnal BP as well as in differentiating between primary and secondary hypertension in pediatric patients.[14,16,19] The ESH recommends 24-hour ABPM to confirm or disprove suspected hypertension in patients with certain comorbidities such as diabetes, renal disease, or solid-organ transplantation and in patients undergoing treatment of refractory hypertension.[15] ABPM may also be useful on diagnosis for evaluation of apparent drug resistance and to assess symptoms of hypotension with antihypertensive therapy. Complementary to the ESH recommendations, the AHA released an official scientific statement regarding the use of ABPM in pediatric patients to guide the diagnosis and treatment of hypertension.[19] In addition, the AHA has published recommended indications for ABPM use in pediatric patients (Box 2), together with normal pediatric ABPM values for girls and boys stratified by age (5–16 years only) and height (boys, 120–185 cm; girls, 120–175 cm).[19]

CLINICAL PRESENTATION

Children with hypertension may have varying underlying etiologies on presentation, categorized as primary or secondary hypertension. *Primary hypertension* is defined as hypertension without a known cause, whereas *secondary hypertension* can be directly linked to a known underlying disorder (e.g., coarctation of the aorta).[14] Although primary hypertension is the most common form of hypertension in adults, the incidence of secondary hypertension in pediatric patients highly outweighs that of primary hypertension.[14,43] In a 2012 study of pediatric patients being treated for hypertension, investigators found that almost two times the number of patients were being treated for secondary hypertension (65%) versus primary hypertension indications (34%).[43] The differences between primary and secondary hypertension in pediatric patients will be described in this section.

PRIMARY HYPERTENSION

Although primary hypertension is relatively uncommon with respect to the distribution of hypertension in pediatric patients as a whole, more attention has been drawn to primary hypertension in children and adolescents because pediatric hypertension may track into adulthood.[8-12,14] The concept of *tracking* when referring to hypertension is illustrated by the likelihood that children who develop hypertension are more likely to be hypertensive in their adult years, thus potentially increasing future risks of individually developing serious cardiovascular disease.[8-12,14] The proportion of adult hypertension specifically thought to be caused by pediatric hypertension is estimated to be about 10%.[13] Investigators have yet to determine if the risk of hypertension in adulthood is decreased as a direct result of the treatment of childhood or adolescent hypertension. The incidence of primary hypertension has been recognized as increasing in children, which explains the AAP Guidelines recommendation for clinicians to increase the frequency of BP screening early in life.[14] Because primary hypertension does not present with obvious clinical signs and symptoms, the disease has the potential to be undiagnosed for months to years and is known as a "silent killer." There is evidence, however, to support that the adoption of a healthy lifestyle, especially reduction or elimination of adiposity, can mitigate the incidence of the hypertension tracking phenomenon.[13] This approach is aimed to curtail the impact of increasing BMI percentile in pediatric patients, which has been directly correlated to increasing BP percentile.[44] Because obesity has been directly linked to primary hypertension in children, preventing and reducing the incidence of obesity in this patient population may be one of the most influential interventions to decrease the incidence of primary hypertension in children.[44]

SECONDARY HYPERTENSION

Unlike primary hypertension, elevated BP in children is typically associated with a directly related underlying disorder. The most common etiologies of childhood hypertension occur secondary to renal/urological diseases or coarctation of the aorta.[45] An underlying etiology should be ruled out for every hypertensive patient, especially when very young children, youths with stage 2 hypertension, or children with severe hypertension and clinical signs of end-organ damage (hypertensive crisis) present with a confirmed diagnosis of hypertension.[14] A comprehensive list of etiologies of pediatric hypertension is shown in Table 3.[46]

Box 2. Indications for Ambulatory Blood Pressure Measurement

- Confirm the diagnosis of hypertension
- Determine the presence of masked hypertension in patients in which a clinical suspicion exists
- Assess blood pressure variability
- Evaluate pharmacologic therapy effectiveness
- More accurately evaluate blood pressure in chronic disease states

---

When ruling out secondary hypertension in children, AAP Guidelines recommend checking BP in an upper and lower extremity.[14] The rationale is to confirm previously measured hypertensive states and potentially detect vascular abnormalities such as coarctation of the aorta.[47] Children with aortic coarctation have decreased lower extremity BP, compared with arm measurements, because of impaired blood flow to the legs.[47] In addition to impaired lower extremity blood flow, left arm BP measurements may be lower than in the right arm if the coarctation is proximal to the left subclavian artery.[48] Although some recommendations guide clinicians to measure two upper extremity BPs followed by one measurement in the legs, many clinicians recommend one upper extremity reading and one lower measurement, especially in younger children, to prevent falsely high measurements caused by discomfort and agitation from repeated BP measurements.

MANAGEMENT

THERAPEUTIC GOALS

The goals of therapeutic management are highly dependent on the clinical presentation and severity of hypertension. For example, BP reduction is needed much more urgently in a patient who presents with hypertensive crisis compared with a patient with stage 1 primary hypertension. This section will review goals of antihypertensive therapies as well as appropriate management strategies of pediatric hypertension, including lifestyle modifications and pharmacologic therapy.

LIFESTYLE MODIFICATIONS

Lifestyle modifications to treat pediatric hypertension include exercise, weight loss, and stress reduction. The goal of using such lifestyle modifications to treat pediatric hypertension is aimed at lowering BP within an acceptable range without the use of medications. When such modifications do not achieve this goal or when medication is required as a first-line treatment option, lifestyle modifications should then be combined with pharmacotherapy. Exercise is a recommended nonpharmacologic therapy for children and adolescents with primary hypertension and may be used as primary or adjunctive treatment.[14] The AHA currently recommends that children 2 years or older participate in at least 60 minutes of developmentally appropriate, moderate-intensity physical activity each day of

Table 3. Common Causes of Pediatric Hypertension

Neonates (0–30 days)	Infant to 6 Years	6–10 Years	10 Years to Adolescence
Renovascular	**Renovascular**	**Renovascular**	**Renovascular**
Renal artery thrombosis	Renal parenchymal disease	Renal artery stenosis	Renal parenchymal disease
Renal venous thrombosis	Pyelonephritis	Renal parenchymal disease	Glomerulonephritis
Renal parenchymal disease	Glomerulonephritis	Glomerulonephritis	End-stage renal disease
Obstructive uropathy	Hemolytic uremic syndrome	Reflux nephropathy	Pyelonephritis
Renal dysplasia	Renal dysplasia	Pyelonephritis	
Polycystic kidney disease	Polycystic kidney disease	Vasculitis	**Primary hypertension**
	Obstructive uropathy		
Neoplasia	Takayasu disease	**Endocrine**	
Neuroblastoma	End-stage renal disease	Corticosteroid excess	
Mesoblastic nephroma	Renal artery stenosis	Hyperaldosteronism	
		(adenoma, hyperplasia)	
Cardiovascular	**Neoplasia**	Pheochromocytoma	
Coarctation of the aorta	Wilm tumor		
		Primary hypertension	
Endocrine	**Primary hypertension**		
Hyperthyroidism			
	Cardiovascular		
Drugs	Coarctation of the aorta		
Corticosteroids			
Phenylephrine eye drops	**Endocrine**		
Theophylline	Corticosteroid excess		
Caffeine	Pheochromocytoma		
Maternal drug use			
(e.g., cocaine)	**Central nervous system**		
	Space-occupying lesions		
Other causes			
Bronchopulmonary dysplasia	**Drugs**		
Intracranial hemorrhage	Amphetamines		
Seizures	Phenylephrine eye drops		
Extracorporeal membrane	Glucocorticoids		
oxygenation	Mineralocorticoids		
Volume overload			
Abdominal wall defect closure	**Other causes**		
	Poisonings (lead, mercury)		

Adapted with permission from Temple ME, Nahata MC. Treatment of pediatric hypertension. Pharmacotherapy 2000;20:140-50.

the week.[49] In many studies, exercise programs lowered both systolic and diastolic BP in children.[50-54] The common factor that reduces BP is aerobic exercise, whereas resistance training alone has not had a therapeutic effect.[50-54] The discontinuation of aerobic activity results in the return of BP to pre-exercise values, so continued commitment to an exercise routine is recommended.[50-53] One exception to exercise as a recommended lifestyle modification, however, pertains to athletes with stage 2 hypertension. For those patients, competitive sports should be restricted until hypertension is controlled.[55]

In addition to exercise, weight loss is an essential lifestyle modification to use when obesity and hypertension coexist.[56] Not only does weight reduction have a BP-lowering effect, but it also minimizes other cardiovascular risk factors such as dyslipidemia and insulin resistance.[14] Diet is an essential part of an adequate weight-loss program, especially in hypertensive patients.[14,57] Salt restriction and other healthy eating habits are recommended for hypertensive adults and children alike.[57] Because excess sodium intake is directly related to hypertension, the AHA recommends a maximum daily sodium intake of 1500 mg for pediatric patients to curb sodium overindulgence.[58] Although the AHA does not stratify sodium intake limits by age, a daily maximum of 1 gram for infants is recommended.[59]

Together with exercise and weight loss, stress reduction may be a key nonpharmacologic intervention to help reduce BP because it has been identified as an environmental factor that may lead to the development of primary hypertension.[46] Although concrete recommendations do not exist regarding the modality in which stress should be reduced in children to prevent or reduce high BP, stress reduction is still thought of as an important potential intervention in pediatric patients.[14] More recent evidence has linked adverse childhood experiences to a more rapid upward BP trajectory in young adulthood.[60]

APPROACH TO PHARMACOLOGIC THERAPY

Because of the potential cardiovascular consequences of prolonged hypertension and the tracking phenomenon of BP into adulthood, BP reduction in children with hypertension is now regarded as an important therapeutic goal to prevent complications associated with the disease.[14] The AAP Guidelines clearly define the indications for pharmacologic treatment of hypertension in children in the following clinical cases: symptomatic hypertension, secondary hypertension, hypertensive target-organ damage, failure of nonpharmacologic BP reduction measures, and type 1 and 2 diabetes mellitus.[14] The goal of pharmacologic therapy in pediatric hypertensive patients is to reduce systolic/diastolic BP to less than the 90th percentile in those age 1–13 years and to less than 130/80 mm Hg in adolescents age 13 years and older.[14] Although adult studies typically aim to reveal differences in morbidity and mortality between treatment groups through long-term follow-up studies, similar high-quality treatment data are unavailable in pediatric patients. Because clinical trials linking improved outcomes to specific antihypertensive agents are nonexistent in pediatric patients, adult data may be extrapolated to this patient population to guide treatment.

Initiation of an antihypertensive agent in a pediatric patient should typically follow a concerted stepwise pattern. In patients for whom lifestyle modifications have been unsuccessful for meeting hypertension treatment goals, pharmacologic interventions should first consist of one of the following medication classes: ACE inhibitors, ARBs, long-acting calcium channel blockers (CCBs), or thiazide diuretics. The recommended strategy for treating pediatric hypertension regardless of the chosen drug class is to start with low doses and titrate slowly to achieve the goal BP and tolerability of the drug.[14] Drug titration should be halted or another agent should be considered for primary or adjunct therapy when the highest recommended dose is reached.[14] When adverse effects develop, medication doses may need to be reduced or discontinued altogether, and another agent may need to be considered.[14] Table 4 provides a comprehensive list of medication doses, including typical pediatric dosing ranges and considerations for antihypertensive agents.

PHARMACOLOGIC THERAPY

Antihypertensive drug classes used in children consist of ACE inhibitors, ARBs, CCBs, diuretics (loop, thiazide, and potassium-sparing diuretics), β-adrenergic receptor blockers (β-blockers), centrally acting sympatholytic agents, peripheral adrenergic blocker, and direct-acting vasodilators. Although a wide range of antihypertensive medication classes exist, the AAP Guidelines have recently established drug class preferences for the treatment of pediatric hypertension that include ACE inhibitors, ARBs, CCBs, and thiazide diuretics.[14] Because treatment-based improvements in morbidity and mortality are generally unavailable in the pediatric population, however, the treatment goal for hypertension in children is simply to lower BP within the range of BP norms while limiting adverse events.[14]

ACE INHIBITORS

Mechanism and use. The therapeutic effect of ACE inhibitors in children is achieved by inhibiting the conversion of AT I to AT II, a potent vasoconstrictor.[61] Because AT II facilitates sympathetic activity, ACE inhibitors reduce BP by decreasing systemic vascular resistance (SVR).[61] In addition, because AT II promotes aldosterone and antidiuretic hormone release while causing vasoconstriction of the efferent arterioles of the kidney, ACE inhibitors decrease intravascular volume by promoting diuresis and natriuresis.[61] In addition, ACE inhibitors prolong the half-life of the vasodilator bradykinin by inhibiting its metabolism.[61] Although ACE inhibitors prevent the cardiac and vascular remodeling associated with chronic hypertension and heart failure in adults, their use for this purpose currently can only be extrapolated to children because pediatric clinical data are unavailable.

Pediatric pharmacokinetics. Captopril is likely one of the most widely used ACE inhibitors in children because of its short half-life, making it an easily titratable drug. This property also enhances safety to the patient and security to the clinician when initiating the drug because its BP-lowering effects will be short-lived if hypotension occurs.

Table 4. Medications Used in Pediatric Hypertension

Drug	Dose by Age or Weight	Interval	Liquid Preparation Available?	Adverse Effects[a]	Removed by Dialysis?	Adjustment for Organ Dysfunction	Notes[14,46,61-64,66-73,78,79,87,91-100,167-185]
ACE INHIBITORS							
Benazepril	Age ≥ 6 yr: 0.2 mg/kg/day or 10 mg Max: 0.6 mg/kg/day or 40 mg	Daily	Yes	Angioedema Cough Dysgeusia Hyperkalemia Neutropenia Orthostatic hypotension Rash	C—Yes HPD—Yes PD—Yes	Renal	Neonates and infants may need lower initial doses and require slow titration Contraindicated in pregnancy
Captopril	Initial: Preterm neonates: 0.01 mg/kg/dose Age < 1 yr: 0.05 mg/kg/dose Age ≥ 1 yr: 0.3–0.5 mg/kg/dose Max: 6 mg/kg/day	TID	Yes		C—Yes HPD—Likely PD—No	Renal	Avoid in patients with bilateral renal artery stenosis Monitor serum potassium and creatinine periodically Incidence of cough is very low in pediatric patients
Enalapril	Initial: 0.08 mg/kg/day up to 5 mg Max: 0.6 mg/kg/day up to 40 mg	Daily–BID	Yes[b]		C—Yes HPD—Likely PD—Yes	Renal	
Fosinopril	Age ≥ 6 yr: 0.1 mg/kg/day up to 5 mg Max: 40 mg/day	Daily	No		C—ND HPD—Minimal PD—No	Renal/Hepatic	
Lisinopril	Initial: 0.07 mg/kg/day up to 5 mg Max: 0.6 mg/kg/day up to 40 mg	Daily	Yes[b]		C—Yes HPD—Likely PD—ND	Renal	
ARBS							
Candesartan	Age 1–6 yr: 0.02 mg/kg/day up to 4 mg/day Max: 16 mg/day > 50 kg: 8mg/day Max: 32 mg/day	Daily—BID	Yes	Cough Hyperkalemia Orthostatic hypotension	C—ND HPD—No PD—ND	No; caution is needed in renal/hepatic impairment	Monitor serum potassium and creatinine periodically Contraindicated in pregnancy Incidence of cough is very low in pediatric patients
Irbesartan	Age 6–12 yr: 75–150 mg/day Age ≥ 13 yr: 150–300 mg/day	Daily	No		C—No HPD—ND PD—ND	No; caution is needed in renal impairment	Use close blood pressure monitoring to guide adjustment for renal or hepatic dysfunction Not recommended in children if creatinine clearance is ≤ 30 mL/min
Losartan	Initial: 0.7 mg/kg/day up to 50 mg Max: 1.4 mg/kg/day up to 100 mg	Daily	Yes		C—No HPD—No PD—No	Not recommended in severe renal or hepatic impairment	Use of valsartan in children age < 6 yr is not recommended Valsartan oral suspension has increased bioavailability vs. tablet formulation
Olmesartan	Age 1–5 yr and ≥ 5 kg: 0.3 mg/kg/day Max: 0.6 mg/kg/day 20 kg to < 35 kg: 10 mg/day up to 20 mg ≥ 35 kg: 20 mg/day up to 40 mg	Daily	Yes		C—No HPD—No PD—Unlikely	No	
Valsartan	Age 6–16 yr: 1.3 mg/kg/day up to 40 mg/day Max: 2.7 mg/kg/day up to 160 mg/day	Daily	Yes		C—No HPD—ND PD—Unlikely	Renal; use caution in hepatic impairment	

(continued)

Table 4. Medications Used in Pediatric Hypertension *(continued)*

Drug	Dose by Age or Weight	Interval	Liquid Preparation Available?	Adverse Effects[a]	Removed by Dialysis?	Adjustment for Organ Dysfunction	Notes[14,46,61-64,66-73,78,79,87,91-100,167-185]
α-BLOCKERS							
Labetalol	Initial: 1–3 mg/kg/day Max: 10–12 mg/kg/day up to 1200 mg	BID	Yes	Bradycardia Bronchospasm Hyperkalemia	C—No HPD—ND PD—No	Potential reduction needed in hepatic impairment	—
β-BLOCKERS							
Atenolol	Initial: 0.5–1 mg/kg/day Max: 2 mg/kg/day up to 100 mg	Daily–BID	Yes	Bradycardia Bronchospasm Drowsiness Exercise intolerance Fatigue Heart block Hypoglycemia Lethargy	C—Yes HPD—Likely PD—No	Renal	Use caution in children with diabetes because β-blockers prevent signs and symptoms of hypoglycemia
Metoprolol	Initial: 1–2 mg/kg/day Max: 6 mg/kg/day up to 200 mg	BID	Yes		C—Yes HPD—Likely PD—ND	Potential reduction needed in hepatic impairment	Hypoglycemia caused by β$_2$-blockade, which inhibits glycogenolysis in the liver and glucagon release from the pancreas
Propranolol	Initial: 0.5–2 mg/kg/day Max: 4 mg/kg/day up to 640 mg	BID–QID	Yes[b]		C—No HPD—Unlikely PD—No	Potential reduction needed in hepatic impairment	Use caution in children with asthma with nonselective agents, although not an absolute contraindication Propranolol is the most lipophilic and has the highest propensity to cause central nervous system-related adverse effects
CCBS							
Amlodipine	Age 1–5 yr: 0.05–0.1 mg/kg/day Age 6–17 yr: 2.5–5 mg/day	Daily–BID	Yes	Constipation Dizziness Flushing Palpitations Tachycardia	C—No HPD—Unlikely PD—No	No; monitor closely in hepatic impairment	Use with caution in patients age < 1 yr Felodipine and nifedipine (extended release only) cannot be crushed or chewed
Felodipine	Initial: 2.5 mg/day Max: 10 mg/day	Daily	No		C—No HPD—Unlikely PD—Unlikely	No; monitor closely in hepatic impairment	
Isradipine	Initial: 0.05–0.1 mg/kg/dose Max: 0.6 mg/kg/day up to 20 mg/day	TID–QID	Yes		C—No HPD—Unlikely PD—No	No; monitor closely in hepatic or renal impairment	
Nifedipine (extended release)	Initial: 0.2–0.5 mg/kg/day Max: 3 mg/kg/day up to 180 mg/day	Daily–BID	No		C—No HPD—Unlikely PD—No	Potential reduction needed in hepatic impairment	
CENTRAL α-AGONISTS							
Clonidine	Initial: 5–10 mcg/kg/day Max: 25 mcg/kg/day OR 0.9 mg/day	BID–TID	Yes[b]	Bradycardia Constipation Drowsiness Dry mouth Orthostatic hypotension Rebound hypertension Sedation	C—No HPD—ND PD—No	Renal	Transdermal dose is equivalent to total daily oral dose Patches should not be cut Should not be abruptly discontinued because of risks of rebound hypertension
Guanfacine	Age ≥ 12 yr: 1 mg Max: 2 mg	QHS	—		C—No HPD—ND PD—No	Use with caution in renal or hepatic impairment	
Methyldopa	Initial: 2.5 mg/kg/dose Max: 65 mg/kg/day OR 3 g/day	BID–QID	Yes		C—Yes HPD—Likely PD—Yes	Renal	

(continued)

Table 4. Medications Used in Pediatric Hypertension *(continued)*

Drug	Dose by Age or Weight	Interval	Liquid Preparation Available?	Adverse Effects[a]	Removed by Dialysis?	Adjustment for Organ Dysfunction	Notes[14,46,61-64,66-73,78,79,87,91-100,167-185]
DIRECT RENIN INHIBITORS							
Aliskiren	Initial: 1.7–2 mg/kg/day Max: 6 mg/kg/day up to 300 mg	Daily	No	Angioedema Diarrhea Dizziness Headache Hyperkalemia	C—ND HPD—ND PD—ND	No; use with caution in renal impairment	Contraindicated in pregnancy Contraindicated in adult patients with diabetes or moderate to severe renal impairment while taking ACE inhibitors or ARBs Reported only in a case series of four patients with chronic kidney disease and in a survey of 10 patients age 4–17 yr Studies are currently enrolling patients, but safety and efficacy data are not known Use caution when using in pediatric patients
DIURETICS: LOOP							
Furosemide	Initial: 0.5–2 mg/kg/dose Max: 6 mg/kg/dose	Daily–QID	Yes[b]	Hypocalcemia Hypochloremic metabolic alkalosis Hypokalemia Hypomagnesemia Hypovolemia Ototoxicity	C—No HPD—Unlikely PD—Unlikely	No	Risk and severity of ototoxicity are directly related to high doses
DIURETICS: THIAZIDE							
Chloro-thiazide	Initial: 10 mg/kg/day Max: 40 mg/kg/day up to 2000 mg/day	Daily–BID	Yes	Dyslipidemia Hypochloremic metabolic alkalosis Hyperglycemia Hypokalemia Hypomagnesemia Hyponatremia Hypovolemia Hyperuricemia	C – No HPD – No PD—No	No	Mechanism behind dyslipidemia and hyperglycemia remains unclear
Hydro-chloro-thiazide	Initial: 1 mg/kg/day Max: 3 mg/kg/day up to 50 mg	Daily	Yes		C—No HPD—ND PD—Unlikely	No	May be ineffective in patients with poor renal function
DIURETICS: POTASSIUM-SPARING							
Amiloride	Initial: 0.4–0.625 mg/kg/day up to 20 mg	Daily	Yes	Gynecomastia (only spironolactone) Hyperkalemia Metabolic acidosis	C—ND HPD—ND PD—ND	Renal	Avoid use in patients with severe renal dysfunction
Spirono-lactone	Initial: 1 mg/kg/day Max: 3.3 mg/kg/day up to 100 mg	Daily–BID	Yes		C—Unlikely HPD—ND PD—Unlikely	Renal	
Triamterene	Initial: 1–2 mg/kg/day Max: 3–4 mg/kg/day up to 300 mg	BID	No		C—ND HPD—ND PD—ND	Renal	
PERIPHERAL α-BLOCKERS							
Doxazosin	Initial: 1 mg/day Max: 4 mg/day	Daily	No	Dizziness Drowsiness Fatigue Headache Muscle weakness Orthostatic hypotension	C—No HPD—ND PD—No	Use with caution in hepatic impairment	Usually not first-line agents — usually used in resistant hypertension
Prazosin	Initial: 0.05–0.1 mg/kg/day Max: 0.5 mg/kg/day or 20 mg/day	TID	Yes		C—No HPD—Unlikely PD—No	No	
Terazosin	Initial: 1 mg/day Max: 20 mg/day	Daily	No		C—No HPD—Unlikely PD—No	No	

Table 4. Medications Used in Pediatric Hypertension *(continued)*

Drug	Dose by Age or Weight	Interval	Liquid Preparation Available?	Adverse Effects[a]	Removed by Dialysis?	Adjustment for Organ Dysfunction	Notes[14,46,61-64,66-73,78,79,87,91-100,167-185]
VASODILATORS							
Hydralazine	Initial: 0.75 mg/kg/day Max: 7.5 mg/kg/day up to 200 mg	Four times/day	Yes	Dizziness Hypertrichosis (minoxidil only) Orthostatic hypotension Sodium and water retention RAAS activation Reflex tachycardia Vivid dreams	C—No HPD—ND PD—No	Renal	Usually not first-line agents — usually used in resistant hypertension or in hypertensive crisis
Minoxidil	Initial: 0.2 mg/kg/dose Max: 50–100 mg/dose	Daily–TID	Yes		C—Yes HPD—Likely PD—Yes	No	Hydralazine may cause rebound hypertension by RAAS activation

[a]All agents may cause hypotension.
[b]Compound is commercially available.
ACE = angiotensin-converting enzyme; ARB = angiotensin receptor blocker; BID = twice daily; C = conventional hemodialysis (KUf ≤ 8 mL/hour/mm Hg); CCB = calcium channel blocker; HPD = high permeability dialysis (KUf > 8 mL/hour/mm Hg); Max = maximum; ND = no data; PD = peritoneal dialysis; QHS = every night; QID = four times daily; RAAS = renin–angiotensin–aldosterone system; TID = three times daily.

This point is important to consider in children, especially infants and neonates, because ACE inhibitor–induced hypotension is more likely to be seen in this age group.[46] Risks of hypotension in this patient population must be respected; thus, low initial doses and slow titration are recommended to avoid these risks, particularly in neonates and infants. For unknown reasons, neonates and infants have an increased sensitivity to ACE inhibitors. Proposed mechanisms include, but are not limited to, higher plasma renin concentrations, developing kidneys, and decreased hepatic drug metabolism in this age group.[46] Other ACE inhibitors with longer half-lives, such as enalapril and lisinopril, are also used in children.[46] Advantages include increased adherence, the availability of a commercially manufactured oral suspension, and improved quality of life with once- or twice-daily administration. Onset of action of ACE inhibitors in children ranges from about 15 minutes for captopril to about 1 hour for enalapril and lisinopril.

Both captopril and enalapril are extensively metabolized and excreted into the urine.[61] Enalapril, which is actually a prodrug, must be metabolized by the liver to its active form, enalaprilat, before it exhibits antihypertensive effects.[61] Lisinopril is not hepatically metabolized and is primarily excreted in the urine as unchanged drug.[61]

Adverse effects. Angiotensin-converting enzyme inhibitors are generally well tolerated in children, making them an attractive therapeutic option. Hypotension and hyperkalemia are generally considered the most likely adverse effects of this drug class in pediatric patients. Many adverse effects caused by ACE inhibitors, particularly ACE inhibitor–induced cough, occur rarely in children compared with the rate of occurrence in adults.[62-64]

AT II RECEPTOR BLOCKERS

Mechanism and use. Because AT II is generated by other pathways, in addition to ACE inhibitors, ARBs were developed to block the final step in this neurohormonal pathway—the binding of AT II to AT II receptor type 1, or AT_1-receptors.[65] By antagonizing this receptor, ARBs cause vasodilation,

aldosterone antagonism, reduction in sympathetic activity, and renal efferent arteriole relaxation.[65] Unlike ACE inhibition, ARBs do not affect the metabolism of bradykinin.[65] Because elevated bradykinin concentrations cause vasodilation, however, this effect may be a drawback to ARB therapy.

Pediatric pharmacokinetics. Many ARBs have been reported to be used in pediatric patients, with several studies recently published at the time of this writing.[66-72] Pharmacokinetic properties of ARBs in pediatric patients vary depending on the agent used.[67,69-72] Onset of action typically occurs within 1–2 hours. Most ARBs are metabolized from an inactive form to an active metabolite, with olmesartan metabolism occurring in the gut.[67,69,71] Elimination of ARBs is primarily through the fecal route as well as the urine.[67,69,71] The half-lives of ARBs are prolonged (6–15 hours), allowing once-daily dosing.[67,69,71] Data in young children (younger than 6 years) are relatively scant, with most available data representing the use of valsartan.[66,67]

Adverse effects. In pediatric randomized controlled trials, ARBs have a pediatric adverse effect profile similar to placebo.[66,70-72] The adverse effects are similar to those of ACE inhibitors, and the class of ARBs as a whole are well tolerated in children, causing minimal episodes of hypotension.[66-71]

DIRECT RENIN INHIBITORS

Mechanism and use. Renin inhibition is not currently an attractive therapeutic option for pediatric hypertension. Aliskiren, the only renin inhibitor to have received label approval from the U.S. Food and Drug Administration, prevents the production of AT I and therefore reduces AT II concentrations, causing vasodilation. As of this writing, the use of aliskiren had only been documented in four pediatric patients with chronic kidney disease in addition to a pharmacokinetic study that enrolled 39 patients age 6–17 years, indicating the paucity of important clinical data to guide prescribers on its safe and effective use.[73]

Pediatric pharmacokinetics. One pharmacokinetic study is available for aliskiren in 39 pediatric patients between age

6–17 years.[73] In these patients, peak absorption occurred between 1–2 hours after dose administration and half-life ranged between 38–45 hours, which is significantly prolonged compared with adults.[73] Onset of action is typically thought to occur between 1–3 hours. Information regarding the extent of hepatic metabolism is still unknown, but hypotheses point to the cytochrome P450 3A4 metabolic pathway with about 20%–25% renal elimination.[74]

CALCIUM CHANNEL BLOCKERS

Mechanism and use. Despite the paucity of clinical data establishing their safety and efficacy, CCBs are being used in the treatment of pediatric hypertension.[75] The classification of CCBs, which identifies drugs in this class as dihydropyridines and non-dihydropyridines, is based on relative cardiac/vascular activity. Cardiac and vascular smooth muscle both rely on intracellular calcium for contraction. By blocking the influx of extracellular calcium, CCBs help decrease SVR and cardiac conduction. At therapeutic doses, the dihydropyridines are relatively safe to use in all age ranges and are the most useful class in the treatment of pediatric hypertension.[75] Their high affinity for vascular calcium channels results in a reduction in BP by decreasing SVR through vasodilation.[75] Non-dihydropyridine CCBs are generally recommended to be avoided in patients younger than 1 year because the inhibition of AV node conduction may cause potent negative inotrope effects and thus can be fatal in young children.[14,75-77] Like the JNC VIII recommendations, AAP Guidelines also include CCBs as an acceptable first-line option in pediatric patients.[14,36]

Pediatric pharmacokinetics. The pharmacokinetics of amlodipine in pediatric patients has been studied in one prospective trial in children as young as 6 months.[78] This study, coupled with other case reports, suggests those younger than 6 years require higher doses per kilogram to maintain adequate BP control.[78,79] This study identified no changes in the pharmacokinetic characteristics of amlodipine or BP control when dosed more than once daily, thus negating claims of previous case studies linking twice-daily dosing to more reliable BP control.[78,79] Nifedipine is used for pediatric hypertension, but most of the available literature addresses its use for hypertensive crisis, which will be discussed later in text.[79] All CCBs are hepatically metabolized and do not require adjustment in the presence of renal dysfunction. Amlodipine is the dihydropyridine with the highest vascular selectivity, greatest oral bioavailability, and longest half-life, allowing once-daily dosing for chronic hypertension.

β-ADRENERGIC RECEPTOR BLOCKERS

Mechanism and use. Reduction in BP with β-adrenergic blockers (β-blockers) is achieved by reducing cardiac output through negative inotropic and chronotropic effects.[80,81] The receptor specificity and relative cardioselectivity vary between β-blockers. Atenolol and metoprolol are very cardioselective (except at high doses), antagonizing only β_1-receptors, whereas propranolol blocks β_1 and β_2. This additional β_2-blockade may result in pulmonary cross-reactivity leading to bronchoconstriction and asthma exacerbations; however, the incidence

in pediatric patients is minimal.[80] In addition to β_1- and β_2-blockade, carvedilol possesses α_1-receptor activity, causing a reduction in SVR.

Pediatric pharmacokinetics. The pharmacokinetics as well as receptor specificity vary widely between β-blockers. All are lipophilic enough to cross the blood-brain barrier and thus have the ability to cause drowsiness and fatigue.[80,81] Propranolol shows the most rapid onset of action (1–2 hours) and has the shortest half-life (4.5 hours), whereas atenolol and metoprolol typically take longer to take effect (3 hours) and have a longer elimination half-life (8 hours). Metoprolol and propranolol are both metabolized in the liver and therefore need not be adjusted in renal dysfunction.[81] Atenolol, however, undergoes minimal hepatic metabolism and is highly eliminated through the urine, leaving patients with renal dysfunction at a higher risk of drug accumulation and accompanying adverse effects.[81]

DIURETICS: MECHANISM AND USE

The AAP Guidelines include thiazide diuretics as an option for first-line antihypertensive therapy in children.[14] By reducing intravascular volume and peripheral vascular resistance, diuretics decrease BP.[46] They may be particularly useful in patients who require several drugs to control hypertension or who have considerable sodium and water retention.

Loop diuretics. Loop diuretics are the most powerful diuretics that may also have effects on hemodynamics. After reaching the tubular lumen of the nephron, their inhibition of the $Na^+/K^+/2Cl^-$ cotransporter in the thick ascending loop of Henle causes increased sodium concentrations in the distal tubule, thus promoting diuresis and natriuresis.[82] Loop diuretics also potentiate the production of prostaglandins in the kidneys, leading to enhanced renal blood flow. As a whole, loop diuretics have no significant effect on hemodynamics, and they are generally not considered potent antihypertensive agents in children.[82] Furosemide is the most commonly used loop diuretic in children. Other loop diuretics, such as torsemide and bumetanide, are not routinely used in the management of hypertension in children.[14,83-86]

Thiazide/thiazide-like diuretics. Thiazide diuretics are recommended by JNC VIII as one of the first-line antihypertensive agent options in adults, and they are used in children as well.[36] By inhibiting the Na^+/Cl^- transporter in the distal tubule, thiazide and thiazide-like diuretics produce mild diuresis and natriuresis by inhibiting about 5% of total sodium reabsorption, showing about one-fifth the diuretic capability of loop diuretics.[87] Although their diuretic actions are mild, the proposed mechanism behind their hemodynamic effects is a reduction in SVR by direct vasodilation caused by vascular potassium channel activation.[87-89] Commonly prescribed thiazide diuretics in children include chlorothiazide and hydrochlorothiazide, whereas thiazide-like diuretics include chlorthalidone and metolazone. Data are unavailable regarding synergistic BP-lowering effects when combining a loop with a thiazide diuretic in children.

Potassium-sparing diuretics. Potassium-sparing diuretics all work to promote diuresis while conserving potassium depletion; however, spironolactone shows slight mechanistic differences compared with amiloride and triamterene. Spironolactone antagonizes aldosterone by competing for binding sites at the distal segment of the distal tubule, causing increased sodium and water excretion into the urine. Its potassium-sparing effects are produced by the inhibition of aldosterone-sensitive sodium reabsorption.[90] By inhibiting this mechanism, fewer potassium and hydrogen ions are excreted in the urine.[90] Amiloride and triamterene, however, directly inhibit sodium channels in the distal convoluted tubule and the collecting duct, thus reducing the activity of the sodium/potassium transporter in the distal renal tubule to produce potassium-sparing diuresis independently of aldosterone.[90]

CENTRALLY ACTING SYMPATHOLYTIC AGENTS

Mechanism and use. α_2-Adrenergic receptor activation in the brain decreases BP through sympathetic tone reduction.[91] Drugs that show this pharmacologic activity include clonidine, guanabenz, guanfacine, and methyldopa.[91] Clonidine is the most commonly prescribed α_2-agonist for the treatment of pediatric hypertension. Guanfacine and methyldopa are also used, but less often.[91] Guanfacine and clonidine are also used for other indications such as attention-deficit/hyperactivity disorder.[92,93] Clonidine is effective in adjunctive analgesia and prevention of withdrawal symptoms associated with opioid weans as well.[94,95]

α_2-Adrenergic receptor agonists are typically not considered first-line therapy for hypertension in adults because of the lack of long-term morbidity and mortality data. Use in pediatric patients is low for the same reasons and may be avoided because of the incidence of adverse effects and subsequent reduction in quality of life. For these reasons, α_2-adrenergic agonists are typically reserved as adjunctive agents to be used in refractory hypertension or single-dose agents for hypertensive emergencies while intravenous agents are being prepared.[91]

Pediatric pharmacokinetics. The onset of action for guanfacine and methyldopa are 1.5–4 hours and 2 hours, respectively.[91] Their duration of action, however, varies widely, with guanfacine showing a half-life of about 17 hours (allowing once-daily dosing), compared with 1.7 hours (dosing up to four times daily) for methyldopa.[91] Both drugs are eliminated primarily by the kidneys.[91] The pharmacokinetic profile of clonidine will be reviewed in detail in the Hypertensive Crisis section later in this chapter.

PERIPHERAL ADRENERGIC BLOCKERS AND DIRECT VASODILATORS

Mechanism and use. These agents are typically used as adjunctive medications for refractory hypertension and are not often selected as first-line agents. Selective α_1-receptor blockade causes peripheral vasodilation and a subsequent reduction in BP. Doxazosin, prazosin, and terazosin make up the α_1-receptor blocker drug class. Minoxidil and hydralazine are direct vasodilators that are also used in the treatment of hypertensive crisis.[46,96-100]

The prescribing of both drug classes for childhood hypertension has dwindled and is associated with the potential for adverse effects.[46] In addition, adult data showing a reduction

in morbidity and mortality with their use are nonexistent and have actually been linked to increases in cardiovascular morbidity, thus preventing pediatric extrapolation and halting subsequent increases in prescribing patterns.[101]

Pediatric pharmacokinetics. The pediatric pharmacokinetic profile of minoxidil and hydralazine will be reviewed in the Hypertensive Crisis section later in the chapter.

MONITORING THERAPEUTIC OUTCOMES

The frequency and intensity of monitoring in patients with pediatric hypertension are highly reliant on the severity of illness at presentation and the presence of underlying disease states. Table 2 highlights the recommended frequency of BP measurement according to severity of hypertension.[14]

HYPERTENSIVE CRISIS

Pediatric hypertensive crisis markedly increases the risks of morbidity and mortality, prompting immediate clinical attention and necessitating emergency treatment.[46,96] Despite many years of available therapeutic treatment options, a paucity of robust pediatric clinical literature exists. Randomized controlled trials enrolling patients with pediatric hypertensive emergencies are nonexistent. This lack of data forces clinicians to make empiric clinical decisions forged from extrapolated adult data and small, observational, pediatric studies. A sound knowledge base of pediatric pharmacology and pathophysiology is needed in conjunction with a thorough understanding of the adult and pediatric clinical literature to guide clinical decision-making.

DEFINITIONS AND CLINICAL PRESENTATION

Both hypertensive urgencies and emergencies are considered types of hypertensive crises. *Hypertensive urgency* is defined as severely elevated BP without signs and symptoms of end-organ dysfunction.[14] A *hypertensive emergency*, however, is severely elevated BP presenting with end-organ damage.[14] An example of the difference between the two diagnoses includes a patient with severely elevated BP and corresponding seizures (hypertensive emergency) compared with a patient with an equivalently elevated BP and less severe symptoms, such as a severe headache (hypertensive urgency).[102,103]

Pediatric hypertensive crises present in a variety of ways, but, by definition, all cases have severely elevated BP. Exceeding stage 2 hypertension in severity, both hypertensive urgencies and emergencies require immediate pharmacologic intervention to reduce BP, even though their clinical presentations differ. Debate is ongoing regarding the necessity to differentiate between the two definitions because each diagnosis equally requires prompt medical intervention with the same pharmacologic agents and treatment strategies.[96] Even more important than being able to differentiate between the definitions of hypertensive *urgency* versus *emergency* on clinical presentation is the ability to grasp the concept that a failure to treat patients with hypertensive crisis sooner leads to end-organ dysfunction that might eventually cause irreversible damage or death.[46,104] Signs and symptoms of end-organ damage may manifest as encephalopathy, seizures, intracerebral hemorrhage, facial palsy, retinopathy, acute renal failure, hematuria, congestive heart failure, and arrhythmias.[14,46,96,104-108]

PATHOGENESIS

As discussed at the beginning of this chapter regarding the pathogenesis of primary and secondary hypertension, hypertensive crises are also a result of the dysfunction of complex neurohormonal and hemodynamic pathways causing dangerous elevations in systemic BP.[96,104] Activation of the RAAS, oxidative and mechanical damage to the microvasculature, fluid overload, severe renal dysfunction, coarctation of the aorta, sympathetic overstimulation, and endothelial dysfunction all may contribute to the pathology of hypertensive crises.[96,104]

PHARMACOLOGIC THERAPY

THERAPEUTIC GOALS

Pediatric guidelines for the treatment of high BP call for controlled antihypertensive therapy in patients with hypertensive crisis.[14] Goals for controlled antihypertensive therapy include a gradual BP decrease of 25% or less within the first 8 hours, followed by a deliberate and gradual lowering of BP throughout the next 40 hours.[14] The rationale for gradual, rather than immediate, reduction of BP over the first 48 hours after hypertensive crisis presentation includes the avoidance of inducing devastating sequelae including stroke, myocardial infarction, and renal insufficiency as a result of end organ hypoperfusion caused by vascular autoregulation failure.[109] Final goals to aim for should include BP at or below the 90th percentile or less for sex, age, and height if age 1–13 years and less than 130/80 mm Hg for adolescents age 13 years and older.[14]

Oral agents may be used for hypertensive crises in pediatric patients, but unlike medications used as rapidly titratable continuous infusions, their utility is generally limited to less severe cases such as hypertensive urgencies.[14,96,99,100,102-108,110-116] Easily titratable continuous infusions are typically preferred because of their superior ability to tightly control BP descent, which allows a rapid reduction in BP while avoiding dangerously fast decreases.[96] Table 5 highlights common intravenous agents, including pediatric dosing ranges and considerations for hypertensive crisis.

SODIUM NITROPRUSSIDE

Mechanism and use. Sodium nitroprusside (SNP) is rapidly metabolized to cyanide and nitric oxide within red blood cells, which directly vasodilates arterial and venous smooth muscle, and this drug is considered a first-line therapeutic agent for hypertensive crises.[80,117] With its initial pediatric data reported in the 1970s, SNP is historically one of the most commonly used agents for hypertensive crisis in children.[118]

Pediatric pharmacokinetics. Pharmacologic assets of SNP include a rapid onset of action (less than 60 seconds) and a short elimination half-life, allowing rapid titration of continuous infusions.[80] Another benefit includes its ability to lower BP by decreasing SVR without increasing preload or causing negative inotropic effects.[119]

Adverse effects. Drawbacks of SNP administration include potential cyanide and thiocyanate toxicity in addition to tachyphylaxis associated with prolonged therapy.[119] Cyanide toxicity results from enzymatic breakdown of SNP within red blood cells.[119,120] Humans are normally able to attenuate cyanide accumulation by forming the thiocyanate molecule, which is then eliminated by the kidneys. This metabolic conversion is accomplished by the enzyme rhodanese in the presence of thiosulfate.

High doses, prolonged infusions, or the presence of hepatic dysfunction causes depletion of endogenous thiosulfate stores, which increases the risk of cyanide toxicity, whereas prolonged infusions and renal dysfunction may cause thiocyanate accumulation and subsequent toxicity.[121] Signs and symptoms of cyanide toxicity include the following: vomiting, headache, hypotension, delirium, psychosis, weakness, muscle spasms, tachypnea, tachycardia, tinnitus, metabolic acidosis, coma, and death.[119,120]

Clinical literature indicates that patients who receive a continuous infusion of 2 mcg/kg/minute or greater for at least 24 hours or those with renal or hepatic dysfunction are at increased risk; however, present evidence has failed to establish reference ranges for cyanide concentrations that correlate to toxicity in pediatric patients.[120,122-127] Nevertheless, the AAP Guidelines recommend monitoring cyanide levels with prolonged use (more than 72 hours) or in renal failure.[14] A more recent study published in 2015 found children to have elevated cyanide levels after a 12-hour infusion without signs and symptoms of toxicity.[128] Focused on combating SNP-induced cyanide toxicity, some institutions add sodium thiosulfate to nitroprusside infusions to take advantage of its ability to reduce serum cyanide concentrations by replacing exhausted thiosulfate reserves.[129-131] Of note, clinical literature describing the safety and efficacy of the prolonged coadministration of the two drugs is lacking. Regardless of the decision to monitor cyanide concentrations in patients receiving SNP, however, clinicians should still be well aware of the signs and symptoms of cyanide toxicity and follow relevant monitoring variables including the following: changes in neurological status, skeletal muscle tone, respiratory rate, heart rate, relative acidosis by way of blood gas monitoring, and venous oxygen saturation.

NICARDIPINE

Mechanism and use. Nicardipine is an intravenous CCB that has recently been studied more often compared with other agents used for hypertensive emergencies in pediatric patients.[132-139] Like SNP, nicardipine is considered a first-line treatment option for pediatric hypertensive crises.[14] Its mechanism of action involves peripheral arterial vasodilation with minimal effects on the myocardium.[14] The relatively high affinity of nicardipine for vascular calcium channels and its lack of activity on myocardial calcium channels causes SVR reduction with a potential to produce reflex tachycardia.[132-134]

Pediatric pharmacokinetics. Much like SNP, nicardipine has a pharmacokinetic profile that includes a rapid onset of action (1–2 minutes) and can be rapidly titrated.[133] Drug elimination is highly driven by hepatic metabolism through cytochrome P450 enzymes. Although a smaller percentage of the

Table 5. Common Intravenous Agents Used in Pediatric Hypertensive Crisis[14,46,75,80,91,96,100,102,103,108,110,111,117-127,129-150,152-155,160-163,186]

Drug	Mechanism of Action	Initial Dose	Maximum Dose	Adverse Effects[a]	Adjustment for Organ Dysfunction	Notes
Esmolol	β_1-Blocker	**B:** 100–500 mcg/kg **C:** 50–500 mcg/kg/hr	**B:** 500 mcg/kg **C:** 1000 mcg/kg/hr	Bradycardia Bronchospasm (potential at high doses) Hypoglycemia	No	Loses β_1-selectivity at higher doses, but dose at which it loses cardioselectivity is unknown Bolus doses as high as 1000 mcg/kg and continuous-infusion rates up to 1000 mcg/kg/min have been used
Hydralazine	Direct vasodilator (arterial)	0.05–0.2 mg/kg/dose every 4–6 hr	1 mg/kg/dose OR 20 mg	Dizziness Headache Palpitations Reflex tachycardia Rebound hypertension Drug-induced lupus-like syndrome	Renal	May be given intravenously or intramuscularly May be given orally (0.25 mg/kg/dose every 6 hr, maximum 25 mg) Activates renin–angiotensin–aldosterone system Prolonged half-life Often used as single dose to control hypertension while continuous agents are being prepared
Labetalol	α_1, β_1, β_2-Blocker	**B:** 0.2–1 mg/kg **C:** 0.25–1 mg/kg/hr	**B:** 20 mg **C:** 3 mg/kg/hr	Bradycardia Bronchospasm Hyperkalemia Hypoglycemia	Potential reduction needed in hepatic impairment	Does not cause reflex tachycardia Longer half-life vs. other agents Young children may require lower doses (~0.6 mg/kg/hr) to achieve a desired antihypertensive effect Bronchospasm occurs infrequently in pediatric patients
Nicardipine	Calcium channel blocker (selective for arterial Ca^{2+} channels)	0.2–0.5 mcg/kg/min	3 mcg/kg/min	Flushing Headache Reflex tachycardia	Renal Potential reduction needed in hepatic impairment	Selective for arterial Ca^{2+} channels with minimal activity on myocardium Doses > 3 mcg/kg/min lack additional benefit in blood pressure reduction
Sodium Nitroprusside	Direct vasodilator (venules and arterioles)	0.3–1 mcg/kg/min	10 mcg/kg/min	Cyanide toxicity Tachyphylaxis Thiocyanate toxicity	Renal Hepatic	Typical maximum dose is 4 mcg/kg/min, but doses as high as 10 mcg/kg/min have been used May administer sodium thiosulfate to prevent or treat cyanide toxicity Tachyphylaxis may develop after prolonged treatment

[a]All agents may cause hypotension.
B = bolus dose; C = continuous infusion.

drug is excreted in urine and feces, no adjustments for renal dysfunction are required. Unlike SNP, its metabolism does not produce toxic metabolites, so it can safely be infused for a prolonged period (e.g., greater than 10 days) without risks of toxicity.[133]

Adverse effects. Common adverse effects of nicardipine include severe hypotension, reflex tachycardia, flushing, headache, and thrombophlebitis.

LABETALOL

Mechanism and use. Labetalol is yet another agent with limited pediatric data that is considered a first-line antihypertensive agent for pediatric hypertensive emergencies and urgencies.[96,117] Unlike nicardipine and nitroprusside, intravenous labetalol reduces BP without causing reflex tachycardia. This effect results from its mechanism of antagonizing both α_1- and β-adrenergic receptors in a 1:7 ratio.[140]

Pediatric pharmacokinetics. The onset of action of labetalol occurs after only 5 minutes, and it can be titrated every 10 minutes.[108] Compared with other continuously infused agents for pediatric hypertensive crisis, labetalol has a relatively long half-life of around 5.5–8 hours.[140] Labetalol is hepatically metabolized by glucuronidation pathways and is unaffected by renal insufficiency.[140-142]

Adverse effects. Adverse effects most commonly seen in patients receiving labetalol are severe hypotension, bradycardia, and bronchospasm.

ESMOLOL

Mechanism and use. As previously stated, esmolol is a cardioselective β_1-adrenergic blocker. Although esmolol may be used in hypertensive emergencies, most pediatric data are specific to use in children with supraventricular tachycardia and hypertension control after repair of aortic coarctation.[143-149]

Pediatric pharmacokinetics. One of the properties that makes esmolol an attractive agent for this indication is its immediate onset of action (less than 1 minute) and specific drug metabolism by red blood cell esterases, resulting in a half-life of 3–9 minutes in pediatric patients.[143-145,147-150] Neonates and infants metabolize esmolol sooner than older children, adolescents, and adults; however, data are conflicting, with a maximum half-life difference of about 6 minutes, which is most likely clinically insignificant.[143-145,148-150]

Adverse effects. Significant adverse effects related to esmolol therapy are most commonly hypotension, bradycardia, thrombophlebitis, and potentially fluid overload because higher doses may be accompanied by a high volume of intravenous fluid administration. Bronchospasm is rarely observed because of its high β-1 receptor selectivity.

HYDRALAZINE

Mechanism and use. Although hydralazine can be used in the treatment of pediatric hypertension, its primary utility resides in the treatment of acute hypertension and hypertensive crisis.[48,96] A direct vasodilator, hydralazine causes a reduction in SVR by inhibiting calcium-dependent adenosine triphosphate and phosphorylation in arteriolar smooth muscle.[97,98,119,151] Recent reports describe the mechanism in more detail as stimulation of the hypoxia-inducible factor-1-α protein by inhibiting prolyl hydroxylase domain enzymes. This mechanism results in the induction of vascular endothelial growth factor, endothelin-1, adrenomedullin, and heme oxygenase 1, all of which cause the intracellular accumulation of cyclic guanosine monophosphate. This effect results in the clinical response of smooth muscle relaxation and arteriolar vasodilation.[151]

Pediatric pharmacokinetics. Typical onset of action for hydralazine occurs between 20 and 40 minutes after an oral dose (not as useful in hypertensive emergencies) and between 5 and 20 minutes after intravenous/intramuscular dosing.[152] Not much is known about the specific pediatric pharmacokinetics of hydralazine aside from methods of drug elimination and onset of action. Hydralazine is highly removed from the body through the first-pass effect. It is mainly metabolized by acetylation in the liver and partly eliminated by the kidneys.[14,96,119] Patients with severe renal dysfunction may exhibit a longer hydralazine half-life and may require dosing less often, depending on their underlying hepatic metabolism rate. Although the reported dosing range varies quite widely, one study noted intravenous doses within the range of 0.08–0.15 mg/kg are more likely to result in optimal BP lowering effects compared with higher doses.[153]

Adverse effects. Common adverse effects of hydralazine therapy include hypotension, rebound hypertension, reflex tachycardia, and headache. Drug-induced lupus-like syndrome has also been reported.

CLONIDINE

Mechanism and use. Oral central α-agonists such as clonidine are also used to treat hypertensive urgencies. Their main effects cause vasodilation through α_2-stimulation and a subsequent reduction in sympathetic tone, which leads to a reduction in SVR and BP.

Pediatric pharmacokinetics. With its rapid onset of action (15–30 minutes after oral ingestion), clonidine is an ideal oral agent for urgent treatment.[91] Clinicians should exercise caution when using clonidine for this indication because its 6- to 8-hour half-life (in adults) could result in a prolonged, dangerous decline in BP.[91,111] The pediatric pharmacokinetics and pharmacodynamics of orally administered clonidine are poorly understood. Rectal and nasal administration of clonidine in infants and children for anesthetic purposes have a half-life of 5–20 hours, possibly indicating prolonged activity in young children.[154,155]

Adverse effects. The adverse effect profile of clonidine includes hypotension, sedation, somnolence, and rebound hypotension and agitation, especially if abruptly discontinued.

ACE INHIBITORS

Mechanism and use. The only intravenous ACE inhibitor used for the treatment of hypertensive crisis is enalaprilat.[156] Although its use has primarily involved pediatric patients with heart failure or hypertension after congenital heart surgery, it is not listed in the AAP Guidelines as a suggested option for the treatment of hypertensive emergencies.[14,157-159]

Pediatric pharmacokinetics. In a small study of pediatric patients with heart failure, the pharmacokinetics of enalaprilat seemed to resemble that of enalapril in pediatrics as well as adults, with the exception of the enteral absorption phase for those receiving enalapril.[158] Of note, significantly lower doses were required for neonates to achieve similar BP-lowering effects, which is similar to other reports of ACE inhibitor use in this age group.[158]

Adverse effects. Significant adverse effects of intravenous enalaprilat include profound hypotension, hyperkalemia, and renal insufficiency. Adverse effects are likely to be pronounced in neonates if dosing is not adjusted accordingly for age.

ORAL CALCIUM CHANNEL BLOCKERS

Mechanism and use. The AAP Guidelines do not include non-dihydropyridines or nifedipine as desirable agents for use in hypertensive crisis.[14] Verapamil and diltiazem use is limited because of their negative inotropic and chronotropic activity through blockade of cardiac electrical conduction. The use of short-acting nifedipine, which has been well documented, is controversial.[75,102,103,160-162] Many authors do not recommend its use because of its overtly potent antihypertensive effects, which may cause significant morbidity and mortality related to a rapid and dangerous decline in BP.[75,102,103,160-162]

Unlike diltiazem and verapamil, dihydropyridines (excluding nifedipine) such as isradipine are more commonly used in children for hypertensive urgencies. Without disturbing myocardial electrical conduction, isradipine produces vasodilation and decreases SVR by exhibiting its primary actions on L-type calcium channels.[160] Pediatric data are available on the use of isradipine for the treatment of acute hypertension; however, information on its use for hypertensive crisis in children is limited.[112-115]

Pediatric pharmacokinetics. Like those of other oral agents used for hypertensive urgencies, the pharmacokinetic profile of isradipine includes a rapid onset of action (30–60 minutes), with peak effects occurring after 2–3 hours.[96] It is metabolized by hepatic enzymes cytochrome P450 3A3 and 3A4 with a half-life of about 3–8 hours.[114] Another CCB, amlodipine, does not have a rapid onset of action but has a long half-life, so it is not used in hypertensive emergencies because of the inability to rapidly titrate its effects on hemodynamics.

MINOXIDIL

Mechanism and use. Minoxidil is a direct arteriolar vasodilator, thus making it a potentially useful agent in the treatment of hypertensive urgencies and emergencies.[96,100] Its use, however, is usually reserved as a single dose to control hypertension while continuous-infusion agents are being prepared or when hypertension is resistant to several drug therapies.[14]

Pediatric pharmacokinetics. Peak drug activity occurs within 60 minutes of ingestion, and a half-life of 4 hours ensures rapid drug clearance.[163] Drug elimination primarily occurs through hepatic glucuronidation with secondary renal elimination.

Adverse effects. Common adverse effects of minoxidil include hypotension, hypertrichosis, pancytopenia, water retention, and weight gain.

FENOLDOPAM

Mechanism and use. Although most reports of fenoldopam use in children are aimed at impacting renal function or reversing or preventing renal insufficiency, often in the pediatric congenital heart disease population, the AAP Guidelines identify it as an agent that could have utility in the management of hypertensive crisis.[14,164-166] Fenoldopam is a rapid, direct-acting, continuously infused vasodilator that is specific for dopamine-1 receptors on the arterial vasculature of most solid organs.[164-166]

Pediatric pharmacokinetics. Only one study to date has examined the pharmacokinetics of fenoldopam in pediatric patients, ranging in age from 3 weeks to 12 years.[166] Whereas the effective dose for BP reduction was higher in pediatric patients compared with adults, the overall pharmacokinetic profiles between the two groups did not differ.[166]

Adverse effects. Typical adverse effects of fenoldopam in the pediatric patient population include hypotension and reflex tachycardia.

MONITORING THERAPEUTIC OUTCOMES

Because hypertensive emergencies have a high propensity to cause marked acute morbidity and mortality, hypertensive emergencies should be monitored very closely in an institutional setting (e.g., intensive care unit), whereas the treatment of less severe forms of hypertension can be followed in an outpatient setting. When patients with hypertension are discharged from the hospital, close follow-up should be scheduled to ensure continued adequate BP control, treatment of any underlying disease states, and limitation of adverse drug effects (Table 2).[14]

CONCLUSIONS

Although pediatric hypertension and hypertensive crisis are relatively rare compared with the incidence in adults, they are both important public health concerns because of their ever-increasing incidence as well as their potential to cause damaging effects on the body, particularly in pediatric patients. Knowledge of pediatric hypertension guidelines, potential lifestyle modifications, and pediatric pharmacology of antihypertensive agents is essential to providing high-quality care that is safe and effective for pediatric patients.

A previously healthy, overweight, 5-year-old girl is assessed by her primary care physician at a well child checkup. She weighs 35.9 kg and is in the 95th percentile for height. Repeat blood pressure (BP) measurements at 5-minute intervals include the following: 116/79 mm Hg, 118/78 mm Hg, and 116/80 mm Hg, which are in the range of stage 1 hypertension. Her caregivers describe her as "very active" and report that she is currently taking no pharmacologic agents, neither prescription nor over-the-counter.

1. What are most common underlying causes linked to this patient's hypertension that her physician should investigate? What relevant interventions should her physician make now? Describe interventions such as further diagnostic work-up and/or treatment, including time span for follow-up appointments if necessary.

Her physician should first investigate potential diagnoses linked to secondary hypertension. Examples include renal abnormalities, cardiovascular lesions such as coarctation of the aorta, endocrine or oncologic etiologies, or potential unreported pharmacologic (prescription or over-the-counter) causes. Secondly, her physician should use ambulatory BP measurement (ABPM) for 24 hours before seeing her in the office again in 1–2 weeks. Final investigations before her leaving this office visit should be queries regarding the type, frequency, and duration of physical activity she partakes in each week in addition to her weekly sodium intake and other diet, such as caffeine intake.

The rationale for this approach is that secondary hypertension is much more common in children and should always be ruled out before moving on with any other workup, which is why her physician should search for an underlying etiology first. The possibility also exists that her in-office hypertension could be linked to white coat hypertension, which is the reason for evaluating 24-hour BP results by ABPM. In addition to white coat hypertension, ABPM could also reveal masked hypertension showing the magnitude of her problem could actually be worse than it seems in the office. Finally, because lifestyle modifications would be the first intervention if an underlying cause (secondary hypertension) is not found, it is important to question her caregivers about her current activity level and diet to gauge if there is room for improvement in exercise and sodium intake if ABPM reveals a true diagnosis of hypertension.

Case (continued). A full workup for secondary hypertension reveals no underlying etiology for her high BP, but the 24-hour ABPM still shows stage 1 hypertension. The patient returns to the pediatrician's office 1 week after the ABPM results. Her BP is consistent with the previous clinic visit and ABPM results. Her caregivers do reveal that her favorite activity is watching television and that she rarely goes outside to play, despite their previous reports of her being "very active."

2. What is the best plan of action, including duration for follow-up, to treat this patient's hypertension?

Lifestyle modifications would be the best choice of action at this time. First of all, her health care provider should recommend a minimum of 60 minutes of active play per day, which would likely result in a reduction in her sedentary television watching time. Next, a daily sodium intake limit of 1500 mg, as recommended

for all pediatric ages by the American Heart Association, would be appropriate to counsel the patient's caregiver on to limit this potential cause of hypertension. Her caregivers should be connected with a registered or licensed dietician to assist with an analysis of the patient's current dietary habits as well as recommendations for diet modifications if necessary. The patient should receive a follow-up visit in 1 month.

The rationale for this approach is that lifestyle modifications such as regular physical activity of at least 60 minutes of active play per day, sodium restrictions, and a healthy diet are the primary interventions recommended by the American Academy of Pediatrics (AAP) Guidelines and the European Society of Hypertension (ESH) for stage 1 hypertension in children. The daily maximum sodium intake recommended by the American Heart Association for children of all ages is 1500 mg.

Case (continued). The initiation of lifestyle modifications over a 3-month time period have not had a positive effect on the child's BP. She still meets criteria for stage 1 hypertension after her third monthly clinic visit.

3. What is the best intervention her health care provider should now make?

Pharmacologic therapy is the best option for the patient at this point. Feasible options include drugs from the following classes: angiotensin-converting enzyme (ACE) inhibitors, angiotensin receptor blocker (ARBs), calcium channel blockers (CCBs), or thiazide diuretics. The drug of choice should include one that has an available and affordable liquid preparation that will best promote patient adherence (e.g., limiting the need for several medication administrations per day) as well as maximize safety (e.g., least likely to cause adverse effects) and efficacy. Doses should be initiated at the lowest reported effective dose and titrated slowly until BP is controlled or adverse effects are seen.

The rationale for this approach is based on the AAP Guidelines and ESH, which recommend pharmacologic therapy for stage 1 hypertension when lifestyle modifications are ineffective. No pharmacologic agents have been proven to reduce morbidity or mortality in children, so there is not an agent of choice that is recommended as first line. Agents should be selected based on pertinent patient characteristics while also considering patient adherence and caregiver socioeconomic status (e.g., the ability to pay for potentially expensive medications). The AAP Guidelines recommend initiating pharmacologic therapy at the lowest reported effective dose followed by a slow titration until BP is controlled or adverse effects are seen.

Case (continued). Her health care provider selects lisinopril as the first-line choice for treatment of her hypertension after lifestyle modifications have failed.

4. Select an initial dose and describe the approach to monitoring, the goals of therapy, the initial follow-up period, and potential medication that may be selected if dose titration to maximum reported dose is ineffective.

The initial dose of lisinopril should be 0.07 mg/kg, or 2.5 mg for this patient at her current weight. The drug can be administered as either liquid or tablet formulation. Monitoring variables include BP, serum potassium, and serum creatinine. Goals of therapy include reducing systolic and diastolic BP to less than the 90th percentile for gender, age, and height. Initial follow-up time should be 1 month after lisinopril therapy is initiated. If lisinopril is titrated to the maximum reported dose and is still ineffective at achieving therapeutic goals without significant adverse effects, then options for additional antihypertensive therapy include the addition of a long-acting CCB or thiazide diuretic.

The rationale for this approach is that the initial dose should be the lowest reported safe dose for pediatric patients and then titrated slowly. The lowest reported safe dose for lisinopril is 0.07 mg/kg, which for this 35.9-kg patient equates to 2.5 mg. This dose could be supplied in liquid or tablet form depending on if the patient is able and prefers to take solid dosage forms. Initial follow-up time after initiating pharmacologic therapy recommended by the AAP Guidelines is 3 months (Table 2). Goals of therapy include reducing systolic and diastolic BP into the normotensive range, which is less than the 90th percentile based on gender, age, and height per the AAP Guideline recommendations (Table 2). Although the next choice of therapy could include any antihypertensive agent, preferable agents with the most data in children per the AAP Guidelines include long-acting CCBs (e.g., amlodipine) or thiazide diuretics (hydrochlorothiazide).

REFERENCES

1. Freis ED. Historical development of antihypertensive treatment. In: Laragh JH, Brenner BM, eds. Hypertension: Pathophysiology, Diagnosis, and Management, 2nd ed. New York: Raven Press, 1995:2741-51.
2. Still JL, Cottom D. Severe hypertension in childhood. Arch Dis Child 1967;42:34-9.
3. Labarthe DR. Overview of the history of pediatric blood pressure assessment and hypertension: an epidemiologic perspective. Blood Press Monit 1999;4:197-203.
4. Esunge PM. From blood pressure to hypertension: the history of research. J R Soc Med 1991;84:621.
5. Rames LK, Clarke WR, Connor WE, et al. Normal blood pressure and the evaluation of sustained blood pressure elevation in childhood: the Muscatine study. Pediatrics 1978;61:245-51.
6. Voors AW, Foster TA, Frerichs RR, et al. Studies of blood pressures in children, ages 5-14 years, in a total biracial community: the Bogalusa Heart Study. Circulation 1976;54:319-27.
7. Londe S. Blood pressure standards for normal children as determined under office conditions. Clin Pediatr 1968;7:400-3.
8. Bao W, Threefoot SA, Srinivasan SR, et al. Essential hypertension predicted by tracking of elevated blood pressure from childhood to adulthood: the Bogalusa Heart Study. Am J Hypertens 1995;8:657-65.
9. Lauer RM, Mahoney LT, Clarke WR. Tracking of blood pressure during childhood: the Muscatine study. Clin Exp Hypertens A 1986;8:515-37.
10. Vos LE, Oren A, Bots ML, et al. Does a routinely measured blood pressure in young adolescence accurately predict hypertension and total cardiovascular risk in young adulthood? J Hypertens 2003;21:2027-34.
11. Sun SS, Grave GD, Siervogel RM, et al. Systolic blood pressure in childhood predicts hypertension and metabolic syndrome later in life. Pediatrics 2007;119:237-46.
12. Nelson MJ, Ragland DR, Syme SL. Longitudinal prediction of adult blood pressure from juvenile blood pressure levels. Am J Epidemiol 1992;136:633-45.
13. Kelly RK, Thomson R, Smith KJ, et al. Factors affecting tracking of blood pressure from childhood to adulthood: The childhood determinants of adult health study. J Pediatr 2015;167:1422-28.
14. Flynn JT, Kaelber DC, Baker-Smith CM, et al. Clinical practice guideline for screening and management of high blood pressure in children and adolescents. Pediatrics 2017;140:1-72.
15. Lurbe E, Cifkova R, Cruickshank K, et al. Management of high blood pressure in children and adolescents: recommendations of the European Society of Hypertension. J Hypertens 2009; 27:1719-42.
16. Parati G, Stergiou G, O'Brien E, et al. European Society of Hypertension practice guidelines for ambulatory blood pressure monitoring. J Hypertens 2014;32:1359-66.
17. Norwood VF. Hypertension. Pediatr Rev 2002;23:197-208.
18. de Moaes ACF, Carvalho HB, Siani A, et al. Incidence of high blood pressure in children—Effects of physical activity and sedentary behaviors: The DEFICS study—high blood pressure, lifestyle and children. Int J Cardiol 2015;180:165-70.
19. Flynn JT, Daniels SR, Hayman LL, et al. Update: Ambulatory blood pressure monitoring in children and adolescents—A scientific statement from the American Heart Association. Hypertension 2014;63:1116-35.
20. Chapleau MW, Hajduczok G, Abboud FM. Mechanisms of resetting of arterial baroreceptors: an overview. Am J Med Sci 1988; 295:327-34.
21. Spyer KM. Central nervous mechanisms contributing to cardiovascular control. J Physiol 1994;474:1-19.
22. Persson PB, Ehmke H, Kirchheim HR. Cardiopulmonary-arterial baroreceptor interaction in control of blood pressure. News Physiol Sci 1989;4:56-9.
23. Hainsworth R. Reflexes from the heart. Physiol Rev 1991;71:617-58.
24. Givertz MM. Manipulation of the renin-angiotensin system. Circulation 2001;104:e14-8.
25. Gereau RW, Conn PJ. Presynaptic enhancement of excitatory synaptic transmission by β-adrenergic receptor activation. J Neurophys 1994;72:1438-42.
26. Gantenbein MH, Bauersfeld U, Baenziger O, et al. Side effects of angiotensin converting enzyme inhibitor (captopril) in newborns and young infants. J Perinat Med 2008;36:448-52.
27. Burnier M. Angiotensin II type 1 receptor blockers. Circulation 2001;103:904-12.
28. Grossman E, Messerli FH. High blood pressure: a side effect of drugs, poisons, and food. Arch Intern Med 1995;155:450-60.
29. Saseen JJ. Hypertension. In: Tisdale JE, Miller DA, eds. Drug-Induced Diseases: Prevention, Detection, and Management, 2nd ed. Bethesda, MD: American Society of Health-System Pharmacists, 2010:517-28.
30. Grinsell MM, Norwood VF. At the bottom of the differential diagnosis list: unusual causes of pediatric hypertension. Pediatr Nephrol 2009;24:2137-46.
31. Butani L, Morgenstern BZ. Casual blood pressure methodology. In: Flynn JT, Ingelfinger JR, Portman RJ, eds. Pediatric Hypertension: Clinical Hypertension and Vascular Diseases, 2nd ed. New York: Humana Press, 2011:113-34.
32. Pickering TG, Hall JE, Appel LJ, et al. Recommendations for blood pressure measurement in humans and experimental

animals. Part 1. Blood pressure measurement in humans: a statement for professionals from the subcommittee of professional and public education of the American Heart Association Council on High Blood Pressure Research. Hypertension 2005;45:142-61.

33. Gillman MW, Cook NR. Blood pressure measurement in childhood epidemiological studies. Circulation 1995;92:1049-57.

34. Clark JA, Lieh-Lai MW, Sarnaik A, et al. Discrepancies between direct and indirect blood pressure measurements using various recommendations for arm cuff selection. Pediatrics 2002;110:920-3.

35. Ogedegbe G, Pickering T. Principles and techniques of blood pressure measurement. 2010;28:571-86.

36. James PA, Oparil S, Carter BL, et al. 2014 Evidence-based guideline for the management of high blood pressure in adults: Report from the panel members appointed to the Eighth Joint National Committee (JNC 8). JAMA 2014;311:507-20.

37. Task Force on Blood Pressure Control in Children. Report of the Second Task Force on Blood Pressure Control in Children—1987. National Heart, Lung, and Blood Institute, Bethesda, MD. Pediatrics 1987;79:1-25.

38. Xi B, Zhang M, Zhang T, et al. Simplification of childhood hypertension definition using blood pressure to height ratio among US youths aged 8–17 years, NHANES 1999–2012. Int J Cardiol 2015;180:210-3.

39. Cantinotti M, Giordano R, Scalese M, et al. Strengths and limitation of current pediatric blood pressure nomograms: a global overview with a special emphasis on regional differences in neonates and infants. Hypertens Res 2015;38:577-87.

40. Falkner B, Gidding SS. Is the SPRINT blood pressure treatment target of 120/80 mmHg relevant for children? Hypertension 2016;67:826-8.

41. Kaelber DC, Pickett F. Simple table to identify children and adolescents needing further evaluation of blood pressure. Pediatrics 2009;123:e972-4.

42. Urbina E, Alpert B, Flynn J, et al. Ambulatory blood pressure monitoring in children and adolescents: recommendations for standard assessment: a scientific statement from the American Heart Association Atherosclerosis, Hypertension, and Obesity in Youth Committee of the Council on Cardiovascular Disease in the Young and the Council for High Blood Pressure Research. Hypertension 2008;52:433-51.

43. Welch WP, Yang W, Taylor-Zapata P, et al. Antihypertensive drug use by children: are the drugs labeled and indicated? J Clin Hypertens (Greenwich) 2012;14:388-95.

44. Parker ED, Sinaiko AR, Kharbanda EO, et al. Change in weight status and development of hypertension. Pediatrics 2016; 137:e20151662.

45. Flynn JT. Neonatal hypertension: diagnosis and management. Pediatr Nephrol 2000;14:332-41.

46. Temple ME, Nahata MC. Treatment of pediatric hypertension. Pharmacotherapy 2000;20:140-50.

47. Rao PS. Coarctation of the aorta. Curr Cardiol Rep 2005;7:425-34.

48. Goudevenos JA, Papathanasiou A, Michalis LK. Coarctation of the aorta with lower blood pressure at the right upper extremity. Heart 2002;88:498.

49. American Heart Association Recommendations for Physical Activity in Kids Infographic. Available at https://www.heart.org/en/healthy-living/fitness/fitness-basics/aha-recs-for-physical-activity-in-kids-infographic. Accessed November 30, 2019.

50. Hagberg JM, Goldring D, Ehsani AA, et al. Effect of exercise training on the blood pressure and hemodynamic features of hypertensive adolescents. Am J Cardiol 1983;52:763-8.

51. Hagberg JM, Goldring D, Heath GW, et al. Effect of exercise training on plasma catecholamines and haemodynamics of adolescent hypertensives during rest, submaximal exercise, and orthostatic stress. Clin Physiol 1984;4:117-24.

52. Hagberg JM, Ehsani AA, Goldring D, et al. Effect of weight training on blood pressure and hemodynamics in hypertensive adolescents. J Pediatr 1984;104:147-51.

53. Danforth JS, Allen KD, Fitterling JM, et al. Exercise as a treatment for hypertension in low-socioeconomic-status black children. J Consult Clin Psychol 1990;58:237-9.

54. Hansen HS, Froberg K, Hyldebrandt N, et al. A controlled study of eight months of physical training and reduction of blood pressure in children: the Odense schoolchild study. BMJ 1991; 303:682-5.

55. Black HR, Sica D, Ferdinand K, et al. Eligibility and disqualification recommendations for competitive athletes with cardiovascular abnormalities: Task Force 6: Hypertension: A scientific statement from the American Heart Association and the American College of Cardiology. Circulation 2015132: e298-302.

56. Chiolero A, Bovet P, Paradis G, et al. Has blood pressure increased in children in response to the obesity epidemic? Pediatrics 2007; 119:544-53.

57. Appel LJ, Brands MW, Daniels SR, et al. Dietary approaches to prevent and treat hypertension: a scientific statement from the American Heart Association. Hypertension 2006;47:296-308.

58. American Heart Association [homepage on the Internet]. Dallas: Sodium and Kids. Available at https://sodiumbreakup.heart.org/sodium_and_kids?utm_source=SRI&utm_medium=Heart-Org&utm_term=Website&utm_content=SodiumAndSalt&utm_campaign=SodiumBreakup. Accessed November 30, 2019.

59. Lava SAG, Bianchetti MG, Simonetti GD. Salt intake in children and its consequences on blood pressure. Pediatr Nephrol 2015;30:1389-96.

60. Su S, Wang X, Pollock JS, et al. Adverse childhood experiences and blood pressure trajectories from childhood to young adulthood: the Georgia Stress and Heart Study. Circulation 2015;131:1674-81.

61. Sinaiko AR. Clinical pharmacology of converting enzyme inhibitors, calcium channel blockers and diuretics. J Hum Hypertens 1994;8:389-94.

62. Moser M, Rosendorff C, White WB. Angiotensin-converting enzyme inhibitors and angiotensin II receptor blockers: is there a difference in response and any advantage to using them together in the treatment of hypertension? J Clin Hypertens 2008;10:485-92.

63. Baker-Smith CM, Benjamin DK Jr, Califf RM, et al. Cough in pediatric patients receiving angiotensin-converting enzyme inhibitor therapy or angiotensin receptor blocker therapy in randomized controlled trials. Clin Pharmacol Ther 2010;87:668-71.

64. Main J. Atherosclerotic renal artery stenosis, ACE inhibitors, and avoiding cardiovascular death. Heart 2005;91:548-52.

65. Burnier M. Angiotensin II type 1 receptor blockers. Circulation 2001;103:904-12.

66. Flynn JT, Meyers KEC, Neto JP, et al. Efficacy and safety of the angiotensin receptor blocker valsartan in children with hypertension aged 1 to 5 years. Hypertension 2008;52:222-8.

67. Blumer J, Batisky DL, Wells T, et al. Pharmacokinetics of valsartan in pediatric and adolescent subjects with hypertension. J Clin Pharmacol 2009;49:235-41.

68. Giordano U, Cifra B, Giannico S, et al. Mid-term results, and therapeutic management, for patients suffering hypertension after surgical repair of aortic coarctation. Cardiol Young 2009; 19:451-5.

69. Wells TG, Portman R, Norman P, et al. Safety, efficacy, and pharmacokinetics of telmisartan in pediatric patients with hypertension. Clin Pediatr 2010;49:938-46.

70. Hazan L, Rodriguez OAH, Bhorat AE, et al. A double-blind, dose-response study of the efficacy and safety of olmesartan medoxomil in children and adolescents with hypertension. Hypertension 2010;55:1323-30.

71. Tocci G, Volpe M. Olmesartan medoxomil for the treatment of hypertension in children and adolescents. Vasc Health Risk Manag 2011;7:177-81.

72. Webb NJA, Wells TG, Shahinfar S, et al. A randomized, open-label, dose-response study of losartan in hypertensive children. Clin J Am Soc Nephrol 2014;9:1441-8.

73. Sullivan JE, Keefe D, Zhou Y, et al. Pharmacokinetics, safety profile, and efficacy of aliskiren in pediatric patients with hypertension. Clin Pediatr (Phila) 2013;52:599-607.

74. Aliskiren tablets [package insert]. Noden Pharma USA Inc., November 2016.

75. Flynn JT, Pasko DA. Calcium channel blockers: pharmacology and place in therapy of pediatric hypertension. Pediatr Nephrol 2000;15:302-16.

76. Radford D. Side effects of verapamil in infants. Arch Dis Child 1983;58:465-6.

77. Epstein ML, Kiel EA, Victorica BE. Cardiac decompensation following verapamil therapy in infants with supraventricular tachycardia. Pediatrics 1985;75:737-40.

78. Flynn JT, Nahata MC, Mahan JD, et al. Population pharmacokinetics of amlodipine in hypertensive children and adolescents. J Clin Pharmacol 2006;46:905-16.

79. Flynn JT. Efficacy and safety of prolonged amlodipine treatment in hypertensive children. Pediatr Nephrol 2005;20:631-5.

80. Kornbluth A, Frishman WH, Ackerman M. β-Adrenergic blockade in children. Cardiol Clin 1987;5:629-49.

81. Haeusler G. Pharmacology of beta-blockers: classical aspects and recent developments. J Cardiovasc Pharmacol 1990;16:S1-9.

82. Eades SK, Christensen ML. The clinical pharmacology of loop diuretics in the pediatric patient. Pediatr Nephrol 1998;12:603-16.

83. Senzaki H, Kamiyama M, Masutani S, et al. Efficacy and safety of torsemide in children with heart failure. Arch Dis Child 2008; 93:768-71.

84. Hein OV, Staegemann M, Wagner D, et al. Torsemide versus furosemide after continuous renal replacement therapy due to acute renal failure in cardiac surgery patients. Ren Fail 2005;27:385-92.

85. Wells TG, Fasules JW, Taylor BJ, et al. Pharmacokinetics and pharmacodynamics of bumetanide in neonates treated with extracorporeal membrane oxygenation. J Pediatr 1992;121:974-80.

86. Sullivan JE, Witte MK, Tamashita TS, et al. Dose-ranging evaluation of bumetanide pharmacodynamics in critically ill infants. Clin Pharmacol Ther 1996;60:424-34.

87. Khan NA, Campbell NR. Thiazide diuretics in the management of hypertension. Can J Clin Pharmacol 2004;11:e41-4.

88. Shah S, Khatri I, Freis ED. Mechanism of antihypertensive effect of thiazide diuretics. Am Heart J 1978;95:611-8.

89. Pickkers P, Hughes AD, Russel FGM, et al. Thiazide-induced vasodilation in humans is mediated by potassium channel activation. Hypertension 1998;32:1071-6.

90. Brater DC. Diuretic therapy: clinical pharmacology of diuretics. Drug Ther 1998;339:387-95.

91. Sica DA. Centrally acting antihypertensive agents: an update. J Clin Hypertens 2007;9:399-405.

92. Jain R, Segal S, Kollins SH, et al. Clonidine extended-release tablets for pediatric patients with attention-deficit/hyperactivity disorder. J Am Acad Child Adolesc Psychiatry 2011;50:171-9.

93. Kollins SH, López FA, Vince BD, et al. Psychomotor functioning and alertness with guanfacine extended release in subjects with attention-deficit/hyperactivity disorder. J Child Adolesc Psychopharmacol 2011;21:111-20.

94. Berde CB, Sethna NF. Analgesics for the treatment of pain in children. N Engl J Med 2002;247:1094-103.

95. Honey BL, Benefield RJ, Miller JL, et al. Alpha2-receptor agonists for treatment and prevention of iatrogenic opioid abstinence syndrome in critically ill patients. Ann Pharmacother 2009; 43:1506-11.

96. Flynn JT, Tullus K. Severe hypertension in children and adolescents: pathophysiology and treatment. Pediatr Nephrol 2009; 24:1101-12.

97. Jacobs M. Mechanism of action of hydralazine on vascular smooth muscle. Biochem Pharmacol 1984;33:2915-9.

98. Bang L, Nielsen-Kudsk JE, Gruhn N, et al. Hydralazine-induced vasodilation involves opening of high conductance Ca2+-activated K+ channels. Eur J Pharmacol 1998;361:43-9.

99. Strife CF, Quinlan M, Waldo FB, et al. Minoxidil for control of acute blood pressure elevation in chronically hypertensive children. Pediatrics 1986;78:861-5.

100. Pennisi AJ, Takahashi M, Bernstein BH. Minoxidil therapy in children with severe hypertension. J Pediatr 1977;90:813-9.

101. The ALLHAT Officers and Coordinators for the ALLHAT Collaborative Research Group. Major cardiovascular events in hypertensive patients randomized to doxazosin versus chlorthalidone: the antihypertensive and lipid-lowering treatment to prevent heart attack trial (ALLHAT). JAMA 2000;283:1967-75.

102. Varon J, Marik PE. The diagnosis and management of hypertensive crises. Chest 2000;118:214-27.

103. Marik PE, Varon J. Hypertensive crises: challenges and management. Chest 2007;131:1949-62.

104. Patel HP, Mitsnefes M. Advances in the pathogenesis and management of hypertensive crisis. Curr Opin Pediatr 2005; 17:210-4.

105. Constantine E, Linakis J. The assessment and management of hypertensive emergencies and urgencies in children. Pediatr Emerg Care 2005;21:391-9.

106. Fivush B, Neu A, Furth S. Acute hypertensive crises in children: emergencies and urgencies. Curr Opin Pediatr 1997;9:233-6.

107. Porto I. Hypertensive emergencies in children. J Pediatr Health Care 2000;14:312-7.

108. Suresh S, Mahajan P, Kamat D. Emergency management of pediatric hypertension. Clin Pediatr 2005;44:739-45.

109. Vaughan CJ, Delanty N. Hypertensive emergencies. Lancet 2000; 356:411-17.

110. Endo H, Shiraishi H, Yanagisawa M. Afterload reduction by hydralazine in children with a ventricular septal defect as determined by aortic input impedance. Cardiovasc Drugs Ther 1994; 8:161-6.

111. Houston MC. Treatment of hypertensive emergencies and urgencies with oral clonidine loading and titration: a review. Ann Intern Med 1986;146:586-9.

112. Flynn JT, Warnick SJ. Isradipine treatment of hypertension in children: a single-center experience. Pediatr Nephrol 2002;17:748-53.

113. Strauser LM, Groshong T, Tobias JD. Initial experience with isradipine for the treatment of hypertension in children. South Med J 2000;93:287-93.

114. Miyashita Y, Peterson D, Rees JM, et al. Isradipine for treatment of acute hypertension in hospitalized children and adolescents. J Clin Hypertens 2010;12:850-5.

115. Johnson CE, Jacobsen PA, Song MH. Isradipine therapy in hypertensive pediatric patients. Ann Pharmacother 1997;31:704-7.

116. López-Herce J, Dorao P, de la Oliva P, et al. Dosage of nifedipine in hypertensive crises of infants and children. Eur J Pediatr 1989;149:136-7.

117. Varon J. Treatment of acute severe hypertension: current and newer agents. Drugs 2008;68:283-97.

118. Davies DW, Greiss L, Kadar D, et al. Sodium nitroprusside in children: observations on metabolism during normal and abnormal responses. Can Anaesth Soc J 1975;22:553-60.

119. Grossman E, Ironi AN, Messerli FH. Comparative tolerability profile of hypertensive crisis treatments. Drug Saf 1998;19:99-122.

120. Benitz WE, Malachowski N, Cohen RS, et al. Use of sodium nitroprusside in neonates: efficacy and safety. J Pediatr 1984; 106:102-10.

121. Moffett BS, Price JF. Evaluation of sodium nitroprusside toxicity in pediatric cardiac surgical patients. Ann Pharmacother 2008;42:1600-4.

122. Kunathai S, Sholler GF, Celermajer JM, et al. Nitroprusside in children after cardiopulmonary bypass: a study of thiocyanate toxicity. Pediatr Cardiol 1989;10:121-4.

123. López-Herce J, Borrego R, Bustinza A, et al. Elevated carboxy-hemoglobin associated with sodium nitroprusside treatment. Intensive Care Med 2005;31:1235-8.

124. Meyer S, Baghai A, Sailer NL, et al. Lactic acidosis caused by sodium nitroprusside in a newborn with congenital heart disease. Eur J Pediatr 2005;164:253-4.

125. Morocco AP. Cyanides. Crit Care Clin 2005;21:691-705.

126. Przybylo HJ, Stevenson GW, Schanbacher P, et al. Sodium nitroprusside metabolism in children during hypothermic cardiopulmonary bypass. Anesth Analg 1995;81:952-6.

127. Thomas C, Svehla L, Moffett BS. Sodium nitroprusside induced cyanide toxicity in pediatric patients. Expert Opin Drug Saf 2009;8:599-602.

128. Hammer GB, Lewandowski A, Drover DR, et al. Safety and efficacy of sodium nitroprusside during prolonged infusion in pediatric patients. Pediatr Crit Care Med 2015;16:397-403.

129. Cole PV, Vesey CJ. Sodium thiosulphate decreases blood cyanide concentrations after the infusion of sodium nitroprusside. Br J Anaesth 1987;59:531-5.

130. Schulz V, Roth B. Detoxification of cyanide in a newborn child. Klin Wochenschr 1982;60:527-8.

131. Vesey CJ, Krapez JR, Varley JG, et al. The antidotal action of thiosulfate following acute nitroprusside infusion in dogs. Anesthesiology 1985;62:415-21.

132. Treluyer JM, Hubert P, Jouvet P, et al. Intravenous nicardipine in hypertensive children. Eur J Pediatr 1993;152:712-4.

133. Flynn JT, Mottes TA, Brophy PD, et al. Intravenous nicardipine for treatment of severe hypertension in children. J Pediatr 2001;139:38-43.

134. Milou C, Debuche-Benouachkou V, Semama DS, et al. Intravenous nicardipine as a first-line antihypertensive drug in neonates. Intensive Care Med 2000;26:956-8.

135. Nakagawa TA, Sartori SC, Morris A, et al. Intravenous nicardipine for treatment of postcoarctectomy hypertension in children. Pediatr Cardiol 2004;25:26-30.

136. Michael J, Groshong T, Tobias JD. Nicardipine for hypertensive emergencies in children with renal disease. Pediatr Nephrol 1998;12:40-2.

137. Gouyon JB, Geneste B, Semama DS, et al. Intravenous nicardipine in hypertensive preterm infants. Arch Dis Child 1997;76:F126-7.

138. McBride BF, White CM, Campbell M, et al. Nicardipine to control neonatal hypertension during extracorporeal membrane oxygen support. Ann Pharmacother 2003;37:667-70.

139. Tenney F, Sakarcan A. Nicardipine is a safe and effective agent in pediatric hypertensive emergencies. Am J Kidney Dis 2000;35:E20.

140. Labetalol hydrochloride injection [package insert]. Bedford, OH: Bedford Laboratories, 2000.

141. Thomas CA, Moffett BS, Wagner JL, et al. Safety and efficacy of intravenous labetalol for hypertensive crisis in infants and small children. Pediatr Crit Care Med 2011;12:28-32.

142. Bunchman TE, Lynch RE, Wood EG. Intravenously administered labetalol for treatment of hypertension in children. J Pediatr 1992;120:140-4.

143. Adamson PC, Rhodes LA, Saul JP, et al. The pharmacokinetics of esmolol in pediatric subjects with supraventricular arrhythmias. Pediatr Cardiol 2006;27:420-7.

144. Tabbutt S, Nicolson SC, Adamson PC, et al. The safety, efficacy, and pharmacokinetics of esmolol for blood pressure control immediately after repair of coarctation of the aorta in infants and children: a multicenter, double-blind, randomized trial. J Thorac Cardiovasc Surg 2008;136:321-8.

145. Wiest DB, Trippel DL, Gillette PC, et al. Pharmacokinetics of esmolol in children. Clin Pharmacol Ther 1991;49:618-23.

146. Vincent RN, Click LA, Williams HM, et al. Esmolol as an adjunct in the treatment of systemic hypertension after operative repair of coarctation of the aorta. Am J Cardiol 1990;65:941-3.

147. Trippel DL, Wiest DB, Gillette PC. Cardiovascular and antiarrhythmic effects of esmolol in children. J Pediatr 1991;119:142-7.

148. Cuneo BF, Zales VR, Blahunka PC, et al. Pharmacodynamics and pharmacokinetics of esmolol, a short-acting beta-blocking agent in children. Pediatr Cardiol 1994;15:296-301.

149. Wiest DB, Garner SS, Uber WE, et al. Esmolol for the management of pediatric hypertension after cardiac operations. J Thorac Cardiovasc Surg 1998;115:890-7.

150. Esmolol hydrochloride [package insert]. Bedford, OH: Bedford Laboratories, 2008.

151. Knowles HJ, Tian Y, Mole DR, et al. Novel mechanism of action for hydralazine: induction of hypoxia-inducible factor-1 alpha, vascular endothelial growth factor, and angiogenesis by inhibition of prolyl hydroxylases. Circ Res 2004;95:162-9.

152. Etteldorf JN, Smith JD, Tharp CP, et al. Hydralazine in nephritic and normal children with renal hemodynamic studies. AMA Am J Dis Child 1955;89:451-62.

153. Flynn JT, Bradford MC, Harvey EM. Intravenous hydralazine in hospitalized children and adolescents with hypertension. J Pediatr 2016;168:88-92.

154. Lönnqvist PA, Bergendahl HTG, Eksborg S. Pharmacokinetics of clonidine after rectal administration in children. Anesthesiology 1994;81:1097-101.

155. Almenrader N, Larsson P, Passariello M, et al. Absorption pharmacokinetics of clonidine nasal drops in children. Pediatr Anesth 2009;19:257-61.

156. Wells TG, Bunchman TE, Kearns GL. Treatment of neonatal hypertension with enalaprilat. J Pediatr 1990;117:664-7.

157. Rouine-Rapp K, Mello DM, Hanley FL, et al. Effect of enalaprilat on postoperative hypertension after surgical repair of coarctation of the aorta. Pediatr Crit Care Med 2003;4:327-32.

158. Nakamura H, Ishii M, Sugimura T, et al. The kinetic profiles of enalapril and enalaprilat and their possible developmental changes in pediatric patients with congestive heart failure. Clin Pharmacol Ther 1994;56:160-8.

159. Sluysmans T, Styns-Cailteux M, Tremouroux-Wattiez M, et al. Intravenous enalaprilat and oral enalapril in congestive heart failure secondary to ventricular septal defect in infancy. Am J Cardiol 1992;70:959-62.

160. Griebenow R, Kaufmann W, Krämer L, et al. Isradipine: a new calcium antagonist with strong vasodilatory but negligible cardiodepressive effects. J Cardiovasc Pharmacol 1990;15:S84-6.

161. Houtman P. Management of hypertensive emergencies in children. Pediatr Perinat Drug Ther 2005;5:107-10.

162. Herbert CJ, Vidt DG. Hypertensive crises. Prim Care Clin Office Pract 2008;35:475-87.

163. Gottlieb TB, Thomas RC, Chidsey CA. Pharmacokinetic studies of minoxidil. Clin Pharmacol Ther 1972;13:436.

164. Strauser LM, Pruitt RD, Tobias JD. Initial experience with fenoldopam in children. Am J Ther 1999;6:283-8.

165. Costello JM, Thiagarajan RR, Dionne RE, et al. Initial experience with fenoldopam after cardiac surgery in neonates with an insufficient response to conventional diuretics. Pediatr Crit Care Med 2006;7:28-33.

166. Hammer GB, Verghese ST, Drover DR, et al. Pharmacokinetics and pharmacodynamics of fenoldopam mesylate for blood pressure control in pediatric patients. BMC Anesthesiol 2008;8:6.

167. Kelland EE, McAuley LM, Filler G. Are we ready to use aliskiren in children? Pediatr Nephrol 2011;26:473-7.

168. Chan JC, Cockram CS, Critchley JA. Drug-induced disorders of glucose metabolism: mechanisms and management. Drug Saf 1996;15:135-57.

169. Hussain T, Greenhalgh K, McLeod KA. Hypoglycaemic syncope in children secondary to beta-blockers. Arch Dis Child 2009;94:968-9.

170. Rybak LP. Pathophysiology of furosemide ototoxicity. J Otolaryngol 1982;11:127-33.

171. Shine NP, Coates H. Systemic ototoxicity: a review. East Afr Med J 2005;82:536-9.

172. Smith SM, Anderson SD, Wen S, et al. Lack of correlation between thiazide-induced hyperglycemia and hypokalemia: subgroup analysis of results from the pharmacogenomic evaluation of antihypertensive responses (PEAR) study. Pharmacotherapy 2009;29:1157-65.

173. Huen SC, Goldfarb DS. Adverse metabolic side effects of thiazides: implications for patients with calcium nephrolithiasis. J Urol 2007;177:1238-43.

174. Carter BL. Preventing thiazide-induced hyperglycemia: opportunities for clinical pharmacists. Pharmacotherapy 2008;28:1425-8.

175. Grimm RH Jr, Leon AS, Hunninghake DB, et al. Effects of thiazide diuretics on plasma lipids and lipoproteins in mildly hypertensive patients: a double-blind controlled trial. Ann Intern Med 1981;94:7-11.

176. Weidmann P, de Courten M, Ferrari P. Effect of diuretics on the plasma lipid profile. Eur Heart J 1992;13:61-7.

177. Flynn JT. Pediatric use of antihypertensive medications: much more to learn. Curr Ther Res Clin Exp 2001;62:314-28.

178. Blowey DL. Antihypertensive agents: mechanisms of action, safety profiles, and current uses in children. Curr Ther Res Clin Exp 2001;62:298-313.

179. Rocchini AP. Childhood hypertension: etiology, diagnosis, and treatment. Pediatr Clin North Am 1984;31:1259-73.

180. Aronoff GR, Berns JS, Brier ME, et al. Drug Prescribing in Renal Failure: Dosing Guidelines for Adults, 5th ed. Philadelphia: American College of Physicians, 2007.

181. Flynn JT. Not ready for prime time: aliskiren for treatment of hypertension or proteinuria in children. Pediatr Nephrol 2011;26:491-2.

182. McMurray JJV, Abraham WT, Dickstein K, et al. Aliskiren, ALTITUDE, and the implications for ATMOSPHERE. Eur J Heart Fail 2012;14:341-3.

183. Baile GR, Mason NA. Dialysis of Drugs: 2012. Saline, MI: Renal Pharmacy Consultants, 2012.

184. Olmesartan medoxomil tablets [package insert]. Tokyo: Daiichi Sankyo, 2009.

185. Valsartan tablets [package insert]. Basel/Novartis Pharmaceuticals, February 2012.

186. Balaguru D, Auslender M. Vasodilators in the treatment of pediatric heart failure. Prog Pediatr Cardiol 2000;12:81-90.

Section IV

Pulmonary Disorders

CHAPTER 11

Neonatal Respiratory Distress Syndrome and Bronchopulmonary Dysplasia

Kimberly Le Dinh, Pharm.D.

INTRODUCTION

Premature neonates commonly have complications with respiratory development and function. Respiratory distress syndrome (RDS) is a respiratory disorder caused by pulmonary surfactant deficiency. Pulmonary surfactant prevents alveolar collapse by facilitating optimal gas exchange and preventing respiratory failure. Neonates with RDS have lung immaturity that often requires oxygen supplementation and mechanical ventilation, both of which are risk factors for the development of bronchopulmonary dysplasia (BPD), a chronic lung disease of infancy in which the lung is characterized by inflammation and fibrosis. Treatment options and supportive therapies for RDS and BPD have significantly improved neonatal outcomes and survival.

RESPIRATORY DISTRESS SYNDROME

Respiratory distress syndrome, historically known as *hyaline membrane disease*, is a lung condition of prematurity. It was a common cause of neonatal morbidity and mortality before the discovery of exogenous pulmonary surfactant several decades ago. Because RDS is considered a developmental disorder, the risk of RDS increases dramatically with decreasing gestational age and birth weight. Maternal steroid use before delivery promotes the maturation of the neonatal surfactant system to decrease the severity and incidence of RDS by up to 60%, depending on gestational age.[1] Even with antenatal interventions, about 50% of infants born before 30 weeks' gestational age and 25% of infants born after 30 weeks' gestational age will develop RDS.[2] Furthermore, surfactant therapy has significantly reduced the incidence of death and BPD in premature infants with RDS.

PATHOPHYSIOLOGY

Pulmonary surfactant acts to lower surface tension at the air–liquid interface in the alveoli to prevent alveolar collapse. A sufficient amount of surfactant to sustain normal lung function is not acquired until the end of the saccular phase (Figure 1) of lung development, which occurs around 36 weeks' gestational age.[3,4] An inadequate production or impaired release of pulmonary surfactant because of prematurity will result in RDS at birth. For comparison, premature infants have one-tenth of the surfactant pool versus term neonates (10 mg/kg vs. 100 mg/kg, respectively).[5] Consequently, inadequate surfactant production leads to atelectasis, a complete or partial collapse of the lung, and impaired gas exchange.

Surfactant consists of highly organized lipid and surfactant proteins in the following concentrations: saturated phosphatidylcholine (50%), unsaturated phosphatidylcholine (20%), natural lipids (8%), phosphatidylglycerol (8%), other phospholipids (6%), and surfactant proteins (8%).[5] Although each surfactant protein has a specific function (Table 1), the critical components required for normal respiratory function are phosphatidylcholine, surfactant protein B, and surfactant protein C. An immature lung has lower percentages of these components, hindering the premature infant from adequately lowering the surface tension to allow adequate gas

Table 1. Functions of Surfactant Proteins

Surfactant Protein	Function
A	Hydrophilic; regulates turnover of pulmonary surfactant, formation of tubular myelin, and immunity
B	Hydrophobic; involved in formation of tubular myelin; facilitates improvement in surfactant surface activity
C	Improves spreadability and surfactant surface activity
D	Involved in bacterial opsonization

exchange within the alveoli. The severity of RDS is dictated by the extent of lung injury as a result of progressive atelectasis and ventilation–perfusion mismatch. The pathogenesis of lung damage may be further complicated by a structurally immature lung, pulmonary edema, and impaired alveolar ventilation.

CLINICAL PRESENTATION

Neonates with RDS usually present soon after birth with signs of respiratory distress such as tachypnea, grunting, retractions, and cyanosis.[6] Physical findings may include the use of accessory breathing muscles, nasal flaring, tachycardia, and increasing oxygen requirements. A characteristic chest radiograph shows diffuse reticular–granular opacification with defined large airways. Other neonatal disorders that may present similarly to RDS include early-onset sepsis, transient tachypnea of the newborn, and spontaneous pneumothorax.[6] The diagnosis of RDS is based on the infant's clinical presentation at birth and is supported by findings on the chest radiograph consistent with surfactant deficiency. Infants who are younger than 30 weeks' gestational age or who did not receive antenatal steroids have the highest risk of RDS. Impaired fetal lung maturity leading to RDS is also observed in neonates born to mothers with diabetes.[7]

The clinical course is dictated by the severity of RDS, birth weight, gestational age, and the extent of lung injury. In uncomplicated cases, RDS is transient, and recovery is expected within several days. However, RDS may be complicated by other common neonatal comorbidities such as patent ductus arteriosus and infection. The infant may require supplemental oxygen or prolonged mechanical ventilation, resulting in extensive lung injury with eventual progression to BPD.

TREATMENT

THERAPEUTIC GOALS

The goal of RDS treatment is aimed at rapidly replacing pulmonary surfactant and minimizing the pathologic sequelae of acute pulmonary injury. The initial management of RDS immediately after birth includes early surfactant administration and establishment of adequate ventilation and oxygenation. The desired outcome is limiting the severity of lung injury and reducing the duration of supplemental oxygen or mechanical ventilation with continued efforts to prevent the development of BPD.

NONPHARMACOLOGIC THERAPY

It is critical to establish ventilation and oxygenation promptly after birth to prevent pulmonary vasoconstriction and subsequent atelectasis. Infants usually require supplemental oxygen, continuous positive airway pressure (CPAP), or mechanical ventilation at any time during the clinical

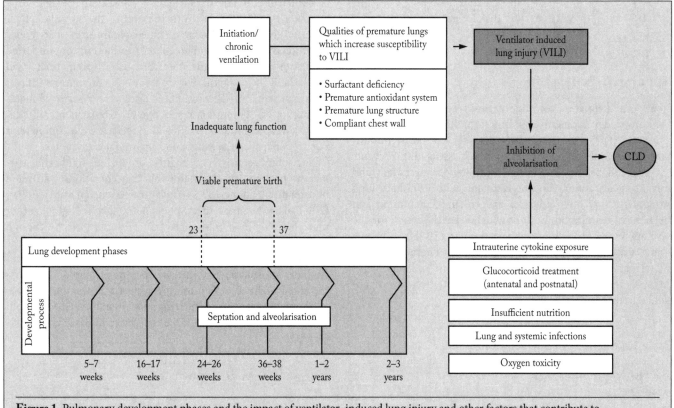

Figure 1. Pulmonary development phases and the impact of ventilator–induced lung injury and other factors that contribute to bronchopulmonary dysplasia (BPD) or chronic lung disease (CLD).

Reprinted with permission from Donn SM, Sinha SK. Minimising ventilator induced lung injury in preterm infants. Arch Dis Child Fetal Neonatal Ed 2006;91:F226-30.

course of RDS. Current evidence indicates that early CPAP is an effective strategy for providing respiratory support for premature infants, even for those who are extremely low birth weight. The early CPAP intervention should be considered as an alternative to routine intubation with surfactant administration and may decrease the need for surfactant administration and mechanical ventilation. However, if the infant subsequently requires surfactant after early CPAP, an increased risk of adverse outcomes has not been demonstrated.[8] In general, CPAP is adequate for mild or moderate RDS and may reduce the need for additional surfactant doses. Supplemental oxygen or mechanical ventilation should be discontinued as soon as tolerated to minimize the risk of BPD.

PHARMACOLOGIC THERAPY

Surfactant replacement therapy. Surfactant therapy is the standard of care for the prophylaxis and treatment of RDS. Systematic reviews have confirmed the many benefits of surfactant replacement, which include decreased ventilation requirements and a reduced incidence in mortality, pneumothorax, and pulmonary interstitial emphysema. Infants younger than 30 weeks' gestational age or with a birth weight of less than 1250 g have the greatest reduction in mortality rates with surfactant therapy.[9] However, the occurrence of other neonatal comorbidities has not changed with the introduction of surfactant.[6,10,11] These comorbidities may include the following: intraventricular hemorrhage, necrotizing enterocolitis, nosocomial infections, retinopathy of prematurity, and patent ductus arteriosus.

Types of surfactant. The two types of exogenous surfactants are *synthetic* and *natural*. Synthetic surfactants contain phospholipids without surfactant proteins.[2] In 2012, the U.S. Food and Drug Administration approved the first synthetic surfactant, lucinactant. However, because lucinactant has been discontinued by the manufacturer and is no longer commercially available, its discussion will not be included in this chapter. Natural surfactants, also known as *animal-derived surfactants*, are modified or purified from bovine or porcine lungs. Systematic reviews show that both synthetic- and animal-derived surfactants are effective in the prophylaxis and treatment of RDS. In addition, neonatal morbidities such as intraventricular hemorrhage, necrotizing enterocolitis and BPD were not significantly different between the two

products.[12] Adverse immunologic or infectious complications with natural surfactant have not been recognized. Animal-derived surfactant is currently considered the mainstay treatment of RDS in clinical practice.[13]

Beractant, calfactant, and poractant alfa are the commercially available animal-derived surfactants in the United States. These products have varying amounts of phospholipids and surfactant proteins B and C. They also differ in viscosity and administration volume (Table 2). All commercially available natural surfactant products are effective for the prevention and treatment of RDS. A systematic literature review of the effectiveness of the animal-derived surfactant identified no significant differences in death or BPD in a comparison of calfactant versus beractant.[14] A meta-analysis showed a significant decrease in mortality with high-dose poractant alfa (200 mg/kg/dose) compared with beractant (100 mg/kg/dose), with the poractant alfa group also requiring fewer total doses.[14,15] Another study demonstrated that treatment with poractant alfa allowed for a quicker weaning of oxygen and ventilatory pressures.[16] In one large database study of 51,282 premature infants, no significant differences were observed between the three animal-derived surfactants when outcomes of air leak syndromes, death, or BPD were adjusted.[17] In another database study of 14,173 subjects evaluating the mortality rate of premature infants with RDS, the unadjusted mortality rate for poractant alfa was 3.61%, beractant was 4.58%, and calfactant was 5.95%. With additional data analysis, the investigators observed that calfactant was associated with a higher mortality compared with poractant alfa and found no statistically significant difference with beractant and poractant alfa.[18] Although conflicting data exist between the animal-derived surfactants, currently no randomized control trials support the superiority of one preparation versus another.

Mechanism of action. Exogenous surfactant replaces deficient or dysfunctional pulmonary surfactant in infants with RDS or premature infants at risk of developing RDS. Surfactant deficiency increases surface tension at the air and alveolar surfaces, leading to alveolar collapse. Because of unopposed surface tension forces, an increase in the work of breathing is required to reinflate the alveoli.[19] Surfactant acts to lower the surface tension at the air–liquid interface to stabilize the alveoli. Once surfactant is instilled and evenly distributed to the distal lung, an acute response occurs within minutes. The exogenous surfactant will decrease the surface tension to allow the lung to inflate at a lower pressure and a

Table 2. A Comparison of the Source, Composition, and Dose of Animal-Derived Surfactants Available in the United States

Surfactant	Animal Source	Phospholipid Concentration (mg/mL)	Initial Dose	Subsequent Doses	Dosing Interval (hr)	Total Number of Doses
			mg of phospholipids/kg (mL/kg)			
Beractant	Bovine	25	100 mg/kg (4 mL/kg)	100 mg/kg (4 mL/kg)	6	4
Calfactant	Bovine	35	105 mg/kg (3 mL/kg)	105 mg/kg (3 mL/kg)	12	4
Poractant alfa	Porcine	80	200 mg/kg (2.5 mL/kg)	100 mg/kg (1.25 mL/kg)	12	3

greater volume, resulting in a rapid oxygenation response. The result is a reduction in the work of breathing, an increase in lung compliance, the resolution of RDS symptoms, and a subsequent reduction in lung injury.

Prophylaxis and rescue therapy. Prophylactic surfactant therapy is surfactant administration within 30 minutes of birth to neonates at high risk of having RDS before the diagnosis of RDS is confirmed. Meanwhile, rescue surfactant therapy is administered to neonates with established RDS within 12 hours of birth. Early rescue therapy is surfactant administration within 1–2 hours of birth, whereas late rescue therapy is administration after 2 hours.[20]

Prophylactic surfactant replacement has the advantage of replacing surfactant before the onset of respiratory symptoms and lung injury. Prophylaxis in premature neonates improves significant clinical outcomes such as death, pneumothorax, and pulmonary interstitial emphysema.[21] However, the impact of prophylactic surfactant administration on the risk of BPD is unclear.[20] A prophylactic approach should be considered in neonates who are at extremely high risk of RDS.[20] The American Academy of Pediatrics strongly recommend that infants born at or earlier than 30 weeks' gestation who have severe RDS requiring mechanical ventilation receive surfactant after initial stabilization.[20] Although these infants will also benefit from rescue surfactant therapy, the prophylactic approach decreases the severity and complications of RDS.[20] Possible clinical risks of a prophylactic approach are unnecessary drug exposure and intubation in infants with respiratory disorders other than RDS (e.g., pulmonary hypoplasia, lung injury).

Few studies have compared prophylactic surfactant therapy with early or late rescue therapy. The limited data show better outcomes with prophylactic administration; however, these therapies were mostly studied in infants who were not exposed to antenatal steroids.[20] Surfactant replacement, either prophylactic or rescue, should occur before or soon after the presentation of RDS to optimize the clinical benefits of drug therapy.

Repeated surfactant doses. Surfactant doses may be repeated up to the recommended maximum number of treatments determined by the surfactant product (Table 2) if persistent respiratory distress is observed 6–12 hours after the initial dose.[22] Infants with lung injury from mechanical ventilation or supplemental oxygen are most likely to benefit from more than a single dose of surfactant because pulmonary edema or inflammation will inhibit surfactant function.[5] A second dose of surfactant may be necessary if the infant continues to need mechanical ventilation with an oxygen requirement (fraction of inspired oxygen [F_{IO_2}]) of greater than 30% or 40%.[23]

Several studies have shown better outcomes with several doses versus a single dose of surfactant in premature infants with RDS.[9,24] A meta-analysis of two trials comparing single versus several doses of surfactant showed a reduction in the incidence of pneumothorax with a trend toward decreased mortality when more than one dose of surfactant was administered.[24] No complications from several surfactant doses were observed in these trials. There is a paucity of data distinguishing the differences in the outcomes of two doses

compared with three or four doses of surfactant. Consensus guidelines recommends subsequent surfactant doses should be administered if the patient demonstrates ongoing RDS with persistent oxygen requirement or a need for mechanical ventilation.[25] Criteria for repeated dosing of surfactant must be further defined to limit unnecessary treatment. The infant should be evaluated after each surfactant administration for signs of clinical improvement, as evidenced by a reduction in oxygen requirement or ventilator support. In general, repeated doses are not indicated if the infant had a favorable improvement in oxygenation and has no significant respiratory distress.

Administration. Surfactant is administered by instilling the solution through a catheter into the endotracheal tube. The volume of medication and number of aliquots depend on the specific surfactant product (Table 2). The neonate may be placed in several positions to facilitate surfactant distribution, which varies according to the manufacturer's guideline for the individual products. For example, each dose of beractant is administered in four 1-mL/kg aliquots with the infant in four different positions as follows: (1) inclined slightly downward with the head turned right, (2) inclined slightly downward with the head turned left, (3) inclined slightly upward with the head turned right, and (4) inclined slightly upward with the head turned left. This administration technique ensures a uniform and rapid distribution of surfactant in the lungs. Mechanical ventilation can be reduced when administering surfactant by using the INSURE technique: INtubate the patient, administer SURfactant and Extubate to CPAP or nasal intermittent positive pressure ventilation or soon after. This method is better tolerated in older and more mature newborns, and the method of administration is selected based on clinical judgement.[25] Complications can occur with transient airway obstruction or inappropriate instillation into the right mainstem bronchus or esophagus, so administration should be performed with the guidance of a trained clinical expert, such as a respiratory therapist.

Monitoring variables and adverse effects. Improvements in lung volume and compliance occur rapidly after surfactant administration. Close observation is critical because the infant may require prompt mechanical ventilation changes to prevent further lung injury and pneumothorax. Although considered a well-tolerated therapy, surfactant may cause adverse effects such as apnea, bradycardia, and oxygen desaturation. An uncommon complication of surfactant therapy is pulmonary hemorrhage, with infants who have an extremely low birth weight at the highest risk.[20,24] Future research should focus on optimizing surfactant preparations, minimizing acute lung injury, and exploring noninvasive administration techniques to reduce short- and long-term complications of RDS, such as the development of BPD.

BRONCHOPULMONARY DYSPLASIA

Bronchopulmonary dysplasia is often the pulmonary sequelae of RDS and the most common cause of morbidity in surviving premature neonates in the United States.[26-28] Also referred to as *chronic lung disease of infancy*, BPD begins with any neonatal disorder that causes postnatal respiratory failure requiring long-term mechanical ventilatory or supplemental oxygen support. Both the underlying condition and the treatment interventions for neonatal respiratory failure contribute to airway inflammation, leading to chronic airflow obstruction and hyperreactivity in the infant with BPD.[29] Neonates born younger than 30 weeks' gestational age or weighing less than 1500 g have the highest risk of BPD. Of the premature neonates born under 1500 g—about 1.5% of all newborns in the United States—around 45% will develop BPD or will die before 36 weeks' postmenstrual age.[30]

PATHOPHYSIOLOGY

The premature lung is most susceptible to lung injury during the saccular stage of lung development between 24 and 36 weeks' gestation. At this stage, lung structure and function are immature, increasing the likelihood of lung injury and disruption of alveolarization.[31] Mechanical ventilation is the primary cause of acute lung injury because of an overdistention of the immature airspaces. This cellular and interstitial lung injury triggers the release of proinflammatory cytokines, resulting in increased alveolar permeability and leakage of protein and water. In addition, high concentrations of oxygen produce free radicals and subsequent damage to the lung parenchyma in the underdeveloped respiratory epithelium and antioxidant defense system.[32] Airway hyperactivity, smooth muscle hypertrophy, and bronchoconstriction are characteristic of the acute stage of BPD. This period occurs during the first few weeks of life after early lung injury, generally around 28–36 weeks' postmenstrual age. The progression to chronic BPD, which occurs after 36 weeks' postmenstrual age, is marked by pulmonary fibrosis and muscularization, leading to a reduction in lung compliance and impairment of gas exchange.[33,34] Other factors that may contribute to the pathophysiology of BPD include the following: infection, steroids, surfactant deficiency, insufficient nutrition, premature lung structure, and oxygen toxicity (Figure 1). Unfortunately, knowledge is very limited regarding the time to complete resolution of BPD, which may last several months to years.[33]

CLINICAL PRESENTATION

Neonates with BPD often present with chronic respiratory signs such as tachypnea, shallow breathing, and retractions. Coarse rhonchi, diffuse rales, and wheezes are heard on auscultation. Chest radiograph often reveals diffuse haziness and lung hypoinflation.[35] The severity of BPD is related to the degree of injury to the airways and distal lung. Neonates with moderate to severe BPD may have acute episodes of pulmonary decompensation, bronchoconstriction, or reversible bronchospasm triggered by worsening pulmonary function. Acute exacerbations are described as a combination of an increased work of breathing or oxygen requirement and the presence of apnea or bradycardia. These episodes may be related to infections, severe airway reactivity, increased pulmonary edema, or the development of tracheobronchomalacia. In addition, BPD may be accompanied by cardiovascular abnormalities (e.g., cardiomegaly), emphysema, pulmonary fibrosis, or lung hyperexpansion.[36] Although BPD is primarily a respiratory disease, short- and long-term complications could involve many systems, including pulmonary hypertension, cardiac dysfunction (e.g., cor pulmonale), poor neurodevelopment, and poor growth in severe cases.[37]

A diagnosis of BPD is made if the neonate continues to require supplemental oxygen or respiratory support at 28 days of life and/or 36 weeks' postmenstrual age.[36] The National Institute of Child Health and Human Development, and the National Heart, Lung and Blood Institute further categorize the disease into mild, moderate, or severe BPD on the basis of gestational age (younger than 32 weeks or age 32 weeks or older), oxygen requirement (FIO_2 of less than 30% or FIO_2 of 30% or greater), or need for positive-pressure ventilation.[38] The greatest risk factors for BPD are prematurity, chronic exposure to mechanical ventilation, and prolonged oxygen supplementation.[39]

TREATMENT

THERAPEUTIC GOALS

Infants often present in acute exacerbation with tachypnea, retractions, or wheezing. The therapeutic goal is an overall improvement in clinical symptoms by minimizing further lung injury and complications, decreasing oxygen requirements, and achieving optimal nutrition for adequate lung growth.

NONPHARMACOLOGIC THERAPY

Mechanical ventilation and supplemental oxygen. Infants with severe BPD often require prolonged ventilator support. Although mechanical ventilation contributes greatly to lung injury, the infant may require respiratory support in the acute phase of BPD during the first several weeks after preterm birth.[40] Ventilator adjustments should be made accordingly to avoid hyperventilation while maintaining appropriate oxygen saturations and adequate gas exchange.[41]

The preferred ventilatory support technique is CPAP because it does not require intubation and mechanical ventilation.[42] Neonates can be weaned off CPAP to supplemental oxygen alone as pulmonary function improves. In the chronic phase and more severe form of BPD, weaning ventilator settings is usually not possible until the neonate shows good growth and a steady weight gain. If the neonate can maintain oxygen saturations at more than 90% during periods of sleep, feedings, and activity, then a trial off supplemental oxygen can be considered. Eventually adequate oxygenation can be maintained with room air as BPD improves or resolves.

Fluid restriction. Pulmonary edema decreases lung compliance and increases the need for mechanical ventilatory support. High fluid intake or inadequate urine output places the neonate at a greater risk of pulmonary edema.[43] Restricting fluid volume from medications or nutrition may help counteract the pulmonary lung injury and capillary leak seen in BPD. In a randomized study of infants weighing less than 1751 g, investigators compared the control group having a fluid intake of 200 mL/kg/day with a restricted group having a fluid intake of 150 mL/kg/day after the first week of life. A significant difference in mortality and BPD, defined by imaging findings, clinical symptoms, and oxygen requirement at

1 month of life, was observed with the group receiving fluid at 150 mL/kg/day.[44] One argument is that the study was quite liberal with the fluid restriction because 150 mL/kg/day could be considered the standard maintenance fluid intake, not a restricted amount in neonate.[36] Although it is uncertain whether fluid restriction less than 150 mL/kg/day provides additional benefit, fluid intake should be kept at the minimum required for optimal growth and adequate urine output to avoid pulmonary edema.[44,45]

PHARMACOLOGIC THERAPY

Most treatment modalities are aimed at improving the clinical symptoms of infants with BPD. Multidrug therapy typically includes diuretics, bronchodilators, and corticosteroids. However, the exact mechanism and safety of these drug therapies are not well studied and have not been shown to reverse pulmonary injury in the BPD population. Currently, there is no optimal agent or regimen for the prevention and treatment of BPD, and an evidence-based treatment guideline does not exist. In addition to the patient's disease severity, the risks of treatment and potential adverse events must be considered before initiating pharmacologic therapy.

Diuretics. Diuretics are often used in neonates with BPD to improve pulmonary function to increase pulmonary compliance by decreasing pulmonary resistance and interstitial lung fluid.[36,46] A transient improvement in gas exchange and reduction in oxygen requirement are observed when diuretics are administered to a neonate with BPD.[47] Diuretics are usually considered when the neonate with BPD cannot be weaned off aggressive respiratory support or has cardiac failure.[48] They are also useful when fluid restriction causes nutritional compromise and inadequate delivery of calories to promote lung growth. The common classes of diuretics used in BPD are loop and thiazide diuretics.[49]

The loop diuretic used most often in neonates is furosemide, a potent diuretic that acts in the ascending loop of Henle and distal tubule.[50] Around 25% of the filtered

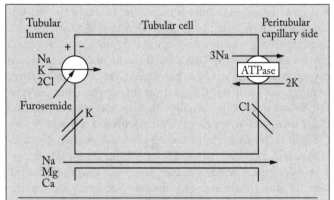

Figure 2. Furosemide binds to the chloride site of the sodium/potassium/chloride cotransporter in the tubule lumen to cause increased excretion of water, sodium, chloride, magnesium, and calcium.

Reprinted with permission from Moghal NE, Shenoy M. Furosemide and acute kidney injury in neonates. Arch Dis Child Fetal Neonatal Ed 2008;93:F313-6.

sodium is reabsorbed to cause significant diuresis (Figure 2). Furosemide is thought to be effective in BPD by increasing plasma oncotic pressure and lymphatic flow while decreasing interstitial edema and pulmonary vascular resistance. A single dose of intravenous furosemide (1 mg/kg/dose) acutely improved pulmonary mechanics compared with placebo in a study of 10 infants with chronic BPD who were not dependent on oxygen. Airway resistance was significantly decreased 1 hour after the furosemide dose. However, this effect returned to baseline values after 2 hours.[51] Age appears to be a contributing factor in the beneficial response of furosemide in infants with BPD. In a systematic study of premature neonates with, or developing, BPD who received intravenous or oral furosemide, no benefits were detectable in neonates younger than 3 weeks. However, in neonates and infants older than 3 weeks, the acute and chronic administration of furosemide improved lung compliance, airway resistance, and oxygenation for at least 1 hour after the furosemide dose.[50] Although short-term improvements in pulmonary mechanics have been observed, there is no current evidence that furosemide improves clinically significant outcomes such as mortality or decreases the incidence of BPD.[46]

Chronic therapy with a loop diuretic may present several complications, including electrolyte disturbances, osteopenia, and ototoxicity.[36] Hypokalemia, hyponatremia, and contractional metabolic alkalosis are often observed in clinical practice, and supplementation with potassium chloride is usually required. Furosemide also increases urinary calcium excretion, which could lead to nephrocalcinosis and nephrolithiasis in infants.[52] Although rare, ototoxicity and transient deafness are possible when furosemide is used chronically or in conjunction with other ototoxic medications such as aminoglycosides. Inhaled furosemide has been studied in BPD as a result of complications seen with systemic diuretics. Because of the limited body of evidence and conflicting results related to pertinent clinical outcomes, the routine use of inhaled furosemide in infants with BPD is not recommended.[53,54]

Thiazide diuretics act in the distal convoluted tubule, where active reabsorption of only 4% to 8% of filtered sodium, chloride, and calcium occurs. Thiazide diuretics also improve pulmonary mechanics in premature neonates and infants with BPD who are older than 3 weeks.[55] The two most extensively studied thiazide diuretics in neonates are chlorothiazide and hydrochlorothiazide. These agents are useful in the pharmacologic armamentarium for neonates or infants experiencing complications or tolerance of furosemide. Electrolyte abnormalities may be observed, but to a considerably lesser degree than with furosemide therapy. Nephrocalcinosis is usually not seen because less calcium resorption occurs with a thiazide than with a loop diuretic.[46] Although less potent and modestly effective compared with furosemide, hydrochlorothiazide or chlorothiazide may be a better alternative for the chronic management of BPD because of its more favorable adverse effect profile.[47,55]

Loop diuretics are most beneficial in the acute BPD phase, and thiazide diuretics are often used in ventilator-dependent infants with chronic BPD when fluid restriction is ineffective. However, whether the chronic use of diuretics improves important clinical outcomes remains to be seen.[46] The duration of diuretic therapy depends on individual responses to diuretics and improvement in symptoms during acute exacerbations. Close monitoring of electrolyte abnormalities is important, and appropriate electrolyte supplementation is required during diuretic therapy.

Inhaled bronchodilators. Bronchodilators act to dilate the small airways caused by muscle hypertrophy observed in moderate or severe BPD.[29,56] They improve airway hyperactivity that causes flow limitation and obstruction through narrowing of the bronchi and may be effective as an adjunctive therapy for the treatment of acute exacerbations to obtain a short-term resolution of symptoms. Two classes of inhaled bronchodilators used in BPD are β-agonists and anticholinergic agents.[1] However, the use of bronchodilators has not been well studied, and their impact on the course of BPD has not been elucidated.[36]

β-Agonists acutely improve pulmonary resistance and lung compliance through bronchial smooth muscle relaxation. Unfortunately, these effects are short term, with a return to baseline 4 hours after drug administration. In a double-blind, placebo-control study of 173 ventilator-dependent neonates younger than 31 weeks' gestation, albuterol did not show any difference in important outcomes such as mortality, chronic lung disease, or duration of ventilator support.[57] Adverse effects of inhaled β-agonists include hypokalemia, tachycardia, hypertension, and arrhythmias.

Inhaled anticholinergic agents such as atropine and ipratropium block the action of acetylcholine in bronchial smooth muscle, resulting in bronchodilation. Adverse effects of inhaled anticholinergic agents are dyspnea, palpitations, dyspepsia, and upper respiratory tract infections. Ipratropium is a more potent bronchodilator than atropine with a more favorable adverse effect profile.[58] Although rarely used in clinical practice, an inhaled anticholinergic may be a therapeutic option in addition to β-agonist therapy to improve symptomatic and reversible airway obstruction. Synergy occurs by interfering with vagal-mediated bronchoconstriction.[58]

In the chronic stage, lung pathology becomes fibrotic and less sensitive to the effects of inhaled therapy; thus, a positive response to inhaled bronchodilators may not be observed in all infants.[56] To ensure optimal drug therapy, a spacer and mask should be used when delivering bronchodilators through a metered dose inhaler. Routine or chronic use of inhaled bronchodilators is not recommended but may be considered if short-term clinical improvements (e.g., resolution of airway obstruction) are observed. The long-term efficacy of bronchodilators in BPD has not been studied, and their effects on lung development, prevention of exacerbations, and improvement of the quality of life remain to be seen.[48]

Corticosteroids. Airway inflammation in BPD suggests a beneficial role for systemic and inhaled corticosteroids. Corticosteroids decrease inflammation by suppressing neutrophil migration and production of inflammatory mediators. Their use in neonatal lung disease was first reported in the 1950s; then in the 1980s and 1990s they became commonly used in practice.[59] The decision to use corticosteroids to treat BPD remains controversial because of their high-risk potential and long-term consequences.

Dexamethasone is the first well-studied corticosteroid in the management of BPD for its potent anti-inflammatory properties. Short-term treatment with dexamethasone reduces the need for supplemental oxygen, with no difference in mortality before hospital discharge.[52] A higher incidence of growth failure, hyperglycemia, hypertension, and hypertrophic cardiomyopathy has been noted in infants treated with dexamethasone. Follow-up data in the late 1990s showed an increased risk of neurodevelopmental consequences. Neonates who received a 4-week course of dexamethasone within 12 hours of birth had twice the risk of cerebral palsy compared with the control group.[60] The most common dexamethasone dosing regimen studied was 0.5 mg/kg/day divided in two doses for 3 days, followed by 0.25 mg/kg/day for 3 days, 0.12 mg/kg/day for 3 days, and 0.05 mg/kg/day for 3 days. These corticosteroid doses were discovered to be relatively high-potency and may have contributed to the harmful neurodevelopmental outcomes.[61-63] The use of dexamethasone for BPD is no longer routinely recommended because of the significant risk of long-term neurodevelopmental sequelae, especially when initiated within the first week of life.

Data on the adverse effects of dexamethasone have led to studies with other corticosteroids, specifically hydrocortisone, for the treatment and prevention of BPD. In a retrospective study evaluating the short- and long-term outcomes of hydrocortisone- and dexamethasone-tapering regimens, both corticosteroids showed effectiveness in decreasing oxygen requirements. Follow-up at age 5–7 years found that children treated with hydrocortisone had better neurodevelopmental outcomes than those treated with dexamethasone and needed less special education resources at school.[64] A double-blind, placebo-control, multicenter, randomized trial evaluated the use of low-dose hydrocortisone (1 mg/kg for 7 days with a 3-day wean) initiated at birth in 573 extremely preterm neonates. Investigators observed that the hydrocortisone group had a higher rate of survival without BPD compared with placebo (60% vs. 51%) but with an increased risk of late onset sepsis in the 24–25 weeks' gestation group who received hydrocortisone (40% vs. 23%); the long-term neurologic outcomes were not evaluated.[65] Although hydrocortisone appears to have a better adverse effect profile and could be a strategy for the prevention of BPD, evidence remains insufficient to establish an evidence-based approach to the use of systemic glucocorticoids in BPD.

Systematic reviews evaluated the use of systemic corticosteroids in the neonatal population at early days of life (7 or less days) and late (more than 7 days) to decrease the risk of BPD in preterm neonates.[66,67] The use of early steroids to prevent BPD demonstrated a reduction of the failure to extubate, BPD, patent ductus arteriosus, and retinopathy of prematurity whereas no difference was found in rates of mortality. Adverse effects reported included the following: gastrointestinal bleeding, intestinal perforation, hyperglycemia, hypertension, hypertrophic cardiomyopathy, and growth failure.[66] The use of steroids after 1 week of life to ameliorate the evolving lung injury sequencing and to facilitate extubation demonstrated a decrease in neonatal mortality at 28 days with no decrease in mortality at 36 weeks, at discharge, or at latest reported age. In addition, a trend toward increased risk of infection and gastrointestinal bleeding was observed.[67] Clinical judgment to balance the potential benefits of corticosteroid treatment and its adverse effects will need to be considered. The routine use of steroids for the prevention and treatment of BPD in preterm infants is not recommended by the American Academy of Pediatrics.[68] Therapy may be reasonable for ventilator-dependent infants with exceptional BPD on maximum support in which hydrocortisone may be lifesaving; however, there is insufficient evidence to recommend the use of systemic corticosteroids for all infants.[68]

Inhaled corticosteroids such as budesonide and fluticasone could improve short-term pulmonary exacerbations with minimal systemic absorption; however, evidence is limited for their role in treating chronic BPD.[69,70] Its use in the prevention of BPD is discussed in the next section.

PREVENTION

The most effective means of preventing BPD is the prevention of prematurity, RDS, and subsequent lung injury. However, several pharmacologic therapies have been investigated to prevent BPD development (Table 3). These therapies remain largely controversial without many control studies, but they could be effective in combination with other preventive strategies. The clinician should weigh the risks and benefits of each preventive modality.

VITAMIN A

Vitamin A is essential for tissue differentiation and cell growth. Premature neonates with extremely low birth weights have inherently low plasma concentrations of vitamin A, possibly predisposing these infants to BPD. In a meta-analysis, supplementation with vitamin A may reduce death or oxygen requirement at age 1 month and the risk of BPD at 36 weeks' postmenstrual age.[71] A multicenter, randomized trial evaluated the effectiveness of vitamin A supplementation in 807 infants with birth weights between 401 g and 1000 g who were ventilator- or oxygen-dependent at 24 hours of life.[72] Vitamin A (5000 international units) was administered three times per week intramuscularly for 4 weeks. The vitamin A group had a significant reduction in mortality or BPD at age 36 weeks (55% vs. 62%). Infants with birth weights less than 1000 g may benefit from vitamin A supplementation to decrease the risk of BPD.

INHALED CORTICOSTEROIDS

Inhaled corticosteroids may enhance the maturation of the pulmonary system with less adverse effects than systemic corticosteroids. In a large, randomized, placebo-control trial in 863 extremely preterm neonates between 23 weeks' and 27 weeks' gestational age, neonates received placebo or inhaled budesonide two puffs (800 mcg) every 12 hours in the first 2 weeks of life and one puff (400 mcg) every 12 hours from day 15 until the neonate no longer required supplemental oxygen and positive pressure support, or until a postmenstrual age of 32 weeks was reached, regardless of ventilator status. The primary outcome was BPD, which was observed in 27.8% of infants in the inhaled budesonide group compared with 38% in the placebo group (p=0.004).[70] In a follow-up study at a corrected age of 18 to 22 months, the investigators found no difference in neurodevelopmental disability in the infants assigned to inhaled budesonide (48.1%) versus placebo (51.4%, p=0.4); however, more deaths were observed in the inhaled budesonide group (19.9% vs. 14.5%, p=0.04).[73] The investigators attributed this finding to nominal statistical significance and observed that most infants had died in the first weeks of life. Based on the current available evidence, the routine use of inhaled corticosteroids for the prevention of BPD is not recommended, especially with the concern for increased mortality.

INHALED NITRIC OXIDE

Inhaled nitric oxide (iNO) may prevent BPD in premature neonates at high risk of developing the disease by decreasing ventilation–perfusion mismatch, reducing inflammation, and restoring normal growth in the premature lung. A multicenter, randomized study involving 793 premature neonates with respiratory failure requiring mechanical ventilation evaluated the effectiveness of low-dose iNO (5 parts per million [ppm]) or placebo for 21 days.[74] There was no difference in the incidence of mortality or BPD between the two groups (71.6% vs. 75.3%). However, neonates with a birth weight greater than 1000 g had a 50% reduction in the incidence of BPD; thus, initiation of low-dose iNO may be beneficial in this weight group. Another randomized study of 294 premature neonates who received decreasing concentrations of iNO for a minimum of 24 days (starting dose of 20 ppm) showed a difference in survival rate without BPD (43.9% vs. 36.8%) when iNO was

Table 3. Medications Studied for the Prevention of Bronchopulmonary Dysplasia

Medication	Administration Route	Dosing	Therapy Duration	Adverse Effects
Vitamin A	Intramuscular	5000 international units 3 times/week	28 days	Allergic reactions (rare)
Nitric oxide	Inhalation	20 ppm for 2–3 days; then decrease to doses of 10, 5, and 2 ppm at weekly intervals	24 days	Hypotension Rebound syndrome
Caffeine citrate	Oral, intravenous	Loading dose: 20–25 mg/kg/dose Maintenance dose: 5–10 mg/kg/day	Until apnea of prematurity resolves	Failure to gain weight Jitteriness Hyperreflexia Seizures

ppm = parts per million.

initiated between age 7 and 21 days.[75] The use of iNO for BPD prevention is not routinely recommended in clinical practice by the National Institutes of Health because of inconclusive evidence and overall cost of therapy.

CAFFEINE CITRATE

Caffeine is a respiratory stimulant in premature neonates and is effective in the treatment of apnea of prematurity (as detailed in the Apnea of Prematurity chapter). A large, international, randomized, placebo-control trial of caffeine citrate was conducted in 2006 infants with birth weights of 500–1250 g.[76] Eligible patients received an intravenous loading dose of caffeine citrate of 20 mg/kg, followed by a maintenance dose of 5 mg/kg or normal saline. The daily maintenance dose was increased to a maximum of 10 mg/kg if apneic episodes persisted. Although BPD was not the primary outcome assessed, a significant reduction in BPD was observed in the caffeine group. Of the 963 infants in the caffeine group who survived at 36 weeks' postmenstrual age, significantly fewer infants in the caffeine group developed BPD compared with infants in the control group (36.3% vs. 46.9%). The investigators speculated that the reduced incidence in BPD was a result of the decreased duration of supplemental oxygen and positive-pressure ventilation observed in the caffeine group. Caffeine citrate should be routinely used in all premature infants at risk of severe apnea. It could prevent the need for invasive mechanical ventilation and progression of BPD.

DISCHARGE PLANNING

Neonates with BPD may be ready for discharge if their respiratory status is stable during periods of sleep, feeding, or activity without significant oxygen desaturation. Although supplemental oxygen is often discontinued before discharge from the neonatal intensive care unit, home oxygen therapy is available and may be offered with periodic assessment of oxygen saturation.[34] Parents should learn about cardiopulmonary resuscitation techniques, signs of decompensation, equipment use, medication administration, and nutritional guidelines before discharge. Infants with BPD are at high risk of long-term pulmonary complications.[76] They should receive routine vaccinations, including pneumococcal and influenza vaccines, and prophylaxis for respiratory syncytial virus with palivizumab (as detailed in the Pediatric Vaccines chapter and the Lower Respiratory Tract Infections chapter).[54]

CONCLUSIONS

The discovery of surfactant has significantly improved the morbidity and mortality of premature neonates with RDS. Because of the improved survival of these neonates, the rate of BPD has also increased.[60] Although several strategies have been proposed to prevent and treat BPD, an evidence-based approach should be used when managing this vulnerable population. Future research should be aimed at identifying optimal treatment strategies to improve the long-term outcomes of premature neonates with RDS and BPD.

Patient Case

RESPIRATORY DISTRESS AND BRONCHOPULMONARY DYSPLASIA IN A PREMATURE NEWBORN

A premature neonate was born at 24 weeks' gestation (birth weight: 780 g) to a 37-year-old mother. At delivery, the neonate had signs of severe respiratory distress and cyanosis. The premature neonate received surfactant and required mechanical ventilation with high ventilator settings. Currently, the patient is age 8 weeks (current weight 1.9 kg) and is having difficulty weaning from mechanical ventilation. A recent chest radiograph shows several cystic regions and lung disease consistent with bronchopulmonary dysplasia (BPD).

Maternal history: Predelivery steroids and magnesium; cesarean delivery because of premature membrane rupture

Medical history: Observed to be limp and nonvigorous at delivery; intubated at delivery and transferred to neonatal intensive care unit for

additional management; Apgar scores at 1, 5, and 10 minutes were 1, 4, and 7, respectively

Family history: No family history available

Allergies: No known drug allergies

Current medications: Caffeine

citrate 19 mg/day (10 mg/kg/day) intravenously

Current nutrition: Donor breast milk at 50 mL/kg/day (advance as tolerated); total parenteral nutrition at 4 mL/hour (50 mL/kg/day); fat emulsion at 1.2 mL/hour (15 mL/kg/day)

1. What is the role of surfactant therapy for this patient at birth? What medication and dosage regimen should be initiated and how should the maximum number of doses be determined?

This patient was born premature at 24 weeks and would benefit from surfactant therapy (i.e., beractant, calfactant, poractant). Surfactant should be administered within 30 minutes of birth because the risk of respiratory distress syndrome (RDS) in this patient is high. Surfactant replacement therapy is the standard of care for the prophylaxis and treatment of RDS. Systematic reviews have confirmed the many benefits of surfactant replacement, which include decreased ventilation requirements and a reduced incidence in mortality, pneumothorax, and pulmonary interstitial emphysema. Infants younger than 30 weeks' gestational age or with a birth weight of less than 1250 g have the greatest reduction in mortality rates with surfactant therapy. Subsequent surfactant doses should be administered if the patient demonstrates ongoing RDS with persistent oxygen requirement or a need for mechanical ventilation.

2. What medication and dosage regimen should be used for the prevention of BPD in this patient and why?

Patient is on caffeine citrate at a dose of 10 mg/kg/day, which may significantly reduce BPD. Vitamin A supplementation is administered for the prevention of BPD. Although vitamin A is not on the patient's current medication list, vitamin A (5000

international units intramuscularly three times per week) would be started at birth for 4 consecutive weeks. Premature neonates with extremely low birth weights have inherently low plasma concentrations of vitamin A, possibly predisposing these infants to BPD. Inhaled nitric oxide (iNO) may prevent BPD in premature patients at high risk of developing the disease by decreasing ventilation–perfusion mismatch, reducing inflammation, and restoring normal growth in the premature lung. These three pharmacologic strategies coupled with respiratory support may lessen the severity or incidence of BPD.

3. What medication should be used for the treatment of BPD in this patient and why?

Furosemide 1.9 mg (1 mg/kg/dose) intravenously once or twice daily is indicated to manage the clinical symptoms of BPD because this patient cannot be weaned off aggressive respiratory support. Furosemide is the most commonly studied diuretic in BPD. The administration of a loop diuretic results in diuresis, a decrease in total lung water, and improvement in lung function. Diuretic therapy should be accompanied by fluid restriction while balancing nutritional requirements and delivery of calories to promote lung growth. This patient is receiving around 115 mL/kg/day of enteral and intravenous nutrition. An evaluation of total parenteral nutrition components may allow for further fluid restriction of the rate of total parenteral nutrition without sacrificing macronutrients.

REFERENCES

1. Roberts D, Brown J, Medley N, et al. Antenatal corticosteroids for accelerating fetal lung maturation for women at risk of preterm birth. Cochrane Database Syst Rev 2017;3:CD004454.
2. Ramanathan R. Surfactant therapy in preterm infants with respiratory distress syndrome and in near-term or term newborns with acute RDS. J Perinatol 2006;26:S51-6.
3. Donn SM, Sinha SK. Minimising ventilator induced lung injury in preterm infants. Arch Dis Child Fetal Neonatal Ed 2006;91:F226-30.
4. Peterson SW. Understanding the sequence of pulmonary injury in the extremely low birth weight, surfactant-deficient infant. Neonatal Netw 2009;28:221-9.
5. Jobe AH. Why surfactant works for respiratory distress syndrome. NeoReviews 2006;7:95-106.
6. Soll RF, Ozek E. Prophylactic protein free synthetic surfactant for preventing morbidity and mortality in preterm infants. Cochrane Database Syst Rev 2010;1:CD001079.
7. Reuter S, Moser C, Baack M. Respiratory distress in the newborn. Pediatr Rev 2014;35:417-29.
8. American Academy of Pediatrics Committee on Fetus and Newborn. Respiratory support in preterm infants at birth. Pediatrics 2014;133:171-4.
9. Liechty EA, Donovan E, Purohit D, et al. Reduction of neonatal mortality after multiple doses of bovine surfactant in low birth weight neonates with respiratory distress syndrome. Pediatrics 1991;88:19-28.
10. Soll RF. Prophylactic natural surfactant extract for preventing morbidity and mortality in preterm infants. Cochrane Database Syst Rev 2000;2:CD000511.
11. Soll RF. Synthetic surfactant for respiratory distress syndrome in preterm infants. Cochrane Database Syst Rev 2000;2:CD001149.
12. Ardell S, Pfister RH, Soll R. Animal derived surfactant extract versus protein free synthetic surfactant for the prevention and treatment of respiratory distress syndrome. Cochrane Database Syst Rev 2015;8:CD000144.
13. Soll RF, Blanco F. Natural surfactant extract versus synthetic surfactant for neonatal respiratory distress syndrome. Cochrane Database Syst Rev 2001;2:CD000144.
14. Singh N, Halliday HL, Stevens TP, et al. Comparison of animal-derived surfactants for the prevention and treatment of respiratory distress syndrome in preterm infants. Cochrane Database Syst Rev 2015;12:CD010249.
15. Singh N, Hawley KL, Viswanathan K. Efficacy of porcine versus bovine surfactants for preterm newborns with respiratory distress syndrome: systematic review and meta-analysis. Pediatrics 2011;128:e1588-95.
16. Ramanathan R. Animal-derived surfactants: where are we? The evidence from randomized, controlled clinical trials. J Perinatol 2009;29:S38-43.
17. Trembath A, Hornik P, Clark R, et al. Comparative effectiveness of surfactant preparations in premature infants. J Pediatr 2013;163:955.
18. Ramanathan R, Bhatia JJ, Sekar K, et al. Mortality in preterm infants with respiratory distress syndrome treated with poractant alfa, calfactant or beractant: a retrospective study. J Perinatol 2013;33:119.
19. Kendig JW, Shapiro DL. Surfactant therapy in the newborn. Pediatr Ann 1988;17:504-7.
20. Polin RA, Carlo WA; Committee on Fetus and Newborn. Surfactant replacement therapy for preterm and term neonates with respiratory distress. Pediatrics 2014;133:156-63.
21. Rojas-Reyes MS, Morley CJ, Soll RF. Prophylactic versus selective use of surfactant in preventing morbidity and mortality in preterm infants. Cochrane Database Syst Rev 2012;3:CD000510.
22. Suresh GK, Soll RF. Overview of surfactant replacement trials. J Perinatol 2005;25:S40.
23. Gal P, Shaffer CL. Acute respiratory distress syndrome. In: DiPiro JT, Talbert RL, Yee GC, et al., eds. Pharmacotherapy: A Pathophysiologic Approach. New York: Elsevier, 2017.
24. Soll R, Ozek E. Multiple versus single doses of exogenous surfactant for the prevention or treatment of neonatal respiratory distress syndrome. Cochrane Database Syst Rev 2009;1:CD000141.
25. Sweet DG, Carnielli V, Greisen G, et al. European consensus guidelines on the management of neonatal respiratory distress syndrome in preterm infants—2016 update. Neonatology 2017; 111:107-25.
26. Walsh MC, Yao Q, Gettner P, et al. Impact of a physiologic definition of bronchopulmonary dysplasia rates. Pediatrics 2004; 114:1305-11.
27. Avery ME, Tooley WH, Keller JB, et al. Is chronic lung disease in low birth weight infants preventable? A survey of eight centers. Pediatrics 1987;79:26-30.
28. Sinkin RA, Cox C, Phelps DL. Predicting risk for bronchopulmonary dysplasia: selection criteria for clinical trials. Pediatrics 1990;86:728-36.
29. Allen J, Zwerdling R, Ehrenkranz R, et al. Statement on the care of the child with chronic lung disease of infancy and childhood. Am J Respir Crit Care Med 2003;1683:356-96.
30. Lapcharoensap W, Gage SC, Kan P, et al. Hospital variation and risk factors for bronchopulmonary dysplasia in a population-based cohort. JAMA Pediatr 2015;169:e143676.
31. Kraybill EN, Runyan DK, Bose CL, et al. Risk factors for chronic lung disease in infants with birth weights of 751 to 1000 grams. J Pediatr 1989;115:115-20.
32. Bonikos DS, Benson KG, Northway WH Jr. Oxygen toxicity in the newborn. The effect of chronic continuous 100 per cent oxygen exposure on the lung of newborn mice. Am J Pathol 1976; 85:623-50.
33. Jobe AH. The new BPD. NeoReviews 2006;7:531-44.
34. Parad RB. Apnea. In: Cloherty JP, Eichenwald EC, Stark AR, eds. Manual of Neonatal Care. Philadelphia: Lippincott Williams & Wilkins, 2016.
35. Toce SS, Farrell PM, Leavitt LA, et al. Clinical and radiographic scoring systems for assessing bronchopulmonary dysplasia. Am J Dis Child 1984;138:581-5.
36. D'Angio CT, Maniscalco WM. Bronchopulmonary dysplasia in preterm infants. Pediatr Drugs 2014;6:303-30.
37. Goodman G, Perkin RM, Anas NG, et al. Pulmonary hypertension in infants with bronchopulmonary dysplasia. J Pediatr 1988; 112:67.
38. Jobe AH, Bancalari E. Bronchopulmonary dysplasia. Am J Respir Crit Care Med 2001;163:1723-9.
39. Northway WH, Rosan RC, Porter DY. Pulmonary disease following respiratory therapy of hyaline membrane disease. N Engl J Med 1967;276:357-68.
40. Deakins KM. Bronchopulmonary dysplasia. Respir Care 2009; 54:1252-62.
41. American Academy of Pediatrics. Supplemental therapeutic oxygen for prethreshold retinopathy of prematurity (STOP-ROP), a randomized, controlled trial. Pediatrics 2000;10:295-310.
42. Ammari A, Suri MS, Milisavljevic V, et al. Variables associated with the early failure of nasal CPAP in very low birth weight infants. J Pediatr 2005;147:341-7.
43. Brown ER, Stark A, Sosenko I, et al. Bronchopulmonary dysplasia: possible relationship to pulmonary edema. J Pediatr 1978; 92:982-4.
44. Tammela OK, Koivisto ME. Fluid restriction for preventing bronchopulmonary dysplasia? Reduced fluid intake during the first weeks of life improves the outcome of low-birth-weight infants. Acta Paediatr 1992;81:207-12.
45. Bell EF, Acarregui MJ. Restricted versus liberal water intake for preventing morbidity and mortality in preterm infants. Cochrane Database Syst Rev 20014;12:CD000503.

46. Ramanathan R. Bronchopulmonary dysplasia and diuretics. NeoReviews 2008;96:260-6.

47. Stewart A, Brion LP. Intravenous or enteral loop diuretics for preterm infants with (or developing) chronic lung disease. Cochrane Database Syst Rev 2011;9:CD001453.

48. Baraldi E, Filippone M. Chronic lung disease after premature birth. N Engl J Med 2007;357:1946-55.

49. Daigle KL, Cloutier MM. Office management of bronchopulmonary dysplasia. Compr Ther 1997;23:656-62.

50. Bestic M, Reed MD. Common diuretics used in preterm and term infant. NeoReviews 2005;6:392-7.

51. Kao LC, Warburton D, Sargent CW, et al. Furosemide acutely decreases airways resistance in chronic bronchopulmonary dysplasia. J Pediatr 1983;103:624-9.

52. Pope JC, Trusler LA, Klein AM, et al. The natural history of nephrocalcinosis in premature infants treated with loop diuretics. J Urol 1996;156:709.

53. Brion LP, Primhak RA, Yong W. Aerosolized diuretics for preterm infants with (or developing) chronic lung disease. Cochrane Database Syst Rev 2006;3:CD001694.

54. Kugelman A, Durand M, Garg M. Pulmonary effect of inhaled furosemide in ventilated infants with severe bronchopulmonary dysplasia. Pediatrics 1997;1:71-5.

55. Stewart A, Brion LP, Abrosio-Perez I. Diuretics acting on the distal renal tubule for preterm infants with (or developing) chronic lung disease. Cochrane Database Syst Rev 2011;9:CD001817.

56. Brundage KL, Mohsini KG, Froese AB, et al. Bronchodilator response to ipratropium bromide in infants with bronchopulmonary dysplasia. Am Rev Respir Dis 1990;142:1137.

57. Denjean A, Paris-Llado J, Zupan V, et al. Inhaled salbutamol and beclomethasone for preventing broncho-pulmonary dysplasia: a randomised double-blind study. Eur J Pediatr 1998;157:926-31.

58. Davis JM, Rosenfeld WN. Bronchopulmonary dysplasia. In: MacDonald MG, Mullett MD, Seshia M, eds. Avery's Neonatology: Pathophysiology & Management of the Newborn. Philadelphia: Lippincott Williams & Wilkins, 2005:578-9.

59. Grier DG, Halliday HL. Management of bronchopulmonary dysplasia in infants. Drugs 2005;65:15-29.

60. Yeh TF, Lin YJ, Huang CC, et al. Early dexamethasone therapy in preterm infants: a follow-up study. Pediatrics 1998;101:E7.

61. Halliday HL, Ehrenkranz RA, Doyle LW. Early postnatal (<96 hours) corticosteroids for preventing chronic lung disease in preterm infants. Cochrane Database Syst Rev 2003;1:CD001146.

62. Halliday HL, Ehrenkranz RA, Doyle LW. Moderately early (7–14 days) postnatal corticosteroids for preventing chronic lung disease in preterm infants. Cochrane Database Syst Rev 2003; 1:CD001144.

63. Halliday HL, Ehrenkranz RA, Doyle LW. Delayed (>3 weeks) postnatal corticosteroids for chronic lung disease in preterm infants. Cochrane Database Syst Rev 2003;1:CD001145.

64. van der Heide-Jalving M, Kamphuis PJ, van der Laan MJ, et al. Short- and long-term effects of neonatal glucocorticoid therapy: is hydrocortisone an alternative to dexamethasone? Acta Paediatr 2003;92:827-35.

65. Baud O, Maury L, Lebail F, et al. Effect of early low-dose hydrocortisone on survival without bronchopulmonary dysplasia in extremely preterm infants (PREMILOC): a double-blind, placebo-controlled, multicenter, randomized trial. Lancet 2016; 387:1827-36.

66. Doyle LW, Cheong JL, Ehrenkraz RA, et al. Early (<8 days) systemic postnatal corticosteroids for prevention of bronchopulmonary dysplasia in preterm infants. Cochrane Database Syst Rev 2017;10:CD001146.

67. Doyle L, Cheong JL, Ehrenkranz R, et al. Late (>7 days) postnatal corticosteroids for chronic lung disease in preterm infants. Cochrane Database Syst Rev 2017;10:CD001145.

68. Watterberg KL, American Academy of Pediatrics. Committee on Fetus and Newborn. Policy statement-postnatal corticosteroids to prevent or treat bronchopulmonary dysplasia. Pediatrics 2010;126:800-8.

69. Shah SS, Ohlsson A, Halliday H, et al. Inhaled versus systemic corticosteroids for the treatment of chronic lung disease in ventilated very low birth weight preterm infants. Cochrane Database Syst Rev 2017;10:CD002058.

70. Bassler D, Plavka R, Shinwell ES, et al. Early inhaled budesonide for the prevention of bronchopulmonary dysplasia. N Engl J Med 2015;373:1497-506.

71. Darlow BA, Graham PJ. Vitamin A supplementation to prevent mortality and short and long-term morbidity in very low birth-weight infants. Cochrane Database Syst Rev 2016;8:CD000501.

72. Tyson JE, Wright LL, Oh W, et al. Vitamin A supplementation for extremely-low-birth-weight infants. N Engl J Med 1999; 340:1962-8.

73. Bassler D, Shinwell ES, Hallman M, et al. Long-term effects of inhaled budesonide for bronchopulmonary dysplasia. N Engl J Med 2018;378:148-57.

74. Kinsella JP, Cutter GR, Walsh WF, et al. Early inhaled nitric oxide therapy in premature newborns with respiratory failure. N Engl J Med 2006;355:354-64.

75. Ballard RA, Truog WE, Cnaan A, et al. Inhaled nitric oxide in preterm infants undergoing mechanical ventilation. N Engl J Med 2006;355:343-53.

76. Schmidt B, Roberts RS, Davis P, et al. Caffeine therapy for apnea of prematurity. N Engl J Med 2006;354:2112-21.

CHAPTER 12

LEARNING OBJECTIVES

1. Describe the clinical presentation and pathophysiology of apnea of prematurity (AOP).

2. Identify nonpharmacologic approaches to the treatment of AOP.

3. Discuss the pharmacologic agents for the treatment of AOP.

4. Evaluate the risks and benefits of treatment modalities aimed at improving the clinical symptoms of infants with AOP.

ABBREVIATIONS IN THIS CHAPTER

AOP   Apnea of prematurity

INTRODUCTION

Apnea, a brief cessation of breathing lasting 5–10 seconds, is common in premature neonates as a manifestation of an immature respiratory control system.[1] These episodes become pathologic when they are prolonged more than 20 seconds.[2] *Apnea of prematurity* (AOP) is defined by the American Academy of Pediatrics as the "cessation of breathing for at least 20 seconds or as a briefer episode of apnea associated with bradycardia, cyanosis, or pallor."[3] Symptomatic neonates may have changes in hemodynamic, ventilation, and oxygenation parameters that are largely dependent on the duration of the apneic episodes.[4-6] If left untreated, AOP has potentially life-threatening or severe neurodevelopmental consequences.[5,7] Nonpharmacologic and pharmacologic treatment strategies have made AOP a manageable condition of prematurity.

EPIDEMIOLOGY

The exact incidence of AOP is unknown because a standardized criterion for the diagnosis of symptomatic apnea is not currently available. However, apnea occurs more often in premature neonates than in term neonates.[8] It is estimated that 70% of premature neonates with a birth weight less than 1500 g will have at least one clinically observed episode of symptomatic apnea while admitted in the neonatal intensive care unit. Around 20% of these neonates will have an identified etiology, and the other 80% will have a nonspecific medical cause of apnea.[9] Because of maturational development, the resolution of apneic episodes typically occurs before 37 weeks' postmenstrual age in neonates born after 28 weeks' gestation. However, infants born before 28 weeks' gestation may have frequent and persistent apnea after 37 weeks' postmenstrual age.[8,10] After 43 weeks' postmenstrual age, severe apneic events are rare and do not occur any more often in premature infants than in healthy term infants.[11]

PATHOPHYSIOLOGY

Three main components are required for normal rhythmic breathing in the neonate: (1) *central respiratory drive*, (2) *maintenance of airway patency*, and (3) *adequate respiratory muscle function*. Consequently, an immature central respiratory drive, a dysfunctional upper airway, and underdeveloped respiratory muscles can precipitate apnea in premature neonates.[12,13] An immature brain stem is the primary reason for hypoventilation and cyanotic episodes in an apneic premature neonate.[14]

Central respiratory control involves a complex interaction of sensory stimulation from the medulla of the brain. The chemoreceptor stimuli are transmitted through the afferent pathways to regulate the respiratory system. In AOP, either an improper transmission of these signals occurs or a lack of appropriate respiratory pump control.[9,15,16]

Maintaining airway patency is challenging in neonates because of immature neuromuscular function and reflexes in the upper airway. This immaturity results in nasal and hypopharyngeal airway obstruction leading to apnea.[17,18]

Overall weakness in the muscles involved in respiration (diaphragm and intercostal muscles) and in the muscles that maintain upper airway patency (larynx and pharynx) can lead to impaired ventilation and oxygenation, resulting in apneic episodes. Because the respiratory system is immature, suck and swallow activity during feeding may also cause apnea and bradycardia, primarily because of inhibitory reflexes triggered by laryngeal receptors.[19] Furthermore, premature neonates have a reduced lung volume, triggering periods of hypoventilation or oxygen desaturation and apnea.[6]

Prolonged apnea will cause a significant decrease in ventilation and subsequent decrease in heart rate. In very premature infants, apnea and bradycardia episodes may precede hypoventilation and oxygen desaturation.[19] *Ventilation-perfusion* match is optimum when the ratio of volume of gas to volume of blood in the lungs is equal. Periods of hypoventilation could lead to ventilation-perfusion mismatching, also resulting in oxygen desaturation. The relationship between apnea, oxygen desaturation, and bradycardia is schematically shown in Figure 1.

CLASSIFICATIONS

The three classifications for apneic episodes are: (1) *central*, (2) *obstructive*, and (3) *mixed*. The absence of airflow movement is observed with central apneas, whereas reduced or no airflow caused by upper airway obstruction is observed with

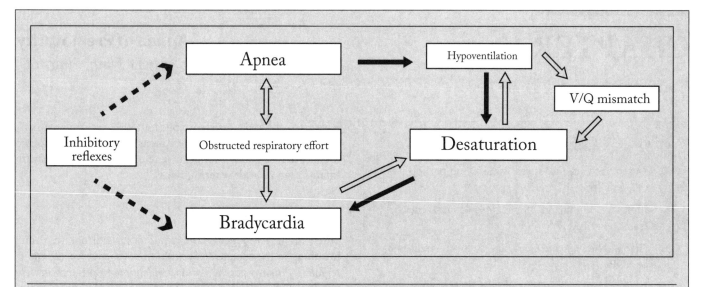

Figure 1. Pathogenesis of apnea of prematurity. The dotted arrows represents the consequences of immature inhibitory reflexes (apnea or bradycardia). Filled arrows represent the most common sequence. Hollow arrows represent pathways that could occur but are not as common.[19]

Reprinted with permission from Macmillan Publishers, Ltd: Mathew OP. Apnea of prematurity: pathogenesis and management strategies. J Perinatol 2001;31:302-10.

obstructive apneas. Mixed apnea is a combination of these effects in which apnea follows airway obstruction with persistent inspiratory efforts.[20] Apnea lasting longer than 20 seconds is very often accompanied by airway obstruction.[21]

One study reviewed 2082 apneic episodes lasting more than 15 seconds in 47 infants younger than 34 weeks' gestational age with idiopathic AOP.[22] The investigators identified that 40% of these episodes were central, 50% were mixed, and 10% were obstructive. A correlation existed with decreased oxygen saturation and increased duration of apnea regardless of the type of apnea or treatment. Infants with central apneas had a higher incidence of bradycardia than infants having mixed or obstructive apneas.

CLINICAL PRESENTATION

The clinical presentation of AOP presents as a transient cessation in respiratory airflow. These short pauses in breathing can persist for 5–20 seconds or more. After about 20 seconds of hypoventilation or apnea, the infant progresses to hypoxemia, and ultimately bradycardia and cyanosis. Pallor and hypotonia may occur after 30–45 seconds of no airflow.[23] All premature infants younger than 35 weeks' gestational age should be monitored for AOP within the first week of life.

Premature infants who are spontaneously breathing without mechanical respiratory support typically present with apnea on the first or second day of life. Infants who require mechanical ventilation at birth may not show symptoms of AOP until ventilator support is discontinued.[24] Apnea presenting after the first week of life in infants who are spontaneously breathing or apnea recurring after 1–2 weeks of an apnea-free period is often associated with a serious underlying condition (such as sepsis or necrotizing enterocolitis), warranting a thorough evaluation for precipitating causes.[10]

DIAGNOSIS

No objective threshold criteria or diagnostic tests currently exist for the diagnosis of AOP. Consequently, the diagnosis is one of exclusion in which causes of secondary apnea should be excluded before initiating treatment for AOP.[9] An extensive evaluation of apneic episodes is required to rule out other conditions (Box 1) to accurately diagnose AOP.[25] Pertinent patient history should include a review of maternal risk factors, medications, and birth history. Findings of lethargy, temperature instability, cyanosis, and respiratory distress are observed through a physical examination. Laboratory studies should include serum electrolytes to rule out metabolic disturbances, a complete blood cell count with differential and platelet count to rule out sepsis and anemia, and an arterial blood gas for evidence of hypoxia. A thorough workup is necessary to identify the precipitating cause of apnea, if present.

Box 1. Common Causes of Neonatal Apnea[6]

Prematurity
Airway abnormalities
Gastroesophageal reflux
Hypoglycemia
Impaired oxygenation
Infection (sepsis, meningitis)
Intracranial pathology (hemorrhage)
Medications (opiates, general anesthesia)
Metabolic disorders (acidosis, electrolyte disturbances)
Maternal drugs (antepartum magnesium sulfate, opiates)
Perinatal asphyxia
Seizures
Temperature instability

If apneic events are persistent and a specific cause has not been identified, electronic cardiorespiratory monitoring may be necessary.[3] Individual apneic episodes are often detected by the presence of three primary symptoms: (1) apnea lasting greater than 20 seconds, (2) bradycardia based on cardiorespiratory monitoring, and (3) oxygen desaturation based on pulse oximetry.[19,20] Evaluation should also include an assessment of breathing regulation while the neonate is sleeping, feeding, and awake. The severity of AOP and the threshold for initiating or adjusting treatment depend on the frequency and severity of clinically observed apneic episodes.[9]

MONITORING AND EVALUATIONS

It is recommended that all premature neonates younger than 35 weeks' gestational age be monitored for at least 1 week after birth because of the higher risk of apneic episodes in this population.[26] Cardiorespiratory monitoring should be performed while the neonate is in the hospital, with assessment during different phases of sleeping, feeding, and alertness. Tactile stimulation usually resolves most apneic episodes in premature neonates. However, some neonates may require assistance with ventilation using a bag and mask when they do not respond to stimulation.[26]

THERAPY GOALS

The primary goal of therapy is to decrease or eliminate the frequency of prolonged apnea lasting greater than 20 seconds or apnea associated with cyanosis and bradycardia. Other causes of apnea must be excluded, and the diagnosis of AOP should be made before initiating an individualized treatment. Treatment is warranted in premature neonates if apneic episodes are frequent and prolonged or if they are associated with hypoxemia and bradycardia.[25] The premature neonate will usually require several weeks of therapy until lung function and central respiratory drive matures until apnea resolves.[8,10] Because apnea is multifactorial in pathophysiology and presentation, a single intervention may not be entirely efficacious, and both nonpharmacologic and pharmacologic therapies may be required for the treatment of AOP.

NONPHARMACOLOGIC THERAPY

Because hypoxemia is a potential cause of apneas, it is reasonable to initiate therapies to improve oxygenation. Supplemental oxygen works to decrease the frequency of hypoxic episodes.[27] Although few approaches have been studied in clinical trials, oxygen saturations generally should be maintained between 85% and 95% to minimize the complications of oxygen toxicity such as retinopathy of prematurity.[28] In addition, transfusion of red blood cells can increase the blood-carrying oxygen capacity, but this treatment approach remains controversial. Cohort studies reporting variable differences in the frequency, severity, or duration of apnea after a blood transfusion are conflicting.[29,30] However, blood transfusions may be considered if the infant also has other comorbidities such as anemia of prematurity, which is common among premature neonates. Therefore, the potential benefits gained from a transfusion should outweigh the complications and hazards of this therapy.

If the cause of apnea is airway obstruction and hypoventilation, strategies to maintain airway patency may be beneficial. For example, positions of extreme flexion or extension of the neck can contribute to upper airway obstruction, and therefore these positions should be avoided.[26] Nasal patency can be preserved by avoiding unnecessary nasal suctioning or nasogastric tubes. Other general measures include preventing reflexes that could trigger apnea and maintaining a stable environmental temperature using a radiant warmer or incubator.[26]

Continuous positive airway pressure, a method of assisted respiratory ventilation often administered with nasal prongs, is effective in decreasing the incidence of mixed and obstructive apnea by opening the upper airways.[27] This method is most useful in neonates younger than 32–34 weeks' postmenstrual age and those with residual lung disease because these groups are most susceptible to pharyngeal collapse.[27,31,32]

If clinically significant apneic episodes accompanied by bradycardia and cyanosis still occur despite optimal drug therapy and continuous positive airway pressure, endotracheal intubation and assisted ventilation may be required as a last-line therapy. This method is not often necessary for the treatment of AOP unless other illnesses such as sepsis or meningitis are present.[26] If significant obstructive or mixed apneic episodes are unresolved, pharmacologic therapy aimed at treating central apneas is essential and should be used in conjunction with nonpharmacologic interventions.

PHARMACOLOGIC THERAPY

METHYLXANTHINES

Methylxanthines, a group of purine alkaloids, have been the mainstay of therapy for AOP since the early 1970s.[33] They stimulate the central respiratory drive to reduce the incidence of apneas and need for mechanical ventilation.[9,34] The most common agents include caffeine citrate, theophylline, and aminophylline (a theophylline salt). Controlled studies comparing aminophylline, theophylline, and caffeine have found them to be comparable in efficacy for the control of AOP.[35,36] However, caffeine remains the standard therapy because of its wide therapeutic index, ease of administration, tolerability, and limited adverse effects. Theophylline and aminophylline are rarely used in clinical practice but are potential alternatives if infants are refractory to caffeine therapy.

MECHANISM OF ACTION

Although methylxanthines are effective and commonly used, their exact mechanism of action in the treatment of AOP is unclear. It is proposed that methylxanthines stimulate the central nervous system, increase carbon dioxide sensitivity, and enhance the force of diaphragmatic contraction.[9] These drugs also initiate some action on the cardiovascular system to increase cardiac output and heart rate while decreasing peripheral vascular resistance.[37]

Methylxanthines are nonspecific inhibitors of adenosine and phosphodiesterase. Adenosine acts to depress the central respiratory drive. Because methylxanthine blocks the action of adenosine, the respiratory drive is enhanced to reduce apneic episodes in neonates.[38] Meanwhile, phosphodiesterase inhibition results in increased levels of cyclic adenosine monophosphate and cyclic guanine monophosphate to relax the airway.[39,40] The combined effects of adenosine and phosphodiesterase inhibition stimulate the central respiratory center to enhance ventilation and blood gas exchange, increase diaphragmatic contractility, and improve upper airway muscle tone.[9]

PHARMACOKINETICS AND DOSING

Pharmacokinetic parameters vary widely in premature and term infants and exhibit high inter-individual variability because of developmental changes in metabolism and excretion.[41] Caffeine and theophylline are extensively metabolized in the liver by cytochrome P450 monooxygenases (CYP1A2) and xanthine oxidase.[37] Metabolism is limited in premature infants because of an immature hepatic enzyme system, but it increases significantly with postnatal age. Metabolic interconversion of active metabolites has been observed in infants. An estimated 3% to 8% of administered caffeine is converted to theophylline, and 25% of administered theophylline is converted to caffeine.[42]

In premature infants, renal excretion is the primary mechanism of elimination for methylxanthines. About 80% of caffeine and its metabolite, theophylline, is excreted unchanged in the urine.[43,44] The half-life of each drug is highly variable and generally decreases in term infants and with postnatal age. Caffeine has an elimination half-life of 52–96 hours compared with theophylline, which has a half-life of 17–43 hours in premature infants.[42,44,45] The longer half-life of caffeine allows for once-daily dosing, which offers an advantage over the multiple-daily dosing required with theophylline and aminophylline. Most studies also recommend a loading dose followed by a maintenance dose. Table 1 lists additional dosing and pharmacokinetic differences between caffeine citrate, theophylline, and aminophylline in neonatal apnea.

THERAPEUTIC DRUG MONITORING

Neonates on theophylline or aminophylline must be closely monitored upon therapy initiation and dose changes. Theophylline at the desired plasma concentrations of 6–12 mg/L provides an adequate clinical response in most infants, although lower concentrations of 3–4 mg/L have also been reported to be effective.[46] The unbound fraction of theophylline is the pharmacologically active compound. Although a neonate and an adult may have the same total theophylline plasma concentration, the unbound concentration is generally higher in the neonate because of reduced protein binding. Therefore, measuring unbound serum theophylline values is recommended in neonates.[47] The narrow therapeutic index requires frequent therapeutic drug monitoring of theophylline to prevent adverse effects or suboptimal therapy.

Theophylline plasma concentrations are recommended before and after a dosage adjustment, after treatment failure, such as an increased frequency of apneas, or with evidence of toxicity.[44,45] Doses should be individualized on the basis of peak levels measured 30 minutes after the end of the bolus infusion and at steady-state concentration, usually after 3 days of therapy. Repeat levels are indicated around 3 days after each dosage titration or weekly if the infant is on a stable maintenance dose.[45] Of importance, patient factors that could potentially affect the clearance and metabolism of theophylline should be carefully observed.[48] For example, anticonvulsants such as phenytoin and phenobarbital are cytochrome P450–inducing agents that can decrease the plasma concentration of theophylline.[49] Because of the substantial individual variability in pharmacokinetics, narrow therapeutic index, and severe toxicity profile with theophylline, therapeutic drug monitoring should be closely followed.

Caffeine, in contrast, exhibits a wide therapeutic index, and therefore routine monitoring of drug concentrations is not typically necessary. Plasma concentrations at usual doses range from 8 mg/L to 20 mg/L. Serious toxicities are rare but have been reported with concentrations greater than 40 mg/L to 50 mg/L.[34,50] Most infants are predicted to reach a therapeutic plasma concentration using the standard recommended caffeine citrate dosing (Table 1). After an oral loading dose of caffeine citrate of 20 mg/kg in preterm neonates, the measured peak plasma concentration for caffeine ranged from 6 mg/L to 10 mg/L.[42] In an observational study of 101 infants, a median caffeine maintenance dose of 5 mg/kg resulted in caffeine concentrations from 3 mg/L to 23.8 mg/L. About 95% of samples resulted in concentrations between 5 mg/L and 20 mg/L, and similar results were observed in patients with renal and liver dysfunction.[51] If clinical response is lacking at high doses or toxicity is suggested, a therapeutic plasma concentration may be considered. The wide therapeutic index without the need to closely follow serum drug values makes caffeine the therapy of choice for AOP.

DURATION OF THERAPY

The optimal time to initiate methylxanthine therapy for AOP has not been established. Some evidence suggests initiating methylxanthine therapy soon after birth in premature infants at high risk of apnea of prematurity. A large retrospective cohort study of premature infants born at less than 31 weeks' gestation found that early caffeine use (within the first 2 days after birth) decreased the odds of a composite outcome of death or bronchopulmonary dysplasia (adjusted odds ratio, 0.81; 95% confidence interval, 0.67–0.98) and patent ductus arteriosus (adjusted odds ratio, 0.74; confidence interval, 0.62–0.89) compared with infants who received caffeine on or after the third day after birth.[52] Further studies are warranted to determine the safety and effectiveness of early prophylactic methylxanthine therapy, especially in infants who require mechanical ventilation. The necessary duration of therapy is highly variable in neonates with AOP and is dependent on the maturity of the brain stem and respiratory control system. Caffeine therapy should be continued until there are no clinically observed apneic episodes for several consecutive days, which is generally observed before 37 weeks' postmenstrual age.[9,26] Because of the long elimination half-life, cardiorespiratory monitoring should continue for about 1 week after discontinuing therapy until the drug is completely eliminated from the body.[26] Consider reinitiating therapy if apnea recurs soon after therapy discontinuation. Clinicians will usually assess postmenstrual age, length of time since the

Table 1. Dosing and pharmacokinetics of caffeine, theophylline, and aminophylline in apnea of prematurity[42,44,45]

Dosing and Pharmacokinetics	Caffeine Citrate	Theophylline and Aminophylline
Route of administration	Oral, intravenous	Theophylline: Oral, intravenous Aminophylline: Intravenous
Loading dose	20–25 (10–12.5 active base) mg/kg/dose	5–6 mg/kg/dose
Maintenance dose	5–10 (2.5–5 active base) mg/kg/day	2–6 mg/kg/day
Dosing interval	Every 24 hours	Every 8–12 hours
Therapeutic plasma concentration (mg/L)	8–20	6–12
Toxic plasma concentration (mg/L)	> 50	> 15
Elimination half-life (hours)	52–96	17–43
Signs of toxicity	Failure to gain weight Restlessness Hyperreflexia Seizures Tachycardia Arrhythmias	Restlessness Vomiting Arrhythmias Seizures Cardiac flutters Tremor

last documented apneic episode, and general clinical status to determine when to discontinue therapy.[9]

ADVERSE EFFECTS

Methylxanthines are generally a safe therapy if caffeine is prescribed within the usual recommended dosing range and theophylline plasma concentrations are carefully monitored. Adverse effects of methylxanthine treatment may include feeding intolerance, sinus tachycardia, diuresis, diaphoresis, and urinary calcium excretion. Severe toxicity can be manifested as hypertonia, cardiac failure, pulmonary edema, metabolic acidosis, and hyperglycemia.[42,44,45] These adverse effects are more commonly observed with theophylline than with caffeine. In addition, dosing changes because of an adverse effect are less likely with caffeine therapy.[53]

CAFFEINE FOR AOP TRIALS

A landmark randomized controlled trial of caffeine citrate in 2006 infants with birth weights of 500–1250 g evaluated the short- and long-term safety and efficacy of methylxanthine therapy.[54] Caffeine citrate was indicated for the prevention or treatment of AOP and the facilitation of endotracheal tube removal. Eligible patients received an intravenous loading dose of caffeine citrate of 20 mg/kg, followed by a maintenance dose of 5 mg/kg or normal saline. The daily maintenance dose was increased to a maximum of 10 mg/kg if apneas persisted. Caffeine was initiated at a median postmenstrual age of 28 weeks and discontinued before 35 weeks' postmenstrual age. The caffeine group discontinued adjunct nonpharmacologic treatments, such as mechanical ventilation and oxygen therapy, 1 week earlier than the placebo group. In addition, the frequency of bronchopulmonary dysplasia, a chronic lung disease of prematurity, was significantly reduced in the caffeine group, 36.3% compared with 46.9%.

The long-term follow-up study at 18–21 months included 937 infants in the caffeine group and 932 infants in the placebo group.[55] Among the primary outcomes assessed were a composite of death, cerebral palsy, cognitive delay, deafness, or blindness at a corrected age of 18–21 months. Significantly fewer infants in the caffeine group died or survived with a neurodevelopmental disability compared with the placebo group (40.2% vs. 46.2%). Treatment with caffeine also showed a reduction in the incidence of cerebral palsy (4.4% vs. 7.3%) and cognitive delay (33.8% vs. 38.3%). There were no differences in rates of death, deafness, and blindness or mean percentiles for height, weight, and head circumference at follow-up between the caffeine and placebo groups.

These trials provide strong evidence that caffeine citrate is a beneficial therapy for AOP. A loading dose of caffeine citrate followed by maintenance dosing has shown favorable short- and long-term outcomes with minimal adverse effects. It also improves survival without neurodevelopmental disability. Although aminophylline, theophylline, and caffeine show similar efficacy for the treatment of AOP, caffeine has been the most rigorously studied and is the mainstay treatment for AOP in clinical practice. It is the preferred pharmacologic treatment for its lower toxicity and longer half-life without the need for routine therapeutic drug monitoring.

DOXAPRAM

Doxapram was one of the first drugs investigated for the treatment of AOP. It is a potent respiratory stimulant that acts on peripheral chemoreceptors and the respiratory center in the medulla.[9] Doxapram has been used in infants with AOP refractory to methylxanthine therapy. Early trials have shown doxapram to be effective in treating infants with neonatal apnea who are unresponsive to methylxanthine therapy.[56,57] However, these studies were small, and additional information is needed to define the role of doxapram in the treatment of AOP. The usual dosing for doxapram infusions ranges from 0.5 to 2 mg/kg/hour. The lowest effective dose of doxapram should be used initially and titrated based on clinical response.

The commercially available intravenous formulation of doxapram contains benzyl alcohol, a preservative associated with a potentially fatal toxicity known as *gasping syndrome* in neonates, and thus this drug should be used with caution.[58] Other important adverse effects include hypertension, seizures, cardiac conduction disorders, hypoglycemia, and gastric irritation.[9] Overall, there is a paucity of data on the tolerability, efficacy, and pharmacokinetics of doxapram. Until larger, controlled trials are available, doxapram should not be used for the treatment of AOP in routine practice.[59]

DISCHARGE PLANNING

Most premature neonates will have resolution of AOP symptoms at 34–36 weeks' postmenstrual age.[9] However, some infants, especially those at gestational ages younger than 28 weeks, may continue to have persistent apneic episodes beyond 38 weeks' postmenstrual age when they may be otherwise ready for discharge.[8] There are no defined treatment guidelines for these infants, but the goal is aimed at reducing the risk and incidence of the apneic episodes so that the infant may be cared for at home. A major dilemma in the management of AOP is deciding whether to continue methylxanthine therapy after discharge or to delay discharge until apnea completely resolves. The decision to provide a home apnea monitor or to continue methylxanthine after discharge should be individualized for each patient. It is difficult to establish the minimum number of symptom- and treatment-free hospital days to ensure an absence of apneic episodes after discharge.

In a retrospective study of premature infants younger than 32 weeks' gestational age and weighing less than 1500 g at birth, the investigators observed that an 8-day absence of symptoms of apnea, bradycardia, and/or color change was a good predictor of AOP resolution.[60] However, published literature does not clearly indicate whether hospital discharge should be delayed or whether AOP treatment and monitoring should be continued at home. The clinician should exert judgment when making this decision on the basis of the infant's history and presentation.

Premature infants may develop apnea or other respiratory symptoms in certain settings such as viral illness or under general anesthesia.[61] Possible apneic exacerbations after discharge should be closely monitored until the infant is at least 44 weeks' postmenstrual age in these situations.

CONCLUSIONS

Apnea is a significant problem for premature infants. Currently, a standard treatment guideline for AOP is unavailable. A careful assessment of the infant is necessary to identify the etiology and an individualized treatment plan. Although several nonpharmacologic and pharmacologic treatment strategies exist, the clinician must carefully weigh the risks and benefits associated with each treatment modality. Caffeine is the first-line pharmacologic treatment strategy for AOP for its favorable pharmacokinetic safety profile and long-term outcomes. Infants treated with caffeine have fewer incidences of bronchopulmonary dysplasia and better neurodevelopmental outcomes. With appropriate management and recognition of symptoms, patients with AOP can have an excellent prognosis.

Patient Case | APNEA OF PREMATURITY IN A PREMATURE NEONATE

A 3-day-old male neonate was delivered at 25 weeks and 5 days of gestation (birth weight: 490 g) by cesarean section. He developed respiratory distress with subcostal retractions, grunting, and cyanosis within minutes after birth. The neonate was also noted to be apneic with poor color and tone. Continuous positive airway pressure was initiated at birth, but he subsequently required endotracheal intubation and initiation of mechanical ventilation.

He received one dose of intratracheal poractant alfa (2.5 mL/kg/dose) for respiratory distress syndrome, intramuscular vitamin K (0.5 mg/dose) for prophylaxis of hemorrhagic disease of the newborn, and topical erythromycin ophthalmic ointment 0.5% to each eye for prophylaxis of neonatal gonococcal or chlamydial conjunctivitis.

The infant was transferred to the neonatal intensive care unit for prematurity, a sepsis workup, and respiratory failure. On the first day of life, antibiotics were initiated, but the sepsis workup was negative after 48 hours of antibiotics. On the third day of life, the patient is still noted to have several episodes of desaturations and bradycardia. His vital signs are otherwise normal.

Maternal history: Mother received dexamethasone and magnesium before delivery. The neonate was delivered by repeat cesarean section for maternal pre-eclampsia and nonreassuring fetal heart tracing with prolonged and severe decelerations.

Epidural anesthesia was administered to the mother.

Current medications:

Sucrose oral solution, 0.2 mL/dose as needed for procedure or pain event

Total parenteral nutrition, 100 mL/kg/day

20% Fat emulsion, 5 mL/kg/day

1. What risk factors does this patient have for the development of apnea of prematurity?

The neonate's prematurity status (25 weeks and 5 days) and extremely low birth weight (490 g) places him at higher risk of apnea of prematurity (AOP). At delivery, the neonate was noted to be apneic with poor color and tone. The neonate also had signs of respiratory distress (retractions, grunting, and cyanosis) requiring continuous positive airway pressure.

2. What are the acute goals of pharmacotherapy in this case?

The primary goal of therapy is to decrease or eliminate the frequency of prolonged apnea lasting greater than 20 seconds or apnea associated with cyanosis and bradycardia. Other causes of apnea must be excluded, and the diagnosis of AOP should be made before initiating an individualized treatment. If AOP is left untreated, decrease oxygen delivery to vital organs could be life threatening.

3. What is the drug of choice for the treatment of this patient's apnea of prematurity? Include the drug, dosage form, dose, schedule, and duration of therapy.

Caffeine citrate is the first-line therapy for the treatment of AOP for its wide therapeutic index eliminating the need for therapeutic drug monitoring, ease of administration, tolerability and limited adverse effects. The patient should be loaded with 20–25 mg/kg/dose of caffeine citrate and initiated on a maintenance dose of 5 mg/kg/day. The dose can be titrated to 10 mg/kg/day to control the apneic episodes. The dosing for oral and intravenous caffeine citrate is equivalent. The necessary duration of therapy is highly variable in neonates with AOP and is dependent on the maturity of the brain stem and respiratory control system. Caffeine therapy should be continued until there are no clinically observed apneic episodes for several consecutive days, which is generally observed before 37 weeks' postmenstrual age. Consider reinitiating therapy if apnea recurs soon after therapy discontinuation.

REFERENCES

1. Gabriel M, Albani M, Schulte FJ. Apneic spells and sleep states in preterm infants. Pediatrics 1976;57:142-7.
2. Perlstein PH, Edwards NK, Sutherland JM. Apnea in premature infants and incubator-air-temperature changes. N Engl J Med 1970; 282:461-6.
3. Task Force on Prolonged Infantile Apnea, American Academy of Pediatrics. Prolonged infantile apnea: 1985. Pediatrics 1985;1:129-31.
4. Perlman JM, Volpe JJ. Episodes of apnea and bradycardia in the preterm newborn: impact on cerebral circulation. Pediatrics 1985; 76:333-8.
5. Jenni OG, Wolf M, Hengartner M, et al. Impact of central, obstructive and mixed apnea on cerebral hemodynamics in preterm infants. Biol Neonate 1996;70:91-100.
6. Martin RJ, Miller MJ, Waldemar A. Pathogenesis of apnea in preterm infants. J Pediatr 1995;127:767-73.
7. Pillekamp F, Hermann C, Keller T, et al. Factors influencing apnea and bradycardia of prematurity—implications for neurodevelopment. Neonatology 2007;91:155-61.
8. Eichenwald EC, Aina A, Stark AR. Apnea frequently persists beyond term gestation in infants delivered at 24 to 28 weeks. Pediatrics 1997;100:354.
9. Thompson WM, Hung CE. Control of breathing: development, apnea of prematurity, apparent life-threatening events, sudden infant death syndrome. In: Macdonal MG, Mullett MD, Seshia MM, eds. Avery's Neonatology, 6th ed. Philadelphia: Lippincott Williams & Wilkins, 2005:535-53.
10. Hofstetter AO, Legnevall L, Herlenius E, et al. Cardiorespiratory development in extremely preterm infants: vulnerability to infection and persistence of events beyond term-equivalent age. Acta Paediatr 2008;97:285-92.
11. Ramanathan R, Corwin MJ, Hunt CE, et al. Cardiorespiratory events recorded on home monitors: comparison of healthy infants with those at increased risk for SIDS. JAMA 2001;285:2199-207.
12. Rigatto H. Maturation of breathing. Clin Perinatol 1992;19:739-56.
13. Alvaro R, Alvarez J, Kwiatkowski K, et al. Small preterm infants (less than or equal to 1500 g) have only a sustained decrease in ventilation in response to hypoxia. Pediatr Res 1992;32:403-6.
14. Henderson-Smart DJ, Pettigrew AG, Campbell DJ. Clinical apnea and brainstem neural function in preterm infants. N Engl J Med 1983;308:353-7.
15. Frantz ID III, Adler SM, Thach BT, et al. Maturational effects on respiratory responses to carbon dioxide in premature infants. J Appl Physiol 1976;41:41-5.
16. Rigatto H, Brady JP, de la Torre Verduzco R. Chemoreceptor reflexes in preterm infants: II. The effect of gestational and postnatal age on the ventilator response to inhaled carbon dioxide. Pediatrics 1975;55:614-20.
17. Reed WR, Roberts JL, Thach BT. Factors influencing regional patency and configuration of the human infant upper airway. J Appl Physiol 1985;58:635-44.
18. Wilson SL, Thach BT, Brouillette RT, et al. Upper airway patency in the human infant: influence of airway pressure and posture. J Appl Physiol 1980;48:500-4.
19. Mathew OP. Apnea of prematurity: pathogenesis and management strategies. J Perinatol 2001;31:302-10.
20. Miller MJ, Martin RJ. Apnea of prematurity. Clin Perinatol 1992;19:789-808.
21. Idiong N, Lemke RP, Lin YJ, et al. Airway closure during mixed apneas in preterm infants: is effort necessary? J Pediatr 1998;133:509-12.
22. Finer NN, Barrington KJ, Hyes BJ, et al. Obstructive, mixed, and central apnea in the neonate: physiologic correlates. J Pediatr 1992;121:943-50.
23. Splaingard ML. Apnea and sudden infant death syndrome. In: Kliegman RM, Nieder ML, Super DM, eds. Practical Strategies in Pediatric Diagnosis and Therapy. Philadelphia: WB Saunders, 2004.
24. Carlo WA, Martin RJ, Versteegh FG, et al. The effect of respiratory distress syndrome on chest wall movements and respiratory pauses in preterm infants. Am Rev Respir Dis 1982;126:103-7.
25. Lawson EE. Nonpharmacological management of idiopathic apnea of the premature infant. In: Mathew OP, ed. Respiratory Control and Disorders in the Newborn. New York: Marcel Dekker, 2003:335-54.
26. Stark AR. Apnea. In: Cloherty JP, Eichenwald EC, Stark AR, eds. Manual of Neonatal Care. Philadelphia: Lippincott Williams & Wilkins, 2016.
27. Miller MJ, Carlo WA, Martin RJ. Continuous positive airway pressure selectively reduces obstructive apnea in preterm infants. J Pediatr 1985;106:91-4.
28. Supplemental therapeutic oxygen for prethreshold retinopathy of prematurity (STOP-ROP), a randomized, controlled trial. Pediatrics 2000;105:295-310.
29. Sasidharan P, Heimler R. Transfusion-induced changes in the breathing pattern of healthy preterm anemic infants. Pediatr Pulmonol 1992;12:170-3.

30. Poets CF, Pauls U, Bohnhorst B. Effect of blood transfusion on apnoea, bradycardia and hypoxaemia in preterm infants. Eur J Pediatr 1997;156:311-6.

31. Durand M, McCann E, Brady JP. Effect of continuous positive airway pressure on the ventilator response to CO_2 in preterm infants. Pediatrics 1983;71:634-8.

32. Martin RJ, Nearman HS, Katona PG, et al. The effect of a low continuous positive airway pressure on the reflex control of respiration in the preterm infant. J Pediatr 1977;90:976-81.

33. Bhatt-Mehta V, Schumacher RE. Treatment of apnea of prematurity. Pediatr Drugs 2003;5:195-210.

34. Henderson-Smart DJ, Steer P. Methylxanthine treatment for apnea in preterm infants. Cochrane Database Syst Rev 2001;3:CD000140.

35. Brouard C, Moriette D, Murat I, et al. Comparative efficacy of theophylline and caffeine in the treatment of idiopathic apnea in premature infants. Am J Dis Child 1985;139:698-700.

36. Bairam A, Boutroy MJ, Badonnel Y, et al. Theophylline versus caffeine: comparative effects in treatment of idiopathic apnea in the preterm infant. J Pediatr 1987;110:636-9.

37. Natarajan G, Lulic-Botica M, Aranda JV. Clinical pharmacology of caffeine in the newborn. NeoReviews 2007;8:214-21.

38. Church MK, Featherstone RL, Cushley MJ, et al. Relationships between adenosine, cyclic nucleotides, and xanthines in asthma. J Allergy Clin Immunol 1986;78:670-5.

39. Torphy TJ, Undem BJ. Phosphodiesterase inhibitors: new opportunities for the treatment of asthma. Thorax 1991;46:512-23.

40. Barnes PJ, Pauwels RA. Theophylline in the management of asthma: time for reappraisal. Eur Respir J 1994;7:579-91.

41. Reiter, P. Neonatal pharmacology and pharmacokinetics. NeoReviews 2002;3:229.

42. Theophylline [product information]. Bethlehem, PA: B. Braun Medical, Inc, 2017.

43. De Carolis MP, Romagnoli C, Muzii U, et al. Pharmacokinetic aspects of caffeine in premature infants. Dev Pharmacol Ther 1991;16:117-22.

44. Taketomo CK, Hodding JH, Krauss DM. Pediatric & Neonatal Dosage Handbook, 24th ed. Hudson, OH: Lexi-Comp, 2017.

45. Caffeine citrate [product information]. Shirley, NY: American Regent, Inc, 2019.

46. Myers TF, Milsap RL, Krauss AN, et al. Low-dose theophylline therapy in idiopathic apnea of prematurity. J Pediatr 1980; 96:99-103.

47. Kato Z, Fukutomi O, Kondo N. Developmental changes of unbound theophylline. Ann Allergy Asthma Immunol 1998;80:517.

48. Spitzer AR, Fox WW. Infant apnea. Pediatr Clin North Am 1986; 33:561-81.

49. Marquis JF, Carruthers SG, Spence JD, et al. Phenytoin–theophylline interactions. N Engl J Med 1982;307:1189-90.

50. Gorodischer R, Karplus M. Pharmacokinetic aspects of caffeine in premature infants with apnea. Eur J Clin Pharmacol 1982;22:47-52.

51. Natarajan G, Botica ML, Thomas R, et al. Therapeutic drug monitoring for caffeine in preterm neonates: an unnecessary exercise? Pediatrics 2007;119:936-40.

52. Lodha A, Seshia M, McMillan DD, et al. Association of early caffeine administration and neonatal outcomes in very preterm neonates. JAMA Pediatr 2015;169:33-8.

53. Henderson-Smart DJ, Steer PA. Caffeine versus theophylline for apnea in preterm infants. Cochrane Database Syst Rev 2010; 1:CD000273.

54. Schmidt B, Roberts RS, Davis P, et al. Caffeine therapy for apnea of prematurity. N Engl J Med 2006;354:2112-21.

55. Schmidt B, Roberts RS, Davis P, et al. Long-term effects of caffeine therapy for apnea of prematurity. N Engl J Med 2007;357:1893-902.

56. Alpan G, Eval F, Sagi E, et al. Doxapram in the treatment of idiopathic apnea of prematurity unresponsive to aminophylline. J Pediatr 1984;104:637-7.

57. Sagi E, Eval F, Alpan G, et al. Idiopathic apnoea of prematurity treated with doxapram and aminophylline. Arch Dis Child 1984;59:281-3.

58. Doxapram [product information]. Bedford, OH: Bedford Laboratories, 2007.

59. Henderson-Smart DJ, Steer P. Doxapram versus methylxanthine for apnea in preterm infants. Cochrane Database Syst Rev 2000;2:CD000075.

60. Darnall RA, Kattwinkel J, Nattie C, et al. Margin of safety for discharge after apnea in preterm infants. Pediatrics 1997;100:795-801.

61. Eichenwald EC, Committee on Fetus and Newborn, American Academy of Pediatrics. Apnea of prematurity. Pediatrics 2016;137:1.

CHAPTER 13

Pediatric Asthma

Jeffrey L. Wagner, Pharm.D., MPH, BCPS

LEARNING OBJECTIVES

1. Define asthma and describe its epidemiologic prevalence based on risk factors, genetics, and population characteristics.

2. Explain the underlying pathology that results in disordered lung function and recognize the associated symptoms and diagnostic criteria of asthma.

3. Classify asthma based on severity and control to develop an approach to effective management.

4. Evaluate nonpharmacologic and pharmacologic therapies for their effect and mechanism in reducing impairment and risk of asthma.

5. Describe selection and monitoring guidelines for pharmacotherapies in the treatment of asthma.

6. Develop an understanding of available therapy and appropriate use of delivery devices to maximize therapeutic outcomes and medication safety, and reduce risk of asthma.

ABBREVIATIONS IN THIS CHAPTER

CYP	Cytochrome P450
FEV₁	Forced expiratory volume in 1 second
ICS	Inhaled corticosteroids
LABA	Long-acting β-agonist
SABA	Short-acting β-agonist

INTRODUCTION

Asthma, the most common chronic disease in childhood, is a chronic, inflammatory disease of the airways caused by a complex interaction of factors. Asthma is characterized by symptoms that occur in paroxysms that are usually related to specific triggering events, airway narrowing that is partially or completely reversible, and increased airway responsiveness to a variety of stimuli.[1] Inflammation and airflow obstruction are often reversible and cause episodes of cough, wheezing, dyspnea, and chest tightness. Despite the long history since the disease was first recognized, recently a greater understanding of asthma etiology and treatment has occurred.

In 1991, the National Heart, Lung, and Blood Institute of the National Institutes of Health published the first Expert Panel Report on asthma, which established guidelines for the diagnosis and management of asthma. Significant advances have been made since the release of the first clinical practice guidelines, with a decrease in the number of deaths caused by asthma despite increasing prevalence, decrease in reports of activity limitation by patients with asthma, and increased proportion of people with asthma who receive formal patient education.[2] However, despite these advances in the care of patients with asthma, the disease continues to pose a significant public health problem because of its unknown cause, complex disease development, and the burden of prevalence, resource use, and mortality.

EPIDEMIOLOGY

The epidemiology of asthma is difficult to define given the lack of a standard definition and methods to identify people with asthma in epidemiologic studies.[3] Despite these epidemiologic challenges and the wide global variation in the prevalence of asthma, it is one of the leading chronic childhood diseases in the United States.[4]

ASTHMA PREVALENCE AND MORTALITY

The estimated worldwide asthma prevalence is 7% to 10% with more than 300 million people affected.[5] Prevalence has more than doubled from 1980 to the mid-1990s in the United States alone according to available and published data.[6] Asthma prevalence among children increased more slowly from 2001 to 2010, from 8.7% to 9.4%, with increasing racial disparity, and then decreased to 8.3% in 2016.[7,8] The number of children who currently have asthma in the United States is estimated to be 6.2 million.[9]

Asthma prevalence across the world is disparate with a trend toward higher prevalence in developed countries. Although westernization may account for some of the difference in prevalence by country, differences in prevalence may be explained by variability in genetic, social, and environmental risk factors.[10] Asthma leads to around 350,000 deaths worldwide each year.[5,11] Annual death rate from asthma in the United States increased from 1982 to 1995, but has declined each year since.[7]

DEMOGRAPHIC CHARACTERISTICS

Asthma affects more male than female children up to age 17 years (9.5% vs. 7.3%, respectively).[9] Asthma prevalence increases with age, although health care use is highest among the youngest children.[12] The racial disparity in asthma prevalence and health care resource utilization is extensive. African American and Puerto Rican children have the highest prevalence rates compared with children of other races, whereas Asian children have the lowest prevalence rates.[9] The higher rates of emergency department visits, hospitalizations, and deaths among minority children have been well documented. The disparity in asthma mortality between African American and white children has increased in recent years, with African American children having higher mortality rates (Table 1).

ETIOLOGY

PATHOPHYSIOLOGY

Asthma is a complex, inflammatory disease process with physiologic reduction in airway luminal diameter, which is critical to the flow of air in the lungs. The relationship between luminal diameter and resistance can be explained with Poiseuille's law (Figure 1), which is based on the physical principle that resistance is inversely proportional to flow; therefore, the greater the resistance, the less the flow.

Given that the viscosity of air (n) and the length of the tube (l) remain relatively constant in the lung, the radius (r) has a dramatic effect on resistance to air flow. For example, if there is a 50% decrease in the radius of an airway, the resistance to airflow increases by a factor of 16. Therefore, an understanding of Poiseuille's law is paramount to understanding the impact of the inflammatory processes and airway narrowing in asthma on airflow.

$$R = \frac{8\,n\,l}{\pi\,r^4}$$

Figure 1. Poiseuille's law.

R = resistance, n= viscosity of air, l = length of tube, r = radius of tube.

The pathophysiology of asthma is characterized by airway and bronchial hyperresponsiveness, bronchoconstriction, and airway inflammation involving inflammatory cells and mediators.[1] *Airway and bronchial hyperresponsiveness*, defined as the degree to which airways narrow in response to a nonspecific stimulus or an environmental trigger, correlates with asthma severity in children.[13,14] Reversible bronchoconstriction and bronchospasm result from bronchial smooth muscle contraction in response to a variety of stimuli. The episodic and sudden onset of bronchoconstriction is commonly referred to as an "asthma attack," and is the dominant physiologic event leading to clinical symptoms. The continuous underlying airway inflammation has a central role in the disease pathophysiology, causing epithelial cell damage and increased mucosal permeability.[15-17] Airway inflammation is evidenced by the presence of the following: (1) inflammatory cells: neutrophils, eosinophils, T cells, alveolar macrophages, and mast cells; (2) mediators: leukotrienes, histamine, prostaglandins, thromboxanes, platelet-activating factor, and adhesion molecules found in bronchoalveolar lavage fluid; (3) immunoglobulin E antibodies, which are linked to progression of lung disease; and (4) exaggerated inflammatory response, which is associated with impaired glutathione homeostasis, a biomarker of oxidant.[18-20]

In addition, many pathologic changes are reflected in the sputum, including *Charcot-Leyden crystals* (eosinophil remnants), *Curschmann spirals* (airway lumen casts of exudate), and *Creola bodies* (clumps of sloughed epithelial cells).[21] A histologic examination of asthmatic lungs shows hyperplasia and hypertrophy of airway smooth muscle, increased airway wall thickness, and mucous gland hypertrophy and mucus hypersecretion.

GENETIC BASIS

Complex interactions between genetics and environmental influences contribute to asthma as an inflammatory disease. Epidemiologic studies suggest a genetic predisposition

Table 1. Asthma Prevalence and Mortality Among Children from Birth to Age 17 Years by Race and Ethnicity in the United States from 2007–2010[12]

Race and Ethnicity	Current Prevalence, % (2008–2010)	Deaths with Asthma as Underlying Cause per 10,000 Persons with Current Asthma (2007–2009)
Race Only		
White	8.2	0.2
Black	16.0	0.6
Other	9.5	0.1
Race/Ethnicity		
Hispanic or Latino	7.5	0.2
Puerto Rican	16.9	—
Mexican	6.5	—
Not Hispanic or Latino	10.0	0.3
Total	**9.5**	**0.3**

to asthma development because twins and families demonstrate patterns of disease consistent with heritable factors.[22-24] In fact, studies of twins suggest that genetic factors account for 50% of susceptibility.[25] Some components of the asthma phenotype appear strongly heritable, although the genes responsible for these components remain to be identified, and inheritance does not follow the Mendelian pattern of genetics. The genetic predisposition for developing an immunoglobulin E-mediated response to common aeroallergens, known as *atopy*, remains the strongest identifiable predisposing factor for developing asthma.[1]

RISK FACTORS

The host and environment play a significant role in the risk for development of asthma. The *hygiene hypothesis* states that lack of exposure to infectious agents and microorganisms in early childhood increases the susceptibility to allergic diseases, including asthma, by suppressing appropriate immune system development and response. Box 1 lists the host factors and environmental factors that have been associated with the development of asthma.[1,6,26-30] In addition to the risk factors for disease, predictors of asthma include family history of asthma, eczema, and/or smoking; history of allergic rhinitis, sinusitis, nasal polyps, eczema, or bronchopulmonary dysplasia; and recurrent cough, bronchitis, and bronchiolitis.[1,31-33]

CLINICAL PRESENTATION AND DIAGNOSIS

SIGNS AND SYMPTOMS

The symptoms of asthma result from airflow obstruction and the cumulative effects of smooth muscle constriction around airways, airway wall edema, intraluminal mucus accumulation, inflammatory cell infiltration of the submucosa, and basement membrane thickening.[15-17] Inflammation causes recurrent episodes of dyspnea, cough, and wheezing that can be nonspecific, making asthma difficult to distinguish from other respiratory diseases in the pediatric patient. About 80% of children with asthma develop symptoms before age 5 years.[34] Older children may experience shortness of breath and chest tightness, whereas younger children may have non-focal chest pain. In addition, younger children may have more subtle symptoms such as decreased physical activity, general fatigue, and difficulty keeping up with peers.

Asthma exacerbations are associated with widespread but variable airflow obstruction and are often reversible with or without treatment. Life-threatening asthma is a constellation of symptoms that can occur in any patient with asthma; these symptoms include the following:[1]

- Marked chest tightness
- Wheezing, severe shortness of breath
- Retractions
- Cyanosis
- Inability to speak or speak in sentences because of dyspnea
- Hunched posture
- Altered mental status (agitation, anxiety, lethargy)

Box 1. Host and Environmental Factors Associated with Asthma

Host Factors

Genetics

Innate immunity

- Atopy: rhinitis and dermatitis
- Hygiene hypothesis: lack of early childhood infection modifies immune response and reduces tendency to produce immunoglobulin E antibodies to environmental allergens

Race/ethnicity

Sex

Environmental Factors

Urbanization and socioeconomic status

Allergens: house dust mites, animal proteins (cat and dog allergens), cockroaches, fungi

Endotoxin exposure: inflammatory lipopolysaccharide molecules from gram-negative bacteria

Respiratory infections, particularly viral infections (RSV and rhinovirus)

Other environmental factors: tobacco smoke, specific pollutants (CO, NO_2, SO_2)

DIAGNOSTIC CRITERIA

The initial diagnosis of asthma in children is often difficult and requires exclusion of other diagnoses. The diagnosis of asthma requires the clinical history or presence of respiratory symptoms consistent with asthma, combined with the demonstration of variable expiratory airflow obstruction. Asthma diagnostic criteria include history, physical examination, pulmonary function testing, and laboratory evaluations.[1] Comorbid conditions that are associated with asthma include gastroesophageal reflux disease, obstructive sleep apnea, obesity, rhinitis, and sinusitis.[1,35-37]

A detailed clinical history involves assessment of the patient for cough, wheeze, shortness of breath, and/or chest tightening that occurs in an "episodic" fashion. These symptoms may occur or worsen with exercise, weather changes, night hours, viral infection, inhalant trigger exposure (e.g., smoke, fur, dust mites, mold, pollen), irritant trigger exposure (e.g., airborne chemicals [aerosols], smoke), strong emotional expressions (e.g., laughing, crying), and menstrual cycles.[1,38-41]

The physical examination should assess for severity of respiratory symptoms, including rhinitis, increased nasal secretions, mucosal swelling, or nasal polyps, and for the presence of airflow obstruction or airway hyperresponsiveness that is partly reversible, for example, spirometry that shows a percent change in forced expiratory volume in 1 second (FEV_1) of 12% or more from baseline or 10% or more of predicted after the patient inhales a short-acting bronchodilator.[1,42] To establish the diagnosis and facilitate severity assessment, the National Education and Prevention Program recommends spirometry in children older than 5 years. In infants and children younger than 5 years, the diagnosis centers on the same evaluation as discussed, although spirometry often cannot be performed in this age group because of developmental ability (e.g., ability to breathe in and exhale fully). Debate is ongoing about how best to diagnose and classify infants and young children with recurrent wheezing. Tests to exclude other diagnoses when the history and physical examination are equivocal include a chest radiograph, bronchoprovocation test, and allergen testing (e.g., eosinophilia, total immunoglobulin E, and, rarely, aspergillosis).[1]

DISEASE COURSE AND PROGNOSIS

The progression of asthma is marked and measured by decline in lung function.[1] Reduction in the FEV_1/forced vital capacity ratio is evidenced in children who have mild or moderate asthma compared with children who do not have asthma. According to longitudinal epidemiologic studies and clinical trials, the characteristic decline in lung function varies by age group. Children with symptoms before age 3 years demonstrate a decline in lung function growth by 6 years, but children age 5–12 years who have mild or moderate persistent asthma usually have no decline in lung function through age 17 years, although a subset of children experience progressive reductions in lung growth.

In addition to the natural progression of asthma, other factors place patients at risk of asthma-related death. These factors include comorbid conditions such as heart or lung disease; previous severe exacerbation (e.g., intubation or intensive care unit admission); two or more hospitalizations or more than three emergency department visits in the past year; use of more than one canister of short-acting β-agonist (SABA) per month; difficulty perceiving airway obstruction or the severity of worsening asthma (parent/caregiver and/or child); low socioeconomic status or urban residence; illicit drug use; and major psychosocial problems or psychiatric disease.[1,40]

ASTHMA SEVERITY AND CONTROL

Asthma severity is determined by a constellation of impairment and risk and is defined along a continuum from *intermittent*, *mild persistent*, *moderate persistent*, and *severe persistent asthma*. In addition to patient history, the tools used to assess severity through measures of lung function for children 5 years and older are spirometry to assess FEV_1, pulmonary function testing, and airway hyperresponsiveness testing using methacholine.[1,42] A patient's level of control is determined at follow-up visits on a scale of well, poorly, and very poorly controlled and is also based on the domains of impairment and risk. In addition, several tools have recently been developed for patient self-assessment to objectively identify those with poorly controlled asthma.[43-49] Asthma severity and control are used to determine the recommended step for initial and stepwise therapy, which are discussed in the following Treatment section of this chapter.

TREATMENT

GOALS OF THERAPY

The National Asthma Education and Prevention Program has defined the primary goal of asthma management as "asthma control," which involves a reduction in both impairment and risk.[1] The reduction in frequency and severity of asthma exacerbations and long-term sequelae should be achieved by maintaining asthma control with the fewest therapeutic

---

Box 2. Key Components of Asthma Education for the Patient and Family[1]

Basic Facts

The contrast between the airways of a person who has asthma and a person who does not have asthma

The role of inflammation

What happens to the airways during an asthma attack?

Role of Medications

Long-term control medications

- Prevent symptoms, often by reducing inflammation

- Must be taken daily

Quick-relief medications

Short-acting β-agonist (SABAs) relax airway muscles to provide prompt relief of symptoms

Use of SABAs > 2 days/wk to relieve asthma symptoms suggests the need to reassess asthma control and consider escalation of therapy

Patient Skill Set

Self-monitoring:

- Self-assessment of level of asthma control

- Monitoring symptoms and, if prescribed, peak expiratory flow measures

- Recognizing symptom patterns and early signs and symptoms of worsening asthma

- Use of a written asthma action plan to know when and how to:
  - Take daily actions to control asthma
  - Adjust medication early in response to signs of worsening asthma
  - Seek medical care as directed
  - Value of adherence and periodic monitoring to adjust therapy

Taking medications correctly

Inhaler technique (demonstration/return demonstration)

Use of devices as prescribed (valved holding chamber or spacer, nebulizer)

Identifying and avoiding triggers that worsen the patient's asthma (allergens, irritants, tobacco smoke)

interventions possible. Intensive education and monitoring are required in caring for all children with asthma and are discussed further in following text.[1,27,28,50]

NONPHARMACOLOGIC THERAPY

The primary principles of nonpharmacologic therapy and the cornerstone to asthma management are patient/caregiver education and self-management. Nonpharmacologic therapy seeks to control exposure to environmental factors, reduce risk from comorbid conditions, and allow for appropriate use of therapy and health care resources. Evidence suggests that educational interventions improve outcomes in asthma. Box 2 lists the key components to asthma education.[1,51-54]

Other suggested nonpharmacologic therapies include the following: (1) breathing techniques: the Buteyko breathing technique, the Papworth method, and yoga breathing, termed pranayama; (2) acupuncture; (3) relaxation techniques: meditation, biofeedback, hypnosis, and progressive muscle relaxation; (4) herbal remedies: butterbur, dried ivy, and ginkgo extract; (5) omega-3 fatty acids; and (6) homeopathy, although not well established.[1]

PHARMACOLOGIC THERAPY

Pharmacologic therapy is used to prevent and control asthma symptoms, improve quality of life, reduce the frequency and severity of asthma exacerbations, and reverse airflow obstruction.[55] Adapted from the National Asthma Education and Prevention Program Guidelines for the Diagnosis and Management of Asthma, Table 2, Table 3, and Table 4 show the classification of asthma severity and assessment of asthma control, each of which guide therapy initiation and subsequent stepwise adjustment of medications for the management of asthma.[1] To initiate pharmacologic therapy, asthma severity is first classified into *intermittent asthma* or *persistent asthma* (Table 2) based on symptoms over the specified time. On the basis of the severity classification, the appropriate step for therapy initiation is determined. Then, on the basis of an assessment of asthma control (Table 3), an action for treatment is recommended within the stepwise management approach. The specific step of therapy gives a preferred and alternate treatment for various age groups (Table 4). When following the stepwise approach to therapy, monotherapy is typically initiated; however, it would not be unreasonable to prescribe a combination product to achieve asthma control.

Table 2. Classifying Asthma Severity and Initiating Therapy by Patient Age (Years)[1]

Components of Severity		Intermittent	Persistent		
			Mild	**Moderate**	**Severe**
Impairment	Symptoms	≤ 2 days/wk	> 2 days/wk	Daily	Throughout day
	Nighttime awakenings	Age < 5: 0	Age < 5: 1–2×/mo	Age < 5: 3–4×/mo	Age < 5: > 1×/wk
		Age ≥ 5: ≤ 2×/mo	Age ≥ 5: 3–4×/mo	Age ≥ 5: >1×/wk	Age ≥ 5: Often, 7×/wk
	SABA use for symptoms	≤ 2 days/wk	> 2 days/wk	Daily	Several times per day
	Limitation of normal activity	None	Minor	Some	Extreme
	Lung function[a]	Age 5–11: FEV$_1$ > 80% FEV$_1$/FVC > 85%	Age 5–11: FEV$_1$ ≥ 80% FEV$_1$/FVC > 80%	Age 5–11: FEV$_1$ 60%–80% FEV$_1$/FVC 75%–80%	Age 5–11: FEV$_1$ < 60% FEV$_1$/FVC < 75%
		Age ≥ 12: FEV$_1$ > 80% FEV$_1$/FVC normal	Age ≥ 12: FEV$_1$ ≥ 80% FEV$_1$/FVC normal	Age ≥ 12: FEV$_1$ 60%–80% FEV$_1$/FVC reduced by 5%	Age ≥ 12: FEV$_1$ < 60% FEV$_1$/FVC reduced > 5%
Risk	Exacerbations requiring oral corticosteroids[b]	0–1×/yr	Age < 5: ≥ 2× in 6 mo requiring steroids or ≥ 4 wheezing episodes in 1 yr and lasting > 1 day AND risk factors for persistent asthma Age ≥ 5: ≥ 2×/yr		
Recommended Step for Initiating Therapy[c]		Step 1	Step 2	Step 3	Age < 5: Step 3 Age 5–11: Step 3 or 4 Age ≥ 12: Step 4 or 5

[a]Note that some people with smaller lungs in relation to their height may NORMALLY have FEV$_1$ < 80% and/or FEV$_1$/FVC < 85%. Lung function measures should be correlated with clinical assessment of asthma severity.
[b]For initial therapy of moderate or severe persistent asthma, consider a short course of oral corticosteroids.
[c]More information about the recommended steps for initiating therapy is provided in this chapter in Table 4: Stepwise Approach to Asthma Management
FEV$_1$ = forced expiratory volume in 1 second; FVC = forced vital capacity; SABA = short-acting β-agonist; × = times.

Table 3. Assessing Asthma Control and Adjusting Therapy for Patients by Age (Years)[1]

Components of Control		Well Controlled	Not Well Controlled	Very Poorly Controlled
Impairment	Symptoms	≤ 2 days/wk	Age < 5: > 2 days/wk Age 5–11: > 2 days/wk or several times on ≤ 2 days/wk Age ≥ 12: > 2 days/wk	Throughout the day
	Nighttime awakenings	Age < 12: ≤ 1×/mo Age ≥ 12: ≤ 2×/mo	Age < 5: > 1×/mo Age 5–11: ≥ 2×/mo Age ≥ 12: 1–3×/wk	Age < 5: >1×/wk Age 5–11: ≥ 2×/wk Age ≥ 12: ≥ 4×/wk
	Interference with normal activity	None	Some limitation	Extremely limited
	SABA use for symptoms	≤ 2 days/wk	> 2 days/wk	Several times per day
	Lung function[a]	Age 5–11: FEV_1 > 80% FEV_1/FVC > 80% Age ≥ 12: FEV_1 > 80%	Age 5–11: FEV_1 60%–80% FEV_1/FVC 75%–80% Age ≥ 12: FEV_1 60%–80%	Age 5–11: FEV_1 < 60% FEV_1/FVC < 75% Age ≥ 12: FEV_1 < 60%
Risk	Exacerbations requiring OCS[b]	0–1×/yr	Age < 5: 2–3×/yr Age ≥ 5: ≥2×/yr	Age < 5: > 3×/yr Age ≥ 5: ≥ 2×/yr
	Reduction in lung growth	Requires long-term follow-up		
	Treatment-related adverse effects	Medication adverse effects do not correlate with specific levels of control, but they should be considered in overall assessment of risk		
Recommended Action for Treatment[c]		Consider step-down if well controlled for ≥ 3 mo	Step up 1 step Reevaluate in 2–6 wk	Consider short-course OCS Step up 1 or 2 steps Reevaluate in 2 wk

[a]Note that some people with smaller lungs in relation to their height may NORMALLY have FEV_1 < 80% and/or FEV_1/FVC < 85%. Lung function measures should be correlated with clinical assessment of asthma severity.
[b]For initial therapy of moderate or severe persistent asthma, consider short course of oral corticosteroids.
[c]More information about the recommended steps for initiating therapy is provided in this chapter in Table 4: Stepwise Approach to Asthma Management
FEV_1 = forced expiratory volume in 1 second; FVC = forced vital capacity; OCS = oral corticosteroids; SABA = short-acting β-agonist; × = times.

It is also important to assess the severity of exacerbations because this factor implicates the clinical course as well as outcomes (Table 5 and Table 6).[1,56] The management of exacerbations depends on the severity, identification of triggers and management of control measures, and therapy initiation and adjustment as appropriate (Figure 2).[1] Management of an asthma exacerbation may occur at home, in the physician's office, or in an urgent care or inpatient setting (Figure 2). Step therapy can be resumed after recovery from an exacerbation.

Several medications are used in the treatment of asthma and exacerbations. Table 7 and Table 8 provide an overview of the classes of medications, including mechanism of action, indication, and adverse effects, as well as medication dosing based on age category.[1,57]

β₂-AGONISTS

The β₂-agonists, both short-acting and long-acting bronchodilators, are the most effective drugs in reversing bronchoconstriction and relaxing airway smooth muscle. Delivery of these medications directly to the airway by inhalation enhances bronchoselectivity, provides a more rapid response, and protects against triggers of bronchospasm. The SABAs albuterol, levalbuterol, isoproterenol, metaproterenol, and terbutaline all have an onset of action within 1–5 minutes and bronchodilation that lasts 2–6 hours. Although their β₂/β₁ potency ratios vary, they are all selective for the β₂ subtype. There is little evidence that intravenous terbutaline has an added benefit for acute exacerbations compared with SABAs, corticosteroids, and ipratropium.

Table 4. Stepwise Approach to Asthma Management by Patient Age (Years)[1]

Step	Preferred Treatments	Alternative Treatments
1	Short-acting β-agonist as needed	N/A
2	Low-dose ICS	Age < 5: Cromolyn or montelukast Age ≥ 5: Cromolyn, nedocromil, LRTA, or theophylline

3	Age < 5:
	  Medium-dose ICS
	
	Age 5–11:
	  Low-dose ICS + LABA, LTRA, or theophylline
	  OR
	  Medium-dose ICS
	
	Age ≥ 12:
	  Low-dose ICS + LABA
	  OR
	  Medium-dose ICS
		Age ≥ 12:
		  Low-dose ICS + LRTA, theophylline, or zileuton

4	Age < 5:
	  Medium-dose ICS + either LABA or montelukast
	
	Age ≥ 5:
	  Medium-dose ICS + LABA
		Age 5–11:
		  Medium-dose ICS + either LTRA or theophylline
		
		Age ≥ 12:
		  Medium-dose ICS + LRTA, theophylline, or zileuton

5	Age < 5:
	  High-dose ICS + either LABA or montelukast
	
	Age 5–11:
	  High-dose ICS + LABA
	
	Age ≥ 12:
	  High-dose ICS + LABA
	  AND
	  consider omalizumab for patients with allergies
		Age 5–11:
		  High-dose ICS + either LRTA or theophylline

6	Age < 5:
	  High-dose ICS + OCS + either LABA or montelukast
	
	Age 5–11:
	  High-dose ICS + LABA + OCS
	
	Age ≥ 12:
	  High-dose ICS + LABA + OCS
	  AND
	  consider omalizumab for patients with allergies
		Age 5–11:
		  High-dose ICS + either LRTA or theophylline + OCS

Note: The stepwise approach is meant to assist in—not replace—clinical decision-making. If clear benefit is not observed within 4–6 weeks when patient technique and adherence are satisfactory, consider adjusting therapy and/or consider alternative diagnoses. Before increasing a step, review patient adherence, inhaler technique, environmental control, and comorbid conditions. When possible, step down if asthma is well controlled for at least 3 months.

ICS = inhaled corticosteroids; LABA = long-acting β-agonist; LTRA = leukotriene receptor antagonist; N/A = not applicable; OCS = oral corticosteroids.

The long-acting-β_2-agonists (LABAs) are used with inhaled corticosteroids (ICS) to prevent symptoms and do not provide quick relief of symptoms. Two of the LABAs, formoterol and salmeterol, have higher lipophilicity compared with the SABAs and act to regulate the diffusion rate from the receptor and allow for longer duration of action of more than 12 hours. Formoterol has an onset of action similar to the SABAs, within 5 minutes, because of its lower lipophilicity compared with salmeterol, which has an onset at 15 minutes.[58] Given the frequency of use of LABAs and ICS, several products combine the two classes of medication into one delivery device.

CORTICOSTEROIDS

Corticosteroids have long been used to treat severe chronic asthma and severe exacerbations by the systemic route, but the development of aerosol formulations has allowed improved safety to extend their use in the treatment of persistent asthma. Systemic steroids are indicated for moderate or severe exacerbations for short-term use. Evidence suggests that currently available therapy controls, but does not modify, the underlying disease process, and evidence supports the immediate use of systemic steroids during an exacerbation.[1,59-62]

Table 5. Classifying Severity of Asthma Exacerbations[1]

Severity	Signs and Symptoms	Initial PEF (or FEV$_1$)[a]	Clinical Course
Mild	Dyspnea only with activity; assess tachypnea in young children	PEF ≥ 70% of predicted or personal best	• Usually cared for at home • Prompt relief with inhaled SABA • Possible short course of OCS • May consider early escalation to high-dose inhaled corticosteroid
Moderate	Dyspnea interferes with or limits usual activity	PEF 40%–69% of predicted or personal best	• Usually requires office or ED visit • Relief from frequently inhaled SABA • OCS • Some symptoms last 1–2 days after treatment begins
Severe	Dyspnea at rest; interferes with conversation	PEF < 40% of predicted or personal best	• Usually requires ED visit and likely hospitalization • Partial relief from frequently inhaled SABA • OCS; some symptoms last for > 3 days after treatment begins • Adjunctive therapies are helpful
Life-threatening	Too dyspneic to speak; perspiring	PEF < 25% of predicted or personal best	• Requires ED hospitalization; possible ICU • Minimal or no relief from frequently inhaled SABA • Intravenous corticosteroids • Adjunctive therapies are helpful

[a]Note that some people with smaller lungs in relation to their height may NORMALLY have FEV$_1$ < 80% and/or FEV$_1$/FVC < 85%. Lung function measures should be correlated with clinical assessment of asthma severity. For infants, assessment depends primarily on physical examination (use of accessory muscles, inspiratory and expiratory wheezing, paradoxical breathing, cyanosis, and a respiratory rate > 60 breaths/minute are key signs of serious distress), although objective measurements, such as oxygen saturation < 90%, also indicate serious distress.

ED = emergency department; FEV$_1$ = forced expiratory volume in 1 second; FVC = forced vital capacity; ICU = intensive care unit; OCS = oral corticosteroids; PEF = peak expiratory flow; SABA = short-acting β-agonist.

METHYLXANTHINES

Methylxanthines are ineffective when aerosolized; they must therefore be administered systemically for effect. Theophylline is primarily eliminated through metabolism by the hepatic cytochrome P450 (CYP) mixed-function oxidase microsomal enzymes, primarily CYP 1A2 and CYP 3A3 isozymes. The inhibition and induction of the hepatic CYP enzymes by environmental factors and drugs alters the metabolism of theophylline, necessitating a review of potential interactions. In addition, intrapatient variability in theophylline clearance is considerable; thus, serum theophylline concentrations should be monitored routinely.

ANTICHOLINERGICS

Inhaled anticholinergic medications are effective bronchodilators but are not as potent as β$_2$-agonists. The use of ipratropium bromide during acute exacerbations in the emergency department setting is well supported by evidence; however, evidence is also available against their routine use as well as their use for in-hospital care.[63,64]

MAST-CELL STABILIZERS

The mast-cell stabilizers, cromolyn and nedocromil, do not produce a bronchodilatory effect and instead are effective only

by inhalation. These medications are limited by their adverse effect profile and dosing frequency. Thus, they are not the first choice for childhood asthma because of their lack of efficacy and safety.

LEUKOTRIENE MODIFIERS

Three of the leukotriene modifiers, montelukast, zafirlukast, and zileuton, may be used as alternatives for mild persistent asthma or as adjuncts to ICS for other asthma severities. They are not indicated for treating acute episodes of asthma and must be taken regularly, even during symptom-free periods.

IMMUNOMODULATORS

Subcutaneous immunotherapy with omalizumab is indicated for adolescents who have a clearly documented allergen relationship with their moderate to severe persistent asthma symptoms.[65]

OTHER MEDICATIONS

Other medications that have been suggested in the treatment of asthma include antihistamines, methotrexate, macrolides, other antibiotics, hydroxychloroquine, dapsone, gold, intravenous gamma-globulin, cyclosporine, colchicine, nonsteroidal anti-inflammatory drugs, inhaled heparin, inhaled

Table 6. Formal Evaluation of Asthma Exacerbation Severity[1]

	Mild	Moderate	Severe	Imminent Risk of Respiratory Arrest
Symptoms				
Breathlessness	While walking	While at rest (infant: softer, shorter cry, difficulty feeding)	While at rest (infant stops feeding)	
	Can lie down	Prefers sitting	Sits upright	
Talks in	Sentences	Phrases	Words	
Alertness	May be agitated	Usually agitated	Usually agitated	Drowsy or confused
Signs				
Respiratory rate	Increased	Increased	Often > 30/minute	
	Guide to rates of breathing in awake children:			

	Age
	  < 2 mo
	  2–12 mo
	  1–5 yr
	  6–8 yr
		Normal rate
		  < 60 breaths/minute
		  < 50 breaths/minute
		  < 40 breaths/minute
		  < 30 breaths/minute		

Use of accessory muscles	Usually not	Commonly	Usually	Paradoxical thoracoabdominal movement
Wheeze	Moderate; often only end expiratory	Loud; throughout exhalation	Usually loud; throughout inhalation and exhalation	Absence of wheeze
Heart rate beats/minute	< 100	100–120	> 120	Bradycardia
	Guide to normal heart rates in children:			

	Age
	  2–12 mo
	  1–2 yr
	  2–8 yr
		Normal rate
		  < 160 beats/minute
		  < 120 beats/minute
		  < 110 beats/minute		

Pulsus paradoxus	Absent < 10 mm Hg	May be present 10–25 mm Hg	Often present > 25 mm Hg (adult) 20–40 mm Hg (child)	Absence suggests respiratory muscle fatigue
Functional Assessment				
PEF % of predicted or % of personal best	≥ 70%	Around 40%–69% or response lasts < 2 hr	< 40%	< 25% Note: PEF testing may not be needed in very severe attacks
Pao₂ (on air)	Normal (test not usually necessary)	≥ 60 mm Hg (test not usually necessary)	< 60 mm Hg: possible cyanosis	
and/or Pco₂	< 42 mm Hg (test not usually necessary)	< 42 mm Hg (test not usually necessary)	≥ 42 mm Hg: possible respiratory failure	
Sao₂ % (on air) at sea level	> 95% (test not usually necessary)	90%–95% (test not usually necessary)	< 90%	
	Hypercapnia (hypoventilation) develops more readily in young children than in adults and adolescents.			

Pao_2 = alveolar oxygen partial pressure; PEF = peak expiratory flow.

furosemide, expectorants, and magnesium sulfate. Information to recommend these therapies routinely for the long-term management and treatment of acute exacerbations is limited, but evidence supports the use of magnesium sulfate only in acute severe exacerbations.[66-70] Heliox, a mixture of helium and oxygen, has also been studied for the treatment of acute exacerbations, but the results to support routine use as an added benefit to β_2-agonists and corticosteroids are lacking.[71-73]

DELIVERY DEVICES

Many delivery devices are used for administering medications to manage and treat asthma. Table 9 lists several different asthma devices, their limitations, and the optimal technique to ensure the best possible delivery for various pediatric patients.[1]

MONITORING THERAPY

Given that asthma is a chronic inflammatory disease with episodes of acute exacerbation, the need to follow therapeutic outcomes through the assessment and monitoring of severity, control, and responsiveness is paramount. In addition to regularly scheduled follow-ups, patients should monitor their asthma control and severity and adhere to their asthma action plan to guide the stepwise approach to therapy escalation (step up) or de-escalation (step down). A peak flow meter is recommended for those with moderate to severe persistent asthma, as well as for those with a history of exacerbations, to regularly monitor lung function and response to treatment. If the patient is unable to use a peak flow meter, a symptom-based action plan is useful in home management of acute exacerbations. Therapeutic outcomes must be balanced against adverse events and toxicity.

FUTURE THERAPIES

Given the significant impact of asthma, advancements are continuously being made to create and identify novel therapies that are effective at reducing impairment and risk as well as the underlying disease pathology. Therapies under evaluation include *bronchial thermoplasty*, which delivers thermal energy to the airway wall to reduce excessive airway smooth muscle; *anticytokine therapies* (interleukin-5, interleukin-4), which reduce inflammation; and *novel steroids*, referred to as *soft steroids*, which are intended to produce an anti-inflammatory effect with minimal adverse effects.

In Home and/or Office

Assess Severity
- Patients at risk of life-threatening asthma require immediate medical attention after treatment
- Symptoms and signs suggesting a more serious exacerbation should result in initial treatment while immediately consulting with a clinician
- Less severe signs and symptoms can be treated initially by assessing response to therapy and taking further steps as listed in this flow chart
- If available, measure PEF
  - 50%–79% of predicted or personal best indicates need for quick-relief medication
  - 50% indicates need for immediate medical care

Initial Treatment: Inhaled SABA
- Up to two treatments 20 minutes apart of 2–6 puffs by MDI or nebulizer treatments
- Children may need fewer puffs

Good Response
- Defined as:
  - No wheezing or dyspnea (tachypnea in young children)
  - PEF ≥ 80% of predicted or personal best
- Management steps
  - Contact clinician for follow-up instructions and further management
  - May continue inhaled SABA every 3–4 hours for 24–48 hours
  - Consider short course of oral systemic corticosteroids

Incomplete Response
- Defined as:
  - Persistent wheezing and dyspnea (tachypnea)
  - PEF 50%–79% of predicted or personal best
- Management steps
  - Add oral systemic corticosteroid
  - Continue inhaled SABA
  - Contact clinician urgently for further instruction

Poor Response
- Defined as:
  - Marked wheezing and dyspnea
  - PEF < 50% of predicted or personal best
- Management steps
  - Add oral systemic corticosteroid
  - Repeat inhaled SABA immediately
  - If distress is severe and unresponsive to initial treatment
    - Call your doctor AND
    - Proceed to emergency department
    - Consider calling 911

Figure 2. Management of asthma exacerbation.[1]

(continued)

Emergency Department and Hospital

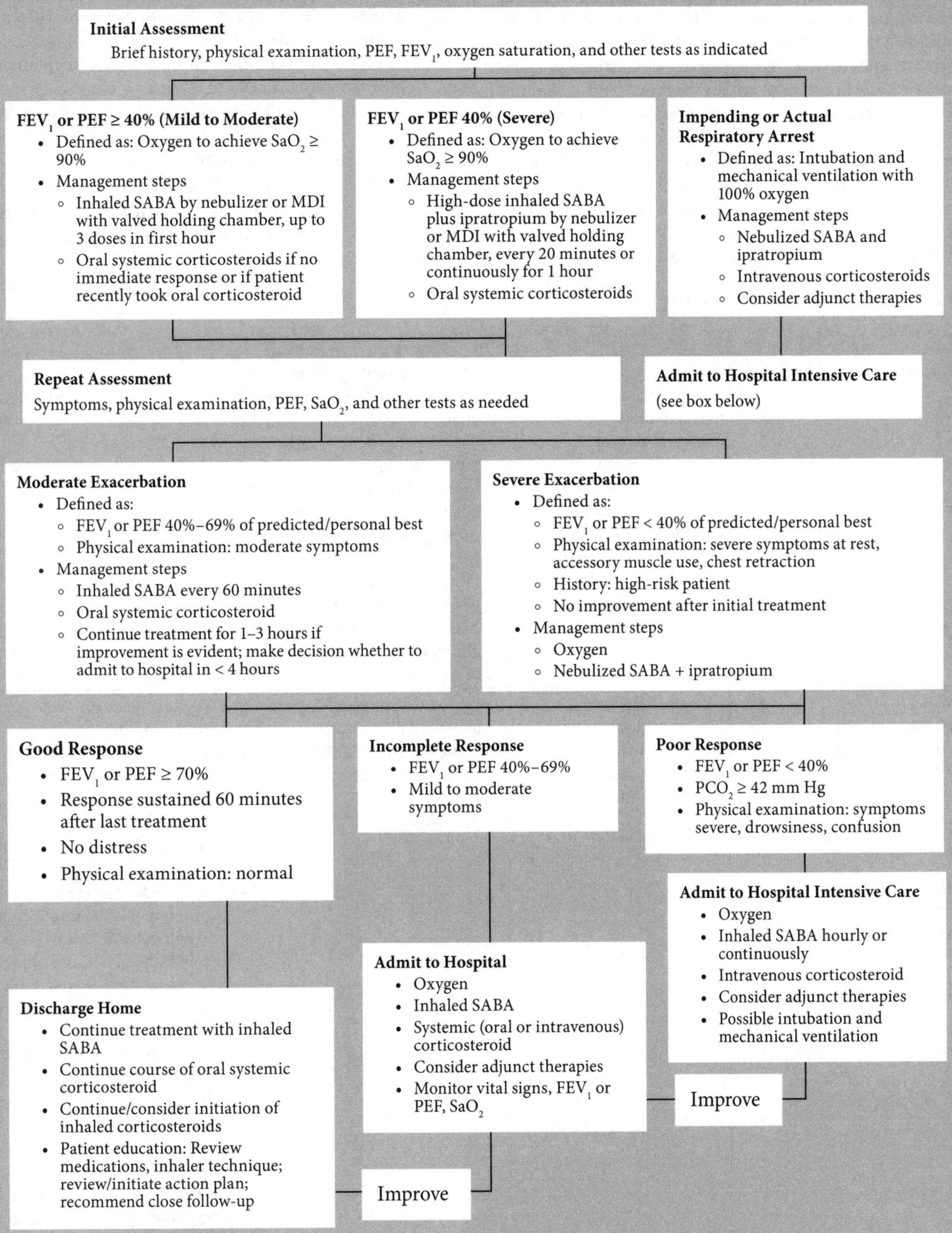

Initial Assessment

Brief history, physical examination, PEF, FEV$_1$, oxygen saturation, and other tests as indicated

FEV$_1$ or PEF ≥ 40% (Mild to Moderate)
- Defined as: Oxygen to achieve SaO$_2$ ≥ 90%
- Management steps
  - Inhaled SABA by nebulizer or MDI with valved holding chamber, up to 3 doses in first hour
  - Oral systemic corticosteroids if no immediate response or if patient recently took oral corticosteroid

FEV$_1$ or PEF 40% (Severe)
- Defined as: Oxygen to achieve SaO$_2$ ≥ 90%
- Management steps
  - High-dose inhaled SABA plus ipratropium by nebulizer or MDI with valved holding chamber, every 20 minutes or continuously for 1 hour
  - Oral systemic corticosteroids

Impending or Actual Respiratory Arrest
- Defined as: Intubation and mechanical ventilation with 100% oxygen
- Management steps
  - Nebulized SABA and ipratropium
  - Intravenous corticosteroids
  - Consider adjunct therapies

Repeat Assessment

Symptoms, physical examination, PEF, SaO$_2$, and other tests as needed

Admit to Hospital Intensive Care
(see box below)

Moderate Exacerbation
- Defined as:
  - FEV$_1$ or PEF 40%–69% of predicted/personal best
  - Physical examination: moderate symptoms
- Management steps
  - Inhaled SABA every 60 minutes
  - Oral systemic corticosteroid
  - Continue treatment for 1–3 hours if improvement is evident; make decision whether to admit to hospital in < 4 hours

Severe Exacerbation
- Defined as:
  - FEV$_1$ or PEF < 40% of predicted/personal best
  - Physical examination: severe symptoms at rest, accessory muscle use, chest retraction
  - History: high-risk patient
  - No improvement after initial treatment
- Management steps
  - Oxygen
  - Nebulized SABA + ipratropium

Good Response
- FEV$_1$ or PEF ≥ 70%
- Response sustained 60 minutes after last treatment
- No distress
- Physical examination: normal

Incomplete Response
- FEV$_1$ or PEF 40%–69%
- Mild to moderate symptoms

Poor Response
- FEV$_1$ or PEF < 40%
- PCO$_2$ ≥ 42 mm Hg
- Physical examination: symptoms severe, drowsiness, confusion

Admit to Hospital Intensive Care
- Oxygen
- Inhaled SABA hourly or continuously
- Intravenous corticosteroid
- Consider adjunct therapies
- Possible intubation and mechanical ventilation

Admit to Hospital
- Oxygen
- Inhaled SABA
- Systemic (oral or intravenous) corticosteroid
- Consider adjunct therapies
- Monitor vital signs, FEV$_1$ or PEF, SaO$_2$

Improve

Discharge Home
- Continue treatment with inhaled SABA
- Continue course of oral systemic corticosteroid
- Continue/consider initiation of inhaled corticosteroids
- Patient education: Review medications, inhaler technique; review/initiate action plan; recommend close follow-up

Improve

Figure 2. Management of asthma exacerbation.[1]

FEV$_1$ = forced expiratory volume in 1 second; MDI = metered dose inhaler; PEF = peak expiratory flow; SABA = short-acting β-agonist.

CONCLUSIONS

The management of asthma involves the interplay of the following four essential components: (1) routine monitoring of symptoms and lung function; (2) patient education; (3) control of trigger factors and comorbid conditions; and (4) pharmacologic therapy. The primary goal of asthma management is centered on the principle of asthma control, through reduction of risk and impairment. Effective asthma management varies based on patient age, and requires a preventive approach, with routine visits to assess symptoms, monitor pulmonary function, adjust medications, and ensure education is provided to allow for self-management and control. Efforts should be made to identify and address environmental triggers and comorbid conditions that impact asthma

management. Pharmacologic therapy varies according to asthma severity and asthma control through a stepwise approach, in which the class and number of medications, dosing, and frequency of administration are increased when necessary and reduced when possible.

Asthma is the most common chronic disease in childhood, and despite the long course of its history, a clear understanding of its etiology is still lacking. This chronic inflammatory disease places a significant burden on those whom it affects and uses a large amount of resources. Until we have a greater understanding of its cause and can identify a means to prevent the development of this disease, pharmacologic and nonpharmacologic therapy to control asthma through reduction of risk and impairment is of extreme importance.

Table 7. Medications Used in the Treatment of Asthma[1]

Class and Medication	Mechanism and Indications	Potential Adverse Effects	Therapeutic Issues
β2-Agonists	*Mechanism* • **Bronchodilation:** Stimulation of β2-adrenergic receptors leads to activation of adenylate cyclase and increase in cyclic adenosine monophosphate, which results in smooth muscle relaxation, producing functional antagonism of bronchoconstriction	• Inhalation route generally causes few systemic adverse effects • Tachycardia, skeletal muscle tremor, hypokalemia, increased lactic acid, headache, hyperglycemia, prolongation of QTc interval in overdose • Diminished bronchoprotective effect may occur within 1 wk of chronic therapy; clinical significance has not been established	
SABAs *Inhaled:* Albuterol Levalbuterol *Systemic (injected):* Epinephrine Terbutaline	*Indications* • Relief of acute symptoms; quick-relief medication • Preventive treatment for EIB before exercise	• In addition to effects noted above for β2-agonists, restlessness, irritability, nervousness, and insomnia	• Drugs of choice for acute bronchospasm • Inhalation route has faster onset, fewer adverse effects, and is more effective than systemic routes • Regularly scheduled daily use is not recommended • Less β2-selective agents (isoproterenol, metaproterenol, and epinephrine) are not recommended because of their potential for excessive cardiac stimulation, especially in high doses • Studies on albuterol (racemic mixture) vs. levalbuterol (active R-enantiomer) does not show a difference in adverse effects or outcomes • Regular use > 2 days/wk for symptom control (not prevention of EIB), increasing use, or lack of expected effect indicates inadequate asthma control and need for anti-inflammatory medication

(continued)

Table 7. Medications Used in the Treatment of Asthma[1] *(continued)*

Class and Medication	Mechanism and Indications	Potential Adverse Effects	Therapeutic Issues
LABAs *Inhaled:* Formoterol Salmeterol	*Indications* • Long-term prevention of symptoms, added to ICS • Prevention of EIB • NOT to be used to treat acute symptoms or exacerbations	• In addition to effects noted above for β2-agonists, potential risk of uncommon, severe, life-threatening, or fatal exacerbation (black box warning for asthma-related deaths)	• Not to be used to treat acute symptoms or exacerbations • Should not be used as monotherapy for long-term control of asthma or as anti-inflammatory therapy • May provide more effective symptom control when added to standard doses of ICS vs. increasing ICS dosage • Clinical significance of potentially developing tolerance is uncertain because studies show symptom control and bronchodilation are maintained
Oral: Albuterol, sustained release			• Inhalation route is preferred because LABAs are longer acting and have fewer adverse effects than oral sustained-release agents • Oral agents have not been adequately studied as adjunctive therapy with ICS

Corticosteroids (Glucocorticoids)	*Mechanism*
	• **Anti-inflammatory**
	  ○ Block late reaction to allergen and reduce airway hyperresponsiveness
	  ○ Inhibit cytokine production, adhesion protein activation, and inflammatory cell migration and activation
	• Reverse β2-receptor down-regulation
	• Inhibit microvascular leakage		

Inhaled (ICS): Beclomethasone dipropionate Budesonide Ciclesonide Flunisolide Fluticasone propionate Mometasone furoate Triamcinolone acetonide	*Indications* • Long-term prevention of symptoms; suppression, control, and reversal of inflammation • Reduce need for oral corticosteroid	• Cough, dysphonia, oral thrush (candidiasis) • In high doses, possible systemic effects (e.g., adrenal suppression, osteoporosis, skin thinning, and easy bruising); studies are inconclusive, and clinical significance has not been established • In low to medium doses, suppression of growth velocity has been observed in children; effect may be transient, and clinical significance has not been established	• Spacer/holding chamber devices with non–breath-activated MDIs and mouth-washing after inhalation decrease local adverse effects • Risks of uncontrolled asthma should be weighed vs. limited risks of ICS therapy; the potential but small risk of adverse events is well balanced by their efficacy

(continued)

Table 7. Medications Used in the Treatment of Asthma[1] *(continued)*

Class and Medication	Mechanism and Indications	Potential Adverse Effects	Therapeutic Issues
Systemic: Methylprednisolone Prednisolone Prednisone	*Indications* • For short-term (3–10 days) "burst" to gain prompt control of inadequately controlled persistent asthma • For moderate or severe exacerbations to prevent progression of exacerbation, reverse inflammation, speed recovery, and reduce rate of relapse • For long-term prevention of symptoms in severe persistent asthma: suppression, control, and reversal of inflammation	• *Short-term use*: reversible abnormalities in glucose metabolism, increased appetite, fluid retention, weight gain, facial flushing, mood alteration, hypertension, peptic ulcer, and rarely aseptic necrosis • *Long-term use*: adrenal axis suppression, growth suppression, dermal thinning, hypertension, diabetes, Cushing syndrome, cataracts, muscle weakness, and impaired immune function • Consideration needed for coexisting conditions possibly worsened by systemic corticosteroids (e.g., herpes virus infections, varicella, tuberculosis, hypertension, peptic ulcer, diabetes mellitus, osteoporosis, *Strongyloides*)	• Other systemic corticosteroids such as hydrocortisone and dexamethasone given in equipotent daily doses are likely to be as effective as prednisolone • Short-term therapy should continue until symptoms resolve; usually 3–10 days but possibly longer; action may begin within 1 hr • Use at lowest effective dose • For long-term use, alternate-day morning dosing produces the least toxicity • No evidence that tapering dose after improvement is useful to prevent relapse in asthma exacerbations

Methylxanthines
Theophylline, sustained-release tablets and capsules
	Mechanism
	• **Bronchodilation**
	  ○ Smooth muscle relaxation from phosphodiesterase inhibition and possibly adenosine antagonism
	  ○ May affect eosinophilic infiltration into bronchial mucosa as well as decreases in T cell numbers in epithelium
	  ○ Increases diaphragm contractility and mucociliary clearance
	
	Indication
	• Long-term control and prevention of symptoms in mild persistent asthma or as adjunctive with ICS, in moderate or persistent asthma
	• NHLBI 2007 guidelines do not recommend oral theophylline for long-term asthma control in children ≤ 5 yr
		• Dose-related acute toxicities include tachycardia, nausea and vomiting, tachyarrhythmias (SVTs), central nervous system stimulation, headache, seizures, hematemesis, hyperglycemia, and hypokalemia
		• Adverse effects at usual therapeutic doses include insomnia, gastric upset, aggravation of ulcer or reflux, and increase in hyperactivity in some children
			• Maintain steady-state serum concentrations 5–15 mcg/mL
			• Routine serum concentration monitoring is essential because of significant toxicities, narrow therapeutic range, and individual differences in metabolic clearance
			• Absorption and metabolism may be affected by several factors that can produce significant changes in steady-state serum theophylline concentrations
			• Patients should be told to discontinue if they experience toxicity
			• Not generally recommended for exacerbations
			• Minimal evidence for added benefit to optimal doses of SABA
			• Serum concentration monitoring is mandatory

(continued)

Table 7. Medications Used in the Treatment of Asthma[1] *(continued)*

Class and Medication	Mechanism and Indications	Potential Adverse Effects	Therapeutic Issues

Anticholinergics
Ipratropium bromide
	Mechanism
	• **Bronchodilation**
	  ○ Competitive inhibition of muscarinic cholinergic receptors
	  ○ Reduces intrinsic vagal tone of the airways
	  ○ May block reflex bronchoconstriction secondary to irritants or to reflux esophagitis
	  ○ May decrease mucous gland secretion
	
	Indication
	• Relief of acute bronchospasm
		• Drying of mouth and respiratory secretions, increased wheezing in some patients, blurred vision if sprayed in eyes
		• If used in ED, produces less cardiac stimulation than SABAs
			• Reverses only cholinergic-mediated bronchospasm; does not modify reaction to antigen; does not block EIB
			• Several doses of ipratropium in ED provide additive effects to SABA
			• May be alternative for patients who do not tolerate SABAs
			• Treatment of choice for bronchospasm because of β-blocker medication
			• Has not proved efficacious as long-term control therapy for asthma

Mast-Cell stabilizers
Cromolyn sodium
nedocromil
	Mechanism
	• **Anti-inflammatory**
	  ○ Blocks early and late reaction to allergen
	  ○ Interferes with chloride channel function
	  ○ Stabilizes mast-cell membranes and inhibits activation and release of mediators from eosinophils and epithelial cells
	  ○ Inhibits acute response to exercise, cold dry air, and SO_2
	
	Indications
	• Long-term prevention of symptoms in mild persistent asthma; may modify inflammation
	• Preventive treatment before exposure to exercise or known allergen
		• Cough and irritation
		• 15%–20% of patients experience an unpleasant taste from nedocromil
			• Therapeutic response to cromolyn and nedocromil often occurs within 2 wk, but a 4- to 6-wk trial may be needed to determine maximal benefit
			• Dose of cromolyn by MDI may be inadequate to affect airway hyperresponsiveness
			• Nebulizer delivery may be preferred for some patients
			• Safety is primary advantage of these agents

LTRAs	*Mechanism* • Selective competitive inhibitor of CysLT1 receptor, a potent constrictor of bronchial smooth muscle		• May attenuate EIB in some patients, but less effective than ICS therapy
Montelukast tablets and granules	*Indication* • Long-term control and prevention of symptoms in mild persistent asthma for patients age ≥ 1 yr • May also be used with ICS as combination therapy in moderate persistent asthma	• Postmarketing reports of behavioral changes in pediatric patients: agitation, aggression, depression, insomnia, tremor • Rare cases of Churg-Strauss; association is unclear	• A flat dose-response curve, without further benefit, if dose is increased beyond recommendations

(continued)

Table 7. Medications Used in the Treatment of Asthma[1] *(continued)*

Class and Medication	Mechanism and Indications	Potential Adverse Effects	Therapeutic Issues
Zafirlukast tablets	*Indication* • Long-term control and prevention of symptoms in mild persistent asthma for patients age ≥ 7 yr • May also be used with ICS as combination therapy in moderate persistent asthma	• Postmarketing reports of reversible hepatitis and, rarely, irreversible hepatic failure resulting in death and liver transplantation	• Administration with meals decreases bioavailability; take at least 1 hr before or 2 hr after meals • Zafirlukast is a microsomal cytochrome P450 enzyme inhibitor that can inhibit the metabolism of warfarin • INRs should be monitored during coadministration • Patients should be warned to discontinue use if they experience signs and symptoms of liver dysfunction (right upper quadrant pain, pruritus, lethargy, jaundice, nausea); monitor patient's ALT values
5-Lipoxygenase Inhibitor	*Mechanism* • Inhibits the production of leukotrienes from arachidonic acid, both LTB4 and the cysteinyl leukotrienes		
Zileuton tablets	*Indication* • Long-term control and prevention of symptoms in mild persistent asthma for patients age ≥ 12 yr • May be used with ICS as combination therapy in moderate persistent asthma in patients age ≥ 12 yr	• Elevation of liver enzymes has been reported • Limited case reports of reversible hepatitis and hyperbilirubinemia	• Zileuton is microsomal cytochrome P450 enzyme inhibitor that inhibits metabolism of warfarin and theophylline; doses of these drugs should be monitored accordingly • Monitor hepatic enzymes (ALT)
Immunomodulators Omalizumab (anti-IgE) For subcutaneous use	*Mechanism* • Binds to circulating IgE, preventing it from binding to the high-affinity (FcεRI) receptors on basophils and mast cells • Decreases mast-cell mediator release from allergen exposure • Decreases the number of FcεRIs in basophils and submucosal cells *Indication* • Long-term control and prevention of symptoms in patients age ≥ 12 yr who have moderate or severe persistent allergic asthma inadequately controlled with ICS	• Pain and bruising of injection sites in 5%–20% of patients • Anaphylaxis in 0.2% of treated patients • Malignant neoplasms in 0.5% of patients vs. 0.2% on placebo; relationship to drug is unclear	• Monitor patients after injection; be prepared and equipped to identify and treat anaphylaxis that may occur • Dose administered either every 2 or 4 wk, depending on patient's body weight and IgE level before therapy • Maximum of 150 mg can be administered in one injection • Must be stored under refrigeration at 2°C–8°C • Unknown whether patients will develop significant antibody titers with long-term administration

ALT = alanine aminotransferase; ED = emergency department; EIB = exercise-induced bronchospasm; ICS = inhaled corticosteroids; IgE = immunoglobulin E; INR = international normalized ratio; LABA = long-acting β_2-agonist; LRTA =leukotriene receptor antagonist; LTB4 = leukotriene B4; MDI = metered dose inhaler; NHLBI = National Heart, Lung, and Blood Institute; SABA = short-acting β_2-agonist; SVT = supraventricular tachyarrhythmia.

Table 8. Asthma Medications and Dosing Based on Age Category[1,39,57]

Medication	< 5 yr			5–11 yr			≥ 12 yr		
	Daily Dose			Daily Dose			Daily Dose		
Inhaled Corticosteroids	Low	Medium	High	Low	Medium	High	Low	Medium	High
Beclomethasone HFA 40 or 80 mcg/puff	N/A	N/A	N/A	80–160 mcg	> 160–320 mcg	> 320 mcg	80–240 mcg	> 240–480 mcg	> 480 mcg
Budesonide DPI 90, 180, 200 mcg/ inhalation	N/A	N/A	N/A	180–400 mcg	> 400–800 mcg	> 800 mcg	180–600 mcg	> 600–1,200 mcg	> 1,200 mcg
Budesonide inhaled Inhalation suspension	0.25–0.5 mg	> 0.5–1 mg	> 1 mg	0.5 mg	1 mg	2 mg	N/A	N/A	N/A
Flunisolide 250 mcg/puff	N/A	N/A	N/A	500–750 mcg	1,000–1,250 mcg	> 1,250 mcg	500–1,000 mcg	> 1,000–2,000 mcg	> 2,000 mcg
Flunisolide HFA 80 mcg/puff	N/A	N/A	N/A	160 mcg	320 mcg	≥ 640 mcg	320 mcg	> 320–640 mcg	> 640 mcg
Fluticasone HFA/MDI 44, 110, 220 mcg/puff	176 mcg	> 176–352 mcg	> 352 mcg	88–176 mcg	> 176–352 mcg	> 176–352 mcg	88–264 mcg	> 264–440 mcg	> 440 mcg
Fluticasone DPI 50, 100, 250 mcg/ inhalation	N/A	N/A	N/A	100–200 mcg	> 200–400 mcg	> 400 mcg	100–300 mcg	> 300–500 mcg	> 500 mcg
Mometasone DPI 100, 200 mcg/inhalation	N/A	N/A	N/A	100 mcga	100 mcg	100 mcg	200 mcg	400 mcg	> 400 mcg
Triamcinolone acetonide 75 mcg/puff	N/A	N/A	N/A	300–600 mcg	> 600–900 mcg	> 900 mcg	300–750 mcg	> 750–1,500 mcg	> 1,500 mcg
Systemic Corticosteroids									
Methylprednisolone (PO/IV)	1–2 mg/kg/day in 1 to 2 divided doses			1–2 mg/kg/day in 2 divided doses			40–60 mg/day in 1 or 2 divided doses		
Prednisolone	Short-course "burst": 1–2 mg/kg/day; maximum 60 mg for 3–10 days			Short-course burst: 1–2 mg/kg/day; maximum 60 mg for 3–10 days			Short-course burst: 40–60 mg/day as a single dose or two divided doses for 3–10 days		
Prednisone									
Intramuscular Methylprednisolone	7.5 mg/kg as a one-time dose			240 mg as a one-time dose			240 mg as a one-time dose		
Short-Acting β-Agonists									
Albuterol HFA 90 mcg/puff	2 puffs every 4–6 hr as needed			2 puffs every 4–6 hr as needed			2 puffs every 4–6 hr as needed		
Albuterol nebulizer 0.63 mg/3 mL 1.25 mg/3 mL 2.5 mg/3 mL 5 mg/mL (0.5%)	0.63–2.5 mg every 4–6 hr as needed			1.25–5 mg every 4–8 hr as needed			1.25–5 mg every 4–8 hr as needed		
Levalbuterol HFA 45 mcg/puff	N/A			2 puffs every 4–6 hr as needed			2 puffs every 4–6 hr as needed		
Levalbuterol nebulizer 0.31 mg/3 mL 0.63 mg/3 mL 1.25 mg/0.5 mL 1.25 mg/3 mL	0.31–1.25 mg every 4–6 hr as needed			0.31–0.63 mg every 8 hr as needed			0.63–1.25 mg every 8 hr as needed		
Pirbuterol Autohaler 200 mcg/puff	N/A			N/A			2 puffs every 4–6 hr as needed		

(continued)

Table 8. Asthma Medications and Dosing Based on Age Category[1,39,57] *(continued)*

Medication	< 5 yr	5–11 yr	≥ 12 yr
	Daily Dose	**Daily Dose**	**Daily Dose**
Systemic (Injected) β-Agonists			
Epinephrine 1 mg/mL	SC: 0.01 mg/kg every 20 min for 3 doses	SC: 0.01 mg/kg (up to 0.3–0.5 mg) every 20 min for 3 doses	SC: 0.3–0.5 mg every 20 min for 3 doses
Terbutaline 1 mg/mL	SC: 0.01 mg/kg every 20 min for 3 doses, then every 2–6 hr as needed	SC: 0.01 mg/kg (up to 0.25 mg) every 20 min for 3 doses, then every 2–6 hr as needed	SC: 0.25 mg every 20 min for 3 doses, then every 2–6 hr as needed
	IV: 4–10 mcg/kg bolus, then continuous infusion of 0.2–0.4 mcg/kg/min, titrate by 0.1–0.2 mcg/kg/min every 30 min based on response or toxicity (Usual maximum: 5 mcg/kg/min; doses of 10 mcg/kg/min reported)	IV: 4–10 mcg/kg bolus, then continuous infusion of 0.2–0.4 mcg/kg/min, titrate by 0.1–0.2 mcg/kg/min every 30 min based on response or toxicity (Usual maximum: 5 mcg/kg/min; doses of 10 mcg/kg/min have been reported)	IV: 4–10 mcg/kg bolus, then continuous infusion of 0.2–0.4 mcg/kg/min, titrate by 0.1–0.2 mcg/kg/min every 30 min based on response or toxicity (Usual maximum: 5 mcg/kg/min: doses of 10 mcg/kg/min have been reported)
Long-Acting β-Agonists			
Salmeterol DPI DPI 50 mcg/blister	N/A	1 blister every 12 hr	1 blister every 12 hr
Formoterol DPI DPI 12-mcg/capsule	N/A	1 capsule every 12 hr	1 capsule every 12 hr
Combined Medication			
Fluticasone/salmeterol DPI 100 mcg/50 mcg (≥ 5 yr) 250 mcg/50 mcg (≥ 12 yr) 500 mcg/50 mcg (≥ 12 yr)	N/A	1 inhalation bid	1 inhalation bid
Fluticasone/salmeterol HFA 45 mcg/21 mcg (≥ 12 yr) 115 mcg/21 mcg (≥ 12 yr) 230 mcg/21 mcg (≥ 12 yr)	N/A	N/A	1 inhalation bid
Budesonide/formoterol HFA/MDI 80 mcg/4.5 mcg (≥ 5 yr) 160 mcg/4.5 mcg (≥ 12 yr)	N/A	2 puffs bid	2 puffs bid
Mometasone/formoterol HFA/MDI 100 mcg/5 mcg (≥ 12 yr) 200 mcg/5 mcg (≥ 12 yr)	N/A	N/A	2 puffs bid
Anticholinergics			
Ipratropium HFA 17 mcg/puff	N/A	1 or 2 puffs every 6 hr	2 or 3 puffs every 6 hr
Ipratropium nebulizer 0.25 mg/mL	0.125–0.25 mg every 8 hr	0.25 mg every 6 hr	0.25 mg every 6 hr
Ipratropium/albuterol nebulizer 0.5–2.5 mg/3 mL	N/A	N/A	3 mL every 4–6 hr
Cromolyn/Nedocromil			
Cromolyn MDI 0.8 mg/puff	N/A	2 puffs qid	2 puffs qid
Cromolyn nebulizer 20 mg/ampule	1 ampule qid (≥ 2 yr)	1 ampule qid	1 ampule qid
Nedocromil MDI 1.75 mg/puff	N/A	2 puffs qid	2 puffs qid

(continued)

Table 8. Asthma Medications and Dosing Based on Age Category[1,39,57] *(continued)*

Medication	< 5 yr	5–11 yr	≥ 12 yr
	Daily Dose	**Daily Dose**	**Daily Dose**
Leukotriene Modifiers			
Leukotriene Receptor Antagonists			
Montelukast 4 mg chew tablet (≥ 1 yr) 4 mg packet (≥ 1 yr) 5 mg chew tablet (> 5 yr) 10 mg tablet (≥ 12 yr)	4 mg every night at bedtime (1–5 yr)	5 mg every night at bedtime (6–14 yr)	10 mg (≥ 15 yr)
Zafirlukast 10-mg tablet (5–11 yr) 20-mg tablet (≥ 12 yr)	N/A	10 mg bid (5–11 yr)	40 mg/day (20-mg tablet bid)
5-Lipoxygenase Inhibitor			
Zileuton 600-mg tablet (≥ 12 yr)	N/A	N/A	2,400 mg/day (600-mg tablet qid)
Methylxanthines			
Theophylline	Starting dose 10 mg/kg/day; usual maximum 16 mg/kg/day (≥ 1 yr)	Starting dose 10 mg/kg/day; usual maximum 16 mg/kg/day	Starting dose 10 mg/kg/day, up to 300 mg maximum; usual maximum 800 mg/day
Immunomodulators			
Omalizumab subcutaneous injection 150 mg/1.2 mL	N/A	N/A	150–375 mg SC every 2–4 wk, depending on weight and serum IgE level

[a]Dosages that are italicized are based on data from clinical trials that support use in patients beyond the FDA-approved labeling.

bid = twice daily; DPI = dry powder inhaler; h = hr; HFA = hydrofluoroalkane; IgE = immunoglobulin E; IV = intravenous; MDI = metered dose inhaler; N/A = not applicable; qid = four times/day; SC = subcutaneously.

Table 9. Delivery Devices for Asthma Drugs[1]

Device/Drugs	Population (Age)	Optimal Technique	Therapeutic Issues

Metered dose inhaler (MDI)
β2-Agonists
  Corticosteroids
  Cromolyn sodium
  Anticholinergics
	≥ 5 yr
	OR
	< 5 with spacer or VHC mask
		Actuation during a slow (3–5 s), deep inhalation, followed by a 10-s breath hold	• Slow inhalation and coordination of actuation during inhalation may be difficult, particularly in young children
			• Patients may incorrectly stop inhalation at actuation
			• Deposition of 50%–80% of actuated dose in oropharynx
			• Mouth washing and spitting is effective to reduce amount of drug swallowed and absorbed systemically

Breath-actuated MDI β₂-Agonists	≥ 5 yr	Tight seal around mouthpiece and slightly more rapid inhalation than standard MDI, followed by a 10-s breath hold	• May be useful for patients unable to coordinate inhalation and actuation • Patients may incorrectly stop inhalation at actuation • Cannot be used with spacer/VHC devices

Dry powder inhaler (DPI)
β₂-Agonists
  Corticosteroids
  Anticholinergics
	≥ 4 yr	• Rapid (1 or 2 s), deep inhalation
		• Minimally effective inspiratory flow is device-dependent
		• Most children < 4 yr do not generate sufficient inspiratory flow to activate the inhaler
			• Dose is lost if patient exhales through device after actuating
			• Delivery may be greater or lesser than MDI, depending on device and technique
			• Rapid inhalation promotes greater deposition in larger central airways
			• Mouth washing and spitting is effective to reduce amount of drug swallowed and absorbed

Spacer or VHC	≥ 4 yr OR < 4 yr VHC with face mask	• Slow (3–5 s), deep inhalation, followed by 10-s breath hold immediately after each actuation • If face mask is used, it should have a tight fit and allow 3–5 inhalations per actuation	• Indicated for patients who have difficulty performing adequate MDI technique • VHC improves lung delivery and response in patients who have poor MDI technique • Facemask allows MDIs to be used with small children, but use of a facemask reduces delivery to lungs by 50% • Spacers and/or VHCs decrease oropharyngeal deposition • Rinse plastic VHCs once a month with dilute household dishwashing detergent

(continued)

Table 9. Delivery Devices for Asthma Drugs[1] *(continued)*

Device/Drugs	Population (Age)	Optimal Technique	Therapeutic Issues

Nebulizer
  β₂-Agonists
    Corticosteroids
    Cromolyn sodium
    Anticholinergics
	Patients of any age who cannot use MDI with VHC and face mask	• Slow tidal breathing with occasional deep breaths
		• Tightly fitting face mask for those unable to use mouthpiece
		• Using the "blow-by" technique (holding the mask or open tube near the infant's nose and mouth) is not appropriate
			• Less dependent on patient's coordination and cooperation
			• May be expensive; time-consuming
			• Use of a facemask reduces delivery to lungs by 50%
			• Nebulizers are as effective as MDIs plus VHCs for delivering bronchodilators in mild to moderate exacerbations
			• Potential for bacterial infections if not cleaned properly

MDI = metered dose inhaler; VHC = valved holding chamber.

Patient Case | PEDIATRIC ASTHMA EXACERBATION

A 6-year-old boy who has asthma is brought by his mother to the emergency department with respiratory distress as evidenced by cough, wheezing, and increasing shortness of breath for 24 hours that began shortly after the onset of a low-grade fever and runny nose. His older sister is also ill with an upper respiratory infection, but she does not have asthma. His mother began treating the boy's exacerbation of asthma with albuterol by metered dose inhaler without a spacer every 4 hours, but he has become increasingly short of breath. He is agitated and talking in short phrases only.

Past medical history is notable for asthma since infancy, with six hospitalizations resulting from upper respiratory infections. The asthma exacerbations have been increasing in frequency and duration, and he also has a history of eczema and environmental allergies. He is prescribed an albuterol by metered dose inhaler with a spacer as needed according to an asthma action plan based on symptoms alone because he does not remember how to test lung function at home. He has been using albuterol daily outside of this exacerbation. His mother is not sure what other medications were prescribed for him because they have recently moved and have not yet found a primary care physician. His mother mentions that he is in first grade and has missed 7 days of school because of asthma; he also has difficulty participating in physical education and sports. His stepfather smokes in the home. The child's vaccinations are up-to-date.

Physical examination reveals moderate respiratory distress with suprasternal and intercostal retractions. His lung examination is notable for decreased breath sounds throughout lung fields with diffuse expiratory wheeze and a prolonged expiratory phase. His weight is 19.8 kg. His vital signs include a Tmax of 100.4°F (38°C), respiratory rate of 44 breaths/minute, heart rate of 124 beats/minute, and an oxygen saturation of 89% on room air. His peak expiratory flow is 38% of predicted. His nasal mucosa is erythematous with clear mucus. His skin is dry with eczema on his arms. The remainder of his examination is unremarkable.

1. How should this patient's underlying asthma severity and control be classified?

This patient is experiencing symptoms daily as evidenced by daily use of albuterol. He has some limitation of normal activity given his challenge in participating in physical education and sports. Given that no information is provided on lung function assessment at home, this patient can be classified as having moderate persistent asthma that is not well controlled.

2. How should the severity of the exacerbation be classified? What initial therapies should be recommended in the emergency department?

Given that this patient's peak expiratory flow is less than 40% of predicted, his exacerbation is considered severe. As a result, oxygen should be initiated to maintain oxygen saturation greater than 90%; albuterol nebulizer solution 2.5 mg/3mL every 20 minutes for 3 doses, then 2.5 mg/3mL every 1 hour as needed; and then ipratropium nebulizer solution 0.25 mg every 20 minutes for 3 doses as needed; and oral systemic corticosteroids should be initiated, with prednisone 10 mg twice daily until peak expiratory flow is 70% of predicted or personal best.

3. What National Asthma Education and Prevention Program Guideline step is the patient on at baseline according to self-report? What step should be recommended on patient discharge?

With a short-acting β-agonist as needed as the only therapy, the patient can be considered to be on Step 1. Given that the patient has moderate persistent asthma that is not well controlled, the recommended action for treatment is to move to Step 2 with initiation of a low-dose inhaled corticosteroid and reevaluation in 2–6 weeks, with fluticasone by metered dose inhaler 44 mcg/puff as 2 puffs twice daily.

REFERENCES

1. National Heart, Lung, and Blood Institute, National Asthma Education and Prevention Program: Expert Panel Report 3: Guidelines for the Diagnosis and Management of Asthma. NIH Publication No. 07-4051. Bethesda, MD: National Heart, Lung, and Blood Institute, 2007.

2. Healthy People 2020. Washington, DC: U.S. Department of Health and Human Services, Office of Disease Prevention and Health Promotion. Available at www.healthypeople.gov/2020/data-search/Search-the-Data#topic-area=3503. Accessed March 1, 2019.

3. Weiss ST, Speizer FE. Epidemiology and natural history. In: Weiss EB, Stein M, eds. *Bronchial Asthma Mechanisms and Therapeutics*. 3rd ed. Toronto, Ontario, Canada: Little Brown, 1993:15–25.

4. Lai CK, Beasley R, Crane J, et al.; International Study of Asthma and Allergies in Childhood Phase Three Study Group. Global variation in the prevalence and severity of asthma symptoms: phase three of the International Study of Asthma and Allergies in Childhood (ISAAC). Thorax 2009;64:476.

5. Masoli M, Fabian D, Holt S, et al.; Global Initiative for Asthma (GINA) Program. The global burden of asthma: Executive summary of the GINA dissemination committee report. Allergy 2004;59:469.

6. Centers for Disease Control and Prevention, National Center for Health Statistics. Summary Health Statistics for U.S. Children: National Health Interview Survey, 2009, Series 10, Number 247. DHHS Publication No. (PHS)-2011-1575. Atlanta: CDC, 2009.

7. Centers for Disease Control and Prevention. Vital Signs: Asthma in Children—United States, 2001–2016. Morbidity and Mortality Weekly Report 2018;67:149–55.

8. Akinbami LJ, Simon AE, Rossen LM. Changing trends in asthma prevalence among children. Pediatrics 2016;137:1–7.

9. Black LI, Benson V. Tables of Summary Health Statistics for U.S. Children: 2017 National Health Interview Survey. 2018. Available at www.cdc.gov/nchs/nhis/SHS/tables.htm. Accessed October 2, 2019.

10. International Study of Asthma and Allergies in Childhood (ISAAC) Steering Committee. Worldwide variation in prevalence of symptoms of asthma, allergic rhinoconjunctivitis, and atopic eczema. Lancet 1998;351:1225–32.

11. World Health Organization (2017, August 31). Asthma. Available at www.who.int/news-room/fact-sheets/detail/asthma. Accessed October 2, 2019.

12. Moorman JE, Akinbami LJ, Bailey CM, et al. National Surveillance of Asthma: United States, 2001–2010. National Center for Health Statistics. Vital Health Stat 3 2012;35:1–58.

13. Larsen GL, Cherniack RM, Irvin CG. Pulmonary physiology of severe asthma in children and adults. In: Szefler SJ, Leung DY, eds. Severe Asthma: Pathogenesis and Clinical Management. New York: Marcel Dekker, 1995:77.

14. Avital A, Noviski N, Bar-Yishay E, et al. Nonspecific bronchial reactivity in asthmatic children depends on severity but not on age. Am Rev Respir Dis 1991;144:36.

15. Laitinen LA, Heino M, Laitinen A, et al. Damage of the airway epithelium and bronchial reactivity in patients with asthma. Am Rev Respir Dis 1985;131:599.

16. Sobonya RE. Quantitative structural alterations in long-standing allergic asthma. Am Rev Respir Dis 1984;130:289.

17. Beasley R, Roche WR, Roberts JA, et al. Cellular events in the bronchi in mild asthma and after bronchial provocation. Am Rev Respir Dis 1989;139:806.

18. Busse WW, Lemanske RF. Asthma. N Engl J Med 2001;344:350.

19. Fitzpatrick AM, Teague WG, Holguin F, et al.; Severe Asthma Research Program. Airway glutathione homeostasis is altered in children with severe asthma: evidence for oxidant stress. J Allergy Clin Immunol 2009;123:146.

20. Barnes PJ. The cytokine network in asthma and chronic obstructive pulmonary disease. J Clin Invest 2008;118:3546.

21. Djukanović R, Roche WR, Wilson JW, et al. Mucosal inflammation in asthma. Am Rev Respir Dis 1990;142:434.

22. Allen M, Heinzmann A, Noguchi E, et al. Positional cloning of a novel gene influencing asthma from chromosome 2q14. Nat Genet 2003;35:258.

23. Van Eerdewegh P, Little RD, Dupuis J, et al. Association of the ADAM33 gene with asthma and bronchial hyperresponsiveness. Nature 2002;418:426.

24. Laitinen T, Polvi A, Rydman P, et al. Characterization of a common susceptibility locus for asthma-related traits. Science 2004;304:300.

25. Sandford A, Weir T, Pare P. The genetics of asthma. Am J Respir Crit Care Med 1996;153:1749–65.

26. van der Hulst AE, Klip H, Brand LP. Risk of developing asthma in young children with atopic eczema: a systematic review. J Allergy Clin Immunol 2007;120:565–9.

27. Global Initiative for Asthma (GINA). Global strategy for asthma management and prevention, 2018. Available at www.ginasthma.org. Accessed October 2, 2019.

28. Scottish Intercollegiate Guidelines Network (SIGN), British Thoracic Society. British guideline on the management of asthma. A national clinical guideline. Edinburgh: SIGN, 2016.

29. Teach SJ, Crain EF, Quint DM, et al. Indoor environmental exposures among children with asthma seen in an urban emergency department. J Pediatr 2006;117:S152–8.

30. Reeves MJ, Lyon-Callo S, Brown MD, et al. Using billing data to describe patterns in asthma-related emergency department visits in children. J Pediatr 2006;117:S106–17.

31. Castro-Rodriguez JA, Holberg CJ, Wright AL, et al. A clinical index to define risk of asthma in young children with recurrent wheezing. Am J Respir Care Med 2000;162:1403–6.

32. Al Sayyad JJ, Fedorowicz Z, Alshimi D, et al. Topical steroids for intermittent persistent allergic rhinitis in children. Cochrane Database Syst Rev 2007;1:CD003163.

33. McCallum GB, Bailey EJ, Morris PS, et al. Clinical pathways for chronic cough in children. Cochrane Database Syst Rev 2014;9:CD006595.

34. Speight AN, Lee DA, Hey EN. Underdiagnosis and undertreatment of asthma in childhood. Br Med J (Clin Res Ed) 1983;286:1253.

35. Gibson PG, Henry RL, Coughlan JL, Gastroesophogeal reflux treatment for asthma in adults and children. Cochrane Database Syst Rev 2003;1:CD001496.

36. Lafond C, Series F, Lemiere C. Impact of CPAP on asthmatic patients with obstructive sleep apnoea. Eur Respir J 2007;29:307–11.

37. Black MH, Zhou H, Takayanagi M, et al. Increased asthma risk and asthma-related health care complications associated with childhood obesity. Am J Epidemiol 2013;178:1120.

38. Kelly KJ, Walsh-Kelly CM, Christenson P, et al. Emergency department allies: a web-based multi-hospital pediatric asthma tracking system. J Pediatr 2006;117:S63–S70.

39. Letz KL, Jain N. Pediatric asthma bridging the gap between knowledge and practice. Clin Advisor 2007;Suppl.:2–14.

40. Murphy KR, Hopp RJ, Kittelson EB, et al. Life-threatening asthma and anaphylaxis in schools: a treatment model for school-based programs. Ann Allergy Asthma & Immunol 2006;96:398–405.

41. Weinberger M, Abu-Hasan M. Pseudo-asthma: when cough, wheezing, and dyspnea are not enough. J Pediatr 2007;120:855–64.

42. Yawn BP, Enright PL, Lemanske RF Jr, et al. Spirometry can be done in family physicians' offices and alters clinical decisions in management of asthma and COPD. Chest 2007;132:1162–8.

43. Patino CM, Okelo SO, Rand CS, et al. The Asthma Control and Communication Instrument: a clinical tool developed for ethnically diverse populations. J Allergy Clin Immunol 2008;122:936.

44. Schatz M, Kosinski M, Yarlas AS, et al. The minimally important difference of the Asthma Control Test. J Allergy Clin Immunol 2009;124:719.

45. Liu AH, Zeiger RS, Sorkness CA, et al. The Childhood Asthma Control Test: retrospective determination and clinical validation of a cut point to identify children with very poorly controlled asthma. J Allergy Clin Immunol 2010;126:267.

46. Meltzer EO, Busse WW, Wenzel SE, et al. Use of the Asthma Control Questionnaire to predict future risk of asthma exacerbation. J Allergy Clin Immunol 2011;127:167.

47. Eisner MD, Yegin A, Trzaskoma B. Severity of asthma score predicts clinical outcomes in patients with moderate to severe persistent asthma. Chest 2012;141:58.

48. Jia CE, Zhang HP, Lv Y, et al. The Asthma Control Test and Asthma Control Questionnaire for assessing asthma control: Systematic review and meta-analysis. J Allergy Clin Immunol 2013;131:695.

49. Rank MA, Bertram S, Wollan P, et al. Comparing the Asthma APGAR system and the Asthma Control Test in a multicenter primary care sample. Mayo Clin Proc 2014;89:917.

50. Coffman JM, Cabana MD, Halpin HA, et al. Effects of asthma education on children's use of acute care services: a meta-analysis. J Pediatr 2008;121:575–86.

51. Kwok MY, Walsh-Kelly CM, Gorelick MH, et al. National Asthma Education and Prevention Program severity classification as a measure of disease burden in children with acute asthma. J Pediatr 2006;117:S71–7.

52. Sockrider MM, Abramson S, Brooks E, et al. Delivering tailored asthma family education in a pediatric emergency department setting: a pilot study. J Pediatr 2006;117:S135–44.

53. Matsui EC, Abramson SL, Sandel MT. Indoor environmental control practices and asthma. Pediatrics 2016;138:e20162589.

54. Janson SL, McGrath KW, Covington JK, et al. Individualized asthma self-management improves medication adherence and markers of asthma control. J Allergy Clin Immunol 2009;123:840.

55. Fanta CH. Asthma. N Engl J Med 2009;360:1002.

56. Thomas A, Lemanske RF Jr, Jackson DJ. Approaches to stepping up and stepping down care in asthmatic patients. J Allergy Clin Immunol 2011; 128:915.

57. Taketomo CK, Hodding JH, Kraus DM. Pediatric & Neonatal Dosage Handbook, 25th ed. Hudson, OH: Lexi-Comp, 2018.

58. Bogie AL, Towne D. Luckett PM, et al. Comparison of intravenous terbutaline versus normal saline in pediatric patients on continuous high-dose nebulized albuterol for status asthmaticus. Pediatr Emerg Care 2007;23:355–61.

59. Rowe BH, Spooner CH, Ducharme FM, et al. Corticosteroids for preventing relapse following acute exacerbations of asthma. Cochrane Database of Syst Rev 2007;3:CD000195.

60. Manning P, Gibson PG, Lasserson TJ. Ciclesonide versus placebo for chronic asthma in adults and children. Cochrane Database Syst Rev 2008;2:CD006217.

61. Manning P, Gibson PG, Lasserson TJ. Ciclesonide versus other inhaled steroids for chronic asthma in children and adults. Cochrane Database Syst Rev 2008;2:CD007031.

62. Murray CS. Can inhaled corticosteroids influence the natural history of asthma? Curr Opin Allergy Immunol 2008;21:877–81.

63. Zorc JJ, Pusic MV, Ogborn CJ, et al. Ipratropium bromide added to asthma treatment in the pediatric emergency department. J Pediatr 1999;103:748–52.

64. Mohapatra SS, Boyapalle S. Epidemiologic, experimental, and clinical links between respiratory syncytial virus infection and asthma. Clin Microbiol Rev 2008;21:495–504.

65. Jacobsen L, Valovirta E. How strong is the evidence that immunotherapy in children prevents the progression of allergy and asthma? Curr Opin Allergy Clin Immunol 2007;7:556–60.

66. Aggarwal P, Sharad S, Handa R, et al. Comparison of nebulised magnesium sulphate and salbutamol combined with salbutamol alone in the treatment of acute bronchial asthma: a randomised study. Emerg Med J 2006;23:358–62.

67. Knightly R, Milan SJ, Knopp-Sihota JA, et al. Inhaled magnesium sulfate in the treatment of acute asthma. Cochrane Database Syst Rev 2017;11:CD003898.

68. Cheuk DK, Chau TC, Lee SL. A meta-analysis on intravenous magnesium sulfate for treating acute asthma. Arch Dis Child 2005;90:74–7.

69. Mohammed S, Goodacre S. Intravenous and nebulised magnesium sulfate for acute asthma: systematic review and meta-analysis. Emerg Med J 2007;24:823–30.

70. Rowe BH, Bretzlaff JA, Bourdon C, et al. Magnesium sulfate for treating exacerbations of acute asthma in the emergency department. Cochrane Database Syst Rev 2000;1:CD001490.

71. Colebourn CL, Barber V, Young JD. Use of helium-oxygen mixture in adult patients presenting with exacerbations of asthma and chronic obstructive pulmonary disease: a systematic review. Anesthesia 2007;62:34042.

72. Ho AM, Lee A, Karmakar MK, et al. Heliox vs air-oxygen mixtures for the treatment of patients with acute asthma: a systematic overview. Chest 2003;123:882–90.

73. Rodrigo G, Pollack C, Rodrigo C, et al. Heliox for non-intubated acute asthma patients. Cochrane Database Syst Rev 2006;4:CD002884.

CHAPTER 14

Cystic Fibrosis

Hanna Phan, Pharm.D., FCCP, FPPA; and
Robert J. Kuhn, Pharm.D., FCCP, FPPA, FASHP

LEARNING OBJECTIVES

1. Describe the incidence and inheritance pattern of cystic fibrosis (CF).

2. List common signs and symptoms of CF, including its initial presentation and multiorgan system effects throughout life.

3. Identify and apply CF-specific pharmacokinetic differences in the selection of antimicrobial therapy.

4. Determine appropriate chronic therapy and accompanying monitoring values to meet efficacy and safety needs of patients with CF.

5. Determine appropriate acute exacerbation therapy and accompanying monitoring values to meet efficacy and safety needs of patients with CF.

6. Discuss the role of a pharmacist as part of the CF interdisciplinary care team and community.

ABBREVIATIONS IN THIS CHAPTER

cAMP	Cyclic adenosine 3',5'-monophosphate
CF	Cystic fibrosis
CFF	Cystic Fibrosis Foundation
CFRD	Cystic fibrosis-related diabetes
CFTR	Cystic fibrosis-transmembrane conductance regulator
Cl⁻	Chloride
CYP	Cytochrome P450
DIOS	Distal intestinal obstruction syndrome
FDA	U.S. Food and Drug Administration
FEV₁	Forced expiratory volume in 1 second
GERD	Gastroesophageal reflux disease
GI	Gastrointestinal
MRSA	Methicillin-resistant *Staphylococcus aureus*
Na⁺	Sodium
PA	*Pseudomonas aeruginosa*
PERT	Pancreatic enzyme replacement therapy
PIVKA-II	Proteins induced by vitamin K absence

INTRODUCTION

Cystic fibrosis (CF) is a genetic, autosomal-recessive, multiorgan disease affecting more than 30,000 in the United States and 70,000 individuals worldwide.[1] Cystic fibrosis is the most common inherited disease in the white population worldwide. This disease has an incidence of 1 in 3500 births in the United States and an overall incidence as high as about 1 in 1300 in European countries such as Ireland.[2,3] Cystic fibrosis also affects a variety of races and ethnicities, with the greatest incidence within the white population (more than 90% of patients with CF in the United States) and a lower incidence among Hispanic (1 in 1900), Asian (1 in 32,000), and African American (1 in 15,000) populations.[3] Without a current cure, CF continues to be a life-shortening, genetic disease most commonly affecting the pulmonary and gastrointestinal (GI) systems with additional effects on the reproductive system, bone, and sudoriferous (sweat) glands. Because of the technological advances of airway clearance, paired with the discovery of effective drug therapies, the median predicted age of survival for people with CF has extended from 10 years in 1960 to 47 years in 2016.[1,2] Given the multifaceted aspect of CF as a disease, an interdisciplinary approach to patient care is needed because of complex drug therapy regimens.

PATHOPHYSIOLOGY AND GENETICS

Cystic fibrosis is the result of a mutation of a single gene in the long arm of chromosome 7. This mutation affects the CF-transmembrane conductance regulator (CFTR), a membrane ion channel in secretory epithelial cells notably found in airway lumens and the pancreatic duct. The CFTR is mediated by cyclic adenosine 3',5'-monophosphate (cAMP). In an individual without CF, cAMP activates the transport of chloride (Cl⁻) from the cell by CFTR, which corresponds with sodium (Na⁺) and water efflux. In individuals with CF, Cl⁻ and Na⁺ movement is significantly decreased or absent, resulting in decreased secretion of Cl⁻ paired with increased Na⁺ retention and water retention in the submucosa (Figure 1). The subsequent loss of volume in epithelial secretions causes them to be thick and viscous, decreasing mucociliary function and causing mucus-associated obstruction and inflammation. This dysfunction usually affects pulmonary epithelia; however, depending on a patient's phenotype, the patient may also exhibit effects to the pancreatic and hepatobiliary ducts as well as to the microvilli of the GI tract.[3]

The five main classes of mutations associated with CFTR include more than 2,000 known mutations (not all disease-causing mutations). The CFTR mutations are classified by the mechanism from which they affect CFTR function (Table 1 and Figure 2). *Class I mutations* affect the synthesis of CFTR, whereas *class II mutations* affect the location of CFTR from the apical membrane surface. Phe508del (aka F508del), a class II mutation, is the most common mutation within the CF population, accounting for almost 70% of mutation alleles in white patients with CF. *Class III* and *class IV mutations* affect the function of CFTR, specifically the regulation of CFTR function in response to cAMP and Cl⁻ transport, respectively. *Class V mutations*, also recognized as "nonsense" mutations, affect the amount of functional CFTR produced.[3,4]

Other ion channels influence the flux of fluid and ions as part of CF and may also present with dysfunction, including the outwardly rectifying Cl⁻ channel, the epithelial Na⁺ channel, and chloride–bicarbonate exchanger.[5-7] Like CFTR, these channels are potential therapeutic targets for future CF therapies.

The phenotype of CF disease varies on the basis of genotype combination (e.g., Phe508del homozygotes vs. Phe508del/R117H); however, phenotypes can also be heterogeneous between siblings with identical mutations.[8] Thus, it is evident that other genetic factors and environmental factors affect phenotype in patients with CF.[3,4] Newborn genetic screening has now made it possible to detect CF at a much earlier age than the historical phenotypic-dependent

screening and presentation of CF-related symptoms at a later age. In the United States, this assessment is now required as part of the newborn screening panel in all 50 states. The use of sweat tests, which measure the dermal excretion of Cl⁻, and advanced DNA analysis have also advanced the ability to confirm diagnosis and identify specific genotype, respectively.[9] Prenatal screening can include CF carrier status testing of parents as well as fetal testing when both parents are carriers. Fetal testing involves chorionic villus sampling through amniocentesis, in which CF gene mutations in the DNA from chorionic villus cells can be identified early in pregnancy (i.e., 11–14 weeks' gestation).[10]

PULMONARY DISEASE IN CF

PHYSICAL MANIFESTATIONS

The accumulation of thick, viscous pulmonary secretions (known as *airway surface liquid*) results in poor mucociliary clearance of debris and mucus by respiratory cilia. Consequently, the dehydrated nature of the airway surface liquid and mucus accumulation result in the obstruction of

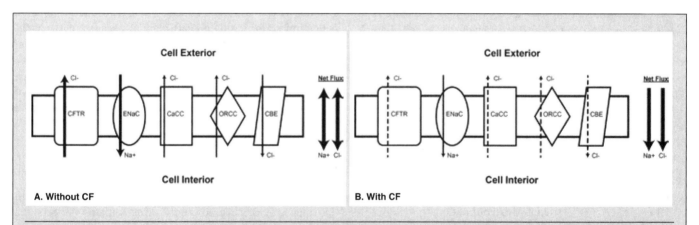

Figure 1. General electrolyte flux and airway lumen/submucosa in an individual (A) without cystic fibrosis (CF), and (B) with CF.

CFTR = cystic fibrosis transmembrane conductance protein; CaCC = calcium activated chloride channel; CBE = chloride bicarbonate exchanger; Cl⁻ = chloride; ENaC = epithelial sodium channel; Na⁺ = sodium.

Table 1. CFTR Mutation Classification, Effect, and Genotype Example[3,4]

Mutation Class	Effect of Mutation on CFTR	Common Genotype Example
I	Premature termination of production, resulting in decreased or no functional CFTR Cl⁻ channels	G542X
II	Defective processing of CFTR; CFTR does not reach apical membrane surface for function	Phe508del[a]
III	CFTR reaches membrane surface but does not respond to cAMP stimulation resulting in defective regulation	G551D
IV	CFTR reaches membrane surface, but Cl⁻ transport is defective	R117H
V	Synthesis of functional CFTR is reduced, resulting in small amount of functional CFTR to the membrane surface	3,849 + 10 kb C→T
VI	Missense mutation resulting in decreased CFTR stability	4326delTC

[a]Most common CF mutation.
cAMP = cyclic adenosine monophosphate; CF = cystic fibrosis; CFTR = CF-transmembrane conductance regulator; Cl⁻ = Chloride.

small and large airways. This obstruction leads to air trapping, bronchiectasis, and atelectasis. Bacteria and other foreign particles remain in the airways, leading to colonization and subsequent infection (e.g., bronchopneumonia) and inflammation (Figure 3). Because of the continued obstruction and inflammatory state, hyperinflammation and dilation of airspaces are often noted in diagnostic imaging. Hemoptysis is also commonly noted in patients with CF, especially as part of pulmonary exacerbations, ranging from streaking in the sputum to massive hemoptysis. Other pulmonary complications include pneumothorax, occurring in about 1 in 167 patients per year.[11]

Patients with CF have distinct phenotypes of their disease, ranging from mild disease with few acute exacerbations to moderate or severe disease more often requiring hospitalization and acute treatment.[12] In addition, patients can be stable for years and then experience a rapid loss of pulmonary function during a relatively short period. With each pulmonary infection and resulting inflammation, pulmonary function is decreased, which is commonly termed the *vicious cycle* of CF pulmonary disease (Figure 3). Percent predicted forced expiratory volume in 1 second (FEV_1) is considered a strong predictor of survival and pulmonary function in patients with CF. Studies have shown that loss of FEV_1 is greatest during adolescence when a nadir of adherence to airway clearance and drug therapy occurs, with an overall average loss of FEV_1 of between 1 and 3 FEV_1 points per year.[13]

Often the lungs of individuals with CF are colonized with gram-positive (e.g., *Staphylococcus aureus*) and/or gram-negative (e.g., *Pseudomonas aeruginosa* [PA]) pathogens in childhood.[3,12,13] Pulmonary colonization and/or infection by other microbes are also noted, which can vary with factors such as age, geographic location, and exposure to pathogens (e.g., hospitalization).[3,14]

THERAPIES FOR PULMONARY DISEASE IN CF

AIRWAY CLEARANCE

The increased viscosity of the mucus of patients with CF, the subsequent obstruction, and even mucus plugging dictate the use of physiotherapy to help loosen this mucus and help with expectoration. First approaches include chest percussion and postural drainage by positioning of the patient in multiple positions to help drain the mucus from the various lobes of the lung while cupping the hands and percussing the chest. This procedure should be done at least two or three times/day and requires about 30 minutes to complete. Because this procedure is very difficult to perform given the considerable requirement for caregiver time to manually provide physiotherapy, mechanical devices have been developed to facilitate this procedure. Chest therapy vests have been developed that use a fitted vest and pneumatic pressure to automate the process and help improve adherence and benefit to the patient. This type of therapy continues today, including the use of physical exercise and other devices that aid in mucus clearance to help maintain airway clearance and prevent clinical deterioration.[15,16]

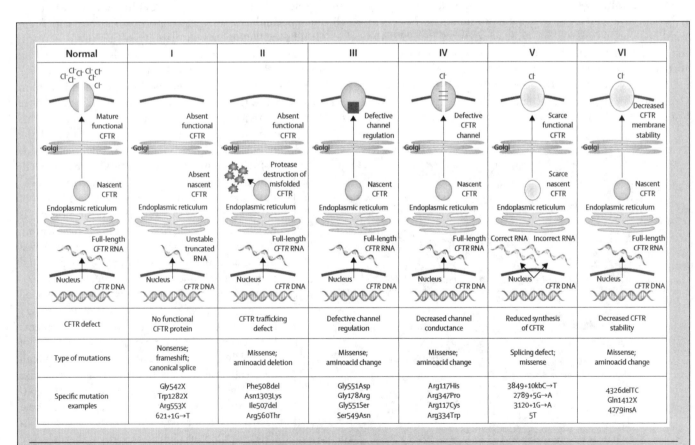

Figure 2. Cystic fibrosis transmembrane conductance protein (CFTR) mutation classes.

Reprinted with permission from Elborn JS. Cystic fibrosis. Lancet 2016;388:2519-31.

PHARMACOTHERAPY

TREATMENT GUIDELINES

In the past 5 years, a concerted effort has been made by the Cystic Fibrosis Foundation (CFF) to help establish guidelines for the treatment of both chronic therapies and acute exacerbations. These key drug therapy findings for chronic therapies and acute exacerbations were based on a level of evidence from the literature as determined by a consensus committee.[15,16]

CHRONIC MAINTENANCE THERAPY

Although CF is a disease of exocrine dysfunction and CFTR abnormalities, the pulmonary manifestations of this disease are the most difficult to treat and account for most of the morbidity and mortality in patients with CF.[17] Because this disease is progressive, therapies to maintain or preserve lung function and quality of life are now the mainstay of treatment. These approaches include the use of mucolytics and long-term inhaled antibiotics as well as chest physiotherapy and other methods to facilitate mucociliary clearance.[15,16,18] Goals for chronic maintenance pulmonary therapy include improving (and/or decreasing loss of) lung function, decreasing frequency of exacerbations, and improving quality of life.

Chronic aerosolized antibiotics. Inhaled antibiotics show long-term benefit in patients with PA colonization.[17,19] For almost 50 years, patients with CF have received inhaled antibiotics. Initially, they were heroic approaches to very ill patients that involved parenteral formulations placed in traditional jet nebulizers by local centers.[20-22] In 1999, the first inhaled aerosolized antibiotic, tobramycin solution for inhalation, was approved with a 300-mg dose twice daily, alternating every 28 days. Because the drug is directly administered to the airway and little systemic absorption occurs, larger doses of aminoglycosides can be used for chronic administration with little risk of long-term nephrotoxicity. Efficacy of this regimen has been shown in children age 6–12 years as well as in those age 13–18 years, with an average improvement in the FEV_1 of almost 10 percentage points.[23] Potential adverse effects of tobramycin solution for inhalation include bronchospasm, hoarseness, and tinnitus. This drug was the only approved nebulized antibiotic until 2011, when aztreonam lysine was approved with a dose of 75 mg three times per day with a similar 28-day alternating-therapy regimen.[24,25] This alternating-day regimen was selected to minimize the development of resistance of PA and other sensitive isolates to these chronic therapies. Potential adverse effects of aztreonam lysine include bronchospasm, sore throat, nasal congestion, and fever (in children). Data from inhaled tobramycin document a rise in the minimum inhibitory concentration of the PA isolated; however, this increase, seen in the first few cycles, seems to plateau with time.[26] Given that the aerosolized concentration in sputum is 50–100 times higher than microbiologic breakpoints and that it has a concentration-dependent killing of this organism, the clinical utility of these breakpoints may not be relevant to patient care.[26] Currently, doses for tobramycin solution for inhalation or aztreonam lysine are standard for all ages of patients requiring therapy. Guidelines currently recommend the chronic use of an inhaled antibiotic (e.g., nebulized or inhaled tobramycin or nebulized aztreonam) in patients age 6 years and older with persistent presence of PA in airway cultures. It should also be considered in patients who are younger (i.e., infants and young children) to eradicate PA at initial acquisition and chronically if cultures are persistently positive for PA.[15,16,18]

In addition, before the availability of approved aerosolized antibiotics, other parenteral formulations were used by aerosolized administration to medically manage patients with CF. Colistimethate has been used for almost 40 years in Europe as well as the United States as an aerosol with a dose of 75–150 mg twice daily.[21,27] Various formulations of this product have been used by centers around the world, and with changing formulations of this natural product, adverse events have occurred, including bronchospasm. Therefore, many centers pretreat with albuterol before a dose of colistin, and careful respiratory monitoring is warranted with the first dose of this medication. Reconstitution of colistin should be done just before administration to minimize the potential formation of broncho-irritative metabolites.

As aerosolized antibiotics have developed during the past decade, nebulizer technology has dramatically changed and improvements have been made to maximize the amount of drug delivered to the patient. Drug delivery can be greatly affected by different devices, and care should be taken to make sure the correct nebulizers are used to deliver the drug. Compressed gas-jet nebulizers were used with most nebulized antibiotics until recently. Piezoelectric cell vibrating-mesh nebulizers (e.g., Trio and Altera, Pari Respiratory Company, Midlothian, VA) now can deliver a uniform particle size

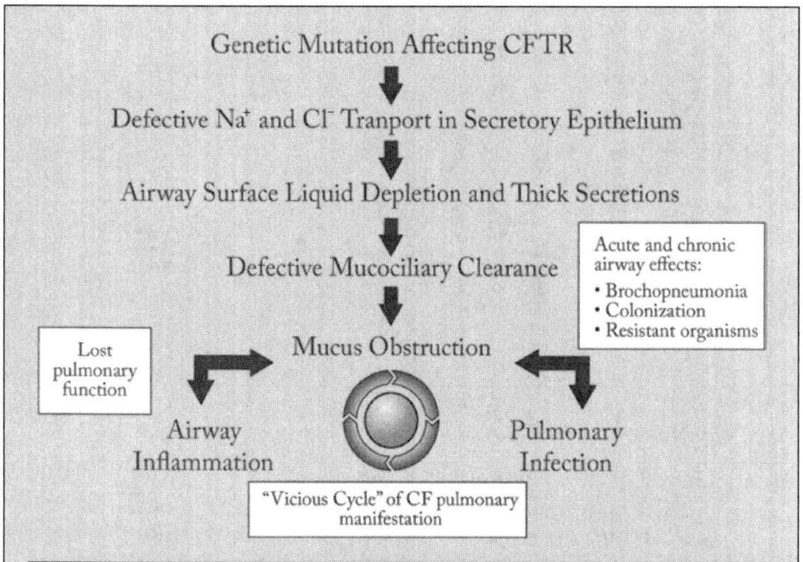

Figure 3. Pulmonary manifestations in CF.

CF = cystic fibrosis; CFTR = CF-transmembrane conductance regulator; Cl⁻ = chloride; Na⁺ = sodium.

aerosol in a very short time.[28] Care must be taken not to universally interchange these devices for antibiotic aerosols or mix them with bronchodilators because performance can be greatly affected. The use of these new improved delivery systems will benefit patients with CF in the coming years, and this technology will help with the delivery of other inhaled medications.

Other aerosolized agents. There are two agents that help increase the removal of the thick sputum produced by patients with CF by breaking down extracellular DNA (dornase alfa) or increasing the amount of fluid in the airway (hypertonic saline). Dornase alfa inhalation has also shown long-term benefit in preserving lung function as part of chronic therapy in CF. This compound works by hydrolyzing extracellular DNA in the sputum to decrease the viscosity of the sputum and improve sputum expectoration by the patient. It has been used for more than a decade with few adverse effects to patients and is one of the first aerosolized therapies initiated in young children with CF. This drug cannot be mixed with other aerosol medications because it often denatures the product, especially with hypertonic solutions.

Since the publication of the latest guidelines, studies with aerosolized 7% hypertonic saline have also shown benefit for chronic therapy, but long-term data (beyond 48 weeks) are currently lacking.[29] Hypertonic saline works by increasing the volume of fluid on the epithelial lining of the airway to maintain normal ciliary flow and increase sputum expectoration. Hypertonic saline concentrations from 3% to 10% were studied, and a 7% solution was found to have the best response with a low rate of bronchospasm, the major adverse effect of this therapy. Some patients may only be able to tolerate 5% solutions, and concentration adjustments may need to be made on an individual basis. To our knowledge, no studies have addressed the concomitant use of these agents for chronic therapy.

The Cystic Fibrosis Foundation recommends use of dornase alfa and hypertonic saline in patients age 6 years and older to help improve lung function, reduce exacerbations, and improve quality of life. It may also be considered in younger patients if they become symptomatic from a pulmonary standpoint.[15,16]

Anti-inflammatory therapy. The vicious cycle of infection and inflammation is now recognized as a key component of the pulmonary manifestations of CF. The focus of therapy has been on long-term anti-inflammatory therapy for patients with CF, although earlier studies with systemic corticosteroids showed improvement in lung function but with an unacceptable toxicity profile, with increases in hyperglycemia, osteoporosis, and growth retardation. Some clinicians use a short course of corticosteroids during an acute pulmonary exacerbation or other illness, but long-term use is not warranted. The use of high-dose, chronic ibuprofen in pediatric patients during a 4-year period showed a decrease in the rate of decline in pulmonary function.[30] This approach, used in only a few patients today, starting at age 6 years and continued until adolescence (age 17 years), requires pharmacokinetic dose monitoring of serum concentrations to maximize the dose. Serum concentrations of 50–100 mcg/mL are required to maximize the effect of this intervention.[16,30,31] Because of concerns about the long-term toxicity of ibuprofen

(e.g., GI irritation and renal dysfunction), this therapy is not widely used. This therapy could be considered in those patients with no known renal dysfunction or bleeding risk and for whom laboratory monitoring (i.e., ibuprofen serum concentration) and pharmacokinetic service is feasible.

In the past decade, the anti-inflammatory properties of azithromycin and other related compounds have been studied, and recent clinical studies have shown benefit in preservation of lung function and decreased pulmonary exacerbations.[32] The benefits of this therapy are from the anti-inflammatory properties of this drug, not its antimicrobial effect. Many patients, including young children, receive this therapy chronically either on a daily or every-other-day basis. According to the CFF guidelines regarding chronic medications, patients with PA consistently in respiratory or sputum cultures should be considered candidates for chronic azithromycin therapy to help improve lung function and reduce exacerbations.[16] Patients without PA positive cultures may also benefit from chronic azithromycin in helping reduce exacerbations.[16] Doses of 250–500 mg given three to seven times/week (not to exceed 10 mg/kg/day) are used by most CF clinicians for long-term therapy. Because the emphasis of this medication is on its anti-inflammatory effects, dosing can be adjusted for convenience because its effect is much longer than its serum half-life. Long-term therapy with azithromycin has not shown any direct adverse reactions. Azithromycin blocks autophagosome clearance, which facilitates the intercellular killing of mycobacteria.[33] Careful follow-up of the CF population receiving azithromycin will help clarify the clinical impact of this observation.

CFTR modulator therapy. Over the past decade, a partnership with the CFF and pharmaceutical industry has produced many new pharmaceuticals for clinical evaluation including aerosolized antibiotics, anti-inflammatory agents, and, most recently, agents that alter the CFTR function. The first novel compound (ivacaftor), a *potentiator*, promotes the channel opening probability of the defective CFTR. The more recent compound (lumacaftor), deemed a *corrector*, increases the number of CFTR proteins that reach the airway surface.[34]

The first agent to treat the underlying defect in CF, ivacaftor, received label approval by the U.S. Food and Drug Administration (FDA) for chronic therapy in patients heterozygous for gating mutations, including the G551D genotype (Table 2). Given that this compound is a potentiator of this "gating" mutation of CF, therapy is limited to about 7% of CF patients. For individuals age 6 years and older, it is given orally at a dose of 150 mg by mouth every 12 hours, taken with a relatively high-fat meal for appropriate absorption. The indication for ivacaftor was expanded to include patients as young as 6 months of age. Dose for individuals age 6 months to 5 years includes 25 mg (for weight 5 to 7 kg), 50 mg (for weight between 7 and 14 kg), or 75 mg (for weight of 14 kg and more) by mouth every 12 hours, with a relatively high-fat meal for appropriate absorption. The original clinical data showed an improvement in FEV_1 of 10.6% and a 55% reduction in the incidence of pulmonary exacerbations.[35] In addition, sweat Cl^- concentrations were reduced by 48.1 mEq/L in this patient population. Liver function monitoring is required in patients on ivacaftor as well as yearly ophthalmic examination for cataracts. A small percentage of patients will have substantial increase in liver function test and may require discontinuation with potential rechallenge.

In 2015, the combination of lumacaftor (a corrector drug) and ivacaftor was approved for patients who are homozygotes for Phe508del mutation, which represents 47% of patients in the United States with CF. This approach to increasing CFTR activity at the airway surface and correcting abnormal CF has the potential to radically change how the disease can be managed, and it may profoundly affect survival and quality of life. On initial FDA approval, the combination drug was indicated in individuals age 12 years and older at a dose of 400 mg lumacaftor and 250 mg ivacaftor (one combination tablet) by mouth every 12 hours with a relatively high-fat meal for appropriate absorption.[36] Since this time, therapy has been expanded to include individuals as young as 2 years. For children between 2 and 5 years, dose is weight dependent, with those weighing less than 14 kg to receive one packet of lumacaftor 100 mg/ivacaftor 125 mg granules and those weighing 14 kg or greater to receive one packet of lumacaftor 150 mg/ivacaftor 188 mg granules, by mouth, mixed with 5 mL of soft food or liquid. For those age 6 to 11 years, the dose is 200 mg lumacaftor and 250 mg ivacaftor (one combination tablet) by mouth every 12 hours. For all patients, doses should be taken with a relatively high-fat meal for appropriate absorption. Unlike with ivacaftor monotherapy, the effect on pulmonary function as measured by FEV_1 was not as impactful, with only an absolute improvement in FEV_1 ranging from 2.6% to 4%.[36] Perhaps the greatest benefit of this combination therapy was a 61% reduction in pulmonary exacerbation requiring hospitalization. In many cases, a pulmonary exacerbation results in a decline in lung function that will not return to baseline even after aggressive therapy so preventing them is an important part of the long-term care of patients with CF. Change in sweat Cl⁻ was evaluated in patients 6 to 11 years, showing a reduction of 24.8 mEq/L at week 24. Monitoring is like that of ivacaftor, with liver function monitoring and ophthalmic examination. For lumacaftor/ivacaftor therapy, abnormal respiration and dyspnea were noted in more than one-third of patients started on this therapy. These symptoms appeared in the first day or week of therapy, and often the symptoms abated as therapy continued. Because these trials were in patients with an FEV_1 greater than 40% predicted, close monitoring of the patients and detailed counseling regarding these symptoms is important. A long-term extension trial demonstrated similar findings including a 42% slower rate of decline in FEV_1 compared with match-controlled patients.[37]

In 2018, a new combination CFTR modulator, tezacaftor/ivacaftor, became available for patients homozygous for the Phe508del or who have at least one mutation responsive to the tezacaftor/ivacaftor combination by clinical evidence or in vitro testing. Currently, it is approved for patients age 6 years and older but studies are ongoing in younger patients. For individuals age 6 to 11 years, the dose is 50 mg tezacaftor and 75 mg ivacaftor (one combination tablet) in the morning

Table 2. CFTR Modulator Therapy with FDA Label Approval for CF Mutations[42-45]

Drug Name	Approved Genotypes			
Ivacaftor	E56K	G178R	S549R	S977F
	F1074L	2789+5G→A	P67L	E193K
	G551D	F1052V	D1152H	3272-26A→G
	R74W	L206W	G551S	K1060T
	G1244E	3849+10kbC→T	D110E	R347H
	D579G	A1067T	S1251N	D110H
	R352Q	711+3A→G	G1069R	S1255P
	R117C	A455E	E831X	R1070Q
	D1270N	R117H	S549N	S945L
	R1070W	G1349D		
Lumacaftor/Ivacaftor	Only Phe508del homozygous			
Tezacaftor/Ivacaftor	E56K	R117C	A455E	S945L
	R1070W	3272-26A→G	P67L	E193K
	Phe508del[a]	S977F	F1074L	3849+10kbC→T
	R74W	L206W	D579G	F1052V
	D1152H	D110E	R347H	711+3A→G
	K1060T	D1270N	D110H	R352Q
	E831X	A1067T 2789+5G→A		
Elexacaftor/Tezactor/Ivacaftor	At least one Phe508del mutation			

[a]Patient must have two copies of the Phe508del mutation or at least one copy of a responsive mutation presented in the table under tezacaftor/ivacaftor to be indicated.
CF = cystic fibrosis; CFTR = CF-transmembrane conductance regulator; FDA = U.S. Food and Drug Administration.

and 75 mg ivacaftor 12 hours later. For those age 12 years and older, the dose is 100 mg tezacaftor and 150 mg ivacaftor (one combination tablet) in the morning and 150 mg ivacaftor 12 hours later in the evening, by mouth, also taken with a relatively high-fat meal for appropriate absorption. In the initial 24-week trial, 504 patients demonstrated a 4% improvement in FEV_1 as well as improvement in Cystic Fibrosis Questionnaire-Revised respiratory score. A 7.4% improvement in FEV_1 and 9.5-point increase in the respiratory domain score of this CF questionnaire was seen in another trial with patients who were heterozygotes for Phe508del and a splice mutation.[38,39] These results are slightly larger than the treatment effect seen in the lumacaftor/ivacaftor trials conducted earlier. It is important to note that the adverse reaction of abnormal respiration was not increased over placebo, and no interaction occurred with oral contraceptives compared with the lumacaftor/ivacaftor combination. These results suggest that these adverse effects could be minimized by using the tezacaftor/ivacaftor combination instead of lumacaftor/ivacaftor therapy.

In 2019, a "triple combination" CFTR modulator agent, elexacaftor/tezacaftor/ivacaftor, became available for patients ages 12 years and older with a least one Phe508del mutation, with studies ongoing in younger patients. This was a huge development in CFTR modulator therapy because it has potential to help treat a greater proportion of persons with CF. The usual dose for age 12 years and older is two orange tablets, each tablet containing elexacaftor 100 mg, tezacaftor 50 mg, and ivacaftor 75 mg, by mouth in the morning and 12 hours later, one blue tablet of ivacaftor 150 mg by mouth, each dose taken with a relatively high-fat meal for appropriate absorption. In a 24-week trial in patients with CF ages 12 years and older with Phe508del and minimal function genotypes, treatment with elexacaftor/tezacaftor/ivacaftor resulted in approximately 14 percentage-point improvement in predicted FEV_1, rate of pulmonary exacerbations that was 63% lower, and improved quality of life with a safe and acceptable side effect profile.[40] For patients homozygous for Phe508del, in a 4-week trial, resulted in approximately 10 percentage-point improvement in predicted FEV_1 and improved quality of life, with a safe and acceptable side effect profile and no treatment discontinuations.[41] CFTR modulator therapy with FDA label approval for CF mutations can be found in Table 2.[42-45]

For CFTR modulators, monitoring of drug–drug interactions is warranted. For example, lumacaftor is a strong inducer

of cytochrome P4503A (CYP3A) and ivacaftor is a substrate of CYP3A4 and CYP3A5. In addition, lumacaftor is a potential inducer of CYP2B6, CYP2C8, CYP2C9, and CYP2C19 enzymes and inhibitor of CYP2C8 and CYP2C9 enzymes. Therefore, it is important to review for potential interactions between a CFTR modulator and concurrent therapy in order to alter or adjust therapy accordingly. A detailed example of dosing guidelines regarding lumacaftor/ivacaftor and drug interactions can be found in Table 3 and Table 4.[42-45]

Studies are ongoing with several compounds to determine whether other genotypes of CF will respond to this class of therapy. For stop mutation (type I), ataluren is in clinical trials to help improve CFTR function in almost 5% of the CF population. If therapy for this population were achieved, then a CFTR modulating therapy would be available to almost 95% of patients with CF.

In addition, the development of novel approaches continues in the delivery of gene therapy (e.g., corrected CFTR delivery) to the airway. Problems with vectors and host response to repeated doses continue to be an issue, but new approaches may be able to overcome these limitations of repeated dosing. Similarly, pharmacologic agents that are not genotype specific are also being developed (e.g., epithelial Na^+ channel modifiers) to create therapies that benefit all patients as well. The promise of these new therapies is indeed exciting and may provide the foundation for a profound change in the outlook of CF in the next decade.[34]

TREATMENT OF ACUTE PULMONARY EXACERBATIONS

Despite the use of daily medications and airway clearance therapies, patients with CF often experience rapid clinical deterioration and increased respiratory symptoms. The increasing cycle of airway inflammation and mucus accumulation in the airway continues, and patients often experience increased work of breathing, fever, increased mucus production, fatigue, and weight loss.[12] This relatively rapid onset of symptoms is referred to as an *acute pulmonary exacerbation*. The hallmark of this disease has been that almost every patient experiences some episodes with variable frequency (e.g., four or five times per year and others, with milder disease, having an exacerbation every 2–3 years). Complete eradication of bacterial and other microbes in the airways becomes more challenging with increased age and/or

Table 3. Dosing and Administration Frequency of Lumacaftor/Ivacaftor with CYP3A Inhibitors[36,37]

Clinical Situation	Dose	Administration Frequency
Initiating lumacaftor/ivacaftor in patients taking strong CYP3A inhibitor[a]	**First Week:** 1 tablet **After First Week:** 2 tablets	**First Week:** once daily **After First Week:** every 12 hours
Initiating CYP3A inhibitors in patients already taking lumacaftor/ivacaftor	No dose adjustments required, standard dose	
Dose Interruptions of lumacaftor/ivacaftor while taking a strong CYP3A inhibitor	• If lumacaftor/ivacaftor is interrupted for > 1 week, and then reinitiated while taking a strong CYP3A inhibitor, reduce dose to 1 tablet daily for first week of treatment reinitiation • Following this period, continue with recommended daily dose	

[a]Strong CYP3A inhibitors are itraconazole and voriconazole.

Table 4. Lumacaftor Drug-Drug Interaction

Drug	Potential Effect of Lumacaftor on Concomitant Drug	Clinical Comment
Montelukast	Decreased	• No dose adjustment recommended • Appropriate clinical monitoring as reasonable
Digoxin	Increased **or** Decreased	• Monitor serum concentration and titrate dose for desired clinical effect
Clarithromycin, Telithromycin, Erythromycin	Decreased	• Consider alternative such as ciprofloxacin, azithromycin, or levofloxacin • No dose adjustments recommended for lumacaftor/ivacaftor when these antibiotics are initiated in patients currently taking lumacaftor/ivacaftor • When initiating lumacaftor/ivacaftor in patients taking these antibiotics, reduce lumacaftor/ivacaftor dose to 1 tablet daily for the first week, then 2 tablets every 12 hours
Warfarin	Increased **or** Decreased	• Monitor INR when co-administration of lumacaftor/ivacaftor is required
Carbamazepine, Phenobarbital, Phenytoin		• Concomitant use **not** recommended • Decreased ivacaftor exposure, may reduce effectiveness of lumacaftor/ivacaftor
Citalopram, Escitalopram, Sertraline	Decreased	• Higher dose of these antidepressants may be required for desired clinical effect
Itraconazole, Ketoconazole, Posaconazole, Voriconazole	Decreased	• Concomitant use **not** recommended • Monitor closely for breakthrough fungal infections if use is necessary • Consider alternative such as fluconazole • No dose adjustment recommended for lumacaftor/ivacaftor when these antifungals are initiated in patients currently taking lumacaftor/ivacaftor • When initiating lumacaftor/ivacaftor in patients taking these antibiotics, reduce lumacaftor/ivacaftor dose to 1 tablet daily for the first week, then 2 tablets every 12 hours
Ibuprofen	Decreased	• Higher dose of ibuprofen may be required for desired clinical effect
Rifabutin, Rifampin		• Concomitant use **not** recommended • Decreased ivacaftor exposure, may reduce effectiveness of lumacaftor/ivacaftor
Midazolam, Triazolam	Decreased	• Concomitant use is **not** recommended • Consider an alternative to these benzodiazepines
Methylprednisolone, Prednisone	Decreased	• Higher dose of these systemic corticosteroids may be required for desired clinical effect
St. John's Wort	Decreased	• Concomitant use **not** recommended • Decreased ivacaftor exposure, may reduce effectiveness of lumacaftor/ivacaftor
Hormonal Contraceptives	Decreased	• Do not rely on hormonal contraceptives, including oral, injectable, transdermal, and implantable, as effective method of contraception • Concomitant use of lumacaftor/ivacaftor with hormonal contraceptives increased menstrual abnormality events • Avoid concomitant use unless benefit outweighs risk
Ranitidine	Increased **or** Decreased	• Dose adjustment may be required for desired clinical effect • No dose adjustment recommended for calcium carbonate antacid
Cyclosporine, Everolimus, Sirolimus, Tacrolimus	Decreased	• Concomitant use is **not** recommended • Avoid use of lumacaftor/ivacaftor
Repaglinide, Sulfonylureas	Increased **or** Decreased	• Dose adjustment may be required for desired clinical effect • No dose adjustment recommended for metformin
Esomeprazole, Lansoprazole, Omeprazole	Decreased	• Dose adjustment may be required for desired clinical effect • No dose adjustment recommended for calcium carbonate antacid

incidence of pulmonary exacerbations; thus, the selection of antimicrobial treatment is a common challenge in the treatment of CF pulmonary exacerbations. Goals for treatment of acute pulmonary exacerbations include recovery or return to baseline lung function, improved symptoms (i.e., reduced cough, sputum production, hemoptysis), improved quality of life, and minimized adverse effects from antimicrobial treatment.

Antibiotic selection. At present, acute pulmonary exacerbation is not well defined, and no clear consensus has been reached regarding what antibiotics should be prescribed or whether the therapy should be inpatient or outpatient. The choice of antibiotics is directed at the most common organisms found in the respiratory tract of each patient because most patients undergo routine quarterly sputum culture collections. Two important caveats in the surveillance and selection of antibiotics should be noted. First, traditional sensitivity results do not predict clinical success of patients with resistant organisms. This finding was described 20 years ago in a study comparing treatment with antibiotics versus placebo for acute pulmonary exacerbations, which found no difference in short-term pulmonary function changes.[46] Other studies have confirmed improvement with antibiotics—usually dual antipseudomonal therapy and additional antibiotics directed at other microbiologic isolates.[47,48] Second, less robust evidence is available to validate the benefit of the duration, number of antibiotics, dosing strategy, and environment of treatment (e.g., inpatient vs. home therapy for the treatment of acute exacerbation).[17] Given this background, most centers still use two-drug antipseudomonal therapies for exacerbation in PA-positive patients for at least 10–14 days. Treatment can be inpatient and/or outpatient in setting, depending on factors including severity and CF center practice trend. The overall improvement in life expectancy and preservation of lung function globally in the CF community for the past 20 years has been an important observation to continue this practice of dual antipseudomonal therapy. Current guidelines from a CFF consensus conference support the use of antibiotics, but they do not endorse two-drug treatments over one susceptible drug. Treatment guidelines have focused on patients with PA, and many patients harbor several other gram-negative organisms and very difficult-to-treat organisms such as *Burkholderia cepacia*, *Stenotrophomonas maltophilia*, and methicillin-resistant *S. aureus* (MRSA), making antibiotic selection complex. Antibiotic selection can be guided, but not dictated, by the results of microbiologic testing. Current practice at most centers would use dual antipseudomonal drug therapy for synergy when treating PA.

During the past 2 decades, several reports of rapid clearance of aminoglycosides and semisynthetic penicillins have been described in patients with CF; therefore, recommended doses of these agents are higher than in patients without CF. Consensus guidelines suggest that once-daily high-dose aminoglycosides like tobramycin at a starting dose of 10 mg/kg/day are warranted.[17,49] As a patient's weight changes with growth, the previous pharmacokinetic guidelines can be used to adjust doses and determine clearance with subsequent serum concentrations. Of importance, given the short half-life of tobramycin and other aminoglycosides, single daily doses will result in a very long time at less than the minimum inhibitory concentration in many pediatric patients. Although the postantibiotic effect of tobramycin against mucoid PA is not clearly understood, it certainly does not exceed 4–6 hours. Therefore, in some patients with very rapid clearances (e.g., with a half-life of less than 2 hours), some centers administer doses of 6–8 mg/kg every 12 hours to shorten this postantibiotic period and still allow substantial clearance of the drug.[48] In any case, careful monitoring of serum concentrations is necessary to prevent accumulation and potential nephrotoxicity and ototoxicity. Once-daily aminoglycoside therapy in CF results in a lower occurrence of nephrotoxicity, as defined by increased serum creatinine and urinary N-acetyl-β-D-glucosaminidase, compared with thrice-daily dosing.[50] No changes in pulmonary function were seen between the once or three times a day therapy strategies. Recent work suggests that patients with CF are indeed candidates for vestibular loss, especially given the many courses of aminoglycosides they have received.[51] With the tremendous increase in life expectancy, the next decade will tell whether total dose or dosing regimens played the most important role in toxicity. Table 5 includes various doses of drugs used for chronic administration and for managing these acute exacerbations in patients.

Because most of the morbidity and mortality with CF is related to lung decline and deterioration, strategies are now being applied to CF from other diseases and conditions. Continuous-infusion antibiotics with time-dependent killing or prolonged infusion of these antibiotics are now being used with intermittent high-dose aminoglycosides to help maximize the treatment of PA exacerbations and other organisms.[52] Practical solutions for ambulatory patients are now available, and many patients can finish their course of antibiotics at home or may receive the entire course at home after a clinic visit. This approach is particularly used for adolescents and adults with CF given their school and/or work demands. No definitive study has been conducted with these approaches to date, but given the success of these strategies in other pulmonary infections, such studies may be of considerable long-term benefit to patients with CF.

Therapy duration is usually determined by careful monitoring of overall symptoms and improvement in pulmonary function (e.g., FEV_1), with treatment often lasting 10–14 days.[17,53] Patients often have a serial pulmonary function test every few days to show improvement as well as symptom improvements and weight gain. Many clinicians monitor biomarkers such as C-reactive protein and procalcitonin to evaluate the progress of an exacerbation, especially for patients in whom pulmonary function testing may be difficult. In one recent study, lower procalcitonin was correlated with patient improvement.[54] Therapy can continue beyond this time if the patient's clinical course does not improve significantly and/or changes in antimicrobial agents are required.

Monitoring of pulmonary therapy. A return to baseline FEV_1 after recovering from a pulmonary exacerbation is ideal, but not always possible, thus the importance of continued suppression of inflammation and infection through airway clearance and accompanying drug therapy.[55]

Because of the aggressive and often-repeated nature of antimicrobial courses, patients with CF require careful monitoring both for long- and short-term events. Initial serum concentrations of aminoglycosides and vancomycin should be obtained within the first 72 hours of therapy unless the patient has a history of delayed clearance or nephrotoxicity. At some CF care centers, it is common to wait 2–3 days to make sure the patient has been adequately rehydrated because many of the patients have had decreased oral intake and increased losses with their increasing symptoms during the previous 5–7 days. Because of the increased incidence of MRSA and PA sputum isolates with pulmonary exacerbation, patients are often treated with intravenous vancomycin in combination with an aminoglycoside. These patients should be monitored often, with care taken for drug accumulation and increased trough concentration during the traditional 10–14 days of therapy. With increasing age and a larger incidence of CF-related diabetes (CFRD), a decrease in aminoglycoside clearance should be anticipated with time. Whether this decrease is caused by age or cumulative toxicity is unclear, but as care moves to adult centers and physicians, previous dosing of drugs should be adjusted accordingly.

Table 5. Antibiotics and Dosing Regimens Commonly Used in the Treatment of Acute Pulmonary Bacterial Exacerbations in Patients with Cystic Fibrosis[a]

Antibiotic	Dosing Regimen[b]
For *Pseudomonas aeruginosa*	
Amikacin	7.5–10 mg/kg/dose intravenous every 8 hours[c] or 30 mg/kg/day
Aztreonam	50–70 mg/kg/dose intravenous every 8 hours (up to 8 g/day)
Cefepime	50–70 mg/kg/dose intravenous every 8 hours (up to 2.5 g/dose)
Ceftazidime	50–70 mg/kg/dose intravenous every 8 hours (up to 8 g/day)[47]
Ciprofloxacin (intravenous)	10 mg/kg/dose intravenous every 8 hours (up to 400 mg/dose)
Ciprofloxacin (oral)	40–50 mg/kg/day oral every 8–12 hours (up to 750 mg/dose)
Colistin	3–6 mg/kg/day intravenous every 8–12 hours
Imipenem/cilastin	25–40 mg/kg/dose intravenous every 6 hours (up to 1 g/dose)
Levofloxacin	Children: 7–10 mg/kg/day intravenous or oral every 24 hours Adults: 500–750 mg/day intravenous or oral every 24 hours
Meropenem	40 mg/kg/dose intravenous every 8 hours (up to 2 g/dose)
Piperacillin/tazobactam	300–500 mg/kg/day intravenous every 4-6 hours (up to 24 g/day)[d]
Ticarcillin/clavulanate	300–500 mg/kg/day intravenous every 6-8 hours (up to 24 g/day)[d]
Tobramycin	10 mg/kg/dose intravenous every 24 hours[c] or 6–7 mg/kg intravenous every 12 hours
For Methicillin-Resistant *Staphylococcus aureus*	
Daptomycin	Should not be used for acute pulmonary exacerbations
Doxycycline	Children: 2.2 mg/kg/dose orally every 12 hours Adults: 100 mg orally every 12 hours
Linezolid	Children: 10 mg/kg/dose intravenous or oral every 8 hours Adults: 600 mg intravenous or oral every 12 hours
Tigecycline	Children: Not applicable Adults: 100 mg loading dose; then 50 mg intravenous every 12 hours
Vancomycin	15–20 mg/kg/dose intravenous every 6-8 hours
Inhaled drugs (used chronically but may be used during acute exacerbations)	
Aztreonam lysine for inhalation	75 mg inhaled three times/day cycling 28 days on/off
Dornase alfa	2.5 mg inhaled daily
Hypertonic saline 7%	4 mL inhaled twice daily
Tobramycin	Solution for inhalation: 300 mg inhaled twice daily, cycling 28 days on/off Dry powder capsules for inhalation: 112 mcg inhaled twice daily, cycling 28 days on/off
Colistin	75–150 mg twice daily (non-labeled use), cycling 28 days on/off

[a]Combination therapy is recommended.
[b]Doses assume normal renal and hepatic function; dose adjustment may be necessary for renal and hepatic impairment.
[c]Use of historical therapeutic milligram-per-kilogram dosage if available.
[d]Based on piperacillin or ticarcillin component.

NUTRITION IN CF

PHYSICAL MANIFESTATIONS

Because of defective CFTR and subsequently impaired transport of Na^+ and Cl^- resulting in viscous epithelial secretions, the pancreatic duct becomes obstructed. This obstruction prevents proper secretion of pancreatic enzymes into the digestive tract, otherwise known as *pancreatic insufficiency*. Chronic pancreatic insufficiency is a common complication affecting around 85% of individuals with CF.[56] Pancreatic insufficiency causes malabsorption of fat and protein, leaving individuals with CF to face challenges in nutritional status. This decrease in nutrient absorption subsequently leads to overall poor growth and, potentially, failure to thrive, especially in infants and younger children. In addition to fat malabsorption, vitamin deficiency is common for fat-soluble vitamins (i.e., vitamins A, D, E, and K). Pancreatic damage, including pancreatitis, can also manifest because of defective pancreatic exocrine secretion.[57,58] Other complications secondary to nutrient malabsorption caused by CF include anemia (often iron-deficient) and osteopenia or osteoporosis.

CALORIC NEEDS AND NUTRITIONAL STATUS IN CF

Individuals with CF often face challenges of poor nutritional status, including poor growth (i.e., weight, stature, and weight-for-stature) and vitamin deficiency. Infants and young children with CF are at increased risk of failure to thrive. Older children and adolescents also face challenges of poor growth because of nutritional risk secondary to CF. Energy needs in this population are increased because of expenditure secondary to their pulmonary condition, including chronic cough, infection, and increased work of breathing. Thus, it is highly recommended that children with CF be provided greater dietary energy intake than children without CF. Weight gain and growth have been shown with intakes from 110% to 200% that of healthy individuals. High-calorie or calorically dense foods are encouraged, such as fortified infant formulas or breast milk for infants and full-fat dairy products and proteins for children and adults. Consistent high-calorie dietary intake can be a challenge in patients with CF because of several physiologic factors, including loss of taste or smell caused by chronic sinusitis and chronic gastroesophageal reflux. In addition, behavioral factors may affect intake, which can require behavioral intervention by dietitians and/or psychologists. For patients of all ages with continued suboptimal growth, use of enteral feeding modes may also be necessary, commonly provided by a gastrostomy tube. With enteral feeding, concentrated, calorically dense formulas may be used to provide more calories with less volume.

THERAPIES FOR NUTRITION CHALLENGES IN CF

PANCREATIC ENZYME REPLACEMENT THERAPY

A diagnosis of pancreatic insufficiency includes genotype evaluation (i.e., two mutations associated with pancreatic insufficiency), growth failure, symptoms including steatorrhea (fatty stool), and measurement of fecal elastase. Measurement of fecal elastase is used for diagnosis versus monitoring of enzyme replacement efficacy. Because fecal elastase involves a general measurement, it is not used for assessing therapy efficacy because it is not a quantitative test. Fecal elastase values less than 200 mcg/g are indicative of pancreatic insufficiency.[59] The 72-hour fecal fat test is an option for quantifying fat malabsorption. However, this approach is not commonly used because it is tedious for caregivers and potentially poor in accuracy.[60]

The mainstay of therapy for pancreatic insufficiency caused by CF is pancreatic enzyme replacement therapy (PERT).[60,61] Although once thought of as dietary supplements and previously poorly regulated in manufacturing and labeling, PERT products for CF are now reviewed for approval by the FDA. Pancreatic enzyme formulations contain different combinations of lipase, protease, and amylase from porcine sources (Table 6).[62-69] The beads or microspheres within the dosage forms (i.e., capsules) are often enteric coated to protect them from acid-mediated destruction in the stomach. This coating dissolves in the less acidic environment of the duodenum, where the enzymes act to aid in digestion and nutrient absorption (i.e., fats, protein, carbohydrates).[61]

Pancreatic enzymes should be taken or administered at meal and snack times, as well as in coordination with enteral feeds if this mode of nutritional provision is used. Pancreatic enzyme formulations contain different combinations of lipase, protease, and amylase from porcine sources (Table 6). Dosing of PERT is weight-based and dependent on the lipase component of dosage forms. The recommended starting dose for infants and children younger than 4 years is lipase 1000 units/kg/meal with infant dosing of lipase 2000–5000 units/kg/meal per feeding of formula or breast milk. For children 4 years and older, a starting dose of lipase 500 units/kg/meal is recommended. Doses should not usually exceed 2500 units/kg/meal, with a maximum of lipase 10,000 units/kg/day.[60,62-69] Dosing for snacks depends on the size and components (i.e., fat content) of the snack. For example, if a snack is about one-half the size of a meal, 50% of the meal dose should be given. However, some patients with CF consume equal-sized portions throughout the day, including both meals and snacks. In these cases, the snack dose would be equivalent to meal dosing. Doses are primarily adjusted on the basis of patient response, with efficacy assessment including patient weight and/or growth markers (e.g., body mass index), frequency of stools, stool consistency (e.g., loose vs. formed), abdominal symptoms (e.g., cramping), and incidence of steatorrhea.

If PERT dosing requirements exceed recommended meal or daily maximums, further investigation about other factors affecting efficacy may be necessary. These factors include adherence, diet, and other comorbidities that may affect GI symptoms such as loose stools, steatorrhea, or abdominal cramping.[60,70] When other possible causes of treatment failure are ruled out, the efficacy of PERT should be considered. The efficacy of PERT can vary because of GI tract pH; thus, comorbidities such as gastroesophageal reflux disease (GERD) may influence therapy outcomes. When maximal dosing is reached, other etiologies are excluded, and the individual continues to present with symptoms of malabsorption (e.g., steatorrhea), the use of long-duration acid suppression by a proton pump inhibitor or histamine H2-receptor blocker may aid in "boosting" the effect of PERT. Studies showing improved growth and decreased incidence of steatorrhea with the addition of a proton pump inhibitor are part of the literature of children as young as 3 years. Dosing is similar to usual starting doses for treatment of GERD (e.g., for a 4-year-old with a weight of 13 kg starting omeprazole 10 mg orally daily) with an indefinite duration because the medication is used to aid in the effect of lifelong PERT.[71]

VITAMIN SUPPLEMENTATION

As part of the malabsorption of nutrients secondary to pancreatic insufficiency, specifically fat, a deficiency in fat-soluble vitamins is a common nutritional complication. Oral supplementation of vitamins A, D, E, and K in individuals with CF, especially those with pancreatic insufficiency, is recommended.[57] For many patients with CF, supplementation by a CF-specific multivitamin containing water-miscible vitamins A, D, E, and K is sufficient for needed supplementation (e.g., AquADEK and DEKA [Callion Pharma, Jonesborough, TN], MVW Complete Formulation [MVW Nutritionals, Huntsville, AL]), with dosing based on age and product formulation. Individuals deficient in these vitamins may be asymptomatic; thus, the use of laboratory tests to assess status is recommended.[60]

Vitamin A is important for several different functions including vision, immune function, and growth. Measurement of the serum concentration of retinol, a marker of vitamin A, is recommended at least annually. Additional oral vitamin A can be provided in doses from 1,500 up to 10,000 units/day, depending on age and deficiency. Excess vitamin A has been associated with bone and liver disease.[72]

Table 6. Examples of Pancreatic Enzyme Replacement Dosage Forms in Cystic Fibrosis[57–65]

Brand Name (dosage form)	Amounts in Units per Dosage Form		
	Lipase	Protease	Amylase
Creon[a] (capsules with enteric-coated, delayed-release microspheres; porcine derived)	3000	9500	15,000
	6000	19,000	30,000
	12,000	38,000	60,000
	24,000	76,000	120,000
	36,000	114,000	180,000
Pancreaze[b] (capsules with enteric-coated, delayed-release microspheres; porcine derived)	2600	6200	10,850
	4200	14,200	24,600
	10,500	35,500	61,500
	16,800	56,800	98,400
	21,000	54,700	83,900
Pertzye[c] (capsules with enteric-coated, bicarbonate buffered, delayed-release capsules; porcine derived)	4000	14,375	15,125
	8000	28,750	30,250
	16,000	57,500	60,500
	24,000	86,250	90,750
Ultresa[d] (capsules with enteric-coated, delayed-release microspheres; porcine derived)	4000	8000	8000
	13,800	27,600	27,600
	20,700	41,400	41,400
	23,000	46,000	46,000
Viokace[e] (tablet; porcine derived)	10,440	39,150	39,150
	20,880	78,300	78,300
Zenpep[e] (capsules with enteric-coated, delayed-release microspheres; porcine derived)	3000	10,000	14,000
	5000	17,000	24,000
	10,000	32,000	42,000
	15,000	47,000	63,000
	20,000	63,000	84,000
	25,000	79,000	105,000
	40,000	126,000	168,000

[a]Abbvie Inc, North Chicago, IL; [b]Vivus, Inc, Campbell, CA; [c]Digestive Care Inc, Bethlehem, PA; [d]Aptalis Pharma, Brookfield, CT; [e]Allergan USA Inc, Irvine, CA.

Vitamin D is necessary for bone health and other functions such as immune function. Deficiency of vitamin D often requires additional oral supplementation with vitamin D_3 (cholecalciferol) ranging from 400–10,000 international units/day, depending on age and 25-hydroxyvitamin-D serum concentration. Although many forms of vitamin D are available for use by prescription or over-the-counter, it has been noted that vitamin D_3 is better absorbed and thus perhaps more efficacious than vitamin D_2 for supplementation in deficiency.[73-75] Measurement of serum concentrations of vitamin D (i.e., 25-hydroxyvitamin-D) are recommended at least annually as part of standard care for patients with CF, with goal concentrations of greater than 30 ng/mL (75 nmol/L).[73-75]

Vitamin E, with its function as an antioxidant, also has a postulated role in suppressing inflammation. Similarly, measurement of a serum level (i.e., α-tocopherol) is recommended at least annually. Because patients with CF often have lower cholesterol levels than individuals without CF, more accurate assessment of vitamin levels may be achieved by use of an α-tocopherol/cholesterol ratio. Additional vitamin E oral supplementation, when levels are low despite standard CF supplementation, can be provided in doses of up to 400 units/day, depending on age and deficiency.[60]

Vitamin K, necessary as a cofactor for the coagulation pathway, is often deficient in individuals with CF because of fat malabsorption as well as changes in GI flora contributed by frequent antimicrobial use. In individuals with CF-associated hepatobiliary disease, this deficiency may be further exacerbated, requiring additional oral supplementation (e.g., phytonadione). Additional oral supplementation of vitamin K may be needed for older children and adults with CF who have chronic deficiency based on laboratory values, who are given long-term antimicrobial therapy, or who have an ongoing history of hemoptysis.[76] Monitoring of serum levels of prothrombin or proteins induced by vitamin K absence (PIVKA-II) is suggested at least annually, with PIVKA-II being more sensitive; however, PIVKA-II may not be easily accessible at all institutions.[60] Additional vitamin K or phytonadione oral supplementation can be provided in doses ranging from 2.5 to 10 mg/day, depending on age.[60]

APPETITE STIMULANTS

For some individuals, dietary intake to reach or maintain nutritional goals in CF is a chronic challenge because of inadequate appetite. Etiology of poor appetite is variable and can be psychological (e.g., depression), result from an adverse effect of a medication (e.g., methylphenidate, bupropion), or be caused by another comorbidity such as poor GI motility (e.g., gastroparesis). Individuals with CF at nutritional risk (i.e., body mass index percentile, 25% or less) should be evaluated appropriately before appetite stimulants are initiated. Dietary intake review (e.g., food diaries), laboratory workup for other comorbidities (e.g., CFRD, GERD), and evaluation of psychosocial or socioeconomic status should be part of the assessment for appropriateness of appetite stimulants.[77]

Treatment of the source of poor appetite or oral intake is ideal (e.g., treatment of depression); however, in certain instances, the employment of appetite stimulants may be considered if the use of primary approaches fails to result in improvement. Agents used as appetite stimulants in CF include those used in patients with cancer (e.g., megestrol acetate, cyproheptadine). These agents each possess useful effects of appetite stimulation and weight gain that are useful for individuals with CF who are challenged in weight gain and poor oral food intake. Choice of agent will depend on patient-specific factors such as age, available data, and dosage form needed (e.g., liquid vs. tablet). Safety and efficacy of agents such as cyproheptadine have been studied for as long as 12 months in some children.[77,78] Dronabinol, the oral dosage form of delta-9-tetrahydrocannabinol, is another potential agent used in patients with cancer and patients with AIDS wasting syndrome. However, documented use of this agent in the CF population as an appetite stimulant is limited, with greater experience in adolescents and adults with CF and use of doses of up to 5 mg by mouth twice daily.[79] Other agents that could be considered for use include the antidepressant mirtazapine at doses of up to 45 mg/day orally, with most experience in adolescents and adults with CF.[80,81] Antipsychotics such as olanzapine, starting at lower doses than used for psychiatric purposes, have also been used in adult patients with CF because they have a strong adverse effect of excessive weight gain.[82]

MONITORING NUTRITIONAL THERAPY

Nutritional status is of utmost importance for children with CF because of the association between normal weight and stature for age and improved FEV_1 and survival. The CFF recommends that children with CF be in at least the 50th percentile in weight-for-length during the first 2 years of life and that individuals with CF who are age 2–20 years maintain at least the 50th percentile or higher for body mass index to optimize FEV_1.[60] Some CF centers have developed color-coded growth charts (Figure 4) to help facilitate the monitoring of nutritional risks on the basis of guidelines and cite specific designated progression of nutritional risk.[57,60,83,84] Additional laboratory monitoring is recommended to assess the nutritional status of individuals with CF. Tests that should be performed on diagnosis and at least annually include vitamin levels, albumin and prealbumin for assessment of protein stores, and hemoglobin and hematocrit for basic assessment of potential iron-deficiency anemia. Additional workups of iron-deficiency anemia (e.g., total iron-binding capacity, total ferritin level) may be considered. Other laboratory tests to consider include serum Na^+ in cases of potential dehydration and essential fatty acids in cases of poor nutritional status. Because patients with CF are at increased risk of osteopenia, the use of tests to assess bone mineral density are warranted, such as DEXA (dual energy x-ray absorptiometry).[60]

OTHER GI DISEASES IN CF

PHYSICAL MANIFESTATION

With the obstruction of the pancreatic duct caused by viscous epithelial secretions, some neonates with CF may exhibit what is known as *meconium ileus*, an early GI manifestation of CF. Meconium ileus is an obstruction of the small intestines by meconium, the early stool of a neonate composed of ingested in-utero material including mucus, amniotic fluid, and bile. With a less common occurrence, meconium ileus presents in only 10% to 15% of patients with CF. Distal intestinal obstruction syndrome (DIOS) is the meconium ileus equivalent in children and adults with CF. Individuals with a history of meconium ileus may be at increased risk of developing DIOS. In DIOS, intestinal contents (e.g., fecal matter) block the small intestinal lumen, and its etiology is not completely understood. Proposed etiologies of DIOS include pancreatic insufficiency, iatrogenic decrease of intestinal motility,

or abnormalities in fluid and electrolyte balance of secretions in the GI tract, resulting in viscous, mucous-like obstruction. Other complications that may or may not accompany DIOS include intussusceptions and rectal prolapse.[85,86] Rectal prolapse, associated with malnutrition, constipation, and diarrhea, is another GI complication reported in about 20% of individuals with CF. This prolapse most commonly occurs in younger children (e.g., 1–3 years), and it is often transient, often resolving at 3–5 years.[87]

Small intestinal bacterial overgrowth is a condition in which bacterial content increases, resulting in damage to enterocytes and worsening malabsorption and malnutrition,

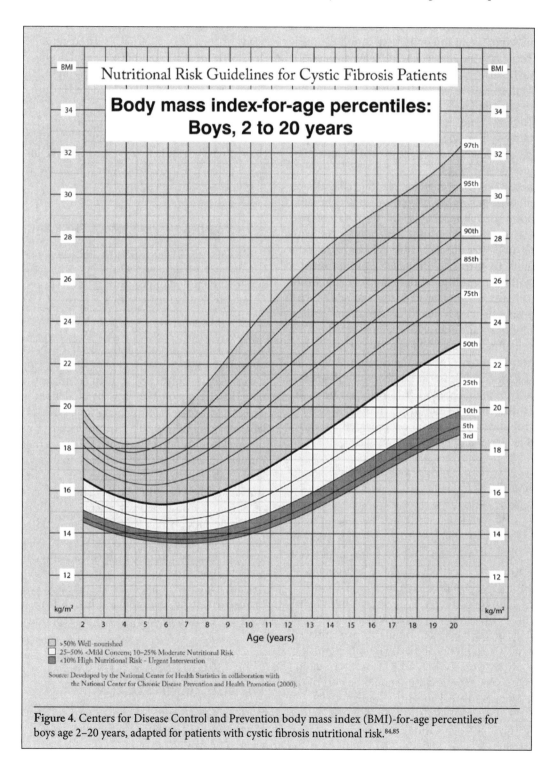

Figure 4. Centers for Disease Control and Prevention body mass index (BMI)-for-age percentiles for boys age 2–20 years, adapted for patients with cystic fibrosis nutritional risk.[84,85]

with an incidence as high as 30%–50% in the CF population.[88] Although small intestinal bacterial overgrowth is also seen in patients without CF, individuals with CF are at risk of this condition because of the potential for poor intestinal motility and use of thrice-weekly azithromycin as part of a chronic pulmonary management regimen.[85,86]

Obstruction of the biliary duct and accumulation of viscous bile can lead to focal biliary cirrhosis in 11% to 70% of individuals with CF; however, this cirrhosis is not always apparent because some individuals may be asymptomatic.[89] Similar to other areas throughout the body where epithelium is located, CFTR is also found in biliary epithelial cells. As a result, bile ducts are obstructed because of viscous bile production, which causes cholelithiasis, cholecystitis, progressive fibrosis, and cirrhosis. In neonates with CF, cholestasis may result, which is sometimes mistaken for biliary atresia. Individuals with CF-associated hepatobiliary disease may also develop steatosis (i.e., fatty liver) because of various factors including essential fatty acid deficiency or malnutrition. Further complications, including portal hypertension, can be found when CF-associated hepatobiliary disease is symptomatic and severe.[89,90] With the increased life expectancy of CF, the incidence of CF-associated hepatobiliary disease may increase because this complication is often found in older children and adults with CF. Evaluation of liver enzymes, including γ-glutamyl transferase at least annually in stable patients with CF, is recommended. For individuals who present with persistent elevations, further investigation is warranted, including an assessment of clinical presentation (e.g., stool pattern, jaundice, abdominal pain) and other possible etiologies such as other GI disorders or medication-induced liver injury. Additional testing including imaging evaluation, upper GI endoscopy, or biopsy may be employed to confirm diagnosis.

Among individuals with CF, GERD is also a common comorbidity, with an incidence as high as 58% to 86%.[91] It is postulated to be attributable to various causes, including transient relaxation of the lower esophageal sphincter and increased intra-abdominal pressure because of chronic cough. Not only does GERD potentiate the risk of poor nutrition in young children with CF, but it may also pose a risk of other complications such as gastric aspiration.[91,92] The diagnosis of GERD in children with CF is similar to the diagnosis of GERD in children without CF.

THERAPIES FOR GI DISEASES IN CF

DIOS AND RECTAL PROLAPSE

Constipation is often associated with DIOS, and definitions separating the two conditions have been outlined in formal guidelines.[93,94] Unlike constipation, in which the use of laxatives (e.g., oral polyethylene glycol, lactulose) often alleviate the condition, DIOS often necessitates the use of more aggressive treatment, including laxatives at higher doses, use of electrolyte intestinal lavage solution (e.g., GoLYTELY, Braintree Laboratories, Braintree, MA), or hyperosmolar enemas. Oral acetylcysteine (5% solution) has also been used for the prevention and treatment of mucus accumulation in the

GI tract of some individuals with DIOS.[93-95] This syndrome is thought to be related to pancreatic insufficiency that is poorly controlled with PERT. Similarly, rectal prolapse may respond to an increase in PERT dose and seldom requires surgical intervention.[88]

SMALL INTESTINAL BACTERIAL OVERGROWTH

Treatment of small intestinal bacterial overgrowth in individuals with CF is also similar to that of individuals without CF, such as the use of oral antibiotics (e.g., rifaximin, metronidazole, norfloxacin). Treatment may help improve the nutritional status of patients with CF. Additional treatment modalities may include dietary manipulation, such as reducing carbohydrate consumption, resulting in a high-fat, low-carbohydrate diet. The use of laxatives and inhaled ipratropium has also been associated with a decreased risk of small intestinal bacterial overgrowth.[96]

HEPATOBILIARY DISEASE

As part of the treatment of hepatobiliary disease in CF, it is imperative to optimize nutrition, especially fat-soluble vitamin and essential fatty acid deficiencies.[60] In addition to nutritional support, treatment with oral ursodeoxycholic acid or ursodiol (20 mg/kg/day divided twice daily) is currently recommended; however, additional outcomes data are necessary to describe its long-term effect on cholestasis, fibrosis, and cirrhosis in CF.[97] Taurine, an organic acid found in bile, has also been proposed for adjunctive treatment of hepatobiliary disease in CF; however, limited data support its routine use for this purpose.[98]

GASTROESOPHAGEAL REFLUX DISEASE

If symptoms of GERD coincide with poor nutritional status (e.g., failure to thrive), treatment is warranted, especially in infants and younger children. Medical management of GERD in children with CF is similar to that in other children without CF, including initial use of histamine-2 receptor blockers (e.g., ranitidine).[99] However, for some patients with CF, management can be more severe, requiring a change to or addition of a proton pump inhibitor (e.g., lansoprazole). Surgical management of GERD by fundoplication is also considered when complications are severe such as erosive esophagitis, uncontrolled pulmonary condition caused by reflux, or failure to thrive despite medical management.[100]

OTHER COMPLICATIONS OF CF

CF-RELATED DIABETES

The pathophysiology of the pancreatic disease also involves endocrine function or insulin regulation. Pancreatic enzyme insufficiency occurs in 85% of patients with CF, and as the cystic changes in the pancreas progress, patients begin to have problems with insulin regulation. Patients with CF develop glucose intolerance as either fasting hyperglycemia or postprandial hyperglycemia. Routine screening is now recommended starting as young as age 10 years, although some centers are starting even earlier in life because of potential variability in the clinical onset of this manifestation.[101] A fasting blood glucose and a 2-hour post-oral glucose load (e.g., glucose tolerance test) are recommended annually. Almost 30% of patients with CF older than 30 years have some form of glucose intolerance. As patients with CF continue to live longer, a higher percentage of them are expected to present with CFRD. This condition is not classic type 1 or 2 diabetes mellitus. Instead, CFRD can often be initially managed with dietary restrictions from concentrated sugars (e.g., soft drinks). If this approach does not work, then insulin is the drug of choice. Insulin therapy for CFRD often involves modest doses of long-acting insulin paired with carbohydrate counting and coverage with rapid-acting insulin.[101] Similar to other patients with diabetes and an infection, an acute pulmonary exacerbation or illness may complicate glucose control, especially when systemic corticosteroids are used during the management of severe pulmonary exacerbations. Addressing issues related to blood glucose control is now paramount in the long-term management of CFRD.[103,104] Another challenge in blood glucose control in CFRD is maintaining high caloric intake without excessive use of carbohydrates as primary source. It is recommended to use a high-calorie, high-protein, and high-fat diet.

CHRONIC SINUSITIS

As part of the upper respiratory tract, the sinuses are also affected in the inflammation and infection processes of CF. This involvement is because of their pseudostratified ciliated epithelium and lack of mucociliary clearance as similarly seen in the airways. Individuals with CF often have hypoplasia of the sinuses, which creates a confined area where respiratory pathogens such as PA can remain, causing chronic infection and inflammation. Sinuses can be assessed by a computed tomography scan to confirm the diagnosis of sinonasal disease before treatment or surgical intervention because the sinuses can appear opacified by age 8 months with conventional sinus radiography.[105] Treatment of the acute exacerbations of sinusitis can include oral and/or intravenous antibiotics, which are also used in pulmonary exacerbations and in intranasal irrigations of antimicrobials such as gentamicin and amphotericin B, although studies defining intranasal irrigation dosing and comparison of approaches are currently lacking.

HYPONATREMIA

The sudoriferous (sweat) glands, an epithelial exocrine system, are also affected by CF. Sweat from individuals with CF contains an abnormally high amount of Na^+ and Cl^- caused by the defective Cl^- impermeability of epithelial cells because of dysfunctional or absent CFTR. Thus, these individuals are at increased risk of electrolyte imbalances (e.g., hyponatremia, hypochloremia) during periods of heavy sweat excretion (e.g., warm weather combined with strenuous exercise).[106]

Because of the excessive loss of Na^+ in sweat, infants with CF are at risk of developing hyponatremic, hypochloremia

dehydration. Infant formulas and breast milk do not provide adequate Na^+ for infants with CF; thus, it is recommended that ⅛ teaspoon of table salt be provided from birth and increased with time to ¼ teaspoon by 6 months through 1 year of age, divided throughout the day by feedings. Additional supplementation may be necessary for any patient with CF living in high-temperature climates, especially those involved in physical activities in these environments (e.g., athletes).[60]

SPECIAL TOPICS RELATED TO CF

CF IN ADULTHOOD

As patients with CF grow older, complications arise, such as progressive respiratory disease and increased incidence of CFRD and insulin therapy. Additional chronic changes in the destructive nature of the lung in CF (e.g., bronchiectasis) develop, and patients often require supplemental oxygen therapy and increased frequency of airway clearance. Osteoporosis is often seen in adult patients with CF because of inadequate intake or absorption or chronic hypoxia. Pharmacists in adult CF centers can be invaluable resources to help manage these complications, together with the CF care team.

Individuals with CF who are male are infertile, but females can conceive and carry children to term. However, the fertility rate of females is reduced compared with that of patients without CF, partly because of the alteration of their cervical mucus, which impairs fertilization. Women with CF and severe lung disease have a higher risk of pregnancy complications.[107] Therefore, it is important to address contraception in CF and explain the options for patients.

ADHERENCE IN CF

Adherence to airway clearance and medication therapy is a lifelong challenge for many individuals with CF. Factors affecting adherence are often variable, making adherence difficult to effectively address in the care of patients with CF. Factors can be age-associated, with different reasons for nonadherence to therapies between an infant or small child compared with an adolescent. In the care of an infant or child, caregivers are primarily responsible for therapy administration. As a result, reasons for nonadherence in these instances include forgetting treatments, becoming confused because of several caregivers' responsibilities, discontinuing treatment in response to lack of symptoms, experiencing resistance from the child, developing concerns about medication adverse effects, and misunderstanding the instructions.[108-111] Conversely, in older patients such as adolescents, self-administration is commonplace, and reasons for nonadherence are more personal and psychosocial. The balance of growing independence and continued parental involvement becomes a challenge for some families. In adolescents, risk-taking behavior, an invincible perspective, or peer influence may negatively affect treatment adherence. When considering the active lifestyles of youth, time can be a limiting factor affecting adherence, especially with respect to airway clearance therapy.[112]

Patient-specific factors including socioeconomic status, culture, and/or caregiver beliefs can also affect adherence to both airway clearance and medication therapies. Studies have shown a potential preference for which therapy patients are adhering to. Medications that may provide perceived immediate relief or results such as pancreatic enzymes, dornase alfa, albuterol, or hypertonic saline may be missed less often than those that provide conceived long-term benefit such as aerosolized antibiotics or even airway clearance.[111,113,114] Many individuals with CF carry a heavy medication burden, which affects patient adherence to regimens. Polypharmacy is often encountered in the treatment of aggressive CF disease; however, despite the good intention of efficacy, combinations of medications can also place patients at increased risk of adverse drug events. Regular assessment of medication regimens is necessary as part of continued care.

Consequences of poor adherence to airway clearance and medication treatment can include increased frequency of exacerbations and increased rate of decline of lung function. Medication adherence has been related to the frequency of use of intravenous antibiotics for exacerbation, and exacerbations have been associated with the failure to return to baseline pulmonary function.[115] Approaches to improve the adherence of individuals with CF include patient and caregiver education, with involvement by a child's school if needed, which should be provided at the start of care and reinforced with each clinic visit and inpatient admission. Interventions to improve adherence can be organizational (e.g., calendars, automated reminders by cell phone alarm), psychoeducational (e.g., reinforced education about disease, treatment, outcomes), or psychotherapeutic or motivational (e.g., therapy diary, setting goals). No single intervention is applicable to all, and because each patient is different, the choice of intervention approach should be a joint, patient-care team decision.[116]

APPROACH TO PATIENT CARE AND THE PHARMACIST'S ROLE ON PATIENT-CARE TEAMS AND IN THE COMMUNITY

The treatment of individuals with CF is often approached in a systematic manner, involving the role of various health care providers including physicians, pharmacists, nurses, respiratory therapists, dietitians, clinical psychologists, physical therapists, and social workers. Patients and their families and caregivers are also fundamental team members in CF care. Patients who are actively involved in their health care often have better outcomes including lower health care utilization and cost. Collaboration and active partnership between patient, family, and health care providers, otherwise known as *coproduction of care*. Not only does this collaboration provide necessary opportunities for patient and caregiver input into clinical decision making, it helps facilitate open communication between patient/caregiver and health care professionals to optimize care and outcomes, thereby optimizing quality of care. Participation by all, from patient, family members, and health care professionals, is essential in successful coproduction of care, as lack of involvement of any one of these parties can result in missed perspective and opportunity.[117]

Information defining the role of a clinical pharmacy specialist in caring for patients with CF is limited, especially in the outpatient setting (e.g., CF centers). A survey of patients with CF conducted by European CF center investigators revealed that only 59% of patients reported access to specialty pharmacists.[114] One of the first descriptions of pharmacist participation in the care of patients with CF described a role involving multidisciplinary rounds in the inpatient setting and the rotation of pharmacy residents in the CF clinic.[114] Inpatient responsibilities of a pharmacist caring for patients with CF should include medication reconciliation, routine assessment of pharmacotherapy, communication with health care colleagues and families, and an active role in preparation for discharge, including home care (e.g., home intravenous antibiotics). Conversely, outpatient or ambulatory care setting responsibilities can include medication reconciliation, assessment of complementary and alternative therapy use, and assessment and intervention of medication adherence. Pharmacists in both inpatient and outpatient settings have a fundamental role in teaching patients and caregivers how to appropriately take or administer medications, including the timing of oral agents such as pancreatic enzymes and the use of metered dose inhalers and nebulized medications. Pharmacists can also play a central role in evaluating the use of dietary supplements, including complementary and alternative medications, because they may interact with prescribed drug therapy.[115]

Interdisciplinary, family-centered care of patients with CF is a care model involving a variety of health care disciplines and has been an increasingly common practice in the inpatient setting. The central focus of this care model, patients and families play an important role in the successful, comprehensive care of patients with CF. Patients and caregivers are encouraged to participate in decision-making with respect to regimen design and approach to overall care. In fact, many CF centers have a family member serve as a representative of patients and families in a role noted as "family liaison." Pediatric Pulmonary Centers, supported by Maternal and Child Health Training grants, are an example of this patient-care model in the outpatient setting. These care centers involve teams composed of various disciplines including medicine, nursing, nutrition, respiratory therapy, social work, family liaisons or representatives, and, the most recent addition, pharmacy. As part of these programs, not only do the various disciplines work together to provide quality patient care to children, but they also provide a way of training future professionals (e.g., residents, interns).

With the complexity of CF drug therapy management given the challenging pharmacokinetics, the combination of acute and chronic drug therapies, and the diversity of patient ages and conditions secondary to medical advances, continuity of care is imperative to optimize medication efficacy while minimizing adverse drug events. A lack of data remains regarding the use and effect of a patient-care model that bridges specialist outpatient care to the management of acute exacerbations and continuation of clinically important maintenance drug therapy for hospitalized patients with CF. A model of continuity of care for these patients should possess elements of optimal drug therapy selection and consistency between outpatient and inpatient care involving an interdisciplinary approach. Additional investigation about effective combined care models will provide clinicians information regarding the active involvement of clinical pharmacy specialists as part of both the outpatient and inpatient care of patients with CF, thereby improving patient outcomes from drug therapy.

Pharmacists, as patient advocates, have a professional responsibility to undergo continued education and training about innovations in therapy to optimize the health of children and adults with CF. In addition to their role as health care providers, pharmacists can play a key role in clinical research, whether as principal investigator or collaborator. Studies of new agents, approaches to dosing, and innovations in therapy adherence interventions are a continued need for advancing patient care and improving quality of life. Advocacy as a clinician, researcher, educator, and/or community leader is a multifaceted role that pharmacists can play in the CF community—it is with this passion and dedication that the care of individuals with CF advances toward a future cure.

Patient Case CYSTIC FIBROSIS

A 6-year-old girl is brought by her mother to the pediatric cystic fibrosis (CF) clinic for her quarterly visit. Her mother is concerned because, "My daughter has been coughing more and can't keep up in school." She reports increased cough, sputum production, and fatigue.

The patient received a diagnosis of CF at age 1 month based on a newborn screening, sweat test, and confirmed CF genotype, Phe508del homozygous; she also has pancreatic insufficiency. She was hospitalized twice in past 12 months for acute CF pulmonary exacerbations. Her other conditions are gastroesophageal reflux and allergic rhinitis. She also has a history of mucoid *Pseudomonas aeruginosa* (PA) and methicillin-resistant *Staphylococcus aureus* (MRSA) in sputum cultures in past 12 months. Her baseline FEV_1 is 95%.

Family history: Notable for her mother having asthma and her father hypertension. She lives with her parents and is currently in the first grade.

Vital signs: HR 105 beats/minute, BP 100/60 mm Hg, RR 22 breaths/minute; Tmax (oral): 99°F (37°C), oxygen saturation is 95%, Wt 21.8 kg, Ht 46 inches

Laboratory findings:

Results of pre-bronchodilator spirometry today are:

FVC	1.29 L
FVC % predicted	92%
FEV_1	1.06 L
FEV_1 % predicted	82%
FEV_1/FVC	82.17
FEV_1/FVC % predicted	89.13%

Results of laboratory tests 1 month ago were:

Na	137 mEq/L
K	4.3 mEq/L
Cl	103 mEq/L
CO_2	22 mEq/L
BUN	10 mg/dL
SCr	0.5 mg/dL
Glucose	82 mg/dL
Ca (total serum)	10.2 mg/dL
Albumin	4.3 g/dL
CRP	7.2 mg/L

Results of laboratory tests 1 month ago were: *(continued)*

AST	29 U/L
ALT	18 U/L
ALK	202 U/L
Total bilirubin	0.5 mg/dL
γ-Glutamyl transferase	10 U/L
Vitamin A (retinol)	30 mcg/dL
Vitamin E (alpha)	4.2 mg/L
Vitamin D (25-hydroxyvitamin)	32 ng/mL
PT	13 sec
INR	1.1

Sputum culture for CF: *Mucoid P. aeruginosa* (moderate growth), 3 months ago

Antibiotic	Minimum Inhibitory Concentration	Result
Amikacin	16	Susceptible
Aztreonam	≤ 2	Susceptible
Cefepime	4	Susceptible
Ciprofloxacin	> 4	Resistant
Levofloxacin	> 4	Resistant
Meropenem	4	Intermediate
Piperacillin/ tazobactam	16	Susceptible
Tobramycin	2	Susceptible

Sputum culture for CF: MRSA (moderate growth), 3 months ago

Antibiotic	Minimum Inhibitory Concentration	Result
Clindamycin	> 4	Resistant
Doxycycline	≤ 0.5	Susceptible
Linezolid	2	Susceptible
Oxacillin	≥ 4	Resistant
Trimethoprim/ sulfamethoxazole	≤ 0.5/9.5	Susceptible
Vancomycin	0.5	Susceptible

Medications:

Pancrelipase (Creon, Abbvie Inc, North Chicago, IL) 12,000-unit capsule: 3 capsules by mouth with meals, 1–2 capsules by mouth with snacks

Dornase alfa 2.5 mg nebulized daily

Hypertonic saline 7% 4 mL nebulized twice daily

CF multivitamin chewable 1 tablet by mouth once daily

Loratadine 10 mg by mouth daily

Lansoprazole 15 mg by mouth daily

Tobramycin solution 300 mg/5mL 1 vials nebulized twice daily, 28 days on/off (currently off cycle)

Albuterol 2.5 mg nebulized twice daily with airway clearance

Epinephrine auto-injector 0.15 mg subcutaneously as needed for anaphylaxis

High-frequency oscillating vest for airway clearance 1 to 2 times daily

Allergies: Bee venom (anaphylaxis); peanuts (hives); sulfa (hives)

Immunizations: All childhood vaccines up to date; last influenza 12 months ago (due)

1. What additional chronic medications can be considered for this patient now that she is 6 years old? Include what the potential patient outcomes are associated with each medication and what monitoring values are required for each medication selected.

Various options can be considered now that the patient is 6 years old. Based on the CF chronic care guidelines, ibuprofen, azithromycin, and lumacaftor/ivacaftor are options and considerations as follows.

High-dose ibuprofen at 20–30 mg/kg/dose by mouth twice daily can be used for this patient (her dose of 600 mg would be 27.5 mg/kg/dose). This approach, used in only a few patients today, starting at age 6 years and continued until adolescence (age 17 years), requires pharmacokinetic dose monitoring of serum concentrations to maximize the dose. Serum concentrations of 50–100 mcg/mL are required to maximize the effect of this intervention. This medication can decrease the rate of decline in pulmonary function in patients with CF. In addition to serum concentration, renal function and signs and symptoms of bleeding, especially GI, should be monitored.

Azithromycin 250 mg by mouth on Mondays, Wednesdays, and Fridays is appropriate for this patient. According to Cystic Fibrosis Foundation guidelines regarding chronic medications, patients with *P. aeruginosa* consistently in respiratory or sputum cultures should be considered candidates for chronic azithromycin therapy to help improve lung function and reduce exacerbations. Doses of 250–500 mg given three to seven times/week (not to exceed 10 mg/kg/day) are used by most CF clinicians for long-term therapy. Because the emphasis of this medication is on its anti-inflammatory effects, dosing can be adjusted for convenience because its effect is much longer than its serum half-life. Appearance of nontuberculous mycobacterium as well as for liver function (as part of annual laboratory tests) and possible drug interactions should be monitored.

Either lumacaftor/ivacaftor 200 mg/250 mg or tezacaftor/ivacaftor 50 mg/75 mg by mouth every 12 hours with high-fat containing food is indicated in this patient because of the confirmed CF genotype, Phe508del homozygous. Monitoring includes liver function tests and ophthalmic examination. For lumacaftor/ivacaftor therapy, abnormal respiration and dyspnea was noted in more than one-third of patients started on this therapy and thus should also be monitored. These symptoms appeared in the first day or week of therapy and often the symptoms abated as therapy continued. For these CFTR modulators, ivacaftor and lumacaftor, monitoring of drug-drug interactions is warranted. Lumacaftor is a strong inducer of CYP3A and ivacaftor is a substrate of CYP3A4 and CYP3A5. In addition, lumacaftor is a potential inducer of CYP2B6, CYP2C8, CYP2C9, and CYP2C19 enzymes and inhibitor of CYP2C8 and CYP2C9 enzymes. Therefore, it is important to review the current list of medications in order to alter or adjust therapy accordingly. It should be noted that, between high-dose ibuprofen and lumacaftor-ivacaftor, only one of the two agents should be used because of drug interaction between lumacaftor and ibuprofen which leads to lower serum ibuprofen (subtherapeutic) levels. Combined use of tezacaftor/ivacaftor and ibuprofen is not well described, thus possible drug interaction risk and clinical benefits should be weighed.

2. What are clinical signs and symptoms that indicate the patient is having an acute pulmonary exacerbation of her CF?

The patient presents with increased cough, sputum production, and fatigue as well as noted clinically significant decrease in her FEV_1 % predicted, being 82% today compared with her baseline value of 95%.

3. What is an appropriate antimicrobial treatment regimen for the patient if she were to need outpatient treatment of an acute pulmonary CF exacerbation? What is an appropriate inpatient treatment of an acute pulmonary CF exacerbation?

Appropriate options for treatment of an acute pulmonary CF exacerbation for the patient could include the following:

Outpatient: Restart her cycling of inhaled tobramycin by nebulizer plus increase frequency of her airway clearance (from twice a day to 3 to 4 times daily). The addition of oral antimicrobials is necessary based on her sputum culture history of mucoid PA and MRSA. Appropriate oral options for treatment of the mucoid PA include oral ciprofloxacin 400 mg by mouth every 12 hours (40–50 mg/kg/day by mouth divided every 8 to 12 hours, up to 750 mg/dose) or levofloxacin 200 mg by mouth every 24 hours (7–10 mg/kg/day by mouth every 24 hours). An appropriate oral option for treatment of MRSA is linezolid 220 mg (10 mg/kg/dose) by mouth every 8 hours. Doxycycline may not be ideal given that she is younger than 8 years because of the risk of staining of teeth.

Inpatient: Increase her airway clearance frequency to 3-4 times daily plus start intravenous or oral antimicrobials based on her sputum culture history of mucoid PA and MRSA. The mucoid PA should be double covered with two antimicrobials of different mechanisms of action (e.g., ß-lactam plus aminoglycoside). Appropriate options for treatment of the patient's mucoid PA include the following example regimen:

- Cefepime 1100 mg intravenously every 8 hours
- Tobramycin 220 mg intravenously every 24 hours

The regimen should consist of the following:

- An antipseudomonal ß-lactam such as piperacillin-tazobactam or cefepime (with doses shown in Table 5)
- Plus one of the following three drugs:
  - Intravenous tobramycin 220 mg every 24 hours: target Cpeak 20–30 mcg/mL, Cmin less than 1 mcg/mL
  - Oral ciprofloxacin 425 mg every 12 hours or intravenous ciprofloxacin 220 mg every 8 hours
  - Oral or intravenous levofloxacin 225 mg every 24 hours
- Appropriate options for treatment of MRSA: include
  - Vancomycin intravenous (e.g., 600 mg intravenous every 8 hours)
  - Linezolid oral or intravenous (e.g., 220 mg by mouth every 8 hours)

REFERENCES

1. Salvatore D, Buzzetti R, Baldo E, et al. An overview of international literature from cystic fibrosis registries. Part 3. Disease incidence, genotype/phenotype correlation, microbiology, pregnancy, clinical complications, lung transplantation, and miscellanea. J Cyst Fibros 2011;10:71-85.
2. Cystic Fibrosis Foundation Patient Registry. 2016 Annual Data Report. Bethesda, MD: Cystic Fibrosis Foundation, 2017.
3. Elborn JS. Cystic fibrosis. Lancet 2016; 388:2519-31.
4. Rowntree RK, Harris A. The phenotypic consequences of CFTR mutations. Ann Hum Genet 2003;67:471-85.
5. Witt H. Chronic pancreatitis and cystic fibrosis. Gut 2003; 52:ii31-41.
6. Hryciw DH, Guggino WB. Cystic fibrosis transmembrane conductance regulator and the outwardly rectifying chloride channel: a relationship between two chloride channels expressed in epithelial cells. Clin Exp Pharmacol Physiol 2000;27:892-5.
7. Rubenstein RC, Lockwood SR, Lide E, et al. Regulation of endogenous ENaC functional expression by CFTR and F508-CFTR in airway epithelial cells. Am J Physiol Lung Cell Mol Physiol 2011;300:88-8.
8. Borgo G, Cabrini G, Mastella G, et al. Phenotypic intrafamilial heterogeneity in cystic fibrosis. Clin Genet 1993;44:48-9.
9. Farrell PM, Rosenstein BJ, White TB, et al. Guidelines for diagnosis of cystic fibrosis in newborns through older adults: Cystic Fibrosis Foundation consensus report. J Pediatr 2008;153:S4-14.
10. American College of Obstetricians and Gynecologists (ACOG). Cystic Fibrosis: Prenatal Screening and Diagnosis. ACOG Frequently Asked Questions Pamphlet FAQ171. Washington, DC: ACOG, 2009. Available at www.acog.org/patient-resources/faqs/pregnancy/cystic-fibrosis-prenatal-screening-and-diagnosis. Accessed July 10, 2018.
11. Flume PA, Mogayzel PJ Jr, Robinson KA, et al. Clinical Practice Guidelines for Pulmonary Therapies Committee; Cystic Fibrosis Foundation Pulmonary Therapies Committee. Cystic fibrosis pulmonary guidelines: pulmonary complications: hemoptysis and pneumothorax. Am J Respir Crit Care Med 2010;182:298-306.
12. Goss CH, Burns JL. Exacerbations in cystic fibrosis. 1. Epidemiology and pathogenesis. Thorax 2007;62:360-7.
13. Liou TG, Elkin EP, Pasta DJ, et al. Year-to-year changes in lung function in individuals with cystic fibrosis. J Cyst Fibros 2010;9:250-6.
14. Lipuma JJ. The changing microbial epidemiology in cystic fibrosis. Clin Microbiol Rev 2010;23:299-323.
15. Lahiri T, Hempstead SE, Brady C, et al. Clinical Practice Guidelines from the Cystic Fibrosis Foundation for Preschoolers with Cystic Fibrosis. Pediatrics 2016;137:e20151784.
16. Mogayzel PJ Jr, Naureckas ET, Robinson KA, et al. Pulmonary Clinical Practice Guidelines Committee. Cystic fibrosis pulmonary guidelines. Chronic medications for maintenance of lung health. Am J Respir Crit Care Med 2013;187:680-9.
17. Mogayzel PJ Jr, Naureckas ET, Robinson KA, et al. Cystic Fibrosis Foundation Pulmonary Clinical Practice Guidelines Committee. Cystic Fibrosis Foundation pulmonary guideline. Pharmacologic approaches to prevention and eradication of initial Pseudomonas aeruginosa infection. Ann Am Thorac Soc 2014;11:1640-50.
18. Borowitz D, Robinson KA, Rosenfeld M, et al. Cystic Fibrosis Foundation evidence-based guidelines for management of infants with cystic fibrosis. J Pediatr 2009;155:S73-93.
19. Flume PA, Mogayzel PJ Jr, Robinson KA, et al. Clinical Practice Guidelines for Pulmonary Therapies Committee. Cystic fibrosis pulmonary guidelines: treatment of pulmonary exacerbations. Am J Respir Crit Care Med 2009;180:802-8.
20. Mendelman PM, Smith AL, Levy J, et al. Aminoglycoside penetration, inactivation, and efficiency in cystic fibrosis sputum. Am Rev Respir Dis 1985;132:761-5.
21. Littlewood JM, Miller MG, Ghoneim AT, et al. Nebulised colomycin for early pseudomonas colonisation in cystic fibrosis. Lancet 1985;1:865.
22. Jensen T, Pedersen SS, Garne S, et al. Colistin inhalation therapy in cystic fibrosis patients with chronic Pseudomonas aeruginosa lung infection. J Antimicrob Chemother 1987;19:831-8.

23. Ramsey BW, Dorkin HL, Eisenberg JD, et al. Efficacy of aerosolized tobramycin in patients with cystic fibrosis. N Engl J Med 1993;328:1740-6.

24. Retsch-Bogart GZ, Burns JL, Otto KL, et al. A phase 2 study of aztreonam lysine for inhalation to treat patients with cystic fibrosis and Pseudomonas aeruginosa infection. Pediatr Pulmonol 2008;43:47-58.

25. McCoy KS, Quittner AL, Oermann CM, et al. Inhaled aztreonam lysine for chronic airway Pseudomonas aeruginosa in cystic fibrosis. Am J Respir Crit Care Med 2008;178:921-8.

26. Moss RB. Long-term benefits of inhaled tobramycin in adolescent patients with cystic fibrosis. Chest 2002;121:55-63.

27. Hodson ME, Gallagher CG, Govan JRW. A randomised clinical trial of nebulised tobramycin or colistin in cystic fibrosis. Eur Respir J 2002;20:658-64.

28. Pitance L, Vecellio L, Leal T, et al. Delivery efficacy of a vibrating mesh nebulizer and a jet nebulizer under different configurations. J Aerosol Med Pulm Drug Deliv 2010;23:389-96.

29. Elkins MR, Robinson M, Rose BR, et al. National Hypertonic Saline in Cystic Fibrosis (NHSCF) Study Group. A controlled trial of long-term inhaled hypertonic saline in patients with cystic fibrosis. N Engl J Med 2006;354:229-40.

30. Konstan MW, Byard PJ, Hoppel CL, et al. Effect of high-dose ibuprofen in patients with cystic fibrosis. N Engl J Med 1995;332:848-54.

31. Konstan MW, VanDevanter DR, Rasouliyan L, et al. Investigators and coordinators of the Epidemiologic Study of Cystic Fibrosis. Trends in the use of routine therapies in cystic fibrosis: 1995–2005. Pediatr Pulmonol 2010;45:1167-72.

32. Saiman L, Anstead M, Mayer-Hamblett N, et al.; AZ0004 Azithromycin Study Group. Effect of azithromycin on pulmonary function in patients with cystic fibrosis uninfected with Pseudomonas aeruginosa. JAMA 2010;303:1707-15.

33. Renna M, Schaffner C, Brown K, et al. Azithromycin blocks autophagy and may predispose cystic fibrosis patients to mycobacterial infection. J Clin Invest 2011;121:3554-63.

34. Kreindler JL. Cystic fibrosis: exploiting its genetic basis in the hunt for new therapies. Pharmacol Ther 2010;125:219-29.

35. Accurso FJ, Rowe SM, Clancy JP, et al. Effect of VX-770 in persons with cystic fibrosis and the G551D-CFTR mutation. N Engl J Med 2010;363:1991-2003.

36. Wainright CE, Elborn JS, Ramsey BW, et al. Traffic and Transport Study Groups Lumacaftor-ivacaftor in patients with cystic fibrosis homozygous for Phe508Del CFTR, N Engl J Med 2015;373:220-31.

37. Konstan MW, McKone EF, Moss RB, et al. Assessment of safety and efficacy of long-term treatment with combination lumacaftor and ivacaftor therapy in patients with cystic fibrosis homozygous for the F508del-CFTR mutation (PROGRESS): a phase 3, extension study. Lancet Respir Med 2017;5:107-18.

38. Taylor-Cousar JL, Munch A, McKone EF et al. Tezacaftor-ivacaftor in patients with cystic fibrosis homozygous for Phe508del. N Engl J Med 2017;377:2013-23.

39. Rowe SM, Daines C, Ringshausen FC et al. Tezacaftor-ivacaftor in residual function heterzygotes with cystic fibrosis. N Engl J Med 2017;377:2024-35.

40. Middleton PG, Mall MA, Drevinek P et al. Elexacaftor–Tezacaftor–Ivacaftor for Cystic Fibrosis with a Single Phe508del Allele. N Engl J Med 2019;381:1809-19.

41. Heijerman HGM, McKone E, Downey D, et al. Efficacy and safety of the elexacaftor plus tezacaftor plus ivacaftor combination regimen in people with cystic fibrosis homozygous for the F508del mutation: a double-blind, randomised, phase 3 trial. Lancet 2019 Oct 30. pii: S0140-6736(19)32597-8. [Epub ahead of print].

42. Kalydeco (ivacaftor) tablets and oral granules [package insert]. Boston: Vertex Pharmaceuticals Inc., 2019.

43. Orkambi (lumacaftor/ivacaftor) tablets [package insert]. Boston: Vertex Pharmaceuticals Inc., 2019.

44. Symdeko (tezacaftor/ivacaftor) tablets [package insert]. Boston: Vertex Pharmaceuticals Inc., 2019.

45. Trikafta (elexacaftor/tezacaftor/ivacaftor) tablets [package insert]. Boston: Vertex Pharmaceuticals Inc., 2019.

46. Gold R, Overmeyer A, Knie B, et al. Controlled trial of ceftazidime vs ticarcillin and tobramycin in the treatment of acute respiratory exacerbations in patients with cystic fibrosis. Pediatr Infect Dis 1985;4:172-7.

47. Richard DA, Nousia-Arvanitakis S, Sollich V, et al. Oral ciprofloxacin vs. intravenous ceftazidime plus tobramycin in pediatric cystic fibrosis patients: comparison of antipseudomonas efficacy and assessment of safety with ultrasonography and magnetic resonance imaging. Pediatr Infect Dis J 1997;16:572-8.

48. Smith AL, Doershuk C, Goldmann D, et al. Comparison of a beta-lactam alone versus beta-lactam and an aminoglycoside for pulmonary exacerbation in cystic fibrosis. J Pediatr 1999; 134:13-21.

49. Flume PA, Mogayzel PJ Jr, Robinson KA, et al. Clinical Practice Guidelines for Pulmonary Therapies Committee. Cystic fibrosis pulmonary guidelines: treatment of pulmonary exacerbations. Am J Respir Crit Care Med 2009;180:802-8 [28-9, online expanded version].

50. Smyth AR, Bratt J. Once-daily versus multiple daily dosing with intravenous aminoglycosides for cystic fibrosis. Cochrane Database Syst Rev 2017;3:CD002009.

51. Al-Malky G. Aminoglycoside antibiotics cochleotoxicity in paediatric cystic fibrosis patients: a study using extended high-frequency audiometry and distortion product otoacoustic emissions. Int J Audiol 2011;50:112-22.

52. Riethmueller J, Junge S, Schroeter TW, et al. Continuous vs thrice-daily ceftazidime for elective intravenous antipseudomonal therapy in cystic fibrosis. Infection 2009;37:418-23.

53. Plummer A, Wildman M. Duration of intravenous antibiotic therapy in people with cystic fibrosis. Cochrane Database Syst Rev 2016;9:CD006682.

54. Gray RD, Imrie M, Boyd AC, et al. Sputum and serum calprotectin are useful biomarkers during CF exacerbation. J Cyst Fibros 2010;9:193-8.

55. Sanders DB, Bittner RC, Rosenfeld M, et al. Failure to recover to baseline pulmonary function after cystic fibrosis pulmonary exacerbation. Am J Respir Crit Care Med 2010;182:627-32.

56. Borowitz D, Baker RD, Stallings V. Consensus report on nutrition for pediatric patients with cystic fibrosis. J Pediatr Gastroenterol Nutr 2002;35:246-59.

57. Tangpricha V, Kelly A, Stephenson A, et al. Cystic Fibrosis Foundation Vitamin D Evidence-Based Review Committee. An update on the screening, diagnosis, management, and treatment of vitamin D deficiency in individuals with cystic fibrosis: evidence-based recommendations from the Cystic Fibrosis Foundation. J Clin Endocrinol Metab 2012;97:1082-93.

58. De Boeck K, Weren M, Proesmans M, et al. Pancreatitis among patients with cystic fibrosis: correlation with pancreatic status and genotype. Pediatrics 2005;115:e463-9.

59. Augarten A, Ben Tov A, Madgar I, et al. The changing face of the exocrine pancreas in cystic fibrosis: the correlation between pancreatic status, pancreatitis and cystic fibrosis genotype. Eur J Gastroenterol Hepatol 2008;20:164-8.

60. Stallings VA, Stark LJ, Robinson KA, et al. Clinical Practice Guidelines on Growth and Nutrition Subcommittee; Ad Hoc Working Group. Evidence-based practice recommendations for nutrition-related management of children and adults with cystic fibrosis and pancreatic insufficiency: results of a systematic review. J Am Diet Assoc 2008;108:832-9.

61. Kraisinger M, Hochhaus G, Stecenko A, et al. Clinical pharmacology of pancreatic enzymes in patients with cystic fibrosis and in vitro performance of microencapsulated formulations. J Clin Pharmacol 1994;34:158-66.

62. Creon (pancrelipase) delayed-release capsules [package insert]. Chicago: AbbVie Inc., 2009.

63. Pancreaze (pancrelipase) delayed-release capsules [package insert]. Titusville, NJ: McNeil Pediatrics Division of Ortho-McNeil-Janssen Pharmaceuticals, 2016.

64. Zenpep (pancrelipase) delayed-release capsules [package insert]. Yardley, PA: Eurand Pharmaceuticals, 2009.

65. Creon (pancrelipase) delayed-release capsules [medication guide]. Chicago: AbbVie Inc., 2015.

66. Zenpep (pancrelipase) delayed-release capsules [medication guide]. Aptalis Pharma, 2017.

67. Ultresa (pancrelipase) delayed-release capsules [package insert]. Aptalis Pharma, 2014.

68. Pertzye (pancrelipase) delayed-release capsules [package insert]. Bethlehem, PA: Digestive Care, 2016.

69. Viokace (pancrealipase) tablet [package insert]. Birmingham: Aptalis Pharma US, 2012.

70. Borowitz DS, Grand RJ, Durie PR, et al. Use of pancreatic enzyme supplements for patients with cystic fibrosis in the context of fibrosing colonopathy. J Pediatr 1995;127:681-4.

71. Tran TM, Van den Neucker A, Hendriks JJ, et al. Effects of a proton-pump inhibitor in cystic fibrosis. Acta Paediatr 1998;87:553-8.

72. Maqbool A, Graham-Maar RC, Schall JI, et al. Vitamin A intake and elevated serum retinol levels in children and young adults with cystic fibrosis. J Cyst Fibros 2008;7:137-41.

73. West NE, Lechtzin N, Merlo CA, et al. Appropriate goal level for 25-hydroxyvitamin D in cystic fibrosis. Chest 2011;140:469-74.

74. Stephenson A, Brotherwood M, Robert R, et al. Cholecalciferol significantly increases 25-hydroxyvitamin D concentrations in adults with cystic fibrosis. Am J Clin Nutr 2007;85:1307-11.

75. Green D, Carson K, Leonard A, et al. Current treatment recommendations for correcting vitamin D deficiency in pediatric patients with cystic fibrosis are inadequate. J Pediatr 2008;153:554-9.

76. Dougherty KA, Schall JI, Stallings VA. Suboptimal vitamin K status despite supplementation in children and young adults with cystic fibrosis. Am J Clin Nutr 2010;92:660-7.

77. Nasr SZ, Drury D. Appetite stimulants use in cystic fibrosis. Pediatr Pulmonol 2008;43:209-19.

78. Homnick DN, Marks JH, Hare KL, et al. Long-term trial of cyproheptadine as an appetite stimulant in cystic fibrosis. Pediatr Pulmonol 2005;40:251-6.

79. Anstead MI, Kuhn RJ, Martyn D, et al. Dronabinol, an effective and safe appetite stimulant in cystic fibrosis. Pediatr Pulmonol 2003;36:343.

80. Boas SR, McColley SA, Danduran MJ, et al. The role of mirtazapine as an appetite stimulant in malnourished individuals with CF. Ped Pulmonol 2000;30:325.

81. Sykes R, Kittel F, Marcus M, et al. Mirtazapine for appetite stimulation in children with cystic fibrosis. Pediatr Pulmonol 2006;40:389.

82. Ross E, Davidson S, Sriram S, et al. Weight gain associated with low dose olanzapine therapy in severely underweight adults with cystic fibrosis. Pediatr Pulmonol 2005;40:350.

83. Settle PJ, Esher MS. CDC Growth Charts for BMI-for-Age Adapted for CF Patient Nutritional Risk. Maternal and Child Health Bureau (in part), HRSA [internal document]. Tucson, AZ: University of Arizona Pediatric Pulmonary Center, 2007.

84. Centers for Disease Control and Prevention Growth Charts. National Center for Health Statistics in collaboration with the National Center for Chronic Disease Prevention and Health Promotion, 2000. Available at www.cdc.gov/growthcharts. Accessed July 10, 2018.

85. Eggermont E, DeBoek K. Small intestinal abnormalities in cystic fibrosis patients. Eur J Pediatr 1991;150:824-8.

86. Eggermont E. Gastrointestinal manifestations in cystic fibrosis. Eur J Gastroenterol Hepatol 1996;8:731-8.

87. Stern RC, Izant RJ Jr, Boat TF, et al. Treatment and prognosis of rectal prolapse in cystic fibrosis. Gastroenterology 1982;82:707.

88. Lisowska A, Wójtowicz J, Walkowiak J. Small intestine bacterial overgrowth is frequent in cystic fibrosis: combined hydrogen and methane measurements are required for its detection. Acta Biochim Pol 2009;56:631-4.

89. Sokol RJ, Durie PR. Recommendations for management of liver and biliary tract disease in cystic fibrosis. Cystic Fibrosis Foundation Hepatobiliary Disease Consensus Group. J Pediatr Gastroenterol Nutr 1999;28:S1-13.

90. Colombo C, Battezzati PM. Hepatobiliary manifestations of cystic fibrosis. Eur J Gastroenterol Hepatol 1996;8:748-54.

91. Bendig DW, Seilheimer DK, Wagner ML, et al. Complications of gastroesophageal reflux in patients with cystic fibrosis. J Pediatr 1982;100:536-40.

92. Blondeau K, Pauwels A, Dupont LJ, et al. Characteristics of gastroesophageal reflux and potential risk of gastric content aspiration in children with cystic fibrosis. J Pediatr Gastroenterol Nutr 2010;50:161-6.

93. Houwen RH, van der Doef HP, Sermet I, et al. ESPGHAN Cystic Fibrosis Working Group. Defining DIOS and constipation in cystic fibrosis with a multicentre study on the incidence, characteristics, and treatment of DIOS. J Pediatr Gastroenterol Nutr 2010;50:38-42.

94. Colombo C, Ellemunter H, Houwen R, et al. ECFS. Guidelines for the diagnosis and management of distal intestinal obstruction syndrome in cystic fibrosis patients. J Cyst Fibros 2011;10:S24-8.

95. Weller PH, Williams J. Clinical features, pathogenesis and management of meconium ileus equivalent. J R Soc Med 1986;79:36-7.

96. Fridge JL, Conrad C, Gerson L, et al. Risk factors for small bowel bacterial overgrowth in cystic fibrosis. J Pediatr Gastroenterol Nutr 2007;44:212-8.

97. Nousia-Arvanitakis S, Fotoulaki M, Economou H, et al. Long-term prospective study of the effect of ursodeoxycholic acid on cystic fibrosis-related liver disease. J Clin Gastroenterol 2001; 32:324-8.

98. Thompson GN. Failure of taurine to improve fat absorption in cystic fibrosis. J Inherit Metab Dis 1988;11:158-60.

99. Malfroot A, Dab I. New insights on gastroesophageal reflux in cystic fibrosis by longitudinal follow up. Arch Dis Child 1991; 66:1339-45.

100. Boesch RP, Acton JD. Outcomes of fundoplication in children with cystic fibrosis. J Pediatr Surg 2007;42:1341-4.

101. Moran A, Brunzell C, Cohen RC, et al. Clinical care guidelines for cystic fibrosis related diabetes. Diabetes Care 2010;33:2697-708.

102. Hameed S, Morton JR, Field PI, et al. Once daily insulin detemir in cystic fibrosis with insulin deficiency. Arch Dis Child 2012;97:464-7.

103. Nathan B, Moran A. Treatment recommendations for cystic fibrosis-related diabetes: too little, too late? Thorax 2011;66:555-6.

104. Suratwala D, Chan JS, Kelly A, et al. Nocturnal saturation and glucose tolerance in children with cystic fibrosis. Thorax 2011;66:574-8.

105. Gysin C, Alothman GA, Papsin BC. Sinonasal disease in cystic fibrosis: clinical characteristics, diagnosis, and management. Pediatr Pulmonol 2000;30:481-9.

106. Sawka MN, Montain SJ. Fluid and electrolyte supplementation for exercise heat stress. Am J Clin Nutr 2000;72:564S-72S.

107. Barak A, Dulitzki M, Efrati O, et al. Pregnancies and outcomes in women with cystic fibrosis. Isr Med Assoc J 2005;7:95-8.

108. Dziuban EJ, Saab-Abazeed L, Chaudhry SR, et al. Identifying barriers to treatment adherence and related attitudinal patterns in adolescents with cystic fibrosis. Pediatr Pulmonol 2010;45:450-8.

109. Zindani GN, Streetman DD, Streetman DS, et al. Adherence to treatment in children and adolescent patients with cystic fibrosis. J Adolesc Health 2006;38:13-7.

110. Bucks RS, Hawkins K, Skinner TC, et al. Adherence to treatment in adolescents with cystic fibrosis: the role of illness perceptions and treatment beliefs. J Pediatr Psychol 2009;34:893-902.

111. Arias Llorente RP, García CB, Díaz Martín JJ. Treatment compliance in children and adults with cystic fibrosis. J Cyst Fibros 2008;7:359-67.

112. Eakin MN, Bilderback A, Boyle MP, et al. Longitudinal association between medication adherence and lung health in people with cystic fibrosis. J Cyst Fibros 2011;10:258-64.

113. Duff AJA, Latchford GJ. Motivational interviewing for adherence problems in cystic fibrosis. Pediatr Pulmonol 2010;45:211-20.

114. Elborn JS, Hodson M, Bertram C. Implementation of European standards of care for cystic fibrosis---provision of care. J Cyst Fibros 2009;8:348-55.

115. Sterner-Allison JL. Management of adolescent and adult inpatients with cystic fibrosis. Am J Health Syst Pharm 1999;56:158-60.

116. Murray KL, Lee CK, Mogayzel PJ Jr, et al. Dietary supplement use in pediatric patients with cystic fibrosis. Am J Health Syst Pharm 2008;65:562-5.

117. Sabadosa KA and Batalden PB. The interdependent roles of patients, families and professionals in cystic fibrosis: a system for the coproduction of healthcare and its improvement. BMJ Qual Saf 2014;23:i90-4.

Section V

Gastrointestinal Disorders

CHAPTER 15

Gastroesophageal Reflux Disease
Kalen Manasco, Pharm.D., BCPS

reflux is simply defined as the passage of stomach contents into the esophagus, with or without regurgitation and vomiting. It is a common occurrence in infancy and is not associated with any pathologic process, but it may be caused by food allergy or colic. Clinical symptoms of GER also vary by age. Gastroesophageal reflux can manifest as spitting up or regurgitation. *Regurgitation* is defined as the passage of gastric contents into the oropharynx or mouth or possibly out of the mouth, commonly referred to as "spitting up." *Gastroesophageal reflux disease* is defined as clinical symptoms and/or complications associated with the passage of stomach contents into the esophagus.[3] These are symptoms that negatively affect a patient's quality of life such as heartburn, excessive regurgitation, food refusal, or abdominal pain. Complications of GERD are reflux esophagitis, hemorrhage, stricture, and Barrett esophagus.[3] *Reflux esophagitis* is inflammation of the esophagus and the presence of damage to the esophageal mucosa (as erosions or ulcerations) as detected by biopsy. *Barrett esophagus* is a disorder in which the epithelial lining of the esophagus is replaced by epithelium similar to the stomach lining secondary to damage from acid reflux. Patients with this disorder are at high risk of developing esophageal adenocarcinoma. Although GERD can be associated with too much acid production, it can also occur in children who present with no acid reflux. *Nonerosive gastroesophageal disease* is defined as the presence of typical symptoms of GERD without any erosive lesions within the esophagus. *Refractory gastroesophageal disease* describes GERD that is unresponsive to optimal treatment after 8 weeks. Optimal treatment occurs when a patient is receiving maximum pharmacologic and/or nonpharmacologic therapy.

INTRODUCTION

Gastroesophageal reflux (GER) is a common clinical manifestation in infancy and childhood. *Gastroesophageal reflux disease* (GERD) is a pathologic condition that may develop from reflux in patients of all ages. The first international consensus guideline on the diagnosis and management of GER and GERD in the pediatric population was published in 2009.[1] A recent update to the consensus guidelines was published in 2018.[2] These guidelines have changed the medical management of patients with GER and GERD.

DEFINITIONS

To better understand the disease process associated with reflux, several definitions are important. The first global, evidence-based consensus definition of GERD in the pediatric population was published in 2009.[3] This definition has been updated with the new 2018 guidelines.[2] *Gastroesophageal*

GER IN INFANTS

EPIDEMIOLOGY AND ETIOLOGY

Gastroesophageal reflux is a normal physiologic process that occurs many times throughout the day in people of all ages. It is most common in infancy and usually resolves by age 12–14 months.[4,5] Up to two-thirds of infants experience recurrent regurgitation and vomiting within the first 4 months of life, but only 5% of infants have symptoms of reflux beyond age 1 year.[6]

Physiologic reflux occurs when the lower esophageal sphincter (LES) relaxes and swallowing does not occur. This process allows the passage of stomach contents into the esophagus. This reflux can occur more often in neonates and infants because of the shorter length of the esophagus, delayed gastric emptying, decreased LES pressure, and immature peristalsis.[7]

Gastroesophageal reflux can be associated with apnea, failure to thrive, and respiratory problems such as recurrent aspiration and wheezing in preterm infants. However, there is no evidence to suggest a causal relationship between GER and these occurrences. One study evaluating the prevalence of infant regurgitation in infants younger than 2 years found no difference in GER between preterm and term infants.[6]

CLINICAL PRESENTATION AND DIAGNOSIS

The most common symptom associated with physiologic reflux in the infant is regurgitation or "spitting up." Reflux can also trigger vomiting. Other signs and symptoms that can be associated with reflux are nonspecific and include irritability, excessive crying, lethargy, feeding refusal, and cough (Table 1), which cannot be distinguished from other causes of reflux such as food allergy or colic. Infants with uncomplicated physiologic reflux are commonly referred to as "happy spitters." These infants can continue to gain adequate weight despite the problematic symptoms associated with reflux.

Reflux episodes can have a temporal relationship with apnea; however, evidence is conflicting whether there is a temporal or causal relationship between apnea and reflux.[1] *Brief resolved unexplained events* (BRUE)—previously categorized as *apparent life-threatening events*—are episodes of apnea, cyanosis, abnormal muscle tone, and/or altered level of responsiveness that usually occur in the first year of life. These events are alarming episodes for parents or caregivers that may result in an admission to the hospital for further diagnostic evaluation. Only when no other explanation is found after obtaining a thorough history and physical examination should BRUEs be diagnosed. A BRUE may be associated with reflux in an infant; however, GER is not thought to cause BRUEs.[1]

The diagnosis of physiologic reflux is often based solely on the parental history and physical examination. Clinicians should perform a thorough examination of the child and obtain a detailed feeding history and description of the exact symptoms, including when they occur in relation to feeding. A feeding history should include information about the volume of liquid consumed, time to completion of feeding, suck/swallow ability, and position of the infant, particularly the infant's head. In addition, a thorough medical and family history should be obtained, including a family history of reflux and other gastrointestinal disorders such as celiac disease and *Helicobacter pylori* infection. Invasive testing is not usually required unless another pathologic diagnosis is suggested that includes GERD.

The Infant Gastroesophageal Reflux Questionnaire Revised is a validated diagnostic questionnaire composed of 14 items that can be used to guide clinicians when obtaining a history; this questionnaire has also been found to help monitor symptom occurrence with time.[8] The items are questions related to the characteristics of regurgitation, crying, feeding refusal, apnea or cyanosis, hiccups, and abnormal body posturing. The Rome III criteria were established to provide diagnostic criteria for infant regurgitation and other functional gastrointestinal disorders. To be diagnosed with infant regurgitation, healthy infants who are age 3 weeks to 12 months must present with both of the following: (1) regurgitation two or more times per day for 3 or more weeks, and (2) no retching, hematemesis, aspiration, apnea, failure to thrive, feeding or swallowing difficulties, or abnormal posturing.[9]

All infants who present with extraesophageal symptoms—apnea, BRUE, arching of the back, failure to thrive—and/or bilious vomiting should undergo a further diagnostic workup. Extraesophageal symptoms are commonly associated with GERD. Bilious vomiting is usually indicative of an obstruction or pyloric stenosis.

PROGNOSIS

Most infants with physiologic reflux have a favorable prognosis because they "outgrow" the symptoms by age 1 year. Children who have persistent symptoms beyond age 18 months, neurologic impairment, prematurity, or a strong family history of GERD have a worse prognosis compared with infants who have physiologic reflux.

TREATMENT

The goals of therapy are to provide parental reassurance and education, alleviate patient symptoms, and prevent complications. The mainstay of treatment in GER is nonpharmacologic. Management strategies include lifestyle changes (feeding and positional changes) and dietary changes. Pharmacologic management is reserved for the management of GERD.

Table 1. Signs and Symptoms Suggestive of Gastroesophageal Reflux[1]

Age group	Infants < 1 year	Children 1–5 years	Older children and adolescents 6–17 years
Symptoms	Regurgitation Vomiting Arching Irritability Poor weight gain Crying	Regurgitation Abdominal pain Cough	Heartburn Epigastric pain Dysphagia
Signs	Sandifer syndrome Food refusal Failure to thrive Brief resolved unexplained event	Food refusal Recurrent pneumonia Dental erosions	Reflux esophagitis

NONPHARMACOLOGIC THERAPY

LIFESTYLE MODIFICATIONS

Lifestyle modifications for infants with physiologic GER include parental reassurance, positional changes, and dietary changes (Box 1). Parental education should include counseling on the management of GER when it occurs, the prevention of reflux episodes, and the natural course and duration of infantile physiologic reflux, as well as counseling on when to seek additional treatment if symptoms persist or complications are noted. Parents should also be counseled on different positioning during and after feeding, burping, and other techniques to reduce the likelihood of reflux episodes.

In infants, the supine position is preferred to the prone position for sleeping. Despite studies showing the prone position can lessen reflux episodes, a significantly increased risk of sudden infant death syndrome exists compared with the supine position.[10,11] For this reason, the prone position is only acceptable when infants are awake and carefully watched after a meal. In addition, holding a sleeping infant in an upright position is acceptable for the first 20–30 minutes if the infant falls asleep after feeding.[1]

DIETARY CHANGES

Potential dietary changes include changing the volume or frequency of feeding, trying a hypoallergenic, hydrolyzed, or antireflux formula, and thickening the formula to increase caloric density. One of the most common situations discovered on questioning parents and caregivers about reflux and regurgitation in their infant is overfeeding. Altering the feeding volume and frequency can be beneficial to infants with GER, as long as the recommended amount per kilogram of body weight per day is maintained (Parenteral and Enteral Nutrition chapter). Studies have shown that smaller-volume feeds can decrease acid reflux.[12] However, clinicians should be cautioned that decreasing the volume or frequency of feeds may lead to inadequate weight gain.

The most common practice when changing the feeding volume is also to add a thickening agent, which will increase the caloric content of the formula. This increase is to ensure adequate weight gain in the infant. The 2018 guidelines

recommend this approach for treating infants for visible regurgitation/vomiting. The efficacy of thickening feeds has recently been evaluated in a systematic review. More than 600 patients were included in eight trials. Formula-fed infants with GER who received thickeners had two fewer regurgitation episodes per day compared with infants with no thickener. The authors concluded that thickeners should be considered in term infants who are formula-fed with persistent GER and regurgitation.[13] Thickening should not be recommended for preterm neonates.

Rice cereal is the most common thickening agent used. One tablespoon of rice cereal per 2 ounces increases the formula from 20 calories per ounce to 27 calories per ounce.[1] The addition of rice cereal does not change the amount of acid reflux, but it does decrease the amount of regurgitation.[13,14] The potential disadvantages of adding rice cereal to formula include increased coughing during feeding and the extra energy expenditure by the infant because of the increased viscosity of the formula.[15] If infants have to suck a thicker substance through the nipple in the bottle, they will use more energy during the feeding process, which can cause an increase in caloric requirements. Infants typically need an enlarged nipple for adequate sucking when using a thickened formula. Recent concerns about the safety of cereal-based thickeners because of inorganic arsenic concentrations has led to action by the U.S. Food and Drug Administration (FDA) to limit the amount of arsenic available in commercial products.

In breastfed infants, carbo bean thickener (Gelmix; Parapharma Tech, Sunrise, FL) is available commercially to thicken breastmilk if needed. Carbo bean thickeners are approved for infants older than 42 weeks' gestation.

Prethickened, anti-regurgitation formulas are commercially available. These formulas include the addition of starch, which thickens only when mixed with the acid in the stomach. These formulas, which do not require the addition of an enlarged nipple, have been found to decrease both the amount of regurgitation and the amount of acid reflux.[16] Theoretically, a potential drug interaction may occur with anti-regurgitation formulas and histamine-2 receptor antagonists (H_2RAs). Because acid content in the stomach is required for the anti-regurgitation formula to work, the effect this formula may be decreased in a patient also taking an H_2RA. Although this interaction occurs only with the H_2RAs, theoretically it could also occur with a proton pump inhibitor (PPI). Before initiating any acid suppression therapy in an infant with GER, first a trial of an anti-regurgitation formula is recommended.

Because it is difficult to distinguish between infants with reflux and those with a milk protein allergy, changing to a hypoallergenic formula may prove beneficial in many patients. Trials of 2-4 weeks of feeding with either protein hydrolysate or amino acid formulas is recommended for infants with suspected GERD after optimal nonpharmacologic measures have failed, according to the current guidelines.[2,17] However, there is no evidence for soy formula in the management of infant reflux.[1]

Box 1. Lifestyle Changes for Patients with Gastroesophageal Reflux and Gastroesophageal Reflux Disease

Infants
Parental reassurance
Dietary changes
Positional changes

Older children and adolescents
Dietary changes
Sleeping position changes
    Elevate head of bed
    Left-sided sleep position
Weight loss
Decreased tobacco smoke exposure

GASTROESOPHAGEAL REFLUX DISEASE

EPIDEMIOLOGY AND ETIOLOGY

The prevalence of GERD has increased during the past several years in both adults and children. The true prevalence in pediatric patients is unknown because of the lack of a consistent definition used in practice. In addition, both the prevalence and incidence vary among the different age groups (neonates, infants, children, and adolescents). The prevalence is highest in infants younger than 2 years (2.2% to 12.6%) compared with children 2–11 years old (0.6% to 4.1%) and adolescents (0.8% to 7.6%).[18] The incidence of GERD in pediatric patients is estimated to be 0.84 per 1000 person-years.[19] Male patients are affected more than female patients. Bottle-fed infants are at an increased risk of GERD compared with breastfed infants.

More than 50% of the pediatric patients who are given a diagnosis of GERD require medical management of their disease. In one study, 4% of all hospital admissions annually were because of GERD.[20] In addition, an estimated $750 million is spent annually on the management of childhood GERD in hospitals.[20]

PATHOPHYSIOLOGY

GERD is caused by transient lower esophageal sphincter relaxations (TLESRs), decreased LES pressure, delayed gastric emptying, and/or hiatal hernia. The movement of reflux from the stomach into the esophagus usually occurs during TLESRs. Normally the LES relaxes very briefly (3–10 seconds) in response to swallowing, whereas TLESRs occur when the LES relaxes for more than 10 seconds and is not induced by the swallowing mechanism. Reflux episodes can also occur because of decreased LES pressure or inability of the LES to increase in response to increased intra-abdominal pressure. Factors that can contribute to decreased LES pressure include tobacco smoke exposure, intake of fatty foods, certain medications (e.g., theophylline, calcium channel blockers), and gastric distention. In addition, normal digestive defense mechanisms can become impaired in the presence of acid reflux and further exacerbate GERD symptoms. Continued exposure of the mucosa and submucosa within the esophagus to refluxate, primarily containing acid, can lead to the development of erosions in the esophagus.

GENETIC BASIS

Evidence suggests that GERD has a genetic component. A specific locus on chromosome 13 (13q14) associated with severe pediatric GERD has been identified.[21] In addition, there are reports of a familial association with GERD. Reflux symptoms, hiatal hernia, erosive esophagitis, Barrett esophagus, and esophageal adenocarcinoma occur more commonly within families.[22,23]

RISK FACTORS

Several pediatric patient populations are at increased risk of severe, chronic GERD and complications associated with GERD. These populations include patients with neurologic impairment (e.g., cerebral palsy), obesity, esophageal atresia, chronic lung disease, and prematurity. These patient populations have a poor prognosis and require long-term treatment of the symptoms associated with GERD.[1]

CLINICAL PRESENTATION

The signs and symptoms of concern associated with GERD include vomiting, irritability, refusal to feed, heartburn, dysphagia, and *Sandifer syndrome*, which is defined as spasmodic dystonia with arching of the neck and back and abnormal posturing.[3] It is important to distinguish between this clinical presentation and similar movements that may be caused by seizures or infantile spasms. Table 1 lists the most common signs and symptoms seen according to age group.

Gastroesophageal reflux disease may or may not lead to erosive esophagitis. This variance is because GERD can be caused by both acid and nonacid reflux. Symptoms most commonly associated with nonacid reflux include regurgitation and cough. Patients with erosive esophagitis typically present with heartburn and belching.

Gastroesophageal reflux disease is associated with both esophageal and extraesophageal symptoms. The most common extraesophageal symptoms in children include respiratory symptoms such as apnea, coughing, and wheezing. Extraesophageal manifestations of GERD include asthma, pneumonia, nocturnal cough, sinusitis, laryngitis, otitis media, and dental erosions. Sections about the clinical presentation and treatment of certain high-risk populations appear in the 2009 guideline, including neurologic impairment (e.g., anoxic brain injury, cerebral palsy, Down syndrome), obesity, esophageal anatomic disorders, chronic respiratory disorders (e.g., cystic fibrosis, bronchopulmonary dysplasia), lung transplantation, and prematurity.[1] This high-risk patient population was not readdressed in the newest update to the guidelines.

DIAGNOSIS

An initial diagnosis of GERD is often based on the clinical presentation of the patient with typical signs or symptoms for reflux. However, because many of the signs and symptoms are nonspecific (e.g., weight loss, dysphagia, cough, irritability), it is difficult to rely only on the clinical presentation for a diagnosis. Other disease states cannot be ruled out on the basis of clinical presentation alone. In addition, children younger than 8–12 years cannot reliably report their subjective symptoms, and children who are unable to communicate (e.g., those with neurologic impairment) will not be able to provide a description of their symptoms.[1] Adolescents who present with typical heartburn symptoms can be given a diagnosis on the basis of symptoms alone, similar to adult patients.[2] This approach to diagnosis is only applicable to adolescents who are verbal and neurologically healthy.

Patients with suspected GERD should undergo a thorough history and physical examination to determine the timing and severity of symptoms and to ascertain whether any complications are present that require further evaluation. Questions should be asked about the feeding history and vomiting, as well as the social, medical, family, and medication history.[24] The history and physical examination can also be used to rule out other disease states such as pyloric stenosis or seizures. Diagnostic questionnaires, such as those previously mentioned for GER, are also helpful for monitoring of symptoms. Unfortunately, there is a poor correlation between symptoms and objective findings in patients with GERD.[25,26]

Many diagnostic tests can be used to aid in the diagnosis of GERD. Esophageal pH monitoring can be used to diagnosis esophagitis and also as an aid in determining the efficacy of anti-secretory therapy. The procedure involves placing a catheter with electrodes along the length through the nose to the LES to measure the frequency and duration of acid reflux episodes.[27] Recordings of the number and frequency of episodes are completed during a 24-hour period. Esophageal pH monitoring alone is not sensitive for the detection of nonacid or weak acid reflux. Normal esophageal pH is 7.0. *Acid reflux* is defined as an esophageal pH less than 4.0 lasting 15–30 seconds.[28] The most reliable marker used during pH monitoring is the *reflux index score*, defined as the percentage of total time that the esophageal pH is less than 4.0. A score greater than 7% is considered abnormal for all patients older than 1 year and 12% or more for infants.[1,29] Additional variables measured by this procedure include the total number of reflux episodes, episodes lasting more than 5 minutes, and duration of pH less than 4.0. Combining pH monitoring with multichannel intraluminal impedance allows the type of reflux to be detected: gas, liquid, solid, or mixed. Thus, it can detect weakly acidic and basic reflux episodes. In addition, it detects the volume and direction of the reflux (antegrade vs. retrograde). The presence of many sensors along the catheter allows impedance to be measured proximally in the esophagus to investigate the relationship between respiratory symptoms and reflux. Of note, pH monitoring does not correlate with severity of reflux.

An upper gastrointestinal endoscopy allows visualization and evaluation of the esophageal mucosa, including distal areas. This test is superior to pH monitoring alone and is useful to determine the presence of esophagitis and complications of GERD such as strictures, hiatal hernia, ulcers, or Barrett esophagus. Biopsies of the mucosa should be obtained during the procedure to evaluate histologic changes in the mucosa. The biopsy can also be used to determine whether there are eosinophils in the tissue, which is consistent with a diagnosis of eosinophilic esophagitis, an allergic inflammatory disorder of the esophagus.

The upper gastrointestinal endoscopy series is a procedure that uses barium contrast radiography to evaluate the upper gastrointestinal tract. This procedure is not specific or sensitive for GERD, but it can be useful in identifying malrotation, pyloric stenosis, hiatal hernia, and anatomic abnormalities such as tracheoesophageal fistula.[30] These diagnoses may also be considered in pediatric patients with symptoms similar to GERD.

Esophageal manometry measures peristalsis, upper and LES pressures, and coordination of swallowing with these functions. Unfortunately, GERD cannot be diagnosed by manometry because of its low sensitivity and specificity.[1] Instead, manometry is used to determine the presence of motility disorders that may have a clinical presentation similar to GERD.

A trial of acid suppression is no longer recommended for infants and young children as a diagnostic test.[1] Older children and adolescents can still have a 4- to 8-week trial to determine whether therapy is beneficial.

TREATMENT

The goals of therapy are to alleviate patient symptoms, heal esophagitis if present, maintain normal growth, prevent complications, and minimize adverse effects of drug therapy. These goals are accomplished with nonpharmacologic interventions such as lifestyle modifications and pharmacologic interventions with acid suppression therapy.

NONPHARMACOLOGIC THERAPY

Nonpharmacologic therapies include lifestyle modifications and antireflux surgery and vary by age. Specific lifestyle modifications are listed in Box 1. Mild symptoms of GERD without complications may be managed by lifestyle changes alone. Strategies for infants include those previously discussed for GER. In rare cases, particularly for patients with recurrent pneumonia and GERD, placement of a nasogastric or nasojejunal feeding tube is required to ensure adequate feeding and growth and to prevent aspiration.[31,32] Older children and adolescents should be encouraged to avoid the ingestion of large meals, as well as to avoid lying down immediately after eating a meal. Of importance, the effectiveness of specific lifestyle modifications, such as positioning during sleep, has not been studied in children and adolescents; rather, data have been extrapolated from adult studies. In adults, only weight loss improves pH profiles and symptoms. Studies have shown that elevating the head of the bed in adults is beneficial (fewer episodes of reflux), so older children and adolescents may also benefit as well. Data on the additive benefit of lifestyle changes to pharmacologic therapy are also lacking for children and adolescents.[1]

Antireflux surgery is recommended only for specific patients as follows: (1) children with GERD whose optimal medical therapy fails; (2) patients with a requirement for long-term medical therapy when adherence or patient preference impedes such use; (3) patients with life-threatening complications (apnea or BRUEs) after failure of optimal medical treatment; and (4) chronic conditions (e.g., neurologic impairment, cystic fibrosis) with a significant risk of complications from GERD.[2] The most common surgical procedure is the Nissen fundoplication. This procedure can be performed laparoscopically or as an open surgery, with the laparoscopic procedure preferred. The fundus of the stomach is wrapped 360 degrees around the lower end of the esophagus and stitched in place to serve as the closure for the LES. This positioning results in increased LES pressure and a decreased number of TLESRs. Surgery can be curative in a subset of patients; however, success rates vary greatly from about 60% to 90%.[33] Complications after surgery can include gas-bloat syndrome, dysphagia, diarrhea, and retching and gagging after feeding. Patients with neurologic impairment are at highest risk of complications after antireflux surgery. In fact, patients with neurologic impairment have twice the postoperative complication rate, a 3-fold higher morbidity (return to preoperative symptoms), and a 4-fold higher reoperation rate compared with patients who are neurologically healthy.[34]

A recent study found a decrease in reflux-related hospitalizations (e.g., aspiration pneumonia, pneumonia, esophagitis, esophageal reflux) in patients who received antireflux surgery at younger than 4 years, but no benefit in older children and an increase in hospitalizations in those older than 4 years with developmental delay.[35] The risks and benefits of antireflux surgery should be carefully considered before recommending this surgery as a treatment option.

PHARMACOTHERAPY

Pharmacotherapeutic options for the chronic management of GERD in pediatric patients include the gastric acid-suppressing agents, H$_2$RAs and PPIs. Use of these agents is considered first-line therapy for managing GERD in pediatric patients. The role of mucosal surface barriers and prokinetic agents will also be discussed in this chapter. Table 2 lists pharmacologic agents used in the management of pediatric GERD, including their advantages, disadvantages, and specific place in therapy. Table 3 includes information on the specific dosing and formulations of various products.

Histamine-2 receptor antagonists. The H$_2$RAs decrease acid production by competitive inhibition of the histamine-2 receptors in gastric parietal cells. They do not inhibit meal-stimulated acid secretion. These agents are most effective for the on-demand relief of GERD symptoms and cases of mild esophagitis, and are less effective than the PPIs for symptom relief and healing of esophagitis.[2] Symptomatic improvement is seen in 70% of patients age 1 to 18 years, and endoscopic healing rates are between 50% and 95% in infants and children older than 1 month.[36,37] One case series in infants age 72 hours to 16 years found endoscopic healing rates of 95% with the use of ranitidine.[38] Although H$_2$RAs are commonly prescribed in neonates and preterm infants, limited efficacy and safety data are available for these patients.[1,39] Studies have been conducted suggesting an association with H$_2$RAs and the development of infections, including necrotizing enterocolitis, in preterm infants.[40,41] The current guidelines recommend H$_2$RAs in the treatment of esophagitis if PPIs are contraindicated or not available and as a 4- to 8-week course in children with GERD.

Drugs in this class include ranitidine, famotidine, nizatidine, and cimetidine. Ranitidine is the most widely used agent because it is well tolerated, with a low potential for drug interactions. Cimetidine is rarely used because of the high incidence of adverse effects such as gynecomastia, increased risk of liver disease, neutropenia, and thrombocytopenia, and because it inhibits cytochrome P450 (CYP), which can lead to significant drug interactions. The H$_2$RAs achieve peak plasma concentrations within 2.5 hours, and the duration of acid suppression is 6 hours, which necessitates dosing two or three times per day.[42] Infants usually require thrice-daily dosing because the gastric pH decreases within 5 hours.[17] One study showed that higher doses of ranitidine (20 mg/kg/day compared with 8 mg/kg/day) were as efficacious as omeprazole.[43]

The H$_2$RAs are associated with some adverse effects, such as irritability, headache, and somnolence in infants. These effects could be mistaken for continual symptoms of GERD in some patients. Tolerance of the acid-suppressive effect of the H$_2$RAs can develop after 6 weeks of therapy.[44,45] This phenomenon is not overcome by a dosage increase.[45]

Proton pump inhibitors. The PPIs inhibit both basal and meal-induced acid secretion by inactivating the H$^+$/K$^+$-ATPase pump in parietal cells (the proton pump). This pump acts as the parietal cell membrane transporter. The PPIs irreversibly inhibit the pump; thus, acid secretion can only return once the parietal cell makes new pumps. These agents also decrease 24-hour intragastric volumes, which helps facilitate gastric emptying and decrease the volume of reflux.[46] The PPIs have superior efficacy to the H$_2$RAs because they have a longer duration of action for acid suppression, inhibit meal-induced acid secretion, and are not associated with the development of tolerance. Drugs in this class include omeprazole, esomeprazole, lansoprazole, dexlansoprazole, pantoprazole, and rabeprazole.

The PPIs are first-line therapy for the management of chronic heartburn in older children and adolescents, reflux esophagitis in infants and children, and on-demand relief of GERD-related symptoms. For the older child or adolescent with heartburn, a 4- to 8-week diagnostic trial of a PPI—in addition to lifestyle changes—is recommended to determine whether an improvement in symptoms occurs. If there is improvement, the PPI can be continued for 8–12 weeks. In the management of reflux esophagitis, PPIs produce mucosal healing in 70% to 100% of patients within 12 weeks and symptom improvement in up to 80% of patients.[47-49] These agents also heal more severe grades of esophagitis and cases refractory to H$_2$RAs. For erosive esophagitis, initial treatment should be continued for 12 weeks.

Currently, only omeprazole and esomeprazole have an FDA indication for use in children younger than 1 year. However, off-label use of PPIs in infants younger than 1 year is quite common. The prevalence of PPI use is increasing among pediatric patients. A 2004 study showed an 11-fold increase in PPI use among infants younger than 12 months during a 6-year period and a shift from omeprazole to lansoprazole as the most commonly prescribed PPI.[50] Evidence exists describing the pharmacokinetics, pharmacodynamics, efficacy, and safety in this age group for both omeprazole and lansoprazole. However, at present, the efficacy data do not support the routine use of PPIs in children younger than 1 year, and concerns have been raised about the safety of these agents in this age group.[1,51]

Omeprazole is the most widely studied PPI in pediatric patients. Data support both its efficacy and long-term safety. Until 2004, it was also the most widely prescribed PPI, used in almost 90% of pediatric patients.[52,53] Pantoprazole has been studied in patients age 5–18 years for both GERD-related symptoms and reflux esophagitis, with healing rates similar to other PPIs (80% to 90%).[54] Esomeprazole has been studied in all pediatric age groups (including preterm infants), and it has been found both safe and efficacious. Researchers have also found similar age-related pharmacokinetics in metabolism and elimination compared with omeprazole and lansoprazole. Rabeprazole has been studied and found to be well tolerated in pediatric and adolescent patients from age 1 year and older.[55,56]

The proton pumps are most active when stimulated by a meal, so the ideal time to take a PPI is 15–30 minutes before the first meal of the day. Because these agents are broken down by gastric acid, most formulations are enteric-coated and delayed release. Administration of delayed-release capsules is challenging in infants and young children. All of the PPIs except rabeprazole can be administered by a nasogastric tube if needed. Both lansoprazole and omeprazole have commercially available compounding kits made using sodium bicarbonate for liquid administration. Immediate-release orally disintegrating tablets of lansoprazole and sprinkle capsules of rabeprazole are available. Esomeprazole and pantoprazole have packets available for administration; however, the pantoprazole packet is only available as a 40-mg packet. The PPIs have a delayed onset of action of up to 4 days.[1] Once administered, the PPI can continue to inhibit acid secretion for up to 15 hours,

Table 2. Therapeutic Management of Pediatric Gastroesophageal Reflux Disease (GERD)[1]

Pharmacologic Class	Advantages	Disadvantages	Approach to Therapy
Histamine-2 receptor antagonist (H$_2$RAs)	Quick onset of acid inhibition and symptom relief Data to support use in pediatric patients Cost-effective No need to taper on discontinuation Availability of liquid formulations Can be added to parenteral nutrition	Tolerance Adverse effects	On-demand therapy Management of erosive esophagitis if PPIs are not available or contraindicated
Proton pump inhibitor (PPIs)	Most potent acid suppression Inhibition of meal-induced acid secretion Greater efficacy than H$_2$RAs in healing esophagitis	Limited formulations available for pediatric patients Cytochrome P450 genetic polymorphisms Adverse effects: constipation, osteopenia, abdominal pain, risk of infections, including necrotizing enterocolitis and *C. difficile* infections Cost Risk of increased community-acquired pneumonia and *Clostridium difficile*-associated diarrhea	First-line maintenance therapy for GERD First-line initial management of erosive esophagitis for 3 months (mild to severe)
Prokinetic agents (metoclopramide, erythromycin, azithromycin, bethanechol)	Facilitate gastric emptying Symptomatic improvement	Significant adverse effects Inferior efficacy to PPIs and H$_2$RAs Limited clinical evidence (except for metoclopramide)	Routine use not recommended May be useful in patients with delayed gastric emptying in combination with an H$_2$RA or PPI
Baclofen	Reduce the frequency of TLESRS and acid reflux Facilitate gastric emptying	Limited formulations available for pediatric patients Adverse effects	Considered as a treatment option before surgery in patients with treatment failures
Antacids	Quick onset Variety of dosage forms available Low risk of adverse effects	Require frequent administration Inferior efficacy to PPIs and H$_2$RAs	On-demand therapy in patients maintained on H$_2$RAs or PPIs
Surface agents	Form a protective coat that may aid in mucosal healing Low risk of adverse effects	Limited clinical evidence	Adjunctive therapy for erosive esophagitis with H$_2$RAs or PPIs

Table 3. Pediatric Doses of Medications Used in the Management of Gastroesophageal Reflux Disease (GERD)

Agent	Dose (Oral)	Formulations
Histamine-2 Receptor Antagonists		
Ranitidine	Neonates: 2 mg/kg/day divided every 12 hours Infants, children, adolescents: 5–10 mg/kg/day divided two to three times (Maximum 300 mg/day; 600 mg/day if erosive esophagitis)	15 mg/mL syrup 75-, 150-, 300-mg tablet 150-, 300-mg capsule 25-mg effervescent tablet for solution
Famotidine	Neonates to 3 months: 0.5 mg/kg/day once daily Infants and children ≥ 3 months to 12 years: 1 mg/kg/day divided twice daily Older children and adolescents > 12–18 years: 20 mg twice daily (GERD) 10–20 mg before meals (heartburn) (Maximum 40 mg/day)	40 mg/5 mL powder for suspension 10-, 20-, 40-mg tablet 20-mg chewable tablet
Cimetidine	Neonates: 5–10 mg/kg/day divided two to three times daily Infants, children, adolescents < 16 years: 20–40 mg/kg/day divided three to four times daily (Maximum 400 mg/dose) Older children and adolescents ≥ 16 years: 400 mg four times daily or 800 mg twice daily (Maximum 1600 mg/day)	300 mg/5 mL solution 200-, 300-, 400-, 800-mg tablet
Nizatidine	Children 6 months to 11 years: 5–10 mg/kg/day divided twice daily Older children and adolescents ≥ 12 years: 150 mg twice daily	15 mg/mL solution 150-, 300-mg capsule
Proton Pump Inhibitors		
Omeprazole	Infants < 1 year: 0.7–1.5 mg/kg/day once daily Children and adolescents 1–16 years, by weight: 5 kg to < 10 kg: 5 mg/day 10 kg to ≤ 20 kg: 10 mg/day > 20 kg: 20 mg/day Alternative: 1 mg/kg/day (range, 0.2–3.5 mg/kg/day) once or twice daily	10-, 20-, 40-mg delayed-release capsule 20-mg delayed-release tablet 2.5-, 10-mg granules for oral suspension packet 2 mg/mL oral suspension (compounding kit)
Omeprazole and sodium bicarbonate	Same as omeprazole	20-, 40-mg immediate-release capsule (contains 1100 mg sodium bicarbonate) 20-, 40-mg of powder for oral suspension packet (contains 1680 mg sodium bicarbonate per packet)
Esomeprazole	Neonates: 0.5 mg/kg/day once daily for 7 days Infants 1–24 months: 0.25–1 mg/kg/day once daily Children 1–11 years: < 20 kg: 10 mg/day for 8 weeks > 20 kg: 10–20 mg/day for 8 weeks 12–17 years: 20–40 mg/day for 8 weeks	20-, 40-mg delayed-release capsule 2.5-, 5-, 10-, 20-, 40-mg granules for suspension packet 20-, 40-mg injection

(continued)

Table 3. Pediatric Doses of Medications Used in the Management of Gastroesophageal Reflux Disease (GERD) *(continued)*

Agent	Dose (Oral)	Formulations
Proton Pump Inhibitors		

Lansoprazole	Neonates:
	    0.2–1 mg/kg/day once daily
	Infants:
	    < 10 weeks: 0.2–0.3 mg/kg/day
	    ≥ 10 weeks: 1–2 mg/kg/day once daily
	Children 1–11 years:
	    ≤ 30 kg: 15 mg/day
	    > 30 kg: 30 mg/day
	    ≥ 12 years: 15 mg/day
	    (Erosive esophagitis: 30–60 mg/day)
		15-, 30-mg delayed-release capsule
		15-, 30-mg orally disintegrating tablet
		15-mg 24-hour tablet
		3 mg/mL oral suspension (compounding kit)

Dexlansoprazole	Children ≥ 12 years:
	    GERD: 30 mg/day for 4 weeks
	    Erosive esophagitis: 60 mg/day for 8 weeks;
	        then 30 mg/day for 6 months
		30-, 60-mg delayed-release capsule
		30-mg orally disintegrating tablets

Pantoprazole	Erosive esophagitis, by weight:
	    15 kg to < 40 kg: 20 mg/day
	    (Alternative: 0.5–1 mg/kg/day)
	    ≥ 40 kg: 40 mg/day
		20-, 40-mg delayed-release tablet
		40-mg granules for suspension
		40-mg injection
		Extemporaneous suspension recipe available

Rabeprazole	Infants and children 1-11 years, by weight:
	    < 15 kg: 5 mg/day for up to 12 weeks
	    ≥ 15 kg: 10 mg/day for up to 12 weeks
	Children and adolescents:
	    ≥ 12 years: 20 mg/day for 8 weeks
		5-, 10-mg oral delayed-release sprinkle capsule
		20-mg delayed-release tablet

Prokinetic Agents		

Metoclopramide	Neonates:
	    0.1–0.15 mg/kg/dose every 6 hours
	Infants, children, adolescents:
	    0.4–0.8 mg/kg/day divided four times daily
	    (Maximum 60 mg/day)
		5 mg/5 mL solution
		5-, 10-mg tablet

Erythromycin	Infants:
	    0.75–3 mg/kg/dose q8h (up to 10 mg/kg/dose)
	Children and adolescents:
	    10–20 mg/kg/day divided two to four times daily
	        before meals
	    (Maximum 250 mg three times daily)
		200 mg/5 mL, 400 mg/5 mL powder for
		    suspension
		250-mg delayed-release capsule
		250-, 500-mg tablet
		400-mg tablet (as ethylsuccinate)
		250-, 333-, 500-mg delayed-release, enteric-
		    coated tablet

Bethanechol	Children: 0.4–0.8 mg/kg/day divided four times daily	5-, 10-, 25-, 50-mg tablet Extemporaneous suspension formula available

Data from Lexi-Comp Online [Internet database]. Hudson, OH: Lexi-Comp.

requiring only one dose per day in most patients.[57] Despite this duration of action, some patients continue to experience heartburn of less severity and may even experience nocturnal acid breakthrough, defined as gastric pH of less than 4.0 for more than 1 hour within 12 hours of a PPI dose.[58]

Pharmacokinetic data show that children age 1–10 years require a higher milligram-per-kilogram dose than adolescents and adults. In addition, infants may require lower milligram-per-kilogram dosing than children and adolescents.[1] A recent study with lansoprazole found that infants 10 weeks and younger had higher plasma concentrations and lower clearance compared with infants older than 10 weeks to 1 year. Thus, a lower dose of lansoprazole is recommended in patients 10 weeks or younger.[51]

The PPIs are metabolized primarily by CYP 2C19 and 3A4. The enzymatic activity of CYP 2C19 varies with age. Low at birth, CYP 2C19 enzymatic activity reaches adult values at age 6–12 months, exceeds adult values between age 1 and 4 years, and then decreases to adult values around puberty.[59] This activity range explains differences in the metabolism and clearance of PPIs among various age groups. There is evidence of reduced metabolism in neonates and preterm infants and increased clearance in children compared with adults. Polymorphisms also exist for *CYP2C19* with three phenotypes: homozygous extensive metabolizers, heterozygous extensive metabolizers, and poor metabolizers. When dosing PPIs in pediatric patients, the clinician must consider interindividual variability caused by the pharmacokinetic and pharmacodynamic relationships that exist, particularly with metabolism and elimination.[60] Rabeprazole metabolism does not appear to be as affected as other PPIs by alterations in the *CYP2C19* genetic polymorphisms because rabeprazole undergoes some nonenzymatic metabolism. The PPIs decrease the absorption of drugs requiring an acidic environment to be absorbed. Drugs that may be affected include itraconazole and griseofulvin. Omeprazole has also been associated with decreased clearance of diazepam and carbamazepine because of its inhibition of *CYP2C19*.[61,62] Close monitoring of carbamazepine concentrations is required when coadministered with omeprazole.

Common adverse effects of PPIs include headache, nausea, constipation, and diarrhea. It is recommended to change to a different agent or decrease the dose if any of these adverse effects occur.[1] These agents can also be associated with some severe adverse effects, including acute interstitial nephritis, parietal cell hyperplasia, fundic gland polyps, enterochromaffin cell–like hyperplasia, vitamin B_{12} deficiency, and bone loss. These severe effects occur more often in patients on prolonged therapy (longer than 2 years) and in adult patients. Because rebound acid secretion is possible after PPI discontinuation, the guidelines suggest that PPIs be tapered over 4 weeks when therapy is complete. However, the evidence supporting this practice is conflicting.[1]

Therapy with a PPI is indicated for 4-8 weeks' duration, with consideration for an additional course if needed. However, patients commonly continue PPI therapy longer than recommended. Long-term acid suppression is not without complications. Gastric acid is protective to the digestive system because it inhibits bacterial flora. Bacterial overgrowth can occur in patients taking gastric acid inhibitors. Both H_2RAs and PPIs have been found to increase the rates of the following: (1) community-acquired pneumonia in children; (2) acute gastroenteritis in children; (3) necrotizing enterocolitis in premature infants; (4) candidemia in premature infants; and (5) *Clostridium difficile*-associated diarrhea in children.[63-68]

Prokinetic agents. Prokinetic therapy used for the management of GERD in pediatric patients includes metoclopramide, erythromycin, bethanechol, and baclofen. A recent systematic review of healthy children age 1 month to 2 years with GER found that metoclopramide produces modest decreases in daily symptoms but is associated with considerable adverse effects.[69] The FDA has issued a black box warning for metoclopramide because of the adverse effects of extrapyramidal reactions and tardive dyskinesia. Erythromycin has been used to increase gastric emptying in some patients because of its action on motilin receptors, but evidence is limited for its use in GERD. The dose for its prokinetic activity is less than that for the treatment of bacteria, thus adverse effects are rare at these lower doses. However, there is still a slight risk of gastrointestinal upset, hepatotoxicity, arrhythmias, and antibiotic resistance with erythromycin use. Bethanechol, a direct cholinergic agonist, has uncertain efficacy and unwanted adverse effects, including headache, malaise, abdominal cramps, belching, nausea, and vomiting. Bethanechol is used to treat urinary retention and so may be considered if comorbid conditions exist as an alternative therapy. Baclofen works to decrease TLESRs and can increase gastric emptying. This agent has been found efficacious in reducing vomiting in children with neurologic impairment and GERD. Because baclofen works directly on the central nervous system, there is a high incidence of adverse effects, such as somnolence, headache, insomnia, and confusion.[70] From the available evidence, the routine use of prokinetic agents for GERD is not recommended. Despite the lack of evidence supporting their efficacy, prokinetic agents are still prescribed in the pediatric population for the management of GERD.[1]

Antacids. Antacids work by buffering gastric acid within the stomach and esophagus, thereby facilitating mucosal healing. Antacid therapy (i.e., magnesium hydroxide, aluminum hydroxide, calcium carbonate) is recommended for on-demand relief of heartburn in older children and adolescents. The advantage to antacid therapy is its quick onset of action; however, because of its short half-life, administration is required more often. All antacids should be used with caution in infants and young children because they increase plasma aluminum concentrations and can cause milk-alkali syndrome, a condition associated with hypercalcemia, alkalosis, and renal failure. In addition, antacids should be avoided in patients with existing renal failure. Chronic antacid therapy for pediatric GERD is not recommended because more effective agents are available.[1]

Surface-protective agents. Surface-protective agents contain either sucralfate or alginate. Sucralfate is a mixture of sucrose, sulfate, and aluminum. In an acidic environment, sucralfate forms a gel that coats the mucosal surface. Alginate alone is useful for on-demand therapy. The commercially available product for infants and young children contains only sodium and magnesium alginate. Older children and adolescents may take the adult formulation that contains both alginate and the buffering agents found in antacids. Surface-protective agents are only recommended as adjunctive therapy for the management of esophagitis and severe GERD-related symptoms. Unfortunately, they need an acidic environment to form the barrier, so they may not be efficacious if used in combination with acid suppressive therapy. They can be used for on-demand therapy in patients with bothersome symptoms despite maximal doses of PPIs, but they are not recommended for chronic therapy.[1]

Combination therapy. Recommendations on the use of combination therapy are unavailable in current guidelines.[1] The most common combination of medication classes is an H_2RA or PPI with a prokinetic agent or an H_2RA and a PPI. In general, changing to a different agent is preferred to adding another agent for chronic maintenance therapy. With many agents, there is a potential for increased adverse effects. In addition, H$_2$RAs and PPIs have a theoretical antagonistic mechanism of action because PPIs require the presence of acid to inhibit proton pumps, and H$_2$RAs directly inhibit acid production. Twice-daily dosing of both an H$_2$RA and PPI would provide potent acid suppression but could further increase the risk of respiratory infections or gastroenteritis.

Adult patients with nocturnal acid breakthrough on PPIs have decreased symptoms with the addition of a bedtime dose of an H$_2$RA, suggesting that nocturnal acid breakthrough is histamine-related. However, the effect is not lasting, secondary to the tolerance that develops to H$_2$RAs. In children, data are limited to one small study of 18 children 1–13 years, which showed no benefit to this strategy.[71] Therefore, adding a bedtime dose of an H$_2$RA to a PPI is not routinely recommended for adult or pediatric patients.

MONITORING GUIDELINES

Patients receiving acid suppression therapy should be monitored for symptom relief, adverse drug reactions, and adherence to the regimen. For the management of chronic heartburn, lifestyle changes and PPIs are recommended for 12 weeks. Patients should be continually monitored during this time to determine whether therapy is providing symptom resolution. If symptoms persist at the end of the treatment period, further diagnostic testing and/or continued maintenance therapy may be required. Patients receiving treatment for reflux esophagitis should be monitored for symptom relief and the presence of any complicating symptoms, such as dysphagia or odynophagia. In addition, because the long-term safety of all medications used for the management of pediatric GERD is unknown, careful and continued monitoring is required throughout the duration of therapy.

Symptoms associated with GERD can have a negative impact on the quality of life of both patients and their caregivers. At present, validated tools to measure the quality of life for children with GERD are limited. Practitioners most often rely on parental reports of symptoms. Assessing improvement in quality of life is important for monitoring the efficacy of treatment strategies.

Special populations: Neurologic impairment. The frequency and severity of GERD in patients with neurologic impairment are increased. An estimated 50% to 70% of children with neurologic impairment such as cerebral palsy have symptoms associated with reflux, and up to 70% have endoscopic evidence of esophagitis.[72] It is more difficult to properly provide a diagnosis for a child with GERD who has neurologic impairment because such children have difficulty communicating their symptoms and may present with atypical symptoms, such as self-injurious behavior, seizures, and dystonia. The most reliable diagnostic tool for GERD in children with neurologic impairment is pH/multichannel intraluminal impedance monitoring.[1] Treatment of GERD in these patients should be individualized and consist of feeding changes, positional changes, muscle spasm control, and antireflux therapy. These patients may benefit from the combination of a PPI and baclofen. Careful monitoring of baclofen's adverse effects is warranted because this agent can cause dizziness, drowsiness, and fatigue, as well as lower the seizure threshold in patients with underlying seizure disorders. Some patients with neurologic impairment improve with medication therapy alone. Antireflux surgery should be considered in patients who do not respond to aggressive medical management and have concomitant respiratory complications. The risks and benefits must be weighed carefully because surgery in these patients has resulted in higher morbidity, mortality, and symptom recurrence.

CONCLUSIONS

Appropriate management of GER and GERD in the pediatric patient is important because symptoms can have a considerable effect on quality of life and may persist into adulthood, causing complications. The recent clinical practice guidelines provide updated information and evidence to help guide the medical management of children with GER and GERD. Many questions remain for these patients because of the lack of large, well-designed clinical trials of different age groups within the pediatric population. Pharmacists should be familiar with current guidelines so that they can provide evidence-based treatment recommendations based on age, risk factors, and family and medical history.

A 2-month-old girl is brought to the pediatrician because of vomiting after feeding. She has a 1-week history of reflux and vomiting after feeds, which have continued despite adequate feeding. She has no significant past medical history and was born at 40 weeks. Her weight today is 4.5 kg (25th percentile for weight, birth weight 3.78 kg). She has been a breastfed infant since birth and receives feedings every 3 hours.

1. What initial nonpharmacologic options are recommended for this patient?

A patient who presents with a 1-week history of reflux and vomiting but has adequate weight gain is likely experiencing physiologic gastroesophageal reflux. The parents or caregivers should be counseled on proper feeding positions and on burping the infant very often throughout the feeding. The infant should remain upright for at least 30 minutes after feeding. Specific positioning recommendations are to make sure that the infant's head remains above the stomach during feeding or having the infant lie across the caregiver diagonally during feeding in a cradle hold. In addition, the parents or caregivers should make sure that the infant is in a straight position and not bent at the stomach. While breastfeeding, it is recommended to burp the infant on each side of the breast before changing to the other side. Positional changes are all that is required at this time.

Case (continued). One month later, the patient returns to the clinic for a routine visit with parental concerns of continued reflux/regurgitation after feeding. Her weight in clinic is 5.1 kg (25th percentile).

2. What is the best treatment at this time? Discuss both pharmacologic and nonpharmacologic recommendations.

The North American Society for Pediatric Gastroenterology, Hepatology, and Nutrition (NASPGHAN) and the European Society for Pediatric Gastroenterology, Hepatology, and Nutrition (ESPGHAN) guidelines recommend a trial of thickened formula/breastmilk, a trial of hydrolyzed formula, or commercially available anti-regurgitation formula in an infant with recurrent regurgitation. To thicken the formula, the addition of one tablespoon of rice cereal to every 2 ounces of formula/breastmilk increases the caloric density of the formula to 20-27 kcal/ounce. This infant has appropriate weight gain despite the reflux; therefore, she may benefit from a trial of one of the commercially available anti-regurgitation formulas. In the first 6 months of life, infants should gain about 20-30 g/day (or 5-7 ounces/week) and double their birth weight around age 4 months. Concerns about thickening agents include increased coughing during feeding and expending extra energy because of the increased viscosity of the formula. In addition, recent safety concerns have arisen about trace amounts of arsenic found in rice cereals. A trial of a hydrolyzed formula is an additional option and may be tried, especially if the infant may have a milk protein allergy. At this point, a trial of a pharmacologic agent is not recommended. A histamine-2 receptor antagonist or proton pump inhibitor (PPI) is appropriate to trial if the infant continues with symptoms despite the previous feeding and positional changes, has weight loss, or symptoms consistent with esophagitis.

Case (continued). Three months later, the infant is still having symptoms of reflux and poor weight gain, so she is referred to a pediatric gastroenterologist. Her current weight is 6.2 kg (10th percentile). She is admitted to the hospital for a 24-hour pH monitoring study with impedance monitoring. The results of this study show a reflux index of 10%.

3. What is the best treatment for the patient at this time? Discuss both pharmacologic and nonpharmacologic recommendations.

This patient has an abnormal 24-hour pH monitoring study with a reflux index greater than 7%. According to the NASPGHAN/ESPGHAN guidelines, acid-suppressive therapy with a proton pump inhibitor is indicated for this patient. Because of the patient's age and need for a liquid dosage form, either lansoprazole or omeprazole suspension is appropriate, with the following approach to using these agents:

- Lansoprazole suspension (3 mg/mL) 6 mg orally every 24 hours (in the morning) or omeprazole suspension (2 mg/mL) 6 mg orally every 24 hours (in the morning): the dose should be given before feeding, administered as a 2-mL dose using an oral syringe after shaking well before administration.

- The parents and caregivers should continue to use positional changes for feeding and feed smaller amounts more often.

- The patient should be re-evaluated in 1 month for change in symptoms with weekly weights to ensure adequate growth. The goal weight gain should be 5-7 ounces/week for the first 6 months of life and 3-5 ounces/week from age 6 months to 1 year.

- Monitoring guidelines should be included for pharmacotherapy agents, such as gastrointestinal adverse effects.

4. How can a PPI be administered to an infant?

All of the PPIs, except rabeprazole, are approved for children younger than age 1 year and have dosage forms available or recipes for extemporaneous preparations. Omeprazole and esomeprazole are available as granule packets to administer to infants. The contents should be mixed with water, stirred to thicken, and administered within 30 minutes of preparation. Alternatively, the 10-mg capsule could be opened and sprinkled onto applesauce and administered to an infant that can take solid foods (usually over 6 months). Omeprazole is also available as a compounding kit that is prepared by the pharmacy and can be administered as a liquid suspension by an oral syringe. Esomeprazole is also available as a granule formulation and administered similarly to omeprazole. Lansoprazole has a commercially available compounding kit (3 mg/mL) and can be administered by an oral syringe as a liquid and also has an orally disintegrating tablet. For infants, the tablet can be placed whole into the bottom of an oral syringe and then the syringe can be filled with water (4 mL for the 15-mg tablet and 10 mL for the 30-mg tablet); after shaking to ensure the tablet has dissolved, the drug can be administered by the oral syringe.

REFERENCES

1. Vandenplas Y, Rudolph CD, Di Lorenzo C, et al. Pediatric gastroesophageal reflux clinical practice guidelines: joint recommendations of the North American Society for Pediatric Gastroenterology, Hepatology, and Nutrition (NASPGHAN) and the European Society for Pediatric Gastroenterology, Hepatology, and Nutrition (ESPGHAN). J Pediatr Gastroenterol Nutr 2009;49:498-547.

2. Rosen R, Vandenplas Y, Singendonk M, et al. Pediatric gastroesophageal reflux clinical practice guidelines: joint recommendations of the North American Society for Pediatric Gastroenterology, Hepatology, and Nutrition (NASPGHAN) and the European Society for Pediatric Gastroenterology, Hepatology, and Nutrition (ESPGHAN). J Pediatr Gastroenterol Nutr 2018;66:516-54.

3. Sherman PM, Hassall E, Fagundes-Neto U, et al. A global, evidence-based consensus on the definition of gastroesophageal reflux disease in the pediatric population. Am J Gastroenterol 2009;104:1278-95.

4. Nelson SP, Chen EH, Syniar GM, et al. Prevalence of symptoms of gastroesophageal reflux during infancy. A pediatric practice-based survey. Pediatric Practice Research group. Arch Pediatr Adolesc Med 1997;151:569-72.

5. Martin AJ, Pratt N, Kennedy JD, et al. Natural history and familial relationships of infant spilling to 9 years of age. Pediatrics 2002;109:1061-7.

6. Campanozzi A, Boccia G, Pensabene L, et al. Prevalence and natural history of gastroesophageal reflux: pediatric prospective study. Pediatrics 2009;123:779-83.

7. Ewer AK, Durbin GM, Morgan MEI, et al. Gastric emptying and gastro-oesophageal reflux in preterm infants. Arch Dis Child 1996;75(suppl):117F-21F.

8. Kleinman L, Rothman M, Strauss R, et al. The Infant Gastroesophageal Reflux Questionnaire Revised: development and validation as an evaluative instrument. Clin Gastroenterol Hepatol 2006;5:588-96.

9. Hyman PE, Milla PJ, Benninga MA, et al. Childhood functional gastrointestinal disorders: neonate/toddler. Gastroenterology 2006;130:1519-26.

10. Corvaglia L, Rotatori R, Ferlini M, et al. The effect of body positioning on gastroesophageal reflux in premature infants: evaluation by combined impedance and pH monitoring. J Pediatr 2007;151:591-6.

11. Oyen N, Markestad T, Skaerven R, et al. Combined effects of sleeping position and prenatal risk factors in sudden infant death syndrome: the Nordic Epidemiological SIDS Study. Pediatrics 1997;100:613-21.

12. Khoshoo V, Ross G, Brown S, et al. Smaller volume, thickened formulas in the management of gastroesophageal reflux in thriving infants. J Pediatr Gastroenterol Nutr 2000;31:554-6.

13. Craig WR, Hanlon-Dearman A, Sinclair C, et al. Metoclopramide, thickened feedings, and positioning for gastroesophageal reflux in children under two years. Cochrane Database Syst Rev 2004;4:CD003502.

14. Horvath A, Dziechciarz P, Szajewska H. The effect of thickened-feed interventions on gastroesophageal reflux in infants: systematic review and meta-analysis of randomized, controlled trials. Pediatrics 2008;122:e1268-77.

15. Orenstein SR, Shalaby TM, Putnam PE. Thickened feeds as a cause of increased coughing when used as therapy for gastroesophageal reflux in infants. J Pediatr 1992;121:913-5.

16. Moukarzel AA, Abdelnour H, Akatcherian C. Effects of a prethickened formula on esophageal pH and gastric emptying of infants with GER. J Clin Gastroenterol 2007;41;823-9.

17. Orenstein S, McGowan J. Efficacy of conservative therapy as taught in the primary care setting for symptoms suggesting infant gastroesophageal reflux. J Pediatr 2008;152:310-4.

18. Mousa H, Hassan M. Gastroesophageal reflux disease. Pediatr Clin N Am 2017;64:487-505.

19. Ruigomez A, Wallander MA, Lundborg P, et al. Gastroesophageal reflux disease in children and adolescents in primary care. Scand J Gastroenterol 2010;45:139-46.

20. Gibbons TE, Stockwell JA, Kreh RP, et al. The status of gastroesophageal reflux disease in hospitalized U.S. children 1995-2000. J Pediatr Gastroenterol Nutr 2001;33:197.

21. Hu FZ, Preston RA, Post JC, et al. Mapping of a gene for severe pediatric gastroesophageal reflux to chromosome 13q14. JAMA 2000;284:325-34.

22. Romero Y, Cameron AJ, Locke GR III, et al. Familial aggregation of gastroesophageal reflux in patients with Barrett's esophagus and esophageal adenocarcinoma. Gastroenterology 1997;113:1449-56.

23. Trudgill NJ, Kapur KC, Riley SA. Familial clustering of reflux symptoms. Am J Gastroenterol 1999;94:1172-8.

24. Michail S. Gastroesophageal reflux. Pediatr Rev 2007;28:101-10.

25. Moore DJ, Tao BS, Lines DR, et al. Double-blind placebo-controlled trial of omeprazole in irritable infants with gastroesophageal reflux. J Pediatr 2003;143:219-23.

26. Heine RG, Jordan B, Lubitz L, et al. Clinical predictors of pathological gastro-oesophageal reflux in infants with persistent distress. J Pediatr Child Health 2006;42:134-9.

27. Francavilla R, Magista AM, Bucci N, et al. Comparison of esophageal pH and multichannel intraluminal impedance testing in pediatric patients with suspected gastroesophageal reflux. J Pediatr Gastroenterol Nutr 2010;50:154-60.

28. Spencer J. Prolonged pH recording in the study of gastro-oesophageal reflux disease. Br J Surg 1969;56:912-4.

29. Higginbotham TW. Effectiveness and safety of proton pump inhibitors in infantile gastroesophageal reflux disease. Ann Pharmacother 2010;44:572-6.

30. Aksglaede K, Pedersen JB, Lange A, et al. Gastro-esophageal reflux demonstrated by radiography in infants less than 1 year of age. Comparison with pH monitoring. Acta Radiol 2003;44:136-8.

31. Srivastava R, Downey EC, O'Gorman M, et al. Impact of fundoplication versus gastrojejunal feeding tubes on mortality and in preventing aspiration pneumonia in young children with neurologic impairment who have gastroesophageal reflux disease. Pediatrics 2009;123:338-45.

32. Ferry GD, Selby M, Pietro TJ. Clinical response to short-term nasogastric feeding in infants with gastroesophageal reflux and growth failure. J Pediatr Gastroenterol Nutr 1983;2:57-61.

33. Gold BD, Freston JW. Gastroesophageal reflux in children: pathogenesis, prevalence, diagnosis, and role of proton pump inhibitors in treatment. Pediatr Drugs 2002;4:673-85.

34. Pearl RH, Robie DK, Ein SH, et al. Complications of gastroesophageal antireflux surgery in neurologically impaired versus neurologically normal children. J Pediatr Surg 1990;25:1169-73.

35. Goldin AB, Sawin R, Seidel KD, et al. Do antireflux operations decrease the rate of reflux-related hospitalizations in children? Pediatrics 2006;118:2326-33.

36. Karjoo M, Kane R. Omeprazole treatment of children with peptic esophagitis refractory to ranitidine therapy. Arch Pediatr Adolesc Med 1995;149:267-71.

37. Kelly DA. Do H2 receptor antagonists have a therapeutic role in childhood? J Pediatr Gastroenterol Nutr 1994;19:270-6.

38. DeAngelis G, Banchini G. Ranitidine in paediatric patients: a personal experience. Clin Trials 1989;26:370-5.

39. Slaughter JL, Stenger MR, Reagan PB, et al. Neonatal histamine-2 receptor antagonist and proton pump inhibitor treatment at United States Children's Hospitals. J Pediatr 2016;174:63-70.

40. Terrin G, Passariello A, DeCurtis M, et al. Ranitidine is associated with infections, necrotizing enterocolitis, and fatal outcome in newborns. Pediatrics 2012;129:e40-5.

41. Guillet R, Stoll BJ, Cotten CM, et al. Association of H2-blocker therapy and higher incidence of necrotizing enterocolitis in very low birth weight infants. Pediatrics 2006;117:e137-42.

42. Orenstein SR, Blumer JL, Faessel HM, et al. Ranitidine, 75 mg, over-the-counter dose: pharmacokinetic and pharmacodynamic effects in children with symptoms of gastro-oesophageal reflux. Aliment Pharmacol Ther 2002;16:899-907.

43. Cucchiara S, Minelia R, Iervolino C, et al. Omeprazole and high dose ranitidine in the treatment of refractory reflux oesophagitis. Arch Dis Child 1993;69:655-9.

44. Nwokolo CU, Smith JT, Gavey C, et al. Tolerance during 29 days of conventional dosing with cimetidine, nizatidine, famotidine, or ranitidine. Aliment Pharmacol Ther 1990;4:S29-45.

45. Wilder-Smith CH, Ernst T, Gennoni M, et al. Tolerance to oral H2-receptor antagonists. Dig Dis Sci 1990;35:976-83.

46. Champion G, Richter JE, Vaezi MF, et al. Duodenogastroesophageal reflux: relationship to pH and importance in Barrett's esophagus. Gastroenterology 1994;107:747-54.

47. Boccia G, Manguso F, Miele E, et al. Maintenance therapy for erosive esophagitis in children after healing by omeprazole: is it advisable? Am J Gastroenterol 2007;102:1291-7.

48. Hassall E, Israel D, Shepherd R, et al. Omeprazole for treatment of chronic erosive esophagitis in children: a multicenter study of efficacy, safety, tolerability and dose requirements. J Pediatr 2000;137:800-7.

49. Tolia V, Ferry G, Gunasekaran T, et al. Efficacy of lansoprazole in the treatment of gastroesophageal reflux disease in children. J Pediatr Gastroenterol Nutr 2002;35:S308-18.

50. Illueca M, Alemayehu B, Shoetan N, et al. Proton pump inhibitor prescribing patterns in newborns and infants. J Pediatr Pharmacol Ther 2014;19:283-7.

51. Chen IL, Gao WY, Johnson AP, et al. Proton pump inhibitor use in infants: FDA reviewer experience. J Pediatr Gastroenterol Nutr 2012;54:8-14.

52. Hassall E, Kerr W, El-Serag HB. Characteristics of children receiving proton pump inhibitors continuously for up to 11 years duration. J Pediatr 2007;150:262-7.

53. Tolia V, Boyer K. Long-term proton pump inhibitor use in children: a retrospective review of safety. Dig Dis Sci 2008;53:385-93.

54. Kearns GL, Blumer J, Schexnayder S, et al. Single-dose pharmacokinetics of oral and intravenous pantoprazole in children and adolescents. J Clin Pharmacol 2008;48:1356-65.

55. James L, Walson P, Lomax K, et al. Pharmacokinetics and tolerability of rabeprazole sodium in subjects aged 12 to 16 years with gastroesophageal reflux disease: an open-label, single- and multiple dose study. Clin Ther 2007;29:2082-92.

56. Haddad I, Kierkus J, Tron E, et al. Efficacy and safety of rabeprazole in children (1-11 years) with gastroesophageal reflux disease. J Pediatr Gastroenterol Nutr 2013;57:798-807.

57. Israel DM, Hassall E. Omeprazole and other proton pump inhibitors: pharmacology, efficacy and safety with special reference to use in children. J Pediatr Gastroenterol Nutr 1998;27:566-79.

58. Hatlebakk JG, Katz PO, Kuo B, et al. Nocturnal gastric acidity and acid breakthrough on different regimens of omeprazole 40 mg daily. Aliment Pharmacol Ther 1998;12:1235-40.

59. Leeder JS, Kearns GL. Pharmacogenetics in pediatrics: implications for practice. Pediatr Clin N Am 1997;44:55-77.

60. Litalien C, Theoret Y, Faure C. Pharmacokinetics of proton pump inhibitors in children. Clin Pharmacokinet 2005;44:441-66.

61. Caraco Y, Tateishi I, Wood AJ. Interethnic difference in omeprazole's inhibition of diazepam metabolism. Clin Pharmacol Ther 1995;58:62-72.

62. Dixit RK, Chawla AB, Kumar N, et al. Effect of omeprazole on the pharmacokinetics of sustained-release carbamazepine in healthy male volunteers. Methods Find Exp Clin Pharmacol 2001;23:37-9.

63. Freedberg DE, Lamousé-Smith ES, Lightdale JR, et al. Use of acid suppression medication is associated with risk for C. difficile infection in infants and children: a population-based study. Clin Infect Dis 2015;61:912-7.

64. Brown KE, Knoderer CA, Nichols KR, et al. Acid-suppressing agents and risk for clostridium difficile infection in pediatric patients. Clin Pediatr 2015;54:1102-6.

65. Canani RB, Cirillo P, Roggero P, et al. Therapy with gastric acidity inhibitors increases the risk of acute gastroenteritis and community-acquired pneumonia in children. Pediatrics 2006;117:e817-e820.

66. Tjon JA, Pe M, Soscia J, et al. Efficacy and safety of proton pump inhibitors in the management of pediatric gastroesophageal reflux disease. Pharmacotherapy 2013;33:956-71.

67. Cohen S, Bueno de Mesquita M, Mimouni FB. Adverse effects reported in the use of gastroesophageal reflux disease treatments in children: a 10 years literature review. Br J Clin Pharmacol 2015;80:200-8.

68. Saiman L, Ludington E, Dawson JD, et al. Risk factors for Candida species colonization of neonatal intensive care unit patients. Pediatr Infect Dis J 2001;20:1119-24.

69. Hibb AM, Lorch SA. Metoclopramide for the treatment of gastroesophageal reflux disease in infants: a systematic review. Pediatrics 2006;118:746-52.

70. Kawai M, Kawahara H, Hirayama S, et al. Effect of baclofen on emesis and 24-hour esophageal pH in neurologically impaired children with gastroesophageal reflux disease. J Pediatr Gastroenterol Nutr 2004;38:317-23.

71. Pfefferkorn MD, Croffie JM, Gupta SK, et al. Nocturnal acid breakthrough in children with reflux esophagitis taking proton pump inhibitors. J Pediatr Gastroenterol Nutr 2006;42:160-5.

72. Pensabene L, Miele E, Del Giudice E, et al. Mechanisms of gastroesophageal reflux in children with sequelae of birth asphyxia. Brain Dev 2008;30:563-71.

CHAPTER 16

Diarrhea and Constipation

Christina L. Cox, Pharm.D., BCPS, BCPPS

INTRODUCTION

Gastrointestinal (GI) disorders in children are a common cause of patient discomfort, family stress, and health care provider and hospital visits each year. These disorders can begin in the first days of life and can be a clinical indicator of an underlying physiologic, anatomic, or metabolic disorder, or even an infectious process. Diarrhea and constipation are two broad categories that encompass many disease or functional GI processes often encountered in the pediatric patient. This chapter seeks not only to outline the impact of diarrhea and constipation on children and their families, but also to provide insight into the diagnosis, treatment, and prevention of these disorders.

DIARRHEA

EPIDEMIOLOGY

Worldwide, diarrhea continues to be a leading cause of morbidity and mortality among infants and children, especially those younger than 5 years. In 2017, the World Health Organization (WHO) reported a worldwide estimate of 1.7 billion cases of childhood diarrheal disease each year. In addition, the WHO reported about 525,000 deaths from diarrheal disease in children younger than 5 years.[1] In 2017, the United States had a reported 806 deaths from diarrheal disease in children younger than 5 years.[2] As evident, these percentages differ greatly in developed versus developing countries, with developing countries accounting for a significant portion of reported deaths.[2] Developing countries struggle with the ability to provide safe drinking water, hygiene, and overall health and nutrition, resulting in an environment ideal for the spread of diarrhea-causing pathogens.[1] Although overall living conditions are more favorable in developed countries, the impact of diarrhea on children should not be underestimated. Diarrhea can result from infectious and noninfectious causes, and can be acute and chronic, all of which contribute to the cost and significant number of hospitalizations associated with this condition.[3-5] This chapter will focus on the noninfectious causes of diarrhea and their respective treatments. Diarrhea related to infectious etiologies is addressed in the Infectious Diarrhea chapter.

ETIOLOGY

Diarrhea is characterized by three or more watery, loose stools per day (or more than an established normal baseline for an individual).[1] Although a precise definition has not been well described, an increased number and changed consistency of stools for less than 1 week is considered *acute diarrhea*. Most diarrheas occurring in infants and children, especially those between age 6 months and 2 years, result from an acute, infectious etiology. Although viral pathogens are the most common, bacterial and parasitic pathogens can also be implicated in diarrhea (Infectious Diarrhea chapter). *Chronic diarrhea* is diarrhea lasting more than 14 consecutive days, usually more than 4 weeks, and is usually associated with chronic medical conditions or GI pathology in the pediatric population.[6,7] Malabsorption syndromes, including cystic fibrosis and celiac disease, often initially present with diarrhea symptoms and should be considered when determining the etiology of new-onset, prolonged diarrhea. In cystic fibrosis, malabsorptive diarrhea is the result of pancreatic insufficiency. With decreased production of pancreatic enzymes, including lipase, fat malabsorption occurs. As a result, undiagnosed or untreated disease can lead to steatorrhea. Celiac disease is an autoimmune condition triggered by gluten intake that damages the small intestine, preventing adequate absorption. Iatrogenic malabsorption secondary to short bowel syndrome is also a significant cause of chronic diarrhea. Short bowel syndrome is the result of surgical removal of portions of the intestines secondary to intestinal ischemia caused by various factors. Irritable bowel syndrome is an example of a functional bowel disorder that can cause diarrhea (Irritable Bowel Syndrome and Celiac Disease chapter).

Nutrition may also play a role in the infant and child with diarrhea, specifically with respect to type of formula used and preparation technique. Hyperosmolar or concentrated formulas can cause fluid shifts, resulting in osmotic diarrhea. Enzyme deficiencies or food sensitivities such as lactase deficiency—or the more common terminology, *lactose intolerance*—make it difficult to digest lactose-containing foods (e.g., milk-containing products), leading to diarrhea. Similarly, food allergies can elicit a diarrheal response when exposure occurs. Often, infants with an allergy to cow's milk protein will present to the health care provider's office because of diarrhea in addition to other allergic symptoms. Ingestion of irritating foods such as nondigestible fibers or insoluble sugar alcohols can also precipitate acute diarrhea. Another well-described etiology in children is medication-induced diarrhea, most commonly with antibiotics. Antibiotic-associated diarrhea does not generally result in severe sequelae and resolves within a few days after the antibiotic course is completed. Recognizing the potential causes of diarrhea, both acute and chronic, can assist in the appropriate management and prevention of morbidity and mortality in the pediatric population.

PATHOPHYSIOLOGY

Diarrhea results when the normal functions of the GI tract for maintaining fluid and electrolyte balance are impaired. The water content of fecal material determines whether stools are too liquid or too dry, which in turn affects bowel function and status. The amount of fluid in stool depends on the amount ingested through diet, the contribution from intestinal secretions in the small intestine, and the amount reabsorbed by the colon. *Chyme*, a semifluid mass of partly digested food and digestive secretions formed during digestion, makes up the remainder of stool content, with the absorption of partly digested fats, carbohydrates, protein and other micronutrients occurring as it passes through the duodenum, jejunum, and ileum. As stool enters the colon past the ileocecal valve, a large amount of water is absorbed, further changing the composition and electrolyte content of the remaining chyme/stool. Normal fecal stool has electrolyte concentrations of sodium 40 mEq/L, chloride 15 mEq/L, potassium 90 mEq/L, and sodium bicarbonate 30 mEq/L.[8,9] Alterations in absorption and secretion of water and electrolytes when GI function is impaired can change these values. Knowledge of normal electrolyte composition is helpful when selecting appropriate replacement therapy for diarrhea. There are four general mechanisms for disruption of water and electrolyte balance and thus four classifications, or types, of diarrhea: *secretory, osmotic, exudative,* and *altered motility*.[8,9]

SECRETORY DIARRHEA

Secretory diarrhea occurs in response to some stimulating substance increasing the secretion of water into the intestinal lumen or decreasing the absorption of water and electrolytes from the intestinal lumen. Causes of secretory diarrhea include unabsorbed dietary fat; laxatives; secretin or other hormones (including those released by tumors); bacterial toxins; or increased bile salts. These agents interrupt the normal cell transport processes by stimulating intracellular cyclic adenosine monophosphate and inhibiting Na^+/K^+-ATPase (sodium/potassium/adenosine triphosphatase), causing the secretion of a large amount of water and indirectly preventing ion (electrolyte) absorption, resulting in an amount of water being secreted into the intestine greater than that absorbed.[8,10] Clinically, this type of diarrhea is identified by large stool volumes with normal electrolyte content.

OSMOTIC DIARRHEA

Water reabsorption in the intestine is a passive process and is dependent on the absorption of other substances. When poorly absorbed substances remain in the lumen, an osmotic gradient is created, resulting in water being pulled into the lumen producing watery, osmotic diarrhea. This type of diarrhea differs from secretory diarrhea because there is no excess secretion of a substance causing changes in the amount; rather, the mechanism for absorption is somehow impaired.[8] Malabsorption, lactose intolerance, and medications, including magnesium (and other divalent ions) and lactulose, are associated with osmotic diarrhea. *Malabsorption*, a collective term, occurs when absorption is decreased because of the inability to digest or absorb a particular nutrient. Altered motility or altered digestion (e.g., pancreatic insufficiency), as previously described, contributes to malabsorption. Decreased absorption of solutes and fluid can also result when intestinal cells along the brush border are damaged by bacterial/viral infection or atrophy after prolonged disuse. Determining the cause of malabsorption can assist with treatment decisions. For example, when osmotic diarrhea is dependent on ingested substances, fasting will decrease or eliminate symptoms. Stools will have an increased osmotic load that can be measured, but clinically, it is often indistinguishable from other types.

EXUDATIVE DIARRHEA

When injury occurs to the mucosal lining of the intestinal tract, exudative diarrhea can occur. Injury can result from inflammation or ulceration, leading to a loss of mucus, serum proteins, or blood into the lumen. The damaged, or inflamed, intestine prevents water and electrolytes from being absorbed, leading to diarrhea. Inflammatory bowel diseases such as Crohn disease and ulcerative colitis are associated with this type of diarrhea. The presence of a large amount of exudates (mucus, proteins, and/or blood) in the stool is characteristic in patients with these inflammatory bowel diseases. Invasive infectious diarrhea can also present with similar symptoms and, on initial presentation, is often indistinguishable from inflammatory bowel disease.[8,10]

ALTERED MOTILITY

Diarrhea caused by altered motility is multifactorial and can involve several mechanisms, including reduction in small intestine contact time, bacterial overgrowth, and/or early emptying of the colon. Decreased exposure of material to the small intestine leads to reduced time for the normal absorption and secretion processes to occur, thus changing the composition of intestinal contents. The resulting changes in osmolarity can lead to diarrhea. Surgical resection of the gut (as in short bowel syndrome) and medications such as erythromycin or metoclopramide can result in a decrease in exposure time to the small intestine. Conversely, if transit time is increased (slowing), bacterial overgrowth may occur, precipitating diarrhea. Diarrhea caused by altered motility is usually associated with sporadic and fast peristaltic waves that impair the absorption of water and prematurely move material into the colon. Sometimes, loose, watery stools may even be associated with chronic constipation. Although this association sounds counterintuitive, chronic constipation leads to a large amount of retained hard, dry stool in the colon and results in stretching of the colon. This state allows soft or liquid stool to leak around the retained stool or loss of control over bowel movements.

CLINICAL PRESENTATION AND DIAGNOSIS

Diarrhea is regarded as either acute or chronic and is differentiated by duration of symptoms. Signs and symptoms can vary depending on the underlying cause, and may be helpful in the diagnostic process. For example, acute diarrheal symptoms secondary to viral gastroenteritis include abrupt onset of nausea, vomiting, abdominal pain, headache, and fever lasting for 10–60 hours (Infectious Diarrhea chapter). Chronic diarrhea is more difficult to diagnose because of the wide range of bowel patterns.[6] The differential diagnosis for diarrhea is lengthy (Table 1), so it is important to qualify presenting characteristics, including the frequency, onset, consistency, and proposed mechanism. A thorough patient history should be completed and should include medication, herbal/nutraceutical, and supplement history, recent travel, drinking water type, and diet, such as consumption of raw meat and increased intake of fruits, fruit juices, and sugar-free food.

CLINICAL AND DIAGNOSTIC EVALUATION CRITERIA

Evaluation of stool characteristics can be helpful in determining the etiology of diarrhea. Frequency, consistency, volume, and even color of stool should be evaluated in a patient

Table 1. Common Causes of Diarrhea

Causes	Examples
Infectious	Viral Cytomegalovirus, adenovirus, rotavirus, norovirus Bacterial *Salmonella, Yersinia, Escherichia coli, Shigella, Campylobacter, Clostridium difficile* Parasitic *Giardia, Entameba histolytica, Cryptosporidium, Microsporidia*
Toxins	*C. difficile* toxin Enterotoxins (from enteric organisms)
Exposures	Radiation enteritis Chemotherapy/Immunosuppressive therapy (e.g., irinotecan, mycophenolate) Laxative abuse Medications (e.g., antibiotics, magnesium-containing antacids) Tumor-associated increased secretion
Malabsorption	Pancreatic insufficiency Celiac disease Chronic liver disease Allergic enteropathy Glucose galactose transport defect
Inflammatory bowel disease	Ulcerative colitis Crohn disease Eosinophilic gastroenteritis Allergic colitis
Genetic-metabolic disorders	Malabsorption syndromes
Chronic nonspecific diarrhea/toddler diarrhea	Usually exacerbated by a low-fat, high-carbohydrate diet in infants to toddler age
Overfeeding	Large quantity of carbohydrate-rich foods in infancy combined with decreased amylase concentration

with diarrhea. A large amount of watery, foul-smelling stool containing undigested food suggests diarrhea originating from the small intestine, whereas diarrhea with red blood present suggests the colon as the origin. The physical examination is important in evaluating disease severity as well as hydration status. Often, the examination will lead to a more focused evaluation and aid in treatment approach. Pertinent findings on physical examination include abdominal tenderness and/or cramping as well as bloating. Vital signs including blood pressure, temperature, and heart rate should be evaluated. The presence of a fever may indicate an infectious etiology, whereas decreased blood pressure could signify the complication of impending shock secondary to dehydration from diarrhea. Assessment of hydration status is an extremely important part of the evaluation in pediatric patients with diarrhea because it can quickly lead to dehydration. In addition to vital signs, hydration status can be assessed by examining urine output (e.g., mL/kg/hr or number of wet diapers per day in infants), mucous membranes, tear production, and physical and mental status changes. A patient who is dehydrated can present with decreased urine output or fewer wet diapers, dry mucous membranes or crying without tears, a sunken appearance around the eyes or cheeks, decreased skin turgor, weight loss, and mental status changes (Fluids and Electrolytes chapter).

Stool studies are generally not required unless the diarrhea persists beyond 24 hours or unless a specific diagnosis (e.g., malabsorption or confirmation of an infectious etiology) is needed. Symptoms including bloody stools and fever, systemic illness, severe dehydration, recent antibiotic use, or need for hospitalization all warrant stool testing. Several studies are available to assist with diagnosis. The presence of fecal leukocytes indicates an inflammatory response, either infectious or inflammatory bowel disease in origin. If positive, a stool culture may be warranted. The stool cultures and testing are completed if an infectious cause is suspected because of clinical findings and patient history. Rotavirus, for example, can be diagnosed within the same day as stool sample collection through specific kits or antibody serologic testing. Antibody serologic tests, however, are not specific and, as with rotavirus, can be time-dependent for accurate results. Together with cultures, the stool can be evaluated for the presence of ova and parasites. Testing for *Clostridium difficile* in patients with diarrhea with recent use of antibiotics or hospital-acquired diarrhea is completed by polymerase chain reaction. A stool analysis can also be evaluated for the presence of mucus, fat, osmolarity, pH, and electrolyte content.[8] Radiographic studies, endoscopy, or a biopsy may be warranted in severe or difficult diagnostic cases, including those in which inflammatory disorders or cancer may be suspected.

COURSE AND PROGNOSIS

The underlying etiology of diarrhea is a key indicator of the duration of symptoms and clinical manifestations. Most acute cases of diarrhea are self-limiting. Acute diarrhea secondary to infectious cases may require antibiotics (Infectious Diarrhea chapter). Diarrhea associated with chronic medical conditions (e.g., Crohn disease) may not be completely resolved, and only temporary symptomatic relief is achieved without treating the primary cause. Although diarrhea itself is uncomfortable, the complications from severe or prolonged diarrhea can be life threatening. Dehydration is the most common complication of diarrhea and should be managed carefully, especially in infants and children younger than 2 years. This population is at particular risk because water constitutes a larger proportion of their body composition compared with adults, in addition to a decreased ability for their kidneys to conserve water. Diarrhea leading to severe dehydration, often associated with a 10% loss of body weight, should be considered a medical emergency. In addition to water loss, severe cases include electrolyte and fluid imbalances leading to additional morbidities that require immediate attention, including, but not limited to, seizures or hypovolemic shock. Malabsorption and related conditions are often linked to chronic diarrhea and should be managed accordingly. This management generally involves supplementation of any electrolyte or nutrient deficiency as well as implementing mechanisms for slowing transit time. Many times, the exact etiology of acute diarrhea is unknown, but a thorough evaluation and differentiation of potential causes are important to provide adequate treatment and predict the clinical course.

NONINFECTIOUS DIARRHEA

ANTIBIOTIC THERAPY

Antibiotic therapy is associated with diarrhea in about 60% of all children prescribed antibiotics.[9] Proposed mechanisms for antibiotic-associated diarrhea include alteration of gut flora leading to decreased carbohydrate transport and increased intestinal lactate levels. Decreased carbohydrate transport from the gut leads to increased osmolarity and increased secretion of water into the stool. Diarrhea associated with antibiotic use is described as *watery*, but it should not have any systemic symptoms. Once the antibiotics are discontinued, the diarrhea should resolve.[9] Although less common in pediatric patients, another consequence of antibiotic therapy that may result in diarrhea is a *C. difficile* infection. *Clostridium difficile* is part of the normal GI flora, but when antibiotic therapy alters the normally balanced flora, the bacteria can become pathogenic. The toxins produced by *C. difficile* can lead to pseudomembranous colitis (Infectious Diarrhea chapter).[11]

MALNUTRITION

Nutrition and diarrhea have a bidirectional relationship. Malnutrition can increase the risk of enteral infections by its effect on host immune function and alterations in the protective barrier of the gut mucosa. Diarrhea, especially chronic diarrhea, can also precipitate malnutrition by decreasing the absorption of nutrients, further worsening the overall clinical effects of both.[12] Large intestinal losses of zinc, an important micronutrient that is involved in intestinal absorption of water and electrolytes and immune function, can lead to deficiency, therefore becoming a focus of treatment, particularly in developing countries. However, the cause of malnutrition may be multifactorial and include frequent infections, bile acid malabsorption, decreased pancreatic enzyme activity, altered motility, decreased intestinal surface area, and changes in intestinal flora. Treatment considerations for malnourished patients with diarrhea should be comprehensive and address both disease states.

DIET

Infant nutrition can be a major factor in diarrhea, caused by overfeeding, type of feeding, or general developmental differences. Overfeeding, particularly in the first few weeks of life, with a high-calorie, hyperosmolar formula, can lead to diarrhea. Diarrhea can occur in infants younger than 6 months who are exposed to cow's milk prematurely or infant-feeding formula. Formula feeding, which is generally associated with firmer stools, may lead to diarrhea, especially with the use of high-calorie formulas or those high in sugar content. If acute diarrheal symptoms are present, providers should perform a thorough history to determine the cause to avoid changing formulas too often or unnecessarily discontinuing breastfeeding.

Developmentally, neonates have a deficiency in the pancreatic enzyme, amylase, which is responsible for the breakdown of carbohydrates. An increase in stool carbohydrate content creates a hyperosmolar environment, leading to diarrhea.[9] Drinks or foods containing a large amount of sorbitol or fructose, including juices, may also cause an osmotic diarrhea. Foods that are spicy; are difficult to break down, such as insoluble fibers in raw vegetables and nuts; or contain or release histamine, such as tomatoes, cheeses, citrus fruits, and fish, may also contribute to diarrhea.[9] In addition, lactase deficiency (lactose intolerance) may lead to diarrhea through the incomplete digestion and/or metabolism of lactose found in milk and milk products. Lactase is produced by the cells lining the small intestine, which break down lactose into the absorbable sugars glucose and galactose. Infants and children younger than 2 years generally do not have diarrhea related to lactase deficiency because this age range is the period of highest production of lactase. In older children and adults, lactase production decreases, causing an increase in the incidence of lactose intolerance.[13] Lactose intolerance is estimated to affect 25% of the American population. Of Americans with lactose intolerance, Asian and African Americans are the most affected (90% and 65%, respectively).[13] This condition can be treated by avoiding high lactose–containing foods and/or taking over-the-counter lactase enzyme–containing medications. Temporary milk intolerance after an acute viral gastroenteritis or diarrhea after antibiotic exposure can also occur. With acute gastroenteritis, the absorptive lining, which also produces lactase, is damaged, causing a transient enzyme deficiency and resulting in intolerance. Short-term use of lactose-free formulas can be used in infants, but any formula changes should be discussed with the provider before changing the diet. Avoidance of high lactose–containing foods and slow reintroduction in children and adolescents can be implemented as antibiotic therapy is discontinued or during acute gastroenteritis.[13]

ALLERGIC DIARRHEA

Diarrhea caused by an allergy to milk proteins is most common in infants younger than 1 year and can be resolved by switching to a soy or elemental formula. However, the overall prevalence of milk protein allergy in infants is only between 2% and 3%.[14] Milk allergies typically resolve by 12 months, and patients can be rechallenged at that time. Breastfeeding mothers should avoid dairy products if a milk protein allergy is confirmed. Flecks of blood in the stool of an otherwise healthy infant may be a defining symptom of milk protein intolerance. Slow introduction of dairy products into the diet and observation of diarrhea symptoms should be noted. If the sensitivity continues in older children (e.g., school-aged children and older), a protein allergy, presenting as a celiac-like disorder, may be considered. Immunoglobulin E–mediated food allergies may include an anaphylactic-type reaction, including vomiting, diarrhea, hypotension, and pallor.[9] Food challenges in these cases should only be done under close provider supervision. Recently, increased awareness of gluten allergy has led to increased availability of gluten-free products. Gluten is a protein contained in wheat, rye, and barley and is implicated in intestinal damage in the autoimmune disorder known as *celiac disease*. It is recommended that patients with celiac disease avoid gluten-containing foods.

CHRONIC NONSPECIFIC DIARRHEA

In healthy children, chronic nonspecific diarrhea, also known as *toddler diarrhea*, is a common reason for loose stools. Occurring most commonly in infants and children between age 9 and 20 months, the otherwise-healthy and thriving toddler may have three to six "runny" stools per day. Clinically, growth is normal and stool tests for blood, bacterial pathogens, white blood cells, and fat are all negative. Usually by the time the child reaches age 3.5 years or after potty training, no other diagnosis is made regarding the etiology, and symptoms subside.[9] Although no definitive cause has been established, several associations have been reported. Low-residue, low-fat, high-carbohydrate diets tend to make stools increasingly loose, which can worsen during stress or illness. Toddlers drinking a large amount of high-sugar fruit juices, parents or caregivers overfeeding or underfeeding the child, and the child's ingestion of irritating foods (including tomatoes and citrus) are other associations. This type of diarrhea is symptomatically similar to irritable bowel syndrome in adults.[9] A slight increase in dietary fat, restriction of osmotic carbohydrates, and changing fiber intake (decreasing if too much fiber and increasing if fiber-deficient) may help control symptoms.

TREATMENT

Although prevention of acute diarrhea secondary to infectious causes plays the biggest role in worldwide efforts to decrease mortality and morbidity, prompt treatment of diarrhea is equally important. The goals of therapy first include prevention and management of water and electrolyte imbalances to restore normal hydration status. Other goals include providing symptomatic relief, treating the underlying cause, and managing the diet or other secondary causes of diarrhea.

NONPHARMACOLOGIC THERAPY

The two main components of nonpharmacologic management of diarrhea are restoring fluid and electrolyte balance and making temporary dietary modifications during the acute illness. Fasting is generally not necessary if the patient can tolerate eating, although the type or amount of food ingested may need to be modified—avoiding excessively fatty, spicy, processed foods, or foods known to upset the stomach, including those high in simple sugars. Guidelines generally recommend early introduction of appropriate food and liquids during the replacement process, if patients can tolerate it.[15] It is not necessary to initiate only clear liquids or the bananas, rice, applesauce, and toast diet, which may, in fact, prolong diarrhea. This "starvation" or nutrition-limited method may delay cellular repair and regeneration of the intestinal lining/brush border. As a result, this diet—as an example of an easily digestible, low-residue, low-fiber diet—is recommended for no more than 24 hours, or when both vomiting and diarrhea are present, unless vomiting is severe enough that aspiration risk is high and nothing should be taken by mouth. In infants with acute diarrhea, current recommendations suggest that feeding should continue, except in a formula-fed infant with severe diarrhea during the initial rehydration period. Because most diarrhea cases are self-limiting and dehydration remains a significant risk in this age group, the benefits of feeding outweigh any risk. Continuation of feeding decreases morbidity and mortality.[15] Maintaining nutrition also plays an important role in the management of chronic diarrhea. Proper caloric intake is important for all age groups and etiologies because feeding will assist in intestinal repair.

Fluid replacement can be with oral or intravenous therapy, depending on the patient's severity/level of dehydration. Determining the severity of dehydration and evaluating the progress of maintaining hydration are particularly important in infants and children younger than 2 years. The combination of risk factors, including being more susceptible to dehydration because of a lack of reserve and the difficulty of determining the effectiveness of rehydration techniques, necessitates close observation and a low threshold for advancing care. Careful clinical observation for signs and symptoms of dehydration and obtaining a good patient history can aid in selecting the best individualized treatment pathway.

Severe dehydration is characterized by dry mucous membranes, loss of skin turgor, delayed capillary refill, tachycardia, and even signs of shock. Mild and moderate dehydration involves dry mucous membranes, increased thirst, sunken eyes and fontanelle, and some loss of skin turgor (Fluids and Electrolytes chapter). For mild and/or moderate dehydration, oral rehydration therapy (ORT) is preferred and is as effective as intravenous therapy in these patients.[15] Patients with severe dehydration, sepsis/shock, or systemic complications require intravenous fluid resuscitation. Fluid management includes both a rehydration and maintenance phase. In the first few hours, the goal of rehydration therapy is to rapidly restore water and electrolytes to normal concentrations. After rehydration has occurred, maintenance therapy is given to replace ongoing losses (i.e., maintain normal body composition) and provide therapy until dietary intake can be initiated (Fluids and Electrolytes chapter). It is important to remember that the reintroduction of feeds, either breastfeeding or formula, is encouraged and supported for infants as a means of maintaining proper fluid balance.

Several commercially available ORT products are available—some are premixed solutions, and others are dry powder packets to which water must be added. The solution is absorbed in the small intestine as a replacement for what is lost in the stool. These products vary in the amount of glucose, sodium, and other electrolytes they contain at specific ratios (Table 2). Products with a sodium content of 75–90 mEq/L are intended for use as rehydration solutions, whereas the sodium content of maintenance solutions is between 40 mEq/L and 60 mEq/L.[15,16] The rationale for the composition of these products is based on the glucose-sodium cotransport system in the GI tract. In this system, the linkage of glucose and sodium molecules allows glucose to carry sodium into the cells of the small intestine. Water then follows sodium into the bloodstream, resulting in increased absorption of both water and sodium.[16] The ORT products also contain potassium and chloride to replace losses, and citrate, which converts to bicarbonate, is added to correct the acidosis associated with dehydration. For these reasons, ORT products are superior to the nonspecific "clear-liquid" diets often prescribed to patients with diarrhea. The composition of many household "clear liquids" is not formulated specifically for

Table 2. Commonly Used Oral Rehydration Fluids and Composition

Solution[a]	Osmolality (mOsm/L)	Glucose (g/L)	Sodium (mEq/L)	Bicarbonate (mEq/L)	Potassium (mEq/L)	Chloride (mEq/L)
Pedialyte[b]	250	25	45	30	20	35
Enfalyte[c]	200	30	50	34	25	45
Rehydralyte[d]	305	25	75	30	20	65
World Health Organization oral rehydration solution	245	13.5	75	30	20	65
Ceralyte[e]	220	40	50–90	30	20	—

[a]Note: Oral rehydration should only be used for mild to moderate dehydration and if the patient can tolerate oral intake.
[b]Abbott Laboratories, Abbott Park, IL;
[c]Mead-Johnson, Chicago, IL;
[d]Ross Products, Columbus, OH;
[e]CERA Products, Hilton Head Island, SC

rehydration or maintenance because the concentrations of electrolytes and glucose-to-sodium ratio are inappropriate, and the amount of sugar is often too high for adequate replacement of stool losses and could further worsen diarrhea.

Specifically, in developing countries where educational levels and languages may vary, WHO and UNICEF (United Nations Children's Fund) recommend using a single oral rehydration solution (the WHO ORS) to avoid mixing errors that would result in the administration of a solution with the incorrect concentration. The high salt content of some ORT products has raised concerns about the use of the higher-sodium solutions in well-nourished children with less severe dehydration who may not need the same level of salt replacement because these solutions may cause hypernatremia. However, in studies ORS is quicker in the correction of dehydration and safer than intravenous fluids.[15-17] Some available ORT products are rice-based oral solutions, which provide glucose for the cotransport system from the breakdown of complex carbohydrates in rice/cereal without increasing the osmotic gradient, as can occur with glucose-based products. Overall, oral rehydration remains safe and effective when using the approved ORT products. Fluids for rehydration in developed countries should also be carefully considered. Many fruit juices are high in sugar content and have a high osmolality with no electrolytes. Higher sugar content and osmolality solutions can precipitate or worsen an osmotic diarrhea, worsening dehydration status. Solutions with no electrolytes will not replace what is lost and can lead to detrimental effects related to the lower serum concentrations of these electrolytes. Examples include hypokalemia causing muscle weakness and hyponatremia resulting in seizures. Lower osmolar fluids that are more like the ORT products are preferred. Overall, water, carbonated sports drinks, caffeinated drinks, and sweetened tea are not acceptable for rehydration because these beverages do not provide adequate electrolytes for replacement or because they are hyperosmolar.[15,16]

PHARMACOLOGIC THERAPY

Outlining the use of pharmacologic therapy as treatment for diarrhea in the pediatric population is challenging because medications and other pharmacologic agents are used solely for supportive care in the management of diarrhea (Table 3). Different classes of medications and supplements have been used to alleviate symptoms including opiates and their derivatives, cholestyramine, psyllium (adsorbents), probiotics, bismuth subsalicylate, zinc, and vitamin A. Although each provides some benefit in alleviating symptoms, guidelines are still lacking for their use in the infant and toddler population. Choosing an agent should include balancing efficacy and safety. Knowing the agent's pharmacologic mechanisms and the related adverse effects can contribute to formulating appropriate recommendations.

OPIOIDS AND DERIVATIVES

Opioids, by acting on the mu receptors in the GI tract, delay GI transit and prolong contact time. Action on these receptors also leads to the well-known adverse effect of constipation (and can lead to ileus). The opioids tincture of opium, paregoric (morphine 2 mg/5 mL), and diphenoxylate—all Schedule II controlled substances—have been studied in the treatment of both acute and chronic diarrhea. Because of drug abuse potential and the risk of ileus, these medications are not widely prescribed for symptomatic treatment of diarrhea. Diphenoxylate is an opioid derivative available in combination with atropine that is used in noninfectious diarrhea, particularly for chronic diarrhea. Atropine is added to the formulation to prevent abuse by causing undesirable anticholinergic effects. Children with malabsorption secondary to short bowel syndrome may benefit from mono- or combination therapy of diphenoxylate/atropine and loperamide.

Loperamide, another opioid derivative, does not cross the blood-brain barrier like other opioids and is thus void of the associated analgesic and central nervous system effects of other opioids. Loperamide acts like other opioids by delaying GI transit time and acts peripherally as an antisecretory agent, regulating chloride secretion. Because water will follow chloride ions, a decrease in water assists in reducing diarrhea. However, loperamide's place in the treatment of acute diarrhea is limited. A meta-analysis of loperamide in pediatric patients found that children younger than 3 years who are malnourished, are severely dehydrated, or have bloody diarrhea are at increased risk of adverse events from loperamide, including lethargy, abdominal distention, and ileus. Loperamide should not be used in most infectious diarrhea cases because decrease in GI transit in patients with infectious diarrhea caused by a toxin-producing bacterium carries the risk of preventing toxins from being cleared from the GI tract. This point is especially important because direct exposure to the toxins is largely responsible for the intestinal damage that occurs. In addition, cases of necrotizing enterocolitis with loperamide use have occurred in children younger than 2 years. Therefore, routine use of loperamide in this population should be avoided. Loperamide may have a use in chronic diarrhea, but is generally not recommended for long-term use. The notable exception in the pediatric population are those with short bowel syndrome to help with malabsorption.[18-20]

OTHER AGENTS

Cholestyramine, a chloride and basic quaternary ammonium anion-exchange–binding resin, has been used in diarrheal disorders involving increased fecal bile acids or pseudomembranous colitis. Cholestyramine forms a nonabsorbable complex with bile acids in the intestines and causes the release of chloride ions during this process. The chloride ions are absorbed, allowing water to follow, thus decreasing diarrhea. Pediatric patients may be at increased risk of hyperchloremic acidosis as a result. However, in studies evaluating the role of cholestyramine in children age 7 months to about 2 years with acute and chronic diarrhea, this approach shortens courses of diarrhea (by about 2 days) and is tolerated without significant adverse effects after adequate hydration with ORT.[21] Dosing and administration of cholestyramine are outlined in Table 3.[20]

Psyllium or other adsorbents are used for symptomatic relief and are nonspecific in their action. As bulking agents,

Table 3. Pediatric Dosing and Clinical Pearls for Select Antidiarrheal Agents[20]

Agent	Dosing by Patient Age, Type of Diarrhea, Timing, and Route of Administration	Comments
Loperamide	**Acute Diarrhea** **2–5 yr, weight 13–20.9 kg** 1 mg with first loose stool; then 1 mg after each subsequent loose stool to 3 mg/day max **6–8 yr, weight 21–27 kg** 2 mg with first loose stool; then 1 mg after each subsequent loose stool to 4 mg/day max **9–11 yr, weight 27.1 to 43 kg** 2 mg with first loose stool; then 1 mg after each subsequent loose stool to 6 mg/day max **≥ 12 yr and adolescents** 4 mg with first loose stool; then 2 mg after each subsequent loose stool to 8 mg/day max **Chronic Diarrhea** 0.08–0.24 mg/kg/day divided BID–TID, to 2 mg/dose max	• Not for use in infectious diarrhea—prevents toxin from being cleared • Risk of bacterial overgrowth • May be used in short bowel syndrome for malabsorption • Risk of ileus increases when max doses exceeded
Paregoric	**Children and adolescents**: 0.25–0.5 mL/kg QD–QID to 10 mL/dose max	• Risk of constipation, ileus • Less preferred because of additives
Diphenoxylate and Atropine	**Initial**: 0.3–0.4 mg/kg/day (10 mg/day max) in 4 divided doses or manufacturer's recommended dosing: **< 2 yr**: not recommended **2 yr, weight 11–14 kg**: 1.5–3 mL QID **3 yr, weight 12–16 kg**: 2–3 mL QID **4 yr, weight 14–20 kg**: 2–4 mL QID **5 yr, weight 16–23 kg**: 2.5–4.5 mL QID **6–8 yr, weight 17–32 kg**: 2.5–5 mL QID **9–12 yr, weight 23–55 kg**: 3.5–5 mL QID **Maintenance**: 25% of initial dose	• Works best before meals/feedings • May be used in short bowel syndrome for malabsorption • Discontinue if no response in 48 hours
Cholestyramine	240 mg/kg/day in 3 divided doses; titrate based on indication	• Risk of hyperchloremic acidosis, but short courses decrease risk • If giving other medications or supplements, give 1 hr before or 4–6 hr after cholestyramine to prevent binding and decreased absorption • Give with plenty of water
Psyllium	**Oral**: Can target normal fiber intake goals; constipation dosing (may require less per day for diarrhea) **Children 6–11 yr**: 1.25–15 g/day in divided doses **Children ≥ 12 yr–adults**: 2.5–30 g/day in divided doses	• Medications or supplements should not be given within 3 hr of psyllium administration • Give with plenty of water to avoid constipation or obstruction
Probiotics	**Lactobacillus** **Children and adults—oral**: Capsules: 1–2 capsules BID–QID Granules: 1 packet added to food/water TID–QID Powder: ¼ to 1 teaspoon QD–TID with liquid Tablet, chewable: 4 tablets TID–QID *Saccharomyces boulardii* **Children**: 250 mg BID (granules and capsule)	• Lactobacillus and Bifidobacterium spp. most studied • S. boulardii most studied in *Clostridium difficile* infections • Sepsis has been reported in neonatal and immunocompromised population

BID = twice daily; max = maximum; QD = daily; QID = four times daily; TID = three times daily.

these drugs absorb liquid in the GI tract, which alters the fluid and electrolyte content and expands the stool, thus forming "bulk." These agents can also absorb irritating digestive juices, nutrients, or medications, which may reduce their bioavailability. Although psyllium can be used as a laxative, its bulk-producing properties may help create a more formed stool and can be beneficial in patients with diarrhea (Table 3).

The use of probiotics for diarrhea in children has recently gained momentum with the introduction of many lactobacillus products and dosage forms. Other bacterial probiotics studied in this population include *Bifidobacterium lactis* and *Streptococcus thermophilus*. *Saccharomyces boulardii* is a generally nonpathogenic yeast that was recently studied for its use in the treatment of infectious diarrhea; however, few data exist in the pediatric population.[22] Probiotics, found in normal gut flora, decrease or prevent diarrhea associated with antibiotic use and benefit children at risk of infectious diarrhea related to malnutrition or pathogen exposure.[23,24] The exact mechanisms of probiotics in the treatment of diarrhea, however, are not well understood. Presumed mechanisms of benefit include enhancement of the immune system, creation of a competitive environment for microbial growth, or extension of antimicrobial action on pathogenic organisms. Despite increased use, controversy exists regarding the potential risk of seeding the organism from the gut into the bloodstream (resulting in bacteremia with lactobacillus or fungemia with *Saccharomyces*), especially in neonatal or immunocompromised populations.[25] A meta-analysis of the use of lactobacillus for acute infectious diarrhea found a reduction in the number of stools and overall safety profile.[23] This analysis predominantly included children age 1–36 months. No studies included the neonatal or premature neonatal populations. The use of probiotic yogurt has also been evaluated for the prevention of antibiotic-associated diarrhea. Results suggest decreased severity of diarrhea and little to no adverse effects.[26] In addition, prebiotics, food, or supplements with nondigestible substances that facilitate microbial growth of indigenous probiotic bacteria have been introduced as a preventive or symptomatic treatment of diarrhea. More studies are needed to assess the true benefit of probiotic and prebiotic use and evaluate the potential for adverse effects in high-risk populations.[24]

The use of zinc and vitamin A has also been described in the treatment of childhood diarrhea. Zinc is an essential mineral that plays a role in immune function; it has been extensively studied in pediatric patients in developing countries.[27,28] These patients may be zinc-deficient secondary to malnutrition, and the extrapolation of these results to use in developed countries may not be as well-founded. The exact mechanism of zinc in the treatment of diarrhea is not fully understood. Zinc may have a role in enhancing cation absorption or suppressing cation secretion. In several studies of children age 1–60 months in developing countries with either acute or persistent diarrhea, zinc provides a reduction in stool frequency and overall incidence of diarrhea without significant adverse effects with short-term use.[29] However, copper deficiency and subsequent anemia has been described with long-term use. Because of the potential concern for copper deficiency with long-term use of zinc (which impairs the absorption of copper), the WHO recommends only a 10- to 14-day course (10 mg for children younger than 6 months; 20 mg for children 6 months or older) for treatment of acute diarrhea.[17]

Vitamin A supplementation has also been investigated in malnourished children of developing countries, with mixed results. Of the children studied, those with a wasting syndrome responded best to vitamin A.[30] As with zinc, those deficient in vitamin A may have better outcomes from supplementation, and routine use for the treatment of diarrhea is not currently recommended.[30]

Bismuth subsalicylate has been used for traveler's diarrhea, for chronic infantile diarrhea, or as an adjunctive treatment for *Helicobacter pylori*–associated gastritis. Bismuth subsalicylate is thought to work by dual mechanisms. Bismuth acts by facilitating the absorption of extra water in the intestines as an antisecretory agent. When the subsalicylate is hydrolyzed into salicylic acid, it inhibits prostaglandins associated with inflammation and possible hypermotility. Bismuth in bismuth subsalicylate may even have antimicrobial effects by binding toxins or because of some inherent bactericidal activity.[8] Because all products contain salicylates, caution should be used in individuals with acute viral illness, such as varicella (chickenpox) or influenza, secondary to the risk of Reye syndrome.

Overall, treatment of diarrhea in the pediatric population consists of rehydration, prevention of dehydration, and provision of symptomatic care when appropriate. Recommending pharmacologic treatment of diarrhea should first include analyzing the etiology and age group. Medication use should be approached with caution and selected according to the clinical condition of the patient, any comorbidities, and potential for adverse effects. Hydration status remains the underlying theme of diarrhea management and thus the recommendation with the most evidence-based support. Most acute, noninfectious diarrhea algorithms will follow a dehydration assessment and treatment plan and suggest antidiarrheal medications only as last-line symptomatic relief.

MONITORING OF THERAPY

The most important monitoring variable with diarrhea is hydration status. Establishing the initial degree of dehydration and evaluating for improvement in hydration status will help direct therapy changes in rehydration fluids. Once initial deficits are accounted for and maintenance therapy is initiated, the decision to reinitiate feeds or trial of oral nutrition should be quickly considered. Symptoms of acute diarrhea should subside within 24–72 hours. Decreased number of and more formed stools, together with decreased clinical symptoms of pain, cramping, and bloating, indicate improvement and response to therapy. Daily examination of body weight with fluid balance totals (input/output) should be monitored, especially in younger patients, because this assessment will help determine hydration status. Serum electrolytes may also need to be monitored to ensure the correction of any deficiencies. For infectious causes, a complete blood cell count, urine analysis, and blood or stool cultures are all appropriate monitoring variable. Chronic diarrhea treatment should focus on treating/managing the underlying cause, together with any symptomatic relief measures. Careful monitoring of hydration status and signs of treatment response is the overriding principle of diarrhea management.

CONSTIPATION

EPIDEMIOLOGY

Worldwide, the estimated prevalence of constipation is 3% among children, with 17% to 40% of cases starting in the first year of life.[31] Between 2006 and 2011, the frequency of constipation-related emergency department visits increased more than 40%.[32] Determining the overall incidence of constipation is difficult because its definitions are multifactorial. The prevalence of childhood constipation, both acute and chronic, has been estimated at anywhere from 0.7% to 29.6% in the general population worldwide.[33] In the United States and United Kingdom, the incidence of chronic constipation is reportedly lower at 1% to 5%.[33] Almost all pediatric chronic constipation cases are a result of withholding behavior (a type of functional constipation), rather than an organic or pathologic cause.[33] Still, constipation consultations represent 25% of pediatric visits to a gastroenterologist.[34]

Even when a general definition of *constipation* is used—such as "the passage of bulky or hard stool at infrequent intervals"—what is "normal" for one patient may not be the same for another, leaving much to subjective interpretation. In addition, different age groups have different stooling habits as well as exposure to different diets, making it difficult to define exactly what constitutes "normal" bowel habits in the pediatric population. For example, breastfed infants are rarely constipated and often have several bowel movements per day, whereas older children typically have fewer per day—although the number can vary markedly, even between children of the same age.[33] It is important to remember that constipation is not based on number of stools alone, but also on stool consistency and complete evacuation of the colon. For example, a child who has several small stools per day and is not completely evacuating the large colon is considered constipated versus a child who regularly has large stools twice a week but completely evacuates the colon. Certain risk factors for constipation in children have been evaluated. One study found a higher incidence of constipation among children with a birth weight less than 750 g and in the presence of neurodevelopmental impairments.[35] A low-fiber diet may also predispose a patient to constipation.[36] In addition, as the number of those with childhood obesity climbs, evidence supports a higher prevalence of constipation and fecal incontinence among these children.[36] Although the mechanism of this link has not been fully elucidated, improper diet and lack of exercise may be contributing factors to the increase in constipation.[37]

DEFINITIONS

Constipation can be generally defined as *having infrequent stools* (less than 3 bowel movements per week), *having hard stools*, *experiencing excessive straining*, or *having a feeling of incomplete evacuation*. Thus, what defines constipation for each case must be individualized for the patient. Whereas the 2014 North American Society for Pediatric Gastroenterology, Hepatology, and Nutrition (NASPGHAN) guidelines use the Rome III criteria (from 2006) to define childhood constipation, the 2016 Rome IV criteria include a similar definition and match the NASPGHAN and European Society for Paediatric Gastroenterology, Hepatology and Nutrition suggestion for quicker attention to symptoms.[38-41] The definition of *functional constipation* is outlined in Table 4.

Table 4. 2016 Rome IV Criteria for Functional Constipation[40,41]

Patient Age	Criteria
Infants and toddlers up to 4 yr	1 mo of ≥ 2 of the following: 1. ≤ 2 defecations/wk 2. History of excessive stool retentions 3. History of painful or hard bowel movements 4. History of large-diameter stools 5. Presence of a large fecal mass in the rectum In toilet-trained children, additional criteria may be used: 1. At least one episode/wk of incontinence after learning toileting skills 2. History of large-diameter stools that may obstruct the toilet
Children > 4 yr and adolescents	≥ 2 of the following six criteria occurring in: Children ≥ 4 yr, who do not meet irritable bowel syndrome criteria, at least once weekly for at least 1 mo 1. ≤ 2 toilet defecations/wk in child of developmental age at least 4 yr 2. At least one episode/wk of fecal incontinence 3. History of retentive posturing or excessive volitional stool retention 4. History of painful or hard bowel movements 5. Presence of a large fecal mass in the rectum 6. History of large-diameter stools that may obstruct the toilet

ETIOLOGY

Constipation, itself, is not a disease, but is a symptom of an underlying problem or disease. Thus, discovering the underlying etiology is important when developing a treatment plan. Constipation can be linked to the following etiologies: *organic/anatomic*, *diet*, *neurogenic*, or *psychogenic*. Organic causes of constipation include neurologic (spina bifida or cerebral palsy), Hirschsprung disease, cystic fibrosis, chronic intestinal pseudo-obstruction, and neuronal intestinal dysplasia.[8] Hirschsprung disease is a condition in which the nerves (or ganglions) at the end of the colon are missing, causing the absence of peristalsis and resulting in obstruction with stool. Treatment of these neurologic causes includes surgery and supportive care, including medications and maintaining an appropriate diet. Irritable bowel syndrome and systemic lupus erythematosus have also been linked to constipation and are managed similarly with medications and diet modifications. Hypothyroidism, diabetes mellitus, and hypercalcemia can also inhibit bowel function and should be ruled out with an appropriate workup and/or managed accordingly if present.[8]

Diet can also be a factor contributing to constipation, particularly in diets low in fiber complicated by the presence of dehydration. In infants, breastfeeding or formula feeding is rarely associated with constipation unless there is an insufficient amount of fluid or improperly prepared food. Constipation in this age group should be evaluated for feeding and anatomic or neurologic etiologies. Changes in diet in older children, particularly an increase in high-fat, low-fiber diets together with dehydration, can precipitate constipation.

Constipation can also occur as a result from use of certain medications. The abuse of cathartics or laxatives, or agents that induce stooling, can begin a cycle of daily or frequent use to maintain "normal" bowel function. Education on the proper use of cathartics and bowel habits is an important part of constipation management. The caregiver should understand that "normal" may not include a daily bowel movement, but instead, if the colon is being fully emptied, then medications are not necessary to facilitate defecation. Other medications that cause constipation, not through dependence but through effects on motility, are outlined in Box 1. In children, one of the primary psychogenic causes of constipation is withholding behavior. Education and guidance on toilet training in children at least age 4 years is recommended to address this behavior.

Neurogenic causes such as brain or spinal cord injury, central nervous system tumors, or cerebrovascular accidents may also contribute to constipation. The link between the brain and GI function is discussed later in text.

PATHOPHYSIOLOGY

The colon functions to absorb fluid and transport waste to the rectum. The rectum stores the waste until defecation. Water and electrolyte active transport are responsible for the consistency of the stool. For example, in cases of dehydration, sodium is actively reabsorbed creating an osmotic gradient and subsequent passive water reabsorption, leading to hard stool. Also, colonic secretion is controlled by chloride channels, such as the cystic fibrosis transmembrane conductance regulator. Inactive channels, in the case of cystic fibrosis, will ultimately lead to an increase of water and electrolyte reabsorption, again causing retained stool to because hard and difficult to pass through the anal canal. (Conversely, overstimulation of this channel would cause secretory diarrhea, as described previously in this chapter.) Colonic motility involves both smaller, nonpropulsive contractions that aid in absorption and mixing of the stool content and larger contractions that move stool along the colon. These larger contractions normally occur in the morning after wakening and can be increased by eating or drinking (infants have this reflex). Motility is greatly decreased during sleep, so special attention should be paid to periods of incontinence during this time period.[42]

Box 1. Medications Known to Cause Constipation

Antidepressants/Antipsychotics

Amitriptyline
Nortriptyline
Doxepin
Haloperidol
Risperidone
Olanzapine
Clozapine
Chlorpromazine

Antihypertensives/Antiarrhythmics

Calcium channel blockers
Clonidine
Verapamil

Antiparkinson agents

Bromocriptine
Trihexyphenidyl
Benztropine

Opioids/Opioid derivatives

Iron-containing products

Ferrous sulfate
Ferrous gluconate

Antihistamines

Chlorpheniramine
Diphenhydramine
Cetirizine

Other medications

Cholestyramine
Loperamide
Sucralfate
Vinblastine
Vincristine

Continence is maintained by muscular contractions of both the internal (involuntary) and external (voluntary) anal sphincter. When stool comes in contact with the mucosa of the lower rectum, an urge to defecate is triggered. Defecation can be controlled by tightening the external sphincter and gluteal muscles, which push the feces away from the lower rectum and eliminates the sensation to have a bowel movement. Withholding causes the rectum to stretch (to accommodate the extra stool), resulting in a decreased ability and sensitivity to pass stool. In addition, because the fecal matter stays in the rectum, it desiccates and becomes harder, and thus the stool is more painful to pass. This pain can lead to a cycle of withholding behavior and increased anxiety in the child. This description is known as *functional constipation*; however, constipation may also result from other causes, as stated previously. The normal colonic transit time varies, but generally follows a 2- to 4-hour period for a meal to pass the pylorus to the ileocolonic junction and 12 to 72 hours to pass through the colon.[43]

CLINICAL PRESENTATION AND DIAGNOSIS

SIGNS AND SYMPTOMS

Painful passage of stools with hard consistency is often described with constipation. In addition to discomfort when stooling, constipation is associated with symptoms such as nausea, abdominal pain, distention, and bloating and can lead to many other complications including rectal fissures, ulcers, rectal prolapse, urinary tract infections, or incontinence. When evaluating for functional constipation, the child may exhibit certain behaviors that aid in suppressing the urge to defecate, which include rocking back and forth, standing on tiptoes, or becoming fidgety. The withholding behavior can lead to painful stooling as well as a decreased appetite or food intake because of a full colon.

DIAGNOSTIC CRITERIA

Evaluating stool history, signs and symptoms may be sufficient for diagnosis of functional constipation. The history should include changes from baseline in the stool pattern: duration of absence of bowel movement; size, number, consistency, and frequency of stools; any rectal or abdominal pain or bleeding; soiling of underwear; having both diarrhea and hard stools; withholding behaviors; any nausea/vomiting, bloating, or decreased appetite; urinary tract symptoms; and weight loss or change in dietary habits. A complete medication and social history should also be performed.

The physical examination should involve evaluation for abdominal distention, tenderness, presence of hard, palpable stool, and physical defects that would be consistent with an underlying cause (e.g., spina bifida).[36] A digital rectal examination will assist in determining whether a mass or fecal impaction is present. *Fecal impaction* is defined as a hard mass in the lower abdomen, a dilated rectum filled with a large amount of stool, or excessive stool in the colon as identified by abdominal radiography.[36] Radiographic studies to aid in diagnosis include abdominal radiography and barium enema. Abdominal radiography is helpful to assess stool volume and rectal dilation, and a barium enema is helpful in the diagnosis of strictures, abnormal bowel shape, and even Hirschsprung disease. When a barium enema is performed, the colon is filled with a barium contrast agent using a rectal tube. A radiograph is taken, and the radiopaque barium will reveal any colonic abnormalities. Biopsies may be performed if abnormalities in histology or neurotransmitters are suspected, as in the diagnosis of Hirschsprung disease, where it is considered the gold standard. The procedure selected is related to the suspected etiology of the constipation.[38]

Laboratory testing can help rule out potential underlying causes. Thyroid function tests can be evaluated for constipation related to hypothyroidism; magnesium levels on the basic metabolic panel rule out or confirm laxative abuse; and a urine analysis can be performed to screen for a urinary tract infection.

In infants, constipation is less common because withholding is unlikely to occur. Diagnosis and workup in this population is geared more toward an organic cause, and presenting signs/symptoms vary from those previously described. A history of delayed passing of meconium, abdominal distention, bilious emesis (suggesting obstruction), and food avoidance indicate an organic cause like Hirschsprung disease. Evaluation for physical signs of congenital defects, like the presence of a sacral dimple, would point to spina bifida. Understanding age-related causes of constipation can help guide the history and physical examination.

COURSE AND PROGNOSIS

Constipation, although uncomfortable, is seldom life threatening. However, significant morbidity can occur if progression to chronic constipation is left untreated. Complications of untreated constipation include impaction or obstruction, urinary retention from ureter obstruction, rectal prolapse, and encopresis. Many children with *encopresis*, defined as the repeated passage of feces in inappropriate locations after the developmental age of 4 years, either have episodes at school or have to wear diaper-type undergarments well past the age-appropriate time. As a result, these patients may undergo social withdrawal, depression, and/or anxiety related to their condition. Medications used to treat depression can compound the problem because they can cause constipation. The social and economic consequences of chronic constipation, including child anxiety and missed days from school or work, should not be overlooked and necessitate the prudent management and prevention of recurrence.[38]

Children age 2–4 years have a higher recurrence rate of constipation than younger infants and children. About one-third of children with constipation continue symptoms beyond puberty.[44] In a recent study, 25% of children with functional constipation had symptoms that persisted into adulthood.[40, 44] Several risk factors were identified, including older age of symptom onset, delay in time from diagnosis to being seen by a gastroenterologist, and lower defecation frequency at first presentation. Women were also more likely to relapse than were men. It has been suggested that quicker follow-up with specialists, especially for those refractory to initial treatment, was an option for relapse prevention.[36, 44]

TREATMENT

GOALS OF THERAPY

The goal of therapy for constipation is multifactorial and should encompass prevention, alleviation of acute symptoms, and formation of a management plan to avoid recurrence. Because the etiology of constipation differs between infants and children, age should be considered in the management of constipation. The NASPGHAN guidelines outline these differences in the diagnosis and treatment of constipation.[38] The first step in therapy is to recognize and provide education on the pathogenesis of constipation. In children and adolescents, social and psychological reasons for the child's constipation should be considered.

Alleviating acute symptoms of constipation through both nonpharmacologic and pharmacologic therapies should be the next step in the management of constipation. Acutely, if impacted stool is present, disimpaction is a priority, either by pharmacologic management or manual measures. Effective disimpaction is necessary before maintenance therapy can begin. When selecting pharmacologic agents, the age of the patient, time to onset of action, and adverse effects should be considered.[38] After acute symptoms are alleviated, any medications used should be weaned to prevent dependence on the medications that would inhibit the development of good bowel habits and act as negative reinforcement for the patient.

Maintenance therapy involving strategies focused on prevention should be initiated once acute alleviation of symptoms has been achieved. This approach generally involves both nonpharmacologic (dietary interventions and behavioral modification) and pharmacologic (laxative) therapy to ensure regular and complete evacuation of stool. When constipation is associated with medications, the dose should be decreased or alternative agents considered, if possible, or concomitant preventive therapy should be initiated.

NONPHARMACOLOGIC THERAPY

In children, nonpharmacologic therapy with both dietary changes and behavioral management contributes largely to the prevention and maintenance therapy strategies. Increased consumption of fluids (water in particular) and intake of fiber in addition to maintaining a balanced diet of whole grains, fruits, and vegetables should be encouraged. Decreasing the intake of constipating foods such as dairy products and starches is also recommended. In infants, juices that contain sorbitol (e.g., prune, pear, and apple juice) are recommended. Fiber can be added in the form of barley malt extract, a natural stool softener. Because of its unpleasant odor, it may be helpful to administer with bottle feeds in infants. Corn syrup and sorbitol act as osmotic laxatives and have been used short term in this population. Small doses, 1–2 teaspoons/day, of corn syrup may serve as an in-home option for constipation treatment. However, in a retrospective study evaluating therapy recommendations made in general pediatric clinics, corn syrup and sorbitol resolved constipation in 25% of children versus 92% of children having resolution with laxatives (milk of magnesia or polyethylene glycol).[45]

Behavioral therapy is an important component of treatment and should be added to any treatment regimen for children and adolescents. Regular toilet habits, which include unhurried time on the toilet, commode positional aids, and maintaining a record of stool frequency, should become part of the daily schedule. Caregivers can institute a positive reinforcement system, or reward system, to record number of stools and foster a relaxed and nurturing environment for the child.

As mentioned previously, digital disimpaction may be used for acute management of impaction, although its use is not widely agreed on in primary care and would most likely occur only if other therapies were unsuccessful as a last-line option.

PHARMACOLOGIC THERAPY

When selecting appropriate therapy, the underlying cause must be considered. Nonpharmacologic and pharmacologic therapy should be used in conjunction to achieve optimal results. The treatment course for constipation can be lengthy. Each phase of treatment (disimpaction and maintenance) has a different duration and expectation for achieving results. For example, treatment of impaction can show results within 2–5 days, whereas maintenance therapy can require 3–12 months of treatment to sustain results. About 40% of children will not respond to initial treatment and will require additional treatment.[36] Treatment duration and outcomes among children are as varied as the child and qualification of constipation. Pharmacologic options and their dosing are generally divided into agents that provide acute relief of impacted stool or maintenance therapy for sustained evacuation or prevention of re-impaction/ reaccumulation (Table 5).

If fecal impaction is present, disimpaction is the first goal of therapy. Disimpaction can be achieved by several methods, which usually include pharmacotherapy. Method and agent chosen depend on patient age, adverse effect profile, route of administration, and severity of impaction. In pediatric practice, agents with the fewest adverse effects, less complicated administration, and high likelihood of adherence are used. Both oral and rectal administration can be used for disimpaction. No studies have identified that one route is superior to the other once obstruction is ruled out; thus the choice depends on the child and caregiver. The oral route is less invasive, but adherence can be challenging (e.g., volume, palatability, frequency). Alternatively, the rectal route is invasive, but it generally has a quick onset. Caution should be used with enema administration to avoid damage to the rectal wall; for this reason, it is not recommended as the first-line option for infants.[38] Pharmacologic treatment options for disimpaction include glycerin or bisacodyl suppositories, enemas, or oral medications (e.g., mineral oil, polyethylene glycol solutions, magnesium citrate).

Osmotic laxatives. Osmotic laxatives have been studied for disimpaction in children.[36,46] Osmotic laxatives prevent the absorption of water or create an osmotic gradient in the gut to pull water into the lumen, thereby increasing the "fluidity" of the stool. Polyethylene glycol is an osmotic laxative with a good safety profile for both infants and children.[47] It is recommended as first-line therapy for initial disimpaction.[38]

Table 5. Pharmacologic Therapy of Constipation[20,38,49]

Agent	Dosing by Patient Age, Type of Diarrhea, Timing, and Route of Administration	Onset (hr)	Comments
Docusate salts: sodium, calcium, potassium (same dosing)	**< 3 yr**: 10–40 mg/day in 1–4 divided doses **3–6 yr**: 20–60 mg/day in 1–4 divided doses **6–12 yr**: 40–150 mg/day in 1–4 divided doses **> 12 yr–adult**: 50–400 mg/day in 1–4 divided doses	12–72	Useful in prevention of constipation, not sole agent for treatment of impaction
Mineral oil	**Disimpaction**: 30 mL/year of age twice daily (240 mL max) **Maintenance: Oral** **5–11 yr**: 5–15 mL once daily or divided **> 12 yr**: 15–45 mL/day once or in divided doses **Maintenance: Rectal** **2–11 yr**: 30–60 mL as single dose **> 12 yr**: 50–150 mL as single dose	6–8	Should not be used for > 1 wk Caution in children < 5 yr because of aspiration risk
Polyethylene glycol	**Disimpaction, oral** 1–1.5 g/kg/day for 3–6 days; 100 g/day max **Maintenance, oral** **Infants, children, adolescents**: 0.2–0.8 g/kg/day; 17 g/day max	At constipation dosing, full results after 2 days–1 wk of therapy	Contraindicated in bowel obstruction Monitor for electrolyte disturbances
Polyethylene glycol-electrolyte solution	**Slow disimpaction, oral/nasogastric** **Children > 2 yr and adolescents**: 20 mL/kg/hr (1 L/hr max) for 4 hr/day for 2 days	1–2	Typically used for bowel cleansing before gastrointestinal procedure or treatment of impactions, and not for long-term use
Lactulose	**Children**: 7.5 mL/day after breakfast **Adults**: 15–30 mL/day; 60 mL/day max	Within 24 hr	After discontinuation of therapy, allow 24–48 hours before normal bowel function resumes
Sorbitol	**Oral as 70% solution** **Children**: 1–3 mL/kg/day in divided doses **Adults**: 30–150 mL as single dose **Enema** **Children 2–< 12 yr**: 30 to 60 mL as single dose **Children ≥ 12 yr and adolescents**: 120 mL as single dose	Within 24 hr	Adjust dose based on number of daily bowel movements (approach similar to lactulose)
Bisacodyl	**Oral** **3–12 yr**: 5–10 mg or 0.3 mg/kg/day as single dose (30 mg/day max) **> 12 yr**: 5–15 mg/day as single dose (30 mg/day max) **Rectal** **< 2 yr**: 5 mg/day as single dose **2–11 yr**: 5–10 mg/day as single dose **> 12**: 10 mg/day as single dose	Oral: 6–10 hr Rectal: 15–60 min	Not recommended for daily use May cause considerable abdominal cramping Do not break or crush enteric-coated tablets
Sennosides	**Syrup** (8.8 mg/5 mL) **1 mo–2 yr**: 1.25–2.5 mL at bedtime (5 mL max) **2–6 yr**: 2.5–3.75 mL at bedtime (3.75 mL max) **6–12 yr**: 5–7.5 mL at bedtime (7.5 mL max) **> 12 yr**: 10–15 mL at bedtime (15 mL max) **Tablet** (8.6 mg): **2–6 yr**: ½ tablet at bedtime (1 tablet BID max) **6–12**: 1 tablet (2 tablets BID max) **> 12 yr**: 2 tablets (4 tablets BID max)	Oral: within 6–24 hr Rectal: evacuation occurs in 30 min–2 hr	Docusate enhances absorption of senna

(continued)

Table 5. Pharmacologic Therapy of Constipation[20,38,49] *(continued)*

Agent	Dosing by Patient Age, Type of Diarrhea, Timing, and Route of Administration	Onset (hr)	Comments
Magnesium citrate	**< 6 yr:** 2–4 mL/kg/dose given once or in divided doses **6–12 yr:** 100–150 mL/dose given once or in divided doses **> 12 yr:** 150–300 mL/dose given once or in divided doses	A few hours after oral administration	Used for acute evacuation, not impaction
Magnesium hydroxide[a]	**< 2 yr:** 0.5 mL/kg/dose **Chewable tablets:** **2–5 yr:** 5–15 mL or 311–622 mg (1–2 tablets) **6–11 yr:** 15–30 mL or 933–1244 mg (3–4 tablets) **> 12 yr–adult:** 30–60 mL or 1866–2488 mg (6–8 tablets)	0.5–6 hr	Use with caution in patients with renal impairment At bedtime or in divided doses
Glycerin	**Neonates:** ½ glycerin suppository as needed **Children:** **< 6 yr:** 1 infant suppository as needed **> 6 yr–adult:** 1 adult suppository as needed	15–30 min	Not useful for impaction; considered a safe laxative
Phosphate soda enemas	**Enema** **Children 2–4 yr:** Administer one half contents of one 2.25-ounce pediatric enema **Children 5–11 yr:** Administer the contents of one 2.25-ounce pediatric enema **Children ≥ 12 yr and adolescents:** Administer the contents of one 4.5-ounce enema as a single dose **Oral** **5–9 yr:** 5 mL as single dose **10–12 yr:** 10 mL as single dose **> 12 yr–adult:** 20–30 mL as single dose	Rectal: 2–5 min Oral: 3–6 hr	For oral administration, mix 1:1 with water Separate doses by 10–12 hr Contraindicated in renal failure May cause electrolyte disturbances

[a]All liquid milliliter doses are based on 400-mg/5-mL magnesium hydroxide, unless noted otherwise.
BID = twice daily; max = maximum.

Electrolyte disturbances should be monitored, however, because osmotic laxatives prevent the absorption of water, and electrolytes follow suit. Polyethylene glycol has also been used in hospital settings for gastric lavage if oral or enema treatment is unsuccessful in disimpaction.[38]

Other osmotic agents that have been used for disimpaction in children, but that have more limited data in pediatric patients, include the following: magnesium citrate, magnesium hydroxide, lactulose, and sorbitol. Magnesium citrate is not commonly used for disimpaction, particularly in those younger than 2 years because of their susceptibility to magnesium toxicity. Toxicity can lead to electrolyte disturbances including hypermagnesemia, hypophosphatemia, and hypocalcemia and their sequelae. Magnesium hydroxide can also be used, but it is indicated more for maintenance therapy. Magnesium hydroxide induces the release of cholecystokinin, which stimulates the secretion of water and motility. Like the citrate salt, it should not be used in infants because magnesium toxicity can occur. In the presence of renal dysfunction, magnesium accumulation can occur, especially when in combination with aluminum salts, and should be avoided in these patients. Magnesium salts can cause considerable cramping and gas; they are therefore less well tolerated in the pediatric population. Lactulose and sorbitol are both osmotic laxatives composed of indigestible sugars. They are generally well tolerated for long-term use, but data are limited on their use for disimpaction. Lactulose and sorbitol cause flatulence and abdominal cramping and should be titrated to balance efficacy with these adverse effects. Sorbitol enemas have also been used for drug overdoses, but they are not routinely used for fecal impaction.

Enemas effective for fecal impaction include phosphate soda and saline enemas. They can be considered as an alternative to polyethylene glycol for disimpaction but should only be used in children older than 2 years. Phosphate soda is an osmotic enema and should not be used in renal impairment because accumulation can occur. The use of soapsuds, tap water, or magnesium enemas is not recommended because of the associated toxicities, including bowel perforations, necrosis, or even water intoxication.[33,38]

Lubricants. Lubricants, such as mineral oil, have been widely described in pediatric and adult literature. Mineral oil works by softening stool and preventing water reabsorption. A dose that is too high results in anal leakage, and it should be titrated accordingly. However, mineral oil should not be used in infants because of the risk of aspiration and resulting lipoid pneumonia. Mineral oil is not recommended for impaction, but may be an alternative agent in maintenance therapy, as appropriate.

Stimulant laxatives. Stimulant laxatives, including glycerin, bisacodyl, and senna, are also effective in the treatment of constipation in children. Glycerin suppositories are perhaps most widely used in the neonatal and infant populations. Glycerin works through osmotic properties, but the direct rectal stimulation in administration often produces the desired results. A stellar safety profile and variety of available dosing sizes make glycerin an ideal choice for infants. However, glycerin's effectiveness may be decreased once rectal distention has occurred.[48] Bisacodyl, a stimulant, can be given orally or rectally in older children (but is not indicated in children younger than 2 years). It works by stimulating the nerves in the colon to cause movement as well as to increase the secretion of water and chloride. Orally, bisacodyl has been used for disimpaction, usually in conjunction with other therapies. Rectal use is generally not as effective because the suppository is usually inserted into the middle of the stool, rather than where it can come into contact with the mucosa, and will not have the desired action. Abdominal cramping, hypokalemia, and diarrhea have all been associated with bisacodyl use. Senna is another stimulant laxative that works by stimulating colonic nerves to produce peristalsis, or movement, in addition to preventing water and electrolyte absorption to soften stools. Senna has a quicker onset of action than bisacodyl (1–3 hours vs. 6–12 hours). Senna is often used in combination with stool softeners, mainly docusate. One specific adverse effect is the presence of melanosis coli, which is a benign darkening of the colon that generally improves within 4–12 months after senna discontinuation.[38]

Stool softeners. Stool softeners such as docusate are generally used in combination with a stimulant in maintenance therapy or as a prevention agent. Softening the stool is helpful to prevent straining and discomfort with defecation. Docusate works by reducing the surface tension of the oil/water interface of stool, causing increased absorption of water in the stool and ultimately softening stools (much like the effects of a soap in changing oil and water interfaces).[49] Docusate is available as several enteral forms and salts, including sodium, calcium, and potassium, which are considered interchangeable.

Other agents. Lubipostone, a chloride channel activator, has been approved for use in chronic idiopathic constipation, irritable bowel with constipation, and opioid-induced constipation in adults. This agent works by opening chloride channels in the gut leading to secretion of chloride-containing fluid and acceleration of gut motility. It also delays gastric emptying by the same mechanism, which can also cause nausea in patients taking this medication. Other reported adverse effects include headache and diarrhea. To date, there are limited studies on using these agents in the pediatric population. In one study, lubiprostone was found to have a dose-dependent increase in stool frequency, similar to adult data. However, this study did not compare to placebo, so caution should be used before widespread use of this agent.[50]

In general, once disimpaction occurs, maintenance therapy involves the combination of dietary and behavioral changes, together with lubricants or osmotic laxatives (or a combination of the two), if pharmacologic therapy is necessary. Guideline recommendations for disimpaction and maintenance therapy are outlined in Box 2. In infants, the maintenance stage can usually be maintained with a stool softener alone. Toddlers—who are stool-withholder experts—may require both stool softeners (e.g., docusate sodium) and stimulants at the beginning of the maintenance phase. Table 4 provides dosing for medications used for the treatment of constipation.

Acute constipation not relieved by these therapies warrants further workup for an underlying disorder. If a patient is unsuccessfully disimpacted, then surgery may be warranted to remove the area of bowel that is not functioning and/or the removal of stool. An ostomy, or surgically created opening from the intestines to the outside of the body, may be needed after surgery. Having an ostomy requires special care and diet considerations because absorption may be affected.

MONITORING OF THERAPY

When evaluating the effectiveness of therapy, the clinician should consider the time of onset for the agent. The type, or class, of agent selected will produce results at different times, and adequate time for these agents to work should be granted before adding or changing therapy (Table 4). Complete evacuation can take 2–5 days. If complete evacuation is not achieved within this time, admission to the hospital for oral gastric lavage with a polyethylene glycol solution can be considered. The patient should have a complete evacuation of stool after treatment, and maintenance therapy begun to reinforce good bowel habits and maintain evacuation to restore normal bowel tone.

During the maintenance phase, stool softeners and, periodically, stimulants, are used to ensure consistent complete evacuation and the return of normal bowel tone. This phase can take from 2 to 6 months. Stimulants and a dependence on laxatives for stooling should be evaluated by the practitioner to prevent dependence.

Weaning of therapy is the final step in the therapeutic plan and should begin when there is a return to the patient's baseline. Weaning agents should be done gradually, and some patients may require regular use of stool softeners even after normal bowel tone returns. If the patient is taking daily medication, the medication may be weaned. One example of a weaning strategy is to decrease by going to every-other-day therapy for 1 month, followed by every 3 days for 1 month until complete evacuation occurs on a regular basis.[51]

Stimulant laxatives may be administered on an as-needed basis if the child does not stool for more than 3 days. Reviewing the patient's stool diary and reinforcement of

---

Box 2. Guideline Recommendations for Initial (Disimpaction) and Maintenance Constipation Therapy[38]

Initial Therapy: Disimpaction

First-line therapy: Polyethylene glycol
Second-line therapy: Age-appropriate enema

Maintenance Therapy

First-line therapy: Polyethylene glycol
Alternative first-line therapy: Lactulose can be first line if polyethylene glycol is not available

Second-line (or additional) therapy:
    Milk of magnesia
    Mineral oil (oral)
    Stimulant laxatives (bisacodyl, senna)

---

good bowel habits may be necessary to recognize the early signs of recurrence including feeling of incomplete evacuation, return of stool-withholding behaviors, or irregular stooling. Throughout therapy, monitoring for drug-specific adverse effects in balance with efficacy should be considered. Introduction of medications or dietary changes that may cause constipation should also be monitored and considered if symptoms of recurrence are present.

CONCLUSIONS

Diarrhea and constipation are common disease states in children. Although diarrhea is a leading cause of morbidity and mortality worldwide, rehydrating with appropriate fluids, such as ORT, and monitoring hydration status considerably affect survival. When treating diarrhea, if an underlying etiology can be identified, then the treatment should be tailored to the specific cause. In many cases, an exact cause of the diarrhea is unknown, but hydration management principles remain the same. Although pharmacologic therapy is not indicated as a cure for most cases of acute diarrhea, treatment with medications may be used for refractory symptoms and for the management of chronic diarrhea. Treatment should be individualized and reassessed often.

Similarly, constipation management should be individualized and guided by the underlying cause, either organic or nonorganic. It is important to identify any underlying etiology because constipation is often recognized as a symptom, so treatment can be specific to the cause. Most cases are functional in origin and should be managed with diet and behavioral and pharmacologic therapy. Ultimately, the goal is to maintain complete evacuation and restoration of good bowel tone and habits. Therapy involves both an acute and maintenance approach and should be continuously monitored for changes in efficacy to step-up or step-down treatment. For both diarrhea and constipation, completion of a careful history, patient evaluation, and close follow-up will ensure appropriate selection and monitoring of therapy.

Patient Case 1 — DIARRHEA

A 4-month-old girl is brought to the clinic by her mother for decreased oral intake, a 2-day history of diarrhea, "dry crying," and irritability. The girl has had no recent changes to her diet and has not changed formulas (currently cow's milk formula). Her mother wonders if her daughter could be allergic to milk. The girl's 3-year-old sister has a recent history of gastroenteritis.

Medical history: Born at 27-week gestation with a neonatal intensive care unit course complicated by necrotizing enterocolitis and resulting removal of a portion of the distal (terminal) ileum and the ileocecal valve; maintained adequate growth (75th percentile for height, weight, and head circumference); meeting developmental milestones

Family history: Maternal grandfather with hypertension and paternal grandmother with diabetes

Social history: Lives at home with mother, father, and 3-year-old sister, 2 dogs, and 1 fish; no smoking in the home; does not attend day care, and is currently at home with her mother while her sister is at preschool

Physical examination:
Oral mucosa moderately dry
Eyes slightly sunken
Skin turgor decreased
Fontanelle slightly reduced
Capillary refill < 2 seconds
Diaper area red, but no broken skin or rash
Scar over abdomen healed

Vital signs: Within normal limits

Medications: None

Immunizations: Up to date for age

1. What is the likely cause of diarrhea in this patient and what is the best initial management?

Based on the short course of symptoms and recent exposure to a family member with gastroenteritis, this patient likely has diarrhea secondary to gastroenteritis. Lactose intolerance may be present in this patient, but only transiently as a result of gastroenteritis. The patient does have a history of necrotizing enterocolitis, but no report of short bowel syndrome. Because gastroenteritis is generally viral in origin, no antibiotics are needed at this time. Hydration and electrolyte balance are important in the management of diarrhea, so this patient would need adequate fluid intake. At this time, the dehydration is mild to moderate, and oral rehydration would be indicated. This patient's diarrhea is classified as mild to moderate because the patient has moderately dry oral mucosa, slightly sunken eyes, decreased skin turgor, and only slightly reduced fontanelle. She also has a good capillary refill. If she were to have severe dehydration, she would have extremely dry mucosa, absent tears, markedly sunken eyes and fontanelle, and a capillary refill of > 8 seconds. Vital sign changes (tachycardia and hypotension) are also signs of severe dehydration. Another reassuring sign that this patient is not severely dehydrated is the weight loss is less than 9% to 15%, which would have indicated severe dehydration. Formula feeding should continue with careful attention to hydration status. If needed, an appropriate oral rehydration fluid for this patient would be Pedialyte (Abbott Laboratories, Abbott Park, IL), but the mother should also discuss with the provider. If needed for mild dehydration, Pedialyte could be initiated at 50 mL/kg/day plus 10 mL/kg for every stool (or emesis) and reassessed every 2 hours. For moderate dehydration, increasing to 100 mL/kg/day plus 10 mL/kg for every stool or emesis, reassessing every hour is recommended. Changing to another formula is not recommended as this time because true milk-protein allergies are rare and the patient does not exhibit signs of a true allergy. In addition, no anti-diarrheal agent is recommended because this agent is not recommended for initial therapy in viral gastroenteritis.

Case *(continued)*. The patient returns to clinic for continued diarrhea 1 month later. She has good oral intake and does not have any signs or symptoms of dehydration at this time. On physical examination, the health care provider notices that her diaper area is red and raw and the stool seems to have a greasy consistency. Her height and weight have decreased on the growth curve, and the provider is concerned about "dumping" as a result of her intestinal surgery.

2. The health care provider asks you to recommend an appropriate therapy for the diarrhea. What are your monitoring and treatment recommendations?

This patient has a physiologic reason for having diarrhea. Because the patient's ileocecal valve has been removed, she is more likely to have decreased intestinal transit time, malabsorption, and "dumping." In addition, the terminal ileum is where bile acids are reabsorbed. Increased bile acids in the stool can cause significant skin irritation with prolonged contact. An agent that would slow intestinal transit time and heal the irritation from increased bile acids would be the best option. Opioids or opioid derivatives would help slow gastrointestinal motility, but may not help with the increased bile acid in stool. Oral cholestyramine would be an appropriate choice for this patient on a short-term basis. The recommended dose for diarrhea secondary to short-bowel syndrome is 240 mg/kg/day in three divided doses (to a maximum of 8 g/day). In this patient, cholestyramine would likely be mixed with formula (at least 60 mL). The duration of therapy may depend on the duration of increased stools. As the number of stools decrease, cholestyramine may be discontinued. The parents should be counseled on appropriate administration as well as potential drug–drug interactions. Cholestyramine will bind with many medications, so other oral agents should be administered 1 hour before and 4–6 hours after cholestyramine administration. Adverse effects include constipation, diarrhea, nausea and abdominal discomfort.

Patient Case 2 | CONSTIPATION

A 6-year-old, 18-kg boy is brought by his parents to clinic for a follow-up appointment. His last visit was 3 months ago. His parents report that the boy is constipated and he has only stooled once a week since his last visit. He has not had any bowel movements the week before this clinic visit. His bowel movements are hard, and he has told them that his stomach hurts.

Medical history: Born at 24-week gestation; has cerebral palsy and developmental delay

Family history: Uncle with seizure disorder

Social history: Adopted from foster family and lives at home with parents, and 2 other children currently in foster care; no pets; no smoking in the home; currently attends first grade

Physical examination: Abdomen soft, but slightly distended; no pain on palpation; all other systems within normal limits

Vital signs: Within normal limits

Laboratory findings: Basic metabolic panel within normal limits; no obstruction on abdominal radiography

Home medications: Multi-vitamins with iron, 1 tablet daily; polyethylene glycol, 17 g daily as needed

Immunizations: Up to date

1. What are the potential risk factors for and causes of this patient's constipation?

This patient likely has issues with constipation based on his underlying neurologic impairment secondary to cerebral palsy. Patients with cerebral palsy are at increased risk of constipation. This patient is also receiving iron supplementation, which can also cause constipation. Although he has been taking as-needed polyethylene glycol, adherence to this regimen is not known.

2. What treatment, both nonpharmacologic and pharmacologic, and monitoring recommendations do you have at this time?

Acute management for constipation is warranted at this time. The North American Society for Pediatric Gastroenterology, Hepatology, and Nutrition recommendation in general are treatment doses of polyethylene glycol as first-line therapy, unless there is a bowel obstruction. This patient should receive 1 g/kg or 18 g daily for 3 to 6 consecutive days; however, dosage form size is generally 17 g/unit, so the patient could receive a maximum of 17 g/dose). Administration is by stirring the powder into 4 to 8 ounces of water or appropriate juice until dissolved for the patient to drink. Monitoring recommendations for this patient include evaluating stool frequency; once the patient begins to stool regularly, then the dose may be decreased and changed to as needed. Other osmotic laxatives are generally not recommended for disimpaction. An enema could be used in this patient because he is older than 2 years, but it may be less comfortable for him. Rectal stimulant laxatives may not be the best choice in this patient because suppositories need to come in contact with the mucosa—if large amounts of stool are present in the distal colon, then the suppository would not come in contact with the mucosa. Senna, especially in combination with docusate (a stool softener) would be an appropriate option for maintenance therapy, but not for disimpaction. When recommending senna and docusate therapy, the best dosage form for this patient should be considered. Depending on whether the patient can swallow tablets and/or if the parents are comfortable crushing the tablet and mixing in food/drink, the patient may require liquids. Because the combination of senna and docusate is only available as a tablet, if liquid is required, then the patient will need to take separate products, which does increase medication "burden." If a tablet can be used, the recommended dose for this patient's age is 1 tablet (docusate 50 mg/8.6 mg sennosides) daily at bedtime, which may be increased to a maximum of 2 tablets twice daily. If liquids are needed, then the recommended dose would be: docusate syrup (60 mg/15 mL) 50–150 mg/day in single or divided doses and senna (8.8 mg sennosides/5 mL) 5–7.5 mL (8.8–13.2 mg sennosides) at bedtime, not to exceed 7.5 mL twice daily. Typically these medications would be initiated at the lowest dose and titrated to effect, not to exceed the maximum dosing. A complete diet history should also be taken. Increase in fiber intake could help with maintenance of normal stool patterns. A stool diary may also be beneficial, although it appears this family is aware of the patient's normal stooling patterns. The parents should be educated on the onset of action and potential adverse effects of therapy, as previously described. The onset of action for polyethylene glycol is typically within 24–96 hours. To avoid dehydration and related electrolyte abnormalities, the parents should discontinue polyethylene glycol after the impaction resolves. This resolution may take 3–6 days for complete evacuation to occur.

REFERENCES

1. World Health Organization. Diarrhoeal Disease [homepage on the Internet]. Available at www.who.int/news-room/fact-sheets/detail/diarrhoeal-disease. Accessed December 12, 2018.
2. World Health Organization. Global Health Observatory Data Repository [homepage on the Internet]. Available at http://apps.who.int/gho/data/view.main.ghe1002015-CH3?lang=en. Accessed December 12, 2018.
3. World Health Organization. 2017. World Health Statistics. Children: Reducing Mortality [homepage on the Internet]. Available at www.who.int/mediacentre/factsheets/fs178/en/. Accessed March 17, 2019.
4. Yen C, Tate JE, Wenk JD, et al. Diarrhea-associated hospitalizations among US children over 2 rotavirus seasons after vaccine introduction. Pediatrics 2011;127:e9-15.
5. Canavan C, West J, Card T. Review article: the economic impact of the irritable bowel syndrome. Aliment Pharmacol Ther 2014;40:1023-34.
6. Schiller LR, Pardi DS, Sellin JH. Chronic diarrhea: diagnosis and management. Clin Gastroenterol Hepatol 2017;15:182-93.
7. Binder HJ. Causes of chronic diarrhea. N Engl J Med 2006;355:236-9.
8. Spruill WJ, Wade WE. Diarrhea, constipation, and irritable bowel syndrome. In: DiPiro JT, Talbert RL, Yee GC, et al., eds. Pharmacotherapy: A Pathophysiologic Approach. New York: McGraw-Hill, 2008:617-31.
9. Hoffenberg EJ, Furuta GT, Kobak G, et al. Gastrointestinal tract. In: Hay WW Jr, Levin MJ, Deterding RR, et al., eds. Current Diagnosis & Treatment: Pediatrics, 24e New York, NY: McGraw-Hill. Available at https://accessmedicine.mhmedical.com/content.aspx?bookid=2390&sectionid=189079593. Accessed March 17, 2019.
10. Access Medicine. Water and Electrolyte Absorption and Secretion. In: Barrett KE. eds. Gastrointestinal Physiology, 2e New York, NY: McGraw-Hill. Available at http://accessmedicine.mhmedical.com/content.aspx?bookid=691&sectionid=45431404. Accessed March 17, 2019.
11. McFarland LV, Ozen M, Dinleyici EC, et al. Comparison of pediatric and adult antibiotic-associated diarrhea and Clostridium difficile infections. World J Gastroenterol 2016;22:3078-104.
12. Brown KH. Diarrhea and malnutrition. J Nutr 2003;133:328S-32S.
13. Eunice Kennedy Shriver National Institute of Child Health and Human Development, NIH and Office of Medical Applications of Research, NIH. Lactose Intolerance and Health: Programs and Abstracts. Available at https://consensus.nih.gov/2010/images/lactose/lactose_abstracts.pdf. Accessed March 16, 2019.
14. De Greef E, Hauser B, Devreker T, et al. Diagnosis and management of cow's milk protein allergy in infants. World J Pediatr 2012;8:19-24.
15. Granado-Villar D, Cunill-De Sautu B, Granados A. acute gastroenteritis. Pediatr Rev 2012;33:487-95.
16. Kleinman RE, Greer FR, eds. Pediatric Nutrition, 7th ed. Chicago: American Academy of Pediatrics, 2013.
17. World Health Organization. 2005. The Treatment of Diarrhoea: A Manual for Physicians and Other Senior Health Workers, 4th rev. Available at https://www.who.int/maternal_child_adolescent/documents/9241593180/en/. Accessed October 23, 2019.
18. Li ST, Grossman DC, Cummings P. Loperamide therapy for acute diarrhea in children: systematic review and meta-analysis. PLoS Med 2007;4:e98.
19. Pulling M, Surawicz CM. Loperamide use for acute infectious diarrhea in children: safe and sound? Gastroenterology 2008;134:1260-2.
20. Lexi-Comp Online, Pediatric and Neonatal Lexi-Drugs Online [Internet database]. Hudson, OH: Lexi-Comp, Wolters Kluwer Clinical Drug Information, Inc. Updated periodically.
21. Isolauri E, Vesikari T. Oral rehydration, rapid feeding, and cholestyramine for treatment of acute diarrhea. J Pediatr Gastroenterol Nutr 1985;4:366-74.
22. Dinleyici EC, Eren M, Ozen M, et al. Effectiveness and safety of Sacharomyces boulardii for acute infectious diarrhea. Expert Opin Biol Ther 2012;12:395-410.

23. Van Niel CW, Feudtner C, Garrison MM, et al. Lactobacillus therapy for acute infectious diarrhea in children: a meta-analysis. Pediatrics 2002;109:678-84.

24. Thomas DW, Greer FR; Committee on Nutrition, Section on Gastroenterology, Hepatology, and Nutrition. Probiotics and Prebiotics in Pediatrics. Pediatrics 2010;126:1217-31.

25. Doron S, Snydman DR. Risk and safety of probiotics. Clin Infect Dis 2015;60:S129-34.

26. Fox MJ, Ahuja KD, Robertson IK, et al. Can probiotic yogurt prevent diarrhea in children on antibiotics? A double-blind, randomized, placebo-controlled study. BMJ Open 2015;5:e006474.

27. Bhutta ZA, Bird SM, Black RE, et al. Therapeutic effects of oral zinc in acute and persistent diarrhea in children in developing countries: pooled analysis of randomized controlled trials. Am J Clin Nutr 2000;72:1516-22.

28. Bhutta ZA, Black RE, Brown KH, et al. Prevention of diarrhea and pneumonia by zinc supplementation in children in developing countries: pooled analysis of randomized controlled trials. Zinc Investigators' Collaborative Group. J Pediatr 1999;135:689-97.

29. Lukacik M, Thomas RL, Arando JV. A meta-analysis of the effects of oral zinc in the treatment of acute and persistent diarrhea. Pediatrics 2008;121:326-36.

30. Fawzi WW, Mbise R, Spiegelman D, et al. Vitamin A supplements and diarrheal and respiratory tract infections among children in Dar es Salaam, Tanzania. J Pediatr 2000;137:660-7.

31. Van den Berg MM, Benninga MA, Di Lorenzo C. Epidemiology of childhood constipation: a systematic review. Am J Gastroenterol 2006;101:2401-9.

32. Sommers T, Corban C, Sengupta N, et al. Emergency department burden of constipation in the United States from 2006 to 2011. Am J Gastroenterol 2015;110:572-79.

33. Tabbers MM, Boluyt N, Berger MY, et al. Constipation in children. BMJ Clin Evid 2010; 0303.

34. Martin BC, Barghout V, Cerulli A. Direct medical costs of constipation in the United States. Manag Care Interface 2006;19:43-9.

35. Hyman PE, Milla PJ, Benninga MA, et al. Childhood functional gastrointestinal disorders: neonate/toddler. Gastroenterology 2006;130:1519-26.

36. Colombo JM, Wassom MC, Rosen JM. Constipation and encopresis in childhood. Pediatr Rev 2015;36:392-402.

37. Olaru C, Diaconescu S, Trandafir L, et al. Some risk factors of chronic functional constipation identified in a pediatric population sample from Romania. Gastroenterol Res and Pract 2016; 2016:3989721.

38. Tabbers MM, DiLorenzo C, Berger MY, et al. Evaluation and treatment of functional constipation in infants and children: evidence-based recommendations from ESPGHAN and NASPGHAN. J Pediatr Gastroenterol Nutr 2014;58:258-74.

39. Simren M, Palsson OS, Whitehead WE. Update on Rome IV criteria for colorectal disorders: Implications for clinical practice. Curr Gastroenterol Rep 2017;19:15.

40. Lacy BE, Mearin F, Chang L, et al. Bowel disorders. Gastroenterology 2016;150:1393-407.

41. Hyams JS, Di Lorenzo C, Saps M, et al. Childhood functional gastrointestinal disorders: Child/Adolescent. Gastroenterology 2016;150:1456-68.

42. Andrews CN, Storr M. The pathophysiology of chronic constipation. Can J Gastroenterol 2011;25:16B-21B.

43. Southwell BR, Clarke MCC, Sutcliffe J, et al. Colonic transit studies: normal values for adults and children with comparison of radiologics and scintigraphic methods. Pediatr Surg Int 2009;25:559-72.

44. Bongers MEJ, van Wijk MP, Reitsma JB, et al. Long-term prognosis for childhood constipation: clinical outcomes in adulthood. Pediatrics 2010;126:e156-62.

45. Loening-Baucke V. Prevalence, symptoms and outcome of constipation in infants and toddlers. J Pediatr 2005;146:359-63.

46. Youssef NN, Peters JM, Henderson W, et al. Dose response of PEG 3350 for the treatment of childhood fecal impaction. J Pediatr 2002;141:410Y4.

47. Bell EA, Wall GC. Pediatric constipation therapy using guidelines and polyethylene glycol 3350. Ann Pharmacother 2004; 38:686Y93.

48. van den Berg MM, van Rossum CH, de Lorijn F, et al. Functional constipation in infants: a follow-up study. J Pediatr 2005;147:700-4.

49. Guo N, Iqbal A. Chapter 12: Gastroenterology. In: Molloy M, McDaniel L, Kleinman K, Shikofski N, eds. The Harriet Lane Handbook, 21st ed. Philadelphia: Elsevier Mosby, 2018:316-32.

50. Hyman PE, Di Lorenzo C, Prestridge LL, et al. Lubiprostone for the treatment of functional constipation in children. J Pediatr Gastroenterol Nutr 2014;58:283-91.

51. Abi-Hanna A, Lake A. Constipation and encopresis in childhood. Pediatr Rev 1998;19:23-31.

CHAPTER 17

Inflammatory Bowel Disease

Brooke L. Gildon, Pharm.D., BCPS, BCPPS;
and Tiffany Kessler, Pharm.D., BCPS

LEARNING OBJECTIVES

1. Describe the epidemiology and pathophysiology of inflammatory bowel disease (IBD) in children and adolescents.

2. Illustrate the typical clinical presentation of a child with ulcerative colitis (UC) and Crohn disease (CD).

3. Define goals of therapy in the management of IBD.

4. Select pharmacologic options for induction of remission and maintenance therapy in children with IBD.

5. Discuss common adverse effects associated with agents used in IBD.

6. Evaluate vaccination status and provide recommendations in pediatric patients with IBD.

ABBREVIATIONS IN THIS CHAPTER

5-ASA	5-Aminosalicylate
6-MP	6-Mercaptopurine
CBC	Complete blood count
CD	Crohn disease
CRP	C-reactive protein
ESR	Erythrocyte sedimentation rate
FDA	U.S. Food and Drug Administration
GI	Gastrointestinal
IBD	Inflammatory bowel disease
IL	Interleukin
PUCAI	Pediatric UC activity index
PCDAI	Pediatric CD activity index
TNFα	Tumor necrosis factor alpha
TPMT	Thiopurine S-methlytransferase
UC	Ulcerative colitis

INTRODUCTION

Inflammatory bowel disease (IBD) includes two major gastrointestinal (GI) disorders: ulcerative colitis (UC) and Crohn disease (CD). *Ulcerative colitis* is described as a chronic disease of the large intestine in which the colon lining becomes diffusely inflamed and ulcerated. *Crohn disease* is manifested by focal, discontinuous, and transmural lesions most commonly at the end of the small intestine and the beginning of the large intestine, but may affect any part of the GI tract from the mouth to the anus. Crohn disease may impact the entire thickness of the bowel wall, whereas UC targets the lining only. Both disorders have distinctive presentations, yet their disease pathogenesis remains poorly understood.

Pediatric-onset IBD is an especially complex condition. Age of onset can impact IBD type and associated genetic features, illness location, disease progression, and response to therapy.[1-3] Furthermore, children with IBD can develop specific complications such as delayed puberty and growth failure. Adolescence is also a time of emotional maturation, and the effect of a chronic disease on social functioning and psychological health can be significant.

This chapter will focus mainly on conventional, polygenic IBD in children and adolescents. However, there is a great need to recognize monogenic disorders and immunodeficiencies associated with pediatric-onset IBD because of their specific treatment strategies.

EPIDEMIOLOGY AND ETIOLOGY

The incidence of IBD peaks in patients between the ages of 15 and 30 years, yet both UC and CD have been reported as early as infancy.[1,4] The incidence of IBD in those younger than 1 year is about 1%, with about 15% of pediatric IBD cases classified as *very early onset IBD*, representing a diagnosis before 6 years.[1,2] This early disease presentation is often called *monogenic IBD* because patients present with a diverse spectrum of rare genetic disorders compared with conventional, polygenic IBD in which hundreds of susceptibility loci add to the collective disease risk.[1] The overall prevalence of CD and UC in the U.S. pediatric population in 2009 was 58 and 34 cases per 100,000, respectively.[5] One study described that IBD was diagnosed before age 20 years in up to 25% of patients, highlighting the importance of IBD recognition by pediatric providers.[6] In addition, the incidence of IBD is increasing—more than doubling over the past 20 years in some geographic areas.[7-10] For example, the crude incidence rate of IBD in U.S. children increased from 1.43 cases per 100,000/year to 4.15 cases per 100,000/year from 1991 to 2002 and then reached 9.5 cases per 100,000/year in 2013.[10-11] Similar rates were also reported from the Netherlands and Scotland.[7-9]

Geographic location may also impact the likelihood of IBD presentation.[12] Of interest, the diagnosis of IBD in developing countries is uncommon and the highest disease rates occur in first-world, Westernized countries.[13-14] In addition, there may also be a North–South gradient evident in the lower rates of IBD in populations closer to the Equator.[15] Genetics and heredity should also be taken into consideration.[12] Pediatric patients of Ashkenazi Jewish descent are at a higher risk of IBD development in general and especially in CD.[12] Historically, white populations had an elevated prevalence of IBD compared with Asian or African American populations. However, new data suggest that environmental factors may now be playing a role in leveling this risk.[12] Environmental factors being investigated include the following: smoking, history of appendicitis, use of oral contraceptives, diet, breast-feeding, infections, vaccinations, and antibiotics.[16] Tobacco smoking is a strong environmental risk factor for IBD, with protective effects for UC and negative consequences for CD.[14] Future studies are necessary to better define these items in the IBD pathogenesis.

The exact cause of UC and CD remains unknown, yet similar elements are thought to be responsible for both disease states. These theories include a combination of the following factors: genetic, infectious, environmental, and immunologic.[12,14,16] Examples include an abnormal regulation of the immune response, reactions to numerous antigens, a GI microflora-induced inflammation, and the impact of psychological factors.[17-20] One proposed theory for IBD etiology includes the hygiene hypothesis.[16,21] Improved sanitation, decreased exposure to pathogens in childhood, smaller family/fewer siblings, younger birth order, and urban environment/housing density may also have an impact on IBD diagnosis.[16] In summary, it is likely that many elements contribute to the development of mucosal inflammation and IBD etiology.

PATHOLOGY OF MUCOSAL INFLAMMATION

Several mechanisms lead to inflammation of the colon. In a typical bowel, the mucosal immune system works to maintain a state of controlled inflammation. Yet in IBD, a trigger alerts neutrophils to a specific insult. These neutrophils play a vital role in the inflammatory process. They infiltrate mucosal tissues, release antimicrobial peptides and reactive oxygen intermediates, and recruit and stimulate other white blood cells, such as macrophages.[14] Neutrophils prompt these white blood cells by the production of chemokines and proinflammatory cytokines, specifically tumor necrosis factor alpha (TNFα), interleukin 1 beta (IL1β), IL-6, and IL-8.[22] Characteristic tissue destruction, intestinal edema, and granuloma formation in IBD is thought to be partially caused by these neutrophil effects.[14] For example, proinflammatory cytokines in the gut can trigger an attack on bowel mucosa, normal immune regulators fail to stop the destruction, and then the disease continues to advance.

The cell-mediated arm of the immune response occurs through different pathways in IBD. T helper cells are sources of inflammation by the production of various cytokines. Crohn disease is described by an excessive T helper 1 response compared with an increased Th2 phenotype in UC.[14,23] The response of T helper 1 is mediated by IL-12 and categorized by the formation of interferon gamma, IL-2, and TNF, which in turn promotes macrophage activation and creation of a delayed-type hypersensitivity response. Interleukin-4, IL-5, IL-13, and the production of other cytokines are associated with an atypical Th2 phenotype seen in UC, which supports a humoral-mediated immune response. Other T helper cells, suppressor cells, and cell defects have also been speculated to impact mucosal inflammation.[14] In summary, this rise in proinflammatory cytokines, chemokines, and prostaglandins leads to increased inflammation and tissue degradation.

CLINICAL PRESENTATION

The clinical picture of IBD can vary widely among patients. Both UC and CD often present with times of exacerbations, or acute flares, and periods of disease remission. This chronic nature of waxing and waning can result in disproportionate morbidity in the pediatric population.[12] Common clinical manifestations in children include GI symptoms, growth failure or delay, physical findings, and extraintestinal manifestations. The GI symptoms of diarrhea and abdominal pain have been described in up to 90% children with IBD.[12] It has also been proposed that the use of nonsteroidal anti-inflammatory drugs, emotional stress, and intestinal infections may exacerbate IBD symptoms.[24-25]

Both UC and CD are associated with extraintestinal manifestations.[23] These complications include hepatobiliary, musculoskeletal, ocular, dermatologic/mucocutaneous, hematologic, coagulation, and metabolic abnormalities. Around 28% of pediatric patients with IBD present with one or more extraintestinal manifestations, with 23.8% and 29.9% in UC and CD, respectively.[26] The most common extraintestinal manifestation is a nonspecific arthralgia in 16.5% of children who receive a diagnosis of IBD.[26] Extraintestinal manifestations do not consistently relate to the degree of intestinal inflammation. Some patients may initially present with these symptoms before any obvious GI involvement is seen.

Children and adults often present with similar clinical features, but pediatric patients can develop specific complications such as impaired growth. Children with IBD often present with a stunted growth at diagnosis, and these height deficits may become permanent.[27] Bone formation and health can be linked to nutritional deficiencies; changes in absorptive processes; physical inactivity; inflammatory cytokines; skeletal mass deficits; and adverse effects of medications, such as corticosteroids used in IBD treatment.[12] Risk factors for bone health compromise in children with IBD include linear growth delays, lean mass deficits, menstrual irregularity, late puberty, and prolonged use of systemic corticosteroids.[28] It is imperative to control inflammation, to improve nutrition, and to encourage physical activity in children to promote bone health.

ULCERATIVE COLITIS

The clinical presentation of UC in an adolescent patient is similar to what is seen in the adult population, including chronic, loose, bloody stools and abdominal pain. Patients with UC typically present with a subacute illness characterized by diarrhea, weakness, anemia, abdominal pain, and weight loss. Some children may have a slower, more insidious clinical presentation (i.e., poor weight gain, nonbloody diarrhea) before the development of more obvious symptoms.[29] An associated rectal bleeding in children is more common with UC (50%–90%) than in CD (15%-60%).[12] Acute, severe UC may be accompanied by more significant abdominal pain, greater bloody diarrhea, tenesmus (a painful spasm of the anal sphincter associated with bowel or bladder urgency and straining), fever, tachycardia, leukocytosis, and hypoalbuminemia. Other signs and symptoms may include blurred vision, eye pain, and photophobia with ocular involvement, arthritis, and raised red, tender nodules on the arms and legs.[23] On physical examination, hemorrhoids, anal fissures, or perirectal abscesses may be present together with ocular and dermatologic findings. A major, infrequent complication of UC is toxic megacolon; however, it is associated with high morbidity and mortality.[30]

CROHN DISEASE

As found with UC, CD has a highly variable presentation. Signs and symptoms associated with CD include: malaise, fever, abdominal pain, frequent bowel movements, hematochezia, weight loss and malnutrition, and arthritis.[23] On physical examination, abdominal mass or tenderness, perianal fissure or fistula, or a bowel obstruction may be found.[23,31] The time between symptom onset and initial diagnosis may be years. Compared with UC, weight loss is more common in children who have a diagnosis of CD, at a rate up to 90%.[12] Impaired linear growth and growth velocity are also observed more often than in UC.[32,33] Furthermore, perianal disease, such as fistulas and anal skin tags, are much more likely in CD.[12] Patients with CD have a 20%–40% lifetime risk for fistula formation.[34] Surgery may be required for small bowel strictures and obstruction. Bleeding is typically less severe, compared with UC; however, development of hypochromic anemia can occur. Because of the impact of intestinal inflammation on appetite, diet selection, and nutrient absorption, patients are increasingly susceptible to iron, zinc, vitamin B_{12}, folate, vitamin D, and calcium deficiencies.[12,35,36] Lastly, pathologic features, such as granulomas (25%–40% of mucosal biopsies), may be a factor indicative of CD.[31]

DIAGNOSIS

There are no specific diagnostic criteria for IBD. Diagnosis is often established by a combination of clinical features or symptoms, family history, laboratory screenings, radiographic studies, and endoscopy, including biopsies. Gastrointestinal tract presentation with UC typically shows a continuous distribution, whereas CD presents with a discontinuous picture including extensive bowel wall injury and narrowing of the intestinal lumen. Pathologic features—such as crypt abscesses commonly found in UC or a cobblestone appearance regularly occurring in CD—highlight further differences between the two diseases. The presence of extraintestinal manifestations may also help in identifying a diagnosis.[37] The North American Society for Pediatric Gastroenterology, Hepatology & Nutrition and the Crohn's & Colitis Foundation of America has published an algorithm to assist clinicians in differentiating childhood UC from CD.[38] Inflammatory bowel disease should be suspected and evaluated for any pediatric patient presenting with one or more of the following symptoms: bloody diarrhea; growth failure or weight loss; chronic watery diarrhea; chronic abdominal pain; perianal abscesses, fistulas, or fissures; oral ulcers; arthritis; or any IBD-related laboratory abnormality, such as anemia, elevated white blood cell count, or depressed albumin level.[39]

Initial laboratory evaluation suggested in suspected IBD includes a complete blood count (CBC) with differential, inflammatory markers (i.e., erythrocyte sedimentation rate [ESR], C-reactive protein [CRP]), liver profile, and albumin level. Abnormal laboratory findings often seen with inflammation associated with IBD include elevations in white blood cell and platelet counts, and ESR and/or CRP elevations. Hemoglobin and hematocrit can be helpful to assess GI blood loss and anemia. Serum albumin is often low in patients with an IBD flare or patients with newly diagnosed disease.[12] Extraintestinal complications, such as hepatobiliary, can be identified with abnormal liver function tests. Stool samples should be examined for *Salmonella*, *Shigella*, *Campylobacter*, *Yersinia* species, *Escherichia coli* 0157, *Clostridium difficile*, ova and parasites, occult blood, and fecal calprotectin or lactoferrin.[12,40,41] Stool studies are recommended to rule out other causes of GI symptoms and/or to detect the presence of intestinal inflammation.

Antibody tests for perinuclear antineutrophil cytoplasmic antibodies, antisaccharomyces cerevisiae antibodies, and antibody to *Escherichia coli* outer membrane porin are periodically used to supplement patient evaluation and diagnosis. A positive test for perinuclear antineutrophil cytoplasmic antibodies is associated with UC whereas a positive result for antisaccharomyces cerevisiae antibodies is linked to CD; however, these tests should not be routinely recommended for differentiating between IBDs or as a sole diagnostic criterion.[31,42] Genetic screening may have an important role in the diagnosis, assessment of prognosis, and proper treatment of monogenic very early onset IBD, yet it is not recommended in conventional IBD.[1]

Regarding imaging studies, testing is individualized based on clinical symptoms, relative cost and availability, and local imaging expertise.[12] Radiographic imaging identifying small bowel disease may be accomplished with abdominal magnetic resonance enterography, computed tomography enterography, and/or an upper GI series with small bowel follow-through. Endoscopic studies, including colonoscopy and upper endoscopy with biopsies, are often also used in the evaluation of a child with suspected IBD.

DISEASE CLASSIFICATION
ULCERATIVE COLITIS

Disease classification and disease severity scoring systems for UC exist for use in the pediatric population. The Paris Classification of IBD in childhood, a pediatric modification of the adult-focused Montreal Classification, was developed specifically for clinical studies involving children with UC or CD.[3] These classification systems look at factors such as age at diagnosis, location, behavior, and growth.[3] Disease involvement in UC is categorized as proctitis, left-sided colitis, or pancolitis. These categories describe the extent of colon involvement, starting with *proctitis*, relating to mucous membrane involvement of the rectum only, up to *pancolitis*, defined as inflammation from the proximal to hepatic flexure.[3] Regarding disease severity, a pediatric UC activity index (PUCAI) (Table 1) has been developed to assess a patient's symptoms.[43] Scoring ranges from 0–85, with 0 to 9 being remission, 10–34 mild disease, 35–64 moderate disease, and 65–85 severe disease.[43] Of these activity index items, rectal bleeding has the most impact on scoring severity. Other factors in the activity index include abdominal pain, stool consistency, number of stools, nocturnal stools that cause wakening, and patient activity level.[43] A decrease of greater than 20 points reflects clinical response.[43]

CROHN DISEASE

In CD, the location and other disease characteristics can be classified with the Paris Classification of IBD, as just described for UC.[3] Localizing the disease (e.g., mouth, stomach, small bowel) allows for medical management to be better targeted. In clinical practice, disease severity is often not standardized in the child with CD. Disease activity may be scored or quantified using the pediatric CD activity index (PCDAI).[44,45] This scoring system is commonly used in clinical trials, but its use may also be valuable in hospitalized

children. Factors addressed in the scoring system include the following: recall history of symptoms such as abdominal pain and stools; laboratory values; and physical examination findings such as abdominal tenderness and extraintestinal manifestations (Table 2).[44,45] Patient history information is 30% of the index, physical examination findings are 30%, laboratory variables account for 20%, and specific weight and height changes are 20%.[45] Activity index scoring ranges from 0–100. Disease activity scores of 0–10 indicate inactive disease, 11–30 represent mild disease, and more than 30 represents moderate to severe disease. A decrease of more than 12.5 points reflects clinical response.[44,45]

NEOPLASTIC COMPLICATIONS

Children with IBD have an increased risk of developing malignancies.[12,31] Colonic dysplasia converting to colorectal carcinoma presents with a 5.7-fold greater risk in UC with colonic involvement compared with the general population.[46] Colorectal carcinoma risk is also increased in CD at a risk of

Table 1. Pediatric Ulcerative Colitis Activity Index[43,52]

Item (Point Range[a])	Response Examples[b]
Abdominal pain (0–10)	No pain to pain cannot be ignored
Rectal bleeding (0–30)	None to large amount in > 50% of stool content
Stool consistency of most stools (0–10)	Formed to completely unformed
Number of stools per 24 hours (0–15)	0–2 to > 8
Nocturnal stools that cause wakening (0–10)	No or yes
Activity level impact (0–10)	No limitation to severe restricted activity

[a]Activity index ranges from 0–85; disease activity scores of 0–9 remission, 10–34 mild, 35–64 moderate, 65–85 severe; a decrease of ≥ 20 points reflects clinical response.
[b]Reflects range of possible responses; the references provide a complete scoring system.[43,52]

Table 2. Pediatric Crohn Disease Activity Index[44,45]

Item (Point Range[a])	Response Examples[b]
Abdominal pain (0–10)	No pain to severe pain
Stools per day (0–10)	0 with no blood to gross bleeding ≥ 6 liquid stools
Patient functioning, general well-being (0–10)	Ranging from no limitations/well to frequent limitation of activity/very poor
Hematocrit (0–5)	Values based on age and gender
Erythrocyte sedimentation rate (0–5)	< 20 to > 50
Albumin (0–10)	≥ 3.5 to ≤ 3
Weight (0–10)	Weight gain/stable to weight loss ≥ 10%
Height at diagnosis (0–10) or Height at follow-up (0–10)	< 1 channel decrease to ≥ 2 channel decrease[c] Height velocity[d] ≥ –1 SD to ≤ –2 SD
Abdomen (0–10)	No tenderness to tenderness with guarding
Perirectal disease (0–10)	None to active fistula or abscess
Extraintestinal manifestations (0–10)	None to ≥ 2

[a]Activity index ranges from 0–100; disease activity scores of 0–10 inactive, 11–30 mild, > 30 moderate to severe; a decrease of ≥ 12.5 points reflects clinical response.
[b]Reflects range of possible responses; the references provide a complete scoring system.[44,45]
[c]*Channel decrease* refers to serial height measurements that deviate across the width of a major curve on standard height-for-age chart.
[d]Height velocity is measured against population standards.

2.5-fold that of the general population.[46,47] The overall cumulative risk of colorectal cancer in CD has been described as 2.9% at 10 years.[48] Disease extent and duration of colonic inflammation are risk factors for colorectal carcinoma. Children with IBD should undergo screening colonoscopies with surveillance biopsies every 1 to 2 years, starting 7–10 years after their initial diagnosis.[12]

GOALS AND PHASES OF THERAPY

Primary goals of therapy are symptom relief and improvement of quality of life. To achieve symptom relief, therapy occurs in two phases that mimic the natural waxing and waning disease course. The two phases are *induction*, targeted at treating times of disease exacerbation to induce remission, and *maintenance*, which aims for maintaining disease inactivity.[12] In general, a patient is in the induction phase of IBD treatment until a sufficient clinical response is seen, defined as a drop in the PUCAI of at least 20 points or a reduction in PCDAI of 12.5 points or more.[43,44] A positive response to induction therapy then triggers the beginning of the maintenance phase and the initiation of maintenance treatment options. If proven to be effective, then maintenance therapy should be continued for a prolonged time, often for several years.[49] The ultimate goal of treatment is disease remission/ inactivity, which can be measured by a PUCAI or PCDAI score of less than 10 points.[43,44] In general, quality of life improves as disease control improves.[49]

Additional goals of therapy include growth optimization and treatment of complications and extraintestinal manifestations. Medication therapy, particularly corticosteroids and immunosuppressive agents, can be associated with significant adverse effects so minimizing drug toxicity is yet another goal. Mucosal healing as a target of treatment outcomes is an evolving goal; the optimal degree and depth of healing still needs further clarification.[49]

TREATMENT

There is no pharmacological cure for IBD. Therefore, treatment should be aimed at decreasing symptoms and minimizing disease complications. The treatment approach is influenced by the location and severity of disease because these features affect medication dose, route, frequency, and formulation. Depending on disease severity and location, providers often follow a step-up approach by starting agents with a more favorable adverse effect profile and then escalating therapy as needed. More recent interest is also emerging regarding a top-down approach of introducing immunosuppressant or biologic agents earlier with the hopes of altering IBD course. More studies are needed regarding the optimal treatment approach in children. Common medication classes used include corticosteroids, aminosalicylates, immunomodulators, biologics, and antibiotics. Other management modalities, such as nutritional considerations (e.g., exclusive enteral nutrition), surgical procedures (e.g., colectomy), and adjunctive therapies to address complications or symptoms are used in children with IBD.

When making therapy decisions, children should have stool cultures completed to rule out infectious etiologies or superimposed infections. For example, a child presenting with an IBD flare may have an underlying *C. difficile* infection that may or may not be the trigger for the IBD exacerbation.[24] All infections should be treated as soon as identified. Overall treatment choices must be individualized for each patient. As a chronic illness requiring lifelong treatment, adherence to IBD therapies is also imperative. Nonadherence has been found to be a common cause of disease exacerbation.[50] Furthermore, adherence has been associated with a decreased risk of colorectal cancer.[50] Simplifying a child's drug therapy regimen is important because it can have a positive impact on adherence.[12]

AMINOSALICYLATES

Oral 5-aminosalicylate (5-ASA) products are a mainstay of treatment for induction of remission in mild to moderate UC.[51,52] They are also used for maintenance therapy in UC and for mild CD.[12,52] The role of 5-ASA products in moderate to severe CD remains unclear.[49,53] Monotherapy with topical, rectal 5-ASA may be effective in some children with UC; however, combination of oral and topical 5-ASA is optimal.[52] This duel therapy of oral and topical 5-ASA has been useful in inducing remission in patients specifically with proctitis.[54] The use of 5-ASA products is also common in conjunction with other IBD drug classes with the goal to adequately control inflammation and prevent complications. A prospective study was conducted in children (age 16 years or younger) newly diagnosed with UC and prescribed 5-ASA products.[55] Study subjects received oral 5-ASA compounds with or without corticosteroids during the first 30 days of treatment. Of these, 40% taking 5-ASA as a primary maintenance therapy at diagnosis were in corticosteroid-free remission after 1 year of treatment. Several 5-ASA products have received label approval from the U.S. Food and Drug Administration (FDA) for IBD, yet efficacy data are often conflicting. Future research is needed with this class of medications in pediatric IBD.

The exact mechanism of action of the 5-ASA products in IBD is unknown. However, these drugs are thought to impact local chemical mediators of the inflammatory response and act as a free radical scavenger.[51,53] This drug class, including oral preparations, can be described as topical because they work directly on the GI mucosa, the drug's site of action.

There are several aminosalicylate preparations and formulations that deliver the active ingredient, mesalamine (5-ASA), to target sites (Table 3).[53] Sulfasalazine was the initial, prototypical aminosalicylate product, yet it is composed of sulfapyridine and mesalamine. Bacteria in the colon cleave these two portions to produce the therapeutically active component in IBD, mesalamine. Sulfapyridine, which is mostly absorbed and excreted in the urine, is thought to be responsible for many of the adverse reactions associated with sulfasalazine. The other aminosalicylate products administer mesalamine alone. These medications include mesalamine, olsalazine, and balsalazide (Table 3).[12] Olsalazine is a dimer of two 5-ASA molecules combined with an azo bond that is separated by gut bacteria in the colon whereas balsalazide is a mesalamine prodrug released in the colon.[56] Pediatric dosing of the aminosalicylates is largely extrapolated from adult studies because pediatric dose-finding trials are not available.[52]

The choice among 5-ASA products depends on delivery system site of action needed, medication formulation, and clinician/patient preference. There is no firm evidence to support superiority of one aminosalicylate product or delivery system over another.[52] Sulfasalazine, olsalazine, and balsalazide are designed to release 5-ASA in the colon, whereas some mesalamine preparations are designed to also deliver medication to the proximal and distal small intestine.[52] Specific enteric coating or timed-release properties affect the medication delivery location. For children who are unable to swallow tablets or capsules, medication formulation is very important. For example, mesalamine capsules may be opened into water or acidic food for immediate consumption.

Typically 5-ASA products are well tolerated with mild adverse effects.[53] Common adverse effects include nausea, anorexia, diarrhea, and headache.[12] Although the 5-ASA agents are considered safe compared with other IBD treatment modalities, rare adverse effects have been described in pediatric case reports, including pneumonitis, pericarditis, and interstitial nephritis.[57-59] Caution should be used with sulfasalazine in patients with a sulfa allergy because symptoms of a generalized allergic reaction have occurred in response to the sulfapyridine component. Recommended medication

monitoring includes CBC, liver chemistries, blood urea nitrogen, and creatinine, and a urinalysis.[12] Some clinicians may also recommend annual blood folate levels with sulfasalazine because it may inhibit the intestinal transport of folic acid.[52,60]

CORTICOSTEROIDS

Oral corticosteroids are effective and recommended for inducing remission in both UC and CD.[49,52] In severe IBD cases when oral corticosteroids have failed to show response, intravenous formulations may be required. Children with UC limited to the rectum, or proctitis, can also be treated using topical corticosteroids, in the dosage forms of suppositories, enemas, and rectal foams. Corticosteroids are not recommended for disease maintenance because of adverse effects. Ideally, a short corticosteroid course will serve as a bridge to long-term maintenance therapy.

Corticosteroids modulate the immune response through interaction with glucocorticoid receptors in the cell nucleus.[61] The corticosteroids (oral, intravenous, and topical) are used to suppress acute inflammation in the treatment of IBD. The steroid effects are important both systemically and locally on the mucosa.

Prednisone and prednisolone are the most commonly used oral corticosteroids. Depending on type and severity of IBD,

Table 3. Aminosalicylates (Derivatives of 5-Aminosalicylate)[12,49,52,77]

Drug	Trade Name	Formulation Considerations	Dosing Per Day	Dosing Intervals	Considerations for Pediatric Administration
Mesalamine: oral	Asacol[a,b]/ Asacol HD[c]	Delayed-release tablet; pH-released	50–100 mg/kg/day; maximum 4 g/day	Multiple daily dosing	Do not break outer coating; do not crush or chew
	Apriso[d]	Extended-release capsule	1.5 g/day	Once daily dosing	Capsules may be opened and sprinkled on soft food
	Delzicol[a,e]	Delayed-release capsule	50–100 mg/kg/day; maximum 4 g/day	Multiple daily dosing	Capsules may be opened and sprinkled on soft food
	Lialda[f]	Delayed-release tablet	2.4 g/day	Once daily dosing	Do not break outer coating; do not crush or chew
	Pentasa[f]	Extended-release capsule; time-released	50–100 mg/kg/day; maximum 4 g/day	Multiple daily dosing	Capsules may be opened and sprinkled on soft food
Mesalamine: suppository	Canasa[g]	Suppository	500 mg/day	Once daily dosing	—
Mesalamine: enema	Rowasa[h]	Enema	4 g/day	Once daily dosing	—
Sulfasalazine	Azulfidine[a,i,j]	Tablet	40–70 mg/kg/day	Multiple daily dosing	Extemporaneous formula available
	Azulfidine EN[a,i,k]	Delayed-release tablet	40–70 mg/kg/day	Multiple daily dosing	Swallow whole; do not crush or chew
Olsalazine	Dipentum[h]	Capsule	25–35 mg/kg/day	Multiple daily dosing	Capsules may be opened and sprinkled on soft food
Balsalazide	Colazal[a,d]	Capsule	2.25–6.75 g/day	Multiple daily dosing	Capsules may be opened and sprinkled on soft food

[a]Has label approval from U.S. Food and Drug Administration (FDA) for pediatric ulcerative colitis; [b]Allergan Inc., Markham, Ontario, Canada; [c]Warner Chilcott, Rockaway, NJ; [d]Valeant Pharmaceuticals, Bridgewater, NJ; [e]Allergan USA, Madison, NJ; [f]Shire US Inc, Lexington, MA; [g]Aptalis Pharma, Bridgewater, NJ; [h]Meda Pharmaceuticals, Somerset, NJ; [i]Has label approval from FDA for pediatric Crohn disease; [j]Pharmacia & Upjohn, New York, NY; [k]Pharmacia & Upjohn, Kalamazoo, MI.

a dose of 1–2 mg/kg/day, up to a maximum of 40–60 mg/day, is recommended.[12,49,52] Oral budesonide has also been suggested as an alternative because of a lower adverse effect profile secondary to its high first-pass hepatic metabolism, which maximizes the amount of corticosteroid at the site of action while minimizing systemic availability.[61] Oral budesonide release is limited to the distal ileum and proximal colon unless budesonide multi-matrix is used, which then extends the release to the entire length of the colon.[62] In adults, oral budesonide has been found to induce remission in active CD, but is less effective than oral corticosteroids and has no benefit in preventing CD relapse.[61] In adults with mild-moderate UC, budesonide multi-matrix was effective versus placebo at inducing combined clinical and endoscopic remission.[62] In children, oral budesonide is slightly less effective compared with prednisone.[63,64] Topical budesonide has been studied in adult patients with active, distal UC and proctitis and may have fewer adverse effects compared with conventional corticosteroids.[65] In patients with severe disease or with insufficient response to oral or topical therapy, intravenous methylprednisolone is used.[49,52] The introduction, dosing, and tapering of corticosteroids is not standardized and is often patient- and provider-specific. It is important to closely evaluate steroid responsiveness during the first weeks of treatment to allow for prompt dosage tapering and reduction in treatment duration.[49,52] A steroid treatment course may look like 2 weeks of prednisone at 1 mg/kg/day followed by a 3-month taper (Table 4).

Commonly reported adverse effects associated with systemic corticosteroids in pediatric IBD include the following: growth disturbance, bone loss, hypertension, hyperglycemia, facial swelling, weight gain, infection, hirsutism, acne, glaucoma, and cataracts.[12,52] Adrenal suppression may also occur and can be seen as early as 1 week after starting therapy.[49] In both adults and children, standard corticosteroids (e.g., prednisone) led to significantly more corticosteroid-related adverse effects compared with budesonide, and budesonide appeared to cause significantly more adverse effects than placebo.[61,63,64] Monitoring variables should consist of growth evaluation, eye examination, tuberculosis skin test/chest radiographic examination, and bone mineral density screening.[12] Growth and development evaluation as well as an inquiry of any visual changes should be assessed at every health care visit. A formal ophthalmologic examination is recommended every 1 to 2 years.[12] Bone mass is most readily measured by DEXA (duel-energy x-ray absorptiometry) with repeat studies no sooner than 6-month intervals, as indicated.[12]

The risk for exacerbation is smaller with prednisone doses greater than 20 mg; however, the risk for adverse events from the drug is elevated.[52] However, steroid dependency should not be accepted and therefore strategies should be used to prevent occurrence. Steroid-tapering schemes have been proposed in both pediatric UC and CD to prevent disease exacerbation and adrenal insufficiency (Table 4).[49,52] Signs and symptoms associated with an abrupt withdrawal of corticosteroids include the following: anorexia, fatigue, nausea, vomiting, dyspnea, fever, arthralgias, myalgias, and orthostatic hypotension to dizziness, fainting, and circulatory collapse. For this reason, tapering should be started early with larger reductions first and slower decreases at lower doses.[52] Patient monitoring should be continued after completion of the steroid taper because adrenal insufficiency can be seen for months after corticosteroid dosing.

ANTIBIOTICS

Antimicrobial agents may have a role in pediatric IBD as an adjunctive therapy option.[12] Increased gut permeability in IBD has been linked to translocation of altered microorganisms in the GI mucosa, therefore worsening chronic inflammation.[66] Furthermore, the microbiome has been proposed as a main factor in IBD occurrence.[66] Antibiotics are used in IBD flares to both treat disease-related intestinal infections and to address this chronic intestinal inflammation.

Because of the limited evidence of efficacy, UC guidelines do not routinely recommend antimicrobials in pediatric patients with UC.[52] Yet more recent studies suggest that broad-spectrum antibiotic cocktails may be effective in this population who are refractory to other therapy options.[66] Antibiotics do have a place in therapy in pediatric CD, especially for patients with perianal and/or colonic disease.[49] In perianal disease, metronidazole- and ciprofloxacin-based treatments have a positive short-term response and may offer a bridge to immunosuppressive agents.[49] One study showed comparable efficacy of antimicrobials to aminosalicylates in the treatment of mild, active CD.[67]

Commonly used antimicrobial agents include metronidazole and ciprofloxacin.[12] Dosing in children is not well established. Consensus recommendations list a dose of 20–30 mg/kg/day in divided doses of oral ciprofloxacin and metronidazole.[12] However, a pediatric CD guideline provides a slightly lower dosing regimen of 10–20 mg/kg/day and 20 mg/kg/day of oral metronidazole and ciprofloxacin, respectively.[49] Rifamycin antibiotics have demonstrated some efficacy in

Table 4. Prednisone/Prednisolone Tapering Plan in Inflammatory Bowel Disease After Induction Therapy Response[49,52]

Starting Dose Options	Week										
	1	2	3	4	5	6	7	8	9	10	11
	Daily Dose (mg)[a]										
A	60	50	40	35	30	25	20	15	10	5	0
B	40	40	30	30	25	25	20	15	10	5	0
C	15	15	15	12.5	10	10	7.5	7.5	5	2.5	0

[a]Table represents three sets of weekly dosing options for tapering; the references provide recommendations for other starting doses.[49,52]

adults with IBD, but more data are needed for routine use in children.[68] The primary adverse effects of these medications are the following: nausea, metallic taste, headache, dry mouth, vaginal/urethral burning, vaginal yeast infection, glossitis, stomatitis, and urticaria.[12] Development of antibiotic resistance, predisposition to *C. difficile* infection, and other medication-related adverse effects are risks associated with long-term antibiotic use.[49]

IMMUNOMODULATORS

THIOPURINES

Azathioprine and 6-mercaptopurine (6-MP) are treatment options for IBD maintenance in children.[12,49,52] The North American pediatric IBD recommendations list 6-MP and azathioprine as potential agents for both disease induction and maintenance of remission.[12] However, European guidelines for pediatric UC and CD state that the thiopurines are ineffective and are not recommended for disease induction because of a delayed time of maximal efficacy (3–6 months).[49,52] In clinical practice, these agents may be started in conjunction with induction agents with the knowledge that by the time induction medications are weaned, azathioprine or 6-MP will be effective in maintaining remission. Azathioprine is metabolized to 6-MP through the reduction by glutathione.[69] Then 6-MP is converted to 6-thiouric acid, 6-methyl-MP, and 6-thioguanine. These compounds inhibit DNA replication by impairing synthesis and they also block the purine pathway.

Clinical remission rates in patients treated with thiopurine agents vary in clinical trials, yet are thought to be around 30%.[70] However, a smaller trial in children with new-onset CD found a much higher maintenance of remission rate of greater than 90% at 18 months when treated with 6–MP and corticosteroids at diagnosis.[71] This study also demonstrated that early introduction of 6-MP (within 8 weeks of diagnosis) reduces corticosteroid exposure and improves the maintenance of clinical remission in pediatric patients with CD.[71] When used in combination, a lower steroid dose may be required and/or corticosteroids may be withdrawn sooner.

The thiopurines are prodrugs that lack intrinsic pharmacologic activity.[72] They undergo extensive metabolic transformation for clinical efficacy and subsequent toxic effects. The key enzyme for this process is thiopurine S-methyltransferase (TPMT).[72] The activity for TPMT varies among patients depending on the polymorphism of the TPMT gene. Adjusting thiopurine dosage based on TPMT status or metabolite blood levels is recommended for optimal therapy and safety.[72] Thiopurines should not be used in patients with homozygous TPMT polymorphisms or children with extremely low or deficient activity because they are at high risk for life-threatening hematologic toxicity at normal doses.[52] A dose reduction should occur in heterozygous children or in those with low activity.[52] Conversely, patients with a high level of TPMT activity may have an elevated risk of poor response. The Clinical Pharmacogenetics Implementation Consortium for Thiopurine Methyltransferase Genotype and Thiopurine Dosing has published a guideline to provide direction on TPMT interpretation and subsequent dosing schemes.[73] Adherence to a standardized approach with TPMT testing and dosing of azathioprine and 6-MP has been shown to improve IBD control and reduce glucocorticoid use.[74]

Standard dosing recommendations for 6-MP and azathioprine in children with IBD are 1–1.5 mg/kg/day and 1.5–2.5 mg/kg/day, respectively.[12] Because of the genetic variation in TPMT status among patients, the optimal dose varies. The thiopurines are generally well tolerated in children. However, toxicities can be significant and frequent monitoring is necessary. Adverse effects include nausea, vomiting, rash, anorexia, hepatotoxicity, bone marrow suppression, pancreatitis, malaise, fever, and stomatitis.[12] Important monitoring variables are TPMT measurements, CBC, liver function tests, amylase, and 6-MP metabolite levels.[12]

As with other immunomodulators and biologic agents, these medications increase a child's susceptibility to bacterial, viral, and fungal infections. Pretreatment screening (e.g., tuberculosis skin testing) and special considerations for vaccines are important (Table 5).[12] Furthermore, these drugs are associated with an increased risk of Epstein-Barr virus-related lymphoma or hemophagocytic lymphohistiocytosis.[12] The absolute risk of lymphoma is 4.5 per 10,000 patient-years in children taking thiopurines compared with 0.6 per 10,000 patient-years in the general pediatric population.[75] Child and family counseling regarding infections, vaccines, and lymphoma is important when starting immunomodulatory therapy.

METHOTREXATE

Methotrexate is recommended as a maintenance therapy option for children with CD.[49] Methotrexate can also be used in patients with thiopurine failure (those for whom treatment has failed or who are intolerant to 6-MP or azathioprine) or as an option for maintenance of steroid-free remission in children at risk of poor CD outcomes (e.g., deep colonic ulcerations on endoscopy, extensive disease, severe osteoporosis).[49] One consensus guideline for the treatment of CD in children describes several cohort studies suggesting a 50%–80% effectiveness rate with methotrexate in children who experienced a failure of response or were intolerant to thiopurines.[49] These studies showed remission rates of 37%–62%, 25%–33%, and 16%–35% at 6, 12, and greater than 12 months, respectively. Experience with methotrexate in pediatric UC is limited and not routinely recommended because of inconsistent or poor outcomes.[52] In patients with UC, its use is limited to those patients who are intolerant to thiopurines or experience treatment failure and when other alternatives are not available.[52]

Methotrexate possesses anti-inflammatory and immune-modifying effects in the treatment of IBD.[76] Methotrexate works as a folate antimetabolite to inhibit DNA synthesis, repair, and cellular replication. Methotrexate dosing in IBD is suggested at 15 mg/m[2]/week subcutaneously to a maximum dose of 25 mg/dose.[12] Adverse effects of methotrexate include nausea, myelosuppression, oral ulcers, infection, pulmonary abnormalities, and hepatitis. Oral administration of folic acid is recommended to help reduce the likelihood of oral ulcers.[49] Finally, methotrexate is strictly contraindicated in pregnancy, as well as in male partners of women who wish to become pregnant.[49] Children or adolescents of reproductive age should be educated regarding effective birth control methods. Important monitoring variables in pediatric patients include the following: CBC, liver function tests, CRP, ESR, chest radiography, pulmonary function tests, and serum creatinine levels.[12,77]

CALCINEURIN INHIBITORS

Immunosuppressants, specifically cyclosporine and tacrolimus, are useful in corticosteroid-refractory pediatric IBD induction.[12,78] They are not recommended for disease maintenance because of their adverse effect profile that includes nausea, hepatitis, nephrotoxicity, seizures, glucose intolerance, infection, and hypertension.[12] A study of adult patients with IBD on cyclosporine reported a frequent incidence of minor adverse events (e.g., paresthesias, hypertension, minor infections) and a 15% incidence of serious adverse events (e.g., nephrotoxicity, death).[79] However, tacrolimus has been used as an alternative to avoid colectomy in pediatric patients with acute severe colitis with short-term success.[52] These agents have also been used as a bridge to thiopurine therapy because they have a rapid onset of action.[52] Most of the data for these immunosuppressant agents are extrapolated from the adult population or from small studies in children. Their proposed mechanism of action in IBD is related to the inhibition of T-cell proliferation through the inhibition of IL-2 production.[80]

BIOLOGICS

Treatment of IBD has evolved considerably with the increasing use of biologic therapies. These treatments include anti-tumor necrosis factor α (TNFα) agents, anti-integrin antibodies, and an anti-IL-12/23 medication, with others under investigation. The anti-TNFα agents include infliximab, adalimumab, certolizumab pegol, and golimumab. The two commonly used biologics that have FDA label approval for use in pediatric patients are infliximab and adalimumab. The anti-integrin antibodies (vedolizumab and natalizumab) and the anti-IL-12/23 agent (ustekinumab) are alternative biologic

Table 5. Evaluation of Vaccine-Preventable Infections in Children with Inflammatory Bowel Disease[88]

Vaccine[a]	Serologic Status Check	Offer Vaccine If: Vaccinations Are Not Current or Patient Is Nonimmune and Vaccine Is Age Appropriate	Subsequent Annual Evaluation
Haemophilus influenzae type b	No	Yes	No
Hepatitis A virus	Consider	Yes	No
Hepatitis B virus	Yes: Hepatitis B surface antigen Anti-hepatitis B core antibody Anti-hepatitis B surface antibody	Yes	Repeat series once if inadequate response; recheck anti-hepatitis B surface antibody 2 mo after 3rd dose
Human papillomavirus	Gynecologic/anal examination if age appropriate	Yes (minimum age 9 years)	Yes, if age appropriate
Influenza virus, inactivated	NA	Yes (annually)	Yes
Polio, inactivated	NA	Yes	No
Measles, mumps, rubella	Yes	Yes[c,d]	No
Meningococcal conjugate A/C/Y/W-135	No	Yes	Yes, if age appropriate or risk factors present[e]
Pneumococcal conjugate (PCV13)	No	Yes[f]	None
Pneumococcal polysaccharide (PPSV23)	No	Yes[g]	Booster once 5 yr after first dose (maximum 2 lifetime doses)
Tetanus, diphtheria (Td), acellular pertussis (Tdap)	NA	Yes	After Tdap, Td booster every 10 yr
Varicella zoster	Yes[b]	Yes[b,c,d]	None

[a]Baseline evaluation should include a review of risk factors, vaccination records, and previous infections.
[b]If evidence of immunity is unknown.
[c]If not receiving immunosuppressive agent or prednisone in past 30 days or any of the following in the past 3 mo: 6-mercaptopurine, methotrexate, azathioprine, or any biologic agent.
[d]Dispense if live virus vaccine can be administered 4 wk before starting immunosuppressive therapy.
[e]Adolescents may require a booster dose in accordance with the Advisory Committee on Immunization Practices vaccine schedule.
[f]For children age 6–18 yr with no previous doses of PCV7 or PCV13, give 1 dose of PCV13, followed 8 wk later by PPSV23.
[g]If both PCV13 and PPSV23 are indicated, then PCV13 should be given first, followed by PPSV23 given 8 wk after.

Adapted with permission from: Ardura MI, Toussi SS, Siegel JD, et al. NASPHGHAN clinical report: surveillance, diagnosis, and prevention of infectious diseases in pediatric patients with inflammatory bowel disease receiving tumor necrosis factor-α inhibitors. J Pediatr Gastroenterol Nutr 2016;63:130–55

agents approved for IBD in adults, but further studies are needed to determine their place in the treatment of pediatric IBD.[81] As agents recommended in pediatric IBD, focus of the biologics in this chapter will highlight the anti-TNFα agents infliximab and adalimumab. The anti-TNFα biologics are administered by infusion (infliximab) or by subcutaneous injection (adalimumab).[40]

ANTI-TUMOR NECROSIS FACTOR AGENTS

Biologic agents that target TNFα, a major proinflammatory pathogenic cytokine present in UC and CD, have become an integral player in the treatment of pediatric IBD induction and maintenance.[12,49,52] They are often used in corticosteroid-refractory IBD or in patients who remain corticosteroid dependent despite immunomodulatory therapy.[40] The anti-TNFα class is more effective compared with thiopurines for inducing complete mucosal healing in the intestine and with perianal fistulas in CD.[82] Furthermore, anti-TNFα agents have shown a positive impact on linear growth in children with an associated growth failure.[83] The anti-TNFα biologic agents are typically at the top of the step-up treatment model, in which a patient has tried a maintenance therapy regimen of 5-ASA agents and immunomodulators without complete success.[84] An exception to this step-up treatment model, in which a patient may start on a biologic agent (i.e., a top-down approach), would be for treatment of CD in children with severe, deep mucosal ulcerations, perianal fistulas, or significant growth failure.[40] In addition, there is evidence that early induction with infliximab (e.g., at diagnosis) is effective for decreasing relapse rates compared with the conventional, step-up approach.[85] Patient-specific risks and benefits must be taken into consideration with the timing of biologic use.

Infliximab is a chimeric monoclonal antibody targeting the cytokine TNFα. Infliximab has demonstrated efficacy in both inducing and maintaining remission in pediatric IBD. Studies have found an 88% response rate to infliximab with 59% in remission at week 10 in children with CD.[83] A clinical response to treatment was defined as a decrease from baseline of the PCDAI score of at least 15 and having a total score of 30 or less. Another study in children with UC used the validated PUCAI scoring system and a more invasive scoring system requiring endoscopy to determine efficacy. This study showed a 73% response rate at 8 weeks in patients for whom conventional therapy failed.[86] Dosing regimens for infliximab in children involve three initial doses (5 mg/kg/dose at 0, 2, and 6 weeks) followed by a maintenance dose (5 mg/kg/dose) every 8 weeks thereafter.[12,49,52] If the response to therapy is incomplete, then the dose can be increased to 10 mg/kg/dose.[12,49] Increasing the frequency of infusions to every 4-6 weeks has also been described.[49,87] Of importance, regularly scheduled treatment can help to optimize efficacy and prevent loss of drug response.

Infliximab is typically well tolerated; however, rare but serious adverse effects are of concern. For example, anti-TNFα medications increase the child's risk for severe infections, specifically with intracellular bacteria, mycobacteria, fungi, and some viruses.[40,88] Before drug initiation, screening for tuberculosis, evaluation of vaccination status, titers for measles, hepatitis B virus serology, and documentation of immunity

to varicella should be completed (Table 5).[88] The North American Society for Pediatric Gastroenterology, Hepatology & Nutrition has published recommendations for surveillance, diagnosis, and prevention of infectious disease in children on anti-TNFα agents.[88] These guidelines should be reviewed before medication initiation for specific recommendations, as applicable, such as prevention and avoidance of risk for IBD patients living in an area endemic for histoplasmosis.[88]

Hepatosplenic T-cell lymphoma (HSTCL) has been reported in very few adolescents and young adults with IBD on infliximab in combination with an immunosuppressant agent (e.g., azathioprine, prednisone).[89] The true long-term risks of lymphoma and other malignancies from anti-TNFα agents alone are unknown. Because of possible increased risks, the FDA performed a review and strengthened warnings in the prescribing information for these agents.[90] A discussion of potential risks and benefits with patients and families is recommended before anti-TNFα initiation.

More common adverse effects from anti-TNFα agents include infusion reactions, nausea, fever/chills, psoriatic rash, fatigue, and hives.[12] One study noted infusion reactions in 15% of children and adolescents on infliximab.[91] Infusion reactions can present with both acute (e.g., chest tightness, vomiting) or delayed (e.g., fever, rash) symptoms. Most reactions are mild and respond to reducing the infusion rate or temporarily stopping the infusion.[49] Premedication with acetaminophen, corticosteroids, or antihistamines are not indicated. Anti-TNFα agents can also induce the appearance of antibodies.[92] These antibodies can lead to acute infusion reactions, delayed hypersensitivity reactions, decreased serum drug levels, and loss of response.[49] Even with adequate serum drug levels, the presence of antibodies has been associated with disease activity.[93] Episodic treatment and low infliximab trough levels may increase the risk of anti-infliximab antibody formation.[81,92] Furthermore, an infliximab trough concentration of more than 3 mcg/mL or more than 5 mcg/mL has been associated with remission.[93-95] The upper limit of the trough target is 8–10 mcg/mL, and a dose reduction may be considered if remission has been achieved.[49,94] Currently, to achieve higher infliximab trough levels the dose can be increased or the administration interval between infusions can be shortened.[81] However, one study found higher infliximab trough levels was associated with interval shortening rather than dose escalation in a retrospective chart review of pediatrics with IBD.[87] The therapeutic drug window during induction and optimal timing to start measurements of serum levels are still evolving.[96]

Recommended routine monitoring for the anti-TNFα class involves infectious diseases screening at therapy onset, routine skin examination, and CBC and liver chemistries every 3–6 months.[12] When a partial or complete loss of response is seen, serum trough levels and the measurement of antibodies may be warranted.[49] Some investigators also call for the consideration of more routine anti-TNFα trough levels and anti-drug antibodies monitoring as part of a tailored program to ensure medication efficacy.[81,97]

Adalimumab is a humanized monoclonal antibody against TNFα. Its use is often reserved for patients who do not respond, those who develop infusions reactions, or those who have lost response to infliximab.[52,81,98] However, available data in pediatric CD suggest that both infliximab and adalimumab show comparable efficacy and safety profiles in anti-TNFα–naive patients.[49] One study found that infliximab-naive patients had greater remission and response rates than infliximab-experienced patients when being treated with adalimumab.[99] This study found adalimumab to successfully induce and maintain remission with more than 80% response to therapy within 4 weeks of treatment.[99] Clinical response and remission were determined based on PCDAI scoring, defined as a decrease of 15 or more points from baseline and PCDAI of 10 or less, respectively. Several adalimumab dosing schemes have been studied in pediatric IBD. The optimal dose remains unknown. For example, some references will recommend an induction dose of 160 mg/dose subcutaneously on week 0, followed by 80 mg on week 2 with a 20- or 40- mg maintenance dose for a child weighing more than or equal to 40 kg to be given every other week.[12,99] However, some newer studies have found weekly dosing to be clinically beneficial in specific pediatric IBD populations.[100] One investigation found that weekly maintenance adalimumab dosing (20 or 40 mg weekly for a child weighing more than or equal to 40 kg) was clinically beneficial for pediatric patients with CD who were nonresponsive or experienced a flare on an every-other-week dosing scheme.[100]

The administration and dosage form of adalimumab provides advantages over infliximab. Adalimumab is given subcutaneously rather than by continuous infusion, which allows home administration. Also, by being a fully humanized antibody, its risk for immune reactions is lessened.[101] General adverse effects and monitoring variables are similar among the anti-TNFα class of medications. As with infliximab, adalimumab trough levels are related to drug efficacy; however, more data are needed to determine the role of measuring drug and antibody levels in clinical practice.[81] Continued study is needed regarding biologic therapy use in pediatrics, including comparative studies of the anti-TNFα agents, combination studies of the anti-TNFα agents plus an immunomodulator, and the newer categories of biologic drugs.

PROBIOTICS

Probiotic use has been investigated in pediatric IBD, with minimal improvements and with mixed results. The European consensus guidelines for UC highlight the need for more evidence, yet they consider probiotic use in children with mild UC intolerant to 5-ASA or as an adjuvant in patients with mild residual activity despite standard treatment.[52] However, some organizations and reviews point to the limited literature that supports probiotic use and thus does not recommend use for maintenance of remission.[49] A recent guideline looking at clinical nutrition in IBD states that probiotics may be useful in UC but not in CD.[102] The pediatric North American recommendations do not endorse probiotic use at this time.[12] Probiotics may modulate intestinal microbial balance, thus improving gut barrier function and improving the local immune response.[103]

Specific probiotic agents that have been studied and have shown some efficacy for mild-moderate UC for induction and maintenance include *Escherichia coli* Nissele 1917 or VSL#3.[102,104] The dosing of VSL#3 is based on age or weight and ranges from 450 billion–1800 billion bacteria/day.[104] Other small trials of probiotics in children suggest possible efficacy with *Lactobacillus ruteri* and *Lactobacillus GG*.[102,105,106] Probiotic studies are ongoing and warranted in pediatric IBD.

TREATMENT ALGORITHMS

The approach to IBD management in children and adolescents is individualized. Treatment paradigms also exist for pediatric CD in a step-up and top-down approach.[49] Initial drug therapy regimens differ based on classification of IBD, either UC or CD, and disease severity (mild, moderate, or severe based on disease activity index scoring). Several guidelines or recommendations are available internationally with management algorithms.[12,49,52] One algorithm in pediatric UC, for example, starts with oral 5-ASA products in mild or moderate disease onset.[52] Oral corticosteroids would be added for patients with an insufficient response. Response is defined as PUCAI drop of at least 20 points with the goal PUCAI less than 10. Once in maintenance, 5-ASA remains a therapy of preference. As disease severity increases, thiopurines are added, with biologics as the last line. This strategy follows the step-up approach in a child with UC. An example of the top-down approach is a child with significant fistulizing CD in the presence of predictors of severe disease course.[49] This patient may be a candidate for anti-TNFα in initial induction therapy. Other approaches and order of therapies are available and appropriate based on the individual child or adolescent with IBD.

The consideration of drug discontinuation or stepping down after a sustained remission is patient specific and should take features such as growth and puberty into account. If a patient is on combination therapy, a step-down approach may be recommended to reduce drug adverse effects and costs.[49] It is also important to confirm complete mucosal healing and to ensure normal hemoglobin, white blood cell count, CRP, and ESR before making drug therapy changes. In CD, for example, stopping all treatments is usually not advisable except in children with very mild disease who have been in a deep, long remission.[49] Even in this situation, a family discussion on the risk of relapse and other complications is advised.

CONCLUSIONS

Inflammatory bowel disease is a chronic inflammatory illness that impacts the GI tract. It is composed of two separate disorders, UC and CD. Both UC and CD are increasingly common in pediatric patients of all ages. In children with IBD it is imperative to recommend positive nutrition and physical activity practices to promote bone health. Nutritional assessments should be ongoing because these children are at risk of macro- and micronutrient deficiencies. Many treatment modalities exist for the management of IBD in children and adolescents. Because there is no pharmacologic cure for IBD, drug therapy is aimed at controlling symptoms and lessening long-term complications. Common medication classes used include aminosalicylates, corticosteroids, antibiotics, immunomodulators, and biologics. Monitoring for drug efficacy and toxicity in addition to providing patient and family education are critical.

A 17-year-old, 51-kg white female received a diagnosis of moderate to severe Crohn disease (CD) about 11 months ago. She is currently on her second corticosteroid burst to induce remission. Her first course of corticosteroids was at diagnosis. Her recent symptoms of abdominal pain, bloody/loose stools, fatigue, and occasional difficulty with daily functions have significantly improved on prednisone therapy. She is being evaluated today for her response to prednisone induction therapy and to determine appropriate maintenance therapy at this time.

Medical history: CD, allergic rhinitis (diagnosed 10 years ago)

Social history: Lives with parents; has an older brother who no longer lives at home. One indoor dog at home. Attends high school as a senior and plans to attend college next fall. Denies sexual activity, tobacco, alcohol, or drug use.

Family history: Father has hypertension, hyperlipidemia, asthma, and allergic rhinitis; mother has osteopenia; brother has type 1 diabetes mellitus (diagnosed at 11 years), allergic rhinitis, and eczema

Allergies: Sulfa allergy (severe rash)

Laboratory findings: Laboratory data were not drawn at the current clinic visit

Current Medications

Medication	Dose	Start Date	Last Dose	Adherence
Cetirizine 10 mg	1 tablet/day (10 mg), oral	4 yr ago	Today	Misses about 2 doses/wk
Mesalamine 250 mg	3 capsules (750 mg) four times per day, oral, for total daily dose of 3000 mg	11 mo ago	Today	No missed doses
Prednisone 20 mg	2 tablets (40 mg) daily in morning, oral	14 days ago	Today	No missed doses

Immunizations

Vaccine	Up-to-Date	Number of Doses and Administration by Patient Age
Haemophilus influenza type b	Yes	3 doses before 18 mo
Hepatitis A virus	Yes	2 doses before 24 mo
Hepatitis B virus	Yes	3 doses before 18 mo
Human papillomavirus	No	None received
Influenza virus, inactivated	Yes	1 dose during October of current year
Polio, inactivated	Yes	4 doses before 7 yr
Measles, mumps, rubella	No	1 dose at 12 mo
Meningococcal conjugate	Yes	Booster at 16 yr
Pneumococcal conjugate (PCV13)	No	None received
Pneumococcal polysaccharide (PPSV23)	No	None received
Diphtheria, tetanus, and acellular pertussis (DTaP) or Tetanus, diphtheria, and acellular pertussis (Tdap)	Yes	DTaP: 5 doses before 7 yr Tdap: at age 12 yr
Varicella zoster	Yes	2 doses before 7 yr

Vital signs:

BP 120/78 mm Hg, HR 65 beats/minute, Wt 51 kg, Ht 63 inches

Peripheral oxygen saturation 98% on room air

Physical examination:

General: Well-developed female in no apparent distress

HEENT: Pupils equal, round, reactive to light and accommodation; extraocular eye movements intact; tympanic membranes clear bilaterally

Pulmonary: Clear to auscultation bilaterally; no retractions or nasal flaring

Cardiovascular: Regular rate and rhythm without murmurs, gallops, or rubs

Abdomen: Mild pain with palpation only

Musculoskeletal: No edema; capillary refill 1 second

Skin: No lesions or rashes

Genital/rectal: One indolent perirectal fistula; two asymptomatic perirectal skin tags

Neuro: Awake, alert, and oriented to person, place, time, and situation; normal upper and lower extremity strength bilaterally; reflexes normal

Pediatric Crohn Disease Activity Index (PCDAI) score: 35 (moderate to severe disease activity) 2 weeks ago, before corticosteroid induction

Assessment

A 17-year-old female with recent, active CD showing clinical response on induction therapy with corticosteroids. PCDAI score today is 20.

1. Using the plan principle of the Pharmacists' Patient Care Process from the Joint Commission of Pharmacy Practitioners, develop a treatment plan for tapering prednisone that will help prevent CD exacerbation and adrenal insufficiency.

Corticosteroid tapering is necessary for CD because patients often require longer treatment durations for induction. One consensus guideline for the management of pediatric CD describes a common practice of decreasing the dose around every 7–10 days. Furthermore, the risk for exacerbation is smaller with prednisone doses greater than 20 mg; however, the threat for adverse effects is higher at elevated doses. Therefore, the taper may be most successful by starting with larger decreases initially and slower decrements at lower doses. An example of a prednisone taper follows:

Prednisone Taper by Weeks 1–11

1	2	3	4	5	6	7	8	9	10	11
40 mg	40 mg	30 mg	30 mg	25 mg	25 mg	20 mg	15 mg	10 mg	5 mg	STOP

To reduce the potential for growth and adrenal suppression, a single total oral dose should be given in the morning. Items such as an exacerbation of symptoms can slow the steroid dosage taper. In the event of disease exacerbations, one option is to increase the corticosteroid dose to that of the previous 1–2 weeks for 1 week and then start weaning again more slowly. The end goal is to successfully wean the patient's prednisone to stop completely while maintaining disease control.

Case (continued). The pediatric gastroenterologist is interested in starting the patient on azathioprine maintenance therapy.

2. Outside of baseline laboratory monitoring (e.g., complete blood count, liver function tests), what testing should be completed before initiation? Why is this testing important? What azathioprine dosage is recommended, assuming that the testing shows normal metabolism?

Thiopurine methyltransferase (TPMT) genotype or phenotype activity testing should be completed before azathioprine initiation. Adjusting the thiopurine dosage based on TPMT status and/or metabolite blood levels is recommended for optimal therapy and safety. Testing for the TPMT activity helps in the identification of patients at risk of early profound myelosuppression. The dose should be reduced in heterozygous patients or in those with low TPMT activity. Thiopurines should not be used in children with homozygous TPMT polymorphisms or those with extremely low TPMT activity. In patients with normal TPMT activity, the starting dosage for azathioprine is 1.5–2.5 mg/kg once daily. In this 51-kg patient, a dose of 100 mg daily would provide about 2 mg/kg/day.

3. Vaccinations are imperative in children and adolescents with inflammatory bowel disease (IBD), especially in patients before starting immunomodulatory or biologic therapies. After review of the patient's immunization record, what vaccines would you recommend at this time?

The patient is not up-to-date with her human papillomavirus (HPV), measles, mumps, and rubella (MMR), and pneumococcal vaccinations. Recommendations for vaccinating this patient follow:

Vaccine	Recommendations
HPV	A 3-dose series as recommended by the Advisory Committee on Immunization Practices (ACIP)
MMR	1 dose as recommended by the ACIP; however, this patient is NOT a candidate at this time because of her current immunosuppressive therapy (prednisone) Also, azathioprine initiation is a contraindication for MMR vaccination at this time
Pneumococcal conjugate (PCV13) Pneumococcal polysaccharide (PPSV23)	1 dose of PCV13 followed by a single dose of PPSV23, with 8 wk between doses

Case (continued). The patient returns to the gastroenterologist about 5 months after initiation of azathioprine. She has had to slow her corticosteroid taper twice and she remains on 20 mg/day of prednisone. Because of the inability to wean her corticosteroids without the return of her previous CD symptoms, a failure of azathioprine therapy is determined. When discussing other maintenance therapy alternatives, the patient wanted to know more about biologic treatment options.

4. What specific biologic drugs could you recommend for this patient for management of her CD? What common adverse effects are of concern with this class of medications? Assuming the most commonly used biologic is selected for her next step in therapy, what regimen and monitoring would you recommend?

The two most commonly used biologic agents that have FDA label approval in pediatric CD are infliximab and adalimumab. There are no head-to-head trials comparing these agents in children. Guidelines state that both infliximab and adalimumab show comparable efficacy and adverse effect profiles in pediatric CD. Because infliximab was the first approved biologic in pediatric IBD, some clinicians may begin with this agent and reserve adalimumab for infliximab nonresponders, those who develop infusion reactions, or those who have lost response to infliximab. However, both are appropriate options for this patient. Points to consider when making a decision should include route of delivery, patient preference, provider experience, and cost/insurance coverage. Common adverse effects linked to this medication class include, infusion/local reactions, nausea, fever/chills, psoriatic rash, fatigue, and hives. The risk of opportunistic infections and the potential risk of malignancy should also be discussed with the patient and her family. If infliximab is selected as her next step in therapy, the dose in children is an initial three doses of 5 mg/kg/dose at 0, 2, and 6 weeks followed by a maintenance dose of 5 mg/kg/dose every 8 weeks thereafter. Therefore, a dose of 250 mg intravenously at weeks 0, 2, and 6 then the same dose every 8 weeks thereafter is recommended for this 51 kg patient. She should be screened for tuberculosis by purified protein derivative (PPD) or chest radiograph and active infection before the initial dose. Also before the first dose of infliximab, she must be evaluated for vaccination status, titers for measles, hepatitis B serology, and immunity to varicella. Before every additional dose, she should be evaluated for active infection. During and after infliximab administration she should be evaluated for acute (e.g., chest tightness, vomiting) and delayed (e.g., fever, rash) infusion reactions. Lastly, routine skin examinations and complete blood count and liver chemistries should be performed every 3–6 months. If partial or complete loss of response to infliximab is seen, a measurement of trough levels and antibodies may be needed.

REFERENCES

1. Uhlig HH, Schwerd T, Koletzko S, et al. The diagnostic approach to monogenic very early onset inflammatory bowel disease. Gastroenterology 2014;147:990-1007.
2. Heyman MB, Kirschner BS, Gold BD, et al. Children with early-onset inflammatory bowel disease (IBD): analysis of a pediatric IBD consortium registry. J Pediatr 2005;146:35-40.
3. Levine A, Griffiths A, Markowitz J, et al. Pediatric modification of the Montreal Classification for inflammatory bowel disease: the Paris Classification. Inflamm Bowel Dis 2011;17:1314-21.
4. Johnston RD, Logan RF. What is the peak age for onset of IBD? Inflamm Bowel Disease 2008;14:S4-5.
5. Kappelman MD, Moore KR, Allen JK, et al. Recent trends in the prevalence of Crohn's disease and ulcerative colitis in a commercially insured US population. Dig Dis Sci 2013;58:519-25.
6. Turunen P, Kolho KL, Auvinen A, et al. Incidence of inflammatory bowel disease in Finnish children 1987-2003. Inflamm Bowel Dis 2006;12:677-83.
7. Armitage E, Drummond H, Ghosh S, et al. Incidence of juvenile-onset Crohn's disease in Scotland. Lancet 1999;353:1496-7.
8. Vander Zagg-Loonen HJ, Casparie M, Taminiau JA, et al. The incidence of pediatric inflammatory bowel disease in the Netherlands: 1999–2001. J Pediatr Gastroenterol Nutr 2004;38:302-7.
9. Armitage E, Drummond HE, Wilson DC, et al. Increasing incidence of both juvenile-onset Crohn's disease and ulcerative colitis in Scotland. Eur J Gastroenterol Hepatol 2001;13:1439-47.
10. Malaty HM, Fan X, Opekun AR, et al. Rising incidence of inflammatory bowel disease among children: a 12-year study. J Pediatr Gastroenterol Nutr 2010;50:27-31.
11. Adamiak T, Walkiewicz-Jedrzejczak D, Fish D, et al. Incidence, clinical characteristics, and natural history of IBD in Wisconsin: a population-based epidemiological study. Inflamm Bowel Dis 2013;19:1218-23.
12. Rufo PA, Denson LA, Sylvester FA, et al. Health supervision in the management of children and adolescents with IBD: NASPGHAN recommendations. J Pediatr Gastroenterol Nutr 2012;55:93-108.
13. Kugathasan S, Judd RH, Hoffmann RG, et al. Epidemiologic and clinical characteristics of children with newly diagnosed inflammatory bowel disease in Wisconsin: a statewide population-based study. J Pediatr 2003;143:525-31.
14. Hanauer SB. Inflammatory bowel disease: epidemiology, pathogenesis, and therapeutic opportunities. Inflamm Bowel Dis 2006;12:S3-S9.
15. Bernstein CN, Blanchard JF, Rawsthorne P, et al. Epidemiology of Crohn's disease and ulcerative colitis in a central Canadian province: a population-based study. Am J Epidemiol 1999;149:916-24.
16. Molodecky NA, Kaplan GG. Environmental risk factors for inflammatory bowel disease. Gastroenterol Hepatol (N Y) 2010;6:339-46.
17. Gersemann M, Wehkamp J, Strange EF. Innate immune dysfunction in inflammatory bowel disease. J Intern Med 2012;271:421-8.
18. Scharl M, Rogler G. Inflammatory bowel disease pathogenesis: what is new? Curr Opin Gastroenterol 2012;28:301-9.
19. Nanau R, Neuman MG. Metabolome and inflammasome in inflammatory bowel disease. Transl Res 2012;160:1-28.
20. Rampton DS. The influence of stress on the development and severity of immune mediated diseases. J Rheumatol 2011;38:43-7.
21. Koloski NA, Bret L, Radford-Smith G. Hygiene hypothesis in inflammatory bowel disease: a critical review of the literature. World J Gasterenterol 2008;14:165-73.
22. Cassatella M. The production of cytokines by polymorphonuclear neutrophils. Immunol Today 1995;16:21-26.
23. Hendrickson BA, Gokhale R, Cho JH. Clinical aspects and pathophysiology of inflammatory bowel disease. Clin Microbiol Rev 2002;15:79-94.
24. Martinelli M, Strisciuglio C, Veres G, et al. Clostridium difficile and pediatric inflammatory bowel disease: a prospective, comparative, multicenter, ESPGHAN study. Inflamm Bowel Dis 2014;20:2219-25.
25. Evans JM, McMahon AD, Murray FE, et al. Non-steroidal anti-inflammatories are associated with emergence admission to hospital for colitis due to inflammatory bowel disease. Gut 1997;40:619-22.
26. Dotson JL, Hyams JS, Markowitz J, et al. Extraintestinal manifestations of pediatric inflammatory bowel disease and their relation to disease type and severity. J Pediatr Gastroenterol Nutr 2010;51:140-5.
27. Pfefferkorn M, Burke G, Griffiths A, et al. Growth abnormalities persist in newly diagnosed children with Crohn disease despite current treatment paradigms. J Pediatr Gasterenterol Nutr 2009;48:168-74.
28. Pappa H, Thayu M, Sylvester F, et al. Skeletal health of children and adolescents with inflammatory bowel disease. J Pediatr Gastroenterol Nutr 2011;53:11-25.
29. Werlin SL, Grand RJ. Severe colitis in children and adolescents: diagnosis, course, and treatment. Gastroenterology 1977;73:828-32.
30. Gan SI, Beck PL. A new look at toxic megacolon: an update and review of incidence, etiology, pathogenesis and management. Am J Gastroenterol 2003;98:2363-71.
31. Baumgert DC, Sandborn WJ. Inflammatory bowel disease: clinical aspects and established and evolving therapies. Lancet 2007;369:1641-57.

32. Heuschkel R, Salvestrini C, Beattie RM, et al. Guidelines for the management of growth failure in childhood inflammatory bowel disease. Inflamm Bowel Dis 2008;14:839-49.

33. Kim SC, Ferry GD. Inflammatory bowel disease in pediatric and adolescent patients: clinical, therapeutic, and psychosocial considerations. Gastroenterology 2004;126:1550-60.

34. Lichtenstein GR, Hanauer SB, Sandborn WJ, The Practice Parameters Committee of the American College of Gastroenterology. Management of Crohn's disease in adults. Am J Gasteroenterol 2009;104:465-83.

35. Hartman C, Eliakim R, Shamir R. Nutritional status and nutritional therapy in inflammatory bowel disease. World J Gasteroenterol 2009;15:2570-8.

36. Filippi J, Al-Jaouni R, Wiroth JB, et al. Nutritional deficiencies in patients with Crohn's disease in remission. Inflamm Bowel Dis 2006;12:185-91.

37. Larsen S, Bendtzen K, Nielsen OH. Extraintestinal manifestations of inflammatory bowel disease: epidemiology, diagnosis, and management. Ann Med 2010;42:97-114.

38. North American Society for Pediatric Gastroenterology, Hepatology, and Nutrition, Colitis Foundation of America, Boustaros A, et al. Differentiating ulcerative colitis from Crohn disease in children and young adults: report of a working group of the North American Society for Pediatric Gastroenterology, Hepatology, and Nutrition and the Crohn's and Colitis Foundation of America. J Pediatr Gastroenterol Nutr 2007;44:653-74.

39. Mack DR, Langton C, Markowitz J, et al. Laboratory values for children with newly diagnosed inflammatory bowel disease. Pediatrics 2007;119:1113-9.

40. Rosen MJ, Dhawan A, Saeed SA. Inflammatory bowel disease in children and adolescents. JAMA Pediatr 2015;169:1053-60.

41. Holtman GA, Leeuwen YL, Day AS, et al. Use of laboratory markers in addition to symptoms for diagnosis of inflammatory bowel disease in children. JAMA Pediatr 2017;171;984-991.

42. Birimberg-Schwartz L, Wilson DC, Kolho KL, et al. pANCA and ASCA in children with IBD-unclassified, Crohn's colitis, and ulcerative—a longitudinal report from the IBD Porto Group of ESPGHAN. Inflamm Bowel Dis 2016;22:1908-14.

43. Turner D, Otley AR, Mack D, et al. Development, validation, and evaluation of a pediatric ulcerative colitis activity index: a prospective multicenter study. Gastroenterology 2007;133:423-32.

44. Hyams J, Markowitz J, Otley A, et al. Evaluation of the pediatric Crohn disease activity index: a prospective multicenter experience. J Pediatr Gastroenterol Nutr 2005;41:416-21.

45. Hyams JS, Ferry GD, Mandel FS, et al. Development and validation of a pediatric Crohn's disease activity index. J Pediatr Gastroenterol Nutr 1991;12:439-47.

46. Velayos F. Managing risks of neoplasia in inflammatory bowel disease. Curr Gastroenterol Rep 2012;14:174-80.

47. Jess T, Gamborg M, Matzen P, et al. Increased risk of intestinal cancer in Crohn's disease: a meta-analysis of population-based cohort studies. Am J Gastroenterol 2005;100:2724-9.

48. Canavan C, Abrams KR, Mayberry J. Meta-analysis: colorectal and small bowel cancer risk in patients with Crohn's disease. Aliment Pharmacol Ther 2006;23:1097-104.

49. Ruemmele FM, Veres G, Kolho KL, et al. Consensus guidelines of ECCO/ESPGHAN on the medical management of pediatric Crohn's disease. J Crohns Colitis 2014;8:1179-207.

50. Kane S, Dixon L. Adherence rates with infliximab therapy in Crohn's disease. Aliment Pharmacol Ther 2006;24:1099-103.

51. Hanauer SB. Oral or topical 5-ASA in ulcerative colitis. Dig Dis 2016;34:122-4.

52. Turner D, Levine A, Escher JC, et al. Management of pediatric ulcerative colitis: joint ECCO and ESPGHAN evidence-based consensus guidelines. J Pediatr Gastroenterol Nutr 2012; 55:340-61.

53. Lim WC, Wang Y, MacDonald JK, et al. Aminosalicylates for induction of remission or response in Crohn's disease. Cochrane Database Syst Rev 2016;7:CD008870.

54. Vecchi M, Meucci G, Gionchetti P, et al. Oral versus combination mesalazine therapy in active ulcerative colitis: a double-blind, double-dummy randomized multicenter study. Aliment Pharmacol Ther 2001;15:251-6.

55. Zeisler B, Lerer T, Markowitz J, et al. Outcome following aminosalicylate therapy in children newly diagnosed as having ulcerative colitis. J Pediatr Gastroenterol Nutr 2013;56:12-8.

56. Campregher C, Gasche C. Aminosalicylates. Best Pract Res Clin Gastroenterol 2011;25:535-46.

57. Kohli R, Melin-Aldana H, Sentongo TA. Mesalamine-induced pneumonitis during therapy for chronic inflammatory bowel disease: a pediatric care report. J Pediatr Gastroenterol Nutr 2005;41:479-82.

58. Sentongo TA, Piccoli DA. Recurrent pericarditis due to mesalamine hypersensitivity: a pediatric case report and review of the literature. J Pediatr Gastroenterol Nutr 1998;27:344-7.

59. Arend LJ, Springate JE. Interstitial nephritis form mesalazine: case report and literature review. Pediatr Nephrol 2004;19:550-3.

60. Selhub J, Dhar GJ, Rosenberg IH. Inhibition of folate enzymes by sulfasalazine. J Clin Invest 1978;61:221-4.

61. Ford AC, Bernstein CA, Khan KJ. Glucocorticosteroid therapy in inflammatory bowel disease: systematic review and meta-analysis. Am J Gastroenterol 2011;106:590-9.

62. Travis SPL, Danese S, Kupcinskas L, et al. Once-daily budesonide MMX in active, mild-to-moderate ulcerative colitis: results from the randomized CORE II study. Gut 2014;63:433-41.

63. Levine A, Weizman Z, Broide E, et al. A comparison of budesonide and prednisone for the treatment of active pediatric Crohn disease. J Pediatr Gastroenterol Nutr 2003;36:248-52.

64. Escher JC, European Collaborative Research Group on Budesonide in Paediatric IBD. Budesonide versus prednisolone for the treatment of active Crohn's disease in children: a randomized, double-blind, controlled, multicentre trial. Eur J Gastroenterol Hepatol 2004;16:47-54.

65. Hanauer SB, Robinson M, Pruitt R, et al. Budesonide enema for the treatment of active, distal ulcerative colitis and proctitis: a dose-ranging study. U.S. Budesonide enema study group. Gastroenterology 1998;115:525-32.

66. Turner D, Levine A, Kolho KL, et al. Combination of oral antibiotics may be effective in severe pediatric ulcerative colitis: a preliminary report. J Crohns Colitis 2014;8:1464-70.

67. Prantera C, Zannoni F, Scribano ML, et al. An antibiotic regimen for the treatment of active Crohn's disease: a randomized, controlled clinical trial of metronidazole plus ciprofloxacin. Am J Gastroenterol 1996;91:328-32.

68. Khan KJ, Ullman TZ, Ford AC, et al. Antibiotic therapy in inflammatory bowel disease: a systematic review and meta-analysis. Am J Gastroenterol 2011;106:661-73.

69. Taylor AL, Watson CJE, Bradley JA. Immunosuppressive agents in solid organ transplantation: mechanisms of action and therapeutic efficacy. Crit Rev Oncol Hematol 2005;56:23-46.

70. Boyle BM, Kappelman MD, Colletti RB, et al. Routine use of thiopurine in maintaining remission in pediatric Crohn's disease. World J Gastroenterol 2014;20:9185-90.

71. Markowitz J, Grancher K, Kohn N, et al. A multicenter trial of 6-mercaptopurine and prednisone in children with newly diagnosed Crohn's disease. Gastroenterology 2000;119:895-902.

72. Chouchana L, Narjoz C, Beaune P, et al. Review article: the benefits of pharmacogenetics for improving thiopurine therapy in inflammatory bowel disease. Aliment Pharmacol Ther 2012; 35:15-36.

73. Relling MV, Gardner EE, Sandborn WJ, et al. Clinical Pharmacogenetics Implementation Consortium for Thiopurine Methyltransferase Genotype and Thiopurine Dosing: 2013 update. Clin Pharmacol Ther 2013;93:324-5.

74. Banerjee S, Bishop WP. Evolution of thiopurine use in a pediatric inflammatory bowel disease in an academic center: role of thiopurine methyltransferase and 6-mercaptopurine metabolite measurements. J Pediatr Gastroenterol Nutr 2006;43:324-30.

75. Dulai PS, Thompson KD, Blunt HB, et al. Risks of serious infection or lymphoma with anti-tumor necrosis factor therapy for pediatric inflammatory bowel disease: a systematic review. Clin Gastroenterol Hepatol 2014;12:1443-51.

76. Egan LJ, Sandborn WJ. Methotrexate for inflammatory bowel disease: pharmacology and preliminary results. Mayo Clin Proc 1996;71:69-80.

77. Lexicomp Online, Pediatric and Neonatal Lexi-Drugs Online [Internet database]. Hudson, OH: Lexi-Comp. Updated periodically.

78. Watson S, Pensabene L, Mitchell P, et al. Outcome and adverse events in children and young adults undergoing tacrolimus therapy for steroid-refractory colitis. Inflamm Bowel Dis 2011; 17:22-9.

79. Sternthal MB, Murphy SJ, George J, et al. Adverse events associated with the use of cyclosporine in patients with inflammatory bowel disease. Am J Gastroenterol 2008;103:937-43.

80. Van Dieren JM, Kuipers EJ, Samsom JN, et al. Revisiting the immunomodulators tacrolimus, methotrexate, and mycophenolate mofetil: their mechanisms of action and role in the treatment of IBD. Inflamm Bowel Dis 2006;12:311-27.

81. Corica D, Romano C. Biological therapy in pediatric inflammatory bowel disease a systematic review. J Clin Gastroenterol 2017;51:100-10.

82. Sands BE, Anderson FH, Bernstein CN, et al. Infliximab maintenance therapy for fistulizing Crohn's disease. N Engl J Med. 2004;350:876-85.

83. Hyams J, Crandall W, Kugathasan S, et al; REACH Study Group. Induction and maintenance infliximab therapy for the treatment of moderate-to-severe Crohn's disease in children. Gastroenterology 2007;132:863-73.

84. Malmborg P, Hildebrand H. The emerging global epidemic of paediatric inflammatory bowel disease—causes and consequences. J Intern Med 2016;279:241-58.

85. Lee YS, Baek SH, Kim MJ. Efficacy of early infliximab treatment for pediatric Crohn's disease: A three-year follow up. Pediatr Gastroenterol Hepatol Nutr 2012;15:243-9.

86. Hyams J, Damaraju L, Blank M, et al. T72 Study Group. Induction and maintenance therapy with infliximab for children with moderate to severe ulcerative colitis. Clin Gastroenterol Hepatol 2012;10:391-9.

87. Hofmekler T, Bertha M, McCracken C, et al. Infliximab optimization based on therapeutic drug monitoring in pediatric inflammatory bowel disease. J Pediatr Gastroenterol Nutr 2017;64:580-5.

88. Ardura MI, Toussi SS, Siegel JD, et al. NASPHGHAN clinical report: surveillance, diagnosis, and prevention of infectious diseases in pediatric patients with inflammatory bowel disease receiving tumor necrosis factor-α inhibitors. J Pediatr Gastroenterol Nutr 2016;63:130-55.

89. Mackey AC, Green L, Leptak C, et al. Hepatosplenic T cell lymphoma associated with infliximab use in young patients treated for inflammatory bowel disease. J Pediatr Gastroenterol Nutr 2007;44:265-7.

90. FDA Drug Safety Communication: UPDATE on Tumor Necrosis Factor (TNF) blockers and risk for pediatric malignancy. Available at www.fda.gov/Drugs/DrugSafety/ucm278267.htm. Accessed September 18, 2019.

91. Lamireau T, Cezard JP, Dabadie A, et al. Efficacy and tolerance of infliximab in children and adolescents with Crohn's disease. Inflamm Bowel Dis 2004;10:745-50.

92. Candon S, Mosca A, Rummele F, et al. Clinical and biological consequences of immunization to infliximab in pediatric Crohn's disease. Clin Immunol 2006;118:11-19.

93. Vande Casteele N, Khanna R, Levesque BG, et al. The relationship between infliximab concentrations, antibodies to infliximab and disease activity in Crohn's disease. Gut 2015;64:1539.

94. Ungar B, Levy I, Yavne Y, et al. Optimizing Anti-TNF-α therapy: serum levels of infliximab and adalimumab are associated with mucosal healing in patients with inflammatory bowel diseases. Clin Gastroenterol Hepatol 2016;14:550-7.

95. Singh N, Rosenthal CJ, Melmed et al. Early infliximab trough levels are associated with persistent remission in pediatric patients with inflammatory bowel disease. Inflamm Bowel Dis 2014;20:1708-13.

96. Papamichael K, Vande Casteele N, Ferrante M, et al. Therapeutic drug monitoring during induction of anti-tumor necrosis factor therapy in inflammatory bowel disease: defining a therapeutic drug window. Inflamm Bowel Dis 2017;23:1510-5.

97. Choi SY, Kang B, Lee JH, et al. Clinical use of measuring trough levels and antibodies against infliximab in patients with pediatric inflammatory bowel disease. Gut Liver 2017;11:55-61.

98. Noe JD, Pfefferkorn M. Short-term response to adalimumab treatment in childhood inflammatory bowel disease. Inflamm Bowel Dis 2008;14:1683-7.

99. Hyams JS, Griffiths A, Markowitz J, et al. Safety and efficacy of adalimumab for moderate to severe Crohn's disease in children. Gastroenterology 2012;143:365-74.

100. Dobinsky MC, Rosh J, Faubion WA. Efficacy and safety of escalation of adalimumab therapy to weekly dosing in pediatric patients with Crohn's disease. Inflamm Bowel Dis 2016;22:886-93.

101. Wyneski MJ, Green A, Kay M, et al. Safety and efficacy of adalimumab in pediatric patients with Crohn disease. J Pediatr Gastroenterol Nutr 2008;47:19-25.

102. Forbes A, Escher J, Hebuterne X, et al. ESPEN guideline: clinical nutrition in inflammatory bowel disease. Clinical Nutrition 2017;36:321-47.

103. Ewaschuk JB, Dieleman LA. Probiotics and prebiotics in chronic inflammatory bowel diseases. World J Gastroenterol 2006; 12:5941-50.

104. Miele E, Pascarella F, Giannetti E, et al. Effect of a probiotic preparation (VSL#3) on induction and maintenance of remission in children with ulcerative colitis. Am J Gastroenterol 2009; 104:437-43.

105. Oliva S, Di Nardo G, Ferrari F, et al. Randomised clinical trial: the effectiveness of Lactobacillus reuteri ATCC 55730 rectal enema in children with active distal ulcerative colitis. Aliment Pharmacol Ther 2012;35:327-34.

106. Bousvaros A, Guandalini S, Baldassano RN, et al. A randomized, double-blind trial of lactobacillus GG versus placebo in addition to standard maintenance therapy for children with Crohn's disease. Inflamm Bowel Dis 2005;11:833-9.

CHAPTER 18

Irritable Bowel Syndrome and Celiac Disease

Shirin Madzhidova, Pharm.D.; and
Kim W. Benner, Pharm.D., FASHP, FPPA, BCPS

LEARNING OBJECTIVES

1. Discuss the epidemiology of irritable bowel syndrome (IBS).

2. Describe the pathophysiology of IBS.

3. Recognize the signs and symptoms of IBS.

4. Discuss the diagnosis and classifications of IBS.

5. Explain the overall management and treatments associated with IBS.

6. Discuss monitoring the efficacy and toxicity of agents used in the treatment of IBS.

7. Describe the prevalence and risk factors associated with celiac disease (CD).

8. Recognize the signs and symptoms of CD.

9. Describe appropriate therapy for a patient with CD, including the role of a gluten-free diet.

10. Evaluate appropriate management of IBS for a pediatric patient case.

ABBREVIATIONS IN THIS CHAPTER

CD	Celiac disease
FODMAPs	Fermentable oligosaccharides, disaccharides, monosaccharides, and polyols
GFD	Gluten-free diet
GI	Gastrointestinal
IBS	Irritable bowel syndrome
IBS-C	Constipation-predominant IBS
IBS-D	Diarrhea-predominant IBS
IBS-M	Mixed IBS
IgA	Immunoglobulin A
IgG	Immunoglobulin G
RCD	Refractory celiac disease
TTG	Tissue transglutaminase

INTRODUCTION

Irritable bowel syndrome (IBS) is the most common cause of functional abdominal pain in children and is prevalent in both developed and developing nations. This syndrome is characterized by changes in stool form and/or frequency that are not explained by structural or biochemical causes and characterized by abdominal pain that is improved by defecation. The exact cause of IBS is not yet well understood; however, it is believed to be a gut–brain axis disorder with multifactorial origins. Children with a family history of IBS are more likely to receive a diagnosis of IBS, although environmental factors such as psychological stress may also play a role. The diagnosis of IBS is based on the presenting symptoms of a child and follows established criteria, such as the Rome IV diagnostic criteria. This syndrome can be distinguished into the following subtypes: diarrhea-predominant IBS (IBS-D), constipation-predominant IBS (IBS-C), mixed IBS (IBS-M), and unspecified IBS (IBS-U). The treatment and management of IBS in children is complex and multifaceted. Because no pharmacologic therapy has yet been established to treat IBS, management is based solely on improvement of symptoms.

Celiac disease (CD) is an immune-mediated reaction to dietary gluten that occurs in the gastrointestinal (GI) tract in patients with a genetic predisposition. This disease is one of the most common causes of chronic malabsorption. Some symptoms overlap between IBS and CD, and patients with IBS are genetically predisposed to CD. Pharmacists can play a crucial role in ensuring that patients and caregivers are adequately educated on proper and effective recognition and management of IBS and CD.

EPIDEMIOLOGY

Irritable bowel syndrome is a subtype of functional GI disorders. It is more common in those who have relatives with the disorder and those of higher socioeconomic status. In a study examining hereditary traits of IBS, authors concluded that having a mother or a father with IBS is a stronger predictor than having a twin, indicating that social learning has an influence.[1] The estimated prevalence of IBS among children and adolescents in the United States overall is 10%, with a prevalence of 6% among middle-school children and 14% among high school adolescents.[1] The most common subtype of IBS in children is IBS-C, followed by IBS-D and IBS-M. Children with IBS may be more likely to carry predisposing genetic factors for CD compared with healthy controls and therefore should be selectively screened for CD.[2]

PATHOPHYSIOLOGY

Despite extensive research to date, no clear mechanism has been identified for the development of IBS. Studies postulate that IBS arises from a state of dysregulation between the brain and the gut, which occurs within the enteric system and central nervous system, leading to changes in gut sensation, motility, and possible immune system dysfunction.[1]

Although colonic motility seems to be the predominant feature in terms of IBS symptomatology, no exact pattern of motor activity is present as a marker for IBS. Certain motor abnormalities of the GI tract are present in some patients. For example, increased frequency and irregular luminal contractions as well as prolonged transit time are observed in IBS-C, whereas exaggerated motor response to cholecystokinin and meal ingestion are present in IBS-D.[3–7] Although the relevance of altered motility to symptoms has not yet been established, pharmacologic stimulation of gut motility can reduce gas retention and improve symptoms.[8] Altered motility used to be thought to be the main contributor in IBS, but current evidence shows that visceral hypersensitivity plays a bigger role.[8]

Visceral hypersensitivity or increased sensation in response to stimuli is commonly found in patients with IBS. Stimulation of various receptors in the gut wall leads to transmission of signals to the dorsal horn of the spinal cord and the brain by afferent neural pathways. Hypersensitivity of nerves in the gut can be triggered by either *distention* (visible or measurable increase in abdominal girth) or *bloating* (person's sensation of abdominal fullness), which are both common in IBS. Studies have shown that IBS patients have increased awareness and pain in response to balloon distention in the intestine compared with controls.[8] In addition, children with IBS have a lower pressure threshold for rectal pain compared with those without IBS, which may be associated with up-regulation of afferent sensitivity to pain.[9]

Intestinal inflammation may also play a role in the etiology of IBS based on studies that have noted alterations in certain immune cells and markers. Lymphocytes, which release mediators such as nitric oxide, histamine, and proteases, have been found in increased amounts in the small intestine and colon. Such mediator release is capable of stimulating the enteric nervous system and triggering a visceral response within the intestine.[10,11] In addition, an increased number of mast cells has also been found in the intestines of patients with IBS, in proximity to colonic nerves. Mast cells are involved in normal immune function and also release mediators.[10] Such proximity of mediators to sensory nerves can lead to the symptoms of abdominal pain and hypersensitivity seen with IBS.

Intestinal flora may also be altered in patients with IBS, which may develop after enteric viral, bacterial, or parasitic infection.[12] This development of IBS may be referred to as *postinfectious IBS* and may have an increased correlation in patients with a history of anxiety.[13] The exact cause of bowel symptoms after an acute enteric infection is not known, although several theories suggest development of bile acid malabsorption and increase in serotonin-containing enteroendocrine cells and T lymphocytes, which can lead to increased GI motility and visceral hypersensitivity.[14,15] In one study, 36% of children with a history of an acute bacterial gastroenteritis developed the abdominal pain symptoms seen with functional GI disorders. Among those children, 87% of their symptoms met the criteria for IBS, and their symptoms persisted for years even after the infection resolved.[16]

Caregivers and children with IBS often report higher level of anxiety and stress as a trigger of their symptoms; therefore, the psychological component may play a role in the pathophysiology of IBS. In addition, these children are less confident in their ability to deal with stress and less likely to use coping strategies.[17] Studies suggest that overactivity in the brain of corticotropin-releasing factor, a major mediator in stress response, contributes to anxiety disorders and depression. When this factor was intravenously administered to patients with IBS, they reported increased abdominal pain and GI motility compared with healthy controls, suggesting a correlation between corticotropin-releasing factor and IBS.[17]

Neurotransmitters such as cholecystokinin, substance P, and 5-hydroxytryptamine (serotonin), found in the brain and intestines, help regulate cortical centers with visceral afferent sensation and intestinal motor function. They can work on the areas of the brain and GI system that have various effects on GI motility, emotions, and pain. Serotonin is a monoamine neurotransmitter found mainly in the GI tract. It plays an important role in gut signaling and function.[18] Serotonin regulates GI motility, secretion, and intestinal sensation. After a meal, serotonin concentrations are elevated in patients with IBS-D, whereas decreased concentrations are seen in patients with IBS-C.[18]

CLINICAL PRESENTATION AND DIAGNOSIS

Children with IBS generally present with recurrent abdominal pain and changes in bowel frequency and/or consistency associated with abdominal pain. The pain is classically relieved by defecation, although many children report feeling of incomplete evacuation. Pain is usually present in the periumbilical region and is poorly defined in children. The pain can last for less than 1 hour and can be unrelated to meals, activity, and stool patterns. Typically, children age 3–10 years report "belly pain" as the most common location, whereas children age 11–17 years most often report headaches in combination with abdominal and back pain.[11] A thorough history and physical examination are very important to diagnose IBS because no biomarkers are present for a definitive diagnosis. Of importance are a family history of IBS, psychosocial factors that may be present, accurate symptom description, and nutritional assessment. Potential organic causes of symptoms should be excluded. In a child with constipation-predominant symptoms, the possibility of functional constipation rather than IBS should be considered. In the case of possible IBS-D, infection, CD, carbohydrate malabsorption, and inflammatory bowel disease should be investigated as the potential source of symptoms.[11] Established criteria, such as the Rome IV diagnostic criteria, should be used to diagnose IBS and exclude most *alarm symptoms,* which could indicate the presence of another disorder not associated with IBS (Box 1).[19,20]

Since the introduction of the Rome IV criteria in early 2016, IBS is characterized under *functional abdominal pain disorders* together with *functional dyspepsia* and *abdominal migraine.*[11] The Manning and Rome criteria provide the standard definitions for IBS in adults and children (Table 1).[21-23] The Manning criteria, introduced in 1978, include abdominal pain relieved by defecation, more frequent stools or looser stools at the onset of pain, visible abdominal distention, passage of mucus, and sensation of incomplete evacuation.[21] The Rome III criteria added the duration and frequency of the stools and symptoms, whereas the Rome IV criteria updated the frequency and added criterion for children with constipation.[22,23] Pediatric IBS can be divided into subtypes analogous to adults reflecting bowel patterns in three main categories:

IBS-D, IBS-C, IBS-M. Those that do not fit into any category are classified under IBS unspecified, as shown in Table 2 and Table 3.[19,24–26]

Invasive diagnostic tests such as barium studies and colonoscopies are not recommended during routine screening in children with suspected IBS, and are rather reserved to rule out other causes in the presence of "red flag" symptoms. Screening for these symptoms, such as blood in the stool, pallor, and growth deceleration, is important because they can indicate an organic disease (Box 2).[20,27]

Laboratory testing is not routinely recommended for diagnosis of IBS and is usually used to rule out organic causes of disease. Recent studies have demonstrated that a negative calprotectin test can rule out inflammatory bowel disease, thus distinguishing this disease from IBS and sparing patients with IBS from invasive studies. A complete blood cell count with differential, C-reactive protein, and erythrocyte sedimentation rate can help confirm an infectious or inflammatory process. Stool studies are not typically done, but they can exclude bacterial, protozoan, or parasitic causes of abdominal pain, such as giardiasis.[13] In addition, a complete metabolic

Table 1. Manning and Rome IV Criteria for Diagnosis of Irritable Bowel Syndrome[21-23]

Manning Criteria	Rome IV Criteria[a]
• Abdominal pain plus ≥ 2 of the following: • Relieved by defecation • More frequent stools at onset of pain • Looser stools at onset of pain • Visible abdominal distention • Passage of mucus • Sensation of incomplete evacuation >25% of the time	• Recurrent abdominal pain or discomfort associated with ≥ 2 of the following[a,b]: • Related to defecation • Onset associated with a change in frequency of stool • Onset associated with a change in form (appearance) of stool
	In children with constipation, pain does not resolve with resolution of constipation[c]
	After appropriate evaluation, symptoms cannot be completely explained by another medical condition

[a]Occurred at least 4 days/month for at least 2 months → at least 1 day/week in the past 3 months. Criteria fulfilled for the past 3 months, with symptom onset at least 6 months prior to diagnosis.
[b]*Discomfort* means an uncomfortable sensation not described as *pain*.
[c]Children for whom the pain resolves with resolution of constipation have functional constipation, not IBS.
IBS = irritable bowel syndrome.

Table 2. Subtype Classifications of Irritable Bowel Syndrome[19,24-26]

Subtype Classification	
Bristol Stool Form Scale	**Description**
Constipation-predominant IBS (IBS-C)	
Bristol Stool Form Scale 1–2	≥ 25% of bowel movements hard or lumpy stools
Bristol Stool Form Scale 6–7	≤ 25% of bowel movements loose/mushy or watery stools
Diarrhea-predominant IBS (IBS-D)	
Bristol Stool Form Scale 6–7	≥ 25% of bowel movements loose/mushy or watery stools
Bristol Stool Form Scale 1–2	≤ 25% of bowel movements hard or lumpy stools
Mixed IBS (IBS-M)	
Bristol Stool Form Scale 1–2	≥ 25% of bowel movements hard or lumpy stools
Bristol Stool Form Scale 6–7	≥ 25% of bowel movements loose/mushy or watery stools
IBS Unspecified	
Patient meets diagnostic criteria for IBS, but bowel habits cannot be accurately categorized into one of three subtypes above.	

IBS = irritable bowel syndrome.

panel that includes a liver function test and amylase or lipase can help exclude metabolic causes or pancreatitis. Depending on the clinical course, some patients need a radiologic evaluation, such as abdominal ultrasonography or computed tomography or an upper GI series with small bowel follow-through, to evaluate structure.[13]

MANAGEMENT

The goal of therapeutic interventions in IBS is to improve the quality of life of the child, which includes minimizing pain and normalizing stool consistency and frequency. The management of IBS in children is based on the predominant symptoms, symptom severity, and specific patient goals. Milder symptoms that are less frequent can generally be managed with education and counseling, dietary restrictions, and bulk laxatives. More persistent disease may require specialized pharmacologic treatment, including antispasmodics and antidiarrheal agents. Most severe forms of IBS may require pharmacologic agents directed at underlying neurohormonal imbalance, such as tegaserod.[20] Regardless of the treatment approach, a positive relationship between the patient and health care provider is important in ensuring treatment success. When the child's biopsychosocial and clinical needs are addressed, parents report higher satisfaction rates with overall care and are more receptive to treatments.[28]

Educating the patient and caregiver can play a vital role in the care of these patients. Caregivers should understand that symptoms that cause pain are not life-threatening but can interfere with the child's life. Caregivers should acknowledge the pain but also encourage daily activities and school attendance.[29]

NONPHARMACOLOGIC MANAGEMENT

Emerging evidence suggests psychosocial interventions may be highly effective in the management of IBS. Such interventions include cognitive behavioral therapy, hypnotherapy, stress management, and written self-disclosure. Children are equipped with learned techniques to help them monitor symptoms, implement relaxation techniques, and use distraction strategies.[30] The main goal of cognitive behavioral therapy is to enable children with strategies to improve coping and problem-solving skills, which can help them better identify their IBS triggers and improve their responses to such triggers. Hypnotherapy uses various self-guided techniques to help reduce colonic contractions and normalize abdominal visceral impulses, thereby improving the child's symptoms and outlook about the condition.[31] The American Academy of Pediatrics guidelines for chronic abdominal pain concluded that these therapies are useful in the short term for improving pain.[20] Other studies have concluded that these approaches decrease pain in 70% to 90% of children and sometimes help reduce school absences and medication use.[32-35]

DIET

Although routine dietary restrictions are not recommended for children with IBS, many caregivers will try an exclusion diet based on the belief that specific foods negatively affect symptoms. Some dietary interventions have been studied extensively and have shown to benefit select patients. However, most dietary interventions require close monitoring by a dietician and strict adherence by the child or caregiver to show efficacy. If the child reports specific dietary triggers, such as lactose, citrus, spicy foods, sorbitol, and gas-producing foods, elimination of such triggers may be warranted.[36] A lactose-free diet may benefit a child who exhibits symptoms of lactose intolerance (e.g., cramping pain and bloating after milk and milk-containing foods). Although patients with IBS do show a higher prevalence of lactose intolerance, routine exclusion is not recommended because the evidence regarding its benefit is inconclusive.[36]

It may be beneficial to exclude gluten in patients with IBS-D who also have CD markers, such as CD-associated serum immunoglobulin G and *HLA-DQ2* allele expression. Gluten is a protein found in wheat and other grains that helps baked foods maintain their shape. In one study symptoms improved in 60% of patients with IBS-D with positive celiac serologies versus 12% in those with negative serologies.[37] The role of gluten in children without CD markers is not yet clearly elucidated; therefore, avoidance of gluten cannot be recommended to all children with IBS. Another group of

Table 3. Bristol Stool Form Scale Subtype Descriptions in Irritable Bowel Syndrome[26]

Type	Description
1	Separate hard lumps, like nuts (hard to pass)
2	Sausage-shaped but lumpy
3	Like a sausage but with cracks on its surface
4	Like a sausage or snake, smooth and soft
5	Soft blobs with clear-cut edges (passed easily)
6	Fluffy pieces with ragged edges, a mushy stool
7	Watery, no solid pieces, entirely liquid

Box 2. Possible Organic Causes of Abdominal Pain[20,27]

Constipation
Carbohydrate malabsorption
Pelvic inflammatory disease
Gastroesophageal reflux disease
Gastrointestinal ulcers
Lactose intolerance
Parasitic infections
Muscle and/or bone pain
Urinary tract infection
Inflammatory bowel disease: Crohn disease or
    ulcerative colitis
Menstruation
Endometriosis

carbohydrates that has been evaluated as a possible cause of IBS are fermentable oligosaccharides, disaccharides, mono-saccharides, and polyols (FODMAPs). Sufficient data are currently lacking to support the use of a diet low in FODMAPs in children and adolescents, although recent reports suggest that strict adherence may affect gut bacterial composition and improve symptoms of IBS.[38] However, FODMAPs are ubiquitous in foods that are essential to a well-balanced diet (e.g., wheat, milk, legumes, various fruits and vegetables, meats, dairy, grains, and bread) in children and requires the help of a dietician.

Nutritional status is of upmost importance in children, especially with IBS-D. If oral intake is inadequate or if malabsorption occurs, then enteral or parenteral nutrition may be considered, although it is not often needed. Sufficient calories should be provided to maintain growth and even allow catch-up weight gain. Micronutrient and vitamin supplementation should also be considered in patients with IBS, with a focus on zinc, vitamin A, folic acid, copper, and selenium because they can be depleted in children with IBS.[39]

PHARMACOLOGIC TREATMENT

CONSTIPATION-PREDOMINANT IBS

Fiber and bulk agents. Fiber is an essential component of a well-balanced diet and helps promote regular bowel movements. The utility of fiber and fiber supplements in children with IBS is somewhat conflicting and should be assessed based on patient-specific symptoms. In a child with IBS-C, fiber and fiber supplementation adds bulk and water content to the stool, making it softer and easier to pass. However, fiber does not improve pain symptoms, and the increased bulk may cause greater distension in the colon, which may worsen flatulence and bloating.[40] Fiber can be found in foods such as whole grains, fruits, and vegetables. Children may also try high-fiber cookies or crackers, granola bars, or dried fruit. Fiber supplementation with soluble fiber, such as psyllium, is the first-line treatment in IBS-C. The American College of Gastroenterology specifically recommends ispaghula husk (i.e., psyllium), but not insoluble fibers (e.g., wheat bran, corn bran) for children with functional GI disorders because insoluble fibers were found to be no more effective than placebo.[13] Fiber supplements are available in several forms, including wafers, chewable tablets, or powdered fiber that can be mixed in juice or made into popsicles. Fiber supplements are usually given twice daily and must be taken with enough water to avoid impaction.

Overall, the daily intake of water should be sufficient, with younger children drinking 2–4 glasses of water and older children drinking at least 6 glasses of water. To decrease the adverse effects of flatulence and bloating, supplementation should be a gradual process in which fiber intake is slowly increased and stool output and frequency are monitored. Fiber supplements can improve global IBS symptoms and reduce symptom severity.[40,41] The additional fiber may exacerbate some symptoms in children; therefore, supplements must be used with caution, especially in children who tend to withhold stools or who have chronic constipation.

Laxatives. The Rome IV criteria clarifies the definition of *functional constipation* versus IBS-C based on studies that show patients with IBS-C often receive a diagnosis of functional constipation. A child who presents with constipation and abdominal pain should initially be treated for constipation. If abdominal pain resolves with such treatment, then the child can be diagnosed with functional constipation; if this pain does not resolve, then the child likely has IBS with constipation, given that possible organic causes of abdominal pain have been ruled out.[12] Laxatives are an appropriate therapy choice for IBS-C because of their relative safety, low cost, and availability. The types of laxatives available are osmotic laxatives (e.g., polyethylene glycol, milk of magnesia, and sorbitol), and stimulant laxatives (e.g., bisacodyl, senna). Osmotic laxatives, particularly polyethylene glycol, are most commonly used in children with IBS-C, and work by increasing water in the intestinal lumen to decrease intestinal transit time. A study of adolescents with IBS-C taking polyethylene glycol alone or in combination with tegaserod, a motility stimulant that works as 5HT-4 agonist, showed an increase in stool frequency; however, abdominal pain remained unchanged.[42] However, tegaserod has since been removed from the market and is only available with special permission from the U.S. Food and Drug Administration for emergencies only. No studies have demonstrated increased efficacy of any particular laxative; all are equally effective and have similar safety profiles. The selection of a laxative depends on the dosage form and frequency to improve adherence to the regimen. The dose of the laxative is titrated slowly and to effect. For example, the dose should be increased every 2 days until the child has one or two soft stools each day. In addition, the dose should be decreased if the patient develops diarrhea.

Lubiprostone. Lubiprostone is a chlorine channel activator that acts locally in the GI tract to increase interstitial fluid secretion and improve fecal transit. It is currently approved for treatment of IBS-C in women older than 18 years and is being evaluated for use in children and adolescents. Lubiprostone has been shown to be well tolerated and provide symptomatic relief when given for 3 to 4 weeks in adults with IBS-C.[43] Because of the similarities in many of the studied symptoms associated with constipation in adults and children, the potential for use of lubiprostone in children is apparent. An open-label, multicenter study conducted in children ages 3–17 years with chronic functional constipation investigated safety and effectiveness of lubiprostone. Patients given lubiprostone at a dose of 0.6–0.8 mcg/kg showed statistically significant improvement from baseline in stool frequency and straining, but experienced no effect on abdominal discomfort and bloating. Although lubiprostone was well tolerated, the study had many limitations, such as a lack of a placebo group, and further studies are needed to establish its use in children with IBS-C.[44]

DIARRHEA-PREDOMINANT IBS

Antidiarrheal agents. Loperamide is an appropriate option for children with IBS-D because it is effective in reducing stool frequency and has a favorable safety profile. It acts on the intestinal mu-opioid receptors, slowing peristalsis and increasing fluid resorption.[45] Loperamide has been found to reduce stool frequency in children with IBS-D, but it does not reduce pain, bloating, or other symptoms.[46]

ABDOMINAL PAIN ASSOCIATED WITH IBS

Antispasmodics. Antispasmodics have varying mechanisms of action depending on the medication; however, all these agents relax GI smooth muscle. Although only limited studies exist, enteric-coated, pH-dependent peppermint oil capsules have been shown to be efficacious in children with IBS to reduce symptom and pain severity. Peppermint oil capsules are available commercially; however, excessive intake can exacerbate GI reflux and has been associated with interstitial nephritis and acute renal failure.[47–49] Other antispasmodics, such as hyoscyamine and dicyclomine, are effective in the treatment of IBS-D in adults; however, data in children are limited.[48] Currently, the American College of Gastroenterology Task Force does not recommend the long-term use of antispasmodics in patients with IBS.[46]

Antidepressants. Antidepressants, particularly tricyclic antidepressant and selective serotonin reuptake inhibitors, are used for the treatment of abdominal pain in adults with IBS. Both classes have analgesic properties independent of their mood improving effects. The theoretical basis for treatment with selective serotonin reuptake inhibitors in IBS is that serotonin is an important neurotransmitter in the GI tract, with 80% of the body's stores located in the enterochromaffin cells of the gut. In addition, antidepressants have anticholinergic effects, and thus may result in improvement of diarrhea, regulation of GI transit and peripheral anti-neuropathic effects. Evidence is limited, however, to support antidepressant use in children with IBS. In two pediatric randomized placebo-controlled trials, amitriptyline was given at 10 mg, 20 mg, or 30 mg (based on weight) for 4–8 weeks of therapy. Amitriptyline improved the overall quality of life from baseline and reduced anxiety scores in patients with IBS. Most of the patients reported feeling better but had inconsistent improvement in pain, with no improvement in other IBS-related symptoms.[50,51] A randomized controlled trial of citalopram in adults with IBS-D showed no significant benefit in symptom improvement, and studies of this drug in children are lacking.[52] Overall, the use of antidepressants in IBS-D may be promising, but their efficacy and safety must still be established in the pediatric population.

Probiotics. Probiotics are live microorganisms that have been shown to confer a health benefit when taken in appropriate amounts. In patients with IBS, probiotics can alter the gut microbiota composition, therefore positively affecting the gut–brain axis.[53] The most commonly used probiotic strain is *Lactobacillus,* and VSL#3 is the most commonly used probiotic blend. Some studies suggest that *Lactobacillus* GG provides a moderate benefit in children by decreasing frequency of pain, but this probiotic does not appear to decrease the severity of pain, whereas other probiotics showed no superiority over placebo.[54,55] Inactive *Escherichia coli* bacteria have also been used with some success and seem to be better tolerated by patients without adverse effects, such as

intestinal flatus.[56] The consensus of physicians and parents is that probiotics are beneficial in children with IBS; however, probiotics are not regulated by the FDA, and efficacy may vary significantly between brands.[57] For a complete list of available treatment options, as well as dosing parameters and common adverse effects, please refer to Table 4[58-60] and Table 5.[50,58]

MONITORING OF THERAPY

Overall monitoring of therapy in children with IBS is related to quality of life. Treatments should be tailored to the individual child's symptoms. It is important that the child's growth parameters, such as height and weight, be monitored to ensure proper growth. Bowel frequency should be monitored, and medications to treat IBS-C and IBS-D should be used to regulate stools to one to two soft stools per day. Adverse drug effects of increasing abdominal distension or abdominal pain as well as medication-specific adverse effects should be monitored. Antidepressants should be closely followed, especially at the initiation of therapy. Patients should be monitored for suicidal ideation and improvement in symptoms of IBS or concomitant anxiety or depression. With appropriate treatment, daily function and quality of life should improve.

CELIAC DISEASE

Celiac disease results from a loss of small intestine surface area, loss of digestive enzymes responsible for the digestion of gluten, and impaired absorption of fat-soluble vitamins, iron, and other nutrients. This disease occurs when a portion of gluten that cannot be completely broken down by the intestines, gliadin, passes through the epithelial layer of the intestine, stimulating an immune response. Once past the epithelial layer, gliadin binds with leukocyte antigens DQ2 or DQ8, activating CD4 T cells in the intestinal mucosa. This immune system activation in the small intestine causes inflammation, resulting in malabsorption, which can manifest as diarrhea.[61]

The incidence of CD has a genetic component, and is more likely to occur in female patients and patients who have a family member with CD, with a stronger association when it appears in first-degree versus second-degree relatives.[61,62] The presence of certain concomitant conditions such as Down syndrome, William syndrome, or Turner syndrome, thyroid disorders, immunoglobulin A deficiency, and type 1 diabetes mellitus have been associated with an increased risk of CD. In children specifically, the risk of CD is higher in patients who have type 1 diabetes than for adults with type 1 diabetes.[61] Other additional risk factors are specific to children. Introducing gluten into a child's diet at age younger than 3 months or after 7 months was noted to increase the risk of acquiring CD compared with exposure at 4–6 months because of unknown mechanisms.[63] Breastfeeding during the period of gluten introduction and continuing to breastfeed during the first year of life has been associated with a decreased risk of CD.[64,65] Finally, birth by cesarean delivery and infection with rotavirus have been reported to be potential risk factors for pediatric patients with CD.[66,67]

CLINICAL PRESENTATION AND DIAGNOSIS

The clinical presentation of CD varies between patients and commonly include diarrhea and flatulence, but can also include abdominal distention, abdominal pain, vomiting, constipation, and weight loss. Symptoms may occur alone or in combination. This disease presents in children between the ages of 6 and 24 months predominantly with manifestations of diarrhea, muscle wasting, weight loss, abdominal distention, and failure to thrive.[61] In more severe cases, children of any age may present with celiac crisis, a rare medical emergency associated with electrolyte imbalances, hypoproteinemia, and vascular compromise. Non-GI symptoms may be more common among adolescents and young adults and include the following: anemia/iron deficiency, aphthous stomatitis, arthritis, ataxia, behavioral problems, dental enamel defects, depression, dermatitis herpetiformis, epilepsy, headaches, hypotonia, infertility, neuropathy, osteopenia/osteoporosis, pubertal delay, and transaminase elevation.[68]

Diagnosis of CD is complicated because it can be difficult to determine which patients to test and when. Guidelines recommend evaluating children for CD if signs, symptoms, or results of laboratory studies are consistent with malabsorption and evaluating children with first-degree relatives who have a diagnosis of CD. Immunoglobulin A (IgA) deficiency

Table 4. Treatment Options for IBS-C and IBS-D[58-60]

Treatments		Patients and Dosing	Common Adverse Effects
IBS-C			
Fiber	Fruits, vegetables, whole grains	Child's age in years plus 5–10 g/day Age 6–11 years: 1.25–15 g/day in two or three divided doses	Rectal distension Colonic distension
	Psyllium	Age > 12 years: 2.5–30 g/day in two or three divided doses Maximum 30 g/day	
Laxatives: Osmotic	Polyethylene glycol (powder)	1 g/kg/day in two or three divided doses Maximum of 17 g/day	Bloating Flatulence
	Lactulose (syrup)	1–3 mL/kg/day in two or three divided doses Maximum 60 mL/day	
Laxatives: Stimulants	Senna (syrup, granules, and tablets)	Age 2–6 years: 2.5–7.5 mL/day in two divided doses Age 6–12 years: 5–15 mL/day in two divided doses Maximum 30 mL/day	Abdominal cramping/pain Discoloration of stool and urine
	Bisacodyl (tablets, suppositories)	Age ≥ 2 years: 0.5–1 suppository or 5- to 10-mg tablet/dose Maximum 30 mg/day	Abdominal cramping/pain
IBS-D			
Antidiarrheals	Loperamide	0.08–0.24 mg/kg/day in two or three divided doses Maximum 2 mg/dose	Abdominal distension Abdominal cramping Urinary retention

IBS-C = constipation-predominant irritable bowel syndrome; IBS-D = diarrhea-predominant irritable bowel syndrome.

Table 5. Treatment Options for Abdominal Pain Associated with Irritable Bowel Syndrome[50,58]

Treatments		Patients and Dosing	Common Adverse Effects
Antispasmodics	Hyoscyamine (elixir, tablets)	Age 2–12 years: 0.0625–0.125 mg per dose every 4 hours as needed Maximum of 0.75 mg/day Age > 12 years: 0.125–0.25 mg every 4 hours as needed Maximum of 1.5 mg/day	Constipation Dry mouth Urinary retention Tachycardia
	Dicyclomine (syrup, tablets)	5–10 mg per dose three or four times/day Maximum of 80 mg/day	
Antidepressants: Tricyclic	Amitriptyline (tablets)	Weight < 35 kg: 10 mg at bedtime Weight > 35 kg: 20 mg at bedtime	Sedation Weight gain

is more common in CD patients than the general population, which is why antibody tests can help confirm a CD diagnosis. For that reason, it is recommended to conduct serology testing every 1 to 3 years. Because of the association with type 1 diabetes, children experiencing CD symptoms who have type 1 diabetes should have yearly or every-other-year CD screening. However, screening is not indicated if HLA-DQ2 and HLA-DQ8 are not present.

In patients younger than 2 years, the IgA anti-tissue transglutaminase (IgA TTG) test should be combined with the immunoglobulin G (IgG)-deamidated-gliadin peptides, which include IgA and IgG. In patients older than 2 years, CD can be detected by serologic testing of celiac-specific antibodies by the IgA TTG test. In patients with a positive serologic test, diagnosis is confirmed by duodenal mucosal biopsies that indicate duodenal villous atrophy. However, a negative serologic test in the presence of villous atrophy does not exclude CD.[69]

The diagnosis of CD must be differentiated from the diagnosis of nonceliac gluten sensitivity. Symptoms alone cannot reliably differentiate CD from nonceliac gluten sensitivity because symptoms often overlap between the two conditions. Patients with gluten sensitivity alone may have celiac symptoms but will not have the diagnostic criteria specific to CD. Because these patients may improve on a gluten-free diet (GFD) alone, resolutions of symptoms with initiation of the GFD diet does not alone warrant the diagnosis of CD. Finally, there is no genetic component related to nonceliac gluten sensitivity.[69]

MANAGEMENT

Nutritional therapy is the only accepted treatment for CD because there are no medications proven to prevent intestinal damage. Removing the antigenic substance accountable for the abnormal immune reaction reverses the manifestations of CD and can improve the quality of life of symptomatic CD patients.[69]

NONPHARMACOLOGIC MANAGEMENT

Individuals who have CD should adhere to a GFD for life. Foods, beverages, and medications have less than 20 part per million of gluten content per serving are labeled "gluten free."[70] Because of trace amounts found in foods, it is not practical to completely eliminate gluten; therefore a gluten intake of less than 10 mg/day is considered safe for patients who have CD because this amount has not been associated with intestinal damage.[71] Sources of dietary gluten include wheat, barley, and rye, so these foods should be avoided in a strictly GFD (Box 3). The consumption of oats has traditionally been controversial because of the possibility that commercially available oats can be contaminated with gluten.[72] Some literature supports no damage despite ingestion of limited quantities of oats in certain patients.[73,74] Patients ingesting oats should be monitored closely for signs of relapse.[69]

If successfully implemented and adhered to, a GFD provides clinical improvement in the majority of CD patients. Although histologic improvement may not be seen for up to 1 year, patients often experience relief of extraintestinal symptoms, such as dyspepsia, within a matter of days or weeks.[68,75]

It is important for children and caregivers to recognize that not only foods contain gluten, but also medications, supplements or vitamins, and other "hidden" sources of gluten. Little available literature provides information related to the exact gluten content in medications[76-78]; this information can also be obtained from the manufacturer of the specific medication. Hidden sources of gluten include not only the previously mentioned items such as medications but also sauces, luncheon meats, communion wafers, and candy.[68]

Pharmacists can educate patients on a GFD and help to stress the importance of adherence, particularly in adolescents, a population that has adherence rates reported to be as low as 52%.[79] In a Canadian survey, 92% of children reported difficulty in determining GF foods, 90% had trouble locating acceptable foods, and 72% were angry for having to follow such a strict diet.[80] An estimated 5% of patients are resistant to a GFD.[61] Strategies for alternative therapy for GFD-resistant patients will be discussed in the Treatment section. Pharmacists can work together with other health care providers, particularly dieticians, to ensure understanding, allowable foods, and hidden sources of gluten.

PHARMACOLOGIC TREATMENT

Currently no treatments exist to correct defects in the digestive enzymes for gluten in patients with CD. However, newly diagnosed patients should be tested and treated for micronutrient deficiencies such as iron, folic acid, and vitamin D, B_6,

---

Box 3. Gluten-Containing Foods to Avoid for Patients with Irritable Bowel Syndrome[68]

Barley
Bran
Bulgur
Couscous
Durum
Einkorn
Emmer
Farina
Faro
Graham flour
Kamut
Malt extract
Matzo flour or meal
Orzo
Panko
Rye
Seitan
Semolina
Spelt
Triticale
Udon
Wheat
Wheat bran/germ
Wheat starch

and B_{12} deficiencies. Copper, zinc, and carnitine concentrations may also be low. Thus, these patients may require treatment with these nutritional supplements.[81] Probiotics, because thought to help maintain intestinal barrier function, have been studied in patients with CD. Although these patients have experienced some benefit in symptom control, no significant reversal of disease occurred.[82,83]

When a GFD alone is insufficient to manage CD, patients may be found to have refractory CD (RCD). *Refractory celiac disease* is defined as persistent or recurrent signs and symptoms of malabsorption together with the presence of villous atrophy in the intestinal wall despite maintaining a GFD for at least 6–12 months and without other contributing factors such as overt lymphoma. Patients with RCD may benefit from adjunctive treatment with medication. For management these patients should be classified as having type 1 or type 2 RCD. Patients with Type 1 RCD have lymphocyte infiltration of the small-intestinal mucosa similar to that seen in patients with untreated CD. These patients may require treatment with oral prednisone, immunosuppressive agents, or even medications such as enteric-coated budesonide or small-intestinal release mesalamine. A trial of azathioprine may benefit patients who do not fully respond to corticosteroid therapy or worsen when the corticosteroid is decreased.[69] Patients with type 2 RCD have intraepithelial CD3-positive T cells that exhibit an abnormal immunophenotype lacking expression of CD8 and other normal cell surface differentiation markers. These patients may require parenteral nutrition support because of malnutrition or treatment with medications such as systemic corticosteroids, enteric-coated budesonide, azathioprine, 6-mercaptopurine, methotrexate, cyclosporine, anti-tumor necrosis factor alpha antibodies (such as infliximab), or cladribine.[84-86] Immunosuppressant medications, such prednisone and azathioprine, should be used with caution in these patients because of the risk of lymphoma.[86]

MONITORING OF THERAPY

Once the diagnosis of CD has been made, patients should be regularly monitored for new or residual symptoms, GFD adherence, laboratory values, and complications. Adherence to a GFD can be monitored using a combination or history and serology testing (IgA TTG or IgA/IgG deamidated-gliadin peptide antibodies). For example, if patients are abiding to a GFD, then the IgA TTG titer should decrease after about 6 months. Titers that remain elevated after 6 months suggest the patient is still consuming gluten-containing foods.[61] Failing to be adherent on a GFD places patients at a higher risk of other adverse health issues such as bone demineralization, tumors, and increased mortality.[68] Patients who continue to be nonadherent are at increased risk of cancers such as B cell and T cell non-Hodgkin lymphomas, esophageal cancer, and small bowel adenocarinomas.[68] Successfully following a GFD can help improve body weight, body mass index, and bone mineralization in children with CD. Children with CD should be monitored for normal growth and development, and any laboratory alterations present at diagnosis should be also be monitored to ensure homeostasis. Consultation with a registered dietitian knowledgeable about CD should be considered for education on maintaining a GFD, related nutritional deficiencies, and alternatives to gluten. Pharmacists can assist in education of patients and caregivers as well as medications to avoid and which nutritional supplements are needed.[69]

CONCLUSIONS

Irritable bowel syndrome in pediatric patients greatly affects quality of life, both for the patient and the family. This syndrome is associated with increased health care and economic burdens. The pathophysiology of IBS is poorly understood and likely multifactorial, with emerging theories leading to better treatments. Finding the optimal treatment for patients with IBS can be challenging, especially given the complexity of the disease. Overall, the treatment for IBS must be patient-centered and individualized to each patient's perception of pain and symptoms, similar to CD. Celiac disease, which is a specific, life-long autoimmune disorder with a varied clinical spectrum, can present similarly to IBS, and the two syndromes must be differentiated. The diagnosis of CD is typically established using serologic testing, duodenal biopsy, and the observation of a response to a GFD. Increasing awareness of the epidemiology, clinical presentation, diagnostic testing, and treatment of CD will lead to earlier diagnosis and a reduction in complications of the disease. Pharmacists can have a pivotal role in the education of patients with either IBS or CD to help maintain a high quality of life.

A 10-year-old girl presents with a 4-month history of recurrent abdominal pain. The symptoms began after a visit to the state fair where she and her grandmother ate homemade ice cream from a vendor's stand. They both became ill with diarrhea and vomiting that lasted 2 days. The grandmother recovered completely and the patient's diarrhea improved, but her abdominal pain never completely resolved. She now has abdominal pain that is localized to the lower abdomen several times a week. She describes the pain as crampy; it is sometimes associated with the passage of loose, mucous stool and other times with hard scybalous stools. Foods such as pizza and candy, tight-fitting clothes, and stress appear to trigger the pain. The pain lasts for a few hours or persists throughout the day, but it does not wake her from sleep. She had lost 4.5 kg since the symptoms began; however, she and her parents attribute the weight loss to not eating much because of a fear that eating may cause pain. She denies chronic fever, blood in her stool, joint swelling or pain, and recurrent mouth ulcers.

The patient's medical history is significant for infectious diarrhea that had self-resolved 4 months ago. She lives with her parents, and her family history is significant for a diagnosis of irritable bowel syndrome (IBS) in her mother; other family history is noncontributory. Review of symptoms is negative for blood in the stool or tarry stools and positive for flatulence and bloating. She states that her abdominal symptoms may improve after the passage of stools, and she is not awakened at night with abdominal pain. She is currently taking no medications.

Vital signs: BP 116/78 mm Hg; HR 96 beats/minute; Tmax 98°F (37°C); Wt 75th percentile; Ht 50th percentile.

Laboratory findings: complete blood count, comprehensive metabolic panel, erythrocyte sedimentation rate and thyroid-stimulating hormone values are all within normal limits. Lactulose hydrogen breath test is negative. Stool culture is negative.

---

1. Based on the Manning and the Rome IV criteria, which subjective findings suggest the diagnosis of IBS in this patient?

Based on the patient's history, her symptoms began after an acute gastrointestinal infection, which suggest a postinfectious etiology of IBS. The history she provides and her normal physical examination satisfy established symptom-based criteria for the diagnosis of IBS. Based on the Manning and the Rome IV criteria, the patient reports recurrent abdominal pain that is relieved by defecation and changes in frequency and form of stool. Organic causes of her symptoms can be excluded by appearance of normal laboratory values and stool cultures.

2. What is the optimal nonpharmacologic and/or pharmacologic management for this patient?

The suspected diagnosis of IBS, the pathophysiology, and the compelling reasons for this diagnosis should be discussed at the initial evaluation of this patient, and realistic goals of therapy should be set. The patient and caregiver should be advised to avoid foods that aggravate her symptoms; however, without a consultation with a dietitian, the clinician must be cautious with diets such as low intake of fermentable oligosaccharides, disaccharides, monosaccharides, and polyols. The patient should be advised to increase her dietary fiber intake with fruits, vegetables, and whole grains. Because the patient reports having hard stools at times, a fiber supplement such as psyllium 15 g/day in two or three divided doses is appropriate. The dose may be

increased every 1 to 2 days based on symptom resolution and titrated to the point when she has one to two soft stools per day. An antispasmodic agent, such as dicyclomine at a dose of 5–10 mg, three to four times per day, is an appropriate pharmacologic agent for a course no longer than 2 weeks to help reduce abdominal pain. Both the patient and caregiver should be advised that the patient should take the medication 30 to 60 minutes prior to meals and at bedtime. A follow-up appointment should be scheduled within 4 to 6 weeks, and the parents should be encouraged to call the physician if symptoms persist.

3. What are the goals of therapy? How should this patient be monitored?

The goals of therapy in a child with diarrhea-predominant IBS should be to minimize abdominal pain and normalize the frequency and consistency of stools to one to two soft stools per day. The patient and caregiver should be educated on proper monitoring of symptoms and potential adverse effects of the medications. The patient should keep a diary of her symptoms to document changes in severity as well as any alleviating factors, such as dietary triggers. Patient and caregiver should be aware of the potential adverse effects associated with the use of psyllium fiber supplement, such as colonic distention, which may exacerbate abdominal pain, as well as dry mouth, urinary retention, and constipation that can be caused by dicyclomine.

REFERENCES

1. Sandhu BK, Paul SP. Irritable bowel syndrome in children: pathogenesis, diagnosis and evidence based treatment. World J Gastroenterol 2014;20:6013-23.

2. Domżał-Magrowska D, Kowalski MK, Szcześniak P, et al. The prevalence of celiac disease in patients with irritable bowel syndrome and its subtypes. Prz Gastroenterol 2016;11:276-81.

3. Kumar D, Wingate DL. The irritable bowel syndrome: a paroxysmal motor disorder. Lancet 1985;2:973.

4. Schmidt T, Hackelsberger N, Widmer R, et al. Ambulatory 24-hour jejunal motility in diarrhea-predominant irritable bowel syndrome. Scand J Gastroenterol 1996;31:581.

5. Agrawal A, Houghton LA, Reilly B, et al. Bloating and distension in irritable bowel syndrome: the role of gastrointestinal transit. Am J Gastroenterol 2009;104:1998.

6. Chey WY, Jin HO, Lee MH, et al. Colonic motility abnormality in patients with irritable bowel syndrome exhibiting abdominal pain and diarrhea. Am J Gastroenterol 2001;96:1499.

7. Nozu T, Kudaira M, Kitamori S, et al. Repetitive rectal painful distention induces rectal hypersensitivity in patients with irritable bowel syndrome. J Gastroenterol 2006;41:217.

8. Faure C, Wieckowska A. Somatic referral of visceral sensations and rectal sensory threshold for pain in children with functional gastrointestinal disorders. J Pediatr 2007;150:66-71.

9. McOmber M, Shulman R. Recurrent abdominal pain and irritable bowel syndrome in children. Curr Opin Pediatr 2007;19:581-5.

10. Chadwick VS, Chen W, Shu D, et al. Activation of the mucosal immune system in irritable bowel syndrome. Gastroenterology 2002;122:1778.

11. Hyams JS, Lorenzo CD, Saps M, et al. Functional gastrointestinal disorders: child/adolescent. Gastroenterology 2016;150:1456-68.

12. Spiller R, Garsed K. Postinfectious irritable bowel syndrome. Gastroenterology 2009;136:1979-88.

13. American College of Gastroenterology Task Force on Irritable Bowel Syndrome, Brandt LJ, Chevy WD, et al. An evidence-based position statement on the management of irritable bowel syndrome. Am J Gastroenterol 2009;104(suppl 1):S1-35.

14. Niaz SK, Sandrasegaran K, Renny FH, et al. Postinfective diarrhoea and bile acid malabsorption. J R Coll Physicians Lond 1997;31:53.

15. Spiller RC, Jenkins D, Thornley JP, et al. Increased rectal mucosal enteroendocrine cells, T lymphocytes, and increased gut permeability following acute Campylobacter enteritis and in post-dysenteric irritable bowel syndrome. Gut 2000;47:804.

16. Saps M, Pensabene L, Di Martino L. Post-infectious functional gastrointestinal disorders in children. J Pediatr 2008;152:812-6, 816.e1.

17. Fukudo S, Nomura T, Hongo M. Impact of corticotropin-releasing hormone on gastrointestinal motility and adrenocorticotropic hormone in normal controls and patients with irritable bowel syndrome. Gut 1998;42:845.

18. Cremon C, Carini G, Wang B, et al. Intestinal serotonin release, sensory neuron activation, and abdominal pain in irritable bowel syndrome. Am J Gastroenterol 2011;106:1290-8.

19. Di Lorenzo C, Colletti RB, Lehmann HP, et al. Chronic abdominal pain in children: a technical report of the American Academy of Pediatrics and the North American Society for Pediatric Gastroenterology, Hepatology and Nutrition. J Pediatr Gastroenterol Nutr 2005;40:249-61.

20. American Academy of Pediatrics Subcommittee on Chronic Abdominal Pain. Chronic abdominal pain in children. Pediatrics 2005;115:812-5.

21. Manning AP, Thompson WG, Heaton KW, et al. Towards a positive diagnosis of irritable bowel. Br Med J 1978;2:653-4.

22. Drossman DA, Corazziari E, Delvaux M, et al., eds. Rome III: The Functional Gastrointestinal Disorders, 3rd ed. McLean, VA: Degnon Associates, 2006: Appendix A 858-98.

23. Drossman DA, Chang L, Chey WD, et al.; The Rome IV Committees, eds. Rome IV functional gastrointestinal disorders – disorders of gut-brain interaction. I. Raleigh, NC: The Rome Foundation; 2016.

24. Rasquin A, Di Lorenzo C, Forbes D, et al. Childhood functional gastrointestinal disorders: child/adolescent. Gastroenterology 2006;130:1527-37.

25. Longstreth GF, Thompson WG, Chey WD, et al. Functional bowel disorders. Gastroenterology 2006;130:1480-91.

26. Lewis SJ, Heaton KW. Stool form scale as a useful guide to intestinal transit time. Scand J Gastroenterol 1997;32:920-4.

27. Lake AM. Chronic abdominal pain in childhood: diagnosis and management. Am Fam Physician 1999;59:1823-30.

28. Schurman JV, Friesen CA. Integrative treatment approaches: family satisfaction with a multidisciplinary paediatric abdominal pain clinic. Int J Integr Care 2010;10:e51.

29. Crushell E, Rowland M, Doherty M, et al. Importance of parental conceptual model of illness in severe recurrent abdominal pain. Pediatrics 2003;112:1368-72.

30. Levy RL, Langer SL, Walker LS, et al. Cognitive behavioral therapy for children with functional abdominal pain and their parents decreases pain and other symptoms. Am J Gastroenterol 2010;105:946-56.

31. Vlieger AM, Rutten JM, Govers AM, et al. Long-term follow-up of gut-directed hypnotherapy vs. standard care in children with functional abdominal pain or irritable bowel syndrome. Am J Gastroenterol 2012;107:627-31.

32. Duarte MA, Penna FJ, Andrade EM, et al. Treatment of non-organic recurrent abdominal pain: cognitive-behavioral family intervention. J Pediatr Gastroenterol Nutr 2006;43:59-64.

33. Sanders MR, Shepherd RW, Cleghorn G, et al. The treatment of recurrent abdominal pain in children: a controlled comparison of cognitive-behavioral family intervention and standard pediatric care. J Consult Clin Psychol 1994;62:306-14.

34. Robins PM, Smith SM, Glutting JJ, et al. A randomized controlled trial of a cognitive-behavioral family intervention for pediatric recurrent abdominal pain. J Pediatr Psychol 2005;30:97-408.

35. Humphreys P, Gevirtz R. Treatment of recurrent abdominal pain: components analysis of four treatment protocols. J Pediatr Gastroenterol Nutr 2000;31:47-51.

36. American Academy of Pediatrics Subcommittee on Chronic Abdominal Pain, North American Society for Pediatric Gastroenterology Hepatology, and Nutrition. Chronic abdominal pain in children. Pediatrics 2005;115:e370.

37. Wahnschaffe U, Schulzke JD, Zeitz M, et al. Predictors of clinical response to gluten-free diet in patients diagnosed with diarrhea-predominant irritable bowel syndrome. Clin Gastroenterol Hepatol 2007;105:859-65.

38. Chumpitazi BP, Hollister EB, Oezguen N, et al. Gut microbiota influences low fermentable substrate diet efficacy in children with irritable bowel syndrome. Gut Microbes 2014;5:165-75.

39. Bhan MK, Bhandari N. The role of zinc and vitamin A in persistent diarrhea among infants and young children. J Pediatr Gastroenterol Nutr 1998;26:446-53.

40. Bijkerk CJ, Muris JWM, Knottnerus JA, et al. Systematic review: the role of different types of fibre in the treatment of irritable bowel syndrome. Aliment Pharmacol Ther 2004;19:245-51.

41. Ford AC, Talley NJ, Spiegel BM, et al. Effect of fibre, antispasmodics and peppermint oil in the treatment of irritable bowel syndrome: systematic review and meta-analysis. BMJ 2008;337:a2313.

42. Khosho V, Armstead C, Landry L. Effect of a laxative with and without tegaserod in adolescents with constipation predominant irritable bowel syndrome. Aliment Pharmacol Ther 2006;23:191-6.

43. Drossman DA, Chey WD, Johanson JF, et al. Lubiprostone in patients with constipation-associated irritable bowel syndrome: results of two randomized, placebo-controlled studies [clinical trial]. Aliment Pharmacol Ther 2009;29:329-41.

44. Hyman PE, Di Lorenzo C, Prestridge LL, et al. Lubiprostone for the treatment of functional constipation in children. J Pediatr Gastroenterol Nutr 2014;58:283-91.

45. Chang L, Lembo A, Sultan S. American Gastroenterological Association Institute technical review on the pharmacological management of irritable bowel syndrome. Gastroenterology 2014;147:1149-72.e2.

46. Brandt LJ, Chey WD, Foxx-Orenstein AE, et al. An evidence-based systematic review on the management of irritable bowel syndrome. Am J Gastroenterol 2009;104(suppl 1): S1-S35.

47. Kline RM, Kline JJ, Barbero GJ. Enteric-coated, pH-dependent peppermint oil capsules for the treatment of irritable bowel syndrome in children. J Pediatr 2001;138:125.

48. Chogle A, Mintjens S, Saps M. Pediatric IBS: an overview on pathophysiology, diagnosis and treatment. Pediatr Ann 2014; 43:e76-82.

49. Kligler B, Chaudhary S. Peppermint oil. Am Fam Physician 2007;75:1027.

50. Saps M, Youssef N, Miranda A, et al. Multicenter, randomized placebo-controlled trial of amitriptyline in children with functional gastrointestinal disorders. Gastroenterology 2009; 137:1261-9.

51. Bahar RJ, Collins BS, Steinmetz B, et al. Double-blind placebo-controlled trial of amitriptyline for the treatment of irritable bowel syndrome in adolescents. J Pediatr 2008;152:685-9.

52. Ladabaum U, Sharabidze A, Levin TR, et al. Citalopram provides little or no benefit in nondepressed patients with irritable bowel syndrome. Clin Gastroenterol Hepatol 2010;8:42-8.e1.

53. Simrén M, Barbara G, Flint HJ, et al. Intestinal microbiota in functional bowel disorders: a Rome foundation report. Gut 2013;62:159-76.

54. Gawronska A, Dziechciarz P, Horvath A, et al. A randomized double-blind placebo-controlled trial of Lactobacillus GG for abdominal pain disorders in children. Aliment Pharmacol Ther 2007;25:177-84.

55. Bauserman M, Michail S. The use of Lactobacillus GG in irritable bowel syndrome in children: a double-blind randomized control trial. J Pediatr 2005;147:197-201.

56. Martens U, Enck P, Ziesenib E. Probiotic treatment of irritable bowel syndrome in children. Geriatr Med Sci 2010;8: Doc07.

57. Vandenplas Y, Benninga M. Probiotics and functional gastrointestinal disorders in children. J Pediatr Gastroenterol Nutr 2009;48:S107-9.

58. Taketomo CK, Hodding JH, Kraus DM. Pediatric & Neonatal Dosage Handbook, 18th ed. Hudson, OH: Lexi-Comp, 2011.

59. Dwyer JT. Dietary fiber for children: how much? Pediatrics 1995; 96:1019-22.

60. Constipation Guideline Committee of the North American Society for Pediatric Gastroenterology, Hepatology and Nutrition. Evaluation and treatment of constipation in infants and children: recommendations of the North American Society for Pediatric Gastroenterology, Hepatology, and Nutrition. J Pediatr Gastroenterol Nutr 2006;43:e1-e13.

61. Pelkowki TD, Viera AJ. Celiac disease: diagnosis and management. Am Fam Physician 2014;89:99-105.

62. Rubio-Tapia A, Van Dyke CT, Lahr BD, et al. Predictors of family risk for celiac disease: a population-based study. Clin Gastroenterol Hepatol 2008;6:983-7.

63. Norris JM, Barriga K, Hoffenberg EJ, et al. Risk of celiac disease autoimmunity and timing of gluten introduction in the diet of infants at increased risk of disease. JAMA 2005;293:2343-51.

64. Akobeng AK, Ramanan AV, Buchan I, et al. Effect of breast feeding on risk of coeliac disease in children: a systematic review and meta-analysis of observational studies. Arch Dis Child 2006; 91:39-43.

65. Radlovic NP, Mladenovic MM, Lekovic ZM, et al. Influence of early feeding practices on celiac disease in infants. Croat Med J 2010;51:417-22.

66. Decker E, Englemann G, Findeisen A, et al. Cesarean delivery is associated with celiac disease but not inflammatory bowel disease in children. Pediatrics 2010;125:e1433-40.

67. Stene, LC, Honeyman MC, Hoffenberg EJ, et al. Rotavirus infection frequency and risk of celiac disease autoimmunity in early childhood: a longitudinal study. Am J Gastroenterol 2006;101:2333-40.

68. Ediger TR, Hill ID. Celiac disease. Pediatr Rev 2014;35:409-16.

69. Rubio-Tapia A, Hill I, Kelly C, et al. ACG clinical guidelines: diagnosis and management of celiac disease. Am J Gastroenterol 2013;108:656-76.

70. Mantegazza C, Zucotti G, Dilillo D, et al. Celiac disease in children: a review. International Journal of Digestive Disease 2015;1:1-7.

71. Akobeng AK, Thomas AG. Systemic review: tolerable amount of gluten for people with celiac disease. Aliment Pharmacol Ther 2008;27:1044-52.

72. Thompson T. Gluten contamination of commercial oat products in the United States. N Eng J Med 2004;351;2021-2.

73. Koskinen O, Villanen M, Korponay-Szabo I, et al. Oats do not produce systemic or mucosal autoantibody response in children with celiac disease. J Pediatr Gastroenterol Nutr 2011;35:459-64.

74. Hogberg L, Luarin P, Falth-Magnusson K, et al. Oats to children with newly diagnosed coeliac disease: a randomised double blind study. Gut 2004;53:649-54.

75. Sugai E, Nachman F, Vaquez H, et al. Dynamics of celiac disease-specific serology after initiation of a gluten-free diet and use in the assessment of compliance with treatment. Dig Liver Dis 2010;42:352-58.

76. King AR. Gluten content of the top 200 medications: follow-up to the influence of gluten on a patients medications choices. Hosp Pharm 2013;48:736-43.

77. Plogsted S. Medications and celiac disease: tips from a pharmacist. Pract Gastroenterol 2007;31:58-64.

78. Mangione RA, Patel PN, Shin E, et al. Determining the gluten content of nonprescription drugs: Information for patients with celiac disease. Am Pharmacists Assoc 2011;51:734-37.

79. Mulder CJ, Wierdsma NJ, Berkenpas M, et al. Preventing complications in celiac disease: our experience with managing adult celiac disease. Best Pract Res Clin Gastroenterol 2015;29:459-68.

80. Fabiani E, Catassi C, Villari A, et al. Dietary compliance in screening-detected coeliac disease adolescents. Acta Pediatr 1996;412:65-7.

81. Botero-Lopez JE, Araya M, Parada, et al. Micronutrient deficiencies in patients with typical and atypical celiac disease. J Pediatr Gastroenterol Nutr 2011;53:265-70.

82. Guandalini S, Assiri A. Celiac disease: a review. JAMA Pediatr 2014;168:272-78.

83. Oliveres M, Castillejo G, Varea V, et al. Double-blind, randomized, placebo-controlled intervention trial to evaluate the effects of bifidobacterium longun cect 7347 in children with newly diagnosed coeliac disease. Br J Nutr 2014;112:30-40.

84. Malamut G, Afchain P, Verkarre V, et al. Presentation and long-term follow-up of refractory celiac disease: comparison of type I with type II. Gastroenterology 2009;136:81-90.

85. Abdallah H, Leffler D, Dennis M, et al. Refractory celiac disease. Curr Gastroenterol Rep 2007;9:401-5.

86. Goerres MS, Meijer JW, Wahab PJ, et al. Azathioprine and prednisone combination therapy in refractory celiac disease. Aliment Pharmacol Ther 2003;18:487-94.

Section VI

Nutritional Disorders

CHAPTER 19

Fluids and Electrolytes
Weng Man Lam, Pharm.D., M.S., BCPS, BCPPS

INTRODUCTION

COMPOSITION OF BODY FLUIDS

In the human body, water is the largest compartment compared with the other nutritional components, including protein, fat, and carbohydrate. As humans age, total body water (TBW), as a percentage of body weight, slowly decreases, as described in Figure 1. The fetus has the highest TBW content, which gradually decreases to about 75% for a full-term infant. During the first year of life, TBW decreases to about 60% and remains steady at this percentage until puberty. In general, TBW is 60% in men and 50% in women.[1] This discrepancy occurs because during puberty the fat content of the female body increases more than that of men, and men tend to have more muscle mass than women. This higher tendency toward muscle affects the TBW of men and women because fat has lower water content and muscle has higher water content.[2]

Water is distributed between two main compartments: intracellular fluid (ICF) and extracellular fluid (ECF). In the adult, the TBW is two-thirds ICF and one-third ECF, which is further divided into three-fourths interstitial fluid and one-fourth plasma.[1] The ECF volume in the fetus and newborn is larger than the ICF volume, but the ECF volume decreases with age. By age 1 year, the ratio of ECF and ICF approaches the adult level because of the postnatal diuresis at birth and the continued expansion of the ICF compartment caused by cellular growth.[2-4] The interstitial fluid, which is about 15% of the body weight, increases in pathologic conditions such as heart failure, liver failure, nephrotic syndrome, and hypoalbuminemia.[2] Plasma is about 5% of total body weight. Plasma is estimated to be 85–100 mL/kg of body weight in neonates compared with 60–70 mL/kg of body weight in adolescents and adults.[3] Plasma volume can be affected by different pathologic conditions, including dehydration, anemia, polycythemia, heart failure, abnormal plasma osmolality, and hypoalbuminemia.

ELECTROLYTE COMPOSITION

The composition of solutes in the ICF differs from that in the ECF. In the ICF, potassium is the predominant cation, and phosphate is the predominant anion.[1] Activity of the Na^+/K^+-ATPase pump (sodium-potassium pump) in plasma membranes is responsible for the low-sodium and high-potassium intracellular concentrations. In the ECF (plasma

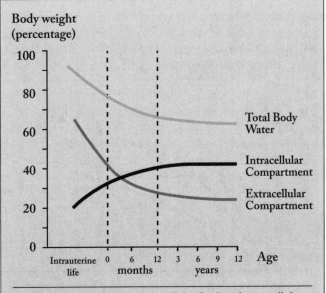

Figure 1. Total body water, intracellular fluid, and extracellular fluid as a percentage of body weight and a function of age.

Reprinted with permission from Winters RW. Water and electrolyte regulation. In: Winters RW, ed. The Body Fluids in Pediatrics. Boston: Little, Brown, 1973.

and interstitial fluid), sodium and chloride are the dominant cations and anions, respectively. Sodium excretion, which can affect the ECF volume, occurs mainly through urine, sweat, and feces. The intake and output of chloride usually parallels that of sodium, and the kidney plays a major role in regulating the reabsorption of filtered chloride. Table 1 describes the approximate electrolyte composition of the ECF and ICF.

Table 1. Approximate Electrolyte Composition of ECF and ICF[1]

Electrolyte	ECF (mEq/L)	ICF (mEq/L)
Na⁺	135–145	10–20
K⁺	3.5–5	120–150
Cl⁻	95–105	0–3
HCO₃⁻	22–30	10
Phosphate	2	110–120

EFC = extracellular fluid; ICF = intracellular fluid.

REGULATION OF OSMOLALITY

Osmolality represents the number of osmoles (solutes) per kilogram. Solutions of higher osmolality have more solute and less water per unit volume whereas solutions of lower osmolality have less solute and more water. Water is the primary factor in maintaining osmotic balance because it moves freely across the cell membrane between the ECF and the ICF. If any disturbance affects the osmolality balance between the body fluid compartments, water will respond to changes in the osmotic shifts.[2,3] For example, in a child with a diagnosis of diabetic ketoacidosis, the body's high blood glucose increases the osmolality of the ECF. This increased osmolality results in a shift in water from the ICF to the ECF to maintain the osmotic equilibrium.

Normal serum osmolality is about 285–295 mOsm/kg. Plasma osmolality is calculated by the following formula with glucose and blood urea nitrogen (BUN):

$$\text{Serum osmolality} = 2[\text{Na}] + \frac{[\text{glucose in mg/dL}]}{18} + \frac{[\text{BUN in mg/dL}]}{2.8}$$

Antidiuretic hormone (ADH) plays a significant role in plasma osmolality, with responses detectable with as small as a 1% change in osmolality.[2] Antidiuretic hormone initiates its physiologic actions by two major types of vasopressin receptors: V1 and V2. The V1 receptors are on the blood vessels, and the V2 receptors are in the basolateral membrane of the collecting tubule cells in the kidney. Osmoreceptors in the hypothalamus sense changes in plasma osmolality. An increase in osmolality leads to ADH secretion. The circulating ADH binds to V2 receptors in the collecting duct cells of the kidney, causing an insertion of water channels (aquaporin-2) into the renal collecting ducts. Thus, ADH increases the permeability of water for reabsorption, resulting in an increased urine concentration and decreased water excretion. Therefore, urine osmolality is an important tool in assessing water homeostasis. Urine osmolality, excluding that in neonates, is 50–1200 mOsm/kg.[1] The high value shows maximally concentrated urine; the low value shows very dilute urine. In a dehydrated patient with normal kidney function, a small volume of highly concentrated urine is produced because the body is trying to retain water; therefore, the urine osmolality has a high value.

FLUID AND ELECTROLYTE MAINTENANCE REQUIREMENTS

Maintenance fluids and electrolytes are required because of normal losses from body basal metabolism. In general, body basal metabolism is divided into two byproducts, solute and heat, which are eliminated to maintain homeostasis.[5,6] Soluble waste byproducts from metabolism are excreted in the urine, which is also known as *urinary water loss*.[6,7] Heat elimination is described as an *insensible water loss* and is a function of basal energy expenditure.[7] Examples of insensible water losses include evaporation of water from the skin surface, elimination of warmed water vapor from the upper respiratory tract during exhalation, and sweating.

In a 1957 study, a child's caloric requirements were estimated to allow a determination of maintenance fluid requirements using weight alone. A comparison of energy expenditure from the basal metabolic rate and the normal activity state is described in Figure 2. The lower line defines the basal metabolic rate at various weights, and the upper line defines the estimated total expenditure with normal activity for various weights.[7] The middle line defines the

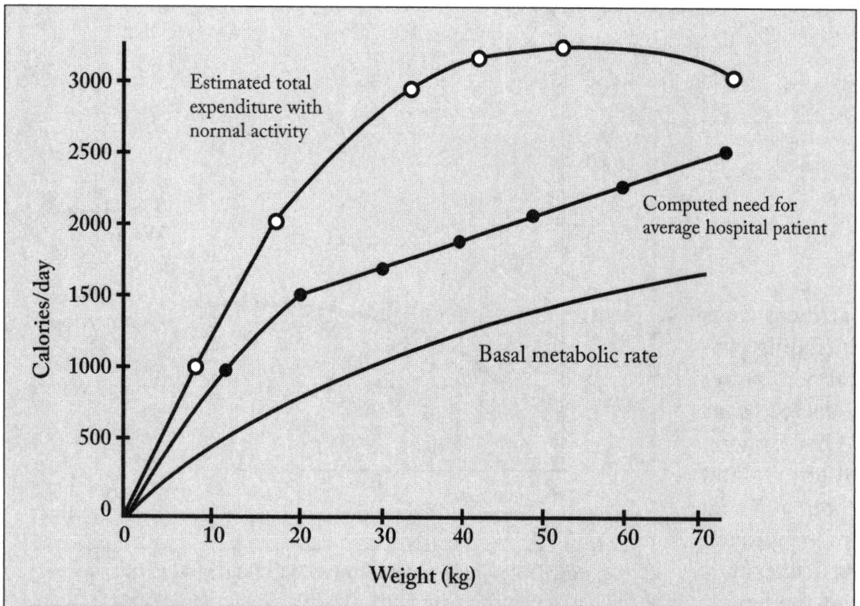

Figure 2. Comparison of energy expenditure in basal and ideal states.

Reprinted with permission from Holliday MA, Segar WE. The maintenance need for water in parenteral fluid therapy. Pediatrics 1957;19:823-32.

calculated energy expenditure for the average hospitalized patient at bed rest. The graph shows that, compared with body weight, the metabolic rate is higher (on a calorie per kilogram basis) in the newborn period than in adulthood. Furthermore, this graph shows that the metabolic rate per unit of body weight declines with increasing age. Adolescents and adults generate less heat and solute from basal metabolism than do children and infants; therefore, they need less fluid and electrolytes per unit of body weight. Similarly, children generate less heat and solute from basal metabolism than infants or neonates and therefore require less fluid and electrolytes per unit of body weight.[6]

These principles dictate how fluid requirements are calculated. Several methods, including the surface area, basal calorie, and Holliday–Segar methods, have been proposed to correlate maintenance requirements to body weight. All three methods work when used appropriately; however, the Holliday–Segar method is commonly used because the formula is easy to apply and remember. The surface area method requires an equation or table to determine the patient's body surface area, as well as the patient's height and weight. The basal calorie method requires a table and information such as weight, height, age, and activity level, and this method also involves more calculations than the other two methods.[6] Therefore, the Holliday–Segar method is commonly used to calculate the 24-hour maintenance fluid requirements in children (Table 2). The 4-2-1 method is also commonly used in a hospital setting; the 24-hour fluid requirement is divided into approximate hourly rates for convenience of calculation. Therefore, the hourly infusion rate can be programmed into the delivery pump.

In general, infants become dehydrated faster than older patients (adolescents); infants therefore have a higher maintenance fluid requirement on a milliliter per kilogram basis. For example, an adolescent can tolerate 12–18 hours without oral intake when preparing for a surgical procedure, but an infant requires intravenous maintenance fluids within 4–6 hours after the last feeding for a morning surgical procedure to avoid developing dehydration. It is very important to recognize the patient populations in need of maintenance fluids versus those who can tolerate an extended period without any fluids.[2]

A premature neonate and a newborn are more susceptible to insensible water losses than are infants. A premature neonate has about five times more body surface area in relation to weight (and a newborn three times more), resulting in a higher fluid loss.[4] A term infant requires 80–120 mL/kg/day of infusion fluid therapy, which may increase to as high as 160 mL/kg/day to meet the infant's needs. Moreover, neonates who are extremely low birth weight or very low birth weight require more fluids than term neonates and infants. For fluid intake, neonates weighing more than 1500 g require 60–80 mL/kg/day, and neonates weighing 1000–1500 g require 80–100 mL/kg/day. The preterm neonates who are extremely low birth weight (less than 1000 g) require fluid volumes of 50–80 mL/kg/day if the neonates are placed inside a double-walled humidified (80%) incubator. If the neonates are under a radiant warmer or in an incubator without humidity, the fluid requirement can be as low as 100 mL/kg/day and as high as 200 mL/kg/day.[8-10] Neonates born with gastroschisis—a birth defect of the abdominal wall in which the neonate's intestines are exposed to the outside of the body by a hole beside the belly button—require an increase in fluid requirement because of the fluid and heat loss from the exposed bowel. In general, once the neonate's weight reaches 3 kg, the Holliday–Segar method is preferred.

The goal of providing maintenance fluids and electrolytes is to prevent dehydration, electrolyte disorders, ketoacidosis, and protein degradation. Maintenance fluids typically consist of water, glucose, sodium, and potassium. Each component of maintenance fluid plays a role in replacing the fluid and electrolyte losses needed by an average individual with normal ICF and ECF volumes over 24 hours.[5]

Maintenance water is designed to provide enough water that the kidney does not need to dilute or concentrate the urine to maintain the fluid balance in the body.[2] The glucose administered to the patient is only sufficient to prevent ketoacidosis and protein degradation. The electrolytes sodium, potassium, and chloride are present in the maintenance fluid to replace normal losses from urine and stool. For most patients, a few days without other electrolyte supplements like calcium, phosphorous, magnesium, or bicarbonate is not problematic; therefore, these supplements are not routinely added to the maintenance fluid therapy. The daily maintenance requirement for sodium is 2–3 mEq/kg/24 hours, potassium is 1–3 mEq/kg/24 hours, and chloride is 2 mEq/kg/24 hours in children.[2,9] Potassium is not required for patients with acute and chronic renal failure or when potassium retention is present.

Maintenance fluids do not provide adequate calories, protein, fat, minerals, or vitamins for normal consumption in children. However, a patient can receive maintenance fluids without additional calories or nutrition for a few days. Nevertheless, the patient's weight should be monitored while receiving maintenance fluid therapy because weight loss may be 0.5%–1% of total weight each day while receiving this therapy alone.[2]

Intravenous fluids that are safe to administer parenterally according to osmolality are shown in Table 3. The solution is selected according to the patient's clinical status and patient's laboratory values. In general, hypotonic fluids theoretically offer enough water and electrolytes to match the maintenance requirements in children based on the Holliday–Segar

Table 2. Methods for Calculating Fluid Requirements in Pediatric Patients[7]

Weight (kg)	24-Hr Maintenance Water Requirement Holliday–Segar Method	Maintenance Water Rate/Hr 4-2-1 Method
≤ 10	100 mL/kg	4 mL/kg/hr
11–20	1000 mL + 50 mL/kg for each kg > 10 kg	40 mL/hr + 2 mL/kg/hr × (weight − 10 kg)
> 20	1500 mL + 20 mL/kg for each kg > 20 kg	60 mL/hr + 1 mL/kg/hr × (weight − 20 kg)

methods.[7] The most hypotonic (lowest osmolality) intravenous solution that can be used safely is 0.45% isotonic sodium chloride (osmolality 154 mOsm/L).[1] Any solution with an osmolality less than 154 mOsm/L is not recommended because cell lysing causes the release of potassium to the extracellular space, resulting in hyperkalemia and potentially cardiac arrhythmias and death.[1] Solutions without dextrose (e.g., 0.45% sodium chloride solution with electrolytes) are administered to patients presenting with diabetic ketoacidosis. Neonates differ from children because neonates tend to have difficulty excreting sodium. Therefore, fluids such as 5% or 10% dextrose in water are used to deliver isotonic fluids without an excessive sodium load while delivering the maintenance water requirements.

In the 1950s, Holliday and Segar published their landmark paper detailing the maintenance fluid volumes required by children, and their method became the basis of intravenous fluid prescribing for the next 50 years.[7] Fluids can be divided into *hypotonic*, *isotonic*, and *hypertonic*. *Tonicity* is defined as the ability of a fluid to exert an osmotic force and influence the movement of fluid across a cell membrane. When the fluid has a similar osmolality to the plasma, it is considered *isotonic* because the osmotic force across the cellular membrane does not change or is not influenced by the tonicity. In contrast, *hypotonic* fluid has a lower osmolality compared with plasma, which means that the osmolality of the intravascular space decreases. This change will create an osmotic gradient, which will drive the intravascular space into the intracellular space. The movement of water into the intracellular space causes its volume to increase. With the limited space available in the brain tissue, this volume increase may potentially result in neurologic damage such as cerebral edema. For a healthy child, the renal system will compensate for the reduced serum osmolality with increased excretion of free water. However, for an ill child, the body will be more likely to release antidiuretic hormone, which reduces the ability of the kidney to excrete free water. For patients who have disease states associated with arginine vasopressin excess, this volume increase can impair the free water excretion, which may put them at risk of developing hyponatremia.[11,12]

Because of the difference between the physiologic processes for healthy or ill children, several studies over the past 20 years have investigated the safest maintenance fluid administration in a hospitalized general pediatric population including age, surgical (postoperative patients), and varying acuity (intensive care unit versus general ward).[13-18] A recent study compared isotonic (sodium chloride 0.9% and dextrose 5%) with hypotonic (sodium chloride 0.45% and dextrose 5%) intravenous maintenance fluid in a hospital setting to evaluate the sodium concentration at 24 and 48 hours from baseline. No clinically significant difference was found between isotonic and hypotonic fluids in the outcome of sodium concentration at 48 hours after intravenous fluid administration. This study supported that the isotonic maintenance fluid was safe in general pediatric patients and may result in fewer cases of hyponatremia.[17] In a meta-analysis that brought attention to the current practice, the investigators assessed the evidence from 10 randomized controlled studies on the safety of isotonic versus hypotonic intravenous maintenance fluid in hospitalized children. A significantly higher risk with hypotonic intravenous fluids for developing hyponatremia and severe hyponatremia was found. Children who received hypotonic fluid during the hospital stay had a greater decrease in plasma sodium concentration. Overall, this meta-analysis showed that isotonic fluids were safer than hypotonic fluids in hospitalized children who required maintenance intravenous fluids. However, there is still no ideal intravenous fluid for all children with respect to composition of fluid (content of sodium), rate, and duration of administration. Therefore, plasma sodium concentrations must be monitored closely when administering intravenous fluids to hospitalized children.[18]

In addition, a recent study evaluated the use of Plasma-Lyte A, pH 7.4 (Baxter Healthcare, Deerfield, IL), a balanced isotonic crystalloid solution in pediatric patients.[19] The osmolarity of Plasma-Lyte A is 294 mOsmol/L, which is within the normal serum osmolality. Plasma-Lyte A is used as a source of water and electrolytes because it contains sodium, chloride, potassium, magnesium, and bicarbonate. Plasma-Lyte A contains chloride 98 mEq/L, making it appropriate to use as a dehydration fluid. This potential for use is because it may

Table 3. Intravenous Fluid Comparison[1,19]

Solution	Osmolality (mOsm/L)	Sodium (mEq/L)	Chloride (mEq/L)	Dextrose (mOsm/L)
Lactated Ringer solution[a]	273	130	109	None
0.9% isotonic NaCl (normal saline)	308	154	154	None
Plasma-Lyte A[b]	294	140	98	None
0.45% NaCl	154	77	77	None
5% dextrose in water	252	None	None	278
5% dextrose + 0.33% NaCl	378	50	50	278
5% dextrose + 0.225% NaCl	329	38.5	38.5	278
5% dextrose + 0.45% NaCl	432	77	77	278

[a]Lactated Ringer solution also contains potassium 4 mEq/L, calcium 3 mEq/L, and lactate 28 mEq/L.
[b]Plasma-Lyte A, Baxter Healthcare, Deerfield, IL.
NaCl = sodium chloride.

reduce the risk of intravenous fluid–induced hyperchloremia metabolic acidosis, which is a common challenge with 0.9% sodium chloride intravenous fluid. In addition, Plasma-Lyte A contains acetate 27 mEq/L and gluconate 23 mEq/L, serving as a buffering agent. Until more studies evaluate the role of Plasma-Lyte A as a maintenance fluid, it is generally considered as another alternative agent.[19]

Maintenance intravenous fluids are used to provide critical supportive care for children who are acutely ill. An American Academy of Pediatrics guideline published in 2018 focuses on administering maintenance intravenous fluids in children in clinical practice. The guideline discusses that hyponatremia (serum sodium concentration less than 135 mEq/L) is the most common electrolyte abnormality in patients who are hospitalized, affecting 15%–30% of children to adult patients. Based on the current literature support, the American Academy of Pediatrics recommends that patients age 28 days to 18 years requiring maintenance intravenous fluids should receive isotonic solutions with appropriate potassium chloride and dextrose because this approach significantly decreases the risk of developing hyponatremia. This guideline clearly states that isotonic solutions have a sodium concentration similar to Plasma-Lyte A or 0.9% sodium chloride, and the guideline only applies to children in surgical (postoperative) and medical acute care settings, including critical care and general inpatient settings. However, because the guidelines do not address the optimal empiric maintenance fluids, additional well-designed trials are needed to determine the needs of the pediatric special population, including patients with the following: neurologic disorders; congenital or acquired cardiac disease; hepatic disease; cancer; renal dysfunction; diabetes insipidus; voluminous water diarrhea; or severe burns, in addition to neonates who are younger than 28 days or in the neonatal intensive care unit and adolescents older than 18 years.[13]

DEHYDRATION

Dehydration is a physiologic disturbance caused by the reduction in or translocation of body fluids, and, if severe, can be considered a type of hypovolemic shock.[20] Dehydration is one of the leading causes of morbidity and mortality in children worldwide. Infants have the highest morbidity and mortality from dehydration because they have a larger water content, a higher metabolic turnover rate of water, renal immaturity, and an inability to independently meet their own needs. In the early process of dehydration, most of the water loss is from the ECF.

In the United States, the main cause of dehydration in children is diarrhea. Other causes of dehydration are gastroenteritis, febrile illness, stomatitis, diabetic ketoacidosis, heat prostration, and burns over 25% of the total body surface area.[14] In many cases, dehydration can be managed with an oral rehydration solution, as discussed in the following section. In more severe cases, intravenous therapy is required, especially when the patient cannot tolerate oral intake or is in hypovolemic shock.[20-22]

CLINICAL EVALUATION OF DEHYDRATION AND SEVERITY OF DEHYDRATION

The first step in treating a child with dehydration is to assess the severity of dehydration. Dehydration is classified as mild, moderate, or severe according to the percentage of body weight loss (Table 4). This estimation is calculated as a percentage of total body weight loss according to pre-illness weight and current (illness) weight (Figure 3). Because infants have a higher percentage of body weight as water, their total percentages of body weight loss are higher than those of older children in moderate and severe dehydration.[5] The history provided by the parents or caregivers is also beneficial

Table 4. Signs and Symptoms Related to Severity of Dehydration[1,2,22,27]

Infants Older Children	Mild 1%–5%[a] 1%–3%[a]	Moderate 6%–9%[a] 4%–6%[a]	Severe > 10% (≥ 15% = shock)[a] > 6% (≥ 9% = shock)[a]
Heart rate	Normal, increased	Tachycardia	Rapid and weak
Systolic blood pressure	Normal	Normal, low	Decreased, very low
Urinary output	Decreased	Little or low < 1 mL/kg/hr	Oliguria < 1 mL/kg/hr
Buccal mucosa	Slightly dry	Dry	Parched
Anterior fontanelle	Normal	Sunken	Very sunken
Eyes	Normal	Sunken	Very sunken
Skin turgor/ capillary refill	Normal	Delayed Cool and pale	Very delayed Cool and mottled
Skin (age < 12 mo)	Normal	Cool	Acrocyanosis
Tears	Normal	Decreased	No tears
Mental status	Normal	Normal to listless	Normal to lethargic or comatose
Thirst	Drinks normally; might refuse liquids	Thirsty; eager to drink	Drinks poorly; cannot drink

[a]The percentage is the amount of body weight loss based on the pre-illness weight and the current (illness) weight.

because it may help describe the child's fluid loss and its origin (Box 1).[20]

When the pre-illness weight is unavailable, it is reasonable to use a scoring system to assess the child's dehydration status. The three validated clinical dehydration scales are the World Health Organization (WHO) scale for dehydration, the Gorelick scale, and the clinical dehydration scale. The clinical dehydration scale is commonly used in children age 1–36 months because it is easy to use and supported by evidence. The clinical dehydration scale has four characteristics: general appearance, eyes, mucous membranes, and tears. Each characteristic is rated 0–2, and the total score is 0–8. A score of 0 is no dehydration, 1–4 is some dehydration, and 5–8 is moderate/severe dehydration (Table 5).[23,24]

PHYSICAL EXAMINATION AND LABORATORY ASSESSMENT

Assessment of vital signs helps evaluate the severity of dehydration. The first vital sign change in mild dehydration is tachycardia. The respiratory rate of a patient with mild to moderate dehydration is usually normal. As the severity of dehydration worsens, the respiratory rate may increase. Severe hypotension is a sign of severe dehydration.

The skin can also be used to reliably assess for signs of peripheral perfusion. Assessment of skin temperature, turgor, and capillary refill is useful in dehydration. For example, cool peripheral extremities are an early sign of poor perfusion, meaning that blood flow to the peripheral part of the body is inadequate. Skin turgor is measured by pinching the skin into folds (tenting) and then promptly releasing it. If there is a delay in the return of skin to its original state, skin elasticity is decreased because of water loss. Capillary refill time is the time needed for vascular reperfusion after blanching pressure is applied to the nail bed.[25,26] Normal capillary refill is usually 2 seconds or less. However, if the capillary refill time is greater than 3 seconds, the patient may have severe fluid loss and impending shock.[20]

A serum electrolyte panel may not be as helpful in predicting the degree of dehydration. Patients presenting with altered mental status, moderate to severe dehydration, or clinical signs of hypokalemia or hypernatremia or infants younger

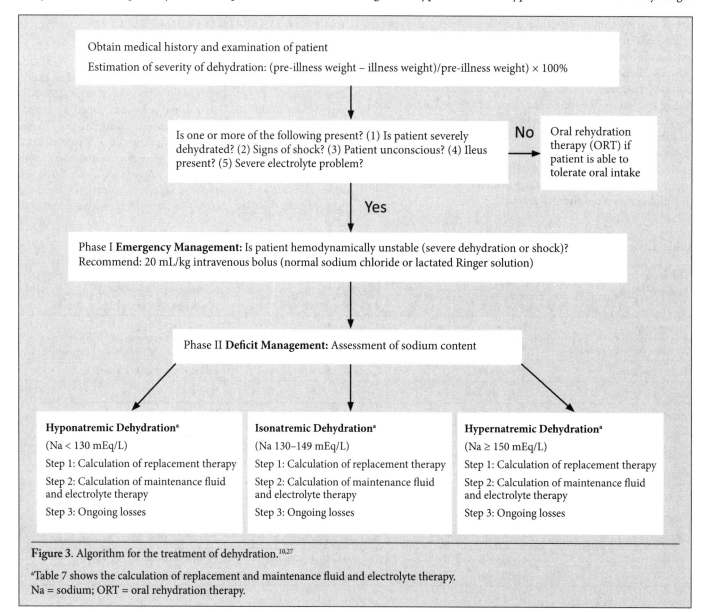

Figure 3. Algorithm for the treatment of dehydration.[10,27]

[a]Table 7 shows the calculation of replacement and maintenance fluid and electrolyte therapy.
Na = sodium; ORT = oral rehydration therapy.

than 6 months warrant an electrolyte panel.[22,27] The serum sodium concentration determines the type of dehydration: hypernatremic, isonatremic, or hyponatremic. Measurement of BUN or serum urea concentration is usually a marker of prerenal uremia and dehydration. Studies have shown a trend toward urea concentration to increase with the degree of dehydration.[28-32] In healthy patients the BUN/serum creatinine ratio is 10:15 to 1; therefore, an elevated BUN/serum creatinine ratio may suggest that the patient is dehydrated.

MANAGEMENT

The severity of dehydration dictates the urgency of the situation and determines whether oral or intravenous therapy is required and indicates the volume of fluid needed to replace the loss. For a patient who can tolerate oral intake, oral rehydration therapy (ORT) is recommended.

Box 1. Examples of Information Obtained from a Parent or Caregiver About Pediatric Patient Dehydration[20]

Volume, type, and frequency of the fluid intake
Amount of urinary output
Frequency of stool output and stool consistency
Frequency and volume of emesis
Recent sick contact with ill people, especially those with gastroenteritis
Use of day care
Appetite pattern
Weight loss
Recent travel history
Absence or presence of tears
Recent use of antibiotics
Possible ingestions
Underlying illnesses (e.g., cystic fibrosis, diabetes, hyperthyroidism, renal disease)
Presence of fever
Presence of sweating
Hyperventilation
Changes in diet[a]
Infant formula

[a]Diluted juices or water can be associated with hyponatremic dehydration, and excess salt intake or low liquid intake can be associated with hypernatremic dehydration

---

ORAL REHYDRATION THERAPY

Oral rehydration therapy is the preferred treatment of fluid and electrolyte losses caused by diarrhea in children with mild and moderate dehydration. Several studies have shown the safety and efficacy of ORT. In addition, ORT has several potential advantages over intravenous therapy. Oral replacement therapy is less expensive, is more convenient, has a low potential for infections, and is less traumatic to the child, and can be given in a variety of settings, such as in a physician's office, in an emergency department, or at home. The ORT solutions have successfully rehydrated more than 90% of dehydrated children and have lower complication rates than intravenous therapy.[33,34] In studies comparing ORT with intravenous therapy, frequency of stools, duration of diarrhea, and rate of weight gain are similar.[27,34-42]

All commercially available rehydration fluids (e.g., Pedialyte, Abbott Laboratories, Columbus, OH) are acceptable for ORT. They contain 2–3 g/dL of glucose; 45–90 mEq/L of sodium; 30 mEq/L of lactate, citrate, or acetate; and 20–25 mEq/L of potassium.[9] A list of commonly used oral rehydration fluids and their composition is in the Diarrhea and Constipation chapter. Rehydration with solutions such as apple juice, ginger ale, sodas, sports drinks, milk, and chicken broth is discouraged because they contain low electrolyte concentrations and high carbohydrate content and they are hypertonic (osmolality 260–700 mOsm/L).[27,41] The high carbohydrate content may worsen diarrhea. In addition, the sodium content is generally too low, which is an important electrolyte that is lost during diarrhea and vomiting.

Correction of mild dehydration includes giving 50 mL of ORT per kilogram plus replacement of any continuing losses over 4 hours. The continuing losses from stools and emesis can be corrected for by giving 10 mL of ORT per kilogram of body weight for each watery stool and 2 mL of ORT per kilogram of body weight for each episode of emesis. The patient is evaluated every 2 hours for progress with ORT and hydration status. As soon as the patient is rehydrated, breastfeeding, formula, milk, or other recommended foods should be resumed, as should continued replacement of ongoing losses with an appropriate ORT solution.[27]

For moderate dehydration, it is recommended to administer 100 mL of ORT per kilogram and to replace continuing losses over 4 hours. The patient's hydration status is assessed on an hourly basis, which is best accomplished in a supervised setting such as the emergency department, urgent care facility, or physician's office. Once rehydration is completed, feeding should be resumed as previously described. Controversy

---

Table 5. Clinical Dehydration Scale Score for Children Age 1–36 Months[23,24]

Characteristics[a]	Scale 0–2		
	0	1	2
General appearance	Normal	Thirsty; restless or lethargic; irritable when touched	Drowsy; limp; cold; or sweaty + comatose
Eyes	Normal	Slightly sunken	Extremely sunken
Mucous membranes	Moist	Sticky	Dry
Tears	Tear	Decreased tears	Absent tears

[a]Assess and score each characteristic according to general appearance, eyes, mucous membranes, and tears of the child.

---

still lies in determining which foods are best for refeeding children. Certain foods, including complex carbohydrates (e.g., rice, wheat, potatoes, bread, and cereals), lean meats, yogurt, fruits, and vegetables are better tolerated in children.[27]

INTRAVENOUS THERAPY

Management of moderate to severe dehydration in children requires acute intervention to ensure adequate tissue perfusion. The care plan for correcting a child's dehydration requires monitoring the patient's clinical status such as vital signs during treatment, modifying the therapy as needed given the clinical situation, and assessing the electrolytes often. Children who are severely dehydrated and in a state of shock or near-shock, as well as those who have severe electrolyte abnormalities, require intravenous fluid therapy. Children who are moderately dehydrated and cannot retain oral liquids because of persistent vomiting should receive intravenous therapy. In addition, children who are unconscious, have an ileus, or have severe electrolyte abnormalities should receive intravenous therapy.[9,27]

Intravenous replacement therapy is generally divided into phase I—*emergency management*, and phase II—*deficit management*, which includes a combination of deficit replacement, maintenance therapy, and ongoing losses. Overall goals of therapy are as follows: restoration of hemodynamic stability, including normal blood pressure, restoration of skin turgor and weight, normal capillary refill; recovery of alertness; tolerance of oral intake of food; and correction of serum chemistry values.[5] Figure 3 provides an algorithm for the treatment of dehydration. The serum sodium concentration determines the type of dehydration: hypernatremic (serum sodium 150 mEq/L or greater), isonatremic (serum sodium 130–149 mEq/L), and hyponatremic (serum sodium less than 130 mEq/L).

Phase I: Emergency management. Volume depletion reduces the blood volume needed to adequately perfuse tissues. If not treated in a timely manner, organ damage may occur. With persistent hypovolemia, shock and death may result. For a hemodynamically unstable patient (severe dehydration or shock), one or more boluses of intravenous fluids are recommended. A common recommendation is to administer 20 mL/kg of 0.9% sodium chloride or lactated Ringer solution in the first 30 minutes of presentation. If the patient

is still unstable after two boluses, 40 mL/kg may be required as a bolus.[9] The main goals of the emergency correction phase are to ensure a return of adequate intravascular volume and to avoid tissue damage.

Phase II: Deficit management. Intravenous rehydration therapy is indicated for deficit management. Selecting the appropriate intravenous therapy (focusing on the sodium content of the fluid) depends on the patient's serum sodium. Patients may present with hyponatremia, isonatremia, or hypernatremia. Steps for calculating the deficit replacement therapy and maintenance therapy of fluids and electrolytes are outlined in the discussion of specific types of dehydration in following text. In general, deficit replacement therapy replaces any current existing water and electrolyte deficits (i.e., sodium and water deficits). The calculated maintenance therapy volume also accounts for expected ongoing losses of water and electrolytes from a normal physiological process.

Replacement therapy is also designed to replace any abnormal ongoing fluid and electrolyte losses. Measuring or estimating the electrolyte content of these losses and replacing them is preferred. Examples of measured losses include continued diarrhea or vomiting and aspirates from a nasogastric tube attached to suction. Other examples of estimated losses from various body fluids include gastric, pancreatic, small bowel, and bile fluids. The electrolyte composition of various body fluids is listed in Table 6.[6] Table 7 details the calculations necessary to determine the amount and type of fluids in the treatment of moderate to severe dehydration. The main goals of the deficit management phase are to replace any existing water and electrolyte deficits; any abnormal ongoing fluid and electrolyte losses; and any abnormal losses from various body fluids.

DISORDERS OF SODIUM HOMEOSTASIS

HYPONATREMIA

Hyponatremia is defined as a serum sodium concentration less than 130 mEq/L. The pathogenesis of hyponatremia is usually a combination of sodium loss and water retention to compensate for volume depletion. The body's primary defense against developing hyponatremia is the kidney's ability to dilute the urine and excrete free water.[6] It is important to determine the patient's volume status: euvolemia, hypovolemia, or hypervolemia. Knowledge of this volume status will help distinguish between hyponatremia caused by low sodium and hyponatremia caused by increased TBW, resulting in a relative dilution of the ECF compartment.[43,44] Hyponatremia can also be linked to renal or nonrenal causes. If the kidney is working properly, normal renal retention of sodium occurs; thus the urinary sodium concentration will be low (less than 10 mEq/L). However, if the kidney is the cause of sodium loss, the urine will have a sodium concentration greater than 20 mEq/L, which reflects a defect in renal sodium retention by the kidney to maintain normal homeostasis. Therefore, assessing the patient's renal function may also play a role in managing hyponatremia.[2] Causes of hyponatremia in children are listed in Box 2.

Table 6. Electrolyte Composition of Various Body Fluids[9,44]

Fluid	Sodium (mEq/L)	Potassium (mEq/L)	Chloride (mEq/L)
Gastric	20–80	5–20	100–150
Pancreatic	120–140	5–15	90–120
Small bowel	100–140	5–15	90–130
Bile	120–140	5–15	80–120
Ileostomy	45–135	3–15	20–115
Diarrhea	10–90	10–80	10–110
Burns	140	5	110
Sweat	10–30	3–10	10–35

HYPOVOLEMIC HYPONATREMIA

Hypovolemic hyponatremia usually occurs in three clinical situations: a net loss of sodium in excess of water, inadequate sodium intake, and movement of sodium into cells.[44] Two common causes of hypovolemic hyponatremia are acute gastroenteritis and administration of loop diuretics (furosemide, bumetanide). Patients with acute gastroenteritis have diarrhea, which may lead to intravascular volume depletion. To compensate for the loss of water, ADH and arginine vasopressin are released. Antidiuretic hormone enhances water reabsorption in the proximal tubule, resulting in renal water retention in the collecting duct. Arginine vasopressin acts on the kidney through the V2 receptors, which leads to the reabsorption of water by the collecting ducts of the kidney, thus decreasing urine formation.[1] Arginine vasopressin also binds to V1 receptors on vascular smooth muscle to cause vasoconstriction and release of prostaglandin, which results in increased arterial pressure. Furthermore, ADH plays a central role in thirst control, which drives the patient to consume water to replace any losses.[2,43]

Loop diuretics (furosemide, bumetanide) cause hypovolemic hyponatremia by inhibiting the $Na^+/K^+/Cl^-$ (sodium/potassium/chloride) cotransporter of the luminal membrane in the ascending limb of the loop of Henle, resulting in decreased reabsorption of sodium, potassium, and chloride ions. Because diuretics affect the reabsorption of sodium ions, hyponatremia will result. The thiazide diuretics (hydrochlorothiazide, chlorothiazide) inhibit the Na^+/Cl^- cotransporter reabsorption at the cortical diluting segments and increase the excretion of sodium and chloride, resulting in the excretion of a hyperosmolar urine. Of note, hypovolemic hyponatremia is caused by loop and thiazide diuretics and requires replacement of both sodium and potassium because both are potassium-depleting agents.[45]

EUVOLEMIC HYPONATREMIA

Euvolemic hyponatremia commonly occurs in patients with the syndrome of inappropriate antidiuretic hormone secretion (SIADH). Common etiologies include renal, adrenal, or thyroid insufficiency; congestive heart failure; nephrotic syndrome; or medication use such as diuretics.[40] In SIADH, ADH secretion is inhibited by neither low-sodium osmolality nor expanded intravascular volume. As a result, children with SIADH cannot excrete water, which causes a dilution of serum sodium and hyponatremia. Retained water causes an expansion of extracellular volume, resulting in the kidney's increase in sodium excretion in an effort to decrease the intravascular volume to normal. In this clinical situation, the patient will present in a hyponatremic state. Fluid restriction is the mainstay of therapy for SIADH. Patients should only receive 50%–75% of their maintenance needs.[44]

Another cause of euvolemic hyponatremia in postoperative patients is the administration of maintenance fluids that are low in sodium (hypotonic fluids). When the patient has stress related to an acute illness, surgical procedures, or trauma, the body will respond by initiating a neurohormonal cascade, maintaining and retaining free water. If the patient receives a low-sodium maintenance fluid and the body fails to maintain the free water balance, hyponatremia can result. Other factors contributing to postoperative hyponatremia include a combination of ADH release, subclinical volume depletion, pain, nausea, and stress.[44,46]

Table 7. Treatment Summary for Dehydration[1,2,9]

Step and Assessment	Hyponatremic Dehydration (< 130 mEq/L)	Isonatremic Dehydration (130–149 mEq/L)	Hypernatremic Dehydration (≥ 150 mEq/L)
Step 1: Calculation of the replacement therapy			
Fluid deficit	Fluid deficit (L) = % dehydration × weight (kg)	Fluid deficit (L) = % dehydration × weight (kg)	TFD = % dehydration × weight (kg) SFD = TFD − FWD
Free water deficit[a]	N/A	N/A	FWD = 4 mL × (actual sodium − desired sodium mEq/L) × body weight (kg)
Sodium deficit[b]	Fluid deficit (L) × 0.6 (L/kg) × normal serum sodium concentration (140 mEq/L)	Fluid deficit (L) × 0.6 (L/kg) × normal serum sodium concentration (135 mEq/L)	SFD (L) × 0.6 (L/kg) × normal serum sodium concentration (140 mEq/L)
Excess sodium deficit	(Desired serum sodium [135 mEq/L] − actual serum sodium) × 0.6 (L/kg) × body weight (kg)	N/A	N/A
Potassium deficit[c]	Fluid deficit (L) × 0.4 (L/kg) × 120 mEq/L	Fluid deficit (L) × 0.4 (L/kg) × 120 mEq/L	SFD (L) × 0.4 (L/kg) × 120 mEq/L
Step 2: Calculation of maintenance fluid and electrolyte therapy: Holliday–Segar method (Table 2)			
Step 3: Assessment of ongoing losses: Table 6 shows the electrolyte composition of various body fluids			

[a]Pure water deficit is part of the TFD.
[b]0.6 L/kg means sodium distribution factor as a fraction of body weight.
[c]0.4 L/kg means potassium distribution factor as a fraction of body weight; 120 mEq/L is the normal value of intracellular potassium concentration.
FWD = free water deficit; N/A = not applicable; SFD = solute fluid deficit; TFD = total fluid deficit.

Hyponatremic encephalopathy is a serious complication of euvolemic hyponatremia that can result in death or permanent neurologic injury. More than 50% of hospitalized children with a serum sodium concentration of less than 125 mEq/L are estimated to develop hyponatremic encephalopathy. Often, this condition is associated with SIADH or occurs during the postoperative period. Therefore, monitoring patients' neurologic status plays a role in preventing this complication.[44,46]

HYPERVOLEMIC HYPONATREMIA

Finally, hypervolemic hyponatremia occurs when the net water retention exceeds the sodium retention. This clinical situation occurs in patients with edema-forming states such as congestive heart failure, cirrhosis, and nephrotic syndrome.[44]

CLINICAL MANIFESTATIONS OF HYPONATREMIA

Hyponatremic dehydration produces more substantial intravascular volume depletion because of the shift of water from the ECF to the ICF. The decreased content of sodium

---

Box 2. Causes of Hypernatremia and Hyponatremia[2]

Hypernatremia
Improperly mixed formula
Excess sodium bicarbonate
Ingestion of seawater or sodium chloride
Intentional salt poisoning
Intravenous hypertonic sodium chloride
Hyperaldosteronism
Nephrogenic diabetes
Central diabetes insipidus
Increased sensible losses
Diarrhea
Emesis/nasogastric suction
Burns
Excessive sweating
Osmotic diuretics (e.g., mannitol)

Hyponatremia
Hyperglycemia
Mannitol
Gastrointestinal (emesis, diarrhea)
Skin (sweating or burns)
Third space losses
Urinary tract obstruction and/or urinary tract infection
Thiazide or loop diuretics
Cerebral salt wasting
Diluted formula
Syndrome of inappropriate antidiuretic hormone
    secretion
Hypothyroidism
Water intoxication
Nephrotic syndrome
Congestive heart failure

---

in the ECF results in the decreased osmolality of ECF. Physiologically, the water will move from the ECF to the ICF to maintain osmotic equilibrium. The increase in water content within the cells will cause the cells to swell. Because the brain is a fixed space in the skull, intracranial pressure increases as the brain cells swell. This brain swelling is the main cause of the neurologic symptoms that occur with hyponatremia. Symptoms suggestive of neurologic complications include anorexia, nausea, emesis, malaise, lethargy, confusion, agitation, headache, seizures, coma, and decreased reflexes. As sodium decreases to less than 125 mEq/L, the patient may have nausea and malaise. If sodium continues to decrease to less than 120 mEq/L, the patient may also develop seizures. Seizures associated with hyponatremia are more refractory to treatment with an antiepileptic and require an increase in serum osmolality to correct the underlying problem.[1,2,45]

CORRECTION OF HYPONATREMIA

The approach to treating hyponatremia in children involves identifying the underlying cause of hyponatremia and administering oral or intravenous therapy to correct the dehydration and hyponatremia. For mild to moderate dehydration, ORT may be used unless the child has persistent vomiting.[1] If intravenous therapy is required, it is very important to avoid rapid correction of hyponatremia in children. Rapid correction of hyponatremia may cause central pontine myelinolysis, an irreversible neurologic injury. Classic features of central pontine myelinolysis include mutism, dysarthria, spastic quadriplegia, pseudobulbar palsy, and ataxia.[46,47] The general recommendation is to avoid correcting the serum sodium concentration by more than 12 mEq/L over 24 hours. The cornerstone of therapy is to replace the sodium and water deficits by applying the formula list included in Table 7. An aggressive initial correction is indicated for the first 3–4 hours of management, with a goal not to exceed an increase in serum sodium of 2 mEq/L per hour. The chemistry panel should be evaluated every 6 hours to determine the progress of sodium and water correction. Intravenous hypertonic sodium chloride (3% hypertonic sodium chloride solution) may be used to rapidly increase the serum sodium in children with active symptoms (e.g., seizures). Hypertonic sodium chloride solution affects serum osmolality, which leads to a decrease in brain edema. During an active seizure associated with acute hyponatremia, administering 6 mL/kg of 3% sodium chloride increases the serum sodium concentration by about 5 mEq/L.[9,45] Hypertonic sodium chloride solution should be administered through a central line because of its high osmolarity (i.e., 1027 mOsm/L). If the solution is to be administered peripherally, it should be infused slowly to minimize venous irritation and avoid infiltration. See Example 1 for a case of a patient with hyponatremia dehydration.

ISONATREMIA (ISOTONIC)

Isonatremic dehydration is defined as a serum sodium concentration of 130–149 mEq/L. Isonatremic dehydration occurs when the degree of water and sodium losses is equal in both ICF and ECF. This condition is the most common type of dehydration in children, and the treatment plan is less complicated than for hyponatremic and hypernatremic dehydration. The treatment formula is listed in Table 7.

CORRECTION OF ISONATREMIA

In phase I—*the emergency management phase*—for a hemodynamically unstable patient, the treatment objective is to expand the ECF volume, thereby preventing circulatory collapse. Acutely, an isotonic fluid (0.9% sodium chloride or lactated Ringer solution) is given as a bolus of 20 mL/kg over 30 minutes and repeated, if necessary. As previously stated, phase II—*the deficit management phase*—requires a calculation of both fluid and sodium deficit to determine the type and amount of fluids needed. In addition, maintenance fluids and ongoing losses must be included in the overall plan. In general, the treatment plan involves providing one-half of the remaining deficit plus one-third of the daily maintenance requirement during the first 8 hours, followed by the other one-half of the remaining deficit plus two-thirds of the daily maintenance during the next 16 hours. Commonly used maintenance solutions are 5% dextrose in 0.2%–0.45% sodium chloride containing 20 mEq/L of potassium chloride. As previously mentioned, these solutions are used because they contain a combination of water, glucose, sodium, and potassium, which are the essential elements of maintenance fluid therapy. In metabolic acidosis, potassium acetate may be used instead of potassium chloride.[42] The acetate portion of potassium acetate will convert to bicarbonate in the liver and help neutralize the acidotic state.

HYPERNATREMIA

Hypernatremic dehydration is defined as a serum sodium concentration of 150 mEq/L or greater. The body has two defense mechanisms to protect against hypernatremia: the ability to produce concentrated urine and a powerful thirst mechanism.[48] When assessing hypernatremia, it is important to distinguish between hypernatremia caused by excessive sodium, by a water deficit, or by a combination of water and sodium deficit.[37] In children, hypernatremia is most likely related to an excess of free water loss (water deficit) because of increased insensible losses from fever, sweating, or gastroenteritis. Causes of hypernatremia in children are listed in Box 2.

An example of the combination of water and sodium deficit is an infant or child presenting with gastroenteritis and mild hypernatremia. However, most children with gastroenteritis do not develop hypernatremia because of their supplemental intake of fluids such as water, juice, or formula, which compensates for the water deficit. If a child develops hypernatremia, it is most likely related to an inadequate intake of water, a lack of access to water, or anorexia.[43]

Excessive sodium administration (also defined as sodium gain greater than water gain) in nonhospitalized patients may stem from improperly mixed formula, consumption of baking soda, intentional salt poisoning, and ingestion of seawater.

The classic causes of hypernatremia from inadequate water administration (water deficit) are nephrogenic diabetes and central diabetes insipidus.[43,48,49] Diabetes insipidus is defined as complete or partial failure of ADH secretion (central diabetes insipidus) or renal response to ADH (nephrogenic insipidus), resulting in the excretion of hypotonic urine.[44] Hypernatremia will occur if patients lack access to water or cannot drink enough water because of neurologic impairment, emesis, or anorexia.[43] Patients with central diabetes insipidus may have a history of head trauma, central nervous system infections, or tumors. However, cases of nephrogenic insipidus may be congenital or acquired.[44]

CLINICAL MANIFESTATIONS OF HYPERNATREMIA

In the hypernatremic state, the ECF is hyperosmolar because of a high serum sodium content. This state promotes water movement from the ICF to the ECF to maintain the osmotic balance. Children may appear less ill because the increased intravascular volume helps maintain their blood pressure and urinary output. Only when children become more symptomatic and dehydrated do they seek medical attention.[43] As a result, this treatment is delayed, and these children have increased morbidity and mortality compared with patients who present with hyponatremia. The mortality rate of hypernatremia is 15% in children.

Hypernatremia can also cause serious neurologic damage. Movement of water from the brain cells to the ECF causes brain cell shrinkage (decrease in brain volume), tearing of blood vessels within the brain (hemorrhages), or cerebral contraction.[37] Seizures and coma are possible sequelae of the brain hemorrhage. Overall, brain cell volume can be decreased as much as 10%–15% in hypernatremia.[46]

Children presenting with mild hypernatremia appear less ill than do children with isotonic dehydration. Children presenting with hypernatremia may have fever, hypertonicity, and hyperreflexia. In severely ill children, cerebral bleeding may develop. Patients with excessive sodium intoxication may have signs of volume overload such as pulmonary edema.[43] On neurologic examination, these children may have increased tone, nuchal rigidity, and brisk reflexes. Other symptoms include myoclonus, asterixis, and chorea. Tonic–clonic and absence seizures have also been described.

CORRECTION OF HYPERNATREMIA

The objectives for correcting hypernatremia are to prevent cerebral edema, identify the underlying causes, limit further water loss, and replace the water deficit.[1] Idiogenic osmoles in the brain require 48–72 hours to adapt to changes in the sodium concentration during the treatment plan; therefore, the free water deficit should not be replaced too rapidly. Rapid lowering of the extracellular osmolality will result in water movement from the ECF to the brain cells, causing cerebral edema. Cerebral edema may lead to seizures, permanent neurologic damage, or death. Hypernatremic dehydration can be treated successfully, but it is difficult to manage and should be approached with caution. Therefore, prevention of any neurologic sequelae is important to emphasize.[49]

The goal of therapy in children is to slowly correct volume deficit while correcting the serum sodium concentration by no more than 12 mEq/L over 24 hours. The general first step is to restore intravascular volume (e.g., administer 0.9% sodium chloride 20 mL/kg within 20–30 minutes). Lactated Ringer solution is avoided because it is a more hypotonic solution (osmolality 273 mOsm/L; sodium content 130 mEq/L), which may lead to a rapid correction of the serum sodium concentration. The correction time varies depending on the initial sodium concentration. If the initial sodium concentration is 150–157 mEq/L, 158–170 mEq/L, 171–183 mEq/L, or 184–196 mEq/L, the correction time is 24 hours, 48 hours, 72 hours, and 84 hours, respectively.[43] The serum sodium concentration should be monitored every 4–6 hours in the initial phases of sodium concentration, thus helping to ensure that the sodium concentration falls slowly and gradually.[50] Typical fluids used for replacement include 5% dextrose in 0.45% sodium chloride or 5% dextrose in 0.2% sodium chloride (both with 20 mEq/L of potassium chloride unless contraindicated). Total volume deficit and free water deficit must be calculated to determine the correct infusion rate and the tonicity of the fluid needed (Table 6).[49,50] See Example 2 for a patient case of hypernatremia. Pharmacists should discontinue all of the patient's medications with high sodium content and avoid solutions with a high sodium content such as 0.9% sodium chloride. If such precautions are not taken, the correction time of the high initial serum sodium concentration may be affected or the patient's risk of developing neurologic complications may be increased.

CONCLUSIONS

The Holliday–Segar formula remains the most popular and universally accepted method for calculating the daily maintenance fluid needs of pediatric patients. The American Academy of Pediatrics recommends that patients age 28 days to 18 years surgical (postoperative) and medical acute care settings (both the critical care and general inpatient ward) requiring maintenance intravenous fluids should receive isotonic solutions with appropriate potassium chloride and dextrose because they significantly decrease the risk of developing hyponatremia. Dehydration is one of the leading causes of morbidity and mortality in children worldwide. Dehydration commonly occurs if a child loses a great deal of fluid from diarrhea or vomiting. In assessing the dehydrated patient, the degree and type of dehydration play a role. For mildly and moderately dehydrated children, ORT is still the mainstay of therapy unless the patient cannot tolerate oral intake, is unconscious, or is in a state of shock. In children with severe dehydration, the key point is to calculate the fluid and electrolyte needs for deficit replacement therapy, maintenance therapy, and ongoing losses. For the hemodynamically unstable patient (severe dehydration or shock), one bolus or more is the initial step to restore an adequate intravascular volume and avoid tissue damage. Depending on the type of dehydration, the correction times are important to prevent any neurologic complications. Overall, the patient must be monitored closely by assessing the sodium concentration, and fluid therapy adjustments must be directed by the laboratory values from the chemistry panel, physical examination (to determine whether the signs of dehydration have improved), weight, and urinary output.

Example 1. Hyponatremic Dehydration Case and Calculations

Presentation: A 12-month-old boy is brought to the emergency department because of diarrhea and intolerance of oral intake.

Vital signs: BP 85/40 mm Hg; weight today 7.5 kg; pre-illness weight 8 kg

Laboratory findings: Serum sodium content 129 mEq/L

Calculation to estimate the severity of dehydration:

[(pre-illness weight – illness weight)/pre-illness weight] × 100 = (8 kg–7.5 kg/8 kg) × 100 = **6% dehydrated = moderate dehydration**

Critical assessment questions: Are one or more of the following present?

- Is the patient severely dehydrated?
- Does the patient have signs of shock?
- Is the patient unconscious?
- Is ileus present?
- Does the patient have a severe electrolyte problem?

None of these findings are present in this patient.

Phase I—Emergency management: No

Phase II—Deficit management: Assessment of sodium content = patient serum sodium content: 129 mEq/L

Step 1: Calculation of the replacement therapy

Fluid deficit (L) = % dehydration × weight (kg) = 6% × 8 kg × 1000 mL/kg = **480 mL**

Sodium deficit = fluid deficit (L) × 0.6 × normal serum sodium concentration (140 mEq/L) = 0.48 L × 0.6 L/kg × 140 mEq/L = 40.3 mEq = **40 mEq**

Excess sodium deficit = (desired serum sodium (135) – actual serum sodium) × 0.6 (L/kg) × body weight (kg) = (135 – 129 mEq/L) × 0.6 L/kg × 8 kg = 28.8 mEq = **29 mEq**

Potassium deficit = fluid deficit (L) × 0.4 (L/kg) × 120 mEq/L = 0.48 L × 0.4 L/kg × 120 mEq/L = **23 mEq**

Step 2: Calculation of maintenance fluid and electrolyte therapy: Holliday–Segar method

- Fluid requirements: 100 mL/kg/day × 8 kg = **800 mL**
- Sodium requirements: 3 mEq/kg/day × 8 kg = **24 mEq**
- Potassium requirements: 2 mEq/kg/day × 8 kg = **16 mEq**

Step 3: Assessment of ongoing losses, if necessary

Management	Water	Sodium	Potassium
Deficit	480 mL	40 mEq + 29 mEq	23 mEq
Maintenance	800 mL	24 mEq	16 mEq
Total	**1280 mL**	**93 mEq**	**39 mEq**
First 8 hr = 1/2 remaining deficit + 1/3 daily maintenance			
1/2 remaining deficit	240 mL	34.5 mEq	11.5 mEq
1/3 daily maintenance	267 mL	8 mEq	5 mEq
Total	**507 mL**	**42.5 mEq**	**16.5 mEq**
Next 16 hr = 1/2 remaining deficit + 2/3 daily maintenance			
1/2 remaining deficit	240 mL	34.5 mEq	11.5 mEq
2/3 daily maintenance	533 mL	16 mEq	11 mEq
Total	**773 mL**	**50.5 mEq**	**22.5 mEq**

Fluid selection:

- **First 8 hours:** 5% dextrose + 0.45% sodium chloride (NaCl)[a] + 20 mEq/L potassium chloride (KCl) at 63 mL/hour
- **Next 16 hours:** 5% dextrose + 0.45% NaCl[b] + 30 mEq/L KCl at 48 mL/hour

[a]Sodium: 77 mEq/L × 507 mL × 1 L/1000 mL = 39 mEq → selection of 0.45% NaCl solution is close to goal of 42.5 mEq.
[b]Sodium: 77 mEq/L × 773 mL × 1 L/1000 mL = 60 mEq → selection of 0.45% NaCl solution is close to goal of 50.5 mEq.

Example 2. Hypernatremia Dehydration Case and Calculations

Presentation: A 12-month-old boy is brought to the emergency department with a 3-day history of illness.

Physical examination: Severe dehydration with a capillary refill of 4 seconds; skin is cool and mottled

Vital signs: BP 70/30 mm Hg; weight today 7.2 kg; pre-illness weight 8 kg

Laboratory findings: Serum sodium content 151 mEq/L

Calculation to estimate the severity of dehydration:

[(pre-illness weight − illness weight)/pre-illness weight] × 100 = (8 − 7.2 kg)/8 kg × 100 = **10% dehydrated** = **severe dehydration**

Critical assessment questions: Are one or more of the following present?

- Is the patient severely dehydrated?
- Does the patient have signs of shock?
- Is the patient unconscious?
- Is ileus present?
- Does the patient have a severe electrolyte problem?

Yes, patient is severely dehydrated with hypotension.

Phase I—Emergency management

Calculation: 20 mL/kg = 20 mL × 8 kg = 160 mL of 0.9% sodium chloride therapy

Phase II—Deficit management: Assessment of sodium content = patient serum sodium content: **151 mEq/L**

Step 1: Calculation of the replacement therapy (round with the nearest number)

Total fluid deficit (TFD) (L) = % dehydration × weight (kg) = 10% × 8 kg × 1000 mL/kg = **800 mL**

Free water deficit (FWD) = 4 mL × (actual sodium − desired sodium mEq/L) × body weight (kg)
4 mL × (151 − 145) × 8 kg = **192 mL**

Solute fluid deficit (SFD) = TFD − FWD = 800 mL − 192 mL = 608 mL = **0.6 L**

Sodium deficit = SFD (L) × 0.6 (L/kg) × normal serum sodium concentration (140 mEq/L) = 0.6 L × 0.6 L/kg × 140 mEq/L = 50.4 mEq = **50 mEq**

Potassium deficit = SFD (L) × 0.4 (L/kg) × 120 mEq/L = 0.6 L × 0.4 L/kg × 120 mEq/L = 28.8 mEq = **29 mEq**

Step 2: Calculation of maintenance fluid and electrolyte therapy: Holliday–Segar method

- Fluid requirements: 100 mL/kg/day × 8 kg = **800 mL**
- Sodium requirements: 3 mEq/kg/day × 8 kg = **24 mEq**
- Potassium requirements: 2 mEq/kg/day × 8 kg = **16 mEq**

Step 3: Assessment of ongoing losses, if necessary

Management[a]	Water	Sodium	Potassium
Deficit	800 mL + 192 mL	50 mEq	29 mEq
Maintenance	800 mL	24 mEq	16 mEq
Total	**1792 mL**	**74 mEq**	**45 mEq**
First 8 hr = 1/2 remaining deficit + 1/3 daily maintenance			
1/2 remaining deficit	496 mL	25 mEq	14.5 mEq
1/3 daily maintenance	267 mL	8 mEq	5 mEq
Total	**763 mL**	**33 mEq**	**19.5 mEq**
Next 16 hr = 1/2 remaining deficit + 2/3 daily maintenance			
1/2 remaining deficit	496 mL	25 mEq	14.5 mEq
2/3 daily maintenance	533 mL	16 mEq	11 mEq
Total	**1029 mL**	**41 mEq**	**25.5 mEq**

[a]The acute phase is usually excluded from the 24-hour calculations.

Fluid selection

- **First 8 hours:** 5% dextrose + 0.225% NaCl[a] + 20 mEq/L KCl at 95 mL/hour
- **Next 16 hours:** 5% dextrose + 0.225% NaCl[b] + 30 mEq/L KCl at 64 mL/hour

[a]Sodium: 38.5 mEq/L × 763 mL × 1 L/1000 mL = 29 mEq → selection of 0.225% NaCl solution is close to goal of 33 mEq.
[b]Sodium: 38.5 mEq/L × 1029 mL × 1 L/1000 mL = 39.6 mEq → selection of 0.225% NaCl solution is close to goal of 41 mEq.

A 3-year-old girl is brought to the emergency department because of diarrhea and vomiting. She has had six episodes of diarrhea and two episodes of vomiting in the past 8 hours. Her mother describes the diarrhea as watery. One hour before the emergency department visit, the mother recorded a rectal temperature of 101°F (38°C) and administered a dose of oral acetaminophen. She also says that her daughter has not wanted to drink anything for the past 12 hours and that she was sick after attending day care yesterday.

Medical history: Febrile seizures at age 9 months

Family history: Nonsignificant

Social history: Has attended day care since age 3 months

Home medications: None

Allergies: No known drug allergies

Immunizations: Up to date

Physical examination:

General appearance: Alert and awake; appears weak; skin appears pale

HEENT: Eyes are slightly sunken; dry buccal mucosa

Pulmonary: Lungs are clear to auscultation

Cardiovascular: No murmurs; capillary refill time is 2 seconds

Gastrointestinal: Soft and nontender; bowel sounds are normoactive

Genitourinary: Nonsignificant

Vital signs: Tmax 100.8°F (38°C) rectal, current weight 13.5 kg, pre-illness weight 14.2 kg, HR 115 beats/minute, RR 35 breaths/minute, BP 90/60 mm Hg, SaO_2 99% room air

Laboratory findings:

Na	125 mEq/L
Cl	100 mEq/L
K	4 mEq/L
HCO_3	19 mEq/L
BUN	10 mg/dL
SCr	0.68 mg/dL
Glucose	89 mg/dL
Ca	8.7 mg/dL

1. Classify this patient's level of dehydration.

Estimation of severity:

[(pre-illness weight – illness weight)/pre-illness weight] × 100) = (14.2 – 13.5 kg)/14.2 kg × 100 = 4.9% moderate dehydration

2. List the signs and symptoms most consistent with dehydration.

- Patient is alert and awake and appears weak
- Eyes are slightly sunken
- Dry buccal mucosa
- Normal capillary refill time
- Tachycardia
- Tachypnea
- Normal blood pressure: The patient's blood pressure is normal, placing her in the moderate dehydration category; however, if the patient's blood pressure had decreased, then she would have been in the severe dehydration category.

3. What are the treatment goals for this patient?

Overall goals of therapy for this patient are the following:

- Restoration of skin color and skin turgor because her current skin is pale
- Tolerance of oral intake of food
- Correction of serum chemistry values
- Normal heart rate and normal respiratory rate

Case (continued). At the emergency department, the patient has a generalized tonic–clonic seizure. The bedside nurse administers a one-time dose of intravenous lorazepam 0.7 mg (0.05 mg/kg/dose intravenously once). The physician wants to prescribe hypertonic sodium chloride solution.

4. What dose of hypertonic sodium chloride solution is recommended?

6 mL/kg of 3% sodium chloride =
6 mL × 14 kg = 84 mL of 3% sodium chloride

Case (continued). After administering hypertonic sodium chloride to the patient for 2 hours, the new sodium concentration is 128 mEq/L. Because this patient cannot tolerate oral intake, the physician decides to initiate intravenous deficit management.

5. Complete the following calculations for deficit and maintenance management and provide a recommendation for intravenous fluid and electrolyte replacement.

Estimation of severity	
Fluid deficit	
Sodium deficit	
Excess sodium deficit	
Potassium deficit	
Calculation of maintenance fluid and electrolyte therapy	
Fluid requirements	
Sodium requirements	
Potassium requirements	

The appropriate calculations and recommendations are as follows.

Estimation of severity	Moderate dehydration
Fluid deficit	Fluid deficit (L) = % dehydration × weight (kg) = 4.9% × 14.2 kg × 1000 mL/kg = 695.8 mL = 696 mL
Sodium deficit	Sodium deficit = fluid deficit (L) × 0.6 × normal serum sodium concentration (140 mEq/L) = 0.696 L × 0.6 L/kg × 140 mEq/L = 58.5 mEq = 59 mEq
Excess sodium deficit	Excess sodium deficit = (desired serum sodium (135) − actual serum sodium) × 0.6 (L/kg) × body weight (kg) = (135 − 129 mEq/L) × 0.6 L/kg × 14.2 kg = 51.1 mEq = 51 mEq
Potassium deficit	Potassium deficit = fluid deficit (L) × 0.4 (L/kg) × 120 mEq/L = 0.696 L × 0.4 L/kg × 120 mEq/L = 33.4 mEq = 33 mEq

Calculation of maintenance fluid and electrolyte therapy	
Fluid requirements	Fluid requirements: 1000 mL + 50 mL/kg for each kg > 10 kg = 1000 mL + 50 mL/kg × 4.2 kg = 1210 mL
Sodium requirements	3 mEq/kg/day × 14.2 kg = 42.6 mEq = 43 mEq
Potassium requirements	2 mEq/kg/day × 14.2 kg = 28.4 mEq = 28 mEq

6. What fluid would you recommend for the first 8 hours of dehydration management for this patient?

Sodium: 77 mEq/L × 751 mL × 1 L/1000 mL = 57 mEq → selection of 0.45% NaCl solution is close to the goal of 69 mEq.

First 8 hours: 5% dextrose + 0.45% NaCl + 20 mEq/L KCl at 94 mL/hour

Management	Water	Sodium	Potassium
Deficit	696 mL	59 mEq + 51 mEq	33 mEq
Maintenance	1210 mL	43 mEq	28 mEq
Total	1906 mL	153 mEq	61 mEq
First 8 hours = 1/2 remaining deficit + 1/3 daily maintenance			
1/2 remaining deficit	348 mL	55 mEq	16.5 mEq
1/3 daily maintenance	403 mL	14 mEq	9.3 mEq
Total	**751 mL**	**69 mEq**	**25.8 mEq**

REFERENCES

1. Feld LG, Friedman A, Massengill SF. Disorders of water homeostasis. In: Feld LG, Kaskel FJ, eds. Fluid and Electrolytes in Pediatrics: A Comprehensive Handbook. New York: Humana Press, 2009:3-46.
2. Greenbaum LA. Maintenance and replacement therapy. In: Kliegman RM, Stanton BF, Geme JW, et al., eds. Nelson Textbook of Pediatrics, 20th ed. Philadelphia: Elsevier, 2016:384-8.
3. Koletzko B, Goulet O, Hunt J, et al. Guidelines on Paediatric Parenteral Nutrition of the European Society of Paediatric Gastroenterology, Hepatology and Nutrition (ESPGHAN) and the European Society for Clinical Nutrition and Metabolism (ESPEN), supported by the European Society of Paediatric Research (ESPR). J Pediatr Gastroenterol Nutr 2005;41:S33-8.
4. Metheny NM. Fluid balance in infants and children. In: Metheny NM, ed. Fluid and Electrolyte Balance: Nursing Considerations, 4th ed. Philadelphia: Lippincott Williams & Wilkins, 2000:341-54.
5. Friedman AL. Pediatric hydration therapy: historical review and a new approach. Kidney Int 2005;67:380-8.
6. Roberts KB. Fluid and electrolytes: parenteral fluid therapy. Pediatr Rev 2001;22:380-6.
7. Holliday MA, Segar WE. The maintenance need for water in parenteral fluid therapy. Pediatrics 1957;19:823-32.
8. Talbert FB. Basal metabolism in children. In: Brennemann's Practice of Pediatrics. Hagerstown, MD: W.F. Prior Company, Inc, 1949:477-517.
9. Nalley CM. Fluids and electrolytes. In: Hughes HK, Kahl LK, eds. The Harriet Lane Handbook, 21st ed. Philadelphia: Elsevier, 2018:290-315.
10. Gomella T, Cunningham M, Eyal FG, et al. Fluid and electrolytes. In: Gomella T, Cunningham M, Eyal FG, et al., eds. Neonatology: Management, Procedures, On-call Problems, Diseases, and Drugs, 7e. New York: McGraw-Hill, 2013.
11. McNab S. Intravenous maintenance fluid therapy in children. J Paediatric Child Health 2016; 52:137-40.
12. Feld LG, Neuspiel DR, Foster BA, et al. Clinical practice guideline: maintenance intravenous fluids in children. Pediatrics 2018;142:e20183083.
13. Kannan L, Lodha R, Vivekanandhan S, et al. Intravenous fluid regimen and hyponatremia among children: a randomized controlled trial. Pediatr Nephrol 2010;25:2303-9.
14. McNab S. Isotonic vs hypotonic intravenous fluids for hospitalized children. JAMA 2015;314:720-1.
15. McNab S, Duke T, South M, et al. 140 mmol/L of sodium versus 77 mmol/L of sodium in maintenance intravenous fluid therapy for children in hospital (PIMS): a randomized controlled double-blind trial. Lancet 2015;385:1190-7.
16. Padua AP, Macaraya JR, Dans LF, et al. Isotonic versus hypotonic saline solution for maintenance intravenous fluid therapy in children: a systematic review. Pediatr Nephrol 2015;30:1163-72.
17. Friedman JN, Beck CE, DeGroot J, et al. Comparison of isotonic and hypotonic intravenous maintenance fluids: a randomized clinical trial. JAMA Pediatr 2015;169:445-51.
18. Wang J, Xu E, Xiao Y. Isotonic versus hypotonic maintenance IV fluids in hospitalized children: a meta-analysis. Pediatrics 2014;133:105-13.
19. Allen CH, Goldman RD, Bhatt S, et al. A randomized trial of Plasma-Lyte A and 0.9% sodium chloride in acute pediatric gastroenteritis. BMC Pediatr 2016;16:117.
20. Spandorfer PR. Dehydration. In: Shaw KN and Bachur RG, eds. Fleisher & Ludwig's Textbook of Pediatric Emergency Medicine, 7th ed. Philadelphia: Lippincott Williams & Wilkins, 2016:128-34.

21. Diggins KC. Treatment of mild to moderate dehydration in children with oral rehydration therapy. J Am Acad Nurse Pract 2008;20:402-6.
22. Colletti JE, Brown KM, Sharieff GQ, et al. The management of children with gastroenteritis and dehydration in the emergency department. J Emerg Med 2010;38:686-98.
23. Guarino A, Ashkenazi S, Gendrel D, et al. European Society for Pediatric Gastroenterology, Hepatology, and Nutrition/European Society for Pediatric Infectious Diseases evidence-based guidelines for the management of acute gastroenteritis in children in Europe: update 2014. J Pediatr Gastroenterol Nutr 2014; 59:132-52.
24. Carson RA, Mudd SS, Madati J. Clinical practice guideline for the treatment of pediatric acute gastroenteritis in the outpatient setting. J Pediatr Health Care 2016;30:610-6.
25. Nager AL, Wang VJ. Comparison of nasogastric and intravenous methods of rehydration in pediatric patients with acute dehydration. Pediatrics 2002;109:566-72.
26. Steiner MJ, DeWalt DA, Byerley JS. Is this child dehydrated? JAMA 2004;291:2746-54.
27. Practice parameter: the management of acute gastroenteritis in young children. American Academy of Pediatrics, Provisional Committee on Quality Improvement, Subcommittee on Acute Gastroenteritis. Pediatrics 1996;97:424.
28. Mackenzie A, Barnes G, Shann F. Clinical signs of dehydration in children. Lancet 1989;ii:605-7.
29. Yilmaz K, Karabocuoglu M, Citak A, et al. Evaluation of laboratory test in dehydrated children with acute gastroenteritis. J Paediatr Child Health 2002;38:226-8.
30. Shaoul R, Okev N, Tamir A, et al. Value of laboratory studies in assessment of dehydration in children. Ann Clin Biochem 2004; 41:192-6.
31. Teach SJ, Yates EW, Feld LG. Laboratory predictors of fluid deficit in acutely dehydrated children. Clin Pediatr 1997; 7:395-400.
32. Wathen JE, MacKenzie T, Bothner JP. Usefulness of the serum electrolyte panel in the management of pediatric dehydration treated with intravenously administered fluids. Pediatrics 2004; 114:1227-34.
33. Reid SR, Bonadio WA. Outpatient rapid intravenous rehydration to correct dehydration and resolve vomiting in children with acute gastroenteritis. Ann Emerg Med 1996;28:318-23.
34. Santosham M, Danum RS, Dillman L, et al. Oral rehydration therapy of infantile diarrhea: a controlled study of well-nourished children hospitalized in the United States and Panama. N Engl J Med 1982;306:1070-6.
35. Tamer AM, Friedman LB, Maxwell SR, et al. Oral rehydration of infants in a large urban US medical center. J Pediatr 1985;107:14-9.
36. Listernick R, Zieserl E, Davis AT. Outpatient oral dehydration in the United States. Am J Dis Child 1986;140:211-5.
37. Vesikari T, Isolauri E, Baer M. A comparative trial of rapid oral and intravenous rehydration in acute diarrhea. Acta Paediatr Scand 1987;76:300-5.
38. MacKenzie A, Barnes G. Randomized controlled trial comparing oral and intravenous rehydration therapy in children and diarrhea. Br Med J 1991;303:393-6.
39. Hartling L, Bellemare S, Wiebe N, et al. Oral versus intravenous rehydration for treating dehydration due to gastroenteritis in children. Cochrane Database Syst Rev 2006;3:CD004390.
40. Bellemare S, Hartling L, Wiebe N, et al. Oral rehydration versus intravenous therapy for treating dehydration due to gastroenteritis in children: a meta-analysis of randomized controlled trials. BMC Med 2004;2:11.
41. Centers for Disease Control and Prevention (CDC). Managing acute gastroenteritis among children. Morb Mortal Wkly Rep 2003;52:16.
42. Spandorfer PR, Alessandrini EA, Joffe MD, et al. Oral versus intravenous rehydration of moderately dehydrated children: a randomized, controlled trial. Pediatrics 2005;115:295-301.
43. Greenbaum LA. Deficit therapy. In: Kliegman RM, Stanton BF, Geme JW, et al., eds. Nelson Textbook of Pediatrics, 20th ed. Philadelphia: Elsevier, 2016:388-91.
44. Bernardo RV, Segeleon JE, Haun SE. Fluids and electrolyte issues, metabolic disorders, tumor lysis syndrome. In: Tobias JD, ed. Pediatric Critical Care: The Essentials. Armonk, NY: Futura Publishing, 1999:287-96.
45. Schneider J, Kelly A. Disorders of water, sodium, and potassium homeostasis. In: Shaffner DH, Nichols DG, eds. Rogers' Textbook of Pediatric Intensive Care, 5th ed. Philadelphia: Wolters Kluwer, 2016:1767-87.
46. Moritz ML, Ayus JC. Preventing neurological complications from dysnatremias in children. Pediatr Nephrol 2005;20:1687-700.
47. Sterns RH. Severe symptomatic hyponatremia: treatment and outcome. A study of 64 cases. Ann Intern Med 1987;107:656.
48. Hanna MG, Bock M. Fluid, electrolyte, and acid-base disorders and therapy. In: Hay WW, Levin MJ, Deterding RR, et al., eds. Current Diagnosis and Treatment: Pediatrics, 22nd ed. Columbus, OH: McGraw-Hill, 2014:742-51.
49. Dudley NC, Mao CS. Glucose and electrolyte disorders. In: Osborn L, DeWitt T, First L, et al., eds. Pediatrics, vol 1. Philadelphia: Elsevier Mosby, 2004:319-25.
50. Goff DA, Higinio V. Hypernatremia. Pediatr Rev 2009;30:412-3.

CHAPTER 20

Parenteral and Enteral Nutrition

Catherine M. Crill, Pharm.D., FCCP, BCNSP; and
Johanna L. Norman, Pharm.D., BCPPS

LEARNING OBJECTIVES

1. Discuss methods to assess adequate nutrition and weight gain in preterm and term infants, children, and adolescents.

2. Determine whether a pediatric patient is a candidate for specialized nutrition support, either with enteral nutrition (EN), parenteral nutrition (PN), or a combination of both EN and PN.

3. Formulate an EN regimen for a pediatric patient given the patient's age, disease state, and clinical status.

4. Formulate a PN regimen for a pediatric patient given the patient's age, type of intravenous access, disease state, and clinical status.

5. Identify common complications associated with EN and PN in pediatric patients and describe monitoring guidelines to minimize these complications.

ABBREVIATIONS IN THIS CHAPTER

ASPEN	American Society of Parenteral and Enteral Nutrition
EFAD	Essential fatty acid deficiency
EN	Enteral nutrition
GI	Gastrointestinal
ILE	Intravenous lipid emulsion
PN	Parenteral nutrition
PNALD	Parenteral nutrition–associated liver disease

INTRODUCTION

The importance of optimal nutrition across the pediatric age spectrum cannot be underestimated. Neonates and infants, particularly those who are born prematurely, and hospitalized pediatric patients are at particular risk of adverse effects from suboptimal nutrition. Pharmacists with skills in pediatric nutrition support play a key role in ensuring that the nutritional needs of pediatric patients are met safely and effectively. This chapter reviews nutrition assessment, requirements, and indications for specialized nutrition support in pediatric patients and outlines specific details related to the optimal provision of enteral nutrition (EN) and parenteral nutrition (PN) therapy in pediatric patients.

NUTRITION ASSESSMENT

Adequate growth should be routinely monitored in healthy and hospitalized infants and children by measuring weight, length or height, and head circumference. These measurements are then used to plot development on growth curves, whereby growth is expressed as an expected percentile for age (based on population standards). Several growth charts are available; the appropriate chart to use varies on the basis of age and sex, and, in infants, whether the infant is fed with human milk or formula (the Introduction to Pediatrics chapter provides more detail).[1,2] Growth charts are used to determine whether infants and children are growing appropriately and are critical in identifying patients with failure to thrive across the pediatric age spectrum. Growth charts using body mass index are useful in identifying children and adolescents at risk of overnutrition or obesity, the prevalence of which has increased significantly during the past few decades.[3,4] Recent evidence suggests the use of body mass index percentiles based on length and weight rather than on weight for length are optimal for assessing adiposity and obesity risk in infants.[5,6] Of note, growth percentiles may increase or decrease in infants, whereas children should generally follow their own growth curves over time. Standard growth charts can be used for preterm infants, provided corrections for gestational age are made for weight until 24 months, length until 40 months, and for head circumference until 18 months postnatal age.[7] Alternatively, the Fenton growth chart may be used for preterm infants from 22 to 50 weeks' gestational age.[8]

Compared with adults, pediatric patients have greater nutrient needs per kilogram and reduced reserves.[9] Significant development related to nutrition occurs during the third trimester and the immediate postnatal period. The maximal period of growth and maturation of the gastrointestinal (GI) tract occurs throughout the third trimester. Nutritive sucking, necessary for oral feeding, is fully developed at 32–34 weeks' gestation. Gastric capacity is limited at birth, causing neonates to feed more often than older infants. Feeding issues, including gastroesophageal reflux, are common in infants and particularly preterm infants. Infants may also present with failure to thrive in which they are not gaining weight according to normal growth curves. Failure to thrive can be the result of inadequate intake or improper reconstitution of formula, or it can be indicative of a pathophysiologic condition such as cystic fibrosis, hypothyroidism, or pyloric stenosis.

Infants have greater total body water per weight than older children or adults, and the percentage of extracellular fluid is even greater in preterm infants. During the first few days after birth, there is contraction of the extracellular fluid and a significant diuresis that is accompanied by a decrease in weight. This weight should be regained within the first to second week of life. Weight gain velocity is greatest during the first few months of life. Term infants should gain about 20–30 g/day, leading to a doubling of their birth weight by about age 4 months.[10] Growth then slows such that infants triple their birth weight by the end of the first year of life.[11] Preterm infants may grow even faster. An infant's length normally increases by 50% during the first year.[11] From 2 to 10 years, children gain about 2–3 kg/year and grow 2.5–3.5 inches/year.[11] Other methods of nutrition assessment in pediatric patients include anthropometric measurements (arm circumference and triceps skinfold thickness), visceral protein measurements (albumin, transferrin, prealbumin or transthyretin, retinol-binding protein), and urine studies for nitrogen balance. With respect to visceral protein status, note that concentrations can also be influenced by other factors including hydration status, metabolic stress, organ dysfunction, and other disease states.[10]

SPECIALIZED NUTRITION SUPPORT

INDICATIONS

In general, specialized nutrition support, to include EN and PN, is necessary in patients who are malnourished or at risk of being malnourished. *Enteral nutrition*, defined as the delivery of nutrition by tube to the GI tract, is indicated in premature neonates younger than 34 weeks' gestation because the suck–swallow reflex has not fully developed, in infants too sick to breast- or bottle-feed, in pediatric patients who are mechanically ventilated, and in any pediatric patient whose needs cannot be met by the oral route.[12] *Parenteral nutrition*, defined as the delivery of nutrition directly to the bloodstream through a peripheral or central venous catheter, is indicated in pediatric patients when nutritional needs cannot be met by EN or when the GI tract is not functioning.

Common examples of indications for PN in infants include the following: prematurity, small bowel resection resulting in short bowel syndrome, abdominal wall defects (gastroschisis and omphalocele), necrotizing enterocolitis, intestinal atresias or webs, malrotation/volvulus, Hirschsprung disease, imperforate anus, diaphragmatic hernia, tracheoesophageal fistula, and meconium aspiration. Other disease states or conditions in which PN therapy may be indicated include the following: critical illness, trauma, extracorporeal membrane oxygenation, appendicitis, pancreatitis, chylothorax, failure to thrive, chronic malabsorption/diarrhea, organ failure, and exacerbations of inflammatory bowel disease. In preterm neonates, particularly those with birth weight less than 1500 g, PN should be initiated promptly after birth.[13] In patients expected to have EN intolerance for an extended period of time, PN should be initiated within 1–2 days in infants and within 4–5 days in older children and adolescents.[13] It is not recommended to begin PN within 24 hours of admission to the pediatric intensive care unit.[14]

FLUID AND CALORIC REQUIREMENTS

When initiating EN or PN support, fluid and caloric needs should be assessed. Table 1 outlines fluid and caloric needs across the pediatric age spectrum.[15] Increased fluid requirements exist with prematurity because of increased losses from evaporation through the skin, immature renal conservation, and the use of radiant warmers and phototherapy. Excess fluid provision may be detrimental with specific disease states such as bronchopulmonary dysplasia, intraventricular hemorrhage, patent ductus arteriosus, heart failure, and liver or renal failure (as described in the Fluid and Electrolytes chapter). Caloric requirements may be increased because of critical

Table 1. Fluid, Caloric, Macronutrient, and Electrolyte Daily Requirements Across Pediatric Weights and Ages[10,15,32,34]

Requirement by Weight and Age					
Fluids	< 1500 g	1500–2000 g	2–10 kg	> 10–20 kg	> 20 kg
	130–150 mL/kg	110–130 mL/kg	100 mL/kg	1000 mL + 50 mL/kg > 10 kg	1500 mL + 20 mL/kg > 20 kg
Calories	Preterm neonate	1–12 mo	1–7 yr	7–12 yr	12–18 yr
	90–120 kcal/kg	80–105 kcal/kg	75–90 kcal/kg	50–75 kcal/kg	30–60 kcal/kg

Macronutrients	Preterm neonate	1–12 mo	1–10 yr	11–17 yr
Protein	3–4 g/kg	2–3 g/kg	1–2 g/kg	0.8–1.5 g/kg
Dextrose	10–14 mg/kg/min	10–14 mg/kg/min	8-10 mg/kg/min	5–6 mg/kg/min
Fat	1–3 g/kg	1–3 g/kg	1–3 g/kg	1–3 g/kg

Electrolytes	Preterm Neonate	Infants/Children	Adolescents
Sodium	2–5 mEq/kg	2–4 mEq/kg	1–2 mEq/kg
Potassium	2–4 mEq/kg	2–4 mEq/kg	1–2 mEq/kg
Calcium	2–4 mEq/kg	0.5–4 mEq/kg	10–20 mEq
Phosphorus	1–2 mmol/kg	0.5–2 mmol/kg	10–40 mmol
Magnesium	0.3–0.5 mEq/kg	0.3–0.5 mEq/kg	10–30 mEq
Acetate/Chloride	Variable	Variable	Variable

illness and disease states such as congenital heart disease or bronchopulmonary dysplasia, or they may be decreased because of developmental delay or immobility. Caloric provision should be reassessed in pediatric patients not gaining appropriate weight or gaining weight too rapidly.

ENTERAL NUTRITION

Enteral nutrition may be provided through a nasogastric, gastric, or jejunal tube. It may be given by bolus administration or by intermittent, continuous, or cyclic enteral infusion.

WHAT TO FEED

Exclusive breastfeeding is recommended by the American Academy of Pediatrics for the first 6 months of life, with support for continued breastfeeding for the first year and beyond. Expressed human milk should be given whenever possible in patients who are receiving their nutrition enterally. In addition, donor breast milk is available through the Human Milk Banking Association of North America.[16] Advantages of human milk feeding include decreased occurrence of the following: upper respiratory infections (particularly otitis media), urinary tract infections, necrotizing enterocolitis, meningitis, diarrhea, sepsis, sudden infant death syndrome, diabetes, cancer, asthma, and obesity. Although there is a risk of jaundice and kernicterus because of the inhibitors of glucuronyl transferase (responsible for bilirubin conjugation) present in breast milk, this potential risk does not outweigh the benefits of human milk feeding in most patients. Infants who are exclusively breastfed are also at risk for vitamin D deficiency because of the low content in breast milk, and the American Academy of Pediatrics recommends supplementation with 400 international units of vitamin D daily.[17]

Infant formulas are available for feeding infants whose mothers are unable to breastfeed or provide expressed human milk. Enteral formulas for administration to children are also commercially available. Formulas come as ready-to-feed products, dry powders, and concentrated liquids. Caregivers should be educated on the proper technique for formula reconstitution and storage.

Most standard infant formulas provide either 19 or 20 kcal/oz (0.63 or 0.67 kcal/mL) of formula; however, some may be available as 22 kcal/oz (0.73 kcal/mL) and 24 kcal/oz (0.8 kcal/mL). The caloric density of a formula may be increased further by concentrating a powdered formula or using protein-, carbohydrate-, or fat-source modular additives. Standard pediatric formulas are typically available as 30 kcal/oz (1 kcal/mL). Table 2 provides examples of standard and therapeutic preterm and term infant formulas and standard and therapeutic child formulas that are commercially available, their indications for use, and their caloric density. Figure 1 outlines examples of calculations for EN feeding regimens based on patient age, caloric goal, and caloric density of formula.

DRUG–NUTRIENT CONSIDERATIONS

Patients with enteral feeding tubes often need to receive medications through the tube. However, several factors must be considered when drugs designed for oral administration are delivered in this manner. Only certain drug formulations should be given through an enteral tube. Modified release dosage forms (e.g., enteric coated or delayed release) or any medications that should not be crushed or opened are not recommended for administration by enteral feeding tube. Administration of liquid medications by enteral tube must be carefully considered because they generally have higher osmolality and contain sugars and other agents feeding. In general, liquid medications with high osmolality or viscosity should be avoided. Immediate-release solid dosage forms may be given after being crushed and mixed with water.

The site of absorption and action of the drug should also be considered. Some drugs have absorption throughout the GI tract, but others have specific sites of absorption that the tube may bypass, depending on the location of the distal tip. Still other medications, such as proton pump inhibitors, are acid labile and rendered ineffective by the lower pH of the GI tract. Finally, patients with enteral feeding tubes may have undergone bowel resection so it is important to consider the length and location of the patient's functional bowel.

To avoid interactions, medications should not be added directly to an enteral feeding formula and should be administered separately from other medications.[18] Even when the formula and medications are given separately, there is still a potential for interactions that can affect the compatibility or stability of the drug or nutrient. If the volume can be tolerated, flushing between each medication will help prevent drug interactions and occlusion of the feeding tube. Caution should be exercised when mixing several medications for administration through a tube because the stability and compatibility of drugs are unknown when tablets are crushed together or liquid formulations are mixed. Safe practices for administration of medications enterally also include the addition of dosage form, route, and access device to the prescriber's order, and pharmacist review of all medication orders as well as the development of policies and procedures for all staff involved in the preparation and administration of medications given enterally.[18] Complete information regarding the potential for interactions between drugs and EN formulations has been reviewed.[19] Table 3 summarizes the most important medications with respect to drug–nutrient interactions.

COMPLICATIONS

Complications associated with EN include the following: mechanical complications, such as feeding tube occlusion and malposition; GI symptoms, such as nausea, vomiting, diarrhea, cramping, aspiration, or constipation; feeding tube site infections; tubing misconnections; and aversion to oral feeding, particularly in enterally fed infants.

Recommendations to prevent feeding tube occlusion include the following: flushing immediately before and after intermittent enteral feedings or at routine intervals with continuous feeding; flushing the tube well before and after medication administration; limiting gastric residual checks (because gastric acid mixing with enteral formula may result in protein precipitates in tube); and using purified water for tube flushes.[18]

Table 2. Commercially Available Enteral Formulas for Infants and Children

Formula Type	Brand Name[a]	Indication	Kilocalories per Ounce (kcal/oz)
Premature Infant Formulas			
Premature	Enfamil Premature Lipil[b] Gerber Goodstart Premature[c] Similac Special Care Advance[d]	Initial formula for low birth weight and premature infants	24–30
Transitional premature	Enfamil EnfaCare[b] Similac NeoSure[d]	Transitional formula for older premature infants or after discharge home	22
Infant Formulas			
Cow milk–based	Enfamil Infant, Newborn[b] Gerber Good Start Gentle[c] Similac Advance, Pro-Advance, Advance 20[d] Similac Pure Bliss[d]	Healthy, term infants	19–20
Organic (cow milk-based)	Similac Organic[d]	Healthy, term infants	20
Pre/probiotic-containing	Enfamil Reguline[b] Gerber Good Start Protect[c] Gerber Good Start Soothe[c] Nutramigen with Enflora LGG[b]	Healthy, term infants	20
Lactose-free	Enfamil Gentlease[b] Gerber Good Start Soothe[c] Similac Sensitive, Pro-Sensitive[d]	Lactose intolerance	19–20
Soy protein–based	Enfamil ProSobee[b] Good Start Soy[c] Similac Soy Isomil[d]	Lactose intolerance or galactosemia	19–20
Protein hydrolysate (semi-elemental)	Nutramigen Lipil, Enflora LGG[b] Pregestimil Lipil[b] Similac Alimentum[d]	Allergy or sensitivity to cow milk or soy protein, impaired digestion or absorption	20
Free amino acid (elemental)	Alfamino[c] Gerber Extensive HA[c] Neocate Infant[e] PurAmino[b] Similac EleCare[d]	Allergy or sensitivity to cow milk or soy protein, impaired digestion or absorption	20
Low-fat, high MCT	Enfaport Lipil[b]	Chylothorax or chylous ascites	30
Low iron	Similac PM 60/40[d]	Renal insufficiency	20
Rice starch/ cereal added	Enfamil AR[b] Similac for Spit-Up[d]	Gastroesophageal reflux	19–20
Other	Similac Total Comfort[d] Similac for Diarrhea[d]	Protein hydrolysate for persistent feeding issues Infants > 6 mo with watery stools	19–20
Infant/Toddler or Children's Formulas			
Cow milk–based	Good Start 2[c] Similac Go and Grow Milk-Based[d] Enfagrow Premium[b] PediaSure[d]	Healthy older infants, toddlers, and children	19–30
Lactose-free	Nutren Junior[c] Boost Kid Essentials[c]	Lactose intolerance	30
Fiber-containing	Nutren Junior Fiber[c] PediaSure with Fiber[d]	Many potential indications (e.g., constipation)	30
Soy protein–based	Bright Beginnings Soy[f] Enfagrow Soy[b] Good Start 2 Soy PLUS[c] Similac Go and Grow Soy-Based[d]	Lactose intolerance or galactosemia	19–20

(continued)

Table 2. Commercially Available Enteral Formulas for Infants and Children *(continued)*

Formula Type	Brand Name[a]	Indication	Kilocalories per Ounce (kcal/oz)
Infant/Toddler or Children's Formulas *(continued)*			
Protein hydrolysate	Peptamen Junior, Peptamen Junior 1.5[c] Vital Jr. [d] PediaSure Peptide, Peptide 1.5[d]	Allergy or sensitivity to cow milk or soy protein, impaired digestion or absorption	30
Free amino acid (elemental)	Alfamino Junior[c] EleCare Jr. [d] Neocate Junior[e] Vivonex Pediatric[c]	Allergy or sensitivity to cow milk or soy protein, impaired digestion or absorption	24–30
Low-fat, high MCT	Portagen[b]	Impaired digestion or absorption of long chain fats, chylothorax or chylous ascites	30
Real food ingredients	Compleat Pediatric[c]	Base for home tube feeding recipes	30
High calorie	Boost Kid Essentials 1.5[c] PediaSure 1.5, PediaSure Peptide 1.5[d] Peptamen Junior 1.5[c]	Increased caloric needs	45

[a]Brand names listed are examples and not a complete list of products in each category.
[b]Abbott Nutrition, Abbott Park, IL; [c]Mead Johnson, Chicago, IL; [d]Nestlé USA Inc, Glendale, CA; [e]Nutricia, Gaithersburg, MD; [f]Perrigo Nutritionals, Allegan, MI
MCT = medium chain triglyceride.

In the event that a feeding tube becomes occluded, applying a gentle back and forth instillation of warm water into the tube by a 30 or 60 mL syringe has been effective. If this action does not work, then a pancreatic enzyme solution may be instilled in the tube for a minimum of 30 minutes. Another option is the use of an enzyme declogging kit or mechanical declogging device.[18]

PARENTERAL NUTRITION

Parenteral nutrition is a formulation composed of dextrose, amino acids, water, minerals, electrolytes, vitamins, and trace elements infused intravenously into the systemic circulation. Intravenous lipid emulsion (ILE) is typically given as a separate infusion in pediatric patients. Parenteral nutrition may be given through peripheral or central venous access. When giving peripheral PN, the osmolarity of the PN solution (which does not include ILE) should be limited to 900 mOsm/L or less, and care should be taken to assess the catheter site regularly for signs of infiltration. Central PN requires the placement of a central catheter (i.e., a peripherally inserted central catheter or tunneled central venous catheter). When PN is initiated in infants and children, it is typically given by continuous infusion over 24 hours. In older infants and children who will be receiving long-term PN, the PN solution may be cycled over a defined period (e.g., a 12-hour PN infusion overnight). Cyclic PN is achieved with a gradual cycle up to a maximum rate for a defined number of hours followed by a gradual cycle down and off. When initiating cyclic PN, monitoring serum glucose after the maximum rate is achieved and during the off-cycle period is recommended.

FORMULA CONSIDERATIONS

Parenteral nutrition solutions may be formulated as a *2-in-1 admixture*, in which the dextrose and amino acid solution infuses separately from the ILE, or as a *total nutrient admixture*, in which all components (dextrose, amino acids, ILE, and additives) are provided in a single solution. The use of a total nutrient admixture in pediatric patients has disadvantages, including lower calcium and phosphorous solubility, inability to use a 0.2-micron filter because of the large particle size of ILE, and inability to visualize particulates, if they exist. For these reasons, the use of a total nutrient admixture is not recommended in neonates and infants.[20-22]

COMPONENTS

PROTEIN

Protein is provided as crystalline amino acids in PN formulations. The standard commercial solutions provide essential, semi-essential, and nonessential amino acids. Pediatric-specific amino acid products (e.g., Aminosyn-PF [ICU Medical (formerly Hospira), Lake Forest, IL], Premasol [Baxter Healthcare Corporation, Deerfield, IL], TrophAmine [B. Braun Medical Inc., Irvine, CA]) were designed to mimic plasma amino acid concentrations of postprandial breastfed infants. These products have lower amounts of methionine, phenylalanine, and glycine, together with supplemental taurine, glutamate, and aspartate. Pediatric-specific amino acid products also have a lower pH, which imparts greater calcium and phosphorus solubility. All amino acid solutions contain varying amounts of electrolytes that should be considered part of the patient's overall electrolyte provision from PN.

Immaturity of the transsulfuration pathway, specifically hepatic cystathionase activity, during infancy prevents optimal conversion of methionine to cysteine. Thus, cysteine becomes a conditionally essential nutrient because it is further metabolized to taurine, which is essential for retinal development, neurodevelopment, and many other critical functions. Addition of cysteine to PN normalizes plasma amino acid patterns (specifically taurine concentrations) of parenterally fed infants.[23] The addition of cysteine also lowers solution pH (160 mg of L-cysteine provides 1 mmol hydrochloric acid), thus enhancing calcium and phosphorus solubility.[24] However, some infants may be more likely to develop metabolic acidosis with higher doses of cysteine. Although as little as 20 mg of cysteine per g of amino acid may be adequate, most institutions use 30–40 mg cysteine per g of amino acid.[24] Higher dosing (40 mg cysteine per 1 g amino acid) may also have positive antioxidant benefits in critically ill neonates.[25] Cysteine supplementation as a conditionally essential nutrient is only recommended during infancy. Its use for enhancing calcium phosphate solubility could be extended across the pediatric age spectrum.

Each gram of protein provides 4 kcal when oxidized for energy; however, controversy exists regarding whether protein calories should be considered in the caloric content of the PN regimen. The argument is that if adequate energy substrate is provided as dextrose and lipids, amino acids should be used for protein synthesis only, not oxidized for energy.[26]

Early initiation of protein is recommended in preterm neonates who are extremely low birth weight or very low birth weight, starting on the first day of life, to decrease protein losses and restore positive protein balances.[27-29] The use of standardized "starter PN" solutions containing limited ingredients (e.g., protein, dextrose, calcium, heparin) allows for early protein provision for preterm neonates admitted to the neonatal intensive care unit after PN compounding has ceased for the day. Preterm neonates have the highest protein needs per kilogram to maintain growth rates similar to what occurs in utero; this protein requirement decreases with age.[30] In infants, 55% of protein intake is used for growth and 45% for maintenance. As the growth rate slows, the balance changes so that only 10% of protein is used for growth by age 4 years.[31]

CARBOHYDRATES

Dextrose serves as the main source of energy in PN, and it is commercially available as dextrose monohydrate in

---

Enteral Nutrition Calculations

Calculate caloric content of formulas:
- 20 kcal/oz of formula (**standard infant formula**) = 20 kcal/30 mL = 0.67 kcal/mL
  - Standard infant formulas contain either 19 or 20 kcal per ounce (depending on the formula manufacturer). In this example, a 20 kcal per ounce formula is used.
- 30 kcal/oz of formula (**standard pediatric formula**) = 30 kcal/30 mL = 1 kcal/mL

Examples of enteral feeding requirements:
- For a 3-kg infant, give 100 kcal/kg or 300 kcal.
- For a 6.5-kg infant, give 100 kcal/kg or 650 kcal.
- For a 19-kg child, give 100 kcal/kg for the first 10 kg, followed by 50 kcal/kg for the next 9 kg (i.e., for each kilogram between 10 and 20 kg): 1000 kcal + 450 kcal = 1450 kcal.

Examples of volume of formula needed and regimen to provide estimated daily caloric needs:
- For a 3-kg infant receiving **standard infant formula** (20 kcal/oz):
  Desired daily calories = 300 kcal
  300 kcal × 30 mL/20 kcal = 450 mL (150 mL/kg)
  - Check to make sure the calories are calculated correctly: 450 mL × 0.67 kcal/mL = 301.5 kcal about 300 kcal).
  Thus, this infant requires about 2 oz (60 mL) of formula every 3 hr to approximate calorie needs.

- For a 6.5-kg infant receiving **standard infant formula** (20 kcal/oz):
  Desired daily calories = 650 kcal
  650 kcal × 30 mL/20 kcal = 975 mL (150 mL/kg)
  - Check to make sure the calories are calculated correctly: 975 mL × 0.67 kcal/mL = 653 kcal (about 650 kcal).
  Thus, this infant requires about 6.5 oz (or 195 mL) of formula every 4 hr during the day to approximate calorie needs (based on the infant sleeping through the night, with only 5 feedings per day).

- For a 19-kg child receiving **standard pediatric formula** (30 kcal/oz or 1 kcal/mL):
  Desired daily calories = 1450 kcal = 1450 mL
  Thus, this child requires about 6 cans of formula (240 mL per can) per day, which can be given by mouth or by tube intermittently during the day.

  Alternatively, it can be given continuously at a rate of 60 mL/hr per tube, or the child can receive an increased amount (milliliters) per hr over less than 24 hr to give the patient time off the tube feeding/pumps.

  This calculation assumes that all caloric needs are being provided with the pediatric formula and the child is not receiving any additional calories from an oral diet.

Figure 1. Examples of enteral nutrition calculations.

concentrations ranging from 5% to 70%. Final concentrations in PN formulations normally vary from 10% (or lower initially in preterm infants) to 35%, depending on the patient's age, nutritional needs, intravenous access, and condition. For example, dextrose should be limited to 12.5% or less in patients with peripheral access.[32]

Each gram of dextrose yields 3.4 kcal when oxidized. Glucose oxidation rates in infants (14–18 mg/kg/minute) are greater than in older children or adults (4-7 mg/kg/minute).[22,32] When the dextrose infusion rate or glucose infusion rate is greater than the glucose oxidation rate, glycogenesis and fat deposition occur.[33] Excess dextrose can lead not only to hyperglycemia, but also to hypertriglyceridemia, excess carbon dioxide production, and hepatic steatosis.[33] Of note, the administration of exogenous insulin will lower the blood glucose, but it will not alter the glucose oxidative capacity.

Preterm infants are more likely to have glucose intolerance, which may result in hyperglycemia or hypertriglyceridemia. Dextrose should be advanced more slowly by about 2–3 g/kg/day (about 1.5–2 mg/kg/min) in these patients. In older infants, dextrose can usually be advanced by 5 g/kg/day (3.5 mg/kg/min).[32,34] Other risk factors for hyperglycemia in pediatric patients include corticosteroid or catecholamine vasopressor therapy, diabetes, pancreatitis, or stress (organ failure,

Table 3. Select Potential Drug–Nutrient Interactions with Enteral Nutrition[19]

Drug or Class	Interaction	Recommendation
Amiodarone	An increased dose may be required when given nasoduodenally	• Administer consistently with respect to timing of enteral feeds • Monitor closely
Carbamazepine	Adsorption to enteral tube feeds may occur	• Dilute suspension 1:1 with water and flush after administration • Monitor closely
Digoxin	Reduced absorption may be possible with fiber-containing enteral feeds	• Administer consistently with respect to timing of enteral feeds • Administer 1 hr before or 2 hr after feeds with high fiber or pectin • Monitor closely
Fluoroquinolones	Reduced absorption may occur because of chelation with cations and/or interactions with the protein content in enteral feeds	• An increased dose of ciprofloxacin and levofloxacin may be needed • Hold enteral feeds 1 hr before and 2 hr after ciprofloxacin administration • Monitor closely
Itraconazole	• Reduced plasma concentrations may occur, even when separated from enteral feeds by 2 hr • An increased dose leads to increased gastrointestinal adverse effects	• Do not administer with enteral feeds
Levothyroxine	Reduced absorption may occur when not in a fasting state	• An increased dose may be needed • Monitor closely
Phenytoin	Reduced plasma concentrations may occur	• An increased dose may be needed • Separate administration by 2 hr • Monitor closely
Proton pump inhibitors	• Active ingredient is acid-labile • Dosage forms include delayed release enteric coated tablets, delayed release capsules with enteric-coated granules, powder packets, or orally disintegrating tablets • Small-bore tubes can be occluded by denatured proteins if powder product contains xanthan gum or is diluted with acidic fluids	• Use of an alkalemic solution for dilution is acceptable for either gastric or small bowel delivery • Follow manufacturer recommendations for diluent for powder packets • Acidic fluids are not recommended • Flush tube well after administration
Sevelamer	High viscosity may clog feeding tubes	• Flush feeding tube well before and after administration
Sucralfate	May complex with protein and clog feeding tubes	• Do not administer by small-bore (i.e., ≤ 12 Fr) feeding tubes
Warfarin	Warfarin resistance may occur because of the vitamin K content of feeds and/or binding to protein in feeds (more recent data)	• Hold enteral feeds 1 hr before and after administration • Monitor the international normalized ratio closely

sepsis, or surgery).[33] Although neonates may develop significant hyperglycemia after surgery, it resolves more quickly in them, with glucose returning to preoperative levels within 12 hours postsurgery.[35]

INTRAVENOUS LIPID EMULSION

Intravenous lipid emulsions provide a concentrated source of calories, prevent or treat essential fatty acid deficiency (EFAD), and extend the life of peripheral intravenous lines. Until recently, commercially available products in the United States have been exclusively based on soybean oil, composed primarily of the long chain fats, linoleic acid (omega-6 fatty acid) and linolenic acid (omega-3 fatty acid). Soybean oil–based ILE have proinflammatory effects secondary to eicosanoid production from omega-6 polyunsaturated fatty acids, and they have been thought to contribute to the development of PN-associated liver disease (PNALD). Two additional ILE products have been approved for use in the United States for adults and recently have become available, a soybean and olive oil emulsion (Clinolipid; Baxter Healthcare Corporation) and a mixed emulsion of soybean, medium chain triglycerides, olive oil, and fish oil (SMOFLipid; Fresenius Kabi, Uppsala, Sweden).[36,37] The ILE products that contain fish oil (with less-inflammatory omega-3 fatty acids) have been shown to improve and potentially prevent PNALD.[38,39] A 100% fish oil product has also recently been approved for use in pediatric patients with PNALD.[40] This product is a 10% ILE, and the maximum daily dose is 1 g/kg/day infused over 12 hours.[40]

With respect to soybean oil–based ILE, the 20% (vs. 10%) product is preferred for use in pediatric patients because of the lower phospholipid-to-triglyceride ratio, which improves triglyceride clearance.[34,41] Whereas the daily requirement for ILE is much greater (up to 3 g/kg/day), the amount of linoleic acid necessary to prevent EFAD can be supplied by providing 2% to 4% of the nonprotein calories, or 0.5–1 g/kg/day, from the ILE.[41,42] Greater daily amounts of mixed oil ILE products may be required to prevent EFAD. In infants receiving only fish oil–based ILE for at least 1 month, EFAD has been prevented.[43] Recent evidence suggests that EFAD may also be prevented by sufficient supply of arachidonic acid and docosahexaenoic acid, which are available in abundant supply in fish oil–based ILE.[44]

Although 1 g of fat provides 9 kcal, the egg phospholipids that are used as emulsifying agents and the glycerol that is added to make the ILE isotonic also provide calories, thereby increasing the caloric content of the 20% ILE to 2 kcal/mL. Product labeling states that patients with severe allergic reactions to eggs should not receive ILE products.[36,37,40,45] However, the occurrence of egg allergy with ILE is rare and in clinical practice, patients are generally observed for hypersensitivity reactions.

Lipid clearance is reduced in premature neonates, and rapid infusion is more likely to result in hypertriglyceridemia. Clearance is further impaired if premature neonates are receiving steroids, are stressed, or have organ dysfunction.[46] Serum triglyceride monitoring is recommended when administering ILE. A longer infusion time of 20–24 hours (rate of 0.15 g/kg/hour) improves ILE tolerance and is recommended in preterm infants.[32,41,42,46,47] Rapid lipid infusions have also been associated with impaired oxygenation in neonates. All ILE products carry a warning regarding preterm infant deaths attributed to pulmonary fat accumulation.[36,37,40,45] These products should be administered with a 1.2-micron in-line filter.[36,37,40,45]

The recommended infusion time per package labeling for ILE is 12 hours. Adherence to this infusion time in pediatric patients is problematic. Commercial ILE products are not available in unit volumes consistent with safe daily doses for infants. In addition, a 3 g/kg/day ILE dose at the recommended infusion rate of 0.15 g/kg/hour requires at least a 20-hour infusion. For these reasons, pediatric institutions have repackaged ILE into smaller units to be infused by syringe pump technology. However, repackaged ILE has resulted in microbial contamination.[21] Aseptic withdrawal of an appropriate ILE volume resulting in a patient-specific dose in the original manufacturer's container (draw down unit) resulted in no contamination in routine clinical practice compared with repackaged syringes, and this approach is recommended by the American Society of Parenteral and Enteral Nutrition (ASPEN) as a potential option.[21] When prolonged ILE infusions are required in neonates and infants, the daily dose should be divided in two separate 12-hour infusions with ILE container and administration tubing replacement every 12 hours. When using repackaged ILE, infusion time should not exceed 12 hours per unit, and the administration tubing should be changed with each new infusion.[21] Figure 2 gives an example of initiating a PN solution in an infant, including caloric calculations.

ELECTROLYTES

Electrolytes added to PN solutions include sodium and potassium (as chloride, acetate, or phosphate salts), calcium, phosphorus (as sodium or potassium phosphate), and magnesium. Requirements vary based on age, disease state, organ function, and concomitant drugs. Based on intravenous access, certain electrolytes should be limited. For example, potassium given through a peripheral line should not exceed 40 mEq/L. Specifics on fluid and electrolyte management can be found in the Fluid and Electrolytes chapter. Table 1 provides typical electrolyte doses per day across pediatric ages.[32] Electrolyte losses from sources other than urine, such as diarrhea or stoma output, should also be replaced.

The provision of calcium and phosphorus in utero during the third trimester approximates 120–150 mg/kg/day of elemental calcium and 70–85 mg/kg/day of elemental phosphorus.[48-51] Supplementation of similar doses through PN is impossible without exceeding solubility limits and causing calcium phosphate precipitation. Despite the inability to supplement with similar in utero mineral doses, the highest retention of both minerals and sufficient bone mineralization has occurred in infants and children on PN when the minerals are given in a 1.7:1 calcium-to-phosphorus (milligram to milligram) ratio.[52-54] This ratio is typically provided throughout the first year of life. Mineral requirements decrease as children age. In older children, an equimolar provision of calcium and phosphorus is optimal. It is important for severely malnourished patients to receive sufficient phosphorus to avoid the refeeding syndrome.

Acetate is provided in PN to help maintain the acid–base balance. Although bicarbonate is not compatible with PN, acetate is converted to bicarbonate in vivo. Premature neonates may be more prone to developing metabolic acidosis caused by reduced renal absorption of bicarbonate, lower pH of pediatric amino acid products, and addition of L-cysteine to PN solutions containing pediatric amino acid products.

Parenteral Nutrition Calculations

Estimate fluid and caloric needs:
For a 3-kg infant, give 300 mL/day parenterally and 300 kcal/day.

Calculate rate of infusion:
300 mL/day ÷ 24 hr/day = 12.5 mL/hr

Carbohydrate (dextrose):
Adjust dose in grams per kilogram.
Advance 2.5–3 g/kg in small, preterm infants.
Advance 5 g/kg in term infants and young children.
In general, advance by 5% per day in older children/adolescents.

Protein:
Begin with desired protein dose on day 1 (no need to titrate protein as done for dextrose and fats).
Include 40 mg cysteine per gram of protein when giving pediatric amino acid products (i.e., Aminosyn-PF[a], Premasol[b], TrophAmine[c]).

Intravenous lipid emulsion (ILE):
Begin at 0.5–1 g/kg/day and advance by 0.25–1 g/kg/day until at desired daily dose.

Total calories:
Add kilocalories per day from dextrose, protein, and ILE.
Divide total by patient weight for kilocalories per kilogram per day.

Total volume:
Add milliliters per day from dextrose/amino acid solution and ILE.
Divide total by patient weight for milliliters per kilogram per day.

Calculate dextrose calories:
Dextrose (g) × 3.4 kcal/g
300 mL of dextrose 10% = 300 mL × 10 g/100 mL = 30 g of dextrose × 3.4 kcal/g = 102 kcal/3 kg = 34 kcal/kg/day

Calculate protein calories:
Protein (g) × 4 kcal/g
2.5 g/kg/day × 4 kcal/g = 10 kcal/kg/day

Calculate ILE calories:
20% fat emulsion provides 2 kcal/mL.
Calculate the volume of fat emulsion per day:
    1 g/kg/day × 3 kg = 3 g/day; 3 g ÷ 20 g/100 mL (i.e., 20% emulsion) = 15 mL; 15 mL/24 hr = 0.625 mL/hr
    Round rate to 0.6 mL/hr × 24 hr/day = 14.4 mL; 14.4 mL/day × 2 kcal/mL = 28.8 kcal/day or 9.6 kcal/kg/day

Final calculations:
3-kg infant receiving parenteral nutrition (10% dextrose and 2.5 g/kg/day protein) at 12.5 mL/hr and 20% ILE at 0.6 mL/hr:

Dextrose	34 kcal/kg
Amino acids	10 kcal/kg
ILE	9.6 kcal/kg
Total	**53.6 kcal/kg**

Continue to advance dextrose and lipid calories to meet the goal of 100 kcal/kg/day.

[a]ICU Medical (formerly Hospira), Lake Forest, IL; [b]Baxter Healthcare Corporation, Deerfield, IL; [c]B. Braun Medical Inc., Irvine, CA.

Figure 2. Examples of parenteral nutrition calculations.

Consequently, these solutions often need acetate added as a sodium or potassium salt. Initial doses for mild acidosis are generally 0.5–1 mEq/kg/day titrated or tapered based on serum bicarbonate and blood gas analysis; however, patients with diarrhea/intestinal losses will receive larger doses.

VITAMINS AND TRACE ELEMENTS

Vitamins are required cofactors in many metabolic processes. They include *lipid-soluble vitamins* (A, D, E, and K) and *water-soluble vitamins* (ascorbic acid and the B-complex vitamins), and both types should be provided in PN. Commercially available multivitamin products are available for use in PN solutions. Infants and young children should receive a pediatric multivitamin product, whereas children/adolescents older than 11 years should receive an adult multivitamin product. Iron is not included in commercially available multivitamin products, so it will need to be supplemented in patients on exclusive long-term PN. An initial trial of oral/enteral iron supplementation is warranted in patients receiving some enteral intake. Intermittent supplementation with parenteral iron products (iron dextran, sodium ferric gluconate, iron sucrose, ferumoxytol) should be initiated in patients failing oral/enteral supplementation.[32] Iron dextran is the only parenteral iron product compatible with PN; none of the parenteral iron products are compatible with ILE.[32]

Chromium, copper, zinc, manganese, and selenium are commonly added to PN solutions to prevent deficiencies. Although pediatric multitrace element products exist for use in PN solutions, they do not contain selenium, and their contents result in the underdosing of zinc in neonates and infants, who thus require additional zinc supplementation. In addition, zinc is important for immune function and wound healing, and supplemental zinc may be needed if abnormal fluid losses are occurring from wounds or increased stooling.[55] Trace element contamination also occurs, primarily with chromium and manganese, in many components of PN, so they may not need to be routinely added. Chromium, selenium, and zinc, which are eliminated renally, may accumulate in patients with renal insufficiency. Similarly, copper and manganese, which are eliminated through the biliary system, accumulate in patients with liver disease. Manganese accumulates in patients with or without liver disease who receive long-term PN, which has been associated with concerns for neurotoxicity. Although iodine supplementation is not needed in patients on short-term PN, deficiency may occur in patients receiving long-term therapy.[56] Given these concerns, some pediatric practitioners individually dose trace elements rather than use the multitrace products. This practice allows the adjustment of trace elements in specific disease states or conditions or for the exclusion of trace elements, such as chromium and manganese, because of contamination. During trace element product shortages, the FDA has allowed temporary importation of alternative multiple trace element products from outside the United States. Clinicians must exercise caution when using imported products as they often differ not only in trace element content, but also in dose per unit and in salt form.

ADDITIVES

Neonates have a reduced biosynthetic capacity for carnitine, a nutrient required for transporting long chain fatty acids into the mitochondria for energy production. Because PN does not contain carnitine, neonates, particularly preterm neonates, will become deficient while receiving exclusive carnitine-free PN. Thus, carnitine supplementation in neonates expected to receive PN for more than 1 week will prevent deficiency and augment their capacity for fatty acid oxidation.[57] Other pediatric patients who may benefit from carnitine supplementation include those with hypertriglyceridemia while receiving ILE, as well as patients with short bowel syndrome, diffuse inflammatory bowel disease, or malabsorption syndromes who are receiving a portion of their calories parenterally.[57]

Parenteral nutrition is not preferred as a drug vehicle because of the risk of interactions with the various components of the admixture; however, several medications can be safely added during compounding. Histamine-2-receptor blockers are often used in patients who are critically ill and in those with short bowel syndrome. Ranitidine, famotidine, and cimetidine have been shown to be compatible with most PN admixtures.[58] These medications should be used judiciously, however, because they have been associated with an increased incidence of necrotizing enterocolitis and sepsis in preterm infants.[59,60] Insulin may also be added to PN solutions to facilitate glucose metabolism, but only regular human insulin should be used. Modified insulin formulations should not be added. Low-dose heparin (0.5-1 unit/mL) may also be added to most PN solutions to help prevent thrombosis of the catheter; however, the addition of heparin to ILE can result in disruption of the emulsion.[61] It is also important to note that heparin addition to PN solutions is not recommended per the ASPEN guidelines.[21] Iron dextran is the only parenteral iron formulation compatible with PN, but it is incompatible with ILE.[32] Dosing strategies for parenteral iron supplementation are available.[32] Table 4 summarizes potential drug–nutrient interactions with commonly used PN additives.

COMPLICATIONS

Although PN is a lifesaving therapy for infants and children who cannot tolerate or absorb EN, it is associated with significant technical, metabolic, and infectious complications.

Technical complications may result with catheters when they are placed or later during their use. Catheters may move or be accidentally removed, or the lumen of the catheter may become occluded with a clot or biofilm. Fibrinolytic agents such as alteplase may be used to dissolve the fibrin and restore the patency of the catheter. Components of the PN solution such as calcium and phosphate may precipitate, causing an occlusion.

Although hyperglycemia and hypoglycemia may both occur, hyperglycemia is seen more often. It often occurs after surgery, when given with concomitant glucocorticoids, when dextrose is advanced too quickly, and in neonates. Hyperglycemia may impair the immune system and make the patient more susceptible to infectious complications.[33] The most serious risk associated with hyperglycemia is the development of a hyperosmolar hyperglycemic state. Blood glucose should be monitored carefully, particularly when PN is initiated, when dextrose is advanced, or in patients who are at increased risk of hyperglycemia because of concomitant medications or their clinical condition. Hypoglycemia may occur if PN is abruptly discontinued.

Hypertriglyceridemia may occur in infants who receive excessive glucose or secondary to the inadequate clearance of ILE. Clearance of the ILE is improved if it is given over 24 hours. Elevated triglycerides may be the result of poor clearance of exogenous chylomicrons or caused by the mobilization of endogenous fat in response to inadequate caloric intake. Assessment of the serum sample is useful; if the ILE is not being adequately cleared from the circulation, the serum sample will be lipemic.

Acid–base disorders are also common in patients receiving PN and may be caused by the underlying condition or, less commonly, by the PN formulation. The acetate and chloride components of PN should be adjusted to prevent or treat metabolic acid–base anomalies.

The refeeding syndrome, which is characterized by hypophosphatemia, hypokalemia, hypomagnesemia, and fluid retention, is a potentially life-threatening complication. It is usually seen in patients who were very undernourished, causing their bodies to mobilize free fatty acids and ketone bodies for energy. If dextrose is started aggressively after a period of undernutrition, hypophosphatemia, hyperinsulinemia (or increased insulin secretion), and other electrolyte abnormalities may develop as energy metabolism is shifted to an anabolic state. Elevated insulin levels may cause fluid retention, which can result in cardiac decompensation in these patients. To prevent the refeeding syndrome, it is imperative

to monitor glucose and other electrolytes in patients who were severely undernourished and to be cautious with advancements of dextrose. The risk may also be reduced in undernourished patients by providing additional phosphorus and potassium above the recommended daily allowance when PN is started.[46]

Parenteral nutrition–associated liver disease, defined as a direct bilirubin equal to 2 mg/dL or more, is a common complication that may develop in 40% to 60% of children receiving long-term PN.[62] In infants, PNALD normally manifests as cholestasis that can progress to liver failure and even death. In older children and adults, hepatic steatosis is more often seen. Risk factors include prematurity, sepsis, lack of enteral feeding, duration of PN, length of bowel remaining, and excessive calories.[62] Components of PN have also been associated with the development of PNALD, including the amino acid composition and soybean oil–based ILE. Fish oil–based ILE reverses PNALD and may help prevent the disease.[38,39] Other treatments include administering ursodiol, cycling PN, restricting the ILE dose (typically to 1 g/kg/day), preventing sepsis, providing trophic feeds, and preventing bacterial overgrowth with the use of antibiotics or probiotics.[39,62] The condition is normally reversible if EN can be advanced and PN discontinued before irreversible liver damage occurs; however, patients may require liver transplantation if the disease progresses.

Metabolic bone disease is also a multifactorial process that is more common in infants on long-term PN. It usually presents as osteopenia in preterm infants, but fractures and rickets can also occur.[63] Preterm infants are at the greatest risk because they missed the third trimester when the highest calcium and phosphorus accretion normally occurs. Metabolic

Table 4. Select Potential Drug–Nutrient Interactions with Parenteral Nutrition[19]

Drug or Class	Interaction	Recommendation
Albumin	Glycosylation of albumin may occur when exposed to dextrose Clogging of 0.2-micron filters may occur Creaming of TNAs may occur	Do not add to PN formulations
Heparin	Lipid instability may occur in presence of high concentrations of heparin	Add low-dose heparin to lipid-free PN formulations only
Histamine-2 receptor blockers	No effect on stability or effectiveness	Histamine-2 receptor blockers may be added to PN formulations (lipid-free or TNA)
Hydrochloric acid	Cracking of TNAs may occur	Add to lipid-free PN formulations only
Insulin	No effect on stability or effectiveness of regular human insulin; other insulins are not compatible Cannot be titrated independently of dextrose if insulin is in PN	Add regular human insulin to PN formulations only in patients with stable insulin requirements
Iron dextran	Lipid instability may occur when iron dextran is added	Add to lipid-free PN formulations only
Octreotide	May be listed as physically compatible, but glycosylation may occur when exposed to dextrose, which leads to inactive metabolites	Do not add to PN formulations
Sodium bicarbonate	Combines with calcium to form a calcium carbonate precipitate	Do not add to PN formulations

PN = parenteral nutrition; TNA = total nutrient admixture.

bone disease may be related to insufficient provision of calcium and phosphorus, increased renal excretion of calcium, or aluminum contamination in the PN solution. To reduce the incidence of metabolic bone disease in infants, calcium and phosphorus should be maximized to amounts that can be safely administered by PN, as well as given in the appropriate ratio; supplemental vitamin D may also be necessary.

Patients receiving PN therapy are at increased risk of infection because of the presence of an intravenous catheter. The most common organisms are coagulase-negative *Staphylococcus*, *Staphylococcus aureus*, *Enterococcus*, and *Candida* spp.[64] Organisms can be introduced from the skin, from the hub of the catheter, or by hematogenous spread from another location in the body. Catheter-related bloodstream infections begin with infection at the catheter site. In addition to systemic antibiotic therapy, treatment may include catheter removal. However, if the child depends on PN for hydration and nutrition, then he or she will continue to require central venous access. Lock therapy may also be used in an effort to salvage the catheter.[65] This approach may include the placement of an antibiotic or ethanol into the catheter lumen where it is allowed to dwell for a time, after which the solution is flushed through the catheter or withdrawn. The use of antibiotic or ethanol lock therapy requires the patient to be cycled off PN and not receiving other systemic medications through the catheter for the duration of the dwell time. Thus, the dwell time can vary from a few hours per day to the entire time the catheter is not in use for PN or other medication administration. If lock therapy is being used for treatment of a catheter-related bloodstream infection, it is commonly given daily, whereas lock therapy for prevention of a catheter-related bloodstream infection is given less often (1–3 times per week). In patients with multi-lumen catheters, lock therapy should be alternated between all the lumens of the catheter for optimal results.

SAFETY CONSIDERATIONS IN NUTRITION SUPPORT

Specialized nutrition support has been associated with several safety issues in which serious harm and/or death have occurred. Commonly reported errors with EN that have resulted in patient death include the contamination of EN formulations and enteral feeding misconnections. Contamination of EN may occur at any point in the compounding, reconstitution, handling, and administration processes. Enteral feeding misconnections have occurred when feeding formulations for enteral delivery have been infused into nonenteral sites, such as a central venous catheter. The EN guidelines published by ASPEN address these

safety issues and give recommendations for preventing EN-related errors.[18]

As a complex formulation of macro- and micronutrients and additives, PN has been associated with several errors that have resulted in serious patient harm and death, including calcium phosphate precipitation, contamination of PN formulation, over- or underdosing of dextrose, omission of dextrose, iron overload, and overdoses of trace elements, electrolytes, and heparin. Errors that have resulted in patient harm have occurred throughout the PN process, including ordering, order entry/verification, compounding and labeling, and handling and administration. The use of computer prescriber order entry or standardized electronic order template for PN ordering and software systems for order review/verification and PN compounding and labeling have resulted in improved efficiency and safety. Software systems for PN compounding should be set up with system and individual additive limits as well as calcium phosphate solubility curve data for optimal order review and patient safety. The guidelines published by ASPEN provide recommendations for the safe provision of PN formulations.[20,21,66] Institutions should develop policies and procedures that support safe PN practices consistent with these guidelines.

Pharmacists in many different practice sites, including home care, institutional pharmacy, and clinical pharmacy, play an integral role in providing specialized nutrition support to patients. Many clinical pharmacists who specialize in nutrition support are directly responsible for ordering PN formulations. Parenteral nutrition solutions are typically compounded in the pharmacy, whereas EN formulations may or may not be dispensed from the pharmacy. Pharmacists are thus responsible for PN order review and verification before compounding. Pharmacy departments responsible for preparing EN and PN formulations should be aware of the safety issues associated with specialized nutrition support, remain current with recommended standards and guidelines for nutrition support, and institute safeguards within their practices to ensure the safe and effective administration of EN and PN to their patients.

CONCLUSIONS

Specialized nutrition support has been lifesaving for many pediatric disease states. Pharmacists practicing in nutrition support should be able to adequately assess nutrition status, understand the appropriate indications for EN and PN use in patients, order and compound EN and PN formulations, avoid drug–nutrient interactions, monitor patients for complications associated with therapy, and ensure the effective and safe use of nutrition therapy in patients.

A 2-day-old preterm male neonate (gestational age 35 weeks; weight 2.5 kg) has a prenatal diagnosis of gastroschisis. He undergoes silo placement on the first day of life with planned surgical closure within 7 days, based on clinical status and regression of intestines back into abdominal cavity. The patient is being managed in the neonatal intensive care unit, is on mechanical ventilation, and has a naso-gastric tube in place with low intermittent suction. He has central access (umbilical venous catheter). His urine output is 4 mL/kg/hr.

Current medications:

7.5% Dextrose in water + 0.22% NaCl	12 mL/hr
Ampicillin	50 mg/kg IV every 6 hr
Gentamicin	5 mg/kg IV every 24 hr
Midazolam	0.05 mg/kg/hr

Laboratory findings:

Test	Result	Normal Values
Na (mEq/L)	136	136–145
K (mEq/L)	3.2	4–6
Cl (mEq/L)	105	95–105
HCO_3 (mEq/L)	21	22–28
BUN (mg/dL)	5	4–15
SCr (mg/dL)	0.6	≤ 0.6
Glucose (mg/dL)	86	< 90

1. Determine this patient's eligibility for nutrition support and formulate an initial nutrition plan for this patient.

This patient is a candidate for parenteral nutrition (PN) given his history of prematurity (35 weeks' gestation), "nothing by mouth" status, and no significant enteral intake likely for at least the next 7–10 days (and potentially much longer). Fluids are providing 115 mL/kg/day (a little more than maintenance volume of 100 mL/kg/day). This volume is acceptable and may actually need to be increased with a silo in place that results in increased water and sodium losses through the exposed abdomen. The blood urea nitrogen value does not suggest dehydration at this time, so it would be appropriate to formulate initial PN to infuse at 12 mL/hr and then add intravenous lipid emulsion (ILE) in addition to this infusion rate. The initial PN should contain 10% dextrose, which is an increase of 2.9 g/kg/day from the current fluids and provides a glucose infusion rate of 8 mg/kg/min. Amino acids can be started at the goal of 3 g/kg/day (target the lower end of goal range given later gestational age). If this patient were started on amino acids at 3 g/kg, it would provide a total of 7.5 g of protein, and then 150–300 mg of cysteine (20–40 mg per gram of protein) should be added. The initial lipid dose of 1 g/kg/day ILE would be appropriate. His serum potassium and bicarbonate values are both low, and his urine output is good. The PN should contain potassium (1 mEq/kg/day initially) and acetate (1 mEq/kg/day as either sodium or potassium acetate). Serum sodium is in the low range of normal and fluids (0.22% sodium chloride equivalent) are providing 4.4 mEq/kg/day sodium. Because a silo is in place (increased losses), this amount of sodium could be continued in the initial PN solution or increased slightly (up to 5 mEq/kg/day) while monitoring serum electrolytes. Standard doses for calcium (3 mEq/kg) and phosphate (1.2 mmol/kg) should be added, maintaining the appropriate ratio for optimal bone mineralization (2.5 mEq calcium:1 mmol phosphorus, which is equivalent to 1.7 mg calcium:1 mg phosphorus). Magnesium (0.4 mEq/kg), pediatric multivitamins, and trace elements should be added.

2. What are the short and long-term nutrition goals for this patient?

Short-term nutrition goals for this patient are to increase dextrose and ILE calories over the first few days of PN to provide about 100 kcal/kg/day. The ILE should be increased by 0.5 to 1 g/kg/day to a maximum of 3 g/kg/day in PN (providing 30 kcal/kg/day). Protein (3 g/kg/day) is providing 12 kcal/kg/day. Thus, dextrose should be increased by 2–3 g/kg/day to achieve approximately 100 kcal/kg/day from the parenteral route. This amount of dextrose in the PN is about 15% and results in a glucose infusion rate of about 11 mg/kg/min. Daily weights should be monitored to ensure the neonate is achieving adequate weight gain. Long-term nutrition goals are to prevent complications, such as PN-associated liver disease (PNALD) and metabolic bone disease, and to prevent macro- and micro-nutrient deficiencies.

3. What laboratory variables should be monitored for this patient when starting PN?

Monitoring is vital to ensure that the patient receives appropriate nutrition with minimal complications. Weight, length, and head circumference should be followed to monitor for adequate growth. Initial laboratory assessments should include a comprehensive metabolic panel, direct bilirubin, magnesium, phosphorus, and triglyceride levels. Patients on long-term PN will need additional laboratory values, including vitamin and trace element levels, carnitine levels, iron studies, and thyroid function.

Case (continued). The patient's serum bicarbonate is now 18 mEq/L (22–28 mEq/L).

4. What can be added to the PN solution to increase the bicarbonate level?

Most drugs should not be added to PN to avoid drug–nutrient interactions. Acetate can be provided as a sodium or potassium salt, and it is converted to bicarbonate in vivo. Since the PN was formulated initially with 1 mE/kg/day acetate, an increase of 1-2 mEq/kg of acetate would be reasonable (for a total acetate of 2-3 mEq/kg/day). Sodium bicarbonate is not compatible with PN.

Case (continued). This patient has uncomplicated surgical closure for gastroschisis at 10 days of life. Three weeks after starting PN, the patient's direct bilirubin is elevated (2.6 mg/dL).

5. How does this direct bilirubin value affect the overall nutrition plan for this patient?

This patient's direct bilirubin value is above the cutoff for PNALD (greater than 2 mg/dL). Overfeeding with macronutrients could worsen existing PNALD. Clinicians should evaluate PN content to determine if macronutrients should be adjusted. Protein should be decreased to 2.5 g/kg/day (neonate is now at more than 38 weeks' postconception age), dextrose should be limited to a maximum glucose infusion of 14 mg/kg/min, and ILE restricted. The ILE restriction could be accomplished by withholding ILE for a few days per week (ILE holidays), by lowering the daily ILE dose, or by both approaches. Macronutrient restriction results in a reduced total caloric intake. Growth should be monitored closely to make sure the neonate is continuing to achieve an acceptable growth rate.

Another consideration would be cyclic PN so the neonate has a PN-free period daily. The neonate is now postsurgical closure, so it would be important to begin enteral feedings if they have not already started or to advance them gradually if they have been initiated. In addition, ursodiol could be initiated. Finally, if the neonate has a prolonged PN course and PNALD progresses, clinicians should consider the use of a mixed-oil ILE (soybean oil, medium chain triglyceride, olive oil, fish oil) rather than the soybean oil–based ILE because it is now commercially available in the United States. Although mixed-oil ILE is not approved for use in pediatric patients, clinical trials are ongoing and the product has been used and studied extensively in pediatric patients outside of the United States. Mixed-oil ILE should be considered interchangeable with the soybean oil–based ILE.

Case (continued). The infant is now age 2 months (weight 4.4 kg) and receiving transitional enteral feeding (expressed breast milk 15 mL every 3 hours) in addition to PN. Direct bilirubin is 3.2 mg/dL. New orders are prescribed for the following medications: cholecalciferol, ferrous sulfate liquid, and ursodiol.

6. What are the indications for these medications?

Infants receiving exclusively breast milk are at risk for vitamin D deficiency, and 400 international units of vitamin D daily is recommended. The patient is currently still receiving PN with a multivitamin containing vitamin D, but the supplemental cholecalciferol will be essential as the patient transitions to full enteral feeds. Iron is not included in PN, and supplementation may be needed given the duration of time that the patient has received PN. Finally, a direct bilirubin greater than 2 mg/dL indicates that the patient still has PNALD. With the initiation of feeds and enteral medications, ursodiol may be beneficial as part of the treatment of PNALD.

REFERENCES

1. National Center for Health Statistics. 2010. CDC Growth Charts: United States. Available at www.cdc.gov/growthcharts/. Accessed May 22, 2019.
2. Grummer-Strawn LM, Reinold C, Krebs NF, Centers for Disease Control and Prevention (CDC). Use of World Health Organization and CDC growth charts for children aged 0-59 months in the United States. MMWR Recomm Rep 2010;59:1-15.
3. Barlow SE, the Expert Committee. Expert committee recommendations regarding the prevention, assessment, and treatment of child and adolescent overweight and obesity: summary report. Pediatrics 2007;120:S164-92.
4. Ogden CL, Carroll MD, Lawman HG, et al. Trends in obesity prevalence among children and adolescents in the United States, 1988–1994 through 2013–2014. JAMA 2016;315:2292-9.
5. Roy SM, Fields DA, Mitchell JA, et al. Body mass index is a better indicator of body composition than weight-for-length at age 1 month. J Pediatr 2018;204:77-83.
6. Woo JG, Daniels SR. Assessment of body mass index in infancy: it is time to revise our guidelines. J Pediatr 2018;204:10-11.
7. American Academy of Pediatrics, Committee on Nutrition. Failure to thrive. In: Kleinman RE, ed. Pediatric Nutrition Handbook, 7th ed. Elk Grove Village, IL: American Academy of Pediatrics, 2014:667.
8. Fenton T, Kim J. A systematic review and meta-analysis to revise the Fenton growth chart for preterm infants. BMC Pediatr 2013; 13:59.
9. Marian M. Pediatric nutrition support. Nutr Clin Pract 1993; 8:171-5.
10. Chessman KH, Kumpf VJ. Assessment of nutrition status and nutrition requirements. In: DiPiro JT, Talbert RL, Yee GC, et al., eds. Pharmacotherapy: A Pathophysiologic Approach, 10th ed. New York: McGraw-Hill, 2017:2323-44.
11. American Academy of Pediatrics, Committee on Nutrition. Feeding the child. In: Kleinman RE, ed. Pediatric Nutrition Handbook, 7th ed. Elk Grove Village, IL: American Academy of Pediatrics, 2014:143.
12. American Academy of Pediatrics, Committee on Nutrition. Enteral nutrition. In: Kleinman RE, ed. Pediatric Nutrition Handbook, 7th ed. Elk Grove Village, IL: American Academy of Pediatrics, 2014:591-605.
13. Worthington P, Balint J, Bechtold M, et al. When is parenteral nutrition appropriate? JPEN J Parenter Enteral Nutr 2017;41:324-77.
14. Mehta NM, Skillman HE, Irving SY, et al. Guidelines for the provision and assessment of nutrition support therapy in the pediatric critically ill patient: Society of Critical Care Medicine and American Society for Parenteral and Enteral Nutrition. JPEN J Parenter Enteral Nutr 2017;41:706-42.
15. Holliday MA, Segar WE. The maintenance need for water in parenteral fluid therapy. Pediatrics 1957;19:823-32.
16. HMBANA [homepage on the Internet]. Fort Worth: Human Milk Banking Association of North America. Available at www. hmbana.org/. Accessed May 23, 2019.
17. Wagner CL, Greer FR, American Academy of Pediatrics Section on Breastfeeding, American Academy of Pediatrics Committee on Nutrition. Prevention of rickets and vitamin D deficiency in infants, children, and adolescents. Pediatrics 2008;122:1142-52.
18. Boullata JI, Carrera AL, Harvey L, et al. A.S.P.E.N. Safe practices for enteral nutrition therapy. JPEN J Parenter Enteral Nutr 2017;41:15-103.
19. Dickerson RN, Sacks GS. Medication administration considerations with specialized nutrition support. In: DiPiro JT, Talbert RL, Yee GC, et al., eds. Pharmacotherapy: A Pathophysiologic Approach, 8th ed. New York: McGraw-Hill, 2010:2494-502.

20. Ayers P, Adams S, Boullata J, et al. A.S.P.E.N. parenteral nutrition safety consensus recommendations. JPEN J Parenter Enteral Nutr 2014;38:296-333.

21. Boullata JI, Gilbert K, Sacks G, et al. A.S.P.E.N. Clinical Guidelines: parenteral nutrition ordering, order review, compounding, labeling, and dispensing. JPEN J Parenter Enteral Nutr 2014;38:334-77.

22. Mattox TW, Crill CM. Parenteral nutrition. In: DiPiro JT, Talbert RL, Yee GC, et al., eds. Pharmacotherapy. A Pathophysiologic Approach, 10th ed. New York: McGraw-Hill, 2014:2345-65.

23. Helms RA, Storm MC, Christensen ML, et al. Cysteine supplementation results in normalization of plasma taurine concentrations in children receiving home parenteral nutrition. J Pediatr 1999;134:358-61.

24. A.S.P.E.N. Parenteral Nutrition L-Cysteine Product Shortage Considerations. Available at www.nutritioncare.org/News/ General News/A S P E N Releases New Parenteral Nutrition L-Cysteine Product Shortage Considerations/. Accessed May 23, 2019.

25. Calkins KL, Sanchez LA, Tseng CH, et al. Effect of high-dose cysteine supplementation on erythrocyte glutathione: a double-blinded randomized placebo controlled pilot study in critically ill neonates. JPEN J Parenter Enteral Nutr 2016;40:224-34.

26. Van Way CW III. Total calories vs nonprotein calories [editorial]. Nutr Clin Pract 2001;16:271-2.

27. Denne SC, Poindexter BB. Evidence supporting early nutritional support with parenteral amino acid infusion. Semin Perinatol 2007;31:56-60.

28. Hay WW Jr. Strategies for feeding the preterm infant. Neonatology 2008;94:245-54.

29. Poindexter BB, Langer JC, Dusick AM, et al., National Institute of Child Health and Human Development Neonatal Research Network. Early provision of parenteral amino acids in extremely low birth weight infants: relation to growth and neurodevelopmental outcome. J Pediatr 2006;148:300-5.

30. Zlotkin SH, Bryan MH, Anderson GH. Intravenous nitrogen and energy intakes required to duplicate in utero nitrogen accretion in prematurely born human infants. J Pediatr 1981;99:115-20.

31. American Academy of Pediatrics, Committee on Nutrition. Protein. In: Kleinman RE, ed. Pediatric Nutrition Handbook, 7th ed. Elk Grove Village, IL: American Academy of Pediatrics, 2014:369-386.

32. Crill CM, Gura KM. Parenteral nutrition support. In: Corkins MR, ed. The A.S.P.E.N. Pediatric Nutrition Support Core Curriculum, 2nd ed. Silver Spring, MD: American Society for Parenteral and Enteral Nutrition; 2015:593-614.

33. Btaiche IF, Khalidi N. Metabolic complications of parenteral nutrition in adults, part 1. Am J Health Syst Pharm 2004; 61:1938-49.

34. American Academy of Pediatrics, Committee on Nutrition. Parenteral nutrition. In: Kleinman RE, ed. Pediatric Nutrition Handbook, 7th ed. Elk Grove Village, IL: American Academy of Pediatrics, 2014:571-90.

35. Elphick M, Wilkinson A. The effects of starvation and surgical injury on the plasma levels of glucose, free fatty acids, and neutral lipids in newborn babies suffering from various congenital anomalies. Pediatr Res 1981;15:313-8.

36. Clinolipid [product information]. Deerfield, IL: Baxter Healthcare Corporation, 2016.

37. SMOFLipid [product information]. Uppsala, Sweden: Fresenius Kabi, 2016.

38. de Meijer VE, Gura KM, Le HD, et al. Fish-oil based lipid emulsions prevent and reverse parenteral nutrition-associated liver disease: the Boston experience. JPEN J Parenter Enteral Nutr 2009;33:541-7.

39. de Meijer VE, Gura KM, Meisel JA, et al. Parenteral fish oil monotherapy in the management of patients with parenteral nutrition-associated liver disease. Arch Surg 2010;145:547-51.

40. Omegaven [product information]. Graz, Austria: Fresenius Kabi, 2018.

41. Kerner JA Jr, Poole RL. The use of IV fat in neonates. Nutr Clin Pract 2006;21:374-80.

42. Barness LA, Dallman PR, Anderson H, et al. Use of IV fat emulsions in pediatric patients. Pediatrics 1981;68:738-43.

43. de Meijer VE, Le HD, Meisel JA, et al. Parenteral fish oil as monotherapy prevents essential fatty acid deficiency in parenteral nutrition-dependent patients. J Pediatr Gastroenterol Nutr 2010;50:212-8.

44. Anez-Bustillos L, Dao DT, Fell GL, et al. Redefining essential fatty acids in the era of novel intravenous lipid emulsions. Clin Nutr 2018;37:784-9.

45. Intralipid [product information]. Uppsala, Sweden: Fresenius Kabi, 2007.

46. Shulman RJ, Phillips S. Parenteral nutrition in infants and children. J Pediatr Gastroenterol Nutr 2003;36:587-607.

47. Cober, MP. Repackaging of intravenous fat emulsions: a clinical conundrum. Nutr Clin Pract 2016;31:642-6.

48. Zeigler EE, O'Donnell AM, Nelson SE, et al. Body composition of the reference fetus. Growth 1976;40:329-41.

49. Shaw JCL. Parenteral nutrition in the management of sick low birth weight infants. Pediatr Clin North Am 1973;20:333-58.

50. Widdowson EM, Dickerson JWT. Chemical composition of the body. In: Comar CL, Bronner F, eds. Mineral Metabolism: An Advanced Treatise. IIA. New York: Academic Press, 1964: 1-214.

51. Kelly HJ, Sloan RE, Hoffman W, et al. Accumulation of nitrogen and six minerals in the human fetus during gestation. Hum Biol 1951;23:61-74.

52. Pelegano JF, Rowe JC, Carey DE, et al. Simultaneous infusion of calcium and phosphorus in parenteral nutrition for premature infants: use of physiologic calcium/phosphorus ratio. J Pediatr 1989;114:115-9.

53. Pelegano JF, Rowe JC, Carey DE, et al. Effect of calcium/phosphorus ratio on mineral retention in parenterally fed premature infants. J Pediatr Gastroenterol Nutr 1991;12:351-5.

54. Koo WWK. Parenteral nutrition-related bone disease. JPEN J Parenter Enteral Nutr 1992;16:386-94.

55. Greene HL, Hambidge M, Schanler R, et al. Guidelines for the use of vitamins, trace elements, calcium, magnesium, and phosphorus in infants and children receiving total parenteral nutrition: report of the Subcommittee on Pediatric Parenteral Nutrient Requirements from the Committee on Clinical Practice Issues of the American Society for Clinical Nutrition. Am J Clin Nutr 1988;48:1324-42.

56. Zimmermann MB, Crill CM. Iodine in enteral and parenteral nutrition. Best Pract Res Clin Endocrinol Metab 2010;24:143-58.

57. Crill CM, Helms RA. The use of carnitine in pediatric nutrition. Nutr Clin Pract 2007;22:204-13.

58. Puzovic M, Hardy G. Stability and compatibility of histamine H2-receptor antagonists in parenteral nutrition mixtures. Curr Opin Clin Nutr Metab Care 2007;10:311-7.

59. Romaine A, Ye D, Fang F, et al. Safety of histamine-2 receptor blockers in hospitalized VLBW infants. Early Hum Dev 2016; 99:27-30.

60. Guillet R, Stoll BJ, Cotton CM, et al. Association of H2-blocker therapy and higher incidence of necrotizing enterocolitis in very low birth weight infants. Pediatrics 2006;117:e137-42.

61. Trissel LA, Gilbert DL, Martinez JF, et al. Compatibility of medications with 3-in-1 parenteral nutrition admixtures. JPEN J Parenter Enteral Nutr 1999;23:67-74.

62. Kelly DA. Preventing parenteral nutrition liver disease. Early Hum Dev 2010;86:683-7.

63. Klein GL. Metabolic bone disease of total parenteral nutrition. Nutrition 1998;14:149-52.

64. Wisplinghoff H, Bischoff T, Tallent SM, et al. Nosocomial bloodstream infections in US hospitals: analysis of 24,179 cases from a prospective nationwide surveillance study. Clin Infect Dis 2004;39:309-17.

65. Kim EY, Saunders P, Yousefzadeh N. Usefulness of anti-infective lock solutions for catheter-related bloodstream infections. Mt Sinai J Med 2010;77:549-58.

66. Ayers P, Adams S, Boullata J, et al. A.S.P.E.N. parenteral nutrition safety consensus recommendations: translation into practice. Nutr Clin Pract 2014;29:277-82.

CHAPTER 21

Pediatric Obesity

Sandra Benavides, Pharm.D., FCCP, FPPA

LEARNING OBJECTIVES

1. Describe the pathophysiology of pediatric obesity.

2. Identify risk factors associated with pediatric obesity.

3. Explain the diagnosis and classification of overweight and obesity in pediatric patients.

4. Discuss treatment goals and strategies for the management of obesity in pediatric patients.

5. List the benefits and limitations of current pharmacologic therapy for the treatment of obesity in pediatric patients.

ABBREVIATIONS IN THIS CHAPTER

AgRP	Agouti-related peptide
BMI	Body mass index
CDC	Centers for Disease Control and Prevention
GLP-1	Glucagon-like peptide 1
NP-Y	Neuropeptide Y
LAGB	Laparoscopic adjustable gastric band
POMC	Pro-opiomelanocortin
RYGB	Roux-en-Y gastric bypass

INTRODUCTION

Pediatric obesity has reached epidemic proportions in the United States. Worldwide the rates of overweight and obesity have increased in children and adolescents, with the highest self-reported rates in the United States.[1] The consequences of pediatric overweight and obesity are leading to increases in chronic health conditions that previously had only occurred in adults. Obesity can lead to many negative health outcomes in children and adolescents and substantially increases the risk of morbidity and mortality in adulthood.

The prevalence of *obesity* (defined as a body mass index [BMI] greater than or equal to 95th percentile for sex and age) in the pediatric population has been increasing since the 1970s, as illustrated in Figure 1.[2] The most dramatic increase was between the 1980s and 2000s, however, when obesity rates tripled in the pediatric population. The most recent estimates of obesity prevalence in youth in the United States is 18.5%, with rates in children age 6–11 years at 18.4% and adolescents slightly more than 20%, as depicted in Figure 2.[3] Although these rates are high, they appear to be remaining stable.[4] Rates for specific sex, racial, and ethnic groups vary as

depicted in Figure 3.[3] The graph illustrates the disproportionate rates of obesity in populations that are underrepresented, such as African American and Hispanic children.

The prevalence of *overweight* in children and adolescents, defined as a BMI greater than or equal to 85th percentile for sex and age, has also increased since the 1970s. More than 15% of children and adolescents between age 2 and 19 years are considered overweight.[5]

PHYSIOLOGIC CONTROL OF WEIGHT

Body weight is determined by many factors including physiologic regulation of appetite and energy expenditure, genetics, and environmental factors, such as diet and physical activity.[6,7] Physiologically, body weight is controlled by the regulation of hunger and satiety and the modulation of energy expenditure and energy storage in adipose tissue. These processes are regulated through the central nervous system (hypothalamus and brain stem) by communication from the gastrointestinal tract, autonomic nervous system, and hormones.[8]

Hunger and appetite control is centrally regulated in the *arcuate nucleus* located in the hypothalamus. The arcuate nucleus contains two sets of neurons that integrate hormonal and nutrient signals from the peripheral circulation and the central and peripheral neurons to control food intake and energy expenditure in the body.[9,10] The pro-opiomelanocortin (POMC)-expressing neurons are *anorexigenic* (appetite-suppressing). In the presence of nutrient ingestion, POMC is cleaved to α-melanocyte-stimulating hormone, which decreases food intake and increases energy expenditure.[9] Another set of neurons are *orexigenic* (appetite-stimulating), and consist of the neuropeptide Y (NP-Y) and agouti-related peptide (AgRP). In response to fasting, the NP-Y neurons stimulate food intake and decreased energy expenditure, whereas the AgRP antagonizes the effects of α-melanocyte-stimulating hormone. In addition, NP-Y/AgRP neurons inhibit POMC

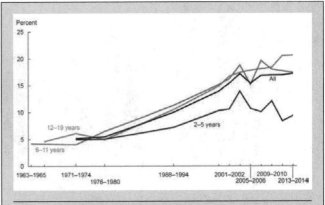

Figure 1. Rising prevalence of obesity in children and adolescents in the United States between 1963 and 2008.[2]

through inhibitory γ-aminobutyric acid, promoting an increase in food intake.[9] The effects of these neuropeptides result from binding to the melanocortin-4 receptor located in the hypothalamic paraventricular nucleus.[10] *Leptin*, a hormone produced by adipose tissue, causes a decrease in food intake and increased energy expenditure by stimulation of the POMC neurons or inhibition of the NP-Y/AgRP neurons. Contrary to leptin, *ghrelin*, a hormone produced in the stomach, increases food intake and decreases energy expenditure through inhibition of POMC and stimulation of NP-Y/AgRP neurons.[11-13]

The brain stem also plays a key role in appetite regulation through its role in detection and response to hunger and satiety signals.[14] The *afferent pathway*, which communicates the energy reserves in the body, consists of neural and hormonal signals that promote the suppression of appetite.[14] The neural signals are received from the vagus nerve that innervates the gastrointestinal tract and transmits mechanical and chemical signals to the nucleus tractus solitarius in the brain stem.[15] In addition to these signals, the vagal afferent neurons express receptors for various hormones involved in the regulation of appetite, such as cholecystokinin, peptide YY, pancreatic peptide, and glucagon-like peptide 1 (GLP-1).[7,26-19] Table 1 describes the various hormones involved in appetite and energy homeostasis.

The hypothalamus works in a negative feedback mechanism to regulate energy stores in the body. After integration of the signals from the afferent pathway and various hormones stimulated by food intake, the hypothalamus produces signals to the sympathetic nervous system and the efferent vagus.[15,20-22] The sympathetic nervous system modulates energy expenditure by increasing lipolysis and promoting the use of energy by cardiac and skeletal muscle. Conversely, to decrease energy expenditure, the hypothalamus activates the efferent vagus. The mechanisms of decreased energy expenditure by the efferent vagus include increasing postprandial insulin secretion resulting in increased fat deposition; increasing insulin sensitivity, leading to increased glucose and free fatty acid into adipose tissue; increasing nutrient absorption through increased gastrointestinal peristalsis and pyloric opening; and decreasing myocardial oxygen use by decreased heart rate.[15,20] Figure 4 illustrates the central and peripheral control of appetite and energy expenditure.

Obesity results from a mismatch between energy consumed and energy expended. Although a genetic component may be causative in some people, the present epidemic of obesity is thought to be secondary to environmental factors, including increased consumption of high-caloric, energy-dense foods; decreased physical activity; and increased screen time.

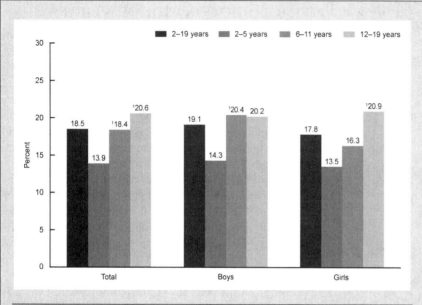

Figure 2. Prevalence of overweight and obesity in children and adolescents for 2015–2016.[3]

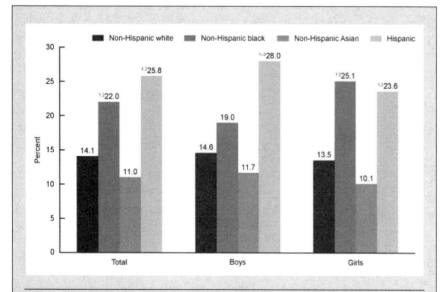

Figure 3. Prevalence of obesity among children and adolescents by sex, age group, and race/ethnicity in the United States for 2007–2008.[2]

GENETICS

Studies for the genetic causes of obesity are ongoing. To date, there is evidence that genetics contribute to obesity; however, the overall contribution to obesity is less than 10%.[23] In twin studies, monozygotic twins share 70%–90% heritability and dizygotic twins 35%–45%.[24] Adoption studies have concluded that children will more closely resemble biological parents rather than adoptive parents with regard to obesity. Also, certain racial groups are more predisposed to obesity (e.g., Pima Indian populations), which may indicate that obesity-causing alleles are present in some populations.[25] To date, genetic causes of obesity

Table 1. Hormones Involved in the Appetite and Energy Expenditure Regulation[12-19,21,22]

Hormone	Location Produced	Cause of Release	Effect
Neuropeptides			
Melanin-concentrating hormone	Expressed in lateral hypothalamus	Behavioral responses to food (e.g., anxiety)	Stimulates appetite
Orexins A and B	Expressed in the lateral hypothalamus	Stimulated by ghrelin	Stimulates NP-Y release, inducing food intake; increases CRF and SNS activity to increase energy expenditure; activates thermogenesis; required for development, differentiation and function of brown adipocytes
Adipokines			
Leptin	White adipose tissue (subcutaneous > visceral)	Stimulated by insulin	Increases expression of POMC; stimulates CRH; stimulates CART; inhibits release of NP-Y/AgRP; catabolic effects
Visfatin	Visceral adipose tissue (visceral > subcutaneous)	Unknown but release regulated by cytokines and hormones that influence glucose homeostasis	Stimulates adipose and muscle glucose transport; decreases hepatic glucose production
Adiponectin	Adipose tissue	Stimulated production by PPAR-γ Inhibited by catecholamines and TNFα	Increases sensitivity to insulin; decreases hepatic glucose production; stimulates fatty acid oxidation
Resistin	Adipose tissue	Unknown	Reduces insulin-stimulated glucose uptake by adipocytes and potentially skeletal muscle
Intestinal Peptides			
Ghrelin	Primarily from gastric endocrine cells, with small amounts in small intestine and hypothalamus	Believed to be released through activation of SNS and through increased efferent vagal tone	Stimulates food intake through activation of the NP-Y/AgRP neurons in the arcuate nucleus
Glucagon-like peptide 1	Primarily from intestine; also expressed in neurons of the NTS	Released by ingestion of carbohydrates, fats, and protein released in response to nutrients, other gastrointestinal hormones (e.g., gastric-inhibitory peptide, gastrin-releasing peptide)	Acts as a satiety signal to reduce food intake; stimulates lipolysis and adiponectin expression; increases energy expenditure; inhibits gastric emptying
Peptide YY	Small intestine and colon	Secreted in postprandial period after exposure to nutrients	Prompts end of a meal; inhibits NPY/AgRP; stimulates POMC/CART; inhibits gastric emptying; decreases gastric acid and pancreatic exocrine secretion
Cholecystokinin	Upper small intestine; enteric nervous system (myenteric and submucosal plexus)	Released in response to food, specifically lipids and proteins	Induces satiety by vagal efferent pathways and activation of cells in the NTS
Pancreatic Hormones			
Insulin	Pancreatic beta cells	Released in response to food, specifically glucose	Peripherally promotes glycogenesis, muscle protein synthesis, fat storage; centrally binds to VMH neurons to regulate food intake by inducing satiety
Amylin	Pancreatic beta cells	Co-released with insulin in response to food, specifically glucose	Reduces food intake; inhibits glucagon secretion; delays gastric emptying; induces satiety
Glucagon	Pancreatic alpha cells	Released in response to low blood glucose or when the body requires additional glucose (e.g., stress, exercise)	Stimulates glucose production; increases lipolysis, fatty acid oxidation, and ketogenesis; increases satiety; increases energy expenditure

AgRP = agouti-related peptide; CART = cocaine- and amphetamine-related transcript; CRF = corticotropin-releasing factor; CRH = corticotropin-releasing hormone; NP-Y = neuropeptide Y; NTS = nucleus tractus solitarius; POMC = pro-opiomelanocortin; PPAR-γ = Peroxisome proliferator-activated receptor gamma; SNS = sympathetic nervous system; TNFα = tumor necrosis factor alpha; VMH = ventromedial nucleus.

are divided into three groups, nonsyndromic monogenic, syndromic monogenic, and polygenic forms.[25]

Both autosomal dominant and recessive mutations have been identified in nonsyndromic monogenic genetic causes. To date, around 200 single point mutations on about 10 genes have been associated with obesity.[25] These mutations are rare and typically result in severe obesity in early childhood. All the mutations have been identified in proteins involved in the hypothalamic signaling pathway that regulates food intake and energy expenditure. Genes that have been identified include those that encode for leptin, the leptin receptor, POMC, proprotein convertase 1, melanocortin-4 receptor, brain-derived neurotrophic factor, neurotrophic tyrosine kinase receptor type 2, and single-minded homolog I.[25]

More than 70 genetic syndromes associated with obesity have been identified.[26] Syndromic monogenic causes of obesity follow Mendelian patterns of inheritance and are associated with distinct clinical presentations such as cognitive impairment, dysmorphic features or organ-specific developmental abnormalities. Common syndromes in pediatrics include Wilms tumor–aniridia–genital anomalies–retardation; Prader–Willi; Bardet–Biedl; Albright hereditary osteodystrophy; Beckwith–Wiedemann; Carpenter; Alstrom; and Cohen syndromes.[27] Children younger than 5 years presenting with extreme obesity, those with features of a genetic obesity syndrome or with a family history of extreme obesity should undergo a full genetic evaluation.[23]

Obesity is polygenic, indicating that several alleles are responsible for the disease phenotype. Genome-wide association studies of obesity have identified more than 80 genetic loci.[24] Each allele has a small effect on obesity and such effects can be additive or nonadditive. Typically, the presence of a polymorphism in these alleles can increase susceptibility to obesity in an obesogenic environment.[25]

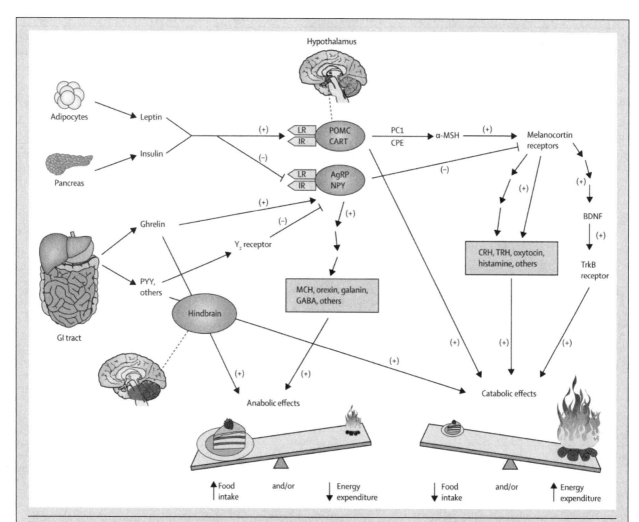

Figure 4. Appetite and energy expenditure regulation.[66]

Peripheral and central factors modulate appetite centers in the brain. Gastrointestinal and fat-derived hormones stimulate specific areas of the hypothalamus and brain stem that sense nutrients and coordinate the response to hunger and the intake of food. The arcuate nucleus in the hypothalamus receives input from brain stem (e.g., vagal) nuclei as well as from direct stimulation by circulating hormones through an incomplete blood-brain barrier. Neurons in the arcuate nucleus are either *orexigenic*—containing neuropeptide Y by way of Y₁ receptors or agouti-related peptide (AgRP)—or *anorexigenic*—containing pro-opiomelanocortin (POMC), cocaine- and amphetamine-related transcript (CART). The anorexigenic neurons containing POMC are a precursor of α-melanocyte stimulating hormone (α-MSH). Ultimately, other regions of the hypothalamus (the paraventricular nucleus and lateral hypothalamus) and higher centers (such as amygdala, limbic system and cerebral cortex) are stimulated to change feeding behavior by influencing the functions of the same hypothalamic nuclei. Reprinted from Han JC, Lawlor DA, Kimm SY. Childhood obesity. Lancet 2010;375:1737-48. With permission from Elsevier.

MEDICAL CONDITIONS AND MEDICATIONS

Obesity can also be a consequence of treatment of medical conditions (i.e., drug induced).[28-35] Children with hypothyroidism, growth hormone deficiency, Cushing syndrome, or a history of trauma to the hypothalamus may present as overweight or obese.[36-38] Medications known to increase weight are listed in Table 2. If weight gain is identified in children or adolescents taking these medications, alternative drug therapy should be considered.

RISK FACTORS

Pediatric obesity has been associated with several risk factors such as intrauterine exposure to gestational diabetes, diet, decreased energy expenditure, increased screen time (e.g., television, video games, smart phones), race/ethnicity, socioeconomic status, and rural residence. Critical times for the development of persistent obesity include prenatal/neonatal and early infancy, the period of adiposity rebound during the early childhood years, and adolescence.

PREGNANCY-RELATED FACTORS

Factors that affect obesity in childhood and adolescence during the prenatal period include maternal pre-pregnancy BMI, gestational weight gain, maternal smoking while pregnant, and gestational diabetes. Infants born to mothers who are obese before pregnancy tend to be large for gestational age, have increased adipose tissue at birth, and be at increased risk of obesity in childhood and adolescence.[39] Equally as important as the mother's BMI before conception is the amount of weight gain during the pregnancy. Studies have reported that excessive weight gain during pregnancy is associated with obesity in children at age 3 years, 7 years, and in adolescence.[40-42] Infants born to mothers with gestational diabetes are typically larger babies, have increased adipose tissue at birth, and have an increased risk of obesity and type 2 diabetes mellitus in adolescence.[43]

Neonates born small for gestational age are also at risk of subsequent obesity. The prenatal period is considered critical in "programming" the metabolic, nutritional, and developmental status for the future of the fetus. This programming

Table 2. Medications Associated with Weight Gain[28-38]

Class	Examples	Mechanism of Weight Gain
Anticonvulsants	Valproic acid, gabapentin, carbamazepine	Controversial, because of potentially decreased oxidation of free fatty acids and gluconeogenesis secondary to carnitine deficiency, resulting in hypoglycemia and activation of hypothalamus to increase feeding; GABA-mediated inhibition in hypothalamus; increase in serum leptin
Antihistamines	Diphenhydramine, cyproheptadine	Antagonist at histamine-1 receptor, which may decrease the effect of leptin; loss of circadian rhythm; increase in fat deposition with a high-fat diet; elevated blood insulin
Antihypertensive agents	Clonidine, propranolol	Decrease in resting energy expenditure; reduced thermic effect of food; decreased exercise tolerance; increased fatigue; decreased nonexercised thermogenesis; inhibition of lipolysis; increased insulin resistance (β-blockers) Increased food intake caused by activation of alpha-2 adrenergic receptors in the paraventricular hypothalamus, which stimulates feeding (clonidine)
Atypical antipsychotics	Olanzapine, risperidone	Antagonist at the histamine-1 receptor, which may decrease the effect of leptin; loss of circadian rhythm; increase in fat deposition with a high-fat diet; elevated blood insulin Antagonism of the serotonin (5-HTc2) receptor, which directly affects NP-Y neurons in the ARC
Glucocorticoids	Prednisolone, prednisone	Activates AMPK, which results in increased appetite and increased deposition of lipids in visceral adipose and hepatic tissue
Hormonal contraceptives	Depot medroxyprogesterone	Estrogen increases the excitatory neurons in POMC in the ARC; estrogen also sensitizes leptin signaling.
Insulin	Regular insulin, insulin aspart, glargine	Inhibits NP-Y/AgRP neurons in the ARC
Insulin secretagogues	Glyburide, glipizide	Inhibits NP-Y/AgRP neurons in the ARC
Mood stabilizers	Lithium	Regulation of the leptin receptor expression
Tricyclic antidepressants	Amitriptyline, imipramine, nortriptyline	Increased plasma leptin concentrations through antagonism at the histaminic receptor

AgRP = agouti-related peptide; AMPK = AMP-activated protein kinase; ARC = arcuate nucleus; GABA = gamma-aminobutyric acid; NP-Y = neuropeptide Y; POMC = pro-opiomelanocortin.

is based on the *thrifty phenotype hypothesis* in which the body learns to store excess fat and decrease energy expenditure when there is a perceived deficiency. Although these infants are born small for gestational age, they often have rapid growth in early infancy. These infants appear to have an increased disposition for obesity, insulin resistance, and cardiovascular disease later in life.[45,46] Malnutrition and maternal smoking during pregnancy have been related to small-for-gestational-age births.

Another potential risk factor for obesity may be the method of delivery at birth. Studies and meta-analysis have found an increased risk of obesity in children delivered by cesarean section, even while controlling for cofounders.[47-49] The biological mechanism for the increase in obesity secondary to a cesarean delivery is proposed to be different intestinal microbiomes in these infants resulting from the exposure to different bacteria and subsequent colonization of the gastrointestinal tract. Two bacteria species, *Bacteroidetes* and *Firmicutes*, have been associated with an increased extraction of nutrients from ingested calories (energy harvest) in animals.[50] The use of antibiotics and the resultant alterations in the microbiome are also theorized to be a risk factor for increased pediatric obesity.[51] Research is ongoing in this area.

INFANCY AND EARLY CHILDHOOD

Breastfeeding is believed to have protective effects against childhood obesity. Infants who are breastfed for at least 1–3 months have a decreased risk of being obese.[52] However, many of the studies that report the benefits of breastfeeding to prevent obesity are observational, and when confounding factors such as socioeconomic status and maternal BMI are considered, the benefits of breastfeeding are minimal.[53,54]

In infants, the BMI increases in the first year of life and peaks at around 1 year of age. After this peak, BMI slowly declines before it begins to increase again, as depicted in the Centers for Disease Control and Prevention (CDC) BMI growth charts in Figure 5.[55] The point at which the BMI begins to increase again is called the *adiposity rebound*. On average, adiposity rebound occurs in children between ages 5 and 7 years. However, if adiposity rebound occurs earlier, such as at ages 2–3 years instead, then the child is at an increased risk of obesity.[56] Dietary factors known to increase the risk of obesity such as the overconsumption of high-calorie, energy-dense foods and sweetened beverages (e.g., soda and fruit juices) may cause an early adiposity rebound.[57] The overconsumption of these foods, coupled with large portion sizes at any age, also contributes to obesity in pediatrics.

PHYSICAL ACTIVITY

Factors that have been associated with increased obesity in pediatric patients are decreases in physical activity and increases in screen time. Studies have proved a relationship between obesity in children and television watching and video game playing.[58] Based on these data, the American Academy

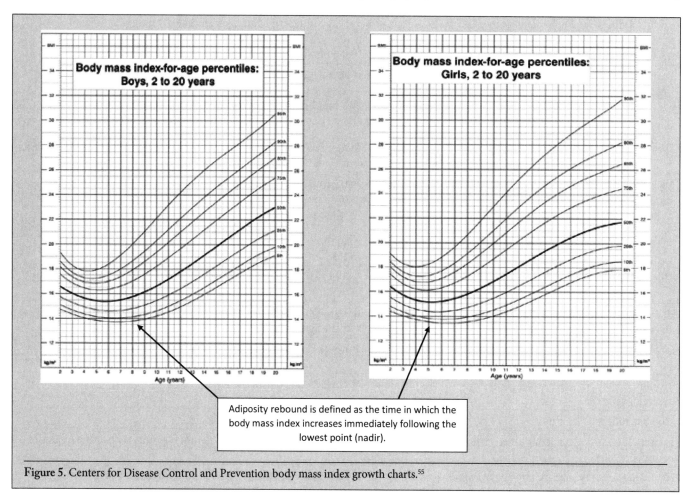

Figure 5. Centers for Disease Control and Prevention body mass index growth charts.[55]

of Pediatrics recommends limiting screen time (e.g., television, computers, mobile devices) to no more than 2 hours/day.[59] The time spent on viewing/gaming, on social media or texting may also replace the time spent on physical activity, which can further increase the risk of becoming obese. Children with sleeping problems—reported as having difficulty falling asleep and awaking several times a night between 6 months and 5 years of age—are also at an increased risk of obesity in early adulthood.[60]

SOCIOECONOMIC STATUS

The National Health and Nutrition Examination Survey examines the relationship between household income and the education level of the head of the household. Between 2011–2014, obesity rates were lowest in the highest income

Table 3. Weight Classifications in Children and Adolescents Age 2–18 Years[64,65]

Weight Category	Criteria
Overweight	BMI-for-age between 85th–95th percentile
Obese	BMI-for-age > 95th percentile
Severely obese	BMI-for-age > 99th percentile or ≥ 120% of 95th percentile BMI-for age or BMI ≥ 35 kg/m²

BMI = body mass index.

Table 4. Cutoff Points for 99th Percentile Body Mass Index for Age and Sex for Children and Adolescents Older Than 5 Years

Age (years)	99th Percentile Body Mass Index Cutoff Point (kg/m²)	
	Male	**Female**
5	20.1	21.5
6	21.6	23.0
7	23.6	24.6
8	25.6	26.4
9	27.6	28.2
10	29.3	29.9
11	30.7	31.5
12	31.8	33.1
13	32.6	34.6
14	33.2	36.0
15	33.6	37.5
16	33.9	39.1
17	34.4	40.8

Reproduced with permission from: Barlow SE. Expert committee recommendations regarding the prevention, assessment, and treatment of child and adolescent overweight and obesity: summary report. Pediatrics 2007;120:S164–92. Copyright 2018 by American Academy of Pediatrics.

group (more than 350% of the federal poverty level) and highest education level (college graduate).[61] In terms of household income, female children between the ages of 2-19 in households of non-Hispanic white adults had a lower prevalence of obesity for the highest income level whereas no other race/ethnicity had differences between income levels. In male children, the prevalence of obesity was lower for Asian non-white and Hispanic non-white heads of household at the highest income level. In terms of level of education for the head of the household, the prevalence of obesity in children decreased with increasing levels of education. Both female and male children of white non-Hispanic and Hispanic races had a lower prevalence of obesity in which the head of the household had a college degree. Although urban residence is attributed to increased obesity rates worldwide, children and adolescents living in rural areas of the United States have the same rates of obesity compared with those living in urban areas.[62] However, the rates of *severe obesity,* defined as a BMI greater than or equal to 120% of the 95th percentile for age and sex, were higher in nonmetropolitan statistical areas (population less than 50,000).

DIAGNOSIS

The identification of obesity is determined on the basis of an increased amount of adipose tissue that can result in adverse health outcomes (e.g., cardiovascular disease). Although excess adipose tissue has been correlated with health risks, specifically cardiovascular disease, the exact amount of obesity necessary to cause disease has not been described.[63] In addition, there is no easy method to quantify the amount of excess adipose tissue in a pediatric patient. For that reason, weight, adjusted for height, is used as a measure of body fat. The accepted and recommended tool to assess body fat is the BMI, which is defined as *weight (in kilograms) divided by the square of height (in meters): BMI = kg/m².* In adults, specific absolute BMI values have been determined to define obesity. In pediatric patients, however, the BMI distribution changes with age, and an absolute BMI would not be appropriate to classify children as obese. For that reason, specific percentile cutoff points, as illustrated in Table 3, have been established to define obesity in children and adolescents. Because of the increase in children and adolescents who are extremely overweight, the "severe obesity" category has been established and defined as a cutoff point greater than the 99th percentile. However, the standard CDC growth charts do not designate the 99th percentile. Table 4 defines the specific cutoff points for the 99th percentile for specific ages and sex for children older than 5 years because data for children younger than 5 years are not available. The American Heart Association (AHA) has recommended an alternate definition for severe obesity, which is a BMI greater than or equal to 120% of the 95th percentile or an absolute BMI equal to or greater than 35 kg/m².[64]

The term *overweight* defines a child or adolescent who has a higher weight for height and sex, but the weight may be not be caused by excess adipose tissue. These children must be further evaluated for risk factors for future obesity. Of note, BMI percentiles are not available and are therefore not included in the CDC growth charts for children younger than 2 years.

In this age group, infants and toddlers weight-for-length on the World Health Organization normative charts are monitored.[59]

All children and adolescents identified as either overweight or obese should be further evaluated for medical and behavioral risks of obesity and subsequent disease. Assessments should include the following: the child's history and physical examination; the child's growth history based on a CDC growth chart; the child's family history (including parental obesity); and the child's activity level, dietary habits, and sedentary time.[65] A complete history will aid in identifying modifiable lifestyle factors. Although no specific laboratory analyses are required for diagnosing obesity, a lipid panel, fasting glucose concentration (or fasting insulin level), and baseline alanine aminotransferase and aspartate aminotransferase should be obtained to assess whether complications of obesity are present.[66] Underlying endocrine and genetic defects or syndromes must be considered when giving a child or adolescent a diagnosis of obesity.

Alternative methods of quantifying adiposity in pediatrics have been described. Direct measurement of adipose tissue using dual-energy x-ray absorptiometry, densitometry, air displacement plethysmography, or bioelectrical impedance can provide a more accurate measure of adipose tissue, but these measurements are not practical in the clinical setting. Other indirect measures of adiposity include waist circumference or skinfold measurement. Waist circumference references are available for children; however, the use of waist circumference does not increase the identification of obesity in children and adolescents versus using BMI.[67] Although the use of skinfold thickness helps identify obesity, the additional benefits are minimal compared with using BMI, and the measurements are more cumbersome to perform.[68]

Childhood obesity has been related to increased morbidity and early mortality in adulthood.[69-72] In obesity, almost all body systems are affected. Table 5 lists complications associated with obesity. During the initial evaluation of an obese pediatric patient, it is important to determine the presence of any comorbidity for early intervention and treatment when necessary.

Preventive strategies in childhood obesity begin in the prenatal period. Pregnant women should be advised to obtain adequate prenatal care, ensure proper nutrition, and stop smoking to minimize the risk of intrauterine growth restriction. In addition, although the data are limited, it is recommended to breastfeed infants for at least 6 months to potentially decrease the risk of obesity. The American Academy of Pediatrics has several obesity-preventive strategies with respect to healthy eating and physical activity.[65] These strategies are listed in Box 1. The American Heart

Table 5. Complications of Obesity in Children and Adolescents[65,66,69-71]

Body System	Complication
Cardiovascular	Atherosclerosis Dyslipidemia Hypertension Left ventricular hypertrophy
Central nervous system	Pseudotumor cerebri
Dermatologic	Acanthosis nigricans Intertrigo Furunculosis Hidradenitis suppurativa Stretch marks
Endocrine	Hyperandrogenism Insulin resistance Polycystic ovary syndrome Pubertal advancement Type 2 diabetes mellitus
Gastrointestinal	Gallbladder disease Gastroesophageal reflux disease Nonalcoholic fatty liver disease
Mental health	Anxiety Decreased quality of life Depression Eating disorders Low self-esteem Social isolation
Orthopedic	Osteoarthritis Slipped capital femoral epiphysis
Pulmonary	Asthma Exercise intolerance Obstructive sleep apnea
Renal	Proteinuria Focal segmental glomerulosclerosis

Box 1. American Academy of Pediatrics Obesity-Preventive Strategies[65]

1. Eat a well-balanced diet regarding fat, carbohydrates, and protein as recommended by the U.S. Department of Agriculture (USDA).
2. Consume the USDA-recommended numbers of fruit and vegetables for each specific age group.
3. Eat a diet rich in calcium.
4. Eat a high-fiber diet.
5. Eat breakfast every day.
6. Limit the amount of sugar-sweetened drinks including sodas, sports drinks, and sweetened fruit juice.
7. Limit the consumption of energy-dense foods.
8. Limit the number of times a family eats at restaurants, especially fast food restaurants.
9. Eat meals together as a family at the dinner table.
10. Pay particular attention to nutrition labels regarding portion sizes in an effort to avoid large portion sizes.
11. Limit television viewing to less than 2 hours/day for children older than age 2 years. Children younger than 2 years should not view any television.
12. Ensure physical activity for at least 1 hour/day.
13. Involve the entire family in healthy lifestyle modifications.

Association also recommends increasing fruits and vegetables to decrease the consumption of energy-dense foods (e.g., fast food, snacks) and limiting high-calorie beverages, refined carbohydrates, excess dietary fat, and large portion sizes.[73] In children younger than 2 years, it is important to provide healthy meals and snacks and to limit sugar-sweetened beverages and energy-dense foods.[65] To date, no medications and/or supplements have been studied or approved for use in healthy-weight children and adolescents for the prevention of obesity.

The treatment goal in obesity is to develop a healthy lifestyle and improve future health status.[65] A study found that children and adolescents who are obese but lose the weight before the onset of adulthood have the same risk of type 2 diabetes mellitus, hypertension, hyperlipidemia, and atherosclerosis as children and adolescents who have never been obese.[74] Such findings underscore the importance of a healthy weight in the pediatric population. However, in pediatric patients, attaining this goal may not always encompass weight loss, but rather maintenance of growth velocity or current weight. In addition, because the stigma of being obese in children can cause poor self-esteem and lead to eating disorders, caution is warranted in the development of treatment plans.

The American Academy of Pediatrics has detailed interventions and goals for treating obesity in children and adolescents based on age and the BMI category (Table 6).

THERAPY GOALS

Specific weight goals for the treatment of obesity differ on the basis of age, initial BMI category, and presence of health risks at diagnosis, as indicated in Table 6. Because children are growing and developing, weight loss is not always a target of therapy. Goals may include *weight velocity maintenance* (weight gain at a stable rate); *weight maintenance*; *slow weight gain*; *gradual weight loss* (defined as a loss of no more than 0.45 kg/month); or *weight loss* (defined as a loss of no more than 0.9 kg/week). Children and adolescents who present with risks of comorbid conditions or those with a BMI above the 99th percentile have more aggressive goals. Health risks include increases in blood pressure, evidence of insulin resistance, abnormal lipid panel, and strong family history of obesity, type 2 diabetes mellitus, or cardiovascular disease. In children younger than 2 years, there is no specific weight goal regardless of the weight-for-height percentile.[65]

Table 6. Interventions for Weight Loss and Weight Goals Based on Age and Body Mass Index Categories[a]

Age, years	BMI Category	Weight Goal	Initial Intervention[b]	Highest Intervention
< 2	Weight-for-height ≥ 95th percentile	N/A	Prevention counseling	Prevention counseling
2–5	85th–94th percentile with no health risks	Weight velocity maintenance	Prevention counseling	Prevention counseling
	85th–94th percentile with health risks	Weight maintenance OR slow weight gain	Stage 1	Stage 2
	≥ 95th percentile	Weight maintenance OR Gradual weight loss (if BMI > 21 kg/m²)	Stage 1	Stage 3
6–11	85th–94th percentile with no health risks	Weight velocity maintenance	Prevention counseling	Prevention counseling
	85th–94th percentile with health risks	Weight maintenance	Stage 1	Stage 2
	95th–99th percentile	Gradual weight loss	Stage 1	Stage 3
	> 99th percentile	Weight loss	Stage 1 (2 or 3 if family motivated)	Stage 4
12–18	85th–94th percentile with no health risks	Weight velocity maintenance; after linear growth is complete weight maintenance	Prevention counseling	Prevention counseling
	85th–94th percentile with health risks	Weight maintenance OR Gradual weight loss	Stage 1	Stage 2
	95th–99th percentile	Weight loss	Stage 1	Stage 4
	> 99th percentile	Weight loss	Stage 1 (2 or 3 if patient and family motivated)	Stage 4

[a]Specific health risks include increased blood pressure, evidence of insulin resistance, dyslipidemia or strong family history of obesity, type 2 diabetes mellitus, or cardiovascular disease.
[b]Stage 1 = Prevention Plus; Stage 2 = Structured Weight Management; Stage 3 = Comprehensive Multidisciplinary Intervention; Stage 4 = Tertiary Care Intervention.
BMI = body mass index; N/A = not applicable.
Reproduced with permission from Barlow SE. Expert committee recommendations regarding the prevention, assessment, and treatment of child and adolescent overweight and obesity: summary report. Pediatrics 2007;120:S164–92. Copyright 2018 by American Academy of Pediatrics.

TREATMENT STAGES

The American Academy of Pediatrics has developed five stages of intervention for the treatment of obesity in children, beginning with prevention counseling and subsequent treatment Stages 1–4.[65] Prevention counseling includes the preventive strategies listed in Box 1. Stage 1 is also known as the *prevention plus* stage. This stage incorporates the prevention counseling strategies with more frequent monitoring. In this treatment stage, it is recommended to allow the child to regulate his or her food intake and not to establish a diet or restriction of food. In implementing this stage, it is important to work with the entire family to determine goals that are reasonable for the family. For example, increasing physical activity to 1 hour/day may not be feasible, whereas starting at 15 minutes and slowly adding time may be more realistic. Also important to consider are the cultural values, financial status, work and school schedule, and motivation of the family. This stage of treatment lasts 3–6 months, and it is reevaluated if goals for the child are not being met.

Stage 2 treatment, *structured weight management*, incorporates many of the same healthy lifestyle strategies as Stage 1, but it differs by providing more structure. In this stage, a planned diet, including daily meals and snacks, and planned physical activity are included. The meals are planned in accordance with the U.S. Department of Agriculture Dietary Reference Intake recommendations, which limit eating and drinking (other than water) in between meal and snack time. Food intake and physical activity are monitored more closely with food recalls and logs of physical activity. The child or adolescent is monitored and reevaluated monthly in this stage of treatment and, if necessary, moves to a different treatment stage. Dietitians, physical therapists, exercise therapists, or clinicians with additional training in these areas are typically involved in the care of these patients.

Stage 3 treatment, referred to as *comprehensive multidisciplinary intervention*, continues to follow the structure of Stage 2, but it becomes more intense in both goal setting and monitoring. Diet and physical activity are set for the child or adolescent with weight loss as a goal. In this stage, a multidisciplinary approach with input from a social worker, psychologist, dietitian, exercise specialist, and physician is recommended. For optimal results, patients are initially monitored weekly for 8–12 weeks and then monthly. Commercial programs (e.g., Weight Watchers) may be suitable at this treatment stage; however, the program should be reviewed to ensure healthy strategies are used.

The highest level of treatment, *tertiary care intervention* (Stage 4), involves more intense interventions such as medications, very low-calorie diets, and weight-loss surgery. This treatment stage is reserved for those who are severely obese, those whose previous stages of treatment have failed, and those who are motivated and committed to the treatment. In addition, this stage requires the child or adolescent to have the maturity to understand the risks associated with medication and surgery. The details of medication use and surgical options for treatment will be discussed later in the chapter.

Treatment recommendations differ for children younger than 2 years. It is important to assess parental status for risk of future obesity. An infant of two obese parents is at high risk of being obese later in life, even if the infant is less than the 95th percentile in weight-for-height. It is not recommended to restrict caloric intake in this age group regardless of weight-for-height. Instead, parents should be counseled on obesity-preventive strategies. Such strategies, as shown in Box 1, include breastfeeding the infant from birth to at least 1 year of age and avoidance of sugar-sweetened beverages and high-fat, energy-dense foods (e.g., chips, french fries). For children between 12 and 24 months, additional nutritional strategies include limiting the amount of milk consumed because more than 24 ounces/day may cause the child not to eat other healthy foods. At this age, it is important not to restrict food intake, but to provide the toddler with healthy meal and snack options. It is advised to provide three meals a day at a table with the family. Young children will typically eat two additional snacks per day.

PHARMACOTHERAPY

Several medications indicated for the treatment of obesity in the adult population have not been studied in the pediatric population, such as phentermine, phentermine/topiramate, lorcaserin, and naltrexone/bupropion. Of the approved medications for obesity in adults, orlistat is presently the only medication approved for the treatment of obesity in the pediatric population. Liraglutide, approved for obesity in adults, has been evaluated for safety in adolescents. Previously, sibutramin was approved for use in adolescents older than 16 years; however, it was removed from the U.S. market in 2010 because of the increased risk of nonfatal myocardial infarctions and strokes associated with its use.[75] The use of metformin has shown some positive results in decreasing weight; however, it is not currently approved or recommended for use in this population. Topiramate, exenatide, and liraglutide also have limited reports of use in the pediatric population. In a systematic review of pharmacotherapy for decrease in BMI, an overall weight loss of 1.3 kg/m^2 (95% confidence interval [CI], –1.9 to –0.8, p<0.00001) was found, with only 5% of all participants discontinuing therapy because of adverse drug reactions.[76] Currently no nonprescription medications or supplements are recommended for use in the pediatric population for the treatment of obesity.

ORLISTAT

Orlistat reversibly inhibits pancreatic lipases in the stomach and small intestine. The inhibition of the enzymes prevents the digestion of dietary fat (in the form of triglycerides) to absorbable free fatty acids and monoglycerides. As a result, orlistat inhibits around 30% of ingested dietary fat, leading to decreased caloric intake and weight loss. Orlistat is minimally absorbed as it exerts its action in the gastrointestinal tract. It is metabolized primarily in the gastrointestinal wall, with 97% excreted in the feces. The elimination half-life of the drug is between 1 and 2 hours.[77]

The efficacy of orlistat has been evaluated in pediatric patients age 10–18 years.[78-83] A meta-analysis showed a decrease in BMI of −0.79 kg/m² (95% CI, −1.08 to −0.51) with a decrease in weight of −0.79 kg (95% CI, −4.31 to −0.65) when used at 120 mg three times daily in combination with lifestyle modifications.[76] About 30% of patients in clinical trials lost more than 5% of body weight, and 15% lost more than 10% of body weight. One study evaluating the long-term efficacy of orlistat found that the BMI decreased by 0.55 kg/m² in the orlistat-treated group and increased by 0.31 kg/m² in the placebo group after 1 year.[79] However, although there was an overall decrease in BMI, participants in both treatment arms gained weight throughout the year. In addition, clinical trials had drop-out rates from 20% to 35% because of adverse drug reactions. The most commonly reported adverse drug effects included mild to moderate gastrointestinal upset in almost all the patients. These effects included nausea, fatty/oily stool, oily spotting, oily evacuation, fecal urgency, frequent stools, diarrhea, abdominal pain, fecal incontinence, and flatulence (with and without discharge). Serious adverse effects reported included systemic cholelithiasis leading to a cholecystectomy in one patient.[79]

Orlistat appears to decrease the absorption of fat-soluble vitamins, resulting in decreases in serum levels of vitamin D.[85] All pediatric patients taking orlistat should receive supplementation with a multivitamin containing vitamin A (5,000 IU), vitamin D (400 IU), vitamin E (300 IU), and vitamin K (25 mcg). The vitamins are best administered at least 2 hours before or after the administration of orlistat. In patients on anticoagulation therapy with warfarin, the decrease in vitamin K absorption may cause an increase in the international normalized ratio. Close monitoring is warranted for patients concomitantly taking orlistat and warfarin. Orlistat also decreases the absorption of levothyroxine and cyclosporine. It is advised to separate orlistat and levothyroxine by at least 4 hours. It is not recommended to use orlistat if the patient is taking cyclosporine. However, if the two drugs are used concomitantly, then they must be separated by at least 2 hours, and careful monitoring of cyclosporine levels is critical.

The recommended dose of orlistat in children older than 12 years is 120 mg orally three times daily with meals. The dose is taken during the meal or up to 1 hour after the meal. It is not recommended to exceed three doses/day. Patients should also be advised to limit fat intake to a maximum of 30% of total caloric intake and to divide between the three meals. If a meal does not contain fat, then it is not necessary to take the medication. Although orlistat is available as an over-the-counter medication (Alli, GlaxoSmith Kline, Warner, NJ), the manufacturer does not recommend its use in anyone younger than 18 years.

METFORMIN

Metformin has been evaluated for weight loss in obese children and adolescents (6–19 years of age) with and without insulin resistance. Metformin decreases hepatic glucose production and intestinal absorption of glucose and improves insulin sensitivity. Although the exact mechanism for weigh loss has not been clearly elucidated, metformin is proven to increase the release of irisin from skeletal muscle.[86] Irisin is a myokine that increases energy expenditure.[87] On

administration, about 50% to 60% of metformin is systemically absorbed. The drug is not bound to plasma proteins. Metformin is excreted unchanged in the urine by tubular secretion. The elimination half-life of metformin is about 17 hours.[88]

In studies with a primary outcome of decreases in BMI, a change in BMI of −1.35 (95% CI, −2.00 to −0.69) and weight of −3.24 kg (95% CI, −5.79 to −0.69) is expected.[76] However, most studies were small, short-term (e.g., less than 6 months), and may not have shown a significant difference over placebo in less than 6 months.[89-99] Further long-term studies and follow-up are necessary to evaluate the role of metformin in weight loss of obese children and adolescents.

Commonly reported adverse effects of metformin in the studies included nausea, dizziness, and loose stools. No reports of serious adverse reactions, such as lactic acidosis, were reported. In addition, only two studies monitoring serum creatinine and liver function enzymes reported elevations in liver function enzymes.[93,99] Minimal clinically significant drug interactions exist with metformin. However, metformin must be discontinued before administering intravenous iodinated contrast materials and not reinitiated until 48 hours after the procedure and adequate renal function is restored. Adolescents should also be cautioned regarding acute or chronic alcohol use because alcohol can increase the risk of lactic acidosis.

The doses used for weight loss ranged from 500 to 1000 mg orally twice daily. In the study using 1 g twice daily, the dose was titrated over a 3-week period.[92] Metformin should be given with meals.

TOPIRAMATE

Topiramate is used in the treatment of seizure disorders and migraine in pediatric patients. Topiramate works by inhibition of voltage-dependent sodium channels, augments the neurotransmission of the γ-aminobutyrate receptor at specific subtypes, antagonizes the AMPA/kainate subtype of the glutamate receptor, and inhibits the isozymes II and IV of the carbonic anhydrase enzyme.[100] The exact mechanism in weight loss is unknown but is thought to affect appetite and satiety.[101]

In pediatric patients using topiramate for seizure disorders and migraine, weight loss has been reported at 1–2 kg versus placebo.[102] A retrospective study of 28 pediatric patients treated with topiramate and lifestyle intervention over 6 months reported a decrease in BMI of −4.9 kg/m² (95% CI, −7.1 to −2.8).[103] A randomized, placebo-controlled pilot study evaluated 30 adolescents (age 12–18 years) with severe obesity, defined as 1.2 times the 95th percentile for sex and age or a BMI greater than 35 kg/m².[104] Participants completed 4 weeks of meal replacements equalling 1,400 kcal/day and then randomized to topiramate or placebo for 28 weeks. Participants were started on topiramate 25 mg once daily for 1 week, 50 mg once daily for 2 weeks, then 25 mg in the morning and 50 mg in the evening. Of all participants 70% completed the study. On completion of the trial, the participants on topiramate had a 1.85% difference in BMI compared with the placebo group (p=0.291). In addition, only 14% of the topiramate group had more than a 5% decrease in BMI compared with 25% in the placebo group; in both groups one participant lost more than 10% of BMI. The most common adverse drug reaction in the topiramate group was paresthesia (25%). Other adverse drug reactions included worsening of depression, resulting in discontinuation of the trial. Participants in the topiramate arm also experienced decreases in visceral fat mass, triglyceride, insulin, glucose, and very low-density lipoprotein cholesterol, although these findings were not clinically significant. The authors did not specify why the participants did not complete the study. The role of topiramate for weight reduction in adolescents requires further investigation.

Qsymia (Vivus Inc, Campbell, CA), a combination of topiramate and phentermine, is approved for treatment of obesity in adults. However, to date, no studies in pediatrics have been conducted. It is not recommended for use in weight loss in children and adolescents at this time.

GLUCAGON-LIKE PEPTIDE-1 RECEPTOR AGONISTS

The glucagon-like peptide-1 receptor agonists are approved for the treatment of type 2 diabetes in adults. In addition, GLP-1 receptor agonists have been studied extensively in the adult population for weight loss with a range of weight loss between 0.9 to 2.9 kg.[105] The GLP-1 agonist binds and activates the GLP-1 receptor in pancreatic beta cells, resulting in increased insulin release and decreased glucagon secretion, in addition to delayed gastric emptying.[106] The mechanism for weight loss is through activation of the POMC/cocaine- and amphetamine-related transcript neurons and inhibition of the NP-Y/AgRP neurons in the arcuate nucleus in the hypothalamus.[107] Two GLP-1 agonists, exenatide and liraglutide, are indicated for weight loss in adults without type 2 diabetes, and these drugs have been studied for weight loss in adolescents.

EXENATIDE

One study has evaluated the efficacy and safety of exenatide in adolescents age 12–19 years with severe obesity not associated with genetic cause or known syndrome.[108] The randomized, double-blind, placebo-controlled trial evaluated exenatide in 26 adolescents with a BMI greater than or equal to 1.2 times the 95th percentile for age and sex or a BMI greater than 35 kg/m². Participants were randomized to exenatide 5 mcg subcutaneously twice daily, titrated to 10 mcg twice daily after 1 month or placebo for 3 months, after which time participants remained in an open-label study for 3 additional months. Exenatide decreased BMI by 2.9% compared with 0.15% with placebo (p=0.025) after the randomized portion of the trial. Exenatide also decreased BMI, weight circumference, total tissue fat, and visceral fat area more than placebo. In terms of weight, exenatide resulted in a mean decrease of 2.04 kg whereas the placebo group had an increase of 0.32 kg. After the additional 3 months in the open-label study, those initially randomized to exenatide had an average decrease in BMI of 4% from baseline.

Common adverse drug reactions included nausea, abdominal pain, diarrhea, headache, and vomiting. During the study, two participants were unable to tolerate the 10-mcg dose secondary to gastrointestinal adverse drug reactions with initial dose increase. However, after a dose reduction for less than 1 week, the participants tolerated the 10-mcg dose. The adverse drug reactions were reported to be mild to moderate and transient in nature. Four patients did not complete the study because of lack of adherence (exenatide group), loss to follow-up, or diagnosis of pseudotumor cerebri (for one patient, unrelated to exenatide). The drug appears to have moderate weight loss after 6 months with good tolerability. Further studies are required to determine the long-term effects.

LIRAGLUTIDE

A randomized, double-blind, placebo-controlled trial assessing safety, tolerability, and pharmacokinetics for liraglutide was conducted in 21 adolescents age 12–17 years.[109] Liraglutide was started at 0.6 mg/week subcutaneously and titrated by 0.6 mg/week up to 3 mg/day as tolerated. The dose was not increased if fasting plasma glucose was less than 70 mg/dL or if the participant experienced hypoglycemia the week before a dose increase. The trial lasted for 6 weeks.

No participants dropped out of the study because of adverse reactions. The most common adverse reaction was mild abdominal pain reported in 85% of participants. Eight participants (with 12 episodes total) experienced hypoglycemia, but only three were confirmed by fasting plasma glucose. About 50% of these episodes occurred 10 hours after a meal. An increase in heart rate (mean 6 beats/minute) was observed. No differences in laboratory analysis were found.

Although benefits in weight, fasting plasma glucose, glycosylated hemoglobin, and fasting serum insulin were seen, these effects were not statistically significant. Further studies are needed to determine the efficacy of liraglutide on obesity in the pediatric population.

SURGICAL THERAPY

The last line of therapy for obesity is surgical intervention. However, careful consideration must be given before electing for weight-loss surgery in pediatric patients. Some factors to consider include BMI, comorbidities, physical and emotional maturity, recovery, surgical complications, cost, and ability to adhere to the lifestyle modifications required after surgery.

In general, pediatric patients considered for weight-loss surgery include those with a BMI greater than or equal to 35 kg/m² with a serious comorbidity such as type 2 diabetes mellitus, moderate or severe obstructive sleep apnea, pseudotumor cerebri, or severe steatohepatitis.[110,111] Many of these comorbidities have been reported to improve or completely resolve after weight-loss surgery.[112,113] Other candidates for weight-loss surgery include children and adolescents with a BMI greater than 40 kg/m² with or without comorbidities such as hypertension, insulin resistance, decreased quality of life, and impaired activities of daily living.[110]

Two types of weight-loss surgery have been successfully performed in pediatric patients: the Roux-en-Y gastric bypass (RYGB) and the laparoscopic adjustable gastric band (LAGB) procedure. The RYGB procedure involves the creation of a 15- to 30-mL gastric pouch to bypass the small intestine.[113]

This form of weight-loss surgery is restrictive and decreases the amount of nutrients absorbed. In adolescents, the RYGB can lead to a weight loss of 18–22 BMI units, with weight loss efficacy rates reported at about 60% in adolescents.[111,112] To date, no in-hospital deaths immediately after the surgery have been reported, although three long-term deaths have been reported.[114] A prospective study reported 9.3% of adolescents undergoing an RYGB experienced a major, life-threatening complication (defined as reoperation for bowel obstruction, bleeding, gastrointestinal leak, sepsis or suspected sepsis, deep vein thrombosis, or splenectomy). In the same study, 16.8% experienced a minor event.[114] Because the RYGB weight-loss surgery often results in nutritional deficiencies, it is recommended to postpone this surgery in children and adolescents until after they have attained at least 95% of adult stature. Two assessments should be completed before surgery: Tanner staging and evaluation of bone age.[111] Because most linear growth spurts occur before puberty, it is advised to defer weight-loss surgery until after Tanner Stage IV is reached in both boys and girls. In addition, bone age can be determined with radiography of the hands and feet. If this criterion is followed, then the child will typically be older than 12 years. The RYGB can still be considered in children not meeting this criterion if they present with severe obesity and comorbidities.

The LAGB procedure involves the placement of a silicone adjustable band on the upper portion of the stomach that results in a small pouch for food.[115] The band is adjusted after surgery and throughout the weight-loss period. This form of weight-loss surgery is not restrictive and does not result in the same nutritional deficiencies as the RYGB. Weight loss in adolescents after the LAGB has ranged from 11 to 14 BMI units with weight-loss efficacy rates from 15% to 87%.[112] To date, no deaths have been reported with LAGB surgery. A prospective study has reported the prevalence of major complications of 7.1% and minor complications of 7.1%.[116] During the perioperative period, only solid organ injury was reported as a minor complication. However, between discharge and 30 days post-operative, major complications included pulmonary embolism. In the same period, minor complications included small bowel obstruction.[116] Other complications of surgery in this population include band slippage, gastric dilation, intragastric band migration, psychological intolerance of band, hiatal hernia, cholecystitis, and cracking of the band. Currently the LAGB is not indicated in pediatric patients and is considered investigational.

Both forms of surgery still require further research to determine long-term efficacy and safety. These forms of surgery should not be considered until all other treatment options have been attempted and failed. It is crucial for any child or adolescent being considered for weight-loss surgery to have the emotional maturity to understand the risks associated with surgery, the motivation to adhere to lifestyle modifications after the surgery, and familial support. In addition, any psychiatric condition should be actively treated and in remission for at least 1 year before the surgery is performed. Typically, the surgery is performed at a center with a multidisciplinary team specializing in obesity.

MONITORING

All children and adolescents should have a yearly height and weight assessment. In those older than 2 years, a BMI should be calculated and plotted on the CDC growth charts to determine the percentile. Any child classified as overweight or obese may require additional laboratory analysis and a physical examination for existing complications of obesity. Weight, height, and BMI are adequate assessments for follow-up; anthropometric measurements, such as skinfold and waist circumference, are unnecessary. Follow-up laboratory values will vary according to the individual child and the child's presenting symptoms. Dietary intake and physical activity should be reviewed at each visit.

For children and adolescents on pharmacotherapy for obesity, additional monitoring is necessary. During treatment with orlistat, a baseline vitamin D level should be obtained. Regardless of whether a multivitamin is also prescribed to the patient, a follow-up vitamin D level should be considered every 3–6 months during orlistat therapy. Patients should be monitored for adverse reactions, which typically subside within 4 weeks of therapy.[85] During treatment with metformin, a baseline serum creatinine level is recommended. Metformin is contraindicated if serum creatinine levels are greater than 1.4 mg/dL and 1.5 mg/dL in female and male patients, respectively.[87] Metformin is also not recommended for use in those with hepatic disease.[87]

CONCLUSIONS

Many challenges exist in the prevention and treatment of pediatric obesity. However, assessing BMI at each encounter with a pediatric patient will assist in identifying those who are overweight and obese for the implementation of lifestyle modifications. Early intervention may halt the progression of complications in this population.

An 8-year-old white boy is brought to the primary physician for his well-visit. His parents have no current concerns, except for some brown patches on his neck and elbows.

His medications are a once-daily multivitamin, and he has no known drug allergies. Medical history is significant for full-term birth at 2.4 kg at 37 weeks (small for gestational age) by cesarean section because of failure to progress during birth, with no other complications. He was formula-fed from 2 weeks of life.

The boy lives with his mother, father, and an older sister (age 10 years). He is in third grade at school, and his grades are mostly Bs and Cs. He has had some fights at school because of other children being "mean" to him. He started participating in Little League Baseball this year. He and his family eat many meals in restaurants, including fast food. The child reports not liking fruits and vegetables. He drinks soda and juice daily and snacks on candy bars and chips.

His family history is as follows: (1) his mother is age 40 years, height 66 inches, and weight 76.2 kg; she received a diagnosis of hypertension less than 1 year ago; (2) his father is age 46 years, height 70 inches, weight 93.4 kg with central obesity; and (3) his sister is age 10 years, height 54 inches, weight 30.8 kg; she has a history of attention deficit hyperactivity disorder.

Vital signs: BP 116/76 mm Hg, HR 76 beats/minute, Wt 44.5 kg, Ht 56 inches

Physical examination:

General: Alert, in no apparent distress, obese
HEENT: Normal
Neck: Supple, no goiter, no nodes
Cardiovascular: Normal, palpable, femoral pulses
Abdomen: Obese, soft, no organomegaly, no bruits
Extremities: Normal
Skin: Mild acanthosis nigricans around neck and on elbows
Neuro: Normal, flat affect

Laboratory findings:

Laboratory Test	Results	Normal References
Fasting blood glucose (mg/dL)	106	70–126
Total cholesterol (mg/dL)	154	127–193
Triglycerides (mg/dL)	80	37–130
HDL-C (mg/dL)	34	32–70
LDL-C (mg/dL)	120	0–130

---

1. What is the patient's body mass index (BMI) and classification for weight?

The patient's BMI is 22 kg/m², which is above the 95th percentile for his age and sex, based on the Centers for Disease Control and Prevention growth charts. This BMI classifies the patient as obese.

2. What risk factors for obesity does this patient have?

Although a full nutrition history has not been obtained, the reports of frequent eating at restaurants, soda and juice consumption, and snacking on energy-dense foods may increase the risk of obesity. The decreased activity also is a risk factor. In addition, this child was small for gestational age, which is associated with an increased risk of obesity. Although conflicting reports exist, the lack of breastfeeding may also be a risk.

Recent studies have found an increased risk of obesity associated with a cesarean delivery. In addition, the mother's weight during pregnancy may be an additional risk factor if she was overweight; also, if gestational diabetes was diagnosed for the mother, then the child would have an additional risk factors for obesity in childhood.

3. What treatment should be initiated for the patient?

The patient would require Stage 1 of treatment as an initial intervention because he is age 8 years and is between the 95th and 99th percentile for sex and age. Stage 1 treatment consists of counseling strategies for weight loss with frequent monitoring. The child should regulate food intake, but not be placed on a diet

or any food restrictions. The counseling should be directed to the entire family to establish reasonable goals and lifestyle habits for the family. Physical exercise should also be increased, as tolerated, to 1 hour/day.

Pharmacotherapy is not recommended at this time. Treatment at Stage 1 would continue for 3–6 months. If treatment goals are not met, then the patient should be re-evaluated, and treatment may be escalated to Stage 2. Pharmacotherapy is not recommended until Stage 4.

4. What is the goal of therapy for the patient?

The goal for this patient, at Stage 1 treatment, is gradual weight loss, which would be no more than 0.45 kg/month. Additional goals include the prevention of complications of diabetes, including monitoring and screening for hypertension, insulin resistance (which is evident by the acanthosis nigricans), and dyslipidemia. The goal is to develop healthy lifestyle habits through diet and physical activity.

5. What health factors should be monitored for this patient? How often is monitoring indicated?

The patient's weight, height, and BMI should be monitored every 3 to 6 months to determine effectiveness of treatment. Physical and laboratory examinations at this time should include blood pressure, lipid panel, status of puberty (Tanner staging), liver function tests, mental health, and albuminuria to determine if complications of obesity are present.

REFERENCES

1. Organisation for Economic Co-operation and Development (OECD). Obesity Update 2017. Available at www.oecd.org/els/health-systems/Obesity-Update-2017.pdf. Accessed September 20, 2019.
2. Fryar CD, Carrol MD, Ogden CL. Prevalence of Overweight and Obesity Among Children and Adolescents: United States, 1963–1965 Through 2011–2012. Centers for Disease Control and Prevention. National Center for Health Statistics, Health E-Stats. Available at www.cdc.gov/nchs/data/hestat/obesity_child_11_12/obesity_child_11_12.pdf. Accessed September 20, 2019.
3. Hales CM, Carroll MD, Fryar CD, et al. Prevalence of Obesity Among Adults and Youth: United States, 2015-2016. NCHS Data Brief, No. 288. Hyattsville, MD: National Center for Health Statistics. 2017. Available at www.cdc.gov/nchs/data/databriefs/db288.pdf. Accessed September 30, 2019.
4. Ogden CL, Carroll MD, Kit BK, et al. Prevalence of obesity and trends in body mass index among US children and adolescents, 1999-2010. JAMA 2012;307:483-90.
5. Fryar CD, Carrol MD, Odgen CL. Prevalence of Overweight and Obesity Among Children and Adolescents Aged 2–19 Years: United States, 1963–1965 Through 2013–2014. Health E-Stats. Hyattsville, MD: National Center for Health Statistics. 2016. Available at www.cdc.gov/nchs/data/hestat/obesity_child_13_14/obesity_child_13_14.pdf. Accessed September 30, 2019.
6. Heymsfield SB, Wadden TA. Mechanisms, pathophysiology, and management of obesity. N Engl J Med 2017;376:254-66.
7. Suzuki K, Jayasena CH, Bloom SR. Obesity and appetite control. Exp Diabetes Res 2012;Article ID 824305.
8. Guarino D, Nannipieri M, Iervasi G, et al. The role of the autonomic nervous system in the pathophysiology of obesity. Front Physiol 2017;8:66.
9. Timper K, Bruning JC. Hypothalamic circuits regulating appetite and energy homeostasis: pathways to obesity. Dis Model Mech 2017;10:679-89.
10. Clemmensen C, Muller TD, Woods SC, et al. Gut-brain crosstalk in metabolic control. Cell 2017;168:758-74.
11. Waterson MJ, Horvath TL. Neuronal regulation of energy homeostasis: beyond the hypothalamus and feeding. Cell Metabolism 2015;223:962-70.
12. Massadi OA, Lopez M, Tschop M, et al. Current understanding of the hypothalamic ghrelin pathways inducing appetite and adiposity. Trends Neurosci 2017;40:167-80.
13. Muller TD, Nogueiras R, Andermann ML, et al. Ghrelin. Mol Metab 2015;4:437-60.
14. Moehlecke M, Canani LH, Oliveira L, et al. Determinants of body weight regulation in humans. Arch Endocrinol Metab 2016;60:152-62.
15. Lustig RH. The neuroendocrine control of energy balance. In: Freedmark MS, ed. Contemporary Endocrinology, Pediatric Obesity: Etiology, Pathogenesis and Treatment. Cham, Switzerland: Springer International Publishing, 2018:15-32.
16. Lee JO, Kim N, Lee HJ, et al. Visfatin, a novel adipokine, stimulates glucose uptake through the Ca^{2+}-dependent AMPK-p38 MAPK pathway in C2C12 skeletal muscle cells. J Mol Endocrinol 2015;54:251-62.
17. Prinz P, Stengel A. Control of food intake by gastrointestinal peptides: mechanisms of action and possible modulation in the treatment of obesity. J Neurogastroenterol Motil 2017;23:180-96.
18. Schmitz O, Broack B, Rungby J. Amylin agonists: A novel approach in the treatment of diabetes. Diabetes 2004;53:S233-38.
19. Habegger KM, Heppner KM, Geary N, et al. The metabolic actions of glucagon revisited. Nat Rev Endocrinol 2010;12:689-97.
20. Camilleri M. Peripheral mechanisms in appetite regulation. Gastroenterology 2015;148:1219-33.
21. Contreras C, Nogueiras R, Dieguez C, et al. Traveling from the hypothalamus to the adipose tissue: the thermogenic pathway. Redox Biol 2017;12:854-63.
22. Bray GA. Afferent signals regulating food intake. Proc Nutr Soc 2000;59:373-84.
23. Styne DM, Arslanian SA, Connor EL, et al. Pediatric obesity—assessment, treatment, and prevention: An endocrine society clinical practice guideline. J Clin Endocrinol Metab 2017;102:709-57.
24. Van der Klaauw AA, Farooqi IS. The hunger genes: Pathways to obesity. Cell 2015;161:119-32.
25. Radha V, Mohan V. Obesity—are we continuing to play the genetic "blame game"? Adv Genomics Genet 2016;6:11-23.
26. Kaur Y, de Souza RJ, Gibson WT, et al. A systematic review of genetic syndromes with obesity. Obes Rev 2017;18:603-34.
27. Kumar S, Kelly AS. Review of childhood obesity: From epidemiology, etiology, and comorbidities to clinical assessment and treatment. May Clin Proc 2017;92:251-65.
28. Greenwood RS. Adverse effects of antiepileptic drugs. Epilepsia 2000;41:S42-52.
29. Matsui-Sakata A, Ohtani H, Sawada Y. Receptor occupancy-based analysis of the contributions of various receptors to antispychotics-induced weight gain and diabetes mellitus. Drug Metab Pharmacokinet 2005;20:368-78.
30. Sharma AM, Pischon T, Hardt S, et al. Hypothesis: Beta-adrenergic receptor blockers and weight gain: A systematic analysis. Hypertension 2001;37:250-4.
31. Wellman PJ, Davies BT, Morien A, et al. Modulation of feeding by hypothalamic paraventricular nucleus alpha 1- and 2-adrenergic receptors. Life Sci 1993;53:669-79.
32. Nasrallah H. A review of the effect of atypical antipsychotics on weight. Psychoneuroendocrinology 2003;28:83-96.
33. Reynolds GP, Hill MJ, Kirk SL. The 5-HT2C receptor and antipsychotic induced weight gain—mechanisms and genetics. J Psychopharmacol 2006;20:15-8.
34. Lee RS, Pirooznia M, Guintivano J, et al. Search for common targets of lithium and valproic acid identifies novel epigenetic effects of lithium on the rat leptin receptor gene. Transl Psychiatry 2015;5:e600.
35. Himmerich H, Minkwitz J, Kirkby KC. Weight gain and metabolic changes during treatment with antipsychotics and antidepressants. Endocr Metab Immune Disord Drug Targets 2015;15:252-60.
36. Christ-Crain M, Kola B, Lolli F, et al. AMP-activated protein kinase mediates glucocorticoid-induced metabolic changes: a novel mechanism in Cushing's syndrome. FASEB J 2008;22:1672-83.
37. Gao Q, Horvath TL. Cross-talk between estrogen and leptin signaling in the hypothalamus. Am J Physiol Endocrinol Metab 2008;294:E817-26.
38. Schwartz MW, Porte D. Diabetes, obesity and the brain. Science 2005;307:375-9.
39. Heerwagen MJ, Miller MR, Barbour LA, et al. Maternal obesity and fetal metabolic programming: a fertile epigenetic soil. Am J Physiol Regul Integr Comp Physiol 2010;299:R711-22.
40. Oken E, Taveras EM, Kleinman KP, et al. Gestational weight gain and child adiposity at age 3 years. Am J Obstet Gynecol 2007;196:322.e1-8.
41. Oken E, Rifas-Shiman SL, Field AE, et al. Maternal gestational weight gain and offspring weight in adolescence. Obstet Gynecol 2008;112:999-1006.
42. Wrotniak BH, Shults J, Butts S, et al. Gestational weight gain and risk of overweight in the offspring at age 7 y in a multicenter, multiethnic cohort study. Am J Clin Nutr 2008;87:1818-24.
43. Catalano PM, Kirwan JP, Haugel-de Mouzon S, et al. Gestational diabetes and insulin resistance: role in short- and long-term implications for mother and fetus. J Nutr 2003;133:1674S-83S.
44. Lucas A. Role of nutritional programming in determining adult morbidity. Arch Dis Child 1994;71:288-90.

45. Ibanez L, Ong K, Dunger DB, et al. Early development of adiposity and insulin resistance after catch-up weight gain in small-for-gestational-age children. J Clin Endocrinol Metab 2006;91:2153-8.

46. Ong KK, Ahmed ML, Emmett PM, et al. Association between postnatal catch-up growth and obesity in childhood: prospective cohort study. BMJ 2000;320:967-71.

47. Kuhle S, Tong OS, Woolcott CG. Association between caesarean section and childhood obesity: a systematic review and meta-analysis. Obes Rev 2015;16:295-303.

48. Darmasseelane K, Hyde MJ, Santhakumaran S, et al. Mode of delivery and offspring body mass index, overweight and obesity in adult life: A systematic review and analysis. PLOS ONE 2014;9:e87896.

49. Yuan C, Gaskins AJ, Blaine AI, et al. Association between cesarean birth and risk of obesity in offspring in childhood, adolescence, and early adulthood. JAMA Pediatr 2016 7;170:e162385.

50. Ley RE, Turnbaugh PJ, Klein S, Gordon JI. Human gut microbes associated with obesity. Nature 2006;444:1022-3.

51. Korpela K, Zijlmans MAC, Kuitunen M, et al. Childhood BMI in relation to microbiotia in infancy and lifetime antibiotic use. Microbiome 2017;5:26.

52. Owen CG, Martin RM, Whincup PH, et al. Effect of infant feeding on the risk of obesity across the life course: a quantitative review of published evidence. Pediatrics 2005;115:1367-77.

53. Gillman MW, Rifas-Shiman SL, Camargo CA, et al. Risk of overweight among adolescents who were breastfed as infants. JAMA 2001;285:2461-7.

54. Grummer-Strawn LM, Mei Z. Does breastfeeding protect against pediatric overweight? Analysis of longitudinal data from the Centers for Disease Control and Prevention Pediatric Nutrition Surveillance System. Pediatrics 2004;113:e81-6.

55. Centers for Disease Control and Prevention, National Center for Health Statistics. CDC Growth Charts: United States. Available at www.cdc.gov/healthyweight/assessing/bmi/childrens_bmi/about_childrens_bmi.html. Accessed November 11, 2017.

56. Rolland-Cachera MF, Deheeger M, Maillot M, et al. Early adiposity rebound: causes and consequences for obesity in children and adults. Int J Obes 2006;30:S11-7.

57. Moreno LA, Rodriguez G. Dietary risk factors for development of childhood obesity. Curr Opin Clin Nutr Metab Care 2007;10:336-41.

58. Marshall SJ, Biddle SJ, Gorely T, et al. Relationships between media use, body fatness and physical activity in children and youth: a meta-analysis. Int J Obes Relat Metab Disord 2004;28:1238-46.

59. American Academy of Pediatrics, Committee on Nutrition. The role of the pediatrician in primary prevention of obesity. Pediatrics 2015;136:e275.

60. Al Mamun A, Lawlor DA, Cramb S, et al. Do childhood sleeping problems predict obesity in young adulthood? Evidence from a prospective birth cohort study. Am J Epidemiol 2007;166:1368-73.

61. Ogden CL, Carroll MD, Fakhouri TH, et al. Prevalence of obesity among youths by household income and education level of head of household—United States 2011–2014. MMWR Morb Mortal Wkly Rep 2018;67:186-9.

62. Ogden CL, Fryar CD, Hales CM, et al. Differences in obesity prevalence by demographics and urbanization in US children and adolescents, 2013–2016. JAMA 2018;319:2410-8.

63. Freedman DS, Khan LK, Dietz WH, et al. Relationship of childhood obesity to coronary heart disease risk factors in adulthood: the Bogalusa Heart Study. Pediatrics 2001;108:712-8.

64. Kelly AS, Barlow SE, Rao G, et al. Severe obesity in children and adolescents: Identification, associated health risks, and treatment approaches. Circulation 2013;128:1689-712.

65. Barlow SE. Expert committee recommendations regarding the prevention, assessment, and treatment of child and adolescent overweight and obesity: summary report. Pediatrics 2007;120:S164-92.

66. Han JC, Lawlor DA, Kimm SY. Childhood obesity. Lancet 2010;375:1737-48.

67. Reilly JJ, Kelly J, Wilson DC. Accuracy of simple clinical and epidemiological definitions of childhood obesity: systematic review and evidence appraisal. Obes Rev 2010;11:645-55.

68. Freedman DS, Wang J, Ogden CL, et al. The prediction of body fatness by BMI and skinfold thicknesses among children and adolescents. Ann Hum Biol 2007;34:183-94.

69. Franks PW, Hanson RL, Knowler WC, et al. Childhood obesity, other cardiovascular risk factors, and premature death. N Engl J Med 2010;362:485-93.

70. Lakshman R, Elks CE, Ong KK. Childhood obesity. Circulation 2012;126:1770-9.

71. Kumar S, Kelly AS. Review of childhood obesity: From epidemiology, etiology, and comorbidities to clinical assessment and treatment. Mayo Clin Proc 2017;92:251-65.

72. Skinner AC, Perrin EM, Moss LA, et al. Cardiometabolic risks and severity of obesity in children and young adults. N Engl J Med 2015;373:1307-17.

73. Daniels SR, Jacobson MS, McCrindle BW, et al. American Heart Association Childhood Obesity Research Summit Report. Circulation 2009;119:e489-517.

74. Juonala M, Magnussen CG, Berenson GS, et al. Childhood adiposity, adult adiposity, and cardiovascular risk factors. N Engl J Med 2011;365:1876-85.

75. James WP, Caterson ID, Coutinho W, et al. Effect of sibutramine on cardiovascular outcomes in overweight and obese subjects. N Engl J Med 2010;363:905-17.

76. Mead E, Atkinson G, Richter B, et al. Drug interventions for the treatment of obesity in children and adolescents. Cochrane Database Syst Rev 2016;11:CD012436.

77. Xenical (Orlistat) [package insert]. San Francisco: Genentech USA, 2016.

78. McDuffie JR, Calis KA, Uwaifo GI, et al. Three-month tolerability of orlistat in adolescents with obesity-related comorbid conditions. Obes Res 2002;10:642-50.

79. Chanoine JP, Hampl S, Jensen C, et al. Effect of orlistat on weight and body composition in obese adolescents: a randomized controlled trial. JAMA 2005;293:2873-83.

80. Ozkan B, Bereket A, Turan S, et al. Addition of orlistat to conventional treatment in adolescents with severe obesity. Eur J Pediatr 2004;163:738-41.

81. Maahs D, de Serna DG, Kolotkin RL, et al. Randomized, double-blind, placebo-controlled trial of orlistat for weight loss in adolescents. Endocr Pract 2006;12:18-28.

82. McDuffie JR, Calis KA, Uwaifo GI, et al. Efficacy of orlistat as an adjunct to behavioral treatment in overweight African American and Caucasian adolescents with obesity-related co-morbid conditions. J Pediatr Endocrinol Metab 2004;17:307-19.

83. Norgren S, Danielsson P, Jurold R, et al. Orlistat treatment in obese prepubertal children: a pilot study. Acta Paediatr 2003;92:666-70.

84. McGovern L, Johnson JN, Paulo R, et al. Treatment of pediatric obesity: a systematic review and meta-analysis of randomized trials. J Clin Endocrinol Metab 2008;93:4600-05.

85. McDuffie JR, Calis KA, Booth SL, et al. Effects of orlistat on fat-soluble vitamins in obese adolescents. Pharmacotherapy 2002;22:814-22.

86. Li DJ, Huang F, Lu WJ, et al. Metformin promotes irisin release from murine skeletal muscle independently of AMP-activated protein kinase activation. Acta Physiol 2015;213:711-21.

87. Perakakis N, Triantafyllou GA, Fernandez-Real JM, et al. Physiology and role of irisin in glucose homeostasis. Nat Rev Endocrinol 2017;13:324-37.

88. Glucophage (Metformin) [package insert]. Princeton, NJ: Bristol-Myers Squibb, 2017.

89. Atabek ME, Pirgon O. Use of metformin in obese adolescents with hyperinsulinemia: a 6-month, randomized, double-blind,

placebo-controlled clinical trial. J Pediatr Endocrinol Metab 2008;21:339-48.

90. Clarson CL, Mahmud FH, Baker JE, et al. Metformin in combination with structured lifestyle intervention improved body mass index in obese adolescents, but did not improve insulin resistance. Endocrine 2009;36:141-6.

91. Freemark M, Bursey D. The effects of metformin on body mass index and glucose tolerance in obese adolescents with fasting hyperinsulinemia and a family history of type 2 diabetes. Pediatrics 2001;107:e55.

92. Kendall D, Vail A, Amin R, et al. Metformin in obese children and adolescents: the MOCA trial. J Clin Endocrinol Metab 2013;98:322-9.

93. Mauras N, DelGiorno C, Hossain J, et al. Metformin use in children with obesity and normal glucose tolerance—effects on cardiovascular markers and intrahepatic fat. J Pediatr Endocrinol Metab 2012;25:33-40.

94. Prado B, Gaete V, Corona F, et al. Metabolic effects of metformin in obese adolescents at risk for type 2 diabetes mellitus. Rev Chil Pediatr 2012;83:48-57.

95. Rezvanian H, Hashemipour M, Kelishadi R, et al. A randomized, triple masked, placebo-controlled clinical trial for controlling childhood obesity. World J Pediatr 2010;6:317-22.

96. Srinivasan S, Ambler GR, Baur LA, et al. Randomized, controlled trial of metformin for obesity and insulin resistance in children and adolescents: improvement in body composition and fasting insulin. J Clin Endocrinol Metab 2006;91:2074-80.

97. Yanoski JA, Krakoff J, Salaita CG, et al. Effects of metformin on body weight and body composition in obese insulin-resistant children: a randomized clinical trial. Diabetes 2011;60:477-85.

98. Weigand S, l'Allemand D, Hubel H, et al. Metformin and placebo therapy both improve weight management and fasting insulin in obese insulin-resistant adolescents: a prospective, placebo-controlled, randomized study. Eur J Endocrinol 2010;163:585-92.

99. Glaser Pediatric Research Network Obesity Study Group. Metformin extended release treatment of adolescent obesity: a 48-week randomized, double-blind, placebo-controlled trial with 48-week follow-up. Arch Pediatr Adolesc Med 2010;164:116-23.

100. Topiramate (Topamax) [package insert]. Titusville, NJ: Janssen Pharmaceuticals, Inc. 2009.

101. Phentermine and topiramate extended release (Qysmia) [package insert]. Mountain View, CA: Vivus, Inc. 2012.

102. Sherafat-Kazemzadeh R, Yanovski SZ, Yanovski JA. Pharmacotherapy for childhood obesity: present and future prospects. Int J Obes 2013;37:1-15.

103. Fox CK, Marlatt KL, Rudser KD, et al. Topiramate for weight reduction in adolescents with severe obesity. Clin Pediatr 2015; 54:19-24.

104. Fox CK, Kaizer AM, Rudser KD, et al. Meal replacements followed by topiramate for the treatment of adolescent severe obesity: a pilot randomized controlled trial. Obesity 2016;24:2553-61.

105. Prasad-Reddy L, Isaacs D. A clinical review of GLP-1 receptor agonists, efficacy and safety in diabetes and beyond. Drugs Context 2015;4:212283.

106. Liraglutide (Victoza) [package insert]. Bagsvaerd, Denmark: Novo Nordisk A/S. 2010.

107. Secher A, Jelsing J, Baquero AF, et al. The arcuate nucleus mediates GLP-1 receptor agonist liraglutide-dependent weight loss. J Clin Invest 2014;124:4473-88.

108. Kelly AS, Rudser KD, Nathan BM, et al. The effect of glucagon-like peptide-1 receptor agonist therapy on body mass index in adolescents with severe obesity: a randomized, placebo-controlled clinical trial. JAMA Pediatr 2013;167:335-60.

109. Danne T, Biester T, Kapitzke K, et al. Liraglutide in an adolescent population with obesity: a randomized, double-blind, placebo-controlled 5-week trial to assess safety, tolerability, and pharmacokinetics of liraglutide in adolescents aged 12-17 years. J Pediatr 2017;181:146-53.

110. Michalsky M, Reichard K, Inge T, et al. ASMBS pediatric committee best practice guidelines. Surg Obes Relat Dis 2012;8:1-7.

111. Inge TH, Krebs NF, Garcia VF, et al. Bariatric surgery for severely overweight adolescents. Concerns and recommendations. Pediatrics 2004;114:217-23.

112. Pratt JS, Lenders CM, Dionne EA, et al. Best practice updates for pediatric/adolescent weight loss surgery. Obesity 2009;17:901-10.

113. Treadwell JR, Sun F, Schoelles K. Systematic review and meta-analysis of bariatric surgery for pediatric obesity. Ann Surg 2008;248:763-76.

114. Lawson ML, Kirk S, Mitchell T, et al. Pediatric Bariatric Study Group. One-year outcomes of Roux-en-Y gastric bypass for morbidly obese adolescents: a multicenter study from the Pediatric Bariatric Study Group. J Pediatr Surg 2006;41:137-43.

115. Inge TH, Zeller MH, Lawson ML, et al. A critical appraisal of evidence supporting a bariatric surgical approach to weight management for adolescents. J Pediatr 2005;147:10-9.

116. Inge TH, Zeller MH, Jenkins TM, et al. Perioperative outcome of adolescents undergoing bariatric surgery: The teen longitudinal assessment of bariatric surgery (Teen-LABS) Study. JAMA Pediatr 2014;168:47-53.

Section VII

Renal Disorders

CHAPTER 22

Acute Kidney Injury

*Elizabeth Farrington, Pharm.D., FCCP,
FCCM, FPPA, BCPS, BCNSP; and
Jeremy Stultz, Pharm.D., BCPPS*

LEARNING OBJECTIVES

1. Evaluate the impact of physiologic development on acute kidney injury (AKI) in the pediatric population.

2. Elucidate risk factors for AKI development in the neonatal and pediatric patient.

3. Compare and contrast different methods for glomerular filtration rate estimation in the pediatric population.

4. Create a plan for the prevention and/or management of AKI in a pediatric patient.

5. Design a medication management and nutrition plan for patients with acute renal failure or those receiving a replacement therapy.

ABBREVIATIONS IN THIS CHAPTER

AKI	Acute kidney injury
AUC$_{0-24}$	24-Hour area under the curve
CRRT	Continuous renal replacement therapy
CVVH	Continuous venovenous hemofiltration
CVVHD	Continuous venovenous hemodialysis
CVVHDF	Continuous venovenous hemodiafiltration
GFR	Glomerular filtration rate
HD	Hemodialysis
ICU	Intensive care unit
IDMS	Isotope dilution mass spectrometry
KDIGO	Kidney Disease Improving Global Outcomes
NICU	Neonatal intensive care unit
NGAL	Neutrophil gelatinase-associated lipocalin
NSAID	Nonsteroidal anti-inflammatory drug
PICU	Pediatric intensive care unit
PD	Peritoneal dialysis
pRIFLE	Pediatric risk, injury, failure, loss, end stage renal disease
RIFLE	Risk, injury, failure, loss, end stage renal disease
RRT	Renal replacement therapy
SCr	Serum creatinine
TPN	Total parenteral nutrition
uNGAL	Urine neutrophil gelatinase-associated lipocalin

INTRODUCTION

Acute kidney injury (AKI), formerly known as *acute renal failure*, is the result of injury that leads to functional or structural changes in the kidney. It is characterized by the failure of the kidneys to adequately regulate electrolyte, acid-base, and fluid homeostasis. Before the 1990s, the most prevalent causes of AKI were hemolytic uremic syndrome and other primary renal diseases, sepsis, and burns.[1-6] The first study to report AKI prevalence in the general and critically ill pediatric populations was published by Sutherland and colleagues in 2013.[7] The authors evaluated a national database consisting of pediatric data from primary and tertiary care centers in rural and urban settings. The study used the coding system of the *International Classification of Diseases*, Ninth Revision to identify patients with AKI. Of 2,644,263 children, 10,322 developed AKI, yielding an incidence of 0.39% (3.9 cases per 1000 admissions). The median age of the AKI cohort was 10.8 years versus 2 years in the non-AKI cohort. The highest incidence was seen in children 15 to 18 years (6.6/1000 admissions). In addition, AKI was more common in African American versus whites (4.5 vs. 3.8/1000). Shock, septicemia, intubation/mechanical ventilation, circulatory disease, congenital heart disease, and extracorporeal support were all associated with AKI. Mortality was the highest in neonates (31.2%) and in children requiring critical care (32.8%) or dialysis (27.1%) whereas children in noncritical care units with AKI had a mortality rate of 9.4%.

Kaddourah and colleagues prospectively reviewed the epidemiology of AKI in pediatric patients admitted to the intensive care unit (ICU).[8] Using the Kidney Disease Improving Global Outcomes (KDIGO) criteria, severe AKI was defined as a maximum stage of 2 or 3. A total of 4683 patients were evaluated; AKI developed in 1261 (26.9%) and severe AKI in 543 (11.5%) for a total of 38.5% during the first 7 days after ICU admission. Severe AKI was associated with an increased risk of death (odds ratio, 1.77), occurring in 60 of 543 patients (11%) versus 105 of 4140 patients (2.5%) without severe AKI (p<0.001). Although the association between the development of AKI and death or new disability has been reported in other small studies with narrow patient populations, this investigation was the first multinational prospective study to confirm the association regardless of the admitting diagnosis.[8-12] It is important to recognize that using the serum creatinine (SCr) alone would not have identified AKI in two-thirds of the patients with low urinary output in this study.

The lack of a consistent definition of AKI in the pediatric literature resulted in variations of reported incidence and morbidity and mortality rates for AKI.[13] This lack of consistency changed with a landmark publication by Chertow and colleagues which demonstrated that an increase in SCr of 0.3 mg/dL in adults was independently associated with increased morbidity and mortality regardless of admitting diagnosis.[14]

Price and colleagues reported a similar association between an increase in SCr of 0.3 mg/dL and poor outcomes in children with acute decompensated heart failure—specifically, an adjusted odds ratio of 10.2 for the combined endpoint of mortality or the need for mechanical circulatory support.[15] In addition, it was recognized that an increase in SCr can be delayed by as much as 48 hours after damage to the kidney has occurred, thus a more specific definition of AKI was needed. In 2000, nephrologists and intensivists formed the Acute Dialysis Quality Initiative, including pediatric representation.[16] This initiative led to the development of the first consensus AKI definition, termed the *Risk, Injury, Failure, Loss and End-Stage Renal Disease (RIFLE) criteria*, which was modified in 2007 by the Acute Kidney Injury Network (AKIN).[17,18] In 2007, a pediatric modified version of the RIFLE (pRIFLE) score was developed and validated.[19] In 2012, an international guideline developed by the KDIGO AKI working group combined the previous definitions into a single standardized definition.[20] A summary of these definitions can be found in Table 1. No data currently recommend the use of one pediatric AKI tool over another, but future recommendations are possible.

Although progress has been made in pediatric AKI, it was not until 2014 when a neonatal specific definition of AKI was published (Table 2) and recommended for defining AKI during the first 120 days of life.[21,22] Assessment of SCr presents a specific challenge in the neonatal population. Neonates are born with their mother's creatinine and may take up to 1 month to decrease to the normal range of 0.2–0.4 mg/dL. Therefore, a change in SCr from the lowest previous SCr was built into the neonatal definition. Risk factors reported to be linked to AKI in neonates include weight < 1500 g, neonates who experience perinatal asphyxia, near-term or term neonates with low Apgar scores, neonates treated with extracorporeal membrane oxygenation, and neonates requiring cardiac surgery and the use of nonsteroidal anti-inflammatory drugs for patent ductus arteriosus. Although the number of neonatal studies evaluating AKI remains small, the data are consistent with adult and pediatric studies in demonstrating neonates with AKI have worse outcomes, including higher mortality rates and longer hospital stays.[23-27]

ESTIMATION OF CREATININE CLEARANCE

Historically, the Schwartz equation, based on SCr determined by the Jaffe assay method, has been the formula to estimate glomerular filtration rate (GFR) in children.[28] At this time, all laboratories in the United States should be using creatinine methods calibrated to the isotope dilution mass spectrometry (IDMS) reference method, which yields blood, serum, and plasma creatinine values that are generally lower compared with SCr obtained by the Jaffe assay method. Therefore, using the original Schwartz equation with a creatinine value from a method calibrated to the IDMS will overestimate GFR by 20% to 40%. The bedside Schwartz equation was developed to account for the IDMS calibration and although many investigators have attempted to develop a new equation to estimate GFR in children,[29-31] none are superior to the new bedside Schwartz equation, as follows:[32-35]

Bedside Schwartz formula to calculate glomerular filtration rate $(mL/min/1.73 \ m^2) = 0.431 \times$ height (cm)/serum creatinine

Table 1. Pediatric Acute Kidney Injury Definitions[18,19,20]

pRIFLE Criteria			AKIN Criteria			KDIGO Criteria		
Stage	SCr Criteria	Urine Output	Stage	SCr Criteria	Urine Output	Stage	SCr Criteria	Urine Output
Risk	> 25% eCrCl decrease	< 0.5 mL/kg/ hr for 8 hr	I	SCr increase ≥ 0.3 mg/dL OR 150%–200% in ≤ 48 hr	< 0.5 mL/kg/ hr for 8 hr	I	SCr increase ≥ 0.3 mg/dL in 48 hr OR 1.5–1.9 times	< 0.5 mL/kg/ hr for 6–12 hr
Injury	> 50% eCrCl decrease	< 0.5 mL/kg/ hr for 16 hr	II	SCr increase 200%–300%	< 0.5 mL/kg/ hr for 16 hr	II	SCr increase 2–2.9 times	< 0.5 mL/kg/ hr for 12 hr
Failure	> 75% eCrCl decrease OR eCrCl < 35 mL/ min/1.73 m²	< 0.5 mL/kg/ hr for 24 hr OR < 0.3 mL/kg/ hr for 12 hr	III	SCr increase 200%–300% OR SCr > 4 mg/dL	< 0.5 mL/kg/ hr for 24 hr OR < 0.3 mL/kg/ hr for 12 hr	III	SCr ≥ 3 times increase OR SCr > 4 mg/dL OR if age < 18 yr, then eCrCl < 35 mL/ min/1.73 m²	< 0.5 mL/kg/ hr for 24 hr OR < 0.3 mL/kg/ hr for 12 hr
Loss	Persistent failure > 4 wk	—	—	—	—	—	—	—
End stage	Persistent failure > 3 mo	—	—	—	—	—	—	—

AKIN = Acute Kidney Injury Network; eCrCl = estimated creatinine clearance; KDIGO = Kidney Disease Improving Global Outcomes; pRIFLE = Pediatric Risk, Injury, Failure, Loss and End-Stage Renal Disease or Pediatric RIFLE criteria.

Table 2. Neonatal Acute Kidney Injury KDIGO Classification[21]

Stage	SCr	Urine Output
0	No change in SCr or rise < 0.3 mg/dL	≥ 0.5 mL/kg/hr
1	SCr increase ≥ 0.3 mg/dL within 48 hr OR 1.5–1.9 times reference SCr[a] within 7 days	< 0.5 mL/kg/hr for 6–12 hr
2	SCr rise ≥ 2–2.9 × reference SCr[a]	< 0.5 mL/kg/hr for ≥ 12 hr
3	SCr rise ≥ 3 × reference SCr[a] OR SCr ≥ 2.5 mg/dL[b] OR Receipt of dialysis	< 0.3 mL/kg/hr for ≥ 24 hr OR Anuria for ≥ 12 hr

[a]Reference SCr is defined as the lowest previous SCr value
[b]SCr value of 2.5 mg/dL represents < 10 mL/min/1.73 m^2
KDIGO = Kidney Disease Improving Global Outcomes.

Table 3. Normal Glomerular Filtration Rate in Neontypeates, Infants, and Young Children[23]

Age	Average GFR mL/min/1.73 m^2	Range of GFR mL/min/1.73 m^2
Gestation < 34 Wk		
2–8 days	11	11–15
4–28 days	20	15–28
30–90 days	50	46–65
Gestation ≥ 34 Wk		
2–8 days	39	17–60
4–28 days	47	26–68
30–90 days	58	30–86
1–6 mo	77	39–144
6–12 mo	103	49–157
12–19 mo	127	62–191
2–12 yr	127	89–165

GFR = glomerular filtration rate.

Table 4. Age-Related Changes of Serum Creatinine Based on the Jaffe Method

Age	SCr (mg/dL)
Birth	Mother's SCr
Infancy–3 yr	0.2 to 0.3
4–7 yr	0.3 to 0.5
8–10 yr	0.6 to 0.8
11–13 yr	0.8 to 0.9
Post-pubertal female adolescents	0.8 to 0.9
Post-pubertal male adolescents	0.9 to 1.2

SERUM CREATININE CONCENTRATIONS AND GFR IN CHILDREN

Nephrogenesis begins at the fifth week of gestation and continues until 34 to 36 weeks.[36] In neonates born at 34 weeks of gestation or later, the development of GFR is linear compared with that for premature neonates with slower GFR development. Table 3 summarizes normal GFR in infants and children. At birth, a neonate's SCr concentration is not reflective of kidney function because of in utero placental transfer of maternal creatinine into the fetus. In a healthy full-term neonate, the SCr drops by approximately 50% during the first 7 to 10 days of life and continues to decrease at a lower rate, stabilizing at 0.2 to 0.3 mg/dL by 4 to 6 weeks of life. Because of these changes occurring in the first weeks of life, urine output between 1 to 2 mL/kg/hr is a better reflection of adequate renal function than a calculated creatinine clearance. One would expect a rise of SCr in the second year of life with the development of muscle mass in children; however, this time is the same period for linear GFR development, which increases creatinine clearance. After the age of 2 to 3 years, further increases in muscle mass are reflected by a rise in SCr concentrations. Table 4 reflects age-related changes in SCr concentrations.

BIOMARKERS FOR EVALUATION OF AKI

Urinary inulin clearance is the gold standard for evaluating renal function, but is not feasible for use in clinical practice; therefore, other biomarkers are used to estimate glomerular filtration and thus renal function. The most commonly used biomarkers for assessing kidney function in general are SCr and urine output, but they are not accurate markers for kidney function, especially in neonates and young infants. A lag between renal injury and abnormalities in SCr makes it a poor marker for timely identification of AKI. By the time that abnormalities in SCr are seen, significant renal damage has already occurred. Patients with lower muscle mass (e.g., patients with cystic fibrosis or cerebral palsy) also may have falsely normal SCr concentrations. In the absence of a urinary catheter in children who are not toilet trained or who are critically ill, urine output is an imprecise estimation. Common practice is to weigh diapers before and after a void to estimate volume, but mixed volume diapers can confound these measurements. In neonates, AKI tends to be nonoliguric because of their inability to concentrate urine. Because of these limitations, current methods of determining the presence of AKI use a combination of urine output and SCr based estimations to detect AKI and have shown increased detection of AKI with incidence ranging from 10%–40%.[7,12,19] Recent research has focused on identification of alternative biomarkers for earlier and more accurate identification of AKI. Summarized in the following text are studied biomarkers that could improve detection of AKI, although most are currently investigational and not consistently used in clinical practice.

Changes in SCr may not be apparent in the early stages of AKI, but monitoring of serum concentrations of medications eliminated by the kidneys (e.g., vancomycin, aminoglycosides) may identify AKI earlier. Although serum concentration monitoring of medications can be used to estimate renal function in addition to other methods of assessing AKI, information correlating drug concentrations and actual kidney function is limited and not well developed.

Cystatin C is a cysteine protease inhibitor produced by all nucleated cells in the body, filtered by the glomerulus, but not secreted by the tubules. Cystatin C may not be affected by body mass or other inflammatory states, but factors affecting cystatin C are not yet fully determined.[37] Use of cystatin C may improve the accuracy of GFR estimations in patients with chronic kidney disease; however, this approach has not been thoroughly evaluated in AKI or in patients with normal renal function and thus is not standard of care.[38] Neutrophil gelatinase-associated lipocalin (NGAL) is a protein responsible for attenuating the extent and severity of renal tissue injury. It is released as an acute phase reactant in inflammatory conditions. In AKI, NGAL is up-regulated and accumulates in the distal nephron leading to higher concentrations in the urine (uNGAL).[39] In pediatric patients after cardiac surgery and in those with critical illness, uNGAL concentrations have been shown to increase 2 days before SCr rises in patients who develop AKI. Sensitivity was higher in the cardiac patients (100%) versus the ICU patients (54%).[40,41] Although not readily incorporated into practice, uNGAL is a promising biomarker for AKI. Kidney injury molecule-1 is another biomarker for renal proximal tubular damage. It is up-regulated in post-ischemic animal kidneys and involved in the clearance of apoptotic debris from the tubular lumen.[41] Two studies evaluating patients in the pediatric intensive care unit (PICU) suggest that NGAL, uNGAL, and/or cystatin C detected AKI faster than SCr.[42,43] In newborns, cystatin C concentrations were different between AKI and non-AKI patients, whereas no significant differences were demonstrated for NGAL and kidney injury molecule-1.[44] This difference may be explained by the immaturity of tubular function in the neonate, with cystatin C being unaffected by this immaturity. The optimal biomarker for AKI determination is yet to be found, but as more literature emerges newer methods may prove useful for AKI detection.

PATHOPHYSIOLOGY OF AKI

The incidence of AKI is increasing because of advances in pediatric medicine, including bone marrow, kidney, hepatic and cardiac transplantation, congenital heart disease surgery, and the care of very low birth weight infants. Despite the differences in risk factors between neonates and pediatric patients, the potential origins can be classified into three categories based on the anatomical location of the injury: prerenal, intrinsic, and postrenal AKI. Prerenal AKI results from a decrease in renal blood flow to the renal parenchyma from either volume depletion or decreased effective circulating blood volume. Causes of prerenal AKI can be found in Box 1. Infants are at increased risk for excessive volume losses because of increased body surface area in relation to body weight. Insensible water loss through the skin can add significantly to volume loss, especially during a febrile illness. Intrinsic renal disease may arise from the glomerular, tubulointerstitial or vascular components of the kidney. The most common cause of intrinsic AKI is transformation of prerenal AKI to acute tubular necrosis after prolonged hypoperfusion.[4] Other common causes are interstitial nephritis, hemolytic uremic syndrome, glomerulonephritis, and nephrotoxins (Box 2). Postrenal AKI results from obstruction to urinary flow. Obstruction can occur anywhere along the urinary tract from the tubules to the ureters and may be congenital or acquired. Some causes of obstruction include renal calculi (e.g., because of nephrocalcinosis or acyclovir), bladder outlet obstruction, and internal or external ureteral obstruction. Other causes of postrenal AKI are summarized in Box 3.

MEDICATION-INDUCED AKI

The cause of most AKI is multifactorial and includes potential nephrotoxins and disease states that can cause kidney injury. Most studies analyzing medication-induced nephrotoxicity sought to identify medication association with nephrotoxicity, but determining independent causation can be difficult. Nephrotoxic medication exposure is a risk factor for AKI in adults, and these medications may also be considered potentially nephrotoxic in the pediatric population. However, compared with the adult population, the rate, underlying causes, and consequences of AKI are different in the pediatric population. Table 5 contains a list of common medications used in the pediatric populations and the likely mechanism by which they could cause AKI. An overview of the specific aspects of AKI in different pediatric subpopulations and detailed descriptions of a few select nephrotoxic medications is provided in the following sections.

Box 1. Causes of Prerenal Acute Kidney Injury

Volume Depletion
Gastrointestinal losses (vomiting, diarrhea)
Hemorrhage
Skin losses
Burns
Osmotic diuresis (mannitol, glycosuria)
Renal losses (diabetes insipidus and diuretic exposure)

Decreased effective circulating volume
Decreased oncotic pressure (cirrhosis or liver disease, nephrotic syndrome, malnutrition, protein-losing enteropathy)
Increased leak from vessels (systemic inflammatory response syndrome, sepsis)
Loss of vascular tone
Sepsis
Anaphylaxis

Decreased blood delivery to the kidneys
Decreased cardiac output (congenital heart disease, heart failure)

Increased resistance to flow
Renal artery stenosis
Abdominal compartment syndrome

As described earlier in this chapter and in the Pediatric Pharmacokinetics chapter, nephrogenesis is usually completed by 36 weeks of gestational age, after which nephron maturation occurs throughout infancy and childhood.[45]

Box 2. Causes of Intrinsic Acute Kidney Injury

Glomerular
Immunoglobulin A nephropathy
Post-infectious glomerulonephritis
Henoch-Schönlein purpura
Membranoproliferative glomerulonephritis
Systemic lupus erythematosus
Antineutrophil cytoplasmic antibody-associated
    vasculitis
Antiglomerular basement membrane syndrome
    (Goodpasture syndrome)

Vascular
Hemolytic uremic syndrome
Polyarteritis nodosa
Renal vascular thrombosis
Nonsteroidal anti-inflammatory drugs
Angiotensin-converting enzyme inhibitors

Tubular (Acute Tubular Necrosis)
Hypoxia/ischemia
Sepsis
Medications
Obstruction by crystals (acyclovir, acute tumor lysis
    syndrome, uric acid)
Pigment nephropathy (rhabdomyolysis, hemolysis)

Interstitial
Infectious
Pyelonephritis
Allergy/drug induced
Infiltrative

Box 3. Causes of Postrenal Acute Kidney Injury

Posterior Urethral Valves
Bilateral upper tract obstruction (ureteropelvic
    junction obstruction,
    ureterovesical junction obstruction)
Nephrolithiasis (bilateral)
Clots
Neoplasm
Trauma (abdominal compartment syndrome)
Prune belly syndrome
Neurogenic bladder
Bilateral renal vein thrombosis (infant of a
    diabetic mother, systemic lupus erythematosus,
    antiphospholipid syndrome, protein C or S
    deficiency)

This physiologic development plays an important role in AKI prevalence in the neonatal and infant population. The prevalence of AKI in the neonatal intensive care unit (NICU) has been reported as 40%, with AKI being positively associated with increasing prematurity.[46] Preterm and low birth weight newborns exposed in utero to nephrotoxic agents (e.g., antibiotics, nonsteroidal anti-inflammatory drugs [NSAIDs], angiotensin-converting enzyme inhibitors) are at high risk for renal failure development.[47,48] After birth, preterm and low birth weight neonates and infants may have a higher incidence of AKI after exposure to nephrotoxic medications.[45,47,48] Historically, AKI has been considered reversible in preterm infants. However, recent literature supports the hypothesis that AKI in the preterm neonatal period before completion of nephrogenesis could alter development of the nephrons and lead to more chronic kidney disease later in life.[49,50] Alternatively, full-term neonates and young infants are believed to have the same or theoretically less risk of AKI compared with adults because nephrogenesis is complete in the pediatric population and their kidneys can recover from nephrotoxic insults as part of the natural maturation process. In addition, immature renal tubular transport in the neonatal and young infant period may prevent the initial toxic pathways of nephrotoxicity from occurring relative to older children.[45,49]

Although it is not clear whether neonatal drug-related AKI causes long-term chronic kidney disease, extrapolated data from AKI overall in preterm neonates and infants may suggest that drug-induced AKI could increase the risk of chronic kidney disease development. This potential risk is important for pharmacists because 86.9% of the neonatal and preterm infant population are exposed to nephrotoxic agents, with aminoglycosides (usually gentamicin), indomethacin, and vancomycin being the most frequent nephrotoxins.[51] All three of these medications are also in the top 20 of overall medications used in the NICU.[52] Other less common nephrotoxin exposures may include acyclovir, amphotericin B, and other antibiotics. It is also important to note that exposure is greater in lower weight neonates and infants and that there is a positive association between number of nephrotoxic medications per day and the maximum SCr increase.[51] This increased exposure and association suggests that NICU patients who are most vulnerable to kidney injury are exposed to the most nephrotoxic medications.

As with most AKI causes, determining which antibiotics are most likely to cause AKI has proven difficult because of the multifactorial nature of AKI. Studies in the NICU using multivariate logistic regression have found that maternal NSAID use and postnatal exposure to ibuprofen, ampicillin, and ceftazidime may increase the risk of AKI.[47,53] Pharmacists in the NICU should be aware of the nephrotoxic medications neonates are exposed to with an aim to minimize exposure as much as possible.

CRITICALLY ILL CHILDREN

In the PICU population, AKI can lead to longer hospitalizations and higher mortality.[54] In this population, multiple risk factors exist for AKI, and the data are conflicting regarding nephrotoxic drug exposure being an independent risk factor for AKI. One study from Canada using a multivariable adjusted regression model suggested nephrotoxic medications both before and during a PICU stay were risk factors for AKI (odds ratio, 3.37). In this analysis, 29 medications were considered nephrotoxins, including diuretics and penicillin.[55] Another study only found a correlation between nephrotoxic medication exposure and AKI on univariate analysis, but not on multivariate analysis after controlling for other factors. The medications considered nephrotoxic in this study were aminoglycosides, vancomycin, acyclovir, foscarnet, and calcineurin inhibitors.[56] The definition of a nephrotoxic medication used in a study appears to affect the independent relationship between nephrotoxic medication exposure and AKI incidence in the PICU. When analyzing medication classes as an independent predictor of AKI, exposure to

Table 5. Nephrotoxins Commonly Used in the Pediatric Population and Their Mechanism of Nephrotoxicity

Drug[a]	Proposed Mechanism	Comments
Antimicrobial Agents		
Acyclovir	Tubular obstruction	Hydration can help reduce incidence; incidence increases with dosage and age
Aminoglycosides	ATN	—
Amphotericin	ATN	Dose related for conventional formulation; lower incidence for lipid formulations
Colistimethate	Renal tubule toxicity because of oxidative stress	Dose related
Penicillins (nafcillin, piperacillin/tazobactam)	AIN, hypersensitivity reactions	Piperacillin/tazobactam and vancomycin combined increased risk of AKI
Trimethoprim/ sulfamethoxazole	AIN, Tubular obstruction, hypersensitivity reactions	Can cause falsely elevated SCr; true causative nephrotoxicity is debatable
Vancomycin	ATN	Widely debated causation as a single agent, but association is well accepted
Cardiovascular Agents		
Angiotensin-converting enzyme inhibitors (enalapril, captopril)	Prerenal	Initial increase SCr will occur, but should return to normal values
Corticosteroids IV	Decreased kidney perfusion	—
Vasopressors	Decreased kidney perfusion	—
Furosemide	AIN	Debated causation because also used to increase diuresis in AKI
Immunosuppressants/Oncologic Agents		
Cisplatin	ATN	—
Cyclosporine	Prerenal	—
Cisplatin	ATN	—
Cyclosporine	Prerenal	—
Ifosfamide	Tubular toxicity because of oxidative stress by metabolite	Higher incidence in children age < 5 years
Methotrexate	Tubular obstruction	—
Tacrolimus	Prerenal	—
Miscellaneous Agents		
IV contrast	ATN	Newer formulations have decreased incidence; dose related
IV immunoglobulin	Osmotic nephrotoxicity	Less toxicity when maltose is not in the formulation
Nonsteroidal anti-inflammatory drugs (e.g., ibuprofen, ketorolac, indomethacin)	Prerenal, ATN, AIN	—

[a]This list is not all inclusive, but more commonly used pediatric medications with high associations with nephrotoxicity were selected.
AIN = acute interstitial nephritis; AKI = acute kidney injury; ATN = acute tubular necrosis; IV = intravenous.

β-lactam antibiotics, glucocorticoids, NSAIDs, and opioids were determined to be medication classes independently associated with AKI occurrence in the PICU. Opioids are generally not considered nephrotoxic, and this finding may reflect a correlation versus causation.[57]

NONCRITICALLY ILL CHILDREN

Children who are not critically ill have a reported AKI rate of 5%–10% of all admitted children, and up to 33% in patients with two or more SCr measurements,[58,59] with medication exposure being an independent risk factor for development of AKI in pediatric patients. One study grouped 62 nephrotoxic medications into two categories: one included single-agent toxic medications; the other group included agents with potential toxicity in combination. Patients with advanced AKI were exposed more often to several of the medications thought to cause nephrotoxicity in combination. There was no difference in exposure between groups when individual agents were analyzed. Of note, regression analysis was not performed in this study.[59] In another study, patients with AKI had more nephrotoxic medication exposures, more days of medication exposure, and more medication doses versus patients without AKI. More nephrotoxic medication exposures also led to increased percentage of patients with nephrotoxicity. Amphotericin B, cisplatin, piperacillin/tazobactam, and vancomycin were commonly used in patients with AKI. On regression analysis, vancomycin and piperacillin/tazobactam were the only medications significantly associated with AKI, with piperacillin/tazobactam only being associated with the injury and failure AKI categories.[58] These studies suggest exposure to multiple nephrotoxic medications (usually three or more) greatly increased the odds of nephrotoxicity in non-critically ill patients and required increased monitoring.

MEDICATIONS THAT CAN INDUCE INJURY

Aminoglycosides. Aminoglycosides are historically thought of as potential nephrotoxins by causing acute tubular necrosis based on collection in the renal tubules. In general, aminoglycosides are not first-line treatment options if safer options are available, and these agents are generally avoided in patients with already apparent renal dysfunction. If used, serum drug monitoring is highly recommended together with use of the shortest effective duration of treatment. Nephrotoxicity is generally associated with serum trough concentrations, although it is difficult to ascertain if an elevated trough is a sign of renal toxicity or a sign that an aminoglycoside is causing renal toxicity. Total drug exposure and duration is also believed to correlate with aminoglycoside nephrotoxicity; however, this correlation is debated. Using once-daily dosing has theoretical advantages of achieving high peak concentration and has been shown in the cystic fibrosis population to potentially decrease nephrotoxicity development.[60] Although this strategy is recommended, the optimal dosage in pediatric patients is unclear.

In the pediatric population, aminoglycosides are still the mainstay of treatment for neonatal sepsis management and cystic fibrosis exacerbation management.[61,62] Nephrotoxicity is of concern for both patient populations and close monitoring should occur with aminoglycoside use. Aminoglycoside monitoring varies between institutions without standardized recommendations. To monitor for nephrotoxicity, trough concentration should be obtained in patients on treatment for more than 2–3 days to ensure that accumulation is not occurring. For conventional dosing and in the neonatal population, concentrations of tobramycin and gentamicin should generally be less than 2 mcg/mL before the next dose (amikacin is usually approximately 3 times higher). In the cystic fibrosis populations, goal troughs are still less than 2 mcg/mL for every 8 hour dosing, but are lower for every 12–24 hour dosing intervals, usually less than 1 mcg/mL.[63] Some institutions may also monitor the 24-hour area under the curve (AUC_{0-24}) to approximate overall drug exposure, but correlation of AUC_{0-24} ranges and nephrotoxicity are not well established.

Vancomycin. Vancomycin as a causative nephrotoxin has been debated for decades. As with aminoglycosides, early reports associated trough concentrations with the development of renal toxicity. However, it is difficult to ascertain if an elevated trough concentration is a sign of renal toxicity or a sign that vancomycin is causing renal toxicity. Others suggest AUC_{0-24} may also be related to nephrotoxicity.[64,65] In vitro models suggest nephrotoxicity can occur because of oxidative damage.[66]

Despite a lengthy debate about nephrotoxicity with vancomycin as a single agent, it is more readily accepted that vancomycin is associated with AKI and can be a cause when administered concomitantly with other nephrotoxins or in other nephrotoxic disease states. For example, the combination of vancomycin and piperacillin/tazobactam has recently been shown to increase the rates of AKI (3.9% with vancomycin alone vs. 23.6% when combined with piperacillin/tazobactam).[67] These two agents were the only medications on multivariate analysis to be risk factors for AKI as previously described in this chapter.[57] A recent study also suggested that AKI can occur with prolonged therapy in children when administered with acyclovir, amphotericin B, and piperacillin/tazobactam. However, on multivariate analysis, age younger than 1 year was the only risk factor significantly associated with AKI.[68] A study has correlated a trough of 15 mcg/mL or more (a commonly recommended trough target for drug efficacy) and an AUC_{0-24} greater than 800 mg/hr/L as possible predictors of nephrotoxicity. This study did control for PICU admission and concomitant nephrotoxins (all combined together), although did not assess the presence of hypotension.[65] Despite conflicting evidence suggesting independent correlations between specific vancomycin concentrations and AKI, general practice is to minimize concomitant nephrotoxin administration when possible and use the lowest effective dosage, concentration, and duration for the indication. At minimum, in patients on vancomycin therapy for more than 2–3 days, trough concentrations should be obtained to assess for potential nephrotoxicity. A definitive goal concentration to prevent toxicity is not currently established, but goals may range from less than 15–20 mcg/mL depending on the indication. Monitoring of vancomycin AUC_{0-24} could also be considered if feasible at a given institution.

Nonsteroidal anti-inflammatory drugs. Nonsteroidal anti-inflammatory drugs can cause AKI in 2.7% of pediatric patients.[69] The mechanism is generally because of decreasing the production of prostacyclin as a response to decreased blood flow, which in turn can lead to acute tubular necrosis or acute interstitial nephritis.[69,70] Some of the most commonly used medications in the pediatric population are NSAIDs such as ibuprofen, naproxen, indomethacin, and ketorolac. In 54% of patients with gastroenteritis and dehydration receiving ibuprofen, AKI occurred; patients with AKI were younger and received ibuprofen more often.[71] Parents who are advised to administer oral rehydration therapy to their children with diarrhea should also be advised to avoid the administration of ibuprofen. In both pediatric inpatients and outpatients, NSAID-induced AKI can occur and thus these agents should be considered nephrotoxic, especially with prolonged use.

PREVENTION AND MANAGEMENT STRATEGIES

The most established AKI prevention and management strategies center around avoiding nephrotoxins, especially combinations; monitoring for nephrotoxicity, such as via serum concentrations or renal function; removing nephrotoxins during AKI; and managing AKI complications. If AKI is suspected, one should avoid nephrotoxic combinations during initiation of drug treatment and remove nephrotoxic agents if possible. If an alternative is not available and nephrotoxin exposure cannot be avoided, then frequent monitoring of renal function markers—potentially daily in critically ill patients—and optimization of dosing based on drug concentrations may be required. Management for prevention and/or treatment of AKI depends on the underlying cause and includes maintaining renal perfusion, fluid and electrolyte balance, controlling blood pressure, treating anemia, providing adequate nutrition, adjusting medications for the degree of renal impairment, and initiating renal replacement therapy (RRT) when indicated. This section will review medications that may be used during AKI and complication-related managements strategies studied in the pediatric population.

PREVENTION OF AKI

There are some disease states and clinical situations in which the risk of AKI is known immediately and the risk factors are not easily modifiable. For some of these situations, treatment-related prevention strategies have been studied to decrease AKI incidence. One of the most common is intravenous contrast-induced AKI. Acetylcysteine, theophylline, and fenoldopam have been studied for the prevention of contrast-induced AKI. Whereas acetylcysteine is recommended by the KDIGO guidelines, data in pediatric patients are limited. Theophylline and fenoldopam have minimal supporting data for their routine use. The most consistent recommendations include using the lowest possible doses of contrast and using the lowest molar contrast media. In addition, appropriate isotonic hydration during and after the exposure is an established method for prevention.[20]

Hypoxic events in newborns also put these patients at a great risk for AKI. Adenosine can cause vasoconstriction in the afferent arterioles, and selective agonism or nonselective antagonism may have a role in preventing hypoxia-related AKI. Specific to the neonatal population, theophylline and aminophylline, which are nonselective adenosine 1- and 2-receptor blockers, have been studied to prevent AKI in newborns who experienced perinatal asphyxiation (e.g., requiring respiratory support shortly after birth). Use has led to significant decreases in SCr, β-2 microglobulin, and sodium excretion. Dosages have ranged from 5–8 mg/kg of theophylline once within the first hour of birth.[72,73] Aminophylline is recommended in the KDIGO guidelines and evidence does support its efficacy, although widespread implementation into practice is currently unknown.[20] Aminophylline given as 8 mg/kg/dose followed by a continuous infusion was also used in patients in the first 72 hours after cardiac surgery to prevent AKI, but this intervention did not find any decrease in AKI occurrence. Thus, use of aminophylline or theophylline for AKI prevention or treatment is currently limited to AKI prevention in asphyxiated newborns.

FLUID MANAGEMENT

Appropriate fluid management is an important aspect for optimal prevention and management of nearly all patients with AKI. Dehydration is considered an independent risk factor for development of AKI. This risk can be illustrated by the high prevalence of AKI in underdeveloped countries caused by severe dehydration with gastrointestinal illnesses.[75,76] For AKI mainly related to dehydration, fluid rehydration with oral rehydration solutions (if possible) or intravenous replacement typically using 0.9% sodium chloride (as a 10–20 mL/kg bolus for 1–2 doses, potentially followed by a maintenance continuous infusion) is the optimal management solution for these patients with additional details in the electrolytes section. Ensuring appropriate fluid intake and preventing dehydration is an AKI prevention strategy when a patient is known to be exposed to nephrotoxic medications or if a planned nephrotoxic event is set to occur (e.g., receiving contrast, acyclovir treatment, or undergoing an invasive surgery).

Alternatively, once an AKI event has started, both inadequate and excessive hydration must be avoided. Fluid overload during AKI has been correlated with worse outcomes and higher mortality in the pediatric and neonatal setting.[77,78] Although the true cause and effect are still uncertain, maintaining euvolemia during AKI is an acceptable practice. At least daily assessments of intake and output ratios and body weight changes must be performed to optimally manage fluid status during AKI. In pediatric critical care settings, the following formula is commonly used to determine the percentage of fluid overload[78,80,81]:

$$[(\text{fluid in [L]} - \text{fluid out [L]})/ \\ (\text{weight on admission to intensive care unit [kg]})] \times 100$$

Fluid overload of more than 15% has been associated with the need for RRT in the ICU setting.[81] For every 1% increase in severity of fluid overload during AKI, there is a 3% increased mortality; furthermore, fluid overload of more than 20%

before initiation of continuous renal replacement therapy (CRRT) has been shown to have an 8.5 times higher odds for mortality compared with fluid overload of less than 20%.[78] Thus, preventing fluid overload is an important measure when AKI occurs.

Minimization of unnecessary fluid intake is an underlying principle for managing fluid in AKI patients. Setting daily fluid intake goals based on intake and output ratios and weight changes should be done with all fluid intakes taken into account. Although no data suggest that this approach will make a difference in the AKI outcome, changing continuous infusion concentrations may impact total daily fluid intake by using higher concentration of medications, such as sedatives, analgesics, and parenteral nutrition.[82]

DIURETICS FOR FLUID MANAGEMENT

If fluid intake monitoring and restriction are not effectively managing the patient's fluid status, then pharmacologic agents may be used to control fluid status. The most commonly used agents are loop diuretics, mainly furosemide and bumetanide. Although treatment with furosemide has not been shown to decrease mortality or outcome, administration of furosemide is a common practice to promote diuresis in patients with AKI. If furosemide is to be used, a test dose is generally recommended to ensure increased diuresis. If there is no increase in diuresis, then treatment is generally not continued. The common intravenous dosage range is 1–2 mg/kg/dose up to 4 doses per day. If the patient is hemodynamically unstable, then continuous infusion furosemide may be preferred. Dosing is initiated at 0.05 mg/kg/hr and titrated to a maximum rate of 0.4 mg/kg/hr. Furosemide is generally not used for long durations during AKI and is only used to promote urine output and manage fluid overload. If third spacing or edema occurs and albumin concentrations are low (less than 2 mg/dL), albumin may be administered followed by furosemide. A common dosage regimen for this treatment is 1 g/kg administered over 1 hour, followed by furosemide 1 mg/kg/dose (maximum initial dose of 40 mg).[83] The data for this intervention in AKI are controversial, although it is common practice at some institutions. Mannitol is usually not used as a diuretic in AKI because of an increased risk of adverse effects, such as worsening AKI and increased plasma osmolality with resultant hyperkalemia and metabolic acidosis.

Although the use of "renal-dose" dopamine has been well established to be ineffective in adult patients, lack of benefit has not been established in pediatric patients. *Renal-dose dopamine* (1–5 mcg/kg/minute) is still used in some centers to promote diuresis in critically ill neonates, infants, and children. The diuretic effect of this intervention has not shown consistent results, with most of the benefits published for neonates.[84-87] This difference in benefit between neonates and adults may be because of the stimulation of β-receptors with lower doses of dopamine in neonates. Therefore, the improved urine output reported from renal-dose dopamine may be the result of improved cardiac output. Retrospective studies suggest benefit of maintaining urine output in the preterm period but no benefits in preventing AKI or AKI outcomes.[86] In the only randomized controlled trial to date, there was not a statistically significant impact on GFR or urine volume.[85] Fenoldopam is a short-acting dopamine-1 agonist that has also been studied to promote diuresis and/or prevent AKI. Most data, coming from the patients receiving cardiac surgery, suggest that fenoldopam administration does not affect the incidence of postsurgical need for RRT or development of AKI, although improvements in AKI biomarkers and diuretic use have been described.[88,89] The most concerning adverse effect of fenoldopam use is systemic hypotension. Although sometimes used in practice, fenoldopam and low-dose dopamine are not recommended by the KDIGO guidelines for AKI management or prevention. Other interventions such as nesiritide and a natriuretic peptide are not recommended by the KDIGO guidelines and generally are not used in the pediatric population.[49]

ELECTROLYTES FOR FLUID MANAGEMENT

Electrolyte management is extremely important in AKI. The two most pertinent electrolytes usually include potassium and sodium. Potassium is eliminated from the body by the kidneys and thus can reach life-threatening concentrations in AKI if not properly managed. Potassium should be removed from maintenance intravenous fluids when AKI is first noticed to prevent hyperkalemia. If a patient is still receiving enteral feedings, then feedings low in potassium should be used, such as Similac PM 60/40 (Abbott Laboratories Inc, Columbus, OH) in infants or Renalcal (Nestle Health Science, Bridgewater, NJ) in children. If hyperkalemia still occurs, then sodium polystyrene sulfonate may be used to prevent excessive potassium intake during AKI. Sodium bicarbonate, furosemide, calcium gluconate or chloride, albuterol, and insulin with dextrose are common agents used alone or in combination in the setting of clinically significant hyperkalemia, such as cardiac rhythm abnormalities (Table 6).[90] Hyponatremia is more common that hypernatremia during AKI, usually because of either renal salt wasting and/or a dilutional hyponatremia caused by fluid overload. If the serum sodium concentration is less than 125 mEq/L but greater than 120 mEq/L, then fluid restriction or water removal with dialysis should be considered and sodium should be corrected to at least 125 mEq/L by using the following equation:

$$[(125 - plasma\ sodium) \times (weight\ in\ kg) \times (0.6)] = mEq\ Na$$

This amount of sodium should be administered over several hours. If the patient is symptomatic or the serum sodium is less than 120 mEq/L, the sodium should be replaced more rapidly using sodium chloride 3% solution. Calcium and phosphate homeostasis may be of concern in AKI, but treatment is usually more pertinent for chronic kidney disease and can be managed with various different phosphate binders.

RENAL REPLACEMENT THERAPY

Renal replacement therapy is considered when all other AKI management options previously discussed in this chapter have been ineffective. The indications for RRT do not include an absolute urine output, but more importantly RRT is considered when patients have volume overload (10% to 20%

fluid excess), severe acidosis, hyperkalemia, uremia (blood urea nitrogen greater than 100 mg/dL), or symptoms of uremia (i.e., changes in mental status, such as confusion, reduced awareness, agitation, psychosis, seizures and coma). In addition, the inability to provide adequate nutrition because of fluid restriction is an indication for RRT. Other pediatric specific indications include inborn errors of metabolism and hyperammonemia. In recent years, the importance of volume overload in critically ill children has been investigated. In all studies, the degree of fluid overload at RRT initiation has been associated with increased mortality, independent of patient severity of illness.[80,91-93]

Modalities of RRT include peritoneal dialysis (PD), hemodialysis (HD), and CRRT. The selection of modality depends on the patient's physical condition, age, size, previous surgical procedures, and overall stability. There are no data to demonstrate that modality choice affects outcome in AKI, but different forms have specific advantages. Solute clearance is superior in HD, then in CRRT, followed by PD. Ultrafiltration can be achieved with all three forms of RRT, yet hemodynamic stability is better maintained with CRRT, followed by PD, then HD. Therefore, the clinician must determine the overall goal of RRT and the patient's individual characteristics to choose the safest modality for the patient. For example, PD is preferred in neonates because it can be technically challenging to obtain vascular access for HD or CRRT. Patients with rapid solute generation and/or urgency for solute removal (e.g., acute tumor lysis syndrome, inborn errors of metabolism, hyperammonemia, symptomatic hyperkalemia, or ingestion of dialyzable toxins) require intermittent HD or CRRT rather than PD. Lastly, patients who are hemodynamically unstable cannot tolerate high flow rates and rapid fluid removal; therefore, CRRT is the preferred modality for this population. A comparison of the primary clearance method between PD, HD, and CRRT is presented in Table 7. The choice of RRT based on indication is summarized in Table 8, and the advantages and disadvantages of each method are summarized in Table 9.

Table 6. Treatment of Hyperkalemia

Drug	Pediatric Dose (Maximum: Adult Dose)	Adult Dose	Route	Administration time (min)	Onset (min)	Length of effect (hr)	Comments	Adverse Effects
Calcium chloride 10%	20 mg/kg/dose	1–2 g	IV, IO	2–5	5	0.5–1	May repeat in 5 min if necessary	Burning at infusion site
Calcium gluconate 10%	60–100 mg/kg/dose	1–2 g	IV, IO	2–5	5	0.5–1	May repeat in 5 min if necessary	Burning at infusion site
Sodium bicarbonate	1–2 mEq/kg/dose	50–100 mEq	IV, IO	2–5	15–60 depending on patient's acid-base status	Various	May repeat every 5–10 min	Hypernatremia, metabolic alkalosis
50% Dextrose	1–2 mL/kg	50 mL	IV, IO	5	20	6	Administer with insulin	Hypoglycemia, hyperosmolarity, volume overload
10% Dextrose	5–10 mL/kg	250 mL	IV, IO	5	20	6	Administer with insulin	Hypoglycemia, hyperosmolarity, volume overload
Regular insulin	0.1–0.2 units/kg	5–10 units	IV, IO	5	20	2–6	Administer with glucose	Hypoglycemia, hyperosmolarity, volume overload
Kayexalate	1 g/kg	60 g	Oral or rectal	—	Oral: 60–120 hr Rectal: < 30 min	4–6	Effective, but slow	Nausea and vomiting
Albuterol	10–20 mg (use concentrated form, 5 mg/mL)	10–20 mg (use concentrated form, 5 mg/mL)	Inhale by nebulizer	10	30	2	Efficacy demonstrated in patients with renal insufficiency	Tachycardia, vasomotor flushing, mild tremor
Furosemide	1 mg/kg	40 mg	IV	1–2	5–30	4	Amount of K excretion is unreliable and does not correlate to furosemide dose	Volume depletion
Hemodialysis	2–4 hr	2–4 hr	—	—	—	—	Hypotension	Volume depletion

IO = intraosseous infusion; IV = intravenous.

PERITONEAL DIALYSIS

Peritoneal dialysis is the least expensive form of dialysis and requires no anticoagulation. It uses the capillaries of the peritoneal membrane for dialysis. The surface of the peritoneal membrane is larger in children versus adults. The dialysis prescription includes exchange volumes of 20 to 50 mL/kg (10 mL/kg at initiation to reduce the risk for leak), dwell times of 25 to 50 minutes, and drain times of 5 to 15 minutes. If a patient needs significant ultrafiltration, then either the volume per pass, the frequency of cycles, or the glucose concentration of the dialysate is increased to have a higher osmolar gradient for ultrafiltration. If a patient needs higher solute clearance in PD, then either the volume per pass is increased or the cycle numbers are decreased to prolong the time in the peritoneum for better solute clearance.[94] Close monitoring is required for patients with preload dependent cardiac physiology. The condition of these individuals will most likely be unstable with filling and draining. In addition, those with pulmonary compromise may have worsening of their symptoms because increased dialytic volumes prevent full diaphragmatic excursion. The biggest risk of PD is the development of peritonitis. However, this condition can be treated with the addition of antibiotics to the PD fluid.

After obtaining PD fluid for microbiologic testing, empiric antibiotic therapy should be started as soon as possible. In the absence of a positive Gram stain, empiric therapy should include antibiotics that cover both gram-negative and gram-positive bacteria. The choice of antibiotics should be determined by the prevalence and types of antibiotic-resistant bacterial isolates from patients with peritonitis in the PD program. Antibiotics should be administered intraperitoneally in most cases. For empiric coverage of gram-positive

bacteria, recommended drugs are cefazolin or vancomycin. In PD programs with a low incidence of methicillin-resistant *Staphylococcus aureus* species and enterococci, cefazolin would be preferred. In many programs, methicillin-resistant coagulase-negative staphylococci and methicillin-resistant *S. aureus* are common pathogens in patients with peritonitis, and vancomycin should be used initially, pending culture results. For empiric coverage of gram-negative bacteria, initial therapy should include a third-generation cephalosporin (ceftazidime or cefepime) or an aminoglycoside (gentamicin, tobramycin, or amikacin). Again, the choice of antibiotics for empiric gram-negative coverage is dependent on the species of bacteria and the prevalence and types of antibiotic-resistant pathogens in the PD program. Dosing of antibiotics in peritoneal fluid is based on the recommendations of the International Society for Peritoneal Dialysis.[95] Their recommendations are summarized in Table 10.

INTERMITTENT HEMODIALYSIS

Hemodialysis produces solute clearance via diffusion across a semipermeable membrane into a dialysate fluid. The high blood flow and dialysate flow rates make it the most rapid solute clearance and removal of extracellular fluid volume. The dialysate composition can easily be adjusted to treat electrolyte abnormalities. Compared with CRRT and PD, HD can provide substantial clearance in several hours, which allows the patient freedom from a machine for most of the day. However, rapid fluid removal over several hours may not be tolerated in the hemodynamically unstable patient. Initially HD is performed daily until the patient's electrolytes and fluid overload stabilize, then can be moved to a schedule of 3 days

Table 7. Predominant Clearance Methods of Renal Replacement Therapies

Technique	Convection	Diffusion	Key Variable Influencing Drug Removal
Intermittent hemodialysis	Negligible	Major	Blood flow rate
CAVH/CVVH	Major	—	Ultrafiltration rate
CAVHD/CVVHD	Negligible	Major	Dialysate flow
CAVHDF/CVVHDF	Marked	Marked	Dialysate flow/ultrafiltration rate

CAVH = continuous arteriovenous hemofiltration; CAVHD = continuous arteriovenous hemodialysis; CAVHDF = continuous arteriovenous hemodiafiltration; CVVH continuous venovenous hemofiltration; CVVHD = continuous venovenous hemodialysis; CVVHDF = continuous venovenous hemodiafiltration.

Table 8. Choice of Renal Replacement Therapy Based on Indication

Indication	Intermittent Hemodialysis	Continuous Renal Replacement Therapy	Peritoneal Dialysis
Hyperkalemia	Negligible	Negligible	Negligible
Symptomatic hyperkalemia	Some	Negligible	—
Uremia	Negligible	Negligible	Negligible
Acute tumor lysis	Negligible	Negligible	—
Inborn errors of metabolism—hyperammonemia	Negligible	Negligible	—
Toxins	Negligible	Negligible	—
Fluid overload	Negligible	Negligible	Negligible
Fluid overload—pulmonary edema/respiratory failure	Negligible	Negligible	—

per week to maintain homeostasis. The biggest risk of HD after hypotension is the development of disequilibrium syndrome. This condition develops because of the rapid removal of urea, which causes an osmotic gradient between plasma and the brain, resulting in cerebral edema and potential death.[94]

CONTINUOUS RENAL REPLACEMENT THERAPY

Advantages to CRRT include the ability to provide RRT in a critically ill child while maintaining hemodynamic stability; the ability to remove a large amount of volume over an extended amount of time; and the ability to limit the need for fluid restriction, which allows provision of essential medications and blood products as well as nutritional supplementation. Several CRRT modalities are available. *Continuous venovenous hemofiltration* (CVVH) refers to the use of replacement fluid for convective clearance. *Continuous venovenous hemodialysis* (CVVHD) is similar to intermittent HD and uses dialysate fluid for diffusion clearance. *Continuous venovenous hemodiafiltration* (CVVHDF) uses a combination of dialysate and replacement fluid for effective diffusion and convection clearance of solutes. A hemofilter may also be placed within an extracorporeal membrane oxygenation circuit to provide CVVH for patients receiving this therapy.

The CRRT circuit requires anticoagulation to maintain patency. This goal can be accomplished by the administration of heparin or citrate. Comparison data by Brophy and colleagues demonstrated similar outcomes in circuit life between the two anticoagulation protocols.[96] Citrate anticoagulation offers a benefit to the patient because it does not affect the bleeding risk. Citrate is delivered before filtering and binds calcium in the extracorporeal blood of the circuit, thus decreasing coagulation in both the intrinsic and extrinsic pathways. Calcium must be administered back to the patient, preferably in the form of calcium chloride, to decrease the risk of hypocalcemia to the patient. The citrate is infused at an infusion rate of 1.5 times the blood pump rate. The rate is adjusted to keep the circuit ionized calcium levels between 0.25 and 0.4 mg/dL whereas the systemic calcium infusion is titrated to maintain the patient's ionized calcium between 1.1 and 1.3 mg/dL. The risks for citrate anticoagulation include metabolic alkalosis and hypocalcemia.[97]

Significant clearance of amino acids can result from CRRT, and patients requiring CRRT typically have an increased protein requirement. One study found an 11% to 12% loss of dietary amino acids and a negative nitrogen balance in pediatric patients receiving CRRT, despite the delivery of 1.5 g/kg/day of protein over the goal for the patient's age and an increased kilocalorie delivery of 20% to 30% above resting

Table 9. Advantages and Disadvantages of Renal Replacement Therapies

Therapy	Peritoneal Dialysis	Hemodialysis	Continuous Venovenous Hemofiltration
Advantages	• Appropriate for patients with hemodynamic instability, multisystem organ failure requiring vasopressors, and congenital heart disease to preserve vascular access • Performed outside of the intensive care unit • Allows long-term dialysis • No anticoagulation required • Least expensive renal replacement therapy • Peritoneal catheter placement may be easier to achieve than reliable vascular access • Avoids use of blood products in potential transplant patients	• Provides rapid ultrafiltration or solute removal • Appropriate for hemodynamically stable patients • Appropriate for patients with toxic ingestions, drug toxicity, acute tumor lysis syndrome, hyperammonemia • Performed outside of the intensive care unit	• Mimics effect of renal function with continual ultrafiltration and solute clearance • Appropriate for patients with hemodynamic instability • Ability to separate ultrafiltration from solute removal
Disadvantages	• Preload dependent on cardiac physiology • Pulmonary compromise • Removal of immune globulins, which leads to increased risk of infection • Manual peritoneal dialysis is labor intensive and requires warm dialysate • Does not provide urgent clearance	• Requires vascular access in the small patient • Blood vessel stenosis or thrombosis possible • Subclavian catheter must be avoided because impossible to prevent fistula formation in the future • Dialysis disequilibrium • Limits nutrition provided to oliguric or anuric patients who need fluid restriction	• Complexity and expense vs. peritoneal dialysis or intermittent hemodialysis • Specialized nursing education required • Additional line required for regional citrate anticoagulation • Blood priming of the circuit required in patients who weigh < 10 kg • Bradykinin reaction possible with activation of complement-coagulation cascade

energy expenditure. Thus, assessment of kilocalorie needs by indirect calorimetry should be performed, and the administration of an additional 1 to 1.5 g/kg/day of protein over those suggested for the patient's age is recommended.[98]

ROLE OF THE PHARMACIST

Pharmacists should be involved at all stages of AKI, particularly in evaluating creatinine clearance in the early stages of AKI and working with the multidisciplinary team to adjust medication doses appropriately, in addition to monitoring serum electrolytes and making appropriate adjustments when necessary. Examples of interventions might include the addition of oral phosphate binders in patients eating a standard diet or changing the enteral formula in patients being fed enterally. It is essential that pharmacists be aware of different RRT modalities. Drug dosing can be significantly different depending on the modality used. For example, vancomycin may be dosed 3 days per week in a patient receiving intermittent HD but may require daily dosing in a patient on CVVH. Close attention to the RRT plan for the patient will allow the pharmacists to change dosing regimens when therapies are changed or discontinued. In addition, the pharmacists should be involved with a multidisciplinary team in setting up computerized provider order entry order sets for nursing and pharmacy orders for different RRTs. Lastly, the pharmacists should assure adequate protein and kilocalorie delivery either by enteral or parenteral nutrition based on the patient status. It is

Table 10. Intraperitoneal Antibiotic Dosing Recommendations for Treatment of Peritonitis

Antibiotics	Intermittent (1 Exchange Daily)	Continuous (All Exchanges)	
		Loading Dose	Maintenance Dose
Aminoglycosides			
Amikacin	2 mg/kg/day	25 mg/L	12 mg/L
Gentamicin	0.6 mg/kg/day	8 mg/L	4 mg/L
Netilmicin	0.6 mg/kg/day	—	10 mg/L
Tobramycin	0.6 mg/kg/day	3 mg/kg	0.3 mg/kg
Cephalosporins			
Cefazolin	10–20 mg/kg/day	500 mg/L	125 mg/L
Cefepime	1000 mg/day	250–500 mg/L	100–125 mg/L
Cefotaxime	500–1000 mg/day	—	—
Ceftazidime	1000–1500 mg/day	500 mg/L	125 mg/L
Ceftriaxone	1000 mg/day 2000 mg/day if > 80 kg	—	—
Penicillins			
Penicillin G	—	50,000 unit/L	25,000 unit/L
Ampicillin	—	—	125 mg/L
Ampicillin/Sulbactam	2 g every 12 hr	750–1000 mg/L	100 mg/L
Piperacillin/Tazobactam	—	4 g/0.5 g/L	1 g/0.125 gL
Others			
Aztreonam	2 g/day	1000 mg/L	250 mg/L
Ciprofloxacin	—	—	50 mg/L
Clindamycin	—	—	600 mg/bag
Daptomycin	—	100 mg/L	20 mg/L
Imipenem/Cilastatin	500 mg in alternate exchange	250 mg/L	50 mg/L
Polymyxin B	—	300,000 unit (30 mg)/bag	300,000 unit (30 mg)/bag
Meropenem	1 g/day	—	—
Vancomycin	15–30 mg/kg/every 5 to 7 days[a]	30 mg/kg OR 1000 mg	25 mg/L OR 1.5 mg/kg
Antifungals			
Fluconazole	IP 200 mg every 24 to 48 hr	—	—
Voriconazole	IP 2.5 mg/kg/day	—	—

[a]Redose vancomycin when levels reach about 15 mcg/mL.

essential that pharmacists work in a multidisciplinary practice model to monitor patients with AKI and provide education when necessary to assure the optimal care of the patient.

CONCLUSIONS

Acute kidney injury in children has many causes and is usually multifactorial. Identification and assessment of AKI is ideally performed by using pediatric- or neonatal-specific methods and tools such as the bedside Schwartz equation and the pRIFLE criteria. Prevention is mainly focused on avoiding multiple nephrotoxin exposures, and the primary treatment generally focuses on managing the underlying cause and removing nephrotoxic medications. Managing complications is a mainstay of AKI treatment, with the highest level of care requiring RRT. The choice of RRT modality depends on patient status and confounders because of the significant advantages and disadvantages for each method of RRT. Teamwork is essential for the provision of safe and efficient management of AKI and RRT in pediatric patients. Drug and nutritional clearance are affected by all degrees of AKI and all forms of RRT, and pharmacists must address these issues.

Patient Case — THE PERFECT STORM FOR ACUTE KIDNEY INJURY

A 3-year-old, 11.5-kg boy was admitted to the hospital 2 days ago and is now being evaluated after transfer to the pediatric intensive care unit (PICU). He has a history of prematurity (born at 25 weeks and 2 days of gestation) and perinatal asphyxiation resulting in acute kidney injury (AKI) and mild spastic cerebral palsy, global neurodevelopmental delay, and tracheostomy dependency. He requires nighttime total parenteral nutrition (TPN) as a result of necrotizing enterocolitis (for which about 25% of his small bowel was removed). His ileocecal valve is intact but he is unable to achieve toleration of full gastric tube enteral feedings.

Before admission, the patient was a permanent resident of a local pediatric long-term care institution because of his extensive daily health care maintenance needs. He has a history of recurrent pneumonias/tracheostomy infections and central line infections. He was transferred from the long-term care facility to the hospital 2 days ago because of inability to tolerate feeds (increased emesis and loose stools) and concerns for an infection/sepsis because of elevated temperature and increased oxygen requirements from baseline. On admission, cultures were drawn before initiation of antibiotics, and he was documented to receive nothing by mouth except medications. Blood pressures initially responded to a fluid bolus, but after 12 hours, the patient went into septic shock and became unresponsive to fluid boluses. He was transferred to the PICU, and a norepinephrine infusion was initiated.

Medications Prior to Admission:

Medication	Dose and Administration	Start Date	End Date	Currently Taking
Cetirizine (1 mg/mL)	2.5 mg (2.5 mL) PO at bedtime	2 yr ago	—	Yes
Fluticasone/Salmeterol 100 mcg/50 mcg	2 inhalations twice daily	2 yr ago	—	Yes
Albuterol nebulizer	4 times a day as needed for wheezing	2 yr ago	—	Yes
Ceftriaxone	800 mg IV every 24 hr for 7 days	5 days before admission	—	Yes
Calcium Carbonate suspension	375 mg calcium carbonate (150 mg elemental calcium) BID	1 yr ago	—	Yes
Clindamycin	150 mg IV every 8 hr for 7 days	5 days before admission	—	Yes
Ferrous sulfate	15 mg elemental iron NG TID	2 yr ago	—	—
Polyethylene glycol 3350	17 g NG BID	1 yr ago	—	—
Baclofen	5 mg NG TID	1 yr ago	—	—
Ciprofloxacin oral suspension	15 mg/kg/dose NG BID for 14 days	4 mo before admission	3.5 mo before admission	Completed
Multivitamin	Daily PO in morning	2 yr ago	—	Yes

BID = twice daily; NG = nasogastric tube; PO = oral; TID = three times daily.

Home nutrition: At baseline, 30% of calories provided by parenteral nutrition and 70% by enteral nutrition; intolerance of enteral nutrition for past 5 days; parenteral nutrition now being titrated to provide adequate caloric needs.

Immunizations: Up to date with receipt of this year's influenza vaccine

Code status: Full

Vital signs:

Sign	On Admission (2 days ago)	Today
BP	75/35 mm Hg	90/55 mm Hg
HR	150 beats/minute (bounding)	100 beats/minute
TMax	Oral: 39°C (102.2°F)	Rectal: 38.4°C (101°F)
RR	22 breaths/minute (ventilated)	20 breaths/minute (ventilated)
Wt	11.5 kg (1 wk before admission: 10.5 kg)	13.5 kg
Ht	34.25 inches	34.25 inches
SpO2	78%	95% (intubated)
Svo_2	71%	85%
Capillary refill	< 1 sec	< 1 sec

Physical examination:

Body System	Values and Findings
Total input/output past 24 hr	1700 mL/130 mL (including other outputs aside from urine)
Urine output past 24 hr	100 mL
Urine output past 12 hr	0 mL
Lines, drains, airways	Intubated, double-lumen peripherally inserted central catheter, arterial line, gastrostomy tube
General appearance	Intubated and sedated
Eyes	Pupils dilated, minimal reactivity to light
Ears	Tympanic membranes clear bilaterally
Throat	Clear mucus membranes, currently intubated
Neck	Moderate lymphadenopathy present
Lungs	Intubated, rails still noted
Heart	Regular rate and rhythm
Abdomen	Distended, bowel sounds faint, but noted
Musculoskeletal	Edematous, warm, dry extremities
Skin	Pitting edema noted; no pressure sores noted
Neurological	Adequately sedated, minimal pain reported per nursing

Laboratory findings:

Component	1 Wk Before Admission	On Admission (2 Days Ago)	Today	Range
Chemistries				
Glucose	95	150	190	60–110 mg/dL
BUN	17	38	75	8–19 mg/dL
Na	142	137	133	138–145 mEq/L
Potassium	4.2	3.5	6.3 (not hemolyzed)	3.4–5.2 mEq/L
Cl	98	99	97	98–107 mEq/L
CO_2	23	18	15	20–28 mEq/L
Anion gap	—	19	21	6–16 mEq/L

Laboratory findings: *(continued)*

Component	1 Wk Before Admission	On Admission (2 Days Ago)	Today	Range
Chemistries *(continued)*				
Creatinine, serum (isotope dilution mass spectrometry traceable)	0.18	0.57	2.1	0.20–0.70 mg/dL
Calcium	9.2	8.6	8.2	8.9–10.1 mg/dL
PO_4	5.3	5.4	6	3.8–5.5 mg/dL
Triglycerides	—	—	120	< 150 mg/dL
Albumin	3.1	3.0	2.9	3.5–5 g/dL
Ionized calcium	—	1.4	1.3	1.2–1.35 mg/dL
pH, arterial	—	7.32	7.29	7.35–7.45
Pco_2, arterial	—	38	36	33–43 mm Hg
Po_2, arterial	—	80	80	80–105 mm Hg
Tco_2, arterial	—	17	16	18–29 mEq/L
LDH	—	290	350	110–295 U/L
CRP	—	13.2	13.8	< 1.2 mg/L
Complete Blood Count With Differential				
WBC	12.1	19.8	18.8	$4.5–11 \times 10^3$ cells/mm^3
RBC	4.8	4.4	4.3	$4.30–5.10 \times 10^6$ cells/mm^3
Hgb	10.1	9.5	9.6	11.4–15.4 g/dL
HCT	41.3	38.8	37.2	36.0–49.0%
MCV	85.2	82.0	81.2	78.0–98.0 fL
MCH	29.0	28.0	26.5	26.0–34.0 pg
MCHC	33.2	34.0	33.1	32.0–35.0 g/dL
RDW	12.3	12.0	11.6	11.5–14.5%
Mean platelet volume	10.5	10.2	10.4	9.4–12.4 fL
Platelets	240	460	470	$150–450 \times 10^3$ cells/mm^3
Neutrophils	—	73.8	75.3	34.0–71.1%
Bands	—	14.9	13.2	5.0–11.0%
Lymphocytes	—	7.2	7.7	19.3–51.7%
Monocytes	—	3.1	2.8	3.0–13.0%
Eosinophils	—	0.8	0.7	0.7–5.8%
Basophils	—	0.2	0.3	0.1–1.2%

Laboratory findings: *(continued)*

Component	1 Wk Before Admission	On Admission (2 Days Ago)	Today	Range
Urinalysis				
Na	—	—	52	< 40 mEq/L
Cr	—	—	22 mg/dL	
Appearance	—	—	Brown, granular casts present	—
WBC	—		3+	Negative
RBC	—	—	2+	Negative
Protein	—	—	+	Negative
Glucose		—	1+	Negative
Toxicology				
Vancomycin serum concentration	—	—	75 ug/mL (5.5 hr after dose 8) 85 ug/mL (15 hr post dose 8; dose 9 held)	—

Diagnostic tests on current admission:

Cultures		
Source	**Organism**	**Resistance, Susceptibilities, and Comments**
Blood: Central line lumen 1	*Pseudomonas aeruginosa*	Resistant to ciprofloxacin, gentamicin Susceptible to colistin, tobramycin, amikacin, meropenem, ceftazidime, cefepime, and piperacillin/tazobactam
Blood: Central line lumen 2	*P. aeruginosa*	Same as for lumen 1
Blood: Peripheral stick	*P. aeruginosa*	Same as for lumen 1
Tracheostomy aspirate	Gram-negative rods and mixed respiratory flora	Preliminary
Other Tests	**Findings and Comments**	
Chest radiograph	Extensive pulmonary edema with new focal infiltrates consistent with right lower lobe and right upper lobe pneumonia	
ECG	Mild peaked T waves noted; QT interval slightly decreased	

Diagnostic tests from previous admissions:

Cultures		
Source	**Organism**	**Resistance, Susceptibilities, and Comments**
Blood: Central line	*P. aeruginosa*, methicillin-susceptible *Staphylococcus aureus*	*P. aeruginosa*: Resistant to aminoglycosides, except amikacin; Susceptible to cefepime, ceftazidime, colistimethate, carbapenems, and piperacillin/tazobactam *S. aureus*: Susceptible to penicillin, nafcillin, clindamycin, vanomycin, and linezolid
Blood: Peripheral lines	Methicillin-susceptible *S. aureus*	Susceptible to penicillin, nafcillin, vancomycin, linezolid
Tracheostomy aspirate	*P. aeruginosa*, methicillin-susceptible *S. aureus*	*P. aeruginosa* and *S. aureus*: same susceptibilities as blood culture

Medications since admission:

Completed Medications	
0.9% NaCl	200-mL bolus times 3 on admission
Piperacillin/Tazobactam	1200 mg piperacillin component IV once over 30 minutes
Vancomycin	5 mg/mL in dextrose 5% in water premixed 175 mg IV once over 1 hr
Midazolam	5 mg/mL IV continuous infusion, maximum rate of 0.16 mg/kg/hr
Fentanyl	10 mcg/mL IV continuous infusion, maximum rate of 4 mcg/kg/hr
Norepinephrine	16 mcg/mL IV continuous infusion, maximum rate of 0.4 mcg/kg/min
Furosemide	10 mg/mL 0.5 mg/kg/dose IV every 6 hr
Albumin	1 g/kg/dose IV over 4 hr administered every 6 hr followed by furosemide
Active Medications	
Acetaminophen	160 mg/5 mL for 150 mg by NG tube every 6 hr as needed for fever > 38°C (100.4°F)
Ibuprofen	100 mg PO every 6 hr
Albuterol 0.083%	2.5 mg/mL nebulization solution by ET tube every 6 hr
Albuterol 0.083%	2.5 mg/mL nebulization solution by ET tube every 3 hr as needed
Baclofen	5 mg by NG tube BID
Calcium chloride	100 mg/mL for 10 mg/kg IV every 3 hr as needed by central line (for ionized calcium < 1.2)
Furosemide	Continuous infusion 2 mg/mL for 0.15 mg/kg/hr
Midazolam	5 mg/mL IV continuous infusion 0.1 mg/kg/hr
Midazolam	5 mg/mL for 0.1 mg/kg/dose, every hour as needed (2 doses in past 24 hours)
Fentanyl	10 mcg/mL in NS as continuous infusion at 2 mcg/kg/hr
Fentanyl	10 mcg/mL in NS for 2 mcg/kg/dose every hour as needed (3 doses in the past 24 hours)
Piperacillin/Tazobactam	1200 mg piperacillin component every 8 hr IV over 30 min
Norepinephrine	16 mcg/mL in dextrose 5% in water for IV continuous infusion at 0.1 mcg/kg/min
Ranitidine	25 mg/mL for 30 mg IV every 8 hr
Vancomycin	5 mg/mL in dextrose 5% in water premixed for 175 mg IV every 6 hr, given over 1 hr
Total parenteral nutrition	Running at 45 mL/hr: Dextrose 15 g/kg/day Amino acids 1.5 g/kg/day Potassium Cl 5 mEq/kg/day Na acetate 2 mEq/kg/day NaPO$_4$ 0.5 mmol/kg/day Ca gluconate 0.5 mEq/kg/day Heparin 1 unit/mL Standard trace elements and multivitamins
Lipids	1.5 g/kg/day

BID = twice daily; ET = endotracheal tube; IV = intravenous; NG = nasogastric; NS = normal saline; PO = oral.

1. What risk factors does this patient have for developing AKI?

This patient's AKI is likely multifactorial. The history of neonatal AKI, prematurity, and birth asphyxiation likely caused this patient to have slightly decreased renal function at baseline, and AKI may be in addition to chronic renal disease. The possible reasons for the acute change are the combination of vancomycin plus piperacillin/tazobactam, sepsis, hypotension, use of vasopressor agents, and possible dehydration because of diarrhea and vomiting.

2. At what stage of AKI was this patient on admission and today?

The bedside Schwartz equation is likely not accurate for this patient because of his underlying chronic disease state, which predisposes him to nutritional deficiencies, creating a falsely decreased SCr because of lack of muscle stores. His SCr on admission is 0.57 mg/dL, which is normal for his age but more than 3 times his baseline (0.18 mg/dL). Thus, Acute Kidney Injury Network or Kidney Disease Improving Global Outcomes criteria may be best used in this patient. Using the Schwartz equation, the patient's clearance would be estimated at about 200 mL/min/1.73 m² at baseline and 63 mL/min/1.73 m² on admission. However, the patient's renal function is likely worse than the equation estimates. On admission, the patient has a more than 3-fold increase in SCr from baseline and a urine output of less than 0.5 mL/kg/hr for 24 hours placing the patient in stage 3 AKI or failure on admission. On day 2, the patient's SCr increases and he is anuric for the past 12 hours, placing him clearly in stage 3 AKI or kidney failure.

3. What medication changes are best to recommend for this patient to manage the AKI?

The following medications and management plan should be considered for this patient.

- Initiate treatment for hyperkalemia.
- Calcium chloride 20 mg/kg/dose (230 mg) intravenous should be administered to stabilize the heart.
- Because the patient's pH is 7.29, the administration of sodium bicarbonate 1 mEq/kg intravenous once will shift the potassium back into the cell. Other options include the following: administration of sodium polystyrene sulfonate 1 g/kg/dose oral or rectal once; albuterol 10 mg nebulized once for removal of potassium, or a combination of dextrose and insulin to also shift potassium back into the cell. Furosemide would be ineffective because the patient is anuric.
- Vancomycin should be discontinued.
- The current TPN should be stopped because it contains potassium and phosphate (which could precipitate with IV calcium when administered). It can be replaced with clear fluids of similar dextrose and sodium content until a new TPN is made. The new fluids and subsequent TPN should likely be decreased to a rate of about 75% maintenance. If anuria persists, and renal replacement therapy (RRT) is not initiated, then the rate should be decreased to insensible or 30% maintenance. For the new TPN, potassium and possibly phosphate should be removed and zinc and selenium dosages should be decreased to prevent accumulation.
- The optimal antimicrobial regimen is likely renally dosed cefepime at 50 mg/kg/dose (575 mg) intravenous every 48 hours or ceftazidime 50 mg/kg/dose (575 mg) every 48 hours. If the tracheostomy aspirate culture is finalized and includes methicillin-susceptible *S. aureus* and there is still a suspicion for pneumonia, cefepime would be preferred to also treat this pathogen. The patient should be treated as having a creatinine clearance of less than 10 mL/min no matter what the bedside Schwartz equation estimates are because his creatinine clearance has been 0 for 12 hours.
- Serum glucose is 190 mg/dL; therefore, if hyperglycemia persists, then an insulin initiation may be considered. Dosing could be started at 0.03–0.05 units/kg/hr to avoid accumulation in renal failure and titrated as needed for a goal glucose of 150–200 mg/dL.

- All continuous infusions should be concentrated. If blood pressure is stable, then vasopressor agents should be weaned to discontinuation if possible.
- Furosemide infusion should be discontinued because the patient has remained anuric for 12 hours, despite the infusion, and there is a risk for ototoxicity with the accumulation of furosemide. Albumin should also be discontinued.
- With acidosis, uremia, and hyperkalemia plus anuria present for 12 hours, RRT should be considered.
- Ibuprofen should be discontinued.
- Ranitidine should be renally adjusted to a dose of 1 mg/kg/dose intravenously every 24 hours.
- Baclofen usage during AKI should be reconsidered based on this patient's spastic issues. It is renally eliminated and can also cause urinary retention. Dosage should be weaned to once daily to avoid baclofen withdrawal seizures.
- The midazolam infusion should be changed to scheduled lorazepam to avoid accumulation of the midazolam active metabolites. This switch will not be necessary if RRT is initiated. Monitoring for propylene glycol toxicity may be needed when using lorazepam.

Case (continued). Now, 24 hours later, the patient is still oliguric. His weight is now 14 kg and SCr is 2.7 mg/dL, and he has not responded to attempts to manage hyperkalemia—his potassium is 6.7 and electrocardiogram abnormalities are worsening. He remains on norepinephrine at 0.1 mcg/kg/min. Because of persistent metabolic abnormalities, severe fluid overload, and progressing AKI, RRT is initiated.

4. Which form of RRT is optimal for this patient?

Continuous renal replacement therapy (CRRT) would be ideal in this patient because he still has some hemodynamic instability. He most likely would not tolerate the rapid fluid changes seen with intermittent hemodialysis.

5. The patient is still receiving the anti-infective agents recommended in Question 3. What dosage would you recommend if the patient is started on RRT?

For cefepime the dosage should be 50 mg/kg/dose intravenously every 12 hours. For ceftazidime the dosage should be 50 mg/kg/dose intravenously every 12 hours. These drugs are the preferred agents for treatment of the infection; other agents are less ideal.

6. What changes in macronutrient nutrition may be needed in the patient's TPN?

Protein needs are increased during CRRT, so the protein component should be increased by 1— 1.5 g/kg/day. Triglycerides typically accumulate in patients on vasopressor infusions; therefore, triglyceride levels should be monitored daily and the fat emulsion decreased if needed. In addition, it is important to continue to monitor point of care glucose and to initiate an insulin infusion if the patient meets the criteria discussed previously.

REFERENCES

1. Ellis D, Gartner C, Galvis AG. Acute renal failure in infants and children: diagnosis, complications and treatment. Crit Care Med 1981;9:607-17.

2. Karlowicz MG, Adelman RD. Acute renal failure in the neonate. Clin Perinatology 1992;19:139-58.

3. Sehie A, Chesney RW. Acute renal failure: diagnosis. Pediatr Rev 1995;16:10-106.

4. Stewart CL, Barnett R. Acute renal failure in infants, children and adults. Crit Care Clin 1997;13:575-90.

5. Airede A, Bello M, Weeraninghe HD. Acute renal failure in the newborn: incidence and outcome. J Paediatr Child Health 1997;33:246-9.

6. Flynn JT. Causes, management approaches, and outcomes of acute renal failure in children. Curr Opin Pediatr 1998;10:184-9.

7. Sutherland SM, Ji J, Sheikhi FH, et al. AKI in hospitalized children: epidemiology and clinical associations in a national cohort. Clin J Am Soc Nephrol 2013;8:1661-9.

8. Kaddourah A, Basu RK, Bagshaw SM, et al. Epidemiology of acute kidney injury in critically ill children and young adults. N Engl J Med 2017;376:11-20.

9. Fitzgerald JC, Basu RK, Akcan-Arikan A, et al. Acute kidney injury in pediatric severe sepsis: an independent risk factor for death and new disability. Crit Care Med 2016;44:2241-50.

10. Brown, JR, Hisey WM, Marshall EJ. Acute kidney injury severity and long-term readmission and mortality after cardiac surgery. Ann Thorac Surg 2016;102:1482-9.

11. Wong JH, Selewski DT, Yu S, et al. Severe acute kidney injury following stage I Norwood palliation: effects on outcomes and risk of severe acute kidney injury at subsequent surgical stages. Pediatr Crit Care Med 2016;17:615-23.

12. Schneider J, Khemani R, Grushkin G, et al. Serum creatinine as stratified in the RIFLE score for acute kidney injury is associated with mortality and length of stay for children in the pediatric intensive care unit. Crit Care Med 2010;38:933-9.

13. Bellomo R, Kellum J, Ronco C. Acute renal failure. Time for consensus. Intensive Care Medicine 2001;27:1685-8.

14. Chertow GM, Burdick E, Honour M, et al. Acute kidney injury, mortality, length of stay, and costs in hospitalized patients. J Am Soc Nephrol 2005;16:3365-70.

15. Price JF, Mott AR, Dickerson HA, et al. Worsening renal function in children hospitalized with decompensated heart failure: evidence for a pediatric cardiorenal syndrome? Pediatr Crit Care Med 2008;9:279-84.

16. Ronco C, Kellum JA, Mehta R. Acute Dialysis Quality Initiative: the New York conference. Curr Opin Crit Care. 2002;8:502-4.

17. Bellomo R, Ronco C, Kellum JA, et al. Acute renal failure—definition, outcome measures, animal models, fluid therapy and information technology needs: the second international consensus conference of the acute dialysis quality initiative (ADQI) group. Crit Care 2004;8:R204-12.

18. Mehta RL, Kellum JA, Shah SV, et al. Acute kidney injury network: report of an initiative to improve outcomes in acute kidney injury. Crit Care 2007;11:R31.

19. Ackan-Arikan A, Zappitelli M, Loftis LL, et al. Modified RIFLE criteria in critically ill children with acute kidney injury. Kidney Int 2007;71:1028-35.

20. Kellum JA, Lamiere N, Aspelin P, et al. Kidney disease: Improving global outcomes (KDIGO) clinical practice guideline for acute kidney injury. Kidney Int 2012;2:1-138.

21. Jetton JG, Askenazi DJ. Acute kidney injury in the neonate. Clin Perinatol 2014;41:487-502.

22. Selewski DT, Charlton JR, Jetton JG, et al. Neonatal acute renal injury. Pediatrics 2015;136:e463-73.

23. Koralkar R, Ambalavanan N, Levitan EB, et al. Acute kidney injury reduces survival in very low birth weight infants. Pediatr Res 2011;69:354-8.

24. Viswsanathan S, Manyam B, Azhibekov T, et al. Risk factors associated with acute kidney injury in extremely low birth weight (ELBW) infants. Pediatr Nephrol 2012;27:303-11.

25. Mathur NB, Agarwal HS, Maria A. Acute renal failure in neonatal sepsis. Indian J Pediatr 2006;73:499-502.

26. Askenazi DJ, Koralkar R, Hadley HE, et al. Fluid overload and mortality are associated with acute kidney injury in sick near-term/term neonate. Pediatr Nephrol 2013;28:661-6.

27. Carmondy JB, Swanson JR, Rhone ET, et al. Recognition and reporting of AKI in very low birth weight infants. Clin J Am Soc Nephrol 2014;9:2036-43.

28. Zachwieja K, Korohoda P, Kwinta-Rybicka, et al. Which equations should and which should not be employed in calculating eGFR in Children? Advances in Medical Sciences 2015;60:31-40.

29. Srivasastava T, Alon US, Althahabi R et al. Impact of standardization of creatinine methodology on assessment of glomerular filtration rate in children. Pediatr Res 2009;65:113-6.

30. Hoste L, Dubourg L, Selistre L, et al. A new equation to estimate the glomerular filtration rate in children, adolescents and young adults. Nephrol Dial Transplant 2014;29:1082-91.

31. Blufpand HN, Westland R, van Wijk JAE, et al. Height-independent estimation of glomerular filtration rate in children: an alternative to the Schwartz equation. J Pediatr 2013;16:1722-7.

32. Schwartz GJ, Haycock GB, Edelmann CM Jr, et al. A simple estimate of glomerular filtration rate in children derived from body length and plasma creatinine. Pediatrics 1976;58:259-63.

33. Schwartz GJ, Munoz A, Schneider MF, et al. New equation to estimate GFR in children with CKD. J Am Soc Nephrol 2009;20:629-37.

34. Schwartz GJ, Work DF. Measurement and estimation of GFR in children and adolescents. Clin J Am Soc Nephrol 2009;4:1832-43.

35. Staples A, LeBlond R, Eatkins S, et al. Validation of the revised Schwartz estimating equation in a predominately non-CKD population. Pediatr Nephrol 2010;25:2321-26.

36. Arant BS. Postnatal development of renal function during the first year of life. Pediatr Nephrol 1987;1:308-13.

37. Pasala S, Carmody JB. How to use… serum creatinine, cystatin C and GFR. Arch Dis Child Educ Pract Ed 2017;102:37-43.

38. Schwartz GJ, Schneider MG, Paula SM, et al. Improved equations estimating GFR in children with chronic kidney disease using an immunonephelometric determination of cystatin C. Kidney International 2012;82:445-53.

39. Mussap M, Noto A, Fanos V, et al. Emerging biomarkers and metabolomics for assessing toxic nephropathy and acute kidney injury (AKI) in neonatology. Biomed Res Int 2014;2014:602526.

40. Mishra J, Dent C, Tarabishi R, et al. Neutrophil gelatinase-associated lipocalin (NGAL) as a biomarker for acute renal injury after cardiac surgery. Lancet 2005;365:1231-8.

41. Zappitelli M, Washburn KK, Arikan AA, et al. Urine neutrophil gelatinase-associated lipocalin is an early marker of acute kidney injury in critically ill children: A prospective cohort study. Crit Care 2007;11:R84.

42. McCaffrey J, Coupes B, Chaloner C, et al. Towards a biomarker panel for the assessment of AKI in children receiving intensive care. Pediatr Nephrol 2015;30:1861-71.

43. Zwiers AJ, de Wildt SN, van Rosmalen J, et al. Urinary neutrophil gelatinase-associated lipocalin identifies critically ill young children with acute kidney injury following intensive care admission: A prospective cohort study. Crit Care 2015;19:181.

44. Askenazi DJ, Koralkar R, Hundley HE, et al. Urine biomarkers predict acute kidney injury in newborns. J Pediatr 2012;161:270-5.

45. Suzuki M. Children's toxicology from bench to bed—drug-induced renal injury (4): Effects of nephrotoxic compounds on fetal and developing kidney. J Toxicol Sci 2009;34:SP267-71.

46. Carmody JB, Swanson JR, Rhone ET, et al. Recognition and reporting of AKI in very low birth weight infants. Clin J Am Soc Nephrol 2014;9:2036-43.

47. Cataldi L, Leone R, Moretti U, et al. Potential risk factors for the development of acute renal failure in preterm newborn infants: A case-control study. Arch Dis Child Fetal Neonatal Ed 2005;90:F514-9.

48. Zaffanello M, Bassareo PP, Cataldi L, et al. Long-term effects of neonatal drugs on the kidney. J Matern Fetal Neonatal Med 2010;23:87-9.

49. Hanna MH, Askenazi DJ, Selewski DT. Drug-induced acute kidney injury in neonates. Curr Opin Pediatr 2016;28:180-7.

50. Carmody JB, Charlton JR. Short-term gestation, long-term risk: Prematurity and chronic kidney disease. Pediatrics 2013;131:1168-79.

51. Rhone ET, Carmody JB, Swanson JR, et al. Nephrotoxic medication exposure in very low birth weight infants. J Matern Fetal Neonatal Med 2014;27:1485-90.

52. Hsieh EM, Hornik CP, Clark RH, et al. Medication use in the neonatal intensive care unit. Am J Perinatol 2014;31:811-21.

53. Cuzzolin L, Fanos V, Pinna B, et al. Postnatal renal function in preterm newborns: A role of diseases, drugs and therapeutic interventions. Pediatr Nephrol 2006;21:931-8.

54. Naik S, Sharma J, Yengkom R, et al. Acute kidney injury in critically ill children: Risk factors and outcomes. Indian J Crit Care Med 2014;18:129-133.

55. Slater MB, Gruneir A, Rochon PA, et al. Risk factors of acute kidney injury in critically ill children. Pediatr Crit Care Med 2016;17:e391-8.

56. Bailey D, Phan V, Litalien C, et al. Risk factors of acute renal failure in critically ill children: A prospective descriptive epidemiological study. Pediatr Crit Care Med 2007;8:29-35.

57. Glanzmann C, Frey B, Vonbach P, et al. Drugs as risk factors of acute kidney injury in critically ill children. Pediatr Nephrol 2016;31:145-51.

58. Moffett BS, Goldstein SL. Acute kidney injury and increasing nephrotoxic-medication exposure in noncritically-ill children. Clin J Am Soc Nephrol 2011;6:856-63.

59. McGregor TL, Jones DP, Wang L, et al. Acute kidney injury incidence in noncritically ill hospitalized children, adolescents, and young adults: A retrospective observational study. Am J Kidney Dis 2016;67:384-90.

60. Smyth A, Tan KH, Hyman-Taylor P, et al. Once versus three-times daily regimens of tobramycin treatment for pulmonary exacerbations of cystic fibrosis—the TOPIC study: A randomised controlled trial. Lancet 2005;365:573-8.

61. Flume PA, Mogayzel PJ Jr, Robinson KA, et al; Clinical Practice Guidelines for Pulmonary Therapies Committee. Cystic fibrosis pulmonary guidelines: treatment of pulmonary exacerbations. Am J Respir Crit Care Med 2009;180:802-8.

62. Polin RA; Committee on Fetus and Newborn. Management of neonates with suspected or proven early-onset bacterial sepsis. Pediatrics 2012;129:1006-15.

63. Prescott WA, Nagel JL. Extended-interval once-daily dosing of aminoglycosides in adult and pediatric patients with cystic fibrosis. Pharmacotherapy 2010;30:95-108.

64. Elyasi S, Khalili H, Dashti-Khavidaki S, et al. Vancomycin-induced nephrotoxicity: Mechanism, incidence, risk factors and special populations. A literature review. Eur J Clin Pharmacol 2012;68:1243-55.

65. Le J, Ny P, Capparelli E, et al. Pharmacodynamic characteristics of nephrotoxicity associated with vancomycin use in children. J Pediatric Infect Dis Soc 2015;4:e109-16.

66. King DW, Smith MA. Proliferative responses observed following vancomycin treatment in renal proximal tubule epithelial cells. Toxicol In Vitro 2004;18:797-803.

67. McQueen KE, Clark DW. Does combination therapy with vancomycin and piperacillin-tazobactam increase the risk of nephrotoxicity versus vancomycin alone in pediatric patients? J Pediatr Pharmacol Ther 2016;21:332-8.

68. Knoderer CA, Gritzman AL, Nichols KR, et al. Late-occurring vancomycin-associated acute kidney injury in children receiving prolonged therapy. Ann Pharmacother 2015;49:1113-9.

69. Misurac JM, Knoderer CA, Leiser JD, et al. Nonsteroidal anti-inflammatory drugs are an important cause of acute kidney injury in children. J Pediatr 2013;162:1153-9.

70. Patzer L. Nephrotoxicity as a cause of acute kidney injury in children. Pediatr Nephrol 2008;23:2159-73.

71. Balestracci A, Ezquer M, Elmo ME, et al. Ibuprofen-associated acute kidney injury in dehydrated children with acute gastroenteritis. Pediatr Nephrol 2015;30:1873-8.

72. Bhat MA, Shah ZA, Makhdoomi MS, et al. Theophylline for renal function in term neonates with perinatal asphyxia: A randomized, placebo-controlled trial. J Pediatr 2006;149:180-4.

73. Jenik AG, Ceriani Cernadas JM, Gorenstein A, et al. A randomized, double-blind, placebo-controlled trial of the effects of prophylactic theophylline on renal function in term neonates with perinatal asphyxia. Pediatrics 2000;105:E45.

74. Axelrod DM, Sutherland SM, Anglemyer A, et al. A double-blinded, randomized, placebo-controlled clinical trial of aminophylline to prevent acute kidney injury in children following congenital heart surgery with cardiopulmonary bypass. Pediatr Crit Care Med 2016;17:135-43.

75. Anochie IC, Eke FU. Acute renal failure in Nigerian children: Port Harcourt experience. Pediatr Nephrol 2005;20:1610-4.

76. Olowu WA, Adelusola KA. Pediatric acute renal failure in southwestern Nigeria. Kidney Int 2004;66:1541-8.

77. Foland JA, Fortenberry JD, Warshaw BL, et al. Fluid overload before continuous hemofiltration and survival in critically ill children: A retrospective analysis. Crit Care Med 2004;32:1771-6.

78. Sutherland SM, Zappitelli M, Alexander SR, et al. Fluid overload and mortality in children receiving continuous renal replacement therapy: The prospective pediatric continuous renal replacement therapy registry. Am J Kidney Dis 2010;55:316-25.

79. Askenazi DJ, Koralkar R, Hundley HE, et al. Fluid overload and mortality are associated with acute kidney injury in sick near-term/term neonate. Pediatr Nephrol 2013;28:661-6.

80. Wald EL, Finer G, McBride ME, et al. Fluid management: Pharmacologic and renal replacement therapies. Pediatr Crit Care Med 2016;17:S257-65.

81. Sinitsky L, Walls D, Nadel S, et al. Fluid overload at 48 hours is associated with respiratory morbidity but not mortality in a general PICU: Retrospective cohort study. Pediatr Crit Care Med 2015;16:205-9.

82. Sutherland A, Jemmett E, Playfor S. The impact of fixed concentrations sedation infusions on fluid overload in critically ill children. Arch Dis Child 2016;101:e2.

83. Duffy M, Jain S, Harrell N, et al. Albumin and furosemide combination for management of edema in nephrotic syndrome: A review of clinical studies. Cells 2015;4:622-30.

84. Jetton JG, Sorenson M. Pharmacological management of acute kidney injury and chronic kidney disease in neonates. Semin Fetal Neonatal Med 2017;22:109-115.

85. Prins I, Plotz FB, Uiterwaal CS, et al. Low-dose dopamine in neonatal and pediatric intensive care: A systematic review. Intensive Care Med 2001;27:206-10.

86. Crouchley JL, Smith PB, Cotten CM, et al. Effects of low-dose dopamine on urine output in normotensive very low birth weight neonates. J Perinatol 2013;33:619-21.

87. Cuevas L, Yeh TF, John EG, et al. The effect of low-dose dopamine infusion on cardiopulmonary and renal status in premature newborns with respiratory distress syndrome. Am J Dis Child 1991;145:799-803.

88. Ricci Z, Stazi GV, Di Chiara L, et al. Fenoldopam in newborn patients undergoing cardiopulmonary bypass: Controlled clinical trial. Interact Cardiovasc Thorac Surg 2008;7:1049-53.

89. Ricci Z, Luciano R, Favia I, et al. High-dose fenoldopam reduces postoperative neutrophil gelatinase-associated lipocaline and cystatin C levels in pediatric cardiac surgery. Crit Care 2011; 15:R160.

90. Andreoli SP. Management of acute kidney injury in children: A guide for pediatricians. Paediatr Drugs 2008;10:379-90.

91. Goldstein SL, Currier H, Graf CD, et al. Outcomes in children receiving continuous venous hemofiltration. Pediatrics 2001; 107:1309-12.

92. Modem V, Thompson M, Gollhofer D, et al. Timing of continuous renal replacement therapy and mortality in critically ill children. Crit Care Med 2014;42:943-53.

93. Selewski DT, Cornell TT, Lombel RM, et al. Weight-based determination of fluid overload status and mortality in pediatric intensive care unit patients requiring continuous replacement therapy. Intensive Care Medicine 2011;37:1166-73.

94. Smoyer WE, Maxvold NJ, Remenapp R. Renal replacement therapy in pediatric critical care. In: Fuhrman BP, Zimmerman JJ, eds. Pediatric Critical Care Medicine, 2nd ed. St Louis, MO: Mosby, 1998:764-78.

95. Li PK, Szeto CC, Piraino B, et al. ISPD peritonitis recommendations: 2016 update on prevention and treatment. Perit Dial Int 2016;36:481-508.

96. Brophy PD, Somers MJ, Baum MA, et al. Multi-center evaluation of anticoagulation in patients receiving continuous renal replacement therapy (CRRT). Nephrol Dial Transplant 2005;20:1416-21.

97. Bunchman TE, Maxvold NJ, Brophy PD. Pediatric convective hemofiltration (CVVH): normocarb replacement fluid and citrate anticoagulation. AM J Kidney Dis 2003;42:1248-52.

98. Maxvold NJ, Smoyer WE, Custer JR, et al. Amino acid loss and nitrogen balance in critically ill children with acute renal failure: a prospective comparison between classic hemofiltration and dialysis. Crit Care Med 2000;28:1161-5.

CHAPTER 23

Nephrotic Syndrome

Adinoyi O. Garba, Pharm.D., BCPS

LEARNING OBJECTIVES

1. Discuss the epidemiology and pathophysiology of the common types of nephrotic syndrome.

2. Recognize the signs, symptoms, and the clinical presentation of nephrotic syndrome as well as the various complications of this disease.

3. Describe the different classifications of nephrotic syndrome based on the response to initial steroid therapy and the evidence-based treatment guidelines for managing each of them.

4. Outline the medications used as adjunct therapies to manage the various complications of nephrotic syndrome.

5. Evaluate a given patient with nephrotic syndrome and recommend evidence- and/or consensus-based treatment strategies.

ABBREVIATIONS IN THIS CHAPTER

ACEI	Angiotensin-converting enzyme inhibitor
ALT	Alanine aminotransferase
AST	Aspartate aminotransferase
CNI	Calcineurin inhibitor
FRNS	Frequently relapsing nephrotic syndrome
FSGS	Focal segmental glomerulosclerosis
KDIGO	Kidney Disease Improving Global Outcomes
MCD	Minimal change disease
SDNS	Steroid-dependent nephrotic syndrome
SRNS	Steroid-resistant nephrotic syndrome
SSNS	Steroid-sensitive nephrotic syndrome
uPCR	Urine protein to creatinine ratio

INTRODUCTION

Nephrotic syndrome is one of the more common childhood kidney diseases. It is characterized by proteinuria, hypoalbuminemia, and edema. These signs and symptoms often cycle through periods of exacerbation and remission. Proteinuria is the hallmark presentation of nephrotic syndrome and is responsible for most of the other clinical signs seen in this disease. Although edema—periorbital, genital, or lower extremity—is usually the first presentation in nephrotic syndrome, an incidental finding of proteinuria on a urine dipstick at a

well-check visit to the pediatrician might be the first indicator of nephrotic syndrome for many patients. Proper diagnosis and treatment of nephrotic syndrome are essential because it is associated with a spectrum of clinically important sequelae that can progress all the way to end-stage renal disease if not properly managed. Nephrotic syndrome can be described as a clinical presentation indicative of damage to the glomerular filtration apparatus. Several glomerular diseases present with this syndrome, and a renal biopsy is usually required to distinguish one disease from another. Some diseases in children that present primarily with nephrotic syndrome include minimal change disease (also called *minimal change nephrotic syndrome*) and focal segmental glomerulosclerosis (FSGS). Membranous nephropathy is another primary nephrotic syndrome, but is relatively rare in children. This goal of this chapter is to evaluate the various forms of idiopathic nephrotic syndrome from both a pathologic perspective and by the response to initial therapy. A summary of the most current evidence-based pharmacotherapeutic approaches used in managing the disease will also be discussed.

EPIDEMIOLOGY AND CLASSIFICATION

Nephrotic syndrome affects 16 in 100,000 children, making it one of the more common childhood kidney diseases. Most children present between age 1 to 7 years.[1] Nephrotic syndrome is divided broadly based on etiology into two classes: *primary* or *idiopathic nephrotic syndrome* and *secondary nephrotic syndrome*. A third form of nephrotic syndrome, *congenital nephrotic syndrome*, is rare and differs from the other classes based on its etiology and management approach.

Primary or idiopathic nephrotic syndrome is the most common variety seen in children, with an incidence of two to seven cases per 100,000 children per year.[1,2] Male children are twice as likely to receive a new diagnosis of nephrotic syndrome compared with female children; however, this difference in incidence disappears by adolescence. The mean age at onset has been reported to be 3.4 years in Asian children and 4.2 years in European children.[3] Ethnicity may also play a role in the histologic variant of nephrotic syndrome. African American and Hispanic children have a higher incidence of steroid-resistant disease and are more likely to have rapid progression to renal failure, and thus have a poorer prognosis.[4]

Idiopathic nephrotic syndrome is further classified based on pathologic findings. The most common classes are: *minimal lesion* or *minimal change disease* (MCD); *focal segmental glomerulosclerosis* (FSGS); and *membranous nephropathy*. The most common form of the disease in children is MCD, accounting for around 85% of cases. Of these children, 75% are younger than 5 years.[2] In MCD, the glomeruli appear normal on examination using light microscopy; however, using electron microscopy shows the fusion of the epithelial foot processes within the glomeruli, which is implicated with the key clinical findings seen in the disease.[3] Of all cases of nephrotic syndrome, FSGS accounts for 10%–15%, with a median age of diagnosis of around 6 years. Pathologically, FSGS is characterized by scar tissue that develops initially in segments of some glomeruli and eventually spreads globally, leading to glomerular sclerosis and tubular atrophy. About 4% of nephrotic syndrome cases in children are membranous nephropathy, which is characterized by diffuse thickening of the glomerular capillary walls.[2,3]

Although most cases of nephrotic syndrome are idiopathic, it can be congenitally acquired or it can develop secondary to other diseases. Diseases that have been associated with causing secondary nephrotic syndrome include the following: Henoch-Schonlein purpura, immunoglobulin A nephropathy, post-streptococcal glomerulonephritis, mesangio-proliferative glomerulonephritis, and systemic lupus erythematosus. The following infectious diseases have also been associated with causing nephrotic syndrome: syphilis, hepatitis B, hepatitis C, and human immunodeficiency virus (HIV). In addition to these pathologic causes, some common medications including nonsteroidal anti-inflammatory drugs and lithium have also been implicated as potential causes of nephrotic syndrome.[3] This chapter primarily focuses on idiopathic nephrotic syndrome and briefly discusses congenital nephrotic syndrome.

PATHOPHYSIOLOGY

Nephrotic syndrome can result from any glomerular injury resulting in proteinuria. To understand the pathophysiology of nephrotic syndrome it is necessary to briefly review the functional units that constitute the glomerulus.

The glomerulus is a specialized capillary composed of three structural components that play key roles in its selective filtration capabilities. These components include the *endothelial cells separated by fenestrae*, the *glomerular membrane*, and the *specialized epithelial cells* (*podocytes*), which have foot processes that form an interlocking network of slit diaphragms. Under normal physiologic conditions, large substances like proteins are prevented from passing through these slits. Podocytes also play a role in maintaining the structural and functional integrity of the glomerular basement membrane and glomerular endothelial cells.

In nephrotic syndrome, an alteration occurs in both the morphology and functioning of the podocyte foot processes. One common biopsy finding in patients with nephrotic syndrome is the presence of effacement of these foot processes.[3] The discovery of mutations in several podocyte proteins identified in families with inherited variants of nephrotic syndrome highlights the central role podocytes play in this disease. Another possibility currently being explored is the possible expression of a plasma factor that may alter glomerular permeability. It is hypothesized that a primary T-cell event could result in the production of a permeability factor that interferes with the expression and/or function of key podocyte proteins resulting in proteinuria.[2] This hypothesis might explain the response of certain variants on the disease to drugs that modulate T-cell function. The pathophysiology of idiopathic nephrotic syndrome is still being studied.

CLINICAL PRESENTATION AND DIAGNOSIS

Patients with nephrotic syndrome typically present with swelling in the periorbital, lower extremity, or genital area. This presentation can range from mild localized edema to anasarca, which tends to be generally worse in the morning because of gravitational shifts and sleep position, but can persist throughout the day. Patients may also report changes in urine appearance, such as "foamy urine." Analysis of the urine is required to complete the work-up for diagnosing nephrotic syndrome. A 24-hour urine collection is considered the gold standard for quantifying proteinuria in nephrotic syndrome because it accounts for the circadian fluctuation in protein excretion. This collection can be difficult to accomplish in young children who are not toilet-trained. A urine protein to creatinine ratio (uPCR) on a random (or spot) urine sample is increasingly being used in practice because of the convenience of these tests. Many studies have suggested that 24-hour collection approach is not superior to a spot-urine collection for measuring proteinuria.[5-7] However, some investigators recommend verifying a spot uPCR with a 24-hour urine protein before making any diagnostic or therapeutic decisions.[8] Whereas most patients with nephrotic syndrome have a urine protein concentration greater than 300 mg/dL, a detectable concentration of protein in the urine lower than 300 mg/dL does not necessarily rule out the diagnosis because dilutional factors can influence this value.

The Kidney Diseases Improving Global Outcomes (KDIGO) 2012 clinical practice guideline for glomerulonephritis has defined the following criteria for diagnosing nephrotic syndrome: proteinuria with a uPCR greater than or equal to 2000 mg/g or urine protein concentration greater than or equal to 300 mg/dL (3+ protein on a urine dipstick); and hypoalbuminemia less than or equal to 2.5 g/dL with edema.[9] Other laboratory analyses including blood urea nitrogen, serum creatinine, cholesterol, antinuclear antibody, and serum complement 3 concentrations should be measured to rule out other causes of proteinuria.[1] Other clinical features associated with nephrotic syndrome include hyperlipidemia, hypertension, and hypercoagulability. Patients with nephrotic syndrome also present with a higher risk of acquiring infections.[9] Some patients may lack one or more of these features; however, both proteinuria and hypoalbuminemia must be present to establish a diagnosis of nephrotic syndrome.

A kidney biopsy is required for definitive diagnosis of nephrotic syndrome and to determine the pathological morphological characteristics such as MCD, FSGS, or membranous nephropathy. An adequate biopsy sample should have at least 20 glomeruli but many biopsies typically do not meet this standard, thus highlighting a key limitation to their diagnostic accuracy. A biopsy is not required for treatment, but may be obtained if the child has an atypical response to treatment. Classification of nephrotic syndrome by response to steroid therapy will be discussed later in this chapter. Repeating the biopsy during treatment is controversial but might be informative in cases of relapsing or treatment-resistant disease.[9]

TREATMENT

The ultimate goals of treatment for nephrotic syndrome are to prevent or delay loss of kidney function and manage disease-related comorbidities. Corticosteroids are the mainstay of treatment for children with nephrotic syndrome. The most common terminology used to describe response to therapy is summarized in Table 1.

Nephrotic syndrome can be further classified based on the response to corticosteroid treatment as *steroid-sensitive nephrotic syndrome* (SSNS) or *steroid-resistant nephrotic syndrome* (SRNS). Steroid sensitive nephrotic syndrome can be further classified into *steroid-dependent nephrotic syndrome* (SDNS) and *frequently relapsing nephrotic syndrome* (FRNS) based on the response of these patients after corticosteroid therapy is tapered or stopped. Table 2 describes the nephrotic syndrome subtypes based on their response to corticosteroid therapy. Treatment response, which can be variable, depends at least partially on the pathologic type of nephrotic syndrome. About 95% of patients with MCD will achieve remission after an 8-week course of steroids compared with a 20% remission rate in patients with FSGS. Of patients with MCD, 75% will achieve remission within 2 weeks. Of all patients with SSNS, 60% will have five or more relapses a year; these patients are classified as having frequently relapsing SSNS or FRNS.[2]

STEROID-SENSITIVE NEPHROTIC SYNDROME

Corticosteroids are the first-line treatment for idiopathic nephrotic syndrome. The guidelines recommend initial therapy with prednisone or prednisolone at 2 mg/kg (60 mg/m^2) per day, up to a maximum of 60 mg/day given once daily for 4 to 6 weeks. On remission, the dose is reduced to 1.5 mg/ kg (40 mg/m^2) up to a maximum of 40 mg/day given every other day for 2 to 6 months while tapering the dose. There is some controversy regarding which approach to steroid dosing—weight-based dosing versus dosing based on body surface area—offers the better outcomes. Dosing prednisone by weight (mg/kg) results in smaller total doses than body surface area (mg/m^2)–based dosing, especially in children weighing less than 30 kg or when the total prednisone dose is less than 60 mg.[10] Studies comparing these approaches have concluded that although the higher total doses with a body surface area–based regimen of steroids may not improve the time to remission, this approach might lead to a reduction in relapse rates.[10-12] It is important to note that, irrespective of the dosing approach, KDIGO guidelines have recommended maximum total doses for daily (60 mg/day) and alternate-day (40 mg/day) regimens. The guidelines recommend corticosteroid therapy for at least 12 weeks in total.

Many practitioners use a 12-week treatment regimen that includes 6 weeks of prednisone or prednisolone at 2 mg/kg (60 mg/m^2) per day, then 6 weeks at 1.5 mg/kg (40 mg/m^2) per day given on alternate days. A study by the Arbeitsgemeinschaft für Pädiatrische Nephrologie Group showed this regimen to be effective in a comparison of the 12-week steroid therapy with the then-standard 8-week steroid course. At 1-year follow up, patients on the 12-week course had a lower relapse rate compared with those on the standard treatment course (38% vs. 65%) but had a higher rate of steroid-induced adverse effects.[13] Therefore, the overall goal in the initial therapy of SSNS is to use the least amount of corticosteroid to achieve and sustain remission, while minimizing the risk of steroid-induced adverse effects.

Response to therapy is determined by monitoring the urine protein concentration, either by 24-hour urine collection, spot

Table 1. Important Clinical Definitions in the Management of Nephrotic Syndrome

Classification	Definition
Complete remission	uPCR < 0.2 (or 200 mg/g) or a negative or trace protein on urine dipstick for 3 consecutive days
Partial remission	Reduction of proteinuria by ≥ 50% from the presenting value and absolute uPCR between 0.2–2 (200–2000 mg/g)
No remission	Failure to reduce urine protein excretion by 50% from baseline or persistent uPCR > 2 (2000 mg/g)
Relapse	uPCR ≥ 2 (2000 mg/g) or at least 3+ protein on a urine dipstick for 3 consecutive days (in a patient who was previously in remission)
Frequent relapse	≥ 2 Relapses within a 6-month period of initial response or ≥ 4 relapses within a 12-month period of initial response

uPCR = urine protein to creatinine ratio.

Table 2. Disease Classification Based on Response to Corticosteroid Therapy

Classification	Definition
Steroid-sensitive nephrotic syndrome (SSNS)	Disease responsive either partially or completely to corticosteroid therapy
Steroid-resistant nephrotic syndrome (SRNS)	Failure to achieve complete remission after 8 weeks of corticosteroid therapy
Steroid-dependent nephrotic syndrome (SDNS)	SSNS with 2 consecutive relapses during corticosteroid therapy or within 14 days of stopping therapy
Frequently relapsing nephrotic syndrome (FRNS)	SSNS with ≥ 2 relapses within 6 months of initial response or SSNS with ≥ 4 relapses in any 12-month period

uPCR, or a urine dipstick. Often the urine protein concentration becomes undetectable within the first few days to weeks of corticosteroid administration. As the corticosteroid dose is tapered, urine protein should be monitored (by urine spot uPCR or dipstick). Recurrence of proteinuria for 3 or more consecutive days or uPCR of 2 (2000 mg/g) or higher from a random or 24-hour urine sample indicates relapse. As noted previously, relapses are common in patients with SSNS and should not be considered a failure of therapy. In patients who experience infrequent relapses, the guidelines suggest treating with prednisone at 2 mg/kg (60 mg/m^2) per day, up to a maximum dose of 60 mg/day until the patient is in complete remission for 3 consecutive days, and then reducing an alternate-day dose of 1.5 mg/kg (40 mg/m^2), up to a maximum of 40 mg/day, for 4 weeks. For patients who experience four or more relapses annually (i.e., patients who have FRNS), the same initial treatment regimen (2 mg/kg [60 mg/m^2] per day) is suggested until remission, and then 1.5 mg/kg (40 mg/m^2) alternate-day dosing for 3 months with taper.[9]

The most common trigger for relapse in nephrotic syndrome is infection. Upper respiratory tract infections and urinary tract infections are by far the most common triggers of relapse.[14] During episodes of respiratory tract infection, children with FRNS or SDNS who are currently on alternate-day steroid therapy should be switched to a daily steroid regimen at the same dose as the alternate-day dose.[9,15,16] Some patients with SSNS are only in remission when they are on full-dose daily steroids and will relapse when switched to alternate-day dosing or soon after steroids are stopped (within 14 days). This subclass is referred to as *steroid-dependent nephrotic syndrome* (SDNS). The KDIGO guidelines suggest that patients with SDNS be treated with the same steroid regimen as in FRNS and be maintained on daily or alternate-day steroids at the lowest dose to maintain remission with minimal adverse effects.

Patients with FRNS or SDNS are at an increased risk of exposure to large amounts of corticosteroids and the accompanying adverse effects. Short-term adverse effects of exogenous corticosteroids include the following: hyperglycemia, hypertension, increased appetite, behavioral changes, and leukocytosis. The long-term effects of using corticosteroids include the following: growth retardation, osteoporosis, peptic ulcer disease, ophthalmic disease (e.g., cataracts), adrenal suppression, and Cushing syndrome. The guidelines recommend that these patients be started on an alternative medication to keep them in remission and lower their total steroid burden. These medications are often referred to as *steroid-sparing agents*. These agents will be discussed in detail later in the chapter. Figure 1 provides a summary of the evidence-based treatment approach for managing SSNS.

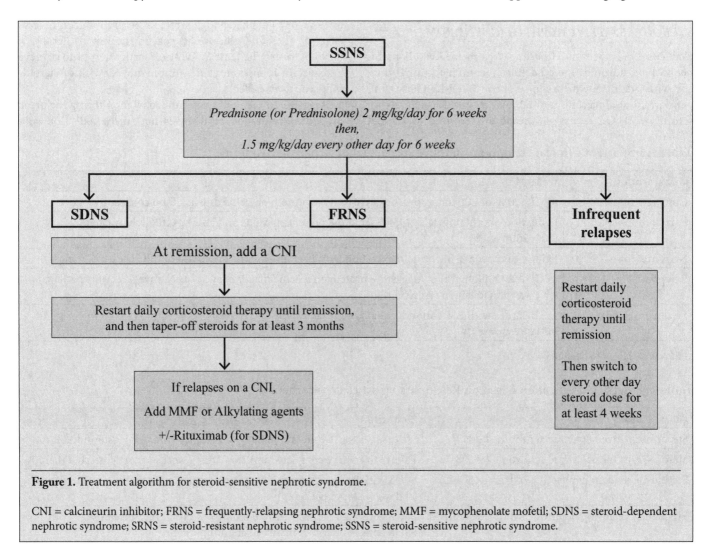

Figure 1. Treatment algorithm for steroid-sensitive nephrotic syndrome.

CNI = calcineurin inhibitor; FRNS = frequently-relapsing nephrotic syndrome; MMF = mycophenolate mofetil; SDNS = steroid-dependent nephrotic syndrome; SRNS = steroid-resistant nephrotic syndrome; SSNS = steroid-sensitive nephrotic syndrome.

STEROID-RESISTANT NEPHROTIC SYNDROME

Some patients with nephrotic syndrome do not respond to corticosteroid therapy. The incidence of this steroid-resistant variant is less than 10%, and these patients typically have a very poor prognosis.[3] Although SRNS may occur as early as at birth, the incidence is higher in children age 2 years or older. About 80% of patients with FSGS do not respond to steroid therapy compared with less than 5% of patients with MCD. This high percentage of lack of response has led many clinicians to expect steroid resistance when FSGS is diagnosed by biopsy; however, a minimum of 8 weeks of corticosteroid therapy is required to confirm steroid resistance. The clinical evaluation of patients with SRNS includes determination of renal function by estimated GFR and quantification of proteinuria. These assessments are useful in determining the rate of regression of renal function, or at the very least they offer a baseline for future comparison.[9] A renal biopsy is recommended for the complete evaluation of SRNS. Figure 2 provides a summary of evidence-based approaches for managing SRNS.

Calcineurin inhibitors (CNIs) are the recommended first-line therapy for children and adolescents with SRNS. These inhibitors should be started for a trial period of at least 6 months and discontinued if the patient does not achieve a partial or complete remission. If the patient experiences at least a partial remission at 6 months, CNIs could be continued for a minimum of 12 months. Relapses have been documented in about 70% of children with SRNS when CNIs have been stopped at or before 12 months of therapy. The optimal duration of CNI therapy is still under investigation, and it is not uncommon for CNI courses to be extended beyond 1 year. In cases in which patients with SRNS relapse after complete remission with CNIs or mycophenolate mofetil, the KDIGO guidelines suggest one of the following approaches: (1) starting oral corticosteroids; (2) returning to the last effective immunosuppressive agent; or (3) using an alternative agent if a risk of cumulative toxicity exists.[5] In addition to CNI therapy, the guidelines suggest adding low-dose steroids. Although the role of low-dose steroids is unclear, this approach is consistent with most of the clinical trials that have reported success in treating SRNS by adding low-dose prednisone 0.3–1 mg/kg daily or on alternate days to a CNI regimen.[17-19] In children who do not experience partial or complete response to CNIs, the following approaches are suggested: mycophenolate mofetil for at least 12 months; high-dose intravenous "pulse" corticosteroids; or a combination of both. Table 3 shows the dosing recommendations for mycophenolate mofetil. Six pulses of high-dose methylprednisolone 30 mg/kg (maximum of 1000 mg) intravenously given on alternate days appeared to be effective in inducing remission in children with SRNS.[20] Evidence backing these approaches

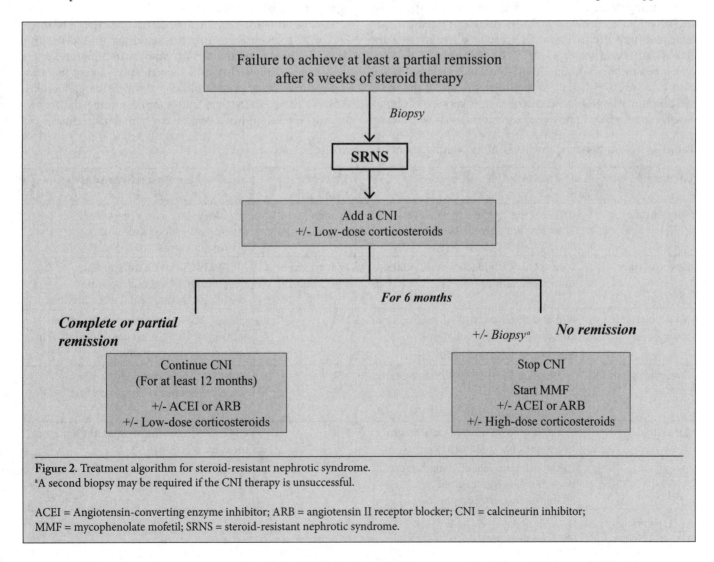

Figure 2. Treatment algorithm for steroid-resistant nephrotic syndrome.
[a]A second biopsy may be required if the CNI therapy is unsuccessful.

ACEI = Angiotensin-converting enzyme inhibitor; ARB = angiotensin II receptor blocker; CNI = calcineurin inhibitor; MMF = mycophenolate mofetil; SRNS = steroid-resistant nephrotic syndrome.

for treating CNI-resistant disease is relatively weak because of the limited number of studies available.

Cyclophosphamide is not recommended for treating SRNS. This conclusion was highlighted by a study of treatment for steroid-resistant FSGS comparing the efficacy of prednisone 40 mg/m² every other day for 12 months with the same steroid regimen plus a 90-day course of cyclophosphamide 2.5 mg/kg/dose by mouth every morning. The primary end point was treatment failure defined as an increase in serum creatinine by 30% or more from baseline or by greater than 0.4 mg/dL or as onset of renal failure defined as serum creatinine greater that 4.0 mg/dL. Treatment failure occurred in 36% of the steroid-only group and 57% of the steroid-plus-cyclophosphamide group (p>0.1). Investigators concluded that adding cyclophosphamide offered no advantage over steroid therapy when treating SRNS and that this medication exposed patients to an increased risk of cytotoxic adverse effects.[21]

The use of medications that block the renin–angiotensin–aldosterone system (RAAS) such as angiotensin-converting enzyme inhibitors (ACEIs) and angiotensin II receptor blockers are recommended for reducing proteinuria, especially in children with SRNS. These medications have been shown to have an anti-proteinuric effect in adults with glomerular diseases.[22] Case series and small studies have shown a reduction in proteinuria in children with nephrotic syndrome using ACEIs.[23,24] The mechanism responsible for the anti-proteinuric effects of ACEIs is not clearly defined, but their ability to decrease intra-glomerular filtration pressure appears to play a major part. In the management of idiopathic nephrotic syndrome, RAAS-blocking medications are used as adjunctive therapy to minimize the use of the more toxic immunosuppressive medications. It is very important to closely monitor blood pressure at regular intervals when using ACEIs or ABRs for their anti-proteinuric function alone, especially in the absence of underlying hypertension. Other monitoring guidelines are discussed later in this chapter.

STEROID-SPARING AGENTS

As mentioned previously, the prolonged steroid use has serious short- and long-term adverse effects, especially in the pediatric population. Other medications may be added to reduce the dose or duration of corticosteroid use in nephrotic syndrome patients who relapse frequently or are steroid-dependent. Some of the common steroid-sparing agents used in the treatment of nephrotic syndrome and their monitoring guidelines are summarized in Table 3.

CALCINEURIN INHIBITORS

Calcineurin inhibitors are drugs that suppress cellular immunity by inhibiting calcineurin phosphatase activity, thereby inhibiting T-cell activation. Two drugs in this class currently have label approval by the U.S. Food and Drug Administration (FDA): cyclosporine and tacrolimus. They have been used for decades as part of anti-graft rejection therapy in patients who have undergone organ transplantation. Over the years these agents have shown efficacy in the management of nephrotic syndrome.

Cyclosporine inhibits the production and release of interleukin II, thereby preventing the activation of T cells. This drug also causes renal arteriolar vasoconstriction and alters glomerular permeability, which might play a role in limiting the amount of protein filtering through the glomerulus. Adverse drug effects from cyclosporine include the following: hypertension, hirsutism, electrolyte abnormalities, and

Table 3. Steroid-Sparing Agents Used in Management of Nephrotic Syndrome

Medication	Initial Dose	Therapeutic Monitoring	Routine Monitoring Assessments
Tacrolimus	0.05–0.3 mg/kg/day, divided every 12 hours (oral formulation)	Trough level: 5–10 ng/mL	BP, CMP, CBC with differential, magnesium, blood tacrolimus, neurologic status
Cyclosporine	3 mg/kg/day, divided every 12 hours (oral formulation)	Trough level: 80–150 ng/mL	BP, CMP, CBC with differential, magnesium, blood cyclosporine, neurologic status, dental examination
Mycophenolate mofetil[a]	600 mg/m²/dose (or 12–18 mg/kg/dose) twice daily (oral formulation) Maximum daily dose: 2000 mg	NR	CMP, CBC with differential, infection signs/symptoms, presence of oral or skin lesions, neurologic status
Cyclophosphamide	2–3 mg/kg/day once daily taken orally for 8–12 weeks Maximum cumulative dose: 168 mg/kg	NR	CMP, CBC with differential, signs/symptoms of hemorrhagic cystitis
Rituximab	375 mg/m²/dose infused intravenously every week for 1–4 doses Initial infusion rate of 50 mg/ hour; if tolerated, then increased by 50 mg/hour every 30 minutes)	NR	CMP, CBC with differential, presence of infusion reactions

[a]Part of the FDA Risk Evaluation and Mitigation Strategies (REMS) program.
BP = blood pressure; CBC = complete blood count; CMP = comprehensive metabolic panel; NR = no recommendations.

nephrotoxicity. Cyclosporine therapy is typically monitored by trough levels. Whereas most studies have targeted cyclosporine trough levels of 80 ng/mL to 150 ng/mL, trough levels ranging from 60 ng/mL and 80 ng/mL have also been shown to be effective and safe in maintaining remission in children with FRNS.[25]

The mechanism of action of tacrolimus in nephrotic syndrome is not completely understood, but, like cyclosporine, tacrolimus inhibits T-cell activation. Tacrolimus inhibits the activation of factors essential for the transcription of cytokine genes in T cells, leading to a decreased production of cytokines. Abnormal T-cell activity is believed to be at least partially implicated in the pathogenesis of nephrotic syndrome.[26] Adverse drug effects associated with tacrolimus include the following: hypertension, hyperglycemia, altered mental status, electrolyte abnormalities, and nephrotoxicity. Like cyclosporine, tacrolimus requires therapeutic drug concentration monitoring because of its narrow therapeutic index; however, target concentrations for nephrotic syndrome have not been properly defined. Most studies have shown efficacy with tacrolimus at trough levels between 5 ng/mL and 10 ng/mL.[9]

A single-center randomized controlled study comparing the safety and efficacy of tacrolimus to cyclosporine in 41 children with SRNS showed similar rates of remission (relative risk 1.14; 95% confidence interval, 0.84–1.55) at 12 months.[27] In this study, patients on cyclosporine had a higher relapse rate than those on tacrolimus, and cosmetic adverse effects such as hypertrichosis and gum hypertrophy were also significantly higher in the cyclosporine group. Several studies have suggested that the better efficacy observed with tacrolimus versus cyclosporine is because of the superior cytokine suppression effect of tacrolimus.[28]

Among various cyclosporine products bioavailability varies, which can affect its efficacy and safety, especially when switching from one formulation to another. Studies have shown significant differences in the bioavailability and other pharmacokinetic values between different formulations of the same brand (solution vs. soft gel capsule) and between brand name versus generic versions of cyclosporine.[29] Similar studies comparing brand name versus generic formulations of tacrolimus in patients after kidney transplantation have found no significant differences in the pharmacokinetic profiles of these formulations.[30,31] Based on this potential variation in bioavailability, clinicians should avoid mixing or switching back and forth between different formulations or brand and generic versions of CNIs to avoid fluctuations in drug concentration and the risk of toxicity. If a switch is necessary, then early and frequent monitoring of drug concentrations in the blood may be required to avoid suboptimal therapy or toxicity.

Cyclosporine and tacrolimus are major substrates of the cytochrome P-450 enzyme, CYP3A4. This status increases the potential for drug–drug interactions. It is necessary to review a patient's medication profile (including supplements) and diet for possible drug–drug or food–drug interactions. This information could be useful in determining the frequency of monitoring the blood concentrations of these drugs.

The duration of CNI therapy remains a controversial issue. The KDIGO guidelines suggest duration of at least 12 months of CNI use in patients who show partial or full remission to CNI therapy. More long-term data are required to ascertain the appropriate duration of CNI therapy in patients with nephrotic syndrome.

MYCOPHENOLIC ACID

Mycophenolate mofetil is another immunomodulatory agent that has shown efficacy in the management of nephrotic syndrome. It has an active metabolite, mycophenolic acid, which inhibits the synthesis of T cells and B cells. In addition, mycophenolate inhibits vascular smooth muscle and mesangial cell proliferation, inhibits nitric oxide synthase, and induces apoptosis in activated T cells. One or more of these actions may be responsible for its efficacy in nephrotic syndrome. In studies comparing the efficacy and safety of mycophenolate to tacrolimus in maintaining remission and preventing relapses in children with FRNS or SDNS, mycophenolate mofetil was found to be as efficacious as tacrolimus.[32,33] Adverse drug effects associated with mycophenolate mofetil include the following: dyspepsia, diarrhea, leukopenia, and rarely lymphoma. The risk of nephrotoxicity is less likely with mycophenolate than with CNIs, which makes it a good alternative in treating patients with nephrotic syndrome and renal insufficiency.

Unlike the CNIs, mycophenolate mofetil has no recommendations for target concentration in treating nephrotic syndrome, and most centers do not monitor drug concentrations when treating this disease in the pediatric population. As mentioned previously with CNIs, there are no recommendations on the appropriate duration of mycophenolate treatment. Similarly, more data are required to determine the most suitable treatment duration when treating nephrotic syndrome with mycophenolate; however, the KDIGO guidelines suggest treatment duration of at least 12 months.[9]

ALKYLATING AGENTS

Alkylating agents such as cyclophosphamide and chlorambucil may also be used as steroid-sparing agent to reduce the risk of relapses. These drugs act by interfering with DNA replication by inserting alkyl chains onto purine bases, thereby interfering with nucleic acid synthesis and cell division. Chlorambucil is less commonly used than cyclophosphamide. Studies have shown that the use of these agents can extend remission by at least 12 months.[34,35] These drugs are no longer popular for treating nephrotic syndrome because of their significant adverse effect profile. Some of the adverse effects common to both drugs include nausea and vomiting and bone marrow suppression. Children receiving alkylating agents are at greater risk of both viral and bacterial infections than with most immunosuppressive medications. Both drugs have also been implicated with causing both male and female infertility. Some adverse effects specifically associated with chlorambucil are seizures and malignancies. Cyclophosphamide has been associated with alopecia, hemorrhagic cystitis, colitis, and myocarditis. Although there are recommendations for drug concentration, patients on these medications should be routinely monitored for myelosuppression and infections by a physical examination and complete blood counts with differential.

ANTI-CD20 AGENTS

The use of B-cell–targeted therapy in the management of nephrotic syndrome has shown some promising results. Rituximab is a chimeric monoclonal antibody with activity against the CD20 surface antigen of B cells. In addition to its immunomodulatory effect, it has been suggested that rituximab may also act directly on podocyte function by preserving sphingolipid-related enzymes that affect cytoskeleton remodeling in podocytes in FSGS.[36] In one study, a single dose of intravenous rituximab of 375 mg/m²/dose was reported to be effective in preventing relapse for an average of about 6 months in children with SDNS.[37] Another study showed that children with SDNS treated with a single 375 mg/m² infusion of rituximab had a median time to relapse of about 18 months compared with 6 months for those on prednisone alone.[38] Although the recommended maximum number of rituximab infusions for treating nephrotic syndrome is not defined, studies have used up to four infusions based on the safety profile of rituximab from experience with treating B-cell lymphoma. A randomized, placebo-controlled, multicenter study of 48 patients, age 2–18 years with either FRNS or SDNS, showed that a rituximab regimen of 375 mg/m²/dose weekly for 4 weeks was well tolerated.[39] Patients on this regimen had a median relapse-free period of 267 days versus 101 days in the placebo group (hazard ratio 0.27; 95% confidence interval, 0.14–0.53; p<0.0001). One consideration for rituximab is that studies to date have had small sample sizes, limiting the generalizability of their results. However, it appears that rituximab may have an important role as a steroid-sparing agent in treating SDNS, although the efficacy of rituximab in treating SRNS is still unclear and data supporting its efficacy are lacking. A systematic review of studies assessing the efficacy of rituximab for managing SDNS and SRNS showed that, although rituximab overall has been effective in managing SDNS, only a few studies have shown any significant success in treating SRNS with rituximab.[40]

The most common serious adverse effects of rituximab include infusion-related reactions and their sequelae such as the following: rash, hypotension, angioedema, hypoxia, bronchospasm, pulmonary infiltrates, acute respiratory distress syndrome, myocardial infarction, ventricular fibrillation, cardiogenic shock, anaphylactoid events, and death. It is recommended that patients receiving rituximab be pretreated with an antihistamine and acetaminophen.[41] Patients on rituximab are also at risk of acquiring infections because of its immunosuppressive properties. A rare but serious adverse effect is rituximab-associated lung injury.[42] Although the pulmonary injury associated with rituximab is often transient and reversible, it can be associated with potentially fatal pulmonary injuries such as interstitial pneumonitis, pulmonary fibrosis, and bronchiolitis obliterans. A chest radiograph should be checked before starting rituximab treatment and periodically during and after treatment because the time to onset of symptoms of rituximab-associated lung injury ranges from 1 to 3 months.[43]

Ofatumumab is another anti-CD20 monoclonal antibody currently suggested for the management of nephrotic syndrome. Although ofatumumab has a similar mechanism of action to rituximab, one major difference is that whereas rituximab is a chimeric anti-CD 20 monoclonal antibody, ofatumumab is a humanized monoclonal antibody. This difference provides ofatumumab the advantage, at least theoretically, of having a lower risk of hypersensitivity reactions. A case report of two children ages 3 and 14 years with SRNS and SDNS, respectively, showed that ofatumumab was well tolerated (they were premedicated with paracetamol [acetaminophen], prednisolone and chlorphenamine). Both patients had a history of hypersensitivity to rituximab and were given a single infusion of 750 mg/1.73 m² ofatumumab together with their CNI regimen. These children remained in remission for 19 and 15 months, respectively.[44] Investigators are currently evaluating the efficacy and safety of ofatumumab in treating children with drug-resistant idiopathic nephrotic syndrome.

CONGENITAL NEPHROTIC SYNDROME

Some infants are born with proteinuria at birth, followed by the clinical symptoms that typify nephrotic syndrome. When these symptoms are observed in an infant younger than 3 months, congenital nephrotic syndrome is suspected. The etiology is usually the result of a mutation, either inherited or acquired in utero; therefore, genetic testing may be needed to fully diagnose this disease. The most common type of congenital nephrotic syndrome is the Finnish type, which has an autosomal recessive inheritance pattern commonly seen in the Finnish population. It has also been identified in several other populations worldwide. For example, in the Mennonite population of Lancaster, Pennsylvania, the incidence is believed to be about 1 in 500 live births.[3]

Several gene mutations have been identified to cause congenital nephrotic syndrome. In this chapter the two most common will be discussed. The common mutations are to the *nephrin gene*, also known as *nephrotic syndrome type-1* or *Finnish type*, and to the *podocin gene* or *nephrotic syndrome type-2*. Both nephrin and podocin play integral roles in the structure and proper functioning of the slit-diaphragms, which play a very important role in the selective filtration process of the glomerulus, as discussed previously in the pathophysiology section of this chapter. There are also nongenetic, secondary forms of congenital nephrotic syndrome that can be caused by infections such as syphilis, toxoplasmosis, malaria, cytomegalovirus, hepatitis B, and rubella.[45]

In contrast to other forms of nephrotic syndrome, steroids and other immunosuppressive therapies are not effective in the management of congenital nephrotic syndrome. The typical management emphasizes supportive therapy. The goals of management include the following: reduction of proteinuria; replacing serum albumin; reducing edema; nutrition support; preventing thrombosis; and infection control.[45] A unilateral (or even a bilateral) nephrectomy is an option that many centers have used as way to reduce protein losses and the frequency of albumin infusions. These approaches have the primary goal of supporting the infant until the child is at least older than 1 year and has attained a body weight and size adequate for a kidney transplant. Offering nutrition support to boost the infant's growth is an important component of patient care. The body weight requirement for kidney transplantation is specific to the health care facility, but most centers prefer the child to be at least 10 kg. This approach takes into account both the physiologic as well as the practical factors necessary for the procedure because the transplanted kidney is often adult-sized. Although a kidney transplant is the only treatment option for these patients, reports have shown a likelihood of recurrence of proteinuria in patients with congenital nephrotic syndrome after transplant.[46]

SUPPORTIVE THERAPY

Children with nephrotic syndrome present with several clinical complications. These complications must be addressed to achieve the best clinical outcomes when treating the primary glomerular pathology. This section discusses a few of these complications as well as the recommended and suggested treatment options in each case.

HYPERTENSION

The recommended blood pressure goal in children with nephrotic syndrome is a value lower than the 90th percentile for their age, gender, and height.[47] First-line antihypertensive options in children with hypertension and proteinuria are ACEIs or angiotensin II receptor blockers unless contraindicated. Enalapril, an ACEI, has been shown to reduce proteinuria in children with SRNS. Enalapril should be initiated at a dose of 0.2 mg/kg/day. Its effectiveness appears to be dose related, which allows for the dose to be increased to a target dose of 0.6 mg/kg/day.[48] Fosinopril is another ACEI studied and shown to reduce proteinuria and renal tubular damage in children with nephrotic syndrome. In this study, patients younger than 5 years received 5 mg/day of fosinopril, patients age 5–10 years received doses 5–7.5 mg/day, and patients older than 10 years received 10 mg/day.[49] Pediatric hypertension guidelines recommend a maximum enalapril dose of 0.6 mg/kg (or 40 mg) daily, in single or twice-daily doses. The recommended fosinopril doses in the pediatric population begin at 0.1 mg/kg/day with a maximum daily dose of 40 mg.[47] Angiotensin II receptor blockers are the recommended alternative in patients who do not tolerate ACEIs because of a dry cough. When initiating an ACEI or an angiotensin II receptor blocker, blood pressure, serum electrolytes, and serum creatinine should be monitored periodically.

NEPHROTIC EDEMA

The goal of supportive therapy is to control edema until remission can be achieved. Edema should be reversed slowly. To begin, dietary sodium intake should be restricted to a maximum of 2000 mg/day.[1,47]

Loop diuretics, such as furosemide, are the preferred choice of diuretics used for managing patients with severe edema or anasarca. Furosemide is initiated at 1 mg/kg/dose; however, higher doses of furosemide are often required to achieve effective intratubular concentrations, which results because furosemide is bound to albumin in the tubular lumen of patients with proteinuria.[50] Adding a second class of diuretics such as thiazides or potassium-sparing diuretics may prevent increased reabsorption in the distal tubule and collecting duct.

Many clinicians use intravenous albumin in combination with intravenous diuretics to aid in fluid removal.[50,51] Albumin is given to increase oncotic pressure, thereby drawing fluid into the intravascular space from the interstitium, and then furosemide is given to remove the fluid from the vasculature via diuresis. Albumin is administered as 25% albumin infusion at doses range from 0.5–1 g/kg per dose infused over 30–60 minutes. Data showing improved diuresis with sequential dosing of albumin and furosemide versus furosemide alone are lacking. Monitoring values when using this approach include the following: vital signs; fluid and electrolyte status; complete blood count; urine volume and specific gravity; and cardiac and pulmonary function.

DYSLIPIDEMIA

Nephrotic syndrome is associated with an increased risk of dyslipidemia. The routine monitoring of lipids in children younger than 8 years is not typically recommended unless the child has an underlying risk of dyslipidemia such as nephrotic syndrome.[47] The pathophysiology of nephrotic syndrome-induced dyslipidemia is complex and beyond the scope of this chapter. A simplistic description of the mechanism involves the urinary loss of high-density lipoprotein and the down-regulation of both low-density lipoprotein and very low-density lipoprotein receptors in the liver. These changes and several other factors lead to a decrease in the catabolism of triglyceride-rich lipoproteins and impaired hepatocyte cholesterol uptake, consequently leading to an increase in serum triglycerides and low-density lipoprotein.[52]

Hyperlipidemia associated with nephrotic syndrome may increase the risk of atherosclerosis and cardiovascular complications. A diet limiting fat to less than 30% of calories, saturated fat to less than 10% of calories, and cholesterol to less than 300 mg/day is recommended.[47] The impact of this dietary approach in nephrotic syndrome has not been fully elucidated, but it is recommended for reducing the risk of cardiovascular disease. Pharmacotherapy for dyslipidemia is not usually recommended in children younger than 10 years, unless they have severe hyperlipidemia (low-density lipoprotein cholesterol greater than or equal to 400 mg/dL or serum triglycerides greater than or equal to 500 mg/dL) or increased risk of cardiovascular disease. Consideration for initiating pharmacologic management of dyslipidemia is based on the average of two or more fasting lipid profiles taken 2 weeks to 3 months apart.[47]

There are several pharmacological options for managing patients with hyperlipidemia. However, statins have been studied in children with nephrotic syndrome. To date, two small prospective studies have assessed the efficacy of statins in treating children with SRNS and hyperlipidemia.[53,54] The larger of these studies assessed the effect of statins in 12 patients between the ages of 8 months and 15 years. Patients were placed on either lovastatin (maximum dose 40 mg) or simvastatin (maximum dose 20 mg), and their lipid profiles were reviewed. At 12-month follow-up, baseline low-density lipoprotein cholesterol decreased from 323 ± 142 mg/dL to 173 ± 65 mg/dL (p<0.001). These investigators also reported that the statins were well tolerated with no symptoms of muscle injury or changes in liver enzymes.[54] Most practitioners use the dosing approach recommended for treating familial hypercholesterolemia. The therapeutic target for children and adolescents on statins with moderate- to high-risk conditions such as nephrotic syndrome is a low-density lipoprotein cholesterol concentration less than 130 mg/dL, but ideally less than 110 mg/dL.[47] Some evidence also suggests that statins may have a role in decreasing proteinuria and preventing further renal injury.[55]

Statins have several adverse effects, including the following: elevation of hepatic enzymes, myopathy that can progress to rhabdomyolysis, and high potential for teratogenicity. Sexually active adolescent females need to be counseled on using contraceptive measures while taking these drugs because statins are contraindicated in pregnancy. Before initiating a statin, it is recommended to obtain a baseline creatinine kinase, alanine aminotransferase (ALT), and aspartate aminotransferase (AST), and then monitor with a fasting lipid panel, creatinine kinase, ALT, and AST after about 4 weeks of initiating therapy. If target low-density lipoprotein cholesterol concentrations are achieved and no apparent adverse effects noted, then these measures should be rechecked in 8 weeks and then every 3 to 6 months thereafter. It is recommended to temporarily withhold the medication and recheck these laboratory results again after 2 weeks if the following occurs: symptoms of myopathy, a 10-fold elevation in creatinine kinase, or a 3-fold or greater elevation in ALT or AST.[47] When these signs and symptoms resolve, then the decision whether to restart the medication or not, and at what dose, is a clinical judgment call, and the medical team must weigh the benefit versus the potential risk.

Some statins are major CYP 3A4 substrates and may interact with other medications used in managing nephrotic syndrome, such as the CNIs. The pharmacist should play a role in initiating more frequent monitoring of laboratory values and assessing clinical results in patients at risk of drug–drug interactions, and, when possible, should offer alternative medication options with less potential of an interaction.

COAGULOPATHY

Patients with nephrotic syndrome are at greater risk of developing thromboembolic complications such as pulmonary embolism and deep venous thrombosis. The incidence of thromboembolism in adults with nephrotic syndrome is about 25% compared with children, for whom the overall risk is about 3%. In children with nephrotic syndrome, the highest risk is in those with membranous nephropathy or similar disease processes such as lupus nephritis (25% of cases). Thrombosis is also common in children with congenital nephrotic syndrome (about 10% of cases) and in secondary nephrotic syndrome, such as renal vasculitis (17.1% of cases). There appears to be a correlation between age and risk of a thrombotic event, with adolescents at the highest risk even within the pediatric population.[56]

The complex pathophysiology of thrombosis in nephrotic syndrome involves the significant loss of both clotting and anti-clotting factors in urine. It is hypothesized that loss of antithrombin III and protein S triggers the synthesis of prothrombotic factors, shifting the hemostatic equilibrium toward a prothrombotic state. The net result includes the following: decreased factor IX and factor XI concentrations; decreased antithrombin III; increased factor V and factor VIII; and increased platelet reactivity.[56] It should be noted that most of the information on nephrotic syndrome-induced thrombosis is from adult data, and it might be difficult to extrapolate this pathophysiology to the pediatric population. As children grow older or if they have other risk factors for thromboembolic complications, such as systemic lupus erythematosus, they may benefit from prophylactic anticoagulant therapy. More studies are required to assess the use of prophylactic anticoagulation in this patient population.

Nephrotic syndrome-related thrombotic events are managed using similar anticoagulation therapy approaches applied to other types of prothrombotic disease states. American College of Chest Physicians guidelines suggest that in patients with active nephrotic syndrome, treatment should include anti-coagulation with unfractionated heparin, low molecular weight heparin, or vitamin K antagonist for at least 3 months, and for a longer duration until the disease is under control or in remission.[57] Detailed information on appropriate anticoagulation management is provided in the Anticoagulation chapter.

It is necessary to review the patient's medication and disease profile before selecting an anticoagulation therapy approach. For example, in patients with poor renal function, a clinician might choose anticoagulation with unfractionated heparin or vitamin K antagonist over low molecular weight heparin, which requires adjustment based on renal function. Another consideration is the potential for drug–drug interactions with vitamin K antagonists, which might rule them out as an option in patients with nephrotic syndrome who are taking many pharmacologic agents.

INCREASED INFECTION RISK

Children with nephrotic syndrome are also at an increased risk of bacterial infections, particularly pneumococcal peritonitis because of low concentrations of endogenous immune globulin. Some investigators suggest that maintaining a serum immunoglobulin G concentration of greater than 600 mg/dL by using intravenously administered immunoglobulin G might help mitigate the risk of infection, which in these patients is further exacerbated by the immunosuppressive management strategies used to control the nephrotic syndrome.[58] Because these patients are at high risk of infection, an increased level of clinical vigilance for infections is recommended.

Children with nephrotic syndrome should be up-to-date on their vaccinations, especially with the pneumococcal immunization series.[59] The most recent pneumococcal immunization recommendations for high-risk children and infants can be found on the Centers for Disease Control and Prevention website.[60] The KDIGO guidelines also recommend that children with nephrotic syndrome receive an influenza vaccination annually. Live vaccines such as measles, mumps, rubella, varicella, and rotavirus are contraindicated in children on immunosuppressive therapy. These vaccines must be deferred until the patient meets the following conditions:

prednisone dose less than 1 mg/kg/day (or 2 mg/kg every other day); off cytotoxic agents for more than 3 months; and off other immunosuppressive agents (e.g., cyclophosphamide, CNIs, or mycophenolate mofetil) for longer than 1 month. Immunosuppressed children who contract chicken pox should be treated with antiviral medications.[9]

VITAMIN D DEFICIENCY

Children with nephrotic syndrome have been found to have a decreased plasma concentration of 25-hydroxyvitamin D, which is at least in part caused by the loss of vitamin D-binding protein in the urine of nephrotic syndrome patients.[61] Because vitamin D plays a key role in bone health, patients with persistently low concentrations are at an increased risk of disorders and fractures. This risk is further enhanced by their prolonged exposure to corticosteroids therapy, which is also a risk factor for bone disorders. An optimal vitamin D concentration of 30 ng/mL or higher is believed to be required for proper bone health.[62] Because of the increased risk of bone disease in these patients 25-hydroxyvitamin D concentrations should be checked periodically. There are no detailed guidelines for preventing bone disease in children on prolonged steroid therapy. Investigators in a prospective, randomized, controlled interventional study of 41 children with new-onset nephrotic syndrome treated with a 12-week course of steroids attempted to address this question.[63] The patients were randomized into a treatment group to receive vitamin D 1,000 IU/day and elemental calcium 500 mg/day and a control group. After the 12-week course of steroids, children in the treatment group showed an increase of 11.2% in bone mineral content measured at the lumbar spine versus the control group children who showed an 8.9% decrease (p<0.0001). In addition, the difference in the change in bone mineral density was significant between these groups. This study suggests that vitamin D and calcium supplementation might help prevent steroid-induced bone degradation in patients on high-dose corticosteroids for treating nephrotic syndrome. The most current guidelines offer no specific recommendations for preventing or treating nephrotic syndrome-related vitamin D deficiency. Although vitamin D supplementation is not a requirement, it might help mitigate the bone disease adverse effects of steroid therapy.

PROGNOSIS

The prognosis for patients depends on the pathologic type of nephrotic syndrome and on their response to initial steroid therapy (steroid-sensitive versus steroid-resistant). Children with MCD generally respond well to treatment, with the best prognosis and the fewest disease-related complications. Conversely, patients with FSGS can develop considerable glomerular scarring, leading to a rapid progression to end-stage renal disease and ultimately resulting in dialysis or transplantation.[64] Similarly, patients with steroid-resistant disease are at greater risk of developing progressive kidney disease than patients with steroid-dependent disease. Regardless of the type of nephrotic syndrome, relapses can occur in most patients throughout life, and some of these patients will eventually become steroid-dependent and possibly steroid-resistant.[65]

CONCLUSIONS

Nephrotic syndrome is a chronic disease that can begin at childhood and usually continues throughout life. It is characterized by periods of remission and relapses. For many patients, nephrotic syndrome can be controlled with the use of corticosteroids; however, in some patients, other medications with significant adverse drug effect profiles are required for disease control. The pharmacist has a role to play in recommending the proper pharmacologic approach, monitoring the patients' response to therapy, identifying adverse effects of these medications, and offering alternative pharmacologic options to the medical team when necessary.

A 4-year-old girl is brought to the nephrology clinic for a follow-up visit because she has had foamy urine, a urine dipstick positive for protein, and periorbital edema.

The patient had received a diagnosis of steroid-sensitive nephrotic syndrome 16 months ago. She went into remission after three doses of prednisolone 2 mg/kg daily and completed the initial 6-week regimen followed by a 1.5-mg/kg every-other-day steroid regimen for another 6 weeks. She has had two relapses within a 5-month period before today's symptoms, which is a total of six relapses since her initial treatment. After each relapse, she was restarted on prednisolone 2 mg/kg daily, she had full remission within 1 week, and was converted to alternate-day steroids, which were then tapered over 8 weeks. She was also started on ranitidine at her last clinic visit after she had abdominal pain suggestive of gastritis secondary to the initiation of steroids.

She had a relapse about 1 week ago after a sinus infection and was brought to the emergency department (ED) with periorbital edema and a urine dipstick showing (2+) protein. Her spot-urine protein to creatinine ratio (uPCR) at the ED was 2.13. She was restarted on prednisolone 60 mg/day at the ED and scheduled for nephrology clinic appointment 1 week later.

At today's nephrology clinic visit, the patient's mother states that the child has been a bit "hyper" lately and is always hungry, especially since she restarted the steroids. On physical examination, her periorbital edema has subsided and no lower extremity or truncal edema is noted. She has gained a substantial amount of weight on her face over the past few months. Her blood pressure is slightly elevated today (above 90th percentile for her age, gender, and height).

Past medical history: None reported

Family history: Negative for renal disease or kidney failure

Social history: Attends preschool and lives with her mother and father; no pets at home

Home medications: Prednisolone 15-mg/5-mL suspension, 20 mL by mouth every morning; ranitidine 75-mg/5-mL syrup, 2 mL by mouth twice daily

Allergies: None reported

Immunizations: Received influenza vaccine this season; all immunizations up to date

Review of systems:
Gastrointestinal: No pain or discomfort
Urinary: No urgency or bed-wetting
Genitalia: Normal
Musculoskeletal: Normal
Extremities: No swelling in lower extremity

Physical examination:
HEENT: Pupils equal, round, reactive to light and accommodation; extraocular eye movements intact; tympanic membranes intact

Neck and lymph nodes: No tenderness to palpitation of the cervical spine

Pulmonary: Clear to auscultation; no wheezes, crackles, or rhonchi

Cardiovascular: No murmurs, rubs, or gallops
Abdomen: Soft, no tenderness or distension, bowel sounds positive, no organomegaly

Vital signs: BP 108/69 mm Hg, HR 109 beats/minute, Tmax 98°F (36.7°C), Wt 31.5 kg, Ht 42 inches, body surface area 0.92 m², and body mass index 27.8 kg/m².

Laboratory findings:

Na	138 mEq/L
K	4.2 mEq/L
Cl	108 mEq/L
CO_2	22 mEq/L
BUN	10 mg/dL
SCr	0.42 mg/dL
Glucose	94 mg/dL
Calcium (total serum)	9.2 mg/dL
RBC	3.2×10^6 cells/mm³
WBC	9.9×10^3 cells/mm³
Hgb	13.1 g/dL
Hct	38.3%
Plt	304×10^3 cells/mm³

Urine dipstick: Leukocyte negative; nitrite negative; trace protein; pH 6.2; blood negative; specific gravity 1.018; glucose negative; ketones negative; bilirubin negative
Other diagnostic tests: uPCR 0.18 (180 mg/g)

---

1. Based on the clinical presentation and other objective data presented, what type and/or subtype of nephrotic syndrome does this patients have?

This patient has *frequently relapsing nephrotic syndrome* (FRNS), also known as *frequently relapsing steroid-sensitive nephrotic syndrome* (FR-SSNS). Based on her history, she has had her third relapse in 6 months and has had a total of six relapses since her initial diagnosis 16 months ago. On each occasion, she responded fully to steroids that were tapered over 8 weeks. During her presentation at the ED, she had a 2+ protein dipstick and a spot-urine uPCR of 2.13. A *relapse* is defined as 3 consecutive days of 1+ or greater on urine dipstick OR a spot urine uPCR of 2 (2000 mg/g) or more. *Frequent relapses* are defined as two or more relapses within 6 months or four or more relapses within 1 year.

---

2. Recommend a suitable pharmacologic regimen to manage this case including the assessments necessary for monitoring.

The approach to this patient should be to taper the steroid and add a steroid-sparing agent, such as tacrolimus or mycophenolate mofetil. The specific approach to ongoing management of this case follows.

Assessment

- The patient is currently taking prednisolone 20 mL of 15-mg/5-mL suspension (2 mg/kg) by mouth every morning and is currently in remission. Today her uPCR is 0.18. In addition she has no peripheral edema on physical examination today.

- Her calculated estimated glomerular filtration rate is 104.7 mL/min/1.73 m² (using the modified-Schwartz equation). This rate classifies her as having stage 1 chronic kidney disease, defined as normal renal function with increased risk factors. Her basic metabolic panel and complete blood count are within normal limits.

- She has an elevated blood pressure of 108/69 mmHg, which is between the 90th to 95th percentile for her age, gender, and height. This value puts her at the prehypertensive stage and is likely a result of her prolonged steroid use.

Plan

- Add tacrolimus 1 mg by mouth every 12 hours (0.05–0.3 mg/kg/day).

- After starting the tacrolimus, revert to alternate-day steroid therapy.

- Start 15 mL of 15-mg/5-mL prednisolone (1.5 mg/kg) every other day and taper over 3 months while optimizing the tacrolimus dose.

- Taper the prednisolone slowly over 3 months. Several recommendations for tapering are available; for this case, the prednisolone dose will be decreased by 5 mg using the following schedule:
  - Prednisolone 40 mg (13 mL) every other day for 2 weeks
  - Prednisolone 20 mg (7 mL) every other day for 2 weeks
  - Prednisolone 15 mg (5 mL) every other day for 2 weeks
  - Prednisolone 10 mg (3 mL) every other day for 2 weeks
  - Prednisolone 5 mg (2 mL) every other day for 2 weeks
  - Prednisolone 2.5 mg (1 mL) every other day for 2 weeks, then off
  - Continue ranitidine 2 mL (75 mg/5 mL) daily while on steroids to prevent gastrointestinal discomfort secondary to steroid use.

- Schedule follow-up visit in one week to assess blood tacrolimus trough levels, comprehensive metabolic panel, and serum magnesium concentrations.

- Monitor blood pressure and apply nonpharmacologic measures such as reduction in salt (sodium) intake (maximum of 2000 mg/day), and encourage physical activity; although no exercise target exists for this age group, a sedentary lifestyle should be discouraged and the family should be counseled to all be active together.

Implementation

- Remind the patient and family about the adverse effects of steroids and counsel them on the steroid taper schedule.
  - Take 13 mL every other day for 2 weeks
  - Take 7 mL every other day for 2 weeks
  - Take 5 mL every other day for 2 weeks
  - Take 3 mL every other day for 2 weeks
  - Take 2 mL every other day for 2 weeks
  - Take 1 mL every other day for 2 weeks, then stop steroids

- Counsel the patient and family on tacrolimus.
  - Take tacrolimus 1 mg by mouth every 12 hours (8 a.m. and 8 p.m.) and remind the patient and family not to take medication before the next visit (if visit is in the morning hours)

- Counsel the patient and family on ranitidine
  - Educate the patient and family about potential adverse reactions from ranitidine, including nausea, vomiting, and diarrhea.
  - Tell the patient and family that if the patient experiences any dizziness, they need to contact the health care provider for further assessment.

- Counsel the patient and family to monitor blood pressure about 2–3 times a week and to report the blood pressure values at next visit.

- Counsel the patient's parents on the need for adherence to her medication schedule. Identify any barriers to proper adherence, and resolve the issues if possible.

Monitoring and Follow-Up

- Schedule follow-up visits weekly until tacrolimus is stable at the desired blood concentration.

- Take these actions at follow-up:
  - Update medication profile to include new prescriptions or over-the-counter medications since the last visit.
  - Order or monitor tacrolimus trough concentration (target 5–10 ng/mL) at this visit, if the patient has not taken her morning dose. Alternatively, order trough concentration to be drawn just before her evening dose. Determine if a dose change is needed.
  - Monitor blood pressure, comprehensive metabolic panel, complete blood count, magnesium, and phosphorus; watch for tremors and other tacrolimus adverse effects.

Justification

- Kidney Disease Improving Global Outcomes (KDIGO) guidelines
  - The 2012 KDIGO guidelines recommend calcineurin inhibitors (CNIs) as a first-line steroid-sparing option in FRNS.[9] Mycophenolate mofetil and alkylating agents are the alternatives. The goal of switching to CNIs is to limit

the use of steroids to reduce their adverse effects. This patient is already beginning to show signs of steroid toxicity: weight gain around her face, elevated blood pressure, behavioral changes, and increased appetite.

○ The KDIGO guidelines recommend a slow taper (over 3 months) based on the strength of data that show that prolonged steroid use even at small doses plus CNIs help extend the period in remission.

○ Follow-up in 1 to 2 weeks because tacrolimus will be at steady state by this time and the trough level would be meaningful. Check the tacrolimus trough level (target of 5–10 ng/mL) to prevent toxicity, basic metabolic panel to estimate kidney function and electrolyte imbalances secondary to tacrolimus, complete blood count, and physical examination to check for tremors and gingival hyperplasia (rare with tacrolimus versus cyclosporine).

• High blood pressure is a significant complication of nephrotic syndrome.

○ In addition to the disease process, several medications used to manage nephrotic syndrome can also cause hypertension, such as corticosteroid and CNIs.

○ For prehypertensive children, the recommendation is lifestyle and dietary modifications and monitoring. The blood pressure goal is below 90th percentile for age, gender, and height.[47]

REFERENCES

1. Gipson DS, Massengill SF, Yao L, et al. Management of childhood onset nephrotic syndrome. Pediatrics 2009;124:747-57.

2. Eddy AA, Symons JM. Nephrotic syndrome in childhood. Lancet 2003;362:629-39.

3. Gordillo R, Spitzer A. The Nephrotic Syndrome. Pediatr Rev 2009; 30:94-104.

4. Ingulli E, Tejani A. Racial differences in the incidence and renal outcome of idiopathic focal segmental glomerulosclerosis in children. Pediatr Nephrol 1991;5:393-7.

5. Lane C, Brown M, Dunsmuir W, et al. Can spot urine protein/creatinine ratio replace 24 h urine protein in usual clinical nephrology? Nephrology (Carlton) 2006;11:245-9.

6. Wahbeh AM, Ewais MH, Elsharif ME. Comparison of 24-hour urinary protein and protein-to-creatinine ratio in the assessment of proteinuria. Saudi J Kidney Dis Transpl 2009;20:443-7.

7. Wahbeh AM. Spot urine protein-to-creatinine ratio compared with 24-hour urinary protein in patients with kidney transplant. Exp Clin Transplant 2014;12:300-3.

8. Akbari A, Fergusson D, Kokolo MB, et al. Spot urine protein measurements in kidney transplantation: a systematic review of diagnostic accuracy. Nephrol Dial Transplant 2014;29:919-26.

9. Kidney Disease: Improving Global Outcomes (KDIGO) Glomerulonephritis Work Group. KDIGO clinical practice guideline for glomerulonephritis. Kidney Int Suppl 2012; 2:163-71.

10. Feber J, Al-Matrafi J, Farhadi E. Prednisone dosing per body weight or body surface area in children with nephrotic syndrome-is it equivalent? Pediatr Nephrol 2009;24:1027-31.

11. Raman V, Krishnamurthy S, Harichandrakumar KT. Body weight-based prednisolone versus body surface area-based prednisolone regimen for induction of remission in children with nephrotic syndrome: a randomized, open-label, equivalence clinical trial. Pediatr Nephrol 2016;31:595-604.

12. Saddeh S, Baracco R, Jain A. Weight or body surface area dosing of steroids in nephrotic syndrome: is there an outcome difference? Pediatr Nephrol 2011;26:2167-71.

13. Ehrich JH, Brodehl J. Long versus standard prednisone therapy for initial treatment of idiopathic nephrotic syndrome in children: Arbeitsgemeinschaft fur Padiatrische Nephrologie. Eur J Pediatr 1993;152:357-61.

14. Uwaezuoke SN. Steroid-sensitive nephrotic syndrome in children: triggers of relapse and evolving hypotheses on pathogenesis. Ital J Pediatr 2015;21:19.

15. Gulati A, Sinha A, Sreenivas V, et al. Daily corticosteroids reduce infection-associated relapses in frequently relapsing nephrotic syndrome: a randomized controlled trial. Clin J Am Soc Nephrol 2011;6:63-9.

16. Abeyagunawardena AS, Trompeter RS. Increasing the dose of prednisolone during viral infections reduces the risk of relapse in nephrotic syndrome: a randomised controlled trial. Arch Dis Child 2008;93:226-8.

17. Bhimma R, Adhikari M, Asharam K, et al. Management of steroid-resistant focal segmental glomerulosclerosis in children using tacrolimus. Am J Nephrol 2006;26:544-51.

18. Tahar G, Rachid LM. Cyclosporine A and steroid therapy in childhood steroid-resistant nephrotic syndrome. Int J Nephrol Renovasc Dis 2010;3:117-21.

19. Kim YC, Lee TW, Lee H, et al. Complete remission induced by tacrolimus and low-dose prednisolone in adult minimal change nephrotic syndrome: a pilot study. Kidney Res Clin Pract 2012; 31:112-7.

20. Hari P, Bagga A, Mantan M. Short term efficacy of intravenous dexamethasone and methylprednisolone therapy in steroid resistant nephrotic syndrome. Indian Pediatr 2004;41:993-1000.

21. Tarshish P, Tobin JN, Bernstein J, et al. Cyclophosphamide does not benefit patients with focal segmental glomerulosclerosis. A report of the International Study of Kidney Disease in Children. Pediatr Nephrol 1996;10:590-3.

22. Jafar TH, Schmid CH, Landa M, et al. Angiotensin-converting enzyme inhibitors and progression of nondiabetic renal disease. A meta-analysis of patient-level data. Ann Intern Med 2001; 135:73-87.

23. Lama G, Luongo I, Piscitelli A, et al. Enalapril: antiproteinuric effect in children with nephrotic syndrome. Clin Nephrol 2000; 53:432-6.

24. Trachtman H, Gauthier B. Effect of angiotensin-converting enzyme inhibitor therapy on proteinuria in children with renal disease. J Pediatr 1988;112:295-8.

25. Ishikura K, Ikeda M, Hattori S, et al. Effective and safe treatment with cyclosporine in nephrotic children: a prospective, randomized multicenter trial. Kidney International 2008;73:1167-73.

26. Kim SH, Park SJ, Han KH, et al. Pathogenesis of minimal change nephrotic syndrome: an immunological concept. Korean J Pediatr 2016;59:205-11.

27. Choudhry S, Bagga A, Hari P, et al. Efficacy and safety of tacrolimus versus cyclosporine in children with steroid-resistant nephrotic syndrome: a randomized controlled trial. Am J Kidney Dis 2009;53:760-69.

28. Loeffler K, Gowrishankar M, Yiu V. Tacrolimus therapy in pediatric patients with treatment-resistant nephrotic syndrome. Pediatr Nephrol 2004;19:281-7.

29. Pollard S, Nashan B, Johnston A, et al. A pharmacokinetic and clinical review of the potential clinical impact of using different formulations of cyclosporin A. Clin Ther 2003;25:1654-69.

30. Alloway RR, Sadaka B, Trofe-Clarke J, et al. A randomized pharmacokinetic study of generic tacrolimus versus reference tacrolimus in kidney transplant recipients. Am J Transplant 2012;12:2825-31.

31. Marfo K, Aitken S, Akalin E. Clinical outcomes after conversion from brand-name tacrolimus (prograf) to a generic formulation in renal transplant recipients: a retrospective cohort study. P&T 2013;38:484-8.

32. Wang J, Mao J, Chen J, et al. Evaluation of mycophenolate mofetil or tacrolimus in children with steroid sensitive but frequently relapsing or steroid-dependent nephrotic syndrome. Nephrology 2016;21:21-7.

33. Choi MJ, Eustace JA, Gimenez LF, et al. Mycophenolate mofetil treatment for primary glomerular diseases. Kidney Int 2002; 61:1098-114.

34. Chiu J, McLaine PN, Drummond KN. A controlled prospective study of cyclophosphamide in relapsing, corticosteroid-responsive, minimal-lesion nephrotic syndrome in childhood. J Pediatr 1973;82:607-13.

35. Grupe WE, Makker SP, Ingelfinger JR. Chlorambucil treatment of frequently relapsing nephrotic syndrome. N Engl J Med 1976;295:746-9.

36. Fornoni A, Sageshima J, Wei C, et al. Rituximab targets podocytes in recurrent focal segmental glomerulosclerosis. Sci Transl Med 2011;3:85ra46.

37. Kamei K, Ito S, Nozu K. Single dose of rituximab for refractory steroid-dependent nephrotic syndrome in children. Pediatr Nephrol 2009;24:1321-8.

38. Ravani P, Rossi R, Bonanni A, et al. Rituximab in children with steroid-dependent nephrotic syndrome: a multicenter, open-label, non-inferiority, randomized controlled trial. J Am Soc Nephrol 2015;26:2259-66.

39. Iijima K, Sako M, Nozu K, et al. Rituximab for Childhood-onset Refractory Nephrotic Syndrome (RCRNS) Study Group. Rituximab for childhood-onset, complicated, frequently relapsing nephrotic syndrome or steroid-dependent nephrotic syndrome: a multicentre, double-blind, randomised, placebo-controlled trial. Lancet 2014;384:1273-81.

40. Safar OY, Aboualhameael A, Kari JA. Rituximab for troublesome cases of childhood nephrotic syndrome. World J Clin Pediatr 2014;3:69-75.

41. Rituxan (rituximab) [prescribing information]. San Francisco, CA: Genentech, Inc. Revised 2016 April.

42. Bitzan M, Anselmo M, Carpineta L. Rituximab (B-cell depleting antibody) associated lung injury (RALI): a pediatric case and systematic review of the literature. Pediatr Pulmonol 2009; 44:922-34.

43. Lands LC. New therapies, new concerns: rituximab-associated lung injury. Pediatr Nephrol 2010;25:1001-3.

44. Vivarelli M, Colucci M, Bonanni A, et al. Ofatumumab in two pediatric nephrotic syndrome patients allergic to rituximab. Pediatr Nephrol 2017;32:181-4.

45. Jalanko H. Congenital nephrotic syndrome. Pediatr Nephrol 2009;24:2121-8.

46. Holmberg C, Jalanko H. Congenital nephrotic syndrome and recurrence of proteinuria after renal transplantation. Pediatr Nephrol 2014;29:2309-17.

47. National Heart Lung and Blood Institute (NHLBI): Expert Panel on integrated guidelines for cardiovascular health and risk reduction in children and adolescents: summary report. Pediatrics 2011;128(suppl 5):S213-56.

48. Bagga A, Mudigoudar BD, Hari P, et al. Enalapril dosage in steroid-resistant nephrotic syndrome. Pediatr Nephrol 2004; 19:45-50.

49. Yi Z, Li Z, Wu XC, et al. Effect of fosinopril in children with steroid-resistant idiopathic nephrotic syndrome. Pediatr Nephrol 2006;21:967-72.

50. Dorhout Mees EJ. Does it make sense to administer albumin to the patient with nephrotic oedema? Nephrol Dial Transplant 1996;11:1224-6.

51. Dharmaraj R, Hari P, Bagga A. Randomized cross-over trial comparing albumin and frusemide infusions in nephrotic syndrome. Pediatr Nephrol 2009;24:775-82.

52. Prescott WA Jr, Streetman DA, Streetman DS. The potential role of HMG-CoA reductase inhibitors in pediatric nephrotic syndrome. Ann Pharmacother 2004;38:2105-14.

53. Coleman JE, Watson AR. Hyperlipidaemia, diet and simvastatin therapy in steroid-resistant nephrotic syndrome of childhood. Pediatr Nephrol 1996;10:171-4.

54. Sanjad SA, Al-Abbad A, Al-Shorafa S. Management of hyperlipidemia in children with refractory nephrotic syndrome: the effect of statin therapy. J Pediatr 1997;130:470-4.

55. Appel GB, Waldman M, Radhakrishnan J. New approaches to the treatment of glomerular diseases. Kidney Int 2006;70:545-50.

56. Kerlin BA, Ayoob R, Smoyer WE. Epidemiology and pathophysiology of nephrotic syndrome-associated thromboembolic disease. Clin J Am Soc Nephrol 2012;7:513-20.

57. Monagle P, Chan AKC, Goldenberg NA, et al. Antithrombotic therapy in neonates and children antithrombotic therapy and prevention of thrombosis, 9th ed.: American College of Chest Physicians Evidence-Based Clinical Practice Guidelines. Chest 2012;141(2 suppl):e737S-801S.

58. Ogi M, Yokoyama H, Tomosugi N, et al. Risk factors for infection and immunoglobulin replacement therapy in adult nephrotic syndrome. Am J Kidney Dis 1994;24:427-36.

59. Fuchshuber A, Kuhnemund O, Keuth B, et al. Pneumococcal vaccine in children and young adults with chronic renal disease. Nephrol Dial Transplant 1996;11:468-73.

60. Pekka Nuorti J, Whitney CG. Prevention of pneumococcal disease among infants and children—use of 13-valent pneumococcal conjugate vaccine and 23-valent pneumococcal polysaccharide vaccine: recommendations of the Advisory Committee on Immunization Practices (ACIP). MMWR 2010;59(RR-11): 1-19. Available at www.cdc.gov/mmwr/pdf/rr/rr5911.pdf. Accessed September 19, 2019.

61. Banerjee S, Basu S, Sengupta J. Vitamin D in nephrotic syndrome remission: a case-control study. Pediatr Nephrol 2013;28:1983-9.

62. Bischoff-Ferrari HA, Giovannucci E, Willett WC, et al. Estimation of optimal serum concentrations of 25-hydroxyvitamin D for multiple health outcomes. Am J Clin Nutr 2006;84:18-28.

63. Choudhary S, Agarwal I, Seshadri MS. Calcium and vitamin D for osteoprotection in children with new-onset nephrotic syndrome treated with steroids: a prospective, randomized, controlled, interventional study. Pediatr Nephrol 2014;29:1025-32.

64. Benfield MR, McDonald RA, Bartosh S, et al. Changing trends in pediatric transplantation: 2001 annual report of the North American Pediatric Renal Transplant Cooperative Study. Pediatr Transplant 2003;7:321-5.

65. Andenmatten F, Bianchetti MG, Gerber HA, et al. Outcome of idiopathic childhood nephrotic syndrome. A 20-year experience. Scand J Urol Nephrol 1995;29:15-9.

Section VIII

Endocrinologic Disorders

CHAPTER 24

Diabetes Mellitus

Sandra Benavides, Pharm.D., FCCP, FPPA

LEARNING OBJECTIVES

1. Differentiate the pathophysiology between type 1 and 2 diabetes mellitus (DM) in pediatric patients.

2. Identify the criteria for the diagnosis of DM in pediatric patients.

3. Describe acute and chronic complications of DM in pediatric patients.

4. Develop an insulin regimen for a pediatric patient.

5. Discuss the available pharmacologic agents for the treatment of type 2 DM in pediatric patients.

ABBREVIATIONS IN THIS CHAPTER

ADA	American Diabetes Association
BG	Blood glucose
CGM	Continuous glucose monitoring
CSII	Continuous subcutaneous insulin infusion
DKA	Diabetic ketoacidosis
DM	Diabetes mellitus
ESRD	End-stage renal disease
GLP-1	Glucagon-like peptide 1
PG	Plasma glucose
SMBG	Self-monitoring of blood glucose

INTRODUCTION

Diabetes mellitus (DM) is one of the most common chronic diseases in pediatrics. Either a lack of insulin release from the pancreas or a resistance to insulin in peripheral tissues, resulting in hyperglycemia, causes DM. Persistent hyperglycemia leads to several acute, microvascular, and macrovascular complications necessitating metabolic control with pharmacologic treatment. Children and adolescents present special challenges in achieving metabolic control. This chapter will focus on such challenges and appropriate pharmacotherapy strategies in pediatric patients.

EPIDEMIOLOGY

Recent prevalence data estimates 1.93 cases of some form of DM per 1000 youths in the United States. The prevalence of DM in children and adolescents up to age 19 years is 1.93 per 1000 youths and 1.20 per 1000 youths for type 1 and type 2 DM, respectively.[1] The overall prevalence of DM increases with increasing age, with rates of any type of DM reaching 3.22 cases per 1000 youths age 15–19 years in 2009.[1] Although

type 1 DM accounts for most diabetes in pediatrics, the number of children and adolescents with type 2 DM is increasing. In 2001, the rates of type 2 DM in youth were 0.34 per 1000 youths, whereas in 2009, the rates increased to 1.20 cases per 1000 youths.[1]

CLASSIFICATION

It is necessary to determine the pathophysiologic basis for diabetes for appropriate pharmacologic treatment. Before the 1990s, most DM cases diagnosed in youth were type 1. However, because of increases in obesity rates, pediatric patients are now presenting with type 2 DM.[2] Youths can also be affected with other forms of diabetes, including maturity-onset diabetes of youth; neonatal diabetes; mitochondrial diabetes; diabetes associated with lipodystrophy; diabetes secondary to other pancreatic, endocrine, or genetic syndromes; or drug induced diabetes (e.g., corticosteroids, immunosuppressants).[3] This chapter will focus on the two most common forms of DM in pediatrics, types 1 and 2. Table 1 highlights the differences between type 1 and type 2 DM.

PATHOPHYSIOLOGY

Type 1 DM is the result of a T-cell–mediated autoimmune attack on the beta cells of the pancreas, resulting in complete insulin deficiency. Before the clinical presentation of DM, autoantibodies and reactive lymphocytes infiltrate the pancreas and destroy beta cells. During this time, the beta cells increase insulin secretion secondary to systemic hyperglycemia, which eventually leads to the destruction of the beta cells. The administration of exogenous insulin at the onset of symptoms provides temporary relief to the beta cells, resulting in increased insulin secretion from the beta cell, referred to as the *honeymoon phase*.[4] The honeymoon phase occurs in about 80% of children and adolescents with type 1 DM.[5]

Individuals with type 1 DM typically have a genetic predisposition, indicated by the presence of human leukocyte antigens. The DR3-DQ2 and DR4-DQ8 alleles are associated with increased risk, whereas the DR2-DQ6 allele is protective against type 1 DM.[6] The T-cell–mediated attack on the beta cells result in an inflammatory process in the islets of Langerhans and the production of antibodies. Antibodies to insulin, glutamic acid decarboxylase, and the protein tyrosine phosphatase are detectable even before the clinical presentation of disease. Zinc transporter autoantibodies can help distinguish those with type 1 diabetes by detecting the zinc transporter protein, which is not found in those with T2DM.[7] The autoimmune process can take months to years to occur. Signs of insulin deficiency do not become evident until about 80% of the beta cells are destroyed. Typically the earlier the onset of destruction, the sooner that insulin deficiency is evident. Although controversial, it is believed that in addition to a genetic predisposition, an environmental toxin contributes to the development of type 1 DM. Environmental factors thought to trigger type 1 DM include certain foods (e.g., cow's milk, nitrosamines) or viral infections (e.g., enterovirus, rotavirus). To date, only exposure to congenital rubella has been associated with the onset of type 1 DM.

Type 2 DM results from both impaired insulin secretion from the pancreas and insulin resistance. Various factors increase the susceptibility to decreased insulin sensitivity, including family history, obesity, physical inactivity, poor dietary choices, and intrauterine factors.[8] Most pediatric patients with a diagnosis of type 2 DM have at least one first- or second-degree relative with type 2 DM. Infants who are born to mothers with gestational diabetes or who are small for gestational age have an increased risk of insulin resistance. The decrease in insulin sensitivity initially leads to an increase in insulin secretion, compensatory hyperinsulinemia, and ultimately beta-cell destruction. Before clinical presentation of type 2 DM, children and adolescents present with hyperinsulinemia or signs of insulin resistance such as acanthosis nigricans. Acanthosis nigricans is a dermatologic disorder characterized by brown to blackish, raised, velvety lesions usually found in skinfolds or creases in the back of the neck, axilla, and genital area.[9] Acanthosis nigricans is thought to be the result of increased insulin levels binding insulin-like growth factor receptors, fibroblasts, and keratinocytes, resulting in the proliferation of epidermal cells.[9,10] During puberty, insulin resistance worsens, precipitating glucose intolerance and, subsequently, the clinical manifestations of type 2 DM.

SCREENING

Typically the time from abnormal glucose control to when the clinical symptoms of disease occur is fairly rapid in type 1 DM; therefore, routine screening is not recommended. However, the American Diabetes Association (ADA) recommends screening for type 2 DM.[11] Children and adolescents who are *overweight*, defined as a body mass index percentile greater than 85 for age and sex, or those who are more than 120% of ideal body weight with two additional risk factors are recommended for screening.[11,12] Additional risk factors include having a family history of type 2 DM in a first- or second-degree relative; being of a racial/ethnic group with high rates of type 2 DM (e.g., American Indian, African American, Hispanic, Asian, Pacific Islander); a mother with a history of gestational diabetes or diabetes during pregnancy with the child or showing evidence of existing insulin resistance.[11,12] Conditions associated with insulin resistance include acanthosis nigricans, hypertension, dyslipidemia, polycystic ovarian syndrome, and a maternal history of gestational diabetes during the child's gestation.[12] Screening consists of a fasting plasma glucose (PG) or an oral glucose tolerance test every 2–3 years starting at age 10 years or at onset of puberty in any child or adolescent meeting these criteria.[11,12]

CLINICAL PRESENTATION AND DIAGNOSIS

The classic signs and symptoms of diabetes are polydipsia, polyuria, polyphagia, and weight loss. Those presenting with type 1 DM may have symptoms for 1 month to several months before diagnosis but often present with acute, severe symptoms of polydipsia, polyuria, polyphagia, weight loss, fatigue, blurred vision, and ketonemia.[13,14] Female patients with type 2 DM might present with candida vulvovaginitis in addition to classic symptoms. Although it is more common for a patient with type 1 DM to present with diabetic ketoacidosis (DKA), patients with type 2 DM are still at risk of developing DKA. Other potential findings on presentation include glycosuria and ketonuria. Of note, however, DM can also present asymptomatically in both type 1 and 2, and its presence can be discovered coincidentally with routine laboratory analysis.

Diagnostic criteria for DM include at least one of the following:[12-14]

1. Hemoglobin A1C of 6.5% or greater;
2. Fasting PG of 126 mg/dL or greater;

Table 1. Characteristics of Type 1 and Type 2 Diabetes Mellitus in Children and Adolescents[8]

Characteristics	Type 1	Type 2
Age of presentation	Throughout childhood	Typically at puberty
Onset	Acute	Insidious to severe
Ketosis at onset	Common	Variable
Affected relative	5%	75%–90%
Female/male sex	1:1	2:1
Human leukocyte antigen *DR3, DR4	Increased association	No association
Ethnicity	All (whites more susceptible)	All
Insulin secretion	Decreased/absent	Variable
Insulin sensitivity	Normal when controlled	Decreased
Insulin dependence	Permanent	Episodic
Obesity	< 24%	> 90%
Acanthosis nigricans	No	Common
Pancreatic autoantibodies	Yes	No

3. 2-hour PG of 200 mg/dL or greater during an oral glucose tolerance test; or

4. Random PG of 200 mg/dL or greater and symptoms of hyperglycemia.

A fasting PG of 126 mg/dL or greater or a 2-hour PG of 200 mg/dL or greater should be repeated for confirming the diagnosis. The diagnosis of diabetes is also confirmed if two of the criteria are met, for example a hemoglobin A1C greater than 6.5% and fasting PG greater than 126 mg/dL. Diagnosis does not need confirmation in children or adolescents with symptoms of diabetes and a random PG greater than 200 mg/dL. To differentiate between type 1 and 2 DM, it is recommended to measure islet autoantibodies, insulin, and C-peptide. The presence of islet autoantibodies is indicative of type 1 DM. Interpretation of insulin and C-peptide can be less conclusive because both may still be present in a person with an early diagnosis of type 1 as well as in those with type 2 DM.[14]

COMPLICATIONS

Diabetes mellitus in children and adolescents is associated with short- and long-term complications. Short-term complications include hypoglycemia, DKA, and hyperosmolar hyperglycemic syndrome. Long-term microvascular complications include retinopathy, nephropathy, and neuropathy. Macrovascular disease, including peripheral, cerebrovascular and cardiovascular disease, are also long-term complications of DM. Common comorbidities with type 1 DM include thyroid and celiac disease.

HYPOGLYCEMIA

Hypoglycemia in patients with DM is defined as an episode of a PG concentration low enough to cause signs or symptoms of harm.[15] In the Diabetes Control and Complications Trial, patients on intensive glycemic control had a three-fold increase in the risk of severe hypoglycemia.[16] Over the past two decades, however, severe hypoglycemia has declined because of the use of insulin analogues, improved insulin delivery systems (e.g., pumps), increased monitoring including the use of continuous glucose monitoring (CGM) technologies, and improved patient education.[15] Children younger than 6 years may be at higher risk of severe hypoglycemia than are adults because of the lack of symptom recognition, their inability to communicate symptoms to the caregiver, and their variable eating and exercise habits.[17] Severe hypoglycemia in children can be associated with seizures, coma, and death. It was previously believed that recurrent or severe hypoglycemia resulted in cognitive impairment in children at an older age. However, long-term follow-up of adolescents enrolled in the Diabetes Control and Complications Trial with severe hypoglycemia did not indicate cognitive impairment.[18] Further follow-up studies have also indicated no *cognitive decline*, defined as decreased full IQ scores; however, severe hypoglycemia at a young age may result in a decrease in executive function, which may be reflected in poorer performance in complex tasks.[19,20] Regardless, because of the potential for death, patients and caregivers are provided education to monitor, treat, and prevent hypoglycemic episodes. Signs, symptoms, and treatment strategies for hypoglycemia will be discussed later in this chapter.

DIABETIC KETOACIDOSIS

Diabetic ketoacidosis results from lack of insulin and increased counterregulatory hormones (e.g., glucagon, catecholamines, cortisol, growth hormone), resulting in a catabolic state.[21] This ketoacidosis is characterized by hyperglycemia, acidosis, ketonemia, and ketonuria.[22] Around 29% and 10% of patients with type 1 and 2 DM, respectively, will present with DKA at initial diagnosis.[23,24] Other factors that precipitate DKA after diagnosis are insufficient exogenous insulin administration, sepsis, trauma, or excessive diarrhea and vomiting.[22] Complications of DKA can include death, usually caused by cerebral edema. Additional causes of death in DKA include other neurologic complications, hypokalemia, hyperkalemia, thrombosis, sepsis, aspiration pneumonia, and pulmonary edema. Long-term complications may include neurologic deficits. Diabetic ketoacidosis will be discussed more thoroughly later in this chapter.

HYPEROSMOLAR HYPERGLYCEMIC SYNDROME

Hyperosmolar hyperglycemic syndrome is a rare but life-threatening complication of uncontrolled type 2 DM. The incidence of this syndrome in pediatric patients is unknown, but it is estimated that 2%–4% will present with hyperosmolar hyperglycemic syndrome at time of diagnosis with type 2 DM.[23]

RETINOPATHY

Retinopathy results from damage to the blood vessels of the retina. It is the most common cause of adult blindness in the United States. Nonproliferative retinopathy (background retinopathy) is transient and consists of microaneurysms and pre- and intraretinal hemorrhages.[25] Nonproliferative retinopathy is not associated with vision loss and does not always progress to proliferative retinopathy. Proliferative retinopathy is a more severe form of retinopathy and is characterized by the development of new blood vessels, which may rupture or bleed into the vitreoretinal space. Visual loss may occur with proliferative retinopathy.[25]

Retinopathy can be present in children and adolescents within 1–2 years after diagnosis of DM, although it is not usually seen for 5–10 years. It occurs in pediatric patients of all ages, but it tends to present post-pubertally. Proliferative retinopathy does not typically present in those younger than 20 years. In those with type 2 DM, the onset and incidence of retinopathy is higher. Prevalence of any form of retinopathy in type 2 DM is 42% within 7 years of diagnosis, whereas in type 1 DM within about the same time the prevalence is 17%.[26] Risk factors for retinopathy include poor glycemic control, longer duration of diabetes, elevated blood pressure, smoking, albuminuria, pregnancy and hyperlipidemia.[14,26] The largest cohort study to date has found a higher risk of retinopathy in those with higher hemoglobin A1C and low-density lipoproteins.[26]

For children and adolescents with type 1 DM, annual ophthalmologic examinations are recommended when the child is at least age 10 years and has diabetes for 3–5 years. After the initial ophthalmologic examination, annual examinations are recommended.[17] In children and adolescents with type 2 DM, the initial ophthalmologic examination should be at diagnosis or shortly thereafter with annual ophthalmologic examinations.[27]

NEPHROPATHY

End-stage renal disease (ESRD) requiring dialysis or transplantation is a microvascular complication of DM. The first clinical signs of diabetic nephropathy are microalbuminuria followed by proteinuria. When coupled with increased blood pressure, proteinuria can result in ESRD. About 20% to 40% of those receiving a diagnosis of type 1 DM will develop ESRD.[28] The incidence of developing ESRD in children and adolescents having a diagnosis of type 2 remains unknown. However, one study evaluating claims of insured children and adolescents with DM reported an overall annual prevalence of nephropathy is 3.44%.[29] After around 7 years of diabetes, the prevalence of nephropathy in type 1 DM was 5.8%, whereas the prevalence in those with type 2 DM was about 20%.[30] Risk factors for the progression of renal disease include poor metabolic control, smoking, and hypertension. Additional risk factors reported in those with type 1 DM include a family history of hypertension or cardiovascular disorders. For patients with type 1 DM, annual screening for albuminuria is recommended beginning at age 10 years or in patients with a history of diabetes for 5 years and then yearly.[17] For type 2 DM, it is recommended to screen for microalbuminuria at the time of diagnosis and then yearly thereafter.[27] In patients with microalbuminuria, treatment with an angiotensin-converting enzyme inhibitor is suggested. In addition, any concomitant hypertension or hyperlipidemia should be treated.

NEUROPATHY

Peripheral and autonomic neuropathies, a complication of DM in adults, are not commonly seen in pediatric patients. Peripheral neuropathies are associated with pain, burning, and diminished sensation to filament testing, typically initially presenting in feet in children and adolescents.[31] With time, peripheral neuropathies result in a loss of motor function, poor wound healing that can result in foot ulceration, infection, and, ultimately, amputation.[31] Children and adolescents suffering from peripheral neuropathies have persistent ongoing pain. Autonomic neuropathies include the cardiovascular, gastrointestinal, and genitourinary systems. Clinical presentation can include postural hypotension, gastroparesis, neurogenic bladder, impotence, and hypoglycemic unawareness. In rare instances, sudden death has been associated with abnormal response and prolonged QT intervals.[31,32] Increased disease duration, particularly with poor metabolic control, is associated with earlier onset of neuropathies. Although the true estimates of the incidence and onset of diabetic neuropathy are not well described, the prevalence of neuropathy in type 1 DM has been reported as 8.2% 6 years after diagnosis and 25.7% in type 2 DM 7 years after diagnosis.[33] The ADA recommends a foot examination for children with type 1 DM beginning at puberty and then yearly thereafter.[17] It is also important to provide patient education on proper footwear and regular monitoring of feet. Although no recommendations exist for children and adolescents with type 2 DM, annual testing from the time of diagnosis and patient education should be considered.

MACROVASCULAR COMPLICATIONS

Macrovascular complications of diabetes include cardiovascular, cerebrovascular, and peripheral vascular disease caused by atherosclerosis. The prevalence of macrovascular complications in children and adolescents is unknown at this time. However, atrial stiffness (measured by pulse wave velocity or carotid-artery media thickness) in children and adolescents with DM is elevated in both type 1 and 2 DM, and is significantly higher in those with type 2 DM (47.4% vs. 11.6%).[30] As such, identifying and modifying the risk factors are important. Risk factors for atherosclerosis include poor glycemic control, hyperlipidemia, smoking, hypertension, obesity, and a family history of cardiovascular disease.[14,32] Screening, and treatment when necessary, of risk factors is critical in children and adolescents with DM to minimize long-term complications.

The American Heart Association recommends a fasting lipid panel in children with type 1 DM older than 2 years up to puberty after 2 years of diagnosis.[34] For pubertal children and adolescents with type 1 DM, a lipid panel should be obtained at diagnosis and subsequently every 3–5 years if the low-density lipoprotein is less than 100 mg/dL.[17,34] For children and adolescents with type 2 DM, a fasting lipid panel should be obtained at diagnosis and every 2 years if results are normal.[27] Pharmacologic treatment is recommended for children older than 10 years if the low-density lipoprotein cholesterol is greater than 130 mg/dL.[35]

THERAPY GOALS

The Diabetes Control and Complications Trial showed a decrease in microvascular complications in patients with type 1 DM when treated with intensive insulin therapy to maintain blood glucose (BG) as close to normal physiologic values as possible.[36] In the trial, adolescents randomized to intensive treatment achieved lower hemoglobin A1C percentages, although were unable to achieve hemoglobin A1C as low as the adults enrolled in the study.[36] Despite being unable to achieve a hemoglobin A1C less than 7%, adolescents in the intensive treatment group had decreases in the onset of retinopathy or improvements in existing retinopathies, improved conduction velocities, and modest improvements in low-density lipoprotein cholesterol levels compared with those in conventional treatment.[36] Long-term outcomes for those enrolled in the trial found that the continuation of intensive therapy (despite not achieving normal hemoglobin A1C levels) provided benefits, such as non-progression to proliferative retinopathy.[37] With the availability of long-acting and rapid-acting insulin, intensive insulin regimens are now the standard of care.[14] However, an intensive insulin regimen predisposes an individual to increased weight gain and an increased number of hypoglycemic episodes; as such, glycemic goals may be adjusted to balance the risk and benefits of tight glycemic control.

Glycemic goals for patients with DM are listed in Table 2. In addition, a decrease in insulin resistance is desired. In all patients with DM, attainment of normal growth and weight, prevention of acute and chronic complications, and minimization of adverse effects secondary to medications are desired.

NONPHARMACOLOGIC THERAPY

Limited data exist on specific nutrition recommendations for children and adolescents with DM. Nutrition recommendations should be aimed at normal growth and development, attainment of glycemic goals, and management or prevention of comorbid conditions such as hypertension and hyperlipidemia.[11,14] In children with type 1 DM, individualized therapy is recommended that considers the child's food preferences, schedule, and activity level.[13] Children and adolescents with type 2 DM should have lifestyle modifications, including diet and exercise incorporated at initial diagnosis.[38] Lifestyle modifications include at least 60 minutes of vigorous exercise each day with strength training at least 3 days a week. Improved eating habits should also be implemented including decrease in energy-dense foods (e.g., chips, cookies), beverages with added sugar, and consumption of nutrient-dense foods (e.g., beans, fruit).[17]

Children and adolescents with diagnosis of type 1 DM have historically been underweight; however, as many as 25% are now classified as overweight at diagnosis.[39] Those presenting with type 2 DM tend to be overweight. However, in both groups, attaining a normal body weight is important. At this time, specific nutritional requirements for pediatric patients with either type 1 or 2 DM are unavailable; therefore, dietitians specializing in DM provide medical nutrition therapy by helping patients develop healthy eating habits as recommended by the U.S. Department of Agriculture. Height, weight, body mass index, and nutrition assessment should be conducted at least yearly.[11,14]

Medical nutrition therapy must consider specific insulin regimens prescribed to the patient. Initially, a consistent carbohydrate content for all meals and snacks is recommended, particularly for those on a fixed insulin regimen. However, this provides a challenge because of the erratic eating habits in this population. Some toddlers and young children may refuse to eat some or all of a meal, leaving them prone to hypoglycemia if insulin has been administered. In children with unreliable eating habits, the caregiver can administer rapid-acting insulin with the first bite of a meal or after a meal. Adolescents also provide a challenge in eating appropriate (i.e., healthy) foods at regular intervals. In these instances, it is crucial for the patient and caregiver to count carbohydrate content in meals. Once a patient and caregiver are able to count carbohydrate content to adjust doses, meals and snacks can be more flexible with respect to carbohydrate content. Other considerations in developing meal plans include increasing the consumption of carbohydrates (in the form of fruits, vegetables, and grains) and fiber and establishing a regular meal pattern because these factors improve glycemic control in children and adolescents with type 1 DM.[40]

Children and adolescents with DM benefit from regular exercise. In type 1 DM, adolescents who exercise regularly had an improved sense of well-being, quality of life, body composition, glycemic control, blood pressure, and lipid profiles.[41-43] Moderate or vigorous physical activity for 60 minutes/day and muscle- and bone-strengthening exercise at least 3 days per week is recommended for children and adolescents with type 1 and 2 DM.[43] However, exercise can increase the risk of hypoglycemia in patients on insulin or an insulin secretagogues, necessitating a decrease in the insulin dose.[43] For children and adolescents with type 2 DM, initially increasing physical activity as tolerated and minimizing sedentary behaviors are recommended. Exercise in this population can improve insulin resistance, glycemic control, and body mass index.[11,38]

PHARMACOLOGIC THERAPY

Because type 1 DM is a result of insulin deficiency, exogenous administration of insulin is required for the patient's survival. Although oral agents are typically used in type 2 DM, insulin is often necessary to achieve glycemic control.

INSULIN

Insulin is a protein composed of 51 amino acids naturally produced by the pancreas. It is made up of two chains, alpha and beta, which are connected with disulfide bonds. Although

Table 2. Glycemic Goals for Diabetes Mellitus[17,38]

Type	Blood glucose goal range		Hemoglobin A1C
	Before Meals	**Bedtime/Overnight**	
Type 1 DM	90–130 mg/dL	90–150 mg/dL	< 7.5%
Type 2 DM	70–130 mg/dL	—	< 7%
Key concepts in setting glycemic goals:			
• Goals should be *individualized,* and lower goals may be reasonable based on a benefit–risk assessment.			
• Blood glucose goals should be modified in children with frequent hypoglycemia or hypoglycemia unawareness.			
• Postprandial blood glucose values should be measured when there is a discrepancy between preprandial blood glucose values and hemoglobin A1C levels to assess preprandial insulin doses in those on basal–bolus regimens.			

porcine and bovine insulin were initially used, insulin products on the market today are manufactured from recombinant DNA technology (using human insulin) and then modified to various insulin analogs. Modifications in the structure allow alterations in the onset, peak, and duration of action of insulin as illustrated in Table 3. Because of pharmacokinetic differences, combinations of different types of insulin are used to mimic the normal physiologic release of insulin. For example, rapid-acting insulin is used with meals to mimic pancreatic release in response to food, whereas long-acting insulin is used to provide basal insulin coverage throughout the day.

EFFICACY OF INSULIN IN PEDIATRIC PATIENTS

To date, no studies have reported increased efficacy of one form of insulin over another; however, various regimens, such as continuous subcutaneous insulin infusion (CSII), may provide improved clinical outcomes (e.g., hemoglobin A1C).[44,45] Many forms of insulin have been studied in pediatric patients and have been efficacious. Table 4 lists advantages and disadvantages of specific insulin types in pediatric patients.

DOSING

The total daily dose of insulin depends on several factors including age, weight, pubertal status, diabetes duration, diet, exercise, BG, daily routines, glycemic control, and concomitant illnesses.[44,45] Dosing guidelines for various populations are listed in Table 5. Insulin dosing decreases during the honeymoon phase, which occurs after the initial onset of type 1 DM while the pancreas increases insulin production before complete cessation of insulin secretion. The honeymoon phase begins several weeks after the diagnosis of type 1 DM and can last from several weeks to months.[46] During puberty,

Table 3. Insulin Types and Pharmacokinetic Parameters[44,47,48]

Insulin Type	Pharmacokinetics			
	Brand (Generic) Names	Onset of Action	Peak of Action	Duration of Action (hr)
Rapid-acting	Fiasp[a] (aspart insulin) NovoLog[a] (aspart insulin) Humalog[b] (lispro insulin) Apidra[c] (glulisine insulin)	10–20 min	1–3 hr	3–5
Short-acting	Novolin-R[a] (regular insulin) Humulin-R[b] (regular insulin)	30–60 min	2–4 hr	5–8
Intermediate-acting	Novolin-N[a] (NPH insulin) Humulin-N[b] (NPH insulin)	2–4 hr	4–12 hr	12–24
Long-acting	Basaglar[b] (insulin glargine) Lantus[c] (insulin glargine)	2–4 hr	No peak	24[d]
Long-acting	Levemir[a] (insulin detemir)	1–2 hr	6–12 hours	20–24
Long-acting	Tresiba[a] (insulin degludec)	30–90 min	No peak	> 42

[a]Novo Nordisk, Bagsvaerd, Denmark; [b]Lily, Indianapolis, IN; [c]Sanofi, Bridgewater, NJ; [d]Duration may be less than 24 hours

Table 4. Advantages and Disadvantages of Insulin Types in Pediatric Patients

Insulin Type	Advantages	Disadvantages
Rapid-acting	Can be given with meals or immediately after meals (useful for young children with variable eating patterns) Treats hyperglycemia faster than regular insulin Can be used in continuous subcutaneous insulin infusion	Expensive
Short-acting	Abundant studies available Inexpensive	Must be given 30 min before meal Child may experience hypoglycemia with incomplete meals
Intermediate-acting	Can be mixed with other insulin without modification of pharmacokinetic parameters	May require more daily injections vs. long-acting insulin
Long-acting	Less intra-patient variability vs. intermediate-acting insulin Fewer hypoglycemia episodes vs. intermediate-acting insulin Greater satisfaction in adolescents vs. intermediate-acting insulin Less weight gain with insulin detemir vs. intermediate-acting insulin	Expensive Glargine may cause a burning sensation on administration because of acidic pH

insulin requirements increase because of insulin resistance secondary to elevated growth and sex hormone secretion.[45]

The total daily dose of insulin can be divided by various methods depending on the ability and needs of the patient and caregiver.[47] Factors dictating which insulin regimen to use include the age of the child or adolescent, duration of diabetes, dietary and exercise patters, school or work schedules, glycemic goals, and preference of the patient and caregiver.[45,48] Types of regimens include split/mixed, multiple daily injections (basal-bolus), CSII, and sensor-augmented therapies.

SPLIT/MIXED REGIMEN

The split/mixed regimen consists of two or three daily injections of a standard insulin dose given as a combination of intermediate- or long-acting insulin and rapid- or short-acting insulin. One common method of calculating the exact insulin doses for a patient using two daily injections follows:

1. Calculate the total daily dose for a patient. For example, a postpubescent adolescent weighing 60 kg would require 1 unit of insulin per kilogram (Table 5) or 60 units of insulin per day.

2. Of the total daily dose, two-thirds of the insulin is administered in the morning and one-third in the afternoon/evening. In the example, the 60 units of insulin per day would be divided into 40 units in the morning and 20 units in the afternoon/evening.

3. When intermediate-acting insulin is used, the total amount of insulin is divided into two-thirds intermediate- and one-third rapid- or short-acting insulin. In the morning, 26 and 13 units of intermediate- and short-acting insulin, respectively, will be given. The afternoon/evening dose would be 13 and 7 units of inter-mediate- and short-acting insulin, respectively.

4. If long-acting insulin is administered, then the dose is given as one-half long-acting and one-half short-acting insulin divided into morning and afternoon/evening doses. The morning dose would be 30 units of long-acting insulin and 15 units of short-acting insulin. The evening dose would be 15 units of short-acting insulin. (Of note, if the patient is stabilized on intermediate-acting insulin and is being converted to glargine, then the dose of glargine must be decreased by 20% to prevent hypoglycemia. The dose need not be decreased if switching to detemir.)

The split/mixed regimen provides basal insulin coverage with the intermediate- or long-acting insulin. This insulin therapy requires the patient to eat at regularly scheduled times and eat a consistent amount of carbohydrates per meal. Additional snacks may also be required to avoid hypoglycemic events, particularly if short-acting insulin is used. The use of intermediate-acting insulin may increase the frequency of nocturnal hypoglycemia. In some cases, replacing the intermediate-acting insulin with long-acting insulin decreases the episodes of nocturnal hypoglycemia. The split/mixed regimen is typically not adequate in most patients to achieve desired hemoglobin A1C.[49] Although administering insulin in this manner may be used on diagnosis of DM for the patient or caregiver to become accustomed to administering insulin, after the honeymoon phase it is standard to switch most pediatric patients to a more intensive control with either multiple daily injections of insulin or a CSII.[14]

MULTIPLE DAILY INJECTIONS (BASAL/BOLUS REGIMEN)

The multiple daily injections (basal/bolus) regimen more closely resembles normal physiologic release of insulin than the split/mixed regimen. Long-acting insulin is administered to emulate normal physiologic basal insulin secretion, whereas postprandial insulin mimics pancreatic secretion in response to meals. Preprandial doses of insulin depend on the BG level before the meal, the anticipated amount of carbohydrates in the meal, and the expected amount of physical activity in subsequent hours.[49]

In the multiple daily injection regimen, 40%–60% of the total daily insulin dose is administered as the basal insulin. Administration at bedtime is common; however, if nocturnal hypoglycemia is experienced, then administration of glargine at dinner or breakfast is preferred. The other 40%–60% of the total daily dose of insulin is divided between meals and snacks. The amount of insulin administered before each meal is calculated by estimating the insulin required to cover the carbohydrates eaten (determined by the carbohydrate factor and the insulin-to-carbohydrate ratio) and to correct a BG outside the goal range (determined by the correction factor). Although the multiple daily injection regimen increases the daily number of injections, it has been associated with lower glucose concentrations, lower rate of long-term complications, and a lower incidence of nocturnal hypoglycemia.

The number of grams of carbohydrates consumed in a meal is calculated with the carbohydrate factor. Carbohydrate

Table 5. Recommended Insulin Dosage for Pediatric Patients[14,44,48]

Stage/Type of Diagnosis	Recommended Total Daily Dose
Initial diagnosis	0.5–1 unit/kg/day
Honeymoon phase	Less than 0.5 unit/kg/day
Prepubertal children (after honeymoon phase)	0.7–1 unit/kg/day
Pubertal adolescents	May require up to 1.2–2 units/kg/day
Type 2 diabetes mellitus initial dosing (basal)	0.1–0.2 units/kg/day
Type 2 diabetes mellitus	May require up to 2 units/kg/day

factors are available online at the U.S. Department of Agriculture website (https://fdc.nal.usda.gov/), or they can be calculated for prepackaged foods using the nutrition facts label. Once the carbohydrate factor is known, it is multiplied by the weight of the food (in grams) to determine the total amount of carbohydrates. The following equation is an example of how to calculate the number of grams in a particular food:

A banana has a carbohydrate factor of 0.23 (meaning 23% of the banana is a carbohydrate).

If the banana weighs 120 g, then a 23% carbohydrate factor equates to 27.6 g of carbohydrates.

The insulin-to-carbohydrate ratio is the amount of insulin required per gram of carbohydrate in a meal. Typically the ratio is 10–15 g of carbohydrates per unit of insulin, but this ratio varies per patient and throughout the day. The insulin-to-carbohydrate ratio is calculated by dividing the total number of carbohydrate grams per day by the total daily dose of insulin. Typically prepubescent children require less insulin per gram of carbohydrate, whereas pubertal adolescents require more. For example, if the total daily dose of insulin is 30 units and the child consumes 450 g of carbohydrates per day, then the insulin-to-carbohydrate ratio is 15. This ratio means that 1 unit of insulin is required for every 15 g of carbohydrates consumed. If this child eats the banana described in the previous equation, then 1.8 units of insulin would be necessary to cover the carbohydrates in the banana.

Another simpler method to determine the insulin-to-carbohydrate ratio is to divide the total daily dose of insulin (long-acting and rapid-acting) by 500. For example, if a child has a total daily dose of 10 units of insulin, then the insulin-to-carbohydrate ratio is 50. This method assumes the individual consumes and produces a total of 500 g of carbohydrates per day. Because of the variability in pediatric patients, the insulin-to-carbohydrate ratio may be an over- or under-estimation of mealtime insulin requirements.

The insulin correction factor is the amount an individual's BG will decrease with 1 unit of insulin. The insulin correction factor is calculated using the 1800 rule (for those using rapid-acting insulin as the bolus insulin). To estimate how much of the BG will decrease per unit of insulin, 1800 is divided by the total daily dose (e.g., if the total daily dose is 20 units, then the correction factor will be 90). A correction factor of 90 requires 1 unit of insulin for every 90 BG points above goal. For patients using short-acting insulin as the bolus insulin, 1500 should be used in place of 1800. With the basal/bolus regimen, the patient and caregiver must keep daily food logs, understand how to read nutrition facts labels, and monitor BG often.

CONTINUOUS SUBCUTANEOUS INSULIN INFUSION

The CSII more closely resembles physiologic insulin secretion from the pancreas. The CSII is a pump with a catheter that is inserted subcutaneously to the patient's buttocks, abdomen, upper leg/hip or arm. The pump can deliver rapid-acting insulin to mimic basal insulin, with the ability to stop or adjust the rate for varying insulin requirements of the child or adolescent

(e.g., acute illness, exercise). In addition, boluses can be programmed to calculate the necessary insulin dose for carbohydrate ingestion and BG levels. The CSII can calculate the necessary insulin dose based on patient's insulin-to-carbohydrate and insulin correction factors.[50-52]

The use of a CSII has demonstrated improved hemoglobin A1C compared with multiple daily injections in pediatric patients.[53-56] Those on CSII require a lower total daily dose indicating the improved glycemic control is related to the delivery of insulin rather than the dose of insulin. Children and adolescents appear to have fewer episodes of severe hypoglycemia with CSII compared with multiple daily injections but increased risk of DKA.[55,57] However, a population-based observational cohort study reported a decrease in severe hypoglycemia and DKA with the use of CSII.[58]

Children and adolescents who should be considered for CSII include those with severe and frequent hypoglycemia, those who have wide fluctuations in glucose levels, those not achieving glycemic goals, and those who may have a lifestyle that is impacted by multiple daily injections. Additional patients that may benefit from CSII include infants, toddlers, and preschool-aged children because of their unpredictable eating habits; the ability to administer small doses of insulin and to overcome the fear of needles or minimize the number of daily injections; adolescents with an eating disorder; children and adolescents with profound dawn phenomenon; pregnant adolescents; ketone-prone patients; and competitive athletes.[59] However, before a child or adolescent begins CSII therapy, the patient and caregiver must be motivated and understand the benefits and limitations of the CSII. At the very least, the patient and caregiver ought to be testing BG at least four times/day and consider the use of real-time CGM.[49] Patient and caregivers should also be able to count carbohydrates and calculate the insulin correction factor. They should also be able to administer insulin by injections in case of pump malfunction.[50] Advantages and disadvantages of CSII are listed in Box 1.

ADMINISTRATION

Insulin is administered subcutaneously into the abdomen, front or lateral thigh, buttocks, or lateral aspects of the arm. In younger children with a small amount of fat, the upper quadrant of the buttocks is the preferred site of injection. Typically, insulin injected into the abdomen will absorb faster than insulin injected into the thigh.[45] Injection in the arm may not work for all children if there is a minimal amount of subcutaneous fat, which increases the chance of injecting the insulin intramuscularly instead of subcutaneously. Site of injection should be rotated to avoid lipoatrophy and lipohypertrophy. Disinfecting the area is not necessary.

When mixing insulin to administer, it is important to instruct the patient or caregiver to draw up the regular insulin (clear) in the syringe before the intermediate-acting insulin (cloudy) to prevent contamination of the short-acting insulin. Although the manufacturer recommends not mixing glargine with any insulin, one study evaluated BG and hemoglobin A1C after the administration of glargine mixed with either lispro or aspart.[60] Although the stability of the mixture remains unknown, there are no differences between BG or hemoglobin A1C compared with being administered separately. Mixing insulin minimizes the number of injections administered into the child or adolescent.

ADVERSE DRUG REACTIONS

Adverse drug reactions associated with insulin include injection-related reactions, hypoglycemia, hypokalemia, and weight gain. Injection-related reactions include local hypersensitivity reactions, lipohypertrophy, lipoatrophy, pain, insulin leakage, and bleeding or bruising.[48]

Hypoglycemia is the most common and serious adverse reaction of insulin in children and adolescents. Hypoglycemia occurs more often in younger children and adolescents; those with a history of recurrent or severe hypoglycemia, excess insulin, decreased food intake, exercise, or alcohol consumption; those with longer duration of diabetes; and those with hypoglycemia unawareness.[15] Adolescents on an insulin pump have a decreased incidence of severe hypoglycemia.[15] Common signs and symptoms of hypoglycemia include tremor, tachycardia, diaphoresis, pallor, impaired vision, dizziness, difficulty concentrating, slurred speech, irritability, inconsolable crying, headache, nausea, and seizures. In younger children, hypoglycemia may present as tantrums.[15] Nocturnal hypoglycemia can lack symptoms or present with nightmares, restless sleep, or confusion on awakening. Patients who have repeated episodes of hypoglycemia or a long duration of diabetes may develop hypoglycemic unawareness. Hypoglycemic unawareness results from the lack of counterregulatory hormones responding to low BG, specifically the lack of an adrenergic response. In these instances, the patient and caregiver must monitor BG more often. In addition, it may be necessary to decrease insulin doses to prevent hypoglycemia.

Hypoglycemia is categorized into mild, moderate, and severe hypoglycemia, although specific BG levels have not been defined for each category. Descriptions of each category of hypoglycemia and recommendations for management are listed in Table 6. Parents and caregivers (and teachers if the child is in school) should be counseled on how to recognize and treat hypoglycemia. In addition, it is necessary to explain when hypoglycemia is more likely to occur, such as during changes in insulin therapy, alterations in diet, increased physical activity, and after alcohol ingestion.[15]

DRUG INTERACTIONS

Several drugs increase or decrease the hypoglycemic effects of insulin as listed in Box 2. In addition, the signs of hypoglycemia can be masked with the concomitant use of a nonselective ß-blocker. If a ß-blocker is required, a cardioselective ß-blocker such as atenolol should be considered.

ORAL ANTIHYPERGLYCEMIC AGENTS

Oral antihyperglycemic agents are indicated for the management of type 2 DM. Currently only one oral medication, metformin, is approved for use in pediatrics. However, other oral agents have been studied. Table 7 summarizes the medications, mechanism of action, available pediatric dosages, adverse drug reactions, and drug interactions of these medications.

Box 1. Advantages and Disadvantages of Continuous Subcutaneous Insulin Infusion[48,52]

Advantages

Allows flexible dosing regimens, including various basal rates

Allows flexibility in meal and snack time

Decreases amount of daily injections

Small doses of insulin can be administered

Allows several boluses throughout meals

Families can download information regarding insulin doses

Increased patient and family satisfaction

"Smart pumps" can automatically calculate meal or correction boluses

Decreases variability in glycemic control

Decreases fear of needles

Ability to adjust for exercise or illnesses

Disadvantages

Larger needles inserted for pump

Must be attached 24 hours per day

Placement of pump may be difficult because of size

Dislodgment and risk of infection

Expensive

Interruptions can lead to increased risk of diabetic ketoacidosis

Can be more demanding for patient and caregivers

Table 6. Categories and Treatment of Hypoglycemia in Children and Adolescents[15]

Category	Symptoms	Management
Mild	Sweating Pallor Palpitations Tremors	10–15 g easily absorbable carbohydrate, such as juice
Moderate	Aggressiveness Drowsiness Confusion	20–30 g of glucose administered by another person
Severe	Altered consciousness Coma Seizure	30 mcg/kg (maximum 1 mg) subcutaneous or intramuscular glucagon OR 0.5 mg for age < 12 yr and 1 mg for age > 12 yr If hospitalized, can administer dextrose 200–500 mg/kg

BIGUANIDES

Metformin was studied in children and adolescents age 10 to 16 years with new-onset type 2 DM in a double-blind, placebo-controlled trial for 16 weeks. Compared with placebo, those in the metformin treatment group had improved fasting BG and hemoglobin A1C, and they were more likely to meet at least one of the ADA glycemic target levels.[61] Subjects taking metformin had improvements in serum cholesterol concentrations compared with those on placebo. Metformin also resulted in weight loss, which is usually indicated in children and adolescents with type 2 DM.

Advantages of treatment with metformin are its proven efficacy (decrease hemoglobin A1C by 1% to 2%), generic

---

availability, improved insulin sensitivity, decrease risk of hypoglycemia, positive impact on weight and serum lipid concentrations, and relative safety.[27,62] Initially, metformin may cause gastrointestinal disturbances, including diarrhea. To minimize this adverse drug reaction, the medication is titrated to the maximal dose slowly, preferably over 3–4 weeks, and administered with food. Although the risk of lactic acidosis is low, metformin is contraindicated in children and adolescents with renal dysfunction or any condition that might predispose them to poor tissue perfusion such as alcohol abuse, radiographic studies with contrast, or surgery with general anesthesia.[63]

THIAZOLIDINEDIONES

Rosiglitazone was compared with metformin in an 8-week, double-blind, controlled, parallel-group trial.[64] The investigators found no difference between rosiglitazone and metformin with respect to lowering hemoglobin A1C. A large, randomized, placebo-controlled trial evaluating the role of monotherapy (metformin) versus combination therapy (metformin and rosiglitazone) enrolled patients age 10–17 years with a diagnosis of type 2 DM for less than 2 years.[65] The participants were initially treated with metformin until glycemic control was obtained. Then the participants were randomized to metformin (100 mg twice daily) monotherapy; metformin with lifestyle intervention (i.e., family-focused weight-loss behavioral changes including diet and exercise); or metformin with rosiglitazone (4 mg twice daily). Those who continued on metformin monotherapy experienced treatment failure 50% of the time, whereas participants treated with metformin and rosiglitazone had significantly lower treatment failures (39%). Those randomized to metformin monotherapy with lifestyle intervention had higher treatment failures (47%) than those on combination therapy. Common adverse effects reported in this study included gastrointestinal disturbances, infection, myalgia, elevation of liver enzymes (metformin), and mild hypoglycemia (metformin and rosiglitazone). One case of nonfatal lactic acidosis was reported in the metformin monotherapy group. Those in the metformin and rosiglitazone arm had a slight increase in body mass index throughout the study. No long-term adverse effects on bone density were reported. Given the results of the study, rosiglitazone may be a viable adjunctive therapy in those who experience treatment failure in response to metformin monotherapy.

The short-term safety of pioglitazone in adolescents was evaluated in a single- and multi-dose pharmacokinetic study.[66] Adverse drug reactions reported in the study included nausea, diarrhea, headache, hypoglycemia, increased glutamyl transferase, and peripheral edema. Efficacy and long-term safety were not established.

A potential advantage of thiazolidinediones is preserving pancreatic beta-cell function.[67] One major disadvantage for this population is the weight gain associated with the thiazolidinediones. The thiazolidinediones have a class black box warning on the relationship between the onset and worsening of congestive heart failure in adults.[68] In addition, in adults, the thiazolidinediones have been associated with hepatotoxicity and bone fractures. Because of the lack of efficacy data in

---

Box 2. Drug Interactions with Insulin[68]

Increases the Effect of Hypoglycemia
Angiotensin-converting enzyme inhibitors
Alcohol (acute use)
α-Blocker
Anabolic steroids
ß-Blocker
Calcium
Fluoxetine
Lithium
Monoamine oxidase inhibitors
Mebendazole
Octreotide
Pentamidine
Pramlintide
Pyridoxine
Sulfonamides
Sulfonylureas
Tetracyclines
Thiazolidinedione

Decreases the Effect of Hypoglycemia
Acetazolamide
Alcohol (chronic use)
Antiretrovirals
Asparaginase
Calcitonin
Corticosteroids
Cyclophosphamide
Diltiazem
Dobutamine
Epinephrine
Lithium
Morphine
Niacin
Nicotine
Oral contraceptives
Phenytoin
Somatropin
Thiazide diuretics
Thyroid hormone

pediatric patients and the associated adverse effects with the thiazolidinediones, rosiglitazone and pioglitazone are not recommended as first-line therapy in type 2 DM at this time.

SULFONYLUREAS

Glimepiride has been studied in children and adolescents between age 8 and 17 years in a 6-month, randomized, single-blind, parallel-group trial with metformin as the control.[69] Both groups had significant decreases in hemoglobin A1C from baseline. Participants taking glimepiride had slight increases in serum cholesterol, low-density lipoprotein, triglycerides, and weight. No differences were reported in adverse drug reactions between the two treatment groups. Adverse reactions included hypoglycemia, abdominal pain, diarrhea, nausea, and headache. Glimepiride may be useful as

adjunctive therapy to metformin in children and adolescents not wanting to use insulin. Disadvantages include the risk of hypoglycemia and weight gain. Glipizide and glyburide do not have any pediatric dosing, efficacy, or safety information.

MEGLITINIDES

Meglitinides are considered short-acting insulin secretagogues. Compared with sulfonylureas, they have a more rapid onset and shorter duration of action. Because of their shorter duration of action, these medications must be taken with meals, which could be advantageous for children and adolescents who do not eat at regularly scheduled times. Nateglinide and repaglinide are two medications in this drug class, but they have not been evaluated for use in the pediatric population.

Table 7. Oral Antihyperglycemic Medications[61,63-66,68-69]

Drug	Drug Class/Mechanism of Action	Dose by Age	Contraindications	Adverse Drug Reactions	Drug Interactions
Metformin (Glucophage[a])	Biguanide ↓ Hepatic production of glucose ↓ Absorption of glucose in gastrointestinal tract Improves insulin sensitivity by increasing peripheral uptake of glucose	10–16 yr: 500 mg BID with meals May titrate by 500 mg weekly to max dose of 2000 mg/day in divided doses	Renal disease or dysfunction (SCr ≥ 1.5 and 1.4 in male and female patients, respectively) Hypersensitivity to metformin Acute or chronic metabolic acidosis (including DKA)	Diarrhea Nausea/vomiting Flatulence Asthenia Indigestion Abdominal discomfort Headache Lactic acidosis	Alcohol Iodinated IV contrast
Rosiglitazone (Avandia[b])	Thiazolidinedione: agonist of PPAR-γ Binding to PPAR-γ improves insulin sensitivity in peripheral tissues	10–17 yr: 2 mg BID titrated to max dose of 8 mg/day after 8–12 weeks	Heart failure	Weight gain Edema Hepatotoxicity	Drugs that inhibit the CYP2C8 may ↑ rosiglitazone concentration whereas inducers may ↓ rosiglitazone concentrations
Pioglitazone (Actos[c])	Thiazolidinedione: agonist of PPAR-γ Binding to PPAR-γ improves insulin sensitivity in peripheral tissues	Adult dose: 15 mg titrated to max dose of 45 mg after 8–12 weeks as monotherapy and 30 mg if used with combination therapy	Heart failure Hypersensitivity to pioglitazone	Weight gain Edema Hepatoxicity	Drugs that inhibit the CYP2C8 may ↑ pioglitazone concentration, whereas inducers may ↓ pioglitazone concentrations If coadministered with a strong inhibitor, max dose of pioglitazone should be 15 mg/day
Glimepiride (Micronase[d])	Sulfonylurea: enhances insulin secretion from the pancreas	8–17 yr: 1 mg/day titrated every 2 weeks by doubling dose to max of 8 mg/day taken 15 minutes before a meal	Hypersensitivity to glimepiride or sulfonamides	Hypoglycemia Weight gain Nausea/vomiting Photosensitivity	Highly protein-bound drugs may ↑ hypoglycemic effects of sulfonylureas

[a]Bristol-Myers Squibb, Princeton, NJ; [b]GlaxoSmithKline, Research Triangle Park, NC; [c]Takeda Pharmaceuticals America, Inc, Deerfield, IL; [d]Pfizer, New York, NY

↓ = decrease(s); ↑ = increase(s); BID = twice daily; CYP=cytochrome P450; DKA = diabetic ketoacidosis; IV = intravenous; max = maximum; PPAR-γ = peroxisome proliferator-activated receptor γ; SCr = serum creatinine

GLUCOSIDASE INHIBITORS

Glucosidase inhibitors inhibit the α-glucosidase enzyme located in the small intestine, resulting in the inhibition of breakdown and absorption of glucose and other monosaccharides. A common adverse reaction with this class of medications is flatulence, which may be unacceptable to adolescents. Drugs in this class include acarbose and miglitol. These medications have not been evaluated for use in the pediatric population.

APPROACH TO PHARMACOTHERAPY IN PEDIATRIC TYPE 1 DM

Children and adolescents with diagnosis of type 1 DM require immediate treatment with insulin. If the patient presents with DKA, intravenous administration is the preferred route. Once stabilized, then the patient may be transitioned to a multiple daily injection regimen to allow the patient and caregiver to become familiar with injecting insulin or started on a CSII. During the honeymoon phase, the split/mixed regimen or the use of intermediate- or long-acting insulin alone is typically adequate for glycemic control. After the honeymoon period, a multiple daily injection regimen can be reinstituted, or the patient can begin to move toward CSII.

SPECIAL CONSIDERATIONS IN PEDIATRIC PATIENTS WITH TYPE 1 DM

SICK-DAY MANAGEMENT

Children and adolescents are prone to hypoglycemia, hyperglycemia, ketosis, and DKA during times of illness. Consulting with the medical team and careful monitoring of hydration status, BG, and urine or blood ketones is necessary. Infants and toddlers, in particular, should have ongoing blood ketone testing during illness. If blood ketone tests are unavailable, urine ketone strips should be used.[70]

Illness can cause an increase or decrease in insulin requirements; however, it is imperative to continue insulin administration during an illness. Discontinuing insulin during an illness predisposes a child or adolescent to DKA.[70] At a minimum, basal insulin should be continued even if dose requirements are less.[70] Lack of appetite, diarrhea, or nausea and vomiting contribute to hypoglycemia with continued insulin therapy. If the child or adolescent is unable to tolerate or eat solid foods, sugar-containing foods and drinks (e.g., soda, juice, ice pops) can be given to avoid hypoglycemia. If the child or adolescent is unable to tolerate such foods and drinks, then glucagon administration is warranted.[70] Because glucagon is associated with nausea and vomiting, a smaller dose of 10 mcg/year of age is typically administered.[71]

Increased levels of stress hormone during an illness can precipitate hyperglycemia and insulin resistance, thus increasing insulin requirements. Ketones can develop, despite euglycemia, in response to low glucose availability for intracellular metabolism. For this reason, monitoring of BG and blood or urine ketones is necessary to determine whether administration of more insulin is needed. Often, smaller doses of insulin are administered more often, such as 5%

to 10% or 10% to 20% (if ketones are present) of the total daily insulin dose every 3–4 hours.[70] Hydration is especially important to aid in the diuresis of glucose and ketoacids.

SCHOOL ADMINISTRATION

Because children and adolescents spend a large part of their day in school or day care, it is important to educate school nurses and teachers about diabetes, monitoring BG, administering insulin, and recognizing the signs, symptoms, and treatment of hypoglycemia. A child or adolescent with diabetes can participate fully in school activities.

ADOLESCENTS AND ADHERENCE

Adolescence becomes a difficult time for glycemic control for several reasons. The onset of puberty increases growth and sex hormones, resulting in increased insulin resistance. In addition, some adolescents seek more independence, may become rebellious, or may experiment with alcohol or illicit substances, which can result in nonadherence to diabetes management.

Adolescents with type 1 DM are at increased risk of psychiatric and behavioral disorders compared with adolescents without type 1 DM.[72] Eating disorders, such as *diabulimia* (defined as the omission of insulin to avoid weight gain), anorexia, bulimia nervosa, and binge eating disorder have been estimated to occur in almost 40% of adolescents with type 1 DM, with female adolescents being more often affected than male adolescents.[72] Ongoing screening for such psychiatric disorders is recommended. In addition, at diagnosis and at follow-up, it is recommended to screen for any new or ongoing psychosocial issues. The ADA has published the first specific guidelines for psychosocial assessments, based on factors including age, type of diabetes, and family support system.[17]

APPROACH TO PHARMACOTHERAPY IN PEDIATRIC TYPE 2 DM

Initial treatment for a child or adolescent who receives a new diagnosis with type 2 DM is dependent on glycemic control at diagnosis. A child or adolescent presenting with ketosis or DKA will require insulin to prevent worsening symptoms or progression to DKA. The administration of exogenous insulin may also benefit the islet beta cell to recover from the toxicity of hyperglycemia.[27] In the absence of ketonuria and ketosis, but poor glycemic control (defined as a BG greater than 250 mg/dL or a hemoglobin A1C greater than 9%), insulin is the recommended first-line agent. In addition, any child or adolescent without a clear differentiation of type 1 or type 2 DM at diagnosis should be treated with insulin until the diagnosis of type 2 DM is confirmed. The use of insulin initially may be short-term, and transition to an oral medication (typically metformin) can occur over 2 to 6 weeks by decreasing the insulin dose by 30%–50% with each dose increase of metformin.[62]

Children and adolescents who present asymptomatically or with symptoms and a hemoglobin A1C less than 9% may start on metformin, insulin, or a combination of both.[27] Regardless of the selected therapy, lifestyle interventions (e.g., diet and exercise) should be initiated together with medication. The benefits of metformin have been described previously; advantages of insulin are the quicker glycemic control and potential to prevent and reverse beta-cell damage.

The TODAY study revealed children and adolescents on monotherapy with metformin experienced treatment failure more than 50% of the time, with treatment failure defined as a hemoglobin A1C greater than 8% for 6 consecutive months or the need for insulin for more than 3 months after an acute event.[73] These results indicate the probable need for treatment with more than one agent to reach glycemic goals. As such, children not achieving a hemoglobin A1C less than 7% must have treatment intensified by addition of another agent. Insulin therapy is an option, however; with limited clinical trials describing efficacy and safety of medication for the use in children and adolescents with type 2 DM, no other recommendations exist for which agent should be added.[73] Other significant findings of the TODAY study indicate that children and adolescents with lower beta-cell function at baseline and a greater decline in beta-cell function after diagnosis predicted worse glycemic control and treatment failure highlighting the importance of early diagnosis and aggressive treatment.[74]

The Restoring Insulin Secretion (RISE) Pediatric Medication Study evaluated the impact of insulin glargine with or without metformin on beta-cell function in children and adolescents age 10 to 19 years. The participants were treated with glargine for 3 months then randomized to metformin alone or metformin plus glargine for 12 additional months.[75] Beta-cell function was not different in either treatment group at 12 or 15 months. At 15 months, beta-cell function was worse than baseline for both regimens.

MONITORING PHARMACOTHERAPY

MONITORING THERAPEUTIC OUTCOMES

Glycemic control in DM is monitored with hemoglobin A1C and BG. Hemoglobin A1C represents glycemic control during a 3-month period. Therefore, it is monitored every 3 months in both type 1 and 2 DM. The ADA recommends that all children and adolescents with type 1 DM, regardless of insulin regimen, consider CGM.[14] This monitoring is a real-time report of interstitial fluid glucose concentrations.[76] Most CGM sensors are inserted transcutaneously and measure glucose concentrations every 5–15 minutes. The sensors will alarm the patient or caregiver of actual or predicted hypo- or hyperglycemia.[77] To date, three CGM devices are approved for use in children older than 2 years. Continuous glucose monitoring decreases hemoglobin A1C more than other methods of BG monitoring when used consistently.[14] Adherence to CGM can be challenging for pediatric patients, with as many as 50% not using the devices consistently (defined as 6 days or more per week for 6 months).[14] Another approach to monitoring BG is self-monitoring of blood glucose (SMBG) by the patient or the caregiver. This type of BG monitoring is performed daily to monitor trends in BG and to adjust insulin doses or food intake. The self-monitoring is ideally performed pre- and postprandially, nocturnally, during dose adjustments of

medications, during illness, or when symptoms of hyper- or hypoglycemia are present.[17] In type 1 DM, at least four tests per day are necessary including before breakfast and dinner, before bedtime, and nocturnally (e.g., between 3:00 a.m. and 4:00 a.m.). The frequency in type 2 DM may be less often. At diagnosis, it is recommended that children and adolescents with type 2 DM monitor BG before meals and at bedtime until stabilized. Children and adolescents prone to hypoglycemia, taking insulin or any medication that may cause hypoglycemia, changing pharmacotherapy, not at glycemic goals, or are ill may need to monitor more often.[49] In type 1 DM, monitoring of BG with CGM or SMBG and blood or urine ketones during an acute illness is necessary to detect early ketosis and subsequent DKA.[70] Blood glucose should be monitored by CGM or every 3–4 hours throughout the day and every 1–2 hours during the night during illness.[70]

Nocturnal monitoring is necessary to differentiate the dawn phenomenon and the Somogyi effect when fasting hyperglycemia occurs in the morning. The *dawn phenomenon* is a result of normal BG increases in the early morning because of increases in growth hormone, increased hepatic glucose production, and increased insulin resistance.[48] The *Somogyi effect* is a rebound hyperglycemia caused by a hypoglycemic event during the night. Management of the dawn phenomenon and Somogyi effect is provided in Table 8.

Continuous glucose monitoring and SMBG allows adjustments in insulin doses and self-management of diabetes by the patient and caregiver. The CGM can calculate the amount of insulin necessary for insulin coverage during a meal. For a patient on a basal/bolus regimen, preprandial SMBG (and carbohydrate content of the meal) dictates the amount of insulin to be administered before a meal. Table 8 provides insulin adjustment recommendations for some situations of hyper- or hypoglycemia.

MONITORING TOXICITIES ASSOCIATED WITH PHARMACOTHERAPY

While on insulin therapy, patients and caregivers must be counseled on recognizing the signs, and treatment of hypoglycemia. Hypoglycemia is also detected with CMG or SMBG. In addition, patients and caregivers should monitor injection sites for local adverse effects including allergic reaction, lipoatrophy, and lipohypertrophy.

Renal and hepatic function and a complete blood cell count are usually obtained before initiating metformin and then yearly. Before initiation of metformin, vitamin B$_{12}$ levels should be obtained and monitored periodically when used long-term, particularly those with anemia or peripheral neuropathy.[44] Metformin alone does not cause hypoglycemia; however, BG monitoring is necessary to assess efficacy. Although lactic acidosis is rare, it is important to monitor for conditions that may predispose the patient to a hypoxic state.

Hepatic function should be evaluated before initiating a thiazolidinedione. If liver enzymes are elevated, the underlying liver disease is treated, or the thiazolidinedione is not used.[78] Monitoring of hepatic function is recommended periodically throughout treatment with a thiazolidinedione. Because of an increased risk of fractures, it is necessary to monitor bone health in pediatric patients and supplement with calcium or vitamin D when indicated. When used as monotherapy, thiazolidinediones do not cause hypoglycemia. However, in combination with insulin or an insulin secretagogue, the risk of hypoglycemia increases. It is not recommended to use rosiglitazone with insulin.[78]

Sulfonylureas can cause hypoglycemia; therefore, patients must be educated about the signs and treatment of hypoglycemia. Patients with G6PD (glucose-6-phosphate dehydrogenase) deficiency are at increased risk of hemolytic anemia if treated with a sulfonylurea.[79] An alternative treatment (e.g., metformin, insulin) is indicated in this population. Other hematologic reactions, such as agranulocytosis, thrombocytopenia, and pancytopenia, are rare. No specific laboratory monitoring is indicated unless an adverse reaction is suspected.

FUTURE PHARMACOTHERAPY/ ADJUNCTIVE PHARMACOTHERAPY

One new ultra-long-acting insulin and three additional classes of medications are approved for adults as adjunctive treatment of DM as follows: insulin degludec, amylin analogs, glucagon-like peptide 1 (GLP-1) receptor agonists, and dipeptidyl peptidase IV (DPP-IV) inhibitors.

INSULIN DEGLUDEC

Insulin degludec is an ultra-long-acting insulin approved for the treatment of type 1 and 2 DM in children older than 1 year. Insulin degludec is a conjugated hexadecenoic acid that forms soluble multihexamers after subcutaneous administration and then slowly disassociates to allow for a slow release.[80] A pharmacokinetic study in children age 6–11 years who had a diagnosis with type 1 DM for at least 1 year found the half-life and duration of action to be similar to adults at 25 hours and 42 hours, respectively.[81] In adults, the use of degludec produces a consistent decrease in BG and low variability at steady state compared to glargine.[82] A 26-week, randomized, controlled, open-label trial comparing insulin detemir was conducted in children and adolescents ages 1–17 years.[83] The

participants randomized to degludec achieved a 30% reduction in basal insulin and lower rates of hyperglycemia with ketosis. No differences in hypoglycemia were found. The use of degludec may be beneficial in children and adolescents with adolescents who may have difficulty administering insulin at the same time each day. Also, degludec can be mixed with short-acting insulin.

AMYLIN ANALOGS

Pramlintide, an amylin analog, is approved as adjunctive therapy in adults with either type 1 or 2 DM on mealtime insulin not achieving glycemic control.[84] Amylin is naturally secreted by the beta cells of the pancreas with insulin in response to food. It is reported to enhance the action of insulin by decreasing glucagon production, slowing gastric emptying, decreasing hepatic glucose production, and increasing satiety.[85] Pramlintide, which is administered subcutaneously before meals, mainly decreases postprandial hyperglycemia. The most common adverse drug reactions include nausea, vomiting, and anorexia. Pramlintide alone does not cause hypoglycemia; however, hypoglycemia can occur (and is listed as a black box warning) when used in combination with insulin, and concomitant use may require dose adjustments of insulin. Weight loss has been associated with pramlintide use.

Short-term pilot studies have been conducted in children and adolescents with type 1 DM older than 12 years.[85] Pramlintide may be beneficial in decreasing postprandial hyperglycemia, hemoglobin A1C, weight and insulin dose. Pramlintide appears to be well tolerated, with nausea being the most common adverse drug reaction. Without dose reductions to insulin, hypoglycemia may occur.

INCRETIN MIMETICS

Incretin mimetics, GLP-1 receptor agonists, are approved for use in adults with type 2 DM. Glucagon-like peptide 1 is an incretin secreted by intestinal L-cells in response to food digestion.[86] Incretins enhance insulin release from the pancreas in response to elevated BG, inhibit glucagon release

Table 8. Insulin Adjustments for Hypo- and Hyperglycemia in Children and Adolescents

Deviation	Adjustment	Precautions
Elevated fasting BG before breakfast (dawn phenomenon)[a]	↑ Evening dose of intermediate- or long-acting insulin OR Administer evening dose of intermediate-acting insulin later	Obtain BG at 3–4 a.m. to ensure nocturnal hypoglycemia does not occur
Elevated fasting BG before breakfast (Somogyi effect)[a]	↓ Evening doses of intermediate- or long-acting insulin	
Elevated BG after meal	↑ Rapid- or short-acting insulin administered before meals	Evaluate carbohydrate content of meal to ensure it is appropriate
Elevated BG before lunch/dinner	↑ Morning basal insulin dose if using intermediate-acting insulin OR ↑ Prebreakfast rapid- or short-acting insulin dose	

[a]Must differentiate between dawn phenomenon and Somogyi effect.
↓ = decrease(s); ↑ = increase(s); BG = blood glucose.

after meals, decrease gastric emptying, and increase satiety.[87] The GLP-1 receptor agonists approved in the adult population that have been studied in children include exenatide and liraglutide.

In adults, exenatide improves postprandial BG, hemoglobin A1C, and weight.[88] Exenatide has been evaluated in a randomized, placebo-controlled, single-blind, dose-escalation, crossover trial in adolescents on metformin. The study included 13 obese children and adolescents age 10–16 years. Exenatide reduced postprandial BG at doses of 2.5 and 5 mcg. No exenatide-related adverse drug reactions were reported. In adults, adverse reactions include nausea, hypoglycemia, diarrhea, dizziness, headache, and dyspepsia.[88] Exenatide has been associated with fatal pancreatitis in adults. The drug is administered subcutaneously before meals.

Liraglutide improves hemoglobin A1C, fasting BG, systolic blood pressure, and body weight.[89] A double-blind, randomized, placebo-controlled, parallel-group trial in children and adolescents age 10–17 years with type 2 DM demonstrated a decrease in hemoglobin A1C. The doses in the study were 0.3 and 0.6 mg once daily. No differences in fasting BG or weight were found.[89] Adverse reactions included diarrhea and nausea.

DIPEPTIDYL PEPTIDASE-IV INHIBITORS (INCRETINS)

Dipeptidyl peptidase-IV enzyme inhibitors, which include sitagliptin, linagliptin, vildagliptin, alogliptin, and saxagliptin, are oral agents approved for use in adults with type 2 DM. The DPP-IV inhibitors block the enzyme responsible for GLP-1 degradation, resulting in increased activity of GLP-1. These agents decrease hemoglobin A1C as well as fasting and postprandial BG. The agents, however, are not associated with weight loss. The DPP-IV inhibitors have been associated with severe arthralgia in adults.[90] Other serious post-marketing adverse reactions include pancreatitis, renal impairment, and serious allergic reactions.[91] No current studies have been published in the pediatric population.

DIABETIC KETOACIDOSIS

Diabetic ketoacidosis is a life-threatening acute complication of DM. It is characterized by hyperglycemia, severe dehydration, electrolyte losses from the intra- and extra-cellular fluid compartment, and acidosis. It results from absolute insulin deficiency, whether from undiagnosed DM, nonadherence to insulin therapy, insulin pump malfunction, illness, infection (particularly gastrointestinal illness with nausea and vomiting), stress, or trauma.

PATHOPHYSIOLOGY

The lack of circulating insulin results in hyperglycemia caused by the inability to uptake glucose into peripheral tissue or into glycogen storage. It also stimulates the release of counterregulatory hormones including glucagon, catecholamines, cortisol, and growth hormone. These hormones further increase serum glucose levels because of increased glycogenolysis and gluconeogenesis. The hyperglycemia results in

serum hyperosmolarity and an osmotic diuresis. The osmotic diuresis results in dehydration, electrolyte loss, and decreased glomerular filtration rates. The lack of insulin also results in increased lipolysis, leading to the release of fatty acids and subsequent production of ketones, particularly ß-hydroxybutyric and acetoacetic acids. The ketones, together with lactic acidosis from poor tissue perfusion, result in a metabolic acidosis. Until exogenous insulin is administered, the counterregulatory hormones continue to be released, resulting in further hyperglycemia and ketone production.[92]

PRESENTING SIGNS AND SYMPTOMS

Common presenting signs and symptoms of DKA include dehydration, polyuria, polydipsia, recent weight loss, rapid, deep sighing (Kussmaul respiration), and fruity-smelling breath. Changes in mental status, such as decreased alertness or loss of consciousness, can also be present. Other nonspecific symptoms, such as nausea, vomiting, or fever, may indicate the presence of an infection that could have precipitated DKA.[22] The physical examination typically includes an evaluation of hydration status, vital signs (cardiovascular and respiratory), and neurologic status. Laboratory tests include BG; blood or urine ketones; electrolytes, including sodium, potassium, calcium, phosphorus, bicarbonate, and blood urea nitrogen; blood gases; serum osmolarity; and a urinalysis for ketone detection.[22] If available, blood levels of ß-hydroxybutyric are measured. Because of potassium abnormalities that occur, an electrocardiogram is obtained.[22]

DIAGNOSIS

The diagnostic criteria for DKA are the following:[22]

1. BG greater than 200 mg/dL

2. Venous pH less than 7.3 or bicarbonate less than 15 mEq/L

3. Ketonemia or ketonuria

The severity of DKA is classified into mild, moderate, and severe depending on the serum pH. A pH between 7.2 and 7.3 is mild, between 7.1 and 7.2 is moderate, and less than 7.1 is severe DKA.[22,92]

THERAPY GOALS

The therapy goals in the management of DKA include the following:[22]

1. Correction of dehydration

2. Correction of acidosis and reversal of ketosis

3. Decreased BG levels

4. Correction of electrolyte abnormalities

5. Prevention of DKA complications

6. Identification and correction of any precipitating factors (e.g., infection, trauma)

TREATMENT OF DKA

TREATMENT OF DEHYDRATION

The initial goal of rehydration in DKA is reperfusion of organs, not complete restoration of fluid lost. For that reason, on initial presentation, a fluid bolus of 10–20 mL/kg over 1 hour with 0.9% saline is recommended.[22] The bolus may be repeated if necessary, but not to exceed 40 mL/kg of total intravenous fluid within the first 4 hours of treatment.[92] After the initial boluses, administration of the estimated fluid deficit is given over a 24–48-hour period to prevent cerebral edema. The total fluid deficit can be difficult to estimate; therefore administering 1.5–2 times the daily maintenance fluid requirements should not be exceeded.[93] The tonicity of the replacement fluid should be at least 0.45% saline. If the serum sodium levels are low, 0.9% saline is recommended, whereas if the sodium levels are high, 0.45% saline is preferred.[22] Despite a variety of sodium chloride content and rates of infusion used in the treatment of DKA, the DKA FLUID study did not find a difference in the neurologic outcomes based on the treatment regimen.[94]

CORRECTION OF ACIDOSIS AND KETOSIS REVERSAL

The initiation of insulin not only decreases BG, but also, of more importance, suppresses lipolysis and ketogenesis, which will reverse the ketoacidosis. Insulin therapy is started 1–2 hours after the initiation of the fluid boluses to minimize the risk of cerebral edema.[92] Regular insulin administered intravenously is the preferred insulin and route of administration. The initial insulin dose is 0.1 unit/kg/hour until the serum pH is greater than 7.3, the bicarbonate is greater than 15 mEq/L, or the anion gap is no longer present. Because BG normalization can occur before the ketoacidosis resolution, dextrose 5% is added to the intravenous fluids once the BG level falls to less than 300 mg/dL to prevent hypoglycemia.[22] A rapid decline in the BG may indicate the child or adolescent is sensitive to insulin, which requires a decrease in the insulin dose to 0.05 unit/kg/hour. Despite BG correction, the insulin is continued until the ketoacidosis is resolved. Once the ketoacidosis is resolved, the patient can be transitioned to a subcutaneous form of insulin. Bicarbonate is not generally recommended for the treatment of DKA.[22]

CORRECTION OF ELECTROLYTE ABNORMALITIES

Although serum potassium levels can appear normal in a child or adolescent with DKA, total body potassium is typically low. Increased levels of serum potassium result from the extracellular shift of potassium secondary to acidosis and hypertonicity. Conversely, at presentation, low serum potassium levels are because of increased elimination caused by osmotic diuresis. In addition, on administration of insulin, serum potassium levels decrease because of the shift of potassium into the cells. Regardless, potassium replacement begins early in the treatment of DKA. If the potassium level is elevated at presentation, adequate renal output is established before initiating potassium replacement.[95] The potassium is generally replaced as potassium chloride, acetate, or phosphate at 40 mEq/L. Potassium acetate or phosphate are preferred over chloride to avoid hyperchloremic metabolic acidosis.[93] However, if potassium phosphate is administered, it is limited to no more than 50% of the total potassium replacement required.[93]

Sodium and phosphate may decrease in DKA. Sodium is typically replaced with intravenous fluids administered for rehydration. Phosphate can be replaced when potassium phosphate is used to treat hypokalemia; however, unless the phosphate concentration is less than 1 mg/dL and the patient is experiencing muscle weakness, it is not recommended to replace phosphate.[92]

MONITORING OF THERAPY

During the treatment of DKA, intensive monitoring is necessary. If possible, vital signs, neurologic status, fluid input and urine output, and capillary BG should be monitored hourly.[22] Electrolyte and blood gases are monitored every 2–4 hours, whereas blood urea nitrogen, creatinine, and hematocrit can be obtained every 6–8 hours. Anion gap and serum osmolality should also be monitored with each laboratory draw.

Children and adolescents with DKA must be closely monitored for signs of cerebral edema. These signs include headache, vomiting, increasing blood pressure, decreasing heart rate, decreasing oxygen saturation, and changes in neurologic status such as confusion and lethargy. Computed tomography may assist in the diagnosis of cerebral edema; however, evidence of cerebral edema is not always present on imaging studies.[22] The onset of cerebral edema is typically within 4–12 hours after the treatment initiation for DKA.

CONCLUSIONS

It has been estimated that a child given a diagnosis of diabetes at age 10 years in the year 2000 will live 20 years less than a child who does not receive a diagnosis of DM at the same age.[96] In addition, the quality of life for these children with DM will be less than for those without DM. However, because of advances in pharmacologic therapy, such as insulin analogs, CGM, and insulin delivery methods (e.g., CSII), improvements in metabolic control in DM can prolong both the quantity and quality of life for pediatric patients with DM. Such care requires full participation of the caregiver and patient, when possible, with a multidisciplinary health care team to optimize pharmacotherapy and minimize complications to prevent complications.

DO I HAVE THE SUGAR DISEASE MY GRANDMOTHER HAS?

A 16-year-old Hispanic girl visits her pediatrician for a physical examination. She is aggravated by her little brothers calling her "chubby," so she plans to try out for the cheerleading team at school this year. On questioning, she indicates that her appetite and thirst have increased lately, which she thinks has made her urinate more often.

Medications: Cetirizine 10 mg every night at bedtime as needed for allergies; albuterol 2–4 puffs every 4–6 hours as needed for wheezing; fluticasone 220 mcg once daily

Allergies: Amoxicillin (rash)

Medical history: Born full term and weighed 4.5 kg at delivery by cesarean section because of mother's gestational diabetes

Social history: She lives with her mother and her 2 younger brothers. She is in tenth grade and does very well in school. Her typical afternoon routine consists of watching YouTube videos, texting, using Snapchat, and eating chocolate chip cookie dough ice cream as a snack.

Family history:

Mother: Age 45 years; weight 120 kg; height 63 inches; has hypertension and hyperlipidemia for 5 years, and asthma since childhood; says she cannot breathe properly when she tries any physical activity

Father: Age 46 years; weight 86 kg; height 73 inches

Maternal grandmother: Age 68 years; obese; wheelchair-bound because of below-knee amputation of left leg; hypertension for 25 years, type 2 diabetes for 25 years; peripheral neuropathy of feet for 15 years

Paternal grandfather: Deceased; history of myocardial infarction at age 55 and 60 years

Brothers: Ages 8 and 10 years; slightly overweight, but play football in school

Vital signs: BP 136/96 mm Hg, HR 84 beats/minute, Wt 81 kg, Ht 65 inches

Physical examination:

General: Alert, no apparent distress, obese

HEENT: White lesions on the back and sides of mouth

Neck: Supple, no goiter, no nodes

Cardiovascular: Normal, palpable, femoral pulses

Abdomen: Obese, soft, no organomegaly, no bruits

Extremities: Normal

Skin: Mild acanthosis nigricans around neck

Neuro: Normal

Laboratory findings:

Test	Results	Normal Values
Fasting blood glucose (mg/dL)	185	70–126
A1C (%)	8.6	3.4%–6.1%
Total cholesterol (mg/dL)	190	127–193
Triglycerides (mg/dL)	250	37–130
HDL–C (mg/dL)	20	32–70
LDL–C (mg/dL)	155	0–130
AST (U/L)	38	10–40
ALT (U/L)	30	10–30
SCr (mg/dL)	0.9	0.5–1.1

1. What subjective and objective information for this patient indicates the presence of type 2 diabetes mellitus (DM)?

Subjective information suggestive of diabetes includes patient-reported polyphagia, polydipsia, and polyuria. Objective findings include laboratory results of fasting blood glucose of 185 mg/dL and hemoglobin A1C of 8.6%. She also has evidence of insulin resistance indicated by the acanthosis nigricans on her neck. The fact that she has evidence of thrush in her mouth may be a result of type 2 DM.

The patient is at high risk for DM because she is Hispanic, an ethnicity that has a higher rate of type 2 diabetes, and she is obese as indicated by her body mass index of 29.6, which is at the 95th percentile for girls her age. Her mother has a history of gestational diabetes, which also increases the patient's risk for type 2 DM. She also has a family history of type 2 DM in her maternal grandmother. In addition, the patient's eating habits and inactivity may also contribute to her obesity, insulin resistance, and subsequent type 2 DM.

2. What treatment should be initiated for this patient?

Because the patient is not presenting in ketosis, has a fasting glucose concentration of 185 mg/dL and a hemoglobin A1C of 8.6%, and has normal renal function, the initial treatment indicated is metformin. To minimize adverse drug reactions, such as gastrointestinal distress, the patient should start on 500 mg twice daily with meals. The dose can be titrated by 500 mg weekly to a maximum dose of 2000 mg/day. Lifestyle modifications should also be started with the patient. She can be referred to a dietician to improve her diet. She should also begin an exercise regimen that she can tolerate and work up to 30–60 minutes per day most days of the week of moderate to vigorous exercise. The patient will also need to be assessed for treatment of hypertension and hyperlipidemia to prevent macrovascular complications.

3. What is the goal of therapy for the patient?

The goal for the patient is a fasting blood glucose between 70–130 mg/dL and a hemoglobin A1C less than 7%. The goal is to prevent long-term micro- and macrovascular complications including retinopathy, nephropathy, neuropathy, and cardiovascular, cerebrovascular and peripheral vascular disease. Other treatment goals are to attain a normal body weight for her age and height. Lastly, prevention of adverse reactions of metformin is a goal, including minimization of gastrointestinal adverse reaction.

4. What clinical assessment and laboratory variables should be monitored in the patient and how often would monitoring be indicated?

The patient should be instructed on self-monitoring blood glucose before meals and at bedtime after the initial diagnosis.

The hemoglobin A1C should be monitored every 3 months. If the patient does not reach the goal of less than 7% in 3 months, intensification of treatment is recommended. The patient may begin on insulin therapy at 0.1–0.2 units/kg/day.

Before starting metformin, the patient should obtain a complete blood count (CBC). Yearly, renal, hepatic and CBC should be monitored to assess toxicity of metformin.

To monitor complications of diabetes, the patient should have an ophthalmologic examination and screening for microalbuminuria at diagnosis, in addition to the blood pressure and lipid screening. The ophthalmologic examination and screening for microalbuminuria should be repeated annually, and the lipid panel every year once it is in normal limits.

REFERENCES

1. Dabelea D, Mayer-Davis EJ, Saydah S, et al. Prevalence of type 1 and type 2 diabetes among children and adolescents from 2001–2009. JAMA 2014;311:1778-86.
2. Pinhas-Hamiel O, Donal LM, Daniels, SR, et al. Increased incidence of non-insulin-dependent diabetes mellitus among adolescents. J Pediatr 1996;128:605-15.
3. American Diabetes Association. 2. Classification and diagnosis of diabetes: standards of medical care. Diabetes 2018;41:S13-27.
4. Van Belle TL, Coppieters KT, Von Herrath MG. Type 1 diabetes: etiology, immunology and therapeutic strategies. Physiol Rev 2011;91:79-118.
5. Cooper JJ, Haller MJ, Ziegler A-G, et al. Phases of type 1 diabetes mellitus in children and adolescents. Diabetes Care 2014;15:18-25.
6. Thornsby E, Ronningen KS. Particular HLA-DQ molecules play a dominant role in determining susceptibility or resistance to type 1 (insulin-dependent) diabetes mellitus. Diabetologia 1993;36:371-7.
7. Wenzlau JM, Frisch LM, Hutton JC, et al. Changes in zinc transporter 8 autoantibodies following type 1 diabetes onset: the type 1 diabetes genetics consortium autoantibody workshop. Diabetes Care 2015;38:S14-20.
8. Botero D, Wolfsdorf JI. Diabetes mellitus in children and adolescents. Arch Med Res 2005;36:281-90.
9. Hermanns-Le T, Scheen A, Pierard GE. Acanthosis nigricans associated with insulin resistance: pathophysiology and management. Am J Clin Dermatol 2004;5:199-203.
10. Rendon MI, Cruz PD Jr, Sontheimer RD, et al. Acanthosis nigricans: a cutaneous marker of tissue resistance to insulin. J Am Acad Dermatol 1989;21:461-9.
11. American Diabetes Association. Type 2 diabetes in children and adolescents. Diabetes Care 2005;23:381-9.
12. American Diabetes Association. Classification and diagnosis of diabetes. Diabetes Care 2016;39:S13-22.
13. Chiang JL, Kirkman MS, Laffel LMB, et al.; Type 1 Diabetes Sourcebook Authors. Type 1 diabetes through the life span: a position statement of the American Diabetes Association. Diabetes Care 2014;37:2034-54.
14. Chiang JL, Maahs DM, Garvey KC, et al. Type 1 diabetes in children and adolescents: a position statement by the American Diabetes Association. Diabetes Care 2018;41:2026-44.
15. Abraham MB, Jones TW, Naranjo D, et al. ISPAD clinical practice consensus guidelines 2018: assessment and management of hypoglycemia in children and adolescents with diabetes. Pediatr Diabetes 2018;19:178-92.
16. Diabetes Control and Complications Trial Research Group. Hypoglycemia in the Diabetes Control and Complications Trial. Diabetes 1997;46:271-86.
17. American Diabetes Association. 12. Children and adolescents: standards of medical care. Diabetes Care 2018;41:S126-36.
18. Musen G, Jacobson AM, Ryan CM, et al. The impact of diabetes and its treatment on cognitive function among adolescents who participated in the DCCT. Diabetes Care 2008;31:1933-8.
19. Strudwick SK, Carne C, Gardiner J, et al. Cognitive functioning in children with early onset type 1 diabetes and severe hypoglycemia. J Pediatr 2005 Nov;147:680-5.
20. Ly TT, Anderson M, McNamara KA, et al. Neurocognitive outcomes in young adults with early-onset type 1 diabetes: a prospective follow-up study. Diabetes Care 2011;34:2192-97.
21. Foster DW, McGarry JD. The metabolic derangements and treatment of diabetic ketoacidosis. N Engl J Med 1983;309:159-69.
22. Wolfsdorf J, Allgrove J, Craig M, et al. Diabetic ketoacidosis and hyperglycemic hyperosmolar state. Pediatr Diabetes 2014; 15:154-79.
23. Klingensmith GJ, Connor CG, Ruedy KJ, et al. Presentation of youth with type 2 diabetes in the Pediatric Diabetes Consortium. Pediatr Diabetes 2016;17:266-73.
24. Rewers A, Klingensmith G, Davis C, et al. Presence of diabetic ketoacidosis at diagnosis of diabetes mellitus in youth: the Search for Diabetes in Youth Study. Pediatrics 2008;121:e1258-66.
25. Glastras SJ, Mohsin F, Donaghue KC. Complications of diabetes mellitus in childhood. Pediatr Diabetes 2005;52:1735-53.
26. Mayer-Davis EJ, Davis C, Saadine J, et al. Diabetic retinopathy in the SEARCH for diabetes in youth cohort: a pilot study. Diabet Med 2012;29:1148-52.
27. Springer SC, Silverstein J, Copeland K, et al. Management of type diabetes mellitus in children and adolescents. Pediatrics 2013;131:e648-64.
28. Brink SJ. Complications of pediatric and adolescent type 1 diabetes mellitus. Curr Diab Rep 2001;1:47-55.
29. Li L, Jick S, Breitenstein S, et al. Prevalence of diabetes and diabetic nephropathy in a large U.S. commercially insured pediatric population, 2002–2013. Diabetes Care 2016;39:278-84.
30. Dabelea D, Stafford JM, Mayer-Davis EJ, et al. Association of type 1 diabetes vs type 2 diabetes diagnosed during childhood and adolescence with complications during teenage years and young adulthood. JAMA 2017;28:825-35.
31. White NH. Long-term outcomes in youth with diabetes mellitus. Pediatr Clin North Am 2015;62:889-909.
32. Donaghue KC, Wadwa RP, Dimeglio LA, et al. Microvascular and macrovascular complications in children and adolescents. Pediatr Diabetes 2014;15:S257-69.
33. Jaiswal M, Lauer A, Martin CL, et al. Peripheral neuropathy in adolescents and young adults with type 1 and type 2 diabetes from the SEARCH for Diabetes in Youth follow-up cohort. Diabetes Care 2013;36:3903-8.

34. Daniels SR, Greer FR. Pediatrics. Lipid screening and cardiovascular health in childhood. Pediatrics 2008;122:198-208.

35. Kavay RW, Allada V, Daniels SR, et al. Cardiovascular risk reduction in high-risk pediatric patients. Circulation 2006;114:2710-38.

36. Diabetes Control and Complications Trial Research Group. Effect of intensive diabetes treatment on the development and progression of long-term complications in adolescents with insulin-dependent diabetes mellitus: Diabetes Control and Complications Trial. J Pediatr 1994;125:177-88.

37. Writing Team for the Diabetes Control and Complications Trial/Epidemiology of Diabetes Interventions and Complications Research Group. Effect of intensive therapy on the microvascular complications of type 1 diabetes mellitus JAMA 2002;287:2563-9.

38. Copeland KC, Silverstein J, Moore KR, et al. Management of newly diagnosed type 2 diabetes mellitus (T2DM) in children and adolescents. Pediatrics 2013;131:364-82.

39. DuBose SN, Hermann JM, Tamborlane WV, et al. Obesity in youth with type 1 diabetes in Germany, Austria, and the United States. J Pediatr 2015;167:627-32.e1-4.

40. Overby NC, Margeirsdottir HD, Brunborg C, et al. The influence of dietary intake and meal pattern on blood glucose control in children and adolescents using intensive insulin treatment. Diabetologia 2007;50:2044-51.

41. Rachmiel M, Buccino J, Daneman D. Exercise and type 1 diabetes mellitus in youth; review and recommendations. Pediatr Endocrinol Rev 2007;5:656-65.

42. Austin A, Warty V, Janosky J, et al. The relationship of physical fitness to lipid and lipoprotein levels in adolescents with IDDM. Diabetes Care 1993;16:421-5.

43. American Diabetes Association. 4. Lifestyle management: standards of medical care in diabetes 2018. Diabetes Care 2018;41:S38-50.

44. American Diabetes Association. 8. Pharmacologic approaches to glycemic treatment: Standards of Medical Care in Diabetes 2018. Diabetes Care 2018;41: S73–85.

45. Danne T, Phillip M, Buckingham BA, at al. ISPAD clinical practice consensus guidelines 2018: insulin treatment in children and adolescents with diabetes. Pediatr Diabetes 2018;19:115-35.

46. Fonolleda M, Murillo M, Vazquez F, et al. Remission phase in pediatrics type 1 diabetes: new understanding and emerging biomarkers. Horm Res Paediatr 2017;88:307-15.

47. Malik FS, Taplin CE. Insulin therapy in children and adolescents in type 1 diabetes. Pediatr Drugs 2014;16:141-50.

48. Bangstad HJ, Deeb L, Jarosz-Chobot P, et al. Insulin treatment in children and adolescents with diabetes. Pediatr Diabetes 2014;15:115-34.

49. Silverstein J, Klingensmith G, Copeland K, et al. Care of children and adolescents with type 1 diabetes: a statement of the American Diabetes Association. Diabetes Care 2005;28:186-212.

50. Tamborlane WV, Sikes KA. Insulin therapy in children and adolescents. Endocrinol Metab Clin N Am 2012;41:145-60.

51. Garvey K, Wolfsdorf. The impact of technology on current diabetes management. Pediatr Clin N Am 2015;62:873-88.

52. Abdullah N, Pesterfield C, Elleri D, et al. Management of insulin pump therapy in children with type 1 diabetes. Arch Dis Child Educ Pract Ed 2014;99:214-20.

53. Szypowska A, Schwandt A, Svensson J, et al.; SWEET Study Group. Insulin pump therapy in children with type 1 diabetes: analysis of data from the SWEET registry. Pediatr Diabetes 2016;17:38-45.

54. Sherr JL, Hermann JM, Campbell F, et al.; T1D Exchange Clinic Network, the DPV Initiative, and the National Paediatric Diabetes Audit and the Royal College of Paediatrics and Child Health registries. Use of insulin pump therapy in children and adolescents with type 1 diabetes and its impact on metabolic control: comparison of results from three large, transatlantic paediatric registries. Diabetologia 2016;59:87-91.

55. Blackman SM, Raghinaru D, Adi S, et al. Insulin pump use in young children in the T1D Exchange clinic registry is associated with lower hemoglobin A1c levels than injection therapy. Pediatr Diabetes 2014;15:564-72.

56. Danne T, Battelino T, Jarosz-Chobot P, et al.; PedPump Study Group. Establishing glycaemic control with continuous subcutaneous insulin infusion in children and adolescents with type 1 diabetes: experience of the PedPump Study in 17 countries. Diabetologia 2008;51:1594-601.

57. Brorsson AL, Viklund G, Örtqvist E, et al. Does treatment with an insulin pump improve glycaemic control in children and adolescents with type 1 diabetes? A retrospective case-control study. Pediatr Diabetes 2015;16:546-53.

58. Karges B, Schwandt A, Heidtmann B, et al. Association of insulin pump therapy vs insulin injection therapy with severe hypoglycemia, ketoacidosis, and glycemic control among children, adolescents, and young adults with type 1 diabetes. JAMA 2017;318:1358-66.

59. Phillip M, Battelino T, Rodriguez H, et al. Use of insulin pump therapy in the pediatric age-group: consensus statement from the European Society for Paediatric Endocrinology, the Lawson Wilkins Pediatric Endocrine Society, and the International Society for Pediatric and Adolescent Diabetes, endorsed by the American Diabetes Association and the European Association for the Study of Diabetes. Diabetes Care 2007;30:1653-62.

60. Kaplan W, Rodriguez LM, Smith OE, et al. Effects of mixing glargine and short-acting insulin analogs on glucose control. Diabetes Care 2004;27:2739-40.

61. Jones KL, Arslanian S, Peterokova VA, at al. Effect of metformin in pediatric patients with type 2 diabetes: a randomized controlled trial. Diabetes Care 2002;25:89-94.

62. Zeitler P, Fu j, Tandon N, et al. Type 2 diabetes in the child and adolescent. Pediatr Diabetes 2014;15:26-46.

63. Glucophage [package insert]. Princeton, NJ: Bristol-Myers Squibb, 2017.

64. Saenger P, Jones K, Dabiri G, et al. Benefits of rosiglitazone in children with T2DM (OR6-90). Horm Res 2005;64:26.

65. The TODAY Study Group. Treatment options for type 2 diabetes in adolescents and youth: a study of the comparative efficacy of metformin alone or in combination with rosiglitazone or lifestyle intervention in adolescents with type 2 diabetes. Pediatr Diabetes 2007;8:74-87.

66. Christensen ML, Meibohm B, Capparelli EV, et al. Single- and multiple-dose pharmacokinetics of pioglitazone in adolescents with type 2 diabetes. J Clin Pharmacol 2005;45:1137-44.

67. Pinhas-Hamiel O, Zeitler P. Clinical presentation and treatment of type 2 diabetes in children. Pediatr Diabetes 2007;8:16-27.

68. Lexicomp Online, Pediatric and Neonatal Lexi-Drugs Online [Internet database]. Hudson, OH: Lexi-Comp, Wolters Kluwer Clinical Drug Information, Inc. Updated periodically.

69. Gottschalk M, Danne T, Vlajnic A, et al. Glimepiride versus metformin as monotherapy in pediatric patients with type 2 diabetes: a randomized single-blind comparative study. Diabetes Care 2007;30:790-4.

70. Laffel LM, Limbert C, Phelan H, et al. ISPAD Clinical Practice Consensus Guidelines 2018: sick day management in children and adolescents with diabetes. Pediatr Diabetes 2018;19:193-204.

71. Haymond MW, Schreiner B. Mini-dose glucagon rescue for hypoglycemia in children with type 1 diabetes. Diabetes Care 2001;24:643-5.

72. Delamater AM, de Wit M, McDarby V, et al. ISPAD Clinical Practice Consensus Guidelines 2018: psychological care of children and adolescents with type 1 diabetes. Pediatr Diabetes 2018;19:237-49.

73. The TODAY Study Group. A clinical trial to maintain glycemic control in youth with type 2 diabetes. N Engl J Med 2012; 366:2247-56.

74. The TODAY Study Group. Effects of metformin, metformin plus rosiglitazone, and metformin plus lifestyle on insulin sensitivity and β-cell function in TODAY. Diabetes Care 2013;36:1749-57.

75. RISE Consortium. Impact of insulin and metformin versus metformin alone on β-cell function in youth with impaired glucose tolerance or recently diagnosed type 2 diabetes. Diabetes Care 2018;41:1717-25.

76. Chan CL. Use of continuous glucose monitoring in youth-onset type 2 diabetes. Curr Diab Rep 2017;17:66.

77. Sherr JL, Tauschmann M, Battelino T, et al. ISPAD clinical practice consensus guidelines 2018: diabetes technologies. Pediatr Diabetes 2018;19:302-25.

78. Avandia [package insert]. Research Triangle Park, NC: Glaxo SmithKline, 2008.

79. Micronase [package insert]. New York, NY: Pfizer, 2015.

80. Tresiba [package insert]. Bagsvaerd, Denmark: Novo Nordisk A/S, 2015.

81. Biester T, Blaesig S, Remus K, et al. Insulin degludec's ultra-long pharmacokinetic properties observed in adults are retained in children and adolescents with type 1 diabetes. Pediatr Diabetes 2014;15:27-33.

82. Heise T, Hermanski L, Nosek L, et al. Insulin degludec: four times lower pharmacodynamic variability than insulin glargine under steady state concentrations in type 1 diabetes. Diabetes Obes Metab 2012;14:859-64.

83. Thalange N, Deeb L, Iotova V, et al. Insulin degludec in combination with bolus insulin aspart is safe and effective in children and adolescents with type 1 diabetes. Pediatr Diabetes 2015;16:164-76.

84. Symlin [package insert]. Wilmington, DE: AstraZeneca Pharmaceuticals LP, 2014.

85. Wood JR, Silverstein J. Incretins and amylin in pediatric diabetes: new tools for management of diabetes in youth. Curr Opin Pediatr 2013;24:502-8.

86. Meehan C, Silverstein J. Treatment options for type 2 diabetes in youth remain limited. J Pediatr 2016;170:20-7.

87. Malloy J, Capparelli E, Gottschalk M, et al. Pharmacology and tolerability of a single dose of exenatide in adolescent patients with type 2 diabetes mellitus being treated with metformin: a randomized, placebo-controlled, single blind, dose-escalation, crossover study. Clin Ther 2009;31:806-15.

88. Byetta [package insert]. San Diego, CA: Amylin Pharmaceuticals, Inc., 2009.

89. Klein DJ, Battelino T, Chatterjee DJ, et al. Liraglutide's safety, tolerability, pharmacokinetics and pharmacodynamics in pediatric type 2 diabetes: a randomized, double-blind, placebo-controlled trial. Diabetes Technol Ther 2014;10:679-87.

90. US Food and Drug Administration. FDA Drug Safety Communication: FDA warns that DPP-4 inhibitors for type 2 diabetes may cause severe joint pain. Available at https://www.fda.gov/drugs/drug-safety-and-availability/fda-drug-safety-communication-fda-warns-dpp-4-inhibitors-type-2-diabetes-may-cause-severe-joint-pain. Accessed October 9, 2019.

91. Onge ES, Miller SA, Motycka C, et al. A review of the treatment of type 2 diabetes in children. J Pediatr Pharmacol Ther 2015;20:4-16.

92. Wolfsdorf J, Glaser N, Sperling MA. Diabetic ketoacidosis in infants, children, and adolescents: a consensus statement from the American Diabetes Association. Diabetes Care 2006;29:1150-9.

93. Rewers A. Current controversies in treatment and prevention of diabetic ketoacidosis. Adv Pediatr 2010;57:247-67.

94. Kuppermann N, Ghetti S, Schunk JE, et al.; PECARN DKA FLUID Study Group. Clinical trial of fluid infusion rates for pediatric diabetic ketoacidosis. N Engl J Med 2018;378:2275-87.

95. Angus MS, Wolfsdorf J. Diabetic ketoacidosis in children. Pediatr Clin North Am 2005;52:1147-63.

96. Narayan KM, Boyle JP, Thompson TJ, et al. Lifetime risk for diabetes mellitus in the United States. JAMA 2003;290:1884-90.

CHAPTER 25

LEARNING OBJECTIVES

1. Illustrate the function of the hypothalamic–pituitary–adrenal axis in the adrenal gland and glucocorticoid homeostasis.

2. Differentiate the etiologies and pathophysiology of primary and secondary adrenal insufficiency in pediatric patients.

3. Describe clinical presentation and different diagnostic approaches to accurately assess primary and secondary adrenal insufficiency.

4. Identify management strategies for adrenal crisis and acute adrenal insufficiency to enable prompt hormone replacement therapy.

ABBREVIATIONS IN THIS CHAPTER

ACTH	Adrenocorticotrophic hormone
AI	Adrenal insufficiency
CAH	Congenital adrenal hyperplasia
CRH	Corticotropin-releasing hormone
HPA	Hypothalamic–pituitary–adrenal

INTRODUCTION

Adrenal insufficiency (AI) describes a dysfunction in the production of glucocorticoids (cortisol) and mineralocorticoids (aldosterone), collectively termed *corticosteroids*, and to a lesser extent describes a dysfunction in the sex steroids from the adrenal gland. This dysfunction may be attributed to pathology existing at one or more sites along the hypothalamic–pituitary–adrenal (HPA) axis, which ultimately affects the secretion of the hormones produced by the adrenal cortex. This chapter will focus on the etiology and pathophysiology of the HPA axis, nomenclature of primary and secondary AI, signs and symptoms in AI, and the diagnosis of AI. Strategies for managing AI are also discussed.

EPIDEMIOLOGY

Primary adrenal insufficiency, known as *Addison disease*, is rare and has a prevalence of about 93–140 cases per 1,000,000 people.[1-3] Although pediatric data are limited, in a Canadian study of 103 pediatric patients younger than 18 years, 13% had autoimmune disease, 72% had congenital adrenal hyperplasia (CAH), and the remaining 15% had a heterogeneous group of disorders such as adrenoleukodystrophy (a rare central nervous system disorder in males) and other rare syndromic

disorders as the cause for primary AI.[4] Whereas autoimmune adrenal disease is the most common cause of primary AI in adults, the most common cause of primary AI in children is CAH, with an incidence of about 1 in 14,000 live births.[5,6] An estimated up to 70% of pediatric patients with primary AI have CAH, whereas autoimmunity accounts for up to 13%–15% of cases.[4]

The term *central adrenal insufficiency*, which collectively refers to *secondary* or *tertiary adrenal insufficiency*, has an estimated prevalence of between 150–280 cases per 1,000,000.[7] Secondary AI usually results from chronic glucocorticoid use, whereas tertiary AI occurs as a result of impaired function of the hypothalamus, usually an inadequate secretion of corticotropin-releasing hormone (CRH).

PATHOPHYSIOLOGY

The production of cortisol from the adrenal gland is stimulated by adrenocorticotrophic hormone (ACTH), which is produced in the pituitary gland. The secretion of ACTH from the pituitary gland is controlled by CRH, which is produced in the hypothalamus. Glucocorticoids, particularly cortisol, may affect the secretion of ACTH by negative feedback. Secretion of ACTH occurs in bursts, primarily between 4:00 a.m. and 10:00 a.m., and contributes to about 75% of the daily cortisol production. This secretion pattern is referred to as the *diurnal* (or *circadian*) *rhythm of ACTH secretion*. With excess cortisol production, both ACTH and CRH release are inhibited, which serves to decrease the output of cortisol produced by the adrenal gland. This negative feedback system, which ultimately results in cortisol production, is collectively termed the *hypothalamic–pituitary–adrenal axis* or *HPA axis* (Figure 1).

In addition to cortisol production, the adrenal gland also produces mineralocorticoids, with aldosterone being the primary mineralocorticoid. Aldosterone production is not controlled by ACTH; however, this production is regulated by the renin–angiotensin–aldosterone system and by the potassium concentration in the extracellular fluid.[8] The stimulus for activating the renin–angiotensin–aldosterone system is linked with the regulation of extracellular fluid volume, blood pressure, as well as sodium and potassium ion concentration. Although ACTH is necessary for secretion of aldosterone, it has little effect on controlling its secretion under normal physiologic conditions.[9]

ETIOLOGY

The causes of primary AI are diverse and may result in isolated adrenal disease or adrenal disease coexisting with other endocrinopathies in a polyglandular syndrome caused by autoimmunity. The most common cause of primary AI in children is CAH, which is caused by a series of enzymatic defects associated with impairment in cortisol production.

Other causes of primary AI, listed in Box 1, include disorders of steroidogenesis, adrenal damage or dysfunction, medications, peroxisomal defects, and abnormal adrenal gland development caused by mutations. Secondary AI is caused by dysfunction of the pituitary gland, affecting the production of cortisol.

Patients with isolated ACTH deficiency or ACTH deficiency in association with other pituitary dysfunction are considered to have secondary AI, whereas those with midline brain defects affecting HPA axis such as septo-optic dysplasia may have AI as a result of CRH deficiency, or tertiary AI. The most common cause of secondary AI is thought to be pharmacotherapy with glucocorticoids. In both secondary and tertiary AI, often referred to as *central adrenal insufficiency*, isolated deficiency of cortisol production may be present or it may occur in combination with other pituitary hormonal deficiencies, alternatively called *hypopituitarism*. The causes of secondary and tertiary AI are listed in Box 2 and in Box 3.

EFFECTS OF GLUCOCORTICOIDS

The physiologic effects of glucocorticoids are diverse, and some are beyond the scope of this chapter. For the purpose of this discussion, however, the effects of glucocorticoids on intermediary metabolism, ACTH section, and resistance to stress will be highlighted.

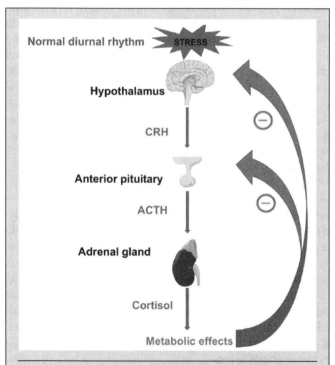

Figure 1. The hypothalamic–pituitary–adrenal (HPA) axis with cortisol-mediated negative feedback.

ACTH = adrenocorticotropin hormone; CRH = corticotropin-releasing hormone.

Figure designed with images from Servier Medical Art (https://smart.servier.com) under a Creative Commons Attribution 3.0 Unported License.

Glucocorticoids increase protein catabolism as well as hepatic glycogenesis and gluconeogenesis. They also result in an increase in glucose 6-phosphatase activity, and their action ultimately results in increased glucose levels. In AI, plasma glucose levels may be normal in the setting of normal calorie intake; however, fasting may result in hypoglycemia.[8]

When the body encounters a stressor (e.g., critical illness, surgery, or trauma), the hypothalamus is activated and releases CRH, which acts on the anterior pituitary gland to stimulate the release of ACTH. ACTH then activates the adrenal gland, which in turn releases cortisol. In production of ACTH, a 39-amino-acid peptide from the anterior pituitary gland, is derived from a precursor, proopiomelanocortin, a 241-amino acid protein. This protein undergoes a series of cleavage reactions, which ultimately result in the production of ACTH. When secreted in excess, such as in untreated Addison disease, ACTH is capable of increased skin pigmentation because these hormones contain a structure similar to melanocyte-stimulating hormone.[10]

CLINICAL PRESENTATION

The clinical presentation of AI depends on whether the patient has primary or secondary AI. The signs and symptoms vary depending on the type of hormonal deficiency present as well as the severity of the possible defect associated with this hormonal deficiency.

In primary AI, both glucocorticoid and mineralocorticoids are deficient. The clinical findings that may occur in glucocorticoid deficiency include the following: fatigue, nausea, fasting hypoglycemia, muscle weakness, and headache. A result of cortisol deficiency is increased production of ACTH- and proopiomelanocortin-related peptides, which include melanocyte-stimulating hormone. The elevation in melanocyte-stimulating hormone is responsible for hyperpigmentation usually seen on sun-exposed areas of the skin or other areas such as the tongue and gingival borders. In mineralocorticoid-deficient states, the deficiency of aldosterone is responsible for symptoms, primarily because of sodium loss. These symptoms include dizziness, hypotension, anorexia, dehydration, and weight loss. Patients may also experience salt craving in addition to electrolyte abnormalities that may include hyponatremia, hypercalcemia, and metabolic acidosis.

In central AI, aldosterone production is not affected because it is regulated by the renin–angiotensin–aldosterone system. Therefore, clinical features associated with mineralocorticoid deficiency, such as dehydration and hypotension, are absent. Hyponatremia and hyperkalemia (both signs of mineralocorticoid deficiency) are usually absent as well, although hyponatremia is occasionally found in patients with central AI because of increased vasopressin secretion.[11,12] Patients with central AI do not experience hyperpigmentation as patients do with primary AI. In isolated ACTH deficiency or in combination with growth hormone deficiency as part of hypopituitarism, hypoglycemia can occur and, if severe, can lead to seizures and coma.[13] In addition to the hypoglycemia that may occur, the symptoms of central AI are often nonspecific, such as poor appetite, fatigue, and dizziness. However, the symptoms may worsen during a stressful event, such as during a fever, infection, trauma, or surgery, and then may include vomiting and dehydration.

In general, patients with AI may present with chronic symptoms that reflect the deficiencies of the hormones involved as previously described. In contrast, patients with AI may also present acutely with dehydration, hypoglycemia, hypotension, or altered mental status. The pathophysiologic basis for this presentation is the sudden loss of both glucocorticoid and mineralocorticoid production by the adrenal gland. This acute presentation, known as *adrenal crisis*, may be triggered by a stressful event such as an infection or trauma. In other instances the precipitating factor may not be identified.[14]

Many clinicians also believe that during periods of critical illness, transient insufficient activation of the adrenal cortex relative to the degree of stress may occur. In this setting, patients present with acute signs of AI, such as hypotension that is refractory to fluid resuscitation and altered mental status. This presentation is a subject of controversy, with some clinicians using the term *relative adrenal insufficiency* or the term *critical illness-related corticosteroid insufficiency*. Factors that have been suggested as likely contributors to this presentation include the release of inflammatory cytokines occurring together with an inhibition of the action of ACTH by these agents; decreased production of cortisol because of factors such as oxidative stress; altered stress-related adrenal blood flow; and also an alteration of the expression of the glucocorticoid receptor during critical illness.[15]

DIAGNOSIS

BASELINE LABORATORY STUDIES

Elevated ACTH and plasma renin activity with low plasma cortisol and/or aldosterone confirms primary AI. A morning cortisol value of less than 3 mcg/dL is indicative of AI, whereas a cortisol value greater than 18 mcg/dL rules out AI.[16] Positive adrenal autoantibodies establish autoimmune AI or Addison disease. All males who receive a diagnosis of primary AI without evidence of autoimmunity should undergo assessment of very long-chain fatty acids in plasma values to rule out X-linked adrenoleukodystrophy.

Box 2. Conditions Associated with Secondary Adrenal Insufficiency in Pediatric Patients

- Chronic glucocorticoids administration: oral, topical, intramuscular, intravenous, intra-articular, and ophthalmic administrations have been reported
- Centrally acting medications, such as opioids (e.g., oxycodone)
- Pituitary disorders
  - Congenital (usually caused by gene mutations) and isolated adrenocorticotrophic hormone deficiency
  - Acquired: brain tumor, brain hemorrhage, surgery, and cranial irradiation
- Adrenal unresponsiveness because of adrenocorticotrophic hormone caused by gene mutations
  - Familial glucocorticoid deficiency
  - Triple A syndrome (also called AAA syndrome or Allgrove syndrome)
- Infiltrative disease
  - Hemochromatosis, sarcoidosis, Langerhans cell histiocytosis

---

Box 3. Conditions Associated with Tertiary Adrenal Insufficiency in Pediatric Patients

- Isolated adrenocorticotrophic hormone deficiency
  - Genetic defects in corticotropin-releasing hormone gene or receptor
- Congenital brain malformations
  - Septo-optic dysplasia
- Infiltrative diseases
  - Hemochromatosis, sarcoidosis, Langerhans cell histiocytosis
- Brain injury
  - Brain tumor, hemorrhage, surgery, cranial irradiation
- Temporary isolated adrenocorticotrophic hormone deficiency because of suppression of hypothalamic corticotropin-releasing hormone secretion
  - Cessation of pharmacologic glucocorticoid therapy
  - Tumor resection

Box 1. Conditions Associated with Primary Adrenal Insufficiency in Pediatric Patients

- Steroidogenic disorders
  - Congenital adrenal hyperplasia
  - Defects in aldosterone production, such as aldosterone synthase deficiency
- Adrenal damage or dysfunction
  - Bilateral adrenal hemorrhage of the newborn
  - Adrenal hemorrhage of acute infection
  - Autoimmunity (isolated or as part of a polyglandular syndrome)
  - Infection, such as tuberculosis, fungal infection, human immunodeficiency virus, cytomegalovirus
  - Transient adrenal insufficiency in premature infants
- Drugs
  - Ketoconazole
  - Etomidate
  - High-dose progestins, such as megestrol acetate
  - Steroid synthesis inhibitors, such as aminoglutethimide and metyrapone
- Peroxisome defects
  - Adrenoleukodystrophy (childhood or neonatal)
- Abnormal adrenal development
  - Congenital adrenal hypoplasia because of gene mutations, such as DAX-1 mutations
  - Critical illness-related corticosteroid insufficiency

When CAH is considered in newborns who present with ambiguous genitalia or salt-losing crisis, random cortisol and androgen hormone studies, particularly 17-hydroxy progesterone, are obtained to confirm or exclude diagnosis. A low random cortisol concentration (less than 18 mcg/dL) obtained at the time of salt-losing or adrenal crisis indicates AI. Patients with mild or early stage of AI or central hypoadrenalism often require additional dynamic testing, as described in following text.

DYNAMIC TESTING TO ASSESS HPA AXIS

ACTH STIMULATION TEST

Administration of cosyntropin (Cortrosyn, Amphastar Pharmaceuticals Inc., Rancho Cucamonga, CA [ACTH 1-24]) to directly stimulate adrenal cortisol release is the most commonly used diagnostic test to evaluate adrenal function. Baseline ACTH and cortisol samples are obtained, with additional tests such as plasma renin activity, aldosterone, or androgen hormones as indicated; then cosyntropin is administered intravenously based on patient age (125 mcg for younger than 2 years; 250 mcg for 2 years or older), followed by cortisol samples drawn 30 and 60 minutes later. Plasma cortisol concentration of 18 mcg/dL or higher, together with a normal baseline ACTH level, rule out primary AI.[17] This test may not be sensitive in identifying patients with mild AI or recent onset secondary AI[18] because adrenal reserve may still be adequate with a normal cortisol response to exogenous ACTH. Therefore, a low-dose ACTH stimulation test using 1 mcg cosyntropin should be used in patients suspected of having secondary AI.

INSULIN-INDUCED HYPOGLYCEMIA

Hypoglycemia provokes a counter-regulatory hormone response and is used to assess the function of the HPA axis. The test is performed by injection of 0.15 international units/kg regular insulin to achieve blood glucose concentrations less than 40 mg/dL and until symptoms of hypoglycemia develop. Blood cortisol samples are taken at 0, 15, 30, 45, 60, 90, and 120 minutes. This test was once considered the gold standard for the diagnosis of AI, but it is no longer used in children because of the risk of hypoglycemic seizures and severe hypokalemia induced by insulin administration.[16,19]

GLUCAGON STIMULATION TEST

The glucagon stimulation test is a sensitive test for evaluating adrenal function. Because this test is not associated with hypoglycemia, it therefore provides an alternative to insulin-induced hypoglycemia in evaluating central hypoadrenalism. Glucagon administration causes an increase in blood glucose, which then evokes an endogenous insulin response, resulting in a decrease in blood glucose. This decrease stimulates a counter-regulatory hormone response, including cortisol.[20] For this test, glucagon at 0.03 mg/kg (maximum 1 mg) is administered subcutaneously. Blood samples for serum glucose and cortisol are obtained at 60, 90, 120, and 150 minutes after glucagon administration. A normal response is achieved if peak cortisol exceeds 20 mcg/dL.

METYRAPONE TEST

Metyrapone inhibits the activity of the enzyme that converts precursors to cortisol. Therefore, low cortisol will increase ACTH secretion, which then stimulates increased production of 11-deoxy-cortisol (the precursor of cortisol) and its urinary metabolites. For this single-dose test, 30 mg/kg to a maximum of 3 g is given orally at midnight, with a snack to decrease the nausea associated with metyrapone ingestion. Cortisol, 11-deoxycortisol, and ACTH are measured at 8 a.m. after the dose. A normal response is the increase in plasma 11-deoxycortisol to greater than 7 mcg/dL.[21] The metyrapone test is an excellent test to evaluate the adrenal function, but is rarely performed because of the difficulty in obtaining metyrapone and the risk of precipitating an adrenal crisis.[16]

TREATMENT

The goal of treatment of AI is to replace the deficient adrenal hormones. In primary AI, both cortisol and mineralocorticoid replacement are needed. In secondary or tertiary AI (central AI), only cortisol replacement is required without the need of mineralocorticoid (aldosterone) replacement.

MANAGEMENT OF ACUTE AI OR ADRENAL CRISIS

Adrenal crisis is a life-threatening emergency that requires prompt diagnosis and treatment to prevent morbidity and mortality associated with acute AI. Cardinal signs of adrenal crisis are hypotension, fever, and altered mental status. Acute AI must be treated urgently with fluid replacement and glucocorticoid administration to restore intravascular volume and electrolyte balance. Treatment of underlying or precipitating conditions such as infection or trauma must also be undertaken.

Normal saline with 5% dextrose is infused at a rate of 1.5 to 2 times maintenance (2250 to 3000 mL/m²/day). If the patient is hypotensive, normal saline at 20 mL/kg should be infused during the first hour of treatment. To quickly replace the deficient cortisol, hydrocortisone should be given as an intravenous bolus of 50 mg/m², followed by 25 mg/m²/dose intravenously every 6 hours. This intravenous hydrocortisone stress dose should be continued in the first 24 hours and tapered over 2 to 3 days (if clinically stable) to oral glucocorticoid maintenance dose. An intravenous isotonic saline with dextrose infusion at maintenance rate should be continued for 24-48 hours after the hydrocortisone dose until patient is hemodynamically stable. Mineralocorticoid replacement is not necessary in the initial period of treatment because the mineralocorticoids provided by the large amount of hydrocortisone and the saline infusion are sufficient. The mineralocorticoid replacement with fludrocortisone should be started in patients with primary AI when they are able to tolerate oral intake. The dose and route of administration of fludrocortisone are described in the chronic maintenance therapy section.

MAINTENANCE THERAPY

GLUCOCORTICOID REPLACEMENT

HYDROCORTISONE

The daily basal cortisol production rate in children is about 6–8 mg/m²/day.[22] When administering orally, the recommended dose for replacement hydrocortisone therapy is higher at about 10–15 mg/m²/day divided two to three times daily, compensating for the incomplete gastrointestinal absorption and hepatic metabolism.[16] In children with AI secondary to CAH with associated androgen excess, a supraphysiologic dose of 12–20 mg/m²/day is required to suppress adrenal androgens in addition to replacing cortisol hormone. Goal of therapy is to control the symptoms of AI without compromising growth and pubertal development that can be seen in overtreatment. Hydrocortisone is the preferred drug of choice in children over other types of glucocorticoid because hydrocortisone has a short half-life, is easier to titrate, and has less adverse effects compared with the more potent longer-acting glucocorticoids. When hydrocortisone is given twice daily in children and adolescents with hypopituitarism, a nonphysiologic nadir of cortisol levels were observed 2-4 hours before the next dose.[23] Therefore, hydrocortisone should be administered three times daily for children with central AI (secondary to hypopituitarism) who are more prone to hypoglycemia or for children with CAH who have additional risk of hyperandrogenism when hydrocortisone is inadequate. It is recommended that glucocorticoids should be administered with food to prolong the half-life of hydrocortisone and to facilitate the production of a more physiological cortisol profile.[24]

In infants and young children, commercial liquid preparations of hydrocortisone or hydrocortisone oral compounded suspension prepared extemporaneously from hydrocortisone tablets can be used.[25,26] Caution must be used to ensure even distribution of the liquid formulation with vigorous shaking before administration. In addition, tablets may be divided and crushed, then sprinkled over applesauce or another food that is pleasant to the child, for administration. When this technique is used, however, the care provider must ensure that the entire contents are consumed so that drug is not accidently left uningested.

DRUG INTERACTION WITH GLUCOCORTICOIDS

Patients taking medications that accelerate hepatic glucocorticoid metabolism by enzyme induction of cytochrome P450 3A4 require an increased hydrocortisone dose to ensure adequate cortisol replacement. Such medications that induce hepatic cortisol metabolism include rifampin, mitotane, and anticonvulsants such as phenytoin, carbamazepine, oxcarbazepine, phenobarbital, and topiramate. Conversely, patients treated with drugs that inhibit cytochrome P450 3A4 such as antiretroviral medication may require reduction of glucocorticoid replacement dose.[27]

OTHER GLUCOCORTICOIDS

Prednisolone and dexamethasone are not recommended as maintenance therapy for AI during childhood because of concerns of growth suppression and weight gain. However, in some circumstances when adherence to hydrocortisone is problematic, oral prednisolone or prednisone can be dosed every 12 hours. The conversion of hydrocortisone to prednisone is a 4:1 ratio (prednisone or prednisolone is 4 times more potent than hydrocortisone). Duration of action and the relative potencies of commonly used glucocorticoids and mineralocorticoids are shown in Table 1.

NOVEL APPROACHES TO GLUCOCORTICOID REPLACEMENT

The current oral replacement regimen for patients with AI does not truly mimic the normal physiologic cortisol rhythm, with a nadir at bedtime and gradually rising levels to the early morning peak between 3 a.m. to 6 a.m. before waking. Many patients continue to have fatigue, nausea, and headaches, despite being on oral glucocorticoid replacement,[34] and some patients have nocturnal hypoglycemia because of very low cortisol levels during the night and early morning.[35]

Table 1. Duration of Action and the Relative Potencies of Commonly Used Glucocorticoids and Mineralocorticoids in Adrenal Insufficiency

Drug Type	Duration of Action	Drug	Potency[a]	Equivalent Doses (mg)
Glucocorticoid	Short-acting (8–12 hr)	Hydrocortisone (cortisol)	1	20
		Cortisone acetate	0.8	25
	Intermediate-acting (12–36 hr)	Prednisone	4	5
		Prednisolone	4	5
		Methylprednisone	5	4
	Long-acting (36–72 hr)	Dexamethasone	30	0.75
		Betamethasone	25–30	0.6
Mineralocorticoid	Intermediate-acting (12–36 hr)	Fludrocortisone	0[b]	0.1–0.2[c]

[a]Glucocorticoid potencies are relative to cortisol, which is arbitrarily assigned a potency of 1.
[b]Mineralocorticoids have no glucocorticoid activity.
[c]Mineralocorticoid replacement dose.

Moreover, a higher prevalence of central adiposity, impaired glucose tolerance, and dyslipidemia occur in patients with Addison disease,[36] with increased use of antihypertensive drugs and lipid-lowering agents compared with the background population, indicating an increased risk of cardiovascular morbidity.[37] A possible explanation for this morbidity may be nonphysiologic dosing with the current oral regimen causing an altered diurnal cortisol profile and supraphysiologic glucocorticoid doses. Increased evening cortisol levels reduce glucose tolerance, insulin secretion, and insulin sensitivity in healthy young adults.[38] Because of all these concerns and unfavorable treatment outcomes, novel therapies have been developed in recent years.

CONTINUOUS SUBCUTANEOUS HYDROCORTISONE INFUSION

Continuous subcutaneous hydrocortisone infusion therapy administered by an insulin pump has been used to deliver hydrocortisone. In several studies, this mode of drug delivery restored a circadian cortisol rhythm and normalized the ACTH levels compared with conventional therapy,[39] and improved quality of life.[40] However, because of high cost, complexity of device usage, and other risks associated with the use of a pump (such as site and pump failures), continuous subcutaneous hydrocortisone infusion has not been used routinely in clinical practice, but can be considered a treatment option in classic CAH poorly controlled on conventional therapy.

SUSTAINED RELEASE HYDROCORTISONE PREPARATIONS

Three modified release hydrocortisone formulations have been developed in Europe with an aim to produce a more physiologic cortisol profile. Chronocort (Diurnal Group PLC, Cardiff, UK) is a hydrocortisone preparation with delayed-release administered twice daily, with a larger dose given at night and a smaller dose given in the morning. The large dose given at night is to suppress the overnight ACTH surge that drives excess androgen production in CAH and to provide a high peak cortisol early in the morning at wakening. Chronocort therapy in adults with CAH resulted in more physiological cortisol profile and was superior to conventional glucocorticoid therapy in controlling androgen levels throughout the day.[41,42]

Plenadren (DuoCort Pharma AB, Helsingborg, Sweden), a dual-release hydrocortisone preparation, is dosed once daily in the morning. Plenadren is formulated with an immediate-release coating that is rapidly absorbed and followed by slow release from the core of the tablet. Studies of this hydrocortisone formulation in adults with Addison disease have been shown to achieve physiologic circadian cortisol rhythm, reduce central adiposity, and improve metabolic and immune-defense profiles as well as improve quality of life.[43-45] Treatment with Plenadren for 36 months in adults with Addison disease and prediabetes improved insulin sensitivity and secretion and also improved anthropometric profiles.[46] Plenadren is not yet licensed for use in the management of AI

in children, but use has resulted in a better cortisol profile in a small case series of children with AI.[47]

Alkindi ([development name: Infacort] Diurnal Group PLC, Cardiff, UK), an immediate-release, oral formulation of hydrocortisone, has been developed specifically for infants and children. Alkindi is provided in capsules containing taste-masked granules that can be sprinkled onto food to obscure the bitter taste of hydrocortisone. The drug is bioequivalent to current hydrocortisone preparations, with flexible low pediatric dosing in units of 0.5 mg, 1 mg, 2 mg, and 5 mg of hydrocortisone.[48] Alkindi is easy to administer to neonates, infants, and children, and has good absorption, achieving cortisol levels at 60 minutes after administration similar to physiologic cortisol levels in healthy children.[48]

FLUDROCORTISONE

In children with primary AI and confirmed aldosterone deficiency, treatment with fludrocortisone at 0.05–0.2 mg/day in two divided doses is recommended. The starting dose for infants with CAH is 0.1 mg/day in two divided doses, and the dose may be reduced to 0.05 mg/day when clinical control of CAH is achieved. The dose adjustment of fludrocortisone for body size is rarely required because the aldosterone secretion rate does not increase from infancy to adulthood. Excessive fludrocortisone can cause hypervolemia, hypertension, and edema; therefore, monitoring the clinical status, weight gain, blood pressure, and serum sodium and potassium values, as well as plasma renin activity, is essential to establish the proper dosage of fludrocortisone. The dose should be increased in patients with salt-wasting CAH with high 17-hydroxy-progesterone levels to avoid too high hydrocortisone dosages.[28] Fludrocortisone may also have glucocorticoid activity,[29] and administration of fludrocortisone significantly inhibited the HPA response to CRH.[30] This inhibition is of particular relevance in newborns and infants to avoid glucocorticoid over-exposure.

SALT SUPPLEMENTATION

Because of low salt content in breast milk and infant formulas and mineralocorticoid resistance in the immature infant kidney, sodium chloride supplements should be given in newborns with salt-wasting CAH, with close monitoring of serum sodium values. Sodium chloride should be started at 1–4 mEq/kg/day, distributed in several feedings, and titrated based on serum sodium values. Sodium chloride supplementation may be up to 1–2 g/day (17–34 mEq/day) in infants with severe salt-wasting CAH, and should be continued until age 8–12 months when salt intake from diet is sufficient.[5,31]

STRESS REPLACEMENT DURING ILLNESS, INJURY OR SURGERY

Cortisol is an important hormone that is essential for human survival, particularly during stress. Surgery, anesthesia, trauma, and illnesses result in increased plasma ACTH and cortisol levels. Many studies have demonstrated increased daily cortisol secretion proportionate to the degree of stress in healthy adults undergoing surgery or in acutely ill individuals.[32,33] According to the recommendations published by the Pediatric Endocrine Society Drug and Therapeutic Committee, the hydrocortisone doses in the setting of stress are 30–50 mg/m²/day in 3 divided doses for mild to moderate stress such as fever or upper respiratory infections, and 100 mg/m²/day given intravenously as a single dose for the most severe stresses, such as major surgery or critical illness.[16] The initial dose is followed by the same dose at a constant rate over a 24-hour period. The stress doses of hydrocortisone are tapered to physiologic or maintenance dose based on the pace of clinical improvement, usually within 2 to 3 days. Patients with diarrhea and vomiting (who are unable to take oral medication by mouth) require parenteral hydrocortisone (100 mg/m² per day), which can be given as a single dose if necessary as the first dose or before a procedure. In an emergency setting if the patient's weight or height is not available, a quick, simple age-based dosing can be used (Table 2).

PATIENT EDUCATION

Patients and their caretakers must be educated about AI, the rationale for replacement therapy, and glucocorticoid stress dosing for stressful events to prevent adrenal crisis. In clinical practice, formal education sessions with written instructions can be provided by health care professionals to the patients and caregivers at diagnosis of AI. Instructions should be reviewed at each clinic visit so that the dose can be increased as the patient grows. Knowledge about AI for both the patients and parents or caregivers should be reassessed at least yearly with re-education as needed during follow-up

clinic visits. Patients and parents/caregivers must be taught how to administer injectable glucocorticoids when the patient is vomiting or unable to take oral stress doses. All patients should wear or carry a medical alert identification and a steroid emergency information card that indicate the diagnosis of "adrenal insufficiency" or "cortisol dependence" to help them receive appropriate steroid stress dose in the event of an emergency.

Table 2. Intravenous or Intramuscular Hydrocortisone Doses During Major Stress (Critical Illness, Surgery) or Adrenal Crisis

Age (years)	Single-Dose Bolus (intravenous/intramuscular)	Maintenance (intravenous mg/day)
0–3	25 mg	25–30
3–12	50 mg	50–75
≥ 12	100 mg	100

CONCLUSIONS

The etiologies of AI in children are diverse, and so are the treatment modalities. Because the signs and symptoms of AI are often nonspecific, clinicians must be aware of the various types of AI and obtain appropriate laboratory investigation for correct diagnosis. Patients with adrenal crisis need to receive a stress dose of hydrocortisone promptly without delay, even before the diagnostic test results are available. Education of the patient and family on the importance of treatment and knowledge of when and how to give hydrocortisone stress dosing is the key to successful therapy of AI.

Patient Case 1

PRIMARY ADRENAL INSUFFICIENCY CAUSED BY ADDISON DISEASE

A 14-year-old white boy is brought to the emergency department with a 6-day history of vomiting. His past medical history is not significant; however, he has a family history of autoimmunity with his mother having systemic lupus erythematosus.

Vital signs: BP 81–93/39–48 mm Hg, HR 120 beats per minute, Tmax 99.1°F (37.3°C), Wt 48.5 kg (37th percentile for age), Ht 61 inches (14th percentile for age), body surface area 1.45 m²

Pertinent findings from his basic metabolic panel showed sodium 114 (normal 135-145 mEq/L) and potassium 5.8 (normal 3.5-5 mEq/L). Of note, he presents with hyperpigmentation to the papillae of his tongue as well as areas of prior bruises to his skin. He is also tanned and of a darker skin complexion as compared to his relatives. In the emergency department, a bolus of 2 L normal saline is administered. Cortisol concentration is 4.7 mcg/dL (normal cortisol at the time of stress is 18 mcg/dL or higher).

Based on the patient's hyponatremia and hyperkalemia, on exploration of his sodium intake, he reveals a 6-month history of profound salt craving with repeated pickle juice consumption.

He was admitted for management of his electrolyte abnormalities and also to undergo a work up. Based on suspicion for an adrenal etiology, a high-dose cosyntropin stimulation test is ordered. His 60-minute cortisol concentration obtained after the administration of a 250-mcg dose of cosyntropin is 3.7 mcg/dL (normal, 18 mcg/dL or greater). He is empirically started on intravenous hydrocortisone 40 mg every 8 hours for 24 hours (83 mg/m²/day) until he is clinically stable. An oral regimen is subsequently started in preparation for his discharge after hospitalization for 5 days.

His adrenal antibodies are markedly elevated at 5000 units/mL (normal, less than 50 units/mL), and ACTH is also markedly elevated at 1670 pg/mL (6–48 pg/mL). In preparation for his discharge, after 24 hours of intravenous hydrocortisone, he was started on oral hydrocortisone 5 mg to be taken each morning, 5 mg in the afternoon, and 5 mg at night (11.5 mg/m²/day), and oral fludrocortisone 0.2 mg daily. Hydrocortisone maintenance dosing is 8–10 mg/m²/day. He is also given a prescription for 100 mg injectable hydrocortisone (76 mg/m²/day) to be given at time of stress when he is unable to take oral hydrocortisone. Education on adrenal insufficiency (AI) and stress-dose hydrocortisone is provided to the patient and his parents.

---

1. What signs and symptoms are consistent with the presentation of AI and what are the reasons for the patient presenting with these symptoms?

The patient presents with hyponatremia, hyperkalemia, and profound salt craving. The latter has developed because of sodium losses. These electrolyte abnormalities can be explained based on the absence of mineralocorticoid activity that occurs in the setting of primary AI. This absence occurs because production of aldosterone—the primary mineralocorticoid—is deficient and this hormone is primarily responsible for sodium reabsorption and potassium excretion.

The patient also presented with skin hyperpigmentation. In primary AI, with the absence of negative feedback caused by cortisol deficiency, ACTH is produced at high levels by the pituitary gland. This hormone has a similar structure to melanocyte-stimulating hormone, and these hormones (both ACTH and melanocyte-stimulating hormone) are derived from a common precursor, proopiomelanocortin.

2. Discuss the rationale for the patient's pharmacotherapy regimen in the ED and at discharge.

In the emergency department the patient was given a normal saline bolus because of his tachycardia, a sign of his dehydration. He was also given intravenous hydrocortisone: 40 mg every 8 hours for 24 hours (83 mg/m²/day), which is considered stress dosing. At stress dosing concentrations, 50–100 mg/m²/day, hydrocortisone has both glucocorticoid and mineralocorticoid activity. This treatment in the emergency setting is important because of decreased production of both glucocorticoids and mineralocorticoids in primary AI.

In preparation for discharge, the patient was started on hydrocortisone 5 mg to be taken each morning, 5 mg in the afternoon, and 5 mg at night (11.5 mg/m²/day) in addition to fludrocortisone. A hydrocortisone dose of close to 10 mg/m2/day is considered to be maintenance dosing. Both hydrocortisone and fludrocortisone serve as replacements for the diminished glucocorticoid and mineralocorticoid production respectively seen in primary AI.

3. Discuss the rationale for stress dose administration under times of stress in the management of this patient.

The patient has Addison disease or AI, which is autoimmune based on the elevated titer of adrenal antibodies, 5000 units/mL (normal, less than 50 units/mL). In patients with Addison disease, a deficiency of both glucocorticoids (cortisol) and mineralocorticoids is secondary to the immune mediated destruction of the gland. Based on these deficiencies, individuals with Addison disease are unable to mount a normal physiologic response that involves increased production of cortisol as a response to stress. As a consequence, the practice of increasing maintenance dosing to 3 times normal oral dosing is done during the times of stress, which includes temperature of 101°F (38.3°C), diarrhea, vomiting episodes, and fractures. Should the patient not be able to tolerate oral stress dosing, intramuscular dosing of hydrocortisone 100 mg (69 mg/m²/day) can be administered and is also considered a stress dose.

An 8-year-old white boy is referred to the endocrinology clinic for a growth evaluation. His parents provided a history of his lack of growth over a 2-year period. Growth chart review showed decreased weight percentile for age, from 10th–25th percentile for age at 3 to 5 years to 5th percentile for age between 5 and 8 years. His annualized height velocity with successive yearly well child visits over the prior 3 years was less than expected. He also had two pediatric intensive care unit admissions over a period of two years. His family history was noncontributory.

His medication history was significant for the use of fluticasone propionate, 110 mcg with 2 actuations inhaled twice daily for 5 years as maintenance therapy for asthma. Albuterol nebulization and inhalation were used to manage acute asthmatic exacerbations.

Based on the patient's history of poor growth and with the use of high doses of inhaled corticosteroids, a morning cortisol screening was done at 8 a.m., showing a concentration of less than 0.09 mcg/dL (normal, 10 mcg/dL or higher), which is well below the lower limit of detection on the assay. His cortisol concentrations at 30 and 60 minutes remained less than 0.09 mcg/dL, after the administration of 1 mcg cosyntropin.

Based on his clinical picture and the results of the low dose cosyntropin stimulation testing, he has steroid-induced adrenal suppression, a form of secondary AI. He is started on maintenance therapy of oral hydrocortisone with doses of 5 mg every morning, 2.5 mg every afternoon, and 2.5 mg night, in addition to stress doses of intramuscular hydrocortisone 10 mg every 8 hours to be administered for the stress-dose indications, which include temperature of 101°F (38.3°C), diarrhea, vomiting episodes, and fractures.

1. Discuss the effect of the inhaled corticosteroids on the etiology of secondary AI.

The patient was prescribed fluticasone propionate 110 mcg with two actuations twice daily for 5 years as a control medication for his asthma. Based on the chronic use of inhaled corticosteroids, he developed secondary AI—more specifically, this patient has *steroid-induced adrenal suppression*. Chronic use of inhaled corticosteroids produces negative feedback on both the pituitary gland and hypothalamus, resulting in decreased cortisol output from the adrenal gland. In this case, unlike in primary AI, the mineralocorticoid axis is not affected. Although inhaled corticosteroids are not commonly associated with adrenal suppression, the patient received such a high daily dose of fluticasone propionate that it resulted in adrenal suppression.

Based on his morning cortisol dose at 8 a.m., concentration was less than 0.09 mcg/dL, well below the normal limits of detection, and steroid-induced adrenal suppression was suspected. This suspicion was later confirmed based on a concentration of less than 0.09 mcg/dL (normal, greater than 18 mcg/dL), 30 minutes after the administration of 1 mcg cosyntropin, in the low dose cosyntropin stimulation test.

2. What are the presenting signs and symptoms and the indications of secondary AI in this patient?

For this patient, his parents provided the history of his linear growth decline over 2 years. In addition, his annualized growth velocity decreased over 3 successive years as noted at his well-child clinic visits. The patient's growth impairment is clinical evidence of the suppressive effect of steroids on his growth.

Aside from the suppressive effects on growth, the use of long-term inhaled high-dose corticosteroids also suppressed his adrenal gland function. The evidence of this suppression is based on the suboptimal response on the low-dose cosyntropin stimulation test with a concentration of less than 0.09 mcg/dL at 30 minutes after the administration of 1 mcg cosyntropin (normal, greater than 18 mcg/dL). The low-dose cosyntropin stimulation test is useful in diagnosing secondary AI, which in this case is steroid-induced adrenal suppression.

3. Discuss the appropriateness of the treatment strategy prescribed for this patient who has secondary AI.

The patient had steroid-induced adrenal suppression. The regulation of glucocorticoid (cortisol) production by the adrenal gland is under the control of ACTH, which is produced by the pituitary gland. Cortisol production is also regulated by corticotropin-releasing hormone, which is produced by the hypothalamus. Use of high-dose corticosteroids produces negative feedback on both the pituitary gland and the hypothalamus. To manage this decreased cortisol output, the patient was placed on physiologic replacement (oral hydrocortisone with doses of 5 mg every morning, 2.5 mg every afternoon, and 2.5 mg every night) with instructions for stress doses of hydrocortisone (intramuscular hydrocortisone 10 mg every 8 hours), which is taken as 2–3 times his maintenance dose.

Fludrocortisone was not added to his treatment regimen because the production of aldosterone is not affected in secondary AI; therefore, aldosterone production from the adrenal gland is not affected by the suppressive effect of the patient's high-dose inhaled steroid.

REFERENCES

1. Kong MF, Jeffcoate W. Eight-six cases of Addison's disease. Clin Endocrinol 1994;41:757-61.

2. Willis AC, Vince FP. The prevalence of Addison's disease in Coventry, UK. Postgrad Med J 1997;73:286-8.

3. Løvås K, Husebye ES. High prevalence and increasing incidence of Addison's disease in western Norway. Clin Endocrinol 2002;56:787-91.

4. Perry R, Kecha O, Paquette J, et al. Primary adrenal insufficiency in children: twenty years experience at the Sainte-Justine Hospital, Montreal. J Clin Endocrinol Metab 2005;90:3243-50.

5. Speiser PW, Azziz R, Baskin LS, et al. Congenital adrenal hyperplasia due to steroid 21-hydroxylase deficiency: an Endocrine Society clinical practice guideline. J Clin Endocrinol Metab 2010;95:4133-60.

6. Morel Y, Miller WL. Congenital adrenal hyperplasia due to 21-hydroxylase deficiency. Adv Hum Genet 1991;20:1-68.

7. Arlt W, Allolio B. Adrenal insufficiency. Lancet 2003;361:1881-93.

8. Hall JE. Adrenocortical hormones. In: Hall J, ed. Textbook of Medical Physiology, 13th ed. Philadelphia, PA: Elsevier; 2016:965-82.

9. Barrett KE, Barman S, Boitano S, et al. The adrenal medulla & adrenal cortex. In: Barrett KE, Barman S, Boitano S, et al., eds. Ganong's Review of Medical Physiology, 25th ed. New York: McGraw-Hill, 2016:353-76.

10. Coll AP, Farooqi IS, Challis BG, et al. Proopiomelanocortin and energy balance: insights from human and murine genetics. J Clin Endocrinol Metab 2004;89:2557-62.

11. Kamoi K, Tamura T, Tanaka K, et al. Hyponatremia and osmoregulation of thirst and vasopressin secretion in patients with adrenal insufficiency. J Clin Endocrinol Metab 1993;77:1584-8.

12. Diederich S, Franzen N-F, Bahr V, et al. Severe hyponatremia due to hypopituitarism with adrenal insufficiency: report on 28 cases. Eur J Endocrinol 2003;148:609-17.

13. Vallette-Kasic S, Brue T, Pulichino A-M, et al. Congenital isolated adrenocorticotropin deficiency: an underestimated cause of neonatal death, explained by TPIT gene mutations. J Clin Endocrinol Metab 2005;90:1323-31.

14. Charmandari E, Nicolaides NC, Chrousos GP. Adrenal insufficiency. Lancet 2014;383:2152-67.

15. Boonen E, Van den Berghe G. Mechanisms in endocrinology: new concepts to further unravel adrenal insufficiency during critical illness. Eur J Endocrinol 2016;175:R1-9.

16. Shulman DI, Palmert MR, Kemp SF. Adrenal insufficiency: still a cause of morbidity and death in childhood. Pediatrics 2007;119:e484-94.

17. Bornstein SR, Allolio B, Arlt W, et al. Diagnosis and treatment of primary adrenal insufficiency: an endocrine society clinical practice guideline. J Clin Endocrinol Metab 2016;101:364-89.

18. Kazlauskaite R, Evans AT, Villabona CV, et al. Corticotropin tests for hypothalamic-pituitary-adrenal insufficiency: a meta-analysis. J Clin Endocrinol Metab 2008;93:4245-53.

19. Binder G, Bosk A, Gass M, et al. Insulin tolerance test causes hypokalaemia and can provoke cardiac arrhythmias. Horm Res 2004;62:84-7.

20. Rao R, Spathis G. Intramuscular glucagon as a provocative stimulus for the assessment of pituitary function: growth hormone and cortisol responses. Metabolism 1987;36:658-63.

21. Fiad TM, Kirby JM, Cunningham SK, et al. The overnight single-dose metyrapone test is a simple and reliable index of the hypothalamic-pituitary-adrenal axis. Clin Endocrinol 1994; 40:603-9.

22. Linder BL, Esteban NV, Yergey AL, et al. Cortisol production rate in childhood and adolescence. J Pediatr 1990;117:892-6.

23. DeVile C, Stanhope R. Hydrocortisone replacement therapy in children and adolescents with hypopituitarism. Clin Endocrinol 1997;47:37-41.

24. Mah PM, Jenkins RC, Rostami-Hodjegan A, et al. Weight-related dosing, timing and monitoring hydrocortisone replacement therapy in patients with adrenal insufficiency. Clin Endocrinol 2004;61:367-75.

25. Fawcett JP, Boulton DW, Jiang R, et al. Stability of hydrocortisone oral suspensions prepared from tablets and powder. Ann Pharmacother 1995;29:987-90.

26. Sarafoglou K, Gonzalez-Bolanos MT, Zimmerman CL, et al. Comparison of cortisol exposures and pharmacodynamic adrenal steroid responses to hydrocortisone suspension vs. commercial tablets. J Clin Pharmacol 2015;55:452-7.

27. Webb EA, Krone N. Current and novel approaches to children and young people with congenital adrenal hyperplasia and adrenal insufficiency. Best Pract Res Clin Endocrinol Metab 2015;29:449-68.

28. Limal J-M, Rappaport R, Bayard F. Plasma aldosterone, renin activity, and 17α-hydroxyprogesterone in salt-losing congenital adrenal hyperplasia. I. Response to ACTH in hydrocortisone treated patients and effect of 9α-fluorotisol. J Clin Endocrinol Metab 1977;45:551-9.

29. Quinkler M, Oelkers W, Remde H, et al. Mineralocorticoid substitution and monitoring in primary adrenal insufficiency. Best Pract Res Clin Endocrinol Metab 2015;29:17-24.

30. Karamouzis I, Berardelli R, Marinazzo E, et al. The acute effect of fludrocortisone on basal and hCRH-stimulated hypothalamic–pituitary–adrenal (HPA) axis in humans. Pituitary 2013;16:378-85.

31. Joint LWPES/ESPE CAH Working Group. Consensus statement on 21-hydroxylase deficiency from the Lawson Wilkins Pediatric Endocrine Society and the European Society for Paediatric Endocrinology. J Clin Endocrinol Metab 2002;87:4048–53.

32. Hume DM, Bell CC, Bartter F. Direct measurement of adrenal secretion during operative trauma and convalescence. Surgery 1962;52:174.

33. Lamberts SW, Bruining HA, de Jong FH. Corticosteroid therapy in severe illness. N Engl J Med 1997;337:1285-92.

34. Erichsen MM, Løvås K, Skinningsrud B, et al. Clinical, immunological, and genetic features of autoimmune primary adrenal insufficiency: observations from a Norwegian registry. J Clin Endocrinol Metab 2009;94:4882-90.

35. Meyer G, Hackemann A, Reusch J, et al. Nocturnal hypoglycemia identified by a continuous glucose monitoring system in patients with primary adrenal insufficiency (Addison's disease). Diabetes Technol Ther 2012;14:386-8.

36. Giordano R, Marzotti S, Balbo M, et al. Metabolic and cardiovascular profile in patients with Addison's disease under conventional glucocorticoid replacement. J Endocrinol Invest 2009;32:917-23.

37. Björnsdottir S, Sundström A, Ludvigsson JF, et al. Drug prescription patterns in patients with Addison's disease: a Swedish population-based cohort study. J Clin Endocrinol Metab 2013;98:2009-18.

38. Plat L, Leproult R, L'Hermite-Baleriaux M, et al. Metabolic effects of short-term elevations of plasma cortisol Are more pronounced in the evening than in the morning. J Clin Endocrinol Metab 1999;84:3082-92.

39. Björnsdottir S, Øksnes M, Isaksson M, et al. Circadian hormone profiles and insulin sensitivity in patients with Addison's disease: a comparison of continuous subcutaneous hydrocortisone infusion with conventional glucocorticoid replacement therapy. Clin Endocrinol 2015;83:28-35.

40. Nella AA, Mallappa A, Perritt AF, et al. A phase 2 study of continuous subcutaneous hydrocortisone infusion in adults with congenital adrenal hyperplasia. J Clin Endocrinol Metab 2016;101:4690-98.

41. Mallappa A, Sinaii N, Kumar P, et al. A phase 2 study of Chronocort, a modified-release formulation of hydrocortisone,

in the treatment of adults with classic congenital adrenal hyperplasia. J Clin Endocrinol Metab 2014;100:1137-45.

42. Jones CM, Mallappa A, Reisch N, et al. Modified release and conventional glucocorticoids and diurnal androgen excretion in congenital adrenal hyperplasia. J Clin Endocrinol Metab 2017;102:1797-806.

43. Giordano R, Guaraldi F, Marinazzo E, et al. Improvement of anthropometric and metabolic parameters, and quality of life following treatment with dual-release hydrocortisone in patients with Addison's disease. Endocrine 2016;51:360-8.

44. Johannsson G, Lennernäs H, Marelli C, et al. Achieving a physiological cortisol profile with once-daily dual-release hydrocortisone: a pharmacokinetic study. Eur J Endocrinol 2016;175:85-93.

45. Isidori AM, Venneri MA, Graziadio C, et al. Effect of once-daily, modified-release hydrocortisone versus standard glucocorticoid therapy on metabolism and innate immunity in patients with adrenal insufficiency (DREAM): a single-blind, randomised controlled trial. Lancet Diabetes Endocrinol 2018;6:173-85.

46. Guarnotta V, Ciresi A, Pillitteri G, et al. Improved insulin sensitivity and secretion in prediabetic patients with adrenal insufficiency on dua-release hydrocortisone treatment: a 36-month retrospective analysis. Clin Endocrinol 2018;88:665-72.

47. Park J, Das U, Didi M, et al. The challenges of cortisol replacement therapy in childhood: observations from a case series of children treated with modified-release hydrocortisone. Pediatric Drugs 2018;20:567-73.

48. Neumann U, Whitaker MJ, Wiegand S, et al. Absorption and tolerability of taste-masked hydrocortisone granules in neonates, infants and children under 6 years of age with adrenal insufficiency. Clin Endocrinol 2018;88:21-9.

LEARNING OBJECTIVES

1. Describe the pathophysiology of osteogenesis imperfecta (OI).

2. Differentiate between the seven types of OI.

3. Identify the signs and symptoms of OI.

4. Discuss the role of bisphosphonates in the treatment of OI.

5. Identify adverse events associated with bisphosphonate use.

ABBREVIATIONS IN THIS CHAPTER

MRC	Metabolic research council
OI	Osteogenesis imperfecta

INTRODUCTION

Osteogenesis imperfecta (OI), also known as *brittle bone disease*, is a genetic disorder primarily caused by defects in type I collagen. This disease is typically characterized by increased bone fragility and low bone mass. The most commonly used classification scheme outlines four distinct types of OI, types I–IV, each categorized in severity according to mutations in the genes encoding type I collagen.[1] Classification schemes have been expanded to include three subtypes, types V–VII, which differ in that they are not associated with type I collagen mutations; these three subtypes are minimally discussed in this chapter.[1] Patients with OI are highly susceptible to recurrent and severe fractures, which place them at risk of deformities and stunted growth in most cases. As a progressive condition, OI requires lifelong management to prevent deformity and complications.

EPIDEMIOLOGY

The overall incidence and prevalence of OI varies among studies. The composite incidence is about 1 in 10,000 births, but it is difficult to assess the true prevalence of the disease because of perinatal deaths resulting from the most lethal forms.[2] An estimated 20,000 to as many as 50,000 individuals in the United States have OI.[3]

Genetics are the most relevant factor in acquiring OI, which can affect individuals of any age, sex, and race. It is often an inherited genetic condition, most often in an autosomal dominant pattern, although autosomal recessive forms have also been reported.[4,5] In autosomal recessive forms of OI, mutations exist in both copies of a gene, which occurs in less than 10% of cases of OI. More than 90% of individuals with OI have an autosomal dominant form of the mutation in the two genes that encode type I collagen that were either inherited from a parent or arose from a new, spontaneous mutation. A parent with an autosomal dominant mutation has a 50% likelihood of passing on a mutated copy of the gene and having a child with OI.[6]

The occurrence of spontaneous mutations, also called *de novo mutations*, varies by severity. About 60% of patients with types I and IV have *de novo* mutations, whereas almost all individuals with types II and III have de novo mutations. A special consideration in the case of *de novo* mutations is mosaicism. *Mosaicism* occurs when a mutation is present in only a portion of an individual's cells, despite the cells originating from the same zygote as normal cells. Thus, if the mutation occurs in germ cells (egg or sperm), it may be passed along to subsequent generations. Mosaicism is presumed when an unaffected parent has more than one child with the same dominant mutation.[6]

PATHOPHYSIOLOGY

The pathophysiology of OI is best understood for forms that are positive for collagen type I mutations because little is known of the pathophysiology for other forms. Type I collagen is the major structural protein of the extracellular matrix of bone, skin, and tendons. In bone, collagen acts as a glue for mineral crystals, provides a template for hydroxyapatite mineral to be deposited, reinforces tissue, and binds molecules essential for normal bone matrix homeostasis and mineralization.[7] A collagen type I molecule is a triple-helical structure composed of three polypeptide chains, two α-1 chains, and one α-2 chain. For the chains to intertwine correctly, a glycine residue must be present at every third position. The most common sequence abnormality associated with OI is a point mutation that affects glycine in *COL1A1* or *COL1A2*, the two genes that encode the α-chains of collagen type I.[1] Cells with this mutation produce a combination of normal and abnormal collagen. Depending on which gene is affected, the position where the substitution arises on the triple helix, and which amino acid was substituted, the arising phenotype can vary from mild, including normal height or mild short stature, and blue sclera, to lethal, including rib and long bone fractures at birth, pronounced deformities, and dark sclera.[1]

CLASSIFICATION AND CLINICAL PRESENTATION

Although there is a wide variety in the clinical severity of OI, classifying patients on a continuum can help assess prognosis and the effects of therapeutic interventions. The Sillence classification system differentiates between four clinical types of OI.[8] An expanded classification system has been further delineated and includes three additional groups with a clinical diagnosis of OI but presenting with distinct features. All types of OI share a common characteristic of bone fragility, which increases in severity as follows: type I < types IV, V, VI, VII < type III < type II.[1]

In addition to bone fragility, other tissues rich in collagen may also be affected by mutations in *COL1A1* and *COL1A2*, leading to extraskeletal manifestations observed in OI such as blue or gray sclera, dentinogenesis imperfecta, hyperlaxity of ligaments and skin, and hearing impairment.[1] *Dentinogenesis imperfecta* is the oral manifestation of deficient collagen formation and is characterized by teeth discoloration (yellow/brown or gray/opalescent blue) and enamel fracture.[9] Because type I collagen is a major component of the sclera, individuals with OI have abnormally thin sclera, which increases transparency of the scleral wall, causing light scattering to be decreased and a bluish hue reflecting from the dark, pigmented choroid within the eye.[10] The presence of dentinogenesis imperfecta as well as blue sclera in OI patients poses a challenge for both dental and ophthalmic care. Dentinogenesis imperfecta places children with OI at risk of abscesses and loss of tooth structure. It is recommended that children see a dentist 6 months after eruption of the first baby tooth to prevent these complications.[9] Blue sclera has been correlated with corneal thinning and decreased ocular rigidity, which are risk factors for glaucoma, retinal detachment, and scleral rupture.[10-12]

The Sillence classification system describes OI types I–IV. The most prevalent type of OI is type I, accounting for 80% of all cases.[13] Type I OI characterizes patients with mild disease without major bone deformities. Vertebral fractures are common in this group and can lead to mild scoliosis, but these patients are typically of normal height or are mildly short in stature. Blue sclera is common in this group, but dentinogenesis imperfecta is not.

Type II characterizes the most severe form of OI. Patients with this type present with severe limb shortening and multiple rib and long bone fractures at birth. Patients with OI type II exhibit pulmonary hypoplasia, possibly secondary to chest wall architecture abnormalities, which results in stunted airway branching and alveolar development, in addition to poor ventilation, which can lead to respiratory failure and death.[14] Because of the severity of the phenotype, few infants with OI type II survive the perinatal period.

Type III is the most severe form of OI for children who survive the neonatal period. These patients are typically very short in stature and have limb and spine deformities from multiple fractures. Patients in this group can present with grayish sclera and dentinogenesis imperfecta. Respiratory complications are the primary cause of death in this group. Chest wall abnormalities caused by kyphoscoliosis, vertebral collapse, rib fractures, and short stature compressing abdominal contents upward, thus producing limited diaphragmatic movement; all these deformities contribute to restricted air movement and poor ventilation.[15] Type IV characterizes patients with mild to moderate bone deformities and variable short stature. Similar to type III, patients with type IV OI can also present with grayish or white sclera and dentinogenesis imperfecta.

From OI type IV, three separate subsets, types V–VII, have been identified based on distinct clinical and bone histological features. All three types share common features that include moderate to severe bone deformity. They differ in their modes of inheritance, and unlike types I–IV, there is no evidence of collagen type I abnormality. Patients with types V–VII are also short in stature, but do not typically present with dentinogenesis imperfecta.[1]

PROGNOSIS

The prognosis for patients with OI varies greatly on the classification and the presence and severity of symptoms. The most common cause of death in patients with OI is respiratory failure, followed by accidental trauma. Although children and adults with OI endure many fractures in their lifetime and are often physically restricted, most have the potential to lead otherwise normal lives.[3]

DIAGNOSIS

The clinical diagnosis of OI is based on the signs and symptoms previously outlined in this chapter. Traditionally, diagnostic emphasis has been placed on the presence of blue/gray sclera and dentinogenesis imperfecta. However, it is important to note that because dark or bluish sclera is common in healthy infants, this diagnostic criterion may not be helpful in this age group.

Diagnosis of OI is usually straightforward in patients who have typical features and/or have a positive family history. Unfortunately, an absence of family history and the bone fragility associated with extraskeletal abnormalities poses a challenge in differentiating between OI and child abuse. Bone mineral density examinations with DEXA (dual-energy x-ray absorptiometry) or CT (computed tomography) have helped in the differential diagnosis.[9,10] In otherwise healthy growing children, bone mineral density increases by 3% to 6% per year before puberty and 14% to 16% per year during puberty.[16] However, information is scarce on the expected bone mineral density of those with mild OI. Analyzing the amount and structure of type I procollagen molecules derived from cultured skin fibroblasts can also be helpful in the diagnosis.[17]

Other diagnostic methods include screening for mutations in the *COL1A1* and *COL1A2* genes by extracting genomic DNA from white blood cells.[17] The majority of collagen type I mutations can be detected using these two methods. A positive study can confirm the diagnosis of OI, but a negative result does not rule it out. If the study is negative, it may still be possible that a mutation is present but was not detected, or the patient has a form that is not associated with type I collagen mutation.[1]

GOALS OF THERAPY

Because there is no known cure for OI, the primary goal of therapy is focused on the management of the disease. Therapeutic goals vary based on phenotype and mobility, but all therapies aim to maximize mobility, prevent long bone deformities, reduce fracture rates, and promote bone strength.[1,7]

NONPHARMACOLOGIC THERAPY

Physical therapy, rehabilitation, and orthopedic surgery have been considered to be the mainstay of treatment for patients with OI. Children with milder forms may have similar activity levels as their healthier peers, so nonpharmacologic therapies may only involve fracture management.[12] In a study that evaluated muscle function and physical activity in children with OI type I, the children had lower muscle force and power but they were as active as their healthy counterparts in terms of volume and distribution of physical activity, time in sedentary activity, number of steps, and the estimated daily energy expenditure.[13] Conversely, children with moderate to severe OI often have long bone deformities, scoliosis, and reduced mobility, which prompt the need for orthopedic and rehabilitation interventions.[12]

PHARMACOLOGIC THERAPY

Despite having understood the molecular causes of OI for some time, specific pharmacologic therapy has lagged behind the science of the disease. Medical treatment for OI has historically been unsuccessful. Treatments involving various hormones, vitamins, minerals, and other therapies have been evaluated, but none have proven to be consistently efficacious.[1]

CALCITONIN

Calcitonin, a hormone secreted by the thyroid gland, was thought to be beneficial in treating diseases with high rates of bone resorption such as Paget disease.[18] Studies then began to consider use of calcitonin for OI. Its role in OI therapy is to inhibit bone resorption by decreasing the number and activity of osteoclasts to improve bone density.[19]

A case report investigated the effect of porcine calcitonin on calcium retention and hydroxyproline excretion in two patients with OI. Hydroxyproline is a component of collagen and is considered an index of bone resorption; urinary excretion is elevated in patients with OI. The patients were started on intramuscular porcine calcitonin 20 metabolic research council (MRC) units twice a day for the first week. The dose was increased to 40 MRC units twice a day in the second week, and then 80 MRC units twice a day in the third week and was continued for 3 more weeks. No calcitonin was given on the seventh week. The results showed a decrease in fecal calcium and an increase in urinary calcium, suggesting that calcitonin increased the intestinal absorption of calcium and the retention of calcium in the skeleton. A decrease in the urinary excretion of hydroxyproline was also observed. The study reported no adverse reactions occurred from porcine calcitonin.[19]

Subsequent studies investigated the use of salmon calcitonin because it was thought to be more potent and longer lasting than porcine on its effects on serum calcium concentrations.[20] One study evaluated long-term therapy using salmon calcitonin on mobility, bone density, and fracture rate in patients with OI. A total of 50 patients (48 children age 6 months to 15 years and two adults age 20 and 22 years) were treated with subcutaneous injections of salmon calcitonin 2 MRC units/kg 3 days per week and with a daily oral calcium supplement equivalent to 230–345 mg of calcium for up to 48 months. Most patients reported increased mobility and strength in the extremities as early as the second week. A decrease in fracture rates from 3.2 fractures per year before therapy to 0.6 fractures per year during therapy was also observed. Bone density was measured using radiographic photodensitometry, which compared patients' bone mineral densities with those of their age- and sex-matched peer norms. An average annual rate of change in bone mineral concentrations was compared between the treatment group and the normal population. Overall, it was determined that the average annual rate of change for the treatment group was less than that of their normal peers, indicating that they did not gain bone mineral as rapidly. Patients 5 years and younger were the only age group found to have a rate of bone mineral deposition that exceeded the norm, suggesting that younger patients respond better to calcitonin than older patients. However, this rate of bone mineral deposition was not sustained for the entire duration of therapy.[16] Adverse effects of calcitonin therapy cited in studies included recurrent nausea and vomiting, flushing of the skin on the hands and feet, and various metabolic disturbances such as hypophosphatemia, hypomagnesemia, hyponatremia, and hypokalemia.[19,21,22]

BISPHOSPHONATES

The class effect of bisphosphonates is to reduce osteoclast activity or cause osteoclast apoptosis, thereby reducing osteoclastic activity. Radiolabeled and fluorescently labeled compounds have been used in studies to confirm the passage of bisphosphonates through the basal membrane of actively resorbing osteoclasts into intracellular vesicles. After absorption, changes in cell morphology occur; borders lose their integrity and cells detach from the bone surface and undergo apoptosis.[15] The resulting structural changes of bisphosphonates on bones of children include increased width of tubular bones, reduced cortical porosity, increased cortical thickness, and widening of the ends of long bones resulting from reduced resorption from trabecular material of the metaphyses. In addition, thickening of the end plate allows for the vertebral structure to be restored. However, formation is favored over resorption, which results in increased bone mass and improved strength.[16]

In addition to these study results, bisphosphonates have become widely used for the treatment of OI after a study that included a series of children and adolescents treated with intravenous pamidronate was published in 1998.[23] The uncontrolled observational study included 30 children age 3 to 16 years with OI type III or IV and evaluated the effects of intravenous pamidronate on bone mineral density and clinical status. Pamidronate was administered for 3 consecutive days per infusion cycle at 4- to 6-month intervals for 1.3 to 5 years. Half of the subjects received a 1.5-mg/kg dose per infusion cycle, which was then increased to 3 mg/kg dosing after the first year of treatment. The other half of the subjects only received a 3-mg/kg dose per infusion cycle. The results showed an increase in bone mineral density by 41.9 ± 29% per year and an improvement in the mean z-score from −5.3

± 1.2 to –3.4 ± 1.5 (p<0.001). In addition, the fracture rate decreased by 1.7% per year (p<0.001), and the cortical width of metacarpals increased by 27.0 ± 20.2% per year, suggesting evidence of new bone formation. A reduction in chronic bone pain was reported as early as 1 week after initiation of therapy, with only an occasional recurrence of pain in the days before a treatment cycle.

A limitation of this study is the study design. Patients, caregivers, and physicians were unblinded and so were aware of treatments being administered, increasing the possibility of bias.[23] It is possible that a placebo effect existed, particularly regarding the relief of bone pain. Despite this limitation, consistent clinical and radiological findings suggested the changes were a result of pamidronate therapy. Since the publication of this study in 1998, bisphosphonates have become the standard of care for the treatment of OI.

Bisphosphonates can be administered orally or intravenously. Cyclical pamidronate is currently the most widely used intravenous option for moderate to severe OI because it has been studied in most detail among all bisphosphonates.[24] Reported dosing regimens are variable; both weight-directed and body surface area-directed dosing regimens have been used. For weight-directed dosing regimens, pamidronate is given in cycles of 3 days, and repeated every 2–4 months depending on age.[25,26] For body surface area-directed regimens, infusions are typically given once a month for 3 months.[27,28] Table 1 provides detailed dosing information. After the first pamidronate infusion, bone resorption immediately decreases and levels of bone formation markers are also reduced.[25,29-31] Within 1–2 weeks after initiating therapy, studies report an increase in well-being and a decrease in chronic bone pain.[23,32-36] Months after initiation of therapy, bone mass and density increase.[30,32,36-40]

Zoledronate is another newer and more potent intravenous bisphosphonate that has been used for the treatment of OI. Studies have shown its efficacy and safety to be similar to that of pamidronate. One small observational study evaluated 17 patients with OI type I treated with 0.05 mg/kg of intravenous zoledronate every 6 months for 1–3.2 years. Results showed that zoledronate therapy decreased the overall fracture incidence from a mean of 0.52 fractures per year before therapy to 0.28 fractures per year after treatment onset. The median bone mineral density z-score increased from –2.0 to –0.7 over the course of 2 years (p=0.011).[41]

An open-label prospective, randomized study assessed the safety and efficacy of zoledronate compared with pamidronate in 23 children with OI. The pamidronate group received 1 mg/kg/day over 2 days and the zoledronate group received 0.025–0.05 mg/kg/day over 2 days every 3–4 months during a 1-year follow-up. After treatment, the bone mineral density of the pamidronate and zoledronate groups increased by 51.8% (p=0.053) and 67.6% (p=0.003), respectively. Improvements in z-scores were also seen in both groups, with the pamidronate group increasing from –5.3 to –3.8 (p=0.032) and the zoledronate group increasing from –4.8 to –2.3 (p=0.007).[42]

Overall, zoledronate was well tolerated. Two patients in the first study experienced mild symptoms of hypocalcemia (fatigue, dizziness, nausea, mild tremor) after the first dose. These symptoms were alleviated after a treatment of intravenous calcium. To avoid a recurrence of these adverse effects, the second zoledronate dose was decreased to 0.025 mg/kg for these two patients with no recurrence of hypocalcemia. The most common adverse effect reported in the study overall was a flu-like reaction after the first infusion, with some patients also experiencing bone pain. One advantage associated with zoledronate is its more favorable administration schedule because it can be given over 45 minutes in 1 day, which can potentially make it a more attractive option over pamidronate in the future.[41-43]

Oral administration of bisphosphonates can be useful for patients who are able to swallow pills. The caveat is that a patient must also be able to take precautions required with oral administration of bisphosphonates, such as drinking a large glass of water and remaining upright after 30 minutes after administration. Compared with intravenous administration, potential challenges with compliance, bioavailability,

Table 1. Intravenous Pamidronate Dosing in Osteogenesis Imperfecta[17,20]

Weight-Directed Dosing	
Infants and Children < 2 years	**Initial:** 0.25 mg/kg once on day 1, then 0.5 mg/kg/dose daily on days 2 and 3 of first cycle
	Subsequent cycles: 0.5 mg/kg/dose once daily for 3 days
	Frequency of cycles: every 2 months for total yearly dose of 9 mg/kg
Children 2–3 years	**Initial:** 0.38 mg/kg once on day 1, then 0.75 mg/kg/dose daily on days 2 and 3 of first cycle
	Subsequent cycles: 0.75 mg/kg/dose once daily for 3 days
	Frequency of cycles: every 3 months for total yearly dose of 9 mg/kg
Children > 3 years and Adolescents	**Initial:** 0.5 mg/kg once on day 1, then 1 mg/kg/dose daily on days 2 and 3 of first cycle
	Subsequent cycles: 1 mg/kg/dose once daily for 3 days
	Frequency of cycles: every 4 months for total yearly dose of 9 mg/kg
Body Surface Area-Directed Dosing	
Infants, Children, and Adolescents	**Initial:** 10 mg/m^2/dose once a month for 3 months, then increase to 20 mg/m^2/dose once a month for 3 months, then increase to 30 mg/m^2/dose once a month for subsequent doses

and gastrointestinal adverse effects may present with oral administration. Oral bisphosphonates that have been used in studies for the treatment of OI include alendronate, risedronate, and olpadronate.[44-49] Several small studies have reported efficacy and tolerability with alendronate, with benefits seen in increased bone density and decreased fracture rates.[44,45]

One double-blind placebo-controlled trial found that oral alendronate given for 2 years was well tolerated and efficacious in 139 children and adolescents with OI type I, III, or IV. Alendronate was administered in doses of 5 mg/day in children who weighed less than 40 kg and 10 mg/day for those who weighed 40 kg or more. A decrease in bone turnover was seen with a 62% decrease in the urinary secretion of bone resorption marker, type I N-telopeptide. There was also an improvement in spine bone mineral density, with a 51% increase in the alendronate group compared with a 12% increase in the placebo group (p<0.001). There was, however, no significant effect on the incidence of fractures, bone pain, or functional status.[46]

Risedronate was used in a single-center, randomized double-blind, placebo-controlled study that included 26 children with OI type I. Patients weighing less than 40 kg were given risedronate 15 mg once per week, and patients weighing 40 kg or more were given 30 mg once per week for 2 years. A 35% decrease in serum concentrations of type I N-telopeptide was seen in the treatment group compared with 6% in the placebo group (p=0.003). Treatment resulted in an increase in lumbar spine bone mineral density, with z-scores increasing by 0.65 compared with a decrease of 0.15 in the placebo group (p=0.002). There was no difference in fracture rate observed. It was also noted that skeletal effects were weaker than those from intravenous pamidronate.[47]

Olpadronate has been used in a randomized, placebo-controlled study in the Netherlands that included 34 children and adolescents with OI. These patients were treated with olpadronate 10 mg/m^2 or placebo for 2 years. Those in the treatment group showed a greater increase in spinal bone mineral density, with an improvement in z-scores from −4.98 to −3.31 with olpadronate compared with −4.84 to −4.70 with placebo (p=0.002). A 31% reduction in long bone fractures was also seen with the olpadronate group (p=0.01); however, there were no differences in functional outcome or changes in urinary markers of bone resorption.[49] Although oral bisphosphonates may have advantages in administration, overall they seem to be generally less effective in treating OI than intravenous bisphosphonates.

Although beneficial in treating OI, bisphosphonate treatment is not without some consequences. Adverse effects from bisphosphonate use can be classified as short term and long term.[24] Short-term adverse effects reported with use of pamidronate included decreased serum calcium concentrations as well as an influenza-like reaction that manifested as fever, rash, and vomiting, and usually presented 12–36 hours after initiation of the infusion. Although the reaction can be easily managed with analgesics, it can be concerning for infants and children in respiratory distress or who have compromised immune systems.

In terms of long-term adverse effects, the antiresorptive properties of bisphosphonates can ultimately diminish bone remodeling and thus interfere with renewal and repair of bone.[1] There are also concerns for delay in post-surgical healing of osteotomy sites for rod insertion and correction of deformities. Therefore, treatment is usually postponed for 4–6 months after evidence of sufficient healing.[50,51]

In addition to these known adverse effects, there are also other effects that remain in question. Osteonecrosis of the jaw has been reported in adult patients receiving high-dose bisphosphonates, which makes it a concern for long-term use in children. However, several studies have not shown evidence of osteonecrosis of the jaw with the use of pamidronate or zoledronate.[52,53] Bisphosphonates also linger in bone tissue for many years, and it is unknown what effects this presence may have on female patients who eventually bear children later in life.[1] There is still much that must be elucidated in terms of the long-term benefit versus risk of bisphosphonate use, particularly for those with mild OI.

OTHER TREATMENTS

The role of growth hormone in treating OI has been investigated. Growth hormone is thought to stimulate the expression of insulin-like growth factor I and insulin-like growth factor binding protein-3 in osteoblasts, which in turn regulates the synthesis of type I collagen and bone formation.[54] Studies have shown that growth hormone may accelerate short-term height velocity.[54,55] In one study that included 14 patients with type I OI, seven patients received human growth hormone 0.2 mg/kg per week (0.6 international units/kg per week) in six injections subcutaneously for 12 months, and the remaining patients were followed as controls. An increase in linear growth velocity was seen in the treatment group compared with the pretreatment period (p<0.05) and the control group (p<0.05); however, these effects were not sustained after treatment stopped. Serum insulin-like growth factor I concentrations were low in the treatment group, but were not statistically different from the control group. Over the course of therapy, concentrations increased, but not significantly. A significant increase in bone density was observed in the treatment group (p<0.05).[54]

Another study involved 26 children with OI types III and IV who were treated with recombinant growth hormone 0.1–0.2 international units/kg/day for 6 days per week for at least 1 year. Of these patients, 14 children had sustained response to growth hormone treatment, achieving a 50% or more increase in their linear growth rate during treatment compared with pretreatment, and 12 children failed to sustain a growth response, even after a dose increase from 0.1 international units/kg/day to 0.2 international units/kg/day. For those children who had a positive response, known as *responders*, the growth rate was 6.4 ± 2.0 cm per year whereas the growth rate for those who did not achieve a positive response, the *nonresponders*, was 4.0 ± 1.7 cm per year. Responders also exhibited a decrease in long bone fractures from an average of 2.0 ± 1.1 fractures per year before treatment to 1.21 ± 0.7 fractures per year during treatment (p=0.030). Fracture rates for nonresponders were unchanged. In addition, bone density improved, with average z-scores increasing after 6 months of therapy (−5.02 ± 0.27 at baseline, −4.73 ± 0.25 6 at 6 months; p=0.01) and stable scores after 12 months (−4.81 ± 0.35; p=0.05).[55]

Adverse effects of growth hormone therapy include pain, discomfort, and bruising with injections. Scoliosis may occur if growth rate is very rapid.[56] In addition, there have also been reports that growth hormone therapy causes an increase in fracture risk.[57,58] In one case, growth hormone was initiated in addition to intravenous pamidronate in a patient with OI type I. After combination therapy was started, the patient's height velocity increased 6 cm/year; however, three bone fractures occurred in the latter 5 months of therapy. Growth hormone therapy was discontinued and pamidronate was continued with no recurrence of fractures for 24 months.[57]

A nonrandomized, interventional clinical trial recently examined the effect of growth hormone therapy on linear growth of children with OI types III and IV. Forty-two children between the ages of 3 and 8 years were included and given the synthetic growth hormone Humatrope (Eli Lilly and Co., LLC, Indianapolis, IN) 0.06 mg/kg/day subcutaneously 6 days per week for one year. The primary outcome was annual growth rate and secondary outcomes include vertebral DEXA and fracture rate. Responders were defined as those who achieved or sustained a 50% increase in growth rate over their baseline in the first year. Those who demonstrated response were continued on treatment for an additional 2 years. After the third year, responders were defined as those who demonstrated a 30% or greater increase above baseline, and will be treated until final adult height is achieved. Preliminary results have been reported for those who completed 1 year of the study. Twenty-five of the 42 (59.5%) participants met the study criteria of at least 50% growth increase from baseline in the first year. One serious adverse event was reported as a suicide attempt by 1 of the 42 participants (2.38%). Results for secondary outcomes have not yet been published.[59]

Parathyroid hormone has also been proposed for OI treatment because it has anabolic properties that have been shown to reduce fractures in postmenopausal osteoporosis.[60] However, risk of developing osteosarcoma, as evidenced in rat studies, makes this option less attractive in children.[61] Teriparatide, a parathyroid hormone analog with bone-anabolic effects, has been studied in adult patients with OI type I. Results showed an increase in bone mineral density at the lumbar spine, but not the hip after 18 months of treatment. Serum markers of bone formation and bone resorption also increased over the course of therapy.[62] Teriparatide has not yet been studied in the pediatric population.

CONCLUSIONS

Osteogenesis imperfecta is a rare genetic disorder that causes brittle bones, leading to recurrent fractures. Special care must be used for these individuals to elude injuries. Treatment goals are directed toward management of the disease with nonpharmacologic therapies including rehabilitation, physical therapy, and orthopedic surgery. Several pharmacologic options have been used to manage OI, but none have been as consistent in improving mobility, preventing deformities, and reducing fracture rates as bisphosphonates. Although the use of bisphosphonates offers benefits in this patient population, many unanswered questions remain and must be delineated including long-term adverse effects.

Patient Case — OSTEOGENESIS IMPERFECTA

A 3-year-old white girl is brought to the emergency department with pain in her right leg. The caregiver is concerned about a possible right tibia fracture after falling. A radiograph of her right lower extremity confirms distal right tibia and fibula fractures with mild posterior displacement.

Medical history: Premature neonate born at 32 weeks' gestation; retinopathy of prematurity after laser therapy; history of multiple fractures in the past 2 years involving right femur and left tibia; severe scoliosis and limb deformities secondary to multiple fractures

Family history: Father with osteogenesis imperfecta

Social history: Lives at home with parents and two brothers; very active

Vital signs: BP 92/58 mm Hg, HR 113 beats/minute, RR 26 breaths/minute, Tmax 99.5°F (37.5°C), Wt 10 kg, pain level 5 on Wong-Baker FACES scale

Review of symptoms: A girl in extreme pain with dentinogenesis imperfecta, grey sclera, short stature, multiple fractures, and severe scoliosis

Physical examination:

General: Awake; alert; crying and in visible distress because of pain

HEENT: Normocephalic, normal tympanic membranes, gray sclera, clear nasal mucosa, moist oral mucosa, no evidence of lesions or thrush, pharynx without erythema or exudates; neck supple with no lymphadenopathy

Respiratory: No retractions; clear to auscultation bilaterally; no rales, rhonchi or wheezes

Cardiovascular: Regular rhythm without murmurs; tachycardic; pulses +2 and symmetrical

Abdomen: Soft, nontender

Extremities: Full range of motion in upper extremities; limited mobility with right lower extremity

Skin: No rashes, lesions, or petechiae

Neuro: Grossly intact

1. What signs and symptoms of osteogenesis imperfecta (OI) are evident in this child's presentation? Based on presentation, what type of OI does this child likely have?

This patient's signs and symptoms characterize her as having type III OI. Her medical history shows that she has had multiple fractures over the past 2 years that have left her with limb deformities and severe scoliosis. These signs are the differentiating characteristic between type III and type IV, which is only moderately deforming. She also presents with gray sclera and dentinogenesis imperfecta.

2. What pharmacologic treatment option is most appropriate at this time?

Because other treatment modalities have been historically inconsistent, the best treatment option is an intravenous bisphosphonate. The most widely used and well-studied intravenous bisphosphonate is pamidronate. Based on this patient's age and weight, the required dose is 0.38 mg/kg intravenous once on day 1, followed by 0.75 mg/kg/dose daily on days 2 and 3 of the first cycle. For subsequent cycles of therapy, the dose is 0.75 mg/kg/dose once daily for 3 days, with each cycle repeated every 3 months for a total yearly dose of 9 mg/kg.

3. What adverse effects may be expected with the use of an intravenous bisphosphonate?

Immediately after infusion, the serum calcium may decrease. The child may also experience the influenza-like reaction (i.e., fever, rash, vomiting) reported 12–36 hours after intravenous pamidronate use that can be alleviated by standard antipyretics. In terms of long-term adverse effects, she may have longer post-surgical healing if she should require osteotomies for rod insertion and correction of deformities.

REFERENCES

1. Rauch F, Glorieux FH. Osteogenesis imperfecta. Lancet 2004; 363:1377-85.
2. Shapiro JR. Clinical and genetic classification of osteogenesis imperfecta and epidemiology. In: Shapiro JR, Byers PH, Glorieux FH, et al., eds. Osteogenesis Imperfecta: A Translational Approach to Brittle Bone Disease. Oxford, UK: Elsevier, 2014:15-22.
3. Osteogenesis imperfecta (OI) Foundation. A Guide for Medical Professionals, Individuals, and Families. Available at https://oif.org/wp-content/uploads/2019/08/Fast_Facts_About_OI.pdf. Accessed December 12, 2019.
4. Ward LM, Rauch F, Travers R, et al. Osteogenesis imperfecta type VII: an autosomal recessive form of brittle bone disease. Bone 2002;31:12-8.
5. Glorieux FH, Rauch F, Plotkin H, et al. Type V osteogenesis imperfecta: a new form of brittle bone disease. J Bone Miner Res 2000;15:1650-8.
6. Cohen JS. Patterns of inheritance in osteogenesis imperfecta. In: Shapiro JR, Byers PH, Glorieux FH, et al., eds. Osteogenesis Imperfecta: A Translational Approach to Brittle Bone Disease. Oxford, UK: Elsevier, 2014:99-101.
7. Makareeva E, Leiken S. Collagen structure folding and function. In: Shapiro JR, Byers PH, Glorieux FH, et al., eds. Osteogenesis Imperfecta: A Translational Approach to Brittle Bone Disease. Oxford, UK: Elsevier, 2014:71-84.
8. Sillence DO, Senn A, Danks DM. Genetic heterogeneity in osteogenesis imperfecta. J Med Genet 1979;16:101-16.
9. Biria M, Abbas FM, Mozaffar S, et al. Dentinogenesis imperfecta associated with osteogenesis imperfecta. Dent Res J 2012;9:489-94.
10. Chau FY, Wallace D, Vajaranant T, et al. Osteogenesis imperfecta and the eye. In: Shapiro JR, Byers PH, Glorieux FH, et al., eds. Osteogenesis Imperfecta: A Translational Approach to the Brittle Bone Disease Oxford, UK: Elsevier, 2014:15-22.
11. Evereklioglu C, Madenci E, Bayazit YA, et al. Central corneal thickness is lower in osteogenesis imperfecta and negatively correlates with the presence of blue sclera. Ophthalmic Physiol Opt 2002;22:511-5.
12. Trejo P, Rauch F. Osteogenesis imperfecta in children and adolescents—new developments in diagnosis and treatment. Osteoporos Int 2016;27:3427-37.
13. Smith R. Osteogenesis imperfecta. Br Med J 1984;289:394-5.
14. Shapiro JR, Burn VE, Chipman SD, et al. Case report: pulmonary hypoplasia and osteogenesis imperfecta type II with defective synthesis of alpha I(1) procollagen. Bone 1989;10:165-71.
15. Sandhaus RA. Pulmonary function in osteogenesis imperfecta. In: Shapiro JR, Byers PH, Glorieux FH, et al., eds. Osteogenesis Imperfecta: A Translational Approach to Brittle Bone Disease. Oxford, UK: Elsevier, 2014:335-42.
16. Davie MWJ, Haddaway MJ. Bone mineral content and density in healthy subjects and in osteogenesis imperfecta. Arch Dis Child 1994;70:331-4.
17. Korkko J, Ala-Kokko L, De Paepe A, et al. Analysis of the COLA1A and COL1A2 genes by PCR amplification and scanning by conformation-sensitive gel electrophoresis identifies only COL1A1 mutation in 15 patients with osteogenesis imperfecta type I: identification of common sequences of null-allele mutations. Am J Hum Genet 1998;62:98-110.
18. Shai F, Baker RK, Wallach S. The clinical and metabolic effects of porcine calcitonin on Paget's disease of bone. J Clin Invest 1971;50:1927-40.
19. Castells S, Inamdar S, Baker RK, et al. Effects of porcine calcitonin in osteogenesis imperfecta tarda. J Pediatr 1972; 80:757-62.
20. Keutmann HT, Parsons HT, Potts JT. Isolation and chemical properties of two calcitonins from salmon ultimobranchial glands. J Bio Chem 1970;245:1491.
21. August GP, Shapiro J, Hung W. Calcitonin therapy of children with osteogenesis imperfecta. J Pediatr 1977;91:1001-5.
22. Castells S, Chakrabarti C, Bachtell RS, et al. Therapy of osteogenesis imperfecta with synthetic salmon calcitonin. J Pediatr 1979;95:807-11.
23. Glorieux FH, Bishop NJ, Plotkin H, et al. Cyclic administration of pamidronate in children with severe osteogenesis imperfecta. N Engl J Med 1998;339:947-52.
24. Rauch F. Bisphosphonate treatment and related agents in children. In: Shapiro JR, Byers PH, Glorieux FH, et al., eds. Osteogenesis Imperfecta: A Translational Approach to Brittle Bone Disease. Oxford, UK: Elsevier, 2014:501-7.
25. Rauch F, Plotkin H, Travers R, et al. Osteogenesis imperfecta types I, III, and IV: effect of pamidronate therapy on bone and mineral metabolism. J Clin Endocrinol Metab 2003;88:986-92.
26. Zeitlin L, Rauch F, Plotkin H, et al. Height and weight development during long-term therapy with cyclical intravenous pamidronate in children and adolescents with osteogenesis imperfecta types I, II and IV. Pediatrics 2003;111:1030-6.
27. Astrom E, Jorulf H, Soderhall S. Intravenous pamidronate treatment of infants with severe osteogenesis imperfecta. Arch Dis Child 2007;92:332-8.

28. Heino T, Astrom E, Laurencikas E, et al. Intravenous pamidronate treatment improves growth in prepubertal osteogenesis imperfecta patients. Horm Res Paediatr 2011;75:354-61.

29. Astrom E, Magnusson P, Eksborg S, et al. Biochemical bone markers in the assessment and pamidronate treatment of children and adolescents with osteogenesis imperfecta. Acta Paediatr 2010;99:1834-40.

30. Arikoski P, Silverwood B, Tillmann V, et al. Intravenous pamidronate treatment in children with moderate to severe osteogenesis imperfecta: assessment of indices of dual-energy X-ray absorptiometry and bone metabolic markers during the first year of therapy. Bone 2004;34:539-46.

31. Cabral de Menezes Filho H, Rodrigues JM, Radonsky V, et al. Decrease of serum alkaline phosphatase after three cycles of pamidronate disodium in children with severe osteogenesis imperfecta. Horm Res 2007;68(Suppl 5):207-8.

32. Lowing K, Astrom E, Oscarsson KA, et al. Effect of intravenous pamidronate therapy on everyday activities in children with osteogenesis imperfecta. Acta Paediatr 2007;96:1180-3.

33. Salehpour S, Tavakkoli S. Cyclic pamidronate therapy in children with osteogenesis imperfecta. J Pediatr Endocrinol Metab 2010;23:73-80.

34. Bhadada SK, Santosh R, Bhansali A, et al. Osteogenesis imperfecta. J Assoc Physicians India 2009;57:33-6.

35. Andiran N, Alikasifoglu A, Gonc N, et al. Cyclic pamidronate therapy in children with osteogenesis imperfecta: results of treatment and follow-up after discontinuation. J Pediatr Endocrinol Metab 2008;21:63-72.

36. Forin V, Arabi A, Guigonis V, et al. Benefits of pamidronate in children with osteogenesis imperfecta: an open prospective study. Joint Bone Spine 2005;72:313-8.

37. Choi JH, Shin YL, Yoo HW. Short-term efficacy of monthly pamidronate infusion in patients with osteogenesis imperfecta. J Korean Med Sci 2007;22:209-12.

38. Rauch F, Plotkin H, Zeitlin L, et al. Bone mass, size, and density in children and adolescents with osteogenesis imperfecta: effect of pamidronate therapy. J Bone Miner Res 2003;18:610-4.

39. Rauch F, Cornibert S, Cheung M, et al. Long-bone changes after pamidronate discontinuation in children and adolescents with osteogenesis imperfecta. Bone 2007;40:821-7.

40. Vallo A, Rodriguez-Leyva F, Rodriguez Soriano J. Osteogenesis imperfecta: anthropometric, skeletal and mineral metabolic effects of long-term intravenous pamidronate therapy. Acta Paediatr 2006;95:332-9.

41. Vuorimies I, Toiviainen-Salo S, Hero M, et al. Zoledronic acid treatment in children with osteogenesis imperfecta. Horm Res Paediatr 2011;75:346-53.

42. Barros ER, Saraiva GL, de Oliveira TP, et al. Safety and efficacy of a 1-year treatment with zoledronic acid compared with pamidronate in children with osteogenesis imperfecta. J Pediatr Endocrinol Metab 2012;25:485-91.

43. Brown JJ, Zacharin MR. Safety and efficacy of intravenous zoledronic acid in paediatric osteoporosis. J Pediatr Endocrinol Metab 2009;22:55-63.

44. Cho TJ, Choi IH, Chung CY, et al. Efficacy of oral alendronate in children with osteogenesis imperfecta. J Pediatr Orthop 2005; 25:607-12.

45. Madenci E, Yilmaz K, Yilmaz M, et al. Alendronate treatment in osteogenesis imperfecta. J Clin Rheumatol 2006;12:53-6.

46. Ward LM, Rauch F, Whyte MP, et al. Alendronate for the treatment of pediatric osteogenesis imperfecta: a randomized placebo-controlled study. J Clin Endocrinol Metab 2011;96:355-64.

47. Rauch F, Munns CF, Land C, et al. Risedronate in the treatment of mild pediatric osteogenesis imperfecta: a randomized placebo-controlled study. J Bone Miner Res 2009;24:1282-9.

48. Bishop N, Harrison R, Ahmed F, et al. A randomized, controlled dose-ranging study of risedronate in children with moderate and severe osteogenesis imperfecta. J Bone Miner Res 2010; 5:32-40.

49. Sakkers R, Kok D, Engelbert R. Skeletal effects and functional outcome with olpadronate in children with osteogenesis imperfecta: a 2-year randomised placebo-controlled study. Lancet 2004;363:1427-31.

50. Munns CF, Rauch F, Zeitlin L, et al. Delayed osteotomy but not fracture healing in pediatric osteogenesis imperfecta patients receiving pamidronate. J Bone Miner Res 2004;19:1779-86.

51. Pizones J, Plotkin H, Parra-Garcia JI, et al. Bone healing in children with osteogenesis imperfecta treated with bisphosphonates. J Pediatr Orthop 2005;25:332-5.

52. Malmgren B, Astrom E, Soderhall S. No osteonecrosis in jaws of young patients with osteogenesis imperfecta treated with bisphosphonates. J Oral Pathol Med 2008;37:196-200.

53. Brown JJ, Ramalingam L, Zacharin MR. Bisphosphonate-associated osteonecrosis of the jaw: does it occur in children? Clin Endocrinol 2008;68:863-7.

54. Antoniazzi F, Bertoldo F, Mottes M, et al. Growth hormone treatment in osteogenesis imperfecta with quantitative defect of type I collagen synthesis. J Pediatr 1996;129:432-9.

55. Marini JC, Hopkins E, Glorieux FH, et al. Positive linear growth and bone responses to growth hormone treatment in children with types III and IV osteogenesis imperfecta: high predictive value of the carboxy-terminal propeptide of type I procollagen. J Bone Miner Res 2003;18:237-43.

56. Germain-Lee E, DiGirolamo DJ, Plotkin H. Growth and growth hormone use in osteogenesis imperfecta. In: Shapiro JR, Byers PH, Glorieux FH, et al., eds. Osteogenesis Imperfecta: A Translational Approach to Brittle Bone Disease. Oxford, UK: Elsevier, 2014:267-80.

57. Kodama H, Kubota K, Abe T. Osteogenesis imperfecta: are fractures and growth hormone treatment linked? J Pediatr 1998; 132:559.

58. Noda H, Onishi H, Saitoh K, et al. Growth hormone therapy may increase fracture risk in a pubertal patient with osteogenesis imperfecta. J Pediatr Endocrinol Metab 2002;15:217-8.

59. Eunice Kennedy Shriver National Institute of Child Health and Human Development (NICHD). Studies of Growth Deficiency and Growth Hormone Treatment in Children With Osteogenesis Imperfecta Types III and IV. ClinicalTrials.gov [Internet database]. Bethesda, MD: National Library of Medicine (US). NLM Identifier NCT00001305. Available at https://clinicaltrials.gov/ct2/show/NCT00001305. Accessed May 28, 2019.

60. Delmas PD. Treatment of postmenopausal osteoporosis. Lancet 2002;359:2018-26.

61. Vahle JL, Sato, M, Long GG, et al. Skeletal changes in rats given daily subcutaneous injections of recombinant human parathyroid hormone (1-34) for 2 years and relevance to human safety. Toxicol Pathol 2002;30:312-21.

62. Gatti D, Rossini M, Viapiana O, et al. Teriparatide treatment in adult patients with osteogenesis imperfecta type I. Calcif Tissue Int 2013;93:448-52.

Section IX

Neurologic Disorders

CHAPTER 27

Seizure Disorders

Shirin Madzhidova, Pharm.D.

LEARNING OBJECTIVES

1. Compare and contrast pediatric seizure types and epilepsy syndromes.

2. Develop an appropriate treatment regimen for different seizure types.

3. Summarize the appropriate treatment approach for febrile seizures.

4. Determine applicable nonpharmacologic treatment options for different seizure types.

5. Describe common toxicities in pediatric patients on antiseizure drug therapy and how to manage these cases.

6. Discuss monitoring variables to ensure effectiveness and safety of antiseizure drug therapies.

ABBREVIATIONS IN THIS CHAPTER

ASD	Antiseizure drug
CNS	Central nervous system
CT	Computed tomography
EEG	Electroencephalographic
FDA	U.S. Food and Drug Administration
GABA	γ-Aminobutyric acid
ILAE	International League Against Epilepsy
KD	Ketogenic diet
MRI	Magnetic resonance imaging

INTRODUCTION

A *seizure* is a transient, involuntary alteration of consciousness caused by hypersynchronous electrical discharge of cortical neurons.[1] During a seizure, a cluster of neurons fires excessively quickly with abnormal electrical activity, which may be related to failure of inhibitory neurotransmitter action, overactive excitatory neurons, or a combination of both. Seizures can present as either generalized or focal, depending on the area of electrical discharge within the brain. Focal seizures generally originate on one side of the brain and may present with or without impaired awareness, whereas generalized seizures involve both sides of the brain and mostly present with impaired awareness.[2] Epilepsy is diagnosed when at least two unprovoked seizures occur more than 24 hours apart without acute provoking factors.[2] Epilepsy syndromes encompass various seizure types, each defined by certain clinical features, signs and symptoms, and neurologic

and electroencephalographic (EEG) findings. *Idiopathic epilepsies* refer to presumed genetic syndromes without structural brain abnormalities. A seizure that lasts more than 30 minutes or two or more seizures that occur without a return to consciousness in between are termed *status epilepticus* and are acute emergencies.[1]

The treatment of seizures and epilepsy are complex and vary by seizure type and syndrome. Certain syndromes do not require treatment with antiseizure drugs (ASDs), whereas others require several agents. Nonpharmacologic treatment options exist for the treatment of seizures, such as the ketogenic diet and vagus nerve stimulation. Such treatments may be beneficial in patients with refractory seizures that are unresponsive to conventional therapies. There are no ideal ASDs because most are associated with adverse effects and many patients do not fully respond to certain therapies. In general, ASDs show efficacy in children with seizures; however, these patients must be closely monitored. Pediatric-specific factors, such as variable pharmacokinetics, availability of dosage forms, and caregiver education must be considered when evaluating and selecting pharmacologic treatment plans.

EPIDEMIOLOGY

Seizures are a common neurologic condition during childhood. Because of the wide spectrum of clinical manifestations and the changing disease classification, it is often difficult to accurately diagnose epilepsy. This difficulty, in turn, poses a challenge when estimating prevalence and incidence of epilepsy and various seizure types. Based on the most current survey, 1.2% (3.4 million people) of the U.S. population reported active epilepsy in 2015. Of those individuals, 470,000 were children who were either physician-diagnosed with epilepsy, were under treatment, or had recent seizures.[1] About 4%–10% of children experience at least one seizure in the first 16 years of life, whereas the cumulative lifetime incidence of epilepsy is 3%.[3] Children in the first year of life have the highest incidence of seizures (144 per 100,000 person-years), which decreases as the child ages (58 per 100,000 at age 10 years).[4] The annual incidence of status epilepticus in children is 18–23 per 100,000, and this disease is most common in children younger than 5 years.[5]

ETIOLOGY

PATHOPHYSIOLOGY

A seizure results from abnormal excessive or synchronous neuronal activity in the brain. Etiology of seizures varies widely because any disruption of the normal homeostasis or stability of neurons can trigger seizures.[6] The causes of seizures and epilepsy are broad and can be categorized as either structural, metabolic, genetic, infectious, immune, or *unknown in origin*. Seizures are classified into four large categories by the International League Against Epilepsy (ILAE) based on clinical and EEG findings: *focal* (formerly known as *partial*), *generalized*, *unknown*, and *unclassified*.[2] Focal seizures may be precipitated by several mechanisms, such as decreased inhibition (defective inhibition of γ-aminobutyric acid [GABA]); defective activation of GABA neurons; alterations in the properties and number of ion channels; or alterations in glutamate-activated channels (*N*-methyl-D-aspartate).[2,7] Generalized seizures mainly arise because of defective T-type calcium channels and hyperpolarization-activated cation channels, which are involved in thalamocortical activity regulation.[7,8]

During a seizure, early systemic changes include tachycardia, hypertension, hyperglycemia, and hypoxemia because of the increased production of carbon dioxide and lactic acid. Cerebral blood flow as well as glucose and oxygen consumption also increases. Although brief seizures rarely cause long-term effects, prolonged seizures can lead to lactic acidosis, rhabdomyolysis, hyperkalemia, hyperthermia, and hypoglycemia, all of which may precipitate neurologic damage.[9]

Many conditions are associated with seizures, and patients with developmental delay, cerebral palsy, head injury, or strokes are at an increased risk for seizures and epilepsy.[10] Some causes of seizures can affect children of any age, and other causes are more likely in certain age groups. In neonates, most seizures can be attributed to symptomatic etiology such as neonatal encephalopathy, intraventricular hemorrhage, a metabolic disturbance, or a central nervous system (CNS) or systemic infection, whereas in older infants and young children febrile seizures are a common cause. Many genetic epilepsies also tend to present during a narrow age range, with most occurring in infancy.[2]

GENETIC BASIS

The role of genetics in seizures and epilepsy have long been contemplated and studied. It is now estimated that genetic factors account for about 40% of the etiologic causes of seizures and epilepsy.[11] A genetic etiology is defined when epilepsy is the direct result of a known or presumed genetic defect and seizures are the core symptom of the disorder. Genetic etiology is primarily based on family and twin studies, whereas only a few patients have a known genetic mutation.[2] Electroclinical syndromes of the genetic generalized epilepsies (previously referred to as *idiopathic generalized epilepsies*) are included in the genetic category and encompass childhood absence epilepsy, juvenile absence epilepsy, juvenile myoclonic epilepsy, and epilepsy with tonic–clonic seizures alone.[2] Other genetic causes, such as Dravet syndrome, are often associated with intellectual disability and poor prognosis for seizure control. A child with a family history of seizures, or those who experience febrile seizures in infancy, may be at greater risk of developing seizures later in life especially in combination with other factors such as trauma or medications that lower the seizure threshold. A *seizure threshold* is defined as a minimum charge required to induce a seizure and is maintained in a balance with inhibitory and excitatory neurotransmitters. Some medications (e.g., opioid analgesics,

stimulants, certain antibiotics) may lower a seizure threshold and thus increase the potential of seizure occurrence in those genetically predisposed.[10]

CLINICAL PRESENTATION AND DIAGNOSIS

SIGNS AND SYMPTOMS

The clinical presentation of various seizure types can differ. In general, during a seizure, extremities may physically convulse, go limp, or stiffen. One extremity or all may be involved in the seizure. The observed symptoms are classified as either *motor onset* or *nonmotor onset*, based on the observer's description. Usually a health care provider will not have witnessed the seizure, and therefore must rely on someone else's description of the event. Specific signs and symptoms of a seizure depend on the type of seizure. Preceding a focal seizure, a child may experience face or extremity twitching, an illusion of a bad smell or taste, and a déjà vu experience, which can be considered as an aura. Others may experience a feeling of fear or epigastric pain and discomfort during an aura; however, children may have difficulty describing this experience.[12] During a seizure, a child may be aware of self and the environment or may experience impaired awareness, which may or may not present with loss of consciousness. After a seizure, a period of fatigue, confusion, or irritability occurs.[13] This state is defined as the *postictal period*. The presence of cyanosis, vocalizations, loss of sphincter tone, and posture of the patient should be noted when describing the seizure.[12] The characteristics for individual seizure disorders are described in more detail later in text.

SEIZURE TYPES

Recently ILAE revised its classification of seizures into four major types: *focal*, *generalized*, *unknown*, and *status epilepticus*.[2] The goal of the revision was to provide health care professionals with a more rational definition of seizure types based on the presenting symptoms. Definitions and characteristics of these seizure types are provided in Figure 1. Focal seizures are characterized into the categories of *aware* and *impaired awareness*, based on the level of awareness during the occurrence. *Awareness* is defined as the knowledge of self and the environment, whereas *impaired awareness* is not synonymous with loss of consciousness. Focal seizures are further subdivided into *motor onset* (e.g., atonic) or *nonmotor onset* (e.g., absence) seizures.[2] In generalized onset seizures, the abnormal electrical activity, based on EEG findings, originates simultaneously on both sides of the brain and mostly presents with impaired awareness. Generalized seizures are also subdivided into motor onset (e.g., tonic–clonic) and nonmotor onset (e.g., absence) seizures based on the clinical presentation. A focal seizure may later spread to both hemispheres of the brain and is termed *focal to bilateral tonic–clonic seizure*, which replaces the previous term *secondarily generalized tonic–clonic seizure*. In cases in which the onset of seizures is unknown, the seizure is classified in *unknown* category, whereas a seizure that cannot be classified into a particular subtype is termed *unclassified*.[2]

The most common childhood seizure type is generalized tonic–clonic.[9] In children experiencing their first unprovoked seizure, focal to bilateral tonic–clonic seizure occurs in 30%, whereas status epilepticus is the presenting seizure in 10% to 12%.[14] The ILAE has identified more than 20 epilepsy syndromes in its classification, and some of the more commonly seen syndromes will be presented in this chapter.

TYPICAL CHILDHOOD EPILEPSY SYNDROMES

Febrile seizures are a common seizure type in children and are classified as a *special syndrome*.[15,16] Studies show that about 4% of children will have at least one febrile seizure by age 7 years. The prevalence of febrile seizures differs among ethnicities in the United States, with African American children occurring at 4.2% versus 3.5% in white children. *Febrile seizures* are defined as a seizure that is accompanied by a temperature of 100.4°F (38°C) or greater in children between ages 6 months and 5 years, with the peak onset at age 14–18 months.[13,17] Independent risk factors for a first febrile seizure occurrence include the following: a first- or second-degree relative with febrile seizures; delayed neonatal discharge of more than 28 days of age; parental report of slow development; and day care attendance.[18] Febrile seizures mostly occur at or above a measured temperature of 100.4°F (38°C), and in some cases can occur when the temperature is between 100.4°F (38°C) and 102.2°F (39°C). Often seizures occur as the temperature is rapidly increasing; however, it is the degree of fever—not the rate of increasing temperature—that is the precipitating factor. The specific mechanism for a febrile seizure is unknown, but it is hypothesized that fever lowers the seizure threshold. For the diagnosis of a febrile seizure, a CNS infection should be ruled out.[17]

Febrile seizures are characterized as *simple* or *complex*. *Simple febrile seizures* are primary generalized seizures that last less than 15 minutes and do not recur within 24 hours.[17] *Complex febrile seizures* are focal, last 15 minutes or longer, and/or recur within 24 hours. Most febrile seizures are benign and self-limited, and 80% are classified as simple. No long-term effects from simple febrile seizures have been identified.[9,17] Children without risk factors are not at a higher risk of developing epilepsy by age 7 years than the general population.[17] Those with risk factors such as many simple febrile seizures, first onset of febrile seizures that occurred at younger than 12 months, and family history of epilepsy are at a 2.4% risk of receiving a diagnosis of generalized afebrile epilepsy by age 25 years.

Neonatal seizures occur in 1.8–3.5 of every 1000 newborns because of the immaturity of the neonatal brain.[13] Most acute and symptomatic neonatal seizures occur as a consequence of a specific identifiable cause, such as the following: neonatal encephalopathy, hypoxic–ischemic encephalopathy, acquired structural brain lesions, metabolic disturbances, and CNS or systemic infections. Signs and symptoms are usually atypical and include eye deviations, lip smacking, or apneic episodes. The mortality and morbidity rate is high among these patients, depending on the underlying cause of the seizures. Neurologic impairment, developmental delay, and epilepsy are common among those children who survive.[19] In addition, neonatal epilepsy syndromes are rare in occurrence, but have distinct characteristics. A *benign familial neonatal seizure* is a syndrome that usually presents within the first 3 days of life and resolves spontaneously by age 6 months. *Fifth-day fits* are known as benign idiopathic neonatal convulsions that appear at day 5 of life and end by day 15 of life.

Infantile spasms is a rare type of epilepsy that usually occurs during the first year of life.[19] They are quick symmetrical contractions of the neck, trunk, and extremities that occur in clusters for less than 5 seconds.[15] Abduction or adduction of the upper extremities can be seen with flexion or extension of the neck, and these clusters may be repeated several times a day.[19] *West syndrome* is a disorder with three specific characteristics: infantile spasms (flexor, extensor, or mixed spasms); a particular EEG pattern (hypsarrhythmia); and developmental arrest or delay.[15] In around 70% of children, developmental delay is seen before

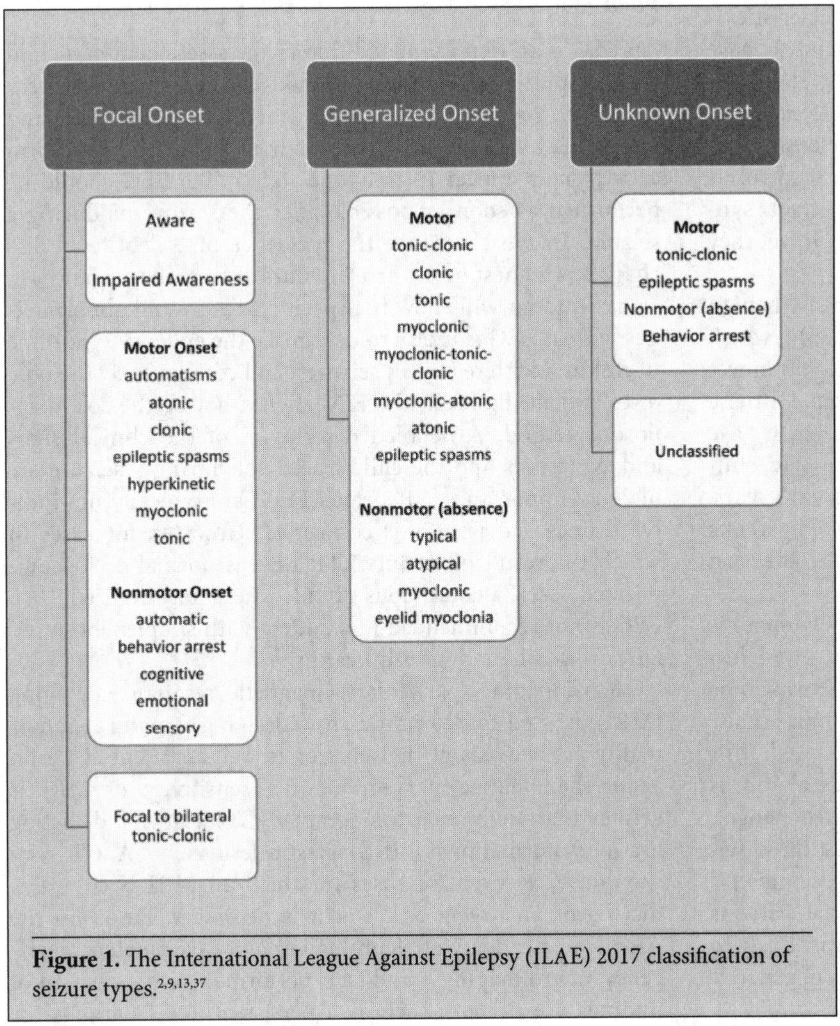

Figure 1. The International League Against Epilepsy (ILAE) 2017 classification of seizure types.[2,9,13,37]

the onset of spasms.[19] Diagnosis usually occurs between age 4 and 18 months, with a peak age of 4–7 months.[9] Male children are affected more than female children, and most patients (95%) have developmental delay. Tuberous sclerosis is seen in 25% of children with infantile spasms, and other causes may include history of hypoxic ischemic encephalopathy and other forms of cerebral insults.[13] Most children with normal development have a good prognosis of becoming seizure free; however, most children with identifiable etiology will have motor and cognitive delay.

Absence seizures is one of the most common childhood benign seizure disorders and accounts for 10% of all childhood seizures.[20] This seizure type generally occurs between age 4 and 10 years and is characterized by sudden pauses in behavior, eye flicker, and staring lasting between 10 and 20 seconds, several times per day.[20] Juvenile onset of absence seizures is less common than childhood onset absence that occurs around puberty. Absence seizures typically do not present with preceding aura, and they end abruptly without a postictal phase. Whereas typical absence seizures resolve over time by age 10–20 years, juvenile onset seizures usually persist to adulthood.[21] Atypical absence seizures occur in children who are developmentally or neurologically atypical.

Lennox-Gastaut syndrome is characterized by a mixture of intractable seizures such as tonic, myoclonic, atonic, and absence, and this syndrome accounts for 2.9% of all epilepsies.[9,13,19] Tonic seizures generally occur during sleep, and absence seizures often are atypical in characteristics.[19] Children with Lennox-Gastaut syndrome also tend to have developmental delay and severe behavioral issues. The onset is usually between age 3 and 10 years, with a peak incidence at 3–5 years.[19] Around 40% of patients have previously been given a diagnosis of infantile spasms. Seizure control is extremely difficult in patients with Lennox-Gastaut syndrome. Most of these patients will take several ASDs, yet they will still experience seizures.

Another syndrome is *benign rolandic epilepsy* (benign childhood epilepsy with centrotemporal spikes), which manifests typically as seizures while sleeping. Clonic movements in the face usually wake the child from sleep. Of these patients 20% have only one seizure, whereas 25% have repeated clusters.[13] This syndrome typically occurs in children age 3–13 years with peak age of onset at age 9–10 years, and it is generally benign, as the name states. Most patients outgrow the seizures by young adulthood with little effect on adult life.[13]

Juvenile myoclonic epilepsy (also termed *Janz syndrome*) is a chronic epilepsy syndrome that usually occurs in adolescents age 12–18 years and presents as brief bilateral myoclonic jerks on waking.[9] Most patients (80%) also have tonic–clonic seizures, and some have absence seizures (25%) as well. This type of epilepsy has no preceding aura but may have a prodromal period of early morning myoclonus. Hormonal changes, stress, alcohol, and sleep deprivation can provoke these seizures. Although, most patients with juvenile myoclonic epilepsy are developmentally and neurologically typical, patients may require lifelong treatment because they are least likely to outgrow their epilepsy compared with other types of generalized epilepsies.[22]

DIAGNOSTIC CRITERIA

LABORATORY DATA

Currently there are no diagnostic laboratory tests for epilepsy. Routine laboratory studies usually are not indicated unless they are performed to rule out treatable causes of seizures, such as metabolic and infectious causes. Serum electrolytes (particularly sodium), glucose, blood urea nitrogen, calcium, and phosphorus tests should be performed in children with the suspicion that one of these values may be abnormal. Blood cultures and complete blood count are not routinely necessary in children with febrile seizures because the incidence of bacteremia is similar to patients with fever alone; however, these tests may be useful if meningitis is suspected.[23] In some cases, particularly after generalized tonic–clonic or complex partial seizures, serum prolactin concentrations may be transiently elevated. Prolactin is thought to be released from the pituitary, which is controlled by the hypothalamus. It is theorized that a seizure can alter the hypothalamus relation.[24] It is best to obtain the prolactin concentration 10–20 minutes after a seizure. An elevated prolactin may help differentiate psychogenic nonepileptic seizures from epileptic seizures in adolescents. Serum prolactin use has not been determined for other types of seizures such as status epilepticus, repetitive seizures, or neonatal seizures.

PROCEDURES

An EEG is an important addition to the assessment of a child with suspected seizures and should be performed for every child with recurrent seizures. In general, both an awake and asleep EEG should always be obtained because epileptiform activity may appear in only one state.[25] The EEG should be performed as soon as possible after the seizure or during a seizure. In most patients, the incidence of epileptiform discharges is highest in the first 24 hours after a seizure; however, some children will show nonspecific background abnormalities.[25,26] An EEG is useful to determine the epilepsy syndrome in children with recurrent seizures, and consequently the type of treatment; however, the EEG should not be the sole diagnostic method. A detailed description of the clinical signs and symptoms and the child's behavior during a seizure are of equal importance.[25] Repeated EEGs are typically not indicated once a diagnosis is confirmed. However, for cases in which the result of an interictal EEG is normal or in complicated cases, a continuous or video EEG may be tried.[13] An EEG is not recommended in a patient with simple febrile seizures who is neurologically healthy.[27]

Neuroimaging, particularly magnetic resonance imaging (MRI), is used to determine an underlying structural abnormality as the basis of the seizures as well as the need for an acute therapeutic intervention. The sensitivity of MRI is greater than computed tomography (CT) scan for detecting brain malformations and dysplastic lesions.[26,28] A CT scan should be reserved for cases in which an MRI is contraindicated or an urgent assessment is necessary. Based on the American Academy of Neurology practice parameters, emergency neuroimaging should be performed only when focal findings are present, such as a persistent Todd paralysis or if the patient does not return to baseline. An MRI should be considered in a patient with cognitive or motor impairment of unknown etiology, with an atypical neurologic examination, with focal seizures, with EEG features that rule out genetic etiology, and in children younger than 1 year.[29]

COURSE AND PROGNOSIS OF DISEASE

Regarding the risk of seizure recurrence, a child who is neurologically normal and has an unprovoked seizure with no evidence of acute cause has a 24% risk of having another seizure in the next year and a 45% risk over the next 14 years. Clinical factors, such as previous neurologic insult and atypical MRI or EEG findings, are associated with an increased risk of recurrent seizures.[30,31] Initiating therapy with an ASD after the first or second unprovoked seizure reduces the risk of recurrence by 35% at 1 to 2 years after a seizure.[32] In a child presenting with status epilepticus as the first seizure, the recurrence rate is similar to those presenting with a brief first seizure. However, if the child experiences a subsequent seizure, the risk of the seizure being prolonged is increased. Children presenting with a first-time febrile seizure have a 30%–35% chance of having another seizure during early childhood.[30,33]

The prognosis of epilepsy is difficult to predict for each child because recurrence and relapse rates differ by type of seizure or syndrome. In the case of the West and Lennox-Gastaut syndromes, patients do not have a favorable prognosis. Benign rolandic epilepsy remits without relapse, whereas absence seizures have a 12% relapse rate, and juvenile myoclonic epilepsy has an 80% rate.[19] Simple febrile seizures are usually outgrown by age 5 years. In addition, children with epilepsy may face psychiatric and other comorbidities that can impact their quality of life. Children commonly have comorbid psychiatric disorders, neurodevelopmental spectrum disorders, and chronic mental illness.[34]

The long-term risk of mortality after a single seizure is low; however, it varies in children with certain seizure types. In children with status epilepticus, the mortality rate varies between 3%–9%, and the risk increases with prolonged duration of the seizure.[35,36] Patients with infantile spasms have a 20% mortality rate, whereas neonates with status epilepticus tend to have the highest mortality and neurologic sequelae.[9]

TREATMENT

THERAPY GOALS

The desired treatment goal for children with seizures is complete elimination of the seizures with limited adverse effects and optimal quality of life. However, less than 50% of patients become seizure free, which is why most pharmacologic therapies are lifelong, and chronic adverse effects must be considered.[37] Single-drug therapy is the goal of epilepsy treatment because it is associated with better compliance, fewer adverse effects, less potential for teratogenicity, and lower associated cost. However, clinical decisions weighing the risks and benefits of ASD therapy must be evaluated on an individual basis. Discontinuation of ASDs should be considered in children with focal epilepsy once they have been seizure free for 2 years on monotherapy. In children with all other seizure types discontinuation can be considered once the patient is seizure free for 5 years on monotherapy.[16] Lowered quality of life is an important factor to consider in children with epilepsy. Presence of cognitive impairment, presence of anxiety, seizures before age 24 months, and past use of three or more ASDs, as well as difficulties with school attendance, are all independently associated with lowered quality of life. This quality-of-life concern highlights the need for comprehensive assessment and management of the condition.[38]

NONPHARMACOLOGIC THERAPY

Few nonpharmacologic therapies exist for seizures. The ketogenic diet (KD) has been widely studied for decades in patients with refractory symptomatic generalized seizures who have failed several ASD therapies. The diet is most beneficial in patients with symptomatic generalized seizures.[39] The diet consists of mainly fat and protein consumption, with very low intake of carbohydrates. Although the exact mechanism of action is not completely understood, it has been proposed that use of ketones for energy metabolism in the brain results in adaptive changes that increase energy reserves and synthesis of GABA (a major inhibitory neurotransmitter), resulting in seizure resistance.[40] The reported efficacy of the KD varies, and was proven to reduce the frequency of seizures by 50% to 70%.[41,42] The diet may also have a positive impact on behavioral and cognitive functioning in children.[43] Patients starting on the classic KD may need to be hospitalized during the initiation of the diet to monitor for hypoglycemia, dehydration, and vomiting. Some children may experience gastrointestinal disturbance and food refusal, which is a common reason for early KD discontinuation.[44] Long-term adverse effects are rare and may include weight loss, hyperlipidemia, hypoproteinemia, nephrolithiasis, renal tubular acidosis, constipation, growth retardation, and increases in hepatic and pancreatic enzymes. Alternative KDs exist, which may make adherence easier for patients. The modified Atkins diet and the low Glycemic Index Treatment may be more tolerable in children and generally do not require inpatient initiation.[42,45] All patients should be monitored routinely and will need vitamin supplementation. Patients on the KD should not be initiated on valproic acid because of the risk of hepatotoxicity, and dextrose should also not be administered intravenously or by medications to a patient on the KD because it may result in increased seizures.[9,46] Many medications, specifically pediatric liquid preparations, have a high carbohydrate content, which may compromise ketosis. Carbamazepine suspension, ethosuximide syrup, phenobarbital elixir, and valproic acid syrup contain the highest amounts of carbohydrates and should be avoided in KD patients.[47] The *Pediatric & Neonatal Dosage Handbook* traditionally provides a table of the carbohydrate amount in medications, which will assist pharmacists in providing information to the patient and caregivers.[48]

Vagus nerve stimulation therapy has received label approval from the U.S. Food and Drug Administration

(FDA) for adults and adolescents older than 12 years with refractory focal seizures. Although randomized studies in other age groups and seizure types are limited, benefits of vagus nerve stimulation therapy may extend to a broad range of seizure types.[49,50] This therapy consists of an implanted device that provides continuous retrograde stimulation to the left vagus nerve. In studies, up to 50% of patients had a decrease in seizures by 50% or greater.[37] Although vagus nerve stimulation is generally well tolerated in children, some of the commonly reported adverse effects are hoarseness, cough, dyspepsia, nausea, and pain. Serious adverse effects such as infections and nerve paralysis have also been seen.[37]

Surgical interventions are considered in children who have persistent, frequent seizures despite optimal management, and this approach may improve functional and cognitive outcomes in children. The precise location of the epileptogenic area in the brain must be known. The average time from diagnosis to surgery ranges from 12 to 15 years.[19] Temporal lobectomy is the most common surgery, with a 78% result of seizure freedom.[51] A hemispherectomy or corpus callosotomy procedure may also be considered to control seizures in certain patients. Each surgery has risks and thus each must be compared with possible benefits for the child.

Recently many case reports have emerged supporting the use of medical cannabis to treat retractable seizures. The cannabis plant includes more than 100 diverse phytocannabinoids, two of which—psychoactive Δ9- tetrahydrocannabinol and nonpsychoactive cannabidiol—have been shown to reduce seizures and reduce mortality in animal models.[52] However, clinical data supporting its efficacy in humans are limited. A recent, open-label, interventional trial investigated the use of oral cannabidiol in patients age 1–30 years with severe, intractable, childhood-onset, treatment-resistant epilepsy, who were receiving stable doses of ASDs before study entry. The researchers reported a reduction in motor seizures at a rate similar to ASDs (median 36.5%), and 2% of patients became seizure free. Only 3% of studied patients dropped out because of adverse events.[53] A double-blind, placebo-control trial had also been recently conducted in patients age 2–55 years for atonic (or "drop") seizures in patients with treatment-resistant Lennox-Gastaut syndrome.[53] Authors reported a decrease in drop seizure frequency by 43.9% in the treatment group versus 21.8% in the placebo group, and determined cannabidiol to be an efficacious add-on treatment option. In June 2018 the FDA approved cannabidiol for the treatment of seizures associated with Lennox-Gastaut syndrome and Dravet syndrome in patients age 2 years and older. With this label approval, cannabidiol (Epidiolex, Greenwich Biosciences, Carlsbad, CA) is administered at the initial dose of 2.5 mg/kg twice daily by mouth and can be increased after 1 week, if needed, up to a maximum of 20 mg/kg/day.[54] The most common reported adverse reactions with cannabidiol are somnolence, decreased appetite, diarrhea, fatigue, sleep problems, infections, and transaminase elevations. Serum transaminases (both alanine aminotransferase and aspartate aminotransferase) and total bilirubin concentrations should be monitored closely, especially when given with other medications that affect the liver.

PHARMACOLOGIC THERAPY

The optimal choice of ASD highly depends on the particular type of seizure and the epilepsy syndrome identified on initial work-up. Some epilepsy syndromes have sufficient data to support the use of a certain ASD, such as ethosuximide or valproate for childhood absence epilepsy or valproate for juvenile myoclonic epilepsy. Other seizure types do not have clear differences in efficacy among ASDs, however, and thus require selection based on various drug-related factors, such as dosing intervals, drug interactions, and cost.[55] Furthermore, certain ASDs may aggravate seizures, such as the use of narrow-spectrum agents (e.g., carbamazepine and phenytoin) in patients with generalized epilepsy syndromes, and should therefore be avoided.[56]

Acute symptomatic seizures in children are caused by an acute illness (e.g., acute trauma, acute infection) and are usually managed by correcting the underlying etiology. Seizures caused early by head trauma seldom require medications.[19] However, phenytoin, carbamazepine, or levetiracetam may be used prophylactically until acute neurologic signs have resolved to prevent early seizures. Seizures with metabolic causes such as hypoglycemia, hyponatremia, or hypocalcemia are treated by correcting the underlying etiology. A first *unprovoked seizure*—defined as unknown in etiology and without acute illness—in a child is generally not treated because of a low risk of seizure recurrence. The ILAE consensus statement advised that it is best to "wait and see" with close follow-up in a child with a first unprovoked seizure until a recurrence pattern has been established.[57] A child presenting with a second unprovoked seizure will most likely require ASD therapy to prevent seizure recurrence, which is epilepsy.

Pharmacologic treatment is typically indicated in patients with epilepsy. Monotherapy is preferred for patients, but combination therapy may be required for seizure control. Several trials of monotherapy with different ASDs may be evaluated for efficacy before using combinations. After therapy is initiated, patients can be categorized into two groups: treatment-responsive or treatment-resistant.[58] After the first or second medication is administered, two-thirds of patients will become seizure free. Unfortunately, 20% to 30% of patients will have uncontrolled or intractable seizures despite therapy, or they will experience significant adverse effects from the ASDs.[58] In patients who experience breakthrough (unprovoked) seizures despite receiving moderate doses on an ASD, it is advised to increase the dose gradually until either seizure control is achieved or unacceptable adverse effects develop. If adverse effects occur before seizure control is reached, the child will require either an alternative ASD or an additional ASD. Selection of the second agent will depend on the same criteria used to select the first agent and on any potential interactions between the two drug groups.

In general the second agent selected will have a different and complementary mechanism of action to the first.[59] All ASDs must be initiated at low dosages and titrated slowly to a therapeutic dose. Fast titration or starting at higher dosages than recommended may cause increased adverse effects in the patient. Table 1 lists ASDs with characteristics focused on pediatrics.

Table 1. Characteristics of Antiseizure Drugs for Pediatric Patients[16,19,47,90,100]

Generic (Trade Name)	Molecular Target	Dosing and Therapeutic Levels by Patient Age, Weight, Regimen	Formulations	Adverse Effects[a]	CYP Drug Interactions	Monitoring
Carbamazepine (Tegretol, Tegretol-XR, Carbatrol, Epitol)[b]	Sodium channel	**< 6 yr:** Initial: 10–20 mg/kg/day BID–TID (suspension: QID) Max: 35 mg/kg/day **6–12 yr:** Initial: 100 mg BID (suspension: 50 mg QID); ↑ by 100 mg/day weekly Maintenance: 400–800 mg/day Max: 1000 mg/day **> 12 yr:** Initial: 200 mg BID (suspension: 100 mg QID), ↑ by 200 mg/day weekly Maintenance: 800–1200 mg/day Max 12–15 yr: 1000 mg/day Max > 15 yr: 1200 mg/day Adjust dose in renal impairment; use with caution in hepatic impairment	ER capsule, suspension, tablet, chewable tablet, ER tablet, extemporaneous suspension	Boxed warnings: aplastic anemia, agranulocytosis, dermatologic reactions (SJS, TEN), use in Asian patients with genotype: *HLA-B*1502* allele Accommodation disorders (blurred vision, diplopia, ataxia, and nausea), SIADH	Major 3A4 and minor 2C8 substrate Strong 1A2, 2B6, 2C8, 2C9, 2C19, 3A4 inducer, P-glycoprotein	Therapeutic levels: 4–12 mcg/mL CBC after 1st mo; repeat every 3–4 wk if WBC is significantly decreased
Clobazam (Onfi)[c]	GABA_A receptor	**< 2 yr:** 0.5–1 mg/kg/day **> 2 yr:** ≤ 30 kg: Initial: 5 mg, ↑ to 10 mg at day 7, ↑ to 20 mg at day 14 > 30 kg: Initial: 10 mg, ↑ to 20 mg at day 7, ↑ to 40 mg at day 14 Divide doses > 30 mg; adjust dose in renal impairment; contraindicated in severe hepatic impairment	Tablet	Rare: somnolence, sedation, drooling, constipation, cough, urinary tract infection, aggression, insomnia, dysarthria, fatigue, SJS, and TEN	Major 2C19 and 3A4 substrate	Respiratory and mental status during initiation
Diazepam (Diastat AcuDial, Diastat Pediatric, Diazepam Intensol, Valium)	GABA_A receptor	**> 30 days–< 5 yr:** 0.2–0.5 mg slow IV every 2–5 min up to max total dose of 5 mg (may be repeated in 2–4 hr for SE) **≥ 5 yr:** 1 mg slow IV every 2–5 min up to a maximum of 10 mg (repeat in 2 –4 hr if needed for SE) Rectal gel formulation: **2–5 yr:** 0.5 mg/kg **6–11 yr:** 0.3 mg/kg **≥ 12 yr:** 0.2 mg/kg	Oral concentrate, solution and tablet; rectal gel; injection; IM auto-injector	Hypotension, skin rash, abdominal pain, neutropenia, injection site reactions, paradoxical reactions (hyperactivity)	Major 3A4 and 2C19 substrate Minor 1A2, 2B6 and 2C9 substrate	Vital signs

(continued)

Table 1. Characteristics of Antiseizure Drugs for Pediatric Patients[16,19,47,90,100] *(continued)*

Generic (Trade Name)	Molecular Target	Dosing and Therapeutic Levels by Patient Age, Weight, Regimen	Formulations	Adverse Effects[a]	CYP Drug Interactions	Monitoring
Eslicarbazepine (Aptiom)[d]	Voltage-gated sodium channels	**≥ 4 yr–≤ 17 yr:** Initial: 200–300 mg once daily based on specific weight Maintenance: 400–1200 mg once daily based on specific weight Max: 600–1200 mg/day based on weight Reduce dose by 50% if CrCL < 50 mL/min; use not recommended in severe hepatic impairment	Tablet	Drowsiness, headache, nausea, blurred vision and other vision changes, ataxia, tremor, constipation; rarely SJS	Moderate CYP2C19 inhibitor Weak 3A4 inducer	Baseline liver enzymes, vision changes Serum sodium and chloride if necessary
Ethosuximide (Zarontin)[e]	Sodium and calcium channels	**< 6 yr:** Initial: 15 mg/kg/day divided BID, ↑ every 4–7 days Maintenance: 15–40 mg/kg/day Max: 1.5 g/day **≥ 6 yr:** 250 mg BID, ↑ by 250 mg/day every 4–7 days Maintenance: 20–40 mg/kg/day Max: 15 g/day Use with caution in renal and hepatic impairment	Capsule, solution, syrup	Nausea, headache, drowsiness, sleep disturbance, hyperactivity Rare: SJS, DRESS, systemic lupus erythematosus, and blood dyscrasias	Major 3A4 substrate	Therapeutic: 40–100 mcg/mL Toxic: > 150 mcg/mL Baseline CBC and platelets Periodic liver enzymes and urinalysis
Felbamate (Felbatol)[f]	Sodium channel, GABA_A, and NMDA receptors	**2–14 yr w/LGS:** 15 mg/kg/day divided TID–QID, ↑ by 15 mg/kg/day weekly Max: 45 mg/kg/day or 3600 mg/day **≥ 14 yr:** Adjunct and conversion to monotherapy: 1200 mg/day divided TID–QID, ↑ by 1200 mg/day weekly Max: 3600 mg/day; Monotherapy: ↑ by 600 mg/day every 2 wk Adjust dose in renal impairment	Suspension, tablet	Boxed warnings: aplastic anemia, acute hepatic failure Somnolence, insomnia, vomiting, weight loss (usually first 3 mo of treatment), nausea, gait abnormality	Minor 2E1 and major 3A4 substrate Weak 2C19 inhibitor Weak 3A4 inducer	Baseline and periodically during treatment: CBC, platelet count and liver function tests (including bilirubin)
Gabapentin (Neurontin)[e]	Calcium channel	**3–12 yr:** Initial: 10–15 mg/kg/day divided TID Maintenance: 3–4 yr: 40 mg/kg/day; 5–12 yr: 25–35 mg/kg/day **> 12 yr:** Initial: 300 mg TID Maintenance: 900–1800 mg/day Max: 3600 mg/day Adjust dose in renal impairment	Capsule, solution, tablet	Somnolence, fatigue, emotional lability, behavior changes, hostility, hyperkinesia, dizziness, fever	Not cytochrome-dependent	Renal function and weight if necessary

Drug	Mechanism	Dosing	Formulations	Adverse effects	Drug interactions	Monitoring
Lacosamide (Vimpat)[g]	Sodium channel	**≥ 17 yr:** Initial: 50 mg BID, ↑ by 100 mg/day weekly Maintenance: 200–400 mg/day Adjust dose in hepatic and renal impairment	Injection, solution, tablet	Prolonged PR interval, dizziness, headache, diplopia (adult data)	Carbamazepine, phenobarbital, and phenytoin may ↓ lacosamide levels	ECG before therapy in cardiac disease Hepatic and renal function if necessary
Lamotrigine (Lamictal, Lamictal ODT, Lamictal XR)[h]	Sodium and calcium channels, inhibits glutamate release	**2–12 yr:** IR: Initial: 0.3 mg/kg/day divided 1–2 doses for wk 1–2; ↑ to 0.6 mg/kg/day divided BID for wk 3–4; ↑ as needed by 0.6 mg/kg/day every 1–2 wk Maintenance: 4.5–7.5 mg/kg/day divided BID Max: 300 mg/day divided BID **Valproic acid–containing regimens:** 0.15 mg/kg/day divided 1–2 doses for wk 1–2; ↑ to 0.3 mg/kg/day divided BID for wk 3–4; ↑ as needed by 0.3 mg/kg/day every 1–2 wk Maintenance: 1–5 mg/kg/day divided BID Max: 200 mg/day divided 1–2 doses; > 6.7 kg–< 14 kg, initial dosing is 2 mg QOD in wk 1–2; then 2 mg/day for wk 3–4 **Enzyme-inducing regimens, without valproic acid:** Initial: 0.6 mg/kg/day divided BID for wk 1–2; ↑ to 1.2 mg/kg/day divided BID for wk 3–4; ↑ as needed by 1.2 mg/kg/day every 1–2 wk Maintenance: 5–15 mg/kg/day divided BID Max: 400 mg/day divided BID **>12 yr:** IR: Initial: 25 mg/day for wk 1–2; ↑ to 50 mg/day for wk 3–4; ↑ as needed by 50 mg/day every 1–2 wk Maintenance: 225–375 mg/day divided BID	Tablet, chewable/dispersible tablet, ER tablet, ODT, extemporaneous suspension	Boxed warning: rash (more common in pediatric population, 0.8%; usually occurs within 8 wk of initiation and resolves after withdrawal; more common with concomitant valproate) Drowsiness, diplopia, dizziness, headache, insomnia, tiredness, fever (with rash as part of hypersensitivity syndrome), agitation, confusion, hallucinations, myoclonus	Carbamazepine and phenytoin may ↑ lamotrigine metabolism Phenobarbital may ↓ lamotrigine levels Valproic acid may ↑ lamotrigine levels	CBC with differential, liver and renal function tests for all patients Rashes; worsening of depressive symptoms or suicidality

(continued)

Table 1. Characteristics of Antiseizure Drugs for Pediatric Patients[16,19,47,90,100] *(continued)*

Generic (Trade Name)	Molecular Target	Dosing and Therapeutic Levels by Patient Age, Weight, Regimen	Formulations	Adverse Effects[a]	CYP Drug Interactions	Monitoring
Lamotrigine *(continued)*		**Valproic acid–containing regimens:** 25 mg QOD for wk 1–2; ↑ to 25 mg/day for wk 3–4; ↑ as needed by 25–50 mg/day every 1–2 wk Maintenance: 100–400 mg/day divided in 1–2 doses Maintenance dose: 100–200 mg/day for patients with lamotrigine and valproic acid alone **Enzyme-inducing regimens, without valproic acid:** Initial: 50 mg/day for wk 1–2; ↑ to 100 mg/day divided BID for wk 3–4; ↑ as needed by 100 mg/day every 1–2 wk Maintenance: 300–500 mg/day divided BID; doses up to 700 mg/day have been used Converting to ER formulation: Daily dose of IR should total the initial daily dose of ER Adjust dose in renal and hepatic impairment				
Levetiracetam (Keppra, Keppra XR)[g]	Calcium channel	**4–15 yr:** Initial: 10 mg/kg/dose BID, ↑ by 10 mg/kg/dose every 2 wk Max: 30 mg/kg/dose BID Clinically, doses > 80 mg/kg/day are used **≥ 16 yr (PO/IV):** IR: 500 mg BID, ↑ by 500 mg/dose every 2 wk Max: 1500 mg BID ER: 1000 mg once daily, ↑ by 1000 mg/day every 2 wk Max: 3000 mg/day IV daily dose = PO daily dose Adjust dose in renal impairment	Injection, solution, tablet, ER tablet	Most common: behavior/ personality changes, irritability, hostility, nervousness, accidental injury, asthenia; others: psychotic symptoms, insomnia, emotional lability, ataxia, tremor, headache, nausea	Not cytochrome-dependent	CBC, renal function, psychiatric/behavioral signs/symptoms Diastolic blood pressure in patients < 4 yr

Drug	Mechanism	Dosing	Formulation	Adverse effects	Metabolism	Monitoring
Lorazepam (Ativan)[j]	GABA$_A$ receptor	**Infants, children, adolescents:** 0.05 mg slow IV infusion over 2–5 min (may repeat in 5–15 min if needed for SE) Max: 4 mg/dose **Children > 12 yr and concomitant valproic acid:** reduce lorazepam dose by 50% Not recommended in severe renal impairment	Oral concentrate and tablet; injection	Hypotension, skin rash, SIADH, blood dyscrasias, paradoxical reactions, visual disturbance, respiratory depression	Not cytochrome-dependent	Vital signs
Midazolam (Versed)[j]	GABA$_A$ receptor	**Infants, children, adolescents:** 0.2 mg/kg IM once Max dose: 10 mg/dose Intranasal: 0.2 mg/kg once Buccal: 0.5 mg/kg once Seizures refractory to standard treatment: 0.2 mg/kg IV loading dose, followed by 0.05–2 mg/kg/hr continuous infusion (must be mechanically ventilated and monitored)	Oral syrup; injection	Boxed warning: respiratory depression and arrest; hypotension in neonates with rapid IV infusion Hypotension, seizure-like activity, nystagmus, apnea, paradoxical reactions	Major 3A4 substrate Minor 2B6 substrate	Vital signs Continuous IV infusion: continuous cardiac monitoring
Oxcarbazepine (Trileptal)[k]	Sodium and calcium channels	**2–16 yr (adjunctive):** < 20 kg: Initiate at 16–20 mg/kg/day divided BID > 20 kg: Initiate at 8–10 mg/kg/day divided BID Max: < 20 kg: 600 mg/day, 20–29 kg: 900 mg/day, 29.1–39 kg: 1200 mg/day, > 39 kg: 1800 mg/day **4–16 yr (monotherapy):** 8–10 mg/kg/day divided BID; ↑ by 5 mg/kg/day every 3rd day Maintenance: 600–2100 mg/day by weight **> 16 yr (adjunctive):** Initial: 300 mg BID, ↑ by 600 mg/day weekly Maintenance: 1200 mg/day divided BID, may ↑, most patients do not tolerate 2400 mg/day (CNS) **> 16 yr (monotherapy):** Initial: 300 mg BID; ↑ by 300 mg/day weekly Maintenance: 1200 mg/day divided BID Adjust dose in renal impairment	Suspension, tablet	More common: somnolence, dizziness, diplopia, headache, nausea, vomiting; others: rash, ataxia, confusion, cognitive changes (difficulty concentrating, speech or language issues), SIADH, and an increased risk of SJS and TEN in HLA-B positive patients	Strong 3A4 inducer Weak 2C19 inhibitor	Baseline CBC and serum sodium Periodic thyroid function tests

(continued)

Table 1. Characteristics of Antiseizure Drugs for Pediatric Patients[16,19,47,90,100] *(continued)*

Generic (Trade Name)	Molecular Target	Dosing and Therapeutic Levels by Patient Age, Weight, Regimen	Formulations	Adverse Effects[a]	CYP Drug Interactions	Monitoring
Perampanel (Fycompa)[l]	AMPA glutamate receptor antagonist	**≥ 12 yr (adjunctive)** **Without enzyme-inducing ASD:** 2 mg/day, may ↑ by 2 mg/wk up to 12 mg **With enzyme-inducing ASD:** 4 mg/day, may ↑ up to 12 mg Adjust dose in hepatic impairment	Suspension, tablet	Boxed warning: serious psychiatric and behavioral changes: aggression, hostility, homicidal ideation and threats Most common: dizziness, somnolence, vertigo, aggression, and slurred speech	Major substrate of CYP3A4 Minor substrate of CYP1A2 and CYP2B6 Alcohol may worsen psychiatric effects	Behavioral changes during initiation and titration
Phenobarbital	Calcium channel, GABA_A receptor	Maintenance: **< 1 yr:** 5–8 mg/kg/day divided in 1–2 doses **1–5 yr:** 6–8 mg/kg/day divided in 1–2 doses **5–12 yr:** 3–6 mg/kg/day divided in 1–2 doses **> 12 yr:** 1–3 mg/kg/day or 50–100 mg 2–3 times/day Adjust dose in renal and hepatic impairment	Elixir; injection, tablet, extemporaneous suspension	Concentration-related effects: 35–80 mcg/mL: slowness, ataxia, nystagmus; 65–117 mcg/mL: coma with reflexes; > 100 mcg/mL: coma without reflexes Drowsiness, lethargy, mental depression, hypotension and hyperkinesia, paradoxical responses (hyperactivity, agitation)	Minor 2C9, 2E1 Major 2C19 substrate Strong 1A2, 2A6, 2B6, 2C8, 2C9, 3A4 inducer	Therapeutic level: 15–30 mcg/mL Toxic: > 40 mcg/mL CBC with differential, liver enzymes, renal function IV: respiratory rate, heart rate, and blood pressure
Phenytoin (Dilantin, Dilantin-125, Phenytek)[e]	Sodium channel	Loading dose (IV/PO): 15–20 mg/kg/dose **Neonates:** Initial: 5 mg/kg/day divided BID; maintenance: 5–8 mg/kg/day divided BID, some patients require TID dosing **Infants/children:** 5 mg/kg/day divided in 2–3 doses Maintenance: 6 mo–3 yr: 8–10 mg/kg/day; **4–6 yr:** 7.5–9 mg/kg/day **7–9 yr:** 7–8 mg/kg/day **10–16 yr:** 6–7 mg/kg/day **> 16 yr:** 300 mg/day or 4–6 mg/kg/day in 2–3 doses Note: 92-mg base phenytoin (suspension/chewable tablet) = 100 mg of phenytoin sodium Note: Obese patients: loading dose based on adjusted body weight; maintenance dose based on ideal body weight	ER capsule, injection, suspension, chewable tablet	Boxed warning: administer IV phenytoin slowly: not to exceed 1–3 mg/kg/min in neonates, 50 mg/min in adults; hypotension and arrhythmias occur with rapid administration Concentration-related effects: > 20 mcg/mL: far lateral nystagmus; > 30 mcg/mL: 45-degree lateral gaze nystagmus, ataxia; > 40 mcg/mL: decreased mental activity; > 100 mcg/mL: death Hypersensitivity reactions and an increased risk of SJS and TEN in HLA-B positive patients Common effects: drowsiness, ataxia, slurred speech (dose related); coarsening of facial features, gingival hyperplasia, hirsutism (rare but with chronic use); anemias (usually respond to folic acid); motor twitching, dyskinesias (rare), tremor (rare), mental confusion	Major 2C9, 2C19 substrate Minor 3A4 substrate Strong 2B6, 2C8, 2C9, 2C19, 3A4 inducer	CBC with differential, liver enzymes, bone growth and vitamin D status with chronic use IV: continuous cardiac monitoring

Fosphenytoin (Cerebyx)[e]	Water soluble prodrug of phenytoin	Always prescribe/dispense in mg of phenytoin Phenytoin 1 mg = fosphenytoin 1 mg phenytoin Loading dose (IV/PO): 15–20 mg phenytoin/kg/dose **Neonates:** maintenance: 4–8 mg phenytoin/kg/day divided BID **Infants/children:** 4–8 mg/kg/day divided in 2–3 doses Maintenance: 8–10 mg phenytoin/kg/day may be necessary in some patients Note: May be substituted for phenytoin at same total daily dose; however, fosphenytoin bioavailability is 100% by IV/IM vs. phenytoin, which is ~90% and serum concentrations may be increased	Injection	Boxed warning: administer IV fosphenytoin slowly: not to exceed 2 mg PE/kg/min; hypotension and arrhythmias occur with rapid administration Hypersensitivity reactions and an increased risk of SJS and TEN in HLA-B positive patients *Purple glove syndrome* may occur with peripheral IV administration: discoloration with edema and pain of distal limb, blood dyscrasias	Major 2C9, 2C19 substrate Minor 2B6, 2C8, 2C9, 2C19, 3A4 inducer	CBC with differential, liver enzymes, platelets, and serum glucose IV: continuous cardiac monitoring
Pregabalin (Lyrica)[e]	Calcium channel	**Adult:** Initial: 150 mg/day in 2–3 doses, titrate as needed Max: 600 mg/day Adjust dose in renal impairment	Capsule	Dizziness, somnolence, ataxia, weight gain, headache, blurred vision (adult data), angioedema, peripheral edema, mild prolongation of the PR interval, rhabdomyolysis and decreased platelet count	Not cytochrome-dependent	Monitor for signs and symptoms associated with adverse effects
Rufinamide (Banzel)[l]	Sodium channel	**≥ 4 yr:** Initial: 10 mg/kg/day divided BID; ↑ by 10 mg/kg/day QOD Maintenance: 45 mg/kg/day or 3200 mg/day divided BID (whichever is lower) If taking valproic acid: initial dose: < 10 mg/kg/day **Adults:** Initial: 400–800 mg/day divided BID; ↑ by 400–800 mg/day every 2 days Max: 3200 mg/day divided BID If taking valproic acid: initial dose: < 400 mg/day Adjust dose in hepatic impairment	Tablet, suspension, extemporaneous suspension	QT-interval shortening (dose-dependent), headache, somnolence, fatigue, dizziness, vomiting	Weak 2E1 inhibitor; Weak 3A4 inducer Valproic acid may ↑ rufinamide levels Carbamazepine, phenobarbital, phenytoin, and primidone may ↓ rufinamide levels Rufinamide may ↑ phenobarbital and phenytoin levels	Baseline CBC Consider ECG if on concurrent medications that can shorten QT interval

(continued)

Table 1. Characteristics of Antiseizure Drugs for Pediatric Patients[16,19,47,90,100] *(continued)*

Generic (Trade Name)	Molecular Target	Dosing and Therapeutic Levels by Patient Age, Weight, Regimen	Formulations	Adverse Effects[a]	CYP Drug Interactions	Monitoring
Tiagabine (Gabitril)[m]	GABA transporter	**12–18 yr:** **With enzyme-inducing regimens:** 4 mg/day for wk 1; 4 mg BID for wk 2; then ↑ by 4–8 mg/day; max: 32 mg/day in two to four doses **Without enzyme-inducing regimen:** lower doses are required Adjust dose in hepatic impairment	Tablet, extemporaneous suspension	Dizziness, tiredness, nervousness (nonspecific), tremor, concentration difficulties, depressed mood	Major 3A4 substrate	Liver function tests periodically
Topiramate (Topamax)[n]	Sodium channel, GABA$_A$ and glutamate receptors, weak carbonic Anhydrase inhibitor	**2–16 yr (adjunctive):** Initial: 25 mg/day or 1–3 mg/kg/day, ↑ by 1–3 mg/kg/day every 1–2 wk Max: 5–9 mg/kg/day divided BID **≥ 17 yr:** Initial: 25 mg/day or BID for 1 wk; ↑ by 25–50 mg/wk Maintenance: 100–200 mg/day Doses > 1600 mg not studied **≥ 10 yr (monotherapy):** Initial: 25 mg BID, ↑ by 50 mg/day weekly; up to 100 mg BID for wk 4; may then ↑ by 100 mg/day weekly Max: 200 mg BID Adjust dose in renal and hepatic impairment	Sprinkle capsule, tablet, extemporaneous suspension	Headache, somnolence, dizziness, paresthesia, oligohidrosis, hyperthermia, weight loss (dose-dependent), behavior problems, difficulty with memory and concentration/ attention, metabolic acidosis (chronic use may lead to decreased growth rates, nephrolithiasis, osteomalacia) Secondary acute angle-closure glaucoma or acute myopia—may present as painful red eye (rare and usually occurs within 1 mo of initiation)	Weak 2C19 inhibitor Weak 3A4 inducer	Baseline serum electrolytes, renal function Body temperature in hot weather
Valproic acid (Depacon, Depakene)[o]	GABA$_A$ and NMDA receptors	**Children and adults:** Initial: 15 mg/kg/day; ↑ by 5–10 mg/kg/day weekly to therapeutic levels, administered in 2–4 doses/day Max: 60 mg/kg/day Adjust dose in hemodialysis and hepatic impairment—see warnings Therapeutic levels; 50–100 mcg/mL, efficacy may improve with higher levels, but toxicity can also occur	Capsule, sprinkle capsule, injection, solution, syrup, delayed-release tablet, ER tablet	Boxed warning: may cause teratogenic effects (neural tube defects), hepatic failure in children (< 2 yr considerable risk), pancreatitis, dose-related thrombocytopenia Occasional: sedation and tremor; transient hair loss (may be dose related—regrowth normally begins within 6 mo); weight gain; gastric disorders (initiation of treatment); hyperactivity, aggression and behavioral deterioration (occasional); transient ↑ in liver enzymes is common, especially at therapy initiation; hyperammonemia; amenorrhea and irregular periods	Minor 2A6, 2B6, 2C9, 2C19, 2E1 substrate Weak 2C9, 2C19, 2D6, 3A4 inhibitor Weak 2A6 inducer	Liver enzymes and CBC with platelets at baseline and at frequent intervals, especially during the first 6 mo

Drug	Mechanism	Dosing	Dosage forms	Adverse effects[a]	Drug interactions	Monitoring
Vigabatrin (Sabril)[c]	GABA transaminase	Restricted access to medication per REMS program, available from SHARE program **1 mo–2 yr:** Initial: 50 mg/kg/day divided BID; ↑ by 25–50 mg/kg/day every 3 days Max: 150 mg/kg/day Adjust dose in renal impairment	Powder for solution, tablet	Boxed warning: permanent vision loss in infants, children, and adults (visual field defects) Very common: somnolence, excitation, agitation; common: nausea, aggression, irritability, depression; fever, vomiting	May ↓ phenytoin levels	Ophthalmologic examination at baseline and periodically during therapy Hemoglobin, hematocrit, and renal function if necessary
Zonisamide (Zonegran)[l]	Sodium and calcium channels, weak carbonic anhydrase inhibitor	**Infants and children:** Initial: 1–2 mg/kg/day divided BID; ↑ by 0.5–1 mg/kg/day every 2 wk Maintenance dose: 5–8 mg/kg/day Max for infantile spasms: 10–13 mg/kg/day in clinical studies **≥16 yr:** Initial: 100 mg/day; ↑ to 200 mg/day after wk 2; may ↑ by 100 mg/day every 2 wk; if no evidence of increased response, >400 mg/day in 1–2 doses Adjust dose in renal and hepatic impairment Zonisamide should not be used in patients with a sulfonamide allergy	Capsule, extemporaneous suspension	Somnolence, dizziness, oligohidrosis, hyperthermia, metabolic acidosis (chronic may lead to decreased growth rates, rash, SJS, nephrolithiasis, osteomalacia), anorexia	Major 3A4 substrate Minor 2C19 substrate	Serum bicarbonate at baseline and periodically Serum creatinine, albumin, BUN and electrolytes periodically Decreased sweating and hyperthermia in hot weather

[a]Adverse effects are pediatric focused and not all inclusive.
[b]Novartis Pharmaceuticals Corporation, East Hanover, NJ (Tegretol, Tegretol-XR); Shire US Inc., Exton, PA (Carbatrol); Teva Pharmaceuticals USA, Inc., North Wales, PA (Epitol).
[c]Lundbeck, Deerfield, IL.
[d]Sunovion Pharmaceuticals Inc., Marlborough, MA.
[e]Pfizer Inc., New York, NY.
[f]MEDA Pharmaceuticals Inc., Somerset, NJ.
[g]UCB, Inc., Smyrna, GA.
[h]GlaxoSmithKline, Research Triangle Park, NC.
[i]Baxter Healthcare Corporation, Deerfield, IL.
[j]Fresenius Kabi, Lake Zurich, IL.
[k]Novartis Pharmaceuticals Corporation, East Hanover, NJ.
[l]Eisai Inc., Woodcliff Lake, NJ.
[m]Cephalon Inc., Malvern, PA.
[n]Janssen Pharmaceuticals Inc., Raritan, NJ.
[o]AbbVie Inc., North Chicago, IL.

↓ = decrease; ↑ = increase; ASD = antiseizure drug; BID = twice daily; CNS = central nervous system; CYP = cytochrome P450; DRESS = drug reaction with eosinophilia and systemic symptoms; ECG = electrocardiogram; ER = extended release; GABA = γ-aminobutyric acid; HLA = human leukocyte antigen; IR= immediate release; IV = intravenous; max = maximum; LGS = Lennox-Gastaut syndrome; NMDA = N-methyl-D-aspartate; ODT = oral disintegrating tablet; PO = by mouth; QID = four times/day; QOD = every other day; REMS = Risk Evaluation and Mitigation Strategies; SE = status epilepticus; SHARE = Support, Help, and Resources for Epilepsy; SIADH = syndrome of inappropriate secretion of antidiuretic hormone; SJS = Stevens-Johnson syndrome; TEN = toxic epidermal necrolysis; TID = three times/day; XR = extended release.

In recent years ASDs have evolved with the addition of second- and third-generation ASDs. The first-generation ASDs are as follows: carbamazepine, phenobarbital, phenytoin, primidone, valproic acid, and ethosuximide. They share many characteristics such as complex pharmacokinetics, which require monitoring, and many drug interactions caused by hepatic induction or inhibition. The first-generation ASDs have FDA label approval for use as monotherapy for particular seizure types. The second-generation ASDs are as follows: felbamate, gabapentin, lamotrigine, topiramate, tiagabine, oxcarbazepine, levetiracetam, and zonisamide. These eight medications came on the market between 1993 and 2000 and have a more favorable drug profile because of fewer drug interactions and kinetics that do not require monitoring. The ASDs approved since 2000 are pregabalin (2004), rufinamide (2008), lacosamide (2008), vigabatrin (2009), clobazam (2011), perampanel (2012), eslicarbazepine (2012), and brivaracetam (2016). Most of these agents have FDA label approval as adjunctive therapies for epilepsy, whereas only oxcarbazepine, lamotrigine, topiramate, and felbamate are approved for use as monotherapy, with some limitations (Table 2).

The ASDs can be divided into three groups, depending on their mechanism of action: those that facilitate GABAergic neurotransmission; those that block neuronal ion channels; and those for which the mechanism of action is unknown. The compounds that act through GABAergic systems can be further divided into three pathways: those that modulate transmission through chloride channels (e.g., barbiturates and benzodiazepines); those that reduce the degradation of GABA by blocking GABA transaminase (e.g., vigabatrin); and those that inhibit the reuptake of GABA into the presynaptic terminal (e.g., tiagabine). The other group of compounds that block neuronal ion channels work by blocking voltage-operated sodium channels leading to decreased electrical activity (e.g., lamotrigine, phenytoin, or carbamazepine), and those that block voltage-operated calcium channels mediate calcium currents in thalamic neurons (e.g., ethosuximide).[60] In addition, ASDs vary by their therapeutic spectrum, with broad-spectrum agents (i.e., lamotrigine, felbamate, or valproate) used to treat both focal and generalized onset, and narrow-spectrum agents (i.e., carbamazepine, phenytoin, or oxcarbazepine) for focal-onset seizures only.

Benzodiazepines are a class of drugs that bind to GABA receptors and facilitate their attachment to its binding site on the receptor, which can rapidly control a seizure. This medication class is commonly used for status epilepticus (i.e., lorazepam, diazepam, midazolam), certain epileptic syndromes (i.e., clobazam), and as a home rescue therapy for emergency treatment of a prolonged seizure (i.e., diazepam, midazolam).[60]

Most of the ASDs are initially approved for use in adolescents and/or adults. Pediatric studies or reports from the literature will eventually emerge, with potential pediatric indications following thereafter. As of today, not all the ASDs listed have received FDA label approval for use in children, but for most medications, pediatric dosing can be located. Table 2 lists recommended medications and corresponding seizure types. Table 1 provides the pediatric dosing of ASDs,

but it does not include all seizure types and ages. Many ASDs are teratogenic; thus, patients of childbearing age must be educated on the possible fetal effects, or select medications may be avoided. Serum pregnancy tests may be obtained in these patients before initiating medication.

Controversy exists over the use of generic ASDs in patients. Bioequivalence studies are conducted comparing a single dose of the generic with the brand formulation, and not comparing generic formulations against other generics.[61] In addition, generic drugs are not required to complete bioequivalence studies in children unless the drug is targeted to this population. Most ASDs have several generic formulations available. However, the "older" ASDs have more variable pharmacokinetics and are narrow therapeutic index drugs, unlike most of the "newer" ASDs. Variability in pharmacokinetics, especially between generic formulations, may cause an alteration of clinical efficacy in the patient. Breakthrough seizures in stable patients could result in harm to themselves or others, emotional distress, or loss of driving privileges or employment in adolescents. Three case-controlled analyses using large national patient medical claims databases found that those who had a recent switch in formulation (brand-to-generic, generic-to-generic, or generic-to-brand) experienced an increase in epilepsy-related events requiring acute care.[62-64]

Cost and supply chain inconsistency also affects the decision to substitute medications. Because of these concerns and the lack of controlled, prospective data, patients should be initiated and remain on the same formulation consistently. Children who are stable on their current regimen should not have their regimen altered.

FEBRILE SEIZURES

In most cases, febrile seizures resolve spontaneously and do not require active treatment with benzodiazepines. Febrile seizures that continue for more than 5 minutes should be treated with an intravenous benzodiazepine (lorazepam 0.05–0.1 mg/kg or diazepam 0.1–0.2 mg/kg).[65] Buccal midazolam (0.2 mg/kg; maximum dose of 10 mg) is an appropriate option if an intravenous access is not available.[65] An additional dose may be given if the seizure persists, and the child's respiratory and circulatory status should be monitored carefully. Treatment with antipyretics at the time of febrile illness may ease discomfort, but it does not affect the recurrence rate of febrile seizures. Although children with febrile seizures are at an increased risk of recurrent febrile seizures and development of afebrile seizures, scheduled ASD therapy is not generally recommended because of the potential adverse effects.[17] In studies, phenobarbital, valproate, or intermittent oral or rectal diazepam were evaluated for prevention of recurrent seizures. Although the risk was reduced in the short term, adverse effects were of concern. Therefore, the guidelines currently neither recommend continuous nor intermittent ASDs in children with one or more simple febrile seizure.[17] Patients in febrile status epilepticus, with prolonged or repetitive seizures despite initial treatment with benzodiazepines, should be treated with additional ASDs such as fosphenytoin at 20 mg phenytoin equivalents/kg intravenously.

Table 2. Seizure Classifications and Medication Options by Type of Seizure[16,19,20,55,58]

Seizure Type	Characteristics of Seizure Type	Signs/Symptoms	Drug of Choice	Alternatives	Drugs That May Worsen Seizure Types
Focal Seizures					
Aware	Seizure begins locally, involves one cerebral hemisphere, and remains localized	• Aware of self and environment • Unilateral movements • Pallor, sweating, flushing, pupillary dilation • Somatosensory symptoms (aura, tingling fear)	**Newly diagnosed** Carbamazepine[b] Gabapentin[b] Lamotrigine[b] Oxcarbazepine[a,b] Phenobarbital[b] Phenytoin[b] Topiramate[b] Valproic acid[b] **Refractory Monotherapy** Lamotrigine Oxcarbazepine Topiramate **Refractory Adjunctive** Gabapentin[a] Lamotrigine[a] Levetiracetam[b] Oxcarbazepine[a] Tiagabine[b] Topiramate Zonisamide[b] Perampanel[b] Lacosamide[b] Eslicarbazepine[b]	Carbamazepine[b] Gabapentin[b] Lamotrigine Oxcarbazepine Phenobarbital[a] Phenytoin[a] Topiramate[a] Valproic acid[a]	—
Impaired Awareness	Seizure begins focally, but may involve other parts of the brain affecting alertness and awareness	• Impaired awareness of self and environment • Unilateral movements, automatisms • Aura, dreamy, distortion of time, anger/irritability			
Focal to Bilateral Tonic–Clonic	Seizure begins focally, then spreads to both hemispheres, producing bilateral seizure discharges and impairing awareness	• Impaired awareness • Aura may or may not be present • Tonic phase: rigidity of all limbs, cyanotic • Motor seizures may be asymmetric • Disoriented afterwards			
Generalized (Motor or Nonmotor) Seizures					
Tonic–Clonic	Seizure begins in both sides of the brain and presents in two phases	• First sign may be groaning and falling down with impaired awareness • Tonic phase: rigidity, teeth clenching, may stop breathing • Clonic phase: rhythmic jerks of arms/legs, pupils dilate and contract • May lose control of bowel or bladder • Usually 1 min, but can be longer • Postictally confused, somnolent	Lamotrigine Topiramate Oxcarbazepine	Carbamazepin[a] Lamotrigine Oxcarbazepine Phenobarbital[a] Phenytoin[a] Topiramate[a] Valproic acid[a]	Tiagabine Vigabatrin Carbamazepine Phenytoin
Absence	Sudden and profound impairment of consciousness without loss of body tone	• Interruption of ongoing activities • Blank stare, unresponsive • Upward eye deviation • Mild clonic or tonic movements • Can recur as many as 10–50 times/day	Lamotrigine Ethosuximide Valproate	Clobazam Clonazepam Levetiracetam Topiramate Zonisamide	Carbamazepine Gabapentin Oxcarbazepine Phenobarbital Phenytoin Tiagabine Vigabatrin
Myoclonic	Single whole-body muscle jerks that occur quickly and often happen in clusters; sometimes associated with other types or generalized seizures	• Repetitious nonrhythmic bilateral jerks • Commonly occurs in morning • Usually without an aura or postictal symptoms	Valproate Levetiracetam Topiramate	Levetiracetam Lamotrigine Topiramate Zonisamide	
Atonic	Sudden drop or loss of muscle tone affecting the head, trunk, or whole body; possible fall to the ground if standing	• Lack of muscle tone • Also called "drop attacks" • Usually < 15 sec • May occur in Lennox-Gastaut or Dravet syndrome	Lamotrigine Topiramate Valproate Felbamate[b] Clobazam		Carbamazepine

[a]Specific recommendation for children.
[b]U.S. Food and Drug Administration has approved this drug for pediatric use; the pediatric age range that has label approval varies by drug

Status epilepticus is a serious and potentially life-threatening medical emergency that requires prompt intervention. *Status epilepticus* is defined as a single seizure that lasts longer than 5 minutes or frequent seizures without return to a baseline clinical state. In an actively seizing patient, termination of the seizure and stabilization of the airway are priorities. Treatment is based on the underlying etiology, patient history, and medication history. Metabolic abnormalities should be corrected. If hypoglycemia is present, dextrose solution should be administered. Sodium and calcium concentrations should also be evaluated, and treatment should be initiated if abnormal values are confirmed. If a CNS infection is hypothesized, antibiotics are warranted. Status epilepticus is aggressively treated with medication if the seizure lasts more than 5 minutes. The ILAE guidelines recommend the use of parenteral benzodiazepines such as lorazepam, diazepam, and midazolam, which can be administered in 5-minute intervals up to two times and generally stop the seizure in 2–3 minutes.[66] In contrast to previous studies, recent guidelines by the American Society of Epilepsy have found intravenous lorazepam and diazepam to have similar efficacy in stopping seizures in children lasting at least 5 minutes.[66] Diazepam has a longer half-life, but lorazepam has a smaller volume of distribution and thus stays longer in the CNS. Diazepam and lorazepam may be administered intravenously and rectally, whereas midazolam can be administered intramuscularly, buccally, or intranasally. If prehospital care is required and intravenous access is unavailable, buccal midazolam or rectal diazepam should be used.[67]

If benzodiazepines are not effective in terminating the seizure after two doses are administered or if seizures recur after successful treatment with a benzodiazepine, then phenytoin, fosphenytoin, phenobarbital, valproate, or levetiracetam can be used as secondary agents. These agents have been shown to be advantageous in preventing recurrence of status epilepticus for extended periods of time; however, because of their delayed onset of action (10 to 30 minutes) a rapidly acting agent should be administered first. Phenytoin must be administered in a large vein to decrease the risk of extravasation. In addition, because of its vehicle (40% propylene glycol), administration-related hypotension and cardiac arrhythmias may occur. Fosphenytoin is a water-soluble prodrug of phenytoin with a lower pH. Fosphenytoin is preferred to phenytoin because of its faster administration rate and ability to be administered intramuscularly. Although fosphenytoin may be an improved agent on the basis of its characteristics, cost as well as its variable pharmacokinetics may limit its use in some health care settings. Phenobarbital is another option used to abate active seizures and has been found to be as efficacious as phenytoin.[68] Phenobarbital must be administered by a slow intravenous infusion and may require several loading doses to achieve desired concentrations. Some of the adverse effects associated with intravenous infusion include sedation and respiratory depression, especially when it is preceded by a benzodiazepine.[69] Some dosage forms of phenobarbital may contain propylene glycol, which is associated with potentially fatal toxicities when administered to neonates in large amounts.

Status epilepticus that fails to cease after two adequate doses of benzodiazepines, phenytoin/fosphenytoin, or barbiturates is deemed refractory. Refractory status epilepticus is more difficult to treat the longer it lasts. Valproate, propofol, levetiracetam, and medically induced comas with pentobarbital or midazolam have all been used for refractory status epilepticus.[70] Use of intravenous valproate and levetiracetam is increasing because of their safety profiles. Propofol should be used with caution, especially if long-term use is warranted, because of the irreversible propofol infusion syndrome seen in children (i.e., hypotension, hyperkalemia, cardiac failure, renal failure, lipidemia, rhabdomyolysis, and severe metabolic acidosis).[48,71] It is generally associated with high-dose, prolonged infusions (greater than 5 mg/kg/hour for more than 48 hours). Monitoring of electrolytes, acid/base status, organ function, and creatine phosphokinase is warranted with propofol infusions. Pentobarbital infusions were found effective in 74% to 100% of refractory status cases in one study.[72] Pentobarbital can be rapidly titrated, but prolonged infusions result in slower elimination because of accumulation in fat stores. Adverse effects such as immunosuppression (high doses) and hypotension resulting in decreased cardiac contractility requiring inotropes may be seen. Pentobarbital contains propylene glycol as a vehicle, and toxicity can result in metabolic acidosis and renal toxicity.[72] Midazolam is the preferred benzodiazepine for continuous infusion because of its short half-life, easy titration, and lack of propylene glycol, which is found in intravenous lorazepam. All patients placed into a medically induced coma should be intubated, provided respiratory support, and monitored by EEG. Hypotension, which is common, should be observed in these patients.[71] A lack of well-controlled studies with these medications limits the ability to state that one medication is superior to another.

SEIZURE SYNDROMES

Many seizure syndromes are treated with specific agents, based on efficacy studies. Description and treatment options of some of the most common syndromes are described in following text.

Infantile spasms. First-line treatment for infantile spasms includes hormonal therapy with corticotropin, ASDs with vigabatrin, and prednisone as an alternative.[73,74] Corticotropin acts by suppressing corticotropin-releasing hormone, which is an endogenous neuropeptide that may provoke convulsions in an immature brain. Corticotropin is the preferred first-line agent in most children with infantile spasms, and its dose may differ in individual patients.[75] The most recent consensus by ILAE concluded that glucocorticoids are probably effective in the short-term control of spasms, but the optimal preparation, dose, and duration are not yet established. In studies, prednisone (2 mg/kg per day orally) is generally reserved for patients who have not responded to initial therapy with corticotropin.[75] Vigabatrin is the only ASD that is considered effective as a first-line treatment for infantile spasms. It raises the concentration of GABA in the CNS by irreversibly inhibiting GABA-transaminase. The optimal dose and duration of treatment with vigabatrin for infantile spasms are unclear.

In studies, children were given either a high-dose of 100–148 mg/kg/day or a low dose of 18–36 mg/kg/day for 14–21 days, with the high-dose treatment being more effective in treating seizures.[76] Valproic acid, lamotrigine, topiramate, and zonisamide also have been used; however, further clinical trials are needed to recommend their use.[77]

Lennox-Gastaut syndrome usually requires several concomitant ASDs to reduce the number of seizure episodes. Typically, valproic acid, felbamate, topiramate, lamotrigine, clobazam, and rufinamide are options in managing these patients, whereas carbamazepine can precipitate drop attacks in some of these children and should be avoided.[78] The recommended first-line therapy in most children with childhood absence epilepsy is ethosuximide. Ethosuximide suppresses the seizure threshold and is usually started at a dose of 5–10 mg/kg/day (divided into two doses) in children younger than 6 years, and 250 mg twice daily for children 6 years and older. Children who experience a failure of response to the maximum tolerated dose of ethosuximide can be switched to valproate monotherapy, or lamotrigine in pediatric patients of childbearing age because of fetal risk.[79] Valproate and other ASDs can be an option for benign rolandic epilepsy. However, agents such as carbamazepine, phenobarbital, and lamotrigine can cause increased seizures.[80] Juvenile myoclonic epilepsy is commonly treated with valproic acid, but lamotrigine, topiramate, levetiracetam, and zonisamide are alternatives.

MONITORING OF THERAPY

THERAPEUTIC OUTCOMES

Because of the complex nature of therapeutic management of seizures, patients should be closely monitored by a neurologist. The follow-up period is individualized to the patient and the treatment modalities. The optimal therapeutic outcomes for these patients are maintaining a quality of life and possible seizure freedom.

Several factors may dictate a successful withdrawal of ASDs. Patients who are seizure-free for 2 to 4 years, or with complete seizure control within 1 year of onset, an onset of seizures after age 2 years but before age 35 years, and those with a normal neurologic examination and EEG results are all candidates for withdrawal. Children who meet these criteria have a 69% chance of successfully remaining off pharmacotherapy.[81] If patients meeting these criteria attempt to discontinue pharmacotherapy, the medications must be tapered slowly for several months.[16] Abrupt discontinuation of medications is not recommended unless the patient is experiencing a severe adverse effect. If the patient is taking more than one ASD, then each medication should be tapered gradually, one at a time. In the case of seizure recurrence, the medication should be increased to the previous effective dose and the withdrawal process should be stopped.

TOXICITY

Most ASDs cause certain toxicities and adverse effects. A few key adverse effects that affect all ASDs will be briefly discussed in this section. Table 1 lists the adverse effects of ASDs that are usually seen in the pediatric population. This list is not inclusive; thus it is critical to consult a drug information resource and literature for a complete list of adverse effects in children and adults.

The most common adverse effects shared by ASDs are those affecting the CNS, which include sedation, dizziness, blurred vision, double vision, ataxia, or difficulty concentrating. Certain agents can have adverse effects on cognition, leading to diminished attention, executive function, intelligence, language skills, memory, and processing speed. Phenobarbital and topiramate have the greatest potential for these problems, although many ASDs may also impair some aspects of cognition. Phenobarbital has also been shown to cause hyperactivity in preschool age children.[82]

Many ASDs have the potential to cause rare but serious adverse effects that may result in death. Although most hypersensitivity reactions to these agents are mild and result in maculopapular rashes, some may progress to Stevens-Johnson syndrome, toxic epidermal necrolysis, or drug reaction with eosinophilia and systemic symptoms, which could be fatal. In those patients who develop a rash, care must be taken to stop the drug and either consider an alternative agent or slow reinitiation and titration.[83] The ASDs that are highly associated with allergic hypersensitivity are phenobarbital, phenytoin, lamotrigine, zonisamide, oxcarbazepine, and carbamazepine, and these agents may also cause higher incidences of rash in children than in adults. Severe hypersensitivity reactions such as Stevens-Johnson syndrome, toxic epidermal necrolysis, or drug reaction with eosinophilia and systemic symptoms are significantly more common in patients of Asian descent with the human leukocyte antigen (HLA)-B*1502, HLA-A*3101, and HLA-A*2402 alleles.[84] Currently, the FDA label recommends screening for certain HLA alleles in patients of Asian ancestry before prescribing carbamazepine. However, screening is only available in specialized centers, which may require a turnaround time of up to 14 days and a high cost of up to $800, depending on insurance coverage.[85]

Children exposed to ASDs have a greater potential of developing adverse events that may differ from those in adults. These differences in pediatric patients result from their immature detoxification mechanisms and a greater variability in dosing pharmacokinetics because of a wider range of body weight and size. Valproate can cause acute hepatic toxicity in children younger than 2 years, whereas topiramate and zonisamide have been associated with nephrolithiasis, oligohydrosis, and metabolic acidosis, which can lead to growth.[86] Levetiracetam may cause behavioral adverse effects, such as irritability and hostility, seen soon after initiation, whereas topiramate, felbamate, and zonisamide may cause weight loss.[87,88]

Serum drug monitoring continues to be important with respect to the first-generation ASDs because specific concentrations correspond to efficacy and toxicity in patients. Therapeutic drug serum concentrations are listed in Table 1. Of note, the targeted therapeutic range may be higher than the normal range if a patient is considered resistant to therapy or placed in a drug-induced coma (phenobarbital). However, the second-generation anticonvulsants have not shown in studies that serum concentrations correspond to efficacy or adverse effects. Serum concentrations are typically not recommended to be drawn for patients taking these medications; however, they may be used to verify adherence.

The risk of major and minor congenital malformation in fetuses exposed to ASDs is increased, particularly with phenobarbital, phenytoin, valproate, and topiramate. However, in many instances the benefit of treatment outweighs the risk because seizures during pregnancy pose an increased risk of fetal mortality. Pregnancy registries are available for patients taking any ASD and should be advised by health care providers regarding their use. The FDA pregnancy ratings for ASDs have been known to change as information on fetal effects have been determined. It is recommended that childbearing women who take ASDs should also supplement with folic acid to prevent birth defects.

Increased suicidality has been linked to several ASDs in children older than 5 years, according to the 2008 FDA report.[89] The elevated risk was observed as early as 1 week after initiating the medication and this elevated risk continued through the 24 weeks of study observation. Although a direct link to a certain drug type has not been established, patients taking these medications should be regularly monitored for emergence or worsening of suicidal ideation or depression. The FDA has required all manufacturers to develop a medication guide to be provided to patients who are prescribed any of these medications.

In addition, certain boxed warnings exist for several ASDs because of potential for serious adverse events. Vigabatrin is currently only available through a restricted program under a risk evaluation and mitigation strategy (called the *Vigabatrin REMS program*) because of the risk of permanent vision loss, and this agent should only be considered for treatment when benefits clearly outweigh the risks.[90] Felbamate has a boxed warning of increased risk of aplastic anemia, and should not be used without consultation from an expert hematologist.[91]

Lastly, hepatic enzyme-inducing ASDs have been implicated for osteoporosis risk because of their effects on lowering vitamin D concentrations. Patients taking chronic ASDs that are hepatic inducers should be supplemented with vitamin D, and their vitamin D concentrations should be evaluated every 2–5 years.[58,92]

DRUG INTERACTIONS

Most clinically relevant drug interactions with ASDs occur from induction or inhibition of drug-metabolizing enzymes, particularly cytochrome P450 (CYP). Phenytoin, phenobarbital, carbamazepine, oxcarbazepine, and felbamate are strong hepatic enzyme inducers and will lower the concentrations of drugs metabolized in the liver, whereas enzyme inhibitors, such as valproate, will decrease the metabolism of the same drugs.[93] Carbamazepine can induce its own metabolism (autoinduction) by stimulating the activity of CYP3A4 component. Autoinduction completes within 3–5 weeks, which increases clearance and reduces the half-life and therapeutic concentrations of carbamazepine by as much as 50%, and thus requires higher doses to maintain steady concentrations in the blood. Lamotrigine also undergoes autoinduction, which is complete

within 2 weeks of initiation, and is associated with a 17% reduction in serum concentrations.[94]

Certain ASDs have the potential to lower the efficacy of hormonal contraceptives, and some contraceptives can lower serum concentrations of ASDs (e.g., lamotrigine). Topiramate, at doses of greater than 200 mg/day; oxcarbazepine; and rufinamide can decrease serum concentrations of ethinyl estradiol.[58] Carbamazepine, phenobarbital, and phenytoin also decrease the estrogen concentrations because of CYP drug interactions. Female patients of childbearing potential should be notified of these interactions and educated on pregnancy and teratogenicity risks.[95]

MEDICATION ADHERENCE

Medication adherence is defined as the extent to which an individual takes medications as prescribed. In the adult population, adherence to medication is very poor, especially in those with chronic conditions. Although, medication adherence among children is generally higher, partly because of the caregiver involvement, in children with chronic conditions, such as seizure disorders, adherence is a major issue. The exact rate of nonadherence among children with seizures is difficult to establish because of variability in study methods conducted. However, most studies have shown that nonadherence rates are around 58% during the first 6 months of therapy and are varied based on seizure type, medication type, and genetic factors, for example.[96] Various barriers to ASD adherence among children have also been identified. Among others, most notable barriers for patients are low socioeconomic status, age, type of seizures, type of medication, taste of medication, refusal to take ASDs, and lack of caregiver involvement.[97,98] Nonadherence to ASDs in children can increase the risk of breakthrough seizures; continued seizures 4 years after diagnosis; higher incidence of emergency department visits and hospital admissions; higher health care costs; motor-vehicle injuries; and fractures.[96,98] Pharmacists can play a crucial role in medication adherence by educating patients about their diseases, explaining adverse effects, encouraging adherence, ensuring accuracy of dosing, and alerting patients and prescribers to potential drug–drug interactions. Beyond community pharmacy, pharmacists can be involved in various health care settings, such as neurology clinics, hospitals, and emergency department, where their expertise can further impact medication adherence. In a survey of adult patients with epilepsy, pharmacists were identified as an important part of disease management, particularly in managing drug interactions, adverse effects, and medication adherence.[99] Pharmacist involvement in the care of children with seizures can significantly improve health outcomes, through medication therapy management, telephone follow-up, and patient/caregiver education to ensure understanding of the disease state and therapy.

FUTURE THERAPIES

Currently, several different therapy categories are under investigation for treatment of epilepsy. These approaches include new medication as well as enhanced drug delivery, dietary supplements, and therapeutic devices. Precision medicine is another prospective treatment of epilepsy for genetic mutations, which involves using knowledge of a patient's specific genotype and targeting specific pathogenic molecular pathways.[100]

CONCLUSIONS

Seizures and epilepsy are common pediatric disease states. Various types of seizures and etiologies exist and are the initial guidance for determining treatment options in patients. However, most patients will be prescribed an ASD. These agents should be used for treatment while balancing the risks and benefits of efficacy and adverse effects. Most patients will be successfully treated with one ASD, but some patients will be classified as treatment-resistant. In general, therapy should be initiated slowly, and monitoring is required for every patient. Febrile seizures are the most common seizure disorder in childhood and is managed based on the presenting etiology. Whereas simple febrile seizures resolve on their own, prolonged seizures may require treatment with benzodiazepines or ASDs. In contrast, convulsive status epilepticus is a serious and potentially life-threatening medical emergency that requires prompt intervention with benzodiazepines, followed by ASDs if seizures persist.

The priority in treating seizures and epilepsy is to improve the patient's quality of life. Pharmacists can play a significant role in optimizing therapy for parents and their children with epilepsy. In the hospital setting, pharmacists review medication profiles for possible drug interactions, dosage adjustments, or the need for alternative agents. Pharmacists can also advise clinicians on appropriate therapeutic drug monitoring. Parents and children should be educated on expected CNS and cognitive adverse effects, potential skin reactions, and the risk for suicidal behavior. It is also important to educate parents on the importance of medication adherence to avoid breakthrough seizures.

Patient Case   FEBRILE SEIZURES

A 2-year-old boy is brought to the pediatrician's office with a fever. His mother reported that his temperature was 38.9°C (102°F) the morning before the office visit, and she had given him acetaminophen. The fever decreased, but was elevated again to 40°C (104°F) the next day, which was again lowered with acetaminophen. The child was playful and eating well until the evening, when the fever returned and the mother observed that he had symmetric stiffening of his upper and lower extremities, abnormal eye movements she described as "rolling back," bluish discoloration around the mouth, and unresponsiveness. This event reportedly lasted for a minute, after which he appeared "drowsy" for the next 10 minutes. The parents then brought the child in to the pediatrician immediately.

Medical history: Uncomplicated caesarian delivery; breastfed for 6 months; achieved all normal milestones; no history of chronic illnesses or antibiotic use in the recent past

Family history: No history of febrile seizures in the family

Social history: Lives with both parents; attends day care

Immunizations: Up to date for age

Vital signs: Tmax 39°C (102.6°F), BP 94/57 mm Hg, HR 127 beats/minute, RR 42 breaths/minute, Wt 12.7 kg, Ht 32 inches

Physical examination: Alert and interactive; all systems normal; no occurrence of another seizure episode in the next 24 hours on observation

Laboratory findings:

Blood glucose: 120 mg/dL by fingerstick

Complete blood cell count: Normal

Electrolytes: Normal

Urine examination: Normal

Lumbar puncture: Negative for bacteremia

1. What is the most likely etiology and characterization of the child's seizure?

Febrile seizures commonly occur in children younger than 5 years and are accompanied by a temperature of 100.4°F (38°C) or greater. This patient suffered a generalized simple febrile seizure that lasted less than 15 minutes and did not recur within 24 hours. Children younger than 3 years should be evaluated for signs of bacterial meningitis and a careful history of risk factors, such as day care attendance, developmental delay, and having first- or second-degree relative with a history of febrile seizure, to identify the risk of developing generalized afebrile epilepsy.

Case (continued). The diagnosis of a central nervous system infection was excluded, and it was determined that the patient does not have additional risk factors for development of epilepsy.

2. What is the most appropriate course of treatment for this patient?

Febrile seizures resolve spontaneously without active treatment in most patients. The child should be managed with an antipyretic, such as acetaminophen, for the fever and discomfort.

3. What pharmacotherapy should the caregiver receive to administer for prevention of a febrile seizure?

The caregivers should be given rectal diazepam gel (Diastat, AcuDial, Valeant Pharmaceuticals, Bridgewater, NJ, or generic) at a dose of 6 mg (0.5 mg/kg), which can be applied rectally in case a seizure recurs and lasts longer than 5 minutes. For administration, the child should be laying on his side with the top leg bent forward. The lubricated rectal tip of the applicator should be inserted into rectum and plunger pushed gently over 3 seconds. It is best for the caregiver to hold the child's buttocks together for 3 seconds to prevent leakage while observing the child. If the child experiences recurrent seizure, he should be brought back to the pediatrician for further evaluation, at which time the need for further treatment should be assessed.

4. What patient education can be provided to the caregiver?

A child who had a febrile seizure is at risk of having another within 1 year of the initial seizure, and the next seizure may or may not occur with an onset of fever. If the parent witnesses a child having a seizure, steps should be taken to prevent the child from self-harm. The parents should be instructed to lay the child on the side of the body without attempting to stop any movement or convulsions, and to not place anything in the child's mouth. If the seizure lasts more than 5 minutes, it requires immediate treatment. While another adult is dialing 911, a parent or caregiver should administer a dose of diazepam gel, 6 mg rectally as instructed. One dose usually is adequate to stop the seizure. If the child is febrile (temperature of 100.4°F [38°C] or greater), an antipyretic agent such as acetaminophen can be given at a dose of 160 mg (5 mL) by an oral syringe, every 4 hours for a maximum of five doses per day, but this administration may not be required in every case.

REFERENCES

1. Zack MM, Kobau R. National and state estimates of the numbers of adults and children with active epilepsy—United States, 2015. MMWR Morb Mortal Wkly Rep 2017;66:821-5.
2. Fisher RS, Cross JH, French JA, et al. Operational classification of seizure types by the International League Against Epilepsy: Position Paper of the ILAE Commission for Classification and Terminology. Epilepsia 2017;58:522-30.
3. McAbee GN, Wark JE. A practical approach to uncomplicated seizures in children. Am Fam Physician 2000;62:1109-16.
4. Aaberg KM, Gunnes N, Bakken IJ, et al. Incidence and prevalence of childhood epilepsy: a nationwide cohort study. Pediatrics 2017;139:e20163908.
5. Chin RF, Neville BG, Peckham C, et al. Incidence, cause, and short-term outcome of convulsive status epilepticus in childhood: prospective population-based study. Lancet 2006;368:222-9.
6. Fisher RS, Boas WV, Blume W, et al. Epileptic seizures and epilepsy: definitions proposed by the International League Against Epilepsy (ILAE) and the International Bureau for Epilepsy (IBE). Epilepsia 2005;46:470-2.
7. Perez-Reyes E. Molecular physiology of low-voltage-activated t-type calcium channels. Physiol Rev 2003;83:117.
8. Robinson RB, Siegelbaum SA. Hyperpolarization-activated cation currents: from molecules to physiological function. Annu Rev Physiol 2003;65:453.
9. Friedman MJ, Sharieff GQ. Seizures in children. Pediatr Clin N Am 2006;53:257-77.
10. Oh A, Thurman DJ, Kim H. Comorbidities and risk factors associated with newly diagnosed epilepsy in the U.S. pediatric population. Epilepsy Behav 2017;75:230-6.
11. Hani AJ, Mikati HM, Mikati MA. Genetics of pediatric epilepsy. Pediatr Clin North Am 2015;62:703-22.
12. Berg AT, Berkovic SF, Brodie MJ. Revised terminology and concepts for organization of seizures and epilepsies: report of the ILAE Commission on Classification and Terminology, 2005-2009. Epilepsia 2010;51:676.
13. Blumstein MD, Friedman MJ. Childhood seizures. Emerg Med Clin North Am 2007;25:1061-86.
14. Hirtz D, Berg A, Bettis D, et al. Practice parameter: treatment of the child with a first unprovoked seizure. Neurology 2003;60:166-75.
15. Subcommittee on Febrile Seizures. Febrile Seizures: Guideline for the Neurodiagnostic Evaluation of the Child with a Simple Febrile Seizure. Pediatrics 2011;127:389-94.
16. National Clinical Guideline Centre (UK). The Epilepsies: The Diagnosis and Management of the Epilepsies in Adults and Children in Primary and Secondary Care: Pharmacological Update of Clinical Guideline 20. London: Royal College of Physicians; 2012 [NICE Clinical Guidelines, No. 137].
17. Steering Committee on Quality Improvement and Management, Subcommittee on Febrile Seizures. Febrile seizures: clinical practice guideline for the long-term management of the child with simple febrile seizures. Pediatrics 2008;121:1281-6.
18. Patel N. Febrile Seizures. BMJ 2015;351:h4240.
19. Guerrini R. Epilepsy in children. Lancet 2006;367:499-524.
20. Jallon P, Latour P. Epidemiology of idiopathic generalized epilepsies. Epilepsia 2005;46:10-4.
21. Bai X. et al. Dynamic time course of typical childhood absence seizures: EEG, behavior, and functional magnetic resonance imaging. J Neurosci 2010;30:5884-93.
22. Hrachovy RA, Frost JD Jr. Infantile spasms. Handb Clin Neurol 2013;111:611-8.
23. Tolaymat A, Nayak A, Geyer JD, et al. Diagnosis and management of childhood epilepsy. Curr Probl Pediatr Adolesc Health Care 2015;45:3-17.
24. Chen DK, So YT, Fisher RS. Use of serum prolactin in diagnosing epileptic seizures: report of the Therapeutics and Technology Assessment Subcommittee of the American Academy of Neurology. Neurology 2005;65:668-75.
25. Sadleir LG, Scheffer IE. Optimizing electroencephalographic studies for epilepsy diagnosis in children with new-onset seizures. Arch Neurol 2010;67:1345.
26. Wilmshurst JM, Gaillard WD, Vinayan KP, et al. Summary of recommendations for the management of infantile seizures: Task Force Report for the ILAE Commission of Pediatrics. Epilepsia 2015;56:1185.
27. Subcommittee on Febrile Seizures. Neurodiagnostic evaluation of the child with a simple febrile seizure. Pediatrics 2011;127:389-94.
28. Hsieh DT, Chang T, Tsuchida TN, et al. New-onset afebrile seizures in infants: role of neuroimaging. Neurology 2010;74:150.
29. Hirtz D, Ashwal S, Berg A, et al. Practice parameter: evaluating a first non-febrile seizure in children: report of the quality standards subcommittee of the American Academy of Neurology, The Child Neurology Society, and The American Epilepsy Society. Neurology 2000;55:616-23.
30. Garcia PJ, Aronoff S, Del VM. Systematic review and meta-analysis of seizure recurrence after a first unprovoked seizure in 815 neurologically and developmentally normal children. J Child Neurol 2017;32:1035-9.
31. Shinnar S, O'Dell C, Berg AT. Mortality following a first unprovoked seizure in children: a prospective study. Neurology 2005;64:880.
32. Krumholz A, Wiebe S, Gronseth GS, et al. Evidence-based guideline: Management of an unprovoked first seizure in adults: Report of the Guideline Development Subcommittee of the American Academy of Neurology and the American Epilepsy Society. Neurology 2015;84:1705.

33. Graves RC, Oehler K, Tingle LE. Febrile seizures: risks, evaluation, and prognosis. Am Fam Physician 2012;85:149-53.

34. Baca CB, Vickrey BG, et al. Psychiatric and Medical comorbidity and Quality of Life Outcomes in Childhood-Onset Epilepsy. Pediatrics 2011;128:e1532-e1543.

35. Chin RF, Neville BG, Peckham C, et al. Incidence, cause, and short-term outcome of convulsive status epilepticus in childhood: prospective population-based study. Lancet 2006;368:222.

36. Kravljanac R, Jovic N, Djuric M, et al. Outcome of status epilepticus in children treated in the intensive care unit: a study of 302 cases. Epilepsia 2011;52:358.

37. Johnson RL, Wilson CG. A review of vagus nerve stimulation as a therapeutic intervention. J Inflamm Res 2018;11:203-213.

38. Reilly C, Atkinson P, Das KB, et al. Factors associated with quality of life in active childhood epilepsy: a population-based study. Eur J Paediatr Neurol 2015;19:308-13.

39. Kossoff EH, Zupec-Kania BA, Amark PE, et al. Optimal clinical management of children receiving the ketogenic diet: recommendations of the International Ketogenic Diet Study Group. Epilepsia 2009;50:304-17.

40. Parakh M, Katewa V. Non-Pharmacologic Management of Epilepsy. Indian J Pediatr 2014.

41. Henderson CB, Filloux FM, Alder SC, et al. Efficacy of the ketogenic diet as a treatment option for epilepsy: meta-analysis. J Child Neurol 2006;21:193-8.

42. Martin K, Jackson CF, Levy RG, et al. Ketogenic diet and other dietary treatments for epilepsy. Cochrane Database Syst Rev 2016;2:CD001903.

43. IJff DM, Postulart D, Lambrechts DAJE, et al. Cognitive and behavioral impact of the ketogenic diet in children and adolescents with refractory epilepsy: A randomized controlled trial. Epilepsy Behav 2016 Jul;60:153-157.

44. Lin A, Turner Z, Doerrer SC, et al. Complications during ketogenic diet initiation: prevalence, treatment, and influence on seizure outcomes. Pediatr Neurol 2017;68:35-39.

45. Kossoff EH, Krauss GL, McGrogan JR. Efficacy of the Atkins diet as therapy for intractable epilepsy. Neurology 2003;61:1789-91.

46. Wheless JW. The ketogenic diet: an effective medical therapy with side-effects. J Child Neurol 2001;16:633.

47. Misiewicz Runyon A, So TY. The use of ketogenic diet in pediatric patients with epilepsy. ISRN Pediatr 2012;2012:263139.

48. Taketomo CK, Hodding JH, Kraus DM. Pediatric & Neonatal Dosage Handbook: An Extensive Resource for Clinicians Treating Pediatric and Neonatal Patients, 2017. Print.

49. Morris GL 3rd, Gloss D, Buchhalter J, et al. Evidence-based guideline update: vagus nerve stimulation for the treatment of epilepsy: report of the Guideline Development Subcommittee of the American Academy of Neurology. Neurology 2013;81:1453.

50. Ryzí M, Brázdil M, Novák Z, et al. Long-term vagus nerve stimulation in children with focal epilepsy. Acta Neurol Scand 2013;127:316-22.

51. Ravindra VM, Sweney MT, Bollo RJ. Recent developments in the surgical management of paediatric epilepsy. Arch Dis Child 2017;102:760-6.

52. Devinsky O, Cilio MR, Cross H, et al. Cannabidiol: pharmacology and potential therapeutic role in epilepsy and other neuropsychiatric disorders. Epilepsia 2014;55:791-802.

53. Devinsky O, Marsh E, Friedman D, et al. Cannabidiol in patients with treatment-resistant epilepsy: an open-label interventional trial. Lancet Neurol 2016;15:270-8.

54. Epidiolex prescribing information. Available at www.accessdata. fda.gov/drugsatfda_docs/label/2018/210365lbl.pdf. Accessed October 7, 2019.

55. Glauser T, Ben-Menachem E, Bourgeois B, et al. ILAE Subcommission on AED Guidelines. Updated ILAE evidence review of antiepileptic drug efficacy and effectiveness as initial monotherapy for epileptic seizures and syndromes. Epilepsia 2013;54:551-63.

56. Arya R, Glauser TA. Pharmacotherapy of focal epilepsy in children: a systematic review of approved agents. CNS Drugs 2013;27:273-86.

57. Wilmshurst JM, Gaillard WD, Vinayan KP, et al. Summary of recommendations for the management of infantile seizures: Task Force Report for the ILAE Commission of Pediatrics. Epilepsia 2015;56:1185-97.

58. French JA, Kanner AM, Bautista J, et al. Efficacy and tolerability of the new antiepileptic drugs I: treatment of new onset epilepsy. Report of the Therapeutics and Technology Assessment Subcommittee and Quality Standards Subcommittee of the American Academy of Neurology and the American Epilepsy Society. Neurology 2004;62:1252-60.

59. St. Louis EK, Rosenfeld WE, Bramley T. Antiepileptic drug monotherapy: the initial approach in epilepsy management. Curr Neuropharmacol 2009;7:77-82.

60. Davies JA. Mechanisms of action of antiepileptic drugs. Seizure 1995;4:267-71.

61. Shaw SJ, Hartman AL. The controversy over generic antiepileptic drugs. J Pediatr Pharmacol Ther 2010;15:81-93.

62. Zachry WM III, Doan QD, Caldwell JD, et al. Case-control analysis of ambulance, emergency room, or inpatient hospital events for epilepsy and antiepileptic drug formulation changes. Epilepsia 2009;50:493-500.

63. Rascati KL, Richards KM, Johnsrud MT, et al. Effects of antiepileptic drug substitutions on epileptic events requiring acute care. Pharmacotherapy 2009;29:769-74.

64. Hansen RN, Campbell JD, Sullivan SD. Association between antiepileptic drug switching and epilepsy-related events. Epilepsy Behav 2009;15:481-5.

65. McTague A, Martland T, Appleton R. Drug management for acute tonic-clonic convulsions including convulsive status epilepticus in children. Cochrane Database Syst Rev 2018;1:CD001905.

66. Brophy GM, Bell R, Claassen J, et al. Guidelines for the evaluation and management of status epilepticus. Neurocrit Care 2012;17:3-23.

67. Alldredge BK, Gelb AM, Isaacs SM, et al. A comparison of lorazepam, diazepam, and placebo for the treatment of out-of-hospital status epilepticus. N Engl J Med 2001;345:631.

68. Phelps SJ, Hovinga CA, Wheless JW. Status epilepticus. In: DiPiro JT, Talbert RL, Yee GC, et al., eds. Pharmacotherapy: A Pathophysiologic Approach, 8th ed. New York: McGraw-Hill Medical, 2011:1007-17.

69. Sofou K, Kristjánsdóttir R, Papachatzakis NE, et al. Management of prolonged seizures and status epilepticus in childhood: a systematic review. J Child Neurol 2009;24:918.

70. Lyttle MD, Gamble C, Messahel S, et al. Emergency treatment with levetiracetam or phenytoin in status epilepticus in children—the EcLiPSE study: study protocol for a randomised controlled trial. Trials 2017;18:283.

71. Shearer P, Riviello J. Generalized convulsive status epilepticus in adults and children: treatment guidelines and protocols. Emerg Med Clin North Am 2011;29:51-64.

72. Owens J. Medical management of refractory status epilepticus. Semin Pediatr Neurol 2010;17:176-81.

73. Go CY, Mackay MT, Weiss SK, et al. Evidence-based guideline update: medical treatment of infantile spasms. Report of the Guideline Development Subcommittee of the American Academy of Neurology and the Practice Committee of the Child Neurology Society. Neurology 2012;78:1974.

74. Elterman RD, Shields WD, Mansfield KA, et al. Randomized trial of vigabatrin in patients with infantile spasms. Neurology 2001;57:1416.

75. Go CY, Mackay MT, Weiss SK. Evidence-based guideline update: medical treatment of infantile spasms. Report of the Guideline Development Subcommittee of the American Academy of Neurology and the Practice Committee of the Child Neurology Society. Neurology 2012;78:1974.

76. Elterman RD, Shields WD, Bittman RM. Vigabatrin for the treatment of infantile spasms: final report of a randomized trial. J Child Neurol 2010;25:1340-7.

77. Song JM, Hahn J, Kim SH, et al. Efficacy of treatments for infantile spasms: a systematic review. Clin Neuropharmacol 2017;40:63-84.

78. Cross JH, Auvin S, Falip M, et al. Expert opinion on the management of Lennox-Gastaut syndrome: treatment algorithms and practical considerations. Front Neurol 2017;8:505.

79. Brigo F, Igwe SC. Ethosuximide, sodium valproate or lamotrigine for absence seizures in children and adolescents. Cochrane Database Syst Rev 2017;2:CD003032.

80. Corda D, Gelisse P, Genton P, et al. Incidence of drug-induced aggravation in benign epilepsy with centrotemporal spikes. Epilepsia 2001;42:754.

81. Beghi E, Giussani G, Grosso S, et al. Withdrawal of antiepileptic drugs: guidelines of the Italian League Against Epilepsy. Epilepsia 2013;54:2-12.

82. Reilly C, Atkinson P, Das KB, et al. Neurobehavioral comorbidities in children with active epilepsy: a population-based study. Pediatrics 2014;133:e1586-93.

83. Cramer JA, Mintzer S, Wheless J, et al. Adverse effects of antiepileptic drugs: a brief overview of important issues. Expert Rev Neurother 2010;10:885-91.

84. Leckband SG, Kelsoe JR, Dunnenberger HM, et al. Clinical Pharmacogenetics. Clin Pharmacol Ther 2013;94:324.

85. Amstutz U, Shear NH, Rieder MJ, et al. Recommendations for HLA-B*15:02 and HLA-A*31:01 genetic testing to reduce the risk of carbamazepine-induced hypersensitivity reactions. Epilepsia 2014;55:496-506.

86. Anderson M, Egunsola O, Cherrill J. A prospective study of adverse drug reactions to antiepileptic drugs in children. BMJ Open 2015;5:e008298.

87. Arif H, Svoronos A, Resor SR Jr, et al. The effect of age and comedication on lamotrigine clearance, tolerability, and efficacy. Epilepsia 2011;52:1905-13.

88. Ben-Menachem E. Weight issues for people with epilepsy—a review. Epilepsia 2007;48:42-5.

89. Mula M, Hesdorffer DC. Suicidal behavior and antiepileptic drugs in epilepsy: analysis of the emerging evidence. Drug Healthc Patient Saf 2011;3:15-20.

90. Sabril (vigabatrin) [prescribing information]. Deerfield, IL: Lundbeck, 2019.

91. Zupanc ML, Roell Werner R, Schwabe MS. Efficacy of felbamate in the treatment of intractable pediatric epilepsy. Pediatr Neurol 2010;42:396-403.

92. Harijan P, Khan A, Hussain N. Vitamin D deficiency in children with epilepsy: Do we need to detect and treat it? J Pediatr Neurology 2013;8:5-10.

93. Patsalos PN, Perucca E. Clinically important drug interactions in epilepsy: general features and interactions between antiepileptic drugs. Lancet Neurol 2003;2:347-56. Review.

94. Patsalos PN, Berry DJ, Bourgeois BF, et al. Antiepileptic drugs— best practice guidelines for therapeutic drug monitoring: a position paper by the subcommission on therapeutic drug monitoring, ILAE Commission on Therapeutic Strategies. Epilepsia 2008;49:1239-76.

95. Curtis KM, Tepper NK, Jatlaoui TC, et al. U.S. Medical Eligibility Criteria for Contraceptive Use, 2016. MMWR Recomm Rep 2016;65:1.

96. Modi AC, Rausch JR, Glauser TA. Patterns of nonadherence to antiepileptic drug therapy in children with newly diagnosed epilepsy. JAMA 2011;305:1669-76.

97. Yang C, Hao Z, Yu D, et al. The prevalence rates of medication adherence and factors influencing adherence to antiepileptic drugs in children with epilepsy: a systematic review and meta analysis. Epilepsy Res 2018;142:88-99.

98. Ramsey RR, Zhang N, Modi AC. The stability and influence of barriers to medication adherence on seizure outcomes and adherence in children with epilepsy over 2 years. J Pediatr Psychol 2017;43:122-132.

99. McAuley JW, Miller MA, Klatte E. Patients with epilepsy's perception on community pharmacist's current and potential role in their care. Epilepsy Behav 2009;14:141-5.

100. Dang LT, Silverstein FS. Drug Treatment of seizures and epilepsy in newborns and children. Pediatr Clin North Am 2017;64:1291-1308.

CHAPTER 28

Migraines

Stacie J. Lampkin, Pharm.D., BCACP, BCPPS, AE-C

LEARNING OBJECTIVES

1. Describe the classification and clinical presentation of migraines in children.

2. Identify nonpharmacologic options for preventing and managing migraine episodes.

3. Compare and contrast medication options for acute treatment of migraine.

4. Summarize the role of preventive medications used for migraines and their associated clinical considerations.

5. List treatment options for managing migraine in the emergency department and inpatient hospital setting.

ABBREVIATIONS IN THIS CHAPTER

CGRP	Calcitonin gene-related peptide
CHAMP study	Childhood and Adolescent Migraine Prevention study
DHE	Dihydroergotamine
ED	Emergency department
ICHD-3	*International Classification of Headache Disorders, 3rd edition*
MOH	Medication overuse headache
NSAID	Nonsteroidal anti-inflammatory drug
PedMIDAS	Pediatric Migraine Disability Assessment Score
PedsQL	Pediatric Quality of Life
SSRI	Selective serotonin reuptake inhibitor
SSNRI	Selective serotonin and norepinephrine reuptake inhibitor

INTRODUCTION

Headaches rank as one of the top five pediatric health problems.[1] Among all types of headaches, migraines are the most common disabling type of headache in children and adolescents.[2] Early and accurate diagnosis and prompt treatment are necessary to improve quality of life and reduce impairment.[2,3] The lack of high-quality evidence in the pediatric population limits adequate management.[4] Nonetheless, when a child receives a diagnosis of migraines, both nonpharmacologic

and pharmacologic options should be optimized to improve and prevent associated pain and symptoms. The focus of this chapter is on acute and preventive outpatient management of migraines in children and adolescents. Emergency department (ED) and inpatient hospital treatment are also discussed briefly.

EPIDEMIOLOGY

About 10% of the pediatric population experiences migraines.[5] Of these children, 60% to 85% have a migraine without aura and 15% to 30% report symptoms consistent with an aura.[3] In children younger than 7 years, migraine is more prevalent in boys. After that age, the prevalence is then similar in boys and girls until adolescence, when the prevalence becomes higher in girls.[2,3] In patients receiving a diagnosis of migraine as a child, 46% of patients may have persistent migraines 10 years after initial diagnosis, and most of these patients have diminished frequency of their headaches.[6] In adolescents, 18% to 34% are reported to experience remission of migraines.[7] However, children who received a diagnosis of migraine after age 11 years are more likely to experience long-term chronic migraine.[6]

QUALITY OF LIFE

Migraines can cause significant disability and negatively impact the quality of life for children and their family or caregivers.[8,9] The degree of disability and impact on quality of life is influenced by migraine severity, duration, and response to therapy.[9] The most common alterations in quality of life are impairment in school and changes in emotional functioning.[8] Specifically, migraines can lead to reduction in school performance and increased absences, decreased home and family interactions, and decreased socialization with friends.[8,9] The unpredictable nature of migraines also makes it difficult for families and children to prepare for missed school days and activities, further contributing to the burden of migraines.[8]

Two tools to assess disability and quality of life in children are the Pediatric Migraine Disability Assessment Score (PedMIDAS) and the Pediatric Quality of Life inventory (PedsQL), respectively. Both can easily be implemented into clinical practice.[2] The PedMIDAS is a modified version of the adult MIDAS questionnaire and more appropriately assesses school-age children and adolescent lifestyles.[9] On an individual basis, the PedMIDAS assesses disability, need for preventive medication, and response to treatment.[2,9] A PedMIDAS score of greater than 30 represents moderate to severe disability, indicating that initiation of preventive medications should be considered. A PedMIDAS score of 0 to 10 is consistent with no disability or limited disability.[9] The PedsQL assesses pediatric quality of life in a disease-independent manner.[2] Changes in disability and quality of life may be the first signs of worsening migraines and/or a positive or negative response to therapy.[1] Thus, early recognition and appropriate management of migraines are needed to prevent long-term disability and enhance quality of life.[2]

PATHOPHYSIOLOGY

Advanced imaging techniques, together with physiological, biochemical, pharmacologic, and genetic studies have enhanced understanding of the mechanisms of migraine headaches. Despite these many advances in knowledge, however, the exact pathophysiology is not fully understood and is still being debated.[10-12] Currently two main theories explain pain and associated symptoms in various migraine phases: vascular theory and neurogenic theory. The *vascular theory* describes migraine as intracranial vasoconstriction followed by rebound vasodilation. This theory is supported by relief of throbbing pain after administration of the vasoconstrictor, ergotamine. The *neurogenic theory* describes migraine as a dysfunction of neuronal networks. This theory explains the neurologic symptoms with aura, but it has yet to explain migraine-associated pain.[2]

Activation of the trigeminovascular system and cortical spreading depression have also been found to contribute to migraine symptoms.[12] The theory of *trigeminovascular system activation* posits that the trigeminovascular system regulates vascular tone and transmission of pain signals. Vasoactive neuropeptides (substance P, calcitonin gene-related peptide, neurokinin A, nitric oxide, and pituitary adenylate cyclase-activating peptide) are stored in the trigeminal sensory nerves, and, once released, cause inflammation and dilation of blood vessels in the cranial meninges. It is unclear what causes the initial activation of the trigeminovascular system.[10,12] *Cortical spreading depression* is an electrophysiological event described as an intense wave that spreads across the cerebral cortex,[12] which is thought to explain the cause of migraine auras.[10]

Eight genes have been identified and associated with migraine as follows: *MTDH, LRP1, PRDM16, MEF2D, ASTN2, PHACTR1, TGFBR,* and *TRPM8.*[10,12] *TGFBR* maintains vascular integrity and function, *TRPM8* is involved in pain signal pathways, and the other six genes are involved in neuronal and glutamatergic pathways. The exact process of how these genetic factors affect migraine symptoms is not known, but their role is supported by the influence of genetics on migraine development. Notably, patients have a 1.9 times higher risk of developing migraine if a first-degree relative has migraines.[10]

Comorbid conditions such as asthma, obesity, epilepsy, and sleep disorders are thought to influence the pathophysiology of migraine pain and associated symptoms. It is hypothesized that migraines and these comorbid conditions share a common neuropathologic pathway, although the exact mechanism is not clearly understood. The patient's experience of difficulty in coping with several other conditions also appears to influence migraine manifestations.[2] It is theorized that stress and environmental factors can lead to cortical activation, and foods can trigger headaches through activation of biochemical mechanisms.[13,14]

CLASSIFICATION AND CLINICAL PRESENTATION OF MIGRAINE

The *International Classification of Headache Disorders, 3rd edition beta* (ICHD-3), published in 2018, is the current standard to classify migraine in children and adults.[11] Compared with previous versions, this edition has been found to have an improved sensitivity for diagnosis of migraine in children and adolescents. However, most pediatric considerations are discussion-based and not listed as specific diagnostic criteria. As research continues, there is a need to develop pediatric specific criteria apart from the adult diagnostic classification to further improve diagnosis of pediatric migraine.[15]

Per the *ICHD-3*, migraine, defined as a *primary headache*, has two main subtypes: *migraine without aura* and *migraine with aura*. The specific ICHD-3 diagnostic criteria are in Table 1.[11] In children and adolescents, *migraine without aura*, previously referred to as *common migraine*, is a recurrent headache that typically lasts 2 to 72 hours. Compared with the common unilateral location of the headache in adults, the headache in children tends to be more bilateral until late adolescence or early adulthood. These headaches are usually frontotemporal. If a child presents with rare occipital headaches, further diagnostic work-up is required to rule-out an alternative diagnosis. The quality of the headache is usually pulsating with the intensity ranging from moderate to severe and is aggravated by routing physical activity.[11] In a recent study, migraines were commonly associated with phonophobia (97%), photophobia (96%), nausea (65%), vomiting (52%), and vertigo (52%).[15] Young children may have difficulty describing certain symptoms, specifically phonophobia and photophobia, so these symptoms may need to be inferred from the child's behavior.[11]

In menstruating patients, migraine without aura can have a menstrual relationship if the migraine occurs anytime between 2 days before and 3 days after the start of menstruation. This headache is further subclassified as *pure menstrual migraine* if the headache occurs only during this time frame or as a *menstrually related migraine* if it occurs during other times of menstruation.[11]

Migraine with aura, previously referred to as *classic migraine*, consists of gradually developing, reversible unilateral visual, sensory, or other central nervous symptoms followed by a headache and migraine symptoms.[11] The typical aura is a transient focal neurological phenomenon that appears gradually over several minutes and usually does not last more than 1 hour.[10] Visual auras are the most common occurring in over 90% of patients, followed by sensory disturbance aura and then auras involving speech disturbance symptoms. If more than one aura symptom is present, then the auras usually start with a visual aura, followed by a sensory aura, then auras involving speech disturbances, but these auras may occur in any order.

Auras should not be confused with *premonitory symptoms*, which can include fatigue, difficulty in concentrating, neck stiffness, sensitivity to light and/or sound, nausea, blurred vision, yawning, and pallor, that start hours or days before the migraine attack. Premonitory symptoms were previously referred to as *prodromes* or *warning symptoms*; however this

Table 1. *International Classification of Headache Disorders, 3rd edition beta* *(ICHD-3)* Diagnostic Criteria[11]

Migraine Without Aura	Migraine With Aura
A. ≥5 Attacks fulfilling criteria B–D	A. ≥2 Attacks fulfilling criteria B and C
B. Headache attacks lasting 4–72 hours (untreated or unsuccessfully treated)[a]	B. ≥1 Fully reversible aura symptom as follows: 1. Visual 2. Sensory 3. Speech and/or language 4. Motor 5. Brainstem 6. Retinal
C. Headache with ≥2 of the following: 1. Unilateral location 2. Pulsating quality 3. Moderate or severe pain intensity 4. Aggravation by or causing avoidance of routine physical activity	C. ≥3 Characteristics as follows: 1. ≥1 Aura symptom that spreads gradually over ≥5 minutes 2. ≥2 Symptoms that occur in succession 3. Each aura symptom lasts 5–60 minutes[b] 4. ≥1 Aura symptom is unilateral 5. ≥1 Aura symptom is positive 6. Aura is accompanied by or followed within 60 minutes by headache
D. During headache, ≥1 of the following: 1. Nausea and/or vomiting 2. Photophobia and phonophobia	
E. Not better classified by another *ICHD-3* diagnosis	D. Not better classified by another *ICHD-3* diagnosis, and transient ischemic attack has been excluded

[a]In children younger than 18 years, attacks may last 2–72 hours.
[b]Motor symptoms may last up to 72 hours.

terminology can be misleading and should be avoided when describing this phase of a migraine attack.

Patients who present with motor weakness as part of their aura are classified separately as *hemiplegic migraine*. Hemiplegic migraine is a separate classification because of differences in pathophysiology compared with migraine with typical aura.[11]

Migraines become classified as *chronic* when the headache occurs on 15 or more days per month for more than 3 months. At least 8 of these 15 days must have features of migraine with or without aura or believed to be a migraine by the patient and relieved by a triptan or ergot derivative.[11] About 3% of pediatric patients with migraines meet the definition of chronic migraines. This subset of patients can be difficult to treat because two or more preventive medications may fail to be effective.[16] Chronic migraines may also be the result of medication overuse in about 50% of patients. According to the *ICHD-3* criteria, chronic migraines and *medication overuse headache* (MOH) are two separate classifications and these patients should receive both diagnoses. After removal of the overused medication, if the headache pattern changes, then the migraine diagnosis should be reclassified appropriately.[11]

The *ICHD-3* reclassified some syndromes specific to pediatric patients that were historically considered manifestations of migraine. These syndromes were previously classified as *childhood periodic syndromes that are commonly precursors of migraines*, and are now reclassified as *episodic syndromes that may be associated with migraine*. These syndromes include the following: recurrent gastrointestinal disturbance, cyclical vomiting syndrome, abdominal migraine, benign paroxysmal vertigo, and benign paroxysmal torticollis. In addition these syndromes usually occur in patients who have migraines or increase the likelihood of developing migraines with or without aura. Less common conditions associated with migraine to consider include motion sickness episodes and periodic sleep disorders, such as sleepwalking, sleep talking, night terrors, and bruxism.[11]

DIAGNOSIS

To ensure accurate diagnosis of migraine, a thorough history is required.[11] The history must include headache pattern, pain quality, location, severity, and associated symptoms. The pattern will help determine if the headaches are acute or chronic.[17,18] Patients and/or caregivers should keep a headache diary to further describe headache manifestations. Minimally, the diary should be a 1-month daily recording of information on pain, associated symptoms, and triggers associated with the headache.[11] In younger patients, pain quality, severity, and associated symptoms are often difficult to describe. Therefore, age-appropriate tools should be used, such as using a Faces Pain Scale for a younger patient versus a numerical scale of 0 to 10 for older children to determine pain severity.[17,18]

A general physical examination together with a neurologic and comprehensive headache examination should also be completed. The comprehensive headache examination consists of additional assessments for symptoms such as tenderness and stability. The neurologic examination aids ruling out other causes of migraines and determining if further evaluation is warranted.[2] If a patient has an abnormal neurologic examination and does not meet diagnostic criteria for migraine, neuroimaging should be considered, but is otherwise not usually necessary. Electroencephalogram, lumbar puncture, and laboratory testing are not routinely recommended unless necessary to rule out other disorders.[17] Medication-specific baseline laboratory tests should be considered before starting preventive medication and to monitor toxicity or adherence throughout treatment.[2,17]

Before an accurate diagnosis of migraines can be made, secondary causes must be ruled out.[2] Conditions such as infections, allergies, and gastrointestinal disorders can mimic symptoms of migraine.[18] Furthermore, secondary causes must be differentiated from episodic syndromes, which may be the first symptoms recognized by the children with migraines until they can communicate head pain.[2,10] Episodic syndromes respond well to migraine medication and may require implementation of both acute and preventive treatments. Treatment options are considered as discussed in following text.[3,10]

ASSOCIATED FACTORS AND COMORBID CONDITIONS

Numerous factors can negatively influence migraines, such as poor lifestyle habits, environmental factors, hormones, and comorbid conditions.[2,11,14,16,17] Stress is the most common lifestyle trigger and has been reported by about 75% of patients with migraines. Changes in school and home environments, bullying, learning disabilities, permissive or strict parents, and lack of friends can contribute to stress in children and adolescents. Other common lifestyle triggers include sleep disturbances, weather, lights, odors, sounds, foods, and interaction with technology.[14,19] Foods commonly implicated in triggering migraines in children and adolescents include chocolate, cheese, citrus fruit, alcohol, and caffeine. The excessive use of electronic media (e.g., watching television, video-gaming), especially when combined with low level of physical activity, has been found to be a risk factor for migraines.[19]

Hormonal changes, especially at the time of menstruation, can lead to migraine symptoms.[2,11] Other comorbid conditions that can contribute to the development of migraines include obesity, asthma and allergic disorders, seizure disorders, sleep disorders, and psychological or emotional disorders. All of these factors can influence response and choice of treatment.[2,17]

GOALS OF THERAPY

The American Academy of Neurology has established long-term goals of migraine treatment and goals for treating an acute migraine attack and chronic migraines. The long-term goals are as follows: (1) reduce attack frequency, severity, and disability; (2) reduce reliance on poorly tolerated, ineffective, or unwanted acute pharmacotherapies; (3) improve quality of life; (4) avoid acute headache medication escalation; (5) educate and enable patients to manage their disease to enhance personal control of their migraine; and (6) reduce headache-related distress and psychological symptoms. The goals of treating an acute migraine attack are as follows: (1) treat attacks rapidly and consistently without recurrence; (2) restore the patient's ability to function; (3) minimize the use of back-up and rescue medications; (4) optimize self-care and reduce subsequent use of resources; (5) be cost-effective for overall management; and (6) have minimal or no adverse events. The goals of therapy for migraine preventive medication are as follows: (1) reduce attack frequency by at least 50%, reduce severity, and reduce duration; (2) improve responsiveness to treatment of acute attacks; and (3) improve function and reduce disability (PedMIDAS score of less than 10).[20]

TREATMENT

To fulfill the goals of therapy, management of migraines in children and adolescents must consist of a balanced and flexible treatment plan tailored to the individual. The treatment plan includes nonpharmacologic therapy, acute treatment, and if needed, preventive medication management.[3,18] To aid in management of pediatric migraines, a practice parameter for pharmacological treatment of migraine headaches in children and adolescents was developed in 2004. Since then, further studies have been published assessing the efficacy and safety of migraine medications in the pediatric population. However, large randomized controlled trials are limited, and most trials are confounded by high placebo-response rates. Most literature used in clinical practice is extrapolated from small pediatric trials and adult studies, creating a wide variation in management practices.[21]

NONPHARMACOLOGIC THERAPY

Many factors may influence the use of nonpharmacologic interventions over pharmacologic treatment. The factors that should be evaluated, if appropriate for a specific patient, include the following: (1) patient/caregiver preference for nonpharmacologic treatments; (2) tolerance or response to pharmaceuticals; (3) adverse effects of medication; (4) actual or planned pregnancy; (5) history of overuse of acute medication; (6) significant stress; (7) inadequate ability to cope with stress or pain; and (8) comorbid psychological disorders (e.g., depression, anxiety). Even if these factors are not identified, nonpharmacologic therapy should be combined with pharmacologic options. In general, nonpharmacologic interventions are not associated with adverse effects and may be often less expensive. Lifestyle modifications, trigger avoidance, use of nutraceuticals, and behavioral therapy are effective and can improve migraine outcomes in children.[14]

LIFESTYLE MODIFICATIONS AND TRIGGER AVOIDANCE

Poor lifestyle habits can trigger migraines. Children and parents should be educated on how to make appropriate lifestyle modifications such as maintaining adequate sleep, hydration, regular exercise, a balanced diet, and limiting use of technology.[14,16,19] In addition, technology can have a negative impact on lifestyle habits by decreasing sleep and reducing time for physical activity.[19]

Additional triggers should be identified through a headache diary, documenting triggers such as stress factors, weather changes, foods, and sensitivity to lights, odors, and sounds. Once identified these triggers should be avoided.[14] A generic recommendation to eliminate common food triggers from a child's diet can lead to child–caregiver conflict and is discouraged. Only patient-specific identified triggers with a temporal relationship to migraine need to be avoided.[3]

NUTRACEUTICALS

Eating foods that are high in certain vitamins and minerals, such as green vegetables rich in riboflavin, has been linked to migraine improvement.[16,22] Alternatively, nutraceuticals and/ or supplements can be considered if conventional medications fail or if the patient or caregiver reports concerns about the effects of prescription medications. Natural products such as riboflavin, magnesium, coenzyme Q10, and butterbur have been reported for use in pediatric migraines. However, all nutraceuticals have limited, inconclusive and low-quality evidence to support their use for migraine management in the pediatric population.[21]

BEHAVIORAL TREATMENTS

Behavioral treatments include relaxation techniques, biofeedback training, and cognitive behavioral therapy, which all may be helpful to reduce headache symptoms.[20] Relaxation techniques are specific to the child or adolescent and are provided after evaluation by a therapist.[13] Biofeedback training and cognitive behavioral therapy provide tools and skills to help patients become more confident in managing stress and coping with migraine pain and associated symptoms.[13,14,16] These approaches are effective and often used in conjunction with pharmacologic management, but are intended to aid in preventing migraines versus alleviating acute symptoms.[13,16,21] Behavioral treatments should be considered; however, their use may be limited by lack of availability of services or access to services; cost, if not covered by insurance; lack of consistent practice of these techniques by the patient and family or caregivers; and length of time to observe a change in response to migraine triggers.

PHARMACOLOGIC THERAPY FOR ACUTE TREATMENT

The purpose of acute treatment is to return the child to normal function within 1–2 hours of medication administration by stopping the pain and associated symptoms of migraine.[5,16] The ideal medication for acute management should provide a consistent response with the fewest and least degree of adverse effects.[17] In addition, acute treatment should prevent the need for further rescue medication.[16]

For the best response, medication should be properly dosed and given as quickly as possible. Ideally, the drug should be given as soon as the headache starts or at onset of aura.[16] Delay of medication can lead to increased pain and disability and can negatively impact quality of life.[20] To ensure quick access to medication and prevent missing school or social activities, acute treatment must be available at school, home, and any other location of the child.[2,16,17] A summary of medication and dosing can be found in Table 2.

OVER-THE-COUNTER (SIMPLE) ANALGESICS

Nonsteroidal anti-inflammatory drugs (NSAIDs). Ibuprofen should be considered the first-line of acute migraine treatment because of its demonstrated safety and efficacy.[16,17] It should be dosed at 7.5 to 10 mg/kg/dose. The maximum dosing and frequency of ibuprofen for migraines varies among

clinical practice. The maximum single dose for migraine ranges from 400 mg to 800 mg. For most indications, including migraine, ibuprofen can be given every 4 to 6 hours as needed for a maximum of daily dose of 2400 mg. However, using NSAIDs more than two or three times per week can lead to MOH. To reduce the risk of MOH, expert opinion has provided an alternative recommendation to prescribe ibuprofen as a single dose with the option to repeat the dose once in 3 to 4 hours for the same headache. For example, a patient weighing 40 kg could be prescribed ibuprofen 400 mg once with instructions to repeat the dose in 3 to 4 hours if the headache persists. The accumulation of these two doses would be considered one treatment and may only be repeated once in a 24-hour period and up to 3 days per week.[16,17]

In adults, naproxen and aspirin have been recommended as effective options for mild to moderate migraines or severe migraines that are known to respond to NSAIDs.[17] However, aspirin should not be used in children because of the risk of Reye syndrome[16] and naproxen only has U.S. Food and Drug Administration (FDA) label approval for pain in children 12 years and older.[23] Combination products containing aspirin, acetaminophen, and caffeine are not recommended in the pediatric population because of lack of evidence for use and risk of worsening headaches. The most common adverse reactions to NSAIDs are hypersensitivity reactions, dyspepsia and gastrointestinal bleeding.[16]

Acetaminophen. Acetaminophen has been shown to be less effective than ibuprofen because of its limited anti-inflammatory properties.[16] In addition, a recent Cochrane review concluded that evidence is insufficient to favor the use of acetaminophen in the treatment of acute migraine.[24] Therefore, this drug should be reserved for patients who are unable use ibuprofen because of hypersensitivity, upper gastrointestinal disease, renal impairment, bleeding disorders, or current oral anticoagulant use.[17] If acetaminophen is used, a dose of 15 mg/kg/dose (maximum 1000 mg/dose) is a safe and well-tolerated option to treat acute migraine attacks. The medication can be given every 4 to 6 hours with a maximum daily dose of 75 mg/kg/day or 4000 mg/day. Because of its adverse effects on the liver, it should not be used in patients who have liver damage, who are chronic alcohol users, or in malnourished patients.[16]

TRIPTANS

Discovery of the role of triptans and their receptor-specific mechanism of action helped provide insight into the pathophysiology of migraines and revolutionized acute treatment of migraines.[11,12] Triptans block the transmission of pain through activation of serotonin (5-HT)1B/1D receptors in the intracranial blood vessels, resulting in vasoconstriction and inhibition of trigeminal nerve terminals.[21] Compared withsimple analgesics, triptans are more expensive and their use is often reserved.[16,21] Nevertheless, about 30% to 60% of children will require triptans as an alternative to simple analgesics.[21] Thus, both simple analgesics and triptans can be considered first-line treatment options.[18] When determining which medication to use, two different strategies, the rescue strategy and stratified strategy, can be considered.

Table 2. Medications for Acute Migraine Treatment[16,23]

Classification	Medication Generic (Brand)	Dosing
Simple analgesics	Ibuprofen (Motrin, Advil)	7.5–10 mg/kg/dose every 4–6 hours Alternate dosing: 7.5–10 mg/kg/dose once; repeat dose in 3–4 hours if headache persists (MSD: 400 to 800 mg; MDD: 2400mg)
	Acetaminophen (Tylenol)	15 mg/kg/dose every 4–6 hours (MSD: 1000 mg; MDD: 75 mg/kg/day not to exceed 4000 mg)
Triptans[a]	Almotriptan[b] (Axert)	Oral tablet: 12–17 years: 6.25–12.5 mg (MDD: 25 mg)
	Rizatriptan[c] (Maxalt/Maxalt MLT)	Oral tablet, oral disintegrating ≥6 years[d]: <40 kg: 5 mg ≥40 kg: 10 mg (Adult MDD: 30 mg)
	Zolmitriptan (Zomig)	Nasal[a]: 12–17 years: 2.5–5 mg (MSD: 5 mg; MDD: 10 mg)
	Sumatriptan (Imitrex/Onzetra/Sumavel/Zembrace)	Nasal: ≥5 years: 5–20 mg (Adult MDD: 40 mg) Subcutaneous: 6–18 years: 3–6 mg (Adult MDD: 12 mg)
	Sumatriptan/naproxen[b] (Treximet)	Oral 12–17 years: 10 mg/60 mg or 85 mg/500 mg (MDD: 1 tablet of 85 mg/ 500 mg)

[a]Dose may be repeated once in 2 hours, if headache is still present.
[b]FDA label approval for children 12 to 17 years.
[c]FDA label approval for children 6 to 17 years.
[d]Requires dose adjustment with concomitant propranolol.
MDD = maximum daily dose; MSD= maximum single dose.

The *rescue strategy* consists of starting with the adequately dosed, patient-preferred, simple analgesic at onset of headache; if relief is insufficient, then a triptan is then used. The *stratified strategy* consists of the patient determining the severity of headache pain at onset and then takes the simple analgesic for less severe pain and the triptan for moderate to severe pain.[5]

In 2016, a Cochrane Review compared 24 prospective, placebo-controlled trials evaluating triptans for acute treatment of migraines in children age 4 to 18 years. The triptans evaluated include almotriptan, rizatriptan, zolmitriptan, sumatriptan, eletriptan, naratriptan, and sumatriptan/naproxen sodium, with more than half of the studies evaluating sumatriptan.[24] Overall these triptans have demonstrated efficacy with minor adverse effects in children and adolescents; however, only almotriptan, rizatriptan, zolmitriptan nasal spray and combination product sumatriptan/naproxen sodium have FDA label approval for use in this population.[16,21,24] Regardless, all of these triptans are widely used in practice, and currently evidence is insufficient to recommend one triptan versus another.[21,24] However, because of variations in pharmacokinetic properties, an alternative triptan should be tried if the triptan chosen initially does not demonstrate efficacy.[5]

Factors to consider when choosing a specific triptan include patient preference, route of administration, palatability, availability, and cost.[24] To maximize efficacy, triptans should be used at onset of headache. The dose may be repeated once in 2 hours, if headache is still present.[21] To enhance appropriate use and ensure efficacy, the most patient-friendly dosage form should be chosen from the variety of available formulations. Oral disintegrating tablets and non-oral dosage forms should be considered in patients who are unable to swallow pills or experience nausea or vomiting with migraines.[16,21]

Overall, minor adverse effects have been reported for all triptans used in the pediatric population. Oral preparations were associated with fatigue, dizziness, asthenia, dry mouth, and nausea or vomiting, whereas nasal preparations were associated with taste disturbance, nasal symptoms, and nausea.[24] Tingling and chest tightness have also been described.[22] To avoid MOH, triptans should be used less than twice per week and six times per month.[5,21] Triptans need to be avoided within 24 hours of administering other triptans or with ergot derivatives. As with use in adults, triptans should be avoided in patients with coronary or cerebrovascular disease, uncontrolled hypertension, severe hepatic impairment, or hemiplegic migraine.[16,21] In addition, they should be avoided in pregnancy and with patients taking monoamine oxidase inhibitors in conjunction.[21]

Almotriptan. Almotriptan gained FDA label approval for acute treatment of pediatric migraine in adolescent patients age 12 to 17 years in 2009.[25] Almotriptan has demonstrated efficacy for treating migraine symptoms and associated photophobia and phonophobia in adolescents, especially when used at the 12.5-mg dose.[16,21]

Rizatriptan. In 2011, rizatriptan received FDA label approval for migraines for children age 6 to 17 years.[25] A study in children 6 years and older found rizatriptan to have efficacy for headache relief at a dose of 5 mg for children weighing less than 40 kg and 10 mg for children weighing 40 kg and more. Patients receiving rizatriptan had lower rates of headache recurrence and used less rescue medication. Another study with the same dose found that children reported the treatment as good or excellent after one or two doses. When stratifying by age, the rate of freedom from pain at 2 hours for rizatriptan was superior to placebo for children age 12 to 17 years. In children 6 to 11 years, statistical significance was not found even though rizatriptan demonstrated greater response then placebo. This lack of statistical significance was likely caused by the lack of power in this subgroup analysis.[5,21]

Zolmitriptan. Zolmitriptan is available as an oral tablet, an oral disintegrating tablet, and a nasal spray. Only the nasal spray received FDA label approval in children age 12 to 17 years in 2015.[23,25] Several studies have demonstrated zolmitriptan nasal spray to be superior to placebo for treatment of migraine in the patient age range approved for use by the FDA.[16,21] Compared with zolmitriptan oral tablet, the nasal spray formulation is absorbed sooner and may especially benefit those who cannot take oral dosage forms.[21]

Sumatriptan. Sumatriptan was the first triptan available in the United States and has been evaluated in numerous studies in pediatrics. It has yet to receive FDA label approval, however, because as studies have failed to show efficacy, likely as a result of the high placebo-response rate. It is available as injection, tablet, and nasal spray formulations.[21] The nasal spray formulation of sumatriptan has been shown to be effective for moderate to severe migraine, with the most common adverse effect being taste disturbance. The subcutaneous form has insufficient data to support efficacy.[16]

Sumatriptan/naproxen sodium. In 2015, sumatriptan/naproxen sodium gained FDA label approval for acute treatment of migraine with or without aura in patients 12 to 17 years.[25] This combination should be considered in patients who do not achieve consistent and rapid headache relief with monotherapy.[5] A study compared various doses of sumatriptan/naproxen to placebo in children 12 to 17 years. The 2-hour pain free rates for sumatriptan/naproxen were significantly higher for the 10/60-mg, 30/180-mg, and 85/500-mg dosages compared with placebo and all dosages were well tolerated. Later in the duration of the headache, the 85/500-mg dose had better efficacy then the lower doses. The authors concluded that the lower doses may be a better choice for younger adolescents and shorter-lasting migraines, whereas the 85/500-mg dose may be better for older adolescents and patients who have migraines of longer duration.[26]

ADDITIONAL CONSIDERATIONS

Because of the unfavorable adverse effect profile, dihydroergotamine (DHE), opioids and dopamine receptor antagonists are generally not recommended for acute treatment.[10] However, dopamine antagonists together with other antiemetic agents should be considered in patients with nausea, vomiting and cyclic vomiting syndrome.[3,20] These symptoms need to be treated appropriately, especially because nausea is a very disabling symptom of migraine.[18,20] Antiemetics to consider include metoclopramide, prochlorperazine, and ondansetron.[3] Both metoclopramide and prochlorperazine have been shown to be helpful with treating nausea and vomiting and have also shown to be effective in treating emergency cases of migraine. In children, their use may be limited by the increased risk of developing extrapyramidal adverse effects.[16] Currently, no pediatric trials specifically assess the efficacy of ondansetron in patients with migraine-associated nausea, but this drug has been found to be an effective and tolerable antiemetic overall.[26]

MEDICATION OVERUSE HEADACHE

All acute medications can cause MOH if used too often.[20] *Medication overuse headaches* is classified as a headache that occurs on 15 or more days per month for more than 3 months and as a result of overuse of acute headache medication. Based on expert opinion, the medication must be taken on at least 15 days per month for simple analgesics (acetaminophen, NSAIDs) or on at least 10 days per month for triptans (in any formulation), DHE, and one or more combinations of analgesics. These headaches usually improve after the overused medication is discontinued. Therefore, education on the causes and consequences of MOH is a key component to its management.[11]

Patients who develop MOHs should be considered for preventive therapy.[20] In addition, the offending agent should be withdrawn. Expert opinion supports abrupt withdrawal compared with tapered withdrawal despite a lack of evidence. This approach is based on the belief that medications used to treat acute migraine do not cause severe withdrawal symptoms and so the offending agent has to be removed from therapy to best treat the MOH.[21]

PREVENTIVE TREATMENT

Similar to acute treatments, pediatric studies to guide choice of preventive medication are limited. Medication information used to aid in choice of therapy is often extrapolated from adult data and combined with clinical expert opinion.[16] Preventive therapy should be considered in children when acute treatments are not working, poorly tolerated, overused, or contraindicated.[17,21] In addition, preventive therapy should be considered when migraines occur more than once per week, cause disability (PedMIDAS score greater than 30, Grade III, or Grade IV) or negatively affect quality of life (a low score on PedsQL). Once preventive therapy is started, a *positive response to treatment* is defined as a reduction in headache frequency (ideally by at least 50%) and decreased disability (PedMIDAS score less than 10) that is sustained for 4 to 6 months.

Table 3. Preventive Medications for Migraine Prophylaxis[16,23]

Classification	Drug	Dosage	Contraindications/ Boxed Warnings	Drug Interactions: Metabolism/ Transport Effects	Briggs Pregnancy Considerations
Antidepressants	Amitriptyline	Initial: 0.25–0.5 mg/kg/day (maximum starting dose: 10–25 mg/dose) at bedtime Titration: every 2 weeks up to 1 mg/kg/day MDD: 150 mg/day	MAO inhibitors; U.S. boxed warning: worsening of depression or suicidal ideations in children with depression	Major 2D6 and minor 1A2, 2B6, 2C19, 2C9, 3A4 substrate; weak inhibitor of 1A2, 2C19, 2C9, 2D6, and 2E1	Human data suggest low risk
Anticonvulsants	Topiramate	Initial: 6 to <12 years and ≥20 kg: 15 mg once daily; ≥12 years: 25 mg once daily Titration: every 1 week up to 2–4 mg/kg/day divided twice daily; usual 50 mg/dose twice daily MDD: 200 mg/day	None for immediate release used for migraine prophylaxis	Weak inhibitor of 2C19	Human and animal data suggest risk
	Valproic acid	Initial: 10–15 mg/kg/day divide twice daily (maximum starting dose: 250 mg/dose) Titration: as needed over 4–6 weeks up to 0-45 mg/kg/day divided twice daily MDD: 1000 mg/day	Liver disease or dysfunction, pregnant women for the prevention of migraine, U.S. boxed warnings: hepatic failure, pancreatitis	Minor 2A6, 2B6, 2C9, 2C19, 2E1 substrate. Weak inhibitor of 2C9; weak/moderate inducer of 2A6	Human data suggest risk
Antihistamines	Cyproheptadine	0.2–0.4 mg/kg/day divided twice daily or 2–8 mg/day MDD: 0.5 mg/kg/day or 32 mg/day	MAO inhibitors, stenosing peptic ulcer, bladder neck and pyloroduodenal obstructions	None	Limited human data; animal data suggest low risk
Antihypertensives	Propranolol (β-blocker)	Initial: 0.5 mg/kg/day or 10 mg/day divided two or three times daily Titration: as needed to 3 mg/kg/day divided two or three times daily MDD: 120 mg/day	Asthma, sinus bradycardia, heart block > 1st degree, sick sinus syndrome	Major 1A2, 2D6 and minor 2C19, 3A4 substrate; weak inhibitor of 1A2, P-glycoprotein	Human data suggest risk in 2nd and 3rd trimester

MDD = maximum daily dose; MAO = monoamine oxidase.

Preventive therapy can also be considered successful when a child has fewer than four migraines per month that respond to acute treatment.[27]

Even if preventive therapy is recommended, parents may be resistant to having their child take medication every day. Lack of migraine prophylaxis can result in a vicious cycle of migraine causing disability and stress, which then causes more migraines. Thus prompt and appropriate treatment is necessary to increase the chance of reducing progression and chronicity of headaches.[27] Details of commonly used preventive medications are in Table 3.

ANTIDEPRESSANTS

Tricyclic antidepressants. Amitriptyline is a widely used medication for migraine prophylaxis in children and adolescents based on assessment of prescribing practices and expert opinion.[17,27] It should be started at a low dosage of 0.25 to 0.5 mg/kg/day in children and titrated every 2 weeks to 1 mg/kg/day with a dose ranging from 10 to 150 mg/day.[27] Previous studies demonstrated efficacy at 1 mg/kg/day, but were limited by the lack of a placebo control.[17,27] The anticipated Childhood and Adolescent Migraine Prevention (CHAMP) study, a randomized double-blind, placebo-controlled trial comparing amitriptyline, topiramate, and placebo in pediatric migraine, was published in January 2017.[28] Notably, at a dosage of 1 mg/kg/day, the percentage of patients who had a reduction of 50% or more in the number of headache days for amitriptyline (52%) was not significantly different from placebo (61%). The implications of this study on clinical practice have yet to be determined.

This CHAMP study also reported higher rates of fatigue and dry mouth in the amitriptyline group.[28] Drowsiness is a known adverse effect; thus the medication should be given at bedtime. For patients with insomnia, this effect may be beneficial. Even if given at bedtime, some patients may experience morning drowsiness that will usually improve over a few weeks.[27] Additional adverse effects to consider include dry eyes, lightheadedness, dizziness, constipation, and increased appetite. QT prolongation is also a potential adverse effect and electrocardiography is recommended, especially at dosages greater than 1 mg/kg/day.[17,27]

An alternative to amitriptyline is nortriptyline. It is often used because sedation has been reported less often with this medication.[27] However, because of an increased risk of arrhythmia when taking nortriptyline, regular electrocardiography may be needed.[17]

Selective serotonin reuptake inhibitors and selective serotonin and norepinephrine reuptake inhibitors. Selective serotonin reuptake inhibitors (SSRIs) have conflicting, but potentially moderate benefit when used for migraine prophylaxis in adults. Based on a study and on expert opinion, the SSRIs fluoxetine, fluvoxamine, and paroxetine have been recommended in adults. Selective serotonin and norepinephrine reuptake inhibitors (SSNRIs), such as venlafaxine or duloxetine, have more evidence then SSRIs to support their use as adult preventive medications.[27] The role of both SSRIs and SSNRIs as medication options for preventive migraine treatment in children and adolescents is yet to be determined.

ANTIEPILEPTICS

Topiramate, valproic acid, levetiracetam, zonisamide and gabapentin are antiepileptics that have been used for migraine prophylaxis.[17,27] Antiepileptic medications are thought to help with migraines by modulating cortical excitation.[27]

Topiramate. In 2014, topiramate was approved for prevention of migraine in pediatric patients 12 years and older.[25] Two double blind randomized placebo-controlled trials demonstrated efficacy of topiramate in migraine prevention for children and adolescents.[29,30] The CHAMP study found no significant difference in the percentage of patients who had a reduction of 50% or more in the number of headache days for 2 mg/kg/day of topiramate (55%) compared with placebo (61%).[28]

Based on all studies, the effective dosage usually ranges from 2 to 4 mg/kg/day or 50 mg/dose twice daily. The topiramate dosage should be titrated slowly, over 8 to 10 weeks, to reduce the potential for adverse effects. Adverse effects are specific to pediatric patients are not reported. However, common adverse effects include decreased appetite, anorexia, abdominal pain, drowsiness, memory or language difficulties, dizziness, and paresthesias. Additional adverse effects reported include hyperthermia, hypohydrosis, metabolic acidosis, renal calculi, and glaucoma.[17,27] Based on its adverse effect profile and alternative indication, patients who may benefit from topiramate include overweight or obese patients and children with seizure disorders.[5]

Valproic acid. Valproic acid may be an effective option for prevention of migraine in pediatric patients based on several open-label and retrospective studies.[17,27] To prevent adverse effects, the dosage should be titrated slowly over 4 to 6 weeks to reported effective dosages of 15 to 20 mg/kg/day and a maximum daily dose of 1000 mg/day.[17] Adverse effects include dizziness, drowsiness, increased appetite, and weight gain. Laboratory monitoring is necessary because of the risk

of thrombocytopenia, lymphopenia, elevated pancreatic enzymes, and potential hyperammonemia. Patients of child-bearing age must be counseled on the significant teratogenic risk,[17,27] and measures should be taken to prevent chance of pregnancy during use.

Other antiepileptics. Less commonly prescribed, levetiracetam and zonisamide have demonstrated some potential for efficacy in preventing migraines in pediatric patients. Both drugs appear to be well tolerated. Adverse effects reported with levetiracetam include irritability, aggressiveness, and mild memory issues. Weight loss and behavioral changes are the most common adverse effects associated with zonisamide. As for gabapentin, efficacy remains limited to adults.[17]

ANTIHISTAMINES

Cyproheptadine, an antihistamine with antiserotonergic properties, has been widely used for migraine prevention, even though efficacy data are sparse. The effective dosing ranges from 0.2 to 0.4 mg/kg/day. Although the maximum daily dose is 32 mg/day, the usual tolerable dosing for migraine ranges from 2 to 8 mg/day. Children older than 6 years or weighing more than 30 kg may require more than 8 mg/day based on the effective milligrams per kilogram dosing. Because of this limitation in dosing and adverse effects, it is most often used in children younger than 6 years or less than 30 kg. The most common adverse effects include sedation and increased appetite, which can contribute to weight gain.[17,27]

ANTIHYPERTENSIVES

Numerous antihypertensives have efficacy in adults with migraines, including propranolol, metoprolol, lisinopril, and candesartan. Verapamil and nimodipine are used but have insufficient evidence in adults. Propranolol has evidence of efficacy for migraines versus other common agents (e.g., amitriptyline, valproic acid) when used in children, despite a lack of placebo-controlled studies.[27] Propranolol can exacerbate clinical depression and is not recommended in patients with asthma.[5,13] In addition, propranolol is known to have an impact on physical activity because if affects the heart rate.[5] Verapamil is commonly used in children; however, no studies are currently evaluating its use in pediatric migraine. The efficacy of lisinopril and candesartan is unknown. Evidence for nimodipine is inconclusive. Compared with metoprolol, behavioral therapy was found to be better at reducing headache frequency and severity. Clonidine has not been found to have efficacy for migraines.[27]

ONABOTULINUMTOXINA

OnabotulinumtoxinA is theorized to interfere with nociceptor up-regulation, thus disrupting the process of central trigeminal sensitization; however, the true mechanism of action is unknown. In 2010, intramuscular injection was approved for chronic migraine in adults. Based on limited evidence, efficacy is suggested in children and the drug may be considered as an off-label treatment option. In general, onabotulinumtoxinA is considered when children have contraindications against using oral therapy options or when two or more preventive medications have failed. Compared with all other preventive medications, benefits of onabotulinumtoxinA appear to include less chance of systemic adverse effects, improved adherence, quicker onset of action, and fewer drug interactions. Its use is limited by cost and patient/caregiver concerns about the multi-injection procedure.[27]

CLINICAL CONSIDERATIONS

Available evidence in pediatric patients does not support the use of one medication versus another. Currently, tricyclic antidepressants, antiepileptic medications, and antihistamines with antiserotonergic properties are the most commonly prescribed agents for prevention of migraines, with topiramate being the only medication with FDA label approval for prophylaxis of migraine headache in adolescents.[17,21] Even though the CHAMP trial did not demonstrate efficacy of amitriptyline or topiramate over placebo, the effects of this study on clinical practice have yet to be determined.

When choosing a preventive treatment option, potential benefits of the migraine medication must be weighed against potential risks. The patient's medication regimen should be evaluated for possible drug interactions.[20] Existing comorbid conditions must be considered with the adverse effects of the migraine medication on that disorder.[20,27] Headache is commonly associated with psychiatric conditions including depression, anxiety, and attention deficit hyperactivity disorder.[14] Patients with depression, anxiety, or emotional disorders can be considered for antidepressant use.[2] However, children with generalized anxiety disorder, attention deficit hyperactivity disorder, and specific phobias are a clinical challenge because it is often unknown which condition is exacerbating which. In severe cases, referral to a psychologist and/or psychiatrist should be considered.[13]

To improve adherence, a medication that requires the least number of doses per day is preferred. Once a medication is started, it will require an adequate trial, which may be 2 to 3 months and should not be stopped prior unless adverse effects are experienced.[17,20] Medications require titration, which should be understood by the patient and caregivers.[17] Patients and caregivers should also be educated on the expectations of treatment to understand that preventive medications take time to work, that the drug must be taken on a daily basis as prescribed, and that the response will not be immediate.[17,18] Patients and family or caregivers should have a clear understanding that migraines will likely not be eliminated and that a reasonable expectation of therapy is a reduction in migraines by 50%.[22] Once headaches are controlled for 3 to 6 months, then tapering the medication can be considered.[20]

EMERGENCY DEPARTMENT TREATMENT

If outpatient management of an acute migraine attack fails and a patient maintains a severe and disabling headache, then more aggressive therapy can be initiated in the ED.[16,17] Numerous medications have been used in various combinations and treatment plans will vary across ED settings. Overall, most clinicians follow a stepwise approach, starting with intravenous hydration.[17,22,31] Medications that have been used include the following: antidopaminergic agents (prochlorperazine, metoclopramide); NSAIDs (ketorolac); triptans; neuroleptics (chlorpromazine); antiepileptics (sodium valproate); magnesium sulfate; dexamethasone; and intravenous DHE. These medications are all off-label and have limited evidence in the pediatric population.[17,22] Despite the fact that many institutions still use narcotics, guidelines and current expert opinion recommend against their use and thus these agents should be avoided.[31]

First-line therapy often consists of a dopamine receptor antagonist, either prochlorperazine or metoclopramide.[22,31] Both have antiemetic properties and can improve migraine symptoms. Prochlorperazine is dosed at 0.15 mg/kg/dose intravenously (maximum of 10 mg/dose) and metoclopramide is 0.1 mg/kg/dose intravenously (maximum of 10 mg/dose). Extrapyramidal symptoms such as akathisia and dystonic reactions are often associated with use. These symptoms can be treated with antihistamines; therefore diphenhydramine is often given at the same time as either medication.[31]

If an antidopaminergic agent fails, second-line agents are usually ketorolac or a triptan.[22,31] Ketorolac can be administered intravenously at a dose of 0.5 mg/kg/dose (maximum of 50 mg/dose). A thorough history of home medication use must be determined because ketorolac cannot be used within 6 hours of another NSAID.[31] If considering use of a triptan, triptans cannot be used within 2 hours of each other and no more than two doses can be used within 24 hours. The choice of triptan depends on the preferred route of administration.[31]

Institutions may also use a combination of therapies also referred to as a *migraine cocktail*. Combinations vary based on the clinical preference of the ED and formulary of the hospital. The only standardized migraine cocktail that has been studied in children includes the combination of intravenous fluid bolus, ketorolac, prochlorperazine, and diphenhydramine.[22,31] This study compared patient outcomes before and after implementation of the standardized treatment and demonstrated that the combination therapy significantly reduced headache pain scores, length of ED stay, and hospital admission rates.[32]

INPATIENT HOSPITAL TREATMENT

About 6% to 7% of patients do not have migraine improvement after treatment in ED and should be considered for a neurology consult.[17,31] In addition, patients with *status migrainosus* (defined as a debilitating migraine attack lasting more than 72 hours), with severe exacerbation of chronic headache, or who did not have a response to ED abortive treatment should be admitted to the hospital.[11,17] The goal of treatment for these patients is to control the disabling headache.[17] Usually DHE is tried first and has been reported to be very effective in children and adolescents with a response rate of at least 75%. Sodium valproate can be considered if DHE is not tolerated or is contraindicated, such as in patients with uncontrolled hypertension, with ischemic heart disease, with severe hepatic or renal disease, who have had administration within the past 24 hours of a triptan or ergot-like agent, or who are pregnant.[16,17,23]

A low-dose protocol or high-dose protocol of DHE can be used based on patient tolerability. Dependent on age, the low-dose consists of 0.1–0.2 mg/dose intravenously every 6 hours and the high-dose is 0.5–1 mg/dose every 8 hours. Regardless of protocol, if a patient does not respond by the fifth dose, then treatment should be stopped. If a patient does respond, then DHE can be continued for a maximum of 20 doses or until the headache resolves. Pretreatment with an antiemetic is recommended because DHE is commonly associated with nausea.[16,22] Valproate can be administered intravenously at 15 mg/kg/dose followed by 5 mg/kg/dose every 8 hours for a maximum of 10 doses or until freedom from headaches.[16,17,22]

FUTURE THERAPIES

Humanized monoclonal antibodies that antagonize calcitonin gene-related peptide (CGRP) are a promising treatment option in development.[33] The discovery of CGRP receptor antagonists and their efficacy in acute migraine attacks helped to further provide insight into the pathophysiology of migraine.[11,12,34] Because of liver toxicity associated with CGRP receptor antagonists, monoclonal antibodies were developed.[34] Phase I, phase II, and preliminary phase III trials of humanized monoclonal antibodies against CGRP have demonstrated a good safety and efficacy profile.[33,34] Although these monoclonal antibodies require intravenous or subcutaneous delivery, only one dose may be needed every 1 to 3 months to prevent or reduce migraine attacks.[33,34] These monoclonal antibodies are not approved for use in adults, and their role in children and adolescents has not been evaluated.[22]

CONCLUSIONS

Pediatric migraine can lead to significant disability and decreased quality of life for both the child and caregivers. Appropriate diagnosis and close follow-up with monitoring is required for all patients. Even with limited and conflicting evidence, management must be optimized to improve patient outcomes. Nonpharmacologic management should be used, consisting of lifestyle modifications, trigger avoidance, nutraceuticals, and behavioral therapy. For acute treatment of migraines, NSAIDs and triptans are considered first-line options and should be taken at onset of headache pain or aura. Prompt implementation of preventive treatment can improve the chance of reducing progression and chronicity of headaches. Numerous preventive treatment options exist and the choice of medication is based on patient and medication specific factors. Abortive treatment in the ED for persistent headaches varies by institution. Patients who have status migrainosus or who did not have a response to ED abortive treatment should be admitted to the hospital and receive intravenous DHE or valproate. Future guidelines and studies need to further stratify management by age range for the school-age child versus adolescents.

Patient Case ADOLESCENT MIGRAINE

A 14-year-old girl is brought to a clinic with a 4-month history of headaches. She reports, "My headaches keep making me miss school." She states the headaches are located over the posterior region and denies neck pain associated with the headache. She reports associated photophobia and phonophobia and often feels nauseous but denies emesis. Onset occurs in the morning or evening with the duration usually lasts at least 12 hours. She reports an intensity of 9/10. Siting in a dark and quiet room helps when she has these attacks. If her headache starts in the morning, she will miss school or spend the day sleeping in the school nurse's office. She doesn't like taking ibuprofen, because says she needs to take at least a few of the 200 mg tablets to get any relief. She tries acetaminophen on occasion, but reports no relief from pain. She reports some headaches turning into a 10/10 pain and these headaches will not respond to ibuprofen. Her frequency of headaches is two or three times per week. She reports that she cannot identify any triggers. She sleeps at least 8 hours per night and consumes a lot of fast food and sugary snacks.

Medical history: Acne, asthma, obesity

Family history: Paternal aunt has migraines; maternal grandfather has hyperlipidemia and diabetes

Social history: She is in ninth grade and lives with her father, mother, and 7-year-old brother

Home medications: Benzoyl peroxide 10% applied to face twice daily; ibuprofen 3 of the 200-mg tablets every 8 hours as needed; fluticasone 110 mcg two puffs twice daily with spacer; albuterol 90 mcg two puffs every 4 hours as needed

Immunizations: Up to date for age; receives annual influenza vaccine

Vital signs: BP 90/55 mm Hg, Wt 106 kg (99th percentile), Ht 66 inches (83rd percentile), BMI 37.9 (99th percentile)

1. What is an appropriate home management plan to treat acute headaches in this patient?

Recommended treatment is ibuprofen 800 mg tablets by mouth once at the onset of headache or almotriptan 12.5-mg tablets by mouth once at onset of headache and once again 2 hours later if the headache persists. Because this patient can identify which headaches will respond to ibuprofen, the stratified strategy is best for prompt treatment. This strategy consists of the patient determining headache severity and taking either the simple analgesic or triptan. Ibuprofen has demonstrated efficacy and can be continued at the maximum dose of 800 mg for the patient's weight. Because she had concerns about the quantity of pills with 200-mg tablets, a prescription should be written. Alternatively, based on her age, naproxen could be considered. For the triptan, no evidence shows one drugs is better than another triptan. Almotriptan, rizatriptan, and zolmitriptan nasal spray have FDA label approval, although any of the triptans are used in practice. The choice is based on preference for dosage form and cost. Although the patient has associated nausea, she did not report any issues with taking pills by mouth, so the oral dosage form can be considered. For this patient, almotriptan was chosen at a dose of 12.5 mg because one study found it to be the most effective dose for 2-hour pain relief.

2. What patient education should be provided to the patient about the home medication plan for acute headaches?

For the best response, medications should be taken as soon as headache is identified. Because the stratified strategy was recommended for this patient, she should take ibuprofen 800 mg by mouth at onset of headache for headaches that have less pain intensity. She should also take almotriptan 12.5 mg by mouth at onset of headache for headaches that are 10/10 pain. Regardless of which medication was taken at start of headache, if headaches persist after 2 hours, she may take almotriptan 12.5 mg once. To prevent medication overuse headaches, ibuprofen should not be taken more than two or three times per week, almotriptan not more than twice per week or six times per month, and the combination of both not more than 10 days per month Adverse effects for ibuprofen include hypersensitivity reactions, dyspepsia, and gastrointestinal bleeding. Almotriptan is associated with fatigue, dizziness, asthenia, dry mouth, and nausea/vomiting. She should keep a daily headache diary for 1 month to track if medications are relieving acute headaches and if she experiences any adverse effects. The headache diary should minimally include pain, associated symptoms, and triggers associated with the headache for 1 month. Common triggers reported include stress, sleep disturbances, weather, lights, odors, sounds, foods (e.g., chocolate, cheese, citrus fruit, alcohol, and caffeine), and hormones.

3. What is an optimal preventive treatment plan for the headaches and how should the patient be counseled regarding the treatment recommendations?

Preventive therapy should be considered when migraines occur more than once per week, cause disability, or negatively impact quality of life—all of which are present in this patient. Studies in the pediatric population are limited to aid in choice of preventive medication, and clinical practice varies widely. Topiramate is the only medication with FDA label approval for prophylaxis of migraine in adolescents. However, a study published in January 2017 found no difference in the percentage of patients who had a reduction of 50% or more in the number of headache days between topiramate (55%), amitriptyline (52%), and placebo (61%). When choosing a treatment, medication-specific factors need to be weighed against the risks and benefits to the patient. Comorbid conditions should be considered. This patient has acne, asthma, and obesity. Topiramate may have benefit for weight loss and is being considered first. Topiramate is recommended at 25 mg/dose by once daily for 1 week, then increased to 25 mg/dose by mouth twice daily. Because of the risk of birth defects with topiramate, preventive measures to prevent pregnancy should be considered. Alternative medications to use include other antiepileptic medications, tricyclic antidepressants, antihypertensives, and antihistamines with antiserotonergic properties. Considerations specific to this patient include the following: valproic acid has the potential for weight gain; tricyclic antidepressants might be used if she has depression; propranolol should not be used because of her asthma; and cyproheptadine is usually used in children younger than 6 years or 30 kg. Once a medication is chosen, patients should be counseled on expectations of treatment and adverse effects. Because topiramate is recommended for this patient, specific education points include the following: (1) it should be taken every day and will not work for acute headaches; (2) it usually takes a 2- to 3-month trial before optimal response; and (3) a reasonable expectation is for the number of headaches per month decrease by 50%; during this time, the dose can be increased if it is not working and if adverse effects are not experienced; (4) common adverse effects include decreased appetite, anorexia, abdominal pain, drowsiness, memory or language difficulties, dizziness, and paresthesias; and (5) if she becomes pregnant while taking this drug, the risk of birth defects increased, therefore measures should be considered to prevent pregnancy.

4. What is an appropriate follow-up and titration schedule for the preventive medication that was recommended?

The patient should return in 1 month for a follow-up. Ideally the patient should be encouraged to keep daily headache diary and bring it with her to her appointment. This diary should keep track of headache frequency and pain and medication adverse effects. If her symptoms have improved, titration of topiramate is not required and she can keep taking same dose. If she is still often having disabling headaches that negatively affect her quality of life, then the medication dose can be increased to topiramate 50 mg/dose in the evening and 25 mg/dose in the morning for 1 week, and then the dose can be increased to topiramate 50 mg/dose twice daily. If needed, topiramate can be increased to a maximum daily dose of 200 mg/day.

REFERENCES

1. Hershey AD, Winner PK. Pediatric migraine: recognition and treatment. J Am Osteopath Assoc 2005;105:2S–8S.
2. Hershey AD. Current approaches to the diagnosis and management of paediatric migraine. Lancet Neurol 2010;9:190–204.
3. Lewis D. Pediatric migraines. Neurol Clin 2009;27:481–501.
4. O'Brien HL, Kabbouche MA, Hershey AD. Treating pediatric migraine: an expert opinion. Expert Opin Pharmacother 2012;13:959-66.
5. Bonfert M, Straube A, Schroeder AS, et al. Primary headache in children and adolescents: update on pharmacotherapy of migraine and tension-type headache. Neuropediatrics 2013;44:3-19.
6. Galinski M, Sidhoum S, Cimerman P. Early diagnosis of migraine necessary in children: 10-year follow-up. Pediatr Neurol 2015;53:319-23.
7. O'Brien HL, Cohen JM. Young adults with headaches: the transition from adolescents to adults. Headache 2015;55:1404-9.
8. Powers SW, Patton SR, Hommel KA, et al. Quality of life in childhood migraines: clinical impact and comparison to other chronic illnesses. Pediatrics 2003;112:e1–e5.
9. Hershey AD, Powers SW, Vockell AL, et al. PedMIDAS: development of a questionnaire to assess disability of migraines in children. Neurology 2001;57:2034–9.
10. Spiri D, Rinaldi VE, Titomanlio. Pediatric migraine and episodic syndromes that may be associated with migraine. Ital J Pediatr 2014;40:92.
11. International Headache Society. The International Classification of Headache Disorders, 3rd ed. Cephalalgia 2018;38:1–211.
12. Gasparini CF, Sutherland HG, Griffiths LR. Studies on the pathophysiology and genetic basis of migraine. Curr Genomics 2013;14:300-15.
13. Green A, Kabbouche MA, Kacperski, et al. Managing migraine headaches in children and adolescents. Expert Rev Clin Pharmacol 2016;9:477-82.
14. Faedda N, Cerutti R, Verdecchia P, et al. Behavioral management of headache in children and adolescents. J Headache Pain 2016;17:80.
15. Lima MM, Bazan R, Martin LC et al. Critical analysis of diagnostic criteria (ICHD-3 beta) about migraine in childhood and adolescence. Arq Neuropsiquiatr 2015;73:1005-8.
16. O'Brien HL, Kabbouche MA, Kacperski J, Hershey AD. Treatment of pediatric migraine. Curr Treat Options Neurol 2015;17:326.
17. Kacperski J, Kabbouche MA, O'Brien HL, et al. The optimal management of headaches in children and adolescents. Ther Adv Neurol Disord 2016;9:53-68.
18. Lewis D, Ashwal S, Hershey A, et al. Practice parameter: pharmacological treatment of migraine headache in children and adolescents: report of the American Academy of Neurology Quality Standards Subcommittee and the Practice Committee of the Child Neurology Society. Neurology 2004;63:2215–24.
19. Russo A, Bruno A, Trojsi F, et al. Lifestyle factors and migraine in childhood. Curr Pain Headache Rep 2016;20:9.
20. Silberstein SD. Practice parameter: evidence-based guidelines for migraine headache (an evidence-based review). Neurology 2000; 55:754–62.
21. Kacperski J, Hershey AD. Newly approved agents for the treatment and prevention of pediatric migraine. CNS Drugs 2016;30:837-844.
22. Merison K, Jacobs H. Diagnosis and Treatment of Childhood Migraine. Curr Treat Options Neurol 2016;18:48.
23. Lexicomp Online, Pediatric & Neonatal Lexi-Drugs[Internet database]. Hudson, OH: Lexi-Comp. Updated periodically.
24. Richer L, Billinghurst L, Linsdell MA, et al. Drugs for the acute treatment of migraine in children and adolescents. Cochrane Database Syst Rev 2016;4:CD005220.
25. US Food and Drug Administration. New pediatric labeling information database. Available at https://www.accessdata.fda.gov/scripts/sda/sdNavigation.cfm?sd=labelingdatabase. Accessed May 20, 2019.
26. Derosier FJ, Lewis D, Hershey AD, et al. Randomized trial of sumatriptan and naproxen sodium combination in adolescent migraine. Pediatrics 2012;129:e1411-20.
27. Hickman C, Lewis KS, Little R, et al. Prevention for pediatric and adolescent migraine. Headache 2015;55:1371-81.
28. Powers SW, Coffey CS, Chamberlin LA, et al. Trial of amitriptyline, topiramate, and placebo for pediatric migraine. N Engl J Med 2017;376:115-24.
29. Winner P, Pearlman EM, Linder SL, et al. Topiramate for migraine prevention in children: a randomized, double-blind, placebo-controlled trial. Headache 2005;45:1304–12.
30. Lewis D, Winner P, Saper J, et al. Randomized, double-blind, placebo-controlled study to evaluate the efficacy and safety of topiramate for migraine prevention in pediatric subjects 12 to 17 years of age. Pediatrics 2009;123:924–34.
31. Sheridan DC, Spiro DM, Meckler GD. Pediatric migraine: abortive management in the emergency department. Headache 2014;54:235-45.
32. Leung S, Bulloch B, Young C, et al. Effectiveness of standardized combination therapy for migraine treatment in the pediatric emergency department. Headache 2013;53:491-197.
33. Burstein R, Noseda R, Borsook D. Migraine: multiple processes, complex pathophysiology. J Neurosci 2015;35:6619-29.
34. Giamberardino MA, Affaitati G, Curto M, et al. Anti-CGRP monoclonal antibodies in migraine: current perspectives. Intern Emerg Med 2016;11:1045-57.

CHAPTER 29

Cerebral Palsy

Mary A. Worthington, Pharm.D.,
FPPA, BCPPS, BCPS

INTRODUCTION

In 2004, an International Workshop on Definition and Classification of Cerebral Palsy was convened in Bethesda, Maryland. Participants emphasized the importance of viewing cerebral palsy (CP) as a clinical descriptive term and defined *cerebral palsy* as a group of permanent disorders of the development of movement and posture, causing activity limitation, that are attributable to nonprogressive disturbances that occurred in the developing fetal or infant brain. The motor disorders of CP are often accompanied by disturbances of sensation, perception, cognition, communication, and behavior; epilepsy; and secondary musculoskeletal problems.[1]

Although CP results from a nonprogressive disturbance, symptoms change over time. This changing clinical course necessitates frequent assessment by health care providers to ensure that treatments are continually evaluated and adjusted to optimize overall function. As drug treatment options expand for motor disorders and other accompanying conditions, pharmacists play an increasing role in selecting optimal medication choices for patients with CP.

EPIDEMIOLOGY AND CLASSIFICATION

Cerebral palsy is one of the most common childhood physical disabilities. A recent meta-analysis estimated an overall worldwide prevalence at 2.11 per 1000 live births, with increased occurrence associated with lower birth weight and gestational age. When reported by birth weight, neonates born weighing 1000–1499 g had the highest prevalence, 59.18 per 1000 live births. The lowest incidence, 1.33 per 1000 live births, was in newborns with a birth weight greater than 2500 g.[2]

Because CP covers a broad range of clinical presentations, the disorder may be classified in several ways on the basis of motor abnormalities and accompanying impairments.[1] Patients may present with more than one movement abnormality, but CP should be classified by the dominant type: *spasticity, dystonia, choreoathetosis,* or *ataxia.*[1] Of all children with CP, 88% are thought to have the spastic type.[3]

How motor abilities in individuals with CP affect their functioning is usually described by the gross motor function classification system (GMFCS).[4] The GMFCS has five levels of classification, which are determined from self-initiated movement, with an emphasis on sitting, transfer, and mobility. Table 1 defines the GMFCS classification levels and estimates the percentage of children with CP who function at each level.[4,5] The GMFCS may be used when considering treatment options.

A newer method of classification centers on better understanding how an individual patient's diagnosis of CP affects the patient more globally, as described by the International Classification of Functioning, Disability and Health (ICF) from the World Health Organization. The ICF model focuses on understanding functioning and disability in the following four areas: *body functions, body structures, activities and participation,* and *environmental factors.* This classification emphasizes biopsychological factors in hopes of better addressing health care and rehabilitative needs in addition to measuring the effects of patients' physical and social environments on the challenges they face.[6]

Accompanying impairments in patients with CP may interfere with functioning and quality of life as much as or more than characteristic motor disabilities. Epilepsy, present in 30%–40% of children with CP,[3] can complicate treatment choices by increasing the risk of drug–drug interactions between therapies for the movement disorder and seizure control. Constipation and urinary incontinence are other common conditions that require concurrent drug therapies. Additional impairments include the following: hearing and vision abnormalities, intellectual disabilities, emotional and behavioral disorders, sleep disturbance, and musculoskeletal problems.

ETIOLOGY AND RISK FACTORS

Because CP is the result of an injury or disturbance in the developing fetal or infant brain, etiology and risk factors are often described as *prenatal*, *perinatal*, or *postnatal*. It is estimated that 80% of CP cases are acquired prenatally. The greatest risks of CP pertain to preterm birth and very low birth weight.[3] The relationship between prematurity and CP is complicated by evolving neonatal intensive care practices. Cystic periventricular leukomalacia and severe intraventricular hemorrhage are independent risk factors for CP in premature patients, and the decreased incidence of CP has been attributed to decreasing cystic periventricular leukomalacia.[7] Cerebral palsy from postnatal causes occurring in infancy has declined, but potential etiologies in this period include meningitis, head trauma, and intentional injury.[3] Box 1 lists factors associated with an increased risk of CP.[3,8]

Prevention of CP typically revolves around decreasing the incidence of premature birth. Additional strategies include avoiding potential causes of injuries to the developing brain such as maternal infections, including the Zika virus.[9] Intrapartum magnesium provides fetal neuroprotection and is recommended for short-term maternal administration if early preterm delivery is anticipated (less than 32 weeks' gestation).[10] Delayed cord clamping of at least 30 seconds is also recommended for neuroprotection. Therapeutic hypothermia administered to term infants with hypoxic-ischemic encephalopathy is associated with reduced brain injuries by neuroimaging and improved neurodevelopmental outcomes.[9]

INITIAL PRESENTATION AND DIAGNOSIS

Most children with CP present as infants and toddlers. Early, careful assessments of motor development, muscle tone, and risk factors are key aspects of diagnosis. A delay in reaching motor developmental milestones is usually viewed as a classic sign of CP in at-risk patients. However, some milestones (e.g., hand preference and even rolling over in select patients) may be achieved before typical ages. Box 2 lists clinical features of CP. The differential diagnosis often focuses on eliminating disorders that are progressive, including metabolic or genetic disorders or central nervous system tumors. Targeted laboratory testing may help rule out these processes.[11]

Diagnosis of CP or identification of high-risk patients in infancy is ideal because this age group benefits from diagnostic-specific early interventions. Before 5 months corrected age, three tools with predictive validity for diagnosis are neonatal magnetic resonance imaging (MRI), the Prechtl Qualitative Assessment of General Movements, and the Hammersmith Infant Neurological Examination (HINE). For older infants, the most predictive tools are MRI, the HINE and the Developmental Assessment of Young Children.[12]

Table 1. Gross Motor Function Classification System Levels and Estimates of Children Who Function at Each Level

Level	General Description in Age 6–12 Yr[4]	Age 8 Yr With Function at Level (%)[5]
I	Walk indoors and outdoors Can climb stairs without limitations Perform gross motor skills such as running and jumping, but speed, balance, and coordination are reduced	38.1
II	Walk indoors and outdoors but have limitations walking on uneven surfaces and inclines or in crowds or confined spaces Can climb stairs holding on to a railing Have minimal ability at best to perform gross motor skills such as running and jumping	16.4
III	Walk indoors or outdoors on a level surface with an assistive mobility device May propel a wheelchair manually or are transported for long distances or outdoors on uneven terrain, depending on upper limb function May climb stairs holding on to a railing	13.2
IV	Require physical assistance for mobility or use powered mobility in most settings May walk short distances at home with a walker and adult supervision but have difficulty turning and maintaining balance on uneven surfaces Are transported in a manual wheelchair or use powered mobility at school, outdoors, and in the community	15.1
V	Have severely limited self-mobility Are transported in a manual wheelchair in all settings Are limited in ability to maintain antigravity head and trunk postures and control leg and arm movements	17.1

ASSESSMENT OF MUSCLE TONE, MOVEMENT, ASSOCIATED CONDITIONS, AND NUTRITION

Muscle tone and movement should be evaluated for patients with CP to determine which motor abnormalities may be present. Symptoms related to motor dysfunction vary greatly from person to person and may be isolated or mixed. Box 2 lists symptom examples on the basis of motor abnormality type. Spasticity, the most common abnormality, describes a form of hypertonia, which is characterized by a velocity-dependent resistance of a muscle to stretch.[13] Dyskinesia describes a movement pattern that is involuntary, uncontrolled, recurring, and occasionally stereotypical.[14] Dyskinetic CP is termed *dystonic* if movements are stiff with increased tone and *choreoathetotic* if movements are slow and writhing with decreased tone.[14] Ataxia in CP describes a loss of orderly muscle contraction with movements that are performed with abnormal force, rhythm, and accuracy.[14]

The motor abnormalities of CP may make it more difficult to recognize other, concurrent impairments. Although epilepsy, intellectual disabilities, and speech and language disorders are not always present, patients should be screened for them.[11] Hearing and vision evaluations may require referral to specialists because some children cannot cooperate and complete typical screenings. Nutrition, growth, and other problems with swallowing function should be monitored.[11] Good nutrition is essential for children with CP, given that it improves general health and participation, neurodevelopmental outcomes, and survival.[15] Children with CP who have the most significant nutritional issues often have poor weight gain at an early age, considerable motor impairments, and feeding or swallowing problems. Assessment of nutritional status should include medical and feeding histories, physical examination, and anthropometric measurements, including weight, height, and triceps skinfold thickness.[15] Height may be challenging to obtain because of physical limitations. In these situations, segmental measurements with specific pediatric calculations can estimate overall length.[15] Enteral nutrition through a gastrostomy tube may be required in some patients, such as in those with poor weight gain and growth despite oral nutritional interventions and patients with aspiration risk during feeding. When gastrostomy tubes are present, oral medications are often given through the tube, and consideration should be given to formulation selection, as described in the Parenteral and Enteral Nutrition chapter. Poor nutrition affects bone health and contributes to low bone mineral density (BMD) in patients with CP, especially in nonambulatory children.[15]

Outcomes measures that help clinicians quantify and monitor overall functioning within the ICF framework are valuable in CP assessment. A toolbox is available that provides recommendations for 25 valid, reliable, age-specific measures to assess ICF components in children and youth with CP.[16] The GMFCS is fundamental in evaluating motor functional abilities in children age 1–18 years with CP.[4] The GMFCS and other instruments that measure outcomes in patients with CP are available on the CanChild Centre website.[17] In patients with spasticity, determining the degree of spasticity is helpful in evaluating response to therapy. The modified Ashworth scale and the modified Tardieu scale can grade spasticity levels.[18,19] The modified Tardieu scale may more effectively quantify a change in spasticity than the modified Ashworth scale.[19]

Box 1. Factors Associated with an Increased Risk of Cerebral Palsy[3,8]

Prenatal
Preterm birth
Low birth weight
Fetal growth restriction
Birth defects
Intracranial hemorrhage
Placental disorders
Multiple pregnancy
Maternal infection
Genetic mutations
Maternal age > 35 yr
Severe maternal iodine deficiency

Perinatal
Birth asphyxia
Maternal infection

Postnatal
Head trauma and hypoxia
Meningitis
Intentional injury

Box 2. Clinical Features of Cerebral Palsy[3,11]

Early clinical features
Slow to reach motor developmental milestones
   (e.g., roll over, sit, crawl, or walk)
Hypotonia (floppy) or hypertonia (stiff, rigid)
Unusual posture
Absent or abnormal fidgety movements at 3 mo
Development of hand preference earlier than 15 mo

Clinical symptoms related to motor abnormalities
Spasticity
   Stiff or tight muscles
   Increased deep tendon reflexes
   Scissored gait with toe-walking
   May be unilateral (one body side) or bilateral (both
      body sides)
   Upper or lower extremities may be more affected

Dyskinesia
   Slow, uncontrollable writhing movements
   Grimacing or drooling caused by hyperactive
      muscles of the face and tongue

Ataxia
   Unsteady wide-based gait
   Difficulty with precise motions such as writing or
      buttoning a shirt

TREATMENT GOALS

The overall treatment goals for patients with CP are to improve function and quality of life, focusing on increasing activity and participation.[3] Care is family centered, and patient treatment plans are individualized and comprehensive. Plans incorporate several components, including physical and behavioral therapy, drug therapy, surgery, and mechanical aids. Drug therapy focuses on managing spasticity and other issues related to the motor aspects of the disorder. Supportive care concerns (e.g., low BMD) also benefit from pharmacotherapy.

TREATMENT OF SPASTICITY

Specific treatment objectives for spasticity are to maximize active function, ease caregiving, relieve pain, and decrease or prevent contractures.[20] First, patients should be assessed for muscle weakness and strength. If weakness is present, it is important to determine whether spasticity is actually helping with function (e.g., with weight bearing or a caregiver's ability to transfer).[20,21] In these patients, treatments should be carefully monitored for worsening weakness and counterproductive effects on function. Second, nonspastic causes of pain and poor positioning should be resolved before other treatments are initiated.[21] Once these issues are addressed, nonpharmacologic management through physical therapy or orthotics is optimized. Regular stretching exercises of affected limbs are prescribed to maintain range of motion and prevent contractures.[20] Typically, caregivers are taught and encouraged to perform these exercises. For patients with unilateral spasticity, constraint-induced movement therapy is a

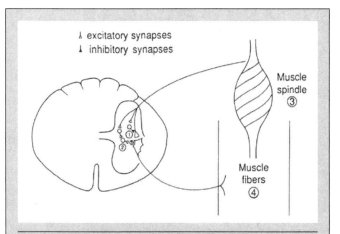

Figure 1. Schematic of presumed sites of action for drugs used to treat generalized spasticity: (1) Clonazepam and diazepam facilitate γ-aminobutyric acid (GABA)-A–mediated presynaptic inhibition; (2) baclofen inhibits activity of polysynaptic reflexes by GABA-B receptor activation; (3) tizanidine acts on α_2-adrenergic receptors; and (4) dantrolene reduces the sensitivity of peripheral intramuscular receptors and reduces release of calcium ions from the sarcoplasmic reticulum, which thus weakens muscle contraction.

Reprinted with permission from: Dietz V, Young R. The syndrome of spastic paresis. In: Brandt T, Caplan L, Dichgans J, et al., eds. Neurological Disorders. Course and Treatment, 2nd ed. San Diego: Academic Press, 2003:1247-57.

rehabilitation option. For example, in a patient with unilateral upper-extremity spasticity, the arm with the greater function is constrained to force the use of the lesser-functioning arm.[22] Ankle-foot orthoses are commonly used to maintain proper foot position and decrease the propensity to toe-walk.[20]

After physical management is maximized, pharmacologic therapy for spasticity is considered. Treatment options include drugs for generalized or localized spasticity. Although not fully elucidated, many spasticity symptoms result from an upper motor neuron lesion causing disinhibition of spinal reflexes or the failure of reciprocal inhibition.[23] Drug effects are aimed at altering these abnormalities. Figure 1 shows the proposed mechanisms of action for the drugs most commonly used to treat generalized spasticity, including the following: oral clonazepam, diazepam, baclofen, tizanidine, dantrolene, and intrathecal baclofen. Botulinum toxin type A blocks acetylcholine release at the neuromuscular junction and is used for localized (focal) spasticity.[3]

Choice of an antispastic drug is often based on experience and trial and error versus evidence-based medicine, particularly with oral medications. Studies using these agents tend to be older, did not use outcomes measures for function or rigorous study design, and were conducted primarily in an adult population.[20] The Quality Standards Subcommittee of the American Academy of Neurology (AAN) and the Practice Committee of the Child Neurology Society addressed these limitations in a practice parameter published in 2010 and reaffirmed in 2013. This parameter evaluates the evidence basis for antispasticity treatments in children and adolescents with CP.[24] In 2012, the National Institute for Health and Care Excellence (NICE) in the United Kingdom published a guideline on managing spasticity in individuals younger than 19 years. It includes recommendations regarding oral drugs, botulinum toxin type A, and intrathecal baclofen.[25] Both resources support diazepam for generalized spasticity (particularly short-term use) and botulinum toxin type A for focal spasticity. The conclusions on baclofen (both oral and intrathecal) are less consistent. The AAN practice parameter finds insufficient data to support or refute its use for generalized spasticity. In contrast, the NICE guideline recommends oral baclofen for generalized spasticity, particularly for sustained effect. It also supports intrathecal baclofen when generalized spasticity is poorly controlled with noninvasive treatments. In practice, baclofen is commonly used concordant with the NICE guideline. The AAN practice parameter provides additional recommendations for dantrolene (insufficient evidence to support or refute use) and tizanidine (may be considered) for generalized spasticity. Table 2 summarizes the AAN practice parameter and the NICE guideline conclusions and recommendations. The following sections review the individual drug therapies in detail.

DIAZEPAM AND CLONAZEPAM

Diazepam, a benzodiazepine, has been used to treat spasticity since the 1960s and is probably effective for short-term management when spasticity causes pain, muscle spasm, or functional disability.[20,24,25] Clonazepam is another benzodiazepine used as an antispastic agent. Their effects on spasticity are mediated through γ-aminobutyric acid (GABA), specifically by increasing the affinity of GABA for GABA$_A$ receptors, resulting in presynaptic inhibition and reduced monosynaptic and polysynaptic reflexes.[26] Both diazepam and clonazepam have anticonvulsant activity, which may provide added benefit in patients with an accompanying seizure disorder. Clonazepam, in particular, has indications as a treatment for absence seizures and myoclonus.

Sedation is the most common, often dose-limiting, adverse effect of the benzodiazepines when they are used for spasticity.[26] However, for patients with insomnia, the benzodiazepines may aid with sleep difficulties if dosed at night. Other adverse effects that limit long-term use include weakness, sialorrhea, and ataxia.[24]

Diazepam and clonazepam are given orally or enterally for spasticity. They are considered long-acting benzodiazepines, with elimination half-lives of up to 48 hours for diazepam

and 60 hours for clonazepam in adults and faster rates in children.[27] Long-acting benzodiazepines are considered to have a decreased risk of withdrawal, but this risk is a known concern with both agents. Because of this risk, abrupt discontinuation should be avoided after prolonged use, and, if possible, intravenous or rectal diazepam should be substituted if oral or enteral cessation becomes necessary.[24,25]

The benzodiazepines should be initiated at a low dose and titrated. Diazepam should be given as a bedtime dose; if response is inadequate, then the dose should be increased or a daytime dose added.[25] The lowest effective maintenance dose should be given to minimize daytime sedation. If a patient's response to diazepam is unsatisfactory at 4–6 weeks of therapy, combined therapy with oral baclofen can be tried. If a patient has a clinical benefit to treatment, then therapy should be reevaluated at least every 6 months.[25] Diazepam is available for oral administration in tablets, a solution, and

Table 2. Evidence-Based Conclusions and Recommendations on Antispasticity Drug Therapy in Children and Adolescents with CP[24,25]

Drug	AAN Practice Parameter Conclusions	AAN Practice Parameter Recommendations	NICE Guideline Recommendations
Generalized Spasticity			
Baclofen (intrathecal)	Inadequate data on continuous intrathecal baclofen as antispasticity treatment; CSF leaks, seromas, catheter-related complications, and wound infections occur often and milder complications occur less often	Insufficient evidence to support or refute use for spasticity (U)[a]	Consider continuous pump administration if, despite use of noninvasive treatments, spasticity or dystonia is causing pain, muscle spasms, or difficulties with posture, function, or self-care (typically GMFCS level IV or V)
Baclofen (oral)	Conflicting evidence regarding effectiveness to reduce spasticity and improve function; some patients have systemic toxicity	Insufficient evidence to support or refute use for spasticity or to improve motor function (U)	Consider if spasticity is contributing to discomfort or pain, muscle spasms, or functional disability. Oral baclofen may help sustain long-term effect
Dantrolene (oral)	Conflicting evidence regarding effectiveness to reduce spasticity; weakness, drowsiness, and irritability are common adverse effects	Insufficient evidence to support or refute use for spasticity (U)	
Diazepam (oral)	Probably effective short-term therapy for spasticity; improved motor function not addressed; ataxia and drowsiness were adverse effects in most studies	Consider a short-term antispasticity treatment (B); insufficient evidence to support or refute use to improve motor function (U)	Consider if spasticity is contributing to discomfort or pain, muscle spasms, or functional disability. Oral diazepam may be useful if a rapid effect is desired
Tizanidine (oral)	Possibly effective spasticity treatment with no toxicity in one small study	May be considered for treatment of spasticity (C); insufficient evidence to support or refute use to improve motor function (U)	
Localized Spasticity			
Botulinum toxin type A	Effective treatment to reduce spasticity in upper and lower extremities; conflicting evidence on functional improvement; generally safe, but severe generalized weakness may occur	For localized/segmental spasticity in upper or lower extremities with CP that warrant therapy, should be offered as an effective and generally safe treatment (A); insufficient evidence to support or refute use to improve motor function (U)	Consider for focal spasticity of the upper limb that impedes fine motor function, the lower limb if impedes gross motor function or if focal limb spasticity compromises care and hygiene, causes pain, disturbs sleep, impedes tolerance of other treatments or causes cosmetic concerns. Consider a trial for focal dystonia that seriously impairs posture or function or causes pain

[a]Classification of recommendations: A = established effective for the given condition in the specified population (requires two or more class I studies), B = probably effective for the given condition in the specified population (requires one class I study or two consistent class II studies), C = possibly effective for the given condition in the specified population (requires one class II study or two consistent class III studies), U = data inadequate or conflicting and treatment is unproved, given current knowledge.

AAN = American Academy of Neurology; CP = cerebral palsy; CSF = cerebrospinal fluid; NICE = National Institute for Health and Care Excellence.

a liquid concentrate for oral use. Clonazepam is available in tablets and orally disintegrating tablets. Although the clonazepam orally disintegrating tablets have increased dosing and administration options for pediatric patients, a compounded oral liquid must sometimes be used.[28] Table 3 lists doses and available products for diazepam and clonazepam.

Table 3. Doses and Formulations for Oral Administration of Antispasticity Drugs

Drug	Oral Dose	Formulations[27,29,36]
Benzodiazepines		
Clonazepam	Infant and child (noted for seizure)[27] **< 10 yr or 30 kg** Initial: 0.01–0.03 mg/kg/day divided as 2–3 doses/day (max initial 0.05 mg/kg/day); ↑ by ≤ 0.5 mg every 3rd day Maintenance: 0.1–0.2 mg/kg/day divided into 3 doses/day (max 0.2 mg/kg/day) **≥ 10 yr (30 kg) or adolescent** Initial: 0.01–0.05 mg/kg/day divided as 2–3 doses/day (max initial 0.5 mg TID); may ↑ by 0.5–1 mg every 3rd to 7th day Maintenance: 0.05–0.2 mg/kg/day divided as 2–3 doses/day (max 20 mg/day)	0.5-, 1-, and 2-mg tablets 0.125-, 0.25-, 0.5-, 1-, and 2-mg ODT Extemporaneous formulation[27] 0.1 mg/mL suspension
Diazepam	**Child** 0.01–0.3 mg/kg/day divided as 2–4 doses/day Low-dose fixed dosing < 8.5 kg: 0.5–1 mg at bedtime 8.5–15 kg: 1–2 mg at bedtime **≥ 5 yr or adolescent** Fixed dosing–Initial: 1.25 mg TID; may titrate to 5 mg QID	2-, 5-, and 10-mg tablets 1 mg/mL oral solution 5 mg/mL oral concentrate
Miscellaneous		
Baclofen	**Child** ≥ 4 mo–< 2 yr: Initial: 2.5 mg every 8 hr[33] Maintenance: 10–20 mg/day in divided doses every 8 hr[27] Max: 40 mg/day in divided doses[27] **2–7 yr** Initial: 5 mg every 8 hr[33] Maintenance: 20–40 mg/day in divided doses every 8 hr[27] Max: 60 mg/day in divided doses[27] **≥ 8 yr** Initial: 5 mg every 8 hr[33] Maintenance: 30–40 mg/day in divided doses every 8 hr[27] Max: 60–80 mg/day in divided doses[27] Titrate dose at 3- to 7-day intervals to effective dose[27] **Adult**[27] Initial: 5 mg TID; increase 5 mg/dose every 3 days Max: 80 mg/day in divided doses	5-, 10- and 20-mg tablets 1 mg/mL solution Extemporaneous formulations[27] 5 mg/mL; 10 mg/mL
Dantrolene	**Child ≥ 5 yr and adolescents < 50 kg**[27] Initial 0.5 mg/kg/dose QD for 7 days; then ↑ to 0.5 mg/kg/dose TID for 7 days; then ↑ to 1 mg/kg/dose TID for 7 days; then ↑ to 2 mg/kg/dose TID **Patient weight ≥ 50 kg** Initial 25 mg QD for 7 days; then ↑ to 25 mg TID for 7 days; then ↑ to 50 mg TID for 7 days; then ↑ to 100 mg TID (max 400 mg/day) Titrate dose to effect; if no benefit with increased dose, decrease to previous lower dose	25-, 50-, and 100-mg capsules Extemporaneous formulation[27] 5 mg/mL
Tizanidine	Limited information available in pediatric patients **Child to 15 yr**[30] 0.05 mg/kg/day Initial 2–< 10 yr: 1 mg/day given at bedtime[33] Initial ≥ 10 yr: 2 mg/day given at bedtime[33] **Adult**[29] Initial: 2 mg/day, may repeat at 6- to 8-hr interval, maximum three doses/day Gradually titrate dose by 2–4 mg/dose with 1–4 days between increases Maximum: 16 mg/dose; 36 mg/day	2-, 4-, and 6-mg capsules 2- and 4-mg tablets

↑ = increase; max = maximum; ODT = orally disintegrating tablet; QD = once daily; QID = four times daily; TID = three times daily.

TIZANIDINE

Tizanidine is a newer oral agent with effectiveness for spasticity primarily in adults with multiple sclerosis or a spinal cord injury.[26] Information is limited on its effectiveness in reducing spasticity in children with CP.[24] As an α_2-adrenergic agonist, tizanidine can reduce muscle tone through the hyperpolarization of motor neurons, with a subsequent decrease in excitability. Tizanidine also has antinociceptive effects mediated through substance P. This ability to reduce pain may contribute to its benefits on tone.[26] Tizanidine is extensively metabolized in the liver. Cytochrome P450 1A2 is the primary enzyme for metabolism, and the potential for drug interactions should be assessed when tizanidine is given with other drugs metabolized through this pathway. Tizanidine is contraindicated with potent inhibitors of the enzyme (e.g., ciprofloxacin or fluvoxamine).[29]

Sedation, hypotension, asthenia, dry mouth, dizziness, hallucinations, and hepatotoxicity are adverse effects in adults.[24] Withdrawal symptoms, including rebound hypertension, have occurred with abrupt discontinuation. Patients taking high doses for long periods or taking concomitant narcotics should have the dosage decreased slowly if discontinuation is desired.[29] Initiating tizanidine as a single daily dose at bedtime may minimize sedation effects on daily function. Dosage is then titrated by adding doses throughout the day. Titration may also help avoid nausea and vomiting in patients.[26] Spasticity was significantly reduced using the Ashworth scale in 10 children given tizanidine at 0.05 mg/kg/day for 6 months compared with 30 children given placebo.[30] Larger studies are needed to determine the optimal dosage in the pediatric population. Tizanidine is available as tablets and capsules. When tizanidine is given with food, the extent of absorption is increased for both tablets and capsules, but to a greater degree with the tablet formulation. Peak plasma concentrations and time to peak are also altered and differ.[29] Pediatric dosing is limited as well by the lack of a commercial or extemporaneous liquid formulation, but the capsules can be opened and the contents sprinkled on applesauce. This administration method increases the peak and extent of absorption and decreases the time to peak concentration.[29] Table 3 summarizes the oral dose and formulation information for tizanidine.

DANTROLENE

Dantrolene is distinct among oral drugs used for spasticity, with a mechanism of action having direct effects on skeletal muscle. Dantrolene inhibits the release of calcium at the sarcoplasmic reticulum, resulting in muscle weakness.[20] Because of its peripheral mechanism, dantrolene may be helpful in patients whose spasticity results from a traumatic brain injury. However, conflicting results on the effectiveness of dantrolene led the AAN practice parameter to conclude that evidence was insufficient to support or refute its use for spasticity in children with CP.[24]

Dantrolene is also limited by its adverse effect profile. Although its therapeutic effects occur outside the central nervous system, dantrolene is often associated with diffuse weakness.[20] Drowsiness and irritability are additional common adverse effects in children with CP.[24] Dantrolene is associated with hepatoxicity. In one series, the risk of fatal hepatic disease was increased in women older than 35 years, patients receiving higher daily dosages, and patients with a diagnosis of multiple sclerosis.[31] Although studies of dantrolene for spasticity in children with CP did not report hepatotoxicity, children being initiated on therapy should undergo baseline and periodic liver function test monitoring.[24] Dantrolene should be avoided in patients receiving additional hepatotoxic therapies.

Dantrolene is extensively metabolized in the liver and has an active metabolite, 5-hydroxy dantrolene. It has potential for interactions with drugs metabolized through the cytochrome P450 3A4 enzyme.[27] Therapeutic benefit for spasticity may take several days for onset, and the dose is titrated to effect at 7-day intervals. When no advantage occurs with a dosage increase, the dose should be lowered to minimize toxicity.[27] Dantrolene is commercially available in capsules that may be opened and mixed with juice or liquid. Extemporaneous oral liquids may be prepared, but these formulations are limited by their complexity in preparation or short time to expiration.[32]

BACLOFEN

Baclofen is a GABA agonist used to treat spasticity by oral and intrathecal administration. Baclofen crosses the blood-brain barrier and binds to $GABA_B$ receptors in laminae I–IV of the spinal cord. It appears to block both monosynaptic and polysynaptic afferents.[26] The mechanism may be as a direct inhibitory neurotransmitter or through hyperpolarization of afferent nerve terminals.[33] Baclofen is rapidly absorbed after oral administration with a bioavailability of 70%–85%. It is primarily eliminated unchanged by the kidneys.[34]

Oral baclofen is often considered the drug of choice for adults with spasticity caused by spinal cord injury.[20] Despite insufficient evidence, baclofen is widely used as a treatment for spasticity in children with CP.[24] The NICE guideline recommends baclofen if spasticity contributes to discomfort, pain, spasms, or functional disability, and it is chosen over diazepam if a sustained long-term effect is needed.[25] Oral baclofen is associated with sedation and confusion, which may lessen after several weeks of therapy.[20] Various oral dosing regimens have been published for baclofen. A modeling study using population pharmacokinetics suggested that dosing could be determined according to body weight (2 mg/kg/day) for children older than 2 years.[34] Baclofen should be initiated at a low dose to avoid serious adverse effects and titrated over about 1 month to achieve the optimal beneficial dose.[25] If a patient's response to baclofen is unsatisfactory at 4–6 weeks of therapy, combined therapy with oral diazepam can be tried. If a patient has a clinical benefit to treatment, therapy should be reevaluated at least every 6 months.[25] If oral baclofen is discontinued, a gradual wean over 1–2 weeks is recommended because abrupt discontinuation may cause withdrawal symptoms, including increased spasms, hallucinations, confusion, fever, and seizures.[24,25,35]

Oral baclofen has historically been commercially available as tablets. In September 2019, the U.S. Food and Drug Administration (FDA) granted approval for labeled use of an oral baclofen solution for patients 12 years of age and older.[36] Until this product becomes readily available, baclofen may still be extemporaneously compounded into a liquid form.[37,38] Because liquid preparations are often compounded in many concentrations, extreme caution should be used to avoid medication errors. Table 3 provides oral dosing and formulation information for oral baclofen.

Intrathecal baclofen is administered through an implantable pump that provides a continuous or variable-rate infusion. The AAN practice parameter concluded that continuous intrathecal baclofen for spasticity in children with CP was not supported by adequate data.[24] A Cochrane Review found limited evidence of short-term efficacy to reduce spasticity in children with CP, but long-term effects were not as clear. The review noted that, although the data required caution, intrathecal baclofen improved gross motor function, ease of care, comfort, and quality of life.[39] A consensus statement from the European Paediatric Neurology Society reviewed the efficacy of intrathecal baclofen and stated that reduced spasticity is best established in patients with severe spasticity in the lower limbs consistent with GMFCS levels IV–V.[40] Reduced spasticity occurs in the upper limbs, but to a lesser extent.[40] The NICE guideline recommends continuous pump–administered intrathecal baclofen if, despite noninvasive treatment, spasticity or dystonia causes pain, muscle spasms, or difficulties in posture, function, or self-care (or ease of care by parents or other providers).[25] Those most likely to benefit are individuals with GMFCS level III, IV, or V and bilateral spasticity affecting the upper and lower limbs.[25]

Although patients have no weight limitations to be considered candidates for therapy, children should have sufficient body mass to allow implantation of the pump, which is about the size of a hockey puck.[20] A local or systemic intercurrent infection is a contraindication for treatment with intrathecal baclofen through a continuous pump. Additional potential complications are certain coexisting medical conditions (e.g., uncontrolled epilepsy or a coagulopathy), previous spinal fusion procedure, malnutrition, and risk of respiratory failure because of a pulmonary disorder.[25]

Figure 2 shows an implanted intrathecal baclofen pump. Because intrathecal baclofen is delivered directly to the subarachnoid space around the spinal cord, the required dosage is less than 1% of an oral dose, which decreases sedation risk.[20] Children and adults (mean age 16 years) administered intrathecal baclofen at doses of 70–1395 mcg/day had cerebrospinal fluid concentrations of 0.2–20 mcg/mL from an intrathecal catheter aspirate.[41] These concentrations did not statistically correlate with the dose of baclofen. In contrast, plasma concentrations of baclofen were at or below the limit of detection (10 ng/mL) in children receiving intrathecal dosages of 77–400 mcg/day in a separate study.[42]

Once selected for therapy, patients and their caregivers should be educated on the treatment, required surgical procedure, possible adverse effects, potential pump-related complications, what will be required of them, and protocols for emergency management.[25,40] Before pump implantation, a screening intrathecal dose should be given as a single injection to assess patient response and determine an initial dose.[25,27] However, this assessment does not reliably predict

functional improvement.[40] Dosage titration is recommended when a patient starts continuous intrathecal infusion to minimize adverse effects.[40] With time, some pumps can be programmed to vary the infusion rate to accommodate the patient's activities throughout the day.[20] Box 3 provides dosing information for intrathecal baclofen.

Careful monitoring by health care professionals experienced with intrathecal baclofen and the infusion device is essential. Patients typically need to have the pump's reservoir transcutaneously refilled by their provider at 2- to 6-month intervals. Pump and battery function should be monitored, and the infusion device should be replaced before the battery expires.[40]

Abrupt withdrawal after unexpected discontinuation and unintentional overdose are challenging complications with intrathecal baclofen. Potential causes of discontinuation include an empty pump reservoir, catheter problems such as kinking or breakage, and pump failure.[20] Withdrawal symptoms consist of elevated temperature, altered mental status, exaggerated rebound spasticity, and muscle rigidity.[43] Severe itching, priapism in males, agitation, tachycardia, hypotension or labile blood pressure, and seizures have been reported.[20] Rarely, symptoms progress to rhabdomyolysis, multi-organ system failure, and death.[43] Early recognition and reinstitution of therapy are essential to manage withdrawal. Benzodiazepines and life support may be needed.[20]

Signs of intrathecal baclofen overdose include excessive hypotonia, drowsiness or decreased arousal, lightheadedness, respiratory depression, and seizures. Coma can occur with acute, massive overdoses.[43] If toxicity is suspected, the patient should be taken to the hospital immediately for assessment

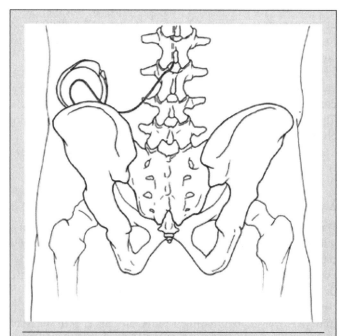

Figure 2. Schematic of an intrathecal baclofen pump implanted in the anterolateral abdominal wall tunneled subcutaneously around the patient to enter the spinal canal.

Reprinted with permission from: Miracle AC, Fox MA, Ayyangar RN, et al. Imaging evaluation of intrathecal baclofen pump-catheter systems. Am J Neuroradiol 2011;32:1158-64.

and emptying of the pump reservoir. Overdose has generally been related to pump malfunction, inadvertent subcutaneous injection, or dosing error.[43] A careful appraisal of the device's programming is an important part of the evaluation. To lessen the risk of complications, patients should be educated on activities that may alter infusion flow. Examples are exposure to considerable changes in altitude or temperatures, excessive twitching or stretching, twiddling with the pump or catheter through the skin, and strong electromagnetic interference.[44]

The potential for infections associated with intrathecal baclofen therapy must be monitored. Infections can occur in the pump area, or, more rarely, meningitis can develop.[24] An analysis of complications in patients treated with intrathecal baclofen showed serious infections in 9.3% of patients. Infection risk was greater when the pump was placed subcutaneously

versus under the fascia. In the subcutaneous group, the probability of infection increased more quickly within the first month after implantation and then increased more slowly.[45]

BOTULINUM TOXIN TYPE A

Botulinum toxin type A is recommended to treat focal spasticity in children and adolescents if the spasticity impedes fine motor function of the upper limb, impedes gross motor function of the lower limb, is a source of pain, disturbs sleep, impairs treatment tolerance, compromises care or hygiene, or causes cosmetic concerns to the patient.[25] Botulinum toxin type A is one of seven serotypes of neurotoxins produced by *Clostridium botulinum*. It inhibits the release of acetylcholine from nerve terminals at the neuromuscular junction, a step critical to initiate muscle response. This inhibition results in a flaccid muscle paralysis and can provide a selective, reversible effect on agonist muscles that can be used to balance forces across joints. Over the following 3–12 months, normal synaptic transmission through acetylcholine release resumes within the neuromuscular junction.[46] Serotype B is available as a pharmaceutical product, but its clinical use is less well established for spasticity because it has a shorter duration of action and an increased rate of adverse effects in children with CP.[47] In the United States, three preparations of botulinum toxin type A and one preparation of botulinum toxin type B are commercially available. In 2009, the FDA issued a safety alert that included a recommendation to modify the established drug names of the botulinum toxin products to emphasize their individual potencies and prevent medication errors.[48] Table 4 lists the revised drug and trade names for botulinum toxin types A and B and product availability.

Licensed use of botulinum toxin products for spasticity varies greatly between countries and is restricted to specific preparations, indications, and dose limits.[49] The FDA has approved labeled uses for abobotulinumtoxinA to treat lower limb spasticity in pediatric patients beginning at age 2 years and upper and lower limb spasticity in adults.[50] OnabotulinumtoxinA has an FDA indication to treat lower and upper limb spasticity in patients 2 years and older although its use for lower limb spasticity has an exclusion for pediatric patients with CP.[51] Although botulinum toxin was unlicensed when the European Paediatric Neurology Society published a consensus statement on it for children with CP, the statement noted that individualized use on the basis of dose, dilution, indication, and muscle group(s) represents appropriate treatment when it is consistent with clinical experience.[49] Specific spasticity indications for botulinum neurotoxin injection for children with CP are recommended by AAN.[52] One recommendation is that injection of botulinum neurotoxin in the calf muscles be offered as treatment for equinus varus, a foot anomaly in which the heel turns inward, and the foot is plantar flexed. Botulinum neurotoxin should be considered a therapeutic option for adductor spasticity, pain control in children undergoing adductor-lengthening surgery, and upper-extremity spasticity.[52]

Box 3. Intrathecal Baclofen Dosing[27,43]

Screening dose for children age at least 4 yr and adolescents: 50 mcg (very small patients 25 mcg) intrathecally with observation for 4–8 hr

- If initial response is less than desired, a second dose of 75 mcg intrathecally may be given after 24 hr with observation for 4–8 hr
- If response is still inadequate, a final dose of 100 mcg intrathecally may be given 24 hr later
- Patients who are unresponsive to the 100-mcg dose are not candidates for an implanted pump for infusion

Initial total daily dose for infusion and titration: Double-screening dose that gave positive effect and administer over 24 hr

- If the efficacy of the screening dose lasted > 8 hr, the initial dose should be the screening dose administered over 24 hr
- After the first 24 hr, the daily dose can be increased slowly by 5% – 15% increments once every 24 hours (usual 50 mcg inpatient, 25 mcg outpatient) until desired clinical response

Daily maintenance dose by patient age:

- 4–12 yr: Average, 274 mcg/day (range 24–1199 mcg/day)
- > 12 yr and adults: Most common, 90–703 mcg/day (range 22–1400 mcg/day)

Table 4. Botulinum Toxin Preparations

Drug Name	Trade Name	Product Availability (unit vials)
AbobotulinumtoxinA	Dysport[a]	300 and 500
IncobotulinumtoxinA	Xeomin[b]	50, 100, and 200
OnabotulinumtoxinA	Botox[c]	100 and 200
	Botox Cosmetic[c]	50 and 100
RimabotulinumtoxinB	Myobloc[d]	2500, 5000, and 10,000

[a]Ipsen Biopharm, Wrexham, UK; [b]Merz Pharmaceuticals, Frankfurt, Germany; [c]Allergan, Dublin, Ireland; [d]Solstice Neurosciences, Louisville, KY.

Botulinum toxin products are distinct with respect to molecular structure, method used to determine biologic activity, and manufacturing process. AbobotulinumtoxinA is contraindicated in individuals with a milk protein allergy because the product may contain trace amounts of the proteins.[50] The products are not interchangeable, and fixed-dose conversion ratios are not applicable in the treatment of spasticity in children with CP.[49] Dosage is individualized per patient. The European Paediatric Neurology Society recommends calculations for the following: "(1) total units per treatment session, (2) total units per kg body weight per session, (3) units per muscle, (4) units per injection site, (5) units per kg body weight per muscle."[49] Box 4 lists patient and muscle factors to consider when dosing botulinum toxin products. The clinical effects of botulinum toxin A typically last 3–6 months, and biochemical and imaging studies have shown effects persisting greater than 12 months.[47] An interval of at least 12 weeks should be maintained between dosing.[27] Twelve-month intervals have been shown to be as effective as 4-month intervals and may be preferred to reduce the risk of possible muscle atrophy or fibrosis.[47]

The most common adverse effects with botulinum toxin type A products in children with CP are injection-site pain, excessive weakness, unsteadiness and increased falls, and fatigue.[24] Common adverse effects of botulinum toxin A in pediatric patients include upper respiratory tract infections, influenza, cough, and fever.[50,51] Botulinum toxin type A should not be recommended if patients have severe muscle weakness, had a previous allergy or reaction to it, or are receiving aminoglycosides. Additional cautions include use in children with bleeding disorders, generalized spasticity, fixed muscle contractures, and significant bony deformities.[25] Strategies to manage injection site reactions include careful injection into the target muscle, using a minimum volume, and slowing the rate of injection.[27] Accurate localization of muscles for injection is aided by electromyography, electrical stimulation, and ultrasonography.

Box 4. Factors to Consider When Dosing Botulinum Toxin Products for Spasticity in Children with Cerebral Palsy[46,49]

Patient Factors
Age
Severity of cerebral palsy
Predominance of movement disorder
Degree of joint deformity
General health
Accompanying impairments
Experience from previous injections

Muscle Factors
Muscle mass
Number of muscles to be injected
Target muscle strength
Activity of muscle
Dynamic vs. fibrotic type
Motor end plate distribution in muscle

Systemic toxicity from the spread of botulinum toxin effects from the injection site has been reported. The 2009 FDA safety alert addressed this concern for pediatric and adult patients. For pediatric patients, the postmarketing case reports were primarily related to its use for spasticity in children with CP.[53] Specifically, the FDA stated: "The reported cases of spread of botulinum toxin effect from beyond the injection site were described as botulism or involved symptoms including difficulty breathing, difficulty swallowing, muscular weakness, drooping eyelids, constipation, aspiration pneumonia, speech disorder, facial drooping, double vision, and respiratory depression."[53]

Cases involving ventilator support and fatality were reported. On the basis of the postmarketing evaluation, the FDA recommended that health care professionals who use botulinum toxin products do the following: (1) recognize that dosage strength expressed in units is different between products and that doses expressed in units are not interchangeable between products; (2) be alert to and educate patients and caregivers about potential adverse effects because of the distant spread of botulinum toxin from the injection site; (3) understand that these adverse events have occurred as early as several hours and as late as several weeks after injection; and (4) advise patients to seek immediate medical attention if they develop any of these symptoms.[53] The FDA safety alert has resulted in revised product names, labeling changes including a black box warning, and implementation of a risk evaluation and mitigation strategy with a medication guide for all products to be given to patients and caregivers. Additional counseling should include reviewing goals related to the treatment and the importance of combining the treatment with recommended physical therapy and orthoses.[3,46] Follow-up assessments should occur 6–12 weeks after injections to assess tone, range of movement, and motor function and over 12–26 weeks after injections to evaluate need for further therapy.[25]

SURGICAL TREATMENTS

Orthopedic surgery and selective dorsal rhizotomy are additional treatment options for spasticity associated with CP.[25] Selective dorsal rhizotomy involves cutting selected sensory (afferent) nerve roots between L2 and S1.[3] This procedure may be considered to improve walking in children and young people in the GMFCS level II and III categories.[25]

TREATMENT OF DROOLING

Drooling is involuntary loss of saliva from the mouth. *Sialorrhea* is often used as a synonym for drooling, referring to excessive flow of saliva. Sialorrhea may be caused by saliva overproduction. However, most patients with CP produce normal amounts of saliva but have difficulty managing it in the oral cavity.[54] Drooling is described as *anterior* if the saliva spills from the mouth and as *posterior* if it pools in the pharynx, posing an aspiration risk. Drooling is considered normal in children up to age 2 years; however, physiologic episodes occur later, particularly with teething.[55]

In a study of children with CP attending special schools, 58% drooled, with 33% described as having severe drooling.[56]

Drooling can negatively affect social interactions, interfere with speech development and communication, and cause skin breakdown around the mouth and chin. Drooling increases the difficulty of oral hygiene for patients and caregivers. In an assessment of participation issues in adolescents with CP, parents identified oral hygiene as their second-highest ranked problem when the adolescent could not communicate.[57]

When a patient or parent presents with concerns about drooling, assessment should include a thorough history, speech pathology examination of the oral region, dental examination if the patient is older than 3 years, and questionnaire to determine severity.[54] The history should determine whether there is evidence of chronic aspiration, gastroesophageal reflux, feeding difficulties, or medications such as cholinergic drugs that could be contributing to the drooling. If present, these problems should be addressed.[55]

In general, nonpharmacologic management is the first step to treat drooling. Patient and caregiver education on oral hygiene, attention to posture and positioning, and oral motor skills training may all provide benefit.[55] After implementing these measures and addressing any dental issues, pharmacotherapy may be justified. Drug treatments include anticholinergic agents and botulinum toxin type A products. Surgical management is another treatment possibility, usually for more severe cases.[55]

Glycopyrrolate and scopolamine are the anticholinergic drugs most commonly used to treat sialorrhea. Their mechanism of action for drooling is to decrease the volume of saliva produced by blocking the cholinergic muscarinic receptors in the salivary glands. However, they lack selectivity and are associated with other undesirable anticholinergic effects such as flushing, urinary retention, and constipation. Glycopyrrolate has the most available evidence on efficacy and a relatively favorable adverse effect profile.[58] A placebo-controlled, double-blind, dose-ranging, crossover study investigated glycopyrrolate in 39 pediatric outpatients with neurodevelopmental conditions and troublesome drooling.[59] Most of the patients had CP and were age 4–19 years. A 4-week dose titration was followed by 4 weeks of maintenance therapy with a 2-week washout before crossover. In the 27 children who completed the study, drooling was significantly reduced according to a 9-point scale. Adverse effects occurred in 69% of the children during the glycopyrrolate arm; seven patients were receiving glycopyrrolate when they withdrew from the study because of an adverse effect. The most common adverse effects were behavioral changes, constipation, excessive oral dryness, and urinary retention.[59] Glycopyrrolate is available in a tablet formulation for oral administration and has FDA-approved labeling for a liquid formulation for chronic severe drooling in children age 3–16 years with neurologic disorders.[60] Dosing recommendations for the oral liquid are to initiate therapy at 0.02 mg/kg/dose three times daily with increases of 0.02 mg/kg/dose at 5- to 7-day intervals, if needed. The maximal recommended dose is 0.1 mg/kg/dose not to exceed 1.5–3 mg. Contraindications are medical conditions that preclude anticholinergic therapy, and patients taking solid oral dosage forms of potassium chloride as glycopyrrolate may extend the time the potassium chloride is in the gastrointestinal tract, increasing the risk of gastrointestinal irritation.[60]

Scopolamine is administered transdermally to treat sialorrhea. Transderm Scop (GlaxoSmithKline, Warren, NJ) is commercially available as a 1.5-mg patch that delivers 1 mg of scopolamine over 3 days.[61] Scopolamine is licensed for adults to prevent motion sickness and for nausea and vomiting associated with recovery from anesthesia and surgery. The patch is placed on a hairless area behind the ear with alternating ear sites within the 3-day interval. The patch should not be cut, and hands should be washed thoroughly after placing and discarding.[61] A study evaluated scopolamine for drooling in a placebo-controlled, double-blind, crossover trial.[62] The study enrolled 30 patients with neurodevelopmental disorders and persistent drooling. Each patient received 2 weeks of transdermal scopolamine and placebo with a 1-week washout before crossover. Scopolamine was administered as a 1.5-mg patch changed every 72 hours. Baseline drooling on a 3-point scale was significantly reduced with scopolamine but not with placebo. Four patients discontinued the study because of adverse effects: one patient had irritability, one patient had agitation, and two patients had skin reactions.[62] Another, smaller trial of 10 patients age 5–18 years with neurodevelopmental disorders and moderate to severe drooling had similar results.[63] Scopolamine significantly reduced scores on a 6-point drooling scale compared with placebo. Pupil dilation was noted in two-thirds of the patients receiving scopolamine.[63] Although transdermal scopolamine may be a reasonable treatment option for drooling in older children and adolescents, questions remain whether it is acceptable to use the dosing form in younger patients and as long-term therapy.

Trihexyphenidyl may be an additional anticholinergic treatment option for drooling in patients who have dystonia. A retrospective chart review of 101 patients treated with trihexyphenidyl for dystonia (28.7%), sialorrhea (5.9%), or both (65.4%) found improvement in drooling in 60.4% of patients. Its benefit in these patients may be a result of both anticholinergic effects and improved central motor control of muscles involved in swallowing. In the study, dosage was initiated at a mean dose of 0.095 mg/kg/day divided into two doses and increased by 10%–20% at a minimum interval of 2 weeks to a mean maximum dose of 0.55 mg/kg/day divided into two or three doses daily. Adverse effects were common, occurring in 69.3% of patients, with the most common concerns being constipation, decreased urinary frequency, and behavioral changes.[64]

The Cerebral Palsy Institute developed an international consensus statement on botulinum toxin for adult and pediatric drooling.[54] For this use, botulinum toxin is given by intraglandular injection into the submandibular and parotid salivary glands. None of the botulinum toxin products have a labeled indication for sialorrhea in pediatric patients, but incobotulinumtoxinA and rimabotulinumtoxinB have indications for chronic sialorrhea in adults.[65,66] Botulinum toxin works for drooling by inhibiting the release of acetylcholine from cholinergic nerve endings in the gland, causing a reduced secretion of saliva. According to a review of clinical trials, the consensus statement recommends botulinum toxin type A in patients with significant drooling. This review recommends excluding patients if they have been given botulinum toxin type A for any reason in the previous 3 months;

have antibodies against botulinum toxin type A; or are unfit for sedation or anesthesia.[54]

Eight studies that investigated botulinum toxin to treat drooling in children with CP were reviewed.[67] Various study designs were used, and the investigations included 122 children age 4–18 years as participants. The GMFCS was reported in one-half of the studies, with most children having GMFCS level V (range I–V). OnabotulinumtoxinA was the most selected product for the studies. Although the review authors noted that a specific protocol for use needed validation, they recommended a dose of onabotulinumtoxinA of 2 units/kg (dilution 1 mL/100 units) divided equally between submandibular and parotid glands. They recommended injections under local or general anesthesia, as tolerated by the child.[67]

The consensus paper and the review recommended ultrasound guidance for injection because this approach helps ensure intraglandular delivery versus injection into surrounding tissue.[54,67] Adverse effects related to trauma at the injection site include pain, hematoma, and fever.[67] Temporary swallowing difficulties may occur because of the swelling of the gland, and patients should be observed for at least 2 hours post-injection. A swallowing problem that persists may be caused by the diffusion of botulinum toxin into surrounding muscle tissue. A follow-up with patients and their caregivers in the first week is recommended to assess for eating and drinking difficulties. Moist food or a pureed diet should be given for the first week after injection. It is important to be alert to thickening of the saliva, which can lead to swallowing or respiratory difficulties.[54] As noted in the Treatment of Spasticity section of this chapter, patients must be monitored and counseled regarding adverse effects caused by the systemic spread of botulinum toxin.

TREATMENT OF LOW BMD

Children with CP, particularly with moderate to severe functional classification of CP, are at risk of developing low BMD. The term *osteoporosis* is used cautiously in children, and it is defined in this population as a BMD z-score of less than -2.0 adjusted for age, sex, and body size plus a clinically significant fracture history as follows: two upper-extremity fractures; a vertebral compression fracture; or one lower-extremity fracture.[68] Risk factors for low BMD in patients with CP include immobilization because of surgery or fracture, feeding difficulties, low calcium and vitamin D intake, use of antiepileptic drugs, and previous fracture.[68] Lack of weight-bearing exercise is an additional contributing factor to low BMD.[69]

Table 5 lists recommendations for preventing osteoporosis in children and young people with physical disabilities and

Table 5. Recommendations for Preventing and Treating Osteoporosis in Children and Young People with Physical Disabilities[69]

Therapeutic Goal	Evaluation	Pharmacologic Interventions[a]	Additional Recommendations[a]

Prevention in children and young people with physical disabilities	Blood and urine analysis at baseline and in 6–12 mo for these goals:
	• 25-OH-D concentration in normal to high range (70–100 nmol/L)
	• Calcium/osmolality ratio spot urine in normal range (< 0.25)
		• (C) Calcium supplementation if dietary intake is less than recommended and cannot be increased
		• Recommended intake of elemental calcium:
		    1–3 yr = 500 mg
		    4–8 yr = 800 mg
		    9–18 yr = 1300 mg
		• (C) Consider vitamin D_2/D_3 supplementation of 800–1000 international units/day
			(U) Promote weight-bearing activities
			
			(U) Provide physiotherapy consult

Treatment fragility fractures, bone pain, or both	• Consider laboratory investigation: calcium, phosphate, PTH, alkaline phosphatase, 25-OH-D, creatinine, calcium/osmolality ratio spot urine • Radiograph of symptomatic area to assess for possible fracture • Consider need for lateral spine radiograph to assess for vertebral compression fractures • Consider wrist radiograph for bone age or rachitic changes • Consider DEXA scans of lateral distal femur or whole body; use z-scores adjusted for age, sex, and height	• (C) Ensure adequate calcium and vitamin D intake • (B) Consider bisphosphonates to increase BMD and (C) possibly decrease fracture rate	Refer to bone health specialist

[a]Classification of recommendations: (B) = probably effective for the given condition in the specified population (requires one class I study or two consistent class II studies); (C) = possibly effective for the given condition in the specified population (requires one class II study or two consistent class III studies); (U) = data inadequate or conflicting and treatment is unproved given current knowledge.
25-OH-D = 25-hydroxyvitamin D; BMD = bone mineral density; DEXA = dual energy x-ray absorptiometry; PTH = parathyroid hormone.

treatment of osteoporosis as defined by fragility fractures, bone pain, or both.[69] Important steps in prevention are reducing modifiable risk factors; ensuring optimal nutritional intake, particularly of calcium and vitamin D; promoting weight-bearing activities; and providing a physiotherapy consult. Class III control studies of calcium and vitamin D supplementation have benefited BMD, but further research is needed to determine their benefit in preventing fractures.[69] Measuring 25-hydroxyvitamin D blood concentrations helps determine whether a patient requires supplemental or treatment doses of vitamin D. Supplementation with vitamin D at 800–1000 international units/day is endorsed for patients with CP to maintain vitamin D concentrations greater than 50 nmol/L.[68,70] Bisphosphonates used with calcium and vitamin D supplementation are a pharmacologic treatment option for osteoporosis in children with CP if they have had a vertebral fracture and/or have a low BMD and two or more long-bone fractures.[71] For patients with CP, biphosphonates increase BMD and possibly lower fracture rate.[69] Evidence for their use is from short-term trials of small numbers of children, and long-term adverse effects, most notably on bone health and structure, are unknown.[70] Thus, they should only be considered after a child has a fragility fracture, and their most judicious use is in patients who have had repeated fractures even after calcium and vitamin D therapy has been optimized.[70] Studies have primarily used intravenous pamidronate, given three or four times a year.[70] Oral alendronate and risedronate have been investigated as treatment of osteopenia in children with CP, but current evidence for their use is considered insufficient.[68] The need for patients to stand or sit for administration of oral bisphosphonates, followed by an upright posture for 30 minutes, may limit their future use in young children and in patients with more severe CP. When a bisphosphonate is initiated, yearly evaluation of bone density is recommended and therapy should be discontinued when height-adjusted BMD z-score exceeds +2.0.[71] Treatment for greater than two years is recommended only if there is ongoing fracture or bone pain.[71] Adverse effects of pamidronate included transient flu-like symptoms and hypocalcemia.[70] Acetaminophen and anti-nausea medications can be used to manage acute reactions. Additionally, using a lower initial dose may reduce the risk of these symptoms.[71] Baseline laboratory monitoring recommendations in children include assessing for electrolyte abnormalities (i.e., decreased calcium, phosphate, potassium, and magnesium), serum creatinine, a complete blood cell count, liver function tests, 25-hydroxyvitamin D level, and parathyroid hormone level.[71] Biphosphonates can cross the placenta and potentially disrupt skeletal development; thus, pregnancy is a contraindication to their use.[71] Osteonecrosis of the jaw is a relatively infrequent, but worrisome, adverse effect associated with bisphosphonates. Although this adverse effect has occurred primarily in patients with cancer, patients with CP have a theoretical increased risk if oral hygiene is poor. In addition, the effects of bisphosphonates on dentition development are unknown.[72] Given these concerns, a patient with CP should have a thorough dental assessment and examination before undergoing treatment with a bisphosphonate, with a primary focus on avoiding invasive and emergency dental procedures.[72] Follow-up dental evaluations are recommended at 6- to 12- month intervals.[71]

CONCLUSIONS

Cerebral palsy is a multifaceted disorder in childhood because of motor disabilities and challenging co-impairments. Children with CP should receive quality care through a primary care medical home model with multidisciplinary and community input.[73] Comprehensive treatment plans optimize function, capabilities, quality of life, and aesthetics. Pharmacotherapy is an important component of treatment. For generalized spasticity, oral diazepam and baclofen are often initial treatment choices, as recommended by the NICE guidelines. Diazepam is typically used for short-term management and baclofen for more sustained treatment periods. The pharmacist can be instrumental in helping with dosing and formulation selection for these therapies and educating patients and families about adverse effects, particularly sedation. Pharmacists also play a pivotal role in education when therapeutic options become more complex, such as with an intrathecal baclofen pump for more severe generalized spasticity or botulinum toxin type A for focal spasticity. Overall, a pediatric pharmacist provides valuable support to the medical care provided in the home or community setting, especially as the number and complexity of treatment options for spasticity and other conditions associated with CP increase.

A 4-year-old white boy with a history of cerebral palsy (CP) with spasticity (gross motor function classification system [GMFCS] level III) and epilepsy is brought by his parents to the physical medicine and rehabilitation clinic for a follow-up. His parents are concerned because he has had increased tightness in his legs over the past month and muscle spasms at night that affect his sleep quality. He primarily uses a power wheelchair in the community setting, and his parents feel his comfort has declined in the chair. His parents report that the patient can sit in a regular chair but usually requires support. He can only stand with support. They have observed that his upper-limb strength is better than his lower-limb strength, and they want to work with physical therapy to help him walk short distances with an assistive device.

Medical history: Born at 29 weeks' estimated gestational age as a twin (birth weight 1300 g); CP diagnosed at 18 months because of delay in meeting developmental milestones, spasticity in lower extremities, and magnetic resonance imaging (MRI) that revealed periventricular leukomalacia; epilepsy diagnosed at 10 months, last seizure 1 year ago

Family history: Twin sister died of sepsis in neonatal intensive care

Social history: Lives with parents and 1-year-old sister; attends an early intervention program three times a week

Vital signs: BP 95/55 mm Hg, HR 100 beats/minute, Tmax 97.7°F (36.5°C) (oral), RR 25 breaths/minute, Wt 14.8 kg (10th–15th percentile), Ht 38 inches (25th percentile)

Physical examination:

General appearance: Thin, pale, pleasant boy in no acute distress; currently seated in his power wheelchair

Eyes: Pupils equal round reactive to light and accommodation, extraocular movements intact, sclera white, conjunctiva clear, wears glasses

Ears: Tympanic membranes clear bilaterally, no known auditory deficits

Throat: Mouth is open, can close with command

Neck: No masses, no lymphadenopathy

Pulmonary: No retractions, breath sounds vesicular and equal

Cardiovascular: Regular rate and rhythm, normal S_1, S_2, no murmurs, rubs, or gallop

Abdomen: Soft, no organomegaly, bowel sounds present all quadrants

Musculoskeletal: 5/5 motor strength in both upper limbs, 3/5 motor strength in both lower limbs; lower-extremity spasticity affects hips, hamstrings, and ankles; equinus varus foot deformity present bilaterally, modified Ashworth scale score of 3 in ankle plantar flexors; stood with support on tiptoe

Skin: Dry, intact, no pressure ulcers

Neuro: Sensory function intact to light touch and pinprick

Diet history: Regular diet, with 8 oz of a pediatric nutritional supplement daily; his parents note that he has difficulty chewing at times, that he more easily eats soft, thicker foods (e.g., mashed potatoes), and that mealtime eating can be slow; no history of aspiration

Immunizations: Up to date; received annual influenza vaccine this year

Allergies: No known allergies

Medication history: Oxcarbazepine 150 mg/2.5 mL by mouth twice daily is the only current medication; at age 2 years he received a 3-month course of baclofen 2.5 mg by mouth three times daily, which was discontinued because of increased sedation

Laboratory findings:

Test	Result	Normal Values
Basic Metabolic Panel		
Glucose (mg/dL)	88	60–105
BUN (mg/dL)	10	8–19
Na (mEq/L)	135	135–145
Potassium (mEq/L)	3.9	3.5–5
Cl (mEq/L)	101	95–105
CO_2 (mEq/L)	23	20–28
SCr (mg/dL)	0.3	0.3–0.7
Calcium (mg/dL)	9.5	9–11
PO_4 (mg/dL)	4.3	3.6–5.6
Liver Function Tests		
Total protein (g/dL)	6.5	6–8
Albumin (g/dL)	3.5	3.5–5.5
Total bilirubin (mg/dL)	0.1 L	0.1–1.5
ALT (U/L)	25	10–30
AST (U/L)	18	15–50
ALK (U/L)	200	85–400
Vitamin D Studies		
25-Hydroxyvitamin D (nmol/L)	35	50–250

1. What risk factors for CP does this patient have, and how do his symptoms relate to GMFCS level III?

The patient's most significant risk of CP is related to his prematurity and low birth weight. His MRI evaluation is consistent with periventricular leukomalacia, which is a common neuroimaging finding when CP is diagnosed in children with a history of prematurity. He has an additional risk because his birth was associated with a twin pregnancy. He has spastic CP, the most common motor abnormality type of CP. His seizure disorder, visual impairment, and insomnia are all potential accompanying diagnoses that can lead to additional challenges for a patient with CP. The patient's functioning in relation to his motor abilities is consistent with GMFCS level III. For example, the patient can sit and stand with support, but he needs a power wheelchair in the community setting. His family's goal for him to walk short distances with an assistive device is also consistent with GMFCS level III and should be attainable.

2. What treatment options are most appropriate to address the patient's spasticity, and how should his parents be counseled on this therapy?

The patient's focal spasticity is affecting his lower extremities, particularly the ankle plantar flexor muscles, as evidenced by the modified Ashworth scale score of 3 for those muscles and the presence of the equinus varus foot deformity. The spasticity is impairing his ability to stand and may be the source of his pain and insomnia, which will need to be addressed to meet his family's goal of physical therapy to help him walk short distances with an assistive mobility device. Because the spasticity is focal, treatment options for generalized spasticity are not indicated, especially because the patient could not tolerate baclofen previously. Because the spasticity is causing functional and physical problems including pain, the patient is a candidate for botulinum toxin type A. AbobotulinumtoxinA is approved for lower limb spasticity in children 2 years and older with CP and can be recommended for this patient. His parents will need to be thoroughly educated on the procedures used to administer abobotulinumtoxinA and its common adverse effects, which include injection-site pain, weakness, fatigue, and unsteadiness with increased falls. In studies, abobotulinumtoxinA was associated with upper respiratory infections, but his up-to-date immunizations and receipt of an annual influenza vaccine may lessen this risk. As part of a risk evaluation and mitigation strategy, the parents will receive a medication guide that reviews the risks and effects of distant spread of botulinum toxin from the injection site. The parents should seek immediate care for the patient if he has difficulty breathing or swallowing, aspiration pneumonia, respiratory depression, muscular weakness, eyelid or facial droop, constipation, speech difficulties, or double vision.

3. How would you assess the patient's risk of low bone mineral density (BMD), and what would you recommend to address this risk?

The patient has an increased probability of low BMD, particularly with his moderate CP functional classification at GMFCS level III, likely lack of weight-bearing exercise with use of the power wheelchair, feeding difficulties, and antiepileptic drug therapy with oxcarbazepine. In the clinic today, his serum vitamin D concentration is 35 nmol/L, which is less than the value recommended for patients with CP at 70–100 nmol/L. A calcium/osmolality ratio spot urine should be obtained to further assess his risk of low BMD. To minimize his risk, a thorough diet history should be obtained to ensure adequate nutritional intake, particularly of calcium. He should receive the recommended intake of 800 mg of elemental calcium per day. If this amount cannot be achieved with diet or nutritional supplement intake, he should be initiated on a calcium supplement. With his serum vitamin D concentration at less than the recommended goal, he should be initiated on vitamin D_2 or D_3 at 800–1000 international units/day. The planned increase in physical therapy and weight-bearing activities may also improve his BMD. He should be carefully monitored for fractures, and, if they occur, he may be a candidate for other therapies such as a bisphosphonate.

REFERENCES

1. Rosenbaum P, Paneth N, Leviton A, et al. A report: the definition and classification of cerebral palsy April 2006. Dev Med Child Neurol 2007;49:8-14.

2. Oskoui M, Coutinho F, Dykeman J, et al. An update on the prevalence of cerebral palsy: a systematic review and meta-analysis. Dev Med Child Neurol 2013;55:509-19.

3. Sewell MD, Eastwood DM, Wimalasundera N. Managing common symptoms of cerebral palsy in children. BMJ 2014;349:g5474.

4. Palisano R, Rosenbaum P, Walter S, et al. Development and reliability of a system to classify gross motor function in children with cerebral palsy. Dev Med Child Neurol 1997;39:214-23.

5. Kirby RS, Wingate MS, Van Naarden Braun K, et al. Prevalence and functioning of children with cerebral palsy in four areas of the United States in 2006: a report from the Autism and Developmental Disabilities Monitoring Network. Res Dev Disabil 2011;32:462-9.

6. World Health Organization (WHO). 2002. Towards a common language for functioning, disability and health ICF. Available at www.who.int/classifications/icf/icfbeginnersguide.pdf. Accessed November 12, 2019.

7. Van Haastert IC, Groenendaal F, Uiterwaal CS, et al. Decreasing incidence and severity of cerebral palsy in prematurely born children. J Pediatr 2011;159:86-91.

8. Nelson KB, Blair E. Prenatal factors in singletons with cerebral palsy born at or near term. N Engl J Med 2015;373:946-53.

9. Jelin AC, Salmeen K, Gano D, et al. Perinatal neuroprotection update. F1000Res 2016;5:1939.

10. American College of Obstetricians and Gynecologists Committee on Obstetric Practice and Society for Maternal-Fetal Medicine. Committee opinion 652: magnesium sulfate use in obstetrics. Obstet Gynecol 2016;127:e52-3.

11. National Institute of Neurological Disorders and Stroke, National Institutes of Health. Cerebral palsy: hope through research. Available at www.ninds.nih.gov/disorders/patient-caregiver-education/hope-through-research/cerebral-palsy-hope-through-research. Accessed November 12, 2019.

12. Novak I, Morgan C, Adde L, et al. Early, accurate diagnosis and early intervention in cerebral palsy advances in diagnosis and treatment. JAMA Pediatr. 2017;171:897-907.

13. Sanger TD, Delgado MR, Gaebler-Spira D, et al.; American Academy of Pediatrics Task Force on Childhood Motor Disorders. Classification and definition of disorders causing hypertonia in childhood. Pediatrics 2003;111:e89-97.

14. Surveillance of Cerebral Palsy in Europe. Surveillance of cerebral palsy in Europe: a collaboration of cerebral palsy surveys and registers. Dev Med Child Neurol 2000;42:816-24.

15. Rempel G. The importance of good nutrition in children with cerebral palsy. Phys Med Rehabil Clin North Am 2015;26:39-56.

16. Schiariti V, Tatla S, Sauve K, et al. Toolbox of multiple-item measures aligning with the ICF core sets for children and youth with cerebral palsy. Eur J Paediatr Neurol 2017;21:252-63.

17. CanChild Centre Cerebral Palsy Diagnosis [homepage on the Internet]. Hamilton, Ontario, Canada: McMaster University. Available at www.canchild.ca/en/diagnoses/cerebral-palsy. Accessed November 12, 2019.

18. Bohannon RW, Smith MB. Interrater reliability of a modified Ashworth scale of muscle spasticity. Phys Ther 1987;67:206-7.

19. Boyd R, Graham HK. Objective measurement of clinical findings in the use of botulinum toxin type A for the management of children with CP. Eur J Neurol 1999;6:S23-35.

20. Tilton A. Management of spasticity in children with cerebral palsy. Semin Pediatr Neurol 2009;16:82-9.

21. Wood E. The child with cerebral palsy: diagnosis and beyond. Semin Pediatr Neurol 2006;13:286-96.

22. Huang HH, Fetters L, Hale J, et al. Bound for success: a systematic review of constraint-induced movement therapy in children with cerebral palsy supports improved arm and hand use. Phys Ther 2009;89:1126-41.

23. Sheean G, McGuire JR. Spastic hypertonia and movement disorders: pathophysiology, clinical presentation, and quantification. PM R 2009;1:827-33.

24. Delgado MR, Hirtz D, Aisen M, et al.; Quality Standards Subcommittee of the American Academy of Neurology, Practice Committee of the Child Neurology Society. Practice parameter: pharmacologic treatment of spasticity in children with cerebral palsy (an evidence-based review). Neurology 2010;74:336-43.

25. National Institute for Health and Care Excellence (NICE). Spasticity in under 19s: management (clinical guideline 145). Available at www.nice.org.uk/guidance/cg145. Accessed November 17, 2019.

26. Krach L. Pharmacotherapy of spasticity: oral medications and intrathecal baclofen. J Child Neurol 2001;16:31-6.

27. Lexicomp Online, Pediatric and Neonatal Lexi-Drugs Online, Hudson, Ohio: Wolters Kluwer Clinical Drug Information, Inc; 2019. Accessed November 17, 2019.

28. Allen LV, Erickson MA. Stability of acetazolamide, allopurinol, azathioprine, clonazepam, and flucytosine in extemporaneously compounded oral liquids. Am J Health Syst Pharm 1996;53:1944-9.

29. Zanaflex [package insert]. Ardsley, NY: Acorda Therapeutics, 2013.

30. Vásquez-Briceño A, Arellano-Saldaña ME, León-Hernández SR, et al. The usefulness of tizanidine: a one-year follow up of the treatment of spasticity in infantile cerebral palsy. Rev Neurol 2006;43:132-6.

31. Chan CH. Dantrolene sodium and hepatic injury. Neurology 1990;40:1427-32.

32. Nahata MC, Pai VB. Pediatric Drug Formulations, 6th ed. Cincinnati: Harvey Whitney, 2011.

33. Edgar TS. Oral pharmacotherapy of childhood movement disorders. J Child Neurol 2003;18:s40-9.

34. He Y, Brunstrom-Hernandez JE, Thio LL, et al. Population pharmacokinetics of oral baclofen in pediatric patients with cerebral palsy. J Pediatr 2014;164:1181-8.

35. Tickner N, Apps JR, Keady S, et al. An overview of drug therapies used in the treatment of dystonia and spasticity in children. Arch Dis Child Educ Pract Ed 2012;97:230-5.

36. Ozobax [package insert]. Athens, GA: Metacel Pharmaceuticals, 2019.

37. Allen LV, Erickson MA. Stability of baclofen, captopril, diltiazem hydrochloride, dipyridamole, and flecainide acetate in extemporaneously compounded oral liquids. Am J Health Syst Pharm 1996;53:2179-84.

38. Johnson CE, Hart SM. Stability of an extemporaneously compounded baclofen oral liquid. Am J Hosp Pharm 1993;50:2353-5.

39. Hasnat MJ, Rice JE. Intrathecal baclofen for treating spasticity in children with cerebral palsy. Cochrane Database Syst Rev 2015; 11:CD004552.

40. Dan B, Motta F, Vles JSH, et al. Consensus on the appropriate use of intrathecal baclofen (ITB) therapy in paediatric spasticity. Eur J Paediatr Neurol 2010;14:19-28.

41. Albright AL, Thompson K, Carlos S, et al. Cerebrospinal fluid baclofen concentration in patients undergoing continuous intrathecal baclofen therapy. Dev Med Child Neurol 2007;49:423-5.

42. Albright AL, Shultz B. Plasma baclofen levels in children receiving continuous intrathecal baclofen infusion. J Child Neurol 1999;14:408-9.

43. Lioresal intrathecal [package insert]. Roswell, GA: Saol Therapeutics, 2019.

44. SynchroMed and IsoMed [prescriber information]. Minneapolis, MN: Medtronic, 2017.

45. Motta F, Antonello CE. Analysis of complications in 430 consecutive pediatric patients treated with intrathecal baclofen therapy: 14-year experience. J Neurosurg Pediatrics 2014;13:301-6.

46. Koman LA, Paterson Smith B, Balkrishnan R. Spasticity associated with cerebral palsy in children, guidelines for the use of botulinum A toxin. Pediatr Drugs 2003;5:11-23.

47. Multani I, Manji J, Hastings-Ison T, et al. Botulinum toxin in the management of children with cerebral palsy. Pediatr Drugs 2019;21:261-81.

48. U.S. Food and Drug Administration (FDA). Information for healthcare professionals: onabotulinumtoxina (marketed as botox/botox cosmetic), abobotulinumtoxinA (marketed as Dysport) and rimabotulinumtoxinB (marketed as Myobloc). FDA Alert. Available at https://wayback.archive-it.org/7993/20170722190448/https://www.fda.gov/Drugs/DrugSafety/PostmarketDrugSafetyInformationforPatientsandProviders/DrugSafetyInformationforHeathcareProfessionals/ucm174949.htm. Accessed November 17, 2019.

49. Heinen F, Desloovere K, Schroeder AS, et al. The updated European consensus 2009 on the use of botulinum toxin for children with cerebral palsy. Eur J Paediatr Neurol 2010;14:45-66.

50. Dysport [package insert]. Wrexham, UK: Ipsen Biopharm, 2019.

51. Botox [package insert]. Dublin, Ireland: Allergan, 2019.

52. Simpson DM, Gracie JM, Graham HK, et al.; Therapeutic and Technology Assessment Subcommittee of the American Academy of Neurology. Assessment: botulinum neurotoxin for the treatment of spasticity (an evidence-based review). Neurology 2008;70:1691-8.

53. U.S. Food and Drug Administration (FDA). Follow-up to the February 8, 2008, early communication about an ongoing safety review of botox and botox cosmetic (botulinum toxin type a) and myobloc (botulinum toxin type b). Available at https://wayback.archive-it.org/7993/20170722190452/https://www.fda.gov/Drugs/DrugSafety/PostmarketDrugSafetyInformationforPatientsandProviders/DrugSafetyInformationforHeathcareProfessionals/ucm143819.htm. Accessed November 18, 2019.

54. Reddihough D, Erasmus CE, Johnson H, et al. Botulinum toxin assessment, intervention and aftercare for paediatric and adult drooling: international consensus statement. Eur J Neurol 2010; 17:109-21.

55. Little SA, Kubba H, Hussain SSM. An evidence-based approach to the child who drools. Clin Otolaryngol 2009;34:236-9.

56. Tahmassebi JF, Curzon ME. Prevalence of drooling in children with cerebral palsy attending special schools. Dev Med Child Neurol 2003;45:613-7.

57. Livingston MH, Stewart D, Rosenbaum PL, et al. Exploring issues of participation among adolescents with cerebral palsy: what's important to them? Phys Occup Ther Pediatr 2011;31:275-87.

58. Tscheng DZ. Sialorrhea—therapeutic drug options. Ann Pharmacother 2002;36:1785-90.

59. Mier RJ, Bachrach SJ, Lakin RD, et al. Treatment of sialorrhea with glycopyrrolate. Arch Pediatr Adolesc Med 2000;154:1214-8.

60. Cuvposa [package insert]. Raleigh, NC: Merz Pharmaceuticals, 2018.

61. Transderm Scop [package insert]. Warren, NJ: GlaxoSmithKline Consumer Healthcare, 2019.

62. Mato A, Limeres J, Tomas I, et al. Management of drooling in disabled patients with scopolamine patches. Br J Clin Pharmacol 2010;69:684-8.

63. Lewis DW, Fontana C, Mehallick LK, et al. Transdermal scopolamine for reduction of drooling in developmentally delayed children. Dev Med Child Neurol 1994;36:484-6.

64. Carranza-del Rio J, Clegg NJ, Moore A, et al. Use of trihexyphenidyl in children with cerebral palsy. Pediatr Neurol 2011;44:202-6.

65. Xeomin [package insert]. Frankfurt, Germany: Merz Pharmaceuticals, 2019.

66. Myobloc [package insert]. Louisville, KY: Solstice Neurosciences, 2019.

67. Porte M, Chaleat-Valayer E, Patte K, et al. Relevance of intraglandular injections of botulinum toxin for the treatment of sialorrhea in children with cerebral palsy: a review. Eur J Paediatr Neurol 2014;18:649-57.

68. Houlihan CM. Bone health in cerebral palsy: who's at risk and what to do about it? J Pediatr Rehabil Med 2014;7:143-53.

69. Ozel S, Switzer L, Macintosh A, et al. Informing evidence-based clinical practice guidelines for children with cerebral palsy at risk of osteoporosis: an update. Dev Med Child Neurol 2016; 58:918-23.

70. Fehlings D, Switzer L, Agarwal P, et al. Informing evidence-based clinical practice guidelines for children with cerebral palsy at risk of osteoporosis: a systematic review. Dev Med Child Neurol 2012;54:106-16.

71. Simm PJ, Biggin A, Zacharin M, et al. Consensus guidelines on the use of bisphosphonate therapy in children and adolescents. J Paediatr Child Health 2018;54:223-33.

72. Bhatt RN, Hibbert SA, Munns CF. The use of bisphosphonates in children: review of the literature and guidelines for dental management. Aust Dent J 2014;59:9-19.

73. Liptak GS; American Academy of Pediatrics Counsel on Children with Disabilities. Providing a primary care medical home for children and youth with cerebral palsy. Pediatrics 2011;128:e1321-29.

CHAPTER 30

Pain Management

Peter N. Johnson, Pharm.D., FPPA, FCCM, BCPS, BCPPS

INTRODUCTION

Pain management in children is a distinct challenge for pharmacists and other health care professionals. Children admitted to the hospital or seen at an emergency department or outpatient clinic may experience several different etiologies of pain including *acute pain*, such as diagnostic and therapeutic procedures and oral/nasal/tracheal suctioning; *established* *pain*, such as thermal/chemical burns and postsurgical pain; *prolonged pain*, such as meningitis and necrotizing enterocolitis; and *chronic pain*, such as sickle cell disease.[1] A recent cross-sectional survey of inpatient pediatric patients found that 76% of children had experienced pain within the previous 24 hours.[2] Most of the pain was attributed to acute pain from procedures, but 12% of children had chronic pain. Another finding of concern was that 50% of children qualified their pain as moderate to severe.[2] Pain pharmacotherapy is associated with many challenges for clinicians, not limited to assessment and treatment. The heterogeneity of the pediatric population makes it difficult for a one-size-fits-all approach. Inadequate pharmacotherapy can be associated with adverse physiologic changes, especially in the neonatal population. In children, analgesics are among the highest class for medication errors, and there are several medication safety concerns that pharmacists should consider when developing pain care plans.

Historically, there have been many misconceptions regarding the definition, recognition, and management of pain in infants and children compared with that of adults. In the 1970s, the International Association for the Study of Pain Subcommittee on Taxonomy defined *pain* as "an unpleasant sensory emotional experience associated with actual or potential tissue damage."[3] Inherent in this definition was the idea that pain is a learned response. Another common misconception was that neonates could not feel pain, and that even if they did feel pain, they would not remember the experience.[4]

Because of these misconceptions, evidence suggests that children have suboptimal pain treatment compared with adults. In the 1980s, a retrospective study was conducted to compare analgesic patterns of use in 90 children and 90 adults matched for sex and diagnosis.[5] The investigators found children received fewer opioid doses compared with adults, but they concluded that knowledge of whether these findings were related to discrepancies in pain assessment or other factors was a challenge. Since then, studies have identified that untreated pain is associated with significant behavioral and biochemical consequences.[6-8] Clinically, these consequences may result in delayed healing, complicated recovery time, and significant stress not only for the patient but also for the patient's caregivers. Because of the emerging research in this population, researchers have proposed a new definition of *pain* that states: "pain perception is an inherent quality of life that appears early in development to serve as a signaling system for tissue damage."[9] The body system is composed of both physiological and behavioral indicators that can adequately depict pain and others can interpret.[9]

PHYSIOLOGY OF PAIN TRANSMISSION

Studies during the past 20 years have explored pain perception among young infants and adults. Research has confirmed that although pain perception is similar among adults and neonates, the differences between the two have been primarily attributed to neurophysiologic and cognitive immaturity.[10] To understand these differences in more detail, it is important to review the physiology of pain stimulation, transmission, perception, and modulation.

The first step in the development of pain involves the sensation of painful or noxious stimuli leading to the excitation of nerve endings called *nociceptors* in the peripheral nervous system. Several different mediators including bradykinin, prostaglandin, histamine, substance P, and serotonin have been associated with the sensitization and activation of nerve transmission in concert with the noxious stimuli. These mediators may be a source for targeted intervention.[11]

Activation of nociceptors results in transmission of nerve impulses along the ascending pain pathway from the peripheral nervous system along A-delta and C-afferent nerve fibers to the dorsal horn of the spinal cord. The *A-delta nerve fibers* are myelinated, large-diameter fibers that allow sharp, localized pain response. The *C-afferent fibers* are unmyelinated fibers, representing the most common path for nociception in both neonates and adults, and result in dull, aching, poorly localized pain.

The nerve impulse is then transmitted along various spinal tracts, including the spinothalamic tract to the thalamus. Once the signal reaches the thalamus, the patient is able to become consciously aware of the source of pain and is able to localize the origin of the pain.[12] Modulation of the pain response occurs through the descending pain pathway when a series of supraspinal structures, including the locus coeruleus and rostral ventromedial medulla, directly or indirectly alter the pain transmission from the brain stem to the spinal dorsal horn.[11] The net result of modulation is that nociception of the painful stimuli is either *inhibited*, leading to pain inhibition, or *facilitated*, leading to exacerbation of the pain response.

DIFFERENCES IN PAIN MANAGEMENT FOR CHILDREN VS. ADULTS

Even though the pathways for pain perception through modulation are essentially the same in all populations, several neurophysiologic factors in neonates make the approach to pain management specific for the neonatal population. The elements of the peripheral and central nervous system necessary for pain transmission and perception develop in the fetus at the end of the first trimester.[13] Evidence suggests the fetus has the ability to perceive pain even before birth; however, the structures necessary for pain modulation through the descending pain pathway are not complete until 30–32 weeks' gestation.[1] The final stage of neural development is complete at 37 weeks' gestation with the integration of a myelin sheath around the spinothalamic tract.[13] In addition to the environmental and disease state factors that may be a source of pain in neonates, the developmental maturity (i.e., gestational age and postnatal age) of the neonate can contribute to differences in pain perception and modulation between neonates and adults. Because premature neonates younger than 32 weeks' gestational age do not have a fully developed descending pain pathway, they experience a lower pain threshold and even

a hypersensitivity that develops as a result of repeated painful procedures.[1,14] In addition, infants have less-precise pain transmission than older infants and children. The touch and pain transmission pathways are close to each other on the spinothalamic tract.[13] Because of the decreased accuracy in pain perception, the infant may lose the ability to differentiate a painful response from a nonpainful response. Research has shown that neonates experience pain and that the early pain responses they experience are associated with long-term changes in pain perception.[13]

In addition to the neurophysiologic factors, other differences in pain management between adults and children must be recognized. There are cognitive and developmental differences in young children that make it difficult to assess and treat pain. Clinicians should also note specific factors in children that may affect the dose of an analgesic medication or even the selection of particular analgesics. Small children may have high oxygen consumption and smaller lung volumes, so they may be more prone to periods of apnea when they are administered opioids or sedative medications to relieve pain and anxiety.[15] In such cases, a dosage adjustment may be required to avoid adverse events. The absorption, metabolism, and excretion of selected pain medications may also be altered in pediatric patients requiring a dosing adjustment compared with adults.

An abundance of data suggests the significance of pain in children. As a result, several different organizations have emphasized the need for pain assessment in children.[16] In 2001, the Joint Commission implemented pain management standards that mandated health care facilities to execute uniform pain assessment and standardized approaches to pain treatment in children.[17] Pain has often been termed "the fifth vital sign," emphasizing the need for continuous reassessment of hospitalized pediatric patients. Despite these recommendations, pediatric pain management continues to be a challenging field with many barriers because of the developmental changes and pharmacokinetic alterations associated with this heterogeneous population.

CLINICAL PRESENTATION AND DIAGNOSIS

GENERAL ASSESSMENT PRINCIPLES

Uniform pain assessment can be very difficult in the pediatric population. Infants may experience nonspecific symptoms of pain with changes in facial expressions and crying; they may also present with autonomic symptoms (e.g., tachycardia, tachypnea), but these symptoms may be associated with their underlying disease state rather than pain by itself.[18] Just like in adults, clinicians should inquire about the character, location, intensity, and duration of painful stimuli in children. Of note, children may not be forthcoming with this information. They may experience a certain level of anxiety with physicians and other health care professionals related to needle sticks, medication injections, and other interventions that they may receive in the clinic, emergency department, or hospital setting.

The ability of a child to describe the experience of pain varies with age, experience, and cognitive developmental states.[19]

In general, clinicians may use self-report, physiologic, and/or behavioral assessments to differentiate between pain and other factors. Because pain is a subjective experience, self-report is generally preferred to make inferences about a patient's pain episodes.[20] Current recommendations call for clinicians to use a child's self-reported pain in conjunction with standardized assessment tools.[20] However, for infants, nonverbal children, or children with cognitive impairment, it may also be difficult to ascertain whether crying and other behavioral manifestations are associated with pain or other factors, such as hunger or fear. In these patients, clinicians should gather a careful history from their caregivers to help differentiate these baseline behavioral manifestations versus the presence of pain.

Table 1 provides a summary of the most common types of assessment tools. Specific vital sign changes including elevation in heart rate and blood pressure may be used in all ages as an indirect measurement of pain. However, the use of these markers alone is questionable because of the effects of the child's underlying disease state or other underlying emotional factors (e.g., anxiety, depression). Other more specific pain assessment tools have been developed, but it is important to understand the role of these tools in relation to the child's age and cognitive developmental stages.

ASSESSMENT METHODS IN PEDIATRIC SUBGROUPS

The most common tools used in this population other than physiologic changes are behavioral/physiologic scales. These scales involve the assessment of a variety of behavioral features including crying, facial expressions, body posture/movements, and, in some cases, vital sign changes (e.g., blood pressure, heart rate).[19] When clinicians evaluate one of the behavioral features alone, they may be unable to assess pain accurately. For example, premature infants and sick full-term infants may be unable to produce an adequate cry when in distress.[19] Many of these scales are available, including the Neonatal Facial Coding System (NFCS), Neonatal Infant Pain Scale (NIPS), and Premature Infant Pain Profile (PIPP). Each scale has been validated in the neonatal population, and each has specific variables that are evaluated. These scales can be time-consuming, and their usefulness in intubated neonates is questionable.[19]

Toddlers have a decreased cognitive ability compared with older children and may not have the ability to differentiate between types of pain. As a result, nonverbal behaviors such as facial expressions, limb movements, and crying may be more accurate than their own self-reports.[19] Children older than 3 years will be able to give a good description of the intensity, location, and severity of their pain, whereas verbal toddlers younger than 3 years will often have a decreased ability to do so.[18,19] Toddlers may have a limited knowledge of numbers and colors, making it difficult to use certain types of pain assessment tools. Thus, age-appropriate behavioral scales such as the Faces Legs Activity Cry Consolability Scale (FLACC) have been developed for children as young as 2 months up to 7 years. The FLACC involves a 0- to 10-point

Table 1. Summary of Pain Measurement Tools in Children[18,19,25]

Name	Recommended Age Range or Groups	Advantages	Disadvantages
Physiologic measures (e.g., heart rate, blood pressure)	All ages	Useful for nonverbal children	Vital sign changes occur unrelated to pain
Neonatal behavioral/ physiologic scales (e.g., NIPS, NFCS, PIPP)	Premature to full-term infants	Evaluate age-appropriate behavioral and physiologic factors; useful for nonverbal children	Nonspecific in some cases; some are time-consuming; questionable validity in selected patients
Other Behavioral/ physiologic scales (e.g., FLACC)	2 mo–7 yr		
Graphic scale (e.g., color analog scale)	≥ 4 yr	Used for preschool children	Limited use in children with cognitive impairment or who are color-blind
FACES scale (e.g., Wong-Baker)	≥ 3 yr	Simple scoring tool used for pain discrimination; used for very young preschool children	Children may confuse their emotional states with pain ratings
Visual Analogue scale	≥ 8 yr	Straightforward, one-dimensional scoring tool for older children	Limited applicability in children with cognitive impairment
Numeric Rating scale	≥ 7 yr	Simple scoring tool that can be given verbally or as a written instrument	Application of scores to treatment decisions is inappropriate
NCCPC-PV	Cognitively impaired children	Validated tool for pain assessment in children with cognitive impairment	Assessment may take substantial time at the bedside to complete (e.g., 10 min)

FLACC = Face Legs Arms Cry Consolability Scale; NCCPV-PV = Non-Communicating Children's Pain Checklist–Postoperative Version; NFCS = Neonatal Facial Coding System; NIPS = Neonatal Infant Pain Scale; PIPP = Premature Infant Pain Profile.

scale that evaluates five key indicators: face, legs, activity, cry, and consolability.[19] Overall, this scale is relatively easy to use and has been validated in the literature.[21]

Preschool children have an increased ability to articulate and discriminate their pain. By age 5 years, most children will be able to rate the severity of their pain.[19] Many different scales have been developed for this age group including the Child Facial Coding System (CFCS), Poker Chip Tool, Graphic Scale, and FACES Pain Scale.[22] These scales, which can be used in children as young as 4 years, involve the use of color and/or drawings. In general, the higher the number and the greater the intensity of color, the more intense the pain. One limitation of this type of tool is its use for children who are color-blind and/or possess developmental disabilities.[18]

The Wong-Baker FACES Pain Rating Scale is one of the most common tools used by several institutions.[23] This scale is recommended for children 3 years and older and requires health care professionals to point to each face and describe the corresponding intensity of pain with the corresponding face.[19] The child is then asked to point to the face that most accurately describes the child's experience of pain. Although the Wong-Baker scale is one of the most common scales used, one disadvantage of it is that the face associated with "no pain" is the "smiling face." Other similar scales involve the use of a "neutral face" instead of a "smiling face." Investigators compared the Wong-Baker scale versus these other types of faces scales.[24] They found that children who saw the smiling face were more likely to report higher pain scores than children who saw the neutral face and suggested that young children may confuse pain ratings with the faces describing different emotional states.[24] For example, an anxious child without a true source of pain may select a face with a corresponding higher pain score because the child is feeling sad rather than experiencing pain.

School-age children have an increased ability to describe their pain compared with younger children. In general, they are more concrete thinkers than are preschool children, and they tend to have a better understanding of measurements, quantitative expressions, and facial expressions.[18,19] Thus, analog scales such as the Visual Analogue Scale and Numeric Rating Scale (NRS) either use faces or numbers to accurately assess their pain. The Visual Analogue Scale is a one-dimensional pain assessment tool that involves a 100-mm horizontal line with corresponding descriptions of pain.[19] The lower end of the spectrum highlights no pain, whereas the highest point score represents severe pain. Children are asked to mark along the continuum the line that best corresponds to the given pain descriptions. One of the main disadvantages of this tool is that it may have questionable usefulness in school-aged children with cognitive impairment.[18]

The NRS is another commonly used scoring tool in older children and adults; one example of this scoring tool is its 0 (no pain) to 10 (severe pain) scale. Few studies have evaluated the validity of this scoring tool in children. In a study that investigated the use of the NRS in 113 children ranging in age from 7 to 16 years who required hospital admission after surgery for postoperative pain management, children with NRS scores greater than 4 had good sensitivity and specificity to predict those who needed additional pain medication.[25]

However, in children with an NRS score greater than 6, less than 50% were somewhat satisfied with their current pain regimen, and another 25% of them were very satisfied with their regimen. The investigators concluded that there was a discrepancy in the relationship of higher pain scores and patient satisfaction with their analgesic regimens. In addition, they concluded that the NRS could be used in this population to assess pain but it might have a limited role in children to correlate the NRS with treatment decisions.

Adolescents tend to have the highest capacity to describe their pain, although in the presence of close family or friends, they may deny their experience of pain.[19] In fact, adolescents may prefer that friends and family are not present when clinicians assess or discuss their pain. Overall, this patient population generally wants the choice to receive interventions for painful procedures; however, in certain situations, adolescents may have regression of their developmental ability to cope with their pain.[19,20] Most, if not all, pain measurement tools would be acceptable in this population.

For children with cognitive impairment, pain assessment can be very difficult. Children with Down syndrome may not adequately describe the character of their pain.[18] Because the sensory perception in children with autism is different from that in other children, it may be difficult to accurately assess painful stimuli versus other stimuli that may exacerbate their underlying disease.[18] It is imperative that clinicians ascertain the patient's neurologic baseline from the parents/caregivers when a child's self-report is not possible. Studies have focused on the development of standardized assessment tools in this population. One study sought to validate the Non-Communicating Child's Pain Checklist-Postoperative Version (NCCPC-PV), a standardized pain assessment scale in the postoperative period for patients younger than 18 years with cognitive impairment.[26] This scale assesses six domains: vocal sounds, social interaction, facial expressions, general activity, body/limb movements, and physiologic signs. The investigators correlated the score on the NCCPC-PV with that of caregivers and found a good correlation between their assessments. It is extremely important for clinicians to use a multiprofessional approach to pain assessment that includes the physician, nursing staff, other allied health care professionals, and parents/caregivers. Evidence suggests that the NCCPV-PV is a useful clinical tool to augment clinical assessment in children with cognitive impairment.

KEY POINT SUMMARY FOR PAIN ASSESSMENT

- Pain should be assessed by patient self-report, together with behavioral/physiologic assessments at regular intervals in hospitalized children.

- Several types of behavioral pain assessment tools are available, and each of them may have advantages and disadvantages over another.

- Pain assessment in children with cognitive impairment requires a multidisciplinary approach and can be augmented with validated assessment tools such as the NCCPC-PV.

TREATMENT

NONPHARMACOLOGIC THERAPY

Many nonpharmacologic interventions can be used to prevent and treat pain in children. An increasing amount of evidence supports the use of these interventions because they have good safety profiles and very few disadvantages.[16,18] One of the proposed mechanisms of these interventions is that they interfere with pain transmission along the ascending pain pathway by introduction of other excitatory messages.[15] Several different types of health care professionals may be needed to incorporate these therapies. One such health care professional is the *child life specialist*—these professionals are trained to use such nonpharmacologic therapies and educate the parents/caregivers and health care professionals on strategies to reduce and eliminate painful stimuli in children.[16] This education will be needed to ensure the success and implementation of these therapies not only for the patient but also for the other members of the health care team.[16] Everything from the "physical" medical environment to the use of child life specialists can be a useful therapeutic intervention to relieve pain and/or anxiety for children in the emergency department and hospital setting.[16]

In recent years, many nonpharmacologic interventions have been suggested for the neonatal population. These nonpharmacologic interventions are useful to decrease pain and discomfort for neonates during procedures (e.g., heel lancing, adhesive removal, intramuscular/subcutaneous injection, venipuncture, lumbar puncture, suctioning).[13,14] Several of these interventions such as swaddling, facilitated tucking, rocking, pacifier use, and positioning have been validated.[13] *Positioning* is a useful intervention that allows the infant to self-adjust after a painful procedure. *Facilitated tucking* is a process by which an infant is wrapped in a blanket and restrained in a tucked position. Practitioners have also focused on targeting environmental factors that may cause neonates pain and anxiety to create a quiet and restful environment. Some neonatal units have taken measures to reduce lighting, decrease the amount of time per day the infant is actually touched, and decrease the volume of alarms and telephones.[13]

The nonpharmacologic therapies in older children can be classified into *cognitive, behavioral,* and *physical interventions.* Cognitive therapies include the use of music, guided imagery, distraction, and hypnosis to reduce or eliminate pain.[15] Distraction techniques can include bubbles, therapeutic play, video games, and television. Behavioral techniques can range from breathing exercises to relaxation techniques and may require education for both the provider and patient to be totally effective.[15] Physical nonpharmacologic interventions may also be used; these interventions may involve the use of acupuncture, massage therapy, and application of transcutaneous electrical nerve stimulation.[15] These therapies may be particularly useful for pain in localized regions.[18]

In summary, nonpharmacologic interventions can be very useful for preventing and treating pain in neonates and children. Some children may respond better to nonpharmacologic interventions than others. In addition, certain therapies may not be appropriate for some children and should not be used in place of analgesic agents. A detailed discussion of these interventions is beyond the scope of this chapter, but these interventions have been published elsewhere.[18,19]

PHARMACOLOGIC THERAPY

PHARMACOKINETIC AND PHARMACODYNAMIC CONSIDERATIONS IN CHILDREN

Developmental pharmacology considerations. Clinicians should consider the pharmacodynamic and pharmacokinetic changes that occur with age when selecting not only medication dosing but also the actual analgesic agent. In the first few years of life, significant changes occur in the absorption, distribution, metabolism, and excretion of various medications. A complete review of these principles in children appears in the Pediatric Pharmacokinetics chapter, but it is necessary to point out some of these considerations pertaining to pain medications in infants and children.

Neonates have a thinner stratum corneum and greater hydration to the epidermis compared with older children.[27,28] As a result, infants may have an excessive exposure of medications administered topically.[29] The application of transdermal medications such as transdermal fentanyl should be avoided in children younger than 2 years because of unpredictability in dosing.[30]

Neonates and infants have a diminished capacity to metabolize medications through the hepatic system. Phase 1 and 2 enzymatic reactions, including oxidation and glucuronidation, respectively, are significantly delayed in neonates compared with older children. As a result, medication regimens in neonates may need to be altered on the basis of decreased hepatic clearance. For example, several studies have noted inadequate efficacy with morphine in preterm infants.[31-33] Morphine is metabolized to an active metabolite by glucuronidation. One study suggests these infants have diminished concentrations of morphine-6-glucuronide, the active metabolite of morphine, and elevated concentrations of morphine-3-glucuronide.[31] Elevated concentrations of morphine-3-glucuronide may antagonize the effects of morphine and morphine-6-glucuronide. These enzyme pathways usually mature by about age 6 months.[34] In fact, children who are age 2–6 years often show increased metabolic clearance and may require doses of nonopioid and opioid medications more often compared with other age groups for a given therapeutic effect.

In addition to knowledge of the developmental changes associated with skin absorption and metabolism, clinicians should be aware of the effects of renal excretion when prescribing certain medications. Specifically, neonates exhibit decreased glomerular filtration and tubular secretion.[34] Morphine-3-glucuronide and morphine-6-glucuronide are both renally excreted, and neurotoxicities such as myoclonus could occur in patients with renal insufficiency.[35] As a result, neonates may require an extension of dosing intervals to prevent the accumulation of a given medication and its metabolites.

Pharmacokinetic alterations in obese children. In addition to the developmental changes related to absorption, distribution, metabolism, and excretion principles in the pediatric populations, other alterations may be noted in obese children. The prevalence of obese children has increased dramatically during the past 30 years. A study recently found that in 2015–2016 around 18.5% of children age 2–19 years were obese.[36] In addition, another study found that obese children accounted for 18.8% of the 15,119 admissions for children age 2–17 years at two academic children's hospitals.[37] A complete review of pediatric obesity may be found in the Pediatric Obesity chapter. Pharmacokinetic alterations have been noted in obese adults, including a higher volume of distribution for lipophilic medications and increased glomerular filtration rates.[38]

There is a paucity of pharmacokinetic studies of obese pediatric patients. Studies of obese adults receiving continuous infusions of fentanyl highlight some possible concerns. Researchers found that optimal dosing of fentanyl continuous intravenous infusions had better correlation with the "pharmacokinetic mass" of the patient rather than an actual, ideal, or adjusted body weight.[39,40] The investigators determined the "pharmacokinetic mass" on the basis of observations of the analgesic effect, serum fentanyl concentrations, and fentanyl dose. Results show that as the actual body weight increased, the pharmacokinetic mass increased logarithmically, suggesting an upper limit to the weight by which fentanyl is dosed.[40] There is a concern in obese patients that if fentanyl is dosed on the basis of actual body weight, there is a higher risk of overdosing and of adverse events such as potential oversedation and respiratory distress. Until more pharmacokinetic studies have been conducted, it is reasonable to use the following recommendations for dosing of pain medications in obese children.[38,41,42]

- For children weighing less than 40 kg and younger than 18 years: Use weight-based dosing (i.e., milligram or microgram for single-dose medications and milligram/kilogram/hour or microgram/kilogram/hour for continuous intravenous medications).
- For children weighing 40 kg or more:
  - Single-dose medications: Use weight-based dosing unless the patient's dose or dose per day exceeds the recommended adult dose for the indication.
  - Continuous intravenous medications: Avoid weight-based dosing strategies; instead, use adult-dosing strategies (i.e., microgram/hour or milligram/hour).

ACUTE PAIN MANAGEMENT

Children who experience acute pain require prompt attention. The World Health Organization (WHO) has recently developed a new algorithm for the management of pain in children that uses two categories: *mild pain* and *moderate to severe pain*.[43] These guidelines specifically address two major changes from the previous guidelines. First, the previous WHO guidelines mainly addressed the management of patients with cancer pain. The new guidelines represent a paradigm shift because the focus is now on children with any type of pain as a result of a medical illness, and the recommendations incorporate findings from recent studies in acute and chronic pain management in children. Second, the new WHO guidelines include a new algorithm to treat pain including a two-step

versus a three-step approach. The driving force behind this recommendation is the de-emphasis by the WHO on the role of codeine for pain management in children.

Nonopioid analgesics remain the mainstay of the treatment of mild pain and should be initiated on a maintenance schedule and titrated to maximum effect. Children with persistent moderate to severe pain should receive a strong opioid analgesic with or without a nonopioid analgesic. In general, patients with severe pain should be initiated on scheduled doses of strong opioids. Intermittent doses of opioids can be useful for patients experiencing acute, breakthrough pain, although this strategy often results in a fluctuation of plasma concentrations. Because several opioid agents have relatively short elimination half-lives, the therapeutic benefit may decrease toward the end of the dosing interval, and the patient may experience breakthrough pain. As a result, patients with severe postoperative pain or other painful episodes should receive continuous intravenous opioid infusions or patient-controlled analgesia (PCA) when appropriate. At any stage, clinicians are encouraged to consider the use of adjuvant agents (e.g., benzodiazepines, antidepressants).

Nonopioid analgesics. Nonopioid analgesics represent an attractive option for patients who may be experiencing mild pain. These agents have been used in patients with acute and chronic pain in a variety of settings, including in children with cancer pain and postoperative pain, and show opioid-sparing effects. In contrast to opioid analgesics, nonopioid analgesics are not associated with respiratory depression, constipation, or urinary retention but may have other risks specific to the individual agents. These agents show a ceiling effect, making their use in patients with moderate to severe pain limited at best. Thus, the efficacy is limited with doses approaching the maximum recommended range but the risk of toxicity is significant.

This group of agents includes both the nonsteroidal anti-inflammatory drugs (NSAIDs) and acetaminophen. The NSAIDs inhibit the cyclooxygenase enzymes' ability to convert arachidonic acid to prostaglandin precursors. Prostaglandins are associated with a wealth of pharmacologic activity including the potentiation of inflammation, protection of the gastrointestinal mucosa, and sensitization of nerves to painful stimuli.[22] Acetaminophen inhibits cyclooxygenase-3, and most experts believe that its main analgesic effects come from inhibiting prostaglandin synthesis in the central nervous system.[44] Unlike NSAIDs, acetaminophen does not inhibit peripheral prostaglandin production, so it is thought not to have any anti-inflammatory activity.

Table 2 includes the most common agents used in an emergency department or inpatient setting.[45-51] There are no studies comparing the efficacy of these agents in children. In addition, a great degree of patient intervariability exists between these agents. Therefore, the rationale for choosing one agent over another would include the dosage form, cost, and adverse effect profile.

Acetaminophen. Acetaminophen represents the most widely used nonopioid analgesic. This agent is available in a variety of formulations including tablets, oral liquid dosage forms (i.e., elixirs, solutions, and suspensions), suppositories, and an intravenous formulation approved in the fall of 2010.

For children younger than 12 years, the usual oral dose of acetaminophen is 10–15 mg/kg with a maximum of 75 mg/kg/day and not to exceed 4 g/day (Table 2).[45] Revised dosing recommendations for obese children or children older than 12 years were made available in fall 2011.[51] At this time, the maker of Extra Strength Tylenol (Johnson and Johnson, New Brunswick, NJ) voluntarily changed the labeling for its acetaminophen product from a maximum of 4 g/day to a maximum of 3 g/day. The new dosing instructions were developed in an attempt to decrease the incidence of hepatotoxicity secondary to accidental overdoses.

Until late in the spring of 2011, acetaminophen was available in a concentrated solution for young infants (i.e., 100 mg/mL) and in another oral solution for older children (i.e., 32 mg/mL). However, the Consumer Healthcare Products Association released a notice of voluntary removal of the concentrated solution from the market beginning in mid-2011, citing concerns with medication safety of self-care use in the community.[51] As a result, only a single-concentration solution (i.e., 32 mg/mL) is commercially available at this time.[52]

Rectal administration of acetaminophen has been used in many different situations for children who may be unable to tolerate oral doses. The recommended doses are found in Table 2. The peak serum concentration is about 2–4 hours.[53] Many sources recommend a loading dose of 20–30 mg/kg/dose to achieve a quicker therapeutic response, given that the rectal absorption of this agent is believed to be erratic and slow. Some studies of children in the postoperative period have shown that children may require doses of 25–45 mg/kg to achieve a therapeutic response, but the optimal dosing remains to be determined.[53]

An intravenous formulation of acetaminophen (Ofirmev; Mallinckrodt Pharmceuticals, Hazelwood, MO) has been released. This agent has a U.S. Food and Drug Administration (FDA)-label indication for moderate pain and fever in children 2 years and older.[46] Of note, this agent has a quicker onset and higher peak concentration than the oral formulation; however, the total area under the curve is similar to oral administration.[45,46] Table 2 lists the FDA-label dosing. Few studies have ascertained the pharmacokinetic profile of intravenous acetaminophen in children younger than 2 years. In general, the area under the curve of intravenous acetaminophen is higher in this population than in older children and adults. The prescribing information lists preliminary recommendations for this population, suggesting that a 33% reduction in dose is required for infants to children younger than

Table 2. Nonopioid Analgesic Agents[45-51]

Medication	Route	Pharmacokinetics	Dose by Age
Acetaminophen	PO	Onset: 0.5 hr (PO) Half-life: 3–7 hr (children to neonates)	< 12 yr: 10–15 mg/kg/dose every 4–6 hr (max dose: < 5 doses/day 75 mg/kg/day or 4 g/day) ≥ 12 yr: 325–500 mg every 4–6 hr or 1 g every 8 hr (max dose: 4 g/day)
Acetaminophen	PR	Onset: Unknown Half-life: Unknown	< 12 yr: 10–20 mg/kg/dose every 4–6 hr (max dose: < 5 doses/day 75 mg/kg/day or 4 g/day) ≥ 12 yr: 325–650 mg every 4–6 hr or 1 g every 6–8 hr (max dose: 4 g/day)
Acetaminophen	IV	Onset: 0.25 hr after 15-min infusion Half-life: 3–7 hr (children to neonates)	2–12 yr or < 50 kg: 15 mg/kg/dose every 6 hr or 12.5 mg/kg/dose every 4 hr (max single dose: 750 mg; max dose/day: 75 mg/kg/day or ≤ 3.75 g) ≥ 50 kg: 1 g every 6 hr or 650 mg every 4 hr (max single dose: 1 g; max dose/day: 4 g)
Ibuprofen	PO	Onset: 1–2 hr Half-life: 1–2 h (children)	< 12 yr: 4–10 mg/kg/dose every 6–8 hr (max dose: 40 mg/kg/day) ≥ 12 yr: 200–400 mg every 4–6 hr (max dose: 2.4 g/day)
Ibuprofen	IV	Onset: N/A Half-life: 1.5–1.8 hr (children)	6 mo to < 12 yr: 10 mg/kg/dose every 4–6 hr (max 40 mg/kg/day or 2.4 g/day) > 12 yr: 400 mg every 4–6 hr (max 2.4 g/day)
Ketorolac	IV/IM	Onset: 0.5 hr Half-life: 3–6 hr (children)	FDA indication for 2–16 yr or < 50 kg: IM: 1 mg/kg/dose (max dose: 30 mg) IV: 0.5 mg/kg/dose; (max dose: 15 mg) 0.5 mg IV every 6 hr for ≤ 5 days ≥ 17 yr or > 50 kg: 30 mg IV every 6 hr (120 mg/day) for ≤ 5 days
Naproxen	PO	Onset: 0.5–1 hr Half-life: 8–17 hr (children)	2–11 yr: 5–7 mg/kg/dose every 8–12 hr > 12 yr: 250–500 mg every 12 hr (max dose: 1250 mg/day initially; then 1000 mg/day)
Choline magnesium trisalicylate	PO	Onset: N/A Half-life: 2–3 hr (adults)	Based on total salicylate content: Children: 10–20 mg/kg/dose every 8–12 hr Adults: 500 mg–1.5 g 1–3 times/day

FDA = U.S. Food and Drug Administration; IM = intramuscular; IV = intravenous; max = maximum; N/A = not available; PO = oral; PR = rectal (refer to text for recommendations on dosing for obese children).

2 years, and a 50% reduction in dose is recommended for neonates.[46] Some additional considerations must be noted. Over the past few years, there has been a 140% increase in the cost of intravenous acetaminophen.[54] Moreover, these vials are intended for single use and short stability after opening (i.e., 6 hours).[46] Because of these factors, pediatric institutions could experience a significant amount of wastage. It seems prudent to restrict the use of this product to children who are unable to take anything by mouth for an extended period, patients in the postoperative care setting, or patients with a contraindication to the rectal administration of medications (i.e., immunocompromised children). In addition, this agent may be considered an alternative to children who have an inadequate response to rectal acetaminophen.

The maximum dosages of acetaminophen products for adults and children are noted in Table 2. The recommendations should especially be noted for children receiving combination opioid analgesic agents because of the propensity for increased hepatic failure with excessive acetaminophen doses. In addition, chronic administration of acetaminophen, with doses at or less than the recommended maximum daily doses, has been noted to cause hepatotoxicity in healthy adult volunteers.[55]

Nonsteroidal anti-inflammatory drugs. The most common NSAIDs used in the emergency department or hospital setting include ibuprofen, naproxen, choline magnesium trisalicylate, and ketorolac. These agents are attractive because they show analgesic and anti-inflammatory activity. Aspirin is classified as an NSAID; however, this agent should generally be avoided for pain in children younger than 12 years because of concerns about the development of Reye syndrome. The common and maximum doses for these agents are shown in Table 2.

Ibuprofen (Caldolor; Cumberland Pharmaceuticals, Nashville, TN) and ketorolac are the only intravenous NSAIDs with an FDA-label indication for pain in the United States. Intravenous ibuprofen (Caldolor) has an FDA-label indication for pain and fever in children as young as age 6 months.[56] This agent should not be confused with the other salt form, ibuprofen lysine (NeoProfen; Lundbeck, Deerfield, IL), which is indicated for closure of the patent ductus arteriosus. However, there are currently no studies supporting the use of ibuprofen lysine (NeoProfen) for pain in pediatric patients, and this agent does not have an FDA-label indication.[47]

Ketorolac is approved for children younger than 2 years for single-dose treatment of 0.5 mg/kg/dose intravenously and 1 mg/kg/dose intramuscularly. Few studies have evaluated the efficacy of several doses of intravenous ketorolac. An observational study reports on 112 children ranging in age from 6 months to 19 years who received usual intravenous doses of 0.5-mg/kg/dose (range 0.17–1.0), most often every 6 hours.[57] Another report describes the use of ketorolac in 53 neonates and infants receiving a multiple dosing regimen.[58] The average dosage regimen included a loading dose of 0.93 ± 0.14 mg/kg followed by a maintenance regimen of 0.44 ± 0.09 mg/kg/dose every 6–8 hours. Although the authors did not specifically evaluate efficacy given the retrospective nature of the study, they proposed that the agent provided beneficial analgesic effects in these children after cardiac surgery. Of note,

this agent has a black box warning and should not be used for adults or children for more than 5 days because of an increased incidence of adverse events (i.e., gastrointestinal bleeding).[48]

The NSAIDs are associated with several adverse events that may limit their use in pediatric patients and are associated with an increased incidence of bleeding secondary to their inhibition of platelet aggregation. If a clinician desires to use an NSAID in a patient with thrombocytopenia or increased bleeding, choline magnesium trisalicylate should be considered because it has no appreciable effects on platelet aggregation. However, this agent is only available in a liquid preparation, which may not be an acceptable alternative for some patients.[50] Other adverse effects of NSAIDs include nephropathy and gastrointestinal bleeding caused by the inhibition of protective prostaglandins in the kidney and stomach, respectively. Ketorolac has been associated with a significant increase in gastrointestinal bleeding, ulceration, and perforation that appears to be related to duration of therapy and dosing.[48] These agents have been associated with fluid retention and edema, especially in patients with congestive heart failure and cardiac decompensation. However, one study suggests ketorolac is a safe option in children after cardiac surgery.[58]

Clinicians should consider two other disease states that may preclude the use of NSAIDs. Because NSAIDs inhibit prostaglandin production, children with asthma could experience an increase in leukotriene production, leading to the development of an asthma exacerbation. It is estimated that 2% of children with asthma are intolerant of aspirin, and another 5% of these patients may have a cross-intolerance with other NSAIDs.[59] A diagnosis of asthma alone should not rule out NSAID use in pediatric patients, but this issue does imply that a complete medication history, including a review of allergies, should be taken before an NSAID is prescribed. Another relative precaution of NSAIDs may be for patients with orthopedic injuries. Some animal research suggests that these agents impair bone healing, but reports are conflicting in this population.[59] One author recommends that the benefits of these agents outweigh the risk of adverse events, except in patient populations for whom bone healing may be a significant issue (e.g., patients recovering from posterior or anterior spinal fusions).[59]

Some clinicians recommend the use of alternating NSAIDs with acetaminophen for pain and/or fever. In addition, alternating agents may allow for use of lower doses of each agent and therefore decrease the risk of exceeding the maximum dose. Theoretically, there may be added benefits of using NSAIDs with acetaminophen because of their anti-inflammatory effects. Despite these perceived benefits, the studies comparing the combination versus single agents had design flaws, which limit their external validity.[60] Currently, the American Academy of Pediatrics (AAP) does not routinely recommend alternation of these agents.[60] In the inpatient setting, this approach may not cause significant concerns. However, in the outpatient setting, alternating NSAIDs and ibuprofen may be associated with caregiver confusion given the different concentrations of the commercially available dosage forms. If this approach is recommended, pharmacists should recommend that acetaminophen and NSAIDs should be alternated every

3 hours, so that they would not exceed the maximum dose or number of doses per day. In addition, caregivers should be encouraged to develop a schedule and keep a diary of medication administration pain to limit confusion.

Opioid analgesics. Opioid analgesics represent the mainstay of treatment for moderate to severe pain in children. These agents are available in several different dosage forms. With oral opioids, the onset of activity may be 45 minutes, with peak activity in 1–2 hours.[61] The intravenous route of administration is favored for patients with an acute onset of severe pain until their pain is under control and for patients who are unable to take oral medications. Some opioids are available for other routes of administration (e.g., transdermal, oral lozenges); however, these products are generally reserved for chronic pain rather than acute pain.

Overall, the mechanism of opioid analgesia is related to the agonism of mu- and kappa-opiate receptors. Coupled with the guanine-nucleotide-binding protein, these receptors modulate nerve activity through these proteins. Opioids inhibit the transmission of nerve impulses through the ascending pain pathway in the spinal cord and higher levels in the central nervous system. However, opioids have no effect on pain transmission through the peripheral nervous system. Unlike acetaminophen and NSAIDs, opioids are not associated with a ceiling effect. These agents can be titrated on the basis of clinical effect until significant adverse events, including respiratory depression, occur.

Table 3 lists the equianalgesic doses for the opioid agents together with suggested equianalgesic potencies.[18,34,35,62-70] Of note, there are significant differences between the potency of the opioid agents. Many different sources provide recommendations for various types of equianalgesic conversions. These conversions are based on potency and on pharmacokinetic guidelines of acute versus chronic administration. Clinicians should choose one set of opioid equianalgesic conversions that they are familiar with and use it consistently in their practice setting.

Specific agents. Intravenous opioids can be delivered by intermittent bolus, continuous infusion, or PCA. Bolus doses may be effective for patients needing immediate relief of pain, but the bolus dose can also be associated with an increase in adverse events. Intermittent dosing has been associated with inadequate pain control as plasma concentrations decrease between doses.[71-72] Continuous infusions are often used in patients requiring more steady-state opioid concentrations. This method of delivery has been found extremely effective in the postoperative setting.[72-73] Of note about continuous infusions is that patients may become tolerant of the effects of opioids and may require intermittent bolus doses of opioids over time or before painful procedures. Table 3 lists common doses for opioids delivered as continuous intravenous infusions including morphine, fentanyl, and hydromorphone.

Morphine is one of the most commonly prescribed opioid agents in children. It is available in several dosage forms including oral elixirs, tablets, and sustained-release products. Intravenous morphine is the most common opioid administered for intermittent bolus dosing. One important consideration about morphine is related to its metabolism. As mentioned previously, morphine is metabolized by glucuronidation to morphine-6-glucuronide (active metabolite) and morphine-3-glucuronide (inactive metabolite). Several studies have shown that morphine continuous infusions are less efficacious in neonates because of a reduced ability to produce the morphine-6-glucuronide metabolite.[31-33] Thus, some experts recommend against using this agent for continuous intravenous infusions.[32] Morphine is renally eliminated with a half-life from 1–3 hours in older infants and children and from 10–20 hours in preterm neonates.[35] With these considerations in mind, the usual dosage recommendations are provided in Table 3.

Morphine produces a significant degree of hypotension that may limit its use. Many different mechanisms for hypotension have been proposed including histamine-mediated vasodilation, negative chronotropic and inotropic effects on the heart, and a decrease in baroreceptor reflex response.[22] This adverse effect has mainly been implicated in patients who are hemodynamically unstable, but it can also occur with all opioids. In addition, the morphine-mediated histamine release may exacerbate episodes of bronchospasm in patients in status asthmaticus.[74] In these cases, it may be prudent to use alternative opioid agents including hydromorphone and fentanyl.

Hydromorphone is a potent opioid available in both oral and intravenous dosage forms. This agent is generally 5 times more potent than morphine. It may be preferred over morphine for intermittent dosing for patients in renal failure because of its decreased amount of metabolites.[22] Hydromorphone has pharmacologic properties similar to morphine. Despite these perceived advantages, there have been few studies describing the efficacy and safety of hydromorphone continuous infusions in children. A retrospective study conducted in 92 critically ill children receiving hydromorphone continuous infusions was found to be an effective analgesic agent.[75] Table 3 lists the common oral, intermittent bolus, and continuous intravenous infusion doses in children.

Fentanyl is a synthetic opioid that is structurally similar to meperidine. In general, it is thought to be 70–100 times more potent for single-dose administration than intravenous morphine. It is more lipophilic than intravenous morphine and has a quicker onset of action, 30 seconds versus 10 minutes.[63] In addition, fentanyl has a short half-life of about 2 hours in children. With the quick onset and short half-life, this agent is very useful for intubation and other procedures including dressing changes and lumbar puncture.

As a continuous infusion, fentanyl has been found to have a "context-sensitive" half-life of 21 hours secondary to its accumulation in peripheral tissue sites.[76] For patients receiving continuous infusions of fentanyl with acute onset of pain, it would be advisable to administer a bolus dose of fentanyl before increasing the rate of the continuous infusion secondary to this increased half-life. One adverse event that may limit the use of intermittent doses of fentanyl is chest wall rigidity. A prospective study of 89 premature and term neonates found that the overall incidence was low, at 4%.[77] Previous reports have noted that this adverse event occurred with fentanyl doses of 25–50 mcg/kg for patients during anesthetic induction, but this study found that chest rigidity occurred with the rapid administration of doses of 3–5 mcg/kg and greater.[76] Chest wall rigidity can be managed with a dose of intravenous naloxone of 10–40 mcg/kg, administration of a dose of an intravenous neuromuscular blocker before the fentanyl bolus, and/or adjustment of the mechanical ventilator for intubated patients.[77]

Methadone is a long-acting opioid often used for chronic pain and detoxification programs for heroin substance abuse. It also is also commonly used in many pediatric intensive care and neonatal intensive care units for iatrogenic opioid withdrawal for neonatal abstinence syndrome.[78] Methadone is metabolized by *N*-demethylation and has an extended half-life of 19 ± 14 hours (range 4–62 hours) in children.[64] It has generally the same potency as morphine, but the peak onset of action for intravenous methadone is 1–2 hours versus 10 minutes for intravenous morphine.[64] Methadone is structurally

Table 3. Opioid Analgesic Agents[18,34,35,62-70]

Medication	Equianalgesic Dose		Initial IV Dosages		IV/PO Ratio	Initial PO Dosages	
	IM/IV (mg)	PO (mg)	< 40 kg	≥ 40 kg		< 40 kg	≥ 40 kg
Morphine	10	Acute: 60 Chronic 10	Bolus: 0.05–0.2 mg/kg/dose every 2–4 hr (max 15 mg/dose) CI: 0.01–0.03 mg/kg/hr	Bolus: 2–5 mg every 2–4 hr CI: 0.8–1.5 mg/hr	Chronic: 1:2.5 Acute: 1:6	0.2–0.5 mg/kg/dose every 4–6 hr IR	10–30 mg every 3–4 hr IR
Hydromorphone	1.5	7.5	Bolus: 0.015 mg/kg/dose every 3–6 hr CI: 0.003–0.005 mg/kg/hr	Bolus: 1–2 mg every 2–4 hr CI: 0.3–0.5 mg/hr	1:3	0.03–0.08 mg/kg/dose every 3–4 hr (max 5 mg/dose)	2–4 mg every 3–4 hr
Fentanyl	0.1	—	Bolus: 1–2 mcg/kg/dose every 1–2 hr CI: 1–2 mcg/kg/hr	Bolus: 25–100 mcg every 1–2 hr CI: 25–100 mcg/hr	—	—	—
Methadone	Acute: 10 Chronic: 2–4	Acute: 20 Chronic: 2–4	Bolus: NR CI: NR	Bolus: NR CI: NR	Chronic: 1:2.5 Acute: 1:6	0.1 mg/kg/dose every 4 hr for 2–3 doses; then 0.1 mg/kg/dose every 6–12 hr (max 10 mg/dose)	5–10 mg every 4–12 hr
Meperidine	75–100	300	Bolus: 0.8–1 mg/kg/dose every 2–3 hr CI: NR	Bolus: 50–100 mg every 3–4 hr CI: NR	1:3	2–3 mg/kg/dose every 3–4 hr	50–150 mg every 3–4 hr
Codeine[a,b]	NR	200	NR	NR	NR	NR	NR
Oxycodone[a]	—	15–30	—	—	—	0.05–0.2 mg/kg/dose every 4–6 hr (max 5 mg/dose of oxycodone)	1–2 tablets (5 mg oxycodone) every 4–6 hr
Hydrocodone[a]	—	30–45	—	—	—	0.1–0.2 mg/kg/dose every 4–6 hr	1–2 tablets (5 mg hydrocodone) every 4–6 hr
Tramadol[a,b]	—	100	—	—	—	NR	IR[c]: 50–100 mg every 4–6 hr (max 400 mg/day) ER[d]: 100 mg/day (max 300 mg/day)
Buprenorphine	0.4	—	Bolus: 2–6 mcg/kg/dose every 4–6 hr CI: NR	Bolus: 0.3 mg every 6–8 hr CI: NR	—	5.3 mcg/kg/dose every 8 hr[e,f]	75–300 mcg/dose every 12 hr[e]

[a]These opioids are available as an oral combination product with acetaminophen. Clinicians should ensure that patients do not exceed 4 g of acetaminophen per day.
[b]Codeine and tramadol now have an FDA black box warning for use in children age < 12 yr, children < 18 yr undergoing a tonsillectomy and/or adenoidectomy, and children 12–18 yr who have a history of obstructive sleep apnea or severe lung disease.
[c]Tramadol is available as: (1) an IR tablet (50 mg) as Ultram (Janssen Ortho LLC, Gurabo, Puerto Rico) with an FDA-label indication for children age ≥ 17 yr for moderate or moderate to severe pain; (2) an IR orally disintegrating tablet (50 mg) as Rybix (Victory Pharma, Inc, San Diego, CA) with an FDA-label indication for age ≥ 17 yr for postoperative, cancer, neuropathic, and low back pain; and (3) an oral combination product with acetaminophen (Ultracet; Janssen Ortho LLC, Gurabo, Puerto Rico) for ≥ 18 yr for short-term (< 5 days) acute pain management.
[d]Tramadol is available as an ER tablet (100, 200, 300 mg) as Ultram ER with an FDA-label indication for children ≥ 18 yr for moderate to moderate to severe pain and as an ER capsule (100, 150, 200, 300 mg) as ConZip (Vertical Pharmaceuticals LLC, Bridgewater, NJ) for ≥ 18 yr with moderate or moderate to severe pain.
[e]Buprenorphine is available as a sublingual tablet or solution.
[f]Dosing recommendations for neonatal abstinence syndrome. No dosing recommendations exist for sublingual buprenorphine for infants and children beyond this indication.
CI = continuous intravenous infusion; ER = extended-release formulation; FDA = U.S. Food and Drug Administration; IM = intramuscular; IR = immediate-release formulation; IV = intravenous; max = maximum; NR = not recommended; PO = oral.

similar to verapamil and may exert calcium channel blockade.[78] All methadone formulations have been associated with bradycardia, hypotension, and cardiac arrhythmias including QT interval prolongation.[64,79] One report highlighted significant bradycardia with a widened QRS complex in an adult after a methadone continuous intravenous infusion.[80] The rapid administration of an intravenous methadone bolus dose in hemodynamically unstable patients could theoretically increase the likelihood of cardiovascular toxicities. Therefore, clinicians should consider avoiding intravenous methadone administration in children who can tolerate enteral administration of medications.

Meperidine is a synthetic opioid that is less potent, with a shorter duration of action than intravenous morphine. This agent is limited in the acute setting because of adverse events secondary to accumulation of its metabolite, normeperidine.[65] This metabolite is associated with adverse events including seizures, agitation, and hyperreflexia. Risk factors for these adverse events include patients receiving higher doses of meperidine or patients in renal failure.[81] This agent may be reserved for prevention of rigors after the administration of blood products or amphotericin and the treatment of postanesthetic shivering. However, its clinical usefulness for acute pain is limited at best.

Tramadol is a centrally acting opiate that binds to mu-opiate receptors to inhibit the ascending pain pathway.[66] It is metabolized by cytochrome P450 2D6 (CYP2D6) to O-desmethyltramadol. This agent also has additional activity beyond its effects with the opioid receptor because it inhibits the reuptake of norepinephrine and serotonin. Tramadol may have a role for some types of pain in the adolescent population. It is available in an immediate-release tablet, an immediate-release orally disintegrating tablet, and an extended-release formulation with FDA-label indications for children 17 years and older with moderate to severe pain and other types of pain syndromes, including neuropathic and postoperative pain (Table 3). The use of this agent may be limited in children with underlying seizure disorders because of its ability to lower the seizure threshold. Prescribers should avoid using tramadol in children who are receiving concomitant selective serotonin reuptake inhibitors (SSRIs) because of the potential for serotonin syndrome.[18]

Codeine is an opioid available in a combination product for patients with mild to moderate pain. The intravenous route of administration is not routinely recommended secondary to hypotension and vasodilation from histamine release. This agent is metabolized by CYP2D6 and demethylated to morphine.[67]

Several studies have noted safety and efficacy concerns with codeine and tramadol as a result of pharmacogenomics differences with the CYP2D6 isoenzyme. One concern is that some children may be "poor metabolizers" because of the decreased activity of the CYP2D6 isoenzyme, resulting in decreased conversion to their active metabolites and decreased analgesic effects.[82] A study investigated the genotype, phenotype, and morphine production in 96 children receiving codeine and diclofenac versus morphine and diclofenac after adenotonsillectomy.[83] The researchers found that 36% of children randomized to codeine and diclofenac

had no evidence of conversion to morphine, suggesting that these patients have deficiencies in 2D6 isoenzymes. An additional concern is that some patients may be "ultra-fast metabolizers" because of the additional activity of the CYP2D6 isoenzyme, which results in high concentrations of morphine and increased incidence of respiratory depression.[82] Several cases of significant respiratory depression and/or death in children receiving codeine and tramadol have been reported because of these pharmacogenomic variations.[84,85] These reports were noted in young children receiving scheduled acetaminophen and codeine or tramadol after adenotonsillectomy.[82] However, no widespread, clinically useful laboratory test is available to identify these pharmacogenomic variations with the CYP2D6 isoenzyme. Based on these concerns, the FDA issued a black box warning for codeine and tramadol for pain and cough for children younger than 12 years and for the treatment of pain after adenotonsillectomy for children younger than 18 years.[86] They also issued a warning for using codeine and tramadol in children 12–18 years with a history of obstructive sleep apnea or severe lung disease because of the increased risk of respiratory depression in these patients.[86] At this time, these agents should not be routinely recommended in patients with moderate to severe pain.

Buprenorphine is a mu opioid agonist, and it also displays properties as a weak kappa-opioid receptor antagonist.[68] It is available as an injection for intravenous or intramuscular use and sublingual tablets for buccal administration. Buprenorphine has a long half-life of about 20 hours in neonates. In adults, buprenorphine has been used for opioid detoxification and moderate to severe pain. Several studies have evaluated the use of buprenorphine for neonatal abstinence syndrome.[87] Because the commercially available sublingual tablets are not appropriate for neonates, many facilities have developed an extemporaneous enteral solution using the intravenous buprenorphine solution.[68] Currently, data are limited for use of buprenorphine for iatrogenic opioid withdrawal in the pediatric intensive care unit and for moderate to severe pain in children.

Hydrocodone and oxycodone are two other opioids available for oral administration. Structurally, these agents are similar to morphine and are considered more potent than codeine. Oxycodone is the most potent oral opioid agent and is used for moderate to severe pain. Table 3 shows the usual dosage. This agent is available in immediate-release tablets, an oral solution, and a controlled-release product.[69] Hydrocodone is an opioid used for moderate pain control and is available solely in combination products. These combination opioid analgesics are available in oral elixir preparations or tablets.[70] Of note, these agents are typically dosed on a "milligram per kilogram" basis according to the opioid analgesic agent. In 2011, the FDA requested that manufacturers of acetaminophen and opioid combination products reduce the acetaminophen content in their dosage forms.[88] Specifically, they have manufacturers reduce the acetaminophen content in these products to 325 mg per tablet, capsule, or other dosage unit to decrease the occurrence of toxicities that have been reported for the past several years. Despite this change, clinicians should still counsel the parents and caregivers receiving these medications to halt the use of other acetaminophen-containing products while taking these combination opioid agents.

It should be noted that there may be additional pharmacogenomic concerns with hydrocodone and oxycodone. These agents are metabolized via CYP2D6 to oxymorphone and hydromorphone, respectively.[69,70] A report described a case of fatal hydrocodone overdose in a child with a CYP2D6 alteration.[89] In 2015, the Clinical Pharmacogenetics Implementation Consortium provided updated recommendations on the use of codeine.[90] Now the consortium recommends that clinicians use an alternative for opioids metabolized through CYP2D6, including buprenorphine, morphine, fentanyl, hydromorphone, and methadone that are not metabolized by CYP2D6. This recommendation can be difficult to implement for pediatric patients because these agents do not all have pediatric dosage forms, and these agents would not be appropriate for children with acute, moderate to severe pain. The AAP has recommended further research must be conducted to identify the most appropriate alternative agents for children with moderate to severe pain.[82]

Other dosage forms of opioids are currently on the market. Rectal dosage forms are available for morphine. Fentanyl is available in a transdermal patch, an oral transmucosal lozenge, and a buccal tablet. These agents are preferred for patients with chronic cancer pain.[30,91] The transmucosal lozenge is generally avoided in most children because there is a risk they could bite down on the lozenge and receive an unintentional bolus of fentanyl. Buprenorphine is available as a transdermal patch for chronic pain.[68] In general, these medications are not used for the management of acute pain and should not be used in patients who are opioid naive or for patients in the postoperative period.

Adverse events. Several adverse events have been implicated with opioids, but a complete review of these events is beyond the scope of this chapter. Table 4 provides an overview to managing these adverse events.[22,92-96] In general, many of the adverse events can be managed by reducing the opioid dose, switching to another opioid agent, or adding another agent. Respiratory depression may be a specific concern in neonates and infants younger than 6 months because of their decreased renal elimination and hepatic immaturity, and they may be at higher risk of significant adverse events including respiratory depression, apnea, and hypoventilation.[34,97] As a result, all infants should receive routine pulse oximetry monitoring when administered opioids. Patients with obstructive sleep apnea or those who are opioid naive may also be at increased risk of respiratory depression and should be considered for cardiorespiratory monitoring by end-tidal carbon dioxide monitoring and/or pulse oximetry.[22]

Other adverse events may be common, including constipation, sedation, nausea/vomiting, and pruritus. Of importance, the rate of adverse events depends largely on the agent and dose used for pain control. All patients receiving long-term opioid agents should receive a scheduled bowel regimen to prevent or decrease the incidence of constipation. For patients who are refractory to the first-line agents in Table 4, other alternatives such as the addition of opioid receptor antagonists (opioid antagonists; e.g., naloxone, methylnaltrexone) have been useful.[22] In patients who experience pruritus, clinicians can consider the administration of oral or intravenous antihistamines to prevent severe itching. One review highlighted the potential benefit that opioid antagonists such as low-dose, continuous naloxone infusions may have for short-term use in patients experiencing a decreased quality of life and comfort associated with profound pruritus.[94] Sedation can be a significant adverse event noted in some patients, especially those with advanced cancer or human immunodeficiency virus.[22] In general, sedation can be managed by

Table 4. Management of Opioid Adverse Events[22,92-96]

Adverse Event	First-Line Intervention	Alternative Interventions
Respiratory depression	Reduce opioid dose if possible	Add low-dose opioid antagonist (e.g., naloxone)
Nausea/vomiting	Reduce opioid dose if possible; add antiemetic agent (e.g., promethazine[a] and/or ondansetron)	Add motility agent (e.g., metoclopramide); alternatively, consider low-dose opioid antagonist (e.g., naloxone)
Sedation	Add nonopioid analgesic to limit use of opioids or switch to opioid agent	Reduce opioid dose or add psychostimulant (e.g., methylphenidate)
Constipation	Add stool softener (e.g., docusate) for all patients, together with stimulant laxative (e.g., bisacodyl)	Add osmotic laxative (e.g., polyethylene glycol) or consider enema; alternatively, consider opioid antagonist (e.g., naloxone, methylnaltrexone)
Pruritus	Switch to different opioid agent (e.g., fentanyl); add antihistamine (e.g., diphenhydramine, hydroxyzine)	Alternatively, consider low-dose opioid antagonist (e.g., naloxone, nalbuphine)
Tolerance	Increase opioid dose or switch to a longer-acting agent	Add nonopioid analgesic or agent that prevents or delays tolerance (e.g., α_2-agonist, low-dose naloxone)
Withdrawal	Taper opioid dose slowly or add long-acting opioid agonist (e.g., methadone, extended-release morphine)	Add a α_2-agonist (e.g., dexmedetomidine, clonidine) or gabapentin

[a]Promethazine for children age > 2 yr because of the U.S. Food and Drug Administration black box warning for respiratory depression in younger children.

switching to another opioid agent, but this approach may not be possible in all patients. Some success has been reported with the use of psychostimulants such as methylphenidate or dextroamphetamine.[22] Clinicians should initiate the lowest dose of these psychostimulants possible and titrate to effect. Nausea and vomiting can also be a significant complication noted with opioid agents. The addition of antiemetics can be a very helpful strategy to manage this adverse event. Promethazine should be avoided in children younger than 2 years because of the black box warning for respiratory depression in this population. Other alternatives such as serotonin-3 receptor blockers, metoclopramide, and low-dose opioid antagonists may also be useful.[22]

Prolonged use of opioids can also be associated with additional complications that require careful consideration. Some children may experience *tolerance*, which refers to a decrease in analgesic effect despite a consistent serum plasma opioid concentration.[92] This complication occurs because of cellular changes at the opioid receptor or another receptor distant to it and can be managed by increasing the opioid dose, switching to another agent within its class, or adding another agent to reduce tolerance from occurring (e.g., ketamine, low-dose naloxone).[92,93] In general, patients receiving an extended duration of synthetic opioids such as fentanyl are more likely to be at risk because of the higher degree of tolerance associated with these agents versus the tolerance of patients receiving natural opioids like morphine.[93] Extended use of opioids can also result in additional complications including psychological dependence, addiction, and physiologic dependence. *Psychological dependence* refers to the individual's need for a substance to obtain euphoric effects. *Addiction* refers to an individual's persistent need to obtain an opioid medication for its euphoric effects, which often involves criminal activity to obtain the agent.[92] Addiction and psychological dependence are rare with acute pain and are topics beyond the scope of this chapter.

Physiologic dependence, more commonly known as *opioid abstinence syndrome*, can also occur in children who are iatrogenically receiving a prolonged duration of opioids. About 35% to 57% of critically ill infants and children develop withdrawal because of receiving long-term opioids in the intensive care unit setting.[93] Opioid abstinence syndrome symptoms fall into three separate categories: *central nervous system irritability*, such as anxiety, agitation, grimacing, and sleep disturbance; *gastrointestinal dysfunction*, such as vomiting and diarrhea; and *autonomic dysfunction*, such as tachypnea, diaphoresis, and hypertension.[98] Several agents have been suggested to treat these symptoms, including α_2-agonists and oral morphine and methadone tapers.[98] It is important for clinicians to have a careful discussion with parents and caregivers to help them understand that children who are experiencing withdrawal from the acute administration of opioids are unlikely to experience psychological dependence.

For children who are discharged on opioids, regardless of the indication, clinicians should perform thorough patient education. Because these agents have many serious adverse events, counseling should include not only a complete review of the agent and indication for use, but also proper instruction on the actual administration of the agent. When possible, all parents and caregivers should be given an oral syringe for children receiving liquid dosage forms of the opioid agents. For patients receiving complex taper schedules, it is the author's opinion that parents/caregivers should be provided a calendar that provides the schedule including the date of administration, the times of administration, and both the medication dose (in milligrams) and corresponding volume (in milliliters).

PATIENT- AND NURSE-CONTROLLED ANALGESIA

For children with severe pain, the use of PCA or nurse-controlled analgesia (NCA) can be quite effective. Patients who are administered intravenous intermittent opioid doses can often experience low opioid trough concentrations before their next scheduled dose, leading to increased pain. In addition, the initial administration of a bolus dose can result in an increased incidence of adverse events such as respiratory depression. With the PCA approach, studies have shown that patients can have similar or even lower pain scores but receive cumulatively fewer opioids than do other children.[22] The PCAs and NCAs involve the use of five components administered through an intravenous delivery pump: *initial dose, basal rate, PCA/NCA bolus dose, lockout time between doses* (e.g., 5–20 minutes), and *maximum opioid dose per hour or per every 4 hours* (i.e., depending on the institution's policy).[99] The three most common agents initiated are morphine, hydromorphone, and fentanyl. Table 5 provides an overview of the initial dosing recommendations for opioid-naive patients.[35,38,62,63,99]

Studies have shown that PCAs can be an effective strategy in children as young as 6 years.[22] Other studies have evaluated the use of PCAs in younger children but have not shown promising results. There have been some concerns that these children may lack the cognitive maturity to understand the relationship between pushing the button on the PCA delivery system and pain relief.[22] For children younger than 6 years, for children with cognitive impairment, or for those who are physically unable to push the button on the delivery system, NCA can be an alternative.

In addition to these strategies, parent- or caregiver-controlled analgesia has been suggested for patients with cognitive impairment or for those unable to push the button on

Table 5. Patient-Controlled Analgesia Dosing Recommendations[35,38,62,63,99]

Opioid Agent	Demand Dose	Lockout Time (min)	Basal Rate
Fentanyl	0.5–3 mcg/kg	6–8	0.5–3 mcg/kg/hr
Hydromorphone	2–5 mcg/kg	10–15	2–5 mcg/kg/hr
Morphine	0.02 mg/kg	10–15	0.02 mg/kg/hr

the delivery system. This approach is quite controversial and may not be an option at some institutions. Some advocates claim that the parents and caregivers of children know their child better and are thus better able to determine whether they are in pain. This method is thought to benefit children who may be unable to receive prompt attention from their nurse to push the bolus dose on their delivery system in hospitals with a higher patient/nurse ratio. The danger with this approach may be of special concern for children with acute onset of pain who are opiate naive (e.g., postoperative surgery). In such cases, the addition of several bolus doses can result in significant adverse events. As a result, some have restricted the use of this strategy to children with cancer or palliative care and have suggested a thorough education program for parents and caregivers involving pain assessment and an overview of opioids.[22]

CHRONIC PAIN MANAGEMENT

Overview. In addition to the acute pain episodes that children experience, there are chronic pain conditions in children that require alternative management, including cancer and burn pain. Many of these children may also experience concomitant psychiatric illnesses such as depression, anxiety disorders, and posttraumatic stress disorder that may also affect their pain.[18] Table 6 has some selected adjuvant agents used in the management of chronic pain.[18,100-111] A review of chronic pain for migraines appears in the Migraines chapter. Most of the medications do not have an FDA-label indication for chronic pain. Dosing information is either extrapolated from adult references, anecdotal case reports, or personal experience. Although these agents are used primarily in the management of chronic pain, the WHO guidelines for pain management clarify that these agents can be used at any stage (i.e., mild, moderate, or severe pain).[43] Because of the lack of compelling data from randomized controlled trials comparing these agents, the selection of these agents should be based on concomitant psychiatric illnesses, drug–drug interactions, and adverse events.

Specific Pain Disorders. Three specific pain disorders are reviewed here: neuropathic pain, cancer pain, and burn pain.

Neuropathic pain. Neuropathic pain refers to a complex type of chronic pain caused by irregular peripheral and central nervous system activity after the resolution of an injury (e.g., posttraumatic or postsurgical nerve injuries) or an inflammatory state.[18] Specific sources of neuropathic pain include solid-organ tumor infiltration of the peripheral nervous system, metabolic disorders, pain after spinal cord injury, and phantom-limb pain.[18,22] Adults often present with symptoms including "burning," "tingling," and "stabbing" pain after a hypersensitive response to even the slightest of touch to their skin, called *allodynia*.[22] Young children may have difficulty describing these symptoms. In these cases, additional tests such as quantitative sensory testing can be conducted to detect sensory abnormalities.[22] Some children and adolescents may also experience a specific type of neuropathic pain called *complex regional pain syndrome type I*, formerly known as *reflex sympathetic dystrophy*. This condition is characterized by several different symptoms including

allodynia, temperature instability, cyanosis, and swelling; it is caused by hyperalgesia in a specific body part (e.g., stomach, esophagus) in patients who have not suffered from a specific nerve injury.[18,22]

Managing neuropathic pain in children can be very difficult. In general, patients with neuropathic pain will not respond to opioid analgesics. Table 6 lists some of the most common agents used to treat neuropathic pain. In adults, the most common agents used as first-line treatment include tricyclic antidepressants and antiepileptics. This practice has been expanded to the management of neuropathic pain in children. The two most common tricyclic antidepressants used in children are nortriptyline and amitriptyline. These agents may be especially useful for children who may have insomnia because of their sedative effects. In general, nortriptyline may be preferred over amitriptyline in young children because of the commercial availability of an oral solution. Both of these agents have the potential to cause QT prolongation.[102,103] Clinicians should perform a thorough physical and family history for cardiac arrhythmias, heart disease, and syncope before these agents are initiated.[18] A baseline electrocardiogram should be conducted on all children.[22] Additional QT monitoring should be considered in patients who require additional increases in dosing for their pain. Children who develop a corrected QT interval greater than 445 milliseconds should be referred to a pediatric cardiologist.[18] Because of the potential toxic effects of these medications, some experts have suggested that clinicians prescribe no greater than a 30-day supply of them to ensure that only limited adverse events occur in children who may attempt suicide. When these agents are discontinued, clinicians should gradually taper the doses of the agents to prevent discontinuation syndrome (i.e., symptoms including agitation, sleep disturbances, and gastrointestinal complications).[18]

Several antiepileptics have been used to treat neuropathic pain. Table 6 lists two antiepileptics that have been used. The antiepileptic with the most available evidence is gabapentin; however, of note, no randomized controlled trials have compared the use of one antiepileptic over another.[22] Gabapentin has a favorable safety profile with less somnolence than other antiepileptics and is available in different dosage formulations for the pediatric population.[104] One important consideration with this agent is that the dosing for neuropathic pain is very patient-specific, and it is difficult to make conclusive recommendations on the dosing range for this indication. Topiramate is another antiepileptic that has been used in select patients with trigeminal neuralgia.[18] One particular concern with this agent is the potential for cognitive impairment. Children with this adverse event may have speech problems, memory difficulties, and significant problems concentrating, rendering this agent not useful for school-aged children.[105] One additional adverse event that should be monitored in patients receiving topiramate is weight loss. This adverse event may be especially difficult in children receiving palliative care who already may have difficulty in receiving adequate nutrition. Other antiepileptics have been used including valproic acid and carbamazepine, but the adverse effect profiles of these agents often limit the routine use for this indication in children.[18]

Table 6. Overview of Adjuvant Analgesic Agents[100-111]

Medication	Indication	Initial Dose by Patient Age	Dosing Formulations	Clinical Pearls
Amitriptyline	Neuropathic pain; adjuvant agent for burn pain	<12 yr: 0.1–2 mg/kg/dose at bedtime; ≥12 yr: 25–200 mg/dose at bedtime	Tablets (10, 25, 50, 75, 100, 150 mg)	Obtain ECG before initiating therapy
Nortriptyline	Neuropathic pain; adjuvant agent for burn pain	<12 yr: 0.05–1 mg/kg/dose at bedtime; ≥12 yr: 10–25 mg/dose at bedtime	Capsule (10, 25, 50, 75 mg); oral solution (2 mg/mL)	Obtain ECG before initiating therapy; preferred TCA in young children
Gabapentin	Neuropathic pain; adjuvant agent for burn pain	<12 yr: Day 1: 5 mg/kg/dose at bedtime; Day 2: 5 mg/kg/dose every 12 hr; Day 3: 5 mg/kg/dose every 8 hr; ≥12 yr: Day 1: 300 mg at bedtime; Day 2: 300 mg every 12 hr; Day 3: 300 mg every 8 hr	Tablet (300, 600, 800 mg); capsule (100, 300, 400 mg); oral solution (50 mg/mL)	Agent with most evidence in neuropathic pain; wide interpatient variability in dosing
Topiramate	Neuropathic pain (e.g., trigeminal neuralgia)	<12 yr: Wk 1: 1 mg/kg/dose at bedtime; Wk 2—1 mg/kg/dose every 12 hr; Wk 3—25 mg bid; ≥12 yr: Wk 1—25 mg at bedtime; Wk 2: 25 mg every 12 hr	IR tablets (25, 50, 100, 200 mg) and capsules (15, 25 mg); ER capsules (25, 50, 100, 150, 200 mg); extemporaneous solution (6 mg/mL)	Cognitive impairment may limit use in school-age children
Fluoxetine	Miscellaneous chronic pain; concomitant depression and anxiety	<12 yr: 0.25 mg/kg/dose or 5 mg/dose daily; ≥12 yr: 10–20 mg/dose daily	Capsule[a] (10, 20, 40 mg); oral solution (4 mg/mL)	Monitor for drug interactions; avoid abrupt discontinuation
Escitalopram	Miscellaneous chronic pain; concomitant depression and anxiety	6–12 yr: 2.5 mg daily; increase by 2.5 mg/dose after 1 wk; >12 yr: 10 mg/daily; titrate by 10 mg/dose after 1 wk	Tablet (5, 10, 20 mg); oral solution (1 mg/mL)	Monitor for drug interactions; avoid abrupt discontinuation
Diazepam	Decrease anxiety	<12 yr: 0.1 mg/kg/dose every 6–8 hr; ≥12 yr: 2–5 mg/dose every 6–8 hr	Tablets (2, 5, 10 mg); oral solutions (1, 5 mg/mL)	Concentrated diazepam solution contains 19% ethanol; prolonged half-life; relies heavily on hepatic metabolism
Lorazepam	Decrease anxiety	<12 yr: 0.05 mg/kg/dose every 4–8 hr; ≥12 yr: 2 mg every 4–8 hr	Tablets (0.5, 1, 2 mg); oral solution (2 mg/mL)	Preferred benzodiazepine for acute pain management
Clonidine	Decrease need for additional opioids; adjuvant agent for burn pain	PO: <12 yr: 2 mcg/kg/dose every 4–6 hr; >12 yr: 0.05–0.1 mg every 6–8 hr; Transdermal: > 12 yr: 0.1 mg/day patch to change every 5–7 days	Tablets (0.1, 0.2, 0.3 mg)[b]; ER tablets (0.1 mg); extemporaneous suspension (0.01, 0.02, 0.1 mg/mL)	Must be tapered before discontinuation to avoid withdrawal symptoms

[a] Also available in tablets (10, 20, 60 mg) as Sarafem (Warner Chilcott Company, Inc., Fajardo, Puerto Rico) with an FDA-label indication for premenstrual dysphoric disorder.
[b] Also available in a 0.1-mg ER tablet (Kapvay; Shionogi Pharma, Inc., Atlanta, GA) for children with attention-deficit/hyperactivity disorder and a 0.17-mg ER tablet (Nexiclon XR; Tris Pharma, Inc., Monmouth Junction, NJ) and 0.09-mg/mL ER oral suspension (Nexiclon XR) with an FDA-label indication for hypertension in adults.
ECG = electrocardiogram; ER = extended-release formulation; FDA = U.S. Food and Drug Administration; IR = immediate-release formulation; TCA = tricyclic antidepressant; PO = oral.

Other antidepressants may be effective adjuvant agents in children experiencing neuropathic pain. The SSRIs have shown some effect in adults to decrease various types of pain episodes.[18] These agents may be especially useful in children with concomitant anxiety and depression in addition to chronic pain. Table 6 lists two of the SSRIs with an FDA indication for depression in the pediatric population.[106,107] Alternatively, venlafaxine and duloxetine have also shown some promise in the management of chronic pain. These agents inhibit the release of norepinephrine and serotonin and may have some direct effect on antagonizing selected pain receptors.[18] In children with chronic pain and concomitant depression, the SSRIs, venlafaxine, and duloxetine may be preferred over tricyclic antidepressants because of the difference in their adverse event profiles. There are special concerns to note, however. Venlafaxine is associated with hypertension and orthostatic hypotension, and, for this reason, children receiving this agent should receive routine blood pressure monitoring.[18] The SSRIs may be associated with serotonin syndrome in children receiving concomitant agents such as tramadol and trazodone.[18]

Cancer pain. Children with cancer experience pain from many different sources. For example, children with a newly diagnosed solid-organ tumor may experience severe pain as a symptom on initial presentation. These tumors can cause significant pain because of infiltration of the viscera, bone, and nerves.[22] Children with hematologic malignancies such as leukemia and lymphoma can also experience infiltration of malignant cells into the viscera and bone marrow and also can present with splenic and hepatic distention.[22] Other children may experience pain from many different etiologies including severe mucositis, distress from painful diagnostic or therapeutic procedures, or pain associated with metastasis to other organs (e.g., bone, lungs).

Mucositis can be a difficult source of acute but also chronic pain in children with cancer. This complication can occur as the result of high-dose chemotherapy or radiation. A complete review of this topic is beyond the scope of this chapter. In general, the mainstay of treatment is preventive care, with good oral hygiene performed to ensure removal of loose tissue and to keep the mucosa moist, which can be accomplished with saline, chlorhexidine, or hydrogen peroxide mouth rinses.[112] For patients experiencing mild cases of mucositis, treatment involves topical therapies consisting of antimicrobial mouthwashes, amino acid rinses, and topical healing agents.[112] For patients with more profound pain, opioid agents should be considered. In patients undergoing bone marrow transplantation in which mucositis may be a profound problem, children may require the use of PCA to control their pain.[22]

The management of advanced cancer pain in children is very difficult and involves the use of pharmacologic and nonpharmacologic approaches. In such cases, the goal should be to keep the patient comfortable and optimize their quality of life. The NSAIDs should be initiated for children experiencing bone pain. Choline magnesium trisalicylate should be first-line therapy in children with profound thrombocytopenia. Scheduled opioids should be initiated for severe pain. In children able to take solid dosage forms, sustained-release or extended-release agents should be initiated, together with an immediate-release product for breakthrough pain. Methadone oral solution may be a suitable alternative in children who are unable to swallow tablets because of its long half-life. Transdermal fentanyl may also be an option in children older than 2 years. The doses of these agents should be escalated on the basis of the patient's response, keeping in mind that both tolerance and the disease itself will have a profound impact on a child's opioid requirement. In refractory cases, PCAs should be considered and titrated to effect until these agents can be switched to a more acceptable long-term alternative. Clinicians should keep in mind that the opioid adverse events might be the rate-limiting step in escalating a child's dose. As a result, they should use the strategies listed in Table 4 and consider using an adjuvant agent listed in Table 6 to reduce the incidence of these adverse events. It has been estimated that 90% of children with advanced cancer will respond to gradual escalation in their opioid therapy.[18] However, another 5% of children may require more than a 100-fold increase in their opioid dose and the use of alternative approaches to pain management including intrathecal administration of anesthetics and opioids, agents targeted at neuropathic pain (e.g., gabapentin), or sedative agents.[22] Nonpharmacologic interventions such as spiritual care and massage therapy should also be considered for children receiving palliative care.

Burn pain. Children with burn injuries can experience both acute and chronic pain. Thermal, electrical, and chemical burns are common in children younger than 10 years.[100] All children with burn injuries will experience pain, no matter the type or severity of the injury. If this pain is untreated in children, they may experience nonadherence to their treatment therapies and have delayed wound healing.[101] They may also develop concomitant psychiatric disease states such as posttraumatic stress disorder because of the untreated pain.[101] Children with acute burn pain may experience background or continuous pain as well as pain associated with procedures.[100] Although the continuous or background pain can be alleviated with scheduled analgesics, the management of procedural pain (e.g., associated with dressing changes) may be difficult to assess. Clinicians may have a difficult time identifying that the procedure itself is a source of a child's pain; thus, many children may have a source of untreated pain during these periods.[101]

Once the burn injuries are healed, children with these injuries may experience chronic pain, often because of neuropathic pain.[101] In such cases, opioid and nonopioid agents will not be entirely effective in diminishing pain. Antidepressants and antiepileptics are useful treatments in these situations. Evidence has suggested that gabapentin has several roles in the management of burn pain. This agent decreases the hyperalgesia associated with acute injury and has shown some positive impact in children with neuropathic pain.[100] In addition, gabapentin has been a useful agent to inhibit the management of refractory pruritus in children after burn injuries.[100]

Anxiety can play a major role in the underlying pain that children face after a burn injury. They may especially be anxious before procedures and treating their anxiety can decrease their anticipatory anxiety before the procedure. Anxiolytic agents also reduce opioid requirements and may have a role in decreasing opioid tolerance.[101] As a result, clinicians have often used benzodiazepines as an adjuvant therapy in burn victims. Table 6 lists two specific benzodiazepines used in maintenance therapy. Diazepam has a long and variable half-life in children that ranges from 15 to 95 hours.[108] It undergoes extensive hepatic metabolism to two active metabolites. Lorazepam has a shorter half-life and is primarily metabolized by glucuronidation to an inactive metabolite.[109] Lorazepam may be preferred to diazepam in patients with burn injuries who may have hepatic or renal insufficiency to avoid the accumulation of active metabolites.

Central α_2-agonists such as clonidine may also be a useful approach to alleviating acute and chronic pain associated with burn injuries. Children with acute burn injuries may require significant escalation in their opioid doses to achieve analgesic effect because of rapidly developing tolerance. In such cases, patients may develop an increased incidence of adverse events, limiting the use of opioids for chronic pain.[100] Central α_2-agonists work to augment the descending pain pathway and thus possess anxiolytic, sedative, and analgesic properties.[93] Studies have noted that these agents can have an opioid-sparing effect in certain types of pain episodes.[100] Clonidine is available as an enteral formulation and as a transdermal patch. The transdermal patch may be suitable in some patients. The lowest dosage form is 0.1 mg, and this dose may exceed the recommended initial dose per kilogram for young children. Some individuals have suggested that these patches be cut into smaller patches; however, this practice is not encouraged. As such, this agent can also be compounded as an extemporaneous formulation that can be suitable for young children because of difficulty in obtaining consistent pharmacokinetic concentrations (Table 6).[110,111] Dexmedetomidine is another commercially available α_2-agonist. This agent is 6–8 times as potent as clonidine; however, it is only available as an intravenous agent and would not be appropriate for long-term administration. Special care must be taken in children who discontinue these agents. Withdrawal symptoms are common and can include rebound hypertension, irritability, and agitation if they are tapered too quickly.[111]

PROCEDURAL PAIN MANAGEMENT

Other nonopioid analgesics may be used for localized administration in children in the emergency department or hospital setting. These agents may be used for many different indications including suture of lacerations, needle procedures, placement of an intravenous line, and prevention of pain associated with laboratory draws.[113,114] The following are recommendations for medications for minor procedures and suture/laceration repair in the emergency department and inpatient settings.

Lidocaine-based agents. Several lidocaine-based agents have been used for minor procedures for placement of intravenous lines and prevention of pain with blood draws including LMX$_4$ (Ferndale Laboratories, Ferndale, MI), Synera (ZARS Pharma, Salt Lake City, UT), and the J-Tip needless injection system (National Medical Products, Irvine, CA). The drug

LMX$_4$ is a 4% topical lidocaine formulation manufactured in an encapsulated lipid layer for greater dermal absorption. It is available over-the-counter in the United States and is recommended for children 2 years and older.[115,116] This product is available over-the-counter for patients with chronic illness who may require frequent trips to the emergency department and has a fast onset of activity, within 15–30 minutes.

Another product, Synera, has an FDA-label indication for children 3 years and older for superficial venous access and dermatologic procedures (e.g., shave biopsy of skin and skin excision).[117] Synera is a combination patch consisting of lidocaine 70 mg and tetracaine 70 mg. This unique disposable patch is composed of an oxygen-activating system to enhance the absorption of the active ingredients through the stratum corneum. After it is removed from its package, its level of heating reaches a maximum skin temperature of 40°C or less.[118] This agent has an onset time of 20 minutes, and, ideally, it should be applied 20–30 minutes before procedures. Of importance, several patches should be applied simultaneously or in immediate succession, and the Synera patch should not be applied to broken or nonintact skin.[117]

In 2001, a needle-free injection of lidocaine, the J-Tip needleless injection system, was introduced to the market. This agent is a disposable, needle-free injection device that uses pressurized carbon dioxide to deliver either 0.25 mL or 0.5 mL of lidocaine into subcutaneous skin.[119] This product, a delivery system, must be filled in the pharmacy with typically 1%–2% buffered lidocaine powder.[119] The product is operated by pressing the device firmly against the skin where the procedure is to take place. Then, subsequently pressing the lever on the device begins the delivery of the lidocaine within seconds and results in an onset of analgesia in 1–3 minutes.[118]

Another topical lidocaine product, Zingo (Anesiva, Inc., South San Francisco, CA), has an FDA-label indication for children 3 years and older for venipuncture or peripheral intravenous line insertion.[120] This agent is a helium-propelled delivery device that provides 0.5 mg of lidocaine hydrochloride monohydrate. One of the main differences between this product and the J-tip delivery system is that this product contains prefilled lidocaine and does not have to be prepared by the pharmacy department.

The AAP Committee on Pediatric Emergency Medicine and Section on Anesthesiology and Pain Medicine has provided recommendations on the role of selected topical agents for procedural pain.[16] They recommend that LMX$_4$ can be many different settings for painful procedures including lumbar puncture, joint aspiration, and abscess drainage.[16] This committee did not specifically address Synera, Zingo, or the J-Tip needle-free injection system. It is difficult to make evidence-based decisions between these agents because there are few clinical trials comparing them. All of these agents have a different onset of action, a variance in cost, and different delivery mechanisms. For pain prevention with procedures, the AAP Committee recommended that the lidocaine-based agents be administered as soon as possible to the affected area to ensure adequate anesthetic effect. One important consideration is that, regardless of the lidocaine-based agent used, it will not provide complete pain relief. Other agents like benzodiazepines and opioids may also have to be administered to complete these procedures. Relative contraindications to the products include allergies to amide anesthetics and non-intact skin.

Other procedural agents. For patients requiring other minor procedures including suture and laceration repair, clinicians may use a combination of topical anesthetics/vasoconstrictor combinations such as lidocaine, epinephrine, and tetracaine (LET). The exact formulation of LET may differ from institution to institution according to the recipe of the pharmacy department. This product has been noted to achieve anesthesia for wound suture repair in 20–30 minutes.[121] The AAP recommends that a maximum dose of 3 mL of LET is indicated for lacerations less than 5 mm on the head, neck, extremities, or trunk. The use of LET is contraindicated in patients who may have an allergy to one of the amide anesthetics, for wounds greater than 5 mm, or for wounds in the ear and genitalia. Of note, the maximum dose of lidocaine administered without epinephrine is 4 mg/kg and, with epinephrine, is 7 mg/kg.[22] Some experts also recommend that intravenous diphenhydramine could be used if a patient receives greater than the maximum dose of lidocaine or LET because of intravenous diphenhydramine's partly local anesthetic effects.[22]

Another unique pharmacologic agent that has been used for minor procedures is vapocoolant spray. This product works by rapidly cooling the skin, with the goal of slowing the initiation and conduction of nerve impulses.[118] Gebauer's Ethyl Chloride (Gebauer's Pain Ease, Cleveland, OH) is recommended for venipuncture and minor procedures.[122] This agent works immediately, but its duration of action is 15 seconds. Gebauer's Pain Ease should be sprayed for 4–10 seconds continuously and at no greater than 7 inches away from the skin.[122] Experts state that if this agent is used, it may take two providers to perform the procedure, with one professional to administer the agent and the other one to perform the procedure.[118] Some children may not tolerate the cooling sensation and may have increased anxiety and perceived pain from the administration of this agent alone. With the availability of other agents for minor procedures, the use of the agents has diminished.[118]

Oral sucrose solutions may be considered for infants for prevention of pain with minor procedures. Sucrose solutions have been associated with a decrease in the production of painful stimuli from heel sticks and venipunctures in neonates.[123] Several institutions have adopted compounded formulations of sucrose. Two commercially available products are available on the market, Sweet-Ease (Koninklijke Philips NV, Andover, MA) and Toot Sweet (Natus Medical, Pleasanton, CA). A study found significant analgesic activity with sucrose combined with the use of a pacifier in neonates.[124] Therefore, the AAP recommends that sucrose solutions be administered to infants younger than 6 months and be used in combination with a pacifier and administered no more than 2 minutes before starting a procedure.[16] The recommended weight-based dosing using the commercially available 24% solution is 0.1 mL/dose for children less than 1 kg, 0.1–0.2 mL/dose for 1–2 kg, and 0.1–0.5 mL/dose for greater than 2 kg.[125] For procedures, it is recommended to be administered 2 minutes before the procedure, repeating up to two additional times as needed.

CONCLUSIONS

Pediatric pain management remains a definite challenge for health care professionals. Many differences exist between the assessment and management of pain in children versus adults. Each health care provider should ensure that pain is assessed on a routine basis with a standardized approach. Several non-pharmacologic interventions are available that should be used in conjunction with pharmacologic treatment. Pharmacists definitely need to be involved in the multidisciplinary pain management in children. As pharmacists, we can play a role in the selection of the appropriate medication for the specific type of pain, monitoring of adverse events, and provision of recommendations for managing these adverse events. In addition, all pharmacists should be involved with the education of parents/caregivers and the patients themselves to ensure that they understand the indication for each pain medication and understand how to safely administer these medications.

A 7-year-old girl (25 kg) with no known drug allergies is brought to the emergency department with fever, right leg pain, and respiratory distress. After fluid resuscitation, she is transferred to the pediatric intensive care unit where vancomycin and ceftriaxone are started. She is placed on oxygen and high-flow nasal cannula to support her respiratory status. Her blood cultures are found to be positive with methicillin-resistant *Staphylococcus aureus*, with susceptibilities pending. Findings on magnetic resonance imaging of her right leg suggest osteomyelitis. She reports moderate to severe pain as noted by her verbalization of her pain with the FACES Scale.

Past medical history: Noncontributory

Physical examination:

General: Mildly dehydrated

Mental status: Alert and oriented × 3

Vital signs: Tmax 102.5°F (39°C), HR 120 beats/minute, BP 80/55 mm Hg, RR 26 breaths/minute, urine output 0.5 mL/kg/hour

Pain scores: Average of 8 based on Face Legs Activity Cry Consolability (FLACC) scale

Laboratory findings:

WBC: 29.3×10^3 cells/mm³; 65% lymphocytes

Platelets: 109×10^3 cells/mm³

Hgb: 12.1 g/dL

Hct: 38%

Basic metabolic panel: Na 136 mEq/L, K 4.4 mEq/L, Cl 107 mEq/L, HCO_3 22 mEq/L, BUN 10 mg/dL, SCr 1.3 mg/dL, glucose 91 mg/dL, Ca (total serum) 8.6 mg/dL

The pediatric intensive care unit team wishes to initiate a pain management regimen. What regimen would you recommend?

Based on the patient's source and pain rating, she would be classified with moderate to severe pain as noted by a score of 8 on the Face Legs Activity Cry Consolability (FLACC) scale, indicating the use of a potent opioid together with a nonopioid. A patient-controlled analgesia (PCA) may be the best choice in treating pain while also limiting the risk of respiratory distress with intermittent dosing. Morphine PCA basal dose 0.5 mg/hour plus 0.5 mg PCA demand dose with a lockout interval of 10 minutes would be an appropriate pain regimen. Intermittent dosing of an opioid, such as morphine, has an increased risk of respiratory distress and may not adequately control the patient's pain. Nonsteroidal anti-inflammatory drugs (NSAIDs) would be a great choice for pain management because the patient has osteomyelitis. However, NSAIDs are contraindicated because of the patient's elevated serum creatinine and decreased urine output. Therefore, acetaminophen would be the best choice as a nonopioid for this patient.

A 12-year-old boy (40.2 kg) was admitted to the hematology/oncology service with worsening mucositis and neutropenic fever. He is initiated on intravenous cefepime and vancomycin. On hospital day 4, he begins to develop significant tingling in his face, arms, thighs, and hands.

Past medical history:

Pre-B cell acute lymphocytic leukemia; patient currently undergoing consolidation regimen

Central-line placement

Home medications:

Fentanyl 12 mcg/hour transdermal patch

Oxycodone 5 mg orally every 4 hours as needed for pain

Ondansetron 6 mg orally every 6 hours as needed for nausea/vomiting

Chlorhexidine 15 mL orally as directed

Physical examination:

General: Ill-appearing, moaning in pain

Mental status: Alert and oriented × 3

Vital signs: Tmax 101.7°F (38°C), HR 100–112 beats/minute, BP 88–127/52–83 mm Hg, RR 20–24 breaths/minute, urine output 3.3 mL/kg/hour

Pain scores: Average of 9–10 based on the Numeric Rating Scale

Laboratory findings:

WBC: 0.44×10^3 cells/mm³; 42% lymphocytes

Platelets: 42×10^3 cells/mm³

Hgb: 12.6 g/dL

Hct: 36%

Basic metabolic panel: Na 139 mEq/L, K 2.7 mEq/L, Cl 109 mEq/L, HCO_3 22 mEq/L, BUN 8 mg/dL, SCr 0.24 mg/dL, glucose 91 mg/dL, Ca (total serum) 8.0 mg/dL

Current medications:

Vancomycin 20 mg/kg intravenously every 6 hours

Cefepime 50 mg/kg intravenously every 8 hours

Morphine patient-controlled analgesia (PCA): basal dose 1.7 mg/hour; 0.7 mg PCA demand dose; lockout 15 minutes

Acetaminophen 650 mg every 6 hours orally as needed for mild pain/fever

The pediatric hematology/oncology team would like recommendations on how to address the patient's pain regimen. What would you recommend?

This patient is experiencing moderate to severe pain despite an opioid PCA and as-needed acetaminophen. Based on the patient's symptoms, he appears to be experiencing neuropathic pain. Opioids and nonopioids are not extremely effective for neuropathic pain; therefore, initiation of an adjunct agent is recommended. Gabapentin and tricyclic antidepressants appear to have the best efficacy for neuropathic pain. Choline magnesium trisalicylate is a useful nonopioid agent for pain in patients with low platelets because it does not inhibit platelet aggregation in low doses. Gabapentin 300 mg every 8 hours orally is also an option for this patient. However, opioids and nonopioids are not extremely effective for neuropathic pain.

REFERENCES

1. Anand KJS. Pharmacological approaches to the management of pain in the neonatal intensive care unit. J Perinatol 2007;27:S4-11.

2. Friedrichsdorf SJ, Postier A, Eull D, et al. Pain outcomes in a US Children's Hospital: A prospective cross-sectional survey. Hosp Pediatr 2015;5:18-26.

3. Merskey H, Albe-Fessard D, Bonica J. Pain terms: a list with definitions and notes on usage. Recommended by the IASP Subcommittee on Taxonomy. Pain 1979;6:249-52.

4. McIntosh N. Pain in the newborn, a possible new starting point. Eur J Pediatr 1997;156:173-7.

5. Schechter NL, Allen A, Hanson K. Status of pediatric pain control: a comparison of hospital analgesic usage in children and adults. Pediatrics 1986;77:11-5.

6. Taddio A, Katz J, Ilersich AL, et al. Effect of neonatal circumcision on pain response during subsequent routine vaccination. Lancet 1997;349:599-603.

7. Taddio A, Shah V, Gilbert-MacLeod C et al. Conditioning and hyperalgesia in newborns exposed to repeated heel lances. JAMA 2002;288:857-61.

8. Walker SM, Franck LS, Fitzgerald M, et al. Long-term impact of neonatal intensive care and surgery on somatosensory perception in children born extremely preterm. Pain 2009;141:79-87.

9. Anand KJS, Craig KD. New perspectives on the definition of pain. Pain 1996;67:3-6.

10. Anand KJS, Hickey PR. Pain and its effects in the human neonate and fetus. N Engl J Med 1982;317:1321-9.

11. Renn CL, Dorsey SG. The physiology and processing of pain: a review. AACN Clin Issues 2005;16:277-90.

12. Golianu B, Krane EJ, Galloway KS, et al. Pediatric acute pain management. Pediatr Clin North Am 2000;47:559-87.

13. Hummel P, Puchalski M. Assessment and management of pain in infancy. Newborn Infant Nurs Rev 2001;1:114-21.

14. Walter-Nicolet E, Annequin D, Biran V, et al. Pain management in newborns: from prevention to treatment. Pediatr Drugs 2010;12:353-65.

15. Bauman BH, McManus JG. Pediatric pain management in the emergency department. Emerg Med Clin North Am 2005;23:393-414.

16. Fein JA, Zempsky WT, Cavero JP; American Academy of Pediatrics Committee on Pediatric Emergency Medicine and Section on Anesthesiology and Pain Medicine. Relief of pain and anxiety in pediatric patients in emergency room systems. Pediatrics 2012;130:1391-405.

17. The Joint Commission. Facts about pain management. Available at https://www.jointcommission.org/topics/pain_management_standards_hospital.aspx. Accessed September 11, 2019.

18. Zeltzer LK, Krane EJ, Palermo TM. Pediatric pain management. In: Kliegman RM, Stanton BF, Geme JW, Schor NF, eds. Nelson's Textbook of Pediatrics, 20th ed. Philadelphia: Saunders Elsevier, 2016:430-48.

19. Srouji R, Ratnapalan S, Schneeweiss S. Pain in children: assessment and nonpharmacological management. Int J Pediatr 2010;2010.

20. Hagan JF, Coleman, Foy JM, et al. The assessment and management of acute pain in infants, children, and adolescents. Pediatrics 2001;108:793-7.

21. Merkel S, Voepel-Lewis T, Malviya S. Pain assessment in infants and young children: the FLACC scale. Am J Nurs 2002;102:55-68.

22. Greco C, Berde C. Pain management for the hospitalized pediatric patient. Pediatr Clin North Am 2005;995-1027.

23. Wong-Baker FACES Foundation [homepage on the Internet]. Available at www.WongBakerFACES.org. Accessed July 15, 2018.

24. Chambers CT, Craig KD. An intrusive impact of anchors in children's faces pain scales. Pain 1998;78:27-37.

25. Voepel-Lewis T, Burke CN, Jeffreys N, et al. Do 0-10 numeric rating scores translate into clinically meaningful pain measures for children? Anesth Analg 2011;112:415-21.

26. Breau LM, Finley GA, McGrath PJ, et al. Validation of the Non-communicating children's pain checklist-postoperative version. Anesthesiology 2002;96:528-35.

27. Rutter N. Percutaneous drug absorption in the newborn: hazards and uses. Clin Perinatol 1987;14:911-30.

28. Okah FA, Wickett RR, Pickens WL, et al. Surface electrical capacitance as a noninvasive bedside measure of epidermal barrier maturation in the newborn infant. Pediatrics 1995;96:688-92.

29. West DP, Worobec S, Solomon LM. Pharmacology and toxicology of infant skin. J Invest Dermatol 1981;76:147-50.

30. Finkel JC, Finley A, Greco C, et al. Transdermal fentanyl in the management of children with chronic severe pain: results from an international study. Cancer 2005;104:2847-57.

31. Carbajal R, Lenclen R, Jugie M, et al. Morphine does not provide adequate analgesia for acute procedural pain among preterm neonates. Pediatrics 2005;115:1494-500.

32. Anand KJS, Hall RW, Desai N, et al. Effects of morphine analgesia in ventilated preterm neonates: primary outcomes from the NEOPAIN randomized trial. Lancet 2004;363:1673-82.

33. Simons SHP, van Dijk M, van Lingen RA, et al. Routine morphine infusion in preterm newborns who received ventilatory support: a randomized controlled trial. JAMA 2003;290:2419-27.

34. Berde CB, Sethna NF. Drug therapy: analgesics for the treatment of pain in children. N Engl J Med 2002;347:1094-103.

35. Lexi-Comp Online, Lexi-Drugs Online [Internet database]. Morphine monograph. Hudson, OH: Lexi-Comp. Updated periodically.

36. Hales CM, Fryar CD, Carroll MD, et al. Trends in obesity and severe obesity prevalence in US youth and adults by sex and age, 2007-2008 to 2015-2016. JAMA 2018;319:1723-5.

37. Johnson PN, Miller JL, Hagemann TM, et al. Assessment of inpatient admissions and top 25 medications for obese pediatric patients at two academic hospitals. Am J Health-Syst Pharm 2016;73:1243-9.

38. Johnson PN, Miller JL, Hagemann TM. Sedation and analgesia in critically-ill children. AACN Advanced Critical Care 2012;23:415-34.

39. Shibutani K, Inchiosa MA Jr, Sawada K, et al. Accuracy of pharmacokinetic models for predicting plasma fentanyl concentrations in lean and obese surgical patients: derivation of dosing weight ("pharmacokinetic mass"). Anesthesiology 2004;101:603-13.

40. Shibutani K, Inchiosa MA Jr, Sawada K, et al. Pharmacokinetic mass of fentanyl for postoperative analgesia in lean and obese patients. Br J Anaesth 2005;95:377-83.

41. Gish EC, Harrison D, Gormley AK, et al. Dosing evaluation of continuous intravenous fentanyl infusions in overweight children. J Pediatr Pharmacol Ther 2011;16:39-46.

42. Johnson PN, Skpepnek GH, Golding CL, et al. Relationship between rate of fentanyl infusion and time to achieve sedation in nonobese and obese critically ill children. Am J Health-Syst Pharm 2017;74e:367-76.

43. World Health Organization (WHO). WHO guidelines on the pharmacological treatment of persisting pain in children with medical illness. Available at https://www.ncbi.nlm.nih.gov/books/NBK138354/. Accessed September 11, 2019.

44. Sciulli MG, Seta F, Tacconelli S, et al. Effects of acetaminophen on constitutive and inducible prostanoid biosynthesis in human blood cells. Br J Pharmacol 2003;138:634-41.

45. Lexi-Comp Online, Pediatric Lexi-Drugs Online [Internet database]. Acetaminophen monograph. Hudson, OH: Lexi-Comp. Updated periodically.

46. Ofirmev [package insert]. Hazelwood, MO: Mallinckrodt Pharmaceuticals, 2014.

47. Lexi-Comp Online, Pediatric Lexi-Drugs Online [Internet database]. Ibuprofen monograph. Hudson, OH: Lexi-Comp. Updated periodically.

48. Lexi-Comp Online, Pediatric Lexi-Drugs Online [Internet database]. Ketoralac monograph. Hudson, OH: Lexi-Comp. Updated periodically.

49. Lexi-Comp Online, Pediatric Lexi-Drugs Online [Internet database]. Naproxen monograph. Hudson, OH: Lexi-Comp. Updated periodically.

50. Lexi-Comp Online, Pediatric Lexi-Drugs Online [Internet database]. Choline magnesium trisalicylate monograph. Hudson, OH: Lexi-Comp. Updated periodically.

51. Consumer Healthcare Products Association (CHPA). Acetaminophen: CHPA supports the current acetaminophen monograph dosing. Available at www.chpa.org/acetaminophen.aspx. Accessed July 15, 2018.

52. Infants' Tylenol oral suspension. Available at www.tylenol.com/products/infants-tylenol-oral-suspension. Accessed July 15, 2018.

53. Buck ML. Perioperative Use of High-Dose Rectal Acetaminophen. Pediatric Pharmacotherapy: A Monthly Newsletter for Health Care Professionals from the Children's Medical Center at the University of Virginia 2001;7. Available at https://med.virginia.edu/pediatrics/wp-content/uploads/sites/237/2015/12/200109.pdf. Accessed July 15, 2018.

54. Prince JS. When IV acetaminophen costs skyrocketed, one health system did some new math. Available at https://www.drugtopics.com/health-system-news/when-iv-acetaminophen-costs-skyrocketed-one-health-system-did-some-new-math. Accessed July 15, 2018.

55. Watkins PB, Kaplowitz N, Slattery JT, et al. Aminotransferase elevations in healthy adults receiving 4 grams of acetaminophen daily: a randomized controlled trial. JAMA 2006;296:87-93.

56. Caldolor [package insert]. Nashville, TN: Cumberland Pharmaceuticals, 2016.

57. Buck ML. Clinical experience with ketorolac in children. Ann Pharmacother 1994;28:1009-13.

58. Moffett BS, Wann TI, Carberry KE, et al. Safety of ketorolac in neonates and infants after cardiac surgery. Pediatr Anaesth 2006;16:424-8.

59. Kokki H. Nonsteroidal anti-inflammatory drugs for postoperative pain: a focus on children. Pediatr Drugs 2003;5:103-23.

60. Section on Clinical Pharmacology and Therapeutics; Committee on Drugs, Sullivan JE, Farrar HC. Fever and antipyretic use in children. Pediatrics 2011;127:580-7.

61. American Pain Society. Principles of analgesic use in the treatment of acute pain and chronic cancer pain. Clin Pharm 1990;9:601-11.

62. Lexi-Comp Online, Pediatric Lexi-Drugs Online [Internet database]. Hydromorphone monograph. Hudson, OH: Lexi-Comp. Updated periodically.

63. Lexi-Comp Online, Pediatric Lexi-Drugs Online [Internet database]. Fentanyl monograph. Hudson, OH: Lexi-Comp. Updated periodically.

64. Lexi-Comp Online, Pediatric Lexi-Drugs Online [Internet database]. Methadone monograph. Hudson, OH: Lexi-Comp. Updated periodically.

65. Lexi-Comp Online, Pediatric Lexi-Drugs Online [Internet database]. Meperidine monograph Hudson, OH: Lexi-Comp. Updated periodically.

66. Lexi-Comp Online, Pediatric Lexi-Drugs Online [Internet database]. Tramadol monograph. Hudson, OH: Lexi-Comp. Updated periodically.

67. Lexi-Comp Online, Pediatric Lexi-Drugs Online [Internet database]. Codeine monograph. Hudson, OH: Lexi-Comp. Updated periodically.

68. Lexi-Comp Online, Pediatric Lexi-Drugs Online [Internet database]. Buprenorphine monograph. Hudson, OH: Lexi-Comp. Updated periodically.

69. Lexi-Comp Online, Pediatric Lexi-Drugs Online [Internet database]. Oxycodone monograph. Hudson, OH: Lexi-Comp. Updated periodically.

70. Lexi-Comp Online, Pediatric Lexi-Drugs Online [Internet database]. Hydrocodone monograph. Hudson, OH: Lexi-Comp. Updated periodically.

71. Lynn AM, Nespeca MK, Bratton SL, et al. Intravenous morphine in postoperative infants: intermittent bolus dosing versus targeted continuous infusion. Pain 2000;88:89-95.

72. Malviya S, Pandit UA, Merkel S, et al. A comparison of continuous epidural infusion and intermittent intravenous bolus doses of morphine in children undergoing selective dorsal rhizotomy. Reg Anesth Pain Med 1999;24:438-43.

73. Esmail Z, Montgomery C, Courtrn C, et al. Efficacy and complications of morphine infusions in postoperative paediatric patients. Paediatr Anaesth 1999;9:321-7.

74. Reisine T, Pasternak G. Opioid analgesics and antagonists. In: Hardman JG, Limbird LE, eds. The Pharmacological Basis of Therapeutics. New York: McGraw-Hill, 1995:521-5.

75. Reiter PD, Ng J, Dobyns EL. Continuous hydromorphone for pain and sedation in mechanically ventilated infants and children. J Opioid Manag 2012;8:99-104.

76. Ginsberg B, Howell S, Glass PS, et al. Pharmacokinetic model-driven infusion of fentanyl in children. Anesthesiology 1996;85:1268-75.

77. Fahnenstich H, Steffan J, Kau N, et al. Fentanyl-induced chest wall rigidity and laryngospasm in preterm and term infants. Crit Care Med 2000;28:836-9.

78. Johnson PN, Boyles KA, Miller JL. Selection of the initial methadone regimen for the management of iatrogenic opioid abstinence syndrome in critically ill children. Pharmacotherapy 2012;32:148-57.

79. Schwinghammer AJ, Wilson MD, Hall BA. Corrected QT interval prolongation in hospitalized pediatric patients receiving methadone. Ped Crit Care Med 2018;19:e403-8.

80. Karir V. Bradycardia associated with intravenous methadone administration for sedation in a patient with acute respiratory distress syndrome. Pharmacotherapy 2002;22:1196-9.

81. Anonymous. American Hospital Formulary Service. In: McVoy GK, ed. Drug Information. Bethesda, MD: American Society of Hospital Pharmacists, 1987, 1991, 1994, 1997, 1999, 2001.

82. Tobias JD, Green TP, Cote CJ; Section of anesthesiology and pain medicine; Committee on Drugs. Codeine: Time to say "no". Pediatrics 2016;138:e20162396.

83. Williams DG, Patel A, Howard RF. Pharmacogenetics of codeine metabolism in an urban population of children and its implications for analgesic reliability. Br J Anaesth 2002;89:839-45.

84. Ciszkowski C, Madadi P. Codeine, ultrarapid-metabolism genotype, and postoperative death. N Engl J Med 2009;361:827-8.

85. Orliaguet G, Hamza J, Couloigner V, et al. A case of respiratory depression in a child with ultrarapid CYP2D6 metabolism after tramadol. Pediatrics 2015;135:e753-5.

86. FDA Drug Safety Communication: FDA restricts use of prescription codeine pain and cough medicines and tramadol pain medicines in children; recommends against use in breastfeeding women. Available at https://www.fda.gov/drugs/drug-safety-and-availability/fda-drug-safety-communication-fda-restricts-use-prescription-codeine-pain-and-cough-medicines-and. Accessed July 13, 2018.

87. Kraft WK, Adeniyi-Jones SC, Chervoneva I, et al. Buprenorphine for the treatment of the neonatal abstinence syndrome. N Engl J Med 2017;376:2341-8.

88. US Food and Drug Administration safety communication. Prescription acetaminophen products to be limited to 325 mg per dosage unit; boxed warning will highlight potential for several liver failure. Available at https://www.fda.gov/drugs/drug-safety-and-availability/fda-drug-safety-communication-prescription-acetaminophen-products-be-limited-325-mg-dosage-unit. Accessed July 15, 2018.

89. Madadi P, Hildebrandt D, Gong I, et al. Fatal hydrocodone overdose in a child: Pharmacogenetics and drug interactions. Pediatrics 2010;126:986-9.

90. Clinical Pharmacogenomics Implementation Consortium (CPIC) guideline information for codeine and CYP2D6 [homepage on the Internet]. PharmGKB: pharmacogenomics, knowledge, and implementation. Available at https://www.pharmgkb.org/guidelineAnnotation/PA166104996. Accessed July 15, 2018.

91. Fine P, Marcus M, De Boer A, et al. An open label study of oral transmucosal fentanyl citrate (OTFC) for the treatment of breakthrough cancer pain. Pain 1991;45:149-53.

92. Tobias JD. Tolerance, withdrawal, and physical dependency after long-term sedation and analgesia of children in the pediatric intensive care unit. Crit Care Med 2000;28:2122-32.

93. Anand KJS, Wilson DF, Berger J, et al. Tolerance and withdrawal from prolonged opioid use in critically ill children. Pediatrics 2010;125:e1208-25.

94. Miller JL, Hagemann TL. Pure opioid antagonists in the management of opioid-induced pruritus. Am J Health Syst Pharm 2011;68:1419-25.

95. Rodriguez A, Wong C, Mattiussi A, et al. Methylnaltrexone for opioid-induced constipation in pediatric oncology patients. Pediatr Blood Cancer 2013;60:1667-70.

96. Lopez J, Fernandez S, Santiago MJ, et al. Methylnaltrexone for the treatment of constipation in critically ill children. J Clin Gasteroenterol 2016;50:351-2.

97. Purcell-Jones G, Dorman F, Summer E. The use of opioids in neonates: a retrospective study of 933 cases. Anesthesia 1987;42:1316-20.

98. Johnson PN. Pain and sedation. In: Eiland L, Todd T, eds. Advanced Pediatric Therapeutics. Memphis, TN: Pediatric Pharmacy Advocacy Group. 2015;433-59.

99. Plate J, Goldstein LB. Post-operative patient-controlled analgesia in pediatric patients. Available at https://www.practicalpainmanagement.com/pain/acute/post-surgical/post-operative-patient-controlled-analgesia-pediatric-patients. Accessed July 15, 2018.

100. Gandhi M, Thomson C, Lord D, et al. Management of pain in children with burns. Int J Pediatr 2010;2010.

101. Richardson P, Mustard L. The management of pain in the burns unit. Burns 2009;35:921-36.

102. Lexi-Comp Online, Pediatric Lexi-Drugs Online [Internet database]. Amitriptyline monograph. Hudson, OH: Lexi-Comp. Updated periodically.

103. Lexi-Comp Online, Pediatric Lexi-Drugs Online [Internet database]. Nortriptyline monograph. Hudson, OH: Lexi-Comp. Updated periodically.

104. Lexi-Comp Online, Pediatric Lexi-Drugs Online [Internet database]. Gabapentin monograph. Hudson, OH: Lexi-Comp. Updated periodically.

105. Lexi-Comp Online, Pediatric Lexi-Drugs Online [Internet database]. Topiramate monograph Hudson, OH: Lexi-Comp. Updated periodically.

106. Lexi-Comp Online, Pediatric Lexi-Drugs Online [Internet database]. Fluoxetine monograph. Hudson, OH: Lexi-Comp. Updated periodically.

107. Lexi-Comp Online, Pediatric Lexi-Drugs Online [Internet database]. Escitalopram monograph. Hudson, OH: Lexi-Comp. Updated periodically.

108. Lexi-Comp Online, Pediatric Lexi-Drugs Online [Internet database]. Diazepam monograph. Hudson, OH: Lexi-Comp. Updated periodically.

109. Lexi-Comp Online, Pediatric Lexi-Drugs Online [Internet database]. Lorazepam monograph. Hudson, OH: Lexi-Comp. Updated periodically.

110. Lexi-Comp Online, Pediatric Lexi-Drugs Online [Internet database]. Clonidine monograph. Hudson, OH: Lexi-Comp. Updated periodically.

111. Capino AC, Miller JL, Johnson PN. Clonidine for sedation and analgesia and drug withdrawal in critically ill infants and children. Pharmacotherapy 2016;36:1290-9.

112. Miller MM, Donald DV, Hagemann TM. Prevention and treatment of oral mucositis in children with cancer. J Pediatr Pharmacol Ther 2012;17:340-50.

113. Kleiber C, Sorenson M, Whiteside K, et al. Topical anesthetics for intravenous insertion in children: a randomized equivalency study. Pediatrics 2002;110:758-61.

114. Berde C. Local anesthetics in infants and children: an update. Paediatr Anesth 2004;14:387-93.

115. Wong D. Topical local anesthetics. Am J Nurs 2003;103:42-5.

116. LMX$_4$ [package insert]. Ferndale, MI: Ferndale Laboratories, 2014.

117. Synera [package insert]. Souderton, PA: Galen US, Inc., 2013.

118. Zempsky WT. Pharmacologic approaches for reducing venous access in children. Pediatrics 2008;122:S140-53.

119. J-Tip Needle-Free Injection System. Available at https://jtip.com. Accessed July 15, 2018.

120. Zingo [package insert]. South San Francisco, CA: Anesiva, Inc., 2007.

121. Ernst AA, Marvez E, Nick TG, et al. Lidocaine adrenaline tetracaine gel versus tetracaine adrenaline cocaine gel for topical anesthesia in linear scalp and facial lacerations in children aged 5 to 17 years. Pediatrics 1995;95:255-8.

122. Gebauer's Pain Ease. Available at www.gebauer.com/ethylchloride. Accessed July 15, 2018.

123. Lewindon PJ, Harkness L, Lewindon N. Randomized controlled trial of sucrose by mouth for the relief of infant crying after immunisation. Arch Dis Child 1998;78:453-6.

124. Carbajal R, Chauvet X, Couderc S, et al. Randomized trial of analgesic effects of sucrose, glucose, and pacifiers in term neonates. BMJ 1999;319:1393-7.

125. Lexi-Comp Online, Pediatric Lexi-Drugs Online [Internet database]. Sucrose monograph. Hudson, OH: Lexi-Comp. Updated periodically.

Section X

Psychiatric Disorders

CHAPTER 31

Attention-Deficit/Hyperactivity Disorder

Joshua Caballero, Pharm.D., FCCP, BCPP

INTRODUCTION

Attention-deficit/hyperactivity disorder (ADHD) is one of the most commonly diagnosed childhood psychiatric disorders. In general, ADHD may display two types of symptoms: inattentive and hyperactive/impulsive types (Box 1). Patients with inattentive symptoms may display careless mistakes or can be easily distracted by external factors. Patients who display symptoms of hyperactivity/impulsivity may have difficulty sitting still, may be unable to play quietly, or may blurt out answers before a complete question is asked.

Consequences of ADHD can include poor school and social functioning for the child. If left untreated, ADHD may lead to increased rates of not completing high school, unemployment, unwanted pregnancy, sexually transmitted diseases, traffic accidents, and incarceration.[1-3] In addition, increased rates of substance abuse and diagnosis of a major psychiatric disorder (e.g., bipolar, anxiety) have been cited in adults with ADHD.[4] Interacting with a child with ADHD can also create a significant amount of stress among caregivers and teachers. Finding the best pharmacologic agent to treat and manage symptoms, together with educational and behavioral therapies, is of utmost importance for this patient population. With many agents available, it is crucial that practitioners select the optimal medication(s) that may serve to appropriately treat symptoms while minimizing adverse events.

EPIDEMIOLOGY

The prevalence of ADHD ranges from 3% to 20% in school-age children, depending on the criteria and sample population used.[5] However, it is estimated that the worldwide prevalence is 5%, although it appears to be almost 9% in the United States.[6,7] The differences in prevalence may be a result of how studies classify "functional impairment" in their patients.[8] Persistence into adolescence and adulthood may reach 85% and 31%, respectively.[9,10] The adult prevalence is estimated at 2.5% because it is believed that some patients "outgrow the disease," undergo neurobiologic maturation, or find better coping mechanisms to adapt to the environment as they grow older.[11] However, caution is warranted because some in the medical community believe that patients do not truly "outgrow the disease"; rather, they outgrow the older diagnostic criteria set forth by the *Diagnostic and Statistical Manual of Mental Disorders, Fourth Edition, Text Revision* (*DSM-IV-TR*).[12,13] Most recently, the *DSM, Fifth Edition* (*DSM-5*) includes symptoms found in older adolescents and adults, such as paying bills, returning phone calls, keeping appointments, and intrusion into or taking over what others are doing. Also, whereas six or more symptoms are required for children, only five or more symptoms are required in either symptom domain (i.e., inattention, hyperactivity/impulsivity) for adolescents and adulthood.

ETIOLOGY

There appears to be a genetic predisposition to ADHD. Studies have shown the heritability of ADHD is about 77% when at least one parent has ADHD.[14] Several genetic/biologic markers in ADHD have been studied, including the 480-bp allele, the dopamine transporter gene, and the dopamine receptor genes.[15] The gene with the strongest association

Box 1. Diagnostic Criteria for Attention-Deficit/Hyperactivity Disorder in the *Diagnostic and Statistical Manual of Mental Disorders, Fifth Edition*[21]

A. A persistent pattern of inattention and/or hyperactivity-impulsivity that interferes with functioning or development, as characterized by (1) and/or (2):

1. **Inattention**: Six (or more) of the following symptoms have persisted for at least 6 months to a degree that is inconsistent with developmental level and that negatively impacts directly on social and academic/occupational activities:

   Note: The symptoms are not solely a manifestation of oppositional behavior, defiance, hostility, or failure to understand tasks or instructions. For older adolescents and adults (age 17 and older), at least five symptoms are required.

   a. Often fails to give close attention to details or makes careless mistakes in schoolwork, at work, or during other activities (e.g., overlooks or misses details, work is inaccurate).

   b. Often has difficulty sustaining attention in tasks or play activities (e.g., has difficulty remaining focused during lectures, conversations, or lengthy reading).

   c. Often does not seem to listen when spoken to directly (e.g., mind seems elsewhere, even in the absence of any obvious distraction).

   d. Often does not follow through on instructions and fails to finish schoolwork, chores, or duties in the workplace (e.g., starts tasks but quickly loses focus and is easily sidetracked).

   e. Often has difficulty organizing tasks and activities (e.g., difficulty managing sequential tasks; difficulty keeping materials and belongings in order; messy, disorganized work; has poor time management; fails to meet deadlines).

   f. Often avoids, dislikes, or is reluctant to engage in tasks that require sustained mental effort (e.g., schoolwork or homework; for older adolescents and adults, preparing reports, completing forms, reviewing lengthy papers).

   g. Often loses things necessary for tasks or activities (e.g., school materials, pencils, books, tools, wallets, keys, paperwork, eyeglasses, mobile telephones).

   h. Is often easily distracted by extraneous stimuli (for older adolescents and adults, may include unrelated thoughts).

   i. Is often forgetful in daily activities (e.g., doing chores, running errands; for older adolescents and adults, returning calls, paying bills, keeping appointments).

2. **Hyperactivity and impulsivity**: Six (or more) of the following symptoms have persisted for at least 6 months to a degree that is inconsistent with developmental level and that negatively impacts directly on social and academic/occupational activities:

   Note: The symptoms are not solely a manifestation of oppositional behavior, defiance, hostility, or a failure to understand tasks or instructions. For older adolescents and adults (age 17 and older), at least five symptoms are required.

   a. Often fidgets with or taps hands or feet or squirms in seat.

   b. Often leaves seat in situations when remaining seated is expected (e.g., leaves his or her place in the classroom, in the office or other workplace, or in other situations that require remaining in place).

   c. Often runs about or climbs in situations where it is inappropriate. (Note: In adolescents or adults, may be limited to feeling restless.)

   d. Often unable to play or engage in leisure activities quietly.

   e. Is often "on the go," acting as if "driven by a motor" (e.g., is unable to be or uncomfortable being still for extended time, as in restaurants, meetings; may be experienced by others as being restless or difficult to keep up with).

   f. Often talks excessively.

   g. Often blurts out an answer before a question has been completed (e.g., completes people's sentences; cannot wait for turn in conversation).

   h. Often has difficulty waiting his or her turn (e.g., while waiting in line).

   i. Often interrupts or intrudes on others (e.g., butts into conversations, games, or activities; may start using other people's things without asking or receiving permission; for adolescents and adults, may intrude into or take over what others are doing).

B. Several inattentive or hyperactive-impulsive symptoms were present prior to age 12 years.

C. Several inattentive or hyperactive-impulsive symptoms are present in two or more settings (e.g., at home, school, or work; with friends or relatives; in other activities).

D. There is clear evidence that the symptoms interfere with, or reduce the quality of, social, academic, or occupational functioning.

E. The symptoms do not occur exclusively during the course of schizophrenia or another psychotic disorder and are not better explained by another mental disorder (e.g., mood disorder, anxiety disorder, dissociative disorder, personality disorder, substance intoxication or withdrawal).

Specify whether:

314.01 (F90.2) Combined presentation: If both Criterion A1 (inattention) and Criterion A2 (hyperactivity-impulsivity) are met for the past 6 months.

314.00 (F90.0) Predominantly inattentive presentation: If Criterion A1 (inattention) is met but Criterion A2 (hyperactivity-impulsivity) is not met for the past 6 months.

314.01 (F90.1) Predominantly hyperactive/impulsive presentation: If Criterion A2 (hyperactivity-impulsivity) is met but Criterion A1 (inattention) is not met over the past 6 months.

Specify if:

In partial remission: When full criteria were previously met, fewer than the full criteria have been met for the past 6 months, and the symptoms still result in impairment in social, academic, or occupational functioning.

Specify current severity:

Mild: Few, if any, symptoms in excess of those required to make the diagnosis are present, and symptoms result in only minor functional impairments.

Moderate: Symptoms or functional impairment between "mild" and "severe" are present.

Severe: Many symptoms in excess of those required to make the diagnosis, or several symptoms that are particularly severe, are present, or the symptoms result in marked impairment in social or occupational functioning.

Reprinted with permission from the *Diagnostic and Statistical Manual of Mental Disorders, Fifth Edition* (Copyright © 2013). American Psychiatric Association. All Rights Reserved.

in ADHD appears to be the 7-repeat allele of the dopamine receptor D4 gene.[16] However, this association has been questioned because it was still small, and there is yet to be an actual gene associated with ADHD.[17] In addition, studies suggest that a genetic predisposition in patients predicts their treatment response.[18] For example, those with a 9-repeat allele show poor response to methylphenidate treatment.[18] Recent data also report that copy number variants, which are submicroscopic chromosomal abnormalities, may be implicated in ADHD (e.g., excess of 16p13.11 duplications).[19]

Environmental triggers associated with ADHD are countless and may include smoking during maternal pregnancy, lead exposure, low birth weight, and severe social deprivation during early infancy.[8] Certain foods (e.g., chocolate, eggs, peanuts) and artificial colors or dyes (e.g., yellow #5, red #3, blue #1) may also exacerbate hyperactive symptoms of ADHD.[20] Of interest, it has been hypothesized that a histamine degradation gene is responsible for hyperactive responses to food dyes.[21]

DIAGNOSIS

The main types of symptoms associated with ADHD include inattention and hyperactivity/impulsivity. The *DSM-5* criteria for diagnosis further describe the common symptoms of

ADHD, which are listed in Box 1. The literature on ADHD may classify patients as predominantly inattentive, predominantly hyperactive/impulsive, or combined type, in which the patient displays a combination of symptoms.

Common features of inattention include difficulty organizing activities, sustaining attention, and following through on instructions, as well as being easily distracted by extraneous stimuli.[22] For example, a young student who sits in the classroom but does not listen attentively in class or successfully complete assignments and often misplaces pencils and books has ADHD of the predominantly inattentive type.

Hallmark features of hyperactivity include often fidgeting with hands or feet, leaving the seat in classroom, and having difficulty engaging quietly in leisure activities. Impulsive symptoms may also be present, which include having difficulty waiting one's turn and interrupting others. For example, a young student who disrupts the classroom by running around at inappropriate times, answering out of turn, and constantly talking with surrounding classmates has ADHD of the predominantly hyperactive/impulsive type. Whereas, for example, another student who has difficulty following directions when spoken to directly (e.g., does not follow orders), avoids completing assignments, talks excessively with classmates, and squirms excessively in the chair has the combined type ADHD.

The female population with ADHD tends to display inattentive symptoms, whereas the male population tends to display hyperactive symptoms.[23] As a result, by comparing the examples just cited, teachers and parents may be more prone to refer male versus female students (at a ratio of 3:1) for diagnosis because hyperactivity will more likely disrupt the classroom or home setting. However, for a proper diagnosis, these behaviors must be present before age 12 years, occur in two or more settings (e.g., home, classroom), and cause significant impairment in the child's social and academic development.

As with most mental health diagnoses, there is a level of subjectivity with diagnosing children with ADHD. Over the past few decades, the diagnosis of ADHD in the pediatric population has increased, and recent data state significant evidence of overdiagnosis in developed countries.[24] One reason for overdiagnosing ADHD includes clinical judgment affected by heuristics because the criteria can be interpreted differently among diagnosticians. Other explanations may include overlapping factors between mental health symptoms; changes added to *DSM-5*, such as lower age of onset for ADHD; diagnosis without using the *DSM* criteria; and health policy limitations, such as a clinician diagnosing a child with borderline symptoms so that the patient may receive insurance coverage.

RATING SCALES

Several scales are used to measure ADHD symptoms.[25] These scales primarily identify specific symptoms that can assist in diagnosing and identifying the subtypes of ADHD. The most commonly known scales include the Conners Rating Scales-Revised (CRS-R); IOWA Conners scale; Swanson, Nolan, and Pelham-IV questionnaire (SNAP-IV); and ADHD Rating Scale-IV. Newer scales, including the Vanderbilt ADHD Rating Scale (VARS) and the ADHD Symptoms Rating Scale (ADHD-SRS), have been developed to capture symptoms/manifestation of conduct disorders, anxiety, or depression (e.g., VARS) and to increase attention to the subtlety of the ways in which ADHD affects social functioning (e.g., ADHD-SRS).[25,26] The time required to complete the scales varies. Some scales such as the CRS-R, SNAP-IV, and ADHD-SRS may take 20–30 minutes to complete, whereas others such as the IOWA Conners, ADHD RS-IV, and VARS may take only 5–15 minutes to complete.[25] All six scales can be completed by parents or teachers. Although some scales (e.g., CRS-R, ADHD RS-IV) may be completed by an adult with ADHD, data are lacking to support whether older adolescents can complete the scales. Some scales (e.g., IOWA Conners, SNAP-IV, ADHD RS-IV, ADHD-SRS) may be divided into two or three subscales, whereas other scales (e.g., CRS-R, VARS) may have four to seven subscales.[25] Of note, most of these scales were derived from *DSM-IV-TR* criteria and therefore predominantly target hyperactive/impulsive symptoms.[25] Thus, caution is needed when using these scales to evaluate female patients who may have more inattentive symptoms.

PATHOPHYSIOLOGY

The pathophysiology of ADHD is complex, with patients showing overall decreased cerebral volume. Specific regions of the brain that consistently show a reduction in size in ADHD include the caudate nucleus, prefrontal cortex white matter, and cerebellar vermis.[27,28] Impairment of the prefrontal cortex and anterior cingulate cortex, which are responsible for controlling appropriate behaviors and inhibitions, appears to be the primary culprit in the manifestation of ADHD.[8,29,30] It is theorized that a prefrontal cortex abnormality exists that causes a dysregulation of two primary neurotransmitters: dopamine and norepinephrine. Dopamine appears to be active in the mesocortical pathways responsible for aspects of cognitive function including verbal fluency, serial learning, executive function, and sustaining attention.[30-31] Norepinephrine appears to be active in the prefrontal pathway responsible for mediating energy/fatigue, motivation, moderation of behavior on the basis of social cues, and sustaining attention.[31] Of note, unlike in other psychiatric illnesses (e.g., depression, schizophrenia, bipolar disorder), serotonin does not seem to play a major role in ADHD. As a result, selective serotonin reuptake inhibitors may be given to those with ADHD who also have a psychiatric comorbidity such as major depression; however, these agents are clinically useless in the treatment of ADHD.

TREATMENT

NONPHARMACOLOGIC TREATMENTS

The best nonpharmacologic treatment available is behavioral therapy, usually given concomitantly with some form of educational session. Behavioral therapy attempts to eliminate or limit inappropriate behaviors by reinforcing desired behaviors. Some short-term studies have shown that behavioral therapy can improve ADHD symptoms, especially in the home environment when used with pharmacologic agents.[32] However, it is not fully clear whether using behavioral therapy as adjunctive treatment will decrease medication dosage. Long-term (3-year) studies show that behavioral therapy may decrease the future incidence of delinquency or substance use.[33] Therefore, behavioral therapy may be considered monotherapy or adjunctive treatment to pharmacologic agents.[34] Behavioral therapy may be used as monotherapy if symptoms are mild, if ADHD diagnosis is unclear, or if parents refuse pharmacologic agents.[8,34] However, therapy sessions can be time consuming (1–3 times a week lasting 30–60 minutes) and can be costly (more than $100/visit); insurance plans may only cover a limited number of sessions. Data suggest that therapy may be more beneficial in preschool children; however, with such variety in treatment (length of sessions, types of behavioral therapy), it is difficult to ascertain who may best respond to behavioral therapy.[35] In addition, there may be a lack of trained professionals (e.g., psychologists, psychiatrists) in certain regions, and identifying a qualified therapist may not be possible.

Diets and certain herbal supplements to treat ADHD have been popular through the years. The Kaiser Permanente or elimination diet (also known as Feingold diet), which works at eliminating foods containing synthetic additives (e.g., benzoate preservatives) or dyes (e.g., yellow #5, yellow #6) has been studied to evaluate its effectiveness in treating symptoms of

ADHD.[36-38] Some trials have shown a significant decrease in behaviors (e.g., hyperactivity) when elimination diets were used.[36] However, the differences might not have been clinically significant and were only noted on the parents' rating scales, with no changes noted on the health care providers' ratings. It also appears that the improvement in behaviors occurred in all children despite ADHD diagnosis, leading to the belief that artificial food dyes and preservatives should be limited in all children.[36,37] Foods containing benzoate preservatives may include soft drinks, fruit juices, sauces (e.g., ketchup, mustard), and pickles. Foods containing dyes may include processed products such as cereals, potato chips, candy, fruit juices, and carbonated beverages. In addition, elimination diets cause a widely varying response among patients, which may be caused by genetic variability (e.g., the histamine degradation gene).[21,36] Therefore, future pharmacogenomic testing may identify those with a higher sensitivity (e.g., greater hyperactive response) to certain foods or additives. Elimination diets may prove highly effective in a small selection of patients; however, these treatment options should not be used to replace prescription therapy (e.g., stimulants). Recent data suggest elimination diets (i.e., gluten-free casein-free, food additive exclusion, oligoantigenic) offer small benefits, and well-controlled trials are still needed.[20] There are also concerns regarding the ability to stay adherent to these diets over long periods of time and during festive events (e.g., holidays, birthdays).

Most diets rich in ω-3 fatty acids have shown no greater efficacy than placebo.[39] However, recent data suggest that a combination of essential fatty acids including eicosapentaenoic acid, docosahexaenoic acid, and γ-linolenic acid provides some benefits for inattention symptoms.[38] The benefits of these fatty acids, although small, may not be seen for at least 3 months. Homeopathy has also been studied, and despite showing some improvements, data appear to be inconsistent and subject to interpretation. As a result, these interventions offer minor relief of symptoms in studies with weak methodologies and prone to bias (e.g., parents vs. physician rating scales).[8,39] Therefore, at this time, vitamin-rich diets and homeopathy are not generally recommended, and further studies are needed.

Vitamins and herbal supplements such as ginkgo biloba and ginseng have been used to improve attention, whereas zinc, valerian root, and lemon balm have been used for symptoms of hyperactivity/impulsivity.[38,40-43] Data supporting other agents (e.g., St. John's wort, L-carnitine, pycnogenol) are weak.[38,40] Despite some benefits in open-label studies (e.g., zinc), adverse events are inadequately measured in most of these studies, and most are subject to bias. In addition, they provide few benefits, and the ingredients are not standardized or monitored by the U.S. Food and Drug Administration (FDA), therefore possibly leading to undesirable consequences.[8,43] In conclusion, the use of herbal supplements should be avoided in the treatment of ADHD.

PHARMACOLOGIC TREATMENTS

TREATMENT GUIDELINES

The Texas Children's Medication Algorithm project revised the ADHD guidelines more than a decade ago; however, core concepts on the guidelines have minimally changed. As new data are disseminated, ADHD guidelines from other organizations have been revised or updated. Table 1 is a guideline based on not only present guidelines but on new published data. As a result, it may differ slightly from older guidelines.[34] Of note, any of these stages can be skipped, if necessary. If

Table 1. Pharmacologic Treatment Guidelines for Attention-Deficit/Hyperactivity Disorder

Stage	Treatment
1	Stimulants: Methylphenidate or amphetamine products
	Although methylphenidate may be preferred because of possibly fewer adverse effects, amphetamines may be chosen because of more favorable kinetics
2	Stimulant class not used in stage 1
3	Atomoxetine
4	Bupropion or guanfacine
	Bupropion may be preferred if a secondary comorbidity of depression exists, whereas guanfacine may be preferred if tics are an issue
	Practitioners may prefer the extended-release formulation of guanfacine, but costs may hinder its use
5	Agent not used in stage 4
6	Tricyclic antidepressant or clonidine
	A tricyclic antidepressant may be preferred if a secondary comorbidity of depression exists, whereas clonidine may be preferred if tics are an issue
	Practitioners may prefer an extended-release formulation of clonidine, but costs may hinder its use
7	Agent not used in stage 6
	Consideration of other agent such as venlafaxine

partial response occurs at a particular stage, some pharmacologic agents may be added adjunctively. In addition, behavioral therapy may be added during any stage. Primary comorbidities of other psychiatric conditions (e.g., Tourette syndrome, psychosis, major depression) may require different pharmacologic treatment principles.

STIMULANTS

Stimulants are controlled substances (Schedule II) in two classes: amphetamines and methylphenidate products. Stimulants are considered first-line agents for the treatment of ADHD, with a response rate of 65% to 75% in double-blind placebo-controlled studies or as high as 90% in other trials.[44,45] When both types of stimulants are tried, efficacy rates increase to 85% to 90%.[44,45] Despite some minor differences in the actual mechanism of action, stimulants are theorized to work by increasing norepinephrine and dopamine concentrations through reuptake inhibition. Methylphenidate is believed to occupy dopamine transporters, resulting in dopamine reuptake inhibition, which causes D_1-receptor activation.[46,47] In addition, recent data indicate that methylphenidate occupies norepinephrine transporters, thereby increasing norepinephrine and dopamine. The literature also supports that norepinephrine transporters actually have more affinity toward dopamine in the prefrontal cortex.[48] Amphetamines increase the release of dopamine through an exchange mechanism (sodium-dependent transport protein) and by binding to dopamine transporter proteins on the exterior of the cell membrane, causing dopamine reuptake inhibition.[47] In addition, amphetamines presynaptically block the reuptake of norepinephrine, thereby increasing the concentration in the synaptic cleft.[47]

There is no clinical preference regarding the stimulant that should be initially selected. Stimulants exist in a variety of formulations, and generics are readily available. Therefore, the selection of an agent will depend on the formulation desired (e.g., onset of action, dosage form). Table 2 lists available stimulants and formulations. Onset of action with stimulants can range from 15 to 120 minutes, and duration may range from 3 to 12 hours, depending on the formulation.[8,49] When selecting an agent, the formulation should be carefully considered. Children weighing less than 16 kg should be initiated on short-acting stimulants.[44,49] Overall, if symptoms are targeted that occur mostly in school, a short-acting agent is preferred. If problems persist after school (e.g., difficulty studying, completing homework), another dose of the short-acting agent can be used. However, this may cause medication burden on teachers or caregivers, especially if the child already has difficulty taking medication.[8,26] Therefore, it is usually better to change to an intermediate-acting formulation (e.g., half-life 5–8 hours). If ADHD symptoms occur throughout the entire day, then a long-acting formulation (e.g., 8–12 hours) is preferred.[26]

In addition, if a child cannot tolerate short-acting formulations, then an intermediate- or long-acting formulation may be used because either of these would provide lower peak concentrations and/or possibly decrease the number or severity of adverse effects (e.g., tics, nausea). Usually the intermediate- and long-acting formulations may take about

1 hour longer than the short-acting agents before efficacy is seen. Therefore, short-acting agents can sometimes be combined with long-acting formulations to provide extra coverage during a specific period (e.g., school hours).[49] Another option may be using formulations that have a short-acting component and a long-acting component (e.g., Ritalin LA [long acting], Novartis, East Hanover, NJ; Adderall XR, Shire, Wayne, PA), which may be preferred rather than using two different formulations. Conversely, if a child is taking a long-acting formulation and he or she is having difficulty sleeping or eating properly, he or she may be changed to an intermediate- or short-acting agent dosed in the morning; therefore, the medication will be mostly eliminated by evening. This should allow the child to eat a large-calorie meal for dinner and sleep better.

Stimulants are usually initiated at low doses and titrated to appropriate efficacy for 2–4 weeks or until unwanted adverse effects occur.[26] For example, a 25-kg child may start dextroamphetamine 5 mg/day in the morning and titrated to 10 mg/day if the child has partial efficacy and mild, if any, adverse effects. After selecting a stimulant, dosing should usually start on a Saturday so that it is easy for the parent to monitor the child for two days before school starts on Monday. With this approach, if any severe adverse effects occur they can be addressed outside of school such as lowering the dose or changing the administration time. Careful dose evaluation should occur over time as the child grows older. As the child grows and gains weight, the dose may need to be increased because stimulants are often dosed according to age and weight. If discontinuing stimulants, tapering is usually not required.

Stimulants increase the amount of monoamines (e.g., dopamine, norepinephrine) into the synaptic cleft; therefore they should not be administered concomitantly or within 2 weeks of discontinuing a monoamine oxidase inhibitor (MAOI).[50] Amphetamines are primarily metabolized by cytochrome P450 (CYP) 2D6.[8,50] Therefore, caution is warranted if strong CYP2D6 inhibitors are used (e.g., desipramine, paroxetine, fluoxetine) because they may increase amphetamine concentrations and increase the potential for cardiac complications.[8,50] Conversely, methylphenidate is metabolized by de-esterification and does not undergo oxidative metabolism. However, the combination of methylphenidate and tricyclic antidepressants (TCAs) may lead to an increase in TCA concentrations through an unknown mechanism.[50] The literature mainly focuses on increased imipramine concentrations with methylphenidate; however, no interactions between desipramine and methylphenidate have been reported.[50,51]

Adverse events. The adverse effects with stimulants for ADHD that are most common (10% to 50%) may include reduced appetite, transient blood pressure changes, dry mouth, headaches, stomach pain/cramps, and insomnia.[8] Overall, the increases in blood pressure are about 2–7 mm Hg and heart rate are about 5 beats/minute.[52-55] Less common adverse effects (1% to 10%) may include dizziness, nausea, irritability, tachycardia, sweating, diarrhea, transient tics, and weight loss. Most children will develop tolerance to these adverse effects over several weeks. Of note, weight loss is about 3 kg during the first year and about 1 kg during the second year of treatment. When addressing appetite suppression/

Table 2. Pharmacologic Treatment of Pediatric ADHD With Stimulants[8,44,49,63]

Brand Name (Generic)	Dosage Forms (mg)	Duration of Action (hr)	Initial Dose (mg); Max Dose (mg) Based on Patient Age	Dosing Range (mg/day)
Amphetamine products				
Adderall[a] (amphetamine/ dextroamphetamine)	Tablets (5, 7.5, 10, 12.5, 15, 20, 30)	Intermediate (4–6)	3–5 yr: 2.5 QAM ≥ 6 yr: 5 QD or 2.5 BID Max: 40	10–40
Adderall XR[a] (amphetamine/ dextroamphetamine)	Capsules (5, 10, 15, 20, 25, 30)	Long (8–12)	6–17 yr: 10 QAM Max dose 6–12 yr: 30	5–30
Dyanavel XR[b] (levoamphetamine/ dextroamphetamine)	Suspension, extended release (2.5 mg/mL)	Long (13)	≥ 6 yr: 2.5–5 QAM Max: 20	2.5–20
Evekeo[c] (levoamphetamine/ dextroamphetamine)	Tablets (5, 10)	Intermediate (4–6)	3–5 yr: 2.5 QAM ≥ 6: 5 QAM–BID Max: 40	2.5–40
Mydayis[d] (levoamphetamine/ dextroamphetamine)	Capsules, extended release (12.5, 25, 37.5, 50)	Long (16)	≥ 13 yr: 12.5 QAM Max: 13-17 yr: 25	12.5-25
Adzenys ER[e] (levoamphetamine/ dextroamphetamine)	Suspension, extended release (1.25 mg/ml)	Long 6–12 yr: (9–11) ≥ 13 yr: (11–14)	6.3 QAM Max: 6–12 yr: 18.8 ≥ 13 yr: 12.5	6.3–18.8
Adzenys XR-ODT[e] (levoamphetamine/ dextroamphetamine)	Tablets, orally disintegrating (3.1, 6.3, 9.4, 12.5, 15.7, 18.8)	Long 6–12 yr: (9–11) ≥ 13 yr: (11–14)	6.3 QAM Max: 6–12 yr: 18.8 ≥ 13 yr: 12.5	6.3–18.8
Dexedrine Spansule[f] (dextroamphetamine)	Spansules (5, 10, 15)	Intermediate (5–8)	≥ 6 yr: 5 QAM–BID Max: 40	5–40
Zenzedi[g] (dextroamphetamine)	Tablets (2.5, 5, 7.5, 10, 15, 20, 30)	Short (4–6)	3-5 yr: 2.5 QAM ≥ 6 yr: 5 QAM Max: 40	5–40
ProCentra[h] (dextroamphetamine)	Solution (5 mg/5 mL)	Short (4–6)	3-5 yr: 2.5 QAM ≥ 6 yr: 5 QAM Max: 40	5–40
Vyvanse[d] (lisdexamfetamine)	Capsules (10, 20, 30, 40, 50, 60, 70) Chewable tablets (10, 20, 30, 40, 50, 60)	Long (10–12)	≥ 6 yr: 30 QAM Max: 70	30–70
Desoxyn[i] (methamphetamine)	Tablet (5)	Short (4–5)	5 QAM–BID Max: 25	5–25
Methylphenidate products				
Ritalin[j] (methylphenidate)	Tablets (5, 10, 20)	Short (3–5)	≥ 6 yr: 5 BID Max: 2 mg/kg or 60	10–60
Ritalin SR[j] (methylphenidate SR)	Tablet (20)	Intermediate (3–8)	≥ 6 yr: 20 QAM Max: 60	20–60
Ritalin LA[j] (methylphenidate LA)	Capsules (10, 20, 30, 40)	Long (8–12)	≥ 6 yr: 20 QAM Max: 60	20–60
Methylin[k] (methylphenidate)	Solution 5 mg/5 mL, 10-mg/5-mL Tablets (5, 10, 20) Chewable tablets[k] (2.5, 5, 10)	Short (3–5)	≥ 6 yr: Tablet: 5 mg BID before breakfast and lunch Solution: 0.3 mg/kg/dose BID Chewable tablet: 2.5 BID Max: 2 mg/kg/day or 60	Tablet 10–60 Solution 10–60 Chewable tablet 0.5–1 mg/kg/day
Methylin ER[k] (methylphenidate ER)	Tablets (10, 20)	Intermediate (3–8)	≥ 6 yr: 10 QAM Max: 60	10–60
Metadate ER[l] (methylphenidate ER)	Tablet (20)	Intermediate (3–8)	≥ 6 yr: 20 QAM Max: 60	20–60

(continued)

Table 2. Pharmacologic Treatment of Pediatric ADHD With Stimulants[8,44,49,63] *(continued)*

Brand Name (Generic)	Dosage Forms (mg)	Duration of Action (hr)	Initial Dose (mg); Max Dose (mg) Based on Patient Age	Dosing Range (mg/day)
Methylphenidate products (continued)				
Relexxii[m] (methylphenidate ER)	Tablets (18, 27, 36, 54, 72)	Long (8-12)	≥ 6 yr: 18 QAM Max:6-12 yr: 54 13-17 yr: 72 not to exceed 2 mg/kg/day	6–12 yr: 18–54 13–17 yr: 18–72
Metadate CD[i] (methylphenidate CD)	Capsules (10, 20, 30, 40, 50, 60) Bimodal drug release 30% IR, 70% ER	Long (8–12)	≥ 6 yr: 20 QAM Max: 60	10–60
Concerta[n] (methylphenidate OROS)	Tablets (18, 27, 36, 54) Bimodal drug release (OROS) 22% IR 78% ER	Long (8–12)	≥ 6 yr: **Not currently taking methylphenidate:** Concerta 18 QAM **Currently taking methylphenidate:** 5 BID–TID or 20 ER QAM: Concerta 18 QAM 10 mg BID–TID or 40 ER QAM: Concerta 36 QAM 15 BID–TID or 60 ER QD: Concerta 54 QAM 20 BID–TID: Concerta 72 QAM Max: 6-12 yr: 54 13-17: 72	6–12 yr: 18–54 13–17 yr: 18–72
Aptensio XR[o] (methylphenidate)	Capsules (10, 15, 20, 30, 40, 50, 60) Bimodal drug release 37% IR, 63% ER	Long (12)	≥ 6 yr: 10 QAM Max: 60	10–60
QuilliChew ER[p] (methylphenidate)	Chewable tablets (20, 30, 40)	Long (8)	≥ 6 yr: 20 QAM Max: 60	20–60
Quillivant XR[p] (methylphenidate)	Suspension, XR (25 mg/ 5 mL)	Long (12)	≥ 6 yr: 20 QAM Max: 60	20–60
Daytrana[q] (methylphenidate)	Transdermal patch (10 mg/9 hr, 15 mg/9 hr, 20 mg/9 hr, 30 mg/9 hr)	Long (12) Wear for 9 hr only	6–17 yr: 10-mg patch daily Wear for up to 9 hr Max: 30 mg/9 hr	10–30 patch/9 hr
Adhansia XR[r] (methylphenidate)	Capsules (25, 35, 45, 55, 70, 85) Bimodal drug release 20% IR, 80% ER	Long (16)	≥ 6 yr: 25 QAM Max: 70	25-70
Cotempla XR-ODT[e] (methylphenidate)	ER orally disintegrating tablets (8.6, 17.3, 25.9)	Long (12)	6-17 yr: 17.3 QAM Max: 51.8	17.3-51.8
Jornay PM[s] (methylphenidate)	DR/ER capsules (20, 40, 60, 80, 100)	Long (12)	≥ 6 yr: 20 QD at 8 PM Max: 100	20–100
Focalin[j] (dexmethylphenidate)	Tablets (2.5, 5, 10)	Short (3–5)	2.5 BID Max: 20	5–20
Focalin XR[j] (dexmethylphenidate)	Capsules (5, 10, 15, 20, 30) Bimodal drug release 50% IR, 50% ER	Long (8–12)	5 QAM Max: 30	10–30

[a]Shire, Wayne, PA; [b]Tris Pharma, Monmouth Junction, NJ; [c]Arbor Pharmaceuticals, Atlanta, GA; [d]Shire, Lexington, MA; [e]Neos Therapeutics, Grand Prairie, TX; [f]Catalent Pharma Solutions, Winchester, KY; [g]Arbor Pharmaceuticals, Atlanta, GA; [h]Independence Pharmaceuticals, Newport, KY; [i]Recordati Rare Disease, Lebanon, NJ; [j]Novartis, East Hanover, NJ; [k]Mallinckrodt, Hazelwood, MO; [l]UCB, Smyrna, GA; [m]Vertical Pharma, Bridgewater, NJ; [n]Alza, Mountain View, CA [o]Rhodes Pharmaceuticals, Coventry, RI; [p]Pfizer, New York, NY; [q]Noven Pharmaceuticals, Miami, FL; [r]Purdue Pharma, Wilson, NC; [s]Ironshore Pharmaceuticals & Development, Durham, NC.
BID = twice daily; CD = controlled delivery of the modified release formulation; ER = extended release; IR = immediate release; LA = long acting; max = maximum; ODT = orally disintegrating tablets; OROS = osmotic-release oral system; QAM = every morning; QD = every day; SR = sustained release; TID = three times/day; XR = extended release.

weight loss, it is recommended to give a high-fat meal in the evening when stimulant effects are lower. Giving a high-fat meal (e.g., during the day) with a stimulant may also be a way to decrease stomachache or nausea; however, certain formulations may have altered kinetics when given with food.[56] For example, amphetamine/dextroamphetamine (e.g., Adderall) may show more than a 50% reduction in plasma concentrations when given with a high-calorie meal.[56]

Rare but severe adverse events include nontransient increased blood pressure and tics. These adverse events may be treated by lowering/splitting the dose or switching agents. Black box warnings for stimulants include sudden death caused by heart-related conditions and new/worsening psychiatric manifestations.[57,58] Sudden death has been reported in around 35 pediatric patients with ADHD.[44] Unknown structural defects are believed to have accounted for these deaths. The risk of sudden death is estimated at 0.2 and 0.5 per 100,000 children for methylphenidate and amphetamine products, respectively.[59] The risk of sudden death in the general untreated population is 0.6–6.[60] There is debate on whether baseline electrocardiograms should be required when prescribing stimulants for ADHD. The American Academy of Pediatrics recommends that practitioners obtain the patient's history and physical examination before initiating therapy.[58]

Psychiatric complications such as mania, hallucinations, aggression, anxiety, and dysphoria are rare but potentially dangerous. The FDA recommends that children who display any psychiatric complications have the stimulant discontinued or lowered as quickly as possible.

The occurrence of growth suppression in stimulant users is high. Among 29 studies, estimated growth suppression of 0.4 inches (1 cm) per year during the first 3 years occurs with stimulants.[61] It is suggested that amphetamines cause a slightly greater effect on growth suppression than methylphenidate.[62] A drug holiday (e.g., during the summer) may be recommended, but an assessment of risk versus benefit for the child is needed.[8] If a drug holiday is initiated, then reinitiation of treatment should not be delayed until the beginning of the school year. Instead, the agent should be restarted a few weeks before school is in session to allow the child and parent to readjust and make any dosing changes if necessary. It is important to remember that the child may grow and gain weight during the drug holiday and therefore may need a dose adjustment.

Amphetamine products. Amphetamine products include amphetamines, dextroamphetamines, and lisdexamfetamine, which is a prodrug to dextroamphetamine. Short-acting amphetamine products include Zenzedi (Arbor Pharmaceuticals, Atlanta, GA), and ProCentra (Independence Pharmaceuticals, Newport, KY). Intermediate-acting products include Adderall, Evekeo (Arbor Pharmaceuticals), and Dexedrine Spansule. Long-acting formulations include Adderall XR, Dyanavel XR (Tris Pharma, Monmouth Junction, NJ), Mydayis (Shire, Lexington, MA), Adzenys ER/XR-ODT (Neos Therapeutics, Grand Prairie, TX), and Vyvanse (Shire, Lexington, MA).[8,49,63] Advantages over methylphenidate products may include more predictable kinetics, possibly because dextroamphetamine is dependent on the liver and/or intestine to cleave the covalent bond instead of a

pH-dependent absorption. As a result, the release and uptake of amphetamine is generally consistent and gradual.[8] General disadvantages of amphetamines over methylphenidate products include possible greater abuse potential, slightly higher rate of causing/worsening tics, and greater growth suppression. Formulations such as Dexedrine Spansule, Adderall XR, Mydayis, or Vyvanse can be opened if the child cannot swallow tablets.[8,49] However, the contents should not be poured over hot food. Adzenys XR-ODT, like other extended release products, should not be crushed or chewed. Although taking this agent with food may decrease maximum concentration (19% reduction) and prolong the time to maximum plasma concentration (about 2 hours), it does not appear to be clinically significant. Vyvanse, a prodrug of dextroamphetamine, may have less abusive potential than other amphetamines because of its longer onset of action.[64]

Methylphenidate products. Methylphenidate products include methylphenidate and dexmethylphenidate. Short-acting methylphenidate products include Ritalin, Methylin (Mallinckrodt, Hazelwood, MO), and Focalin (Novartis, East Hanover, NJ). Intermediate-acting products include Ritalin SR (sustained release), Methylphenidate SR, Methylin ER (extended release), and Metadate ER (UCB, Smyrna, GA).[8,49] Long-acting formulations include Concerta (ALZA, Mountain View, CA), Aptensio XR (Rhodes Pharmaceuticals, Coventry, RI), Relexxii (Vertical Pharma, Bridgewater, NJ), Metadate CD, Ritalin LA, Focalin XR, Jornay PM (Ironshore Pharmaceuticals & Development, Durham, NC), Cotempla XR ODT (Neos Therapeutics), QuilliChew (Pfizer, New York, NY), Quillivant XR (Pfizer), Adhansia XR (Purdue Pharma, Wilson, NC), and Daytrana (Noven Pharmaceuticals, Miami, FL).[49,63] Advantages over amphetamines may include less likelihood to suppress appetite, worsen tics, and cause insomnia. General disadvantages of methylphenidate products may include more erratic kinetics, especially with short-acting agents, and greater differences reported between brand and generic formulations.[49] The Daytrana patch should be rotated daily at different sites. Jornay PM is dosed in the evening (starting at 8:00 p.m., then administration timing may be adjusted between 6:30 and 9:30 p.m. to maximize efficacy and tolerability) compared to the vast majority of stimulants which are typically dosed in the morning or mid-day.[63] Formulations such as Ritalin LA, Metadate CD, Focalin XR, Adhansia XR, Jornay PM, and Aptensio XR may be opened.[8,63] In addition, caution with gastrointestinal obstruction may be needed with Concerta, and parents should be counseled that the capsule will appear intact in the stool.[49]

NONSTIMULANTS

Atomoxetine. Atomoxetine is a nonstimulant, noncontrolled agent that has FDA label approval for the treatment of ADHD.[65] It acts by selectively inhibiting the presynaptic reuptake of norepinephrine. Clinical trials have shown that atomoxetine is 63%–80% effective in stimulant-naive patients and can treat all symptoms of ADHD.[65,66] It also appears to be around 55% effective in patients whose stimulant therapy has failed.[67]

Atomoxetine is usually initiated at 0.5 mg/kg/day and titrated to reach a target daily dose of 1.2 mg/kg (Table 3).

Titration should occur over a minimum of 3 days, with most patients waiting at least 1–2 weeks before titrating. Dosing can be increased to a maximum of 1.8 mg/kg/day. Efficacy may not be seen for 2–4 weeks, and some data suggest that 6 weeks is needed for optimal benefits.[44,65,66] Some patients may respond to the lower doses, whereas others may benefit from higher doses. Therefore, patience is warranted when this agent is titrated. Atomoxetine is considered a second-line agent after stimulants have failed. It can be used as monotherapy or in combination with other agents.[34] It may also be preferred in those who have high abuse potential or those who are afraid

of using stimulants. It may also be useful in those with a comorbidity of anxiety because it may help by either not exacerbating symptoms or by decreasing anxiety symptoms.[44]

Atomoxetine can be administered once or twice daily. When considering once-daily dosing, there is debate regarding whether to administer in the morning or at bedtime.[45] Morning doses will provide higher concentrations in the morning, thereby increasing efficacy, but they may predispose patients to a higher risk for adverse effects. Single bedtime dosing may be used for those who are experiencing adverse effects, especially sedation; however, drug concentrations may

Table 3. Pharmacologic Treatment of Pediatric ADHD With Nonstimulants[8,44,49,64,73–75,79]

Brand Name (generic)	Dosage Forms (mg)	Initial Dose (mg); Max Dose (mg/day) Based on Patient Age	Dosing Range (mg/day)	Notes and FDA-Label Approval
Strattera[a] (atomoxetine)	Capsules 10, 18, 24, 40, 60, 80, 100	≥ 6 yr ≤ 70 kg: 0.5 mg/kg/day Max: 1.4 mg/kg/day > 70 kg: 40 QD Max: 100	≤ 70 kg: 1.2 mg/kg/day > 70 kg: 80	Approved Norepinephrine reuptake inhibitor Fewer weight/growth concerns vs. stimulants
Wellbutrin[b] (bupropion)	Tablets 75, 150 XL 150, 300 SR 100, 150, 200	≥ 6 yr: 1.4–6 mg/kg/day Max: 300	50–300	Not approved Dopamine and norepinephrine reuptake inhibitor. Can worsen tics, irritability
Intuniv[c] (guanfacine)	Tablets, ER 1, 2, 3, 4	≥ 6 yr: 1 AM Max: 4	1–4	Approved for Intuniv/Kapvay Adjust Intuniv in increments of no more than 1 mg/wk
Tenex[d] (guanfacine)	Tablets, SA 1, 2	≥ 6 yr: 0.5–1 HS Max: 27–40 kg: 2 41–45 kg: 3 > 45 kg: 4	1–4	Intuniv and Kapvay are long-acting formulations Sedation may be helpful for sleep Agents helpful for tic comorbidities Tenex brand recently discontinued
Kapvay[e] (clonidine)	Tablets, ER 0.1	≥ 6 yr: 0.1 HS; Max: 0.4	0.1–0.4	
Catapres[f] (clonidine)	Tablets 0.1, 0.2, 0.3 Patch (TTS) 0.1/24 hr, 0.2/24 hr, 0.3/24 hr	≥ 6 yr: < 45 kg: 0.05 HS > 45 kg: 0.1 HS; Max: 27–40 kg: 0.2 41–45 kg: 0.3 > 45 kg: 0.4	0.1–0.4	
Pamelor[g] (nortriptyline)	Capsules 10, 25, 50, 75	≥ 6 yr: 0.5 mg/kg/day; Max: 100	50–100	Not approved: TCA Give in divided doses with higher dose at bedtime
Tofranil[g] (imipramine)	Capsules 75, 100, 125, 150 Tablets 10, 25, 50	≥ 6 yr: 1 mg/kg/day; Max: 200	75–200	Sedation may be helpful for sleep Sudden death reported with desipramine TCAs are last-line therapy
Norpramin[h] (desipramine)	Tablets 10, 25, 50, 75, 100, 150	6–12 yr: 1 mg/kg/day; > 12 yr: 25–50 Max: 150	25–150	
Effexor[i] (venlafaxine)	Tablets 25, 37.5, 50, 75, 100	5-17 yr: 12.5-25 mg/day Max: 150	37.5–150	Not approved Give in divided doses Brand discontinued; however, brand extended release products available

[a]Eli Lilly, Indianapolis, IN; [b]GlaxoSmithKline, Research Triangle Park, NC; [c]Shire, Lexington MA; [d]Pantheon PR, Manati, Puerto Rico; [e]Concordia Pharmaceuticals, St. Michael, Barbados; [f]Boehringer Ingelheim Pharmaceuticals, Ridgefield, CT; [g]Mallinckrodt, Hazelwood, MO; [h]Validus Pharmaceuticals LLC, Parsippany, NJ; [i]Wyeth Pharmaceuticals, Philadelphia, PA.
FDA = U.S. Food and Drug Administration; HS = at bedtime; max = maximum; QD = every day; TCA = tricyclic antidepressant.

be low by the morning, thus limiting its efficacy. Therefore, providers may choose twice-daily dosing because of more stable plasma concentrations and possibly better tolerability. Atomoxetine can be taken with or without food and can be discontinued without tapering.

Atomoxetine is highly metabolized by the CYP2D6 pathway.[65] The half-life of atomoxetine is about 5 hours, but in poor metabolizers of CYP2D26, it can be as long as 20 hours. As a result, plasma concentrations can increase 5- to 10-fold in poor metabolizers, and dose adjustment is warranted.[65] In addition, dose adjustment or slower titration may be needed with the coadministration of other potent CYP2D6 inhibitors such as paroxetine and fluoxetine.[65] Of note, atomoxetine is highly protein bound (98%); therefore, interactions with other highly protein-bound drugs are possible, although data are lacking. Finally, atomoxetine should not be administered with MAOIs, and a minimum of 2 weeks is needed before initiating atomoxetine after MAOI discontinuation or vice versa.

Common adverse events of atomoxetine include abdominal pain (18%), decreased appetite (16%), vomiting (12%), somnolence (10%), irritability (7%), fatigue (7%), dizziness (5%), and dyspepsia (5%).[65] Somnolence, fatigue, and dizziness are more common with atomoxetine than with a stimulant. An increased heart rate of about 8 beats/minute and mild increased blood pressure (around 2–3 mm Hg) are also noted with atomoxetine.[65] However, studies show the adverse effects are usually mild and well tolerated, with discontinuation rates caused by adverse events between 4% and 10%.[65] Growth suppression is about 0.4 inches during a 2-year period, which is smaller than that with stimulants.[68] Black box warnings for atomoxetine include hepatic failure (in two cases: one adult, one adolescent, both fully recovered), new-onset suicidal ideations (0.4%), and sudden death caused by heart complications (risk 0.5/100,000).[44,66] Abuse potential is also much lower than with stimulants.

Atomoxetine is only available in capsule form at this time, and generic formulations were recently approved. Although the manufacturer of atomoxetine (Eli Lilly) states the capsule cannot be opened, the data on file suggest the contents may be dissolved in 60 mL of juice (i.e., Tropicana 100% apple juice, 100% Welch's grape juice, fruit punch–flavored Gatorade). After waiting 5 minutes for dissolution to occur, it may be stable at room temperature for 6 hours. However, atomoxetine has a very bitter taste that, despite attempts to mask, may cause an increase in gastrointestinal complications. In addition, atomoxetine is an ocular irritant, so extreme caution is warranted when opening the capsule.

Bupropion. Bupropion is a norepinephrine and dopamine reuptake inhibitor used off-label for the treatment of ADHD. Bupropion is extensively hepatically metabolized. The usual starting dose for ADHD treatment is about 1.5 mg/kg/day and dose adjusted based on commercially available doses. Titration should occur over 7 days to a target dose of 3 mg/kg/day; however, it may be titrated to 6 mg/kg/day, not to exceed 300 mg/day (Table 3).[8,69] Efficacy rates range from 60% to 70%, mostly treating symptoms of hyperactivity. Bupropion can be given once or twice daily; however, data suggest twice-daily dosing is more tolerable and efficacious.[70] Most common adverse events reported include nausea, irritability, and insomnia.[8,71]

In addition, rash has been reported in a few cases.[71] There are some reports of decreased appetite, but they appear to be less severe compared with stimulants; however, tremors and/or tics may also occur similar to stimulants. Seizures may occur in doses exceeding 400–450 mg/day.[49] Efficacy is not seen for a minimum of 2 weeks at the therapeutic doses, and it may take up to 6 weeks for optimal results to be seen. Bupropion is contraindicated in those with seizure or eating disorders (e.g., bulimia, anorexia), and it carries a black box warning for new-onset suicidality for children, adolescents, and young adults age 24 years or younger.[49] Bupropion may have use in those who have a comorbidity of depression or in patients who are high-risk substance users.[34] It can be used adjunctively or as monotherapy after first- and second-line agents have failed. Currently, it may be preferred over TCAs because of its safer cardiovascular profile and better tolerability.

Bupropion is available as immediate release and various extended-release formulations, and generic alternatives exist. Bupropion, similar to other antidepressants, should not be administered with MAOIs, and a minimum of 2 weeks is needed before initiating bupropion after MAOI discontinuation, or vice versa. Food does not affect absorption, so it can be administered with food if nausea occurs. Tapering of bupropion is recommended if it is being discontinued.

Tricyclic antidepressants. Even though TCAs are serotonin and norepinephrine reuptake inhibitors, the primary neurotransmitter involved in the treatment of ADHD with these agents is norepinephrine.[47] As noted previously, serotonin does not play a role in ADHD, which is why selective serotonin reuptake inhibitors are ineffective. Imipramine, nortriptyline, and desipramine are the most commonly used TCAs. However, desipramine has been associated with cardiac-related sudden death in pediatric patients and is generally avoided.[44] The usual starting dose for treatment of ADHD is 0.5–1 mg/kg/day with titration to 2–3 mg/kg/day up to a maximum of 2–4 mg/kg/day (Table 3).[44] Therapeutic range is usually between 50 and 150 mg/day, and doses are usually divided into two or three daily doses. Regardless of whether patients are stimulant-naive or if their treatment with stimulants has failed, efficacy rates among TCAs are about 70%, mostly targeting symptoms of hyperactivity. Benefits are not seen for at least 2 weeks, and maximal efficacy may not be reached for at least 4 weeks.

The most common adverse effects (about 10% to 20%) include thirst/dry mouth, headaches, and sedation. Dizziness, constipation, and weight gain occur in about 5% to 10% of cases.[44,47,72] Caution with heart complications (e.g., increased heart rate, arrhythmias) and cardiac toxicity is warranted. As a result, an electrocardiogram should be done at baseline and with each dose increase.[44] Tricyclic antidepressants also carry a black box warning for new-onset suicidality, similar to all antidepressants (for patients younger than age 25 years). Because of the adverse event profile of TCAs, they are usually reserved as third-line agents. They may be used adjunctively and may have use in patients with comorbidity of tic disorders, depression, or enuresis. Tricyclic antidepressants are available as capsules, tablets, and solution. These agents should not be administered with MAOIs, and a minimum of 2 weeks is needed before initiating a TCA after MAOI discontinuation or vice versa. If discontinuing, tapering of these agents is recommended.

α₂-Adrenergic agonists. Guanfacine and clonidine are the two most commonly used α₂-agonists to treat ADHD (Table 3). Most data suggest that these agents primarily block norepinephrine presynaptically, acting as an autoreceptor-release modulator; however, some studies also support the postsynaptic blockade of norepinephrine.[47] These agents may also increase blood flow to the prefrontal cortex.[73]

Guanfacine and clonidine have been used for many years with documented efficacy. Extended-release tablet formulations have recently become available in an attempt to offer greater adherence, less kinetic fluctuations, and better tolerability.[74,75] Even though the extended-release formulations are supposed to offer greater tolerability than the immediate-release formulations, adequate studies are lacking to compare the formulations of these agents.[76] Currently, both guanfacine (Intuniv, Shire, Wayne, PA) and clonidine extended release (Kapvay, Shionogi Pharma, Atlanta, GA) have FDA indications as monotherapy or adjunctive therapy for ADHD. Of note, a few deaths have been reported with the coadministration of clonidine and immediate-release stimulants, leading to concerns regarding whether these agents can be concomitantly administered safely.[49] Deaths in these cases could have been attributed to etiologic confounders (e.g., congenital malformation).[77] Other studies have shown that the combination can be safely used. Nonetheless, if this coadministration should occur, assessing cardiac risk factors before treatment and monitoring for cardiac adverse effects during treatment may be useful. Optimal efficacy may not be reached for at least 2–4 weeks with these agents.[74] Despite data showing efficacy in all symptoms of ADHD, there appears to be more efficacy toward hyperactivity/impulsivity. These agents may be especially useful in those who have a comorbidity of tics and aggressive/oppositional disorders. In addition, these medications should be tapered by weekly increments if they are to be discontinued.[74]

Guanfacine is metabolized and eliminated equally by hepatic and renal elimination.[76,78] It is primarily metabolized by CYP3A4. Although studies in children are lacking, adult studies show dose adjustments may be needed in those with severe renal or hepatic impairment. Immediate-release formulations may be initiated at 0.5 mg/day or twice daily and may be increased to 1–4 mg/day in divided doses.[8,74] The extended-release formulation is initiated at 1 mg/day and titrated weekly by 1 mg/day to a target of 2–4 mg/day.[76] Even though the extended-release formulation of guanfacine should not be crushed, the short-acting formulation may be crushed. High-fat meals should be avoided with the extended-release formulation because of increased concentration. Efficacy rates range from 60% to 80%, and adverse effects include the following, at around these percentages of occurrence: somnolence (40%), headache (25%), fatigue (15%), upper abdominal pain (10%), hypotension (8%), irritability (6%), nausea (6%), and dizziness (6%).[74,76] Serious, less common adverse events include syncope (2%) and convulsions (0.4%). Most of the adverse events appear to be dose related.[74,75,79] Guanfacine may be theoretically preferred to clonidine because of its longer half-life and its higher selectivity at the α₂ₐ-receptor, thereby leading to less

dizziness and less sedation.[8] However, no comparison studies exist at this time.

Clonidine is 40% to 50% hepatically metabolized and 50% to 60% renally eliminated. Although pediatric data are lacking, dose adjustments may be needed in those with renal impairment. Immediate-release formulations may be initiated at 0.05 mg/day and titrated weekly by 0.05 mg/day to a target of 0.1–0.4 mg/day in divided doses two to four times/day. The extended-release formulation is initiated at 0.1 mg and titrated weekly by 0.1 mg to a target of 0.2–0.4 mg/day.[80] Twice-daily dosing is still needed for extended-release clonidine, especially with doses greater than 0.1 mg, with the higher dose given in the evening.[81] Efficacy rates range from 60% to 70%; adverse events are similar to those of guanfacine and appear to be dose related. The short-acting formulation of clonidine may be crushed; however, the extended-release formulation should not be crushed or chewed. Food has no effect on any formulation.

Miscellaneous agents. Serotonin norepinephrine reuptake inhibitors such as venlafaxine and duloxetine have been studied in ADHD because their mechanism of action is similar to TCAs. Based on recent studies, venlafaxine (initiated at 12.5–25 mg/day and titrated to 150 mg/day) has the most supporting data and may be considered in patients who cannot tolerate TCAs or bupropion or for whom these therapies have failed.[82] Other agents for the treatment of ADHD have been used, including modafinil, mood stabilizers, and antipsychotics. Modafinil at 300 mg (dosed daily or in divided doses) has shown benefits over placebo. Modafinil has been mostly studied in late adolescents, and although it has proven to be effective, the potential for skin reactions (e.g., Steven Johnson Syndrome) and overconfidence in self-assessing efficacy are a concern.[39,83] In addition, adverse effects such as severe rashes and psychiatric complications make this agent a last-line alternative. Those with a comorbidity of bipolar or severe aggressive behaviors may be treated with divalproex or carbamazepine.[8] Low-dose antipsychotics may also be used; of these agents, most of the literature is focused on haloperidol, risperidone, and quetiapine. These agents should be used with caution and reserved as last-line agents because they mostly treat the symptoms of these co-occurring disorders and not necessarily ADHD symptoms.

CONCLUSIONS

Behavioral therapy used with educational sessions appears to be the best nonpharmacologic treatment. Elimination diets may be useful in a few patients; however, such diets should not be used to replace pharmacotherapy. Studies with vitamins and herbal products have shown some possible benefits; nevertheless, most trials are subject to bias, and adverse events have not been adequately addressed or evaluated. As a result, the primary treatment of ADHD focuses on pharmacotherapy with prescription medications. There are many pharmacologic agents and both short- and long-acting formulations to choose from in the treatment of ADHD. Stimulants (i.e., amphetamines, methylphenidate) are considered to be first-line treatment and have a much faster onset and higher efficacy rates than nonstimulants.

Atomoxetine is a noncontrolled agent that may be used as an alternative in patients who have experienced a partial or failed response to stimulants or in those who refuse to use a controlled substance. The literature suggests antidepressants (e.g., bupropion, TCAs) can be considered treatment options for ADHD, especially in those with depressive symptoms. However, bupropion is preferred over TCAs because of its tolerable and safer adverse effects. Increasing data indicate that α_2-agonists, especially with long-acting formulations, have shown good efficacy and may be considered alternative agents in ADHD. Among α_2-agonists, it appears guanfacine is the preferred agent because of its higher selectivity to receptors and because a daily formulation is available. Miscellaneous agents (e.g., mood stabilizers, antipsychotics) may be used if the comorbidity of other psychiatric illnesses is present. Despite the agent chosen, careful monitoring is recommended for any changes in efficacy or for the development of rare but potentially serious adverse events.

Patient Case | SWITCHING BETWEEN PHARMACOLOGIC AGENTS

A 10-year-old boy with attention-deficit/hyperactivity disorder (ADHD) has been receiving stimulant treatment for 3 years. His mother comes into the pharmacy to drop off a new prescription for amphetamine/dextroamphetamine (Adderall XR, Shire, Wayne, PA) 10-mg capsules orally every morning. She is concerned about possible adverse effects. The patient's medication profile shows he is taking methylphenidate (Ritalin LA, Novartis, East Hanover, NJ) 40 mg/day orally every morning, and this prescription was last picked up two weeks ago for a 30-day supply.

1. In counseling the patient's mother, how would you explain the proper steps to take for initiating this new medication, and how would you answer her question about adverse effects?

A possible script for counseling the patient follows: "First, we need to confirm if your son is currently still taking Ritalin LA. If so, he will need to discontinue this medication before starting Adderall XR. If discontinuing Ritalin LA, no tapering is required—he can just stop taking that medication. Adverse effects of the new medication may include headache, dizziness, nausea, and loss of appetite, which usually go away after a few weeks. Nausea can be minimized by administering Adderall XR with food. Rare adverse effects include mild tremor of the hands, increased blood pressure, or tics. These adverse effects may also go away after a couple of weeks; however, contact your prescriber so that they are aware your child is experiencing these symptoms. Adderall XR can be opened and sprinkled on applesauce if your son has a hard time swallowing pills. If sprinkling, make sure they eat all of the content and do not heat or save food for later use. It is best to start the new medication on the weekend on Saturday so you can see if he develops any side effects and how severe they may be. There may be some growth suppression, which is on average about 0.4 inches per year during the first 3 years. If the growth suppression is severe or is a concern for you, you can provide a drug holiday over the summer. If you want to do a drug holiday, talk with your physician and make sure to restart a few weeks before the school semester starts in the fall so the physician can assess if any dosing adjustment is needed."

Case (continued). The child is now 13 years old and weighs 102 lb. He has tried several different stimulants for his ADHD, but now wants to take another medication. His symptoms mostly include inattentiveness, but he still displays some hyperactivity.

2. Which agent would you recommend, how would you approach the initiation/titration of any agent, and what counseling would you provide?

Atomoxetine is second-line treatment for ADHD, and a trial in this patient is warranted. Because he weighs 102 lb, he would start 24 mg/day (his weight is 102 lb/2.2 lb/kg = 46.4 kg × 0.5 mg/kg/day = 23.2 mg/day which rounds up to the 24-mg capsule). Although titration may occur between 3 to 14 days, it would be best to wait 2 weeks because the next capsule dose is 40 mg. This approach will allow the patient to get used to the adverse effects, if any. At atomoxetine 40 mg/day (assuming the patient does not gain any weight in 2 weeks) will average about 1.2 mg/day, which is the target for this patient. The dose can be further increased until a maximum of 1.8 mg/kg/day (80 mg/day). However, these increases should be done at least every 6 to 8 weeks because efficacy may not be fully seen until 6 weeks. The patient and caregivers should be aware that as the patient ages and gains weight (once the patients weighs more than 70 kg), the dose may need to be further increased. Counseling points should include the following: efficacy will take longer than that seen for stimulants (about 6 weeks), and common side effects include abdominal pain, decreased appetite, vomiting, and irritability. Also, somnolence, fatigue, and dizziness are more common with atomoxetine than with a stimulant. However, most side effects are mild and typically last a few weeks, making atomoxetine generally well tolerated. Also, height suppression is lower with atomoxetine. More importantly, because the patient is now an adolescent, it is important to educate the patient and caregivers on the rare but potential risk for suicidal ideations.

Case (continued). After another 2 years, the patient returns for a follow-up visit. He is now 15 years old, weighs 57 kg, is taking atomoxetine 80 mg/day, and reports only mild hyperactivity. The higher dose did not provide additional efficacy; however, he experienced vomiting that did not resolve even with food or bedtime dosing.

3. What other agents would you recommend?

An α_2-agonist may be initiated for this patient. Both guanfacine and clonidine may assist with mild hyperactivity. Guanfacine may be preferred because it would likely cause fewer side effects. However, clonidine may be used if the mild hyperactivity occurs more often during a specific part of the day because even the extended formulation of clonidine has a shorter half-life than that for guanfacine.

REFERENCES

1. Barkley RA, Guevremont DC, Anastopoulos AD, et al. Driving-related risks and outcomes of attention deficit hyperactivity disorder in adolescents and young adults: a 3- to 5-year follow-up survey. Pediatrics 1993;92:212-8.

2. Hechtman L, Weiss G, Perlman T. Hyperactives as young adults: past and current substance abuse and antisocial behavior. Am J Orthopsychiatry 1984;54:415-25.

3. Barkley RA, Fischer M, Smallish L, et al. Young adult outcome of hyperactive children: adaptive functioning in major life activities. J Am Acad Child Adolesc Psychiatry 2006;45:192-202.

4. Biederman J, Monuteaux MC, Mick E, et al. Young adult outcome of attention deficit hyperactivity disorder: a controlled 10-year follow-up study. Psychol Med 2006;36:167-79.

5. Faraone SV, Sergeant J, Gillberg C, et al. The worldwide prevalence of ADHD: is it an American condition? World Psychiatry 2003;2:104-13.

6. Polanczyk G, de Lima MS, Horta BL, et al. The worldwide prevalence of ADHD: a systematic review and metaregression analysis. Am J Psychiatry 2007;164:942-8.

7. Froehlich TE, Lanphear BP, Epstein JN, et al. Prevalence, recognition, and treatment of attention-deficit/hyperactivity disorder in a national sample of US children. Arch Pediatr Adolesc Med 2007;161:857-64.

8. Dopheide JA, Pliszka SR. Attention-deficit-hyperactivity disorder: an update. Pharmacotherapy 2009;29:656-79.

9. Biederman J, Faraone S, Milberger S, et al. A prospective 4-year follow-up study of attention-deficit hyperactivity and related disorders. Arch Gen Psychiatry 1996;53:437-46.

10. Gittelman R, Mannuzza S, Shenker R, et al. Hyperactive boys almost grown up. I. Psychiatric status. Arch Gen Psychiatry 1985;42:937-47.

11. Simon V, Czobor P, Balint S, et al. Prevalence and correlates of adult attention-deficit hyperactivity disorder: meta-analysis. Br J Psychiatry 2009;194:204-11.

12. Polanczyk G, Rohde LA. Epidemiology of attention-deficit/hyperactivity disorder across the lifespan. Curr Opin Psychiatry 2007;20:386-92.

13. Asherson P. Review: prevalence of adult ADHD declines with age. Evid Based Ment Health 2009;12:128.

14. Biederman J. Attention-deficit/hyperactivity disorder: a selective overview. Biol Psychiatry 2005;57:1215-20.

15. Ilott NE, Saudino KJ, Asherson P. Genetic influences on attention deficit hyperactivity disorder symptoms from age 2 to 3: a quantitative and molecular genetic investigation. BMC Psychiatry 2010;10:102.

16. Faraone SV, Doyle AE, Mick E, et al. Meta-analysis of the association between the 7-repeat allele of the dopamine D(4) receptor gene and attention deficit hyperactivity disorder. Am J Psychiatry 2001;158:1052-7.

17. Pittelli SJ. Meta-analysis and psychiatric genetics. Am J Psychiatry 2002;159:496-7.

18. Stein MA, Waldman ID, Sarampote CS, et al. Dopamine transporter genotype and methylphenidate dose response in children with ADHD. Neuropsychopharmacology 2005;30:1374-82.

19. Williams NM, Zaharieva I, Martin A, et al. Rare chromosomal deletions and duplications in attention-deficit hyperactivity disorder: a genome-wide analysis. Lancet 2010;376:1401-8.

20. Ly V, Bottelier M, Hoekstra PJ, et al. Elimination diets' efficacy and mechanisms in attention deficit hyperactivity disorder and autism spectrum disorder. Eur Child Adolesc Psychiatry 2017;26:1067-79.

21. Stevenson J, Sonuga-Barke E, McCann D, et al. The role of histamine degradation gene polymorphisms in moderating the effects of food additives on children's ADHD symptoms. Am J Psychiatry 2010;167:1108-15.

22. American Psychiatric Association. Diagnostic and Statistical Manual of Mental Disorders, 5th ed. (DSM-5). Washington, DC: American Psychiatric Association, 2013.

23. Biederman J, Mick E, Faraone SV, et al. Influence of gender on attention deficit hyperactivity disorder in children referred to a psychiatric clinic. Am J Psychiatry 2002;159:36-42.

24. Merten EC, Cwik JC, Margraf J, et al. Overdiagnosis of mental disorders in children and adolescents (in developed countries). Child Adolesc Psychiatry Ment Health 2017;11:5.

25. Collett BR, Ohan JL, Myers KM. Ten-year review of rating scales. V: Scales assessing attention-deficit/hyperactivity disorder. J Am Acad Child Adolesc Psychiatry 2003;42:1015-37.

26. Rader R, McCauley L, Callen EC. Current strategies in the diagnosis and treatment of childhood attention-deficit/hyperactivity disorder. Am Fam Physician 2009;79:657-65.

27. Tripp G, Wickens JR. Neurobiology of ADHD. Neuropharmacology 2009;57:579-89.

28. Valera EM, Faraone SV, Murray KE, et al. Meta-analysis of structural imaging findings in attention-deficit/hyperactivity disorder. Biol Psychiatry 2007;61:1361-9.

29. D'Agati E, Casarelli L, Pitzianti MB, et al. Overflow movements and white matter abnormalities in ADHD. Prog Neuropsychopharmacol Biol Psychiatry 2010;34:441-5.

30. Curatolo P, D'Agati E, Moavero R. The neurobiological basis of ADHD. Ital J Pediatr 2010;36:79.

31. Stahl S. Essential Psychopharmacology: Neuroscientific Basis and Practical Applications, 2nd ed. New York: Cambridge University Press, 2000.

32. Waxmonsky JG, Waschbusch DA, Pelham WE, et al. Effects of atomoxetine with and without behavior therapy on the school and home functioning of children with attention-deficit/hyperactivity disorder. J Clin Psychiatry 2010;71:1535-51.

33. Molina BS, Flory K, Hinshaw SP, et al. Delinquent behavior and emerging substance use in the MTA at 36 months: prevalence, course, and treatment effects. J Am Acad Child Adolesc Psychiatry 2007;46:1028-40.

34. Pliszka SR, Crismon ML, Hughes CW, et al. The Texas Children's Medication Algorithm Project: revision of the algorithm for pharmacotherapy of attention-deficit/hyperactivity disorder. J Am Acad Child Adolesc Psychiatry 2006;45:642-57.

35. Sonuga-Barke EJ, Brandeis D, Cortese S, et al. Nonpharmacological interventions for ADHD: systematic review and meta-analyses of randomized controlled trials of dietary and psychological treatments. Am J Psychiatry. 2013;170:275-89.

36. Kanarek RB. Artificial food dyes and attention deficit hyperactivity disorder. Nutr Rev 2011;69:385-91.

37. Stevens LJ, Kuczek T, Burgess JR, et al. Dietary sensitivities and ADHD symptoms: thirty-five years of research. Clin Pediatr 2011;50:279-93.

38. Hurt EA, Arnold LE, Lofthouse N. Dietary and nutritional treatments for attention-deficit/hyperactivity disorder: current research support and recommendations for practitioners. Curr Psychiatry Rep 2011;13:323-32.

39. Keen D, Hadijikoumi I. ADHD in children and adolescents. BMJ Clin Evid 2008;2008:0312.

40. Rucklidge JJ, Johnstone J, Kaplan BJ. Nutrient supplementation approaches in the treatment of ADHD. Expert Rev Neurother 2009;9:461-76.

41. Larzelere MM, Campbell JS, Robertson M. Complementary and alternative medicine usage for behavioral health indications. Prim Care 2010;37:213-36.

42. Berdonces JL. [Attention deficit and infantile hyperactivity]. Rev Enferm 2001;24:11-4.

43. Arnold LE. Alternative treatments for adults with attention-deficit hyperactivity disorder (ADHD). Ann N Y Acad Sci 2001;931:310-41.

44. Pliszka S. Practice parameter for the assessment and treatment of children and adolescents with attention-deficit/hyperactivity disorder. J Am Acad Child Adolesc Psychiatry 2007; 46:894-921.

45. Wigal SB. Efficacy and safety limitations of attention-deficit hyperactivity disorder pharmacotherapy in children and adults. CNS Drugs 2009;23:21-31.

46. Arnsten AF. Toward a new understanding of attention-deficit hyperactivity disorder pathophysiology: an important role for prefrontal cortex dysfunction. CNS Drugs 2009;23:33-41.

47. Wilens TE. Mechanism of action of agents used in attention-deficit/hyperactivity disorder. J Clin Psychiatry 2006;67:32-8.

48. Hannestad J, Gallezot JD, Planeta-Wilson B, et al. Clinically relevant doses of methylphenidate significantly occupy norepinephrine transporters in humans in vivo. Biol Psychiatry 2010;68:854-60.

49. Daughton JM, Kratochvil CJ. Review of ADHD pharmacotherapies: advantages, disadvantages, and clinical pearls. J Am Acad Child Adolesc Psychiatry 2009;48:240-8.

50. Markowitz JS, Patrick KS. Pharmacokinetic and pharmacodynamic drug interactions in the treatment of attention-deficit hyperactivity disorder. Clin Pharmacokinet 2001;40:753-72.

51. Cohen LG, Prince J, Biederman J, et al. Absence of effect of stimulants on the pharmacokinetics of desipramine in children. Pharmacotherapy 1999;19:746-52.

52. Samuels JA, Franco K, Wan F, et al. Effect of stimulants on 24-h ambulatory blood pressure in children with ADHD: a double-blind, randomized, cross-over trial. Pediatr Nephrol 2006;21:92-5.

53. Wilens TE, Hammerness PG, Biederman J, et al. Blood pressure changes associated with medication treatment of adults with attention-deficit/hyperactivity disorder. J Clin Psychiatry 2005;66:253-9.

54. Weisler RH, Biederman J, Spencer TJ, et al. Long-term cardiovascular effects of mixed amphetamine salts extended release in adults with ADHD. CNS Spectr 2005;10:35-43.

55. Findling RL, Biederman J, Wilens TE, et al. Short- and long-term cardiovascular effects of mixed amphetamine salts extended release in children. J Pediatr 2005;147:348-54.

56. Auiler JF, Liu K, Lynch JM, et al. Effect of food on early drug exposure from extended-release stimulants: results from the Concerta, Adderall XR Food Evaluation (CAFE) Study. Curr Med Res Opin 2002;18:311-6.

57. Wilens TE, Prince JB, Spencer TJ, et al. Stimulants and sudden death: what is a physician to do? Pediatrics 2006;118:1215-9.

58. Perrin JM, Friedman RA, Knilans TK. Cardiovascular monitoring and stimulant drugs for attention-deficit/hyperactivity disorder. Pediatrics 2008;122:451-3.

59. Villalba L. Safety Review: Follow-up review of AERS search identifying cases of sudden death occurring with drugs used for the treatment of attention deficit hyperactivity disorder (ADHD). 2006. Available at https://wayback.archive-it. org/7993/20170405072639/https://www.fda.gov/ohrms/dockets/ ac/06/briefing/2006-4210b_07_01_safetyreview.pdf. Accessed October 21, 2019.

60. Wren C. Sudden death in children and adolescents. Heart 2002;88:426-31.

61. Poulton A. Growth on stimulant medication; clarifying the confusion: a review. Arch Dis Child 2005;90:801-6.

62. Pliszka SR, Matthews TL, Braslow KJ, et al. Comparative effects of methylphenidate and mixed salts amphetamine on height and weight in children with attention-deficit/hyperactivity disorder. J Am Acad Child Adolesc Psychiatry 2006;45:520-6.

63. Steingard R, Taskiran S, Connor DF, et al. New formulations of stimulants: An update for clinicians. J Child Adolesc Psychopharmacol 2019;29:324-39.

64. Cowles BJ. Lisdexamfetamine for treatment of attention-deficit/ hyperactivity disorder. Ann Pharmacother 2009;43:669-76.

65. Caballero J, Nahata MC. Atomoxetine hydrochloride for the treatment of attention-deficit/hyperactivity disorder. Clin Ther 2003;25:3065-83.

66. Hammerness P, McCarthy K, Mancuso E, et al. Atomoxetine for the treatment of attention-deficit/hyperactivity disorder in children and adolescents: a review. Neuropsychiatr Dis Treat 2009;5:215-26.

67. Hammerness P, Doyle R, Kotarski M, et al. Atomoxetine in children with attention-deficit hyperactivity disorder with prior stimulant therapy: a prospective open-label study. Eur Child Adolesc Psychiatry 2009;18:493-8.

68. Spencer TJ, Newcorn JH, Kratochvil CJ, et al. Effects of atomoxetine on growth after 2-year treatment among pediatric patients with attention-deficit/hyperactivity disorder. Pediatrics 2005;116:e74-80.

69. Barrickman LL, Perry PJ, Allen AJ, et al. Bupropion versus methylphenidate in the treatment of attention-deficit hyperactivity disorder. J Am Acad Child Adolesc Psychiatry 1995;34:649-57.

70. Daviss WB, Perel JM, Rudolph GR, et al. Steady-state pharmacokinetics of bupropion SR in juvenile patients. J Am Acad Child Adolesc Psychiatry 2005;44:349-57.

71. Conners CK, Casat CD, Gualtieri CT, et al. Bupropion hydrochloride in attention deficit disorder with hyperactivity. J Am Acad Child Adolesc Psychiatry 1996;35:1314-21.

72. Otasowie J, Castells X, Ehimare UP, et al. Tricyclic antidepressants for attention deficit hyperactivity disorder (ADHD) in children and adolescents. Cochrane Database Syst Rev 2014;9:CD006997.

73. Avery RA, Franowicz JS, Studholme C, et al. The alpha-2A-adrenoceptor agonist, guanfacine, increases regional cerebral blood flow in dorsolateral prefrontal cortex of monkeys performing a spatial working memory task. Neuropsychopharmacology 2000;23:240-9.

74. Scahill L. Alpha-2 adrenergic agonists in children with inattention, hyperactivity and impulsiveness. CNS Drugs 2009;23:43-9.

75. Sallee FR, Lyne A, Wigal T, et al. Long-term safety and efficacy of guanfacine extended release in children and adolescents with attention-deficit/hyperactivity disorder. J Child Adolesc Psychopharmacol 2009;19:215-26.

76. Sallee FR, McGough J, Wigal T, et al. Guanfacine extended release in children and adolescents with attention-deficit/ hyperactivity disorder: a placebo-controlled trial. J Am Acad Child Adolesc Psychiatry 2009;48:155-65.

77. Ming M, Mulvey M, Mohanty S, et al. Safety and efficacy of clonidine and clonidine extended-release in the treatment of children and adolescents with attention deficit and hyperactivity disorders. Adolesc Health Med Ther 2011;2:105-12.

78. Kiechel JR. Pharmacokinetics and metabolism of guanfacine in man: a review. Br J Clin Pharmacol 1980;10:25S-32S.

79. Biederman J, Melmed RD, Patel A, et al. A randomized, double-blind, placebo-controlled study of guanfacine extended release in children and adolescents with attention-deficit/ hyperactivity disorder. Pediatrics 2008;121:e73-84.

80. Jain R, Segal S, Kollins SH, et al. Clonidine extended-release tablets for pediatric patients with attention-deficit/hyperactivity disorder. J Am Acad Child Adolesc Psychiatry 2011;50:171-9.

81. Kollins SH, Jain R, Brams M, et al. Clonidine extended-release tablets as add-on therapy to psychostimulants in children and adolescents with ADHD. Pediatrics 2011;127:e1406-13.

82. Park P, Caballero J, Omidian H. Use of serotonin norepinephrine reuptake inhibitors in the treatment of attention-deficit hyperactivity disorder in pediatrics. Ann Pharmacother 2014;48:86-92.

83. Bagot KS, Kaminer Y. Efficacy of stimulants for cognitive enhancement in non-attention deficit hyperactivity disorder youth: a systematic review. Addiction 2014;109:547-57.

CHAPTER 32

Autism Spectrum Disorder

Jose Valdes, Pharm.D., BCPP; and
Jose A. Rey, Pharm.D., M.S., BCPP

LEARNING OBJECTIVES

1. Explain the clinical presentation and diagnostic criteria for autism spectrum disorder (ASD).

2. Discuss the application and efficacy of pharmacotherapeutic interventions for symptom-specific treatment and the limitations of pharmacotherapy in ASD.

3. Recommend and monitor pharmacotherapy for ASD for therapeutic outcomes and adverse drug effects, together with considerations of possible comorbid conditions.

ABBREVIATIONS IN THIS CHAPTER

ABC-I	Aberrant Behavior Checklist—Irritability subscale
ADHD	Attention-deficit/hyperactivity disorder
ASD	Autism spectrum disorder
CARS	Childhood Autism Rating Scale
CGI-I	Clinical Global Impression Scale-Improvement Scale
DSM-5	*Diagnostic and Statistical Manual of Mental Disorders, Fifth Edition*
DSM-IV-TR	*Diagnostic and Statistical Manual of Mental Disorders, Fourth Edition, Text Revision*
FDA	U.S. Food and Drug Administration
M-CHAT-R/F	Modified Checklist for Autism in Toddlers–Revised with Follow-Up
PDD	Pervasive developmental disorder
PDD-NOS	Pervasive developmental disorder–not otherwise specified
SSRI	Selective serotonin reuptake inhibitor

INTRODUCTION

Neurodevelopmental disorders can be characterized by deficits in a child's development that impairs the child's personal, academic, social, or occupational functioning.[1] Although neurodevelopmental disorders can coexist, clinical presentation generally involves symptoms of not only deficits and delays (e.g., reaching expected developmental milestones) but of excess as well (e.g., repetitive patterns).[1] Autism spectrum disorder (ASD) is grouped in the broad category of neurodevelopmental disorders in the *Diagnostic and Statistical*

Manual of Mental Disorders, Fifth Edition (DSM-5) together with intellectual disabilities, communication disorders, attention-deficit/hyperactivity disorder, specific learning disorder, motor disorders, tic disorders, and other neurodevelopmental disorders.[1] Although the classification of ASD changed since it was first formally classified in the *DSM, Fourth Edition, Text Revision (DSM-IV-TR)* under the pervasive developmental disorders (PDDs), what has not changed are the considerable challenges for patients, families, caregivers, and health care providers. Using the *DSM-IV-TR*, patients who once could receive a diagnosis with one of the five PDDs—Asperger disorder, autistic disorder, childhood disintegrative disorder, Rett disorder, and pervasive developmental disorder-not otherwise specified (PDD-NOS)—now fit in the catch-all diagnosis of ASD.[1,2]

In 1943, the psychiatrist Dr. Leo Kanner described children who withdrew, disregarded people, avoided eye contact, lacked social awareness, had limited language, displayed stereotyped motor movements, and showed a preservation of sameness as having a disorder called early infantile autism.[3,4] At the time, Dr. Kanner proposed that autism resulted from an inborn inability to form loving relationships with other people and described the parents of these children as "cold" and "detached." Today, the general behavioral description of the disorder has not changed significantly, but the proposed causes of autism are now believed to be more neurobiologic in etiology, although they are still not definitively known.[4]

The most significant clinical features of a child with an ASD often include qualitative impairments in the major domains of social interaction and social communication, and repetitive or restricted patterns of behavior interests or activities.[1] Other challenging and maladaptive behaviors that may prompt the use of pharmacotherapy include irritability, tantrums, aggression, and attention-deficit/hyperactivity symptoms.[2]

EPIDEMIOLOGY

The prevalence of ASD has been a matter of debate in recent years. Some estimate the numbers to be 1 or 2 per 1000, whereas other reports estimate the prevalence to be as high as 1 or 2 per 100.[5-13] The Centers for Disease Control and Prevention estimate the prevalence of ASD to 14.6 per 1000 children age 8 years (one in 68) living in catchment areas of Autism and Developmental Disabilities Monitoring Network sites, using *DSM-IV-TR* diagnostic criteria.[14] Estimates of prevalence using the newer *DSM* classification, from the *DSM-5*, are not yet widely available, thus the impact of changing diagnostic criteria has not been determined. However, studies comparing the proportion of patients who had a diagnosis of ASD based on the *DSM-IV-TR* classification who also meet diagnostic criteria for ASD under the *DSM-5* criteria range from 38% to 93%.[15]

A 2009 study by the psychiatrist Dr. Eric Fombonne published in *Nature* proposed that the increased prevalence of ASD within the past 15–20 years may be a result of the increase in awareness of ASD, expansion of diagnostic criteria, and development of services for those affected by ASD, although other factors may also have contributed.[5] The criteria for infantile autism was provided in the *DSM-III*, but has since changed through the years, which may have affected how the disorder is identified. Another event that may have affected the diagnosis rate of ASD is the passage of the Individuals with Disabilities Education Act in 1990.[9] With this Act, services could be billed for ASD. Until the Act was passed, ASD did not become a diagnosis for which children became eligible to receive special education services.[9] Internationally, the World Health Organization estimates that 0.76% of the world's children had a diagnosis of ASD in 2010, although this estimate is based on countries that represent 16% of the global population of children.[16]

The reported ratio of male to female individuals with ASD in the United States is about 4.5:1.[5,8,14] There may be racial differences in prevalence, with non-Hispanic white children identified more often than non-Hispanic African American children or Hispanic childrens.[6,17] The gender, racial, and ethnic differences may be culturally based, with less reporting in certain groups. Other countries may also have differences in prevalence because of the reporting of neuropsychiatric disorders or limited diagnostic and treatment resources. No evidence exists for a socioeconomic boundary, with similar rates across social status and cultures.[9] Children having siblings with an ASD also have a higher likelihood of receiving a diagnosis of an ASD, with the risk being around 10-fold.[9,18-22]

ETIOLOGY AND PATHOPHYSIOLOGY

The etiology of ASD is unknown. The earliest proposed cause of ASD—dysfunctional attachment as a result of parenting style—is no longer accepted. Today, ASD is thought to have a heterogeneous etiology that is neurobiologically based with a complex genetic, and therefore possibly heritable, component. Estimates in studies on twins place heritability from 50% to 95%, with a higher risk in monozygotic twins versus dizygotic twins. This range means that half or more of the liability for ASD rests in the genetic make-up, and the other half in other factors (e.g., environmental risk factors).[23-25] Genetic mutations are being evaluated in research, but no specific causes have been identified; however, several have been identified to be associated with ASD (e.g., *SHANK3*, *ADNP*, *SCN2A* genes).[9,18-22,26-29] The discovery of copy number variations and the clinical and behavioral similarities of ASD to other syndromes with recognized genetic deletions or mutations reinforce the proposed genetic abnormalities that may underlie ASD.[9,27,28] Fragile X syndrome (*FMR1* gene), Angelman syndrome (*UBE3A* gene), and tuberous sclerosis (*TSC1* and *TSC2* genes) are examples of syndromes with recognized genetic mutations that also have behaviors similar to ASD.[9,21,30] Increasing evidence suggests that *polygenic risk*, defined as the cumulative effect of several genetic variants, may be important in the risk factors for ASD and other psychiatric disorders.[31,32]

Determining the biochemical markers for ASD (e.g., abnormal neurotransmitter concentrations) in both the periphery and central cerebrospinal fluid has been extensively researched; however, data are inconclusive. A dysfunction in serotonin has the strongest support for explaining the behaviors associated with ASD.[33-35] Earlier hypotheses that endogenous opioids or norepinephrine was implicated in the pathology of ASD are not consistently supported.[34] Dopamine dysfunction is still a target of research, given the efficacy of the antipsychotics, with both older and newer atypical agents demonstrating the ability to reduce ASD symptoms.[33,34] Various hormones and neuropeptides (e.g., cortisol, oxytocin, vasopressin) have also been suggested as factors in the etiology of ASD; however, these hypotheses have minimal support.[9,33,35] Other biomarkers (more than 70 others) identified in unusual concentrations in patients with ASD are carnitine, glutamine, glutamic acid, GABA (γ-aminobutyric acid), DPP-IV (dipeptidyl peptidase-4), C4B, interferon-γ, interleukin-12, melatonin, testosterone, cysteine, glutathione, and MT-2 (metallothionein-2).[36,37] Evidence continues to accumulate linking oxidative stress as an important manifestation of autism in addition to mitochondrial dysfunction and inflammation in the brain.[38]

Claims put forth in the early 1990s—subsequently determined to have been based on fraudulent data (and retracted by the publisher of the data, *The Lancet*)—that vaccinations were related to the development of ASD have been disproved by several investigations.[9,39-43] Despite the evidence that vaccinations do not contribute to ASD, many parents continue to believe that vaccinations caused their child to develop ASD.[43,44] One hypothesis for the relationship between vaccines and ASD was that some vaccines contained thimerosal as a preservative; however, this compound has been removed, or greatly reduced to only trace amounts, from most vaccine products. Although this action by the pharmaceutical industry took place about 15 years ago, ASD rates have not decreased since then, supporting the lack of relationship between thimerosal exposure and ASD.[43,45] Exposure to heavy metals such as lead and mercury remains a potential causal factor in some cases of neurodevelopmental deficits.[9,46] Abnormal immune responses have also been proposed to be related to ASD. This theory may still be connected to vaccine exposure as a form of immune system activation, although further research is needed in this area before accepting the existence of a connection between vaccinations or infections and abnormal immune responses leading to ASD.[9,47,48]

Neuroimaging studies indicate the involvement, and possible dysfunction, of various areas of the brain, including the cortical, subcortical, and limbic regions, which may reflect early pathology.[9,49-53] Increased head circumference in early years (accelerated growth in the first year) will approach normal to less than normal after childhood (deceleration).[52] Together with increased head size in 20% to 30% of children with ASD, imaging reveals a general increased brain volume.[9,49-52] Certain neuronal cells (e.g., Purkinje cells in the cerebellum, forebrain cells, frontal and temporal lobe cortical mini-column cells, and cells in the area of Broca) are smaller.[9,50-52] In addition, compared with age-matched controls, patients with ASD have global reductions in white matter volume leading to atypical structural connectivity (hypoconnectivity), confirmed by functional connectivity MRI.[54-56] Brain stem abnormalities have also been observed.[51,52] One explanation for the impairments in empathy, imitation, and language could be a dysfunction in mirror neurons.[53] Whereas neuroimaging studies are mostly focused on major structural abnormalities in the brain, its connectivity and function, little is known about what may be occurring at the microscopic level.[57]

Other proposed risk factors for ASD include maternal and fetal exposure to teratogenic medications, selective serotonin reuptake inhibitor (SSRI) antidepressants, neurotoxins, smoking, alcohol, infection, and prenatal malnutrition.[9,35,46,58,59] These environmental factors may act as modulators to the expression of preexisting genetic factors. Although smoking and consumption of alcohol are known to increase the risk of adverse neonatal outcomes, evidence currently does not show an association to ASD.[60,61] Older parents (older than 35–40 years) have a higher risk of having children with ASD, which may be related to spontaneous genetic mutations, such as a copy number variant related to age.[62-64] In addition a short interpregnancy interval (of 12 months or less) has been consistently reported to increase the risk of ASD, as well as long interpregnancy intervals (more than 60–84 months) in limited reports.[65-71] Furthermore, infection during pregnancy (bacterial or viral) and other immune factors such as a family history of autoimmune disorders may increase the risk of ASD.[72,73] Various metabolic maternal conditions (e.g., diabetes), lower gestational age at birth (e.g., premature infant), and abnormal infant size at birth (large or small) all independently have been reported to increase the risk of ASD.[73]

CLINICAL PRESENTATION AND DIAGNOSIS

Simultaneously with the rise in the diagnosis of ASD, early screening and diagnosis has become increasingly important over the years. It was not long ago that children with ASD did not receive a diagnosis and subsequent treatment until their school-age years. However, because of increased awareness and improved diagnostic tools, it is possible to identify children earlier, as noted in one study with a mean age of 34 months at diagnosis.[74] Another study found that a diagnosis by an experienced professional by age 2 can be considered very reliable.[75] Data support early identification and intensive interventions to improve optimal outcomes and achieve normal cognitive function and behavior.[76] Evidence is mounting to support interventions being most effective when started early, and that such interventions may even help to reduce or avoid behavioral issues.[77] Screening should be provided using validated tools, such as the Infant Toddler Checklist, the Modified Checklist For Autism In Toddlers–Revised with Follow-Up (M-CHAT-R/F), and the Childhood Autism Rating Scale, 2nd edition (CARS-2), at the 9-, 18-, and 24- or 30-month visits because signs of ASD are generally present before age 2 years.[78] These signs can be seen as early as the first year of life, with disruptions in communication, temperament, social interest, and attention that may be subtly noticed by parents.[79]

In addition, for children who are losing skills they once had, the lack of pointing/gestures or lack of pretend/symbolic play by 12 and 18 months, respectively, may be important early signs and symptoms of ASD.[9,80] Furthermore, the American Academy of Neurology and the Child Neurology Society suggest being aware of the following "red flags," which are indicators to evaluate further and immediately for ASD[81]:

- No babbling, pointing, or other gestures by 12 months
- No single words by 16 months
- No two-word spontaneous (not echolalia) phrases by 24 months
- Loss of language or social skills at any age

The diagnosis of ASD requires the presence of persistent impairments and deficits in the following: (1) social communication and interaction (e.g., social–emotional reciprocity, nonverbal communicative behaviors, and developing, maintaining, and understanding relationships), and (2) repetitive or restricted patterns of behavior (e.g., ritualized patterns, inflexible to change in routines, hypo- or hyper-reactivity to sensory input), interests (e.g., fixated abnormal intensity or focus), or activities (e.g., repetitive or stereotyped movements, use of objects or speech), as listed in Box 1. These impairments and deficits may be current or in the person's history, and severity may be used to classify level of support needed (Table 1) based on symptomatology. Severity may fluctuate over time after diagnosis and even fall below Level 1 on subsequent assessment. Specifiers are used to provide additional detail if an individual presents with or without the following: (1) an accompanying intellectual impairment or (2) accompanying language impairment, or is (3) associated with a known medical, genetic, or environmental factor, and has (4) catatonia. Based on the recent change in diagnostic criteria from the *DSM-IV-TR* to the *DSM-5*, those with an established diagnosis using the *DSM-IV-TR* criteria for autistic disorder, Asperger disorder, or PDD-NOS should receive a diagnosis of ASD. Those with deficits in social communication but no other symptoms that would meet the criteria for ASD should be evaluated for social (pragmatic) communication disorder, newly added to the *DSM-5*.[1]

Cognitive deficits that may qualify as mental retardation (IQ of 70 or less) are often present in children with ASD.[2,9] Also seen commonly in this population are electroencephalogram abnormalities and epilepsy.[82] Many children with ASD also present with comorbidities or associated symptoms of attention-deficit/hyperactivity disorder (ADHD), anxiety, catatonia, and depression, together with the co-occurring maladaptive behaviors and symptoms of aggression, irritability, tantrums, poor impulse control, and self-injurious behavior.[1-4,9,80] Individuals with ASD may have psychiatric symptoms that do not fulfill the criteria for a separate disorder. However, when criteria for a disorder (e.g., ADHD, anxiety disorder, depressive disorder) are met, each diagnosis should be given.[1] A clinical syndrome requiring more research into etiology and treatment that may be rarely encountered with some clinical presentations similar to ASD is the group of pediatric autoimmune neuropsychiatric disorders associated with streptococcal infections. A child with this diagnosis may demonstrate new-onset stereotypic or ritualistic and obsessive-compulsive behaviors. However, this set of autoimmune neuropsychiatric disorders can reverse with time and antibiotic treatment, whereas ASD does not.[83,84]

Some children with ASD may present with gastrointestinal symptoms such as constipation or diarrhea, whereas others may have difficulties with sleep patterns. Appropriate evaluation of these symptoms is recommended to rule out other reversible causes of the other diagnoses just discussed, and appropriate symptomatic management is recommended. The clinician should also consider that the patient's behavioral changes may be secondary to disturbances in sleep or gastrointestinal distress.[85] Although pharmacotherapy is sometimes used for the gastrointestinal or sleep disturbances in ASD, these issues should be addressed and treated according to recommended pediatric guidelines for such symptoms. Some of

---

Box 1. Diagnostic Criteria for Autism Spectrum Disorder[1]

Diagnostic Criteria

A. Persistent deficits in social communication and social interaction across many contexts, as manifested by the following, currently or by history[a]:
   1. Deficits in social-emotional reciprocity, ranging from, for example: abnormal social approach and failure of normal back-and-forth conversation; to reduced sharing of interests, emotions, or affect; to failure to initiate or respond to social interactions
   2. Deficits in nonverbal communicative behaviors used for social interaction, ranging from, for example: poorly integrated verbal and nonverbal communication; to abnormalities in eye contact and body language or deficits in understanding and use of gestures; to a total lack of facial expressions and nonverbal communication
   3. Deficits in developing, maintaining, and understanding relationships, ranging from, for example: difficulties adjusting behavior to suit various social contexts; to difficulties in sharing imaginative play or in making friends; to absence of interest in peers

Specify current severity: Severity is based on social communication impairments and restricted repetitive patterns of behavior[b]

B. Restricted, repetitive patterns of behavior, interests, or activities, as manifested by at least two of the following, currently or by history[a]:
   1. Stereotyped or repetitive motor movements, use of objects, or speech, for example: simple motor stereotypies, lining up toys or flipping objects, echolalia, idiosyncratic phrases
   2. Insistence on sameness, inflexible adherence to routines, or ritualized patterns of verbal or nonverbal behavior, for example: extreme distress at small changes, difficulties with transitions, rigid thinking patterns, greeting rituals, need to take same route or eat same food every day
   3. Highly restricted, fixated interests that are abnormal in intensity or focus, for example: strong attachment to or preoccupation with unusual objects, excessively circumscribed or perseverative interest
   4. Hyper- or hyporeactivity to sensory input or unusual interests in sensory aspects of the environment, for example: apparent indifference to pain/temperature, adverse response to specific sounds or textures, excessive smelling or touching of objects, visual fascination with lights or movement

Specify current severity: Severity is based on social communication impairments and restricted, repetitive patterns of behavior[b]

C. Symptoms must be present in the early developmental period, but may not become fully manifest until social demands exceed limited capacities, or may be masked by learned strategies in later life

D. Symptoms cause clinically significant impairment in social, occupational, or other important areas of current functioning

E. These disturbances are not better explained by intellectual disability (intellectual developmental disorder) or global developmental delay. Intellectual disability and autism spectrum disorder often co-occur; to make comorbid diagnoses of autism spectrum disorder and intellectual disability, social communication should be less than that expected for general developmental level

Specify if:

- With or without accompanying intellectual impairment
- With or without accompanying language impairment
- Associated with a known medical or genetic condition or environmental factor
- With catatonia

[a]Examples are illustrative, not exhaustive; chapter text provides further detail.
[b]Table 1 in this chapter provides the severity levels for autism spectrum disorder.

---

the psychotropic medications selected for disturbed behaviors in this population will carry the adverse effects of sleep disturbances (i.e., sedation or insomnia) and gastrointestinal disturbances (i.e., constipation or diarrhea), and these issues should be considered during pharmacotherapy selection and monitoring. Evaluations to aid in diagnosing ASD include neuropsychological, medical, speech–language, audiologic, neurologic, and laboratory analysis to rule out other, better-explained diagnoses and environmental factors such as heavy metal exposure (e.g., lead).[1,2,8,9,80]

TREATMENT

TREATMENT GOALS

The overall goal of treatment for ASD is not to cure or prevent this condition, but to manage symptoms. Pharmacologic treatment strategies target a core aspect of ASD (e.g., a disruptive behavior) that is interfering with the individual's ability to participate in other treatments designed to achieve maximum functional ability. When a child with ASD demonstrates disruptive, irritable, aggressive, or agitated behaviors that do not respond to nonpharmacologic behavioral interventions, targeted pharmacotherapy may be warranted (Figure 1).[85,86] A clinically meaningful reduction in behavioral symptoms (e.g., irritability, aggression, self-injury) is the desired outcome so

that the individual can then engage in the nonpharmacologic treatments intended to improve overall functioning in all the affected domains and identified deficits.[85]

NONPHARMACOLOGIC TREATMENTS FOR ASD

Nonpharmacologic treatments for ASD should be implemented in a coordinated manner before pharmacologic treatment.[85] Therapies that may be beneficial in the management of a child with ASD include occupational therapy, physical therapy, educational interventions, behavioral therapy (e.g., applied behavior analysis), speech–language therapy, and possibly diet modification in those who are responsive to such an intervention.[87-89] Common dietary changes include reducing or eliminating dairy protein intake (casein-free) and certain protein-containing cereals (gluten-free).[88] Dietary modifications in research provide inconsistent results; however, many parents of children with ASD will attempt this intervention, with mixed outcomes, before more costly or medically warranted interventions. Given the case-based lay and medical literature of benefit and the mixed results of dietary modification in formal research studies, this practice of dietary modification continues. If this approach successfully reduces some of the behaviors or symptoms in a particular child with ASD so that the child may engage in other treatments, then it also

Table 1. Severity Levels for Autism Spectrum Disorder[1]

Severity Level	Social Communication	Restricted, Repetitive Behaviors
Level 3: Requiring very substantial support	• Severe deficits in verbal and nonverbal social communication skills cause severe impairments in functioning, very limited initiation of social interactions, and minimal response to social overtures from others • For example, a person with few words of intelligible speech who rarely initiates interaction and, when he or she does, makes unusual approaches to meet needs only and responds to only very direct social approaches	• Inflexibility of behavior, extreme difficulty coping with change, or other restricted/repetitive behaviors that markedly interfere with functioning in all spheres • Great distress/difficulty changing focus or action
Level 2: Requiring substantial support	• Marked deficits in verbal and nonverbal social communication skills; social impairments apparent even with supports in place; limited initiation of social interactions; and reduced or abnormal responses to social overtures from others • For example, a person who speaks simple sentences, whose interaction is limited to narrow special interests, and who has markedly odd nonverbal communication	• Inflexibility of behavior, difficulty coping with change, or other restricted/repetitive behaviors that appear often enough to be obvious to the casual observer and interfere with functioning in a variety of contexts • Distress and/or difficulty changing focus or action
Level 1: Requiring support	• Without supports in place, deficits in social communication cause noticeable impairments • Difficulty initiating social interactions, and clear examples of atypical or unsuccessful response to social overtures of others • May appear to have decreased interest in social interactions • For example, a person who is able to speak in full sentences and engages in communication but whose to- and-fro conversation with others fails, and whose attempts to make friends are odd and typically unsuccessful	• Inflexibility of behavior causes significant interference with functioning in one or more contexts • Difficulty switching between activities • Problems of organization and planning hamper independence

serves to empower and offer a level of control by the family and caregivers regarding the child's total treatment.[90]

About 50% of parents of children with ASD use complementary and alternative treatments, despite the lack of evidence for their efficacy. Such treatments include the use of dietary supplements (e.g., vitamins B and C, ω-3 fatty acids, probiotics, magnesium, melatonin), acupuncture, sensory integration, and aromatherapy.[85,89-93] The use of microbiota (fecal) transplantation is a relatively new area of investigation for ASD; however, further research is needed in this area.[94]

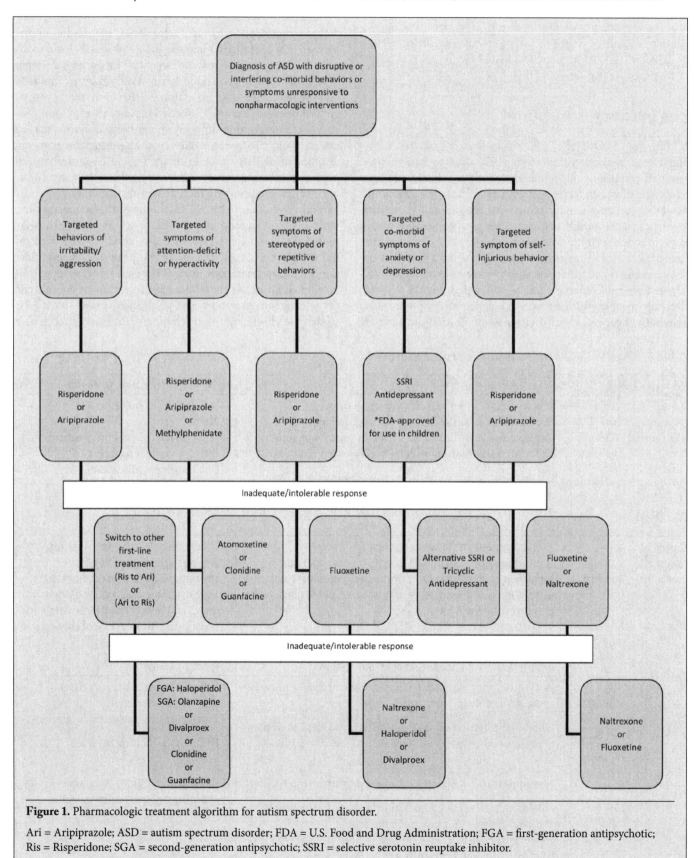

Figure 1. Pharmacologic treatment algorithm for autism spectrum disorder.

Ari = Aripiprazole; ASD = autism spectrum disorder; FDA = U.S. Food and Drug Administration; FGA = first-generation antipsychotic; Ris = Risperidone; SGA = second-generation antipsychotic; SSRI = selective serotonin reuptake inhibitor.

PHARMACOTHERAPY

Pharmacotherapy is best used to allow the child to better engage in treatment plans such as speech–language plans, occupational therapy plans, or those that are educationally, behaviorally, or socially oriented for maximum benefit to the child with an ASD. The impairments in social interaction and communication are generally unresponsive to pharmacotherapy. Even maladaptive behavioral problems should be managed without medications, if possible. Use of psychotropic medications should be reserved for moderate to severe problems with specific behaviors such as irritability and aggression.[85,95,96] Pharmacotherapeutic interventions may also be used for a comorbid symptom of the disorder such as inattention, hyperactivity, or repetitive/stereotypic behaviors that are also interfering with the child's overall treatment plan and that are not responding adequately to the nonpharmacologic interventions. Medical treatment of comorbid diagnoses such as epilepsy, gastrointestinal symptoms, or sleep disorders may also be required in many children with ASD.[85]

Steps to determine the need for, and implementation of, pharmacotherapy for ASD should include those listed in Box 2.[85,86]

The pharmacologic management of children with ASD includes many medications that are indicated for other disorders and have not received label approval for ASD from the U.S. Food and Drug Administration (FDA) (Table 2). Only two antipsychotics are approved with established efficacy and safety for irritability associated with ASD.[97-108] Research indicates that most subjects receiving pharmacotherapy for irritability can have some clinically recognized improvement. However, because a target symptom may be similar to symptoms encountered in other disorders for which these agents have established efficacy, or that are co-occurring because of another diagnosed disorder, the use of certain medications (e.g., SSRIs, psychostimulants) is accepted practice. Published research also supports the use of certain medications for targeted symptom management. These behaviors or symptoms may include repetitive or stereotyped behaviors that resemble the symptoms of obsessions and compulsions and therefore may respond to the medications approved for obsessive-compulsive disorder, such as some of the SSRIs.[109,110] Symptoms of inattention and hyperactivity may respond to prescribed psychostimulant medications, although these agents may exacerbate irritability and agitation.[111] In addition, other agents used in attention-deficit disorder and ADHD (e.g., clonidine, guanfacine) may be beneficial for certain targeted symptoms such as hyperactivity and aggression.[112-115]

The use of various medications for ASD management has been increasing during the past 2 decades. A 1995 study indicated about 30% of children with ASD were receiving a psychotropic medication. Studies of children with ASD published from 1995–2017 indicated that up to 42%-56% of the children with ASD were receiving at least one psychotropic medication, and 20% of the children were receiving three or more medications concurrently.[116-119] Antipsychotic medications were the most commonly prescribed class of psychotropics in

---

Box 2. Steps to Determine the Need for and Implementation of Pharmacotherapy for Autism Spectrum Disorder[85,86]

- Identify and perform a baseline assessment of target behaviors through several sources (e.g., parents, teachers), in addition to factors and triggers modifying the behaviors

- Assess the degree of interference with functioning and consider using rating scales and clinical judgment (by the clinician) to establish baseline functioning both before the intervention and at follow-up to determine positive and negative outcomes

- Determine the efficacy achieved with behavioral interventions and other psychosocial supports and education

- Identify potential medical factors through physical assessment and testing that may be causing or exacerbating the target behavior(s) (e.g., pain, gastrointestinal discomfort, sleep disorders, menstruation)

- Consider psychotropic medication given the evidence that the target symptoms are interfering with learning/academic progress, socialization, and health/safety (self and others) or the patient's quality of life and that the patient had a suboptimal response to nonpharmacologic interventions

- Choose a medication on the basis of known efficacy for the specific target symptoms, its potential adverse effects, formulations available, dosing schedule, and need for laboratory or other monitoring (e.g., electrocardiographic)

- Acquire informed consent from the parent/guardian (required in certain instances) and, when possible, from the patient

- Establish a plan for monitoring and following up all treatment outcomes and the desired or expected timeframe for such outcomes, including laboratory and physical monitoring for changes in weight, glucose, lipids, and other potential laboratory values affected by the chosen medication

- If outcomes are less than desired or expected, and adequate dosing and length of treatment was achieved, then consider alternative treatment options, including switching to another agent or augmentation with a different medication

- If the patient has responded favorably for the past 6–12 months, consider tapering and discontinuing treatment to reassess the need for pharmacotherapy

---

this population, with psychostimulants and antidepressants being the second and third most commonly used, respectively, in children based on a recent meta-analysis of more than 300,000 individuals with ASD.[119]

ANTIPSYCHOTICS

Historically, first-generation antipsychotics have been used in the management of maladaptive behaviors associated with ASD. Although not approved for treating ASD, haloperidol was the most commonly used and studied agent before the atypical antipsychotics were developed. While haloperidol is efficacious in treating the irritability, aggression, and stereotypes associated with ASD in several small studies, its risk of extrapyramidal adverse effects such as dystonias, tremors, and the potentially irreversible tardive dyskinesia significantly limits its use today.[120-125] In 40 autistic children age 2–7 years, haloperidol was effective in reducing behavioral symptoms and producing general clinical improvement.[120] Based on published research, the optimal dose may be no more than 1–2 mg/day. In addition to extrapyramidal symptoms, other adverse effects including increased appetite, weight gain, and sedation may also limit its use in this population. Sustained and higher-than-average prolactin levels secondary

Table 2. Pharmacotherapy Options for Autism Spectrum Disorder

Medication	Target Symptoms with Level of Evidence[a]						
	Core Domains				Associated Behaviors		
	Social Interaction	C/L	S/RB	Irritability/ Aggression	Attention	Hyperactivity	SIB
Antipsychotics							
Risperidone[b]	B		A	A	B	B	B/C
Aripiprazole[b]			A	A	B	B	B/C
Haloperidol[b]	C		C	A		B	
Olanzapine				B			
Quetiapine				C			
Ziprasidone				C			
SSRIs							
Fluoxetine[b]			B				C
Fluvoxamine			D				D
Citalopram			D				D
Clomipramine			C	C/D			C/D
α1-RAs							
Clonidine			C/D	C		C	
Guanfacine			C/D	C		C	
Psychostimulants							
Amphetamine[b]				F		F	
Methylphenidate[b]					C	B	
Others							
Naltrexone	C/D		B/C	C		C	C
Divalproex[b]			B/C	B/C			
Lamotrigine	D	F	F	F	D		
Oxcarbazepine[b]				D			D
Levetiracetam[b]			D	D	D	D	
Topiramate				F		F	
Atomoxetine						B	

[a]A = Many DBPC studies with positive efficacy; B = one DBPC study (moderate to large) with positive efficacy (or two small studies); C = open-label studies with positive efficacy; D = questionable efficacy with limiting ADRs/positive efficacy through case reports/series; F = negative efficacy studies with problematic ADRs.
[b]Denotes availability as a liquid formulation option. Valproic acid is available as liquid formulation.
ADR = adverse drug reaction; ASD = autism spectrum disorder; C/L = communication/language impairments; DBPC = double-blind, placebo-controlled (study); RA = receptor agonist; SIB = self-injurious behavior; S/RB = stereotypy/repetitive behaviors; SSRI = selective serotonin reuptake inhibitor.

to antipsychotic use may have adverse effects on development in both female and male individuals with ASD.[99,126] Clinically, manifestations of high prolactin levels can include gynecomastia, galactorrhea, amenorrhea, and possibly osteoporosis; thus, monitoring for these adverse effects is warranted.

In 2006, risperidone became the first medication to receive FDA label approval for the treatment of irritability associated with ASD in children and adolescents age 5–16 years. Risperidone has well-established efficacy in many double-blind, placebo-controlled, and open-label trials.[85,97-104] The two principal double-blind, placebo-controlled trials used for FDA approval established the efficacy of risperidone using the outcome measurements of the Clinical Global Impression Scale (CGI) and the Aberrant Behavior Checklist (ABC).[97,100,101,105] Up to 75% of subjects in the trials had a CGI score of either 1 ("very much improved") or 2 ("much improved") compared with only 11% of subjects receiving placebo. At least 50% of the subjects had a reduction in the ABC-Irritability subscale (ABC-I) of at least 25%. The mean reduction in the ABC-I for risperidone was 57% compared with the mean reduction in the placebo group of 14%.[100] The maladaptive behaviors of irritability, aggression, tantrums, and self-injury are the principal targets when using risperidone; however, research indicates that other symptoms such as hyperactivity and stereotypy may improve as well. The core domains of communication impairment and issues with social interaction are not considered principal targets of pharmacotherapy with risperidone, although these symptoms may occasionally improve with pharmacotherapy. The manufacturer-recommended dosage range is 0.25–3 mg/day, with higher doses sometimes needed for individuals weighing more than 45 kg. The recommended starting dose and range are based on weight (0.01–0.06 mg/kg/day), with 0.25 mg/day for children weighing less than 20 kg and 0.5 mg/day for children weighing 20 kg or more. Titration to the effective dosage should take place every 2 weeks in increments of 0.25–0.5 mg/day, with a target dose of 0.5 mg/day for children weighing less than 20 kg and 1 mg/day for children weighing 20 kg or more.[104,105] Common adverse effects during the clinical trials include fatigue (42%), somnolence (67%), increased appetite (49%), weight gain (5%), hypersalivation (22%), and extrapyramidal symptoms (7%-12%) such as dystonias, tremors, and dyskinesias.[96,99,100,102,104] Increases in prolactin levels have been observed during clinical trials and should be monitored for in children and adolescents receiving risperidone, as well as possible clinical manifestations of hyperprolactinemia such as gynecomastia and galactorrhea.[99,126]

In 2009, aripiprazole became the second agent to receive FDA label approval for the treatment of irritability associated with ASD in children and adolescents age 6–17 years.[106] Like risperidone, the approval was based on two studies, with results indicating that aripiprazole was superior to placebo in reducing the symptom of irritability associated with ASD in children and adolescents, age 6–17 years, by at least 25% as well as in achieving a "much-improved" or "very much-improved" score on the CGI for more than 50% of the subjects taking medication compared with 16% of the subjects receiving placebo who achieved a "much-improved" or "very much-improved" rating. The mean reduction in the ABC-I for aripiprazole was 44% compared with the mean reduction in the placebo group of 16%.[107,108] The recommended treatment dosage range is 2–15 mg/day. A once-daily dose of 2 mg is the recommended starting dose; 5–10 mg/day is the recommended treatment dose; and 15 mg/day is the maximum recommended dose for children age 6–17 years.[106] Common adverse events during the trials included sedation (21%), fatigue (17%), vomiting (14%), tremor (10%), hypersalivation (9%), decreased appetite (7%), dizziness (3%), and extrapyramidal symptoms (6%).[105,106,127,128] Only one head-to-head comparison of aripiprazole and risperidone has been performed in a randomized, double-blind trial. No significant difference was seen between the two medications in their reduction of ABC-I subscale scores or rates of adverse effects or over a period of 2 months.[129] Aripiprazole appears to have a lower risk of significant weight gain and hyperprolactinemia than other atypical antipsychotic agents that may be used in ASD.[105,127,128] One recent Cochrane Review on aripiprazole for ASD concluded that aripiprazole can be effective at reducing irritability, hyperactivity, and stereotypies in the short term (8 weeks); however, relapse rates in the long term (16 weeks) did not differ compared with placebo, suggesting that after stabilization of target symptoms, re-evaluation of use is warranted.[130]

Other atypical antipsychotic agents have also been researched in ASD. In one placebo-controlled, double-blind study, olanzapine had positive efficacy for the treatment of aggression and irritability in children and adolescents age 6–14 years with a PDD (n=11; 6 with ASD, 1 with Asperger disorder, and

Table 3. Select Dosing and Formulation Availability

Medication[a]	Dosing	Formulations
Haloperidol	≤ 1–2 mg/day	Oral tablets Oral solution Intramuscular injection
Risperidone	0.25–3 mg/day	Oral tablets Oral solution Orally disintegrating tablets
Aripiprazole	2–15 mg/day	Oral tablets Oral solution Orally disintegrating tablets
Fluoxetine	2.5 mg/day starting dose; then up to daily total dose of 0.8 mg/kg/day	Oral capsules Oral tablets Oral solution
Clomipramine	25 mg/day starting dose; then up to total daily dose of 3 mg/kg/day or 200 mg/day maximum	Oral capsules

[a]Monitoring: All of these agents can cause changes in weight, extrapyramidal symptoms, insomnia/sedation, and prolactin changes; therefore, the clinician must periodically assess for efficacy and adverse drug reactions.

4 with PDD-NOS).[130] Clozapine, ziprasidone, and quetiapine have been evaluated in small open-label studies or case reports, with modest efficacy in reducing irritability, aggression, and tantrums.[132-134] Further research is required with these agents and with the more recently approved atypical antipsychotics (paliperidone, asenapine, iloperidone, lurasidone, ziprasidone) to establish their potential roles in treating children with ASD.

On the basis of early experiences with antipsychotic medications in ASD and the established efficacy and approval of risperidone and aripiprazole, these two agents should be considered first-line treatment; after treatment failure or the inability to use one of these two agents because of intolerability, other antipsychotics should be considered (Table 3).

ANTIDEPRESSANTS

Stereotypic behaviors present with symptoms similar to obsessions and compulsions. The SSRIs have been studied and used in clinical practice for the repetitive behaviors in ASD; however, their overall efficacy appears inconsistent. Medications such as fluoxetine, sertraline, escitalopram, fluvoxamine, and clomipramine have been evaluated for their ability to reduce repetitive behaviors with limited and mixed results.[109,110,135-137] Although fluoxetine has proved to have some efficacy in reducing the repetitive behaviors associated with ASD when using the Child-Yale Brown Obsessive Compulsive Scale, agents such as fluvoxamine have minimal efficacy in children.[109,110,131]

Other SSRIs such as sertraline and paroxetine have only been studied in case reports and open-label trials, which do not consistently support their use in children with ASD.[110] Citalopram was studied at a mean dose of 16.5 mg/day in a relatively large placebo-controlled, double-blind trial (n=149) of children and adolescents age 5–17 years with ASD. Citalopram was no different from placebo in clinical outcomes; however, it caused significant adverse events including activation, impulsiveness, hyperactivity, stereotypies, diarrhea, and insomnia.[137] If the decision is made to use an SSRI, then the prescriber should consider using agents with established safety and tolerability in children and adolescents from data generated from other approved indications such as obsessive-compulsive disorder or depression. These agents include fluoxetine, sertraline, escitalopram, and fluvoxamine.

Clomipramine, a highly serotonergic tricyclic agent, was the first agent to receive FDA label approval for adults for obsessive-compulsive disorder. Clomipramine has been studied in trials (dosage range 25–250 mg/day; mean 150 mg/day) of both child and adult populations and has modest efficacy compared with desipramine (n=24; patients age 6–18 years and showing superior efficacy to desipramine) and haloperidol (n=36 patients age 10–36 years and showing efficacy similar to haloperidol). The areas of improvement were generally related to obsessive-compulsive behaviors and stereotypies, but they also included reductions in anger and hyperactivity, as well as an overall general improvement, as reflected in the CGI-Improvement Scale (CGI-I) of the subjects. However, the tolerability and general adverse effect profile (e.g., dizziness, drowsiness, insomnia, nervousness, diaphoresis, xerostomia, constipation, difficulty in micturition, tremor, and visual disturbance) of clomipramine suggest it should be used after other agents such as antipsychotic agents and SSRIs have failed.[121,136]

PSYCHOSTIMULANTS

For ADHD-like symptoms that accompany ASD, psychostimulants such as methylphenidate have been used with mixed results.[138-140] The amphetamines also have limited efficacy data in ASD, with no controlled studies since the 1970s, which is before current diagnostic criteria were used. Two small placebo-controlled crossover studies using methylphenidate resulted in positive data showing improved hyperactivity, noting adverse effects of social withdrawal and irritability.[140,141] In addition, in a larger placebo-controlled trial of 72 children with ASD investigating the effects of methylphenidate 0.125-0.5mg/kg/day, 49% of participants noted mild to moderate improvement in hyperactivity and global severity using the ABC-Hyperactivity subscale and CGI-I scale; however, similar to the aforementioned smaller studies, social withdrawal and irritability were seen.[138] The response to psychostimulants in the ASD population may be less than that experienced by someone with ADHD without ASD.[139,142] Psychostimulants may be an option in treating symptoms of hyperactivity in ASD; however benefits must be carefully weighed against the potential adverse effects, including a worsening of ASD symptoms.[85]

Clonidine and guanfacine, both approved for ADHD treatment, have been studied in children and adolescents with ASD with reports of moderate efficacy in reducing symptoms of stereotypy, hyperactivity, irritability, sleep, inappropriate speech, and oppositionality.[112-115,143] One recent randomized, placebo-controlled trial investigated the effects of extended-release guanfacine in 62 children with ASD and found a 43.6% decline in scores on the ABC-Hyperactivity subscale compared with 13.2% in the placebo group. Improvement on the CGI-I was also noted to be 50% in the guanfacine group compared with 9.4% in the placebo group. Overall, a reduction in hyperactivity, impulsivity, and distractibility was seen.[144] Sedation and fatigue are common adverse effects of α_2-agonists. Atomoxetine has also been studied for the treatment of ADHD in children with ASD in a number of placebo-controlled, open-label, and retrospective studies, showing improvements in ADHD symptoms and causing adverse effects such as nausea, decreased appetite, and mid-nocturnal awakenings.[145]

OTHER PHARMACOTHERAPIES

Anticonvulsants used for their mood-stabilizing properties have been investigated to determine their potential role in the treatment of aggression, affective dysregulation, and impulsivity in individuals with ASD.[145] Divalproex sodium is the most widely investigated, with mixed results. Early reports identified improvements in language and maladaptive behaviors in children with ASD and seizures/abnormal EEGs.[146-148] Two double-blind, placebo-controlled trials in children and adolescents with ASD were performed to investigate early claims of improvement; one study found significant improvement in irritability (62% responder rate vs. 9% in placebo), whereas the other study did not find differences between groups for aggression and irritability using CGI-I, ABC-I, and Overt Aggression Scale scores.[149,150] A third study of 13 individuals in a double-blind, placebo-controlled group showed improvements in reducing repetitive behaviors.[151] Lamotrigine was also investigated in a randomized, double-blind, placebo-controlled trial for treating aberrant behaviors and core symptoms of ASD in children, and found no difference from placebo using ABC subscales, Vineland Adaptive Behaviors Scales, and other measures.[152] Studies on levetiracetam, oxcarbazepine, and topiramate showed similar findings with intolerable adverse effects.[153-157] Controlled trials are needed to determine the benefit of anticonvulsants in children with ASD.

Naltrexone continues to be questionable in efficacy and utility. Many studies have been done, both open label and placebo controlled, and the results are mixed. Although naltrexone may not be very effective for self-injurious behaviors and social interaction, as originally postulated, it may have some effect on hyperactivity and is generally well tolerated.[111,112,158,159]

Oxytocin, memantine, riluzole, D-cycloserine, acetylcysteine, acamprosate, arbaclofen, buspirone, mirtazapine, lithium, and other agents are being investigated; much is still to be learned about their potential psychopharmacologic benefits and roles in treating core symptoms and/or aberrant behaviors in ASD.[143,145,160,161]

MONITORING OF THERAPY

Monitoring of ASD in clinical practice is generally through parental and observer reports, in addition to teacher and other caregiver input. Assessment tools such as the ABC, Childhood Autism Rating Scale (CARS), or CGI are used in research, but not commonly in practice. The ABC-I is a 15-item parent-rated or primary caregiver–rated assessment focusing on agitation, aggression, tantrums, self-injury, and unstable mood with a possible 0–45 score; higher scores indicate greater severity of symptoms. In research, a common outcome goal is achieving at least a 25% reduction in symptoms of irritability compared with baseline. As a clinician assessment tool, CARS assists with both diagnostics and the monitoring of individuals with ASD. This tool has 15 items assessing several areas including social interactions and relationships, communication, and behaviors. The CGI is rated for severity (1 = not at all ill up to 7 = extremely ill) or improvement (1 = very much improved vs. 7 = very much worse) with clinicians generally using these versions in research to provide a simplified and global rating of severity or level of change at baseline and follow-up, respectively.[162-164]

Specialty-specific outcomes (e.g., speech–language) are measured differently, depending on the type of deficits or behaviors being addressed through treatment and the type of treatment or therapy being used.[9,85,86] When the ABC, CARS, or CGI are used in research, improvements can be observed as early as 1 week of treatment in some individuals. However, an adequate trial of the appropriate medication at the appropriate daily dose may require up to 8 weeks or more before that intervention is declared a success or failure, with the exception of early discontinuation because of intolerable adverse effects to the patient.

In addition to clinical monitoring for efficacy outcomes, the use of the antipsychotics and other psychotropics warrants the monitoring of laboratory values that assess metabolic values such as lipids and glucose control. Prolactin levels should be assessed at baseline and periodically, in addition to observable manifestations of hyperprolactinemia such as gynecomastia and galactorrhea. Regular monitoring for weight changes in patients taking antipsychotics, psychostimulants, mood stabilizers, and antidepressants is also recommended. Many agents for treating ASD may also cause movement disorders in the form of extrapyramidal symptoms (dystonic reactions, pseudoparkinsonism, akathisia, tardive dyskinesia), motor tics, or tremors. Clinicians should consider a baseline assessment of clinical symptoms, laboratory values, and physical examination findings, with a follow-up in 1 month, and then provide a quarterly assessment as indicated unless caregiver or patient input or monitoring data warrant assessments more often.

PHARMACOTHERAPEUTIC OUTCOMES

The desired outcomes of pharmacotherapy are best described as reductions in the maladaptive and challenging behaviors so that the child with ASD can then engage in nonpharmacologic treatments such as speech–language therapy or educational treatment plans.[86] The sometimes-limited efficacy of the psychotropics discussed in this chapter should be considered, in addition to their liabilities of adverse effects such as weight gain, sedation, or even the possible worsening of some of the behaviors of ASD. Given that ASD is a chronic condition, some children with ASD may require long-term treatment with medications, and the risks of long-term exposure to some of the medications discussed are not well known. Nonpharmacologic interventions should be the first-line treatment with psychotropics held in reserve for more severe cases.[85,86] The atypical antipsychotic medications risperidone and aripiprazole, which have been approved for use in ASD, were approved for use in 2006 and 2009, respectively (Table 3). Some adverse effects of medications may take years to manifest, such as problems secondary to significant weight gain or the development of tardive dyskinesia with antipsychotics or, yet undetermined, the long-term negative effects with other psychotropics such as SSRIs or psychostimulants. The type of symptom identified as challenging or disruptive and thus targeted to be addressed with pharmacotherapy will influence the medication selected. The antipsychotics are best suited for the disruptive behaviors of aggression, irritability, tantrums, and stereotypic/repetitive behaviors. If the patient has a recognized comorbid attention deficit or hyperactivity, a psychostimulant may be warranted, although caution should be taken not to exacerbate preexisting irritability or agitation. If comorbid obsessive-compulsive disorder is occurring, an antidepressant that is approved for child and adolescent use is recommended. Self-injurious behaviors may respond not only to antipsychotics, but also to SSRIs and possibly naltrexone. Some practitioners, who may associate the repetitive behaviors with obsessive-compulsive symptoms, could consider prescribing an SSRI or clomipramine for such behaviors, given their efficacy for obsessive-compulsive disorder. Again, it is important to consider pharmacotherapy as a targeted symptomatic treatment approach to assist in the patient's total treatment plan to maximize functioning that may be inhibited by his or her disruptive and aggressive behaviors, thereby making the patient unable to engage in the equally important nonpharmacologic interventions designed to address the other core areas of ASD.

CONCLUSIONS

The use of medications to treat the maladaptive behaviors and comorbid symptoms of ASD is a common practice, according to surveys of prescribers and parents.[116-118] With only two medications that currently have FDA label approval for the treatment of irritability related to ASD, most pharmacologic agents are being used off-label, although with some research supporting their use and thus with some evidence for their positive benefit in reducing certain behavioral issues. The prescriber should keep in mind, and discuss with the patient's family and caregivers, that pharmacotherapy in ASD is for symptomatic management only. Because improvements in the core features of ASD can be made through other interventions and over time, the need for pharmacotherapy should be reassessed periodically. If the maladaptive and other co-occurring behaviors such as irritability, tantrums, agitation, and hyperactivity are addressed, then ideally the child with ASD can better engage in the other treatments and therapies that can address the core domains of the ASD and improve overall outcomes.

Patient Case — NEWLY SUSPECTED AUTISM SPECTRUM DISORDER

A 28-month-old white boy is brought by his mother to the pediatrician's outpatient office. The mother has noticed that over the past few weeks the child is less verbal and communicative than she believes he should be (and less than his brother was at the same age) and that he is not pointing at the items he wants from his mother; he will not repeat anything that is said to him; he does not call out for his "mama" or "papa," and he does not often play with his older brother. His mother was not previously concerned about these behaviors because she has been spending less time with the child since she recently began working part-time. However, after 2 weeks of caring for the boy for what she thought was a simple stomach virus with foul-smelling diarrhea, and thus spending more time with the child to maintain hydration and other care, she grew concerned that his behaviors were not improving and may not be related to the recent illness. She then made an appointment to see the pediatrician as early as possible for evaluation. The pediatrician assessed the child using a Modified Checklist for Autism in Toddlers-Revised (M-CHAT-R) screening tool.

The patient's medical history, surgical history, and family history are noncontributory. His mother had a full-term pregnancy, with vaginal delivery at 36 weeks and no complications. The boy lives with both biological parents and one 5-year-old brother with no history of medical illness. At the patient's previous follow up at 24 months, he was determined to be developmentally on target. He has no special dietary restrictions. His immunizations are up to date, and he has no known allergies.

Vital signs: BP 101/65 mm Hg, HR 97 beats/minute, oral Tmax 98.7°F (37°C), RR 18 breaths/minute, Wt 14.1 kg, Ht 36 inches, oxygen saturation SpO_2 99%

Physical examination:

General: Well developed, well nourished

Eyes: Pupils reactive; extraocular movements intact; fundi normal; vision grossly intact

Ears: External auditory canals and tympanic membranes clear; hearing grossly intact

Throat: Oral cavity and pharynx normal; no inflammation, swelling, exudate, or lesions; teeth and gingiva in good general condition

Neck: No lymphadenopathy; supple with no meningismus, masses or thyromegaly; trachea midline

Pulmonary: Clear to auscultation bilaterally with good aeration, no retractions, no nasal flaring

Cardiovascular: Sinus rhythm; normal S1 and S2; no S3, S4 or murmurs; no peripheral edema, cyanosis or pallor; extremities warm to the touch and well perfused; capillary refill is less than 2 seconds; no carotid bruits

Abdomen: Soft, nontender; positive bowel sounds, nondistended; no hepatosplenomegaly

Musculoskeletal: Adequately aligned spine; range of motion intact for spine and extremities; no joint erythema or tenderness; normal muscular development; normal gait

Skin: Flushed and sweating; no rashes, petechiae, or purpura

Neurologic: No gross deficits; unable to assess strength in upper and lower extremities; cranial nerves II-XII intact; sensation symmetric and intact throughout; reflexes 2+ throughout; the child does not look at the face of others

Laboratory findings:

Basic Metabolic Panel		
Test	Result	Normal Values
Glucose	100	60–110 mg/dL
BUN	10	7–17 mg/dL
Na	139	138–145 mEq/L
K	4.2	3.4–5.2 mEq/L
Cl	103	98–107 mEq/L
CO_2	21	20–28 mEq/L
Anion gap	15	6–16 mEq/L
Creatinine	0.51	0.2–0.7 mg/dL
Calcium (total serum)	9.4	8.9–10.1 mg/dL

Calculated Osmolality		
Calculated osmolality	265	263–273 mOsm/kg
Complete Blood Count with Differential		
WBC	6.7	$4.5–11 \times 10^3$ cells/mm³
RBC	5.9	$4.30–5.10 \times 10^6$ cells/mm³
Hgb	13.6	11.4–15.4 g/dL
Hct	45%	36%–49%
MCV	82	78–98 fL
MCH	31	26–34 pg
MCHC	33	32–35 g/dL
Red cell distribution width	12.9%	11.5%–14.5%
Plt	345	$150–450 \times 10^3$ cells/mm³
Mean platelet volume	11.5	9.4–12.4 fL
Neutrophils	35%	34.0%–71.1%
Immature granulocytes	0.2%	0.0%–0.5%
Neutrophils, absolute	2.94	$1.56–6.13 \times 10^3$ cells/mm³
Lymphocytes	34.2%	19.3%–51.7%
Lymphocytes, absolute	2.75	$1.18–3.74 \times 10^3$ cells/mm³
Monocytes	8.2%	3%–13%
Monocytes, absolute	0.47	$0.24–0.86 \times 10^3$ cells/mm³
Eosinophils	1.2%	0.7%–5.8%
Eosinophils, absolute	0.19	$0.04–0.36 \times 10^3$ cells/mm³
Basophils	0.9%	0.1%–1.2%
Basophils, absolute	0.04	$0.01–0.08 \times 10^3$ cells/mm³

Diagnostic Test: M-CHAT-R

Administered to the mother, the patient's score was 15 of possible 20. Scored options follow:

1. Child does not look at objects you point to across the room
2. Parent has wondered if the child might be deaf
3. Child does not play pretend or make-believe
4. Child makes unusual finger movements near his face/eyes
5. Child does sometimes point to objects to ask for something but not usually
6. Child does not point to show parent something interesting
7. Child does not appear interested in other children or actively plays with his older brother
8. Child does respond to his name but not usually
9. Child does get upset by everyday noises like the vacuum cleaner and garbage disposal unit
10. Child does not look the parent or pediatrician in the eye
11. Child does not mimic others, such as copying a parent when they turn their head to look at something
12. Child does not try to get parents' or sibling's attention
13. Child does understand when you tell him to do something but not usually
14. Child does not look to parent when something new happens
15. Child does not like to be swung or bounced on a knee

1. What symptoms described throughout the case raises concerns of autism spectrum disorder (ASD)?

Although the patient was believed to be reaching developmental milestones, some assessments are more thorough than others when the clinician is expecting normal results and no collateral information is provided to warrant a more in-depth assessment. Per the mother's report, the patient is less verbal and communicative, no longer points, no longer calls out, and no longer plays with his older brother. These behaviors were not obvious at all times. Only when an illness caused more attention to be provided to the patient were some behaviors then thought to be abnormal, and not necessarily caused by an illness, such as a stomach flu. On further investigation after providing the M-CHAT-R screening tool, additional red flags are revealed, indicating the following for this child:

- Does not look at objects the parent points to across the room
- Does not play pretend or make-believe
- Makes unusual finger movements near his face/eyes
- Does sometimes point to objects to ask for something but not usually
- Does not point to show parent something interesting
- Does not appear interested in other children or actively plays with his older brother
- Does respond to his name but not usually

- Does get upset by everyday noises like the vacuum cleaner and garbage disposal (hypersensitivity)
- Does not look the parent or pediatrician in the eye (also noted in physical examination)
- Does not mimic others, such as copying a parent when they turn their head to look at something
- Does not try to get parents' or sibling's attention
- Does understand when you tell him to do something but not usually
- Does not look to parent when something new happens
- Does not like to be swung or bounced on a knee

A total score of 15 of possible 20 indicates a high risk for ASD and should be referred immediately for diagnostic evaluation. The M-CHAT-R is 85% sensitive and 99% specific, validated on more than 15,000 children in primary care practices.

2. What are the nonpharmacologic and/or pharmacologic treatment strategies that could be recommended for this child after a diagnosis is confirmed by a referred specialist(s) and other disorders, such as specific communications disorders, have been ruled in or ruled out?

Nonpharmacologic and pharmacologic options should be carefully considered after the diagnosis of ASD is confirmed. Therapies of benefit for the patient include the following:

- Speech therapy to assess/assist with the patient's verbal and nonverbal communication symptoms

- Occupational therapy to:
  - Assess/assist the home and patient and maximize the environment to reduce excessive stimuli
  - Enhance the patient's ability to feed, dress, and groom himself as appropriate for his age
  - Enhance his other activities of daily living (e.g., play, social participation)
  - Maximize the patient's ability to function independently as appropriate for his age
  - Collaborate with the family to identify safe methods of community mobility

Behavior therapy is not indicated at this time because the patient does not display any aberrant behaviors. Although dietary modifications (e.g., gluten-free, casein-free) have inconsistent results in clinical studies, parents of children may attempt this intervention before other costly or medically warranted interventions. Some case reports identify the change in a patient's diet to resolve symptoms of severe foul-smelling diarrhea with great improvement in ASD symptoms. In this case, the patient's gastrointestinal symptoms (believed to be caused by a stomach virus) may have simply been coincidental to the observed behaviors. Other complementary and alternative treatments can be explored, although the lack of compelling evidence of efficacy should warrant a pragmatic approach. Pharmacotherapy is not indicated at this time because the parent did not describe any symptoms such as irritability, aggression, hyperactivity, repetitive/stereotypic behaviors, depression, obsessive/compulsive disorder, oppositionality, or impulsivity treated with antipsychotics, psychostimulants, antidepressants, anticonvulsants, or other psychopharmacotherapies. Only if symptoms prevent a patient from engaging in physical, occupational, educational, speech, or behavioral therapy should pharmacotherapy be used judiciously and for short periods of time.

Case (continued). The patient is now age 5 years and has had some meaningful improvements in communication and occupational activities. However, he is also now more irritable and aggressive when therapists and parents are attempting to engage him in various therapies, to the point that many appointments have had to be canceled. His physical aggression is also demonstrated toward his sibling. Behavioral interventions have had some improvement; however, because the child is also beginning to spend more time in structured environments such as pre-kindergarten educational settings with larger groups of children, his irritability and aggression could jeopardize and interfere with his ongoing therapies and educational activities.

3. What recommendations for pharmacologic treatment could you provide now at follow-up to address behaviors of irritability and aggression?

Risperidone has U.S. Food and Drug Administration (FDA) label approval for children with ASD and symptoms of irritability who are age 5 years or older. This patient is now age 5 years with symptoms of irritability that are interfering with his overall treatment and educational plans. Monitoring for efficacy and adverse effects, such as greater than desired or expected weight gain, sedation, and extrapyramidal symptoms, should be ongoing on a regular basis. If the patient can engage in his other therapies and improve his behaviors through those interventions, then periodic reduction in doses, and even the reevaluation for the need of pharmacotherapy, should be done on a regular basis. A starting dose for this patient should be considered at 0.25 mg/day or 0.5 mg/day, based on his new weight and assess for efficacy and adverse drug reactions. The doses based on patient weight are as follows:

Dose Timing and Target	Body weight < 20 kg	Body weight ≥ 20 kg
Day 1	0.25 mg/day to start	0.5 mg/day to start
Up to Day 4	Can increase to 0.5 mg/day by Day 4	Can increase to 1 mg/day by Day 4
After Day 4, at intervals of > 2 wk	Titrate by 0.25 mg/day	Titrate by 0.5 mg/day
Target dose	0.5 mg/day	1 mg/day
	Daily doses may range from 0.5 to 3 mg/day based on response	

Counseling

The irritability and aggressiveness should improve with a decrease in frequency and severity for the patient within 1-2 weeks. If no improvement in these target behaviors is occurring, then the family or caregiver should report lack of response to the pharmacist and prescriber for possible adjustment. If the medication treatment is sedating or causes fatigue to child, then the family or caregiver may give the daily dose at bedtime. The clinician should also tell the family or caregiver that the patient's appetite may increase and they should consider healthy dietary choices (i.e., not all carbohydrates, which are usually the preferred food in many patients taking antipsychotics); also, they should monitor the patient's growth on a monthly basis to ensure it is within desired ranges. Movement disorders may present as muscle pain, tremors in hands, or increased restlessness and should be reported to the pharmacist and prescriber for management.

If the patient is intolerant to the first treatment option, aripiprazole may be considered as an FDA-approved drug for this patient's symptoms in children age 6 years and older.

Dosing for aripiprazole

- Dosing should be initiated at 2 mg/day
- Dose should be increased to 5 mg/day, with subsequent increases to 10 or 15 mg/day if needed
- Dose adjustments of up to 5 mg/day should occur gradually, at intervals of no less than 1 week
- Recommended dosage range for the treatment of pediatric patients is 5 to 15 mg/day

Counseling and monitoring for efficacy and adverse drug reactions with aripiprazole is the same as it was for risperidone. However, with aripiprazole the child may possibly have a higher risk for insomnia or stomach upset. The family or caregiver may give this medication with food, and if insomnia is observed, then they may give the medication in the morning. Finally, other treatments that do not have FDA label approval for ASD could be considered if these first two treatment options are found to be ineffective or intolerable to the patient.

REFERENCES

1. American Psychiatric Association. Diagnostic and Statistical Manual of Mental Disorders, 5th ed. Washington, DC: American Psychiatric Association, 2013.

2. American Psychiatric Association. Diagnostic and Statistical Manual of Mental Disorders, 4th ed., text revision. Washington, DC: American Psychiatric Association, 2000.

3. Kanner L. Autistic disturbances of affective contact. Nerv Child 1943;2:217–50.

4. Kanner L. Follow-up study of eleven autistic children originally reported in 1943. J Autism Child Schizophr 1971;1:119-45.

5. Fombonne E. Epidemiology of pervasive developmental disorders. Pediatr Res 2009;65:591–8.

6. U.S. Centers for Disease Control and Prevention. Prevalence of autism spectrum disorders: Autism and Developmental Disabilities Monitoring Network, United States, 2006. MMWR Surveill Summ 2009;58:1–20.

7. Yeargin-Allsopp M, Rice C, Karapurkar T, et al. Prevalence of autism in a US metropolitan area. JAMA 2003;289:49–55.

8. Kim YS, Leventhal BL, Koh YJ, et al. Prevalence of autism spectrum disorders in a total population sample. Am J Psychiatry 2011;168:904-12.

9. Johnson CP, Myers SM; American Academy of Pediatrics Council on Children with Disabilities. Identification and evaluation of children with autism spectrum disorders. Pediatrics 2007; 120:1183-215.

10. Centers for Disease Control and Prevention. Mental health in the United States: parental report of diagnosed autism in children aged 4–17 years—United States, 2003–2004. MMWR Morb Mortal Wkly Rep 2006;55:481-6.

11. Fombonne E, Zakarian R, Bennett A, et al. Pervasive developmental disorders in Montreal, Quebec, Canada: prevalence and links with immunizations. Pediatrics 2006;118:e139-50.

12. Autism and Developmental Disabilities Monitoring Network Surveillance Year 2000 Principal Investigators; Centers for Disease Control and Prevention. Prevalence of autism spectrum disorders—Autism and Developmental Disabilities Monitoring Network, Six Sites, United States, 2000. MMWR Surveill Summ 2007;56:1-11.

13. Autism and Developmental Disabilities Monitoring Network Surveillance Year 2002 Principal Investigators; Centers for Disease Control and Prevention. Prevalence of autism spectrum disorders: Autism and Developmental Disabilities Monitoring Network, 14 sites, United States, 2002. MMWR Surveill Summ 2007;56:12-28.

14. Christensen DL, Baio J, Braun KV, et al. Prevalence and characteristics of autism spectrum disorder among children aged 8 years—Autism and Developmental Disabilities Monitoring Network, 11 Sites, United States, 2012. MMWR Surveill Summ 2016;65:1-23.

15. Smith IC, Reichow B, Volkmar FR. The effects of DSM-5 criteria on number of individuals diagnosed with autism spectrum disorder: a systematic review. J Autism Dev Disord 2015;45:2541-52.

16. Baxter AJ, Brugha TS, Erskine HE, et al. The epidemiology and global burden of autism spectrum disorders. Psychol Med 2015; 45:601-13.

17. Mandell DS, Wiggins LD, Carpenter LA, et al. Racial/ethnic disparities in the identification of children with autism spectrum disorders. Am J Public Health 2009;99:493-8.

18. Risch N, Spiker D, Lotspeich L, et al. A genomic screen of autism: evidence for a multilocus etiology. Am J Hum Genet 1999;65:493-507.

19. Kumar RA, Christian SA. The genetics of autism spectrum disorders. Curr Neurol Neurosci Rep 2009;9:188-97.

20. Folstein SE, Rosen-Sheidley B. Genetics of autism: complex etiology for a heterogeneous disorder. Nat Rev Genet 2001;2:943-55.

21. Abrahams BS, Geschwind DH. Advances in autism genetics: on the threshold of a new neurobiology. Nat Rev Genet 2008; 9:341-55.

22. Bailey A, Phillips W, Rutter M. Autism: towards an integration of clinical, genetic, neuropsychological, and neurobiological perspectives. J Child Psychol Psychiatry 1996;37:89-126.

23. Colvert E, Tick B, McEwen F, et al. Heritability of autism spectrum disorder in a UK population-based twin sample. JAMA Psychiatry 2015;72:415-23.

24. Sandin S, Lichtenstein P, Kuja-Halkola R, et al. The familial risk of autism. JAMA 2014;311:1770-7.

25. Hallmayer J, Cleveland S, Torres A, et al. Genetic heritability and shared environmental factors among twin pairs with autism. Arch Gen Psychiatry 2011;68:1095-102.

26. Simons Foundation Autism Research Initiative. SFARI Gene. New York: Simons Foundation. 2017. Available at www.sfari.org/resource/sfari-gene/. Accessed December 9, 2019.

27. Sanders SJ, Ercan-Sencicek AG, Hus V, et al. Multiple recurrent de novo CNVs, including duplications of the 7q11.23 Williams syndrome region, are strongly associated with autism. Neuron 2011;70:863-85.

28. Levy D, Ronemus M, Yamrom B, et al. Rare de novo and transmitted copy number variation in autistic spectrum disorders. Neuron 2011;70:886-97.

29. Gilman SR, Iossifov I, Levy D, et al. Rare de novo variants associated with autism implicate a large functional network of genes involved in formation and function of synapses. Neuron 2011;70:898-907.

30. Weaving LS, Ellaway CJ, Gecz J, et al. Rett syndrome: clinical review and genetic update. J Med Genet 2005;42:1-7.

31. de la Torre-Ubieta L, Won H, Stein JL, et al. Advancing the understanding of autism disease mechanisms through genetics. Nat Med 2016;22:345-61.

32. Gaugler T, Klei L, Sanders SJ, et al. Most genetic risk for autism resides with common variation. Nat Genet 2014;46:881-5.

33. Lam KSL, Aman MG, Arnold LE. Neurochemical correlates of autistic disorder: a review of the literature. Res Dev Disabil 2006; 27:254-89.

34. McDougle CJ, Erickson CA, Stigler KA, et al. Neurochemistry in the pathophysiology of autism. J Clin Psychiatry 2005;66:9-18.

35. Hadjikhani N. Serotonin, pregnancy and increased autism prevalence: is there a link? Med Hypotheses 2009;74:880-3.

36. Ratajczak HV, Sothern RB. Measurement in saliva from neurotypical adults of biomarkers pertinent to autism spectrum disorders. Future Sci OA 2015;1:FSO70.

37. Ratajczak HV. Theoretical aspects of autism: biomarkers—a review. J Immunotoxicol 2011;8:80-94.

38. Rossignol DA, Frye RE. Evidence linking oxidative stress, mitochondrial dysfunction, and inflammation in the brain of individuals with autism. Front Physiol 2014;5:150.

39. Hviid A, Stellfeld M, Wohlfahrt J, et al. Association between thimerosal-containing vaccine and autism. JAMA 2003; 290:1763-6.

40. Parker SK, Schwartz B, Todd J, et al. Thimerosal-containing vaccines and autistic spectrum disorder: a critical review of published original data. Pediatrics 2004;114:793-804.

41. Stratton K, Gable A, Shetty P, et al., eds. Institute of Medicine, Immunization Safety Review Committee. Immunization Safety Review: Measles-Mumps-Rubella Vaccine and Autism. Washington, DC: National Academies Press, 2001.

42. DeStefano F, Karapurkar B, Thompson WW, et al. Age at first measles-mumps-rubella vaccination in children with autism and school-matched control subjects: a population-based study in metropolitan Atlanta. Pediatrics 2004;113:259-66.

43. Baker JP. Mercury, vaccines, and autism: one controversy, three histories. Am J Public Health 2008;98:244-53.

44. Harrington JA, Rosen L, Garneco A, et al. Parental perceptions and use of complementary and alternative medicine practices for children with autistic spectrum disorders in private practice. J Dev Behav Pediatr 2006;27:S156-161.

45. Newschaffer CJ, Croen LA, Daniels J, et al. The epidemiology of autism spectrum disorders. Annu Rev Public Health 2007; 28:235-58.

46. Mendola P, Selevan SG, Gutter S, et al. Environmental factors associated with a spectrum of neurodevelopmental deficits. Ment Retard Dev Disabil Res Rev 2002;8:188-97.

47. Ashwood P, Willis S, Van de Water J. The immune response in autism: a new frontier for autism research. J Leukoc Biol 2006; 80:1-15.

48. Connolly AM, Chez M, Streif EM, et al. Brain-derived neurotrophic factor and autoantibodies to neural antigens in sera of children with autistic spectrum disorders, Landau-Kleffner syndrome, and epilepsy. Biol Psychiatry 2006;59:354-63.

49. Redcay E, Courchesne E. When is the brain enlarged in autism: a meta-analysis of all brain size reports. Biol Psychiatry 2005;58:1-9.

50. Sparks BF, Friedman SD, Shaw DW, et al. Brain structural abnormalities in young children with autism spectrum disorder. Neurology 2002;59:184-92.

51. Bauman ML, Kemper TL. Structural Brain Anatomy in Autism: What is the Evidence? In: Bauman ML, Kemper TL, eds. The Neurobiology of Autism, 2nd ed. Baltimore: Johns Hopkins University Press, 2005:121-35.

52. Lainhart JE. Advances in autism neuroimaging research for the clinician and geneticist. Am J Med Genet C Semin Med Genet 2006;142:33-9.

53. Ramachandran VS, Oberman LM. Broken mirrors. Sci Am 2006;295:62-9.

54. Koshino H, Carpenter PA, Minshew NJ, et al. Functional connectivity in an fMRI working memory task in high-functioning autism. Neuroimage 2005;24:810-21.

55. Koshino H, Kana RK, Keller TA, et al. fMRI investigation of working memory for faces in autism: visual coding and underconnectivity with frontal areas. Cereb Cortex 2008;18:289-300.

56. Andrews DS, Avino TA, Gudbrandsen M, et al. In vivo evidence of reduced integrity of the gray-white matter boundary in autism spectrum disorder. Cereb Cortex 2017;27:877-87.

57. Ecker C, Murphy D. Neuroimaging in autism—from basic science to translational research. Nat Rev Neurol 2014;10:82-91.

58. Arndt TL, Stodgell CJ, Rodier PM. The teratology of autism. Int J Dev Neurosci 2005;23:189–99.

59. Croen LA, Grether JK, Yoshida CK, et al. Antidepressant use during pregnancy and childhood autism spectrum disorders. Arch Gen Psychiatry 2011;68:1104–12.

60. Rosen BN, Lee BK, Lee NL, et al. Maternal smoking and autism spectrum disorder: a meta-analysis. J Autism Dev Disord 2015;45:1689-98.

61. Eliasen M, Tolstrup JS, Nybo AM, et al. Prenatal alcohol exposure and autistic spectrum disorders—a population-based prospective study of 80,552 children and their mothers. Int J Epidemiol 2010;39:1074-81.

62. Croen LA, Najjar DV, Fireman B, et al. Maternal and paternal age and risk of autism spectrum disorders. Arch Pediatr Adolesc Med 2007;161:334–40.

63. Reichenberg A, Gross R, Weiser M, et al. Advancing paternal age and autism. Arch Gen Psychiatry 2006;63:1026-32.

64. Gardener H, Spiegelman D, Buka SL. Prenatal risk factors for autism: comprehensive meta-analysis. Br J Psychiatry 2009; 195:7-14.

65. Cheslack-Postava K, Liu K, Bearman PS. Closely spaced pregnancies are associated with increased odds of autism in California sibling births. Pediatrics 2011;127:246-53.

66. Cheslack-Postava K, Suominen A, Jokiranta E, et al. Increased risk of autism spectrum disorders at short and long interpregnancy intervals in Finland. J Am Acad Child Adolesc Psychiatry 2014; 53:1074–81.e4.

67. Coo H, Ouellette-Kuntz H, Lam YM, et al. The association between the interpregnancy interval and autism spectrum disorder in a Canadian cohort. Can J Public Health 2015;106:e36-42.

68. Dodds L, Fell DB, Shea S, et al. The role of prenatal, obstetric and neonatal factors in the development of autism. J Autism Dev Disord 2011;41:891-902.

69. Durkin MS, DuBois LA, Maenner MJ. Inter-pregnancy intervals and the risk of autism spectrum disorder: results of a population-based study. J Autism Dev Disord 2015;45:2056-66.

70. Gunnes N, Suren P, Bresnahan M, et al. Interpregnancy interval and risk of autistic disorder. Epidemiology 2013;24:906-12.

71. Zerbo O, Yoshida C, Gunderson EP, et al. Interpregnancy interval and risk of autism spectrum disorders. Pediatrics 2015; 136:651-57.

72. Lee BK, Magnusson C, Gardner RM, et al. Maternal hospitalization with infection during pregnancy and risk of autism spectrum disorders. Brain Behav Immun 2015;44:100-5.

73. Lyall K, Croen L, Daniels J, et al. The changing epidemiology of autism spectrum disorders. Annu Rev Public Health 2017; 38:81-102.

74. Rutter M. Autism: its recognition, early diagnosis, and service implications. J Dev Behav Pediatr 2006;27:S54-8.

75. Lord C, Risi S, DiLavore PS, et al. Autism from 2 to 9 years of age. Arch Gen Psychiatry 2006;63:694-701.

76. Orinstein AJ, Helt M, Troyb E, et al. Intervention for optimal outcome in children and adolescents with a history of autism. J Dev Behav Pediatr 2014;35:247-56.

77. Volkmar F, Siegel M, Woodbury-Smith M, et al.; American Academy of Child and Adolescent Psychiatry (AACAP) Committee on Quality Issues (CQI). Practice parameter for the assessment and treatment of children and adolescents with autism spectrum disorder. J Am Acad Child Adolesc Psychiatry 2014;53:237-57.

78. Robins DL, Casagrande K, Barton M, et al. Validation of the modified checklist for Autism in toddlers revised with follow-up (M-CHAT-R/F). Pediatrics 2014;133:37-45.

79. Webb SJ, Jones EJ. Early Identification of autism: early characteristics, onset of symptoms, and diagnostic stability. Infants Young Child 2009;22:100-18.

80. Richards M, Mossey J, Robins DL. Parents' concerns as they relate to their child's development and later diagnosis of autism spectrum disorder. J Dev Behav Pediatr 2016;37:532-40.

81. Filipek PA, Accardo PJ, Ashwal S, et al. Practice parameter: screening and diagnosis of autism: report of the Quality Standards Subcommittee of the American Academy of Neurology and the Child Neurology Society. Neurology 2000;55:468-79.

82. Tuchman R, Rapin I. Epilepsy in autism. Lancet Neurol 2002; 1:352-8.

83. Swedo SE, Leonard HL, Rapoport JL. The pediatric autoimmune neuropsychiatric disorders associated with streptococcal infection (PANDAS) subgroup: separating fact from fiction. Pediatrics 2004;113:907-11.

84. Moretti G, Pasquini M, Mandarelli G, et al. What every psychiatrist should know about PANDAS: a review. Clin Pract Epidemiol Ment Health 2008;4:13.

85. Myers SM, Johnson CP; American Academy of Pediatrics Council on Children with Disabilities. Management of children with autism spectrum disorders. Pediatrics 2007;120:1162-82.

86. Myers SM. The status of pharmacotherapy for autism spectrum disorders. Expert Opin Pharmacother 2007;8:1579-603.

87. Matson JL, Smith KRM. Current status of intensive behavioral interventions for young children with autism and PDD-NOS. Res Autism Spectrum Disord 2008;2:60-74.

88. Mulloy A, Lang R, O'Reilly M, et al. Gluten-free and casein-free diets in the treatment of autism spectrum disorders: a systematic review. Res Autism Spectrum Disord 2010;4:328-39.

89. Rossignol DA. Novel and emerging treatments for autism spectrum disorders: a systematic review. Ann Clin Psychol 2009; 21:213-36.

90. Wong HHL, Smith RG. Patterns of complementary and alternative medical therapy use in children diagnosed with autism spectrum disorder. J Autism Dev Disord 2006;36:901-9.

91. Elder JH, Kreider CM, Schaefer NM, et al. A review of gluten- and casein-free diets for treatment of autism: 2005-2015. Nutr Diet Suppl 2015;7:87-101.

92. Horvath A, Łukasik J, Szajewska H. ω-3 Fatty acid supplementation does not affect autism spectrum disorder in children: a systematic review and meta-analysis. J Nutr 2017;147:367-76.

93. Navarro F, Liu Y, Rhoads JM. Can probiotics benefit children with autism spectrum disorders? World J Gastroenterol 2016; 22:10093-102.

94. Kang DW, Adams JB, Gregory AC, et al. Microbiota transfer therapy alters gut ecosystem and improves gastrointestinal and autism symptoms: an open-label study. Microbiome 2017;5:10.

95. Goldstein H. Communication intervention for children with autism: a review of treatment efficacy. J Autism Dev Disord 2002; 32:373-96.

96. White SW, Keonig K, Scahill L. Social skills development in children with autism spectrum disorders: a review of the intervention research. J Autism Dev Disord 2007;37:1858-68.

97. Research Units on Pediatric Psychopharmacology Autism Network (RUPPAN). Risperidone treatment of autistic disorder: longer-term benefits and blinded discontinuation after 6 months. Am J Psychiatry 2005;162:1361-9.

98. Aman MG, Arnold LE, McDougle CJ, et al. Acute and long-term safety and tolerability of risperidone in children with autism. J Child Adolesc Psychopharmacol 2005;15:869-84.

99. Anderson GM, Schahill L, McCracken JT, et al. Effects of short- and long-term risperidone treatment on prolactin levels in children with autism. Biol Psychiatry 2007;61:545-50.

100. McCracken J, McGough J, Shah B, et al. Research Units on Pediatric Psychopharmacology Autism Network. Risperidone in children with autism and serious behavioral problems. N Engl J Med 2002;347:314-21.

101. McDougle CJ, Scahill L, Aman MG, et al. Risperidone for the core symptom domains of autism: results from the study by the Autism Network of the Research Units on Pediatric Psychopharmacology. Am J Psychiatry 2005;162:1142-8.

102. Troost PW, Lahuis BE, Steenhuis MP, et al. Long-term effects of risperidone in children with autism spectrum disorders: a placebo discontinuation study. J Am Acad Child Adolesc Psychiatry 2005;44:1137-44.

103. Shea S, Turgay A, Carroll A, et al. Risperidone in the treatment of disruptive behavioral symptoms in children with autistic and other pervasive developmental disorders. Pediatrics 2004; 114:634-41.

104. Chavez B, Rey JA, Chavez-Brown M. Role of risperidone in children with autism spectrum disorder. Ann Pharmacother 2006; 40:909-16.

105. Risperdal [package insert]. Titusville, NJ: Ortho-McNeil-Janssen Pharmaceuticals.

106. Abilify [package insert]. Tokyo: Bristol-Myers Squibb & Otsuka Pharmaceutical.

107. Owen R, Sikich L, Marcus RN, et al. Aripiprazole in the treatment of irritability in children and adolescents with autistic disorder. Pediatrics 2009;124:1533-40.

108. Marcus RN, Owen R, Kamen L, et al. A placebo-controlled, fixed-dose study of aripiprazole in children and adolescents with irritability associated with autistic disorder. J Am Acad Child Adolesc Psychiatry 2009;48:1110-9.

109. McDougle CJ, Kresch LE, Posey DJ. Repetitive thoughts and behavior in pervasive developmental disorders: treatment with serotonin reuptake inhibitors. J Autism Dev Disord 2000; 30:427-35.

110. Leskovec TJ, Rowles BM, Findling RL. Pharmacological treatment options for autism spectrum disorders in children and adolescents. Harv Rev Psychiatry 2008;16:97-112.

111. Posey DJ, McDougle CJ. The pharmacotherapy of target symptoms associated with autistic disorder and other pervasive developmental disorders. Harv Rev Psychiatry 2000;8:45-63.

112. Fankhauser MP, Karumanchi VC, German ML, et al. A double-blind, placebo-controlled study of the efficacy of transdermal clonidine in autism. J Clin Psychiatry 1992;53:77-82.

113. Jaselskis CA, Cook EH, Fletcher KE, et al. Clonidine treatment of hyperactive and impulsive children with autistic disorder. J Clin Psychopharmacol 1992;12:322-7.

114. Posey DJ, Putney JI, Sasher TM, et al. Guanfacine treatment of hyperactivity and inattention in pervasive developmental disorders: a retrospective analysis of 80 cases. J Child Adolesc Psychopharmacol 2004;14:233-41.

115. Scahill L, Aman MG, McDougle CJ, et al. A prospective open trial of guanfacine in children with pervasive developmental disorders. J Child Adolesc Psychopharmacol 2006;16:589-98.

116. Aman M, Van Bourgondien M, Wolford P, et al. Psychotropic and anticonvulsant drugs in subjects with autism: prevalence and patterns of use. J Am Acad Child Adolesc Psychiatry 1995; 34:1672-81.

117. Aman M, Lam K, Collier-Crespin A. Prevalence and patterns of use of psychoactive medicines among individuals with autism in the Autism Society of America. J Autism Dev Disord 2003;33:527-33.

118. Mandell DS, Morales KH, Marcus SC, et al. Psychotropic medication use among Medicaid-enrolled children with autism spectrum disorders. Pediatrics 2008;121:441-8.

119. Jobski K, Höfer J, Hoffmann F, et al. Use of psychotropic drugs in patients with autism spectrum disorders: a systematic review. Acta Psychiatr Scand 2017;135:8-28.

120. Anderson LT, Campbell M, Grega DM, et al. Haloperidol in the treatment of infantile autism: effects on learning and behavioral symptoms. Am J Psychiatry 1984;141:1195-202.

121. Remington G, Sloman L, Konstantareas M, et al. Clomipramine versus haloperidol in the treatment of autistic disorder: a double-blind, placebo-controlled, crossover study. J Clin Psychopharmacol 2001;21:440-4.

122. Joshi PT, Capozzoli JA, Coyle JT. Low-dose neuroleptic therapy for children with childhood-onset pervasive developmental disorder. Am J Psychiatry 1988;145:335-8.

123. Cohen IL, Campbell M, Posner D, et al. Behavioral effects of haloperidol in young autistic children: an objective analysis using a within-subjects reversal design. J Am Acad Child Psychiatry 1980;19:665-77.

124. Campbell M, Anderson LT, Small AM, et al. The effects of haloperidol on learning and behavior in autistic children. J Autism Dev Disord 1982;12:167-75.

125. Anderson LT, Campbell M, Adams P, et al. The effects of haloperidol on discrimination learning and behavioral symptoms in autistic children. J Autism Dev Disord 1989;19:227-39.

126. Findling RL, Kusumakar V, Daneman D, et al. Prolactin levels during long-term risperidone treatment in children and adolescents. J Clin Psychiatry 2003;64:132-69.

127. Stigler KA, Potenza MN, Posey DJ, et al. Weight gain associated with atypical antipsychotic use in children and adolescents: prevalence, clinical relevance, and management. Pediatr Drugs 2004;6:33-44.

128. Fleischhaker C, Heiser P, Hennighausen K, et al. Weight gain in children and adolescents during 45 weeks treatment with clozapine, olanzapine and risperidone. J Neural Transm 2008;115:1599-608.

129. Ghanizadeh A, Sahraeizadeh A, Berk M. A head-to-head comparison of aripiprazole and risperidone for safety and treating autistic disorders, a randomized double blind clinical trial. Child Psychiatry Hum Dev 2014;45:185-92.

130. Hirsch LE, Pringsheim T. Aripiprazole for autism spectrum disorders (ASD). Cochrane Database Syst Rev 2016;6:CD009043.

131. Hollander W, Wasserman S, Swanson E, et al. A double-blind, placebo-controlled pilot study of olanzapine in childhood/adolescent pervasive developmental disorder. J Child Adolesc Psychopharmacol 2006;16:541-8.

132. Malone RP, Delaney MA, Hyman SB, et al. Ziprasidone in adolescents with autism: an open-label pilot study. J Child Adolesc Psychopharmacol 2006;17:779-90.

133. Martin A, Koenig K, Scahill L, et al. Open-label quetiapine in the treatment of children and adolescents with autistic disorder. J Child Adolesc Psychopharmacol 1999;9:99-107.

134. Chavez B, Chavez-Brown M, Sopko MA, et al. A review of the literature on atypical antipsychotics in children with pervasive developmental disorders. Pediatr Drugs 2007;9:249-66.

135. Hollander E, Phillips A, Chaplin W, et al. A placebo controlled crossover trial of liquid fluoxetine on repetitive behaviors in childhood and adolescent autism. Neuropsychopharmacology 2005;30:582-9.

136. Gordon CT, State RC, Nelson JE, et al. A double-blind comparison of clomipramine, desipramine, and placebo in the treatment of autistic disorder. Arch Gen Psychiatry 1993;50:441-7.

137. King BH, Hollander E, Sikich L, et al. Lack of efficacy of citalopram in children with autism spectrum disorders and high levels of repetitive behavior. Arch Gen Psychiatry 2009;66:583-90.

138. Research Units on Pediatric Psychopharmacology Autism Network (RUPPAN). Randomized, controlled, crossover trial of methylphenidate in pervasive developmental disorders with hyperactivity. Arch Gen Psychiatry 2005;62:1266-74.

139. Stigler KA, Desmond LA, Posey DJ, et al. A naturalistic retrospective analysis of psychostimulants in pervasive developmental disorders. J Child Adolesc Psychopharmacol 2004;14:49-56.

140. Handen BL, Johnson CR, Lubetsky M. Efficacy of methylphenidate among children with autism and symptoms of attention-deficit hyperactivity disorder. J Autism Dev Disord 2000;30:245-55.

141. Quintana H, Birmaher B, Stedge D, et al. Use of methylphenidate in the treatment of children with autistic disorder. J Autism Dev Disord 1995;25:283-94.

142. Greenhill LL, Swanson JM, Vitiello B, et al. Impairment and deportment responses to different methylphenidate doses in children with ADHD: the MTA titration trial. J Am Acad Child Adolesc Psychiatry 2001;40:180-7.

143. Politte LC, Henry CA, McDougle CJ. Psychopharmacological interventions in autism spectrum disorder. Harv Rev Psychiatry 2014;22:76-92.

144. Scahill L, McCracken JT, King BH, et al. Extended-release guanfacine for hyperactivity in children with autism spectrum disorder. Am J Psychiatry 2015;172:1197-206.

145. Accordino RE, Kidd C, Politte LC, et al. Psychopharmacological interventions in autism spectrum disorder. Expert Opin Pharmacother 2016;17:937-52.

146. Anagnostou E, Esposito K, Soorya L, et al. Divalproex versus placebo for the prevention of irritability associated with fluoxetine treatment in autism spectrum disorder. J Clin Psychopharmacol 2006;26:444-6.

147. Childs JA, Blair JL. Valproic acid treatment of epilepsy in autistic twins. J Neurosci Nurs 1997;29:244-8.

148. Plioplys AV. Autism: electroencephalogram abnormalities and clinical improvement with valproic acid. Arch Pediatr Adolesc Med 1994;148:220-2.

149. Hellings JA, Weckbaugh M, Nickel EJ, et al. A double-blind, placebo-controlled study of valproate for aggression in youth with pervasive developmental disorders. J Child Adolesc Psychopharmacol 2005;15:682-92.

150. Hollander E, Chaplin W, Soorya L, et al. Divalproex sodium vs placebo for the treatment of irritability in children and adolescents with autism spectrum disorders. Neuropsychopharmacology 2010;35:990-8.

151. Hollander E, Soorya L, Wasserman S, et al. Divalproex sodium versus placebo in the treatment of repetitive behaviors in autism spectrum disorder. Int J Neuropsychopharmacol 2006;9:209-13.

152. Belsito KM, Law PA, Kirk KS, et al. Lamotrigine therapy for autistic disorder: a randomized, double-blind, placebo-controlled trial. J Autism Dev Disord 2001;31:175-81.

153. Wasserman S, Iyengar R, Chaplin WF, et al. Levetiracetam versus placebo in childhood and adolescent autism: a double-blind placebo-controlled study. Int Clin Psychopharmacol 2006;21:363-7.

154. Douglas JF, Sanders KB, Benneyworth MH, et al. Brief report: retrospective case series of oxcarbazepine for irritability/agitation symptoms in autism spectrum disorder. J Autism Dev Disord 2013;43:1243-7.

155. Canitano R. Clinical experience with topiramate to counteract neuroleptic induced weight gain in 10 individuals with autistic spectrum disorders. Brain Dev 2005;27:228-32.

156. Rugino TA, Samsock TC. Levetiracetam in autistic children: an open-label study. J Dev Behav Pediatr 2002;23:225-30.

157. Kapetanovic S. Oxcarbazepine in youths with autistic disorder and significant disruptive behaviors. Am J Psychiatry 2007;164:832-3.

158. Bouvard MP, Leboyer M, Launay JM, et al. Low-dose naltrexone effects on plasma chemistries and clinical symptoms in autism: a double-blind, placebo-controlled study. Psychiatry Res 1995;58:191-201.

159. Campbell M, Anderson LT, Small AM, et al. Naltrexone in autistic children: behavioral symptoms and attentional learning. J Am Acad Child Adolesc Psychiatry 1993;32:1283-91.

160. Arnold LE, Aman MG, Cook AM, et al. Atomoxetine for hyperactivity in autism spectrum disorders: placebo-controlled crossover pilot trial. J Am Acad Child Adolesc Psychiatry 2006;45:1196-205.

161. Baribeau DA, Anagnostou E. Social communication is an emerging target for pharmacotherapy in autism spectrum disorder—a review of the literature on potential agents. J Can Acad Child Adolesc Psychiatry 2014;23:20-30.

162. Marshburn EC, Aman MG. Factor validity and norms for the Aberrant Behavior Checklist in a community sample of children with mental retardation. J Autism Dev Disord 1992;22:537-73.

163. Schopler E, Reichler RJ, Renner BR. The Childhood Autism Rating Scale (CARS). Los Angeles: Western Psychological Services, 1988.

164. Guy W. ECDEU Assessment Manual for Psychopharmacology, revised ed. (DHEW Publication No. [ADM] 76-338). Rockville, MD: National Institute of Mental Health, 1976.

CHAPTER 33

Pediatric Depression
Tiffany-Jade M. Kreys, Pharm.D., BCPP; and
Stephanie V. Phan, Pharm.D., BCPP

INTRODUCTION

Major depressive disorder (MDD) can occur in children as young as preschool age and is associated with an increased risk of morbidity and mortality. Psychotherapy and pharmacotherapy are the mainstays of treatment for pediatric depression. This chapter will highlight important concepts in the diagnosis and management of depression in children and adolescents and evaluate key studies and controversies surrounding the use of antidepressant therapy in this patient population. The clinical course and duration of depression in pediatric patients, together with a review of treatment phases and pharmacologic options, are also discussed.

EPIDEMIOLOGY OF PEDIATRIC DEPRESSION

MDD IN CHILDREN

Major depressive disorder may present in children as young as preschool age.[1] There is a lack of current epidemiologic data available regarding the prevalence of childhood depression; however, earlier studies have described a prevalence rate for preadolescents (age 6–11 years) ranging from 0.6% to 2.7%.[2] According to the Centers for Disease Control and Prevention National Health and Nutrition Examination Survey (NHANES), there is a 3.7% prevalence of mood disorders in children age 8–15 years, with higher prevalence rates in girls and older children.[3]

MDD IN ADOLESCENTS

According to the adolescent supplement of the National Comorbidity Survey, the lifetime prevalence rate of MDD in adolescents age 13–18 years is 11.0% and the 12-month prevalence rate is 7.5%.[4] Severe MDD, which is characterized by high levels of distress and impairment on questionnaire items, has a lifetime and 12-month prevalence rate of 3.0% and 2.3%, respectively.[5] Disease prevalence estimates show that MDD increases with progressing age, with almost double the rate for older adolescents versus younger children.[4,5] About 60% of adolescents who had a diagnosis of MDD received treatment, and about 34% received disorder-specific treatment or treatment from the mental health center or provider.[6] In 2015, National Survey on Drug Use and Health reported about 3 million adolescents age 12–17 years had one or more major depressive episodes in the previous 12 months, representing 12.5% of the U.S. population in this age range.[7] Although the depression rate is equal in female and male children before puberty, depression is twice as common in female versus male adolescents after puberty, which is consistent with the rates observed in adulthood.[6] Female adolescents have almost a 4-fold risk of severe MDD compared with males.[5] Aside from sex and age, there were no other major differences in other sociodemographic factors (e.g., poverty index ratio, parent education, urbanicity).[5] Greater than 60% of adolescents with MDD had a co-occurring mental disorder.[5] Children and adolescents with MDD have at least one other psychiatric condition, with dysthymia and anxiety disorders (both at 30% to 80%), disruptive disorders (10% to 80%), and substance use disorders (20% to 30%) being the most commonly occurring psychiatric comorbidities.[6] In addition, it has been found that depressive symptoms below the threshold for meeting diagnostic criteria for MDD in adolescents are predictive of a major depressive episode in adulthood.[8]

MDD AND SUICIDE

Major depressive disorder is associated with an increased risk of morbidity and mortality.[9] According to the National Center for Health Statistics, suicide was the third leading cause of death in 2014 in children age 5–14 years and the second leading cause of death in those age 15–24 years.[10] When looking more specifically at the 10–14 year age range, suicide becomes the second leading cause of death.[10] In the National Comorbidity Survey, almost 30% of adolescents with MDD reported suicidality in the past year, with about 10% reporting a suicide attempt.[4] In a secondary analysis of the 28-week Adolescent Depression Antidepressants and Psychotherapy Trial, predictors of suicidality and nonsuicidal self-injury (e.g. cutting, scratching, burning) found that family dysfunction, high levels of suicidality, and recent self-harm increase the risk of future suicide attempts and that recent nonsuicidal self-injury is the strongest predictor of future nonsuicidal self-injury.[11] In another study of pediatric suicide, difficulty with relationships was the most common precipitating factor in children age 5 to 14 years.[12]

About 50% to 75% of children and adolescents who commit suicide have had a mood disorder, with MDD being the most common.[13] Additional risk factors for suicide, as reported by the Centers for Disease Control and Prevention, include previous suicide attempts, family history of suicide, history of depression or other psychiatric disorder, substance abuse, stressful life event or loss, easy access to lethal methods, exposure to the suicidal behavior of others, and incarceration.[14] Although adolescent boys are more likely to complete suicide (male/female ratio of 4:1) as a result of using more lethal methods for suicide, female adolescents have a higher rate of suicide attempts.[6] Suicide attempts are also increased in those with several psychiatric comorbidities.[15] Because depression is strongly associated with suicidal thoughts and behaviors, it is recommended that clinicians evaluate for the presence of these symptoms and risk factors on initial presentation and subsequent assessments.[9]

ETIOLOGY AND PATHOPHYSIOLOGY

The exact etiology of depression remains unknown but is thought to be caused by genetic, biochemical, and environmental influences.[6] Twin studies support a genetic component to depression, with a concordance rate for a major affective disorder of 76% and 19% in monozygotic and dizygotic twins, respectively.[6] Studies show that a family history of depression is a major risk factor for the development of depression in children.[6] The presence of serotonin gene transporter variants may also contribute to the development of pediatric MDD.[16]

According to the "monoamine hypothesis"—one of the most researched depression theories—depression results from a deficiency or imbalance in monoamine neurotransmitters such as serotonin, dopamine, and norepinephrine.[17] Supporting this hypothesis is that antidepressant medications enhance monoamine function, thereby treating symptoms of depression. However, because the clinical benefits of the medication may take weeks to manifest, other neurochemical or neuroplasticity hypotheses or cognitive neuropsychological approaches are likely to explain the development of depression.[17,18]

The pathophysiology of depression is likely caused by a variety of factors, with recent research focusing on molecular mechanisms of depression.[19] Hypercortisolemia, brain-derived neurotrophic factor, hippocampal neurogenesis, circadian rhythm changes, and functional and structural brain imaging are among the various proposed factors contributing to the pathogenesis of depression.[17]

In one study, children of parents with an affective disorder had a 2.6 times greater rate of developing MDD than children whose parents had no disorder.[19] In the Sequenced Treatment Alternatives to Relieve Depression (STAR*D) Child study, the relationship between remission or amelioration of maternal depression and its impact on psychiatric and social functioning in children was assessed.[20] Women age 25–60 years and their biological children 7–17 years were eligible for inclusion. This analysis showed remission in maternal depression was associated with lower levels of internalizing (e.g., depression, anxiety) and externalizing (e.g., behavioral) problems in pediatric patients. In addition, remission of maternal depression predicted changes in mothers' expressions of warmth and acceptance, which led to changes in tendencies by pediatric patients to internalize symptoms. These findings suggest that short-term treatment with an antidepressant induces maternal remission of depression, thereby affecting the mother's expression of warmth and acceptance, leading to decreased depressive and anxiety symptoms in children. Additional risk factors for child and adolescent depression include the following: psychosocial stressors, such as childhood neglect or abuse; psychiatric comorbidities, such as attention-deficit/hyperactivity disorder (ADHD) and anxiety; chronic illness, such as diabetes; female sex; hormonal changes during puberty; and use of certain medications.[16]

DIAGNOSTIC CRITERIA AND CLINICAL PRESENTATION

According to the *Diagnostic and Statistical Manual of Mental Disorders, Fifth Edition (DSM-5)*, the diagnostic criteria for MDD in children and adolescents are similar to those in adults. To meet the diagnostic criteria for a major depressive episode, at least five of nine depressive symptoms must be present during the same 2-week period. At least one of the five symptoms must be depressed mood or *anhedonia*, defined as an inability to experience pleasure in normal pleasurable acts; however, an irritable mood may be considered equivalent to depressed mood in children or adolescents. Depressive symptoms should be present almost every day for most of the day and include the following:

- Depressed or irritable mood
- Anhedonia or lack of interest/pleasure
- Significant weight loss or weight gain or, specifically, failure to meet expected weight gains in children
- Sleep disturbances
- Psychomotor agitation or retardation
- Fatigue or low energy
- Feelings of worthlessness or undue or inappropriate guilt
- Difficulty concentrating or inability to make decisions
- Repeated thoughts of death or suicidality

To further meet diagnostic criteria, these depressive symptoms must cause clinically significant distress or impairment in social, occupational, or other areas of functioning. In addition, the symptoms must not be caused by illicit drug use, a medication, a general medical condition, and/or bereavement.[21]

Although the diagnostic criteria for depression in children and adolescents are similar to those for adults, some differences in the clinical presentation of depression may exist based on the physical, emotional, cognitive, and social developmental stage of the pediatric patient.[9] Because data are conflicting with respect to the symptom presentation of depression in children and adolescents, a database study of children and adolescents who were referred to an outpatient mood and anxiety disorders clinic was conducted.[22] This study evaluated clinical characteristics of depression in this patient population. Adolescents with depression showed more hopelessness/helplessness, fatigue/lack of energy/tiredness, hypersomnia, weight loss, and suicidality compared with children with depression. Comorbid substance abuse/dependence was also more prevalent in depressed adolescents, whereas comorbid separation anxiety, oppositional defiant disorder, and ADHD occurred more often in depressed children. A depressed or irritable mood in children was often associated with specific events or preoccupations compared with adolescents. Other depressive symptoms, including feelings of guilt, negative self-image, anhedonia, delusions/hallucinations, weight gain, increased appetite, anorexia, psychomotor agitation/retardation, social withdrawal, and insomnia, were observed to occur at similar rates in both children and adolescents.

DIFFERENTIAL DIAGNOSIS

The presence of specific medical and psychiatric conditions that may occur with or show symptoms similar to depression should be assessed before confirming an MDD diagnosis.[9] These medical conditions include the following: hypothyroidism, mononucleosis, anemia, certain cancers, autoimmune disease, premenstrual dysphoric disorder, and chronic fatigue syndrome; these psychiatric conditions include the following: anxiety, dysthymia, ADHD, and oppositional defiant disorder, pervasive developmental disorder, and substance abuse. The use of certain medications that may cause symptoms of depression, such as stimulants, corticosteroids, and contraceptives, should also be evaluated.[9] Patients with bipolar disorder, a cyclic mood disorder characterized by alternating episodes of mania and depression, will often experience an acute depressive episode before any periods of mania, making it difficult to distinguish between unipolar and bipolar depression. About 20%–40% of children and adolescents initially presenting with depression develop bipolar disorder within 5 years after the onset of depression.[9] Characteristics associated with an increased risk of developing bipolar disorder in adolescents with MDD include early-onset depression, depression accompanied by psychomotor retardation or psychotic features, family history of bipolar or other mood disorders, and drug-induced mania.[23] Thus, it is important to monitor for the presence of hypomanic symptoms, such as a decreased need for sleep, excessive talking, distractibility, and flight of ideas, which often tend to worsen with antidepressant therapy.[23] The Pediatric Bipolar Disorder chapter provides more detailed information in children and adolescents.

Under the Depressive Disorders diagnosis and within the *DSM-5*, the new diagnosis Disruptive Mood Dysregulation Disorder was added to address concerns with over-diagnosing bipolar disorder in the pediatric population. Characteristics of this new diagnosis include temper outbursts and irritability. Additional diagnoses that include depressive symptoms, yet not meeting criteria for MDD, include both the Adjustment Disorder diagnosis and Persistent Depressive Disorder (dysthymia) diagnosis.[2] Adjustment disorder with depressed mood involves low mood, tearfulness, and hopeless within the context of a stressor in the previous 3 months and persistent depressive disorder involves fewer MDD criteria, lower severity of symptoms, and the presence of symptoms for at least 1 year.[2]

SCREENING FOR MDD

Although evidence supporting the use of depression-screening instruments in pediatric patients is limited, it is recommended that clinicians screen all children and adolescents for depressive symptoms using checklists derived from the *DSM, Fourth Edition, Text Revision (DSM-IV-TR)*, clinician-based instruments, and/or child/parent depression self-reports.[9,24] An update to the 2009 U.S. Preventive Services Task Force recommendation statement for screening for depression in children and adolescents recommends screening for MDD in all children age 12–18 years, whereas no recommendation exists for children 11 years and younger.[24] The patient evaluation should also include interviews with the child and parent/caregiver and an interview alone with the adolescent, if possible.[9] The Patient Health Questionnaire-9 Item (PHQ-9) is a self-administered depression-screening tool, based on *DSM-IV-TR* criteria, developed for use in adults in primary care settings.[18] Its usefulness in screening for adolescent depression was recently highlighted: the PHQ-9 has greater sensitivity but lower specificity in detecting depression in adolescents compared with adults. Thus, the tool is unlikely to miss detecting depression in adolescents; however, false positives—possibly caused by an overlap of symptoms among mental health disorders or subthreshold symptoms of depression combined with adjustment disorder—may occur, thereby warranting further inquiry by providers. A limitation of the PHQ-9 is that it does not include an item for irritability, a symptom of depression included as part of the diagnostic criteria for MDD in children and adolescents but not adults. Therefore, providers may need to specifically inquire about the presence of irritability when screening for depression. The PHQ-2 (Patient Health Questionnaire 2), which is a 2-item depression screening scale consisting of questions relating to depressed mood and anhedonia from the PHQ-9, has also been validated in adolescents.[25] This tool could be used as a first-line screening tool to identify those needing further assessment because it is brief and accessible, although similar limitations exist compared with the PHQ-9.[25,26] Other instruments evaluated for use in adolescent depression screening in the primary care setting include the Beck Depression Inventory–Primary Care Version, a 7-item self-rated questionnaire, and the Patient Health Questionnaire for Adolescents, a 67-item self-rated questionnaire.[27,28] The Strength and Difficulties Questionnaire has been studied in children age 4–16 years but has a lower sensitivity in detecting depression in this population (33% to 54% sensitivity) compared with the other instruments just discussed to detect depression in adolescents.[11] The Children's Depression Inventory, a 27-item self-rated scale, can also be used to assess for depressive symptoms in children age 7–17 years and is the most commonly used inventory for childhood depression.[29] In addition, the Children's Depression Rating Scale (CDRS), a 16-item clinician-rated instrument based on parent, child, and school-teacher interviews, can be used to determine the severity of depression in children age 6–12 years.[30] All of these screening tools are self-rated and/or parent/caregiver- or teacher-rated with the exception of the CDRS. The CDRS could be administered by a pharmacist clinician with an understanding of the terms through training.[30] Although it is not clear which screening tools are preferred or should be done first or routinely, it may be more time-efficient to use a shorter scale initially to screen for depression and consider longer scales for added clarification of specific symptoms, including frequency and severity.

CLINICAL COURSE AND DURATION

Five major terms are used to describe the clinical course of MDD: response, remission, recovery, relapse, and recurrence. *Response* is defined as significant improvement, usually considered a 50% reduction in symptom severity from baseline, during the initial or acute treatment phase. *Remission* is a period of at least 2 weeks and less than 2 months characterized by the presence of no or very few depressive symptoms (i.e., PHQ-9 less than 5). *Recovery* is defined as either an asymptomatic period lasting 2 months or more or the presence of no more than one or two depressive symptoms for at least 2 months. *Relapse* is an episode of depression during the remission period. *Recurrence* is the emergence of MDD symptoms during the recovery period.[9]

A major depressive episode persists for about 7–9 months in clinically referred pediatric patients. Although around 90% of major depressive episodes remit within the first 1–2 years of onset, the likelihood of recurrence is between 20% and 60% and further increases to 70% after 5 years. Risk factors for recurrence include younger age at onset, increased number of past episodes, severe current episode, psychosis, and psychosocial stressors.[9]

TREATMENT

TREATMENT PHASES

The three main phases of treatment for MDD are *acute*, *continuation*, and *maintenance*. The main goal of acute-phase treatment, which typically lasts 6–12 weeks, is to achieve symptom response and remission. Medication-related adverse effects typically occur shortly after therapy initiation, whereas symptom improvement is often not observed until at least 2–4 weeks of treatment at a therapeutic dose. Adequate antidepressant dose has been associated with better adherence, thus the delay in effect as well as slow dose titration recommended in pediatric patients may affect adherence.[31]

After remission has been achieved, patients enter the continuation phase of treatment, which typically lasts at least 6–12 months. Continuation-phase treatment is recommended for all patients who have responded to acute-phase treatment, with the goal of this treatment phase being relapse prevention. The dose used to achieve remission should be continued during the continuation phase of therapy. In a study evaluating continuation treatment and relapse prevention, patients age 7–18 years with MDD and responding to fluoxetine treatment at 12 weeks were randomized to receive fluoxetine or placebo for an additional 6 months.[32] Patients treated with fluoxetine had lower rates of relapse and an increased time to relapse compared with placebo. This study supports the continuation of antidepressants for at least 6 months after remission is achieved.

Patients with at least two previous depressive episodes, one severe episode, and/or chronic episodes of depression may require maintenance therapy. Other patient-specific factors that should be considered when assessing the need for maintenance therapy include comorbidities, psychosocial stressors, and family psychiatric history. During the maintenance phase of treatment, the antidepressant is continued for an additional 1–2 years or longer. The therapy goal during this treatment phase is to reduce the risk of recurrence.[9]

Regardless of the treatment phase, psychoeducation, supportive management, and family and school involvement are recommended. *Psychoeducation* is a term used to describe the education that family and the patient receive regarding the cause of depression, symptoms, course of the disease, available treatment options, adverse effects, and consequences of untreated depression. Supportive management consists of psychotherapy, which entails self-reflection, problem solving, and the learning of coping skills. Through family and school involvement, the disorder will be better understood, and treatment can be monitored more closely.[9]

TREATMENT OPTIONS

The two main treatment options for pediatric depression include nonpharmacologic and pharmacologic therapy. The following factors should be considered when selecting treatment modality: age, cognitive development, symptom severity and duration, comorbidities, family history of medication response, family and social environment, impact on functioning, and suicide risk. Service availability and patient or family preference may further guide treatment selection. For example, cognitive behavioral therapy (CBT) may be unavailable in the patient's geographic area, or the child's parents may object to medication treatment.[9]

PSYCHOTHERAPY

A meta-analysis published in 2006 of 35 randomized controlled trials showed psychotherapy has only modest effects on adolescent depression compared with previous trials reporting substantial benefit from psychotherapy.[33] This meta-analysis identified that many important characteristics which might impact the efficacy of psychotherapy were not consistently reported, such as severity of depression, other demographic traits, or specific intervention (e.g., frequency or duration of psychotherapy). The lack of this information prevents clinicians from accurately identifying the best candidates for psychotherapy or the true effects of psychotherapy. It was noted, however, that treatment benefit was robust in some samples, such as those with an actual depressive disorder diagnosis and those with depression symptom measures; therefore, the modest effect size of psychotherapy for pediatric patients may be confounded by many other factors.[33] The practice guideline for children and adolescents with depressive disorders published by the American Academy of Child and Adolescent Psychiatry (AACAP) in 2007 provides a brief review of studies assessing the effectiveness of psychotherapy in pediatric depression. The AACAP practice guideline states:

> It is reasonable, in a patient with a mild or brief depression, mild psychosocial impairment, and the absence of clinically significant suicidality or psychosis, to begin treatment with education, support, and case management related to environmental stressors in the family and school.

As stated by AACAP, supportive therapy is as effective as CBT or interpersonal psychotherapy. However, AACAP mentions that in those with moderate to severe depression, chronic or recurrent depression, significant psychosocial impairment, suicidality, agitation, and/or psychosis, supportive therapy and case management are not usually effective and that specific types of psychotherapy or pharmacotherapy are warranted.[9] These recommendations are in line with the National Institute for Health and Care Excellence guidance (NICE), which recommends against medications for mild depression and concurrent psychotherapy and pharmacotherapy, specifically fluoxetine, in moderate to severe depression.[6] Whereas CBT is centered on addressing inaccurate or negative thinking patterns or behaviors that contribute to the patient's emotional distress, interpersonal psychotherapy focuses on the patient's social functioning and relationship with others.[34,35] Although AACAP states that moderate depression may respond to CBT or IPT alone, it also specifies that more severe depressive episodes generally require antidepressant treatment, either alone or in combination with psychotherapy. If monotherapy with psychotherapy or antidepressants is ineffective, AACAP recommends a combination of the two treatment modalities.

In the Adolescent Depression Antidepressants and Psychotherapy Trial, 208 patients age 11–17 years with moderate to severe depression and for whom a psychosocial brief initial intervention failed were randomized to receive treatment with a selective serotonin reuptake inhibitor (SSRI) plus CBT or an SSRI alone.[36] All patients received routine mental health services together with active clinical care. No difference in treatment effectiveness was observed at any time. In moderately to severely depressed adolescents, the addition of CBT to an SSRI did not result in improved outcomes or prevent adverse events and was not cost-effective. The authors concluded that if psychosocial interventions do not elicit a response within 2–4 weeks, then an SSRI should be prescribed. Thus, in patients with more severe depression who are undergoing psychotherapy but do not experience a response, clinicians should have a low threshold for initiating antidepressant therapy.

PHARMACOTHERAPY

There are four main antidepressant drug classes, which includes tricyclic antidepressants (TCAs), monoamine oxidase inhibitors (MAOIs), SSRIs, and serotonin norepinephrine reuptake inhibitors (SNRIs). Of these drugs, TCAs and MAOIs are older antidepressants that are not recommended for use in pediatric depression because of their adverse effect profile, toxicity in overdose, and lack of data supporting their use in this patient population.[37] The TCAs inhibit the reuptake of both serotonin and norepinephrine, thereby increasing serotonin and norepinephrine in the synapse. A meta-analysis of 12 randomized, controlled trials evaluating TCA efficacy in children age 6 to 18 years showed no benefit compared with placebo.[38] The MAOIs block monoamine oxidase, the enzyme responsible for the breakdown of monoamines, including serotonin, norepinephrine, and dopamine.[39]

Newer antidepressants include SSRIs, SNRIs, bupropion, and mirtazapine. The SSRIs block the reuptake of serotonin, whereas the SNRIs block the reuptake of both serotonin and norepinephrine.[39] Bupropion is a norepinephrine and dopamine reuptake inhibitor.[39] Mirtazapine increases the release of norepinephrine and serotonin through presynaptic α_2-blocker.[39,40] Mirtazapine also shows action as a serotonin-2 and -3 blocker, which is associated with decreased serotonin-mediated adverse effects, such as gastrointestinal disturbances or sexual dysfunction.[39]

Most controlled studies have evaluated SSRIs for the treatment of pediatric depression. The U.S. Food and Drug Administration (FDA) label-approved SSRIs for acute and maintenance treatment of depression in adults include citalopram, escitalopram, fluoxetine, paroxetine, and sertraline. Although only fluoxetine and escitalopram are indicated for treatment of depression in pediatric patients, all of these SSRIs have some data supporting their use in this patient population.[39,41-44] Fluoxetine is FDA approved for use in patients age 8–18 years, whereas escitalopram is FDA approved for use in patients age 12–17 years.[45,46]

For the treatment of adult depression, recommended first-line therapies include SSRIs, SNRIs, bupropion, and mirtazapine.[47] Although no SNRIs have received FDA label approval for use in pediatric depression, venlafaxine has efficacy data supporting its use for the treatment of adolescent depression.[48] Moreover, some open-label trials support the use of bupropion sustained release (SR) and mirtazapine in adolescent depression.[49,50]

The more recently approved antidepressants, levomilnacipran and vilazodone, have not been studied in pediatric patients. One open-label study of vortioxetine was found to be effective in patients age 7 to 17 years with depressive or anxiety disorders.[51] Case studies found benefit in the use of adjunctive quetiapine for treatment-resistant adolescent depression; however, no other antipsychotics approved as adjunctive therapy for adult unipolar depression have been found to be effective in the pediatric population.[52] Thus, antipsychotics should not be used to treat MDD in pediatric patients.

To further assist with treatment selection and sequencing, two multisite, randomized controlled trials have been published. The Treatment for Adolescents with Depression Study was a randomized controlled trial of 439 outpatients age 12–17 years with an MDD diagnosis. Most patients included in this study were considered to have moderate to severe depression. For 12 weeks, this study assessed the effectiveness of fluoxetine in combination with CBT compared with treatment with fluoxetine or CBT alone, as well as the effectiveness of fluoxetine or CBT alone compared with placebo. Fluoxetine in combination with CBT produced the greatest improvement in depressive symptoms. Combination therapy also elicited an earlier treatment response compared with CBT or fluoxetine alone. Fluoxetine alone was more efficacious than CBT alone, and CBT was no more effective than placebo.[47] Response rates at 12 weeks for fluoxetine with CBT were 71%, whereas fluoxetine alone produced a response in 60.6% of patients. About 43% of patients responded with CBT alone compared with a response rate of 34.8% with placebo. However, by week 36 of therapy, no significant differences in response rates were observed between treatments (86% combination therapy, 81% fluoxetine, 81% CBT).[39] Although high-risk suicidal patients were excluded from the study, about 29% of patients at baseline were described as having at least minimal to severe suicidal ideation. Suicidal thinking significantly improved in all of these patients at 12 weeks, with the greatest reduction occurring in the fluoxetine plus CBT cohort. In addition, there were no completed suicides in this study. By 36 weeks of treatment, patients treated with fluoxetine alone were more likely to show suicidal ideation and treatment-emergent suicidal events than were patients receiving combination therapy or CBT alone.[39] Investigators concluded fluoxetine alone or in combination with CBT hastens the improvement of depression compared with CBT alone and that CBT added to fluoxetine decreases suicidal ideation and treatment-emergent adverse events in adolescents. Alternatively, another study found that sequential treatment with CBT added in children 8–17 years with response, defined as a 50% reduction in symptoms, to fluoxetine after 6 weeks reduced the risk of relapse, but did not increase the time to remission.[53]

The Treatment of SSRI-Resistant Depression in Adolescents trial (TORDIA) was a randomized controlled trial of 334 patients age 12–18 years with a primary MDD diagnosis who did not respond to an adequate dose and duration (2 months) of an SSRI. Patients were randomized to 12 weeks of the following: (1) a different SSRI; (2) venlafaxine, an SNRI; (3) a different SSRI plus CBT; or (4) venlafaxine plus CBT. It was found that CBT plus a switch to either another SSRI (e.g., paroxetine, citalopram, fluoxetine) or venlafaxine produced a higher response rate (54.8%) compared with either medication alone (40.5%). No significant difference in response rates existed with venlafaxine (48.2%) compared with a second SSRI (47%). Although response rates were comparable, venlafaxine was not as well tolerated as the SSRIs. Skin adverse effects occurred more often in patients in the venlafaxine cohort. Significant increases in diastolic blood pressure and heart rate were also observed in patients receiving venlafaxine. Therefore, because SSRIs are equally effective and better tolerated than venlafaxine, investigators concluded that patients whose response to initial SSRI therapy failed should be switched to another SSRI rather than to venlafaxine. No statistically significant difference in self-harm adverse events or suicidality between treatments was observed, and no subjects in this study completed suicide. Contrary to findings from the Treatment for Adolescents with Depression Study, the addition of CBT to antidepressant therapy did not reduce suicidal adverse events. This finding may have been because patients in the TORDIA study had higher suicidality at baseline and often underwent intense safety monitoring. Overall, given the results obtained in these two trials, combination therapy with CBT and an antidepressant may produce the greatest symptom improvement in adolescents.[54]

In a follow-up study of the TORDIA sample, remission and relapse rates were evaluated at 48 and 72 weeks from intake.[54] Remission was defined as 3 weeks or more with one or no clinically significant symptoms and no functional impairment, and relapse was defined as 2 weeks or more with probable or definite depressive disorder. About 61% of children reached remission by 72 weeks. Random treatment assignment did not affect remission rate or time to remission. Factors associated with higher rates of remission included less severe depression, shorter depressive episode, lower functional impairment, less nonsuicidal self-harm behavior, and less drug and alcohol abuse. Of the 130 subjects who achieved remission by week 24, about 25% relapsed by 72 weeks. No statistically significant difference was observed between random treatment assignments. Only non-white race was associated with higher rates of relapse.

In the past several years, meta-analyses have been published evaluating the efficacy and tolerability of antidepressants in children and adolescents. A Cochrane Database

Systematic Review on the use of "newer" antidepressants (considered largely to be the SSRIs in this review, but also including SNRIs, bupropion, mirtazapine, reboxetine, and agomelatine) compared with placebo in treating depressive disorders showed a minimal benefit and increased risk of suicide-related outcome, although trials of children and adolescents at a high risk of suicide, with comorbidities, and a higher severity of illness were excluded.[55] A 2016 network meta-analysis showed only fluoxetine to be of benefit compared with placebo and with better tolerability compared with other antidepressants.[56] Limitations of these meta-analyses include strict inclusion and exclusion criteria, particularly exclusion of pediatric patients with severe symptoms or at high risk for suicide and the variable quality and heterogeneity of studies included. (The Antidepressants and Suicidality section of this chapter provides more detail.)

TREATMENT GUIDELINES

The NICE guidelines (which are directed toward children and adolescents ages 5 to 18 years) recommend that antidepressants not be used in pediatric patients with mild depression, but that they should be offered to those with moderate to severe depression only in combination with some form of psychotherapy.[57] In early 2018, the American Academy of Pediatrics published the Guidelines for Adolescent Depression in Primary Care, aimed at the pediatric and young adult population age 10 to 21 years.[58,59] In 2007, the Texas Children's Medication Algorithm Project published updated consensus guidelines focusing on medication management in pediatric depression, specifically in patients age 6–17 years. No recommendations for children younger than 6 years are provided, given the lack of evidence available. This publication makes no recommendations regarding combination therapies versus medication management alone, but instead focuses on a stepwise approach to medication management in pediatric patients with depression significant enough to warrant medications, such as depressive symptoms causing impairment in social or school performance and/or risk of harm to the patient or others. Based on the published literature, it is recommended that patients receive treatment with an SSRI such as fluoxetine, sertraline, or citalopram in stage I of therapy if they have not received an antidepressant for their current depressive episode or if they have received an inadequate trial of an antidepressant. The Guidelines for Adolescent Depression in Primary Care recommend using SSRIs in adolescents and make no recommendations toward other classes of antidepressants.[59] Most studies have evaluated fluoxetine for the treatment of pediatric depression. Therefore, fluoxetine has the most evidence to support its use, and thus is considered the antidepressant of choice unless drug interactions, history of poor response, or family resistance preclude its use.

In addition, the NICE guidelines and the Canadian Network for Mood and Anxiety Treatments 2016 guidelines on treating MDD in pediatric patients support the use of fluoxetine as a first-line agent.[57,60] The NICE guidelines recommend more cautious use in children 5 to 11 years versus 12 to 18 years because of lack of robust studies.[57] Citalopram and sertraline are also considered reasonable treatment alternatives in cases of fluoxetine inefficacy or intolerability.[57,61] Escitalopram is approved for depression in adolescents age at least 12 years.[59] Paroxetine is not recommended as first-line therapy because of the increased number of study dropouts caused by adverse effects (e.g., exacerbation of depressive symptoms, agitation, hostility, epistaxis) occurring in the children treated with paroxetine compared with placebo.[62,63]

If the patient does not respond to SSRI treatment or is unable to tolerate the current SSRI, it is recommended that the patient be switched to a different SSRI, including fluoxetine, sertraline, citalopram, escitalopram, or paroxetine (only adolescents can be switched to paroxetine). The new antidepressant should be cross-tapered with the initial antidepressant in patients not switching from fluoxetine. Fluoxetine does not need to be tapered because of its long half-life. Patients who experience adverse effects from the initial agent should have that antidepressant discontinued, and a new antidepressant should be initiated at a lower dose. For those showing partial response to the initial antidepressant, an augmentation agent can be added to the medication regimen. Augmentation permits partial responders to continue receiving benefit from the initial antidepressant and enables the targeted treatment of symptoms not responding to the initial agent. It is unclear which augmentation strategies are most efficacious and best tolerated in the pediatric population because of the lack of evidence. Some augmentation strategies that have evidence for effectiveness in the adult population include bupropion SR and mirtazapine; thus, these agents are recommended as possible augmentation strategies for pediatric depression. Although selected antipsychotics are approved for treatment-resistant depression in adults, antipsychotics should generally be avoided for MDD in pediatric patients (with no other psychiatric comorbidities) because of the tolerability profile.

In some cases, patients who have not responded to at least two adequate SSRI trials may then try a different antidepressant class (e.g., bupropion, venlafaxine, mirtazapine, duloxetine).[62,63] The guidelines do not provide further recommendations for subsequent stages of treatment because of the lack of data available in the pediatric population. The NICE guidelines do not recommend venlafaxine or TCAs, although the 2016 Canadian guidelines mention that TCAs could be used in the adolescent population; this choice should be done cautiously.[57,60]

In patients not responding to antidepressant therapy, the following factors should be evaluated: medication adherence, dose of antidepressant, duration of antidepressant trial, diagnosis—re-examine the appropriateness of primary diagnosis and evaluate for the presence of psychiatric comorbidities, and psychosocial stressors. It is also recommended that psychotherapy, specifically CBT or interpersonal psychotherapy, be tried in patients who have not responded to other psychotherapeutic interventions. If psychotherapy has not previously been tried, it is advised that a trial of psychotherapy be recommended to the child and family.[61]

In patients with severe depression that fails to respond to antidepressant trials, electroconvulsive therapy should be considered. This therapy entails sending electric currents to the brain to induce a seizure, which subsequently leads to neurotransmitter release. State statutes may differ regarding the age requirement for electroconvulsive therapy. According to an executive summary published by AACAP, the administration of electroconvulsive therapy in adolescents should be considered only if the depression is severe, persistent, and significantly disabling and if it has failed to respond to at least two adequate trials of pharmacologic agents that have been accompanied by other treatment modalities. Electroconvulsive therapy may be considered earlier in the treatment of patients who either cannot tolerate pharmacologic treatment or cannot physically take medications or in high-risk patients when waiting for a pharmacologic response may endanger their life.[64]

The Texas Children's Medication Algorithm Project (TCMAP) also provides information on treating pediatric depression in children with other psychiatric comorbidities including psychosis, anxiety disorders, ADHD, and other disruptive behavior disorders. A review of treatments for these conditions is beyond the scope of this chapter but can be found in the TCMAP publication.[61]

DOSING

No dose-response studies of antidepressants have been performed in pediatric patients.[65] Antidepressant dosing in the pediatric population is thought to be similar to that in adults; however, some studies report that the half-lives of SSRIs (paroxetine, sertraline, citalopram) and other, newer antidepressants (bupropion) in children are much shorter than in adults.[66] These studies infer that antidepressants may need to be dosed twice daily; however, more studies are needed to support this dosing recommendation.[65] Thus, monitoring for the presence of withdrawal symptoms should occur, specifically 8–12 hours after the last dose.[61]

Most antidepressants should be initiated at a lower dose than recommended for adults to minimize the occurrence of adverse effects. The dose should subsequently be titrated on the basis of efficacy and tolerability. The SSRIs and SNRIs are typically dosed once daily in the morning or evening with or without food. Because only escitalopram and fluoxetine have received FDA label approval for pediatric depression, specific dosing recommendations for other antidepressants in this patient population are lacking in the literature. Adolescents being treated with escitalopram should be initiated on a dose of 10 mg/day, which can be titrated to 20 mg/day after a minimum of 3 weeks. Those treated with fluoxetine should be initiated on 10 mg/day, which can be increased after a minimum of 1 week.[66] Because of the long half-life of fluoxetine compared with that of other antidepressants, patients who have difficulty with medication adherence may benefit from using this agent.[65] The extended-release formulation of venlafaxine is dosed once daily compared with the twice or three times daily dosing of the immediate-release formulation.[67] Immediate-release and SR formulation of bupropion should be administered twice daily, with no single dose exceeding 200 mg/day, to avoid high peak concentrations. In addition, the dose of bupropion SR should not exceed 400 mg/day because of an increased risk of seizures associated with higher doses.[68] To further reduce seizure risk, dose titration should

be gradual. In addition, bedtime administration of bupropion should be avoided to prevent insomnia from occurring. Conversely, it is recommended that mirtazapine be administered at bedtime because of its sedating properties; however, in adults, it has been found that the drowsiness and sedation observed at lower doses diminishes in frequency and severity with higher mirtazapine doses.[69] Thus, in children and adolescents receiving higher mirtazapine doses at bedtime and experiencing insomnia, a switch to morning administration of mirtazapine may be warranted.

Table 1 shows the doses and dose ranges of antidepressants studied in pediatric depression trials, as well as the major metabolic pathways and half-lives of these agents.[70-73] Of the antidepressants listed in Table 1, citalopram, escitalopram, fluoxetine, paroxetine, and sertraline are available in liquid dosage form. Mirtazapine is available as an orally disintegrating tablet and may be beneficial for use in children unable to swallow tablets and capsules.[74] In children who have difficulty swallowing and who are prescribed venlafaxine immediate or extended release, the contents of the capsule can be sprinkled on a spoonful of applesauce and swallowed immediately without chewing.[67] A glass of water should then be administered to ensure that all pellets have been swallowed. Bupropion SR is only available in tablet form, and to minimize the risk of seizures it should not be crushed, divided, or chewed.[68]

OPTIMIZING PHARMACOTHERAPY

Therapy response should be assessed at 4-week intervals. It is recommended that the patient receive treatment with a therapeutic dose of an antidepressant for a minimum of 4 weeks, if tolerated. If, at 4–8 weeks, the patient shows minimal to no response to medication therapy, or for those unable to tolerate the antidepressant, the antidepressant should be discontinued, and a new antidepressant should be tried. Patients showing partial response to therapy at weeks 4–8 of treatment may benefit from an increase in dose, or, if the patient is already taking the maximum recommended dose, then augmentation therapy may be used. In patients who continue to be partial responders at week 12 of therapy, the next stage of treatment should be tried.[9] Patients with residual symptoms at week 12 are more likely to relapse during the next 6 months of treatment compared with patients having no residual symptoms at this time.[32] Thus the treatment goal should be remission of symptoms rather than response to therapy.

DRUG INTERACTIONS

Fluoxetine, bupropion, and paroxetine are potent cytochrome P450 (CYP) 2D6 inhibitors, thereby predisposing these agents to clinically significant drug interactions.[75] Sertraline has been found to inhibit 2D6 in a dose-dependent manner, with doses greater than 150 mg/day causing moderate to potent 2D6 inhibition.[75] Thus, plasma levels of medications metabolized by the CYP2D6 enzyme, such as TCAs and antipsychotics (i.e., risperidone or aripiprazole), may be increased, resulting in adverse effects and toxicity. Citalopram and escitalopram have minimal CYP enzyme activity and few drug interactions. The MAOIs irreversibly inhibit enzymes responsible for dopamine, norepinephrine, and serotonin metabolism. To prevent serotonin syndrome, MAOIs should not be given within 5 weeks of discontinuing fluoxetine or within 2 weeks of discontinuing other antidepressant agents. In addition, antidepressants should not be administered within 2 weeks after discontinuing an MAOI.

ADVERSE EFFECTS

Overall, SSRIs and other antidepressants are well tolerated by the pediatric patient population.[9] Common adverse effects associated with SSRIs and SNRIs include gastrointestinal disturbances, sleep changes (insomnia, somnolence, vivid dreams, and nightmares), restlessness, diaphoresis, headaches, akathisia, appetite changes, and sexual dysfunction. These adverse effects are usually dose-dependent and typically resolve with time; however, many adverse effects can be treated by either lowering the antidepressant dose or switching to a different antidepressant.[65,76] Venlafaxine has been associated with causing dose-related increases in blood pressure; thus, routine monitoring of blood pressure is recommended. Mirtazapine may cause an increase in appetite, weight gain, and somnolence.[9] The use of bupropion

is contraindicated in patients with a seizure disorder, in patients with a history of anorexia/bulimia, and in patients undergoing abrupt discontinuation of alcohol or sedatives. Antidepressants also cause behavioral activation, characterized by impulsivity, irritability, agitation, and/or silliness in about 3% to 8% of patients.[65] Antidepressants may also cause rare adverse effects such as bleeding and serotonin syndrome.[9]

WITHDRAWAL SYMPTOMS/ DISCONTINUATION SYNDROME

After the continuation or maintenance phase of treatment is complete, and if lifelong antidepressant therapy is unwarranted, then antidepressants should be slowly tapered rather than abruptly discontinued to prevent the occurrence of withdrawal symptoms. *Antidepressant discontinuation syndrome* is diagnosed if the patient has been taking a medication for at least 1 month and is experiencing withdrawal symptoms on discontinuation of the antidepressant.[22] Withdrawal symptoms include flu-like symptoms such as nausea, headache, light-headedness, chills, and body aches, together with neurologic symptoms such as paresthesias, insomnia, and "electric shocks."[47] Some patients may develop symptoms similar to

Table 1. Antidepressant Dosing in Pediatric Depression Trials and Pharmacokinetic Values

Antidepressant	Patient Age (yr)	Starting Dose (mg/day)	Dose Range[a] (mg/day)	Major Metabolic Pathway[54]	Half-life[54]
Selective Serotonin Reuptake Inhibitors (SSRIs)					
Citalopram (Celexa[b])[41,70,71]	7–18	10–20	10–40	2C19, 3A4	24–48 hr
Escitalopram[c] (Lexapro[d])[42]	12–17	10	10–20	2C19, 3A4	27–32 hr
Fluoxetine[c] (Prozac[e])[32,39,47,72]	8–18	10–20[f]	10–20	2C19, 2D6 3A4 for norfluoxetine	4–6 days Active metabolite: 9.3 days
Paroxetine (Paxil[g])[43,70]	7–18	10–20	10–50	2D6	21 hr
Sertraline (Zoloft[h])[44]	6–17	25[f]	50–200	2C19, 2D6	26 hr
Serotonin Norepinephrine Reuptake Inhibitors (SNRIs)					
Venlafaxine (Effexor[h])[48]	12–18	37.5	150–225	2D6	5 ± 2 hr Active metabolite: 11 ± 2 hr
Other Agents					
Bupropion SR (Wellbutrin SR[g])[49]	12–17	100	150–400 (administer in 2 divided doses if ≥ 300 mg/day)	2B6	12 ± 3 hr[62]
Mirtazapine (Remeron[i])[50]	12–18	30	30–45	1A2, 2C9, 2D6, 3A4	20–40 hr

[a]Dose range information from Lexi-Comp, Lexi-Drugs Online. Hudson, OH: Lexi-Comp. Updated periodically.
[b]Allergan, Madison, NJ
[c]Drug has received U.S. Food and Drug Administration label approval for depression in children and adolescents.
[d]Lundbeck, North Ryde, Australia
[e]Eli Lilly, Indianapolis, IN
[f]In children younger than 12 years, consider initiating antidepressant at half the listed starting dose.[73]
[g]GlaxoSmithKline, Brentford, United Kingdom
[h]Pfizer, New York, NY
[i]Remeron: Merck, Whitehouse Station, NJ
SR = sustained release.

those consistent with a relapse in or recurrence of a depressive episode.[9] Withdrawal symptoms can occur after receiving antidepressant treatment for only 6–8 weeks and can begin as early as 24–48 hours after treatment discontinuation.[9] Symptoms typically resolve without treatment during a 1- to 2-week period.[47] To prevent the occurrence of withdrawal symptoms, it is recommended that the antidepressant dose be decreased by no more than 25% per week, with tapering usually occurring during a 2- to 3-month period.[61] With its longer half-life, fluoxetine may not require a slow taper.

ANTIDEPRESSANTS AND SUICIDALITY

In October 2004, the FDA issued a black box warning for all antidepressants, describing the increased risk of suicidal thinking and behavior in children and adolescents (younger than 18 years) with MDD and other psychiatric disorders when treated with antidepressants. This warning was extended in 2007 to include young adults up to age 25 years.[77] The black box warning recommends evaluating the benefits and risks associated with antidepressant therapy when considering antidepressants for use in this patient population. Because short-term studies did not show an increase in suicidality in adults older than 24 years and actually showed a decrease in suicidality in adults older than 65 years, this warning applies only to patients younger than 25 years. Also mentioned in this warning is that depression itself is associated with an increased risk of suicide, making it difficult to determine whether suicidality is a result of antidepressant treatment or a consequence of the disease. After the first black box warning in 2004, antidepressant prescription rates decreased by 18% from July 2003 to July 2004, whereas teen suicide rates increased for the first time in more than a decade, highlighting the consequence of untreated depression.[78] A population-based observational study of children age 6–18 years enrolled in health care with Tennessee State Medicaid showed no difference between suicide attempt risk leading to death or medical intervention among new users of commonly prescribed SSRIs and SNRIs.[79] In a cohort study of depressed patients age 10–18 years initiated on antidepressant therapy, the risk of suicidal acts did not vary within the class of SSRIs or between antidepressants (SNRIs, TCAs, mirtazapine, nefazodone, trazodone), thereby supporting the inclusion of all antidepressant agents in the black box warning.[80]

Regardless of whether suicidality is because of antidepressant therapy or the disease itself, health care providers should educate patients of all ages and caregivers about the possibility of increased suicidal symptoms, especially early in treatment, and monitor patients for clinical worsening, suicidality, and unusual changes in behavior during the first few months of therapy and during dosage adjustments. Pharmacists can participate in suicide prevention training programs that allow them to detect signs of suicide, respond to patients with suicidal ideation, and understand resources available to and when to refer patients.[81] At a minimum, pharmacists should be aware of the National Suicide Prevention Lifeline (1-800-273-8255), as well as local suicide prevention hotlines or resources in the area to provide to patients, and when patients should be referred for emergency psychiatric evaluation. The FDA guidelines specifically recommend the clinician should meet face-to-face with the patient weekly during the first 4 weeks of antidepressant treatment. For the next 4 weeks of therapy, the FDA advises biweekly visits, followed by a visit at 12 weeks. Thereafter, the patient can be seen as clinically indicated. In addition, symptoms such as anxiety, agitation, panic attacks, insomnia, irritability, hostility, aggressiveness, impulsivity, akathisia, hypomania, and mania may be indicative of suicidality. Thus, family and caregivers should be educated on the importance of monitoring for the presence of these symptoms and of the subsequent need to contact a health care provider if any of these symptoms arise.

CONCLUSIONS

Major depressive disorder can present as early as childhood and is associated with an increased risk of morbidity and mortality. To restore optimal functioning and prevent recurrence, it is necessary to identify symptoms of depression early in their course and provide effective treatment through psychotherapy and/or pharmacotherapy. More studies are required to further evaluate the efficacy and tolerability of antidepressant agents as monotherapy or in combination with psychotherapy in the pediatric patient population. Because of the risk of suicidality associated with antidepressant use, close monitoring for clinical worsening, behavioral changes, and suicidality is recommended when initiating antidepressants in patients younger than 25 years.

Patient Case | PEDIATRIC DEPRESSION

A 13-year-old girl is brought by her mother to the pediatrician. Her mother reports that her daughter appears to have been experiencing a loss of energy, irritability, and poor concentration over the past few months. She also mentions her daughter's academic performance has declined this past semester; she used to be on the honor roll each semester but more recently has received grades of all Cs and Ds in her courses. The patient used to be very social and enjoyed spending time with her friends but lately she has been spending more time alone in her room. The Patient Health Questionnaire-9 Item (PHQ-9) results today are consistent with severe depression. The patient's father was diagnosed with major depressive disorder (MDD) 5 years ago and was treated with citalopram. The patient has not received treatment for depression in the past, and she denies use of any other medications or illicit substances.

1. The patient's symptoms are consistent with what diagnosis? What are appropriate treatment options?

The patient meets *Diagnostic and Statistical Manual of Mental Disorders, Fifth Edition* criteria for MDD based on her symptoms of loss of energy, poor concentration, and anhedonia (isolating herself and not enjoying time with her friends), in addition to scoring as severely depressed on the PHQ-9. She also is functionally impaired (declining academic performance) as a result of these symptoms. Concurrent psychotherapy and pharmacotherapy should be considered. If the patient and her mother agree to psychotherapy, then interpersonal or cognitive behavioral therapy is preferred. Regardless, the patient should receive pharmacotherapy because of the classification of "severe depression" for which studies support medication management with or without psychotherapy. Although the patient's father responded to citalopram, fluoxetine is considered first-line therapy by many guidelines and has the most evidence for efficacy and safety in the treatment of MDD in pediatric patients. Fluoxetine should be initiated at a low dose of 10 mg/day to avoid adverse effects and may be increased by increments of 10 mg every 1–4 weeks, based on medication effectiveness and tolerability. An appropriate dose might be considered fluoxetine 20–40 mg/day for at least 12 weeks. Failure of this treatment could include inability to reach the dosage range because of intolerabilities or lack of efficacy at the dosage range after 12 weeks. If improvement in symptoms throughout the 12 weeks is not evident, then increasing dosage to the maximum tolerated dose should be considered. If no change in symptoms results despite dosage titration, then the patient should be assessed for medication adherence. If treatment fails for this patient after an adequate trial of fluoxetine (appropriate dose and duration), then alternative treatment options include citalopram (preferentially based on family history), escitalopram (s-isomer of citalopram racemic mixture), or sertraline.

2. What are the three phases of treatment and goals in each phase for this patient?

The three phases of treatment for this patient consist of acute, continuation, and maintenance treatment. The goal of acute phase treatment (up to 12 weeks) includes obtaining remission, characterized by an alleviation of depressive symptoms such that the patient returns to baseline functioning, and/or loses the diagnostic status for MDD.

On obtaining remission, then the patient enters continuation phase treatment for at least 6 months, with the goal to sustain remission and prevent relapse. In clinical practice, this goal is generally accomplished by continuation of the antidepressant used by the patient to meet remission. Any residual symptoms that were not completely resolved in the acute phase may also be targeted.

On completion of the continuation phase, the patient may be assessed for maintenance treatment, with the goal to prevent recurrence. Because this patient is considered to have severe depression, she may be a candidate for maintenance therapy. Other factors, such as depression chronicity and treatment efficacy (whether all symptoms are completely treated), may be considered when determining the duration of therapy.

Because it appears that this episode of depression is the patient's first, it is possible that she could later be evaluated for antidepressant discontinuation, which should only be attempted if the patient is not experiencing current stressors or life changes. If discontinuation of an antidepressant is considered, a dose taper is necessary to prevent withdrawal symptoms or discontinuation syndrome (although the taper is unnecessary if the patient is treated with fluoxetine). A taper can also identify the return of depressive symptoms that might signify that the patient is not a candidate for antidepressant discontinuation (the patient should resume the effective dose of the medication). Throughout each phase, treatment tolerability and adherence should also be evaluated.

3. Describe monitoring guidelines for this patient's antidepressant therapy.

The patient should be monitored for effectiveness, tolerability, and adherence to the antidepressant. The response of MDD to the antidepressant can be monitored using several MDD rating scales studied in pediatric patients. In this case, the PHQ-9 was completed at baseline and can be used to monitor effectiveness of fluoxetine in treating MDD. Desired treatment goals include obtaining remission, preventing relapse, and the return of baseline functioning. For this patient, these goals would include increased energy and concentration, reduced isolation, increased interest in activities she previously found pleasurable, and a reduction in irritability. Her academic performance should also concurrently or subsequently improve with treatment. If the patient is started on a selective serotonin reuptake inhibitor, such as fluoxetine, then she should be educated on and monitored for short-term adverse effects, including gastrointestinal upset or symptoms, sleep changes, restlessness or akathisia, headaches, appetite changes, or diaphoresis. Long-term adverse effects include sexual dysfunction. Behavioral activation may occur and should also be monitored. Less common adverse effects may include bleeding or serotonin syndrome. Fluoxetine has a long half-life; therefore, the patient would be at less risk of discontinuation syndrome or symptoms with missed doses. The patient and her mother should also be educated on the risk of suicidality after starting the antidepressant. If the patient experiences an increase in suicidal thoughts or behavior, closer monitoring by the health care provider is warranted, including an increased level of care (e.g., inpatient admission) or change in treatment. Adherence can be monitored by asking the patient and/or her mother open-ended questions regarding antidepressant use or perceptions at appointments. Doing so may help health care providers identify potential barriers to adherence and strategies to overcome partial or non-adherence.

REFERENCES

1. Luby JL. Early childhood depression. Am J Psychiatry 2009; 166:974-9.

2. Fleming JE, Offord DR, Boyle MH. Prevalence of childhood and adolescent depression in the community. Ontario Child Health Study. Br J Psychiatry 1989;155:647-54.

3. Merikangas KR, He JP, Brody D, et al. Prevalence and treatment of mental disorders among US children in the 2001–2004 NHANES. Pediatrics 2010;125:75-81.

4. Avenevoli S, Swendsen J, He JP, et al. Major depression in the national comorbidity survey-adolescent supplement: prevalence, correlates, and treatment. J Am Acad Child Adolesc Psychiatry 2015;54:37-44.e32.

5. Merikangas KR, He JP, Burstein M, et al. Lifetime prevalence of mental disorders in U.S. adolescents: results from the National Comorbidity Survey Replication—Adolescent Supplement (NCS-A). J Am Acad Child Adolesc Psychiatry 2010;49:980-9.

6. Jellinek MS, Snyder JB. Depression and suicide in children and adolescents. Pediatr Rev 1998;19:255-64.

7. National Institute of Mental Health. Major depression among adolescents [monograph on the Internet]. Available at https://www.nimh.nih.gov/health/statistics/major-depression.shtml. Accessed July 25, 2018.

8. Pine DS, Cohen E, Cohen P, et al. Adolescent depressive symptoms as predictors of adult depression: moodiness or mood disorder? Am J Psychiatry 1999;156:133-5.

9. Birmaher B, Brent D, Bernet W, et al. Practice parameter for the assessment and treatment of children and adolescents with depressive disorders. J Am Acad Child Adolesc Psychiatry 2007; 46:1503-26.

10. National Center for Health Statistics, National Vital Statistics System. Deaths, percent of total deaths, and death rates for the 15 leading causes of death in selected age groups, by race and sex: United States, 2014. Available at www.cdc.gov/nchs/data/dvs/lcwk3_2014.pdf. Accessed July 25, 2018.

11. Wilkinson P, Kelvin R, Roberts C, et al. Clinical and psychosocial predictors of suicide attempts and nonsuicidal self-injury in the Adolescent Depression Antidepressants and Psychotherapy Trial (ADAPT). Am J Psychiatry 2011;168:495-501.

12. Sheftall AH, Asti L, Horowitz LM, et al. Suicide in elementary school-aged children and early adolescents. Pediatrics 2016; 138:e20160436.

13. Pelkonen M, Marttunen M. Child and adolescent suicide: epidemiology, risk factors, and approaches to prevention. Paediatr Drugs 2003;5:243-65.

14. National Center for Health Statistics, National Vital Statistics System. 10 leading causes of death by age group, United States–2014. Available at www.cdc.gov/injury/images/lc-charts/leading_causes_of_death_age_group_2014_1050w760h.gif. Accessed July 25, 2018.

15. Lewinsohn PM, Rohde P, Seeley JR. Major depressive disorder in older adolescents: prevalence, risk factors, and clinical implications. Clin Psychol Rev 1998;18:765-94.

16. Bhatia SK, Bhatia SC. Childhood and adolescent depression. Am Fam Physician 2007;75:73-80.

17. Lee S, Jeong J, Kwak Y, et al. Depression research: where are we now? Mol Brain 2010;3:8.

18. Harmer CJ, Duman RS, Cowen PJ. How do antidepressants work? New perspectives for refining future treatment approaches. Lancet Psychiatry 2017;4:409-18.

19. Beardslee WR, Keller MB, Lavori PW, et al. The impact of parental affective disorder on depression in offspring: a longitudinal follow-up in a nonreferred sample. J Am Acad Child Adolesc Psychiatry 1993;32:723-30.

20. Foster CE, Webster MC, Weissman MM, et al. Remission of maternal depression: relations to family functioning and youth internalizing and externalizing symptoms. J Clin Child Adolesc Psychol 2008;37:714-24.

21. American Psychiatric Association. Diagnostic and Statistical Manual of Mental Disorders, DSM-5, 5th ed. Washington, DC: American Psychiatric Association, 2013.

22. Yorbik O, Birmaher B, Axelson D, et al. Clinical characteristics of depressive symptoms in children and adolescents with major depressive disorder. J Clin Psychiatry 2004;65:1654-9; quiz 1760-1.

23. Birmaher B, Ryan ND, Williamson DE, et al. Childhood and adolescent depression: a review of the past 10 years. Part II. J Am Acad Child Adolesc Psychiatry 1996;35:1575-83.

24. Siu AL. Screening for Depression in Children and Adolescents: US Preventive Services Task Force Recommendation Statement. Pediatrics 2016;137:e20154467.

25. Richardson LP, Rockhill C, Russo JE, et al. Evaluation of the PHQ-2 as a brief screen for detecting major depression among adolescents. Pediatrics 2010;125:e1097-103.

26. Borner I, Braunstein JW, St Victor R, et al. Evaluation of a 2-question screening tool for detecting depression in adolescents in primary care. Clin Pediatr (Phila) 2010;49:947-53.

27. Williams SB, O'Connor EA, Eder M, et al. Screening for child and adolescent depression in primary care settings: a systematic evidence review for the US Preventive Services Task Force. Pediatrics 2009;123:e716-35.

28. Johnson JG, Harris ES, Spitzer RL, et al. The patient health questionnaire for adolescents: validation of an instrument for the assessment of mental disorders among adolescent primary care patients. J Adolesc Health 2002;30:196-204.

29. Sajatovic M, Ramirez LF, eds. Rating Scales in Mental Health, 2nd ed. Hudson, OH: Lexi-Comp, 2003.

30. Poznanski EO, Cook SC, Carroll BJ. A depression rating scale for children. Pediatrics 1979;64:442-50.

31. Fontanella CA, Bridge JA, Marcus SC, et al. Factors associated with antidepressant adherence for Medicaid-enrolled children and adolescents. Ann Pharmacother 2011;45:898-909.

32. Emslie GJ, Kennard BD, Mayes TL, et al. Fluoxetine versus placebo in preventing relapse of major depression in children and adolescents. Am J Psychiatry 2008;165:459-67.

33. Weisz JR, McCarty CA, Valeri SM. Effects of psychotherapy for depression in children and adolescents: a meta-analysis. Psychol Bull 2006;132:132-49.

34. Stahl SM. Stahl's Essential Psychopharmacology: Neuroscientific Basis and Practical Applications. New York: Cambridge University Press, 2008.

35. Reinecke MA, Ryan NE, DuBois DL. Cognitive-behavioral therapy of depression and depressive symptoms during adolescence: a review and meta-analysis. J Am Acad Child Adolesc Psychiatry 1998;37:26-34.

36. Goodyer IM, Dubicka B, Wilkinson P, et al. A randomised controlled trial of cognitive behaviour therapy in adolescents with major depression treated by selective serotonin reuptake inhibitors. The ADAPT trial. Health Technol Assess 2008;12:iii-iv, ix-60.

37. Smiga SM, Elliott GR. Psychopharmacology of depression in children and adolescents. Pediatr Clin North Am 2011;58:155-71, xi.

38. Hazell P, O'Connell D, Heathcote D, et al. Efficacy of tricyclic drugs in treating child and adolescent depression: a meta-analysis. BMJ 1995;310:897-901.

39. March JS, Silva S, Petrycki S, et al. The treatment for adolescents with depression study (TADS): long-term effectiveness and safety outcomes. Arch Gen Psychiatry 2007;64:1132-43.

40. de Boer T. The effects of mirtazapine on central noradrenergic and serotonergic neurotransmission. Int Clin Psychopharmacol 1995;10 Suppl 4:19-23.

41. Schirman S, Kronenberg S, Apter A, et al. Effectiveness and tolerability of citalopram for the treatment of depression and anxiety disorders in children and adolescents: an open-label study. J Neural Transm (Vienna) 2010;117:139-45.

42. Emslie GJ, Ventura D, Korotzer A, et al. Escitalopram in the treatment of adolescent depression: a randomized placebo-controlled multisite trial. J Am Acad Child Adolesc Psychiatry 2009;48:721-9.
43. Keller MB, Ryan ND, Strober M, et al. Efficacy of paroxetine in the treatment of adolescent major depression: a randomized, controlled trial. J Am Acad Child Adolesc Psychiatry 2001;40:762-72.
44. Wagner KD, Ambrosini P, Rynn M, et al. Efficacy of sertraline in the treatment of children and adolescents with major depressive disorder: two randomized controlled trials. JAMA 2003;290:1033-41.
45. Prozac [package insert]. Indianapolis, IN: Eli Lilly and Company, 2011.
46. Lexapro [package insert]. St. Louis, MO: Forest Pharmaceuticals, 2011.
47. March J, Silva S, Petrycki S, et al. Fluoxetine, cognitive-behavioral therapy, and their combination for adolescents with depression: treatment for adolescents with depression study (TADS) randomized controlled trial. JAMA 2004;292:807-20.
48. Brent D, Emslie G, Clarke G, et al. Switching to another SSRI or to venlafaxine with or without cognitive behavioral therapy for adolescents with SSRI-resistant depression: the TORDIA randomized controlled trial. JAMA 2008;299:901-13.
49. Glod CA, Lynch A, Flynn E, et al. Open trial of bupropion SR in adolescent major depression. J Child Adolesc Psychiatr Nurs 2003;16:123-30.
50. Haapasalo-Pesu KM, Vuola T, Lahelma L, et al. Mirtazapine in the treatment of adolescents with major depression: an open-label, multicenter pilot study. J Child Adolesc Psychopharmacol 2004;14:175-84.
51. Findling RL, Robb AS, DelBello MP, et al. A 6-month open-label extension study of vortioxetine in pediatric patients with depressive or anxiety disorders. J Child Adolesc Psychopharmacol 2018;28:47-54.
52. Pathak S, Johns ES, Kowatch RA. Adjunctive quetiapine for treatment-resistant adolescent major depressive disorder: a case series. J Child Adolesc Psychopharmacol 2005;15:696-702.
53. Kennard BD, Emslie GJ, Mayes TL, et al. Sequential treatment with fluoxetine and relapse–prevention CBT to improve outcomes in pediatric depression. Am J Psychiatry 2014;171:1083-90.
54. Vitiello B, Emslie G, Clarke G, et al. Long-term outcome of adolescent depression initially resistant to selective serotonin reuptake inhibitor treatment: a follow-up study of the TORDIA sample. J Clin Psychiatry 2011;72:388-96.
55. Hetrick SE, McKenzie JE, Cox GR, et al. Newer generation antidepressants for depressive disorders in children and adolescents. Cochrane Database Syst Rev 2012;11:CD004851.
56. Cipriani A, Zhou X, Del Giovane C, et al. Comparative efficacy and tolerability of antidepressants for major depressive disorder in children and adolescents: a network meta-analysis. Lancet 2016;388:881-90.
57. National Collaborating Centre for Mental Health (UK). Depression in Children and Young People: Identification and Management in Primary, Community and Secondary Care. NICE Clinical Guidelines [CG28]. Leicester, UK: British Psychological Society, 2005.
58. Zuckerbrot RA, Cheung A, Jensen PS, et al.; GLAD-PC Steering Group. Guidelines for Adolescent Depression in Primary Care (GLAD-PC): Part I. Practice preparation, identification, assessment, and initial management. Pediatrics 2018;141:e20174081.
59. Cheung AH, Zuckerbrot RA, Jensen PS, et al.; GLAD-PC Steering Group. Guidelines for Adolescent Depression in Primary Care (GLAD-PC): Part II. Treatment and ongoing management. Pediatrics 2018;141:e20174082.
60. MacQueen GM, Frey BN, Ismail Z, et al. Canadian Network for Mood and Anxiety Treatments (CANMAT) 2016 Clinical Guidelines for the Management of Adults with Major Depressive Disorder: Section 6. Special Populations: Youth, Women, and the Elderly. Can J Psychiatry 2016;61:588-603.
61. Hughes CW, Emslie GJ, Crismon ML, et al. Texas Children's Medication Algorithm Project: update from Texas Consensus Conference Panel on medication treatment of childhood major depressive disorder. J Am Acad Child Adolesc Psychiatry 2007;46:667-86.
62. Emslie GJ, Wagner KD, Kutcher S, et al. Paroxetine treatment in children and adolescents with major depressive disorder: a randomized, multicenter, double-blind, placebo-controlled trial. J Am Acad Child Adolesc Psychiatry 2006;45:709-19.
63. Cheung AH, Emslie GJ, Mayes TL. Review of the efficacy and safety of antidepressants in youth depression. J Child Psychol Psychiatry 2005;46:735-54.
64. Ghaziuddin N, Kutcher SP, Knapp P, et al. Practice parameter for use of electroconvulsive therapy with adolescents. J Am Acad Child Adolesc Psychiatry 2004;43:1521-39.
65. Boylan K, Romero S, Birmaher B. Psychopharmacologic treatment of pediatric major depressive disorder. Psychopharmacology 2007;191:27-38.
66. Findling RL, McNamara NK, Stansbrey RJ, et al. The relevance of pharmacokinetic studies in designing efficacy trials in juvenile major depression. J Child Adolesc Psychopharmacol 2006;16:131-45.
67. Effexor XR [package insert]. Collegeville, PA: Wyeth Pharmaceuticals, 2009.
68. Wellbutrin SR [package insert]. Research Triangle Park, NC: GlaxoSmithKline, 2010.
69. Fawcett J, Barkin RL. Review of the results from clinical studies on the efficacy, safety and tolerability of mirtazapine for the treatment of patients with major depression. J Affect Disord 1998;51:267-85.
70. Hetrick S, Merry S, McKenzie J, et al. Selective serotonin reuptake inhibitors (SSRIs) for depressive disorders in children and adolescents. Cochrane Database Syst Rev 2007;3:CD004851.
71. von Knorring AL, Olsson GI, Thomsen PH, et al. A randomized, double-blind, placebo-controlled study of citalopram in adolescents with major depressive disorder. J Clin Psychopharmacol 2006;26:311-5.
72. Hemeryck A, Belpaire FM. Selective serotonin reuptake inhibitors and cytochrome P-450 mediated drug-drug interactions: an update. Curr Drug Metab 2002;3:13-37.
73. Southammakosane C, Schmitz K. Pediatric psychopharmacology for treatment of ADHD, depression, and anxiety. Pediatrics 2015;136:351-9.
74. RemeronSolTab [package insert]. Eden Prairie, MN: Schering Corporation, 2010.
75. Sandson NB, Armstrong SC, Cozza KL. An overview of psychotropic drug–drug interactions. Psychosomatics 2005;46:464-94.
76. Gelenberg AJ, Freeman MP, Markowitz JC, et al. Practice Guidelines for the Treatment of Patients with Major Depressive Disorder. Washington, DC: American Psychiatric Association, 2010.
77. U.S. Food and Drug Administration. Medication guide: about using antidepressants in children and teenagers [monograph on the Internet]. Available at http://criticalthinkrx.org/pdf/m5/Module-5-FDA-guidelines-for-kids-on-ADs.pdf. Accessed July 25, 2018.
78. Friedman RA, Leon AC. Expanding the black box—depression, antidepressants, and the risk of suicide. N Engl J Med 2007;356:2343-6.
79. Cooper WO, Callahan ST, Shintani A, et al. Antidepressants and suicide attempts in children. Pediatrics 2014;133:204-10.
80. Schneeweiss S, Patrick AR, Solomon DH, et al. Comparative safety of antidepressant agents for children and adolescents regarding suicidal acts. Pediatrics 2010;125:876-88.
81. Painter NA, Kuo GM, Collins SP, et al. Pharmacist training in suicide prevention. J Am Pharm Assoc (2003) 2018;58:199-204.e2.

CHAPTER 34

Pediatric Bipolar Disorder

Andria Farhat Church, Pharm.D., BCPS, BCPP; and
Alberto Augsten, Pharm.D., M.S., BCPP, DABAT

Andria Farhat Church, Pharm.D., BCPS, BCPP; and
Alberto Augsten, Pharm.D., M.S., BCPP, DABAT

LEARNING OBJECTIVES

1. Describe the theories that support the etiology and pathophysiology of pediatric bipolar disorder (PBD).

2. Explain the signs, symptoms, and diagnostic criteria for PBD.

3. Describe the treatment goals of PBD.

4. Evaluate pharmacologic therapy for the treatment of PBD to determine the best treatment for individual patients, including mood stabilizers, antipsychotics, and adjunctive treatments.

5. Recognize common monitoring variables, including common adverse effects, for the pharmacologic treatments of PBD.

ABBREVIATIONS IN THIS CHAPTER

AACAP	American Academy of Child and Adolescent Psychiatry
BPD	Bipolar disorder
BPI	Bipolar I disorder
BPII	Bipolar II disorder
CANMAT	Canadian Network for Mood and Anxiety Treatments
CDRS-R	Child Depression Rating Scale-Revised
CYP	Cytochrome P450
DA$_2$	Dopamine receptor
DSM-IV	*Diagnostic and Statistical Manual of Mental Disorders, Fourth Edition*
DSM-5	*Diagnostic and Statistical Manual of Mental Disorders, Fifth Edition*
ECT	Electroconvulsive therapy
EPS	Extrapyramidal symptoms
FDA	U.S. Food and Drug Administration
GABA	γ-Aminobutyric acid
ISBD	International Society for Bipolar Disorders
K-SADS	Kiddie Schedule for Affective Disorders and Schizophrenia
LOCF	Last observation carried forward
SGA	Second-generation antipsychotic
TSH	Thyroid-stimulating hormone
PBD	Pediatric bipolar disorder
YMRS	Young Mania Rating Scale

INTRODUCTION

Bipolar disorder (BPD) is a type of mood disorder that consists of mania, depression, hypomania, and periods of normal mood. This disorder can affect children, adolescents, and adults, and it is categorized into two main subtypes, depending on the prominent moods displayed. Bipolar I disorder (BPI), which was formerly referred to as *manic depression*, includes mood episodes of mania and can also include episodes of hypomania and/or major depression.[1] A person must experience at least one manic episode to meet the diagnosis of BPI.[1] Bipolar II disorder (BPII) includes mood episodes of hypomania and major depression; at least one episode of each is required for diagnosis. A switch between moods can occur spontaneously or can be the result of a trigger, such as secondary to a medication. Although these descriptions refer to the symptom criteria required for bipolar diagnosis, how those symptoms present in children and adolescents can vastly differ from how adults present with the disorder. This point will be discussed more in depth in the Clinical Presentation section later in this chapter. Cyclothymic disorder, although related, differs from BPD in that the person does not meet the full criteria required for either diagnosis of BPI or BPII (i.e., major depression, hypomania, or mania).[1] Therefore, cyclothymia will not be discussed within this chapter. Other forms of BPD that will not be discussed in this chapter include those induced by medications or by underlying health conditions because these forms can be patient specific and vary greatly. More information on mood-induced changes secondary to substance use or abuse (e.g., alcohol, cocaine) is presented in the Substance Use Disorder chapter. Bipolar disorder pervades throughout an individual's life and necessitates both pharmacologic and nonpharmacologic treatment strategies to obtain mood stabilization. This chapter will review the treatment options available to the pediatric population for management of this disorder.[1,2]

EPIDEMIOLOGY

Based on lack of clear diagnostic guidelines, mental health disorder comorbidities confounding the BPD diagnosis, and possible underreporting of pediatric bipolar disorder (PBD) cases, the epidemiologic statistics vary depending on the resource used. Per the National Alliance on Mental Illness, the average age of onset for BPD is 25 years; however, onset of illness can occur at any point throughout a lifespan.[1,3] The age range of BPD onset most commonly spans from 15 to 30 years.[4] In the case of early-onset BPD, the diagnosis is more common in male patients, particularly if occurring before age 13 years.[4] When assessing age of onset, some researchers have speculated that individuals have an earlier onset (i.e., childhood diagnosis) if they experienced psychosocial adversity (e.g., abuse) as a child and/or have a parent or grandparent with psychiatric illness; each of these elements is referred to as a *vulnerability factor*.[5] Within the United States, 2.9% of the population receives a diagnosis of BPD annually.[1,3] A national survey found a 14.3% lifetime prevalence of any mood disorder in pediatric patients age 13–18 years, with a higher occurrence in older children and female patients.[6] The survey data ranges from 2001–2004 and is based on criteria in the *Diagnostic and Statistical Manual of Mental Disorders, Fourth Edition (DSM-IV)*. Overall, the prevalence is an estimated 1% of the population, which increases with age.[4] It is estimated that in a patient with BPD, the lifetime suicide risk is 15 times greater than reported in the general population.[1] One study specifically addressed suicidal ideation and suicide attempts in PBD.[7] In a systematic review of 14 studies in nonoverlapping PBD studies, the researchers found that at least one of two children or adolescents had current or lifetime history of suicidal ideation, and one of four or five children or adolescents had current or lifetime history of suicide attempts. The review also mentions that in the four prospective studies reviewed throughout a mean follow-up of 3.5 years, incidence rates were 27% and 15% for suicidal ideation and suicide attempts, respectively.[7] In addition, an association between recovery and long duration of BPD illness exists, and the probability of recovery declines by 20% for each year the patient remains ill.[8]

ETIOLOGY AND PATHOPHYSIOLOGY

The cause of BPD remains unknown; however, various theories exist regarding the etiology of the disorder. Some explanations for BPD include genetic inheritance, individual brain structure, and secondary results from a stressful incident or environmental factor (e.g., illicit substance use, trauma).[3,9] Although not absolute, a person is more susceptible to developing BPD if they have a relative who also has the disorder, particularly a first-degree relative.[1,3] Neurochemical theories suggest involvement from various body pathways for bipolar symptom onset and the cause of switching from one mood to the other.[9,10] The first of these is the monoamine theory, which proposes an imbalance in the neurotransmitters dopamine, serotonin, and norepinephrine, which results in manic (elevated neurotransmitters) or depressive (depleted neurotransmitters) symptoms.[10] Secondly, BPD may also be the result of imbalances between glutamate and γ-aminobutyric acid (GABA).[10] Lastly, the kindling model, which is used to explain the development of epilepsy, is also a theory that explains mood episodes in BPD.[9] Kindling coincides with structural and functional alterations within the brain that have an extended duration and are potentially permanent.[9] The kindling theory asserts that when an individual is genetically susceptible to developing BPD, experiences such as using illicit substances, taking particular medications, or undergoing a traumatic life event can decrease the "threshold" for mood changes. Moreover, a mechanism called *episodic sensitization* illustrates that each episode further decreases the threshold, leaving the individual at greater risk of mood fluctuations.[9] Neuroendocrine systems (e.g., those involving thyroid hormones, cortisol) and neuropsychological triggers (e.g., psychosocial stress) may also be involved in BPD.[10]

CLINICAL PRESENTATION AND DIAGNOSIS

Bipolar disorder is most often diagnosed in late adolescence and early adulthood, with BPI often diagnosed earlier than BPII.[11] Special consideration should be taken when making a diagnosis for a pediatric or adolescent patient. Although there is some controversy regarding this point in the literature, a child or adolescent may present similarly or differently from an adult with BPD. In addition, an adult presentation of BPD is usually similar among adults (e.g., presenting with grandiosity); however, that is less common when comparing bipolar onset between children. More often, children may grow at different developmental paces; therefore, two children at the same age might show different maturity levels.[4] Thus, challenges in diagnosis arise when classic behaviors for a child (e.g., high energy) are the same behaviors used to denote mania (e.g., increased activity or energy).[1] This similarity exemplifies why it is so vital to evaluate each child against the child's own baseline and against expectations for that child's developmental level.[1]

In a practice guideline that addresses PBD assessment and treatment, adolescent mania is noted to coincide with noticeably labile moods, psychotic symptoms, and/or a mixture of both mania/depression symptoms.[4] Whereas euphoria is a common adult presentation of mania, children may more often show signs of aggression, irritability, volatility, and manic/depressive symptom mix; these variations in behavior, mood, and energy are considerably labile and unpredictable.[4,12] Regarding bipolar depressive symptoms, children may potentially display dysphoria and anger.[4] The practice guideline also mentions that compared with adult onset of BPD, the adolescent onset may be more chronic and treatment refractory, and the long-term prognosis is analogous to or worse than adults. The guideline goes on to state that in both children and adolescents the mood episodes are recurrent, with high rates of rapid cycling and low rates of recuperation between episodes. Conversely, some literature states the term "rapid cycling" does not best describe PBD because these patients do not have defined episodes of mania; instead their mood dysregulation is described as several profound, acute, and prolonged mood swings, occurring daily.[12] The common comorbidities in PBD are anxiety, disruptive behavior disorders, substance use disorders, pervasive developmental disorders and attention-deficit/hyperactivity disorder.[4,12-15] In general, comorbidities can mask bipolar symptoms. Furthermore, comorbidities can increase the individual's impairment and can make treatment of the disorders more challenging.[15]

However, despite all these differences between adolescents and adults with BPD, some argue that adolescents do present similarly to adults; furthermore they argue that age has little to no impact on mania symptoms (i.e., presentation does not change from youths to adults), but that depression symptoms do change with age.[16] Even with conflicting information on the presentation of symptoms, it is still recommended to use the *Diagnostic and Statistical Manual of Mental Disorders, Fifth Edition (DSM-5)* criteria for diagnosing children, adolescents, and adults.[16] Elements regarded as hallmark symptoms for adults may not apply to children and adolescents. Table 1

Table 1. Bipolar Disorder Symptom Comparison Between Adults and Children/Adolescents[1,12,65,66]

Adult Presentation	Child/Adolescent Presentation
Mania Symptoms • *Key symptom criteria:* An irritable, expansive, or elevated mood and increased energy or goal-directed activity • *Additional symptom criteria:* At least 3 other symptoms must be present[a,b] • *Time frame:* The key symptoms must be present throughout the majority of the day, almost daily, and last for at least 1 week; the additional symptoms must occur during the same 1-week period and be present to a significant degree[c] • *Important notes:* Hypomania criteria are the same as for mania, but duration is only 4 consecutive days and hospitalization is not warranted	
Reduced need for sleep[a]	Reduced need for sleep by ≥ 2 hours a night with no sign of fatigue the next day; wandering in the middle of the night
Grandiosity or inflated self-esteem[a]	Bragging, exaggerating; acting on grandiose beliefs; inability to distinguish imaginary play from reality
Flight of ideas[a]	Flight of ideas may be more easily observed by others vs. self-report, or topic changes coincide with noted difficulty in following what the patient is saying; not to be confused with difficulty in following the limited vocabulary of a younger child (e.g., age 3 yr)
Racing thoughts[a]	May need to ask if brain/thoughts is/are "going too fast"; racing thoughts are impairing function or activities
Expansive, elevated mood	Extremely silly, giggly, cheerful mood
Irritability[b]	Irritability, plus possibly displaying: severe rage over something insignificant, aggression, and/or self-injurious behavior
Increased energy	No significant differences from adults
More talkative or pressure to keep talking[a]	Talkativeness marks a change from baseline; may be invasive, loud, and hard to interrupt
Distractibility[a]	Distraction marks a change from baseline and coincides with manic mood (cannot be the result of another underlying disorder, such as attention-deficit/hyperactivity disorder); may fully lose ability to focus in school and/or may become "flighty" at home, easily forgetting a task they were doing
Increased goal-directed activity	Increased goal-directed activity (e.g., marked increase in drawing or building structures with blocks) is more revealing of mania than psychomotor agitation; may also present with disorganization and a lack of productivity or have unrealistic plans
Psychomotor agitation[a]	Psychomotor agitation may appear as though the patient might "jump out of their skin" and usually has a "pressured" character to the agitation (i.e., intense need to fulfill the agitated urge)
Overly involved in risky/dangerous activities[a]	Often presents as hypersexual actions (must rule out sexually explicit exposure and sexual abuse)
Psychosis	Same as adult (presenting with delusions, hallucinations); assess whether psychotic features coincide with mood changes (otherwise may signify a different psychiatric disorder)
Depression Symptoms • *Key symptom criteria:* Loss of interests/pleasure or depressed mood • *Additional symptom criteria:* At least 4 other depressive symptoms must be present • *Time frame:* Symptoms must be present during the same 2-week period	
Depressed mood[d]	Same as an adult, but may also present with: • Irritable mood/low frustration tolerance • Labile mood • Temper tantrums • Crying, becomes tearful, or expresses sadness • Social withdrawal/difficulty with relationships and/or increased awareness of social failure and/or rejection • Poor communication • Somatic symptoms • Rumination • Talk of running away or attempts to run away
Significant, unintentional weight loss or gain; or appetite increase/decrease[e]	Same as an adult, but instead may not meet predicted weight gain goals (per a growth chart)

(continued)

Table 1. Bipolar Disorder Symptom Comparison Between Adults and Children/Adolescents[1,12,65,66] *(continued)*

Adult Presentation	Child/Adolescent Presentation
Thoughts of death occur repeatedly; repeated suicidal ideation without a plan, or a specific plan for committing suicide or a suicide attempt	High risk of suicidal ideation, intent, plans, and/or attempts during periods of psychosis, depression, and mixed mood episodes; may also display self-harm behavior
Hypersomnia or insomnia[e]	Same as an adult; may also lie in bed for extended periods
Substantial decrease in pleasure/ interest in activities[d]	Same as an adult
Indecisiveness, or decreased ability to think/focus[e]	Same as an adult; may also demonstrate poor academic performance or often be absent from school
Decreased energy or fatigue[e]	Same as an adult; may also present with lethargy or persistent boredom
Excessive or inappropriate guilt, or feeling worthless[e]	Same as an adult
Psychomotor retardation or agitation[e]	Same as an adult; may also present with a "nervous habit" such as nail biting

[a]These are the potential symptoms needed to meet the additional ≥ 3 symptom criteria for a manic episode. In the *DSM-5* some symptoms are paired together as a single criterion (e.g., flight of ideas or racing thoughts). They have been separated within this table for a more specific comparison to child/adolescent clinical presentation. See *DSM-5* for the precise criteria.
[b]Irritability requires 4 additional symptoms to meet manic episode criteria.
[c]In mania, symptoms can be for any duration if the patient warrants hospitalization for management; hospitalization is not part of hypomania criteria.
[d]Occurs majority of the day, almost daily
[e]Occurs almost daily

provides a detailed comparison of adult versus pediatric presentation of symptoms, and the required timeframes for symptom development. When assessing for PBD, it is important to consider the following: (1) hyperactivity or dangerous play are common symptoms in childhood disorders, and therefore, other underlying causes of the behavior/mood changes should be ruled out; (2) a lively imagination, having high energy, and bragging/exaggerating are common, normal childhood behaviors; and (3) as previously stated, behavior should always be compared against a child's individual baseline and what is expected for that child's developmental level.[4] Apart from the *DSM-5* criteria, a gold standard for diagnosis in PBD is still lacking.[4]

Two diagnostic questionnaires are extensively used: Kiddie Schedule for Affective Disorders and Schizophrenia (K-SADS) and Washington University in St. Louis K-SADS.[4] Another questionnaire, the Young Mania Rating Scale (YMRS), is reserved for symptom and treatment response assessments and is not considered a diagnostic tool.[4] The general diagnosis for BPI requires that the individual meets the criteria for at least one manic episode (Table 1). For BPII, the diagnosis requires that the individual meets at least one major depressive and one hypomanic episode, with no occurrence of a manic episode (Table 1). The symptoms that an individual experiences from depression, or interchange between hypomania and depression, must either cause clinically significant distress or debilitate the patient's ability to function in an important area of life (e.g., socially/relationally, academically, professionally). Furthermore, any manic, hypomanic, or major depressive episode(s) cannot be the result of schizophrenia, schizoaffective or schizophreniform disorders, or psychotic or delusional disorders.[1] An additional specifier, "with rapid cycling," should be added to an individual's bipolar diagnosis if they have four or more mood changes (e.g., mania to depression) within a 1-year period.[1]

TREATMENT

TREATMENT GOALS

Therapy goals include the following: (1) treating the current mood symptoms, such as acute mania, acute depression; (2) preventing or decreasing the frequency of future mood episodes by the use of maintenance pharmacotherapy, which also includes decreasing subthreshold symptoms, affective cycling, unstable mood, and risk of suicide; (3) educating the patient and family regarding the course of the mental disorder and potential pharmacotherapy and nonpharmacotherapy options; (4) emphasizing medication adherence for optimal treatment success; (5) supporting the patient's normal growth, development, and overall wellness; (6) decreasing morbidity (including morbidity related to social and vocational settings); and (7) improving psychosocial function.[4,12]

TREATMENT ALGORITHMS FOR ACUTE AND MAINTENANCE THERAPIES

When selecting a pharmacotherapy option for a child or adolescent, the clinician should choose from the pediatric treatments that have label approval from the U.S. Food and Drug Administration (FDA), if possible; however, it is also appropriate to choose a medication approved for BPD in adults.[4] These medications include mood stabilizers, such as divalproex and lithium, and second-generation antipsychotics (SGAs), such as risperidone and quetiapine. Table 2 provides a list of treatment options for PBD that have FDA label approval. As mentioned in the treatment goals, there are two phases of BPD to consider: acute treatment and maintenance treatment. Therapy selection depends on the patient's symptom phase. For example, lithium can be used to treat both the acute phase of mania and serve as a maintenance therapy, versus aripiprazole, which can be used for the acute treatment of mania or mixed mood episodes.[17,18]

Table 2. Medications with FDA Label Approval for Pediatric Bipolar Disorder[17,18,22,25,37-41,67-69]

Generic Name	Brand Name	Indications by Patient Age	Formulations	Dosage and Administration	Common Adverse Effects in Pediatrics
Atypical Antipsychotics					
Aripiprazole	Abilify,[a] Abilify Discmelt[b]	Bipolar I disorder: acute treatment of mania or mixed episodes as monotherapy or adjunct to lithium or valproate in children and adolescents 10–17 yr	Oral tablet: 2, 5, 10, 15, 20, 30 mg Orally dissolvable tablet: 10, 15 mg Oral solution: 1 mg/mL	Titration schedule: 2 mg/day for 2 days, 5 mg/day for 2 days, and then 10 mg/day; titrate by 5 mg/day increments when needed Recommended target dose: 10 mg/day Maximum dose: 30 mg/day	Somnolence, nausea, extrapyramidal symptoms, fatigue, weight gain, akathisia, dizziness, blurred vision, salivary hypersecretion
Olanzapine	Zyprexa,[c] Zyprexa Zydis[c]	Bipolar I disorder: acute treatment of mania or mixed episodes and maintenance treatment, as monotherapy in children and adolescents 13–17 yr	Oral tablet: 2.5, 5, 7.5, 10, 15, 20 mg Orally dissolvable tablet: 5, 10, 15, 20 mg	Initial dose: 2.5–5 mg/day, titrate by 2.5–5 mg increments when needed Recommended target dose: 10 mg/day Maximum dose: 20 mg/day	Weight gain, increased appetite, sedation, fatigue, dry mouth, headache, dizziness, abdominal pain, pain in extremity
Olanzapine/ fluoxetine	Symbyax[d]	Bipolar I disorder: acute treatment of depressive episodes in children and adolescents 10–17 yr	Oral capsule: olanzapine 3 mg/fluoxetine 25 mg, 6 mg/25 mg, 6 mg/50 mg, 12 mg/50 mg	Initial dose: 3 mg/25 mg daily Recommended target dose: 6 mg/25 mg - 12 mg/50 mg Maximum dose: 12 mg/50 mg daily	Sedation, weight gain, appetite increase, triglyceride increase, hepatic enzyme increase, tremor
Quetiapine	Seroquel,[e] Seroquel XR[e]	Bipolar I disorder: acute treatment of manic episode as monotherapy in children and adolescents 10–17 yr	Oral tablet: 25, 50, 100, 200, 300, 400 mg Oral tablet, extended release: 50, 150, 200, 300, 400 mg	Titration schedule: Using *immediate-release* formulation: *Day 1:* 25 mg BID; *day 2:* 50 mg BID; *day 3:* 100 mg BID; *day 4:* 150 mg BID; *day 5:* 200 mg BID; increase by no more than 100 mg/day thereafter Recommended dose: 400–600 mg/day (may be administered in divided doses three times daily) Maximum dose: 600 mg/day Titration schedule: Using *extended-release* formulation: *day 1:* 50 mg/day; *day 2:* 100 mg/day; *day 3:* 200 mg/day; *day 4:* 300 mg/day; *day 5:* 400 mg/day Recommended dose: 400–600 mg/day Maximum dose: 600 mg/day	Somnolence, dizziness, increased appetite, weight gain, dry mouth, tachycardia, fatigue, nausea, vomiting
Risperidone	Risperdal,[f] Risperdal M-tab[f]	Bipolar I disorder: acute treatment of mania or mixed episodes as monotherapy in children and adolescents 10–17 yr	Oral tablet: 0.25, 0.5, 1, 2, 3, 4 mg Orally dissolvable tablet: 0.25, 0.5, 1, 2, 3, 4 mg Oral solution: 1 mg/mL	Initial dose: 0.5 mg/day, titrating by 0.5–1 mg increments per day Target dose: 1–2.5 mg/day Effective dose range: 1-6 mg/day Maximum dose: 6 mg/day	Sedation, somnolence dizziness, fatigue, nausea, extrapyramidal symptoms, weight gain, hyperprolactinemia

(continued)

Table 2. Medications with FDA Label Approval for Pediatric Bipolar Disorder[17,18,22,25,37-41,67-69] *(continued)*

Generic Name	Brand Name	Indications by Patient Age	Formulations	Dosage and Administration	Common Adverse Effects in Pediatrics
Atypical Antipsychotics *(continued)*					
Asenapine	Saphris[g]	Bipolar I disorder: acute treatment of manic or mixed episodes as monotherapy in children and adolescents 10–17 yr	Oral sublingual tablet: 2.5, 5, 10 mg	Initial dose: 2.5 mg BID Recommended dose: 2.5–10 mg BID Maximum dose: 10 mg BID	Somnolence, fatigue dizziness, dysgeusia, oral paresthesia, nausea, increased appetite, increased weight
Lurasidone	Latuda[h]	Bipolar I disorder: treatment of depressive episode as monotherapy in children and adolescents 10-17 yr	Oral tablet: 20, 40, 60, 80, 120 mg	Initial dose: 20 mg/day; may titrate dose after one week Recommended dose: 20-80 mg/day Maximum dose: 80 mg/day	Weight gain, nausea, insomnia
Mood Stabilizers					
Lithium	Lithium carbonate, lithium citrate, Eskalith CR,[i] Lithobid[j]	Bipolar I disorder: acute treatment of manic or mixed episodes or maintenance treatment in children and adolescents ≥ 7 yr	Oral capsule, as lithium carbonate: 150, 300, 600 mg capsule Oral tablet, controlled release as lithium carbonate: 300, 450 mg Oral syrup, as lithium citrate: 8 mEq/5 mL (equivalent to 300 mg of lithium carbonate immediate release capsules/tablets)	*Dosing based on lithium carbonate capsules* For patients weighing 20-30 kg Initial dose: 300 mg BID Dose titration: 300 mg/week Acute treatment goal: serum level 0.8 - 1.2 mEq/L (usual dose: 600 - 1500 mg/day in divided doses) Maintenance treatment goal: serum level 0.8 - 1 mEq/L (usual dose: 600 - 1200 mg/day in divided doses) For patients weighing > 30 kg Initial dose: 300 mg TID Dose titration: 300 mg every 3 days Acute treatment goal: serum level 0.8 - 1.2 mEq/L (usual dose: 600 mg two to three times daily) Maintenance treatment goal: serum level 0.8 - 1 mEq/L (usual dose: 300 - 600 mg two to three times daily)	Nausea, tremor, diarrhea, weight gain, sedation

[a]Otsuka, Tokyo, Japan or Bristol-Myers Squibb Co., Princeton, NJ; [b]Bristol-Myers Squibb Co., Princeton, NJ; [c]Lilly USA, LLC, Indianapolis, IN; [d]Lilly USA, LLC, Indianapolis, IN; [e]AstraZeneca, Wilmington, DE; [f]Janssen Ortho, LLC, Gurabo, Puerto Rico; [g]Allergan USA, Inc., Irvine, CA; [h]Sunovion Pharmaceuticals Inc., Marlborough, MA; [i]GlaxoSmithKline, manufactured by Cardian Health, Winchester, KY; [j]ANU Pharmaceuticals, Inc., Baltimore, MD.
BID = twice daily; CR = controlled release; FDA = U.S. Food and Drug Administration; XR = extended release

The child/adolescent treatment guidelines published in 2005 and 2007, both by the American Academy of Child and Adolescent Psychiatry (AACAP), mainly focus on BPI because it is the most studied in children and adolescents and because of the lack of evidence of BPII in this population.[4,12] Furthermore, it is noted in the AACAP 2005 guidelines that the recommendations are not to serve as "an absolute standard of medical or psychological care."[12] The Canadian Network for Mood and Anxiety Treatments (CANMAT) and International Society for Bipolar Disorders (ISBD) released a guideline in early 2018 for the treatment of BPD. Within this text is a specific section that addresses children and adolescents. Given the roughly 11- to 13-year gap between the AACAP and CANMAT/ISBD guidelines, there are some differences in treatment recommendations and therapeutic approaches, such as the first-line and second-line therapies. To differentiate between the guidelines, Table 3 provides the 2018 CANMAT/ISBD recommendations and Figure 1 provides the 2005 AACAP recommendations. The therapeutic approaches are based on varying degrees of evidence, ranging from placebo-controlled, randomized clinical trials to expert/clinical opinion/adult treatment experience. The evidence levels are defined within each respective guideline, and readers are encouraged to review them because the details are beyond the scope of this chapter. The treatments discussed in this section are derived from these guidelines.

Commonly, it is recommended that a medication trial lasts 6 to 8 weeks at therapeutic blood concentrations or adequate doses to determine treatment efficacy; this trial should be done before changing or adding a medication.[4] Figure 1 provides a treatment algorithm for BPI (acute, manic or mixed) in the pediatric population. It is divided into two parts: with psychosis and without psychosis, and each algorithm progresses through six stages of treatment. It is important to note that the guidelines do not provide a definitive conclusion regarding which agents in stage 1 should be first- or second-line; however, most authors in the guideline panel recommend divalproex or lithium as a first-line agent for nonpsychotic mania.[12] The CANMAT/ISBD guideline divides treatment recommendations based on bipolar symptoms and phases: acute mania, acute depression, and maintenance therapies. Within each symptom category are the medication recommendations beginning with first line.

In Figure 1, part 1, which shows treatment for patients *without psychosis*, three primary atypical antipsychotics are suggested (risperidone, quetiapine, olanzapine) and three primary mood stabilizers are suggested (carbamazepine, lithium, valproic acid). The premise is that a patient begins monotherapy with one of the two drug classes. How the patient responds will guide further treatment decisions. In the case of no response or if the therapy is intolerable, then it is recommended to switch to an alternate agent (either within the same drug class or from the other drug class). For example, in the case of a child on a trial of lithium for 8 weeks at therapeutic blood concentrations who achieves no improvement in bipolar symptoms, the clinician and parents could now decide to switch the child to valproic acid or risperidone. Conversely, if the child achieved partial improvement with lithium, the clinician and parents may decide to add a second medication (either a mood stabilizer or atypical antipsychotic) to help augment the lithium therapy and ultimately achieve a better symptom response. The AACAP guideline recommends alternative therapies outside of the six main drugs listed once a patient reaches stage 5, having not achieved desired response with the first-line recommended agents. At this point, ziprasidone, aripiprazole, and oxcarbazepine are potential options. Lastly in stage 6, if all other recommended treatment options fail, electroconvulsive therapy (ECT) can be considered for adolescents *only*, and clozapine therapy can be considered for children or adolescents. Clozapine has demonstrated potential efficacy in a small, open-label trial of 10 adolescents; however, because of adverse effects and the need for further study, it should be reserved for cases in which first-line pharmacotherapy was ineffective.[13]

In cases of BPI *with psychosis* (Figure 1, part 2), the initial therapy options change. The guidelines recommend a mood stabilizer *plus* atypical antipsychotic (vs. monotherapy in cases without psychosis). In fact, throughout stages 1–4, combination therapy is recommended. Stages 5 and 6 have the same recommendations as the algorithm for without psychosis. The evidence available in the earlier guidelines is limited by small sample sizes or the lack of placebo-controlled randomized clinical trials. The CANMAT/ISBD guidelines also make note of limited evidence, with particular paucity for the treatment of acute bipolar depression.[19] There remains more research to be

Table 3. Summary of Treatment Recommendations for Children and Adolescents from the 2018 CANMAT/ISBD Guidelines[19]

Symptom	Treatment Choice	Recommendation[a]	
Acute mania	First line	Lithium	
		Risperidone	
		Aripiprazole	
		Asenapine	
		Quetiapine	
	Second line	Olanzapine	
		Ziprasidone	
		Quetiapine as adjunct treatment	
	Third line	Divalproex	
	NOT recommended	*Oxcarbazepine*	
Acute depression	First line	Lurasidone	
	Second line	Lithium	
		Lamotrigine	
	Third line	Olanzapine/fluoxetine	
		Quetiapine	
	NOT recommended	*Oxcarbazepine*	
Maintenance	First line	Aripiprazole	
		Lithium	
		Divalproex	
		Lamotrigine as adjunct treatment for age ≥ 13 years	
	Second line	*No current therapy meets the sufficient evidence threshold to make recommendation*	
	Third line	Asenapine	
		Risperidone	
		Quetiapine	
		Ziprasidone	

[a]Only treatments with a stated level evidence in the guideline are listed; review guideline for full list of treatments discussed in this population for acute mania, acute depression, and maintenance

CANMAT = Canadian Network for Mood and Anxiety Treatments; ISBD = International Society for Bipolar Disorders.

conducted for PBD, particularly in regard to safety and as new medications are developed and approved for the treatment of BPD.

Since the publication of the earlier AACAP guidelines, there have been new studies and new atypical antipsychotics released into the market. Aripiprazole, asenapine, olanzapine, quetiapine, and risperidone have all received FDA label approval for the acute treatment of manic or mixed episodes in BPI.[13] One of the authors of the AACAP guidelines published an article in 2016 reviewing these five antipsychotics, noting their favorable efficacy in PBD symptom reduction.[13] In addition, although ziprasidone does not have

FDA label approval, preliminary data may show some efficacy.[13] Atypical antipsychotics tend to be the preferred first-line choice (vs. mood stabilizers) because of the supportive evidence of efficacy; however, their adverse effect profiles can be worse.[13,20] The CANMAT/ISBD guideline addresses these newer antipsychotic agents, placing asenapine, for example, as a first-line option for acute mania.[19] Combination therapy is commonly seen in practice for the treatment of PBD; however, this approach excludes the use of combination antipsychotics because this therapy has no data to support it and may increase the risk of adverse drug reactions.[20] However, data from large, controlled studies are needed to assess atypical

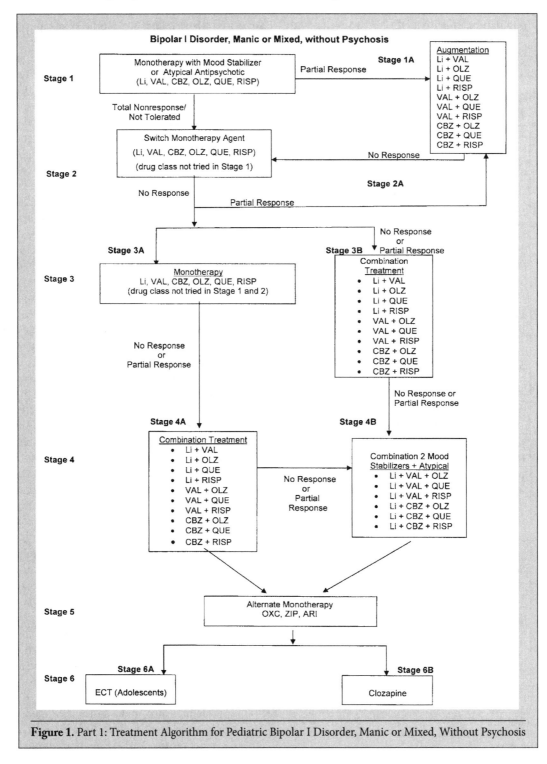

Figure 1. Part 1: Treatment Algorithm for Pediatric Bipolar I Disorder, Manic or Mixed, Without Psychosis

antipsychotic plus mood stabilizer combination to further support initial evidence of safety and efficacy.[20]

ACUTE THERAPIES

For the acute treatment of BPI depressive episodes, antidepressants are not typically recommended because of the risk of inducing mania, particularly if they are used as monotherapy. Use of these agents to treat depression in BPD is controversial overall because of scarcity of evidence.[12,21] One article cites that antidepressant use in BPD is simply data extrapolation from their efficacy and use in unipolar depression.[21] Although the data are contradictory, some studies have found patients are at risk of switching into mania with use of tricyclic antidepressants, selective serotonin reuptake inhibitors, or serotonin/norepinephrine reuptake inhibitors.[21] Because of this risk and the lack of data, it is not recommended to use an antidepressant as monotherapy in

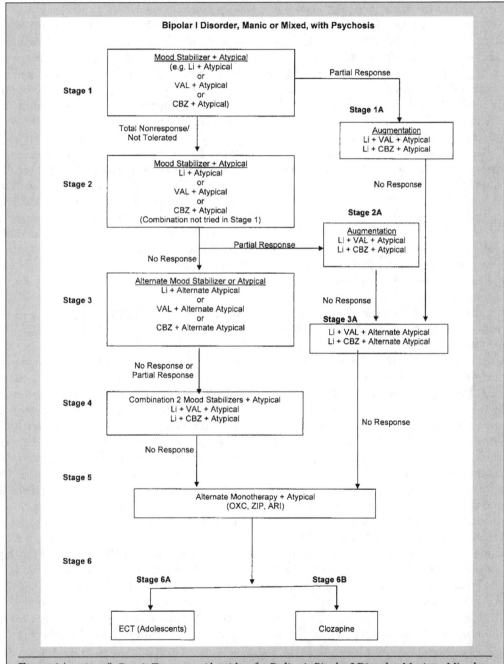

Figure 1 (*continued*). Part 2: Treatment Algorithm for Pediatric Bipolar I Disorder, Manic or Mixed, With Psychosis

ARI = aripiprazole; CBZ = carbamazepine; ECT = electroconvulsive therapy; Li = lithium; OLZ = olanzapine; OXC = oxcarbazepine; QUE = quetiapine; RISP = risperidone; VAL = valproate; ZIP = ziprasidone.

Reprinted with permission from Kowatch RA, Fristad M, Birmaher B, et al. Treatment guidelines for children and adolescents with bipolar disorder. J Am Acad Child Adolesc Psychiatry 2005;44:213-35.

adults, children, or adolescents with BPD; however, if use is necessary, an antidepressant should be concomitantly prescribed with an antimanic medication (e.g., mood stabilizer) to decrease risk of mania.[12,13,19,21] No treatment algorithm for bipolar depression was created for the AACAP 2005 guideline because of insufficient evidence; however, the CANMAT/ISBD 2018 guideline does provide some treatment guidance for acute depression.[12,19] Currently the only antidepressant with FDA label approval for use in BPD is fluoxetine in combination with the atypical antipsychotic, olanzapine. This combination is approved for the acute treatment of depressive disorders in BPI for both adults and children and adolescents.[22] This combination has demonstrated efficacy in children and adolescents.[13] Based on the AACAP guideline, other potential options for treatment include lithium with or without divalproex for children and adolescents, and ECT for adolescents if their bipolar depression is severe and treatment resistant.[12] The CANMAT/ISBD guideline suggests lurasidone, lithium, lamotrigine, olanzapine/fluoxetine, and quetiapine (Table 3).[19] More studies need to be conducted that assess pharmacotherapy (and nonpharmacotherapy) options for the treatment of PBD-related depression.

MAINTENANCE THERAPIES

Recall the treatment goals mentioned at the beginning of the treatment section, in particular that the goal of maintenance therapy is to reduce patient relapse/mood episode recurrence, ultimately keeping the patient stable. Maintenance therapy may include continuation of the patient's current acute treatment (if the patient is tolerating it and has had improvement).[12] One recent study assessed various medications for maintenance treatment in PBD in 210 patients age 10 to 17 years who were randomized to aripiprazole (10 mg/day or 30 mg/day) or placebo.[13] Investigators found that although only one-third of patients completed the study, more patients in the aripiprazole arms continued versus placebo, and those in the aripiprazole arms had a statistically significant improvement in YMRS scores (p<0.001). In addition, an aripiprazole maintenance discontinuation study of 60 patients age 4 to 9 years determined a statistically significant greater length of time until discontinuation for the aripiprazole versus placebo arm; also, no patient stopped aripiprazole secondary to an adverse drug event.[13] In a study with 60 patients stabilized on acute combination therapy with divalproex and lithium, investigators randomized patients age 5 to 17 years to receive either divalproex or lithium monotherapy for maintenance.[13] Results illustrated comparable efficacy between the two therapies, with median time to relapse of 112 days for divalproex and 114 days for lithium. Lastly, researchers evaluated the use of lamotrigine or placebo as adjunct therapy for 36 weeks in 173 patients age 10 to 17 years. In evaluating time to occurrence of a bipolar event, investigators found no statistically significant difference in efficacy between placebo and treatment arms.[13] However, in patients age 13 to 17 years, the treatment arm postponed the time to mood episode recurrence.[13]

In adults, once the individual is stabilized, maintenance therapy is recommended to continue for at least 18 months.[12] For children/adolescents, the AACAP guidelines recommend that once remission has been achieved for *at least* 12 to 24 consecutive months, the clinician can consider tapering the medication to discontinuation; however, lifelong or longer term therapy may be warranted for some patients on an individual basis.[4,12] Discontinuing pharmacotherapy can place the patient at increased risk of a relapse.[4] However, the risk of emerging adverse drug reactions, particularly in children younger than 10 years, must also be considered.[13] Therefore, the risks versus benefits for each patient should be considered before discontinuation or the decision for long-term therapy. A specific subpopulation at greater risk of relapse includes children and adolescents with a history of psychosis, severe aggression, and/or suicidality.[12] On deciding to stop pharmacotherapy, the AACAP guidelines recommend the following approach: (1) taper to discontinuation, and do not cease abruptly because this approach can prompt medication withdrawal; (2) begin medication taper when it is deemed that the patient is at the least risk of negative consequences, such as possible academic or social dysfunction; and (3) monitor closely for any signs of a potential change in mood, together with a stable environment for the patient.[12] To help prevent the child or adolescent from relapsing, family and friends should be aware that environmental and emotional triggers can play a role; therefore, involving these individuals to monitor for the patient's stress, lack of sleep, and any other harmful factors can help keep the environment stable and lower risk of relapse or recurrence.[12]

MEDICATIONS FOR PBD

ANTIPSYCHOTICS

Atypical antipsychotics, otherwise known as *second-generation antipsychotics*, are a large class of medications used in PBD. The mechanism of action of SGAs in the treatment of PBD is not fully understood, but it is likely that dopamine and serotonin-receptor blockade contributes to their efficacy in the acute treatment of mania or mixed states. This blockade results in decreased dopamine receptor (DA_2) transmission in the mesolimbic pathway and increased DA_2 transmission in the mesocortical pathway. Although the SGAs with FDA label approval are all in the same drug *class*, they do not all possess exactly the same mechanisms of action. Notably, their receptor binding affinities to serotonin-2A and DA_2 are different. For example, olanzapine has higher affinity for serotonin-2A than for DA_2, but aripiprazole has higher binding affinity for DA_2 than for serotonin-2A.[23,24] This distinction is a brief example of the differing mechanisms of action because the pharmacology of this drug class is quite complex. In fact, SGAs bind to a host of different serotonin and dopamine receptor subtypes (e.g., serotonin-1A, D_3) in addition to histaminic, adrenergic, and muscarinic receptors, the details of which go beyond the scope of this chapter.[23,24] Not all antipsychotics are approved for use in BPD or PBD. Some SGAs have indications for specific symptoms (e.g., lurasidone used for bipolar depression in adults, adolescents, and children) whereas others within the same class do not (e.g., aripiprazole used for manic or mixed episodes in adult and pediatric BPD).[17,25]

Two different studies looked at the impact of aripiprazole in both the acute treatment phase and maintenance phase. In the acute phase, a 4-week study enrolled 296 participants age 10 to 17 years randomized to aripiprazole or placebo.[26] At the end of week four, aripiprazole demonstrated statistically significant changes in YMRS scores from baseline (primary efficacy end point) of –14.2 (10-mg dose) and –16.5 (30-mg dose). Adverse drug reactions that occurred in more than 10% of participants in the aripiprazole 10-mg arm of 98 patients included somnolence, fatigue, headache, and extrapyramidal disorder; adverse drug reactions in the aripiprazole 30-mg arm of 99 patients included somnolence, headache, extrapyramidal disorder, akathisia, and nausea. The most common extrapyramidal symptoms (greater than 10%) were Parkinsonism (both doses), and akathisia (30-mg dose). In the second study, some participants from the acute, 4-week study were continued into the 26-week extension trial to assess long-term efficacy, safety and tolerability.[27] A similar adverse drug reactions profile was noted in these patients, together with improvement in the mean change of the YMRS scores. The investigators did note, however, that there was a high dropout rate, making data analysis more challenging.

In a 3-week, double-blind, randomized trial in patients age 13 to 17 years with BPI, olanzapine in 107 patients was compared against placebo in 54 patients.[28] This trial aimed to assess the efficacy of olanzapine through mean change in YMRS from baseline to end point. Investigators found that the mean change in YMRS (last observation carried forward [LOCF] end point) was improved in the olanzapine arm versus placebo (p<0.001).[28] Regarding safety, olanzapine illustrated significantly higher rates of weight gain (3.66 kg, SD=2.18, p<0.001), appetite increase, somnolence, and sedation; other negative metabolic effects associated with olanzapine also occurred in the trial, including increased blood pressure, increased fasting blood glucose, and elevated prolactin.[28] In another trial that was open label and lasted 8 weeks, 23 patients age 5 to 14 years with BPI were given olanzapine monotherapy, with significant improvement in the YMRS total score from baseline to end point (LOCF; p<0.001).[29] The most common adverse drug events included somnolence, increased appetite, weight gain (mean increase of 5 ± 2.3 kg, p<0.001), and abdominal pain. In addition, there was a statistically significant mean change from baseline to end point in prolactin (p=0.002).[29]

In a pediatric study of patients age 10 to 17 years, quetiapine demonstrated efficacy over placebo for the treatment of BPI.[30] In this study, quetiapine treatment arms demonstrated significant improvement in the total YMRS score versus the placebo arm (p<0.001). Most common adverse effects in those treated with quetiapine included sedation, somnolence, headache, and dizziness.[30] Of note, however, the trial duration was only 3 weeks. Another study assessed the use of quetiapine monotherapy in participants age 4–15 years with a bipolar spectrum disorder.[31] Participants were divided into two age groups: 4–6 years and 6–15 years. The prospective, open-label study spanned 8 weeks, and the mean dose of quetiapine at the end of week eight was 175.8 ± 63.8 mg/day and 248.7 ± 153.1 mg/day, respectively. Investigators found statistically significant improvement in mean YMRS scores (LOCF analysis) for those on quetiapine (p<0.001 for preschool and school-age children), and the drug was well tolerated; however, quetiapine did cause statistically significant weight gain, with a mean change of 3.4 ± 3.5 kg (p<0.001).[31]

Risperidone was evaluated for the treatment of acute mania in a randomized, double-blind study.[32] Individuals age 10 to 17 years were randomized to either risperidone 0.5–2.5 mg/day or 3–6 mg/day (n=111 both arms), or placebo (n=58) for 3 weeks (intent to treat population). Investigators aimed to evaluate the efficacy and safety or risperidone. They found statistically significant improvement in the YMRS total score from baseline with the risperidone arms (p<0.001). Most commonly noted adverse events were fatigue, somnolence, and headache. Risperidone versus placebo showed similarity in the percentage of subjects with at least one reported extrapyramidal symptom (EPS) adverse event (5% placebo, 8% in risperidone 0.5–2.5 mg group), with notably higher EPS reports in the risperidone 3–6 mg group (25%). There was a dose-dependent elevation in prolactin concentrations (reported by 2% in placebo, 4% in 0.5–2.5 mg risperidone, and 5% in 3–6 mg risperidone arms).[32]

A study comparing asenapine versus placebo for the acute treatment of mania or mixed episodes in PBD was completed in patients age 10 to 17 years.[33] In this study asenapine had statistically significant changes in YMRS scores: –3.2 (2.5 mg twice daily), –5.3 (5 mg twice daily), and –6.2 (10 mg twice daily); however, numerous adverse effects occurred in the asenapine arms, notably metabolic changes such as weight gain. A second, open-label, extension trial, including some patients from the first trial, addressed the safety of asenapine over 50 weeks.[34] Although no pre-specified end points were indicated, the investigators mainly sought to examine key safety events from baseline to study's end. Most common adverse drug reactions in this trial were somnolence, weight gain, sedation, and headaches. Investigators recommended metabolic monitoring when using this medication, which is in keeping with the SGA class (i.e., the potential for metabolic syndrome).[34]

To date, the only SGA long-acting injectables that carry an FDA label approval for BPD are Risperdal Consta (Janssen Pharmaceuticals Inc., Titusville, NJ) and Abilify Maintena (Otsuka Pharmaceutical Co., Tokyo, Japan). Both are indicated as maintenance therapy for BPI in adults, with Risperal Consta used as monotherapy or adjunct to lithium or valproate, and Abilify Maintena used as monotherapy.[35,36] Neither have FDA label approval for the use of PBD. Originally, lurasidone had only FDA label approval for bipolar depression in adults, but in 2018 the approval was extended to include pediatric patients.[25] Clozapine has significant adverse effects that require monitoring more often, and it does not have FDA label approval for PBD but may be useful in the treatment of refractory patients who have a diagnosis of PBD.[4,12] Lower doses of atypical antipsychotics are used in pediatric patients than in adult patients, and dose titration is more conservative (Table 2).

In general SGAs are well absorbed when administered orally; they are also highly lipophilic and highly bound to plasma proteins. In addition, they have long half-lives, which allow once-daily administration for most of the medications.

A few of the SGAs have multiple formulations, such as a dissolvable tablet, which may be potentially helpful in children and adolescents who prefer not to or are unable to swallow tablets or capsules (Table 2). The SGAs approved for PBD—plus clozapine because it is used off-label but considered as a last-line agent—have various metabolism pathways. They are mostly metabolized in the liver by the cytochrome P450 (CYP) pathways, and most have major and minor pathways through several CYPs. A few examples of those metabolized through different pathways include: CYP2D6 (risperidone, aripiprazole, olanzapine, clozapine), CYP3A4 (aripiprazole, quetiapine, clozapine, lurasidone), and CYP1A2 (asenapine, clozapine and olanzapine). In addition to CYP metabolism, asenapine and olanzapine also undergo glucuronidation. In the combination drug olanzapine/fluoxetine, fluoxetine is a known inhibitor of CYP2D6 and olanzapine is minorly metabolized by that enzyme; therefore, fluoxetine does slightly decrease olanzapine clearance, but it was not deemed to be clinically significant.[22] Other medications can affect the blood concentrations of the SGAs through induction or inhibition the CYP system. When combined with lithium or valproic acid/divalproex, which is common in the treatment of mania associated with PBD, these medications do not affect the metabolism of the antipsychotics, but additive adverse effects may be seen.[4,17,18,25,37-44]

The major pediatric adverse effects for antipsychotics that have FDA label approval for PBD are listed in Table 2. In this section, we will discuss common adverse effects associated with the SGA drug class. Although the SGAs have similar adverse effects overall (e.g., sedation and weight gain), certain medications may be more likely to cause specific adverse effects, particularly in the pediatric population. For example, risperidone is more likely to cause increases in prolactin (leading to gynecomastia, amenorrhea, and sexual dysfunction) and EPS.[45] Olanzapine and clozapine are more likely to cause increased weight, increased appetite, hyperglycemia, and hyperlipidemia.[45] Quetiapine is more likely to cause dizziness or somnolence, and aripiprazole is more likely to cause nausea and restlessness, such as akathisia.[17,39] In 2016, an additional warning of pathological gambling and other compulsive behaviors was added to all prescribing information for aripiprazole.[17] Clozapine causes hyperlipidemia, hyperglycemia, sedation, and orthostatic hypotension, and carries several black box warnings.[42] In addition, patients receiving clozapine need to be monitored for severe neutropenia weekly for the first 6 months, every other week for the next 6 months, and then once a month. Although rare, all atypical antipsychotics confer some risk of tardive dyskinesia and neuroleptic malignant syndrome, and should be monitored in all patients. Antidepressants have a black box warning for increased risk of suicidal thinking and behavior for children and adolescents. Given that there does exist a combination therapy of olanzapine/fluoxetine for the treatment of PBD, parents, guardians, and clinicians should monitor for this behavior.[22] Of note, Health Canada published safety alerts in September 2017 and April 2018 on several SGAs regarding the risk of sleepwalking/sleep-related–eating disorder and drug reaction with eosinophilia and systemic symptoms.[46] It will be important to follow these risks and any other safety changes that arise.

MOOD STABILIZERS

LITHIUM

The mechanism of action for lithium in the treatment and prevention of mania and depression is largely unknown, but it may have a positive effect on many of the theorized pathophysiologies in PBD such as normalizing second-messenger systems and regulating neurotransmitters and gene expression. Lithium has FDA label approval for BPD in patients age 7 years and older.[4,18] The decision to approve lithium was based on data extrapolated from adult studies.[4,13] One article discusses the studies in the Collaborative Lithium Trials, which were conducted to assess lithium's safety and efficacy in pediatric patients age 7 to 17 years with BPI.[13] Those studies found the drug was generally well tolerated, with the most common adverse effects being nausea and vomiting. In terms of efficacy, the investigators found that lithium versus placebo had improvements in clinical global impressions, as well as amelioration of mania symptoms. The drug has also been evaluated for the use of bipolar depression. A study of 28 patients 12 to 18 years with a depressive episode in BPI received open-label lithium dosed at 30 mg/kg (divided twice a day) with target serum concentrations (1.0–1.2 mEq/L).[47] Results showed tolerability and a decrease from baseline in the Child Depression Rating Scale-Revised (CDRS-R) and YMRS scores; however, the response rate (50% or more reduction from baseline to end point in CDRS-R) was 48% (n=13).[47] However, the trial had a small sample size and a short duration (6 weeks). Further studies are warranted before considering lithium for the management of bipolar depression.

Whereas lithium is one of the oldest antimanic agents available, it is not without significant adverse drug reactions and clinically significant drug interactions. Lithium is mostly renally excreted and susceptible to changes in the glomerular filtration rate and sodium concentration. Specifically, a decrease in glomerular filtration rate may result in lithium accumulation. In addition, sodium depletion may result in lithium reabsorption and potential toxicity. Although children and adolescents may not use the following medications as often as adults, it is important to note the drug–drug interactions in the event that these agents are prescribed. Medications such as nonsteroidal anti-inflammatory drugs, thiazide diuretics, angiotensin-converting enzyme inhibitors, and angiotensin receptor blockers may result in an increase in lithium serum concentrations because of a decrease in the renal elimination of lithium.[18,48] Medications such as loop diuretics and acetaminophen are less likely to cause this interaction. When concomitant administration cannot be avoided, assessment of serum lithium concentrations at steady state is recommended to determine the effect of these medications and if a decrease in lithium dosing is warranted. Caffeine and medications such as theophylline and acetazolamide may cause a decrease in lithium serum concentrations because of increased renal excretion. Use of these products while on lithium require additional monitoring to ensure therapeutic serum concentrations are maintained with adequate therapeutic response.[49] Table 2 provides more details on target lithium concentration levels.

Lithium is a monovalent cation that is rapidly absorbed when administered orally. It has no protein binding or metabolism and is excreted unchanged through the urine. The half-life of lithium depends on renal function, but it is generally about 24 hours. Although lithium has a half-life that would dictate once-daily dosing, it is divided two or three times per day to improve tolerability and decrease adverse effects when administered as immediate release. Extended-release can be dosed one or two times per day. Drug interactions occur with a change in renal elimination of lithium as described in the Monitoring Guidelines section of this chpater.[18,49]

Adverse effects of lithium are usually dose related and most common when first initiated and 1–2 hours after a dose. Nausea, somnolence, diarrhea, tremor, headache, confusion, poor concentration, polydipsia, polyuria, and weight gain are common adverse effects.[18] Lithium has negative effects on the kidney as well, such as morphologic changes with long-term use. Another organ affected by long-term lithium administration is the thyroid gland because lithium can cause hypothyroidism.[18] This effect may be especially problematic for pediatric patients because thyroid hormone is essential to proper growth and development. Long-term studies to assess safety in the pediatric population are needed to differentiate possible adverse outcomes in this population versus adults.[12,49,50]

DIVALPROEX SODIUM AND VALPROIC ACID

The mechanism of action of divalproex in PBD is unclear, but it may be related to its modulating effect on sodium and calcium channels and its enhancing action on GABA. Divalproex has been studied in PBD with generally positive results, but does not have FDA label approval for PBD.[43,44,51] The FDA granted divalproex approval to treat adults for certain seizure disorders, migraine headache prophylaxis, and BPD. Divalproex is recommended for acute mania and maintenance therapy because of its efficacy in adults. Divalproex also has shown to be efficacious in the treatment of mixed states or rapid cycling patients because of its antikindling effect. Valproic acid (the nonenteric-coated formulation) may also be used, but it has the potential to cause more adverse effects than divalproex, such as worse gastrointestinal adverse drug reactions, which can ultimately lead to nonadherence. In general, the therapeutic serum drug concentration for PBD is thought to be 50–125 mcg/mL and dosing is based on weight.[4,37] The Seizure Disorders chapter provides for more information on divalproex and valproic acid.

CARBAMAZEPINE

Carbamazepine (both immediate-release and extended-release formulations) has FDA label approval for adults in the treatment of epilepsy and trigeminal neuralgia. Its mechanism of action in epilepsy involves blocking voltage-sensitive sodium channels.[23,52,53] It has a tricyclic antidepressant-like structure and thus has many potential adverse effects related to its antimuscarinic properties, resulting in poor tolerance.[54] The epoxide metabolite of carbamazepine can result in serious toxicities, particularly bone marrow suppression. Carbamazepine also causes many drug interactions (e.g., with

oral contraceptives) because it is a potent CYP3A4 inducer. In addition, carbamazepine induces its own metabolism, and dosage adjustments may be needed after 4 weeks when induction effects have been maximized.[52] As such, carbamazepine is recommended only for pediatric patients whose other options in the management of their PBD have failed.[37] A study evaluated the safety and efficacy of the extended-release formulation in 27 patients age 6 to 12 years with BPI, BPII, or BPD not otherwise specified. The study showed a modest change in the YMRS score (–10.1 ± 10.2, p <0.001), which predicted that mania symptoms were not fully resolved.[55] Investigators noted that although the change in score was statistically significant and that the drug was generally well tolerated, other controlled trials need to be conducted for more conclusive evidence.[55] Therapeutic concentrations of carbamazepine are 4–12 mcg/mL, which is the reference range used in epilepsy.[52] The Seizure Disorders chapter provides more information on carbamazepine.

OTHER STUDIED MEDICATIONS

OXCARBAZEPINE

Oxcarbazepine is a structural analog of carbamazepine with an FDA label indication for seizures in adults and children.[56] At first the drug was praised for having an improved adverse effect profile and fewer drug interactions than carbamazepine, but this claim is controversial. Oxcarbazepine is not a potent CYP inducer nor is it prone to autoinduction as seen with carbamazepine. Adverse effects include dizziness, somnolence, diplopia, rash, and hyponatremia.[50,56] A small study on this drug was conducted in 116 patients age 7 to 18 years with BPI, of which 73 completed the trial.[57] Investigators compared oxcarbazepine against placebo to assess the mean change of the YMRS (primary end point) from baseline to end and safety. Investigators found no difference between the drug and placebo in the primary end point (YMRS adjusted mean change was –10.90 oxcarbazepine and –9.79 placebo). There was a 90% incidence of adverse drug reactions in the oxcarbazepine arm versus 79% in placebo. In addition, 11 patients discontinued the study because of oxcarbazepine adverse effects (vs. two discontinuations in the placebo arm).[57] The Seizure Disorders chapter provides more information on oxcarbazepine.

LAMOTRIGINE

Lamotrigine has FDA label approval for the maintenance treatment of BPI in adults to delay the onset time of a mood episode in patients already being treated for an acute mood episode. It is not recommended for the use of acute treatment, and is not approved for the use of PBD.[58] The mechanism of action of lamotrigine involves inhibiting voltage-sensitive sodium channels; of importance, this drug has a specific dose titration based on the risk of a life-threatening rash (e.g., Stevens-Johnson syndrome, toxic epidermal necrolysis).[58] Dose adjustments are also required if the patient receives concomitant carbamazepine, divalproex, or any other medication that can induce or inhibit enzyme metabolism of lamotrigine.[58] A PBD study in the age range of 8 to 18 years enrolled 48 patients (46 treated) to evaluate lamotrigine for maintenance treatment in manic and depressive symptoms.[59] Improvement in the manic symptoms using YMRS (primary efficacy measure) resulted in a response rate of 72% at 14 weeks; and the depressive symptoms using the CDRS-R resulted in a response rate of 82%. Remission rate at the end of 14 weeks was 56% with a mean lamotrigine dose of 1.8 mg/kg. Whereas lamotrigine was used in combination with an SGA (for acute stabilization), lamotrigine illustrated positive results for maintenance control evidenced by the results from week eight to 14. Moreover, during the monotherapy phase patients continued to improve with their depressive symptoms as an additional 34.8% of subjects reached remission.[59] The Seizure Disorders chapter provides more information on lamotrigine.

TOPIRAMATE

Topiramate carries an FDA label approval for epilepsy and migraine prophylaxis in both adults and children.[60] This drug has four properties that assist in seizure control and may also help with mood stabilization: (1) enhances GABA at some of the GABA-A receptor subtypes, (2) blocks voltage-dependent sodium channels, (3) inhibits carbonic anhydrase, and (4) blocks one of the glutamate receptor subtypes.[60] In a pilot study, topiramate monotherapy was assessed against placebo for treatment efficacy in acute mania for children age 6 to 17 years.[61] Investigators claim the drug was well tolerated; however, data were inconclusive because of early termination secondary to another study illustrating lack of adult efficacy. Regarding the pharmacokinetic data and adverse reactions with topiramate, the Seizure Disorders chapter provides for more information.

COMBINATION TREATMENTS

Both SGAs and mood stabilizers can be combined to achieve optimum symptom control for the acute treatment phase and the maintenance treatment phase.[12] A small prospective study (fewer than 100 patients) addressed the combination of risperidone plus either divalproex or lithium, for manic or mixed episodes in PBD in participants age 5 to 18 years.[62] Both pharmacotherapy combinations were well tolerated with statistically significant improvements in the YMRS, CDRS-R, and Clinical Global Impression Scale for Bipolar Disorder mean scores from baseline. As discussed in the Treatment Algorithm section of this chapter, combination treatment can be considered when monotherapy provides no response or only a partial response, and in cases of psychosis.

OTHER TREATMENTS: ELECTROCONVULSIVE THERAPY

Electroconvulsive therapy (ECT) may be considered for those patients where pharmacotherapy fails or is intolerable; however, literature support is lacking.[4,12] The following should be considered before initiating ECT in an adolescent patient: (1) pharmacotherapy treatment failure/intolerance (defined per the AACAP guideline, failure of Stages 1–5), (2) severe mania or depression symptoms, and (3) the individual's BPD is well defined (i.e., cannot be a diagnosis of BPD not otherwise specified or an atypical presentation of the disorder).[4] After ECT the patient may present with adverse effects such as disinhibition, short-term cognitive impairment, anxiety, and altered seizure threshold.[4]

TREATMENT MONITORING

The pediatric population is more prone to certain adverse effects—and, in some cases, different adverse effects—than adults, particularly metabolic adverse effects, and in patients younger than age 10 years.[13,19] Just as it is important to monitor for adverse effects for any adult patient, one could argue that monitoring in children and adolescents is even more vital, particularly in cases of combination therapy.[20] Given a lack of data on long-term safety for BPD pharmacotherapy, especially in children and adolescents, careful monitoring is essential, as well as a need for long-term studies.[12] Patients treated with SGAs should be monitored for metabolic adverse effects, such as elevations in blood pressure, fasting blood glucose and triglycerides, weight gain, and high-density lipoprotein cholesterol. Whereas the American Diabetes Association (ADA) has a consensus statement on antipsychotics that details the monitoring frequencies of each metabolic parameter, there is also an article that provides more specific details for pediatrics.[4,45,63] In addition, CANMAT/ISBD notes an increased risk of early cardiovascular disease and accelerated atherosclerosis, highlighting the importance of routine health evaluations in pediatric patients receiving an SGA.[19]

Researchers assessed endocrine and metabolic adverse effects of psychotropic medications in the pediatric population.[45] The article outlines the criteria for metabolic syndrome in children and adolescents as the following: (1) fasting glucose greater than or equal to 110 mg/dL (the same for adults); (2) blood pressure greater than or equal to the 90th percentile for age/sex; (3) fasting high-density lipoprotein cholesterol less than 40 mg/dL in both the male and female population; (4) fasting triglycerides greater than or equal to 110 mg/dL; and (5) waist circumference greater than or equal to the 90th percentile *or* a body mass index greater than or equal to the 95th percentile.[45,63] Body mass index is an important objective value for body fat that is based on height and weight, and normal ranges are determined by a patient's age and sex. Therefore, in children and adolescents the body mass index should be compared against growth charts to determine if the individual is within or outside the expected growth.[45] The article provides extensive detail for the timeline of assessments for all recommended laboratory tests and vital signs, and a few will be discussed here. It is important to evaluate family and personal history *before selection* of an SGA or mood stabilizer, in addition to monitoring the following: baseline height, weight, blood pressure and pulse; the values for prolactin, complete blood cell count with differential, thyroid-stimulating hormone (TSH) for quetiapine, valproate, or lithium, and serum calcium for lithium or valproate; daytime sedation; appetite; dietary/exercise habits; and sexual function.[45] Prolactin can also assist in providing objective information in the event that the patient presents with abnormal sexual signs/symptoms (e.g., erectile dysfunction, amenorrhea or oligomenorrhea).[45]

At follow up, *before initiation* of an SGA or mood stabilizer, assessment of vital signs, fasting blood work, and prolactin should be repeated. At each follow-up visit, height and weight should be assessed. Weight gain is associated with many of the SGAs, lithium, and valproic acid/divalproex. Of note, the article recommends that blood pressure and pulse be checked every 3 months; however, all vital signs are usually part of a standard physician visit so it is likely that blood pressure and pulse will be assessed each time. Blood work should be repeated at 3 months, and then every 6 months thereafter. For quetiapine, it is recommended that TSH be checked at 3 months and then annually. Other monitoring variables such as sexual function, appetite, sedation, and diet and exercise are recommended for monthly assessment for the first 3 months, and then every 3 months moving forward. Again, these are also areas that will likely be checked at every visit as part of basic mental health assessments. In addition to the aforementioned laboratory variables, other pertinent baseline assessments for lithium include urinalysis, serum creatinine, and blood urea nitrogen.[4] For valproic acid/divalproex, another baseline assessment includes liver function tests because of the medication's potential to cause hepatotoxicity.[4,43] For female patients of child-bearing age, which includes some children and adolescents, a pregnancy test should be conducted before the initiation of any medications, in addition to continued monitoring of pregnancy status throughout the duration of treatment.[4,64] Of course, these are general guidelines to follow, and evaluations of these points can occur more often, particularly if a patient develops any metabolic or endocrine abnormalities or weight gain.[45]

Although the SGAs carry less risk of EPS than typical antipsychotics (i.e., first-generation antipsychotics), there is still a potential risk, such as with risperidone, which has had reports of tardive dyskinesia in pediatric patients.[23,40] Therefore, the patient should be monitored for abnormal/involuntary movements at each visit. The abnormal involuntary movement scale is one of a few movement evaluations (especially useful in early detection of tardive dyskinesia) that can be easily conducted at follow-up visits. Risk of hyperprolactinemia is mostly associated with risperidone treatment. However, postpubertal children and adolescents may be at an increased risk of developing this condition compared with adults.[45]

After initiation of a mood stabilizer, laboratory values, including drug concentrations (i.e., for lithium and valproic acid) should occur every 3 to 6 months.[4] The lithium concentration should be checked more often if there is a dose change, renal function becomes impaired, or a drug–drug interaction affects renal clearance of lithium (e.g., nonsteroidal anti-inflammatory drugs). Because lithium is renally excreted, checking kidney function throughout therapy is vital. Lithium has a narrow therapeutic window, and blood concentrations should be monitored often.[18,37] A higher concentration of lithium (greater than 1.5 mEq/L) in the blood can lead to mild toxicity, evidenced by increased or more severe adverse effects such as nausea, vomiting, ataxia, coarse tremor, or confusion. A lithium concentration more than 2.0 mEq/L constitutes severe toxicity, and patients at this concentration could potentially experience severe gastrointestinal effects, decreased coordination, seizures, slurred speech, muscle twitching, kidney failure, cardiac arrhythmias, or death.[18,37] However, some patients may be more sensitive to lithium and experience toxic symptoms at lower concentrations.[18] In addition to these laboratory assessments, TSH and calcium values should be checked again at 1 month, 6 months, and then annually.[45]

For valproic acid/divalproex, the laboratory values and drug concentrations should be checked every 3 to 6 months after initiating therapy.[4] In addition, TSH must be checked at 3 months and then annually afterwards.[45] Like lithium, the valproate drug concentration can be checked more often if there is a dose change, liver impairment, or drug interaction affecting metabolism. Also, because divalproex has been linked to polycystic ovarian syndrome, it is important to monitor menstrual cycles as well as encourage a healthy diet and regular exercise.[45] Overall, the maintenance of a healthy lifestyle is encouraged in conjunction with medications and/or psychotherapy; including monitoring for substance use and smoking, physical exercise, and proper diet.[19]

CONCLUSIONS

There is still a need for research on the safety and efficacy of pharmacotherapy in the PBD population. Future areas of growth may involve the SGAs if existing agents are studied in pediatric trials or as new agents enter the market. Appropriate pharmacotherapy for management of bipolar symptoms while reducing the risks for adverse effects is critical in all patients, but especially in pediatric patients who may be at increased risk of adverse drug reactions. Before using pharmacotherapy, a confirmed diagnosis of BPD should be documented, and the patient, family, and health care professional(s) should make a joint decision to move forward with both medication and nonmedication therapy. Additional resources are provided in Box 1. This mental health disorder is serious because it may cause impairment and negatively impact daily functioning. If the disorder remains untreated, the risk of health deterioration and other comorbidities increases. Through adherence and informed decisions, BPD can be successfully treated with a combination of pharmacotherapy and psychotherapy.

Box 1. Additional Resources

American Academy of Child and Adolescent Psychiatry: www.aacap.org

Mental Health America: (800) 969-6642, www.mhanational.org

National Alliance on Mental Illness: (800) 950-6264, www.nami.org

Bipolar Network News: www.bipolarnews.org—under "Child Network"

A 10-year-old boy is referred to the psychiatrist by his pediatrician after his parents noted extreme and consistent changes in his behavior. These behaviors have occurred over the past 3 months at least four times a week throughout the day. The changes began when he repeatedly got in trouble at school because of his excessive silliness during quiet reading time and becoming increasingly talkative. His parents and teacher noted that he has always been a very joyful child, but over the past few months he has been increasingly energetic. Other pertinent changes include irritable mood, loss of some friendships at school because of his behavior, and a decrease in the number of hours of sleep. He normally slept 10 hours each night, but within the past 6 months his total sleep has diminished to around 6 hours. His parents recall that in the past 3 months he has been aggressive towards his little brother, more so than what is deemed appropriate for regular sibling play. They cited two incidences where he used a pair of scissors as a sword while playing and almost stabbed his brother in the arm. At first his parents had considered the likelihood of attention-deficit/hyperactivity disorder, but given the family history of BPD and the other disturbing behavior, they are concerned his behavior is a sign of another condition that may be more severe.

Medical history: Type 1 diabetes (T1DM; onset 2 years ago)

Social history: Unremarkable

Family history: Father and mother are both alive and well, age 38 and 36 years, respectively; maternal grandfather had history of bipolar I disorder and died at age 54 years from liver failure secondary to alcohol abuse

Medications: Uses an insulin

pump with insulin aspart with the pump setting maintained by his pediatric endocrinologist; no herbals, supplements, or over-the-counter medications used

Allergies: No known allergies to medications, foods, or substances

Immunizations: Up to date on all childhood vaccines

Vital signs: Ht 58 inches, Wt 45 kg, body mass index: 20.9, considered

overweight for a boy his age, height, and weight

Physical examination: Last pediatrician visit was 1 month ago, when the patient was noted to be overweight; all other physical findings were normal or unremarkable

Laboratory findings: Within normal limits, except for the following:

A1C 8.5%

Fasting blood glucose 145 mg/dL

---

1. What are the signs and symptoms that support a diagnosis of pediatric bipolar disorder in this patient?

The *Diagnostic and Statistical Manual of Mental Disorders, Fifth Edition (DSM-5)* provides very specific criteria regarding mood and behavioral changes for the diagnosis of bipolar 1 disorder. However, as discussed within this chapter, a child or adolescent may present differently than an adult. Based on this patient's presentation, the initial thought would be bipolar I disorder because he is displaying signs of mania. His behavior changes began 3 months ago and have been extreme and consistent, occurring throughout the day most days of the week. In addition, his caregivers noted irritability and increased energy. He has had a marked decrease in nightly sleep, increased talking, inappropriate silliness, and dangerous aggression towards his brother. He has lost some friendships at school secondary to his behavior, and based on his medical and social history there is no other physiological or substance-related problem to which these changes can be attributed. This patient meets criteria for diagnosis of pediatric bipolar disorder.

2. What are three potential pharmacotherapy recommendations (including dose and duration) that you would make to the psychiatrist for the treatment of pediatric bipolar disorder?

First, lithium monotherapy—based on extensive studies and proven efficacy as a mood stabilizer—should be considered as a potential first-line agent. Lithium is the only agent with FDA label approval for children age 7 years and older. Lithium can also be continued for maintenance therapy. This agent is also

known to cause weight gain, so the patient should be closely monitored, especially considering that he is currently overweight. Based on his weight of 45 kg, the initial dose would be 300 mg orally three times daily, and then titrating by 300 mg every three days to achieve an acute serum concentration goal of 0.8-1.2 mEq/L. The drug should be continued for at least 12 months, but 24 months may be warranted.

Second, risperidone monotherapy should be considered because it has FDA label approval for acute treatment of mania in children age 10–17 years. Although risperidone is a second-generation antipsychotic (SGA), it shares characteristics of first-generation antipsychotics (the adverse effects of extrapyramidal symptoms) more than other SGAs. Given this patient's diabetes and overweight status, it may be more appropriate to consider this SGA over some of the newer agents (e.g., quetiapine, olanzapine) to decrease the likelihood of metabolic syndrome. The approach is to begin with 0.5 mg/day orally and then slowly titrate to 2.5 mg/day as needed. If the patient experiences continued somnolence, the daily dose can be split in half and administered twice daily. However, as previously discussed, all SGA medications need to be monitored for metabolic changes. In addition, it would not be incorrect to select other SGA agents approved for the treatment of this patient's acute mania, such as aripiprazole. The drug should be continued for at least 12 months, but 24 months may be warranted.

Third, aripiprazole monotherapy should be considered because it has FDA label approval for the acute treatment of mania in children age 10–17 years. This approach is another viable treatment option. It is important to recall that SGAs carry the risk of metabolic syndrome, and this patient has T1DM and is overweight. Although it is not contraindicated to use these agents in diabetes, it is vital to closely monitor any changes in weight, fasting blood glucose, and hemoglobin A1C secondary to SGA use. The approach is to begin with aripiprazole 2 mg/day orally daily for 2 days, then 5 mg/day for 2 days, then 10 mg/day. The drug can be increased by 5 mg daily if needed thereafter. This therapy should be continued for at least 12 months, but 24 months may be warranted.

Additional considerations of other agents are important to note. Given the high propensity for weight gain with the use of olanzapine, it would be best to avoid this drug as a first-line option in a growing child, particularly in a patient with T1DM and one who is overweight. Other potential SGAs to consider for treatment include quetiapine and asenapine, both of which carry FDA label-approved indications in pediatric and adolescent patients. Divalproex monotherapy does not currently carry an FDA indication for use in pediatric and adolescent patients; however, based on data it is a viable option. Divalproex is recommended over valproic acid because the latter medication is nonenteric coated and can cause more gastrointestinal upset.

3. Based on your previous answers and the recommended treatments in Question 2, describe what laboratory values need to be monitored and how often for each treatment.

Lithium: All metabolic and endocrine values as outlined in the chapter should be evaluated at baseline. Most vital signs will be assessed at every visit. Fasting blood work should be repeated in 3 months and then every 6 months. Remember that it is important to assess diet and exercise, sedation, appetite, and sexual signs and symptoms at least monthly for the first 3 months and then every 3 months thereafter. In addition, baseline TSH and serum calcium should be evaluated before initiating lithium; then TSH should be checked again at 3 months, and then annually. Lastly, a serum lithium concentration should be checked once the drug has reached steady state, to ensure it is at the goal trough level. Recall that the goal concentration varies depending on acute or maintenance treatment. Monitor for signs and symptoms of lithium toxicity throughout treatment.

Risperidone: Given this medication's propensity to induce hyperprolactinemia, prolactin should be evaluated at baseline before drug initiation. It is recommended to check prolactin again only if the patient is symptomatic. In addition, all metabolic and endocrine values outlined in this chapter should be evaluated at baseline. Most vital signs will be assessed at every visit. Fasting blood work should be repeated in 3 months and then every 6 months. Remember that it is important to assess diet and exercise, sedation, appetite, and sexual signs and symptoms at least monthly for the first 3 months and then every 3 months thereafter. It is also important to check for any movement abnormalities at each follow-up visit.

Aripiprazole: The same monitoring of metabolic and endocrine values in addition to movement abnormalities apply to aripiprazole as stated for risperidone.

REFERENCES

1. Bipolar and related disorders. In: American Psychiatric Association: Diagnostic and Statistical Manual of Mental Disorders, 5th ed. Arlington, VA: American Psychiatric Association; 2013:123-54.
2. Drayton SJ, Pelic CM. Drayton S.J., Pelic C.M. Drayton, Shannon J., and Christine M. Pelic.Bipolar Disorder. In: DiPiro JT, Talbert RL, Yee GC, et al., DiPiro J.T., Talbert R.L., Yee G.C., Matzke G.R., Wells B.G., Posey L Eds. Joseph T. DiPiro, et al.eds. *Pharmacotherapy: A Pathophysiologic Approach, 9e.* New York: McGraw-Hill, 2014. Available at http://accesspharmacy.mhmedical.com/content.aspx?bookid=1861&sectionid=134127982. Accessed July 18, 2018.
3. National Alliance on Mental Illness (NAMI) [homepage on the Internet]. Bipolar disorder. Available at www.nami.org/Learn-More/Mental-Health-Conditions/Bipolar-Disorder. Accessed July 19, 2018.
4. McClellan J, Kowatch R, Findling RL, et al. Practice parameter for the assessment and treatment of children and adolescents with bipolar disorder. J Am Acad Child Adolesc Psychiatry 2007;46:107-25.
5. Post RM, Altshuler LL, Kupka R, et al. Age of onset of bipolar disorder: combined effect of childhood adversity and familial loading of psychiatric disorders. J Psychiatr Res 2016;81:63-70.
6. National Institute of Mental Health (NIMH) [homepage on the Internet]. Any mood disorder in children. Available at www.nimh.nih.gov/health/statistics/prevalence/any-mood-disorder-in-children.shtml Accessed July 19, 2018.
7. Hauser M, Galling B, Correll C, et al. Suicidal ideation and suicide attempts in children and adolescents with bipolar disorder: a systematic review of prevalence and incidence rates, risk factors, and targeted interventions. Bipolar Disord 2013;15:507-23.
8. Birmaher B, Axelson D, Goldstein B, et al. Four-year longitudinal course of children and adolescents with bipolar spectrum disorders: the course and outcome of bipolar youth (COBY) study. Am J Psychiatry 2009;166:795-804.
9. Mula M, Marotta AE, Monaco F. Epilepsy and bipolar disorders. Expert Rev Neurother 2010;10:13-23.
10. Chen J, Fang Y, Kemp DE, et al. Switching to hypomania and mania: differential neurochemical, neuropsychological, and pharmacologic triggers and their mechanisms. Curr Psychiatry Rep 2010;12:512-21.
11. Baldessarini RJ, Bolzani L, Cruz N, et al. Onset-age of bipolar disorders at six international sites. J Affect Disord 2010;121:143-6.
12. Kowatch RA, Fristad M, Birmaher B, et al. Treatment guidelines for children and adolescents with bipolar disorder. J Am Acad Child Adolesc Psychiatry 2005;44:213-35.
13. Findling RL. Evidence-based pharmacologic treatment of pediatric bipolar disorder. J Clin Psychiatry 2016;77:e02.
14. Moreno C, Gonzalo L, Blanco C, et al. National trends in the outpatient diagnosis and treatment of bipolar disorder in youth. Arch Gen Psychiatry 2007;64:1032-9.
15. Frias A, Palma C, Farriols N. Comorbidity in pediatric bipolar disorder: prevalence, clinical impact, etiology and treatment. J Affect Disord 2015;174:378-89.
16. Demeter C, Youngstrom E, Carlson G, et al. Age differences in the phenomenology of pediatric bipolar disorder. J Affect Disord 2013;147:295-303.
17. Abilify (aripiprazole) [package insert]. Tokyo, Japan: Otsuka Pharmaceutical, 2019. Revised August 2019.
18. Lithium carbonate [package insert]. Colvale-Bardez, India: Glenmark Pharmaceuticals, 2019. Revised February 2019.

19. Yatham LN, Kennedy SH, Parikh SV, et al. Canadian Network for Mood and Anxiety Treatments (CANMAT) and International Society for Bipolar Disorders (ISBD) 2018 guidelines for the management of patients with bipolar disorder. Bipolar Disord 2018;20:97-170.

20. Chang K. Pediatric bipolar disorder: combination pharmacotherapy, adverse effects, and treatment of high-risk youth. J Clin Psychiatry 2016;77:e03.

21. Goodwin GM, Haddad PM, Ferrier IN, et al. Evidence-based guidelines for treating bipolar disorder: Revised third edition, Recommendations from the British Association for Psychopharmacology. J Psychopharmacol 2016;1:1-59.

22. Symbyax (olanzapine/fluoxetine) [package insert]. Indianapolis, IN: Eli Lilly and Co.; 2019. Revised November 2019.

23. Stahl S, ed. Stahl's Essential Psychopharmacology. 4th ed. Cambridge, United Kingdom: Cambridge University Press, 2013: 370-87.

24. Miyamoto S, Duncan GE, Marx CE, et al. Treatments for schizophrenia: a critical review of pharmacology and mechanisms of action of antipsycotic drugs. Mol Psychiatry 2005;10:79-104.

25. Latuda (lurasidone) [package insert]. Malborough, MA: Sunovion Pharmaceuticals, 2019. Revised March 2018.

26. Findling RL, Nyilas M, Forbes R, et al. Acute treatment of pediatric bipolar I disorder, manic or mixed episode, with aripiprazole: a randomized, double-blind, placebo-controlled study. J Clin Psychiatry 2009;70:1441-51.

27. Findling RL, Correll CU, Nyilas M, et al. Aripiprazole for the treatment of pediatric bipolar I disorder: a 30-week, randomized, placebo-controlled study. Bipolar Disord 2013;15:138-49.

28. Tohen M, Kryzhanovskaya L, Carlson G, et al. Olanzapine versus placebo in the treatment of adolescents with bipolar mania. Am J Psychiatry 2007;164:1547-56.

29. Frazier J, Biederman J, Tohen M, et al. A prospective open-label treatment trial of olanzapine monotherapy in children and adolescents with bipolar disorder. J Child Adolesc Psychopharmacol 2001:11:239-50.

30. Pathak S, Findling RL, Earley WR, et al. Efficacy and safety of quetiapine in children and adolescents with mania associated with bipolar I disorder: a 3-week, double-blind, placebo-controlled trial. J Clin Psychiatry 2013;74:e100-e109.

31. Joshi G, Petty C, Wozniak J, et al. A prospective open-label trial of quetiapine monotherapy in preschool and school age children with bipolar spectrum disorder. J Affect Disord 2012; 136:1143-53.

32. Haas M, DelBello M, Pandina G, et al. Risperidone for the treatment of acute mania in children and adolescents with bipolar disorder: a randomized, double-blind, placebo-controlled study. Bipolar Disord 2009;11:687-700.

33. Findling RL, Landbloom R, Szegedi A, et al. Asenapine for the acute treatment of pediatric manic or mixed episodes of bipolar I disorder. J Am Acad Child Adolesc Psychiatry 2015;54:1032-41.

34. Findling RL, Landbloom RL, Mackle M, et al. Long-term safety of asenapine in pediatric patients diagnosed with bipolar I disorder: a 50-week open-label, flexible-dose trial. Pediatr Drugs 2016;18:1367-78.

35. Risperdal Consta (risperidone long-acting injectable) [package insert]. Titusville, NJ: Janssen Pharmaceuticals, 2007.

36. Abilify Maintena (aripiprazole long-acting injectable) [package insert]. Tokyo, Japan: Otsuka Pharmaceutical Co., Ltd., 2017.

37. Thomas T, Stansifer L, Findling RL. Psychopharmacology of pediatric bipolar disorders in children and adolescents. Pediatr Clin N Am 2011;58:173-87.

38. Zyprexa (olanzapine) [package insert]. Indianapolis, IN: Eli Lilly and Co., 2019.

39. Seroquel (quetiapine) [package insert]. Wilmington, DE: AstraZeneca Pharmaceuticals LP, 2019. Revised November 2019.

40. Risperdal (risperidone) [package insert]. Titusville, NJ: Janssen Pharmaceuticals, 2007. Revised January 2019.

41. Saphris (asenapine) [package insert]. Irvine, CA: Allergan USA, 2017. Revised January 2017.

42. Clozaril (clozapine) [package insert]. Rosemont, PA: Novartis Pharmaceuticals, 2017.

43. Divalproex sodium [package insert]. Bachupally, India: Dr. Reddy's Laboratories, 2018.

44. Valproic acid [package insert]. St. Petersburg, FL: Catalent Pharma Solutions, 2017.

45. Correll C, Carlson H. Endocrine and metabolic adverse effects of psychotropic medications in children and adolescents. J Am Acad Child Adolesc Psychiatry 2006;45:771-91.

46. Recent Summary Safety Reviews. Government of Canada [homepage on the Internet]. Available at https://www.canada.ca/en/health-canada/services/drugs-health-products/medeffect-canada/safety-reviews.html. Updated August 3, 2018. Accessed August 4, 2018.

47. Patel N, DelBello MP, Bryan HS, et al. Open-label lithium for the treatment of adolescents with bipolar depression. J Am Acad Child Adolesc Psychiatry 2006;45:289-97.

48. Atherton JC, Doyle A, Gee A, et al. Lithium clearance: modification by the loop of Henle in man. J Physiol 1991;437:377-91.

49. Finley PR, Warner MD, Peabody CA. Clinical relevance of drug interactions with lithium. Clin Pharmacokinet 1995;29:172-91.

50. Liu HY, Potter MP, Woodworth KY, et al. Pharmacologic treatments for pediatric bipolar disorder: a review and meta-analysis. J Am Acad Child Adolesc Psychiatry 2011;8:749-62.e39.

51. Findling RL, McNamara NK, Youngstrom EA, et al. Double-blind 18-month trial of lithium versus divalproex maintenance treatment in pediatric bipolar disorder. J Am Acad Child Adolesc Psychiatry 2005;44:409-17.

52. Carbamazepine [package insert]. Detroit, MI: Caraco Pharmaceutical Laboratories, 2008.

53. Carbamazepine extended-release [package insert]. Parsippany, NJ: Validus Pharmaceuticals, 2009.

54. French JA, Pedley TA. Initial management of epilepsy. N Engl J Med 2008;359:166-76.

55. Joshi G, Wozniak J, Mick E, et al. A prospective open-label trial of extended-release carbamazepine monotherapy in children with bipolar disorder. J Child Adolesc Psychopharmacol 2010;20:7-14.

56. Oxcarbazepine [package insert]. East Hanover, NJ: Novartis Pharmaceuticals Corporation, 2018.

57. Wagner KD, Kowatch RA, Emslie GJ, et al. A double-blind, randomized, placebo-controlled trial of oxcarbazepine in the treatment of bipolar disorder in children and adolescents. Am J Psychiatry 2006;163:1179-86.

58. Lamotrigine [package insert]. Salisbury, MD: Jubilant Cadista Pharmaceuticals, 2017.

59. Pavuluri MN, Henry DB, Moss M, et al. Effectiveness of lamotrigine in maintaining symptom control in pediatric bipolar disorder. J Child Adolesc Psychopharmacol 2009;19:75-82.

60. Topiramate [package insert]. North Wales, PA: Teva Pharmaceuticals USA, 2017.

61. Delbello MP, Findling RL, Kushner S, et al. A pilot controlled trial of topiramate for mania in children and adolescents with bipolar disorder. J Am Acad Child Adolesc Psychiatry 2005;44:539-47.

62. Pavuluri MN, Henry DB, Carbray JA, et al. Open-label prospective trial of risperidone in combination with lithium or divalproex sodium in pediatric mania. J Affect Disord 2004;82S:S103-11.

63. American Diabetes Association, American Psychiatric Association, American Association of Clinical Endocrinologists, and North American Association for the Study of Obesity. Consensus development conference on antipsychotic drugs and obesity and diabetes. Diabetes Care 2004;27:596-601.

64. U.S. Food and Drug Administration [homepage on the Internet]. FDA Drug Safety Communication. Antipsychotic Drug Labels Updated on Use During Pregnancy and Risk of Abnormal Muscle Movements and Withdrawal Symptoms in Newborns.

Available at www.fda.gov/Drugs/DrugSafety/ucm243903.htm. Updated August 2017. Accessed August 3, 2018.

65. Birmaher B, Brent D, et al. Practice parameter for the assessment and treatment of children and adolescents with depressive disorders. J Am Acad Child Adolesc Psychiatry 2007;46:1503-26.

66. Depression in children and teens. American Academy of Child and Adolescent Psychiatry [homepage on the Internet]. Available at https://www.aacap.org/AACAP/Families_and_Youth/ Facts_for_Families/FFF-Guide/The-Depressed-Child-004.aspx. Updated March 2018. Accessed July 19, 2018.

67. Lithium carbonate extended release [package insert]. Colvale-Bardez, India: Glenmark Pharmaceuticals, 2014.

68. Lithium solution [package insert]. Columbus, OH: Roxanne Laboratories, 2013.

69. Seroquel XR (quetiapine extended-release) [package insert]. Wilmington, DE: AstraZeneca Pharmaceuticals, 2019. Revised November 2019.

CHAPTER 35

Eating Disorders in Children and Adolescents

Cherry W. Jackson, Pharm.D., FCCP, FASHP, BCPP

INTRODUCTION

Eating disorders in children and adolescents are complex disease states with high rates of morbidity and mortality. The number of children and adolescents with eating disorders has steadily increased during the past 60 years,[1-3] whereas the age of onset has steadily declined.[1,4,5] Hospitalizations for children younger than 12 years with diagnoses of eating disorders have increased by 119% since the late 1990s.[5] The typical patient with an eating disorder has changed as well. At one time, eating disorders were considered an illness primarily in wealthy young white women; however, these disorders are now increasing in minorities,[6-8] males,[9,10] and countries where eating disorders were once relatively unknown.[11,12]

EPIDEMIOLOGY

Eating disorders must be recognized and treated at their earliest stage to achieve positive outcomes. The lifetime prevalence of eating disorders in adolescents in community samples in the United States is estimated to be 13%.[13-15] Eating disorders are more common in females than males at a 10:1 ratio.[16] The diagnostic criteria for the two most common eating disorders, anorexia nervosa (AN) and bulimia nervosa (BN), in the *Diagnostic and Statistical Manual of Mental Disorders, Fifth Edition* (*DSM-5*) have been expanded, which increases the prevalence of these disorders from 0.1% in the *Diagnostic and Statistical Manual of Mental Disorders, Fourth Edition, Text Revision*.[16] The estimated lifetime prevalence of AN and BN in adolescents is 0.8%–1.7% and 0.8%–2.6%, respectively. Binge eating disorder (BED) is a new diagnosis in *DSM-5* and has a prevalence of 2.3%–3% in adolescents.[15,17] Avoidant-restrictive food intake disorder is a new diagnosis in *DSM-5* that replaces feeding disorders of early infancy and childhood.[16] Prevalence studies for this new diagnosis are limited, but the diagnosis is currently estimated to occur at a rate of 5%–23%.[18] Feeding disorders are beyond the scope of this chapter and will not be discussed.

ETIOLOGY

The etiology of the various eating disorders is still unknown, but many factors appear to contribute to the development of an eating disorder.[19] Although debated, dieting, especially severe dieting, may lead to the onset of these disorders.[20,21] Other etiologic factors include genetic, biological, and psychological predispositions as well as environmental, social, and cultural factors.

Social, cultural, and environmental factors regarding ideal weight and shape and their relationship to what is culturally considered beautiful often influence the way females think and feel about their bodies. Dieting is not uncommon in industrialized countries; in fact, most women admit that they have tried a diet. Although dieting is considered an entry point into developing an eating disorder, less than 3% of all females will actually develop an eating disorder.[21] In one study, severe dieters were 18 times more likely to develop an eating disorder than were non-dieters.[22] In nations that are less industrialized and less exposed to Western culture, the prevalence of eating disorders is much lower.[23]

Studies of twins and families with at least one member having an eating disorder suggest a genetic link in the development of eating disorders. Studies of monozygotic and dizygotic twins have had high concordance rates, though the studies themselves have had differing results. Some studies have shown that the greatest concordance is between monozygotic twins, whereas others have shown higher rates with dizygotic twins.[24-27] Heritability for AN is estimated to be 24%–74%, with environmental factors rounding out the remainder of the estimate for AN, and heritability for BN is estimated to be 28%–83%.[28-30] In families having at least two members with either AN or BN, genomic studies show initial linkage regions on chromosomes 1, 3, 4, and 13 in AN and on chromosome 10p and 14 in BN.[31,32] Additional genomic studies are under way.[33] Together with genetic risk, psychological factors are believed to influence eating disorder development. Traits such as perfectionism, inflexibility, a drive to be thin, a need for control, and interpersonal distrust have all been proposed to affect the onset of eating disorders.[34] Traits common in eating disorders are also associated with several psychiatric conditions. The incidence of depression and other mood disorders is 50%–80% in patients with both AN and BN. Individuals with eating disorders have a 30%–65% incidence of anxiety, and obsessive-compulsive disorder is especially common in individuals with AN; patients with eating disorders have a 20%–80% incidence of personality disorders, especially borderline personality disorder.[26,35,36]

The neurotransmitters serotonin, dopamine, and norepinephrine increasingly appear to play a role in the etiology of eating disorders. Serotonin is known to play a role in satiety, anxiety, mood, sleep, and obsessive-compulsive behaviors. Serotonin antagonists increase food cravings and intake, which leads to weight gain. The serotonin metabolite 5-hydroxyindoleacetic acid (5-HIAA) concentration is often low in those who are underweight but corrects itself once normal weight is achieved. Deficiencies in 5-HIAA can lead to suicidality, aggression, and impulsive behaviors.[37-39] In patients who have recovered from AN, norepinephrine concentrations are lower than in control populations. Lower norepinephrine concentrations as the result of starvation can lead to bradycardia, hypotension, and hypothermia.[40] Dopamine may also be related to the etiology of eating disorders. Common symptoms that may be linked to dopamine dysregulation include distorted body image, decreased energy, decreased motivation, and reduced response to rewards.[41,42]

Leptin, a hormone produced in adipose tissue, is related to weight regulation and energy balance. In addition, leptin appears to play a significant role in mediating eating disorders. Patients with AN tend to have decreased leptin concentrations because of low levels of circulating fat. These low leptin concentrations signal low energy levels to the brain. Patients who have recovered from eating disorders continue to have lower concentrations of serum leptin than the concentrations required on the basis of their body mass index (BMI). Both leptin and norepinephrine may serve as trait markers for patients with eating disorders, but more research is needed to confirm this association.[43,44]

Ghrelin is a hormone that suppresses appetite, and its concentrations are increased in females with AN.[45,46] Studies suggest that weight restoration can be achieved with a ghrelin gene variant in females who have the TT genotype of the T3056C variant. Those with the ghrelin-activating gene, ghrelin O-acyltransferase or GOAT, are 1.5 times more likely to have AN.[31,45]

MEDICAL COMPLICATIONS

Eating disorders have the highest mortality rates of all the psychiatric disorders at 4%.[47-49] Medical complications associated with these disorders are especially lethal in children and adolescents. Suicidality is a risk factor associated with eating disorder–related mood changes and dissatisfaction with body image.[49] Anorexia nervosa is more often associated with mortality than are BN and BED. The most common causes of mortality as a result of AN include cachexia, organ failure, and circulatory collapse.[50]

According to the Agency for Healthcare Research and Quality, the hospitalization rate for children younger than 12 years with malnutrition rose by 119% in 1999–2006.[5] Long-term consequences are often associated with eating disorders, even once disordered eating behaviors have resolved. These consequences include osteopenia, structural changes to the gray and white matter of the brain, growth retardation, and pubertal delay.[51] With time, the body cannot compensate for long-term nutritional deficits, causing metabolic rate declines and inhibition of temperature regulation. Ultimately, almost all of the body's organ systems are affected by malnutrition.[52-54]

Malnutrition and starvation lead to dysfunction of the endocrine system, including hyperactivity of the hypothalamic-pituitary-adrenal axis. These changes affect thyroid function and the reproductive system, leading to hypothyroidism, hypogonadism, hypercortisolism, and amenorrhea. In addition, endocrine dysfunction can lead to growth retardation and a delay in the onset of puberty in children and adolescents. These effects on the hypothalamic-pituitary-adrenal axis as well as the inability of growth hormone to bind to insulin-like growth factor-1 may be part of the mechanism of growth retardation.[41-54] Unfortunately, the effects on growth, especially on short stature, may be a permanent manifestation of malnutrition.[55]

Weight loss causes a decrease in the volume of the gray and white matter of the brain and cerebrospinal space.[56] Cognitive dysfunction often occurs in patients with eating disorders secondary to hypercortisolism and hypogonadism.[57] Magnetic resonance imaging has revealed changes in brain activity. From neuroimaging, it appears that the volumetric decreases in gray matter caused by malnutrition may be permanent, whereas white matter may improve with refeeding.[57,58]

Hypogonadism, amenorrhea, and nutritional deficiencies lead to low bone marrow density. This is a significant problem for children and adolescents because bone mineralization is important in patients this age during these periods of growth. It is unclear whether refeeding will reverse these changes on bone mineral density.[59,60]

Eating disorders cause significant damage to the gastrointestinal (GI) tract. Effects on the GI tract include delays in gastric emptying, gastroesophageal reflux, and GI bleeding. Constipation is commonly caused by nutritional deficits. Enlargement of the salivary glands is associated with hyperemesis.[61] Self-induced vomiting can cause a callus on the dorsum of the hand called Russell's sign. Repeated forced emesis can also cause a separation of the mucosal membrane between the esophagus and the stomach that may lead to extensive bleeding called a Mallory-Weiss tear. Stomach acid from hyperemesis may also cause dental erosion.

Dehydration from purging behaviors leads to imbalances in fluids and electrolytes. In addition, hyperemesis may lead to a hypochloremic metabolic alkalosis because of the loss of hydrochloric acid. The body's attempt to conserve fluid in the face of dehydration can lead to hypokalemia-causing cardiac arrhythmias. Hypomagnesemia from malnutrition can lead to sudden cardiac death. Similarly, malnutrition and laxative abuse can induce hypoproteinemia, which can lead to significant edema and, potentially, congestive heart failure. Dehydration caused by laxative abuse may induce a hyperchloremic metabolic acidosis. Dilutional hyponatremia may occur in patients who try to improve their weight before visiting their health care provider.[53-55,61,62]

Finally, malnutrition can lead to stomatitis; dry, cracked, scaly skin; and hair and nail changes. The development of lanugo, a fine soft hair that covers the body, and yellow skin are not uncommon in patients with eating disorders.[54,55]

PATIENT ASSESSMENT

Eating disorders can adversely affect every organ system of the body, so patients with these disorders should have a thorough medical and psychosocial evaluation. In addition to a complete physical examination, laboratory values should be obtained, including an electrolyte panel, liver function tests, a complete blood cell count, thyroid function tests, and glucose, calcium, and magnesium concentrations. In patients with amenorrhea, a serum pregnancy test, serum estradiol, serum prolactin, and follicle-stimulating hormone should be measured. In addition, in female patients with amenorrhea, a bone scan should be completed to check for osteopenia. An electrocardiogram should be considered for those with electrolyte abnormalities or cardiovascular symptoms. Neuroimaging of the brain should be considered for those with severe malnutrition.[63]

Of importance, clinicians should assess patients on the basis of their symptoms, given that laboratory results may be normal in patients with eating disorders. Clinicians also need to be aware that patients with AN and BN tend to be ambivalent about treatment, and it is common for them to hide their illness. Thus, denial by the patient does not exclude the possibility of an eating disorder. With time, these disorders can become egosyntonic, meaning that the behaviors provide positive reinforcement for the patient, and changing the behavior is more frightening than living with it.[63,64]

Psychosocial evaluations should include an assessment of how patients view food, nutrition, and their current body image. Social factors such as their relationships with significant others, including parents, siblings, friends, and other support systems, should be assessed. Because eating disorders often co-occur with other psychiatric conditions such as mood, anxiety, and personality disorders, these psychiatric disorders should be assessed for as well. As many as 50% of individuals with an eating disorder also use alcohol or another illicit drug. Patients with BN are most likely to have a substance use disorder, followed by those with BED, with the lowest risk in patients with AN.[65] A complete medical history, including use of illicit drugs and over-the-counter medications such as laxatives, stimulants, and diuretics, should be obtained. It is important to discuss with patients whether they have any history of sexual, physical, or emotional abuse because such factors can play a role in developing eating disorders. It is not uncommon for patients with an eating disorder to complete a suicide, so evaluating the patient's risk is an important part of an initial patient evaluation and ongoing clinical care.[64]

STANDARDIZED RATING SCALES

A variety of assessment measures exist for evaluating eating disorders. These measures vary and may include semistructured interviews, self-reporting, symptom checklists, and clinical rating scales. The most commonly used assessment measures are the Eating Disorder Examination, the Yale-Brown-Cornell Eating Disorder Scale, the Eating Attitudes Test, and the Eating Disorder Inventory. Any member of the eating disorder treatment team, including psychiatrists, psychologists, pharmacists, dietitians, nurses, and social workers, can be trained to provide interviews for the various scales.

The Eating Disorder Examination is a semistructured interview with four subscales (restraint, eating concern, shape concern, and weight concern). This examination evaluates eating behaviors over the previous 28 days. The examination is validated for adults and children older than 9 years. The children's version of the Eating Disorder Examination is typically used for those 9 years and younger. This examination allows the clinician to develop a diagnosis, which is selective for certain eating behaviors such as binge eating. Disadvantages of this scale are that it should be administered by a trained interviewer and can take up to 1 hour to complete.[66]

The Yale-Brown-Cornell Eating Disorder Scale is also a semistructured interview and has a 65-item checklist and questions that cover the ritualistic and obsessive behaviors that sometimes occur in patients with eating disorders. This scale is validated in adolescents and adults (ages 14–39; average age 16.2 years) with AN and BN. There is no child version of this scale. An advantage of this scale is that it takes 15 minutes to complete.[67] Another advantage is that it measures the degree of impairment caused by the eating disorder. Although this scale is preferred for individuals with an eating disorder with obsessive-compulsive symptomatology, a disadvantage is that it is not a comprehensive eating disorder scale.[68]

The Eating Attitudes Test is one of the two most commonly used eating disorder measures. This test is a self-report measure that includes a full-scale 50-item test and a brief 26-item measure that evaluates for global eating disorder symptoms. The Eating Attitudes Test is sensitive to treatment effects[69] and is validated in adolescents and adults with an average age of 22 years. This test for children is called the Children's Eating Attitudes Test and is validated in individuals 8–13 years of age. The Eating Attitudes Test contains 26 items, and scores greater than 20 are considered associated with developing an eating disorder.[70] The test measures an individual's concern about weight and food intake and is specific to AN. A disadvantage is that it is not designed for individuals with BN or BED. In addition, the Eating Attitudes Test scale does not measure the degree of impairment caused by the eating disorder.

Another standardized self-report measure, the Eating Disorder Inventory is the other most commonly used measure to evaluate patient attitudes and their behaviors around food, body image, and weight. The Eating Disorder Inventory also measures patient attitudes concerning perfection, effectiveness, trust, and maturity. The Eating Disorder Inventory is sensitive to treatment effects and has been validated in individuals age 13–20, with a mean age of 15.6.[71] An advantage of the Eating Disorder Inventory is that it is also a self-report measure. Another advantage is that one of its subscales measures core eating disorder symptoms and demographic information.[72] However, like the Eating Attitudes Test, it does not measure the degree of impairment caused by the eating disorder.

Self-reports are simple and take minimal time to complete. They are also inexpensive and objective, avoiding rater bias. The primary disadvantage of these scales is that they may be less accurate than the semistructured interviews, given that individuals filling out the scale may exaggerate or minimize symptoms according to what they believe is expected by the person providing the test.

ANOREXIA NERVOSA

Anorexia nervosa is one of the most serious psychiatric disorders in children and adolescents. Anorexia nervosa has occurred in children as young as 7 years.[73] Patients with AN are often perfectionists and high achievers who, under stress-induced situations, use caloric restriction as a means of controlling situations in which they otherwise have no control.[74] Initially, this weight loss may be reinforced by positive comments from friends and family admiring it. However, continued weight loss is associated with obsessions and compulsions that provide secondary reinforcement, which then becomes a vicious cycle.[74]

EPIDEMIOLOGY

The incidence of AN is highest in adolescent females age 15–19 at 0.48%–0.7%.[75] Early-onset AN (i.e., AN in prepubertal children or children younger than 14 years) occurs in 5% of all cases.[73-77] Although AN may be thought of as a disease of females, in the prepubertal population, boys and girls have an equal incidence of this disorder, with some studies theorizing that at very young ages, boys actually have a greater incidence of AN.[78] At least one-third of individuals with AN develop a chronic disorder marked by relapse and recurrent hospitalizations.[79]

CLINICAL PRESENTATION

The DSM-5 lists three essential features to meet the criteria for AN: restriction of energy intake, an intense fear of becoming fat or gaining weight, and body dysmorphism.[16] The core feature of AN involves a refusal to maintain adequate body weight for age and height. Body dysmorphism, a distortion in one's body image, is a primary reason for the refusal to maintain weight. Once weight is lost, the patient has a fear of gaining weight or becoming overweight or obese. In children and adolescents, this level of malnutrition prevents normal growth patterns, including a delay in sexual maturation, which sometimes leads to amenorrhea in females. Patients

with AN may either restrict their intake of food or binge and purge. Patients with AN can meet the diagnostic criteria for BN (e.g., having binge/purge behaviors). In addition to restricting caloric intake and developing extensive food rituals, patients with AN often participate in excessive exercise to inhibit weight gain.[80,81]

DIAGNOSTIC CRITERIA

The DSM-5 diagnostic criteria for AN involve individuals who have an extreme fear of weight gain, and although these individuals are underweight, they develop specific behaviors to prevent an increase in weight. In addition, these individuals are extremely underweight for their sex and age, according to normal growth scales. In children and adolescents with AN, weight is less than the minimum weight that would be expected for others in the same peer group. Finally, individuals with AN cannot recognize the significant impact of their weight on their physical health. Patients with AN perceive their weight or shape much differently from how others perceive it. The two distinct types of AN are the restricting type and the binge eating/purging type. The restricting type of AN is defined as either limiting intake or exercising to incur weight loss. To meet the criteria for restricting type, the individual cannot have had binge eating or purging in the previous 3 months. The binge eating/purging type of AN is defined as binge eating together with vomiting or use of drugs like laxatives to maintain low body weight. In addition, during the past 3 months, the individual must have engaged in recurrent episodes of binge eating or purging behavior (i.e., self-induced vomiting or the misuse of laxatives, diuretics, or enemas).[16]

RISK FACTORS

One risk factor for developing AN is a family history of an eating disorder. Family studies have shown that individuals with a first-degree relative with AN are 11 times more likely to have AN themselves.[21,82] Parental eating behavior and weight may also play a role. A recent study showed that families who sat down to dinner most days in the week were less likely to develop AN than families who did not.[83] Personality traits such as a "type A personality" or perfectionism may also be a risk factor. Mood symptoms in patients and their first-degree relatives may also place patients at an increased risk of developing AN. Many patients with AN were mildly overweight before developing the disorder.[83]

COURSE AND PROGNOSIS

Anorexia nervosa is rare before puberty and after age 40. The course of AN varies, with some individuals recovering after one episode and others experiencing relapse or recurrence. Most individuals will have remission of their symptoms within 5 years of disorder presentation.[80] As noted earlier, AN has the highest mortality rate of all the eating disorders. The mortality risk is estimated to be 10% within 10 years of an AN diagnosis and is primarily caused by starvation or suicide.[47,84,85]

Anorexia nervosa has significant comorbidity with other psychiatric disorders. In patients who restrict food intake, obsessive behaviors such as repetitive and/or intrusive thoughts, perfectionism, and inflexibility are common. In patients with AN who purge, suicidality and self-harm are common. Mood disorders and anxiety disorders are common to both AN subtypes.[86]

If AN is treated in the early stages of development, especially in prepubertal adolescents in whom weight restoration has been achieved, outcomes appear good. Patients with AN who continue to refuse to maintain their minimum weight tend to start using binging and purging behaviors that may evolve into a diagnosis of BN.[86,87]

TREATMENT

INITIAL TREATMENT GOALS

The initial treatment goals in AN are to restore the patient's nutritional status and treat the medical complications. The degree of malnutrition dictates how best to medically manage the patient. In the initial approach, the degree of electrolyte and nutrient loss must be determined before the patient's nutritional status can appropriately be restored. Electrolytes (e.g., potassium, sodium, and magnesium) and calcium, folic acid, zinc, and iron must be restored early in the process of refeeding.[88] Once patients are at less than 75% of their ideal body weight, are medically unstable, or have a heart rate of less than 50 beats/minute, they should be hospitalized.[88]

Because these patients have been in starvation mode, it is important to improve their energy deficits early by slowly titrating energy calories. Restoring deficits in children is of greater concern than in adolescents and adults. Children may have lower energy or fat stores, and they may dehydrate more rapidly. Body mass index is unreliable in children and young adolescents who have not finished growing. Growth may be stunted, and assessing appropriate weight gain in the still-growing youth is difficult.[88,89]

The initial goal for inpatients is to eat 30–40 kcal/kg/day, and the initial goal for outpatients is to eat 20 kcal/kg/day, with the subsequent goal of gaining 1 kg/week (inpatient) and 0.5 kg/week (outpatient). Recommendations on how to achieve this weight gain vary, but it is considered reasonable to start refeeding with 1400–2000 calories daily with close medical monitoring and to titrate slowly, as tolerated. Later in the refeeding process, the goal is to gain 1–1.5 kg/week (inpatient) and 0.5 kg/week (outpatient). Most patients will begin to achieve adequate weight gain with an intake of 2200–2500 calories daily. As energy requirements are replaced and the level of physical activity resumes, the metabolic rate normalizes, and the rate of weight gain declines.[88-92]

Anorexia nervosa is associated with an increased risk of fractures throughout the period of energy deficit into adulthood. Weight gain and return of menses can improve bone mineral density, but not in all individuals. Current recommendations include supplemental calcium and vitamin D and treatment of vitamin D deficiency. Serum 25-hydroxyvitamin D concentrations of less than 30 ng/mL (75 nmol/L) should be treated with vitamin D 50,000 international units weekly or 2000 international units daily for 6–8 weeks. For low bone mineral density in AN, treatment should include weight restoration with resumption of spontaneous menses, optimal intake of calcium (1300 mg/day of elemental calcium) and vitamin D (600 international units/day), and treatment of vitamin D deficiency. If amenorrhea has lasted more than 6 months, a dual-energy x-ray absorptiometry scan should be obtained.[90,91,93]

The clinician must take care not to cause refeeding syndrome. Refeeding syndrome occurs when an individual is fed normal quantities of food too quickly after a long period of starvation. When a patient is in starvation mode, insulin secretion declines because of a reduced intake of carbohydrates. Protein stores are broken down first, followed by fat stores to provide energy to the individual. During this level of starvation, intracellular electrolytes are reduced. Intracellular phosphate concentrations are at particular risk of depletion, though extracellular phosphate, which is typically measured in laboratory results, appears normal. Once normal feeding resumes, the body shifts from breaking down fat to breaking down carbohydrates once again. The cycle is reversed: insulin is secreted, and phosphates are shifted intercellularly. This leads to a profound extracellular hypophosphatemia. The serum phosphate concentration, usually less than 0.5 mmol/L, causes refeeding syndrome. Refeeding syndrome is characterized by hypotension, arrhythmias, seizures, cardiac failure, respiratory failure, rhabdomyolysis, coma, and sudden death. Refeeding syndrome can occur not only with oral feeding, but also with parenteral or enteral feeding.[94]

Once patients have stopped losing weight, their weight has begun to trend upward to at least 75% of their ideal body weight, and their laboratory results have normalized, they can go to a supportive home, where they can continue to work with a dietitian and therapist on a regular basis. If a supportive environment is not available, patients may go to a day treatment program, where they can be monitored for progress toward their weight gain goals.

NONPHARMACOLOGIC TREATMENT

Once the patient is stabilized medically, the next stage in treatment is to focus on developing new dietary habits as well as changing cognitive response to eating, weight, and the underlying psychopathology that led to the eating disorder.

At one time, environmental factors in families were thought to cause eating disorders, but this theory has been dismissed. In the past decade, research suggests that family therapy is the most beneficial treatment for AN. In family therapy – also called family-based treatment or family-based therapy (FBT) – parents/caregivers initially take responsibility for the child's or adolescent's eating behaviors. It is the family's job to ensure that the patient is eating adequately and avoiding eating disorder behavior. Once patients have regained at least 85% of their normal weight, they slowly become responsible for their own eating. In the last treatment phase, the patient and family work toward resuming what would be a normal developmental stage for the child or adolescent.[87] At least five controlled trials of FBT show promise for this treatment, especially in children or adolescents with a short illness.[95-100] Family-based therapy typically takes 6–12 months to complete, and the outcomes have been durable at the 5-year follow-up.[96-101]

Family-based therapy is typically advised for intact, supportive families. In families where the affected child has been abused, or in the most nutritionally and medically compromised patients, FBT is not the treatment of choice.[87] In these patients, enhanced cognitive behavioral therapy (CBT-E), interpersonal psychotherapy, or adolescent-focused therapy should be considered.

More than one-half of patients treated with cognitive behavioral therapy (CBT) do not recover. To improve response to CBT, a therapy called *enhanced cognitive behavioral therapy,* or CBT-E, assists with issues such as perfectionism, mood, interpersonal problems, and low self-esteem.[102] *Enhanced cognitive behavioral therapy* teaches the patient strategies to cope with the feelings and events that initially led to the eating disorder. In addition, CBT-E improves self-esteem and helps the patient correct body image distortions.[103,104] Interpersonal psychotherapy typically focuses on interpersonal problems that may play a role in eating disorder behaviors. However, few studies have been completed with interpersonal psychotherapy, and it is less effective than FBT, adolescent-focused therapy, and CBT-E.

Adolescent-focused therapy trains adolescents to cope with age-appropriate challenges and negative emotions. Studies show outcomes similar to FBT, though longitudinally at 6- and 12-month time intervals, individuals actually had improved outcomes with FBT. Adolescent-focused therapy may be beneficial in adolescents with fractured family situations or when families cannot commit time to therapy.[105,106]

PHARMACOLOGIC TREATMENT

There are no randomized controlled trials of any pharmacologic agent for the treatment of AN in children or adolescents alone. Although trials have been completed in adolescents and adults, most were either too short or used medication doses that today would be considered insufficient for treating an eating disorder. In addition, studies that have been published typically lack the statistical power required to make evidence-based decisions.

If medications are used in AN, they should be considered for the co-occurring psychiatric conditions common with AN, rather than for the eating disorder alone.

Pharmacologic treatments for AN have included antidepressants, antipsychotics, cyproheptadine, hormones, and zinc. Most randomized controlled trials completed in adults have been with antidepressants. The tricyclic antidepressants clomipramine and amitriptyline have been studied for the treatment of AN. Clomipramine 50 mg/day increased appetite, which did not carry over to weight gain in patients.[107] Amitriptyline has been studied in two trials. In the first trial, there was no significant difference between amitriptyline 160 mg/day and placebo, though patients had adverse effects with amitriptyline.[108] In the second trial, amitriptyline 160 mg/day was compared with cyproheptadine 32 mg/day and placebo. Patients taking amitriptyline had no improvement in weight gain or depression scores, whereas patients taking

cyproheptadine had improvement in both areas.[109] Tricyclic antidepressants may cause several cardiac adverse effects, including prolongation of the QT interval and sudden death in children and adolescents; thus, they should be used cautiously under direct medical supervision only.

The selective serotonin reuptake inhibitors (SSRIs) fluoxetine and citalopram have been studied in randomized controlled trials of AN. The SSRIs have efficacy for depression and obsessive-compulsive disorder symptoms in children and adolescents and are safer than the tricyclic antidepressants; however, no studies using SSRIs in doses up to 60 mg/day have shown patient improvements in weight restoration or eating disorder symptoms.[76] In addition, use of SSRIs in children and adolescents has a black box warning (see the Pediatric Depression chapter), so these medications should only be used when benefits outweigh risks.

Most information regarding the use of antipsychotics for the treatment of AN has revolved around either case reports or case series. Although most studies with these agents have been completed in adults, there are some studies of atypical antipsychotics in children and adolescents. The most-studied atypical antipsychotics in children and adolescents are olanzapine, quetiapine, risperidone, and aripiprazole.

Open-label trials and a case series have documented BMI improvements in children and adolescents taking olanzapine 2.5 mg/day.[110,111] In addition, patient anxiety and agitation around eating meals was reduced. In randomized controlled trials using olanzapine 2.5–5 mg in adults with AN, one study found improvements in weight gain and obsessive thinking. However, weight gain, a common adverse effect of olanzapine, led to treatment refusal by one-half of the patients in the trial. Patients forced to gain weight without concomitant improvements in anxiety around gaining the weight typically have difficulty adhering to treatment. In the other trial, olanzapine 5 mg/day and CBT did not separate out significantly from CBT alone.[110] The first double-blind, placebo-controlled trial of olanzapine found no difference in weight, eating behaviors, or resting energy expenditure in adolescents taking olanzapine compared with those taking placebo.[112] In an 8-week, double-blind, placebo-controlled study of a mean dose of 8.5 mg of olanzapine versus placebo, investigators found a statistically significant improvement in BMI compared with placebo.[113]

Quetiapine has been used in two open-label studies of individuals with AN.[114,115] In these studies, quetiapine at 150–300 mg/day improved depression and anxiety scores but did not significantly improve weight gain. In a third randomized controlled open-label pilot study of quetiapine at 200–400 mg/day, adolescents' outcomes were similar to those in the previous open-label trials regarding improving depression and anxiety scores, together with improvements in other psychological and physical well-being measures, with few adverse effects. However, this study was not powered to determine statistical significance.[116] In a case series of children and adolescents who used quetiapine for AN, patients reported improvements in body dysmorphism.

Two case reports used risperidone 1.5 mg/day in adolescents.[117,118] Patients had no significant improvements in eating or weight gain in these reports but did have a decline in anxiety and obsessions surrounding food. A double-blind, placebo-controlled trial of risperidone (mean dose 2.5 mg/day) for the treatment of AN in adolescents showed no benefit for weight restoration.[119]

One case series of five patients with AN showed some improvements in anxiety and depression that may have led to improvements in BMI when aripiprazole was added to patients' medication regimens. Patients, observed for between 4 and about 40 months, seemed to have fewer obsessive symptoms and less distress around eating when aripiprazole was added.[120] The National Institute of Mental Health completed a clinical trial of aripiprazole for the treatment of AN; however, the results have not been published.

Common adverse effects of antipsychotics include sedation and the potential for extrapyramidal adverse effects, which, in the long term, can lead to tardive dyskinesia. These agents can also cause metabolic syndrome, including hypertension, diabetes, and hyperlipidemia, and should be used with caution in children and adolescents.

Hormones have also been used in adolescents and adults with AN. Growth hormone has been compared with placebo in adolescents with AN.[121] In one study, patients taking growth hormone became medically stabilized 10 days faster than patients not taking growth hormone. None of these patients had any significant improvement in weight. Studies of testosterone use in adults with AN have shown mood improvement but no specific improvements in weight compared with placebo.[122]

One open-label trial using elemental zinc 100 mg/day showed improvements in weight gain in patients with AN. Similar to the patients in the growth hormone study, the patients receiving elemental zinc were hospitalized for about 7 days less than the patients who did not receive zinc.[123]

SUMMARY

Medications should not be a first-line treatment in AN. Although medications may benefit co-occurring depression, anxiety, or obsessive-compulsive symptomatology, evidence is insufficient that they improve weight gain or eating disorder symptoms. After medical stabilization and refeeding, non-pharmacologic therapy, especially FBT, is the most appropriate treatment.

BN AND BED

Both BN and BED, as opposed to AN, are often characterized by a loss of control in food intake. Whereas patients with AN try to take charge of their lives by limiting food intake, patients with BN and BED often feel that they have lost control. Children and adolescents with AN who start binge and purge behaviors may eventually develop BN, though BN typically occurs independently of AN.

EPIDEMIOLOGY

Although AN may occur in children and adolescents, BN usually occurs in adolescence or early adulthood, with a peak onset at age 15.7–18.1 years.[124] Bulimia nervosa seldom occurs in premenarchal females. The lifetime prevalence of BN is 0.8%–2.6%; the incidence of BN is 1%–2%.[15,17,125,126] The lifetime prevalence of BED is 2.3%–3% in adolescents.[15,17] In one national study, less than one-third of all BN/BED cases were recognized by a clinician because of the secretive nature of the disorders.[126] Mortality rates of 3.9% for patients with BN are much lower than for patients with AN and are often associated with suicidality and medical complications, primarily electrolyte imbalances.[127] Binge eating disorder is associated with obesity and morbid obesity, which place an individual at an increased risk of mortality, but the incidence is difficult to quantify. In a study of suicide in individuals with BED, no suicides had occurred in 246 patients after 5 years.[128-131]

CLINICAL PRESENTATION

Both BN and BED are characterized by disinhibited eating of large quantities of food during a short time. The difference between BN and BED presentations depends on whether an individual participates in compensatory purging, either by self-induced vomiting, diuretics, laxatives, or all of these to reduce the potential weight gain associated with the binge. Individuals with BN are typically of normal weight or overweight, whereas individuals with BED do not purge, and about two-thirds are overweight. Although the calories taken in during a binge vary per individual, as many as 2000–5000 calories can be taken in during a discrete period. When individuals binge, they typically do so until they have significant abdominal discomfort. In BN, vomiting helps decrease the stomach discomfort caused by the binge and, for some patients, allows them to continue the binge. Often, patients with this disorder have obesity in childhood and early adolescence. The disorder itself is often not recognized by family, friends, or even health care professionals because the patient is typically within a normal weight range for age and height.[73] Patients with BN often have over-idealistic views of what body weight and shape should be, leading them to feel conflicted about eating. Fluctuations in weight are common because of binge/purge behaviors.[74]

Binge eating disorder is characterized by binging without the commensurate purging behaviors such that patients with this disorder gain a great deal of weight and typically develop obesity. Unlike the sex ratios with AN and BN, the ratio of males to females with BED is similar. Personality traits common to BED are low self-esteem and dissatisfaction with body shape and image. In addition to obesity, depression commonly co-occurs with BED.[74]

DIAGNOSTIC CRITERIA

The DSM-5 criteria for BN include repeated periods of overeating, at least weekly over 3 months, that feel outside the individual's control. These binge eating episodes are followed by behaviors that are specifically designed to prevent weight gain, such as vomiting, using laxatives, or using diuretics. Bulimia nervosa cannot occur if the individual meets the criteria for AN.[16]

The *DSM-5* criteria for BED include distress caused by repeated periods of overeating that feel outside the individual's ability to control and occurring at least weekly for 3 months. In addition, individuals with BED must do three of the following four things: eat more rapidly than would be considered normal, eat until they feel uncomfortably full, binge eat when they do not feel hungry, and eat by themselves because of embarrassment over their eating behaviors. To fully meet the criteria for BED, individuals cannot meet the criteria for either AN or BN.[16]

RISK FACTORS

Like the risk factors for AN, those for BN include having a family history of an eating disorder. Often, the parents of patients with BN have obesity, and the relative risk of developing BN is 4.2% for first-degree female relatives with AN and 4.4% for first-degree relatives of patients with BN.[131] A history of physical or sexual abuse and low self-esteem are also risk factors for BN. Personality traits such as impulsivity and self-harm are common in this population. Patients with BN often have a history of excess dieting, often skipping meals, and dissatisfaction with their body image. Performers like models, actors, jockeys, and athletes in certain sports such as ballet, gymnastics, dance, running, wrestling, and racing are at greater risk of developing BN because of stringent weight and body shape requirements.[132,133] Risk factors for BED include obesity in both first-degree family members and the patient, as well as low self-esteem, unhappiness with current body weight and shape, and a history of depression.

COURSE AND PROGNOSIS

Bulimia nervosa has a chronic course with periods of recovery and recurrence. Although the 5-year clinical recovery rate is 55%,[127] as many as 46% will continue to have eating disorder symptoms 6 years after treatment. Although treatment can improve long-term outcomes, BN symptoms diminish over time without treatment. As stated previously, the mortality risk associated with BN is estimated to be 3.9%.[51] Bulimia nervosa has a better outcome than AN, and a shorter illness before treatment is associated overall with improved outcomes. Premorbid obesity, poor family and peer relationships, and excessive exercise are all associated with poorer outcomes.[134] Although research on the course and prognosis of BED is limited, the prognosis appears good. In one 5-year study, 72% of patients fully or partly recovered without treatment.[134]

TREATMENT OF BN

INITIAL GOALS OF TREATMENT

Initial goals in BN treatment include addressing any medical complications and decreasing and eventually eliminating binging and purging behaviors. It is important to provide patient education regarding adequate nutrition and to rectify incorrect thinking regarding body shape and size, eating, and weight. Treatment of co-occurring psychiatric conditions

is imperative. Support systems should be used to prevent relapse.

The goal of treating BED is to eliminate binging and help the patient lose weight in a healthy manner.

NONPHARMACOLOGIC TREATMENT

Outside psychotherapy, much less is known about the nonpharmacologic treatment for BN and BED than for AN. Evidence is substantial regarding the use of CBT-E in patients with BN. Patients should receive CBT-E on a weekly basis for 4–5 months.[132] Interpersonal psychotherapy also plays a role in helping patients with BN work through interpersonal issues that may affect their eating disorder.

There are two controlled trials of FBT in adolescents and one trial of FBT in combination with CBT-E.[135] Family-based therapy has slightly better short-term outcomes than CBT-E but is equivalent long term.[136]

Like for BN, both CBT-E and interpersonal psychotherapy are the most effective nonpharmacologic treatments for BED. Treatments target normalizing eating by using food diaries, problem solving, and reframing how patients view interpersonal issues.

PHARMACOLOGIC TREATMENT

Antidepressants are the most-studied medications for the treatment of BN. The first antidepressant trials used the tricyclic antidepressant desipramine 200–300 mg/day, the tetracyclic antidepressant trazodone 400 mg/day, and the monoamine oxidase inhibitor brofaromine (mean dose 175 mg/day).[137-140] All were randomized controlled trials, and all found improvements in binging and purging behaviors distinct from treatment of mood. However, these studies had small sample sizes and a short duration, as well as inadequate follow-up trials. In addition, adverse effects of these medications include sedation, dry mouth, and weight gain. Monoamine oxidase inhibitor use is limited by dietary restrictions.

Bupropion at doses of 450 mg/day or greater was studied in one clinical trial, and although it decreased binge and purge behaviors, it also caused grand mal seizures in 4 of 55 patients, after which an advisory against its use in eating disorders was released. The mechanism of this interaction in BN is because bupropion is highly protein bound, with the immediate-release formulation of the drug affecting patients with eating disorder and low albumin concentrations. Seizures are not as significant an issue with the sustained- and extended-release formulations of bupropion.[141] Fluoxetine is the only medication to be U.S. Food and Drug Administration (FDA) label approved for treating BN. Moreover, six randomized controlled trials support the use of fluoxetine for treating BN. Most of these trials support the use of fluoxetine 60 mg/day, a much higher dose than used for treating depression. Although binge/purge behaviors begin to respond in as few as 3 weeks, most studies suggest that at least 8 weeks are needed to allow a response, and treatment should be continued for at least 1 year.[142-147] Both venlafaxine and fluvoxamine (mean dose of 182 mg/day) have shown promise in treating BN. An adequate dose for an adequate time appears to be imperative for use of any of the antidepressants in BN treatment.[148-150] Topiramate (mean dose 100 mg/day), naltrexone (50–300 mg/day), and ondansetron 24 mg/day have all been used in small trials for BN, and all three have successfully treated core symptoms. However, further study in larger trials needs to be completed to recommend these medications in BN.[141-154]

The SSRIs, including fluoxetine, fluvoxamine, sertraline, citalopram, and escitalopram, together with the tricyclic antidepressant imipramine, have the most studies supporting their use in BED. The SSRIs appear to help decrease binge frequency but not weight loss. In a 10-week randomized trial comparing fluoxetine 60 mg, fluvoxamine 200 mg, and sertraline 100 mg, fluoxetine and fluvoxamine caused significant differences in body weight, purging episodes, and caloric intake.[155] Medications studied for BED have been in short-term trials (less than 12 weeks), which have had high dropout rates. Like SSRI use in BN, doses must be in the high-end range to be effective. The SSRIs do not appear to be better for BED than behavioral therapy.[74]

Other medications helpful for binge eating in adults include topiramate, atomoxetine, zonisamide, lamotrigine, acamprosate, orlistat, and lisdexamfetamine.[74] Lisdexamfetamine, at doses of up to 70 mg/day, was FDA approved for treating BED in adults in 2015. In a 12-week randomized, double-blind, placebo-controlled trial, lisdexamfetamine at a dose of 70 mg/day significantly improved binging episodes in the last 4 weeks of the trial.[156] However, adverse effects from these agents, in addition to the lack of studies in children and adolescents, indicate these treatments are not currently recommended first line for pediatric BED.

SUMMARY

Although fluoxetine has an FDA label–approved indication in adults for the treatment of BN because research on fluoxetine has primarily been completed in adults, treatment response may not translate to children and adolescents. Because information about children and adolescents is limited and because of the black box warning for antidepressant use in these age groups, antidepressants should be used with caution in this population. In addition, because CBT-E has been found beneficial in BN, medication is not considered first-line treatment. When medications are used, they should be used to help treat eating disorder comorbidities, and the patient should be closely monitored by a clinician.

Antidepressants, especially the SSRIs, improve BED by reducing binge eating. Antidepressants do not seem to cause significant long-term weight loss. Lisdexamfetamine also appears to reduce the incidence of binge eating but has not yet been studied to see whether it benefits individuals younger than 18 years. Topiramate may also help with binging and weight loss in adults, but further study must be completed to confirm the results of current trials.

CONCLUSIONS

Anorexia nervosa, BN, and BED are all complex, serious, life-threatening disorders that should be viewed as such by clinicians. Mortality associated with eating disorders ranks highest among all the psychiatric disorders, especially regarding suicidality and starvation.

Data analyses on the use of medications for the treatment of AN are especially weak. Managing AN with medications alone is inappropriate. Some evidence suggests that, after medical stabilization and refeeding, FBT and CBT-E are beneficial, which may decrease the risk of relapse.

The binging and purging behaviors of BN and the binging behaviors of BED respond to the SSRIs. Fluoxetine 60 mg/day is the only FDA label–approved treatment for BN in adults. Evidence suggests that CBT-E and interpersonal psychotherapy are effective for BN and BED. Of importance, patients are often nonadherent to medications because of the associated adverse effects.

Medication studies of the treatment of eating disorders in children and adolescents have several limitations. Many lack scientific rigor. Many are also poorly designed, have insufficient sample sizes, and lack sufficient power. Moreover, as with most psychiatric research, the dropout rate is high, which affects study outcomes.

The long-term prognosis of eating disorders is improved if appropriate and adequate treatment is provided as early as possible.

A 16-year-old patient with a 5-year history of AN presents with her mother to her pediatrician's office with severe weakness, tiredness, and an emaciated appearance. She has a reported 22-kg weight loss over the past 3 months. She states that when she looks in the mirror, she feels like her stomach, hips, and thighs are fat. Her medical history includes treatment of AN for the past 5 years. She has taken sertraline 25 mg by mouth daily for the past 2½ years.

Family history: Mother with history of AN with purging as a young woman, evolving into BN in her 20s; father with history of major depressive disorder

Social history: Lives at home with parents; is a sophomore in high school; when not in school, practices ballet for 6 hours daily, including before and after school; neither smokes nor drinks alcohol; denies the use of illicit drugs

Home medications: Sertraline 25 mg orally daily

Vital signs: BP 90/72 mm Hg, HR 76 beats/minute, RR 20 breaths/minute, Tmax 96.8°F (36°C), Wt 40.8 kg, Ht 65 inches, BMI 14.97 kg/m^2

Laboratory findings:

Hgb: 15.2 g/dL

Hct: 40%

Absolute neutrophil count: 2130 cells/mm^3

Na: 132 mEq/L

K: 4.1 mEq/L

BUN: 12 mg/dL

SCr: 0.5 mg/dL

Glucose: 86 mg/dL

ALT: 26 U/L

AST: 22 U/L

On review of the patient's physical and laboratory findings, the pharmacist develops a treatment plan.

1. What criteria does the patient meet for the diagnosis of AN?

The patient meets the *DSM-5* criteria for restriction of energy intake, low body weight, fear of gaining weight, or fear of becoming fat as well as behavior that interferes with weight gain (i.e., excess time exercising [ballet]), even though she is at a significantly low weight and has binge eating/purging behaviors.

2. The patient restricts her caloric intake but also binges and purges. She self-induces vomiting. What are some of the signs of self-induced vomiting that would be noticed on physical examination?

Russell's sign, parotiditis, and eroded enamel on teeth would be caused by self-induced vomiting. Russell's sign is a callus on the dorsum of the hand from chronic contact of the hand with the upper teeth when inducing vomiting. Parotiditis is a swelling of the parotid glands along the jaw, which gives a "chipmunk-like" appearance to the face. Chronic exposure of the teeth to gastric acid will cause an erosion of the tooth enamel.

3. The patient's mother asks whether any medical complications are associated with AN. How would you respond?

Malnutrition can prevent normal growth, which can lead to amenorrhea in females because of a delay in sexual maturation.

Depending on her nutritional status, her electrolytes may be out of balance and may need to be restored (potassium, sodium, magnesium, calcium, folic acid, zinc, iron). If her ideal weight falls below 75% or her heart rate falls below 50 beats/minute, she will be considered medically unstable and will need to be hospitalized. When individuals have to be hospitalized because of malnutrition, they must be medically stabilized, and if they are feeding too quickly, hypotension, arrhythmias, seizures, cardiac and respiratory failure, rhabdomyolysis, coma, and death can result. In addition, malnutrition can lead to the risk of fractures; weight gain and return of a menstrual cycle can improve bone strength, but not in all individuals.

4. Assume there is no psychiatric comorbidity, what medication would be indicated to treat the patient's AN?

The patient currently takes sertraline. Had she been given a diagnosis of depression or had symptoms of depression, antidepressants might have been beneficial once her weight was restored to a normal range. Optimum treatment of depression would require a minimal effective dose of an antidepressant. The minimum dose of sertraline for treatment of depression is 50 mg, but many individuals with depression require doses of 100–200 mg/day. In this case, the patient has no psychiatric comorbidity, so sertraline would not likely be beneficial.

REFERENCES

1. Childress AC, Brewerton TD, Hodges EL, et al. The kids eating disorder survey (KEDS): a study of middle-school students. J Am Acad Adolesc Psychiatry 1993;32:843-50.

2. Lucas RA, Beard CM, O'Fallon WM, et al. Fifty year trends in the incidence of anorexia nervosa in Rochester, Minn: a population-based study. Am J Psychiatry 1991;148:917-22.

3. Whitaker AH. An epidemiologic study of anorectic and bulimic symptoms in adolescent girls: implications for pediatricians. Pediatr Ann 1992;21:752-9.

4. Krowchuk DP, Kreiter SR, Woods CR, et al. Problem dieting behaviors among young adolescents. Arch Pediatr Adolesc Med 1998;152:884-8.

5. Agency for Healthcare Research and Quality (AHRQ). Eating Disorders Sending More Americans to the Hospital. AHRQ News and Numbers. April 1, 2009. Available at https://archive.ahrq.gov/news/newsroom/news-and-numbers/040109.html. Accessed November 2, 2018.

6. Gard C, Freeman CP. The dismantling of a myth: a review of eating disorders and socioeconomic status. Int J Eat Disord 1996; 20:1-12.

7. Pike KM, Walsh BR. Ethnicity and eating disorders: implications for incidence and treatment. Psychopharmacol Bull 1996; 32:265-74.

8. Crago M, Shisslak CM, Estes LS. Eating disturbances among American minority groups: a review. Int J Eat Disord 1995; 19:239-48.

9. Carlat DJ, Camargo CA, Herzog DM. Eating disorders in males: a report on 135 patients. Am J Psychiatry 1997;154:1127-32.

10. Rosen DS. Eating disorders in adolescent males. Adolesc Med 2003;14:677-89.

11. Lai KY. Anorexia nervosa in Chinese adolescents: does culture make a difference? J Adolesc 2000;23:561-8.

12. Le Grange D, Telch CF, Tibbs J. Eating attitudes and behaviors in 1435 South African Caucasian and non-Caucasian college students. Am J Psychiatry 1998;155:250-4.

13. Ornstein RM, Rosen DS, Mammel KA, et al. Distribution of eating disorders in children and adolescents using the proposed DSM-5 criteria for feeding and eating disorders. J Adolesc Health 2013;53:303-5.

14. Stice E, Marti CN, Rohde P. Prevalence, incidence, impairment, and course of the proposed DSM-5 eating disorder diagnoses in a community cohort of young women. J Abnorm Psychol 2013; 122:445-57.

15. Smink FR, van Hoeken D, Oldehinkel AJ, et al. Prevalence and severity of DSM-5 eating disorders in a community cohort of adolescents. Int J Eat Disord 2014;47:610-9.

16. American Psychiatric Association (APA). Diagnostic and Statistical Manual of Mental Disorders, 5th ed. Washington, DC: APA, 2013.

17. Hoek HW. Incidence, prevalence and mortality of anorexia nervosa and other eating disorder. Curr Opin Psychiatry 2006; 19:389-94.

18. Micali N, Hagberg KW, Petersen I, et al. The incidence of eating disorders in the UK in 2000-2009: findings from the general practice research database. BMJ Open 2013;3:e002646.

19. Garner DM. Pathogenesis of anorexia nervosa. Lancet 1993; 341:1631-5.

20. Patton GC, Selzer R, Coffey C, et al. Onset of eating disorders: population based cohort over 3 years. BMJ 1999;318:765-8.

21. Hoek HW. Lack of relation between culture and anorexia nervosa—results of an incidence study in Curacao. N Engl J Med 1998;338:1231-2.

22. Fichter MM, Elton M, Sourdi L, et al. Anorexia nervosa in Greek and Turkish adolescents. Eur Arch Psychiatry Neurol Sci 1988;237:200-8.

23. Holland AJ, Hall A, Murray R, et al. Anorexia nervosa: a study of 34 twin pairs and one set of triplets. Br J Psychiatry 1984;145:414-9.

24. Walters EE, Kendler KS. Anorexia nervosa and anorexic-like syndromes in a population-based female twin sample. Am J Psychiatry 1995;152:64-71.

25. Gershon ES, Schreiber JL, Hamovit JR, et al. Clinical findings in patients with anorexia nervosa and affective illness in their relatives. Am J Psychiatry 1984;141:1419-22.

26. Strober M, Freeman R, Lampert C, et al. Controlled family study of anorexia nervosa and bulimia nervosa: evidence of shared liabilities and the development of partial syndromes. Am J Psychiatry 2000;157:393-401.

27. Lilenfeld LR, Wonderlich S, Riso LP, et al. Eating disorders and personality: a methodological and empirical review. Clin Psychol Rev 2006;26:299-320.

28. Kortegaard LS, Hoerder K, Joergensen J, et al. A preliminary population-based twin study of self-reported eating disorder. Psychol Med 2001;31:361-5.

29. Klump KL, Miller KB, Keel PK, et al. Genetic and environmental influences on anorexia nervosa syndromes in a population-based twin sample. Psychol Med 2001;31:737-40.

30. Bulik CM, Sullivan PF, Wade TD, et al. Twin studies of eating disorders: a review. Int J Eat Disord 2000;27:1-20.

31. Trace SE, Baker JH, Penas-Lledo E, et al. The genetics of eating disorders. Annu Rev Clin Psychol 2013;9:589-620.

32. Bulik CM, Devlin B, Bacanu SA, et al. Significant linkage on chromosome 10p in families with bulimia nervosa. Am J Hum Genet 2003;72:200-7.

33. Scherag S, Hebebrand J, Hinney A. Eating disorders: the current status of molecular genetic research. Eur Child Adolesc Psychiatry 2010;19:211-26.

34. Jimerson DC, Lesem MD, Kaye WH, et al. Eating disorders and depression: is there a serotonin connection? Biol Psychiatry 1990;28:443-54.

35. Ulfvebrand S, Birgegard A, Norring C, et al. Psychiatric comorbidity in eating disorders. Results from a large clinical database. Psychiatry Res 2015;230:294-9.

36. Sansone RA, Sansone LA. The relationship between borderline personality and obesity. Innov Clin Neurosci 2013;10:36-40.

37. Kaye WH, Gwirtsman HE, George DT, et al. Altered serotonin activity in anorexia nervosa after long-term weight restoration: does elevated cerebrospinal fluid 5-hydroxyindoleacetic acid level correlate with rigid and obsessive behavior? Arch Gen Psychiatry 1991;48:556-62.

38. Jimerson DC, Lesem MD, Kaye WH, et al. Low serotonin and dopamine metabolite concentration in cerebral spinal fluid from bulimic patients with frequent binge episodes. Arch Gen Psychiatry 1992;49:132-8.

39. Urwin RE, Bennetts B, Wilcken B, et al. Anorexia nervosa (restrictive subtype) is associated with a polymorphism in the novel norepinephrine transporter gene promoter polymorphic region. Mol Psychiatry 2002;7:652-7.

40. Barry VC, Klawans HL. On the role of dopamine in the pathophysiology of anorexia nervosa. J Neural Transm 1976;38:107-22.

41. Kaye WH, Bulik CM, Thornton L, et al. Comorbidity of anxiety disorders with anorexia and bulimia nervosa. Am J Psychiatry 2004;161:2215-21.

42. Hebebrand J, Muller TD, Holtkamp K, et al. The role of leptin in anorexia nervosa. Mol Psychiatry 2007;12:23-35.

43. Chan JL, Mantzros CS. Role of leptin in energy deprivation states: normal human physiology and clinical implications for hypothalamic amenorrhea and anorexia nervosa. Lancet 2005;366:74-85.

44. Haas V, Onur S, Paul T, et al. Leptin and body weight regulation in patients with anorexia nervosa before and during weight recovery. Am J Clin Nutr 2005;81:889-96.

45. Hotta M, Ohwada R, Akamizu T, et al. Ghrelin increases hunger and food intake in patients with restricting-type anorexia nervosa: a pilot study. Endocr J 2009;56:1119-58.

46. Himmerich H, Schonknecht P, Heitmann S, et al. Laboratory parameters and appetite regulators in patients with anorexia nervosa. J Psychiatr Pract 2010;16:82-92.

47. Muller TD, Greene BH, Bellodi L, et al. Fat mass and obesity-associated gene (FTO) in eating disorders: evidence of association of the rs9939609 obesity risk allele with bulimia nervosa and anorexia nervosa. Obes Facts 2012;5:408-19.

48. Sullivan PF. Mortality in anorexia nervosa. Am J Psychiatry 1995;152:1073-4.

49. Crow SJ, Peterson CB, Swanson SA, et al. Increased mortality in bulimia nervosa and other eating disorders. Am J Psychiatry 2009;166:1342-6.

50. Fichter MM, Quadflieg N. Mortality in eating disorder – results of a large prospective clinical longitudinal study. Int J Eat Disord 2016;49:391-401.

51. Katzman DK. Medical complications in adolescents with anorexia nervosa: a review of the literature. Int J Eat Disord 2005;37:S52-S59.

52. Misra M, Aggarwal A, Miller KK, et al. Effects of anorexia nervosa on clinical, hematologic, biochemical, and bone density parameters in community-dwelling adolescent girls. Pediatrics 2004;114:1574-83.

53. Brambilla F, Monteleone P. Physical complications and physiological aberrations in eating disorders: a review. In: Maj M, Halmi K, Lopez-Ibor JJ, et al., eds. Eating Disorders, vol. 6. Chichester, UK: John Wiley & Sons, 2003.

54. Mehler PS, Birmingham LC, Crow SJ, et al. Medical complications of eating disorders. In: Grilo CM, Mitchell JE, eds. The Treatment of Eating Disorders: A Clinical Handbook. New York: Guilford, 2010.

55. Swenne I. Weight requirements for catch-up growth in girls with eating disorders and onset of weight loss before puberty. Int J Eat Disord 2005;38:340-5.

56. Katzman DK, Zipursky RB, Lambe EK, et al. Longitudinal magnetic resonance imaging study of the brain changes in adolescents with anorexia nervosa. Arch Pediatr Adolesc Med 1997;151:793-7.

57. Chui HT, Christensen BK, Zipursky RB, et al. Cognitive function and brain structure in females with a history of adolescent-onset anorexia. Pediatrics 2008;122:e426-e437.

58. Van den Eynde F, Treasure J. Neuroimaging in eating disorders and obesity: implications for research. Child Adolesc Psychiatr Clin North Am 2009;18:95-115.

59. Wong JCH, Lewindon P, Mortimer R, et al. Bone mineral density in adolescent females with recently diagnosed anorexia nervosa. Int J Eat Disord 2001;29:11-6.

60. Golden NH, Shenker IR. Amenorrhea in anorexia nervosa: etiology and implications. Adolesc Med 1992;3:503-18.

61. Mitchell JE, Crow S. Medical complications of anorexia nervosa and bulimia nervosa. Curr Opin Psychiatry 2006;19:438-43.

62. Casiero D, Frishman WH. Cardiovascular complications of eating disorders. Cardiol Rev 2006;14:227-31.

63. Rosen DS; and the Committee on Adolescence. Identification and management of eating disorders in children and adolescents. Pediatrics 2010;126:1240.

64. Kleifield E, Wagner S, Kalami KA. Cognitive-behavioral treatment of anorexia nervosa. Eating disorders. Psychiatr Clin North Am 1996;19:715-34.

65. Fouladi F, Mitchell JE, Crosby RD, et al. Prevalence of alcohol and other substance use in patients with eating disorders. Eur Eat Disord Rev 2015;23:531-6.

66. Fairburn CG, Cooper Z. The Eating Disorder Examination, 12th ed. In: Fairburn CG, Wilson GT, eds. Binge Eating: Nature Assessment and Treatment. New York: Guilford, 1993:317-60.

67. Sunday SR, Halmi KA, Einhorn AN. The Yale-Brown-Cornell Eating Disorder Scale: a new scale to assess eating disorder symptomatology. Int J Eat Disord 1995;18:237-45.

68. Mazure CM, Halmi KA, Sunday SR, et al. The Yale-Brown-Cornell Eating Disorder Scale: development, use, reliability and validity. J Psychiatr Res 1994;28:425-45.

69. Garner DM, Olmstead MP, Bohr Y, et al. The Eating Attitudes Test: psychometric features and clinical correlates. Psychol Med 1982;12:871-8.

70. Maloney MJ, McGuire JB, Daniels SR. Reliability testing of a children's version of the Eating Attitude Test. J Am Acad Child Adolesc Psychiatry 1988;27:541-3.

71. Pike KM, Woll SL, Gluck M, et al. Eating disorder measures. In: American Psychiatric Association Handbook of Psychiatric Measures. Washington, DC: American Psychiatric Association, 2000:647-71.

72. Mitchell JE, Hatsukami D, Eckert E, et al. The Eating Disorders Questionnaire. Psychopharmacol Bull 1985;21:1025-43.

73. Bostic JQ, Muriel AC, Hacks S, et al. Anorexia nervosa in a 7-year-old girl. J Dev Behav Pediatr 1997;18:331-3.

74. Jackson CW, Cates M, Lorenz R. Pharmacotherapy of eating disorders. Nutr Clin Pract 2010;25:143-59.

75. Halmi KA. Perplexities and provocations of eating disorders. J Child Psychol Psychiatry 2009;50:163-9.

76. Hoek H, Hoeken DV. Review of prevalence and incidence of eating disorders. Int J Eat Disord 2003;34:383-96.

77. Arnow B, Sanders MJ, Steiner H. Premenarcheal versus postmenarchal anorexia nervosa: a comparative study. Clin Child Psychol Psychiatry 1999;4:403-14.

78. Thunder S. Anorexia nervosa with an early onset: selection, gender, outcome, and results of a long-term follow-up study. J Youth Adolesc 1996;25:419-25.

79. Pike KM. Long-term course of anorexia nervosa: response, relapse, remission and recovery. Clin Psychol Rev 1998;18:4437-75.

80. American Psychiatric Association (APA). Diagnostic and Statistical Manual of Mental Disorders, 4th ed.; text rev. Washington, DC: APA, 2000.

81. Dittmer N, Voderholzer U, von der Muhlen M, et al. Specialized group intervention of compulsive exercise in inpatients with eating disorders: feasibility and preliminary outcomes. J Eat Disord 2018;6:27.

82. Strober M, Freeman R, Lampert C, et al. Controlled family study of anorexia nervosa and bulimia nervosa: evidence of shared liability and transmission of partial syndromes. Am J Psychiatry 2000;157:393-401.

83. Haines J, Gillman MW, Rifas-Shiman S, et al. Family dinner and disordered eating behaviors in a large cohort of adolescents. Eat Disord 2010;18:10-24.

84. Keel PK, Dorer DJ, Eddy KT, et al. Predictors of morality in eating. Arch Gen Psychiatry 2003;60:179-83.

85. Arcelus J, Mitchell AJ, Wales J, et al. Mortality rates in patient with anorexia nervosa and other eating disorders: a meta-analysis of 36 studies. Arch Gen Psychiatry 2011;68:724-31.

86. Steinhausen HC. The outcome of anorexia nervosa in the 20th century. Am J Psychiatry 2002;159:1284-93.

87. Wentz E, Gillberg IC, Anckarsater H, et al. Adolescent-onset anorexia nervosa: 18 year outcome. Br J Psychiatry 2009;194:168-74.

88. Winston AP; and the Working Group Council Report CR 130. Guidelines for the Nutritional Management of Anorexia Nervosa. London: Royal College of Psychiatrists, 2005. Available at http://www.mazi.org.cy/mazi/userfiles/Guidelines-for-the-nutritional-management-of-anorexia-nervosa.pdf. Accessed February 16, 2019.

89. American Psychiatric Association (APA). Treatment of Patients with Eating Disorders, 3rd ed. In: American Psychiatric Association Practice Guidelines for the Treatment of Psychiatric Disorders. Washington, DC: American Psychiatric Publishing, 2004.

90. Golden NH, Katzman DK, Sawyer S, et al. Update on the medical management of eating disorders in adolescents. J Adolesc Health 2015;56:370-5.

91. Golden NH, Katzman DK, Sawyer S, et al. The Society for Adolescent Health and Medicine. Position paper of the society for adolescent health and medicine: medical management of restrictive eating disorders in adolescents and young adults. J Adolesc Health 2015;56:121-5.

92. Marzola E, Nasser JA, Hashim SA, et al. Nutritional rehabilitation in anorexia nervosa: review of the literature and implications for treatment. BMC Psychiatry 2013;13:290.

93. Golden NH, Abrams SA. Committee on Nutrition. Optimizing bone health in children and adolescents. Pediatrics 2014; 134:e1229e43.

94. Hearing SD. Refeeding syndrome is underdiagnosed and undertreated, but treatable. BMJ 2004;328:908-9.

95. Le Grange D, Eisler I. Family interventions in adolescent anorexia nervosa. Child Adolesc Psychiatr Clin North Am 2009;18:159-73.

96. Lock J, Agras WS, Bryson S, et al. A comparison of short- and long-term family therapy for adolescent anorexia nervosa. J Am Acad Child Adolesc Psychiatry 2005;44:632-9.

97. Le Grange D, Eisler I, Dare C, et al. Evaluation of family treatments in adolescent anorexia nervosa: the results of a controlled comparison of two family interventions. J Child Psychol Psychiatry 2000;41:727-36.

98. Robin AL, Siegel PT, Koepke T, et al. Family therapy versus individual therapy for adolescent females with anorexia nervosa. J Dev Behav Pediatr 1994;15:111-6.

99. Robin AL, Siegel PT, Moye AW, et al. A controlled comparison of family versus individual therapy for adolescents with anorexia nervosa. J Am Acad Child Adolesc Psychiatry 1999;38:1482-9.

100. Russell GFM, Szmukler GI, Dare C, et al. An evaluation of family therapy in anorexia nervosa and bulimia nervosa. Arch Gen Psychiatry 1987;44:1047-56.

101. Eisler I, Dare C, Hodes M, et al. Family therapy for adolescent anorexia nervosa: the results of a controlled comparison of two family interventions. J Child Psychol Psychiatry 2000;41:727-36.

102. Fairburn CG, Cooper Z, Shafron R. Enhanced cognitive behavioral therapy for eating disorders ("CBT-E"): an overview. In: Fairburn CG, ed. Cognitive Behavior Therapy and Eating Disorders. New York: Guilford, 2008:23-34.

103. Lock J, Le Grange D, Agras WS, et al. Randomized clinical trial comparing family-based treatment with adolescent-focused individual therapy for adolescents with anorexia nervosa. Arch Gen Psychiatry 2010;67:1025-32.

104. Fitzpatrick K, Moye A, Hoste R, et al. Adolescent focused psychotherapy for adolescents with anorexia nervosa. J Contemp Psychother 2010;40:31-9.

105. Cooper Z, Stewart A. CBT-E and the younger patient. In: Fairburn CG, ed. Cognitive Behavior Therapy and Eating Disorders. New York: Guilford, 2008:221-30.

106. Dalle Grave R, Calugi S, Doll HA, et al. Enhanced cognitive behaviour therapy for adolescents with anorexia nervosa: an alternative to family therapy? Behav Res Ther 2013;51:R9-12.

107. Lacey J, Crisp A. Hunger, food intake and weight: the impact of clomipramine on a refeeding anorexia nervosa population. Postgrad Med J 1980;56:79-85.

108. Biederman J, Herzog DB, Rivinus TM, et al. Amitriptyline in the treatment of anorexia nervosa: a double-blind, placebo-controlled study. J Clin Psychopharmacol 1985;5:10-6.

109. Halmi KA, Eckert E, LaDu TH, et al. Anorexia nervosa: treatment efficacy of cyproheptadine and amitriptyline. Arch Gen Psychiatry 1986;43:177-81.

110. Brambilla F, Garcia C, Fassino S, et al. Olanzapine therapy in anorexia nervosa: psychobiological effects. Int Clin Psychopharmacol 2007;22:197-204.

111. Bissada H, Tasca G, Barber A, et al. Olanzapine in the treatment of low body weight and obsessive thinking in women with anorexia nervosa: a randomized, double-blind, placebo-controlled trial. Am J Psychiatry 2008;165:1281-8.

112. Kafantaris V, Leigh E, Hertz S, et al. A placebo controlled pilot study of adjunctive olanzapine for adolescents with anorexia nervosa. J Child Adolesc Psychopharmacol 2011;21:207-12.

113. Attia E, Kaplan AS, Walsh BT, et al. Olanzapine versus placebo for out-patients with anorexia nervosa. Psychol Med 2011; 41:2177-82.

114. Powers P, Bannon Y, Eubanks R, et al. Quetiapine in anorexia nervosa patients: an open-label outpatient pilot study. Int J Eat Disord 2007;40:21-6.

115. Bosanac P, Kurlender S, Norman T, et al. An open-label study of quetiapine in anorexia nervosa. Hum Psychopharmacol 2007;22:223-30.

116. Court A, Mulder C, Kerr M, et al. Investigating the effectiveness, safety and tolerability of quetiapine in the treatment of anorexia nervosa in young people: a pilot study. J Psychiatr Res 2010;44:1027-34.

117. Fisman S, Steele M, Short J, et al. Case study: anorexia nervosa and autistic disorder in an adolescent girl. J Am Acad Child Adolesc Psychiatry 1996;35:937-40.

118. Newman-Toker J. Risperidone in anorexia nervosa. J Am Acad Child Adolesc Psychiatry 2000;39:941-2.

119. Hagman J, Gralla J, Sigel E, et al. A double-blind placebo-controlled study of risperidone for the treatment of adolescents and young adults with anorexia nervosa: a pilot study. J Am Acad Child Adoles Psychiatry 2011;50:915-24.

120. Trunko ME, Schwartz TA, Duvvurs V, et al. Aripiprazole in anorexia nervosa and low weight bulimia nervosa. Int J Eat Disord 2011;44:269-75.

121. Hill K, Bucuvalas J, McClain C, et al. Pilot study of growth hormone administration during the refeeding of malnourished anorexia nervosa patients. J Child Adolesc Psychopharmacol 2000;10:3-8.

122. Miller KK, Grieco KA, Klibanski A. Testosterone administration in women with anorexia nervosa. J Clin Endocrinal Metab 2005;90:1428-33.

123. Birmingham CL, Goldner EM, Bakan R. Controlled trial of zinc supplementation in anorexia nervosa. Int J Eating Disord 1994;15:251-5.

124. Stice E, Agras WS. Predicting onset and cessation of bulimic behaviors during adolescence. Behav Ther 1998;29:257-76.

125. Fairburn CG, Beglin SJ. Studies of the epidemiology of bulimia nervosa. Am J Psychiatry 1990;147:401-8.

126. Binford R, Le Grange D. Adolescents with bulimia nervosa and eating disorder not otherwise specified-purging only. Int J Eat Disord 2005;28:157-61.

127. Keski-Rahkonen A, Hoek HW, Linna MS, et al. Incidence and outcomes of bulimia nervosa: a nationwide population-based study. Psychol Med 2009;39:823-31.

128. Ogden CE, et al. The epidemiology of obesity. Gastroenterology 2007;132:2087-102.

129. Solomon CG, Manson JE. Obesity and mortality: a review of the epidemiologic data. Am J Clin Nutr 1997;66:1044S-1050S.

130. Preti A, Rocchi MB, Sisti D, et al. A comprehensive meta-analysis of the risk of suicide in eating disorders. Acta Psychiatr Scand 2011;124:6-17.

131. Strober M. Family-genetic studies of eating disorders. J Clin Psychiatry 1991;52:9-12.

132. Sundgot-Borgen J. Eating disorders in female athletes. Sports Med 1994;17:176-88.

133. Nichols JF, Rauh MJ, Lawson MJ, et al. Prevalence of the female athlete triad syndrome among high school athletes. Arch Pediatr Adolesc Med 2006;160:137-42.

134. Rome ES, Ammerman S, Rosen DS, et al. Children and adolescents with eating disorders: the state of the art. Pediatrics 2003; 111:e98.

135. Lock J. Adjusting cognitive behavioral therapy for adolescent bulimia nervosa: results of a case series. Am J Psychother 2005;59:267-81.

136. Murray SB, Anderson LK, Cusack A, et al. Integrating family-based treatment and dialectical behavioral therapy for adolescent bulimia nervosa: preliminary outcomes of an open pilot trial. Eat Disord 2015;23:336-44.

137. Walsh BT, Hadigan CM, Devlin MJ, et al. Long-term outcome of antidepressant treatment for bulimia nervosa. Am J Psychiatry 1991;148:1206-12.

138. Agras WS, Rossiter EM, Arnow B, et al. Pharmacologic and cognitive-behavioral treatment for bulimia nervosa: a controlled comparison. Am J Psychiatry 1992;149:82-7.

139. Walsh BT, Wilson GT, Loeb KL, et al. Medication and psychotherapy in the treatment of bulimia nervosa. Am J Psychiatry 1997;154:523-31.

140. Wilson GT, Loeb KL, Walsh BT, et al. Psychological versus pharmacological treatments of bulimia nervosa: predictors and processes of change. J Consult Clin Psychol 1999;67:451-9.

141. Horne RL, Ferguson JM, Pope HG, et al. Treatment of bulimia with bupropion: a multicenter controlled trial. J Clin Psychiatry 1988;49:262-6.

142. Fluoxetine Bulimia Nervosa Collaborative Study Group. Fluoxetine in the treatment of bulimia nervosa: a multicenter, placebo controlled, double-blind trial. Arch Gen Psychiatry 1992;49:82-7.

143. Goldstein DJ, Wilson MG, Thompson VL, et al. Long-term fluoxetine treatment of bulimia nervosa. Fluoxetine Bulimia Nervosa Research Group. Br J Psychiatry 1995;166:660-6.

144. Kanerva R, Rissanen A, Sarna S. Fluoxetine in the treatment of anxiety, depressive symptoms, and eating-related symptoms in bulimia nervosa. Nord J Psychiatry 1994;49:237-42.

145. Beaumont PJ, Russell JD, Touyz SW, et al. Intensive nutritional counseling in bulimia nervosa: a role for supplementation with fluoxetine? Aust N Z J Psychiatry 1997;31:514-24.

146. Goldstein DJ, Wilson MG, Ashcroft RC, et al. Effectiveness of fluoxetine therapy in bulimia nervosa regardless of comorbid depression. Int J Eat Disord 1999;25:19-27.

147. Romano SJ, Halmi KA, Sarkar NP, et al. A placebo-controlled study of fluoxetine in continued treatment of bulimia nervosa after successful acute fluoxetine treatment. Am J Psychiatry 2002;159:96-102.

148. Malhotre S, King JL, Welsh JA, et al. Venlafaxine treatment of binge eating disorder: a series of 35 patients. J Clin Psychiatry 2002;63:802-6.

149. Fichter MM, Kruger R, Rief W, et al. Fluvoxamine in prevention of relapse in bulimia nervosa: effects on eating-specific psychopathology. J Clin Psychopharmacol 1996;16:9-18.

150. Fichter MM, Leibel C, Kruger R, et al. Effects of fluvoxamine on depression, anxiety and other areas of general psychopathology in bulimia nervosa. Pharmacopsychiatry 1997;31:514-24.

151. Faris PL, Kim SW, Meller WH, et al. Effect of decreasing afferent vagal activity with ondansetron on symptoms of bulimia nervosa: a randomized double-blind trial. Lancet 2000;355:792-7.

152. Hoopes SP, Reimherr FW, Hedges DW, et al. Treatment of bulimia nervosa with topiramate: a randomized, double-blind placebo-controlled trial. Part 1: improvement in binge and purge measures. J Clin Psychiatry 2003;64:1335-41.

153. Hedges DW, Reimherr FW, Hoopes SP, et al. Treatment of bulimia nervosa with topiramate in a randomized, double-blind placebo controlled trial. Part 2: improvement in psychiatric measures. J Clin Psychiatry 2003;64:1449-54.

154. Steffen KL, Roerig JL, Mitchell JE, et al. Emerging drugs for eating disorder treatment. Expert Opin Emerg Drugs 2006;1:315-36.

155. Milano W, De Rosa M, Milano L, et al. A comparative study between three different SSRIs in the treatment of bulimia nervosa. Curr Neurobiol 2013;4:39-43.

156. McElroy S, Hudson J, Ferreira-Cornwell M, et al. Lisdexamfetamine dimesylate for adults with moderate to severe bind eating disorder: results of two pivotal phase 3 randomized controlled trials. Neuropsychopharmacology 2015;41:1251-60.

CHAPTER 36

Substance Use Disorder
Lisa Lubsch, Pharm.D., FPPA, BCPPS, AE-C

INTRODUCTION

The consequences of substance use disorder (SUD) during childhood negatively impacts all aspects of the adolescent's current and future life. The harms to the adolescent and family range among biological, psychological, social, spiritual, and financial problems. The status continuum varies between healthy, substance misuse, and SUD. Addiction is a chronic brain disease, the most severe form of SUD, and is associated with compulsive or uncontrolled use of one or more substances.[1] Adolescent SUD is treatable, but often becomes more difficult to manage as it progresses to a chronic problem.

DEFINITIONS

A *substance* is a psychoactive compound that may be broadly categorized as a depressant, stimulant, and/or hallucinogen. The use of any substance in a manner, situation, amount or frequency that can cause harm to the user or to individuals around them is known as *substance misuse*.[1] *Intoxication* is a reversible, substance-specific syndrome causing significant problematic behavior or psychological changes during or shortly after use.[2] *Withdrawal* is a syndrome that occurs once the concentration of a substance decreases after heavy and prolonged use.[2] Repeated misuse of a substance or substances leads to *substance use disorder* or *SUD*. According to the *Diagnostic and Statistical Manual of Mental Disorders, Fifth Edition*, SUDs are characterized by a problematic pattern of substance use leading to clinically significant impairment in cognitive, behavioral, and physiological function.[2] Substance use disorders vary in severity (*mild, moderate, severe*) and duration of remission (*early, sustained*). The American Society of Addiction Medicine defines *addiction* as a primary, chronic disease of brain in the areas that process reward, motivation, and memory characterized by the inability to consistently abstain, impairment in behavioral control, craving, diminished recognition of significant problems with one's behaviors and interpersonal relationships, and a dysfunctional emotional response.[3]

EPIDEMIOLOGY

Although several national surveys measure differing rates of substance use among adolescents, all show widespread use of alcohol and other drugs. The Youth Risk Behavior Survey (YRBS) is a national survey administered every 2 years to representative samples of ninth- to 12th-grade students. The 2017 survey showed that 60.4% of students had consumed at least one alcoholic drink in their lifetime. The present rate of *alcohol use* (defined as at least one drink in the previous 30 days) among high school students is 29.8%. A significant decrease in both the prevalence of ever drinking or current alcohol use has occurred over the past two decades.[4] The National Survey on Drug Use and Health (NSDUH), an interview of individuals 12 years or older, has shown similar long-term trends, with lower prevalence rates compared with the YRBS. In 2018, 9% of people age 12 to 17 years reported current consumption of alcohol.[5] According to the NSDUH, the past year illicit drug use, including misuse of prescription drugs, among those age 12 to 17 years is 16.7%.[5] Marijuana is the most widely used substance, with a present rate of 12.5%. However, the YRBS showed a higher current use rate for marijuana among adolescents of 19.8%.[4]

Another survey of students in the eighth, 10th, and 12th grades shows long-term trends similar to those in the previously mentioned studies. In the 2018 Monitoring the Future (MTF) report, alcohol and marijuana use declined, with recent peaks in marijuana use, among all three grades. However, alcohol and marijuana use more than doubled between eighth and 10th grade.[6]

Prescription drugs, including pain relievers, tranquilizers, stimulants and sedatives, are subsequent to marijuana with 1.9% of children age 12 to 17 years misusing these substances in the year, and with 2.8% of the misuse representing opioids. The NSDUH reports the percentage of current heroin use (0.1%) in adolescents was similar to previous years' estimates.[5]

Tobacco is another commonly misused substance among adolescents. According to the YRBS, 8.8% of adolescents currently smoke traditional cigarettes and 13.2% use an electronic vapor product including e-cigarettes, e-cigars, e-pipes, vape pipes, vaping pens, e-hookahs, and hookah pens.[4] The current cigarette use rate (2.7%) is lower in the NSDUH, and use of electronic vapor products were not assessed in the NSDUH.[5] Of current concern, data from the National Youth Tobacco Survey revealed current e-cigarette use increased from 11.7% in 2017 to 20.8% in 2018.[7] This finding is consistent with the MTF survey, which showed the largest ever recorded increase in vaping of all substances (nicotine, marijuana, and flavoring) among eighth-, 10th-, and 12th-grade students.[6] This rapid rise is likely the result of increasing use of "pod mod" vapor products (e.g., Juul [JUUL Labs, Inc., San Francisco, CA]), which are discrete and contain a higher concentration of nicotine.[8]

NEUROBIOLOGY OF ADDICTION

Addiction progresses over the course of three stages, with each stage corresponding to alterations to neurobiologic circuits in the central nervous system (Figure 1). The first stage, *binge and intoxication*, involves the reward pathway of the basal ganglia. The neurotransmitters or neuromodulators with key roles in reinforcing the pleasurable effects of substances are primarily mesolimbic dopamine together with opioid peptide, γ-aminobutyric acid (GABA), and endocannabinoid. Further neuroadaptation results in incentive salience by which associated cues (e.g., people, places) trigger substance-seeking because of an increase in glutamate. A second stage—*withdrawal and negative effect*—results from activation of the extended amygdala. The neurotransmitters involved in stress at this stage are corticotropin-releasing factor, norepinephrine, and dynorphin. A widely distributed network, including the prefrontal cortex and hippocampus, mediates the third stage—*preoccupation and anticipation*. Executive function is impaired including disruption of decision-making and behavioral inhibition. Glutamate is the main neurotransmitter involved in this phase of craving leading to relapse.[1,9]

A PERIOD OF VULNERABILITY

Adolescents may be particularly vulnerable to the exposure to alcohol and other drugs because the brain is still developing throughout this period into young adulthood. A recent review of prospective studies suggests that the following changes over this age period predispose adolescents to initiate substance use: poorer neuropsychological functioning on tests of inhibition and working memory; smaller gray and white matter volume; changes in white matter integrity; and altered brain activation during inhibition, working memory, reward, and resting state. The effects of alcohol and marijuana use during adolescence include poorer cognitive functioning on tests of the following: verbal memory, visuospatial functioning, psychomotor speed, working memory, attention, cognitive control, and overall IQ. Studies show heavy alcohol use in adolescence leads to a decrease in gray matter, a decrease in white matter development and integrity, and increased brain activation during tasks of inhibition and working memory. Adolescents may be more susceptible to negative and chronic effects of substance use.[10]

RISK VERSUS PROTECTIVE FACTORS

Addiction has a strong genetic component.[11] Environmental influences from the community, caregiver, and/or the adolescent may increase or decrease the probability of substance use. Risk or protective factors affecting adolescent SUDs are listed in Table 1.[1] With the interaction of genetic predisposition and environment, the more risk factors an adolescent has, the greater the chance of substance use progressing to addiction.

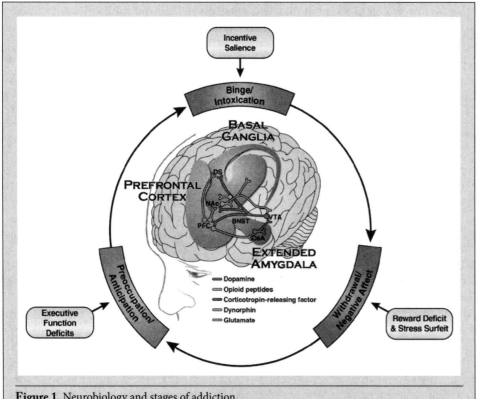

Figure 1. Neurobiology and stages of addiction.

Reprinted from Center for Substance Abuse Treatment. Detoxification and Substance Abuse Treatment. Treatment Improvement Protocol (TIP) Series 45. HHS Publication No. (SMA) 06-4131. Rockville, MD: Substance Abuse and Mental Health Services Administration, 2006.

CLINICAL PRESENTATION AND DIAGNOSIS

The NSDUH revealed 946,000 adolescents had an SUD in 2018, which represents a rate of 3.8%, or about 1 in 26 adolescents.[5] Addiction cycles through signs and symptoms of impulsivity, positive reinforcement or pleasure from the substance (which decreases with tolerance), negative reinforcement or needing relief, and compulsivity from withdrawal.

SCREENING

A recent policy statement and clinical report from the American Academy of Pediatrics (AAP) supports the approach recommended by the Substance Abuse and Mental Health Services Administration for screening for substance use.[12-14] This approach—*screening, brief intervention, and referral to treatment*—is defined as a comprehensive, integrated, public health approach to the delivery of early intervention for individuals with risky alcohol and drug use, and the timely referral to more intensive substance abuse treatment for those who have an SUD.

The process shown in Box 1 is suggested by AAP for screening adolescents for an SUD.[15-19] Routine drug testing is not currently recommended by AAP for screening of an adolescent SUD.[20] Voluntary drug testing may supplement information obtained by history and should not be used alone for diagnosing an SUD.

DIAGNOSIS

Box 2 lists 11 criteria used to diagnose an SUD. These criteria may be grouped by impaired control, social impairment, risky use, and pharmacologic variables (tolerance and withdrawal). A mild SUD is suggested by the presence of two to three symptoms, moderate by four to five symptoms, and severe by six or more symptoms, also known as *addiction*. Severity may improve or worsen over time, and, if remission is attained, the duration should be specified.[2]

Table 1. Factors Influencing Substance Use Disorder in Adolescents

Risk Factors	Protective Factors
Individual and Peer	
Early initiation of substance use Early and persistent problem behavior Rebelliousness Favorable attitudes toward substance use History of sexual or physical abuse History of mental health disorder Transition (puberty, change in school, graduation) Peer substance use	Social, emotional, behavioral, cognitive, and moral competence Self-efficacy Spirituality Resiliency
Family	
Family management problems Family conflict Favorable parental attitudes toward substance use Family history of substance misuse Parental history of mental health disorder Transition (divorce, military deployment) Parental crime and incarceration	Healthy beliefs and standards for behavior Parental recognition for positive behavior Bonding
School and Community	
Academic failure beginning in late elementary school Lack of commitment to school Low cost of alcohol High availability of substances Community laws and norms favorable to substance use Media portrayal of alcohol use Low neighborhood attachment Community disorganization Low socioeconomic status Transitions and mobility	Opportunities for positive social involvement Recognition for positive behavior Attachment to school

Adapted from U.S. Department of Health and Human Services (HHS), Office of the Surgeon General, Facing Addiction in America: The Surgeon General's Report on Alcohol, Drugs, and Health. Washington, DC: HHS, 2016.

COMMON SUBSTANCES

The more commonly abused drugs, together with common "street names" and health risks, are listed in Table 2. The signs and symptoms of intoxication or withdrawal are specific to the type of substance used and are described in the following text.

CANNABINOIDS

The active ingredient of marijuana, delta-9-tetrahydrocannabinol, is available from the *Cannabis sativa* plant together with other cannabinoids. This agent is a partial agonist at cannabinoid receptors. Cannabinoids are currently used to treat chronic pain, spasticity, nausea, and vomiting caused by chemotherapy, weight gain in HIV infection, sleep disorders, and Tourette syndrome.[21] The use of synthetic cannabinoids, named *K2* and *spice*, are marketed as herbal incense products and continue to be widely available. As listed in Box 3, the intoxicating effects of cannabis occur within 2 hours of use, and the withdrawal signs and symptoms may be apparent several days after last use. Evidence on the impact of recreational and/or medical marijuana state laws and adolescent use is conflicting. Currently, AAP opposes legalization of marijuana.[22]

DEPRESSANTS

Alcohol acts as a central nervous system depressant by activating $GABA_A$. The AAP considers alcohol use a pediatric

Table 2. Common Substances in Substance Use Disorder[32,33]

Substances	Street Names	DEA Schedule	Administration	Health Risks
Marijuana				
Marijuana	Weed, blunt, chronic, dope, ganja, grass, green, herb, hydro, joint, bud, mary jane, pot, reefer, sinsemilla, skunk, smoke	I	Swallowed, smoked	Cough, frequent respiratory infections, anxiety, depression, schizophrenia
Synthetic marijuana	K2, spice, bliss, black mamba, Bombay blue, fake marijuana, fake weed, genie, Yucatan fire, skunk, moon rocks, zohai	I	Smoked	Hallucinations, anxiety, heart attack, long-term effects unknown
Depressants				
Alcohol		Not scheduled	Swallowed	Increased risk of injuries, violence, fetal damage in pregnant women, depression, neurologic deficits, hypertension, liver and heart disease, fatal overdose
Opioids (oxycodone/ hydrocodone)	Oc, ox, oxy, oxycotton, oxycet, roxy, hillbilly heroin, percs/Vike, Watson-387	II	Swallowed, snorted, smoked, injected	Respiratory depression and arrest, nausea, confusion, constipation, sedation, unconsciousness, coma
Heroin	Big H, black tar, brown sugar, chiva, dope, hell dust, horse, junk, negra, smack, thunder	I	Injected, smoked, snorted	Constipation, endocarditis, hepatitis, HIV, fatal overdose
GHB	G, Georgia home boy, goop, grievous bodily harm, liquid ecstasy, soap, scoop, goop, liquid X	I	Swallowed	Unconsciousness, seizures, coma
Flunitrazepam	Circles, forget-me pill, la rocha, lunch, Mexican valium, money drug, R2, reynolds, roach, roche, roofies, roofinol, rope, rophies, row-shay, ruffies, wolfies	IV	Swallowed, snorted	Confusion, fatigue, impaired coordination, memory, judgment, respiratory depression and arrest
Stimulants				
Amphetamines/ methylphenidate	Bennies, black beauties, crosses, hearts, LA turnaround, speed, truck drivers, uppers/JIF, MPH, R-ball, skippy, the smart drug, vitamin R	II	Swallowed, snorted, smoked, injected	Weight loss, insomnia, cardiac or cardiovascular complications, stroke, seizures Also, for amphetamines: tremor, loss of coordination, irritability, anxiousness, restlessness, delirium, panic, paranoia, impulsive behavior, aggressiveness

(continued)

Table 2. Common Substances in Substance Use Disorder[32,33] *(continued)*

Substances	Street Names	DEA Schedule	Administration	Health Risks
Stimulants *(continued)*				
Mephedrone/ MDPV/methylone	Bath salts, bliss, blue silk, cloud nine, drone, energy-1, ivory wave, lunar wave, meow meow, ocean burst, pure ivory, purple wave, red dove, snow leopard, stardust, vanilla sky, white dove, white knight, white lightening	I	Swallowed, snorted, injected	Hallucinations, insomnia, breakdown of skeletal muscle tissue, kidney failure
Cocaine	Blow, bump, C, candy, charlie, coke, crack, flake, rock, snow, toot	II	Snorted, smoked, injected	Weight loss, insomnia, cardiac or cardiovascular complications, stroke, seizures, nasal damage from snorting
Methamphetamine	Batu, bikers coffee, black beauties, chalk, chicken feed, crank, crystal, fire, glass, go-fast, hiropon, ice, meth, methlies quick, poor man's cocaine, shabu, shards, speed, stove top, tina, trash, tweak, uppers, ventana, vidrio, yaba, yellow bam	II	Swallowed, snorted, smoked, injected	Weight loss, insomnia, cardiac or cardiovascular complications, stroke, seizures, irreversible neurologic damage, impaired memory and learning, severe dental problems
Tobacco	Cigarettes, cigars, bidis, hookahs, smokeless tobacco (snuff, spit tobacco, chew) e-cigarettes, e-cigars, e-pipes, vape pipes, vaping pens, e-hookahs, hookah pens	Not scheduled	Smoked, snorted, chewed	Chronic lung disease, cardiovascular disease, stroke, cancers of the mouth, pharynx, larynx, esophagus, stomach, pancreas, cervix, kidney, bladder, and acute myeloid leukemia, adverse pregnancy outcomes
Hallucinogens				
MDMA	Ecstasy, adam, beans, clarity, disco biscuit, E, eve, go, hug drug, lover's speed, peace, STP, X, XTC	I	Swallowed, snorted, injected	Sleep disturbances, depression, impaired memory, hyperthermia
PCP (phencyclidine)	Angel dust, boat, hog, love boat, peace pill	I, II	Swallowed, snorted, smoked, injected	Memory loss, difficulties with speech and thinking, depression, weight loss
Ketamine	Cat valium, jet K, K, kit kat, purple, special K, super acid, super K, vitamin K	III	Snorted, smoked, injected	Anxiety, tremors, numbness, memory loss, nausea
Dextromethorphan	CCC, dex, DXM, poor man's pcp, robo, robotripping, skittles, triple C, velvet	Not scheduled	Swallowed	Hypoxic brain damage from severe respiratory depression
LSD	Acid, blotter, blue heaven, cubes, dots, mellow yellow, window pane	I	Swallowed, absorbed through mouth tissues	Flashbacks, hallucinogen persisting perception disorder
Psilocybin	Magic mushrooms, purple passion, shrooms, little smoke	I	Swallowed	Flashbacks, risk of psychiatric illness, impaired memory
Salvia divinorum	Salvia, shepherdess's herb, maria pastora, magic mint, sally-d	Not scheduled	Smoked, swallowed, chewed	Hallucinations, long-tern effects unknown
Other Substances				
Inhalants	Laughing gas, gluey, huff, poppers, rush, snappers, whippets	Not scheduled	Inhaled through nose or mouth	Cramps, muscle weakness, depression, memory impairment, damage to cardiovascular and nervous systems, unconsciousness, sudden death
Anabolic steroids	Arnolds, juice, gym candy, pumpers, roids, stackers, weight gainers	III	Injected, swallowed, applied to skin	Hypertension, blood clotting and cholesterol changes, liver cysts, hostility and aggression, acne, premature stoppage of growth; in males: prostate cancer, reduced sperm production, shrunken testicles, breast enlargement; in females: menstrual irregularities, development of beard and other masculine characteristics

DEA = Drug Enforcement Agency; GHB = γ-hydroxybutyrate, LSD = lysergic acid diethylamide, MDMA = methylenedioxymethamphetamine, MDPV = methylenedioxypyrovalerone.

health concern because alcohol can interfere with brain development during adolescence.[23] Also, binge drinking is a major issue and alcohol misuse is associated with the leading causes of death and serious injury at this age (i.e., motor vehicle accidents, homicides, and suicides).[24] Withdrawal may develop after several hours to a few days after alcohol cessation. γ-Hydroxybutyrate (GHB) and flunitrazepam are typically used as an adjunct to sleep, and these agents are also commonly the drugs used for date rape. γ-Hydroxybutyrate acts at the GHB and $GABA_B$ receptors, and flunitrazepam, like other benzodiazepines, acts at the $GABA_A$ receptor. The intoxication and withdrawal effects of these substances mimic those of alcohol (Box 4).

Opioid drugs interact with several opioid receptors, but the μ-receptor is primarily responsible for analgesia and addiction. Although nonmedical prescription opioids, heroin misuse, and subsequent SUD are major concerns for young adults, their use in adolescents continues to decline.[5,6] These trends highlight the continued need for targeting preventive strategies for opioid misuse in adolescents. Withdrawal may develop within a few minutes to several days after last opioid use or after administration of an opioid blocker (Box 5).

STIMULANTS

Stimulants (amphetamines, cocaine) work by either increasing the release or inhibiting the uptake of dopamine and norepinephrine. Synthetic stimulants, commonly marketed as "bath salts" and "glass cleaner," are sold over the counter. Withdrawal may occur within a few hours (typical for cocaine) to several days (typical for amphetamines or related substances) after cessation from stimulants (Box 6).

Box 3. Cannabis: Intoxicating Effects and Withdrawal Effects

Intoxicating Effects
Conjunctival injection
Increased appetite
Dry mouth
Tachycardia

Withdrawal Effects
Irritability, anger, or aggression
Nervousness or anxiety
Sleep difficulty (insomnia, disturbing dreams)
Decreased appetite or weight loss
Restlessness
Depressed mood
Abdominal pain, shakiness or tremors, sweating, fever, chills, headache

---

Box 4. Alcohol: Intoxicating Effects and Withdrawal Effects

Intoxicating Effects
Slurred speech
Incoordination
Unsteady gait
Nystagmus
Impairment in attention or memory
Stupor or coma

Withdrawal Effects
Autonomic hyperactivity (sweating or heart rate greater than 100 beats/minute)
Increased hand tremor
Insomnia
Nausea or vomiting
Transient visual, tactile, or auditory hallucinations or illusions
Psychomotor agitation
Anxiety
Generalized tonic–clonic seizures

Box 5. Opioids: Intoxicating Effects and Withdrawal Effects

Intoxicating Effects
Pupillary constriction
Drowsiness or coma
Slurred speech
Impairment in attention or memory

Withdrawal Effects
Dysphoric mood
Nausea or vomiting
Muscle aches
Lacrimation or rhinorrhea
Pupillary dilation, piloerection, or sweating
Diarrhea
Yawning
Fever
Insomnia

Box 6. Amphetamines and Cocaine: Intoxicating Effects and Withdrawal Effects

Intoxicating Effects
Tachycardia or bradycardia
Pupillary dilation
Elevated or lowered blood pressure
Perspiration or chills
Nausea or vomiting
Weight loss
Psychomotor agitation or retardation
Muscular weakness, respiratory depression, chest pain, or cardiac arrhythmias
Confusion, seizures, dyskinesias, dystonias, coma

Withdrawal Effects
Dysphoric mood
Fatigue
Vivid and unpleasant dreams
Insomnia or hypersomnia
Increased appetite
Psychomotor retardation or agitation

The AAP considers tobacco use disorder a pediatric disease because misuse almost always starts in childhood or adolescence.[25] Nicotine is primarily the addictive component in tobacco and acts on the nicotinic acetylcholine receptors in the peripheral nervous system and central nervous system. Tobacco use increases the risk of pulmonary disease, cardiovascular disease, various cancers, and premature death. Withdrawal begins within 24 hours of last nicotine use (Box 7).

Adolescent use of traditional cigarettes has dramatically decreased since 2014. Today the most common method for tobacco use is with an electronic vapor product.[26] The AAP is now concerned that the previous progress with tobacco control is being threatened because children who use e-cigarettes are more likely to go on to use traditional cigarettes. Therefore, AAP is calling for the regulation, legislative action, and counterpromotion of e-cigarettes to protect children.[27] The U.S. Food and Drug Administration (FDA) recently issued a draft guidance that will require tobacco manufacturers to acquire authorization for flavored products by 2021.[28]

Caffeine is likely the most widely used substance, but is not included in the previous surveys of adolescents. Caffeine competitively blocks receptors for the inhibitory neurotransmitter, adenosine. Of concern are the effects of the energy drinks that contain unregulated amounts of caffeine and ingredients that lack evaluation in adolescents.[29] The withdrawal symptoms occur within 24 hours after last caffeine use (Box 8).

HALLUCINOGENS

Methylenedioxymethamphetamine (MDMA), commonly referred to as *ecstasy*, works mainly by inhibiting the reuptake of serotonin. Common symptoms of intoxication include mild hallucinogenic effects, increased tactile sensitivity, empathic feelings, lowered inhibition, anxiety, chills, sweating, teeth clenching, and muscle cramping. Often sold in combination with other drugs, MDMA often results in unpredictable effects when it is misused.

Phencyclidine (PCP) works mainly as a glutamate receptor blocker. Within 1 hour of use the following may occur: vertical or horizontal nystagmus; hypertension or tachycardia; numbness or diminished responsiveness to pain; ataxia; dysarthria; muscle rigidity; seizures or coma; and hyperacusis. The actions of ketamine and high-dose dextromethorphan are similar to PCP in causing the dissociative feeling separate from one's body and environment.

Lysergic acid diethylamide (LSD) is a partial agonist at serotonin receptors. Psilocybin, better known as *mushrooms*, has LSD-like properties. *Salvia divinorum* is a plant with potent activity at the κ-opioid receptors. In a state of full wakefulness and alertness, perceptual changes occur after recent use of a hallucinogen, including the following: subjective intensification of perceptions, depersonalization, derealization, illusions, hallucinations, and synesthesias. Other signs that develop are pupillary dilation, tachycardia, sweating, palpitations, blurred vision, tremors, and incoordination.

OTHER SUBSTANCES: INHALANTS

Inhalants are next to marijuana as the most common drug initially used by adolescents. Inhalants include solvents (e.g., paint thinners, gasoline, glues), gases (e.g., butane, propane, aerosol propellants, nitrous oxide), and nitrites (e.g., isoamyl, isobutyl, cyclohexyl). The mechanism of action of inhalants is not fully understood. Of primary concern is the risk of sudden sniffing death syndrome, which may occur with any use of inhalants (Box 9).[30]

Anabolic steroids and other performance-enhancing substances (protein supplements and creatine) have few to no intoxicating effects. However, the AAP strongly objects to the use of performance-enhancing substances because of the potential for adverse health problems and the lack of principle and fairness.[31] Adolescent athletes who are "doping" are at risk of the many consequences listed in Table 2.

COMORBIDITIES

The coexistence of an SUD and another mental health disorder is often referred to as *dual diagnosis*. Adolescents often have more psychiatric comorbidity. Common adolescent comorbidities associated with addiction are mood disorders, attention-deficit/hyperactivity disorder, and conduct disorder. It is important to establish whether the SUD preceded the

---

Box 7. Tobacco: Withdrawal Effects

Irritability, frustration, or anger
Anxiety
Difficulty concentrating
Increased appetite
Restlessness
Depressed mood
Insomnia

Box 8. Caffeine: Intoxicating Effects and Withdrawal Effects

Intoxicating Effects
Restlessness
Nervousness
Excitement
Insomnia
Flushed face
Diuresis
Gastrointestinal disturbance
Muscle twitching
Rambling flow of thought and speech
Tachycardia or cardiac arrhythmia
Periods of inexhaustibility
Psychomotor agitation

Withdrawal Effects
Headache
Marked fatigue or drowsiness
Dysphoric mood, depressed mood, or irritability
Difficulty concentrating
Flulike symptoms (nausea, vomiting, or muscle pain/ stiffness)

---

mental health condition, or if the reverse is true—the adolescent may either be experiencing a health consequence of the SUD or be self-medicating to treat the psychiatric illness, respectively.

TREATMENT

About 159,000 adolescents in 2018 received treatment for an SUD which represents a rate of 0.6%.[5] The overall goals for managing an adolescent with an SUD are to help them reduce harmful substance misuse or abstain, to improve their health and social function, and to manage their risk for relapse. The suggested treatment for adolescent SUD is listed in Table 3.[32,33] According to the National Institute on Drug Abuse (NIDA), treatment should be individualized and should consider an adolescent's level of psychological development, gender, relations with family and peers, how well they are doing in school, the larger community, cultural and ethnic factors, and any special physical or behavioral issues.[34] There are a variety of settings for treatment that provide differing intensity of clinical and environmental support services. The level and length of care the adolescent may need are determined by the severity of the SUD (Box 10). Treatment is recommended for a minimum of 3 months.[34,35]

NONPHARMACOLOGIC THERAPY

After assessment in the model of screening, brief intervention, and referral to treatment, a conversation encouraging healthy choices to prevent, reduce, or stop risky behaviors should occur. Brief intervention may range from positive reinforcement for adolescents reporting no substance use; advice to abstain for those reporting use but showing no evidence of an SUD; brief motivational interventions when a mild or moderate SUD is revealed; and referral to treatment of those with a severe SUD.[13] Motivational interviewing is widely recommended but has mixed evidence for treating adolescent SUD.[36] Other interventions for adolescent SUD are motivational enhancement therapy, cognitive–behavioral therapy, family therapy, 12-step facilitation therapy, and contingency management.

PHARMACOLOGIC THERAPY

Pharmacologic therapy for SUD is divided into medications used in the intoxication phase to stabilize the patient,

---

Box 9. Inhalants—Solvents, Gases, and Nitrites: Intoxicating Effects

Dizziness
Nystagmus
Incoordination
Slurred speech
Unsteady gait
Lethargy
Depressed reflexes
Psychomotor retardation
Tremor
Generalized muscle weakness
Blurred vision or diplopia
Stupor or coma
Euphoria

Box 10. Substance Use Disorder Inpatient and Outpatient Treatment

Inpatient
Detoxification
Acute residential treatment
Residential treatment
Therapeutic boarding school

Outpatient
Individual counseling
Group therapy
Family therapy
Intensive outpatient program
Partial hospital program

Table 3. Management Options for Adolescent Substance Use Disorder[32,40-42,44-49,59-60,62]

Substances	Intoxication Management	Maintenance Medications	Behavioral Therapies
Marijuana		Acetylcysteine	Cognitive-behavioral therapy Contingency management or motivational incentives Motivational enhancement therapy
Alcohol	Benzodiazepines	Acamprosate Naltrexone (oral) Ondansetron Topiramate Disulfiram	Cognitive-behavioral therapy Contingency management or motivational incentives Motivational enhancement therapy 12-Step facilitation therapy
Opioids: oxycodone, hydrocodone, heroin	Buprenorphine (+/- naloxone) Clonidine (patch)	Buprenorphine/naloxone Methadone Naltrexone (intramuscular)	Contingency management or motivational incentives 12-Step facilitation therapy
Tobacco		Nicotine replacement therapy Bupropion Varenicline	Cognitive-behavioral therapy Self-help materials Mail, phone, and Internet quit resources

detoxification to manage the signs and symptoms during the withdrawal phase, and maintenance of recovery. Most medications do not have FDA label approval for adolescent SUD. The risk–benefit ratio must be balanced before initiating pharmacologic therapy in those adolescents who do not respond adequately to psychosocial interventions. Data on SUD treatment in adolescents are limited, and management strategies are often extrapolated from adult recommendations. Table 4 lists the available dosing information for the drug therapies reviewed in detail in the following text.

INTOXICATION MANAGEMENT

The management of intoxication should focus on respiratory, cardiac, and neurologic stabilization, together with administration of an antidote when indicated and available. Life support to maintain cardiorespiratory function and fluid replacement for hydration may be necessary. Comatose adolescents at risk of aspiration may require intubation and ventilation. Adolescents exhibiting psychosis may need sedation and antipsychotics. Medications recommended for reversal are naloxone (given repeatedly as needed) for acute opioid intoxication, and flumazenil for acute intoxication with benzodiazepines, including flunitrazepam but not GHB. Physostigmine may have a role in GHB toxicity.[37] Decontamination may be indicated for the gastrointestinal tract by activated charcoal and gastric lavage or clothes and skin because of inhalant use. Other substance-specific problems are methemoglobinemia from inhalant intoxication, needing methylene blue treatment, and hyperthermia from MDMA, requiring management with rapid cooling, antipyretics, dantrolene, and benzodiazepines for shivering or seizures.[30,38]

WITHDRAWAL MANAGEMENT

Detoxification for adolescents is uncommon for most substances, but depressants may require therapy to manage the signs and symptoms of withdrawal. Long-acting benzodiazepines, although seldom needed, together with vitamin replacement, are appropriate for treatment of alcohol withdrawal. Opioid detoxification is more complicated in adolescents than in adults, and use of opioid agonists may be indicated. Methadone is a full receptor agonist with no controlled studies in adolescents. Buprenorphine is a partial agonist approved for opioid dependence in those 16 years and older used as monotherapy or combined with naloxone. A Cochrane Review provides no conclusion regarding opioid

Table 4. Medications for Treatment of Adolescent Substance Use Disorder[40-42,44-47,59,60,62]

Acute Intoxication	
Flumazenil	0.01 mg/kg (maximal dose 0.2 mg) intravenously, repeat every minute to maximal cumulative dose 1 mg
Naloxone	2 mg intravenously, repeat every 2–3 min Evzio[a]: 2 mg intramuscularly, repeat every 2–3 min Narcan[b]: 4 mg intranasally, may repeat every 2–3 min
Detoxification	
Buprenorphine/naloxone	6–8 mg sublingually, fixed taper dosing up to 14 mg/day for 2 wk
Clonidine patch	0.1 mg on day 1, add 0.1 mg on day 2, add an optional 0.1 mg on day 4 Remove all patches on day 7 and replace with 0.2-mg doses Remove all patches on day 14 and replace with 0.1-mg doses Remove all patches on day 21
Methadone	Flexible dosing orally daily for 4 wk
Maintenance	
Acetylcysteine	1200 mg orally twice daily for 8 wk
Naltrexone	25–50 mg orally daily for 6 wk
Acamprosate	666 mg orally in morning, 333 mg in afternoon, 333 mg in evening for 12 wk
Topiramate	Escalating dose orally up to 200 mg/day orally for 5 wk
Buprenorphine/naloxone	Fixed taper dosing sublingually up to 24 mg/day for 9 wk, taper to wk 12
Methadone	Flexible dosing orally daily for up to 24 wk
Nicotine patch	> 20 cigarettes/day: 21 mg/day for 3 wk, 14 mg/day for 3 wk, 7 mg/day for 3 wk ≤ 20 cigarettes/day: 14 mg/day for 3 wk, 7 mg/day for 3 wk
Bupropion extended release	150 mg orally daily for 7 days, 300 mg orally daily for 7 wk
Varenicline	≥ 55 kg: 0.5 mg orally daily for 3 days, 0.5 mg twice daily for 4 days, and then 1 mg twice daily for 7 wk < 55 kg: 0.5 mg orally daily for 7 days, 0.5 mg twice daily for 7 wk

[a]Kaleo, Inc., Richmond, VA; [b]Adapt Pharma, Inc., Radnor, PA.

detoxification from the two controlled trials using buprenorphine in adolescents.[39] The findings from these trials are that 8 weeks of buprenorphine–naloxone maintenance is more effective in reducing positive urine screens and reported use than 2 weeks of buprenorphine alone, and buprenorphine is more effective than clonidine for opioid treatment.[40,41] Clonidine may be used early on for control of early autonomic withdrawal symptoms from opiates.

MAINTENANCE OF RECOVERY

Acetylcysteine is a cysteine prodrug that modulates glutamate. A large, randomized controlled trial (RCT) in adolescents with cannabis use disorder showed a decrease in use and positive urine screens during treatment.[42] Topiramate has also been evaluated in an RCT of adolescents age 15 to 24 years with marijuana addiction and resulted in inconsistent effects with poor tolerability.[43]

Maintenance therapies may be considered in treatment-resistant adolescents for alcohol use disorder. Naltrexone, an oral opioid receptor blocker, was found to reduce alcohol consumption and craving in two small pilot trials of adolescents.[44,45] Acamprosate works by activating $GABA_A$ receptors and blocking glutamate receptors. This agent increased abstinence compared with placebo in adolescents with alcohol addiction at 90 days.[46] Topiramate, ondansetron, and disulfiram have also been evaluated in adolescents but are seldom recommended over the previously noted therapies for alcohol addiction.[47-49]

A recent AAP policy recommends that medication-assisted treatment should be offered to adolescents with severe opioid use disorder; however, evidence to support pharmacotherapy is limited.[50] A Cochrane Review of adolescents with opiate use disorder was unable to draw conclusions about maintenance treatments.[51] There are no controlled trials of methadone maintenance therapy for pediatric patients, and adolescents must fail drug-free treatment twice before referral to a specialty clinic. As stated previously, buprenorphine is effective for increasing abstinence from opiates at week 8, but the effect is not long term.[40] A small feasibility study in adolescents age 16 to 20 years found clinical improvement with monthly naltrexone intramuscular injections for opiate addiction.[52] In a large national retrospective cohort of adolescents and young adults with opioid use disorder, claims for buprenorphine or naltrexone increased from 2001 to 2014, but only one in four individuals received medication.[53] Timely prescribing of buprenorphine, naltrexone, or methadone for youth with opioid use disorder was associated with greater retention in treatment.[54]

The use of pharmacotherapy in adolescents with tobacco use disorder is debatable. Although nicotine replacement therapy is safe, a meta-analysis of six RCTs in pediatric patients age 12 to 20 years found little evidence that such medications are effective in promoting smoking cessation. Moreover, the evidence does not support the use of bupropion either alone or as an adjunct to nicotine replacement therapy, and adherence to these treatments is poor.[55] A Cochrane Review of tobacco cessation interventions concluded similar findings.[56] A more recent RCT of the nicotine patch in adolescent smokers found it associated with increased cessation at week 2; however, there was no difference at 6- or 12-month follow up.[57,58] A secondary analysis did find a higher abstinence rate from the nicotine patch in more adherent adolescents at 6 months.[59] In another recent trial, adherence to bupropion 300 mg/day also resulted in higher rates of smoking cessation in adolescents with tobacco use disorder.[60] Varenicline is a α4β2 nicotinic receptor agonist approved for tobacco cessation in those 17 years and older. In a RCT of 157 adolescents age 12–19 years, varenicline did not significantly increase abstinence rates compared with placebo.[61] In a small RCT comparing varenicline with bupropion in adolescent smokers, the number of cigarettes per day decreased in both groups.[62] However, the FDA recently updated the label recommending the drug not be used in children age 16 years or younger because of the lack of efficacy data.[63]

COMORBIDITY TREATMENT

Adolescents with an SUD and a co-occurring psychiatric illness may benefit from programs that integrate treatment of both disorders. Because of overlapping signs and symptoms, a brief period of abstinence of the substance(s) is recommended first to further assess for psychiatric comorbidities.

Medications for mental health disorders that are considered nonaddictive would be more appropriate treatments for adolescents with dual diagnosis. For example, long-acting methylphenidate, atomoxetine, and bupropion may be considered over short-acting stimulant medications for the treatment of attention-deficit/hyperactivity disorder in an adolescent who also has an SUD.[64-66] Medications used in studies of adolescents with a coexisting SUD and another mental health disorder include fluoxetine or sertraline for depression and alcohol or other drug use disorder, lithium for bipolar disorder and alcohol or other drug addiction, and bupropion for attention-deficit/hyperactivity disorder with nicotine use disorder.[67-72]

MONITORING AND PROGNOSIS

Drug testing may be an important component in the ongoing assessment of substance use during and after treatment. The opportunity for detection from a urine drug test may be small because the more common substances used by adolescents, except for marijuana, are fully excreted within 72 hours or less. Other important limitations are that standard panels do not detect some of the drugs, such as alcohol and inhalants, and false-positive results may occur, which require follow-up.[22] Other monitoring for efficacy may include self-reported substance use, adherence to therapies, and behavioral changes. Adolescents may also need screening for sexually transmitted disease, including *Chlamydia trachomatis*, *Neisseria gonorrhoeae*, and HIV, as well as HIV and hepatitis B and C if using substances intravenously.

Untreated adolescents who use substances may progress to have addiction and/or another mental illnesses in adulthood. Treatment may effectively lead to abstinence; however, relapse is common in adolescents. Continuing care with a provider, which may even include sessions at the adolescent's home, is necessary to prevent relapse. With continued treatment and encouragement to abstain from alcohol and other drugs, the adolescent may lead a full and healthy life.

PREVENTION

In an analysis of the MTF survey, complete abstinence by high school students increased over the past four decades and mostly from nonuse of alcohol and cigarettes.[73] Prevention is thought to be essential to promoting abstinence and reducing the risk of progression to later SUD. The identification of a child's risk and protective factors is the basis for prevention programs (Table 1). Beyond the universal interventions such as minimum legal drinking age or taxation, several evidence-based prevention interventions are available for schools and caregivers (Box 11).[1]

In addition to participating in community prevention programs, pharmacists are able to assist adolescents and their families with other harm reduction interventions. Pharmacists should oppose the sale of alcohol and tobacco products in pharmacies. Adolescents using nonmedical prescription opioids commonly report the availability from a friend or relative. Pharmacists should educate caregivers about the correct storage and disposal of medications and encourage participation in prescription take-back initiatives. Pharmacists should participate in their state prescription drug monitoring programs and discourage prescribing practices that enable misuse. Pharmacists should provide care to adolescents being treated for SUD. Specific examples include appropriately treating acute pain or comorbid disorders and distributing and educating on naloxone.[74,75]

CONCLUSIONS

Alcohol and other drug use is common among adolescents, but progression to later addiction may be preventable. Screening along the substance use continuum, followed by the suggested treatment of brief intervention to referral, is an appropriate management strategy for adolescent SUD. At minimum, adolescents should be advised that even casual use of substances, regardless of amount or frequency, is likely illegal and has the potential for adverse consequences. Pharmacists should educate adolescents and their families about addiction and should intervene and assist those who misuse substances or have an SUD.

Box 11. Evidence-Based Prevention Interventions for Substance Use Disorder in Pediatric Patients[1]

Birth to 10 years

School
Good Behavior Game
Classroom-Centered Intervention
Raising Healthy Children
The Fast Track Program

Family
Nurse–Family Partnership

10–18 years

School
LifeSkills Training
keepin' it REAL
Project Toward No Drug Abuse

Family
Strengthening Families Program: For Parents and Youth 10–14
Strong African American Families
Familias Unidas
Coping Power

Internet-based programs
I Hear What You're Saying
Project Chill

A 15-year-old boy is admitted to the emergency department because of redness, swelling, and pain in both of his elbows for the past 5 days. He says that 10 to 14 days ago he obtained new needles from a pharmacy and attempted to inject oxycodone intravenously in veins around his elbows. The oxycodone was obtained from "a friend." No changes were present until about 5 days ago when he noted increasing redness, swelling, and pain, and then streaking up both arms. He denies any other intravenous drug abuse and denies injecting in any other areas. He reports having a temperature up to 101°F (38°C). He currently denies suicidal ideation or thoughts.

Medical history: Major depressive disorder and generalized anxiety disorder with cutting; previously hospitalized for suicidal ideation; severe stimulant and cannabis use disorder for past year; recent residential treatment over the summer, with discharge about 2 months ago

Immunizations: Up to date except human papillomavirus vaccines

Family history: Cancer in paternal grandfather

Social history: Lives at home with father, mother, and sister; attends high school as a sophomore with C grades; no employment and no extracurricular activities; history of methamphetamine, marijuana, tobacco, and oxycodone use; not sexually active and has never had a sexually transmitted infection

Home medications: Aripiprazole 5 mg/day orally, recently initiated

Emergency Department medications: Vancomycin 1000 mg intravenously once; ketorolac 30 mg intravenously once; acetaminophen 500 mg orally once; 0.9% sodium chloride intravenously bolus

Allergies: Amoxicillin (rash)

Review of systems:

Constitutional: Positive for chills, fatigue, fever; negative for weight gain, weight loss

Eyes: Negative for eye redness, vision loss

Ears, nose, and throat: Negative for congestion, rhinorrhea, sore throat

Respiratory: Negative for cough, dyspnea on exertion, shortness of breath

Cardiovascular: Positive for chest pain; negative for palpitations, cyanosis, dyspnea on exertion

Gastrointestinal: Negative for abdominal pain, change in bowel habits, vomiting

Hematologic: Positive for chills; negative for swollen nodes

Musculoskeletal: Positive for joint pain, joint swelling

Neurologic: Positive for headaches; negative for dizziness, seizures, weakness, syncope

Psychiatric: Positive for agitation, anxiety, depressed mood, illicit drug use, sleep disturbance

Vital signs: BP 108/60 mm Hg, HR 56 beats/minute, Tmax 96.8°F (36°C), RR 14 breaths/minute, Wt 70.8 kg

Physical examination:

General: Well developed and well nourished; in distress; pain and redness over bilateral antecubital fossa

Head: Normocephalic, atraumatic

Eyes: No periorbital edema, no injection, no discharge

Nose: Clear discharge

Oropharynx: Moist mucous membranes

Neck: Supple

Cardiovascular: Regular rate and rhythm, normal S1 and S2, no murmurs

Pulmonary: Clear to auscultation bilaterally; normal respiratory effort

Abdomen: Soft, nontender, nondistended, normal bowel sounds, hepatosplenomegaly or masses

Musculoskeletal: Moves all extremities well, no peripheral edema, no pain to palpation, no splinter hemorrhages or Janeway lesions noted

Skin: Right antecubital fossa with old needle marks; minimal erythema and mild warmth to touch; left antecubital fossa with coalescing erythema and mild streaking toward axilla, warm to touch, not fluctuant; healing linear cuts and designs on bilateral volar aspect of forearms

Neurologic: Awake, alert, deep tendon reflexes, normal, motor and sensory normal bilaterally

Laboratory findings:

Test	Results
WBC	12.3×10^3 cells/mm³
Hgb	11.9 g/dL
Hct	34.9%
Plt	180×10^3 cells/mm³
Na	131 mEq/L
K	3.4 mEq/L
Cl	97 mEq/L
CO_2	26 mEq/L
BUN	11 mg/dL
SCr	1.01 mg/dL
Glucose	100 mg/dL
Calcium (total serum)	8.1 mg/dL
Albumin	3.4 g/dL
ALK	104 U/L
ALT	28 U/L
AST	26 U/L
Bilirubin (total)	0.6 mg/dL
Protein (total serum)	7.1 g/dL
Urine drug screen	In process
Blood culture	Pending

Imaging:

Ultrasound: Subcutaneous tissues are thickened, without focal mass or fluid collection

Doppler scan: Negative

1. In addition to infection, what are the patient's psychiatric disorders, including his risk factors for substance use?

The patient likely has severe substance use disorder (SUD), with the specific substances yet to be determined. According to the *Diagnostic and Statistical Manual of Mental Disorders, Fifth Edition*, six or more of the 11 symptoms are needed to diagnosis severe SUD. Continued use despite physical or psychological problems is a symptom detailed in this patient (infection and recent hospitalization, respectively). Other signs and symptoms need to be further evaluated. His risk factors are history of mental health disorder, early initiation of substance use, peer substance use, and lack of protective factors (i.e., lack of attachment to school grades). The patient has a history of depression and generalized anxiety disorder, which, if left untreated, could lead to substance misuse and/or his SUD will worsen the other psychiatric illnesses. Family and school or community information is unknown in the setting but contributes to the risk of SUD and should be assessed during continuing care sessions.

2. What signs and symptoms of intoxication or withdrawal is the patient experiencing?

Patient Case Table 1 shows intoxication and withdrawal signs and symptoms for opiates, stimulants, cannabis, and tobacco; criteria that the patient is experiencing are shown in bold. The patient is not intoxicated from opiates; however, all other substances should be assessed. If the patient was experiencing clinically significant problematic behavior or psychological changes, then he may meet the diagnostic criteria for stimulant intoxication because only two or more signs and symptoms are necessary after use.

The withdrawal effects may be caused by a separate medical problem and need to be monitored further. Specifically, for opiate withdrawal, three or more criteria need to develop within minutes to several days of use. For cannabis withdrawal, three or more criteria, plus at least one physical symptom (i.e., fever, chills, headache), need to occur within 1 week of use. Four or more criteria are needed within 24 hours of last use for tobacco withdrawal.

Patient Case Table 1. Patient Case Study: Intoxication and Withdrawal Signs and Symptoms for Opiates, Stimulants, Cannabis, and Tobacco[a]

Intoxicating Effects	Withdrawal Effects
Opiates	
Pupillary constriction	Dysphoric mood
Drowsiness or coma	Nausea or vomiting
Slurred speech	Muscle aches
Impairment in attention or memory	Lacrimation or rhinorrhea
	Pupillary dilation, piloerection, or sweating
	Diarrhea
	Yawning
	Fever
	Insomnia

Patient Case Table 1. *(continued)*

Intoxicating Effects	Withdrawal Effects
Stimulants	
Tachycardia or bradycardia	**Dysphoric mood**
Pupillary dilation	Fatigue
Elevated or lowered blood pressure	Vivid and unpleasant dreams
Perspiration or chills	**Insomnia or hypersomnia**
Nausea or vomiting	Increased appetite
Weight loss	Psychomotor retardation or agitation
Psychomotor agitation or retardation	
Muscular weakness, respiratory depression, **chest pain**, or cardiac arrhythmias	
Confusion, seizures, dyskinesias, dystonias, coma	
Cannabis	
Conjunctival injection	Irritability, anger, or aggression
Increased appetite	**Nervousness or anxiety**
Dry mouth	**Sleep difficulty (insomnia, disturbing dreams)**
Tachycardia	Decreased appetite or weight loss
	Restlessness
	Depressed mood
	Abdominal pain, shakiness or tremors, sweating, **fever, chills, headache**
Tobacco	
—	Irritability, frustration, or anger
	Anxiety
	Difficulty concentrating
	Increased appetite
	Restlessness
	Depressed mood
	Insomnia

[a]Criteria that the patient is experiencing are shown in bold font.

3. What pharmacotherapy and monitoring should the patient receive for his psychiatric problems?

For SUD, the patient does not require any specific intoxication management and needs supportive care. Frequent clinical monitoring for withdrawal must continue with follow-up on the urine drug screen. Buprenorphine/naloxone may be considered for opiate withdrawal, or it may be preferable to initiate medication-assisted treatment based on further assessment. Patient Case Table 2 shows the 12-week regimen for buprenorphine–naloxone sublingual.

Patient Case Table 2. Supportive Care Plan for Pharmacotherapy and Monitoring

Induction	Day 1: 2 mg, may repeat 2–6 mg after at least 2 hr if withdrawal symptoms are not relieved
	Day 2: Repeat total daily dose from day 1, may repeat 2–6 mg after at least 2 hr if withdrawal symptoms are not relieved
	Day 3: Repeat total daily dose from day 2, may repeat 2–6 mg after at least 2 hr if withdrawal symptoms are not relieved
Stabilization	Up to 24 mg per day; then begin taper at wk 9

Naloxone (Evzio) 2-mg auto-injector should be provided at discharge, and the patient and his family should receive education on naloxone technique and signs of opioid overdose, specifically respiratory or central nervous system depression. An HIV enzyme-linked immunosorbent assay and Western blot and hepatitis panel should be obtained secondary to intravenous drug use risk.

Additional maintenance therapy to consider after further evaluation is acetylcysteine for cannabis use disorder and nicotine replacement therapy with nicotine patches or bupropion for tobacco use disorder. The aripiprazole should be further investigated for indication and likely discontinued. Aripiprazole is only approved as an adjunctive therapy for depression in adults, and worsening agitation and anxiety are common adverse effects. Fluoxetine (or escitalopram) 10 mg orally once daily should be initiated after a brief period of abstinence because selective serotonin reuptake inhibitors are first-line treatments for adolescent depression and anxiety. The dose should be increased to 20 mg daily at week 1 and, if necessary, increased to a maximum of 40 mg per day. Fluoxetine is approved with the most evidence in children for treatment of depression and generalized anxiety disorder. Escitalopram is approved for treatment of depression in children and has less activation, which may benefit comorbid anxiety. The patient should be monitored for worsening depression and suicidality during initiation and when doses are increased.

REFERENCES

1. U.S. Department of Health and Human Services (HHS), Office of the Surgeon General, Facing Addiction in America: The Surgeon General's Report on Alcohol, Drugs, and Health. Washington, DC: HHS, 2016.
2. American Psychiatric Association (APA). Substance-Related and Addictive Disorders. Diagnostic and Statistical Manual of Mental Disorders, Fifth Edition. Washington, DC: APA, 2013.
3. American Society of Addiction Medicine [homepage on the Internet]. Public Policy Statement: Definition of Addiction. Available at https://www.asam.org/quality-practice/definition-of-addiction. Accessed January17, 2020.
4. Kann L, McManus T, Harris WA, et al. Youth Risk Behavior Surveillance—United States, 2017. MMWR Surveill Summ 2018;67:1-114.
5. Center for Behavioral Health Statistics and Quality. Key Substance Use and Mental Health Indicators in the United States: Results from the 2018 National Survey on Drug Use and Health. HHS Publication No. PEP19-5068, NSDUH Series H-54. Rockville, MD: Center for Behavioral Health Statistics and Quality, 2019. Available at http://www.samhsa.gov/data/. Accessed January 21, 2020.
6. Johnston LD, O'Malley PM, Miech RA, et al. Monitoring the Future National Survey Results on Drug Use, 1975-2018: 2018 Overview, Key Findings on Adolescent Drug Use. Ann Arbor, MI: Institute for Social Research, University of Michigan, 2019.
7. Cullen KA, Ambrose BK, Gentzke AS, et al. Use of electronic cigarettes and any tobacco product among middle and high school students-United States, 2011-2018. MMWR 2018;67:1276-7.
8. Barrington-Trimis JL, Leventhal AM. Adolescents' use of "Pod Mod" e-cigarettes- urgent concerns. N Engl J Med 2018. 379;12: 1099-102.
9. Koob GF, Volkow ND. Neurocircuitry of addiction. Neuropsychopharmacol Rev 2010;35:217-38.
10. Squeglia LM, Gray KM. Alcohol and drug use and the developing brain. Curr Psychiatry Rep 2016;18:46.
11. Wang JC, Kapoor M, Goate AM. The genetics of substance dependence. Annu Rev Genomics Hum Genet 2012;13:241-61.
12. American Academy of Pediatrics, Committee on Substance Abuse. Substance use screening, brief intervention, and referral to treatment [policy statement]. Pediatrics 2016;138.
13. Levy S, Williams JF; American Academy of Pediatrics, Committee on Substance Abuse. Clinical report: substance use screening, brief intervention, and referral to treatment. Pediatrics 2016;138.
14. Substance Abuse and Mental Health Services Administration. Screening, Brief Intervention and Referral to Treatment (SBIRT) in Behavioral Healthcare [monograph on the Internet]. Available at https://www.samhsa.gov/sites/default/files/sbirtwhitepaper_0.pdf. Accessed January 17, 2020.
15. Hagan JF, Shaw JS, Duncan P, eds. Bright Futures: Guidelines for Health Supervision of Infants, Children, and Adolescents, 4th ed. Elk Grove Village, IL: American Academy of Pediatrics, 2017.
16. Goldenring JM, Rosen D. Getting into adolescent heads: an essential update. Contemp Pediatr 2004;21:64-90.
17. National Institute on Alcohol Abuse and Alcoholism. Alcohol Screening and Brief Intervention for Youth: A Practitioner's Guide. Bethesda, MD: National Institute on Alcohol Abuse and Alcoholism; 2011. NIH Publication 11-7805 [monograph on the Internet]. Available at https://www.niaaa.nih.gov/sites/default/files/publications/YouthGuide.pdf. Accessed January 17, 2020.
18. Kelly SM, Gryczynski J, Mitchell SG, et al. Validity of brief screening instrument for adolescent tobacco, alcohol, and drug use. Pediatrics 2014;133:819-26.
19. Levy S, Weiss R, Sherritt L, et al. An electronic screen for triaging adolescent substance use by risk levels. JAMA Pediatr 2014;168:822-8.
20. Levy S, Siqueira MM; American Academy of Pediatrics, Committee on Substance Abuse. Clinical report: testing for drugs of abuse in children and adolescents. Pediatrics 2014;133:e1789-807.
21. Whiting PF, Wolff RF, Deshpande S, et al. Cannabinoids for medical use: a systematic review and meta-analysis. JAMA 2015; 313:2456-73.
22. American Academy of Pediatrics, Committee on Substance Abuse. The impact of marijuana policies on youth: clinical, research, and legal update [policy statement]. Pediatrics 2015; 135:584-7.
23. American Academy of Pediatrics, Committee on Substance Abuse. Alcohol use by youth and adolescents: a pediatric concern [policy statement]. Pediatrics 2010;125:1078-87. [Reaffirmed December 2014.]
24. Siqueira L, Smith V; American Academy of Pediatrics, Committee on Substance Abuse. Clinical report: binge drinking. Pediatrics 2015;136:e718-26.
25. Farber HJ, Walley SC, Groner JA, et al.; American Academy of Pediatrics, Section on Tobacco Control. Clinical practice policy to protect children from tobacco, nicotine, and tobacco smoke. Pediatrics 2015;136:1008-17.
26. U.S. Department of Health and Human Services. E-Cigarette Use Among Youth and Young Adults. A Report of the Surgeon General. Atlanta, GA: U.S. Department of Health and Human Services, Centers for Disease Control and Prevention, National Center for Chronic Disease Prevention and Health Promotion, Office on Smoking and Health, 2016.
27. Jenssen BP, Walley SC, American Academy of Pediatrics, Section on Tobacco Control. E-Cigarettes and Similar Devices [policy statement]. Pediatrics 2019;143:e20183652.

28. U.S. Food & Drug Administration. Modifications to Compliance Policy for Certain Deemed Tobacco Products [monograph on the Internet]. Available at https://www.fda.gov/regulatory-information/search-fda-guidance-documents/enforcement-priorities-electronic-nicotine-delivery-system-ends-and-other-deemed-products-market. Accessed April 1, 2019.

29. Seifert SM, Schaechter JL, Hershorin ER, et al. Health effects of energy drinks on children, adolescents, and young adults. Pediatrics 2011;127:511-28.

30. Williams JF, Storck M; Committee on Substance Abuse and Committee on Native American Child Health. American Academy of Pediatrics. Inhalant abuse. Pediatrics 2007;119:1009.

31. Committee on Sports Medicine and Fitness. American Academy of Pediatrics. Use of performance-enhancing substances. Pediatrics 2005;115:1103-6.

32. National Institute on Drug Abuse. Commonly Abused Drugs Charts [monograph on the Internet]. Available at https://www.drugabuse.gov/drugs-abuse/commonly-abused-drugs-charts. Accessed January 17, 2020.

33. Drug Enforcement Administration. Drugs of Abuse: A DEA Resource Guide. Washington, DC: U.S. Department of Justice, 2015.

34. National Institute on Drug Abuse. Principles of Adolescent Substance Use Disorder Treatment: A Research-Based Guide [monograph on the Internet]. Available at https://www.drugabuse.gov/publications/principles-adolescent-substance-use-disorder-treatment-research-based-guide/acknowledgements. Accessed January 17, 2020.

35. Mee-Lee D, Shulman GD, Fishman MJ, et al., eds. The ASAM Criteria: Treatment Criteria for Addictive, Substance-Related, and Co-Occurring Conditions, 3rd ed. Carson City, NV: Change Companies, 2013.

36. Li L, Zhu S, Tse N, et al. Effectiveness of motivational interviewing to reduce illicit drug use in adolescents: a systematic review and meta-analysis. Addiction 2016;111:795-805.

37. Traub SJ, Nelson LS, Hoffman RS. Physostigmine as a treatment for gamma hydroxybutyrate toxicity: a review. J Toxicol Clin Toxicol 2002;40:781-7.

38. Hall AP, Henry JA. Acute toxic effects of 'ecstasy' (MDMA) and related compounds: overview of pathophysiology and clinical management. Br J Anaesth 2006;96:678-85.

39. Minozzi S, Amato L, Bellisario C, et al. Detoxification treatments for opiate dependent adolescents. Cochrane Database Syst Rev 2014;4:CD006749.

40. Woody GE, Poole SA, Subramaniam G, et al. Extended vs short-term buprenorphine-naloxone for treatment of opioid-addicted youth: a randomized trial. JAMA 2008;300:2003-11.

41. Marsch LA, Bickel WK, Badger GJ, et al. Comparison of pharmacological treatments for opioid-dependent adolescents. Arch Gen Psychiatry 2005;62:1157-64.

42. Gray KM, Carpenter MJ, Baker NL, et al. A double-blind randomized controlled trial of N-acetylcysteine in cannabis-dependent adolescents. Am J Psychiatry 2012;169:805-12.

43. Miranda R Jr, Treloar H, Blanchard A, et al. Topiramate and motivational enhancement therapy for cannabis use among youth: a randomized placebo controlled pilot study. Addict Biol 2017;22:779-90.

44. Deas D, May MP, Randall C, et al. Naltrexone treatment of adolescent alcoholics: an open-label pilot study. J Child Adolesc Psychopharmacol 2005;15:723-8.

45. Miranda R, Ray L, Blanchard A, et al. Effects of naltrexone on adolescent alcohol cue reactivity and sensitivity: an initial randomized trial. Addict Biol 2014;19:941-54.

46. Niederhofer H, Staffen W. Acamprosate and its efficacy in treating alcohol dependent adolescents. Eur Child Adolesc Psychiatry 2003;12:144-8.

47. Monti PM, Miranda R, Justus A, et al. Biobehavioral mechanisms of topiramate and drinking in adolescents: preliminary findings. Neuropharmacology 2010;35:S164.

48. Dawes MA, Johnson BA, Ait-Daoud N, et al. A prospective, open-label trial of ondansetron in adolescents with alcohol dependence. Addict Behav 2005;30:1077-85.

49. Niederhofer H, Staffen W. Comparison of disulfiram and placebo in treatment of alcohol dependence of adolescents. Drug Alcohol Rev 2003;22:295-7.

50. American Academy of Pediatrics, Committee on Substance Abuse. Medication-assisted treatment of adolescents with opioid use disorder [policy statement]. Pediatrics 2016;138:e20161893.

51. Minozzi S, Amato L, Bellisario C, et al. Maintenance treatments for opiate dependent adolescents. Cochrane Database Syst Rev 2014;6:CD007210.

52. Fishman MJ, Winstanley EL, Curran E, et al. Treatment of opioid dependence in adolescents and young adults with extended release naltrexone: preliminary case-series and feasibility. Addiction 2010;105:1669-76.

53. Hadland SE, Wharam JF, Schuster MA, et al. Trends in receipt of buprenorphine and naltrexone for opioid use disorder among adolescents and young adults, 2001-2014. JAMA Pediatr 2017;171:747-55.

54. Hadland SE, Bagley SM, Rodean J. Receipt of timely addiction treatment and association of early medication treatment with retention in care among youths with opioid use disorder. JAMA Pediatr 2018;172:1029-37.

55. Kim Y, Myung SK, Jeon YJ, et al. Effectiveness of pharmacologic therapy for smoking cessation in adolescent smokers: meta-analysis of randomized controlled trials. Am J Health Syst Pharm 2011;68:219-26.

56. Stanton A, Grimshaw G. Tobacco cessation interventions for young people. Cochrane Database Syst Rev 2013;8:CD003289.

57. Scherphof CS, van den Eijnden RJ, Engels RC, et al. Short-term efficacy of nicotine replacement therapy for smoking cessation in adolescents: a randomized controlled trial. J Subst Abuse Treat 2014;46:120-7.

58. Scherphof CS, van den Eijnden RJ, Engels RC, et al. Long-term efficacy of nicotine replacement therapy for smoking cessation in adolescents: a randomized controlled trial. Drug Alcohol Depend 2014;140:217-20.

59. Scherphof CS, van den Eijnden RJ, Lugtig P, et al. Adolescents' use of nicotine replacement therapy for smoking cessation: predictors of compliance trajectories. Psychopharmacology 2014;231:1743-52.

60. Leischow SJ, Muramoto ML, Matthews E, et al. Adolescent smoking cessation with bupropion: the role of adherence. Nicotine Tob Res 2016;18:1202-5.

61. Gray KM, Baker NL, McClure EA, et al. Efficacy and safety of varenicline for adolescent smoking cessation: a randomized clinical trial. JAMA Pediatr 2019;173:1146-53.

62. Gray KM, Carpenter MJ, Lewis AL, et al. Varenicline versus bupropion XL for smoking cessation in older adolescents: a randomized, double-blind pilot trial. Nicotine Tob Res 2012;14:234-9.

63. U.S. Food & Drug Administration. FDA in Brief: FDA updates label for Chantix with data underscoring it's not effective in children 16 and younger [news brief]. Available at https://www.fda.gov/news-events/fda-brief/fda-brief-fda-updates-label-chantix-data-underscoring-its-not-effective-children-16-and-younger. Accessed April 1, 2019.

64. Riggs PD, Winhusen T, Davies RD et al. Randomized controlled trial of osmotic-release methylphenidate with cognitive-behavioral therapy in adolescents with attention-deficit/hyperactivity disorder and substance use disorder. J Am Acad Child Adolesc Psychiatry 2011;50:903-14.

65. Thurstone C, Riggs PD, Salomonsen S, et al. Randomized controlled trial of atomoxetine for ADHD in adolescents with substance use disorder. J Am Acad Child Adolesc Psychiatry 2010;49:573-82.

66. Riggs PD, Leon SL, Mikulich SK, et al. An open trial of bupropion for ADHD in adolescents with substance use disorder

and conduct disorder. J Am Acad Child Adolesc Psychiatry 1998;37:1271-8.

67. Cornelius JR, Bukstein OG, Wood DS, et al. Double-blind placebo-controlled trial of fluoxetine in adolescents with comorbid major depression and an alcohol use disorder. Addict Behav 2009;34:905-9.

68. Riggs PD, Mikulich-Gilbertson SK, Davies RD, et al. A randomized controlled trial of fluoxetine and cognitive behavioral therapy in adolescents with major depression, behavior problems, and substance use disorders. Arch Pediatr Adolesc Med 2007;161:1026-34.

69. Deas D, Randall C, Roberts J, et al. A double-blind, placebo controlled trial of sertraline in depressed adolescent alcoholics: a pilot study. Hum Psychopharmacol 2000;15:461-9.

70. Riggs PD, Mikulich SK, Coffman, LM, et al. Fluoxetine in drug-dependent delinquents with major depression: an open trial. J Child Adolesc Psychopharmacol 1997;7:87-95.

71. Geller B, Cooper T, Sun K, et al. Double-blind and placebo-controlled study of lithium for adolescent bipolar disorders with secondary substance dependence. J Am Acad Child Adolesc Psychiatry 1998;37:171-8.

72. Upadhyaya H, Brady K, Wang W. Bupropion SR in adolescents with comorbid ADHD and nicotine dependence: a pilot study. J Am Acad Child Adolesc Psychiatry 2004;43:199-205.

73. Levy S, Campbell MD, Shea CL, et al. Trends in abstaining from substance use in adolescents: 1975–2014. Pediatrics 2018; 142:e20173498.

74. American Society of Health-System Pharmacists. ASHP statement on the pharmacist's role in substance abuse prevention, education, and assistance. Am J Health-Syst Pharm 2016; 73:e267-70.

75. Matson KL, Johnson PN, Tran V, et al.; Pediatric Pharmacy Advocacy Group, Advocacy Committee. Opioid use in children [position paper]. Pediatr Pharmacol Ther 2019;24:72-5.

Section XI

Infectious Diseases

CHAPTER 37

Meningitis in Infants and Children

Anita Siu, Pharm.D., BCPPS

INTRODUCTION

Meningitis is defined as an inflammation of the meninges that, when suspected, is considered a medical emergency. Meningitis can be caused by a variety of pathogens, including bacteria, viruses, fungi, and parasites. This chapter will focus on bacterial meningitis with a brief overview of viral meningitis. Bacterial meningitis, when untreated, is associated with a mortality rate approaching 100%.[1] With appropriate treatment, the mortality rate decreases to 20% to 30% in neonates and 1% in infants and children.[2] Before the availability of immunizations against common bacterial meningitis pathogens such as *Streptococcus pneumoniae* (pneumococcus) and

Haemophilus influenzae, bacterial meningitis occurred in almost 6000 infants and children annually, with 70% of these cases caused by *H. influenzae*.[3] The introduction of the *H. influenzae* type b (Hib) and 7-valent pneumococcal conjugate (PCV7) vaccines has reduced the incidence of disease caused by these pathogens. In 2000—13 years after the introduction of the Hib conjugate vaccine—the incidence of meningitis caused by Hib decreased by 99%.[4] Similarly, in 2010—10 years after the introduction of PCV7—the incidence of invasive pneumococcal disease caused by the seven serotypes contained in the vaccine also decreased by 99%.[5] Because of the emergence of pneumococcal serotypes not covered by the PCV7, *S. pneumoniae* continues to be one of the most prevalent meningitis pathogens. Thus, in early 2010, the U.S. Food and Drug Administration approved a 13-valent pneumococcal conjugate vaccine (PCV13) that covers the serotypes found in PCV7, such as 4, 6B, 9V, 14, 18C, 19F, and 23F, plus protects against serotypes 1, 3, 5, 6A, 7F, and 19A. At this time, it is unclear how the introduction of PCV13 will affect the incidence of pneumococcal meningitis.

Despite reductions in mortality, morbidity associated with bacterial meningitis remains high. In neonates, the risk of neurologic sequelae and disabilities after bacterial meningitis is as high as 56%, and up to 25% of childhood meningitis survivors are at risk of developing major disabilities.[6,7] Common meningitis-induced neurologic impairments include behavior and adjustment disorders, hearing or visual loss, intellectual impairment, motor abnormalities, and seizures.[7] Risk factors associated with poor outcomes include young age, delay in presentation, presence of seizures for more than 72 hours, coma, need for inotropes, leukopenia, and pneumococcal etiology.[6,8,9] Fortunately, for meningitis caused by some bacteria, the timely addition of dexamethasone to antibiotic treatment has resulted in a decreased incidence of certain neurologic impairments.

Aseptic meningitis occurs in the absence of bacterial isolation from the cerebrospinal fluid (CSF). Viruses are the most common cause of aseptic meningitis. Viruses can also cause encephalitis, with inflammation that extends beyond the meninges and involves brain parenchyma, often referred to as *viral meningoencephalitis*. Viral meningitis and meningoencephalitis account for more central nervous system (CNS) infections in the United States than all other pathogens combined.[10] Despite recent advances in molecular diagnostics, a thorough understanding of viral CNS infections is lacking, which leads to delayed diagnosis and underreporting.[10]

ETIOLOGY

Although many pathogens have the potential to cause meningitis, few are responsible for most cases. The most common community-acquired bacterial pathogens depend on the age of the patient. Table 1 lists the most common pathogens based on age group and other predisposing factors.[11]

Bacterial meningitis acquired early in the neonatal period, at 72 hours of age or younger, is usually the result of colonization from vaginal delivery. *Streptococcus agalactiae*, otherwise known as group B *Streptococcus*, is a gram-positive organism commonly found in the vaginal canal. Because of vertical transmission from mother to newborn, *S. agalactiae* is a common pathogen in neonatal early-onset sepsis and meningitis. *Escherichia coli*, an enteric gram-negative bacillus, is the second leading cause of bacterial meningitis in neonates and the most common isolated organism from infected urine in pregnant woman.[12] Most *E. coli* isolates responsible for meningitis in this age group possess the K1 capsular antigen, which is associated with higher morbidity and mortality rates than other *E. coli* isolates.[13] *Listeria monocytogenes* is a gram-positive bacillus that can be acquired by the mother, most commonly through the consumption of contaminated food, and transmitted vertically to the fetus. Although not the most common cause of bacterial meningitis in neonates, *L. monocytogenes* has the potential to cause more morbidity and mortality than other common pathogens. Because of these risks, empiric coverage of *L. monocytogenes* should always be considered in infants younger than 1 month.[14] Other gram-negative enteric organisms, such as *Klebsiella* spp., can also cause meningitis during the neonatal period.

Late-onset neonatal bacterial meningitis, neonatal age older than 72 hours of life, and meningitis in all other pediatric age groups are more likely to be caused by a community-acquired pathogen.[12] Bacterial meningitis in patients age 1–23 months is caused by several different pathogens. The most commonly reported causes in this age group are *S. pneumoniae* and *Neisseria meningitidis*, also known as *meningococcal meningitis*. In this age group, *S. agalactiae*, *H. influenzae*, and *E. coli* are also potential pathogens. As discussed previously, the incidence of *H. influenzae* meningitis decreased dramatically after the introduction of the Hib conjugate vaccine. In fact, the mean age of recorded *H. influenzae* meningitis increased from age 15 months to 25 years.[15] Meanwhile, *S. pneumoniae* serotypes not found in PCV7 have increased by 275% and are now the leading cause of meningitis in the 1- to 23-month age group.[16] There are many different strains of *N. meningitidis*, a gram-negative diplococci, but the most common in the United States are serotypes B, C, and Y. Serotype B is the most common in infants younger than 1 year. Currently, three licensed meningococcal vaccines cover four serotypes (A, C, W-135, and Y), and two products cover for serotype B.[17-19]

The most common bacterial pathogen reported in patients age 2–18 years is *N. meningitidis*.[15] The most common meningococcal serotypes in children 11 years and older are C, Y, and W-135.[17,18] The quadrivalent meningococcal vaccine licensed for use in the United States that includes serotypes A, C, Y, and W-135 is recommended for all children between age 11 and 12 years, followed by a booster at age 16 years. In addition, routine meningococcal vaccination is recommended for those 2 years and older with specific disease states or medical conditions that result in reduced immune response (Pediatric Vaccines chapter).[18] Serogroup B meningococcal vaccine may

Table 1. Common Pathogens by Pediatric Age Group and Recommended Empiric Therapy for Bacterial Meningitis

Predisposing Factor	Bacteria	Empiric Therapy
Age		
< 1 mo	*Streptococcus agalactiae*, *Escherichia coli*, *Listeria monocytogenes*, *Klebsiella* spp.	Ampicillin plus cefotaxime, or ampicillin plus an aminoglycoside
1–23 mo	*Streptococcus pneumoniae*, *Neisseria meningitidis*, *S. agalactiae*, *Haemophilus influenzae*, *E. coli*	Vancomycin plus a third-generation cephalosporin
2–18 yr	*N. meningitidis*, *S. pneumoniae*	Vancomycin plus a third-generation cephalosporin
Head Trauma[a]		
Basilar skull fracture	*S. pneumoniae*, *H. influenzae*, group A β-hemolytic streptococci	Vancomycin plus a third-generation cephalosporin
Penetrating trauma	*Staphylococcus aureus*, coagulase-negative staphylococci (especially *Staphylococcus epidermidis*), aerobic gram-negative bacilli (including *Pseudomonas aeruginosa*)	Vancomycin plus cefepime, vancomycin plus ceftazidime, or vancomycin plus meropenem
Postneurosurgery[a]	Aerobic gram-negative bacilli (including *P. aeruginosa*), *S. aureus*, coagulase-negative staphylococci (especially *S. epidermidis*)	Vancomycin plus cefepime, vancomycin plus ceftazidime, or vancomycin plus meropenem
Cerebrospinal fluid shunt[a]	Coagulase-negative staphylococci (especially *S. epidermidis*), aerobic gram-negative bacilli (including *P. aeruginosa*), *S. aureus*, *Propionibacterium acnes*	Vancomycin plus cefepime, vancomycin plus ceftazidime, or vancomycin plus meropenem

[a]Empiric treatment of pathogens associated with these predisposing factors should be considered in combination with empiric treatment of pathogens based on age. Adapted with permission from Oxford University Press. Tunkel AR, Hartman BJ, Kaplan SL, et al. Practice guidelines for the management of bacterial meningitis. Clin Infect Dis 2004;39:1267-84.

be administered in adolescents and young adults (age 16–23 years), preferably at age 16–18 years. Routine administration of serogroup B meningococcal vaccine is recommended for people 10 years and older identified as being at increased risk because of either a serogroup B meningococcal disease outbreak or certain medical conditions.[19] The second leading cause of meningitis in this age group is *S. pneumoniae*, and similar to younger children, the most common serotypes found in this age group that now cause meningitis are not found in PCV7.

As discussed previously, viral meningitis and meningoencephalitis account for more cases of meningitis than all other pathogens combined. The most common viral pathogen isolated is the enterovirus, which accounts for more than 50% of all cases each year.[20] More than 50 serotypes of enterovirus have been associated with meningitis.[20] In addition, respiratory viruses such as influenza and adenoviruses, arboviruses such as West Nile virus, and herpes simplex viruses (HSVs) can cause viral meningitis.[20,21]

ANATOMY AND PHYSIOLOGY OF THE CNS

MENINGES AND CSF

The CSF suspends the brain within the protective layers of the meninges. The meninges are composed of three layers: the pia mater, arachnoid mater, and dura mater.[22,23] The choroid plexuses, which are located in the lateral third and fourth ventricles, produce 85% of the CSF. This fluid is secreted from the choroid plexus and flows outward into the subarachnoid space. The CSF then circulates around the brain and the spinal cord by bulk flow; complete exchange of CSF occurs every 3–4 hours.[23] The fluid is normally clear, and in infants, children, and adults, it contains less than 50 mg/dL of protein (less than 170 mg/dL in neonates).[24,25] A CSF glucose concentration of 50% to 55% of the peripheral serum concentration (75% to 80% in neonates) is a normal finding in the CSF of infants and children without CNS disease. In addition, in children a normal CSF can contain less than 5 white blood cells (WBCs) per cubic millimeter (less than 20 WBCs in neonates).[26,27] These values change in the presence of infection with bacteria or viruses as shown in Table 2.[28]

BLOOD-BRAIN BARRIER

The interface between the brain and the bloodstream, although commonly referred to as the *blood-brain barrier* (BBB), consists of two components: the BBB and the blood-CSF barrier. For this chapter, the combination of the BBB and blood-CSF barrier will be referred to as the *BBB*. The BBB is a functional barrier composed of brain microvascular endothelial cells that regulate the passage of molecules to and from the brain and protect the brain from microbes and toxins.[29] The main functional component of the BBB is the tight junctions that exist between the brain microvascular endothelial cells and restrict the passage of virtually all molecules. Because of the makeup of the BBB, molecules that are small and lipophilic are more likely to cross the BBB and enter the brain. The presence of transport proteins in the endothelial cells allows the transfer of essential nutrients and molecules to the brain that might not otherwise pass through the tight junctions.[30] During bacterial meningitis, bacteria cause the release of proinflammatory cytokines and toxic compounds, resulting in pleocytosis, increased WBCs in the CSF, and increased permeability of the BBB.[29]

PATHOGENESIS

Most cases of meningitis occur spontaneously. Although the exact mechanism of CNS invasion is unknown, many cases begin with nasopharyngeal colonization.[31] After mucosal colonization of the nasopharynx, bacteria must overcome the host defense mechanisms to invade the bloodstream and penetrate the CNS, thereby eliciting meningitis and neuronal damage.[29]

Bacterial colonization of the nasopharyngeal mucosa and systemic invasion are more likely when the bacteria possess fimbriae or a polysaccharide capsule. *Fimbriae* are organelles found on the surface of many bacterial cells that enhance the adhesion to host cells.[31] One species known to possess fimbriae is *N. meningitidis*. Of *N. meningitidis* isolates in the nasopharyngeal mucosa and CSF of patients with meningitis, 80% are fimbriated.[32] By inhibiting neutrophil phagocytosis and resisting complement-mediated bactericidal activity, bacterial polysaccharide capsules promote systemic invasion. The

Table 2. CSF Findings in Pediatric Bacterial and Viral Meningitis[24-28]

CSF Finding	Normal for Age	Bacterial Meningitis	Viral Meningitis
Opening pressure (mm H_2O)	50–80	100–300	80–150
Glucose (ratio of CSF to serum)	Neonates: 0.75–0.8 All other ages: 0.5–0.55	Neonates: ≤ 0.6 All other ages: ≤ 0.4	Normal[a]
Protein (mg/dL)	Neonates: < 170 All other ages: < 50	100–500	30–150
WBC (cells/mm³)	Neonates: 0–25 Infants: 0–8 Children-adults: 0–5	1000–5000	100–1000[b]
Differential (%)	> 90 monocytes	80–95 neutrophils	50 lymphocytes[c]

[a]Lower-than-normal glucose has been observed in some patients.
[b]High red blood cell count can be markedly raised in patients with HSV meningoencephalitis.
[c]Initial CSF may reveal a predominance of neutrophils.
CSF = cerebrospinal fluid; HSV = herpes simplex virus.

most common meningeal pathogens, *H. influenzae, S. pneumoniae, N. meningitidis,* and *S. agalactiae,* are examples of encapsulated bacteria. Before the routine use of the Hib vaccine, all strains of encapsulated *H. influenzae* accounted for only 5% of nasopharyngeal isolates; however, more than 95% of meningeal and systemic infections were caused by type b strains.[31,33]

The mechanism of meningeal invasion has not been well elucidated. One theory is that a high concentration of bacteria in the bloodstream for a sustained period (at least 6 hours in animal models) increases the likelihood of bacterial penetration into the CNS.[34] Other studies evaluating *E. coli,* Hib, and *S. pneumoniae* in neonates and children show an increased likelihood of developing meningitis with high bacterial blood counts (greater than 100–1000 colony-forming units/mL).[35-37]

The site at which bacteria cross the BBB is also debated. Studies of infant rats and primates have shown that the choroid plexus, the site of the blood-CSF barrier, is the entry site because of its high blood flow rate compared with other areas, although other evidence points toward the dural venous sinus system as the point of entry.[31] To further support the choroid plexus theory, studies have shown that meningeal pathogen receptors are present on choroid plexus cells, facilitating the passage of pathogens across the blood-CSF barrier and into the subarachnoid space.[31] Another hypothesis is that bacteria gain access to the CNS in association with monocytes migrating along normal pathways.[38]

Once in the CNS, host defense mechanisms are usually unable to prohibit bacterial survival and replication, resulting in concentrations as high as 10^7 colony-forming units/mL.[39] The presence of bacteria in the CNS signals the release of proinflammatory cytokines and reactive oxygen species, which promote the migration of WBCs across the BBB. In turn, inflammation weakens the tight junctions of the BBB, allowing easier entry of bacteria and other substances from the bloodstream into the CNS.[29] Bacterial replication, cytokine production, and inflammation continue until appropriate antibiotic therapy is administered. The cycle of inflammation that ensues increases the risk of neuronal damage, increased intracranial pressure, decreased cerebral vascular perfusion, thrombus formation, and hydrocephalus. Not only do replicating bacteria in the CNS lead to inflammation and neuronal damage, but also the byproducts of bacterial lysis caused by antibiotic therapy result in subarachnoid inflammation, further increasing the risk of neurologic sequelae.[40,41]

RISK FACTORS

As true for patients having many other infectious diseases, immunocompromised patients are at increased risk of developing meningitis. In addition, the incidence and severity of meningitis are increased in young children, with the highest incidence occurring in the first year of life.[42,43] The incidence remains high until age 2 years and then declines dramatically.[44] Other risk factors include the following: asplenia or splenosis; sickle cell disease and other hemoglobinopathies; terminal complement deficiencies; and recent exposure to someone with meningococcal or *H. influenzae* meningitis. Any situation in which a direct route exists for bacteria to enter the CSF (e.g., surgical procedures, penetrating head trauma, neurosurgical procedures, presence of CSF leak, presence of a CSF shunt, cochlear implants) increases the risk of bacterial meningitis. When meningitis occurs under these circumstances, the most common bacteria found are from the environment (*Staphylococcus* spp. and gram-negative organisms such as *Pseudomonas* spp.).[44-46] The focus of this chapter is community-acquired meningitis in the nonsurgical, nontrauma patient; therefore, discussion regarding the treatment of these organisms is limited to the information presented in Table 1 and Table 3.

CLINICAL MANIFESTATIONS

SIGNS AND SYMPTOMS

The signs and symptoms of meningitis in the pediatric population, unlike the adult population, are generally subtle and nonspecific and can lead to misdiagnosis, especially in young children. Infants and young children often present with the following signs and symptoms: fever; poor feeding; vomiting; lethargy; apnea; irritability; nuchal rigidity (neck stiffness); and seizures, which are more common in pediatric patients than in adults. In addition, a bulging fontanel can often be seen in neonates and young infants. A study of 110 pediatric patients with bacterial meningitis found that the most common presenting symptoms were irritability and impaired consciousness in patients age 1–5 months and 6–11 months, respectively. In children 12 months or older, vomiting and nuchal rigidity were the most common signs and symptoms of meningitis.[47] These findings support the premise that older children and adolescents are more likely to present with classic meningeal signs and symptoms of nuchal rigidity, headache, and photophobia than are infants and young children. In addition, compared with infants and children younger than 18 months, older children and adolescents are more likely to present with a positive physical diagnosis of the Kernig and/or Brudzinski sign.[28,48,49] The Kernig sign produces pain when the patient flexes the hips at a 90-degree angle and cannot extend the knee angle any further, usually around 135 degrees. The Brudzinski sign includes positive findings in the leg or neck. The Brudzinski neck sign is produced when flexing the patient's neck forward causes flexion of the hips and knees. The Brudzinski leg sign is exhibited when the examiner flexes the patient's leg and the contralateral leg flexes or the reciprocal contralateral leg extends spontaneously.

In a systematic review, including 10 studies with children from birth to age 17 years, the following were associated with an increased likelihood of meningitis: a history of bulging fontanel; nuchal rigidity; seizures, if patient is out of the age range for febrile seizures; and poor feeding. According to the same article, the presence of the following findings on physical examination was also associated with increased likelihood of meningitis: jaundice; bulging fontanel; toxic appearance; positive Kernig and/or positive Brudzinski sign; and increased muscle tone.[50]

DIAGNOSIS

Although most diagnostic signs and symptoms of meningitis can be debated, it is well known that many are nonspecific and that diagnosis can be missed, resulting in greater morbidity and mortality. A definitive diagnosis of meningitis can only be determined through a laboratory evaluation of the CSF; therefore, in most cases, a lumbar puncture (LP) is obtained as soon as possible. After the removal of CSF by LP, it is normal to have mild, transient lowering of the CSF pressure.[11] In some patients with certain intracranial lesions, this decrease in CSF pressure could precipitate brain herniation. The time required for neuroimaging to determine abnormalities in the head can delay treatment with antibiotics; therefore, computed tomography scans should not be performed routinely.[51] The Infectious Diseases Society of America (IDSA) recommends that only infants and children with certain signs and symptoms receive a head computed tomography scan before an LP (Figure 1).[11]

Once an LP has been performed, CSF should be sent to the laboratory for cell counts (WBC and red blood cell [RBC]), glucose and protein content, and Gram stain and culture.

In addition, measuring the opening CSF pressure during LP may provide diagnostic information. Table 2 summarizes the CSF findings in patients with bacterial and viral meningitis. Although CSF RBC count is not used for direct diagnosis of meningitis, it is routinely used to determine occurrence of a traumatic LP or presence of subarachnoid or intracerebral hemorrhage. If RBCs are present in the CSF, the WBC count could be falsely elevated because of WBCs introduced from the bloodstream. Performing a Gram stain on the CSF allows an accurate identification of the causative organism in most community-acquired bacterial meningitis cases with a specificity of 97%.[52] The accuracy by which a Gram stain detects a bacterial pathogen is directly related to the concentration of bacteria in the CSF: the higher the concentration, the greater the chance of pathogen detection.[53] In addition, it is exceedingly important to note whether the patient received antibiotic therapy before LP. Sterilization of the CSF can occur after the administration of one dose of intravenous antibiotic therapy. The speed at which the CSF will become sterile depends on the bacterial pathogen present and the antibiotic used.[54]

Table 3. Recommendations for Specific Therapy Based on Isolated Pathogen and Susceptibility

Microorganism, Susceptibility	Standard Therapy	Alternative Therapies
Streptococcus agalactiae	Penicillin G or ampicillin	Third-generation cephalosporin[a]
Escherichia coli and *Klebsiella* spp.	Third-generation cephalosporin	Aztreonam, fluoroquinolone, meropenem, trimethoprim/sulfamethoxazole[b]
Listeria monocytogenes	Penicillin G or ampicillin	Meropenem
Streptococcus pneumoniae Penicillin MIC		
< 0.1 mcg/mL	Penicillin G or ampicillin	Third-generation cephalosporin[a]
0.1–1 mcg/mL[c]	Third-generation cephalosporin[a]	Cefepime, meropenem
≥ 2 mcg/mL	Vancomycin plus third-generation cephalosporin[a]	Fluoroquinolone[d]
Cefotaxime/ceftriaxone MIC ≥ 1 mcg/mL	Vancomycin plus third-generation cephalosporin[a]	Fluoroquinolone[d]
Haemophilus influenzae		
β-Lactamase negative	Ampicillin	Third-generation cephalosporin,[a] cefepime, fluoroquinolone
β-Lactamase positive	Third-generation cephalosporin[a]	Cefepime, fluoroquinolone
Neisseria meningitides Penicillin MIC		
< 0.1 mcg/mL	Penicillin G or ampicillin	Third-generation cephalosporin[a]
0.1–1 mcg/mL	Third-generation cephalosporin[a]	Fluoroquinolone, meropenem
Staphylococcus aureus		
Methicillin susceptible	Nafcillin or oxacillin	Vancomycin, meropenem
Methicillin resistant	Vancomycin	Trimethoprim/sulfamethoxazole,[b] linezolid
Staphylococcus epidermidis	Vancomycin	Linezolid
Pseudomonas aeruginosa	Cefepime or ceftazidime	Aztreonam, ciprofloxacin, meropenem

[a]Cefotaxime or ceftriaxone (avoid the use of ceftriaxone in the first 28 days of life).
[b]Avoid the use of trimethoprim/sulfamethoxazole in the first 28 days of life.
[c]Cefotaxime/ceftriaxone-susceptible isolates.
[d]Guidelines recommend gatifloxacin or moxifloxacin, but there are no dosing recommendations for use in pediatric patients.
MIC = minimum inhibitory concentration.
Adapted with permission from Oxford University Press. Tunkel AR, Hartman BJ, Kaplan SL, et al. Practice guidelines for the management of bacterial meningitis. Clin Infect Dis 2004;39:1267-84.

Other laboratory tests that may help determine the presence of bacterial meningitis include latex agglutination, limulus lysate assay, and polymerase chain reaction (PCR). Latex agglutination is a rapid test that uses either a serum that contains bacterial antibodies or commercially available antisera that are directed against the capsular polysaccharides of meningeal pathogens.[11] The limulus lysate assay is designed as a test to determine the presence of gram-negative meningitis and works by giving a positive result in the presence of endotoxin from gram-negative bacteria.[55] For patients with meningitis, IDSA does not recommend the routine use of latex agglutination and limulus lysate assay.[11]

As a primer-mediated technique for the enzymatic amplification of specific DNA sequences, PCR can be used to detect the presence of many pathogens, including the most common causes of bacterial meningitis, including the following: *N. meningitidis*, *S. pneumoniae*, Hib, *S. agalactiae*, and *L. monocytogenes*. Compared with traditional microbiology cultures, PCR allows for quicker detection of pathogens such as enterovirus, reducing the identification time from days to hours.[56] The sensitivity and specificity of PCR vary depending on the test, but when a broad range of bacterial primers are used, the sensitivity is 100% with a specificity of 98%, a positive predictive value of 98%, and a negative predictive value of 100%.[57] The IDSA guidelines suggest PCR is useful for excluding the diagnosis of bacterial meningitis and that it potentially plays an influential role in the decision to initiate or discontinue antibiotic therapy.[11]

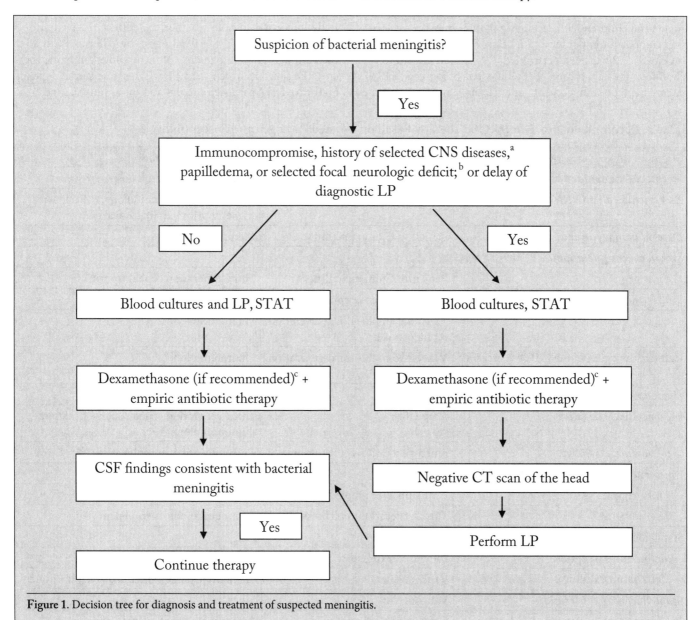

Figure 1. Decision tree for diagnosis and treatment of suspected meningitis.

[a]Includes diseases associated with CSF shunts, hydrocephalus, or trauma; diseases occurring after neurosurgery; or space-occupying lesions.
[b]Palsy of cranial nerves VI or VII is not an indication to delay LP.
[c]See chapter text for adjunctive dexamethasone recommendations.
CNS = central nervous system; CSF = cerebrospinal fluid; CT = computed tomography; LP = lumbar puncture; STAT = immediately.
Adapted with permission from Oxford University Press. Tunkel AR, Hartman BJ, Kaplan SL, et al. Practice guidelines for the management of bacterial meningitis. Clin Infect Dis 2004;39:1267-84.

Clinicians are often faced with the diagnostic dilemma of differentiating between bacterial and viral meningitis, especially when Gram stain and culture of CSF yield negative results. Several tests have been shown to be somewhat helpful in differentiating bacterial from viral meningitis, including CSF lactate concentration, serum C-reactive protein concentration, and serum procalcitonin. Although these tests have not yet replaced standard measures for the diagnosis of bacterial versus viral meningitis, high concentrations of CSF lactate and serum C-reactive protein, and serum procalcitonin greater than 2 ng/mL have been found to be indicators of bacterial rather than viral meningitis.[58-60] In addition, the presence of a CSF glucose concentration of less than 34 mg/dL; a ratio of CSF to serum glucose of less than 0.23; a CSF protein concentration of greater than 220 mg/dL; a CSF leukocyte count of more than 2000 leukocytes/mm³; or a CSF neutrophil count of greater than 1180 neutrophils/mm³ is an individual predictor of bacterial, rather than viral, meningitis with 99% or higher certainty.[61,62]

The diagnosis of viral meningitis, in most clinical settings, involves the exclusion of bacterial meningitis. In addition to CSF cell counts, glucose and protein concentrations, and viral culture, PCR has become an important diagnostic tool to determine the cause of meningitis. Commercial PCR kits are available for the detection of various HSVs as well as enteroviruses.[63-65]

TREATMENT

Empiric therapy for the treatment of community-acquired bacterial meningitis depends on the age of the patient and should cover all commonly encountered organisms for that age group (Table 1). Once cultures and sensitivities are reported, then the antimicrobial therapy should be narrowed for treatment of the specific isolated organism (Table 3). For maximum penetration into the CSF, antibiotics should be administered intravenously; recommended antimicrobial doses are summarized in Table 4.[66,67] The duration of antibiotic therapy depends on the offending pathogen. The IDSA recommends a 7-day treatment course for meningitis caused by *N. meningitidis* and *H. influenzae*; a 10- to 14-day course for *S. pneumoniae* meningitis; a 14- to 21-day course for *S. agalactiae* meningitis; 21 days for *E. coli* and other aerobic gram-negative bacilli; and 21 days or more for *L. monocytogenes* meningitis.[11] In addition, guidelines recommend that neonates with gram-negative meningitis be treated for 2 weeks after the first sterile CSF culture or for 3 weeks or more, whichever is longer.[11] The remainder of this section focuses on the treatment of specific community-acquired bacterial meningitis, adjunctive treatment, and supportive care.

STREPTOCOCCUS AGALACTIAE (GROUP B STREPTOCOCCI)

Streptococcus agalactiae is susceptible to various antibiotics with the goal of achieving adequate CNS penetration using narrow-spectrum agents such as penicillin, ampicillin, or a cephalosporin. Ampicillin is typically the drug of choice for empiric coverage of *S. agalactiae*. Once *S. agalactiae* has been identified and clinical and microbiologic response has been documented, penicillin or ampicillin alone can be used. To minimize the potential development of antibiotic resistance, penicillin should be used, if possible, because of its narrow spectrum of activity.[12,68] Although higher-than-normal doses of antibiotics are routinely used in the treatment of meningitis because it is a sequestered infection site, use of these high doses is even more important with *S. agalactiae* meningitis in neonates. Neonates often present with a higher CSF bacterial load than older age groups, and *S. agalactiae* has a minimum bactericidal concentration that is 10-fold higher than other *Streptococcus* spp., warranting more aggressive doses of antibiotics than in infants and children.[65]

LISTERIA MONOCYTOGENES

As discussed previously, *L. monocytogenes* is a potentially devastating meningeal pathogen in neonates. The mainstay of treatment for *L. monocytogenes* is the combination of ampicillin and gentamicin. Although ampicillin is typically the drug of choice for treatment, the combination of ampicillin and an aminoglycoside is typically used initially because of improved survival observed in animal models.[14,70] Gentamicin is typically the preferred aminoglycoside, whereas tobramycin and amikacin are typically reserved for more resistant organisms.

ESCHERICHIA COLI AND KLEBSIELLA SPP.

Although the combination of ampicillin and an aminoglycoside is adequate for most empiric treatments of *E. coli* and *Klebsiella* infections in neonates, emerging ampicillin resistance, coupled with the relatively poor CSF penetration of aminoglycosides, warrants the use of a different agent. The most commonly used antibiotic in this setting is cefotaxime, a third-generation cephalosporin. Although second- and third-generation cephalosporins have similar spectra of activity against common meningeal pathogens, the use of third-generation cephalosporins for the treatment of meningitis results in better outcomes.[69] For several reasons, cefotaxime is preferred to other intravenous third-generation cephalosporins such as ceftazidime and ceftriaxone. Ceftazidime provides unnecessarily broad gram-negative coverage for community-acquired meningitis, including *Pseudomonas aeruginosa*, and less gram-positive activity than cefotaxime. Unlike cefotaxime, ceftriaxone is up to 95% protein bound and has the ability to displace bilirubin from albumin-binding sites. In neonates, increased free bilirubin increases the risk of kernicterus, a neurologically devastating condition in which bilirubin deposits in the basal ganglia of the brain; therefore, cefotaxime is preferred in this population. In addition, concomitant use of ceftriaxone and intravenous calcium-containing products is contraindicated in neonates in the first month of life because of the precipitates found in the lungs and kidneys. Although cefotaxime has a broader spectrum of activity than aminoglycosides, which may lead to an increased incidence of antibiotic resistance, it safely reaches much higher CSF concentrations than aminoglycosides. Cefotaxime may decrease the risk of prolonged infection and treatment failure, so it should be considered for empiric coverage of suspected neonatal meningitis caused by *E. coli* and *Klebsiella* spp.[12]

STREPTOCOCCUS PNEUMONIAE

Historically *S. pneumoniae* was best treated by penicillin. In the 1960s, the first case of penicillin-resistant *S. pneumoniae* was documented; since then, the emergence of resistant pneumococcus has increased around the world. More recently, pneumococcal isolates resistant to third-generation cephalosporins have become more common.[15,71] In 1998, data published from the Active Bacterial Core Surveillance program in the United States showed that as many as 35% of invasive *S. pneumoniae* isolates were resistant to penicillin, and 14% of isolates were resistant to cefotaxime.[72] For this reason, vancomycin should always be given with a third-generation cephalosporin, either ceftriaxone or cefotaxime, for empiric treatment of suspected meningitis in patients 1 month and older for adequate coverage of *S. pneumoniae*.[11] Of note, the use of ceftriaxone in patients older than 1 month is safe because the risk of kernicterus is greatly decreased after this time. As is true with all other isolated pathogens, if *S. pneumoniae* is isolated, the antibiotic therapy selection is narrowed on the basis of susceptibility results.

Table 4. Antimicrobial and Antiviral Dosing for Meningitis[11,24,45,66,67]

Antimicrobial Agent	CSF Penetration[a]	Dose (mg/kg/dose), Dosing Interval		Infants–Children	Maximum Single Dose	Comments
		Neonates, Age in Days (> 2000 g)				
		0–7	8–28			
Acyclovir	+	20 mg/kg, every 8 hr	20 mg/kg, every 8 hr	20 mg/kg, every 8 hr	N/A[b]	Ensure adequate hydration
Ampicillin	+	100 mg/kg, every 8 hr	75 mg/kg, every 6 hr	75 mg/kg, every 6 hr	2000 mg	
Aztreonam	+	30 mg/kg, every 8 hr	30 mg/kg, every 6 hr	30 mg/kg, every 6 hr	2000 mg	
Cefepime	+	50 mg/kg, every 12 hr	50 mg/kg, every 12 hr	50 mg/kg, every 8 hr	2000 mg	
Cefotaxime	+	50 mg/kg, every 8–12 hr	50 mg/kg, every 6–8 hr	75 mg/kg, every 6 hr	2000 mg	
Ceftazidime	+	50 mg/kg, every 8–12 hr	50 mg/kg, every 8 hr	50 mg/kg, every 8 hr	2000 mg	
Ceftriaxone	+	—	—	50 mg/kg, every 12 hr	2000 mg	Not for neonates[d] Avoid use with calcium-containing IV fluids[e]
Ciprofloxacin	+	—	—	10–15 mg/kg, every 12 hr	800 mg/day	
Meropenem	+	20 mg/kg, every 12 hr	20 mg/kg, every 8 hr	40 mg/kg, every 8 hr	2000 mg	
Nafcillin	+	25 mg/kg, every 8 hr	25–35 mg/kg, every 6 hr	50 mg/kg, every 6 hr	12 g/day	
Oxacillin	+	50 mg/kg, every 8 hr	50 mg/kg, every 6 hr	50 mg/kg, every 6 hr	12 g/day	
Penicillin G	+	50,000 units/kg, every 8 hr	50,000 units/kg, every 6 hr	66,000 units/kg, every 4 hr	24 million units/day	
Rifampin	++	—	10 mg/kg, every 12 hr	10 mg/kg, every 12 hr	600 mg	Do not use as monotherapy
Trimethoprim/ sulfamethoxazole	++	—	—	5 mg/kg TMP, every 6–8 hr	20 mg/kg/ day	Do not use in neonates[d]
Vancomycin	+	15 mg/kg, every 8–12 hr	15 mg/kg, every 6–8 hr	15 mg/kg, every 6 hr	N/A[b,c]	Goal trough: 15–20 mcg/mL[11]

[a]+ = Therapeutic concentrations in the CSF with inflammation of the meninges; ++ = therapeutic concentrations in the CSF with or without inflammation of the meninges.
[b]Maximum dose has not been established.
[c]Monitor serum concentrations; doses should be adjusted to achieve appropriate serum concentrations.
[d]Highly protein bound; risk of bilirubin displacement and development of kernicterus.
[e]Avoid this use because of the risk of precipitation.
CSF = cerebrospinal fluid; IV = intravenous; N/A = not applicable; TMP = trimethoprim.
Adapted with permission from Oxford University Press. Tunkel AR, Hartman BJ, Kaplan SL, et al. Practice guidelines for the management of bacterial meningitis. Clin Infect Dis 2004;39:1267-84.

HAEMOPHILUS INFLUENZAE

Despite the routine use of the Hib conjugate vaccine in the United States, *H. influenzae* remains a potential and important cause of meningitis in infants age 1–23 months. In the 1970s, β-lactamase–producing *H. influenzae* resulted in penicillin treatment failures. In some areas of the United States, the incidence of β-lactamase–positive *H. influenzae* is now approaching 50%.[71] To overcome this resistance and to reduce the risk of treatment failures, a third-generation cephalosporin, either cefotaxime or ceftriaxone, is recommended for empiric treatment of patients age 1–23 months who are at risk of *H. influenzae* meningitis.[11] If *H. influenzae* is isolated from the CSF and the β-lactamase enzyme is not present, ampicillin would be an appropriate choice.

NEISSERIA MENINGITIDIS

Penicillin is the treatment of choice for *N. meningitidis*, the most common meningeal pathogen isolated in patients older than 2 years. Although penicillin-resistant strains of *N. meningitidis* are rare, a third-generation cephalosporin, either ceftriaxone or cefotaxime, should be used empirically until susceptibilities are reported. If a penicillin-susceptible strain of *N. meningitidis* is isolated, therapy should be changed to penicillin for the duration of treatment. Although *N. meningitidis* is a highly pathogenic organism, it is easily treated with appropriate antibiotic therapy. In one study, after the single dose of a third-generation cephalosporin, all CSF cultures were negative after 2 hours compared with other pathogens that took longer.[54] The treatment duration required for meningococcal meningitis is 7 days, much shorter than for other pathogens. In fact, some evidence, although limited, supports even shorter durations with no increased incidence of relapse.[73]

VIRAL PATHOGENS

Therapy for viral meningitis pathogens is limited; therefore, supportive care is typically the mainstay of treatment. Unfortunately, no antiviral treatment is available for enterovirus, the most common viral pathogen isolated in viral meningitis cases. If HSV is suspected, especially in neonates, parenteral acyclovir should be initiated and continued for 14–21 days until HSV infection is ruled out, at which point acyclovir can be discontinued. Acyclovir dosing in neonates, infants, and children younger than 12 years with suspected HSV meningitis or encephalitis is 20 mg/kg/dose intravenously administered every 8 hours. Of note, some experts recommend 15 mg/kg/dose every 8 hours for children older than 2 months to younger than 12 years. For children 12 years and older, a dose of 10 mg/kg intravenously administered every 8 hours is recommended.[74] Acyclovir has the potential to cause nephrotoxicity; therefore, pharmacists should ensure patients receive adequate hydration as well as proper monitoring of urine output and renal function, especially when acyclovir is combined with other nephrotoxic agents. Currently no effective therapies are available for the other potential viral causes of meningitis, such as respiratory viruses or arboviruses.

SUPPORTIVE CARE

The maintenance of normal temperature and blood pressure, adequate cerebral perfusion pressure, and management of increased intracranial pressure are paramount in preventing the most life-threatening complications of bacterial meningitis. Strategies used to reduce intracranial pressure include bed head elevation of 30 degrees, avoidance of frequent vigorous procedures, hypertonic saline administration, and, potentially, administration of high-dose barbiturates.[45] In addition, patients who become obtunded and unable to protect their airway often require intubation and mechanical ventilation.

ADJUNCTIVE TREATMENT WITH DEXAMETHASONE

As discussed previously, bacterial meningitis remains an important and significant cause of morbidity and mortality in children. The neurologic sequelae associated with this disease are mainly a result of the inflammatory processes from bacterial proliferation and bacterial lysis in the CSF. For this reason, dexamethasone, a corticosteroid with potent anti-inflammatory effects, has been studied in patients with bacterial meningitis to decrease the incidence of morbidity and mortality. Dexamethasone, when used in the appropriate pediatric patient, can decrease hearing loss and neurologic sequelae but does not seem to affect overall mortality.[11,75,76]

Dexamethasone use in neonatal meningitis is not well studied; therefore, it is not recommended for treatment of bacterial meningitis in this population. According to a recent meta-analysis, in children older than 1 month with bacterial meningitis mainly caused by *H. influenzae*, administration of dexamethasone decreased the risk of hearing loss.[75] Because of the potential for increased inflammation as a result of bacterial lysis after antibiotic therapy, dexamethasone should be administered before the first dose of antibiotic therapy to be most effective. The latest IDSA treatment guidelines for meningitis recommend the use of dexamethasone, at a dose of 0.15 mg/kg every 6 hours for 2–4 days, in infants and children with *H. influenzae* meningitis as long as it is initiated before the administration of antibiotic therapy.[11]

The use of adjunctive dexamethasone treatment for pneumococcal meningitis showed to reduce mortality.[75] Current IDSA guidelines state dexamethasone therapy should be considered in patients with pneumococcal meningitis and that the potential risks and benefits should be weighed before initiating treatment.[11,77] More recently, it was found that dexamethasone treatment has a protective effect against the development of hearing loss in non–*H. influenzae* meningitis in children.[75] There is no benefit for the use of adjunctive dexamethasone in meningococcal or gram-negative meningitis.

ADJUNCTIVE TREATMENT WITH RIFAMPIN

Rifampin is an agent commonly used synergistically in combination with other antibiotics for the treatment of *Staphylococcus* spp. Although rifampin may be an attractive agent for the treatment of CNS infections because of its excellent BBB penetration, resistance to rifampin develops quickly as monotherapy. Therefore, rifampin should always be used in combination with another agent when treating bacterial meningitis. On the basis of its activity against *Staphylococcus* spp., it is recommended that rifampin be considered in addition to vancomycin in patients with CNS shunt infections, particularly if the shunt is not going to be removed.[11] Although data are limited, some experts recommend the addition of rifampin to either cefotaxime or ceftriaxone for the treatment of *S. pneumoniae* meningitis in the following circumstances: the patient's condition continues to deteriorate after 24–48 hours of therapy; a repeat CSF culture shows continued growth or does not show a significant reduction in the number of organisms growing; or the *S. pneumoniae* isolate has a cefotaxime/ceftriaxone MIC greater than 2 mcg/mL.[11,78]

MONITORING TREATMENT

Patients should be monitored for improvement in signs and symptoms of meningitis. For patients who respond appropriately to treatment, repeat LP is not routinely recommended. For patients in whom symptoms do not improve after 48 hours of therapy, repeat LP should be considered.[11] This approach is especially true for patients with pneumococcal meningitis that is resistant to penicillin or cephalosporins, neonates with meningitis caused by gram-negative bacteria, or those who have received adjunctive dexamethasone therapy. Patients should also be monitored for adverse effects of antibiotic/antiviral treatment (Table 5).

CHEMOPROPHYLAXIS

Chemoprophylaxis for *H. influenzae* should be provided for specific household contacts. *Household contact* is defined as people residing with the index patient or nonresidents who spent 4 or more hours with the index patient for at least 5 of the past 7 days before the day of hospital admission. Any household with at least one child who is younger than 4 years and unimmunized or incompletely immunized, or any household with a person who is immunosuppressed (regardless of immunization status), should also receive chemoprophylaxis. Chemoprophylaxis is also recommended for nursery school and day care center contacts when two or more *H. influenzae* cases have occurred in the past 60 days.[79]

Chemoprophylaxis is recommended in several situations if a documented case of meningococcal meningitis occurs in the following: a household contact (as previously defined), especially children younger than 2 years; a day care or preschool contact at any time during the previous 7 days from the onset of illness; anyone who has had direct exposure to the index patient's secretions through kissing, sharing toothbrushes, or sharing eating utensils; and markers of close social contact at any time during the previous 7 days leading up to illness. In addition, people who have slept several times in the same dwelling as the index patient during the 7 days preceding the illness or any passenger seated directly next to the index case during airline flights lasting more than 8 hours during the 7 days before illness should receive chemoprophylaxis for meningococcal disease. Routine chemoprophylaxis for health care providers is not recommended; however, health care providers who have provided mouth-to-mouth resuscitation or had unprotected contact during endotracheal intubation at any time within 7 days before the onset of illness should receive chemoprophylaxis.[80] Table 6 provides a list of recommended chemoprophylaxis agents and dosage.

VACCINATION

Vaccination is the most effective way to prevent bacterial meningitis in infants and children.[81] The Pediatric Vaccines chapter provides further information on specific vaccinations.

CONCLUSIONS

Bacterial meningitis is a medical emergency requiring prompt diagnosis and treatment. The exact pathophysiology of the disease has yet to be elucidated, but evidence supports the theory of nasopharyngeal colonization leading to bacteremia

Table 5. Common Adverse Effects of Therapy[66]

Agent	Adverse Effects
Acyclovir	Rash, nausea, phlebitis, nephrotoxicity, elevated liver function tests
Aztreonam	Neutropenia, elevated liver function tests, pain at injection site, elevated serum creatinine
Cephalosporins (ceftriaxone, cefotaxime, ceftazidime, cefepime)	Hypersensitivity reactions, nausea, vomiting, diarrhea, pain at injection site, biliary sludging (ceftriaxone), contraindicated with concomitant calcium intravenous solutions (ceftriaxone)
Ciprofloxacin	Neurologic events (dizziness, nervousness), rash, photosensitivity, nausea, vomiting, tendon rupture
Meropenem	Hypersensitivity reactions, headache, rash, nausea, vomiting, diarrhea, phlebitis, seizures (rare)
Penicillins (ampicillin, nafcillin, oxacillin, penicillin G)	Hypersensitivity reactions, seizures (with high concentrations), bone marrow suppression, elevated liver function tests, interstitial nephritis (rare)
Trimethoprim/sulfamethoxazole	Nausea, vomiting, rash, jaundice/kernicterus in neonates, blood dyscrasias (rare), hepatotoxicity (rare)
Vancomycin	Red man syndrome, nephrotoxicity, hypotension, fever, neutropenia

and eventual penetration of the meninges. Without a true understanding of the development of the disease, regardless of improvements in diagnostic testing, early recognition of bacterial meningitis remains a challenge. Nevertheless, the timely use of appropriate antibiotic therapy has resulted in improved outcomes through the years, but morbidity and mortality in young infants and children remain high. The most effective means of reducing morbidity and mortality from the disease is prevention of the disease through the development and implementation of effective conjugate vaccines.

Table 6. Chemoprophylaxis Agents and Dosing[79,80]

Meningeal Pathogen	Rifampin[a]	Ceftriaxone	Ciprofloxacin[a,b]
Haemophilus influenzae type b	< 1 mo: 10 mg/kg PO every day for 4 days ≥ 1 mo: 20 mg/kg (max 600 mg) PO every day for 4 days	Not recommended	Not recommended
Neisseria meningitidis	< 1 mo: 5 mg/kg PO every 12 hr for 2 days ≥ 1 mo: 10 mg/kg (max 600 mg) PO every 12 hr for 2 days	< 15 yr: 125 mg IM once ≥ 15 yr: 250 mg IM once	≥ 1 mo: 20 mg/kg (max 500 mg) PO once

[a]Not recommended for use in pregnant women.
[b]Use only if fluoroquinolone-resistant strains of *N. meningitidis* have not been identified in the community.
IM = intramuscularly; max = maximum; PO = orally.

Patient Case PEDIATRIC MENINGITIS

A 2-year-old girl is admitted to the general pediatric unit for a temperature of 102°F (39°C), lethargy, and decreased appetite for the past 3 days. Her mother noted that she had poor intake and refusal of feeding, and since then she has had limited solid and liquid intake. At an appointment with her pediatrician 2 days before hospital admission, an ear infection was diagnosed. She was prescribed amoxicillin 600 mg orally twice daily for 10 days. Despite receiving antibiotics for 2 days, she continues to have persistent fevers, lethargy, and decreased interactions.

Medical history: Significant history of recurrent ear infections, for which her pediatric ear, nose, and throat physician recently recommended placement of myringotomy tubes; however, the surgical date is pending

Medications: Amoxicillin 600 mg orally twice daily started 2 days before admission for acute otitis media

Immunizations: Incomplete, pending the last doses of the vaccine series including 13-valent pneumococcal conjugate vaccine, *Haemophilus influenzae* type b, inactivated polio virus, and annual influenza

Family history: Mother has diabetes; father has hypertension; her two siblings (sister age 8 years and brother age 5 years) are currently healthy

Social history: Lives at home with her mother, father, and two siblings; attends day care and plays well with other children; attends weekly dance classes

Vital signs on admission: Tmax 102°F (39°C), HR 100 beats/minute, RR 20 breaths/minute, BP 100/80 mm Hg, Wt 15 kg

Physical examination: All within normal limits, except the neurologic examination and a positive Kernig sign

Laboratory findings:

Chemistry	Value
Na	135 mEq/L
K	3.5 mEq/L
Cl	101 mEq/L

CO_2	20 mEq/L
Glucose	98 mg/dL
BUN	20 mg/dL
SCr	0.4 mg/dL
Hematology	**Value**
WBC	22×10^3 cells/mm³
Hgb	13 g/dL
Hct	43%
Plt	320×10^3 cells/mm³
Segmented neutrophils	45%
Band neutrophils	22%
Lymphocytes	33%

Cerebrospinal fluid (CSF) analysis:

WBC	1550 cells/mm³
Neutrophils	65%
Glucose	15 mg/dL
Protein	165 mg/dL
RBC	2 cells/mm³

Blood culture: Pending

CSF culture: Pending

Imaging: Chest radiography within normal limits

1. What clinical signs and symptoms of meningitis are attributed to this patient? Is the patient likely to have bacterial or viral meningitis?

The patient presents with clinical manifestations consistent with meningitis: She has a fever, lethargy, poor appetite, and a recent ear infection, and her immunization status is incomplete. Based on the lumbar puncture, viral meningitis does not appear to be the primary cause of infection (Table 2). Laboratory findings are consistent with bacterial meningitis with elevated leukocytes greater than 1000 cells/mm^3, glucose ratio of 0.4 or less (patient's ratio is 0.15), and elevated protein greater than 100 mg/dL.

2. What is the pharmacologic agent(s) of choice for the initial empiric treatment of suspected meningitis in this patient?

Neisseria meningitides is the most common bacterial pathogen reported in patients between age 2 and 18 years. *Streptococcus pneumoniae* is the second leading cause of meningitis in this age group. Based on the lack of complete immunization status, *Haemophilus influenzae* is another pathogen of concern, although typically this pathogen affects infants age 1–23 months. Penicillin is the treatment of choice for *N. meningitides*; however, penicillin-resistant strains are increasing. A third-generation cephalosporin, either ceftriaxone or cefotaxime, should be used empirically until susceptibilities for *N. meningitides* are reported. With the increase of pneumococcal isolates resistant to third-generation cephalosporins, vancomycin should always be given with a third-generation cephalosporin for empiric treatment. The incidence of β-lactamase–positive *H. influenzae* is also increasing. To overcome this resistance and to reduce the risk of treatment failures, a third-generation cephalosporin is recommended for empiric treatment. Based on the predisposing factor age between 2 and 18 years and the most common pathogens of *N. meningitides and S. pneumoniae*, the recommended empiric therapy should be vancomycin plus a third-generation cephalosporin. Appropriate doses include vancomycin 225 mg (15 mg/kg) intravenously every 6 hours and ceftriaxone 750 mg (50 mg/kg) intravenously every 12 hours for 14 days. Because *S. agalactiae, E. coli, and L. monocytogenes* meningitis are unlikely in this patient, treatment duration beyond 14 days is not necessary.

Case (continued). The patient receives the empiric pharmacologic treatment indicated. The CSF culture and Gram stain returns on day two as gram-positive cocci in chains and shows *S. pneumoniae*, with no other pathogens noted. Antibiotic testing reveals susceptibility to all agents except penicillin.

3. Which regimen and duration is best to treat the patient's meningitis?

As described earlier in the chapter, *S. pneumoniae* is best treated by penicillin. This case is an example of the emergence of resistant pneumococcus increasing globally. Although pneumococcal isolates resistant to third-generation cephalosporins have become more common, the patient's susceptibility results showed no resistance of these agents against *S. pneumoniae*. Because *S. pneumoniae* was isolated, the antibiotic therapy selection is narrowed to a third-generation cephalosporin, such as ceftriaxone 750 mg (50 mg/kg) intravenously every 12 hours for a total of 10 to 14 days, with the discontinuation of vancomycin. Adjunctive dexamethasone treatment for pneumococcal meningitis may be considered to reduce mortality. Current Infectious Diseases Society of America guidelines state that dexamethasone therapy, 2.3 mg (0.15 mg/kg) intravenously every 6 hours for 2 to 4 days, should be considered in patients with pneumococcal meningitis and that the potential risks and benefits should be weighed before initiating treatment. Controversy on the use of dexamethasone for pneumococcal meningitis remains, and a clear benefit is not well established. Because the patient has already received 2 days of antibiotics, the addition of dexamethasone is unlikely to improve her outcome. Monitoring variables for ceftriaxone include hypersensitivity reactions, nausea, vomiting, diarrhea, and biliary sludging. Clinical signs of improvement to monitor include the patient's resolution of fever, improvement of feeding, and negative blood and CSF cultures.

REFERENCES

1. Kim KS. Acute bacterial meningitis in infants and children. Lancet Infect Dis 2010;10:32-42.
2. Saez-Llorens X, McCracken GH Jr. Bacterial meningitis in neonates and children. Infect Dis Clin North Am 1990;4:623-44.
3. Schuchat A, Robinson K, Wegner JD, et al. Bacterial meningitis in the United States in 1995. Active Surveillance Team. N Engl J Med 1997;337:970-6.
4. Centers for Disease Control and Prevention (CDC). Progress toward elimination of Haemophilus influenzae type b invasive disease among infants and children: United States, 1998-2000. MMWR Morb Mortal Wkly Rep 2002;5:234-7.
5. Nuorti JP, Whitney CG; Centers for Disease Control and Prevention (CDC). Prevention of pneumococcal disease among infants and children—use of 13-valent pneumococcal conjugate vaccine and 23-valent pneumococcal polysaccharide vaccine—recommendations of the Advisory Committee on Immunization Practices (ACIP). MMWR Recomm Rep 2010;59:1-18.
6. Klinger G, Chin CN, Beyene J, et al. Predicting the outcome of neonatal bacterial meningitis. Pediatrics 2000;106:477-82.
7. Grimwood K, Anderson VA, Bond L, et al. Adverse outcomes of bacterial meningitis in school-age survivors. Pediatrics 1995; 95:646-56.
8. Roine I, Peltola H, Fernandez J, et al. Influence of admission findings on death and neurological outcome from childhood meningitis. Clin Infect Dis 2008;46:1248-52.
9. Chang C, Chang W, Huang L, et al. Bacterial meningitis in infants: the epidemiology, clinical features, and prognostic factors. Brain Dev 2004;26:168-75.
10. Romero JR, Newland JG. Viral meningitis and encephalitis: traditional and emerging viral agents. Semin Pediatr Infect Dis 2003;14:72-82.
11. Tunkel AR, Hartman BJ, Kaplan SL, et al. Practice guidelines for the management of bacterial meningitis. Clin Infect Dis 2004; 39:1267-84.
12. Heath PT, Yusoff NKN, Baker CJ. Neonatal meningitis. Arch Dis Child Fetal Neonatal Ed 2003;88:F173-8.
13. Kinberlin DW. Meningitis in the neonate. Curr Treat Options Neurol 2002;4:239-48.
14. Lorber B. Listeriosis. Clin Infect Dis 1997;24:1-9.
15. Short WR, Tunkel AR. Changing epidemiology of bacterial meningitis in the United States. Curr Infect Dis Rep 2000;2:327-31.
16. Hsu HE, Shutt KA, Moore MR, et al. Effect of pneumococcal conjugate vaccine on pneumococcal meningitis. N Engl J Med 2009;360:244-56.
17. Brigham KS, Sandora TJ. Neisseria meningitidis: epidemiology, treatment, and prevention in adolescents. Curr Opin Pediatr 2009;21:437-43.
18. Centers for Disease Control and Prevention (CDC). Updated recommendations for the use of meningococcal conjugate vaccines—Advisory Committee on Immunization Practices (ACIP) 2010. MMWR Morb Mortal Wkly Rep 2011;60:72-6.
19. Centers for Disease Control and Prevention (CDC). Updated recommendations for use of MenB-FHbp Serogroup B meningococcal vaccine—Advisory Committee on Immunization Practices (ACIP) 2016. MMWR Morb Mortal Wkly Rep 2017;66:509-13.
20. Kumar R. Aseptic meningitis: diagnosis and management. Indian J Pediatr 2005;72:57-63.
21. Solomon T, Hart IJ, Beeching NJ. Viral encephalitis: a clinician's guide. Pract Neurol 2007;7:288-305.
22. Kristensson K. Microbes' roadmap to neurons. Nat Rev Neurosci 2011;12:345-57.
23. Weller RO, Sharp MM, Christodoulides M, et al. The meninges as barriers and facilitators for the movement of fluid, cells and pathogens related to the rodent and human CNS. Acta Neuropathol 2018;135:363-85.
24. Sarff LD, Platt LH, McCracken GH. Cerebrospinal fluid evaluation in neonates: comparison of high-risk infants with and without meningitis. J Pediatr 1976;88:473-7.
25. Biou D, Benoist JF, Nguyen-Thi C, et al. Cerebrospinal fluid protein concentrations in children: age-related values in patients without disorders of the central nervous system. Clin Chem 2000;46:399-403.
26. Elshaboury RH, Hermsen ED, Holt JS, et al. Chapter 84. Central nervous system infections. In: DiPiro JT, Talbert RL, Yee GC, et al., eds. *Pharmacotherapy: A Pathophysiologic Approach, 9e.* New York, NY: McGraw-Hill; 2014.
27. Gray LD, Fedorko DP. Laboratory diagnosis of bacterial meningitis. Clin Microbiol Rev 1992;5:130-45.
28. Janowski AB, Hunstad DA. Central nervous system infections. In: Kliegman RM, Behrman RE, Jenson HB, et al., eds. Nelson Textbook of Pediatrics, 21st ed. Philadelphia: Saunders Elsevier, 2019:3222-36.
29. Kim KS. Pathogenesis of bacterial meningitis: from bactaeremia to neuronal injury. Nat Rev Neurosci 2003;4:376-85.
30. Rubin LL, Staddon JM. The cell biology of the blood-brain barrier. Annu Rev Neurosci 1999;22:11-28.
31. Tunkel AR, Scheld WM. Pathogenesis and pathophysiology of bacterial meningitis. Clin Microbiol Rev 1993;6:118-36.
32. Stephens DS, McGee ZA. Attachment of Neisseria meningitidis to human mucosal surfaces: influence of pili and type of receptor cell. J Infect Dis 1981;143:525-32.
33. Smith AL. Pathogenesis of Haemophilus influenzae meningitis. Pediatr Infect Dis J 1987;6:783-6.
34. Ostrow PT, Moxon ER, Vernon N, et al. Pathogenesis of bacterial meningitis. Studies on the route of meningeal invasion following Haemophilus influenzae inoculation in infant rats. Lab Invest 1979;40:678-85.
35. Dietzman DE, Fischer GW, Schoenknecht FD. Neonatal Escherichia coli septicemia—bacterial counts in the blood. J Pediatr 1974;85:128-30.
36. Bell LM, Alpert G, Campos JM, et al. Routine quantitative blood cultures in children with Haemophilus influenzae or Streptococcus pneumoniae bacteremia. Pediatrics 1985;76:901-4.
37. Sullivan DT, LaScolea LJ, Neter E. Relationship between the magnitude of bacteremia in children and the clinical disease. Pediatrics 1982;69:699-702.
38. Williams AE, Blakemore WF. Pathogenesis of meningitis caused by Streptococcus suis type 2. J Infect Dis 1990;162:474-81.
39. Scheld WM. Bacterial meningitis in the patient at risk: intrinsic risk factors and host defense mechanisms. Am J Med 1984; 76:193-207.
40. Scheld WM, Dacey RG, Winn HR, et al. Cerebrospinal fluid outflow resistance in rabbits with experimental meningitis: alterations with penicillin and methylprednisolone. J Clin Invest 1980;66:243-53.
41. Tauber MG, Khayam-Bashi H, Sande MA. Effects of ampicillin and corticosteroids on brain water content, cerebrospinal fluid pressure, and cerebrospinal fluid lactate levels in experimental pneumococcal meningitis. J Infect Dis 1985;151:528-34.
42. Feigin RD, McCracken GH Jr, Klein JO. Diagnosis and management of meningitis. Pediatr Infect Dis J 1992;11:785-814.
43. Bedford H, deLouvois J, Halket S, et al. Meningitis in infancy in England and Wales: follow up at age 5 years. BMJ 2001;323:533-6.
44. Oliver LG, Harwood-Nuss AL. Bacterial meningitis in infants and children: a review. J Emerg Med 1993;11:555-64.
45. Chavez-Bueno S, McCracken GH. Bacterial meningitis in children. Pediatr Clin North Am 2005;52:795-810.
46. Odio C, McCracken GH, Nelson JD. CSF shunt infections in pediatrics. A seven-year experience. Am J Dis Child 1984; 138:1103-8.
47. Valmari P, Peltola H, Ruuskanen O, et al. Childhood bacterial meningitis: initial symptoms and signs related to age, and reasons for consulting a physician. Eur J Pediatr 1987;146:515-8.
48. El Bashir H, Laundy M, Booy R. Diagnosis and treatment of bacterial meningitis. Arch Dis Child 2003;88:615-20.

49. Verghese A, Gallemore G. Kernig's and Brudzinski's signs revisited. Rev Infect Dis 1987;9:1187-92.

50. Curtis S, Stobart K, Vandermeer B, et al. Clinical features suggestive of meningitis in children: a systematic review of prospective data. Pediatrics 2010;126:952-60.

51. Kaplan SL. Clinical presentation, diagnosis, and prognostic factors of bacterial meningitis. Infect Dis Clin North Am 1999;13:579-94.

52. van de Beek D, Brouwer MC, Tunkel AR. Advances in treatment of bacterial meningitis. Lancet 2012;380:1693-702.

53. La Scolea LJ Jr, Dryja D. Quantitation of bacteria in cerebrospinal fluid and blood of children with meningitis and its diagnostic significance. J Clin Microbiol 1984;19:187-90.

54. Kanegavye JT, Soliemanzadeh P, Bradley JS. Lumbar puncture in pediatric bacterial meningitis: defining the time interval for recovery of cerebrospinal fluid pathogens after parenteral antibiotic pretreatment. Pediatrics 2001;108:1169-74.

55. McCracken GH Jr, Sarff LD. Endotoxin in cerebrospinal fluid: detection in neonates with bacterial meningitis. JAMA 1976;235:617-20.

56. Ramers C, Billman G, Hartin M, et al. Impact of a diagnostic cerebrospinal fluid enterovirus polymerase chain reaction test on patient management. JAMA 2000;283:2680-5.

57. Saravolatz LD, Manzor O, VanderVelde N, et al. Broad-range bacterial polymerase chain reaction for early detection of bacterial meningitis. Clin Infect Dis 2003;36:40-5.

58. Abro AH, Abdou AS, Ustadi AM, et al. CSF lactate level: a useful diagnostic tool to differentiate acute bacterial and viral meningitis. J Pak Med Assoc 2009;59:508-11.

59. Sormunen P, Kallio MJ, Kilpi T, et al. C-reactive protein is useful in distinguishing Gram stain-negative bacterial meningitis from viral meningitis in children. J Pediatr 1999;134:725-9.

60. Alkholi UM, Abd Al-Monem N, Abd El-Azim AA, et al. Serum procalcitonin in viral and bacterial meningitis. J Glob Infect Dis 2011;3:14-8.

61. Spanos A, Harrell FE Jr, Durack DT. Differential diagnosis of acute meningitis: an analysis of the predictive value of initial observations. JAMA 1989;262:2700-7.

62. McKinney WP, Heudebert GR, Harper SA, et al. Validation of a clinical prediction rule for the differential diagnosis of acute meningitis. J Gen Intern Med 1994;9:8-12.

63. Glaser CA, Gilliam S, Schnurr D, et al. In search of encephalitis etiologies: diagnostic challenges in the California Encephalitis Project, 1998-2000. Clin Infect Dis 2003;36:731-42.

64. Kumar R. Aseptic meningitis: diagnosis and management. Indian J Pediatr 2005;72:57-63.

65. Lee BE, Davies HD. Aseptic meningitis. Curr Opin Infect Dis 2007;20:272-7.

66. Taketomo CK, Hodding JH, Kraus DM. Pediatric & Neonatal Dosage Handbook, 26th ed. Hudson, OH: Lexi-Comp, 2019.

67. Bradley JS, Jackson MA; Committee on Infectious Diseases, American Academy of Pediatrics. The use of systemic fluoroquinolones. Pediatrics 2011;128:e1034-45.

68. American Academy of Pediatrics. Group B streptococcal infections. In: Pickering LK, ed. Red Book: 2018 Report of the Committee on Infectious Diseases, 31st ed. Elk Grove Village, IL: American Academy of Pediatrics, 2018:762-8.

69. Schaad UB, Suter S, Gianella-Borradori A, et al. A comparison of ceftriaxone and cefuroxime for the treatment of bacterial meningitis in children. N Engl J Med 1990;322:141-7.

70. Edmiston CE, Gordon RC. Evaluation of gentamicin and penicillin as a synergistic combination in experimental murine listeriosis. Antimicrob Agents Chemother 1979;16:862-3.

71. Klugman KP, Madhi SA. Emergence of drug resistance: impact on bacterial meningitis. Infect Dis Clin North Am 1999;13:637-46.

72. Whitney CG, Farley MM, Hadler J, et al. Increasing prevalence of multidrug-resistant Streptococcus pneumoniae in the United States. N Engl J Med 2000;343:1917-24.

73. Viladrich PF, Pallares R, Ariza J, et al. Four days of penicillin therapy for meningococcal meningitis. Arch Intern Med 1986; 146:2380-2.

74. American Academy of Pediatrics. Herpes simplex. In: Pickering LK, ed. Red Book: 2015 Report of the Committee on Infectious Diseases, 30th ed. Elk Grove Village, IL: American Academy of Pediatrics, 2015:432-44.

75. Brouwer MC, McIntyre P, Prasad K, et al. Corticosteroids for acute bacterial meningitis. Cochrane Database Syst Rev 2015; 9:CD004405.

76. Mongelluzzo J, Mohamad Z, Ten Have TR, et al. Corticosteroids and mortality in children with bacterial meningitis. JAMA 2008; 299:2048-55.

77. American Academy of Pediatrics. Pneumococcal infections. In: Pickering LK, ed. Red Book: 2015 Report of the Committee on Infectious Diseases, 30th ed. Elk Grove Village, IL: American Academy of Pediatrics, 2015:626-37.

78. Kaplan SL. Management of pneumococcal meningitis. Pediatr Infect Dis J 2002;21:589-91.

79. American Academy of Pediatrics. Haemophilus influenzae infections. In: Pickering LK, ed. Red Book: 2015 Report of the Committee on Infectious Diseases, 30th ed. Elk Grove Village, IL: American Academy of Pediatrics, 2015:368-75.

80. American Academy of Pediatrics. Meningococcal infections. In: Pickering LK, ed. Red Book: 2015 Report of the Committee on Infectious Diseases, 30th ed. Elk Grove Village, IL: American Academy of Pediatrics, 2015:547-57.

81. Saez-Llorens X, McCracken GH Jr. Bacterial meningitis in children. Lancet 2003;361:2139-48.

CHAPTER 38

Acute Otitis Media and Upper Respiratory Tract Infections

Jennifer Le, Pharm.D., MAS, FCCP, FIDSA, FCSHP, BCPS-AQ ID

LEARNING OBJECTIVES

1. Compare and contrast the etiologic pathogens causing acute otitis media (AOM) and upper respiratory tract infections (URTIs), including rhinosinusitis and pharyngitis.

2. Identify and assess the risk factors associated with, and the need for treatment of, AOM or URTIs in a case study.

3. Develop scenarios for which a cephalosporin would or would not be recommended in a child with a penicillin allergy.

4. Formulate a therapeutic plan for a case study of a patient with an AOM or URTI, including rhinosinusitis and pharyngitis.

5. To ensure antimicrobial stewardship in the outpatient setting, counsel parents and caregivers on judicious antibiotic use for AOM and URTIs, on appropriate use of adjunctive medications for symptomatic relief (including antipyretics, decongestants, and antihistamine) by pediatric age groups, and on prevention through immunization.

ABBREVIATIONS IN THIS CHAPTER

ABRS	Acute bacterial rhinosinusitis
AOM	Acute otitis media
GAS	Group A β-hemolytic *Streptococcus*
OM	Otitis media
RADT	Rapid antigen detection test
URTI	Upper respiratory tract infection

INTRODUCTION

Acute otitis media (AOM) and upper respiratory tract infections (URTIs), including rhinosinusitis and pharyngitis, are common infections affecting different pediatric groups.[1] Whereas AOM and rhinosinusitis peak in infants and young children, pharyngitis is more common in children older than 5 years. *Both viruses and bacteria may cause these infections; therefore,* antibiotic therapy should be carefully selected for those with true infection of bacterial origin or those at risk of serious complications. The most common bacterial etiologies for AOM and rhinosinusitis are *Streptococcus pneumoniae, Haemophilus influenzae,* and *Moraxella catarrhalis. Streptococcus pyogenes* (also known as group A β-hemolytic *Streptococcus,* or GAS) is the most common bacterial cause of pharyngitis. Some infections may be self-limiting and resolve

without treatment. Watchful waiting to delay or minimize the use of antibiotics is a prudent strategy for these infections, particularly AOM, without adversely influencing the clinical course. However, because pharyngitis caused by GAS can progress to potentially fatal complications (e.g., toxic shock syndrome), antibiotic treatment should ensue after a confirmed diagnosis.

ACUTE OTITIS MEDIA

Acute otitis media is an infection of the middle ear characterized by middle ear effusion, inflammation, and acute onset of symptoms. It is the most common diagnosis leading to antibiotic prescription in children.[2,3] However, antibiotic prescriptions and clinic visits for otitis media (OM) decreased in 2005–2006 compared with 1995–1996.[4] Because the incidence of AOM peaks in infants and young children age 6 months to 2 years, 80%–90% of children will have at least one episode by age 2–3 years.[5-8] Complications of AOM may occur and include the following: temporary hearing impairment that may delay speech, language, and cognitive abilities; perforation of the tympanic membrane; and intracranial suppurative complications such as meningitis and brain abscess.[9] Temporary hearing loss, caused by fluid in the middle ear, is the most common complication. In contrast, intracranial complications seldom occur.

Immature immune systems and function of the eustachian tube predispose young children to AOM. In particular, the angle of the opening of the eustachian tube is decreased in young children, which allows nasopharyngeal bacteria to ascend to the middle ear cavity and prevents adequate drainage of middle ear fluid, both resulting in infection. The anatomic features of the eustachian tubes, together with other risk factors, are associated with the development of OM (Box 1).[5,8,10] Around 37% of children with recent viral URTIs, particularly caused by rhinovirus and adenovirus, will subsequently develop AOM, showing that a viral URTI is an important risk factor for AOM.[7] In addition, exposure to tobacco smoke, allergies to food or airborne particles, and attendance in day care should be evaluated in every child with AOM. If modifiable, exposure to these risk factors should be minimized.

Although viruses, including respiratory syncytial virus, rhinoviruses, influenza, and adenoviruses, cause AOM, the most common etiologies in the United States are bacterial in up to 56% of cases and include *S. pneumoniae,* nontypeable *H. influenzae,* and *M. catarrhalis.*[4,11] The advent of pneumococcal vaccinations has resulted in the decline of OM cases in children younger than 3 years and in the alteration in the distribution of these bacteria, particularly a decrease in *S. pneumoniae* and a potential increase in nontypeable *H. influenzae* and *M. catarrhalis.*[8,12,13] Bacteria that rarely cause AOM are atypical pathogens, GAS, and gram-negative

---

organisms, including *Pseudomonas aeruginosa*.[4,10] Mixed infections caused by both bacterial and viral respiratory tract pathogens can occur in up to two-thirds of cases.[14]

Universal immunization in 2000 with the 7-valent pneumococcal conjugate vaccine, which covered 60%–70% of the pneumococcal serotypes isolated in AOM, has contributed to the changing epidemiology of bacterial AOM. Certain *S. pneumoniae* serotypes not contained in this vaccine, like serotypes 6C and 19A, became more prevalent in the United States and worldwide.[15-20] As a result, the 13-valent pneumococcal vaccine was introduced in the United States in 2010 to provide coverage against all the serotypes available in the 7-valent vaccine, with additional coverage against 19A and potentially 6C through cross-protection.[15] In addition to a decline in penicillin nonsusceptibility since the use of this 13-valent vaccine, decreased rates of 19A serotypes, visits related to OM, recurrent OM, mastoiditis, and ventilating tube insertion have occurred.[21,22] The 13-valent pneumococcal vaccine, together with vaccines for *M. catarrhalis* that are under development, will continue to change the microbiology of AOM.[23] In addition, nontypeable *H. influenzae* strains have now become the predominant pathogen and will contribute to the changing microbiology of AOM.[16,17] Furthermore, *H. influenzae* has been associated with severe tympanic membrane inflammation.[11]

Although some studies found that *S. pneumoniae* causes more severe AOM, others refute this finding by associating *H. influenzae* with bilateral disease and increased severity of inflammation.[3] Conflicting studies show that the causative pathogen cannot be predicted by clinical presentation alone, and culture data are necessary only if the pathogen must be identified. However, AOM associated with conjunctivitis is likely caused by nontypeable *H. influenzae*.[3]

Antimicrobial resistance among the common bacterial respiratory tract pathogens has continued to evolve over the past decades. In the 1960s, *S. pneumoniae*, *H. influenzae*,

and *M. catarrhalis* were susceptible to penicillin. Today, all of these bacteria have developed resistance to penicillin at varying degrees over time since the introduction of routine childhood immunization. Alteration of the penicillin-binding proteins, a resistance mechanism acquired by pneumococci, renders the organism resistant to penicillins, cephalosporins, and other β-lactam antibiotics. In the United States, the prevalence of penicillin-nonsusceptible (including resistant and intermediately susceptible) strains of *S. pneumoniae* was 10% in 2011–2012.[24] The introduction of the 13-valent pneumococcal vaccine has been correlated with a decrease in penicillin nonsusceptibility (i.e., minimum inhibitory concentration of greater than 2 mcg/mL), especially among the 19A serotype in children with OM or mastoiditis.[25-27] Even in the presence of resistance, high-dose amoxicillin at 80–90 mg/kg/day achieves elevated drug concentrations in the middle ear to consequently provide activity against intermediately susceptible and many resistant *S. pneumoniae*.[4,28] Because oral agents are most commonly used for the treatment of AOM, the susceptibility of oral penicillins should be evaluated by local surveillance to show their clinical usefulness.

Streptococcus pneumoniae has developed resistance beyond just penicillin. Termed *drug-resistant S. pneumoniae*, resistance or reduced susceptibility has developed to other antibiotics, namely trimethoprim/sulfamethoxazole, macrolides (including clarithromycin and azithromycin), tetracyclines, and clindamycin.[29-31] Cross-resistance between erythromycin and clindamycin, which is mediated by the *erm*B ribosomal methylation mechanism (MLS$_B$ phenotype) that inhibits binding of the antibiotic to the target site, occurred in 32% of *S. pneumoniae* isolates in the United States.[29,32] Resistance to fluoroquinolones has emerged (partly because of their extensive use for community-acquired respiratory tract infections in adults), but the incidence remains extremely low.[24,33] Since the introduction of the 13-valent pneumococcal vaccine, resistance to penicillin, erythromycin, and clindamycin, particularly among the 19A serotype, has declined in children with OM or mastoiditis.[27]

CLINICAL PRESENTATION AND DIAGNOSIS

Middle ear effusion and acute onset of symptoms—including fever, rhinorrhea, irritability, otalgia (or ear pain), tugging or rubbing of the ear, and other nonspecific symptoms—are the presenting attributes of AOM. In contrast to AOM, *OM with effusion* refers to uninfected middle ear effusion (i.e., fluid in the middle ear cavity) without acute onset of symptoms, and it can precede or follow AOM.

On otoscopic examination for AOM, the tympanic membrane typically appears erythematous, cloudy, white, or pale yellow. Middle ear effusion is evident by changes in the tympanic membrane, including bulging or fullness into the external auditory canal, impaired or absent mobility, and otorrhea.[4,34] A bulging tympanic membrane is most characteristic of acute inflammation and therefore AOM.[34] Acute perforation with purulent otorrhea is diagnostic for AOM once otitis externa has been excluded.

The diagnosis of AOM is primarily based on clinical presentation with otoscopic examination. Diagnosis should

---

Box 1. Risk Factors Associated with Otitis Media

Young age, especially < 2 yr
Day care attendance
Recent viral upper respiratory illness
Nasopharyngeal colonization with middle ear bacterial pathogens
Tobacco smoke exposure
Bottle-feeding
Pacifier use
Sick sibling(s) in household
Native American, Eskimo, and Australian ethnicities
Non-Hispanic white race
Allergies to foods or airborne particles
Familial predisposition or family history of acute otitis media
Immunodeficiency
Cleft palate or other craniofacial abnormalities
Male sex
Low socioeconomic status

---

follow the stringent criteria outlined in the 2013 American Academy of Pediatrics guideline to ensure diagnostic accuracy and judicious antibiotic use.[4] Two significant challenges in diagnosing AOM are establishing the presence of middle ear effusion and distinguishing it from OM with effusion.[4] Consequently, some uncertainty exists when diagnosing AOM centered on clinical signs and symptoms. To determine the actual etiology, aspiration of the middle ear fluid (also called *tympanocentesis*) for culture can be performed. However, this approach is reserved for special cases, including children who appear toxic or are unresponsive to several courses of empiric antibiotic therapy.

TREATMENT

Therapeutic goals for AOM include alleviating symptoms (excluding middle ear effusion), preventing recurrence, using antibiotics judiciously, ensuring patient adherence, and preventing adverse drug reactions. In many cases, particularly in those infected with *H. influenzae* or *M. catarrhalis*, the presenting symptoms of AOM usually resolve within 2–3 days after onset. Even in the case of inappropriate therapy, 75% of children with specifically *M. catarrhalis* infection had bacteriologic resolution.[4] Although most symptoms resolve without antibiotic therapy, middle ear effusion can persist for weeks to months in up to 70% of children.[35] Middle ear effusion has been associated with temporary hearing loss; however, clinicians must be aware that prolonged middle ear effusion alone is not AOM and does not require the use of antibiotics. Furthermore, immediate antimicrobial treatment of AOM does not significantly affect the resolution of middle ear effusions.[14] If antibiotics are used, medication nonadherence likely because of poor taste is an issue that should be considered when treating a pediatric patient. Several methods are suggested to improve adherence to prescribed therapies (Box 2).[36]

NONPHARMACOLOGIC THERAPY

Mild cases are self-limiting. Even when left untreated, clinical symptoms improve in the first 24 hours and with no major adverse sequelae in most of these cases.[4] Most cases of AOM spontaneously resolved in patients living in high-income countries.[37] As such, initial observation, with proper pain control, has been widely accepted by the medical community to promote judicious antibiotic use.[38] Initial observation allows a delay in antibiotic therapy, if even necessary, for up to 48–72 hours in some children with AOM.[4] The American Academy of Pediatrics endorses initial observation based on the child's age and severity of illness. Initial observation is warranted in those 6 months to 2 years presenting with unilateral AOM and mild symptoms.[4,39] Appropriate follow-up mechanisms should be in place to monitor children, especially in those 6 months to 2 years who experience a high rate of treatment failures, if initial observation is used.[4,39]

A primary concern with initial observation in AOM is its effect on the clinical course of infection. Mild infections in most children resolve spontaneously without the need for antibiotic therapy. However, children with AOM who do not improve must subsequently receive antibiotic treatment, with a potential delay of up to 3 days. Compared with those receiving immediate therapy, children with nonsevere AOM who received delayed antibiotic therapy had more pain initially and took longer to recover from symptoms.[40,41] However, these symptoms resolved, regardless of antibiotic use, within 7–10 days. As such, in children with symptomatic improvement during initial observation, a routine, in-person, follow-up visit may not be necessary; a telephone call to parents or caregivers may be sufficient.[42]

Although symptomatic control may be achieved faster than with delayed therapy, immediate antibiotic treatment resulted in more drug-related adverse events and nasopharyngeal carriage of multidrug-resistant *S. pneumoniae* on day 12.[41] In fact, one child in every 14 children treated with antibiotics experienced drug-related adverse effects, including vomiting, diarrhea, or rash.[37] Clinic and emergency department visits, days of missed work or school, and parent satisfaction were unaffected by delayed antibiotic therapy.[40,41] Furthermore, delayed therapy was not associated with an increase in mastoiditis in children older than 2 years.[43] Notably, a meta-analysis showed no difference in complication rates and patient satisfaction when antibiotic therapy was delayed for the treatment of respiratory infections, with reduction in antibiotic use (from 93% to 31%).[44] In children with severe AOM admitted to the emergency department, reduced antibiotic prescribing for AOM because of the initial observation strategy was not associated with any adverse outcomes.[45]

PHARMACOLOGIC THERAPY

Antibiotic treatment should be initiated immediately in children with severe disease, manifesting as the following: toxic appearance, bulging tympanic membrane with apparent pus, perforated tympanic membrane, severe otalgia, bilateral infection, or temperature of 102.2°F (39°C) or higher. In addition, a child younger than 6 months is usually at increased risk of a more serious infection and therefore should always be initiated on antibiotic therapy, even if the diagnosis is uncertain.[4] Most clinical symptoms, except for middle ear effusion, usually resolve within 48–72 hours after antibiotic initiation. Of note, persistent middle ear effusion does not indicate treatment failure.

Antibiotic therapy is generally empiric and usually involves the use of oral agents. High-dose amoxicillin, defined as 80–90 mg/kg/day, is the first-line treatment for children without recent exposure to a β-lactam antibiotic, concomitant purulent conjunctivitis, and history of recurrent AOM.[46] The response rate in studies has been greater than 80% (Table 1).[4,47] In children younger than 2 years, amoxicillin was the most cost-effective immediate treatment.[48] High-dose amoxicillin achieves elevated drug concentrations in the middle ear to consequently provide activity against intermediately susceptible and many resistant *S. pneumoniae*. However, with evidence supporting reduced resistance to penicillin, the use of high-dose amoxicillin versus the standard dose warrants further investigation.[13] The most common adverse effects are gastrointestinal, including nausea and diarrhea. The incidence of adverse effects associated with high-dose amoxicillin is similar to that with standard-dose amoxicillin.[49]

Adding clavulanic acid 6.4 mg/kg/day to high-dose amoxicillin or changing to ceftriaxone (intramuscular injection), cefuroxime, or cefpodoxime can be considered if the patient does not respond to high-dose amoxicillin.[4,13,50] Appropriate candidates for these broad-spectrum antibiotics include children with antibiotic exposure within the previous 30 days or children in whom *H. influenzae* or *M. catarrhalis* infection (i.e., AOM with accompanying conjunctivitis) is suspected. Despite the addition of clavulanic acid, or substitution with a cephalosporin—enhancing the activity against β-lactamase–producing *H. influenzae* and *M. catarrhalis*—patients infected by *H. influenzae* may respond to high-dose amoxicillin, and those with *M. catarrhalis* may self-resolve without the need for antibiotic therapy. Further studies are needed to elucidate the use of these broader-spectrum antibiotics versus amoxicillin as first-line therapy.[51] The ratio of amoxicillin to clavulanate that maximizes the amoxicillin dose is 14:1, administered in two divided doses.[4,52] However, this ratio has been associated with significant diarrhea caused by the increased amoxicillin component, despite the reduction in clavulanate.[53] Oral cephalosporins, including cefdinir (more palatable than the other two cephalosporins listed), cefuroxime axetil, and cefpodoxime, are other treatment options, but these agents are not as effective as high-dose amoxicillin against pneumococcus.[4]

The standard duration of antibiotic therapy is 10 days, particularly for children who are younger than 2 years, have perforated tympanic membranes, or have recurrent AOM.[39,54] However, a shorter course of 5–7 days is an option for children with mild disease, particularly those 6 years and older or who have had tympanocentesis.[4,50,55] The only exceptions are ceftriaxone for 1–3 days and azithromycin for 3–5 days, depending on the severity of disease and persistence of symptoms.[56] One day of ceftriaxone is a reasonable option for patients who are vomiting or unable to tolerate oral medications; however, multiple daily doses may be necessary to prevent recurrence.[4]

Box 2. Medication Adherence and Counseling Tips

Tips to improve adherence to oral medications in children
- Use flavoring services offered by pharmacies or mix with small amounts of juice or milk to improve palatability; consider chocolate or strawberry flavoring for cefuroxime, cefpodoxime, and clindamycin suspensions
- Use oral syringes to easily extract the medication dose by quickly pushing in the plunger so that the liquid squirts on the inner cheek; blowing on the child's face can facilitate swallowing
- Use oral suspensions for a child age < 2 yr; some children age 2 years may tolerate chewable tablets, but most children will be unable to swallow tablets or capsules until age 8 years
- Acetaminophen suppositories should be considered for an uncooperative child

Important counseling points for parents and caregivers
- Antibiotics do NOT cure viral infections (like the cold or flu), nor do they relieve fever or pain
- Mild cases of acute otitis media will resolve without antibiotic use
- Observation for 48–72 hr is an acceptable alternative to antibiotic treatment in older children with mild symptoms of acute otitis media; however, if the child does not improve within 48–72 hr, then follow-up with the pediatrician is needed
- When an antibiotic is prescribed, provide dosing instructions and emphasize the importance of completing the full course of antibiotic to successfully treat the infection and prevent the development of antibiotic resistance; also provide instruction on the common adverse effects of the prescribed antibiotic (as noted in Table 1)
- Ensure that the duration of antibiotic therapy is 10 days for a child age < 2 yr
- Relieve anxiety about a febrile child by explaining that fever is a natural body response to infection and that it will not harm the child
- When recommending acetaminophen or ibuprofen for fever or ear pain, provide clear instructions on the following points:
  - Use weight-based dosing to enhance the effective and safe use of these drugs
  - Ensure that parents understand how much to give, expressed in both milligrams and milliliters, to prevent accidental overdose; also note that infant formulations are more concentrated and thus require less volume per dose
  - Optimize the dose for fever control: ibuprofen 10 mg/kg is about equal to acetaminophen 15 mg/kg; acetaminophen can be administered as often as every 4 hr (not to exceed five doses in 24 hr) and ibuprofen as often as every 6 hr[36]
  - Discourage methods of alternating acetaminophen and ibuprofen unless clear verbal and written instructions are provided
- Encourage routine childhood vaccinations using the schedule recommended by the Centers for Disease Control and Prevention
  - Be prepared to recommend local clinics and pharmacies that provide immunizations
  - Identify and recommend the annual flu vaccine for all people at high risk of complications from influenza infection

Resources for additional information
- Recommended "Be Antibiotics Aware" on the Centers for Disease Control and Prevention website (www.cdc.gov/getsmart/)
- Check the official website of the American Academy of Pediatrics (www.healthychildren.org)

Table 1. Common Causative Bacterial Pathogens and Antibiotic Treatment Options for Upper Respiratory Tract Infections in Children[a]

Pathogens and Therapy	Dose	Common Adverse Effects
Acute Otitis Media		
Streptococcus pneumoniae, *Haemophilus influenzae*, and *Moraxella catarrhalis*		
Recommended	High-dose amoxicillin 80–90 mg/kg/day divided in 2 doses[b]	Diarrhea and allergic reactions, including Stevens-Johnson syndrome
Alternative	High-dose amoxicillin 80–90 mg/kg/day with clavulanate 6.4 mg/kg/day divided in 2 doses[b]	Diarrhea and allergic reactions, including Stevens-Johnson syndrome
	Ceftriaxone 50 mg/kg/day IM once daily for 1–3 days —OR— PO cephalosporins[c]	Injection-site pain, allergic reactions, diarrhea, gallbladder sludging
	Azithromycin 10 mg/kg/day once daily for 3 days (max 500 mg/day) —OR— 15 mg/kg on day 1 (max 500 mg), followed by 5 mg/kg/day as a single dose for 4 days (max 250 mg/day) —OR— 30 mg/kg as one dose on single day (max 1500 mg)[d]	Diarrhea, abdominal pain, nausea, vomiting
	Clarithromycin 15 mg/kg/day divided in 2 doses (max 1000 mg/day)[d,e]	Diarrhea, abdominal pain, nausea, vomiting, drug interactions
	Clindamycin 30–40 mg/kg/day divided in 3 doses (max 1.8 g/day)[d,f]	Diarrhea, pseudomembranous colitis
	Erythromycin/sulfisoxazole 50 mg/kg/day of erythromycin divided in 3–4 doses (max 2 g/day erythromycin or 6 g/day sulfisoxazole)	Check local susceptibility pattern; often rejected by patients because of taste and frequency of dosing
	Levofloxacin, by patient age: 6 mo–5 yr: 20 mg/kg/day divided in 2 doses > 5 yr: 10 mg/kg/day once daily (max 500 mg/day)[g]	Musculoskeletal disorders: arthralgia, arthritis, tendinopathy, and gait abnormality Vomiting, diarrhea
Acute Bacterial Rhinosinusitis		
S. pneumoniae, *H. influenzae*, and *M. catarrhalis* (less common anaerobic bacteria, *Streptococcus* spp., and *Staphylococcus aureus*)		
Recommended	Amoxicillin 45 mg/kg/day with or without clavulanate, divided in 2 doses[b,h] (max 1.75 g/day)	Diarrhea and allergic reactions, including Stevens-Johnson syndrome
Alternative	Amoxicillin/clavulanate 80–90 mg/kg/day with 6.4 mg/kg/day of clavulanate, divided in 2 doses[b,h] (max 4 g/day of amoxicillin)	Diarrhea and allergic reactions, including Stevens-Johnson syndrome
	Ampicillin/sulbactam 200–400 mg/kg/day IV divided every 6 hr	Rash, diarrhea
	Ceftriaxone 50–75 mg/kg/day IV or IM once or BID[i]	Injection-site pain, allergic reactions, diarrhea, gallbladder sludging
	Cefotaxime 100–200 mg/kg/day IV or IM divided every 6–8 hr[i]	Rash, diarrhea
	Clindamycin 30–40 mg/kg/day in 3 divided doses <u>plus</u> cefixime 8 mg/kg/day in 2 divided doses —OR— Cefpodoxime 10 mg/kg/day in 2 divided doses[f]	Diarrhea and pseudomembranous colitis (clindamycin); rash and diarrhea (cephalosporins)
	Levofloxacin 10–20 mg/kg/day every 12–24 hr[d] IV route recommended for hospitalized patients	Tendinopathy, arthritis, arthralgia of weight-bearing joints
Acute Pharyngitis		
Group A β-hemolytic *Streptococcus* [j]		
Recommended	PO penicillin V (phenoxymethylpenicillin), by patient weight: ≤ 27 kg: 250 mg (400,000 units) BID or TID for 10 days > 27 kg: 250 mg (400,000 units) QID or 500 mg (800,000 units) 2 times/day	Allergic reactions, including anaphylaxis; injection-site pain (if applicable); serum sickness–like reactions; diarrhea
	Amoxicillin 50 mg/kg/day PO as single dose or in 2 divided doses (max 1000 mg) Age ≥ 12 yr: 775-mg ER tablet once daily with meals; 875 mg BID, or 500 mg TID	Diarrhea and allergic reactions, including Stevens-Johnson syndrome
	Ampicillin 50–100 mg/kg/day in 3–4 divided doses	Diarrhea and allergic reactions, including Stevens-Johnson syndrome

(continued)

Table 1. Common Causative Bacterial Pathogens and Antibiotic Treatment Options for Upper Respiratory Tract Infections in Children[a] *(Continued)*

Pathogens and Therapy	Dose	Common Adverse Effects
Acute Pharyngitis		
Group A β-hemolytic *Streptococcus* [j]		
Alternative	Intramuscular benzathine penicillin[k] ≤ 27 kg: 600,000 units as a single dose > 27 kg: 1,200,000 units as a single dose	Allergic reactions, including anaphylaxis; injection-site pain (if applicable); serum sickness–like reactions; diarrhea
	Cephalexin 40 mg/kg/day in 2 divided doses (max 1,000 mg/day)[l]	Rash, diarrhea
	Cefadroxil 30 mg/kg once daily (max 1,000 mg)[l]	Rash, diarrhea
	Azithromycin 12 mg/kg once daily for 5 days (max 500 mg/day)[d,m]	Diarrhea, abdominal pain, nausea, vomiting
	Clindamycin 20 mg/kg/day in 3 divided doses (max 900 mg/day)[d,f]	Diarrhea, pseudomembranous colitis

[a] All antibiotic dosing regimens are based on normal renal and hepatic functions. All antibiotics are available in oral formulations except for ceftriaxone, cefotaxime, and penicillin G benzathine.

[b] To minimize diarrhea, the maximum recommended daily dose of amoxicillin is 3–4 g, and twice-daily administration is preferred for high-dose amoxicillin with clavulanic acid. High-dose amoxicillin with clavulanic acid may be considered in children with antibiotic exposure within the previous 30 days or who have acute otitis media with accompanying conjunctivitis.

[c] Ceftriaxone may be useful for nonadherent patients, with duration from 1–3 days. Ceftriaxone provides sufficient antibiotic concentrations in the middle ear for activity against penicillin-nonsusceptible *S. pneumoniae*. Oral cephalosporins, including cefuroxime axetil 30 mg/kg/day, cefdinir 14 mg/kg/day, and cefpodoxime 10 mg/kg/day, can alternatively be used, but these agents may not achieve adequate concentrations.

[d] Safe alternatives for severe or type I hypersensitivity reactions to penicillin or cephalosporins.

[e] Together with reduced activity against *H. influenzae* among macrolides, resistance limits their clinical utility. Clarithromycin has many significant drug interactions.

[f] Although clindamycin is active against drug-resistant *S. pneumoniae*, 22%–31% of strains are resistant.[24,35]

[g] Because levofloxacin is not approved for acute otitis media, it should be reserved for persistently recurrent otitis media.

[h] High-dose amoxicillin with clavulanate should be reserved for children with antibiotic exposure within the past 30–90 days, recent hospitalization, severe symptoms, age < 2 yr, day care attendance, or residing in regions with penicillin-nonsusceptible *S. pneumoniae* ≥ 10%.

[i] For children with vomiting that precludes the use of oral antibiotics. Conversion to an oral antibiotic should be instituted within 24 hr or on resolution of vomiting (whichever is earlier).

[j] Although viruses and other bacteria may cause acute pharyngitis, antimicrobial treatment is indicated for group A β-hemolytic *Streptococcus* (GAS). To successfully eradiate GAS, oral antibiotics should be administered for 10 days (unless otherwise indicated).

[k] Indicated for those who cannot complete or tolerate a 10-day course of oral therapy, or those at increased risk of acute rheumatic fever. The formulation of benzathine penicillin G 900,000 units (562.5 mg) with procaine penicillin G 300,000 units (187.5 mg) is recommended for children who weigh ≤ 27 kg. Efficacy of this combination for adolescents weighing > 27 kg and adults has not been shown. Sites for intramuscular administration are the mid-lateral aspect of the thigh for infants and small children and the upper, outer quadrant of the buttock for adolescents and adults.

[l] Other oral cephalosporins are acceptable alternatives, including cefprozil, cefaclor, cefuroxime, cefdinir, cefpodoxime, cefixime, and ceftibuten. Therapy duration is 5 days for cefpodoxime and cefdinir and 10 days for all other cephalosporins.

[m] Use should be based on local resistance patterns. Erythromycin or clarithromycin for 10 days is an alternative. However, erythromycin is associated with a high incidence of gastrointestinal adverse effects.

BID = twice daily; ER = extended-release; IM = intramuscularly; IV = intravenously; max = maximum; PO = oral; QID = four times daily; TID = three times daily.

PENICILLIN ALLERGY

Use of β-lactam antibiotics may present a dilemma in a child with penicillin or cephalosporin allergy. The risk of cross-reactivity to cephalosporins is increased in children with a history of penicillin allergy and between different cephalosporins, particularly those with similar side chains.[57,58] A prospective study of children reported a 30% cross-reactivity to cephalosporins among those with penicillin allergy.[57] However, based on a review of seven studies, the cross-reactivity to cephalosporins in patients with positive penicillin skin tests was 4.4%.[59] Cross-sensitivity appears significant with primarily first- (vs. second- or third-) generation cephalosporins.[58] These data suggest that most children with a history of mild reactions to penicillin will tolerate cephalosporins.

Although most children with a mild penicillin allergy will tolerate cephalosporins, the safety of administering cephalosporins still requires systematic assessment. Assessing the timing (including first-dose response) and nature of the penicillin allergy to determine the presence of potentially life-threatening reactions (including type I, immunoglobulin

E-mediated hypersensitivity) is critical in making the clinical decision of whether to expose a child to a cephalosporin.[60] If a child has a non–life-threatening or mild reaction to penicillin (including morbilliform rashes, commonly reported with amoxicillin), a cephalosporin (e.g., cefdinir, cefpodoxime, cefuroxime, or ceftriaxone) may be considered because serious reactions to cephalosporins are rare.[4,61] In contrast, if the child develops an immunoglobulin E-mediated hypersensitivity reaction (i.e., anaphylaxis), which is considered life threatening, then both amoxicillin and cephalosporins should be avoided.

In evaluating an antibiotic allergy, obtaining an accurate medical history is essential to distinguish true hypersensitivity reactions from other, less severe adverse reactions.[60] A non–β-lactam antibiotic should be used in children with severe immunoglobulin E-mediated hypersensitivity reactions or in cases in which the type of reaction or history of penicillin allergy is uncertain. Treatment options include macrolides (specifically azithromycin and clarithromycin) and clindamycin. Clarithromycin and azithromycin have activity against *M. catarrhalis* and atypical respiratory pathogens. A study showed similar effectiveness, but with fewer adverse effects and improved adherence, between a single 60-mg/kg dose of azithromycin extended-release suspension (although not recommended by current guidelines) and a 10-day course of high-dose amoxicillin with clavulanate in children with AOM.[4,62] However, the macrolides have limited efficacy against *S. pneumoniae* and *H. influenzae*.[4,62]

Although not a β-lactam, these antibiotics are hindered in usefulness by the high prevalence of resistance to trimethoprim/sulfamethoxazole and erythromycin by drug-resistant *S. pneumoniae*.[28] At least 80% of drug-resistant *S. pneumoniae* are resistant to trimethoprim/sulfamethoxazole and 50% to erythromycin.[63] In addition, trimethoprim/sulfamethoxazole has limited activity against GAS, which can cause AOM associated with perforation of tympanic membranes. Pediazole (Abbott Nutrition, Columbus, OH), which contains erythromycin and sulfisoxazole, may be considered in geographic regions with a low prevalence of drug-resistant *S. pneumoniae* and may be a safe alternative in children with a history of hypersensitivity reactions to penicillin. Nonetheless, these agents are not recommended in children for whom high-dose amoxicillin therapy has failed.

In addition, the risk of cartilage toxicity and concern for resistance associated with fluoroquinolones (particularly levofloxacin) limit their usefulness in children with AOM. However, levofloxacin may play a role in children with persistent and recurrent AOM, although it is not an approved indication. Tympanocentesis should be performed first to determine the causal pathogen; subsequently, tympanostomy tube placement or therapy with levofloxacin, especially for susceptible isolates, can be considered.[64]

ADJUNCTIVE THERAPY

A child with AOM may present with fever; therefore, the parents should be instructed on the appropriate use of antipyretic medications (Box 2). A *fever* is defined as an elevation in body temperature exceeding 100°F (37.8°C) by mouth (100.4°F [38°C] rectally) and is mediated by an increase in the hypothalamic heat regulatory set point regulated by prostaglandins. Acetaminophen 10–15 mg/kg given every 4–6 hours can be administered orally to children of all ages and is considered the agent of choice for infants younger than 6 months. Alternatively, ibuprofen 5–10 mg/kg administered orally every 6–8 hours can be used for children older than 6 months.

According to one meta-analysis, ibuprofen may be more effective than acetaminophen as an antipyretic, particularly in sustaining this effect.[36] However, this speculation was based on studies with small sample sizes and assessing the effect of a single dose. Another meta-analysis found no difference between ibuprofen and acetaminophen in relieving pain in children with AOM, except that the use of either drug is more effective than placebo.[65] Although acetaminophen can be administered in infants younger than 6 months, it does not have an anti-inflammatory effect, which is present in ibuprofen. The black box warnings for ibuprofen are potentially fatal cardiovascular, thrombotic, and gastrointestinal events; for acetaminophen, the warning is the life-threatening hepatic failure that most often arises from exceeding the maximum

daily dose or the use of several acetaminophen-containing products. Weight-based dosing is recommended for those weighing less than 50 kg.

Several methods exist for alternating antipyretics, such as interchanging acetaminophen and ibuprofen every 2–3 hours, or acetaminophen every 4 hours with ibuprofen every 6 hours. However, these methods contain inherent flaws, including surpassing the five-dose daily allowance of acetaminophen, inappropriately shortening the frequency of ibuprofen at every 4 hours, and administering both medications at two same time points within 24 hours.[66] Together with the lack of evidence for efficacy, the primary concern for alternating antipyretics is potential dosing errors. Dosing errors can lead to intoxication or hepatotoxicity from acetaminophen or nonoliguric renal dysfunction from ibuprofen. Thoroughly educating parents and caregivers on appropriate antipyretic use is imperative for preventing dosing errors and is a critical role for health care professionals (Box 2).

A common feature of AOM is ear pain. Assessment and treatment of pain should be provided for all patients with AOM, and analgesics should be used regardless of whether antibiotics are initiated. With the limited effect of antibiotics on pain, clinical management of AOM should focus on adequate analgesia.[37] Acetaminophen and ibuprofen are equally effective in treating mild to moderate ear pain. Topical benzocaine, procaine, or lidocaine preparations (if available) may be considered for children 2 years and older with no tympanic membrane perforation. Codeine is effective for moderate to severe pain but requires a prescription and is accompanied by a risk of adverse effects, including gastrointestinal upset, constipation, and respiratory depression. For a heavy middle ear effusion, draining this fluid may relieve the pain caused by the fluid pressure.

Antihistamines and decongestants for symptomatic relief of AOM have not been well studied. In fact, their use has been associated with increased medication adverse effects.[67] Furthermore, over-the-counter cough and cold medications should not be given to infants and children younger than 2 years because of the risk of life-threatening adverse effects, and the evidence for use in children younger than 6 years is limited.[68]

PREVENTION THROUGH IMMUNIZATION

The two vaccines effective in preventing AOM are the pneumococcal and influenza vaccines. The influenza vaccine may reduce AOM occurrence by 50%, particularly in young children attending day care.[53,69] The injectable influenza formulations are indicated for infants at least age 6 months, and the intranasal spray is recommended for children older than 2 years. For any child age 6 months to 9 years who receives the vaccine for the first time, two doses are recommended to enhance immunity.[39,70]

The 7-valent pneumococcal conjugate vaccine, introduced in the United States in 2000, only modestly decreases AOM occurrence compared with the flu vaccine.[55] However, widespread use of the 13-valent vaccine since 2010 has been correlated with a decrease in 19A serotype colonization, penicillin nonsusceptibility, visits related to OM, recurrent

OM, mastoiditis, and ventilating tube insertion.[21,22,25,26] Furthermore, colonization of 13-valent vaccine serotypes was reduced in children who were appropriately immunized, but colonization increased with recent antibiotic use.[22]

PREVENTION OF RECURRENCE

Recurrence, defined as three or more documented episodes within 6 months or four or more episodes within 12 months, can occur in some children, particularly those who first had AOM at younger than 6 months and those with immune deficiencies (e.g., IgG deficiency) or craniofacial abnormalities (e.g., cleft palates).[4] Antibiotic prophylaxis is not recommended by the American Academy of Pediatrics because the benefit is modest, decreasing AOM episodes only during the administration of prophylactic antibiotic.[4] Furthermore, prolonged antibiotic use may select for infections caused by resistant nasopharyngeal bacteria.[71] Because of these concerns for modest effectiveness and selection for resistant bacteria, surgical intervention by placing tympanostomy tubes to drain the copious middle ear fluid should be considered in children with recurrent AOM.

SUMMARY

The treatment modality for AOM does not necessitate its use in all cases. In fact, because AOM is self-limiting, initial observation is warranted for mild cases, and antibiotic therapy should be reserved for those with severe disease or young infants. Although antibiotic therapy improves patient response within 3 days, adverse drug effects may occur. More studies are needed to discover the characteristics of children who will most benefit from antibiotic therapy. Parent or caregiver education on the proper use of antibiotics, if warranted, and other medications for symptomatic relief, including their adverse effects, is critical to ensure optimal management of AOM.

RHINOSINUSITIS

Sinusitis, an inflammatory process that involves the mucous membranes of both the nose and the paranasal sinuses, is more properly termed rhinosinusitis, also called the common cold. Rhinosinusitis is classified as acute (sudden symptom onset with a duration of less than 30 days), subacute (duration of 30 days or more and less than 90 days), or chronic (duration greater than 90 days). The viruses that are responsible for most acute cases of rhinosinusitis include the following: human rhinovirus, influenza A and B viruses, parainfluenza virus, respiratory syncytial virus, adenovirus, and enterovirus. Most cases are self-limiting and resolve without treatment within 5–10 days after symptom onset.

Acute bacterial rhinosinusitis (ABRS) is a secondary infection that occurs in 8% of children with a viral URTI and peaks in the second year of life.[72] In addition to inhibiting macrophage and lymphocyte function, viruses induce inflammatory changes to block the sinus ostia, impair mucous drainage, and cause poor aeration, leading to increased susceptibility to secondary bacterial infection. Day care attendance and allergic rhinitis may also predispose children to ABRS.[73-75] Because ABRS requires appropriate management to facilitate recovery and prevent orbital and intracranial complications, the following discussion will focus strictly on the etiology and management of ABRS, excluding viral rhinosinusitis.

By early childhood, most children are colonized by at least one of three respiratory tract pathogens, including H. influenzae (nontypeable), S. pneumoniae, and M. catarrhalis. These respiratory tract bacteria are the most common causes of ABRS.[76-78] The prevalence of H. influenzae has increased and that of S. pneumoniae has decreased after routine pneumococcal vaccination in children in the United States.[26,47] As such, the production of β-lactamases, which is common in H. influenzae, limits the clinical usefulness of amoxicillin alone compared with amoxicillin with clavulanate. Similar to AOM, anaerobic bacteria, Staphylococcus aureus, and GAS can also cause ABRS, although less commonly. The clinical significance of atypical pathogens, including Chlamydia pneumoniae and Mycoplasma pneumoniae, in the pathogenesis of ABRS remains unclear.

Inflammation of the paranasal sinuses exceeding 90 days is considered chronic rhinosinusitis and should be distinguished from ABRS. In contrast to ABRS, the pathogenesis of chronic rhinosinusitis is believed to be multifactorial, with potential causes including the following: microorganisms (i.e., bacteria, fungi); inflammatory agents, such as allergens, pollutants, and smoke; asthma; cystic fibrosis; gastroesophageal reflux; immunodeficiency; and nasal polyposis.[74,77,78] These factors may appear concurrently to cause persistent inflammation of the nose and paranasal sinuses.

CLINICAL PRESENTATION AND DIAGNOSIS

Evidence of respiratory symptoms, including nasal discharge and congestion with or without daytime cough are the clinical features of ABRS. The nasal discharge may be watery, serous, or purulent. Of importance, purulent nasal secretions and a change in the color of nasal discharge are not specific indicators of ABRS. Purulent discharge can also occur in patients with viral rhinosinusitis. When cough is present, it may be wet or dry, occur during the day, and possibly worsen at night. Fever, sore throat, headache, and malodorous breath may occur together with these cardinal respiratory symptoms.[79] The fever usually subsides within 48 hours when the nasal symptoms become more evident.

A diagnostic challenge of ABRS is that no single sign or symptom clinically distinguishes it from viral rhinosinusitis. Although the clinical presentations of ABRS and viral URTIs are similar, the distinctive characteristics of ABRS are the persistence, severity, and progression (or worsening) of symptoms.[80] Respiratory symptoms in children with ABRS persist without improvement beyond 10 days, unlike viral URTIs, in which symptoms usually abate within 5–10 days.[47,78] In addition, a slight improvement that precedes the considerable worsening of symptoms on the sixth or seventh day of illness, known as "double sickening," suggests ABRS.[80] Another indicator of ABRS is a fever (defined as a temperature of 102.2°F [39°C] or higher) with purulent nasal discharge, or facial pain for 3 or more consecutive days.[47]

Diagnosis of ABRS is generally based on clinical presentation with persistent, worsening, or severe symptoms that extend beyond 10 days. Although no single sign or symptom is highly sensitive or specific, the presumptive diagnosis of ABRS based on the overall constellation of clinical findings is generally sufficient for treatment. Viral or allergic etiologies that may present similarly to ABRS should be excluded. Sinus aspiration with positive microbiological culture results definitively confirms a diagnosis of ABRS. However, because this procedure is invasive and requires a skilled specialist, it is not routinely performed.

Imaging studies—radiography, computed tomography, or magnetic resonance imaging—are unnecessary to confirm the diagnosis because abnormal findings indicate inflammation without providing the cause (i.e., virus, bacteria, or allergy).[78] Radiologic examination is recommended only in children with suspected orbital or intracranial complications associated with ABRS, or in those with persistent or recurrent infection who are unresponsive to therapy.[47,78] A sinus contrast-enhanced computed tomography scan is the imaging study of choice because it is more sensitive and specific than plain radiographs.[47,78]

In children with inadequate treatment, complications of ABRS may occur and can range in severity from mild, such as periorbital cellulitis, to serious, including orbital cellulitis, osteomyelitis of the frontal bone, meningitis, and epidural or brain abscess.[76,78,81] Immediate aggressive medical therapy, which may include surgery, is necessary, especially if abnormal vision, altered mental status, and periorbital edema are presenting symptoms.[82]

TREATMENT

Providing symptomatic relief, preventing complications, and minimizing adverse drug effects are the primary goals of antibiotic therapy in children with ABRS. Although the effectiveness of antibiotic therapy in preventing complications remains uncertain, it does appear to improve clinical cure rates.[47,83] A meta-analysis showed no difference in complication rates and patient satisfaction, with reduction in antibiotic use (from 93% to 31%) when antibiotic therapy was delayed for the treatment of respiratory tract infections.[44]

PHARMACOLOGIC THERAPY

Antibiotic treatment of ABRS should target the common etiologic culprits, particularly H. influenzae (nontypeable including β-lactamase–positive isolates), S. pneumoniae, and M. catarrhalis, and account for resistance patterns among these pathogens (as described in the previous section on AOM). Overuse of antibiotics has contributed to the emergence and increased prevalence of resistance in the United States. To address resistance, the most recent guidelines for the treatment of acute rhinosinusitis focus on judicious antibiotic use.[78] For children experiencing 10 days of symptoms that are neither severe nor worsening, immediate antimicrobial therapy or a 3-day period of observation can be considered.

Because of its safety, palatability, and low cost, amoxicillin with or without clavulanate is recommended by the American Academy of Pediatrics as first-line therapy in children with ABRS (Table 1).[78] The Infectious Diseases Society of America recommends amoxicillin with clavulanate because of concerns for an increased prevalence of H. influenzae, including β-lactamase–producing strains.[47] Dosing of the amoxicillin component should depend on the potential for drug-resistant pneumococci (e.g., recent antibiotic exposure, day care attendance, and geographic region) and severity of illness. High-dose amoxicillin with clavulanate is recommended for children with the following: severe symptoms (including a temperature of 102.2°F [39°C] or higher with concurrent purulent nasal discharge for at least 3–4 consecutive days); recent hospitalization or antibiotic exposure; age younger than 2 years; day care attendance; or residence in regions with penicillin-nonsusceptible S. pneumoniae at 10% or greater.[47,78] The ratio of amoxicillin to clavulanate that maximizes the amoxicillin dose is 14:1, administered in two divided doses.[4,52] However, this ratio has been associated with significant diarrhea, potentially caused by the increased amoxicillin component, despite the reduction in clavulanate.[53]

When H. influenzae or M. catarrhalis is highly suspected, amoxicillin alone is less likely to be effective because most isolates produce β-lactamases. Treatment options consist of amoxicillin with clavulanate or cephalosporins. Alternatives to amoxicillin with clavulanate are third-generation cephalosporins (specifically cefixime and cefpodoxime), in addition to clindamycin (which should not be used as monotherapy). When a liquid formulation is necessary, cefdinir tastes better, but it possesses reduced activity against H. influenzae compared with cefpodoxime. Otherwise, a single dose of ceftriaxone can be administered either intravenously or intramuscularly when oral therapy is not possible. Although treatment usually occurs in the outpatient setting, seriously ill children with ABRS should be hospitalized for intravenous antibiotics, including ampicillin/sulbactam, cefotaxime, ceftriaxone, or levofloxacin.

Concern for musculoskeletal adverse effects and the increased nonsusceptibility of pneumococcus associated with levofloxacin limits its use to children with immediate type I hypersensitivity to β-lactam antibiotics.[84] As such, the use of fluoroquinolones in children should be limited as an alternative to parenteral antimicrobial therapy or for cases that lack other safe and effective options.

Except for those with a history of true type I hypersensitivity to β-lactams, children with other types of reactions to one specific β-lactam antibiotic may tolerate another β-lactam. Macrolides, doxycycline, and trimethoprim/sulfamethoxazole are not routinely used in children because of concern about treatment failure, given susceptibility patterns. Doxycycline is also relatively contraindicated in children 8 years and younger because of the risk of permanent teeth discoloration.

Patients usually respond to appropriate treatment within 48–72 hours.[83] The recommended therapy duration for ABRS is 10–14 days, or at least 7 days after clinical improvement begins.[47,78] Antibiotic therapy in children with ABRS who are unresponsive 72 hours after treatment initiation should be broadened to high-dose amoxicillin with clavulanate or other second-line alternatives, including intravenous formulations, if deemed necessary. If orbital or intracranial complications are suspected, or the use of intravenous antibiotics is contemplated, then the diagnosis of ABRS should be confirmed with sinus imaging. In addition, sinus aspiration with subsequent cultures can help identify the causative pathogen and thus tailor therapy appropriately under these circumstances.

ADJUNCTIVE THERAPY

Symptomatic relief is one of the goals in the treatment of ABRS. Intranasal budesonide provides a modest reduction in nasal discharge and cough.[85] Similarly, the combination of an antihistamine and decongestant offers minimal symptomatic relief.[86] As such, these adjunctive therapies are not recommended for routine use in children, especially in those without an allergic component.[47,78] However, saline nasal drops, spray, or irrigation helps to dissolve secretions and prevent crust formation.[87] The water used for irrigation should be distilled, sterile, or previously boiled. Because it possesses minimal risk, saline topical therapy may be used in children for symptomatic relief of nasal symptoms. A systematic review reported lack of randomized, placebo-controlled trials of antibiotic treatment for ABRS, particularly those incorporating the quantitative assessment of sinus aspirate cultures. As such, the true efficacy of antihistamines, decongestants, and nasal irrigation in children with acute sinusitis requires further research.[88]

SUMMARY

Appropriate management of ABRS requires an understanding of its distinctive pathogenesis and clinical features. In contrast to the common cold and chronic rhinosinusitis, ABRS does not have viral or allergic etiologies. In addition, the symptoms of ABRS persist without improvement beyond 10 days and usually completely resolve by 30 days. Even though ABRS is a secondary infection caused by respiratory tract bacterial pathogens, it is judicious to treat it with antibiotics to limit the development of resistance.

PHARYNGITIS

Pharyngitis, characterized by inflammation of the mucous membranes and structures of the throat, encompasses tonsillitis, tonsillopharyngitis, and nasopharyngitis. It is common in children and therefore accounts for many annual clinic visits.[89] Although a sore throat accompanies pharyngitis, objective findings of erythema, exudates, or ulceration are required for diagnosis. Many etiologic agents or factors have been implicated for pharyngitis, including infectious vehicles, aphthous stomatitis, Behçet syndrome, and Kawasaki disease.[90] Nonetheless, viruses, followed by bacteria, are the most common infectious causes of pharyngitis in children and adolescents. Viral pharyngitis is predominant in the summer and fall seasons, whereas bacterial pharyngitis occurs in the late autumn, winter, and spring in temperate climates.[91]

Certain viruses, including the Epstein-Barr virus, cytomegalovirus, adenoviruses, herpes simplex virus, influenza viruses, and enterovirus, directly insult the pharynx to cause inflammation.[92] Other viruses, including rhinoviruses, coronaviruses, respiratory syncytial virus, and parainfluenza viruses, cause nasopharyngitis. In these cases, the sore throat is not because of direct pharyngeal insult, but because of irritation related to mouth breathing or cough caused by rhinorrhea.

Among bacterial pathogens, GAS accounts for up to 37% of all pharyngitis cases in children and adolescents.[93,94] As such, it is the most common bacterial cause of pharyngitis, particularly in children older than 5 years.[1,94] Penicillin resistance has not been a significant issue for GAS; however, macrolide resistance (including azithromycin) has been reported in school-age children.[95-97] Erythromycin resistance and biofilm formation appear to be similar between recurrent and reinfection GAS isolates; however, pili and fibronectin-binding proteins may be associated with recurrence.[98] Other bacterial culprits of pharyngitis are non–group A *Streptococcus*, *M. pneumoniae*, *Neisseria gonorrhoeae* (particularly in adolescents who engage in oral–genital sex), *Arcanobacterium haemolyticum*, and *Corynebacterium diphtheriae*.[90]

The following sections will focus on the clinical presentation and therapeutic management of bacterial pharyngitis, particularly streptococcal pharyngitis. However, distinctive clinical features of viral and bacterial pharyngitis will also be presented because differentiating between the two etiologies is critical to justify antibiotic therapy initiation.

CLINICAL PRESENTATION AND DIAGNOSIS

Evidence of erythema, edema, or exudates of the pharynx on physical examination is mandatory for diagnosing acute pharyngitis caused by either viruses or bacteria. Pharyngitis caused by GAS often occurs in school-age children and adolescents. Symptom onset is usually abrupt in children 3 years and older. Sore throat, fever, tonsillar exudates, cervical adenopathy, headache, abdominal pain, nausea, and vomiting are clinical characteristics of GAS pharyngitis.[91,99,100] An inflamed uvula may also be present. Symptom inception is abrupt, and symptoms usually resolve without antibiotic treatment within 3–5 days. In fact, sore throat persisting for more than 7 days suggests other causes of pharyngitis. Nonetheless, antibiotic treatment is indicated for clinical cases of GAS pharyngitis to minimize its progression to serious complications.

Although uncommon, GAS pharyngitis may occur in infants and children younger than 3 years, particularly as outbreaks in childcare settings. The clinical presentation in this age group is generally nonspecific and subtle and includes fever, irritability, and anorexia. However, the finding of close contacts (e.g., siblings and day care attendants) with recent GAS infection strongly suggests GAS pharyngitis.

The common features of viral pharyngitis are concurrent conjunctivitis, cough, coryza, diarrhea, anterior stomatitis, ulcerative lesions, and rash.[89,91,97] Certain viruses have distinct clinical attributes. For example, infectious mononucleosis caused by Epstein-Barr virus and cytomegalovirus that commonly occurs in adolescents manifests as prolonged exudative pharyngitis, cervical lymphadenopathy, hepatitis, and rash that develops when treated with ampicillin or amoxicillin. Pharyngoconjunctival fever is highly indicative of adenovirus, and herpangina with small vesicles appearing in the posterior pharynx indicates coxsackie A viruses (a type of enterovirus). Pharyngitis caused by herpes simplex virus generally presents with ulcerative lesions of the mouth and lips in young children and adolescents. Finally, the seasonality of infection, in addition to fever, cough, and myalgias, is typical of influenza infection.

Although clinical signs and symptoms may provide evidence for a GAS etiology, diagnosis should be validated by throat culture, rapid antigen detection test (RADT), or both, ideally before therapy is begun.[101,102] In the absence of indicators for a viral URTI, candidates likely to have GAS pharyngitis are those in recent contact with an individual infected by GAS (including a history of acute rheumatic fever or poststreptococcal glomerulonephritis) or those residing in a region with a high prevalence of GAS.[103] In addition, age 5–15 years, the winter season, enlarged anterior cervical lymph nodes (greater than 1 cm), and temperature of 101°F–103°F (38.3°C–39.4°C) are predictive factors for positive GAS throat cultures and scarlatiniform rash.[93,97] Laboratory confirmation should be performed in children who present with acute onset of sore throat with pharyngeal exudates or pain on swallowing and who have these predisposing factors.

Throat culture for diagnostic workup is the gold standard and is more cost-effective than RADT.[99,104] Neither test can differentiate between infection and carrier state; however, throat cultures are highly sensitive and specific in identifying GAS as well as other bacteria. The throat culture should thus be used in primary testing to confirm GAS. Even if RADT is used initially, negative RADT, with its limited sensitivity, should always be confirmed with throat cultures in children and adolescents.[89,97] The use of RADT may be beneficial when throat culture results are unavailable for more than 48 hours (i.e., because RADT results are available in minutes) and when children who are highly likely to have positive throat cultures are tested. Because RADT is very specific (95%–98%), a positive test is adequate for antibiotic initiation. A reduced sensitivity of 86% indicates some cases of GAS pharyngitis will be missed by RADT.[105] Serologic testing for antistreptococcal antibody titers can validate true streptococcal infection.[89,103] However, positive titers occur 2–3 weeks after infection; therefore, they have no value during the diagnostic process for acute GAS pharyngitis.

Complications caused by GAS pharyngitis consist of acute rheumatic fever (with an incidence of two or fewer cases per 100,000 school-age children in the United States), acute glomerulonephritis, streptococcal toxic shock syndrome, and scarlet fever. Some of these sequelae are serious and potentially life threatening and are caused by certain types of GAS such as nephritogenic strains for glomerulonephritis.[91,106] Other complications, particularly those that are purulent, include OM, sinusitis, peritonsillar and retropharyngeal abscesses, necrotizing fasciitis, and bacteremia.

TREATMENT

Antibiotic treatment is indicated for symptomatic GAS pharyngitis because GAS pharyngitis can progress to serious complications. In particular, antibiotic therapy eradicates certain GAS strains that can elicit an immune response,

leading to acute rheumatic fever.[99] Viral pharyngitis, in contrast, can self-resolve with or without adjunctive remedies for symptomatic relief. Laboratory confirmation of GAS as the etiologic agent during diagnostic workup is essential to appropriately managing the infected patient as well as ensuring judicious antimicrobial use (i.e., avoiding antibiotics in patients with viral infections).

Preventing the subsequent development of acute rheumatic fever is the primary goal of antibiotic treatment. Symptomatic recovery, eradication of GAS from the pharynx, prevention of suppurative and nonsuppurative complications, and prevention of transmission are other therapeutic goals. Symptom resolution generally occurs within 3–4 days but can occur as soon as 2 days with appropriate antibiotic therapy. To expedite clinical recovery, antibiotics should be initiated promptly within the first 2 days of infection, if possible.[107] However, prevention of rheumatic fever requires antibiotic initiation within 9 days after illness onset.[108] Eradication of GAS from the upper respiratory tract is an indicator of successful prevention of rheumatic fever. Prevention of glomerulonephritis through antibiotic use remains unclear.[107] Although the risk of transmitting GAS pharyngitis peaks during acute infection, communicability decreases markedly after 24 hours of appropriate antibiotic therapy.[91,109]

PHARMACOLOGIC THERAPY

Penicillin, available in oral and injectable formulations, is the treatment of choice for GAS pharyngitis because penicillin is effective, safe, and relatively inexpensive (Table 1).[89,91,99] Injectable benzathine penicillin G is beneficial for children at greater risk of rheumatic fever, including those who live in crowded conditions or have a history of rheumatic heart disease. In addition, benzathine penicillin G is a prudent choice for children who are nonadherent to oral penicillin, which is a major contributing factor to treatment failure. Because one dose provides bactericidal levels for about 2 weeks, benzathine penicillin G is administered as a single intramuscular dose for the treatment of GAS pharyngitis.[110] Benzathine penicillin G should be warmed to room temperature before intramuscular injection to minimize pain. The combination product containing benzathine penicillin G and procaine penicillin G can be considered to minimize discomfort.[91]

Predominantly for young children, amoxicillin is a reasonable oral alternative to penicillin because of its enhanced palatability and activity against GAS. Because GAS is highly susceptible to amoxicillin, once- or twice-daily dosing is effective for the treatment of pharyngitis (Table 1).[111] Other oral antibiotics are reserved for patients with penicillin allergies (Table 1). With their enhanced microbiological and clinical cure rates in children, cephalosporins are excellent substitutes for those with mild penicillin allergies.[112-114] However, first-generation cephalosporins are preferred because of their cost-effectiveness and because of concerns about antibiotic resistance with second- and third-generation cephalosporins.[112]

Cephalosporins should be avoided in children with life-threatening immediate or type I hypersensitivity to β-lactams. Oral clindamycin and macrolides, including azithromycin, are appropriate options in these patients, but their selection for use should be based on local susceptibility patterns (Table 1). Azithromycin requires higher doses to overcome GAS resistance, which varies regionally and temporally.[97] Furthermore, based on a meta-analysis, children with GAS pharyngitis experienced more adverse events with macrolides, including azithromycin, compared with amoxicillin.[115] Because of their reported high resistance rates and failure to eradicate GAS, sulfonamides and tetracyclines should not be used for treating pharyngitis.[91]

Empiric antibiotic initiation while waiting for confirmatory laboratory results remains controversial. The decision to initiate antibiotics empirically should be based on patient circumstances, although prevention of rheumatic fever allows antibiotic initiation as late as the ninth day of illness, when laboratory results should be available.[102,108] Antibiotics should be discontinued in the absence of positive throat cultures or RADT, except in patients with acute rheumatic fever who may initially have negative throat cultures. The duration of oral penicillin or amoxicillin therapy to achieve pharyngeal GAS eradication and thereby prevent acute rheumatic fever is 10 full days, even in the presence of clinical resolution. Shorter courses of oral therapy, with efficacy similar to a 10-day course of penicillin, are available for cefpodoxime, cefdinir, cefixime, cefadroxil, and azithromycin.

A post-treatment throat culture to confirm cure is recommended for patients and their domestic contacts, even if asymptomatic, who developed pharyngitis during an outbreak of acute rheumatic fever or poststreptococcal glomerulonephritis; who have a history or are at high risk of rheumatic fever; or who have several family members in whom GAS infection has occurred.[91,116] More importantly, in these circumstances, asymptomatic household contacts with positive laboratory results should be treated with a standard course of antibiotic therapy.

Complications, including acute rheumatic fever, are unlikely to occur from pharyngitis caused by bacteria other than GAS; therefore, antimicrobial therapy is unnecessary in many of these situations, except in rare cases of acute pharyngitis caused by *C. diphtheriae*, *N. gonorrhoeae*, and *A. haemolyticum*. In addition, antibiotics (usually for 5 days) may improve clinical response to non–group A streptococcal pharyngitis and so may be considered in this situation.[99] Pharmacologic and nonpharmacologic therapies for other causes of acute pharyngitis may be warranted, including activity restriction for Epstein-Barr virus mononucleosis to prevent splenic rupture, acyclovir for herpes simplex virus, and other antiviral agents for influenza.

RECURRENT INFECTION AND PHARYNGEAL CARRIAGE

Acute pharyngitis may recur in some children, particularly those who are nonadherent to prescribed antibiotics, those who are streptococcal pharyngeal carriers with concurrent viral infection, those acquiring a new infection from GAS-infected close contacts, or those with a history of rheumatic fever. Streptococcal carriage occurs in 20% of asymptomatic school-age children and may persist for months in the

pharynx. Because throat culture and RADT cannot differentiate between carrier state and infection, these diagnostic tests are indicated to confirm pharyngitis caused by GAS. Carriers can be identified by positive GAS laboratory tests between episodes of acute pharyngitis when carriers are asymptomatic or by serologic response to GAS extracellular antistreptolysin O antigen (even though titers are generally low).[91] Transmission of GAS to close contacts and development of suppurative complications are low in GAS carriers. However, eradicating GAS presents a therapeutic challenge.[117,118] Nonetheless, antibiotic therapy is indicated for GAS pharyngeal carriers only under special circumstances, including an outbreak of acute rheumatic fever, a case of poststreptococcal glomerulonephritis, or a family history of acute rheumatic fever.[91]

A repeated course of antibiotics, using any of the therapeutic options other than the one prescribed initially, is indicated for those with a second incident of laboratory-confirmed pharyngitis. Intramuscular benzathine penicillin G is a practical selection for those with medication adherence issues. Injection-site pain may be minimized by icing the area and keeping the muscle relaxed. To eliminate chronic carriage state, which may contribute to recurrent infections, clindamycin and amoxicillin/clavulanate may be effective, given their high eradication and clinical cure rates.[97,119] These agents are reasonable options for patients with several recurrent episodes, which are likely caused by nonstreptococci (i.e., viral) in GAS pharyngeal carriers. Rifampin for the last 4 days of treatment, together with penicillin, is an alternative for chronic streptococcal carriage.[91,97] Tonsillectomy is not recommended if used only to reduce the episodes of GAS pharyngitis.[97]

ADJUNCTIVE THERAPY

Nonprescription remedies for sore throat, including lozenges and mouthwashes, provide few benefits.[91] Similarly, antihistamines and decongestants offer minimal symptomatic relief. With their potential risks of adverse drug effects, these adjunctive therapies are not recommended for routine use in children and adolescents with URTIs. Acetaminophen or ibuprofen can be advantageous for their analgesic and antipyretic effects and thus can be considered as adjunct to antibiotic therapy.[97]

PREVENTION

Secondary prevention of recurrent rheumatic fever using prophylactic antibiotics is recommended for individuals with a documented history of acute rheumatic fever or rheumatic heart disease.[91] Penicillin, including penicillin G benzathine administered every 3–4 weeks, is recommended for secondary prophylaxis. Otherwise, sulfadiazine, sulfisoxazole, or macrolides can be substituted for patients with anaphylactic reactions to penicillin. Leukopenia associated with sulfonamides may occur after 2 weeks of prophylaxis and should be monitored.

Chemoprophylaxis should be initiated at the time of diagnosis and continued indefinitely for children with rheumatic heart disease. For individuals with rheumatic fever, antibiotic prophylaxis should be continued for at least 5 years, or until these individuals are age 21 years (whichever duration is longer). Although not well studied under controlled environments, tonsillectomy may be considered for patients with six or more GAS infections per year—or five or more episodes each year in 2 consecutive years.[120] Research is currently ongoing for a vaccine against GAS.[121,122]

SUMMARY

Acute pharyngitis can be caused by viruses or bacteria. Discerning the clinical manifestations for each form of acute pharyngitis is imperative for identifying pediatric patients with GAS pharyngitis, an infection that can progress to serious complications, including acute rheumatic fever. Patients with GAS pharyngitis are usually age 5–15 years and acutely present with exudative sore throat, fever, and cervical lymphadenitis. Diagnosis should be confirmed with laboratory testing before initiating antibiotic therapy to ensure the appropriate use of these therapies.

OUTPATIENT ANTIMICROBIAL STEWARDSHIP

Use of antibiotics presents risks, which must be carefully considered and recognized by both health care professionals and parents or caregivers (Table 1). In addition to contributing to an increased prevalence of antimicrobial resistance, antibiotic use can lead to adverse drug reactions. In fact, antibiotics are the leading cause of adverse drug reactions in hospitalized children.[123] Among specific antibiotics, penicillins and cephalosporins most often contribute to the adverse events. Specifically, children with AOM treated with antibiotics have more adverse effects than those who are untreated.[50]

Although hospitals have implemented antimicrobial stewardship programs to optimize antimicrobial use, these efforts in the outpatient and community settings can be improved.[124] The role of community pharmacists in outpatient antimicrobial stewardship is critical to ensure judicious antibiotic use, appropriate use of over-the-counter medications for symptomatic relief, and prevention through immunization. Not all infections require antibiotics, an important concept embraced and promoted by the Centers for Disease Control and Prevention through its Get Smart campaign. Viruses are responsible for most acute cases of rhinosinusitis and pharyngitis; therefore, antibiotics are ineffective. For AOM, initial observation should be considered in certain cases (i.e., older children or those presenting with mild symptoms) to increase efforts toward judicious antibiotic use. If antibiotics are prescribed, the drug, dose, and duration should be reviewed to ensure the appropriateness for age. Pharmacists should ensure the duration is appropriate (i.e., 5–7 vs. 10 days for AOM) and educate patients and parents or caregivers on the importance of completing the prescribed course of therapy.

In addition to antibiotic therapy, recommendations may be necessary for over-the-counter medications to control symptoms such as fever or ear pain. When recommending these products, providers must give clear instructions on dosing and ensure that parents and caregivers understand that the various nonprescription drug formulations are not interchangeable (Box 2). Weight-based dosing and standardized concentrations are strategies to ensure the effective and safe use of a common drug, acetaminophen.[125] In fact, a black box warning accompanies the use of weight-based dosing of acetaminophen for children weighing less than 50 kg. Finally, immunization, particularly the pneumococcal and influenza vaccines for AOM, is imperative for prevention. Immunization status should be monitored at each patient encounter.

An 18-month-old previously healthy, full-term boy is brought to the clinic with 2 weeks of intermittent dry cough, congestion, and fever. Two days before presentation, he had intermittent daily oral temperatures of up to 102°F (38.9°C), with slight improvement on acetaminophen. The parents were concerned about his continued fevers and brought their son to the pediatrician for antibiotic therapy. The parents denied that he has had any vomiting, altered mental status, and change in feeding or appetite. The patient tugs on both ears and cries loudly during the office visit.

Birth history: Born at 37 weeks' gestation by normal spontaneous vaginal delivery

Medical history: Episode of acute otitis media (AOM) at age 11 months

Surgical history: None

Development history: Not significant

Social history: No siblings, pets at home, or recent travel; attends a day care center; no significant exposures

Family history: Father smokes cigarettes, 5 packs/day

Diet: Normal appetite, bottle-feeds with strong suck response, uses pacifier often

Immunizations: Up-to-date, including two doses of the current season's influenza vaccine

Allergies: No known drug or food allergies

Current medications history: Parent-initiated acetaminophen 160 mg (5 mL) orally every 6 hr

Vital signs: BP 110/65 mm Hg, HR 145 beats/minute, Tmax 102.4°F (39.1°C), RR 40 breaths/minute, Wt 13 kg, Ht 33 inches

Physical examination:

General: Well developed and well nourished; active with a strong cry; no apparent distress

Eyes: Normal conjunctivae; pupils are equal, round, and reactive to light; no sign of discharge

Ears: Bilateral: External ear and pinna normal; no foreign bodies; tympanic membranes are abnormal, erythematous, and cloudy; middle ear effusion is evident

Nose: Nasal discharge

Throat: Oropharynx is clear

Neck: Normal range of motion; supple

Pulmonary: Normal effort; no stridor, respiratory distress, wheezes, rhonchi, rales, or retraction

Cardiovascular: Normal rate and regular rhythm

Abdomen: Soft without extension or tenderness

Musculoskeletal: No signs of injury; free range of motion from all extremities

Skin: Warm; no petechiae, purpura, or rash; no diaphoresis, cyanosis, mottling, jaundice, or pallor

Neuro: Alert; normal muscle tone

Laboratory findings: None available

A diagnosis of bilateral AOM is made.

1. What risk factors associated with AOM are present in this patient?

This patient's first episode of AOM was at age 11 months. Infants and young children are at increased risk of developing AOM because of the decreased angle of the opening of the eustachian tube, which allows nasopharyngeal bacteria to ascend to the middle ear cavity and prevents adequate drainage of middle ear fluid. This anatomic feature of the eustachian tubes, together with other risk factors, is associated with the development of otitis media (OM). Other risk factors for AOM evident in this patient are as follows. If modifiable, exposure to these risk factors should be minimized.

- Young age (younger than 2 years)
- Recent upper respiratory tract infection, particularly caused by rhinovirus and adenovirus, because they promote bacteria replication and increase inflammation in the nasopharynx and eustachian tube, which then facilitates bacterial entry into the middle ear space
- Exposure to secondhand tobacco smoke
- Day care attendance

2. What would you recommend to manage this patient's AOM? Provide a justification, and, if pharmacologic treatment is warranted, devise a plan for managing his AOM.

Antibiotic treatment should be initiated immediately in children with severe disease, as evidenced in this patient by bilateral AOM, persistent otalgia for more than 48 hours (i.e., "tugs on both ears and cries loudly"), and a temperature of 102.2°F (39°C) or higher. Even if those symptoms were attenuated without pharmacologic treatment, bilateral AOM in a child younger than 2 years would warrant treatment of some type, given the possible sequelae of untreated disease such as hearing loss and mastoiditis in a developing infant.

Antibiotic therapy should target activity against the three most common organisms: *Streptococcus pneumoniae*, nontypeable *Haemophilus influenzae*, and *Moraxella catarrhalis*. The patient had his first episode of AOM 7 months ago and likely received antibiotic therapy for that infection. High-dose amoxicillin with clavulanic acid may be considered in children who have antibiotic exposure within the previous 30 days or have AOM with accompanying conjunctivitis. However, this patient has not been exposed to amoxicillin in the past 30 days, nor does he have purulent conjunctivitis or a penicillin allergy. As such, the first-line treatment is oral high-dose amoxicillin 80–90 mg/kg/day twice daily for 10 days administered as 550 mg of oral suspension twice daily (versus three times daily, to prevent diarrhea), which can be provided as the 400 mg/5 mL suspension.

Adjunctive therapy should address fever and otalgia. Acetaminophen at the dose that the patient currently takes (i.e., 160 mg [5 mL] orally every 6 hours) is effective as needed for ear pain and fever. If no improvement is evident within 48–72 hours, then an evaluation for viral disease or a change in antibiotic therapy may be warranted.

3. What educational points should you provide to the anxious parents to optimize the care of the patient's current and potential future infections?

The parents should be educated on the differences between AOM and OM with effusion. Typically, AOM is caused by bacteria and is treatable by antibiotics (but for only certain diagnoses or severe disease), whereas OM with effusion is usually caused by viruses, thus making antibiotics ineffective. For the current infection, the presenting symptoms (e.g., fever) usually resolve within 2–3 days after initiating antibiotics. Middle ear effusion can persist for weeks to months in up to 70% of children.

Notably, immediate antimicrobial treatment of AOM does not significantly affect the resolution of middle ear effusions.

Other educational recommendations include finishing the 10-day antibiotic therapy course, avoiding day care attendance (if possible), and having the father engage in smoking cessation or having the child avoid secondary smoke; for example, after smoking and before contact with the child, the father would wash his hands and face. The parents were concerned about the patient's fevers, prompting them to initiate acetaminophen. A *fever* is defined as an elevated body temperature exceeding 100°F (37.8°C) by mouth (or 100.4°F [38°C] rectally) and is part of the natural human body response to infection. Fevers do not harm the patient and can be managed using appropriate doses of acetaminophen. Finally, the two vaccines with effectiveness in preventing AOM are the pneumococcal and influenza vaccines. Immunizations are up to date in this patient, but the parents should be reminded of the annual influenza vaccine.

REFERENCES

1. Danchin MH, Rogers S, Kelpie L, et al. Burden of acute sore throat and group A streptococcal pharyngitis in school-aged children and their families in Australia. Pediatrics 2007;120:950-7.

2. McCaig LF, Besser RE, Hughes JM. Trends in antimicrobial prescribing rates for children and adolescents. JAMA 2002; 287:3096-102.

3. Grijalva CG, Nuorti JP, Griffin MR. Antibiotic prescription rates for acute respiratory tract infections in US ambulatory settings. JAMA 2009;302:758-66.

4. Lieberthal AS, Carroll AE, Chonmaitree T, et al. The diagnosis and management of acute otitis media. Pediatrics 2013;131:e964-99.

5. Daly KA, Giebink GS. Clinical epidemiology of otitis media. Pediatr Infect Dis J 2000;19:S31-6.

6. Teele DW, Klein JO, Rosner B. Epidemiology of otitis media during the first seven years of life in children in greater Boston: a prospective, cohort study. J Infect Dis 1989;160:83-94.

7. Chonmaitree T, Revai K, Grady JJ, et al. Viral upper respiratory tract infection and otitis media complication in young children. Clin Infect Dis 2008;46:815-23.

8. Kaur R, Morris M, Pichichero ME. Epidemiology of acute otitis media in the postpneumococcal conjugate vaccine era. Pediatrics 2017;141:pii.

9. Teele DW, Klein JO, Chase C, et al. Otitis media in infancy and intellectual ability, school achievement, speech, and language at age 7 years. Greater Boston Otitis Media Study Group. J Infect Dis 1990;162:685-94.

10. McKee C, Giddon B, Ibach B. Common Pediatric Illnesses. In: Zeind CS, Carvalho MG, eds. Applied Therapeutics: The Clinical Use of Drugs. 11th ed. Philadelphia, PA: Wolters Kluwer, 2018:Chapter 104.

11. Van Dyke MK, Pircon JY, Cohen R, et al. Etiology of acute otitis media in children less than 5 years of age: a pooled analysis of 10 similarly designed observational studies. Pediatr Infect Dis J 2017;36:274-81.

12. Ben-Shimol S, Givon-Lavi N, Leibovitz E, et al. Impact of widespread introduction of pneumococcal conjugate vaccines on pneumococcal and nonpneumococcal otitis media. Clin Infect Dis 2016;63:611-8.

13. Wald ER, DeMuri GP. Antibiotic recommendations for acute otitis media and acute bacterial sinusitis: conundrum no more. Pediatr Infect Dis J 2018;37:1255-7.

14. Ruohola A, Meurman O, Nikkari S, et al. Microbiology of acute otitis media in children with tympanostomy tubes: prevalences of bacteria and viruses. Clin Infect Dis 2006;43:1417-22.

15. Green MC, Mason EO, Kaplan SL, et al. Increase in prevalence of Streptococcus pneumoniae serotype 6C at Eight Children's Hospitals in the United States from 1993 to 2009. J Clin Microbiol 2011;49:2097-101.

16. Stamboulidis K, Chatzaki D, Poulakou G, et al. The impact of the heptavalent pneumococcal conjugate vaccine on the epidemiology of acute otitis media complicated by otorrhea. Pediatr Infect Dis J 2011;30:551-5.

17. Casey JR, Adlowitz DG, Pichichero ME. New patterns in the otopathogens causing acute otitis media six to eight years after introduction of pneumococcal conjugate vaccine. Pediatr Infect Dis J 2010;29:304-9.

18. Dupont D, Mahjoub-Messai F, Francois M, et al. Evolving microbiology of complicated acute otitis media before and after introduction of the pneumococcal conjugate vaccine in France. Diagn Microbiol Infect Dis 2010;68:89-92.

19. Bardach A, Ciapponi A, Garcia-Marti S, et al. Epidemiology of acute otitis media in children of Latin America and the Caribbean: A systematic review and meta-analysis. Int J Pediatr Otorhinolaryngol 2011;75:1062-70.

20. Sierra A, Lopez P, Zapata MA, et al. Non-typeable Haemophilus influenzae and Streptococcus pneumoniae as primary causes of acute otitis media in Colombian children: a prospective study. BMC Infect Dis 2011;11:4.

21. Marom T, Tan A, Wilkinson GS, et al. Trends in otitis media-related health care use in the United States, 2001–2011. JAMA Pediatr 2014;168:68-75.

22. Lee GM, Kleinman K, Pelton S, et al. Immunization, antibiotic use, and pneumococcal colonization over a 15-year period. Pediatrics 2017;140:pii.

23. O'Brien MA, Prosser LA, Paradise JL, et al. New vaccines against otitis media: projected benefits and cost-effectiveness. Pediatrics 2009;123:1452-63.

24. Mendes RE, Costello AJ, Jacobs MR, et al. Serotype distribution and antimicrobial susceptibility of USA Streptococcus pneumoniae isolates collected prior to and post introduction of 13-valent pneumococcal conjugate vaccine. Diagn Microbiol Infect Dis 2014;80:19-25.

25. Centers for Disease Control and Prevention. Active Bacterial Core Surveillance (ABCs) Report—Surveillance: Streptococcus pneumoniae, 1998-2016. Available at https://www.cdc.gov/abcs/reports-findings/surreports/spneu-types.html. Accessed October 8, 2019.

26. Kaplan SL, Barson WJ, Lin PL, et al. Early trends for invasive pneumococcal infections in children after the introduction of the 13-valent pneumococcal conjugate vaccine. Pediatr Infect Dis J 2013;32:203-7.

27. Kaplan SL, Center KJ, Barson WJ, et al. Multicenter surveillance of Streptococcus pneumoniae isolates from middle ear and mastoid cultures in the 13-valent pneumococcal conjugate vaccine era. Clin Infect Dis 2015;60:1339-45.

28. Pottumarthy S, Fritsche TR, Sader HS, et al. Susceptibility patterns of Streptococcus pneumoniae isolates in North America (2002–2003): contemporary in vitro activities of amoxicillin/clavulanate and 15 other antimicrobial agents. Int J Antimicrob Agents 2005;25:282-9.

29. Jacobs MR, Felmingham D, Appelbaum PC, et al. The Alexander Project 1998-2000: susceptibility of pathogens isolated from community-acquired respiratory tract infection to commonly used antimicrobial agents. J Antimicrob Chemother 2003;52:229-46.

30. Thornsberry C, Sahm DF, Kelly LJ, et al. Regional trends in antimicrobial resistance among clinical isolates of Streptococcus pneumoniae, Haemophilus influenzae, and Moraxella catarrhalis in the United States: results from the TRUST Surveillance Program, 1999–2000. Clin Infect Dis 2002;34 Suppl 1;S4-16.

31. Farrell DJ, Mendes RE, Ross JE, et al. LEADER Program Results for 2009: an activity and spectrum analysis of linezolid using 6,414 clinical isolates from 56 medical centers in the United States. Antimicrob Agents Chemother 2011;55:3684-90.

32. Farrell DJ, Morrissey I, Bakker S, et al. Molecular characterization of macrolide resistance mechanisms among Streptococcus pneumoniae and Streptococcus pyogenes isolated from the PROTEKT 1999–2000 study. J Antimicrob Chemother 2002;50 Supple S1:39-47.

33. Jacobs MR. Worldwide trends in antimicrobial resistance among common respiratory tract pathogens in children. Pediatr Infect Dis J 2003;22:S109-19.

34. Rothman R, Owens T, Simel DL. Does this child have acute otitis media? JAMA 2003;290:1633-40.

35. Teele DW, Klein JO, Rosner BA. Epidemiology of otitis media in children. Ann Otol Rhinol Laryngol Suppl 1980;89:5-6.

36. Perrott DA, Piira T, Goodenough B, et al. Efficacy and safety of acetaminophen vs ibuprofen for treating children's pain or fever: a meta-analysis. Arch Pediatr Adolesc Med 2004;158:521-6.

37. Venekamp RP, Sanders SL, Glasziou PP, et al. Antibiotics for acute otitis media in children. Cochrane Database Syst Rev 2015;6:CD000219.

38. Chao JH, Kunkov S, Reyes LB, et al. Comparison of two approaches to observation therapy for acute otitis media in the emergency department. Pediatrics 2008;121:e1352-6.

39. Hoberman A, Paradise JL, Rockette HE, et al. Treatment of acute otitis media in children under 2 years of age. N Engl J Med 2011;364:105-15.

40. Little P, Gould C, Williamson I, et al. Pragmatic randomised controlled trial of two prescribing strategies for childhood acute otitis media. BMJ 2001;322:336-42.

41. McCormick DP, Chonmaitree T, Pittman C, et al. Nonsevere acute otitis media: a clinical trial comparing outcomes of watchful waiting versus immediate antibiotic treatment. Pediatrics 2005;115:1455-65.

42. Uitti JM, Tahtinen PA, Laine MK, et al. Close follow-up in children with acute otitis media initially managed without antimicrobials. JAMA Pediatr 2016;170:1107-8.

43. Groth A, Enoksson F, Hermansson A, et al. Acute mastoiditis in children in Sweden 1993–2007—no increase after new guidelines. Int J Pediatr Otorhinolaryngol 2011;75:1496-501.

44. Spurling GK, Del Mar CB, Dooley L, et al. Delayed antibiotic prescriptions for respiratory infections. Cochrane Database Syst Rev 2017;CD004417.

45. Spiro DM, Tay KY, Arnold DH, et al. Wait-and-see prescription for the treatment of acute otitis media: a randomized controlled trial. JAMA 2006;296:1235-41.

46. Dickerson LM, Mainous AG, 3rd, Carek PJ. The pharmacist's role in promoting optimal antimicrobial use. Pharmacotherapy 2000;20:711-23.

47. Chow AW, Benninger MS, Brook I, et al. IDSA clinical practice guideline for acute bacterial rhinosinusitis in children and adults. Clin Infect Dis 2012;54:e72-e112.

48. Shaikh N, Dando EE, Dunleavy ML, et al. A cost-utility analysis of 5 strategies for the management of acute otitis media in children. J Pediatr 2017;189:54-60.e3.

49. White AR, Kaye C, Poupard J, et al. Augmentin (amoxicillin/clavulanate) in the treatment of community-acquired respiratory tract infection: a review of the continuing development of an innovative antimicrobial agent. J Antimicrob Chemother 2004;53 Suppl:i3-20.

50. Tahtinen PA, Laine MK, Huovinen P, et al. A placebo-controlled trial of antimicrobial treatment for acute otitis media. N Engl J Med 2011;364:116-26.

51. Frost HM, Gerber JS, Hersh AL. Antibiotic recommendations for acute otitis media and acute bacterial sinusitis. Pediatr Infect Dis J 2019;38:217.

52. Hoberman A, Paradise JL, Burch DJ, et al. Equivalent efficacy and reduced occurrence of diarrhea from a new formulation of amoxicillin/clavulanate potassium (Augmentin) for treatment of acute otitis media in children. Pediatr Infect Dis J 1997;16:463-70.

53. Kuehn J, Ismael Z, Long PF, et al. Reported rates of diarrhea following oral penicillin therapy in pediatric clinical trials. J Pediatr Pharmacol Ther 2015;20:90-104.

54. Hoberman A, Paradise JL, Rockette HE, et al. Shortened antimicrobial treatment for acute otitis media in young children. N Engl J Med 2016;375:2446-56.

55. Pichichero ME. Shortened antimicrobial treatment for acute otitis media. N Engl J Med 2017;376:e24.

56. Kozyrskyj A, Klassen TP, Moffatt M, et al. Short-course antibiotics for acute otitis media. Cochrane Database Syst Rev 2010; 9:CD001095.

57. Atanaskovic-Markovic M, Velickovic TC, Gavrovic-Jankulovic M, et al. Immediate allergic reactions to cephalosporins and penicillins and their cross-reactivity in children. Pediatr Allergy Immunol 2005;16:341-7.

58. Pichichero ME, Casey JR. Safe use of selected cephalosporins in penicillin-allergic patients: a meta-analysis. Otolaryngol Head Neck Surg 2007;136:340-7.

59. Kelkar PS, Li JT. Cephalosporin allergy. N Engl J Med 2001; 345:804-9.

60. Gruchalla RS, Pirmohamed M. Clinical practice. Antibiotic allergy. N Engl J Med 2006;354:601-9.

61. Apter AJ, Kinman JL, Bilker WB, et al. Is there cross-reactivity between penicillins and cephalosporins? Am J Med 2006; 354:e11-9.

62. Arguedas A, Soley C, Kamicker BJ, et al. Single-dose extended-release azithromycin versus a 10-day regimen of amoxicillin/clavulanate for the treatment of children with acute otitis media. Int J Infect Dis 2011;15:e240-8.

63. Dowell SF, Butler JC, Giebink GS, et al. Acute otitis media: management and surveillance in an era of pneumococcal resistance—a report from the drug-resistant Streptococcus pneumoniae Therapeutic Working Group. Pediatr Infect Dis J 1999;18:1-9.

64. Pichichero ME, Casey JR. Emergence of a multiresistant serotype 19A pneumococcal strain not included in the 7-valent conjugate vaccine as an otopathogen in children. JAMA 2007;298:1772-8.

65. Sjoukes A, Venekamp RP, van de Pol AC, et al. Paracetamol (acetaminophen) or non-steroidal anti-inflammatory drugs,

66. Mayoral CE, Marino RV, Rosenfeld W, et al. Alternating anti-pyretics: is this an alternative? Pediatrics 2000;105:1009-12.

67. Flynn CA, Griffin GH, Schultz JK. Decongestants and antihistamines for acute otitis media in children. Cochrane Database Syst Rev 2004;3:CD001727.

68. American Academy of Pediatrics. Use of codeine- and dextromethorphan-containing cough remedies in children. American Academy of Pediatrics. Committee on Drugs. Pediatrics 1997; 99:918-20.

69. Manzoli L, Schioppa F, Boccia A, et al. The efficacy of influenza vaccine for healthy children: a meta-analysis evaluating potential sources of variation in efficacy estimates including study quality. Pediatr Infect Dis J 2007;26:97-106.

70. Smith NM, Bresee JS, Shay DK, et al. Prevention and Control of Influenza: recommendations of the Advisory Committee on Immunization Practices (ACIP). MMWR Recomm Rep 2006; 55:1-42.

71. Brook I, Gober AE. Prophylaxis with amoxicillin or sulfisoxazole for otitis media: effect on the recovery of penicillin-resistant bacteria from children. Clin Infect Dis 1996;22:143-5.

72. Revai K, Dobbs LA, Nair S, et al. Incidence of acute otitis media and sinusitis complicating upper respiratory tract infection: the effect of age. Pediatrics 2007;119:e1408-12.

73. Furukawa CT. The role of allergy in sinusitis in children. J Allergy Clin Immunol 1992;90:515-7.

74. Slavin RG, Spector SL, Bernstein IL, et al. The diagnosis and management of sinusitis: a practice parameter update. J Allergy Clin Immunol 2005;116:S13-47.

75. Wald ER, Dashefsky B, Byers C, et al. Frequency and severity of infections in day care. J Pediatr 1988;112:540-6.

76. Cherry, JD, Shapiro, NL. Sinusitis. In: Textbook of Pediatric Infectious Diseases, 6th ed., Feigin, RD, Cherry, JD, Demmler-Harrison, et al., eds. Philadelphia: Saunders, 2009:201.

77. Wald ER. Microbiology of acute and chronic sinusitis in children and adults. Am J Med Sci 1998;316:13-20.

78. Wald ER, Applegate KE, Bordley C, et al. Clinical practice guideline for the diagnosis and management of acute bacterial sinusitis in children aged 1 to 18 years. Pediatrics 2013;132:e262-80.

79. Wald ER, Milmoe GJ, Bowen A, et al. Acute maxillary sinusitis in children. N Engl J Med 1981;304:749-54.

80. Meltzer EO, Hamilos DL, Hadley JA, et al. Rhinosinusitis: establishing definitions for clinical research and patient care. J Allergy Clin Immunol 2004;114:155-212.

81. Bair-Merritt MH, Shah SS, Zaoutis TE, et al. Suppurative intracranial complications of sinusitis in previously healthy children. Pediatr Infect Dis J 2005;24:384-6.

82. Germiller JA, Monin DL, Sparano AM, et al. Intracranial complications of sinusitis in children and adolescents and their outcomes. Arch Otolaryngol Head Neck Surg 2006;132:969-76.

83. Wald ER, Nash D, Eickhoff J. Effectiveness of amoxicillin/clavulanate potassium in the treatment of acute bacterial sinusitis in children. Pediatrics 2009;124:9-15.

84. Jackson MA, Schutze GE. The use of systemic and topical fluoroquinolones. Pediatrics 2016;138:pii.

85. Barlan IB, Erkan E, Bakir M, et al. Intranasal budesonide spray as an adjunct to oral antibiotic therapy for acute sinusitis in children. Ann Allergy Asthma Immunol 1997;78:598-601.

86. McCormick DP, John SD, Swischuk LE, et al. A double-blind, placebo-controlled trial of decongestant-antihistamine for the treatment of sinusitis in children. Clin Pediatr (Phila) 1996;35:457-60.

87. Wang YH, Yang CP, Ku MS, et al. Efficacy of nasal irrigation in the treatment of acute sinusitis in children. Int J Pediatr Otorhinolaryngol 2009;73:1696-701.

88. Shaikh N, Wald ER. Decongestants, antihistamines and nasal irrigation for acute sinusitis in children. Cochrane Database Syst Rev 2014;10:CD007909.

89. Bisno AL, Gerber MA, Gwaltney JM, Jr., et al. Practice guidelines for the diagnosis and management of group A streptococcal pharyngitis. Infectious Diseases Society of America. Clin Infect Dis 2002;35:113-25.

90. Cherry, JD. Pharyngitis. In: Textbook of Pediatric Infectious Diseases, 6th ed, Feigin, RD, Cherry, JD, Demmler-Harrison, GJ, et al., eds. Philadelphia: Saunders, 2009:160.

91. American Academy of Pediatrics. Group A Streptococcal Infections In: Red Book: 2009 Report of the Committee on Infectious Diseases, 28th ed, Pickering, LK, ed. Elk Grove Village, IL: American Academy of Pediatrics, 2009.

92. Gerber MA. Diagnosis and treatment of pharyngitis in children. Pediatr Clin North Am 2005;52:729-47, vi.

93. Wald ER, Green MD, Schwartz B, et al. A streptococcal score card revisited. Pediatr Emerg Care 1998;14:109-11.

94. Shaikh N, Leonard E, Martin JM. Prevalence of streptococcal pharyngitis and streptococcal carriage in children: a meta-analysis. Pediatrics 2010;126:e557-64.

95. Horn DL, Zabriskie JB, Austrian R, et al. Why have group A streptococci remained susceptible to penicillin? Report on a symposium. Clin Infect Dis1998;26:1341-5.

96. Martin JM, Green M, Barbadora KA, et al. Erythromycin-resistant group A streptococci in schoolchildren in Pittsburgh. N Engl J Med 2002;346:1200-6.

97. Shulman ST, Bisno AL, Clegg HW, et al. Clinical practice guideline for the diagnosis and management of group a streptococcal pharyngitis: 2012 update by the Infectious Diseases Society of America. Clin Infect Dis 2012;55:1279-82.

98. Wozniak A, Scioscia N, Geoffroy E, et al. Importance of adhesins in the recurrence of pharyngeal infections caused by Streptococcus pyogenes. J Med Microbiol 2017;66:517-25.

99. Gerber MA, Baltimore RS, Eaton CB, et al. Prevention of rheumatic fever and diagnosis and treatment of acute Streptococcal pharyngitis: a scientific statement from the American Heart Association Rheumatic Fever, Endocarditis, and Kawasaki Disease Committee of the Council on Cardiovascular Disease in the Young, the Interdisciplinary Council on Functional Genomics and Translational Biology, and the Interdisciplinary Council on Quality of Care and Outcomes Research: endorsed by the American Academy of Pediatrics. Circulation 2009;119:1541-51.

100. Pfoh E, Wessels MR, Goldmann D, et al. Burden and economic cost of group A streptococcal pharyngitis. Pediatrics 2008; 121:229-34.

101. Arguedas A, Dagan R, Pichichero M, et al. An open-label, double tympanocentesis study of levofloxacin therapy in children with, or at high risk for, recurrent or persistent acute otitis media. Pediatr Infect Dis J 2006;25:1102-9.

102. Steele, RW. Pharyngitis and Tonsilitis. In: Textbook of Pediatric Care, 6th ed, McInery TK, Adam HM, Campbell DE, et al., eds. Elk Grove Village, IL: American Academy of Pediatrics, 2009:308.

103. Stollerman GH. Rheumatic fever. Lancet 1997;349:935-42.

104. Edmonson MB, Farwell KR. Relationship between the clinical likelihood of group a streptococcal pharyngitis and the sensitivity of a rapid antigen-detection test in a pediatric practice. Pediatrics 2005;115:280-5.

105. Cohen JF, Bertille N, Cohen R, et al. Rapid antigen detection test for group A streptococcus in children with pharyngitis. Cochrane Database Syst Rev 2016;CD010502.

106. Batsford SR, Mezzano S, Mihatsch M, et al. Is the nephritogenic antigen in post-streptococcal glomerulonephritis pyrogenic exotoxin B (SPE B) or GAPDH? Kidney Int 2005;68:1120-9.

107. Del Mar CB, Glasziou PP, Spinks AB. Antibiotics for sore throat. Cochrane Database Syst Rev 2000;4:CD000023.

108. Catanzaro FJ, Stetson CA, Morris AJ, et al. The role of the streptococcus in the pathogenesis of rheumatic fever. Am J Med 1954; 17:749-56.

109. Snellman LW, Stang HJ, Stang JM, et al. Duration of positive throat cultures for group A streptococci after initiation of antibiotic therapy. Pediatrics 1993;91:1166-70.

110. Peloso UC, De Souza JC, Botino MA, et al. Penicillin concentrations in sera and tonsils after intramuscular administration of benzathine penicillin G to children. Pediatr Infect Dis J 2003;22:1075-8.

111. Bradley JS, Dudley MN, Drusano GL. Predicting efficacy of anti-infectives with pharmacodynamics and Monte Carlo simulation. Pediatr Infect Dis J 2003;22:982-92; quiz 93-5.

112. Casey JR, Pichichero ME. Meta-analysis of cephalosporin versus penicillin treatment of group A streptococcal tonsillopharyngitis in children. Pediatrics 2004;113:866-82.

113. Pichichero ME. A review of evidence supporting the American Academy of Pediatrics recommendation for prescribing cephalosporin antibiotics for penicillin-allergic patients. Pediatrics 2005;115:1048-57.

114. Kaplan EL, Oakes JM, Johnson DR. Unexpected individual clinical site variation in eradication rates of group a streptococci by penicillin in multisite clinical trials. Pediatr Infect Dis J 2007;26:1110-6.

115. van Driel ML, De Sutter AI, Habraken H, et al. Different antibiotic treatments for group A streptococcal pharyngitis. Cochrane Database Syst Rev 2016;CD004406.

116. Gerber MA. Treatment failures and carriers: perception or problems? Pediatr Infect Dis J 1994;13:576-9.

117. Kaplan EL. The group A streptococcal upper respiratory tract carrier state: an enigma. J Pediatr 1980;97:337-45.

118. Kaplan EL, Gastanaduy AS, Huwe BB. The role of the carrier in treatment failures after antibiotic for group A streptococci in the upper respiratory tract. J Lab Clin Med 1981;98:326-35.

119. Mahakit P, Vicente JG, Butt DI, et al. Oral clindamycin 300 mg BID compared with oral amoxicillin/clavulanic acid 1 g BID in the outpatient treatment of acute recurrent pharyngotonsillitis caused by group a beta-hemolytic streptococci: an international, multicenter, randomized, investigator-blinded, prospective trial in patients between the ages of 12 and 60 years. Clin Ther 2006;28:99-109.

120. Alho OP, Koivunen P, Penna T, et al. Tonsillectomy versus watchful waiting in recurrent streptococcal pharyngitis in adults: randomised controlled trial. BMJ 2007;334:939.

121. Burlet E, HogenEsch H, Dunham A, et al. Evaluation of the potency, neutralizing antibody response, and stability of a recombinant fusion protein vaccine for streptococcus pyogenes. AAPS 2017;19:875-81.

122. Nordstrom T, Pandey M, Calcutt A, et al. Enhancing vaccine efficacy by engineering a complex synthetic peptide to become a super immunogen. J Immunol 2017;199:2794-802.

123. Le J, Nguyen T, Law AV, et al. Adverse drug reactions among children over a 10-year period. Pediatrics 2006;118:555-62.

124. Dellit TH, Owens RC, McGowan JE, Jr., et al. Infectious Diseases Society of America and the Society for Healthcare Epidemiology of America guidelines for developing an institutional program to enhance antimicrobial stewardship. Clin Infect Dis 2007;44:159-77.

125. Tamur S, Gosselin S. A call for advocacy: standardized concentration and weight-based dosing of acetaminophen may enhance the therapeutic benefit and reduce the risk for harm. Paediatr Child Health 2015;20:235-6.

CHAPTER 39

Lower Respiratory Tract Infections
Kristin C. Klein, Pharm.D., FPPA, BCPPS

LEARNING OBJECTIVES

1. List the risk factors associated with development of severe bronchiolitis, pertussis, acute bronchitis, influenza, and community-acquired pneumonia.

2. List the goals of therapy for the treatment of bronchiolitis, pertussis, acute bronchitis, influenza, and community-acquired pneumonia.

3. Describe the role of palivizumab in the prevention of bronchiolitis.

4. Describe when post-exposure prophylaxis would be beneficial for a child exposed to pertussis.

5. Describe situations in which the use of antivirals might be beneficial for the treatment of influenza in pediatric patients.

6. Formulate an appropriate antibiotic regimen for a pediatric patient with pertussis, community-acquired pneumonia, lung abscess, empyema, or necrotizing pneumonia on the basis of age, infecting organism, and severity of illness.

ABBREVIATIONS IN THIS CHAPTER

AUC	Area under the curve
CAP	Community-acquired pneumonia
CDC	Centers for Disease Control and Prevention
LRTI	Lower respiratory tract infection
MIC	Minimum inhibitory concentration
MRSA	Methicillin-resistant *Staphylococcus aureus*
PCR	Polymerase chain reaction
RSV	Respiratory syncytial virus

INTRODUCTION

Lower respiratory tract infections (LRTIs) are a significant cause of morbidity and mortality in pediatric patients. A survey of Medicaid enrollees showed that close to 20% of pediatric enrollees were hospitalized for LRTIs.[1] Of these patients, 64% had a diagnosis of pneumonia, 38% had bronchiolitis, and 7.7% had influenza. This chapter will discuss the management of LRTIs commonly observed in pediatric patients.

BRONCHIOLITIS

Bronchiolitis is the most common LRTI in infants younger than 12 months and is usually the result of a viral infection.[2] Bronchiolitis is characterized by inflammation of the bronchioles and is often associated with wheezing.[3] In addition to inflammation, bronchiolitis is associated with airway edema, epithelial lining necrosis, mucous production, and bronchospasm.[3] Infection occurs after exposure to infected respiratory droplets. The incubation period is generally 4–6 days, but it may last up to 4 weeks in young infants.[2]

EPIDEMIOLOGY

In the United States, bronchiolitis usually occurs during winter months, spanning from November through April. Many viruses have been implicated as causing bronchiolitis, but respiratory syncytial virus (RSV) has been most closely associated.[2-4] In addition to RSV, viruses associated with bronchiolitis include rhinovirus, human metapneumovirus, human bocavirus, influenza A and B, adenovirus, and parainfluenza viruses.[2,5,6]

It is estimated that more than 2 million children younger than age 5 years require medical intervention each year in the United States because of bronchiolitis from RSV.[7,8] Bronchiolitis is a significant cause of hospitalization, with an estimated cost of $1.7 billion to the U.S. health care system during 2009.[2] By age 2 years, almost 100% of children will contract RSV.[8] Reinfection with RSV can occur throughout a person's lifetime.[3] An estimated 100 children die of RSV bronchiolitis annually in the United States.[2] In one study, an overall mortality rate of 0.9% for RSV infection was reported.[9] All the infants who died in this study had underlying medical conditions, such as chronic lung disease, cardiac abnormalities, chromosomal abnormalities, or immunodeficiency. None of the deaths occurred in previously healthy children.

Children who develop RSV bronchiolitis are also at higher risk of recurrent wheezing episodes throughout childhood and adolescence.[10,11] The link between wheezing and RSV bronchiolitis is not fully understood. One theory is that children who are predisposed to developing asthma are more likely to have severe RSV disease. Alternatively, severe RSV infections may cause lung damage, making a child more susceptible to developing asthma later in life. In one study, children who developed RSV bronchiolitis before age 1 year were followed until age 18 years to determine whether recurrent wheezing or asthma persisted into early adulthood.[10] Recurrent wheezing or asthma occurred in 39% of the RSV-infected group compared with 9% of the control group at age 18 years. A Kaplan-Meier plot measuring time free from an asthma or recurrent wheezing diagnosis demonstrated significantly shorter time to diagnosis in the RSV group at age 18 years, showing that this effect persists at least through late adolescence.[10]

ETIOLOGY

Children at highest risk of developing severe RSV bronchiolitis include those with prematurity (especially younger than 29 weeks' gestation), chronic lung disease, bronchopulmonary dysplasia, or congenital heart disease.[12,13] Additional risk factors associated with contracting RSV include birth within 6 months of the RSV season, product of multiple births, attendance at day care, school-age siblings, exposure to cigarette smoke, neuromuscular disease, and low socioeconomic status.[4,9,13]

CLINICAL PRESENTATION

For most children, bronchiolitis initially presents with cold-like symptoms, such as low-grade fever, rhinorrhea, and cough.[3,13] Tachypnea, wheezing, retractions, and nasal flaring may also be present later in the disease course.[3,13] Bronchiolitis is generally a self-limited condition. Most children with bronchiolitis experience complete resolution of their symptoms within 8–15 days without needing medical intervention, although cough may persist for up to 3 weeks.[14] Those who experience more severe disease might present with the additional symptoms of hypoxia, cyanosis, apnea, and respiratory distress.[3,13] Infants with more severe disease will likely require hospitalization, may require mechanical ventilation, and, in extreme cases, may require extracorporeal membrane oxygenation until the lung injury has improved.

DIAGNOSIS

The American Academy of Pediatrics recommends diagnosing bronchiolitis based on clinical presentation, a thorough history and physical examination, and investigation of known risk factors in a child presenting with probable bronchiolitis.[3] To make a diagnosis of RSV bronchiolitis, one should also consider the time of year and the respiratory viruses circulating in the community. Infants presenting with probable bronchiolitis should be evaluated for risk factors for severe disease (e.g., history of premature birth, younger than 12 weeks, chronic lung disease, congenital heart defect, immunodeficiency) to help determine whether hospitalization is warranted. Other non-specific indicators of infection, such as white blood cell count, are not clinically useful in diagnosing bronchiolitis.

Viral cultures and antigen testing of nasopharyngeal swabs and chest radiography are of limited benefit in diagnosing bronchiolitis because their results do not help predict the severity of illness. The polymerase chain reaction (PCR) tests for many of the viruses that commonly cause bronchiolitis are now available commercially, which may allow faster, more reliable identification of these viruses; however, routine use is not recommended because the results will not influence decisions regarding treatment or isolation practices in hospitalized patients.

PREVENTION

Palivizumab is a humanized monoclonal antibody specific for RSV. It is labeled for prevention of LRTIs from RSV in high-risk pediatric populations.[15] Palivizumab is currently the only product licensed for the prevention of RSV infection in the United States.

Palivizumab is administered at a dose of 15 mg/kg intramuscularly every month during the RSV season for high-risk populations. The RSV season generally occurs from late October or early November to late March or early April; however, prophylaxis should not be initiated until the local RSV season has begun. The season officially starts when the average RSV positivity rate is 10% or greater in the community for 2 consecutive weeks.[16] The season ends when the community's positivity rate drops to less than 10%.[16] The American Academy of Pediatrics recommends a maximum of five doses of palivizumab, although children born during the RSV season will need fewer doses.[17] Prophylaxis should continue until a child has received the maximum number of doses recommended, even if the community positivity rate drops to less than 10%. Palivizumab is generally well tolerated. The most common adverse effects include fever and injection site reactions, such as pain, redness, or swelling.[18]

The American Academy of Pediatrics recommends palivizumab prophylaxis for the following pediatric populations during the first year of life: all infants born before 29 weeks, 0 days' gestation; infants born before 32 weeks, 0 days' gestation who require more than 21% oxygen for at least the first 28 days of life; and infants with a "hemodynamically significant" congenital heart defect.[17] Prophylaxis for RSV during the second year of life may be considered for children with chronic lung disease who continue to require medical therapy (e.g., supplemental oxygen, corticosteroids, diuretics) within 6 months of the RSV season. Palivizumab may also be considered for infants younger than 12 months who are profoundly immunocompromised or who have a congenital or anatomical anomaly that makes clearing of respiratory secretions difficult (e.g., muscular dystrophy). Table 1 provides more information regarding the use of palivizumab for prophylaxis of RSV bronchiolitis.

TREATMENT

The goals of therapy for bronchiolitis are to maintain oxygenation, maintain adequate hydration, and reduce fever. The treatment of bronchiolitis is primarily supportive. Children with bronchiolitis may exhibit a decrease in oxygen saturations because of airway

Table 1. Indications for Palivizumab Prophylaxis[17]

Indication by Age	Max Doses per Season
Premature infants < 29 wk, 0 days' gestation during 1st yr of life	5
Premature infants < 32 wk, 0 days' gestation during 1st yr of life[a,b]	5
Infants < 24 mo with chronic lung disease[b,c]	5

[a]Indicated if the infant required oxygen for at least 28 days after birth.
[b]Indicated if the child has a "hemodynamically significant" cardiac lesion (e.g., cyanotic heart disease, moderate or severe pulmonary hypertension, receiving therapy for congestive heart failure).
[c]Indicated if the child requires oxygen or pharmacologic treatment of lung disease within 6 mo of respiratory syncytial virus season.
Max = maximum.

edema, excessive mucous production, and bronchospasm. Children with signs or symptoms consistent with bronchiolitis may receive supplemental oxygen if their oxygen saturations decrease to less than 90%.[3] Intravenous fluids may also be necessary to avoid dehydration. Chest physiotherapy and heliox (a blend of helium and oxygen) are unlikely to improve outcomes in infants with bronchiolitis, and should not be used.[3,19]

PHARMACOLOGIC THERAPY

Both α-adrenergic (e.g., racemic epinephrine) and β-adrenergic (e.g., albuterol) bronchodilators have been used in the management of bronchiolitis. A 2014 Cochrane review evaluated 30 studies to determine the effectiveness of bronchodilators for children with bronchiolitis.[20] For children who received bronchodilators as outpatients, there was no significant reduction in hospitalization rates.[20] For children who received bronchodilators as inpatients, there was no significant reduction in length of hospital stay.[20] The American Academy of Pediatrics does not recommend the routine use of bronchodilators for children with bronchiolitis.[3]

Corticosteroids such as dexamethasone and methylprednisolone have been theorized to reduce inflammation associated with bronchiolitis. A 2013 Cochrane review evaluating the use of corticosteroids for bronchiolitis did not show a significant reduction in hospitalizations, nor did they show a significant decrease in length of hospital stay.[21] Corticosteroids combined with nebulized racemic epinephrine decreased length of stay; however, more data are necessary before this combination can be recommended.[3,21] The American Academy of Pediatrics does not recommend the routine use of corticosteroids in children with bronchiolitis.[3]

The use of nebulized hypertonic saline (3%–12%) was identified as a treatment modality for clearing mucous plugs in individuals with cystic fibrosis in the mid-2000s. In recent years, its use has been studied in bronchiolitis. A Cochrane review found that children who received 3% hypertonic saline had significantly shorter lengths of hospital stay and significantly lower clinical severity scores during the first 3 days of therapy (lower scores indicate less severe response to disease).[22] The authors concluded that the use of nebulized hypertonic saline 3% may be beneficial in reducing length of hospital stay and severity scores for infants with bronchiolitis, although they comment that the level of evidence is only low to moderate. A major confounder of studies evaluating the use of hypertonic saline is that many of the studies also used bronchodilators concomitantly with hypertonic saline, limiting the applicability of the data.

Antibiotics have been used in children with bronchiolitis; however, their use does not result in significant clinical improvement.[23] Bronchiolitis is primarily the result of a viral infection. As such, antibiotics should be reserved for children with a concomitant bacterial infection.[3]

SUMMARY

Treatment of bronchiolitis remains supportive in nature. Because smoking exposure is a modifiable risk factor for bronchiolitis, parents and caregivers should be counseled to quit smoking. If that is not possible, they should be counseled not to smoke in the home, car, or other locations where their children are present, and they should change clothing after smoking. Families should also be counseled regarding proper hand hygiene, including washing hands before and after contact with a sick child.

PERTUSSIS

Pertussis, commonly known as *whooping cough*, is a respiratory tract infection caused by the gram-negative organism *Bordetella pertussis*. Pertussis is highly contagious. Infection occurs through exposure to contaminated respiratory droplets after close contact with an infected individual. The incubation period for pertussis is usually 7–10 days after exposure but may last as long as 21 days.[24] Infected individuals are most contagious during the first 1–2 weeks of infection (known as the *catarrhal phase*) and within 2 weeks of the onset of cough.[24]

EPIDEMIOLOGY

Before a pertussis vaccine became available in the 1940s, more than 200,000 people became infected with *B. pertussis* annually in the United States.[25] Pertussis infections decreased dramatically after routine use of the pertussis vaccine; however, the number of pertussis infections reported to the Centers for Disease Control and Prevention (CDC) has been increasing since the 1980s, reaching a high of more than 48,000 cases in 2012.[25,26]

Before the availability of a vaccine, pertussis was a disease primarily found in school-age children. Since the early 2000s, the incidence of pertussis has increased in infants (younger than 12 months), adolescents, and adults.[25] From January 1, 2000, through December 31, 2016, almost 340,000 cases of pertussis were reported in the United States.[27] About 75% of the cases were in children younger than 18 years, with the highest percentage of cases (27.7%) in children age 11–18 years. It is important to note that 15.1% of the reported cases of pertussis were in children younger than age 1 year because this population is at the highest risk of hospitalization (49.9% of reported hospitalizations) and death (88.8% of reported deaths).[27]

For several reasons, a shift in disease burden away from school-age children has been observed. First, an improvement in the ability to reliably diagnose pertussis and an increase in its awareness—both in the lay public and in health care practitioners—likely contributed to an increase in the diagnosis of pertussis in other populations.[28] Additional factors that have been suggested include a decrease in vaccine coverage (i.e., fewer people receiving the vaccine) and waning of vaccine-induced immunity over time.[28] One study demonstrated that effectiveness of the tetanus, diphtheria, acellular pertussis vaccine declined significantly in recipients who were more than 2 years post-vaccination compared with those who were less than 2 years from receipt of the vaccine (34% vs. 69%, p<0.01).[29] Unvaccinated or undervaccinated adolescents and adults often serve as the reservoir for infants infected with *B. pertussis*.

The most common complication of pertussis in infants is pneumonia. Of infants who are hospitalized for complications of pertussis, 23% will have pneumonia.[26] Pneumonia is far less common in adolescents and adults, with only 2% of each population developing pneumonia.[26] Other pulmonary complications that have been described with pertussis include cyanosis, apnea, pulmonary hypertension, hypoxia, and need for oxygen supplementation or mechanical ventilation.[25,30,31] Other complications reported in infants include poor feeding, anorexia, seizures, and encephalopathy, possibly because of hypoxia caused by coughing.[25,30]

Infants are at the highest risk of death from pertussis infection, especially those who are too young to be vaccinated (or completely vaccinated) against pertussis. A total of 72 deaths were reported to the CDC from 2008–2011, 60 (83%) of which occurred in infants younger than 3 months.[25] Hispanic ethnicity has also been identified as a risk factor for death from pertussis.[30,31]

Adolescents and adults are much less likely to exhibit significant morbidity because of pertussis. Pertussis also has a much lower mortality rate in adolescents and adults, occurring in only 0.1% of infected individuals in these age ranges.[32] The most common complications of pertussis reported in adolescents and adults include loss of bladder control, rib fractures, pneumothoraces, anorexia, and weight loss.[25,26,32] Rib fracture is more likely to occur in individuals with profound paroxysmal coughing and in those with osteoporosis.[32] Intracranial hemorrhages have also been reported but are more common in individuals who receive anticoagulants.[32] Seizures and encephalopathy have also been reported in this population, but they occur in less than 1% of those infected.[32]

ETIOLOGY

Disease from pertussis is primarily caused by toxin production by the organism, which causes impaired mucociliary function and lung inflammation.[33] This impairment and inflammation leads to an inability to clear respiratory secretions and the associated cough.

CLINICAL PRESENTATION

Pertussis infection has three phases: *catarrhal*, *paroxysmal*, and *convalescent*. The catarrhal phase usually lasts 1–2 weeks, and symptoms generally mimic those of the common cold (e.g., rhinorrhea, sneezing, cough, and low-grade fever).[25] Infected individuals are most likely to be contagious during this phase of the disease. The next phase, the paroxysmal phase, may last between 1 and 6 weeks and is when the classic paroxysmal cough occurs, followed by an inspiratory whoop.[25] The cough is characterized by a burst of persistent, rapid coughs (known as *paroxysms*) and the accompanying whoop that is caused by a narrowed glottis during a prolonged inspiratory period. Children, especially young infants, can become cyanotic and may appear visually ill during these episodes.[25] The paroxysms occur more often at night and increase in frequency throughout this phase of the disease. Post-tussive emesis is also common during this phase, especially in adolescents.[26,34] The convalescent, or recovery, phase, during which symptoms slowly improve as the paroxysms begin to resolve, may last weeks to months.[25] Unvaccinated infants and children are more likely to have severe disease. Older children who have been vaccinated, adolescents, and adults typically have less severe disease and may not present with the classic symptoms of pertussis, although they often present with a nagging cough that has persisted for several weeks.[25,34]

DIAGNOSIS

The diagnosis of pertussis is often made using a combination of clinical presentation and microbiologic tests. Pertussis should be highly suspected in any child or adolescent who presents with a cough of more than 2 weeks' duration.[14] White blood cell counts are often elevated during pertussis and show lymphocyte predominance on a differential.[25,34]

Several laboratory tests may be used to confirm the presence of *B. pertussis*. Bacterial culture has historically been the gold standard for diagnosing pertussis; however, isolating *B. pertussis* by culture is often difficult because it is a fastidious organism. Cultures can be negative once an infected individual has been symptomatic for 2 weeks, if antimicrobial therapy has been started, or if the individual was previously vaccinated.[24] A more sensitive testing method is PCR assay, especially if the individual presents later in the disease course.[24,25,34] The PCR assay also has the advantages of being readily available in the community setting and a rapid turnaround time because it does not measure the presence of living organisms.

PREVENTION

The primary mode for preventing the spread of pertussis is through vaccination of susceptible individuals against *B. pertussis*, especially those who may be exposed to infants who are not fully vaccinated. In an attempt to address the issue of providing protection against pertussis to young infants, some institutions have implemented immunization clinics to administer the tetanus, diphtheria, acellular pertussis vaccine to pregnant women, household members, and other close contacts who may care for young infants.[35]

Several vaccines are available to protect against pertussis. Confusion regarding the various acronyms used to discuss the available pertussis vaccines is common, so it is important for health care practitioners to understand the differences and indications for each vaccine. Further information regarding the pertussis-containing vaccines may be found in the Pediatric Vaccines chapter.

TREATMENT

The primary goal of treatment for pertussis is to reduce transmission to infants and children at high risk of significant morbidity or mortality, such as infants younger than 4 months and children who are immunocompromised. Antimicrobial therapy initiated during the catarrhal phase of pertussis can hasten recovery from the disease. Once a cough has developed, antimicrobial therapy will not contribute to symptomatic improvement, but it can limit the spread of disease to susceptible individuals.[24] Macrolide antibiotics are the treatment of choice for pertussis. Information regarding the dose and duration of antibiotics for pertussis treatment is available in Table 2.

Erythromycin is the oldest macrolide antibiotic on the market in the United States and has, historically, been used as a first-line approach in the treatment of pertussis. Erythromycin is the only macrolide antibiotic labeled for use in infants younger than 6 months; however, when used in young infants, it has been associated with an increased risk of infantile hypertrophic pyloric stenosis.[24,36] This risk appears to be highest during the first 2 weeks of life and when given for 14 or more days.[36] Erythromycin, which should be administered four times daily, has a high rate of gastrointestinal adverse effects, including abdominal cramping, nausea, vomiting, and diarrhea. Erythromycin is a potent inhibitor of the cytochrome P450 3A subclass with many drug–drug interactions.[37] Although QT prolongation has been associated with all the macrolide antibiotics, erythromycin has the highest risk of QT prolongation.[37] Because of these factors, erythromycin is no longer the macrolide antibiotic of choice for pertussis.

Azithromycin is generally better tolerated than the other macrolide antibiotics. Azithromycin has the advantages of once-daily dosing and a shortened length of therapy. The most common adverse effects include gastrointestinal upset, diarrhea, vomiting, headache, and dizziness. Azithromycin is a less potent inhibitor of the cytochrome P450 system than the other macrolide antibiotics and has fewer drug–drug interactions. Although pyloric stenosis in young infants has been reported with azithromycin, the incidence appears to be much lower than that associated with erythromycin.[24] For these reasons, azithromycin is often used as the first-line agent for pertussis, even in infants younger than 6 months. Infants younger than 6 months receiving azithromycin therapy should be closely monitored for signs of pyloric stenosis.[36,37]

For children or adolescents allergic to or intolerant of macrolide antibiotics, trimethoprim/sulfamethoxazole may be used as an alternative.[37] Infants younger than 2 months should not receive this combination drug unless the benefits of therapy outweigh the risks of hyperbilirubinemia and kernicterus that can result from the displacement of bilirubin from its protein-binding site.

POST-EXPOSURE PROPHYLAXIS

Pertussis is a highly contagious, infectious disease. Up to 80% of people who have close contact with an infected person also contract pertussis; as a result, preventive antibiotics should be considered in certain situations.[37] The CDC considers a close contact anyone who has face-to-face contact within 3 feet of an infected person.[37] Anyone who has been exposed to an infected person's oral, nasal, or respiratory secretions (e.g., nurse, parent, day care provider) also qualifies as a close contact.[37] Anyone who shares a confined space (e.g., car, bed, crib) with an infected person for at least 1 hour also qualifies as a close contact.[37] If a household contact of an infected person develops a cough, then the contact should receive a course of antibiotics for pertussis.[37] If a person develops pertussis in a household with an infant younger than 12 months or a pregnant woman in her third trimester, then all members of the household should receive preventive antibiotics.[37] Preventive antibiotics may also be considered in close contacts at high risk of developing severe disease or complications from pertussis, such as children who are immunocompromised or who have chronic lung disease.[37] Preventive antibiotics may be considered in other individuals who have had close contact with an infected person, but the benefits of therapy should be weighed against the risks of adverse effects before therapy is initiated. Antimicrobial therapy and duration of antimicrobials used for post-exposure prophylaxis are the same as those used to treat pertussis.

SUMMARY

Anyone with a cough lasting more than 2 weeks should be presumed to have pertussis until proven otherwise. Macrolide antibiotics, especially azithromycin, are the mainstay of treatment for pertussis. Therapy duration ranges from 5 to 14 days, depending on the antibiotic selected. Preventing pertussis transmission to at-risk populations is the most important step in treating pertussis. Parents and caregivers should be encouraged to have their children vaccinated against pertussis on time and according to schedule. If a household contact of an infant younger than 12 months or a pregnant woman in her third trimester contracts pertussis, then all members of the household should receive preventive antibiotics.

ACUTE BRONCHITIS

Acute bronchitis is a self-limited respiratory tract infection characterized by a cough that can last up to 2–3 weeks.[38] Acute bronchitis is usually triggered by a viral infection and is associated with inflammation of the bronchioles, airway hyperresponsiveness, and mucous production.[39]

Table 2. Antibiotics for Pertussis: Dosing and Duration of Therapy by Age[37]

Antibiotic	Infants ≤ 5 Mo	Infants/Children ≥ 6 Mo	Adolescents/Adults	Duration (days)
Azithromycin	10 mg/kg/day	10 mg/kg on day 1; then 5 mg/kg/day on days 2–5	500 mg on day 1; then 250 mg/day on days 2–5	5
Erythromycin[a]	10 mg/kg/dose QID	10 mg/kg/dose QID	500 mg QID	14
TMP/SMZ[b,c,d]	4 mg/kg/dose BID	4 mg/kg/dose BID	160 mg (1 double-strength tablet) BID	14

[a]Not recommended for infants younger than 1 month.
[b]Alternative agent for infants, children, or adolescents with an allergy or intolerance to macrolide antibiotics.
[c]Dosing is based on the trimethoprim component.
[d]Not recommended for infants younger than 2 mo.
BID = twice daily; QID = four times daily; TMP/SMZ = trimethoprim/sulfamethoxazole.

EPIDEMIOLOGY

Cough is one of the most common reasons for seeking care in the ambulatory setting, accounting for about 5% of outpatient visits.[40] It is estimated that 5%–10% of children have a chronic cough.[41] Although acute bronchitis is largely caused by a viral infection, the CDC estimates that patients with viral respiratory tract infections inappropriately receive antibiotics 50% of the time.[42] More than $2 billion is spent on over-the-counter cough medications per year in the United States.[41]

ETIOLOGY

Acute bronchitis is usually the result of infection from respiratory viruses, such as influenza A and B, parainfluenza, and RSV; however, cultures are rarely performed at the time of diagnosis.[38] Although *Mycoplasma pneumoniae*, *Chlamydophila pneumoniae*, and *B. pertussis* have also been associated with bronchitis, bacterial causes have been implicated in less than 10% of those with a diagnosis of bronchitis.[38]

CLINICAL PRESENTATION

Children who present with acute bronchitis typically have a cough with or without phlegm production. Because acute bronchitis is predominantly caused by respiratory viruses, its symptoms are often difficult to distinguish from those of the common cold. Acute bronchitis is a self-limited condition that should resolve within about 3 weeks.[38] A child who presents with a cough lasting more than 3 weeks should be evaluated for other conditions (e.g., pertussis).

DIAGNOSIS

In making a diagnosis of acute bronchitis, other explanations for the cough need to be evaluated and excluded.[38] A child with a cold may present with a cough; however, other symptoms, such as rhinorrhea and congestion, are often present.[43] Symptoms of a cold also usually resolve within 10–14 days. A child presenting with pneumonia usually has additional signs or symptoms, such as fever, tachycardia, tachypnea, or diminished breath sounds on auscultation, which rule out acute bronchitis as the cause of the cough.[38] A child with a history of asthma who presents with a cough should be evaluated for an acute asthma exacerbation. Once other possible explanations for a cough have been excluded, the diagnosis of acute bronchitis can be made. Viral and bacterial cultures should not be performed routinely in children with the presumed diagnosis of acute bronchitis.[38]

TREATMENT

The primary treatment goal for acute bronchitis is to keep the child comfortable by ameliorating symptoms until the infection subsides. Antibiotic therapy is not warranted for individuals with the presumptive diagnosis of acute bronchitis.[38] The overuse of antibiotics for conditions including acute bronchitis led to a campaign by the CDC called "Be Antibiotics Aware," designed to educate the public and health care practitioners regarding the appropriate use of antibiotics. More information about the Be Antibiotics Aware campaign is available at the campaign website at https://www.cdc.gov/antibiotic-use/index.html.

Medications used to alleviate the symptoms associated with acute bronchitis have largely been proven ineffective and may cause more harm than good in children. Antitussive agents, such as dextromethorphan or codeine, should not be used in children.[38,44] These agents have not shown efficacy; moreover, they have been associated with unintentional overdoses.[44,45] Infants and young children are also at increased risk of adverse effects from codeine because of immature hepatic function. The performance of the glucuronidation pathway, which is necessary to metabolize codeine, is highly variable in children younger than 10 years.[44,46] Decongestants and other cough or cold products should also be avoided in children, especially those younger than 4 years. In January 2008, the U.S. Food and Drug Administration issued a Public Health Advisory stating that over-the-counter cough and cold products should not be used in children younger than 2 years because of serious adverse effects reported in this population.[47] Later that year, members of the Consumer Healthcare Products Association voluntarily agreed to change the package labeling of pediatric over-the-counter cough and cold products to state that they should not be used in children younger than 4 years.[47,48] An alternative to over-the-counter cough products, honey, when administered before bedtime to a child with an acute cough, has shown some success in decreasing the frequency and severity of cough and in improving the sleep of both the child and the parent.[49] However, honey should not be given to infants younger than 12 months because of the risk of developing infant botulism.

SUMMARY

Acute bronchitis is generally a self-limited condition that resolves on its own within 3 weeks of symptom development. Other possible explanations for cough (e.g., asthma, common cold, pneumonia) should be ruled out before a diagnosis of acute bronchitis is made. Antibiotic therapy is not warranted for children with acute bronchitis. Over-the-counter cough and cold products are not useful in children and are considered unsafe in children younger than 4 years. Parents and caregivers should be counseled that acute bronchitis is the result of a viral infection and that antibiotic therapy will not help relieve their child's symptoms.

INFLUENZA

Influenza is transmitted through close contact with infected respiratory droplets. Infection usually occurs within 3–4 days of exposure.[50] Infected individuals may remain symptomatic for up to 7 days.[50,51] Children who contract influenza may shed virus for 10 or more days.[50] School-age children have the highest attack rate and serve as the primary source of infection during influenza outbreaks.[51] Influenza follows a seasonal pattern and typically occurs during the winter months.

EPIDEMIOLOGY

During the 2018–2019 influenza season, the viruses circulating predominately were the 2009 pandemic H1N1 and H3N2, both influenza A strains.[52] Although adults older than 65 years are at highest risk of hospitalization because of influenza, children younger than 4 years had a hospitalization rate of 73.6/100,000 people (through Week 18 of 2019).[52] A total of 186 pediatric influenza deaths were reported in the United States during the 2017–2018 season, and 108 pediatric deaths were reported through Week 18 of 2019 during the 2018–2019 season.[52]

Children younger than 2 years and those with comorbid conditions, such as asthma or immunosuppression, are at highest risk of secondary complications from influenza.[50] Children with a history of asthma and those younger than 5 years have a higher risk of developing pneumonia after infection with influenza.[50] Children with influenza-associated pneumonia are at higher risk of admission to an intensive care unit, respiratory failure, and death. Other complications of influenza infection in children include febrile seizures, myocarditis, pericarditis, encephalopathy, and Reye syndrome.[50] Reye syndrome has been described in children younger than 18 years who were infected with influenza or varicella and who received aspirin therapy.[51]

ETIOLOGY

Most influenza infections worldwide are caused by influenza A or B.[53] Influenza A causes moderate to severe disease in individuals of all ages.[51] Influenza B typically causes milder disease and primarily affects children.[51] Over time, gene mutations in the surface proteins of influenza result in subtle changes to the influenza subtypes, which circulate worldwide; this evolution is known as *antigenic drift*.[53] These drifts can result in community epidemics and require annual changes to the influenza A and B subtypes contained within the influenza vaccine. Another type of gene mutation, known as *antigenic shift*, occurs only in influenza A viruses and results in dramatic changes in the hemagglutinin or neuraminidase surface proteins of the virus.[53] This shift results in a new viral strain that can lead to a pandemic if the virus is able to sustain person-to-person transmission. An antigenic shift occurred in 2009 with the novel influenza A H1N1 pandemic, in which it was estimated that 60 million individuals contracted this strain in the United States.[51] This pandemic resulted in more than 270,000 hospitalizations and 12,500 deaths in both children and adults.[51]

CLINICAL PRESENTATION

The most common symptoms associated with influenza are fever, myalgias, sore throat, cough, rhinorrhea, and general malaise.[50] Children infected with influenza may also present with otitis media, nausea, and vomiting. Children younger than 5 years are less likely to present with the classic symptoms of fever or cough.[50] Signs and symptoms of influenza generally resolve within 3–7 days in uncomplicated cases.

DIAGNOSIS

Diagnosis of influenza in the outpatient setting may be made on the basis of clinical presentation and knowledge of the respiratory viruses circulating in the community. Clinical diagnosis is nonspecific and may be of limited benefit because many respiratory viruses present with similar signs and symptoms. Microbiologic testing to confirm the diagnosis of influenza is useful to guide therapy. Microbiologic tests for influenza include viral culture, antigen testing, and PCR. The most common microbiologic tests used to detect influenza in the community are the rapid diagnostic tests, which can detect the presence of influenza from a nasopharyngeal swab within 15–30 minutes.[54] Many of the rapid diagnostic tests can be used in any outpatient setting, making them convenient to use in a physician's office. The rapid diagnostic tests are immunoassays, which have a high degree of specificity but a sensitivity of only 50% to 70% compared with viral culture or PCR.[54] As a result, there is a higher possibility of yielding a false-negative result, especially when community rates of influenza are high.[54] During community outbreaks of influenza, practitioners should consider using a molecular test, such as reverse transcription-PCR, to confirm negative rapid diagnostic tests.[54]

PREVENTION

Vaccination of all individuals older than 6 months, including adults, against influenza is the most effective way to prevent transmission of the disease. Parents, caregivers, and children should also be instructed to wash their hands frequently to prevent the spread of disease. The Pediatric Vaccines chapter provides a more detailed discussion of the influenza vaccines.

TREATMENT

The goals of therapy for treating influenza in children are to alleviate the associated symptoms and prevent the spread of infection. Analgesic antipyretics such as acetaminophen are useful for managing fever and myalgias associated with influenza. Antiviral agents may also be beneficial in reducing the duration of symptoms in some children.

Two classes of antivirals have activity against influenza: the adamantanes and the neuraminidase inhibitors. The adamantanes (amantadine and rimantadine) do not have activity against influenza B, but until recently they did exhibit activity against influenza A.[50] Influenza resistance to the adamantanes has been increasing for the past 10 years. During the 2009–2010 influenza season, 100% of the seasonal influenza A H3N2 viruses were resistant to the adamantanes, and 99.8% of the pandemic influenza A H1N1 viruses tested were resistant to them.[55] Adamantanes also have unfavorable adverse effect profiles, including irritability, anxiety, hallucinations, and abnormal dreams. For these reasons, the use of adamantanes is not appropriate for the treatment or prevention of influenza infections.

The neuraminidase inhibitors (oseltamivir, zanamivir, and peramivir) have good activity against both influenza A and B (more than 99% susceptibility), although influenza A resistance to oseltamivir has been documented.[56] The neuraminidase inhibitors are the agents of choice for the treatment and prevention of influenza in children.

Many children with suspected influenza infections who present with minor febrile illnesses will not require antiviral therapy. The use of oseltamivir in children age 1–3 years reduced the duration of influenza symptoms to a median of 3.5 days when therapy was initiated within 24 hours of symptom onset.[57] Because antiviral therapy may shorten the duration of influenza symptoms by only about 1 day on average, the decision to initiate antiviral therapy should consider the respiratory viruses circulating in the community, the individual's risk of developing complications of influenza infection, the severity of the individual's disease, and the duration of symptoms. The CDC recommends outpatient antiviral therapy be considered for previously healthy, symptomatic individuals who are at low risk of serious sequelae from influenza if therapy can be initiated within 48 hours of symptom onset.[50] Once the decision to initiate therapy has been made, the antiviral should be continued for 5 days.[50]

Individuals who are at highest risk of serious complications from influenza infection should receive antiviral therapy as early as possible after symptom onset, ideally within 48 hours.[58] This group includes the following: all children younger than 2 years; children with other comorbid conditions (e.g., asthma, sickle cell disease, diabetes, seizure disorders, mental retardation, HIV); children 18 years and younger receiving chronic aspirin therapy; American Indians or Native Americans; women who are pregnant or within 2 weeks after delivery; and children who are residents of chronic care facilities. Early initiation of antiviral therapy for influenza may also reduce the risk of serious complications, such as influenza-associated pneumonia or death. Children who have severe, progressive disease or who have been hospitalized because of influenza should also receive antiviral therapy.[50] A longer therapy duration may be warranted for critically ill children who have been admitted to the hospital or for immunocompromised children.[58]

Oseltamivir is an oral agent that is generally well tolerated. Oseltamivir is available as an oral solution, which makes it the treatment of choice for influenza in infants and young children. Oseltamivir is labeled for treatment of influenza in infants and children age 2 weeks and older, and for prophylaxis in children age 1 year or older. Table 3 describes appropriate oseltamivir dosing for children. During times of shortage, an extemporaneous product may be compounded from oseltamivir capsules using a recipe from the package insert with the final concentration that is the same as the commercial solution (6 mg/mL). The most common adverse effects associated with oseltamivir use in children are nausea, vomiting, and diarrhea.[59] Children and adolescents may also be at increased risk of neuropsychiatric disorders, such as hallucinations and abnormal behaviors that may result in harm, after oseltamivir administration.[59,60]

Zanamivir is available as a powder for inhalation and is packaged in its own specific delivery device called a Rotadisk (GlaxoSmithKline, Research Triangle Park, NC).[61] It is labeled for the treatment of influenza in children 7 years or older and for prophylaxis of influenza in children 5 years or older. Because of the device in which zanamivir is packaged, it cannot be nebulized into ventilators. The Rotadisk for zanamivir is also difficult for young children to use. It is not a pressurized canister and requires the recipient to inhale a forceful breath, which is difficult for young children to perform. Zanamivir is generally well tolerated. Phase III studies of children showed no significant difference in the adverse effects of zanamivir compared with placebo.[61] Post-marketing surveillance of zanamivir use has shown a risk of bronchospasm after administration.[61] As a result, zanamivir should not be used in children with preexisting pulmonary disease, such as asthma. Table 4 describes appropriate zanamivir dosing for children.

Peramivir is only available as solution for intravenous injection. It is labeled for the treatment of influenza in children 2 years and older.[62] For children age 2–12 years, peramivir should be administered at a dose of 12 mg/kg. Children and adolescents 13 years or older should receive 600 mg. A safety study evaluating a single dose of peramivir administered to children age 2–17 years versus 5 days of oseltamivir demonstrated that the drug was generally well tolerated; however, the study was not powered to detect significant differences in efficacy end points.[62] A study of patients 6 years and older hospitalized for influenza compared 5 days of peramivir to standard

Table 3. Dosing of Oseltamivir for Treatment and Prevention of Influenza in Children[50]

Age		Treatment	Post-Exposure Prophylaxis
< 14 days		3 mg/kg/dose daily	Not recommended unless critical
14 days–2 mo		3 mg/kg/dose BID	Not recommended unless critical
3–5 mo		3 mg/kg/dose BID	3 mg/kg/dose daily
6–11 mo		3 mg/kg/dose BID	3 mg/kg/dose daily
≥ 12 mo	≤ 15 kg	30 mg BID	30 mg/day
	15.1–23 kg	45 mg BID	45 mg/day
	23.1–40 kg	60 mg BID	60 mg/day
	> 40 kg	75 mg BID	75 mg/day

BID = twice daily.

Table 4. Dosing of Zanamivir for Treatment and Prevention of Influenza in Children[50]

Age	Treatment	Post-Exposure Prophylaxis
< 5 yr	Not recommended	Not recommended
5–6 yr	Not recommended	10 mg (2 inhalations) daily
≥ 7 yr	10 mg (2 inhalations) twice daily	10 mg (2 inhalations) daily

of care, which may have included a neuraminidase inhibitor.[63] No differences were observed between the peramivir and standard of care groups in terms of clinical end points, such as resolution of symptoms, fever defervescence, or survival. For this reason, peramivir should only be considered for use in patients who are unable to receive oseltamivir. Peramivir should not be used for treatment of influenza B because limited data support its use.[58]

Baloxavir, a new agent that does not belong to either the adamantanes or neuraminidase inhibitors, works by inhibiting cap-dependent endonuclease, thereby inhibiting viral replication. Baloxavir is labeled for use in children and adults 12 years and older with uncomplicated influenza.[64] A single dose of 40 mg is administered to individuals who weigh 40 to less than 80 kg, whereas individuals who weigh 80 kg or more should receive a single dose of 80 mg. In a randomized clinical trial in individuals 12 years or older with influenza symptoms for less than 48 hours, a single dose of baloxavir (40 mg or 80 mg) was compared with 5 days of oseltamivir (75 mg twice daily) or placebo.[65] Baloxavir shortened the duration of symptoms by about 1 day (26.5 hours) compared with placebo. Duration of symptoms was comparable between the baloxavir and oseltamivir groups. One concern arising from trials of baloxavir is the emergence of resistance. Polymerase acidic protein variants with I38T/M/F substitutions leading to decreased baloxavir susceptibilities occurred in 2.2% of baloxavir recipients in a phase II study and 9.7% of recipients in the previously described phase III study.[65] Baloxavir has no data to support its use in hospitalized patients. Baloxavir should only be considered for use in children 12 or older with uncomplicated influenza within 48 hours of symptom onset. Its use is likely to be limited, but it may be beneficial in individuals for whom adherence to 5 days of oseltamivir therapy is a concern.

PROPHYLAXIS

Some children may benefit from antiviral prophylaxis with either oseltamivir or zanamivir when a community outbreak of influenza occurs. Children who should receive antiviral prophylaxis during community outbreaks (i.e., pre-exposure prophylaxis) include the following: children at high risk of influenza complications with a contraindication to influenza vaccine; children at high risk of influenza complications if an outbreak occurs within 2 weeks of influenza vaccination; household contacts of unimmunized children at high risk of influenza complications; and household contacts of infants and children younger than 2 years.[66] Once initiated, pre-exposure prophylaxis is most beneficial if administered for the duration of influenza activity in the community.[50] When contemplating the initiation of post-exposure prophylaxis, the practitioner should consider the exposed individual's risk of developing serious complications from influenza infection and the length of exposure to the infected individual. Post-exposure prophylaxis should only be considered if antiviral therapy is initiated within 48 hours of exposure to the infected individual.[50] Once post-exposure prophylaxis is initiated, it is generally continued until 10 days after the last known exposure to an infected individual.

SUMMARY

Otherwise healthy children will receive only limited benefit, if any, from antiviral therapy. Antiviral therapy should be initiated in all children at high risk of complications from influenza infection, including those younger than 2 years and those with other comorbid conditions, such as chronic lung disease, diabetes, or congenital heart disease. Only the neuraminidase inhibitors (oseltamivir and zanamivir) should be used for the treatment or prophylaxis of influenza. Oseltamivir is the preferred antiviral agent in young children because it is available in an oral solution.

COMMUNITY-ACQUIRED PNEUMONIA

EPIDEMIOLOGY

According to the World Health Organization, pneumonia is the most common illness worldwide to cause death in children younger than 5 years, with an estimated 1.8 million deaths from pneumonia in children worldwide in 2009.[67] Mortality is highest in impoverished children who lack adequate resources to provide good nutrition or health care. Pulmonary complications that may result from pneumonia include pleural effusion, empyema, lung abscess, and necrotizing pneumonia. These complications often result in the need for admission to the intensive care unit and mechanical ventilation. Children infected with typical bacterial organisms, such as *Streptococcus pneumoniae*, and those with mixed bacterial and viral infections are more likely to develop pleural effusions.[68] Bacteremia can also result from pneumonia and lead to metastatic complications, such as meningitis, pericarditis, and septic arthritis.[69] Adults who had childhood pneumonia before age 7 years have been noted to have reduced pulmonary function.[70] Factors that increase the risk of developing pneumonia in children include the following: age younger than 5 years; recurrent upper respiratory tract infections; otitis media before age 2 years; a history of wheezing; and race, including American Indians, Native Alaskans, and African Americans.[71,72]

ETIOLOGY

The most common organism responsible for causing community-acquired pneumonia (CAP) in children varies by the child's age. Table 5 describes the most common organisms that cause pneumonia in children.

VIRAL PNEUMONIA

Viruses that commonly cause pneumonia in children include the following: influenza A and B, RSV, human metapneumovirus, parainfluenza, adenovirus, coronaviruses, and rhinoviruses.[73] Viral and bacterial coinfection is common in children with pneumonia.[68]

BACTERIAL PNEUMONIA

During the neonatal period, group B *Streptococcus* and gram-negative enteric organisms, especially *Escherichia coli*, are the most common causes of pneumonia.[69] *S. pneumoniae* is the most likely bacterial cause of pneumonia in infants and children.[69] *M. pneumoniae* and *C. pneumoniae* are common causes of bacterial pneumonia in children older than 5 years.[74] Other, less common bacteria associated with pneumonia in children include *Staphylococcus aureus*, *B. pertussis*, group A *Streptococcus*, *Moraxella catarrhalis*, *Haemophilus influenzae*, and *Mycobacterium tuberculosis*.[69,74] Tuberculosis will not be discussed in this chapter. The CDC guidelines at https://www.cdc.gov provide information regarding the proper assessment and medical management of a child with tuberculosis.

CLINICAL PRESENTATION

The most common symptoms associated with pneumonia in children are fever and cough, with fever present in more than 90% of children with pneumonia.[69,74,75] Bacterial pneumonia usually has a rapid onset and may include productive cough and chest pain.[69] Other signs or symptoms of pneumonia that may be present include tachypnea, difficulty

breathing, retractions, grunting, wheezing, and crackles.[69,75] In children, tachypnea is defined as greater than 50 breaths/minute in infants age 2–12 months, greater than 40 breaths/minute in children age 1–5 years, and greater than 20 breaths/minute in children 6 years and older.[74] Some children with pneumonia may have nonspecific symptoms of nausea, vomiting, and abdominal pain.[69] Children who develop pneumonia from atypical organisms may present with symptoms of fever, cough, sore throat, and malaise that develop slowly, usually over 3–5 days.[76]

DIAGNOSIS

The presence of infiltrates on chest radiograph is considered the gold standard for diagnosing pneumonia.[75] For an afebrile child with a clinical presentation strongly suggestive of pneumonia, radiography is not necessary for determining proper outpatient management. Chest radiography is recommended for infants and children with hypoxia or respiratory distress,

Table 5. Empiric Treatment of Community-Acquired Pneumonia in Children[69,74,76]

Age	Causative Organisms	First-Line Therapy	Second-Line Therapy
Birth–3 wk	*Escherichia coli*	Ampicillin + gentamicin	Ampicillin + cefotaxime
	Group B *Streptococcus*		
	Listeria monocytogenes		
	Haemophilus influenzae	3rd-generation cephalosporin	—
3 wk–3 mo	Viruses	Supportive care	—
	Chlamydia trachomatis	Azithromycin	—
	Streptococcus pneumoniae	High-dose amoxicillin	Azithromycin, oral 3rd-generation cephalosporin, clindamycin
		3rd-generation cephalosporin in hospitalized infants	Vancomycin
	H. influenzae	3rd-generation cephalosporin	—
4 mo–4 yr	Viruses	Supportive care	—
	Chlamydophila pneumoniae *Mycoplasma pneumoniae*	Azithromycin	Doxycycline,[a] fluoroquinolone[b]
	S. pneumoniae	High-dose amoxicillin	Azithromycin, oral 3rd-generation cephalosporin, clindamycin, levofloxacin[b]
		3rd-generation cephalosporin in hospitalized infants	Vancomycin, levofloxacin[b]
≥ 5 yr	*C. pneumoniae* *M. pneumoniae*	Azithromycin	Doxycycline,[a] fluoroquinolone[b]
	S. pneumoniae	High-dose amoxicillin	Azithromycin, oral 3rd-generation cephalosporin, clindamycin, levofloxacin[b]
		3rd-generation cephalosporin in hospitalized infants	Vancomycin, levofloxacin[b]
Empyema, lung abscess, necrotizing pneumonia	*S. pneumoniae*	Vancomycin Clindamycin	Ceftriaxone,[c] doxycycline,[a] levofloxacin[b]
	Staphylococcus aureus (including MRSA)	Vancomycin Clindamycin	Doxycycline,[a] linezolid

[a]Doxycycline should not be used in children < 8 yr because of discoloration of permanent teeth.
[b]Use of fluoroquinolones in children should be avoided unless no other safe alternatives are available.
[c]Ceftriaxone should only be used if cultures show the absence of MRSA.
MRSA = methicillin-resistant Staphylococcus aureus.

Pediatric Pharmacotherapy, 2nd Ed

for infants or children who do not respond to an initial course of antibiotics, and for all infants or children admitted to the hospital with pneumonia.[76] Bacterial pneumonias often exhibit lobar infiltrates, whereas atypical pneumonias often exhibit perihilar infiltrates, although these findings are nonspecific and can also be seen in viral pneumonias.[69] Pneumonias caused by atypical organisms may exhibit patchy infiltrates bilaterally.[74] Children with pneumonia often have elevated white blood cell counts and C-reactive protein; however, these laboratory findings are nonspecific and not helpful in differentiating bacterial from viral pneumonia.[69,74,75]

Blood cultures are positive less than 10% of the time when pneumococcal pneumonia is present.[74] As a result, they should not be obtained routinely in children who are treated for CAP as outpatients. Blood cultures should be performed if a child does not experience improvement on antimicrobial therapy, shows clinical deterioration, or has disease progression.[76]

Sputum cultures are not routinely performed in children. Obtaining a culture of the throat or respiratory secretions may not accurately reflect the organisms that are causing LRTI and may result in the inappropriate use of antimicrobials.[77] Unfortunately, for most bacteria, the only way to confirm the causative organism is to obtain a bacterial culture from pleural fluid or an empyema, if present. For some organisms, such as *M. pneumoniae*, PCR tests that measure the presence of DNA are available and should be used when a child presents with symptoms consistent with pneumonia from atypical organisms.[76,77] Viral antigen testing is not helpful in differentiating bacterial from viral pneumonia because the presence of a virus does not exclude a bacterial process, although it may be useful for infection control in a hospital setting.

PREVENTION

Vaccination against influenza, *S. pneumoniae*, and *H. influenzae* type b can markedly decrease a child's risk of developing pneumonia. Since the introduction of the pneumococcal conjugate vaccine in 2000, the incidence of hospitalization because of pneumonia from any cause has decreased by 33% in children, and the incidence of hospitalization from pneumococcal pneumonia has decreased by 61%.[78] The Pediatric Vaccines chapter provides a more detailed discussion of these vaccines.

TREATMENT

The primary goals of therapy for CAP are to eradicate the infection and prevent the development of complications. Children who are afebrile and not critically ill (e.g., without hypoxia or signs of respiratory distress) may be treated as outpatients. Infants and children with suspected pneumonia in the following situations should be hospitalized: those younger than 6 months; those who appear dehydrated or cannot tolerate oral liquids; those with respiratory distress or persistent hypoxia; those with CAP caused by a highly virulent organism, such as community-acquired methicillin-resistant *S. aureus* (MRSA); and those who may have unstable family or social situations that make follow-up difficult.[69,74,76] Hospital admission should also be considered for children with underlying chronic medical conditions or children for whom outpatient

management has failed. Because recovery of the causative organism is rare in children with CAP, treatment is usually empiric and should include coverage of the organisms most likely to cause pneumonia in the child's age group.

VIRAL PNEUMONIA

Children who are younger than 5 years typically develop pneumonia from viral pathogens. A child with viral pneumonia should be treated with supportive care because antibiotics are not effective in this situation. Antipyretics such as acetaminophen or ibuprofen may be useful for children with a low-grade fever. Children with viral pneumonia should be encouraged to maintain good fluid intake to avoid dehydration. Antivirals should be used in infants or children infected with influenza who are at high risk of complications from infection.

NEONATAL PNEUMONIA

During the neonatal period (up to age 1 month), pneumonia is typically caused by pathogens that colonize the genitourinary tracts of pregnant women, specifically group B *Streptococcus* and *E. coli*. Neonates with bacterial pneumonia should be hospitalized to manage potential respiratory distress and facilitate the use of intravenous antibiotics. Empiric therapy should consist of ampicillin and an aminoglycoside (usually gentamicin) or a third-generation cephalosporin (usually cefotaxime). Ceftriaxone should not be used in this population because of the risk of kernicterus.

PNEUMOCOCCAL PNEUMONIA

The treatment of choice for pneumococcal CAP in children receiving outpatient therapy is amoxicillin.[74,76,77] Amoxicillin should be administered at a dose of 90 mg/kg/day divided twice daily to adequately treat penicillin-resistant *S. pneumoniae*.[76] *S. pneumoniae* exhibits resistance to β-lactam antibiotics by alterations to penicillin-binding proteins, which often can be overcome by high doses of β-lactams.[79] Because pneumococci do not produce β-lactamases, amoxicillin/clavulanate has no additional benefit in the treatment of pneumococcal pneumonia.[77] For children with an allergy or intolerance to amoxicillin, a second- or third-generation cephalosporin (e.g., cefuroxime, cefprozil, cefpodoxime) may be used unless the child has had a type 1 hypersensitivity reaction to β-lactam antibiotics (e.g., angioedema, hives, anaphylaxis).[76] Other alternatives for outpatient management of CAP include levofloxacin (if susceptible) or linezolid. Clindamycin is another viable alternative if community resistance rates are low (typically, less than 10%). Once treatment is initiated, symptomatic improvement should occur within 48–72 hours. If a child does not respond to therapy, further evaluation is warranted to rule out other causes of the child's symptoms. Therapy duration for outpatient management of CAP in children is typically 7–10 days.

For children who require hospitalization, intravenous antibiotics should be used. If *S. pneumoniae* has been isolated in a child with CAP, therapy should be selected on the basis of the penicillin minimum inhibitory concentration (MIC) for the organism. For *S. pneumoniae* isolates with a penicillin MIC of

2 mcg/mL or less, ampicillin or aqueous penicillin G is preferred.[76] Alternatives for *S. pneumoniae* with a penicillin MIC of 2 mcg/mL or less are ceftriaxone, cefotaxime, clindamycin (if susceptible), or vancomycin. For *S. pneumoniae* isolates with a penicillin MIC of 4 mcg/mL or higher, ceftriaxone is the preferred agent. Alternative agents for isolates of *S. pneumoniae* with a penicillin MIC of 4 mcg/mL or higher include high-dose ampicillin, clindamycin (if susceptible), vancomycin, levofloxacin, or linezolid. For children hospitalized with CAP, the therapy duration is typically 10–14 days. Longer treatment durations may be necessary in children who develop complications, such as lung abscesses or necrotizing pneumonia.

PNEUMONIA CAUSED BY ATYPICAL ORGANISMS

Empiric coverage of atypical organisms should be added to pneumococcal coverage in both the inpatient and outpatient management of CAP beyond the neonatal period whenever there is a high degree of suspicion that an atypical organism is present. Macrolide antibiotics are generally the preferred treatment for the atypical organisms (*M. pneumoniae*, *C. pneumoniae*, and *Chlamydia trachomatis*). Azithromycin is the preferred macrolide antibiotic in children because of its tolerability and shorter treatment duration. Azithromycin should be administered at a dose of 10 mg/kg on day 1 and then 5 mg/kg/day on days 2–5.[74,77] For children who may be at risk of not adhering to therapy, azithromycin may alternatively be administered at 10 mg/kg/day for 3 days. For children unable to tolerate oral medications, azithromycin is also available in an injectable form. Because of increasing resistance rates of *S. pneumoniae* to macrolides, empiric therapy for pneumonia beyond the neonatal period should include a β-lactam antibiotic in addition to azithromycin. For children in whom coverage of atypical organisms is warranted but who have an allergy or intolerance to macrolide antibiotics, doxycycline or a fluoroquinolone may be used.[76] Doxycycline should not be used in children younger than 8 years because of the risk of permanent tooth staining. Fluoroquinolones have shown joint toxicities in studies of juvenile animals. A review of available literature reporting use of fluoroquinolones in more than 7000 children demonstrated that the rate of arthralgia in children is no higher than the level expected in the general population.[80] In addition, no adverse effects on growth were found. Although permanent joint damage has not been observed in children, black box warnings have been issued for the serious adverse effects that have mostly been reported in adult or elderly patients (e.g., tendon rupture, peripheral neuropathy, lowered seizure threshold, exacerbation of myasthenia gravis).[81-83] As a result, the American Academy of Pediatrics recommendation is that the use of fluoroquinolones be reserved for situations when safe alternative therapies are not available.[84,85]

SUMMARY

Children who have viral pneumonia should be treated with supportive care. Antibiotics offer no benefit to children with viral pneumonia. Pneumococcus is a common cause of bacterial pneumonia in children and can be treated using high-dose amoxicillin in an ambulatory setting, even for penicillin-resistant *S. pneumoniae*. Empiric therapy for pediatric CAP should include amoxicillin and azithromycin when there is a high degree of suspicion that an atypical organism is contributing to disease.

LUNG ABSCESS, EMPYEMA, AND NECROTIZING PNEUMONIA

EPIDEMIOLOGY

Lung abscess, empyema, and necrotizing pneumonia are some of the more serious complications associated with CAP in children. The incidence of these complications of CAP in children has increased during the past 20 years.[78,86-88] An increase in the incidence of complications of CAP from pneumococcal serotypes not contained in the heptavalent vaccine has also been reported.[72,78,89] One study reported that children who had been treated with antibiotics or ibuprofen for CAP before hospitalization had an increased risk of developing an empyema. In addition to having more severe disease, children with an empyema were more likely to have a fever lasting more than 7 days and the presence of chest pain, which suggests a more prolonged disease course.[86] Additional risk factors for empyema include children age 3 years and older and children with varicella infection within 1 month of hospitalization.[86]

ETIOLOGY

Organisms most commonly associated with empyema and necrotizing pneumonia are *S. pneumoniae*, *S. aureus* (including MRSA), and group A *Streptococcus*.[74,78,86-91] Other organisms that have been isolated in children with an empyema or necrotizing pneumonia include the following: *M. pneumoniae*, *Streptococcus milleri*, viridans streptococci, *H. influenzae*, *Fusobacterium* spp., *Eikenella* spp., *Pseudomonas aeruginosa*, other gram-negative organisms, and *M. tuberculosis*.[74,87,91-95]

CLINICAL PRESENTATION

Symptoms of empyema or necrotizing pneumonia may be similar to those seen with CAP and include fever, tachypnea, and chest pain.[74,91] The development of symptoms in a person with an empyema or necrotizing pneumonia is generally a more insidious process than what is typically seen with CAP. A child with an empyema or necrotizing pneumonia will generally be more ill-appearing than will a typical child with CAP and may present with chest pain and splinting.[74] On physical examination, absent or diminished breath sounds may be noted, as well as dullness on percussion of the chest wall.[74,91] Empyema rarely causes increased mortality in children.[94]

DIAGNOSIS

Chest radiographs are often performed to document the presence of pneumonia, but they are not sensitive enough to confirm the presence of an empyema.[94] Necrotizing pneumonia and cavitation may be detected by chest radiograph. Any child who presents with a cavitary lesion on chest radiography should be evaluated for tuberculosis. Ultrasonography may be useful for differentiating a pleural effusion from a loculated fluid collection, which may require surgical intervention.[94] Chest computed tomography may also be helpful for diagnosing an empyema; however, it should not be used routinely for children with pneumonia because of the high-radiation exposure dose associated with computed tomography scan.[94] Sputum and throat cultures are not helpful in identifying the organism responsible for causing empyema or necrotizing pneumonia in children. If surgical drainage of a fluid collection, empyema, or abscess is performed, the material should be sent to the microbiology laboratory for Gram stain and culture to provide targeted antimicrobial therapy.

TREATMENT

The goals of therapy for the treatment of empyema, lung abscess, or necrotizing pneumonia are to limit the destruction of lung tissue and prevent further morbidity or mortality. Empiric therapy for children with an empyema or necrotizing pneumonia should include coverage of *S. pneumoniae* and *S. aureus*, including MRSA.[96] If surgical drainage is performed and bacterial cultures are obtained, then definitive antibiotic therapy should be targeted at the specific organisms identified once final identification and sensitivity results are known. The typical duration of therapy for an empyema or necrotizing pneumonia is 2–4 weeks.

THIRD-GENERATION CEPHALOSPORINS

Ceftriaxone is most commonly used as monotherapy for the treatment of empyema and necrotizing pneumonia caused by *S. pneumoniae*, even when the penicillin MIC is 4 mcg/mL or greater (Table 6).[76] Cefotaxime is an acceptable alternative to ceftriaxone at institutions where ceftriaxone is not on formulary. Ceftriaxone has only moderate activity, at best, against *S. aureus*, and no activity against MRSA.[74] As a result, it should not be used as monotherapy for empiric therapy in a child with an empyema or necrotizing pneumonia. Ceftriaxone also shows good activity against many gram-negative organisms, except for *P. aeruginosa*, *Enterobacter* spp., and *Citrobacter* spp. Ceftriaxone should be administered at a dose of 50–100 mg/kg/day intravenously given once or twice daily and is generally well tolerated. Adverse effects may include cholelithiasis and gallbladder sludging. The second- and third-generation cephalosporins (e.g., cefpodoxime, cefuroxime, cefprozil) are acceptable agents for step-down oral therapy when a child with an empyema is stable enough to transition to outpatient therapy. Ceftriaxone is contraindicated in neonates with a post-menstrual age of less than 41 weeks' with hyperbilirubinemia because of a risk of kernicterus and in those who are up to 28 days of life receiving calcium-containing solutions because of a risk of precipitation of calcium-ceftriaxone crystals that may accumulate in organs, such as lungs or kidneys.[97]

VANCOMYCIN

Vancomycin is typically used empirically in combination with a third-generation cephalosporin for the treatment of empyema and necrotizing pneumonia. Vancomycin has good coverage against *S. pneumoniae*, *S. aureus*, and MRSA.[79] Vancomycin has lower tissue penetration and slower antibacterial activity than other antibiotics typically used for pneumonia. As a result, vancomycin should be discontinued if an organism other than MRSA is identified and the child can tolerate the antibiotic of choice, or a reasonable alternative, for the identified organism. Vancomycin should be initiated at a dose of 60–80 mg/kg/day intravenously divided every 6 hours for children age 3 months to 12 years, and at a dose of 60–70 mg/kg/day divided every 6 hours for children age 12 years or older.[98] Area under the curve (AUC) monitoring of vancomycin is becoming the standard of care over trough monitoring. Maintaining an AUC:MIC ratio of more than 400 is no longer recommended. Instead, an AUC—versus an AUC:MIC ratio—should be maintained between 400–600 mcg/hour/mL to maximize efficacy and minimize the risk of toxicity.[98] An AUC can be estimated using two concentrations, generally a vancomycin peak and a trough, or through software that uses Bayesian modeling.

The most common adverse effect associated with vancomycin is red man syndrome, which may include flushing of the face and neck from histamine release. Extending the vancomycin infusion time generally prevents further episodes of red man syndrome. Nephrotoxicity has also been associated with vancomycin administration. This effect is more common at trough concentrations higher than 15 mcg/mL, with the concurrent administration of other nephrotoxic agents, including piperacillin/tazobactam, or in children who become dehydrated.[98,99]

CLINDAMYCIN

Clindamycin is a reasonable alternative to vancomycin for the treatment of empyema and necrotizing pneumonia caused by *S. pneumoniae* or *S. aureus* (if susceptible). It can be used in combination with a third-generation cephalosporin for empiric therapy or as monotherapy, if the causative organism is susceptible. Clindamycin has excellent oral bioavailability, so it has the advantage of offering an oral dosage form in children who are stable and can tolerate oral therapy. Clindamycin has good activity against staphylococci and streptococci; however, community-acquired MRSA resistance is increasing. The Infectious Diseases Society of America recommends clindamycin not be used empirically when community resistance rates for MRSA are greater than 10%.[96] If *Staphylococcus* is identified from a child with an empyema or necrotizing pneumonia, the practitioner should note the erythromycin susceptibility results in addition to the clindamycin susceptibility results. Methicillin-resistant *S. aureus* has the potential to carry a gene (*erm*) that codes for inducible clindamycin resistance.[100] If an MRSA strain shows erythromycin resistance but is susceptible to clindamycin during the initial susceptibility testing, then a disk diffusion test (also called a *D test*) should be performed to rule out the presence of inducible clindamycin resistance.[96,100] Clindamycin is an acceptable choice for step-down therapy in children ready to transition to oral therapy, if the organism is susceptible. Clindamycin is typically administered at a dose of 40 mg/kg/day intravenously divided every 6–8 hours. The most common adverse effects associated with clindamycin are diarrhea (including *Clostridium difficile*–associated diarrhea) and taste intolerance for children who receive the oral liquid. Many techniques can be used to improve the tolerance of poor-tasting medications, including coating the tongue with peanut butter before administering the dose or mixing the dose with chocolate syrup.

DOXYCYCLINE

Doxycycline generally has good coverage against *S. aureus*, including MRSA. Historically, it has not been an acceptable empiric choice for empyema or necrotizing pneumonia in most children because of the risk of tooth discoloration and possible resistance. Recent data evaluating the use of doxycycline for Rocky Mountain spotted fever in children younger than 8 years have shown no increase in tooth discoloration in children exposed to doxycycline compared with children without doxycycline exposure for courses ranging from 7 to 10 days.[101] As a result, if an MRSA isolate sensitive to doxycycline is recovered in a child with an empyema, doxycycline is a reasonable alternative to vancomycin for step-down oral monotherapy. It is also a reasonable alternative to macrolides if coverage of atypical organisms is desired in a child who is allergic or intolerant. Doxycycline also has excellent

Table 6. Dosing of Antibiotics Used for Pediatric Respiratory Tract Infections[76]

Antibiotic	Neonates[a]	Infants and Children
Amoxicillin	30 mg/kg/day divided BID	80–100 mg/kg/day divided BID
Amoxicillin/ Clavulanate	30 mg/kg/day divided BID	80–100 mg/kg/day divided BID
Ampicillin	50–100 mg/kg/day divided BID or QID	150–200 mg/kg/day divided QID 300–400 mg/kg/day divided QID for PRSP
Azithromycin	10 mg/kg/day	10 mg/kg on day 1; then 5 mg/kg day on days 2–5 OR 10 mg/kg/day for 3 days
Aztreonam	60–90 mg/kg/day divided BID or TID	90–120 mg/kg/day divided TID or QID
Cefazolin	40–60 mg/kg/day divided BID or TID	50–100 mg/kg/day divided TID
Cefepime	30 mg/kg/dose BID	50 mg/kg/dose BID
Cefotaxime	100 mg/kg/day divided BID	100–200 mg/kg/day divided TID
Ceftazidime	100 mg/kg/day divided BID	100–150 mg/kg/day divided TID
Ceftriaxone	Avoid	50–100 mg/kg/day QD or divided BID
Ciprofloxacin	Avoid	20–30 mg/kg/day divided BID
Clindamycin	15–30 mg/kg/day divided TID or QID	30 mg/kg/day divided TID or QID
Doxycycline	Avoid	2–4 mg/kg/day QD or BID
Gentamicin	3.5–5 mg/kg/day QD	2.5 mg/kg/dose TID or 5–7.5 mg/kg/day QD
Levofloxacin	Avoid	10 mg/kg/dose BID for children age <5 yr 10 mg/kg/dose QD for children ≥5 yr
Linezolid	10 mg/kg/dose BID or TID	10 mg/kg/dose TID for children age <12 yr 10 mg/kg/dose BID for children ≥12 yr
Meropenem	20 mg/kg/dose BID or TID	20 mg/kg/dose TID
Nafcillin	75–140 mg/kg/day divided TID or QID	100–200 mg/kg/day divided QID
Oxacillin	100–200 mg/kg/day divided TID or QID	150–200 mg/kg/day divided QID
Piperacillin/ Tazobactam	150–300 mg/kg/day divided TID or QID	200–300 mg/kg/day divided TID or QID
Ticarcillin/ Clavulanate	225–300 mg/kg/day divided TID	200–300 mg/kg/day divided QID
TMP/SMZ[b]	Avoid	10–12 mg/kg/day divided BID
Tobramycin	3.5–5 mg/kg/day QD	2.5 mg/kg/dose TID OR 5–7.5 mg/kg/day QD

[a]Dosing for full-term neonates.
[b]Dosed based on TMP component.
BID = twice daily (or every 12 hours); PRSP = penicillin-resistant *Streptococcus pneumoniae*; QD = daily; QID = four times daily (or every 6 hours); TID = three times daily (or every 8 hours); TMP/SMZ = trimethoprim/sulfamethoxazole.
Adapted from Lexi-Comp Online, Pediatric and Neonatal Lexi-Drugs Online. Hudson, OH: Lexi-Comp, 2019.

Pediatric Pharmacotherapy, 2nd Ed

oral bioavailability, and when the child can tolerate oral antibiotics, treatment can easily be transitioned to oral therapy. Doxycycline should be administered orally or intravenously at a dose of 2 mg/kg every 12 hours.

LINEZOLID

Linezolid has good activity against most staphylococcal and streptococcal species, including MRSA, penicillin-resistant *S. pneumoniae*, and vancomycin-resistant enterococci. It has excellent oral bioavailability and offers an acceptable alternative to oral monotherapy on an outpatient basis. Although resistance to linezolid is rare, its use is limited by its high cost and high rate of thrombocytopenia, especially when used for more than 2 weeks.[96] The average wholesale price of linezolid is about $820 for a 240-mL bottle of 100 mg/5 mL suspension and around $184 per tablet (600 mg).[102] For children younger than 12 years, linezolid is typically administered at a dose of 10 mg/kg every 8 hours. For children 12 years and older, it is typically administered at a dose of 10 mg/kg every 12 hours.

FLUOROQUINOLONES

Fluoroquinolones have broad-spectrum activity against many gram-positive and gram-negative organisms, with the exception of ciprofloxacin, which predominantly has gram-negative activity. Levofloxacin is the fluoroquinolone with gram-positive activity that is most often used in children because of its well-established dosing information. Levofloxacin generally has good activity against *S. pneumoniae* and may exhibit in vitro activity against MRSA; however, it should not be used routinely for MRSA because resistance develops when used as monotherapy.[96] Ciprofloxacin is a reasonable choice for the treatment of an empyema or necrotizing pneumonia caused by gram-negative organisms such as *P. aeruginosa*; however, it lacks activity against *S. pneumoniae*. The fluoroquinolones also have very good oral bioavailability and may be used as step-down therapy for children who are transitioning to outpatient therapy. For children 5 years and older, levofloxacin is typically administered at 10 mg/kg once a day. Ciprofloxacin may be administered at a dose of 10–15 mg/kg/dose every 12 hours, regardless of the child's age.

SUMMARY

Empiric therapy for empyema, lung abscess, and necrotizing pneumonia should include coverage of the organisms most commonly associated with these processes—*S. pneumoniae*, group A *Streptococcus*, and *S. aureus*, including MRSA. Many treatment options exist for these complications of CAP. Vancomycin in combination with a third-generation cephalosporin is often the mainstay of therapy until a definitive organism and its susceptibilities are identified. Therapy duration for these complications of CAP is not well defined and should be individualized on the basis of the child's response. Treating a child with 3–4 weeks of antibiotics for an empyema, lung abscess, or necrotizing pneumonia is common.

CONCLUSIONS

Lower respiratory tract infections are a significant cause of hospitalizations in children and are among the most common reasons for a child to be seen in a primary care physician's office. Many LRTIs that are caused by viral infections respond well to symptom management. Bacterial LRTIs often require antibiotic therapy to prevent the transmission of the disease to other susceptible individuals and to limit the development of complications.

An otherwise healthy 6-year-old boy is brought to the emergency department by his mother because of a 2-day history of cough, wheezing, poor appetite, vomiting, lethargy, irritability, and fever.

Medical history: No significant illnesses

Immunizations: Up to date

Allergies: No known drug allergies

Social history: Attends kindergarten 5 days per week at a school where many children have recently been ill; no recent travel and no exposure to anyone who has travelled recently

Vital signs: BP 100/62 mm Hg, HR 89 beats/minute, Tmax 101°F (38.3°C), pulse oximetry 94% oxygen on room air; RR 41 breaths/minute, Ht 44 inches, Wt 21.3 kg.

Physical examination:

Breathing: Mild dyspnea, but no apnea, no retractions, no nasal flaring, no grunting

Cough: Productive (purulent)

Skin: Not cyanotic

Chest: Left lower lobe rales and crackles

Laboratory findings: Complete blood count with differential as follows:

WBC	17×10^3 cells/mm³
Hgb	12.5 g/dL
Hct	37%
Plt	300×10^3 cells/mm³
Segmented neutrophils	48%
Bands	11%
Lymphocytes	34%
Monocytes	5%
Eosinophils	2%

Imaging studies: On chest radiography, patchy infiltrates in left lower lobe; no evidence of pleural effusion

Diagnostic studies: Rapid influenza diagnostic test is negative

Cultures of blood and sputum: No growth to date

1. What pathogens are the most likely cause of the child's pneumonia?

Based on the patient's age, clinical presentation, elevated white blood cell count (with a left shift), and chest radiography results, he most likely has a bacterial pneumonia. *Streptococcus pneumoniae* is the most likely pathogen.

2. Would you recommend treatment as an outpatient, as an inpatient on a general care ward, or as an inpatient in an intensive care unit?

The child does not appear to be in respiratory distress. As long as his dyspnea does not worsen, and he is able to tolerate oral fluids so he is not at risk of dehydration, he can be safely monitored as an outpatient.

3. How should the pneumonia be treated?

Because *S. pneumoniae* is the most likely pathogenic cause of the child's pneumonia, he should be treated with a β-lactam antibiotic. Because there are no significant concerns regarding respiratory distress, and the patient has no medication allergies, amoxicillin would be the drug of choice. Given the concern for penicillin-resistant *S. pneumoniae,* the child should be treated with amoxicillin 1000 mg orally twice daily (around 94 mg/kg/day). If the child experiences improved symptoms and a lower fever curve after initiation of amoxicillin, a 7–10 day treatment course should be sufficient.

REFERENCES

1. Greenbaum AH, Chen J, Reed C, et al. Hospitalizations for severe lower respiratory tract infections. Pediatrics 2014;134:546-54.

2. Meissner HC. Viral bronchiolitis in children. N Engl J Med 2016;374:62-72.

3. Ralston SL, Lieberthal AS, Meissner HC, et al. Clinical practice guideline: the diagnosis, management, and prevention of bronchiolitis. Pediatrics 2014;134:e1474-502.

4. Dawson-Caswell M, Muncie HL. Respiratory syncytial virus infection in children. Am Fam Physician 2011;83:141-6.

5. Calvo C, Pozo F, Garcia-Garcia ML, et al. Detection of new respiratory viruses in hospitalized infants with bronchiolitis: a three-year prospective study. Acta Paediatr 2010;99:883-7.

6. Antunes H, Rodrigues H, Silva N, et al. Etiology of bronchiolitis in a hospitalized pediatric population: prospective multicenter study. J Clin Virol 2010;48:134-6.

7. Hall CB, Weinberg GA, Iwane MK, et al. The burden of respiratory syncytial virus infection in young children. N Engl J Med 2009;360:588-98.

8. Centers for Disease Control and Prevention. Respiratory Syncytial Virus [monograph on the Internet]. Atlanta: Centers for Disease Control and Prevention, 2019. Available at www.cdc.gov/rsv. Accessed May 23, 2019.

9. Thorburn K. Pre-existing disease is associated with a significantly higher risk of death in severe respiratory syncytial virus infection. Arch Dis Child 2009;94:99-103.

10. Sigurs N, Aljassim F, Kjellman B, et al. Asthma and allergy patterns over 18 years after severe RSV bronchiolitis in the first year of life. Thorax 2010;65:1045-52.

11. Bont L, Ramilo O. The relationship between RSV bronchiolitis and recurrent wheeze: the chicken and the egg. Early Hum Dev 2011;87S:S51-4.

12. Weisman LE. Populations at risk for developing respiratory syncytial virus and risk factors for respiratory syncytial virus severity: infants with predisposing conditions. Pediatr Infect Dis J 2003;22:S33-9.

13. Checchia P. Identification and management of severe respiratory syncytial virus. Am J Health Syst Pharm 2008;65:S7-12.

14. Shields MD, Thavagnanam S. The difficult coughing child: prolonged cough in children. Cough 2013;9:11.

15. Synagis [package insert]. Gaithersburg, MD: MedImmune, 2017. Available at https://dailymed.nlm.nih.gov/dailymed/drugInfo.cfm?setid=8e35c4c8-bf56-458f-a73c-8f5733829788. Accessed May 23, 2019.

16. Centers for Disease Control and Prevention. Respiratory syncytial virus seasonality—United States, 2014-2017. MMWR 2018; 67:71-6.

17. Committee on Infectious Diseases and Bronchiolitis Guidelines Committee. Updated guidance for palivizumab prophylaxis among infants and young children at increased risk of hospitalization for respiratory syncytial virus infection. Pediatrics 2014; 134:415-20.

18. Scott LJ, Lamb HM. Palivizumab. Drugs 1999;58:305-11.

19. Liet JM, Ducruet T, Gupta V, et al. Heliox inhalation therapy for bronchiolitis in infants. Cochrane Database Syst Rev 2015;9:CD006915.

20. Gadomski AM, Scribani MB. Bronchodilators for bronchiolitis. Cochrane Database Syst Rev 2014;6:CD001266.

21. Fernandes RM, Bialy LM, Vandermeer B, et al. Glucocorticoids for acute viral bronchiolitis in infants and young children. Cochrane Database Syst Rev 2013;6:CD004878.

22. Zhang L, Mendoza-Sassi RA, Wainwright C, et al. Nebulized hypertonic saline solution for acute bronchiolitis in infants. Cochrane Database Syst Rev 2017;12:CD006458.

23. Farley R, Spurling GKP, Eriksson L, et al. Antibiotics for bronchiolitis in children under two years of age. Cochrane Database Syst Rev 2014:10: CD005189.

24. American Academy of Pediatrics. Pertussis (whooping cough). In: Kimberlin DW, Brady MT, Jackson, MA, et al., eds. Red Book: 2018 report of the Committee on Infectious Diseases. American Academy of Pediatrics, 2018:620-34.

25. Centers for Disease Control and Prevention. Pertussis. In: Hamborsky J, Kroger A, Wolfe S, eds. Epidemiology and Prevention of Vaccine-Preventable Diseases, 13th ed. Washington, DC: Public Health Foundation, 2015:261-78. Available at www.cdc.gov/vaccines/pubs/pinkbook/index.html. Accessed November 1, 2019.

26. Centers for Disease Control and Prevention. Pertussis (whooping cough) [monograph on the Internet]. Atlanta: Centers for Disease Control and Prevention, 2017. Available at www.cdc.gov/pertussis/index.html. Accessed May 24, 2019.

27. Skoff TH, Hariri S. The epidemiology of nationally reported pertussis in the United States, 2000-2016. Clin Infect Dis 2019; 68:1634-40.

28. Mooi FR. Bordetella pertussis and vaccination: the persistence of a genetically monomorphic pathogen. Infect Genet Evol 2010; 10:36-49.

29. Briere EC, Pondo T, Schmidt M, et al. Assessment of Tdap vaccination effectiveness in adolescents in integrated health-care systems. J Adolesc Health 2018;62:661-6.

30. Greenberg DP, Wirsing von Konig CH, et al. Health burden of pertussis in infants and children. Pediatr Infect Dis J 2005;24:S39-43.

31. Falcon M, Rafael M, Garcia C, et al. Increasing infant pertussis hospitalization and mortality is south Texas, 1996-2006. Pediatr Infect Dis J 2010;29:265-7.

32. Rothstein E, Edwards K. Health burden of pertussis in adolescents and adults. Pediatr Infect Dis J 2005;24:S44-7.

33. Nuolivirta K, Koponen P, He Q, et al. Bordetella pertussis infection is common in nonvaccinated infants admitted for bronchiolitis. Pediatr Infect Dis J 2010;29:1013-5.

34. Leung AKC, Robson WLM, Davies HD. Pertussis in adolescents. Adv Ther 2007;24:353-61.

35. Jakubecz MA, Temple-Cooper ME, Philipson EH. Development of an outpatient clinic to provide pertussis vaccinations to maternity patients and family members. Am J Health Syst Pharm 2016;73:e54-8.

36. Maheshwai N. Are young infants treated with erythromycin at risk for developing hypertrophic pyloric stenosis? Arch Dis Child 2007;92:271-3.

37. Centers for Disease Control and Prevention. Recommended antimicrobial agents for treatment and postexposure prophylaxis of pertussis: 2005 CDC guidelines. MMWR 2005;54:1-20.

38. Kincade S, Long NA. Acute bronchitis. Am Fam Physician 2016; 94:560-5.

39. Knutson D, Braun C. Diagnosis and management of acute bronchitis. Am Fam Physician 2002;65:2039-44.

40. Centers for Disease Control and Prevention. National Center for Health Statistics: ambulatory health care data [monograph on the internet]. Atlanta: Centers for Disease Control and Prevention, 2019. Available at https://www.cdc.gov/nchs/ahcd/web_tables.htm#2015. Accessed November 1, 2019.

41. Kasi AS, Kamerman-Kretzmer RJ. Cough. Pediatr Rev 2019; 40:157-67.

42. Centers for Disease Control and Prevention. Antibiotic use in the United States, 2017: antibiotic use by healthcare setting [monograph on the Internet]. Atlanta: Centers for Disease Control and Prevention, 2019. Available at www.cdc.gov/antibiotic-use/stewardship-report/outpatient.html. Accessed November 1, 2019.

43. Centers for Disease Control and Prevention. Common cold [monograph on the Internet]. Atlanta: Centers for Disease Control and Prevention, 2017. Available at www.cdc.gov/antibiotic-use/community/for-patients/common-illnesses/colds.html. Accessed May 24, 2019.

44. American Academy of Pediatrics Committee on Drugs. Use of codeine- and dextromethorphan-containing cough remedies in children. Pediatrics 1997;99:918-20.

45. Tobias JD, Green TP, Cote CJ; AAP Section on Anesthesiology and Pain; AAP Committee on Drugs. Codeine: time to say "no." Pediatrics 2016;138:e20162396.

46. Kearns GL, Abdel-Rahman SM, Alander SW, et al. Developmental pharmacology-drug distribution, action, and therapy in infants and children. N Engl J Med 2003;349:1157-67.

47. U.S. Food and Drug Administration. FDA statement following CHPA's announcement on nonprescription over-the-counter cough and cold medicines in children [FDA statement on the Internet]. Silver Spring, MD: U.S. Food and Drug Administration, 2008. Available at https://www.pharmaceuticalonline.com/doc/fda-on-nonprescription-otc-medicines-children-0001. Accessed May 24, 2019.

48. Centers for Disease Control and Prevention. Revised product labels for pediatric over-the-counter cough and cold medicines. MMWR 2008;57:1180.

49. Paul IM, Beiler J, McMonagle A, et al. Effect of honey, dextromethorphan, and no treatment on nocturnal cough and sleep quality for coughing children and their parents. Arch Pediatr Adolesc Med 2007;161:1140-6.

50. Centers for Disease Control and Prevention. Antiviral agents for the treatment and chemoprophylaxis of influenza: recommendations of the Advisory Committee on Immunization Practices (ACIP). MMWR 2011;60:1-24.

51. Centers for Disease Control and Prevention. Influenza. In: Hamborsky J, Kroger A, Wolfe S, eds. Epidemiology and Prevention of Vaccine-Preventable Diseases, 13th ed. Washington, DC: Public Health Foundation, 2015:187-208. Available at www.cdc.gov/vaccines/pubs/pinkbook/flu.html. Accessed May 24, 2019.

52. Centers for Disease Control and Prevention. Weekly US Influenza Surveillance Report [monograph on the Internet]. Atlanta: Centers for Disease Control and Prevention, 2019. Available at www.cdc.gov/flu/weekly/summary.htm. Accessed November 1, 2019.

53. Clark NM, Lynch JP III. Influenza: epidemiology, clinical features, therapy, and prevention. Semin Respir Crit Care Med 2011;32:373-92.

54. Centers for Disease Control and Prevention. Overview of influenza testing methods [monograph on the Internet]. Atlanta: Centers for Disease Control and Prevention, 2019. Available at https://www.cdc.gov/flu/professionals/diagnosis/overview-testing-methods.htm. Accessed May 24, 2019.

55. Centers for Disease Control and Prevention. Update: influenza activity—United States, 2009–10 season. MMWR 2010;59:901-8.

56. Centers for Disease Control and Prevention. Weekly US influenza surveillance report [monograph on the Internet]. Atlanta: Centers for Disease Control and Prevention, 2019. Available at https://www.cdc.gov/flu/weekly/index.htm. Accessed May 24, 2019.

57. Heinonen S, Silvennoinen H, Lehtinen P, et al. Early oseltamivir treatment of influenza in children 1–3 years of age: a randomized controlled trial. Clin Infect Dis 2010;51:887-94.

58. Centers for Disease Control and Prevention. Influenza antiviral medications: summary for clinicians [monograph on the Internet]. Atlanta: Centers for Disease Control and Prevention, 2018. Available at https://www.cdc.gov/flu/professionals/antivirals/summary-clinicians.htm. Accessed May 24, 2019.

59. Tamiflu [package insert]. San Francisco: Genentech USA, 2016. Available at https://dailymed.nlm.nih.gov/dailymed/drugInfo.cfm?setid=ee3c9555-60f2-4f82-a760-11983c86e97b. Accessed May 24, 2019.

60. Toovey S, Prinssen EP, Rayner CE, et al. Post-marketing assessment of neuropsychiatric adverse events in influenza patients treated with oseltamivir: an updated review. Adv Ther 2012; 29:826-48.

61. Relenza [package insert]. Research Triangle Park, NC: GlaxoSmithKline, 2017. Available at https://dailymed.nlm.nih.gov/dailymed/drugInfo.cfm?setid=d7c3bcc3-0c0d-4068-fd80-88cf54a376ef. Accessed May 24, 2019.

62. Rapivab [package insert]. Summit, NJ: Seqirus USA, 2008. Available at https://dailymed.nlm.nih.gov/dailymed/drugInfo.cfm?setid=7fdedaec-9e53-4a37-a4e4-a301c8a251b8. Accessed May 24, 2019.

63. de Jong MD, Ison MG, Monto AS, et al. Evaluation of intravenous peramivir for treatment of influenza in hospitalized patients. Clin Infect Dis 2014;59:e172-85.

64. Xofluza [package insert]. San Francisco, CA; Genentech, 2018. Available at https://dailymed.nlm.nih.gov/dailymed/drugInfo.cfm?setid=e49e1a61-1b7c-4be5-ac84-af6240b511e7. Accessed May 24, 2019.

65. Hayden FG, Sugaya N, Hirotsu N, et al. Baloxavir marboxil for uncomplicated influenza in adults and adolescents. N Engl J Med 2018;379:913-23.

66. American Academy of Pediatrics, Committee on Infectious Diseases. Policy statement—recommendations for prevention and control of influenza in children, 2016–2017. Pediatrics 2016;138:e20162527.

67. World Health Organization, The United Nations Children's Fund (UNICEF). Global Action Plan for Prevention and Control of Pneumonia (GAPP) [monograph on the Internet]. Geneva: World Health Organization, 2009. Available at https://apps.who.int/iris/bitstream/handle/10665/70101/WHO_FCH_CAH_NCH_09.04_eng.pdf?sequence=1. Accessed November 1, 2019.

68. Michelow IC, Olsen K, Lozano J, et al. Epidemiology and clinical characteristics of community-acquired pneumonia in hospitalized children. Pediatrics 2004;113:701-7.

69. Shah S, Sharieff G. Pediatric respiratory infections. Emerg Med Clin North Am 2007;25:961-79.

70. Johnston IDA, Strachan DP, Anderson HR. Effect of pneumonia and whooping cough in childhood on adult lung function. N Engl J Med 1998;338:581-7.

71. Heiskanen-Kosma T, Korppi M. Risk factors of community-acquired pneumonia in children. Eur Respir J 2010;36:1221-2.

72. Tan TQ. Pediatric invasive pneumococcal disease in the United States in the era of pneumococcal conjugate vaccines. Clin Microbiol Rev 2012;25:409-19.

73. Jain S, Williams DJ, Arnold SR, et al. Community-acquired pneumonia requiring hospitalization among US children. N Eng J Med 2015;372:835-45.

74. Durbin WJ, Stille C. Pneumonia. Pediatr Rev 2008;29:147-60.

75. Don M, Canciani M, Korppi M. Community-acquired pneumonia in children: what's old? what's new? Acta Paediatr 2010;99:1602-8.

76. Bradley JS, Byington CL, Shah SS, et al. The management of community-acquired pneumonia in infants and children older than 3 months of age: clinical practice guidelines by the Pediatric Infectious Diseases Society and the Infectious Diseases Society of America. Clin Infect Dis 2011;53:e25-76.

77. McIntosh K. Community-acquired pneumonia in children. N Engl J Med 2002;346:429-37.

78. Grijalva CG, Nuorti JP, Zhu Y, et al. Increasing incidence of empyema complicating childhood community-acquired pneumonia in the United States. Clin Infect Dis 2010;50:805-13.

79. von der Poll T, Opal SM. Pathogenesis, treatment, and prevention of pneumococcal pneumonia. Lancet 2009;374:1543-56.

80. Burkhardt JE, Walterspiel JN, Schaad UB. Quinolone arthropathy in animals versus children. Clin Infect Dis 1997;25:1196-204.

81. Cipro [package insert]. Whippany, NJ: Bayer Healthcare Pharmaceuticals, 2019. Available at https://dailymed.nlm.nih.gov/dailymed/drugInfo.cfm?setid=888dc7f9-ad9c-4c00-8d50-8ddfd9bd27c0. Accessed May 24, 2019.

82. Levaquin [package insert]. Titusville, NJ: Janssen Pharmaceuticals, 2019. Available at https://dailymed.nlm.nih.gov/dailymed/

drugInfo.cfm?setid=a1f01e8e-97e9-11de-b91d-553856d89593. Accessed May 24, 2019.

83. Avelox [package insert]. Whippany, NJ: Bayer Healthcare Pharmaceuticals, 2019. Available at https://dailymed.nlm.nih.gov/dailymed/drugInfo.cfm?setid=64b6763e-e6c6-4d7d-a0eb-e4bd6a5eed3a. Accessed May 24, 2019.

84. Bradley JS, Jackson MA; AAP Committee on Infectious Diseases. The use of systemic and topical fluoroquinolones. Pediatrics 2011;128:31034-45. Available at https://pediatrics.aappublications.org/content/128/4/e1034. Accessed May 24, 2019.

85. American Academy of Pediatrics. AAP publications reaffirmed or retired. Pediatrics 2015;136:e730. Available at https://pediatrics.aappublications.org/content/pediatrics/136/3/e730.full.pdf. Accessed May 24, 2019.

86. Byington CL, Spencer LY, Johnson TA, et al. An epidemiological investigation of a sustained high rate of pediatric parapneumonic empyema: risk factors and microbiological associations. Clin Infect Dis 2002;34:434-40.

87. Francois P, Desrumaux A, Cans C, et al. Prevalence and risk factors of suppurative complications in children with pneumonia. Acta Paediatr 2010;99:861-6.

88. Moffett K, Tantoco AM. Report of increased number of children with parapneumonic empyema as a complication of bacterial pneumonia in West Virginia in 2005. W V Med J 2011;107:14-9.

89. Kalaskar AS, Heresi GP, Wanger A, et al. Severe necrotizing pneumonia in children, Houston, Texas, USA. Emerg Infect Dis 2009;15:1696-8.

90. Schultz KD, Fan LL, Pinsky J, et al. The changing face of pleural empyemas in children: epidemiology and management. Pediatrics 2004;113:1735-40.

91. Langley JM, Kellner JD, Solomon N, et al. Empyema associated with community-acquired pneumonia: a pediatric investigator's collaborative network on infections in Canada (PICNIC) study. BMC Infect Dis 2008;8:129. Available at https://bmcinfectdis.biomedcentral.com/articles/10.1186/1471-2334-8-129. Accessed November 1, 2019.

92. Li STT, Tancredi DJ. Empyema hospitalizations increased in US children despite pneumococcal conjugate vaccine. Pediatrics 2010;125:26-33.

93. Leonardi S, Miraglia del Guidice M, Spicuzza L, et al. Lung abscess in a child with Mycoplasma pneumoniae infection. Eur J Pediatr 2010;169:1413-5.

94. Calder A, Owens CM. Imaging of parapneumonic pleural effusions and empyema in children. Pediatr Radiol 2009;39:527-37.

95. Kunyoshi V, Cataneao DC, Cataneo AJM. Complicated pneumonias with empyema and/or pneumatocele in children. Pediatr Surg Int 2006;22:186-90.

96. Liu C, Bayer A, Cosgrove SE, et al. Clinical practice guidelines by the Infectious Diseases Society of America for the treatment of methicillin-resistant Staphylococcus aureus infections in adults and children. Clin Infect Dis 2011;52:1-38.

97. Ceftriaxone [package insert]. Schaumburg, IL: SAGENT Pharmaceuticals, 2018. Available at https://dailymed.nlm.nih.gov/dailymed/drugInfo.cfm?setid=9bcf7973-54fa-487c-99da-db8a92b5e074. Accessed May 24, 2019.

98. Rybak MJ, Le J, Lodise TP, et al. Therapeutic monitoring of vancomycin: a revised consensus guideline and review of the American Society of Health-System Pharmacists, the Infectious Diseases Society of America, the Pediatric Infectious Diseases Society, and the Society of Infectious Diseases Pharmacists [draft guideline]. Available at https://www.ashp.org/-/media/assets/policy-guidelines/docs/draft-guidelines/draft-guidelines-ASHP-IDSA-PIDS-SIDP-therapeutic-vancomycin.ashx. Accessed November 1, 2019.

99. Rybak M, Lomaestro B, Rotschafer JC, et al. Therapeutic monitoring of vancomycin in adult patients: a consensus review of the American Society of Health-System Pharmacists, the Infectious Diseases Society of America, the Society of Infectious Diseases Pharmacists. Am J Health Syst Pharm 2009;66:82.

100. Nemerovski CW, Klein KC. Community-associated methicillin-resistant Staphylococcus aureus in the pediatric population. J Pediatr Pharmacol Ther 2008;13:212-25.

101. Todd SR, Dahlgren FS, Traeger MS, et al. No visible dental staining in children treated with doxycycline for suspected Rocky Mountain spotted fever. J Pediatr 2015;166:1246-51.

102. Linezolid. In: REDBOOK Online [online database]. Greenwood Village, CO: Truven Health Analytics, 2019. Available at: www.micromedexsolutions.com/home/dispatch. Accessed May 23, 2019.

CHAPTER 40

Urinary Tract Infections in Infants and Children

Juan Carlos Rodriguez, Pharm.D., BCPPS

LEARNING OBJECTIVES

1. Identify prevalence and risk factors for the development of urinary tract infections (UTIs) in infants and children.

2. Recognize uropathogens associated with pediatric UTIs and the mechanisms leading to infection.

3. Describe UTI classification systems, signs and symptoms, and diagnostic criteria in children.

4. Review potential complications and long-term sequelae associated with pediatric UTIs.

5. List pharmacotherapeutic options available to treat UTIs in infants and children.

6. Discuss controversies surrounding the use of antibiotic prophylaxis in pediatric UTI patients.

ABBREVIATIONS IN THIS CHAPTER

AAP	American Academy of Pediatrics
CFU	Colony-forming unit
CRP	C-reactive protein
DMSA	Dimercaptosuccinic acid
LE	Leukocyte esterase
MRI	Magnetic resonance imaging
SPA	Suprapubic aspiration
US	Ultrasonography
UTI	Urinary tract infection
VCUG	Voiding cystourethrography
VUR	Vesicoureteral reflux
WBC	White blood cell

INTRODUCTION

Urinary tract infections (UTIs) are common in the pediatric population and occur when pathogenic organisms colonize any of the structural components of the urinary tract (e.g., kidney, ureters, bladder, urethra), leading to acute illness.[1] These infections can potentially lead to serious complications in infants and children. Bloodstream infections are associated with pediatric UTIs and are more common in infants, affecting up to 18% of infants younger than 3 months, 6% of infants age 4–8 months, and, uncommonly, in patients older than 1 year. Urosepsis may progress to decompensated septic shock and/ or meningitis, especially in patients younger than 3 months.[2,3] Renal scarring (i.e., irreversible parenchymal damage) secondary to UTIs is a potential long-term complication in children and is associated with a subsequent risk of chronic kidney disease, hypertension, and pre-eclampsia.[1,4] Risk factors for renal scarring include urinary tract anomalies and recurrent UTIs. The risk of renal damage is higher as the number of UTI recurrences increases and is greater in infants and young children than in other age groups.[1,2,5-7] Less common UTI sequelae include pyonephrosis, renal, perirenal, and retroperitoneal abscesses, emphysematous and xanthogranulomatous pyelonephritis, and infective calculi.[6] Therefore, prompt and appropriate management of UTIs is indicated in infants and children to minimize the risk of developing serious complications.[8,9]

EPIDEMIOLOGY

The overall incidence of UTIs in prepubescent children is reported to be 3% for female and 1% for male children. However, UTI incidence varies with patient age, sex and, in male children, circumcision status. Table 1 summarizes UTI incidence for the different subgroups.[1,10] The factors accounting for variability in UTI incidence also influence its prevalence. In addition, UTI prevalence increases in children presenting with fever and is highest in infants, particularly in uncircumcised male infants younger than 3 months. Table 2 summarizes UTI prevalence in infants according to patient characteristics. Overall pooled UTI prevalence for pediatric patients younger than 19 years presenting with urinary symptoms and/or fever is 7.8% (confidence interval [CI], 6.6–8.9).[11]

ETIOLOGY

The most common pathogens causing UTI are bacteria of enteric origin. *Escherichia coli*, a gram-negative rod bacterium, is the most prevalent pathogen, accounting for more than 80% of primary pediatric UTIs. Other less commonly isolated gram-negative urinary pathogens include *Citrobacter* spp., *Enterobacter* spp., *Klebsiella* spp., *Morganella morganii*, *Proteus mirabilis*, *Providencia stuartii*, *Pseudomonas aeruginosa*, *Serratia* spp., and *Neisseria gonorrhea*. Gram-positive organisms causing UTIs in children include *Enterococcus* spp., *Staphylococcus aureus*, *Staphylococcus saprophyticus*, *Staphylococcus epidermidis*, and group B and D streptococci. Less common uropathogens include *Candida albicans*, *Chlamydia trachomatis*, *Ureaplasma urealyticum*, and *Mycoplasma hominis*.[1,5,12,13] Patient characteristics increasing the probability of recovering non-*E. coli* UTI pathogens include presence of functional or structural urinary tract anomalies (discussed later in this chapter), previous antibiotic exposure, younger age, recurrent UTIs, afebrile status, circumcision in male infants, and Hispanic ethnicity. Nosocomial UTIs are associated with more resistant pathogens such as *Pseudomonas, Enterobacter, Citrobacter, Proteus, Providencia,* or *Enterococcus* spp. *Staphylococcus saprophyticus* is second to *E. coli* as a cause of cystitis in young women. Candiduria is increasingly common in immunosuppressed patients receiving broad-spectrum antibiotics for presumptive or definitive management of systemic infections. Candidal infections may also occur in catheterized children.[14-17]

INFECTION PATHWAYS

Infection of the urinary tract typically occurs by one of four pathways. The most common pathway is retrograde ascent. Uropathogens associated with retrograde ascent usually originate from the host's gastrointestinal tract and colonize periurethral or vaginal areas. Vaginal flora may also serve as a reservoir for organisms causing UTIs. The pathogens enter the urinary tract through the urethra and migrate to the bladder, where they multiply and potentially progress to infect the upper urinary tract (i.e., kidney).[1,18] Specific bacterial virulence factors are necessary to colonize cells of the urinary tract and facilitate ascension into the bladder and upper urinary tract while evading the host defense mechanisms. Adhesins commonly present in uropathogenic *E. coli* that promote urinary tract colonization include type 1 fimbriae and P fimbriae. Type 1 fimbriae are often found in *E. coli* strains that cause acute cystitis whereas the presence of P fimbriae in *E. coli* is strongly associated with acute pyelonephritis. After attachment to the uroepithelial mucosal surface, additional virulence factors (e.g., ureases, iron-scavenging proteins, α-hemolysin, bacterial toxins) are produced to support continued bacterial growth within the urinary tract. Release of bacterial toxins and proteases induce host cell damage.[5,19]

A second UTI pathway is nosocomial infection. Introduction of a foreign body or instrumentation (e.g., urethral catheterization) into the urinary tract increases the risk of UTI, particularly with longer durations of catheterization.[1,6] Catheterization generates a robust immune response. Accumulation of fibrinogen on the catheter provides a favorable growth medium for bacteria that express fibrinogen-binding proteins. Once attached, bacteria multiply and ascend the urinary tract as previously described.[19]

A third infection pathway is the hematogenous route. The infecting organisms disseminate from their original nidus outside of the urinary tract, resulting in a systemic infection with subsequent urinary tract seeding (e.g., staphylococcal bacteremia or endocarditis, neonatal sepsis).[8] This pathway is more common in infants and immunocompromised patients.[1,5]

A fourth pathway involves the development of a fistula between the urinary tract and the gastrointestinal tract or vagina (e.g., vesicointestinal, urethrorectal, or vesicovaginal fistulae). This mechanism is rarely encountered.[1]

HOST FACTORS

The primary host defense mechanism against UTI is the continuous flow of urine from the kidneys to the bladder, ultimately resulting in micturition and complete bladder emptying through the urethra. Normal urinary flow typically clears urinary tract pathogens. In addition, several antibacterial inhibitory factors in urine play protective roles against UTIs. Inhibitory substances in urine include urea, organic acids, and salts. Urine pH and osmolarity also contribute to antibacterial activity. Low osmolarity inhibits bacterial growth; high osmolarity, if associated with low pH, is also inhibitory. Other substances that inhibit bacterial adherence to urinary tract mucosa include the Tamm-Horsfall protein, bladder mucopolysaccharide, low–molecular weight oligosaccharides, secretory immunoglobulin A, and lactoferrin. The inflammatory response (e.g., polymorphonuclear neutrophils, cytokines) as well as humoral and cell-mediated immunity are other components involved in the urinary tract's host defense mechanism against invading pathogens.[1,5,18]

Other host factors are associated with increased UTI risk. Vesicoureteral reflux (VUR) is an anatomic disorder that predisposes children to UTIs. The prevalence of VUR ranges between 18% and 35% among children with UTIs.[20] Primary VUR (the most common type) is a congenital defect that results in the shortening of the longitudinal muscle in the submucosal ureter; this shortened muscle length compromises closure of the ureter with bladder filling and limits urination, thus facilitating the retrograde ascent of urine from the bladder into the ureter(s) and potentially the kidney(s).[1,2,5,21] Vesicoureteral reflux is classified into grades I through V. Grade I describes reflux into the ureter(s); grade II flow into the kidney(s) without dilation of the renal pelvis; grade III dilation of ureter(s) and renal pelvis; grade IV dilation of ureter(s), renal pelvis, and calyces; grade V severe dilation of uterer(s), renal pelvis, and calyces.[22] Grades I–III are more likely to resolve spontaneously by age 5 years than grades IV and V reflux. Probability of spontaneous resolution is lower in patients presenting at an older age and in those with bilateral reflux. More rapid resolution of VUR has been observed in African American children.[2,21] Other host factors increasing susceptibility to bacteriuria are listed in Table 3.[1,5,18,23] Surgical intervention may be necessary to manage urinary tract abnormalities.

CLASSIFICATION

There are several methods to classify UTIs. One common method is based on the

Table 1. Incidence of Urinary Tract Infection in Pediatric Patients[1,10]

Sex	Age < 12 mo	Age 1–5 yr	Age > 5 yr (prepubescent)
Female	0.4%–1%	0.9%–1.4%	0.7%–2.3%
Male	0.19% (circumcised) 0.7% (uncircumcised)	0.1%–0.2%	0.04%–0.2%

Table 2. Pooled Prevalence of Urinary Tract Infection in Febrile Infants[11]

Age (mo)	Female	Male	Circumcised	Uncircumcised
< 3	7.5%	8.7%	2.4%	20.1%
3–6	5.7%	3.3%	—	—
6–12	8.3%	1.7%	0.3%	7.3%

infection site. The infection may be localized in the *bladder (cystitis)*, *urethra (urethritis)*, *urine (bacteriuria)*, or *kidney (pyelonephritis)*. The infection site in the urinary tract may be more broadly classified as a *lower UTI* or *upper UTI*. Cystitis and urethritis are examples of lower UTIs whereas pyelonephritis is classified as an upper UTI.[1,10,21]

A second method classifies UTIs as either uncomplicated or complicated. An *uncomplicated UTI* occurs in normal urinary tracts without previous instrumentation (e.g., catheterization).[10] A *complicated UTI* describes patients with structural or functional urinary tract abnormalities, genitourinary obstruction (e.g., stones), immunosuppression, diabetes mellitus, renal insufficiency, or with indwelling and intermittent catheter use, or who are pregnant or a neonate, in addition to most patients with clinical evidence of pyelonephritis or renal abscess. Patients initially diagnosed with an uncomplicated

UTI who do not experience a response to appropriate therapy or for whom the organism is not eradicated after appropriate therapy are reclassified as a complicated UTI.[24,25]

A third strategy to classify pediatric UTIs is based on episode. Using this method, UTIs are categorized as either a *first infection* or a *recurrent infection*. The first infection is the initial UTI diagnosed by a reliable urine culture. Recurrent infections are further subcategorized as *unresolved bacteriuria*, *bacterial persistence*, or *reinfection*.[25,26]

Unresolved bacteriuria is defined as persistent positive cultures with the same uropathogen isolated in the original culture. Unresolved infection is commonly the result of inadequate therapy (e.g., uropathogen resistance to selected antibiotic, patient nonadherence to prescribed antibiotic, intestinal malabsorption, subtherapeutic antibiotic concentrations in urine). Once culture and antibiotic susceptibility results are

Table 3. Host Factors Associated with Increased Risk of Urinary Tract Infection in Pediatric Patients[1,5,18,23]

Host Risk Factor	Proposed Mechanism/Supporting Observations
Younger age group (neonates and infants)	Incompletely developed immune system
	Breastfeeding may be protective by supplementing maternal IgA, lactoferrin, and anti-adhesive oligosaccharides
Female sex	Periurethral and vaginal moisture promotes uropathogen growth
	Shorter urethra increases probability of ascending infection
Uncircumcised infants	Increased concentration of uropathogens in boys with foreskin
Fecal and perineal colonization	Colon and urogenital flora expressing specific virulence factors
Antibiotic exposure	Alters normal microbiota of urogenital mucosa, thus increasing relative risk of UTI and resulting in isolation of more resistant microbial strains
Constipation	Distended rectum presses on bladder wall to produce outflow obstruction and dysfunctional voiding
Anatomic anomalies (posterior urethral valves, VUR, ureteropelvic junction obstruction)	Inadequate clearance of uropathogens
Functional abnormalities (dysfunctional voiding, neurogenic bladder)	Urinary retention, urinary stasis, and incomplete bladder emptying result in decreased urinary bacterial clearance
Female sexual activity	Bowel and vaginal bacterial transfer to urethral meatus, leading to postcoital bacteriuria
Spermicide use	Alteration of vaginal flora facilitating adherence of *Escherichia coli* to epithelial cells
HIV disease	Immunocompromised state
Renal transplantation	Immunocompromised state
Diabetes mellitus	Urine glucose supplies a growth medium for pathogens
Genetic predisposition	Epidemiologic studies show a higher incidence of cystitis and pyelonephritis in female patients whose female relatives reported a history of UTIs, with higher risk reported as the number of affected relatives increased
	White female patients are more likely to develop a UTI than their African American counterparts
	Associations between specific blood group phenotypes and recurrent UTIs have been reported
	Host cell receptors facilitating bacterial adherence to uroepithelium have been identified (e.g., α-Gal(14) β-Gal receptor)

Gal = galactosidase; HIV = human immunodeficiency virus; IgA = immunoglobulin A; UTI = urinary tract infection; VUR = vesicoureteral reflux.

available, unresolved bacteriuria is typically treated successfully if uropathogen resistance is identified.[26]

In *bacterial persistence*, negative urine cultures are documented after treatment of the initial UTI; however, because of incomplete eradication of the infection, the original infecting organism is isolated in subsequent episodes. Patients with documented bacterial persistence may have an underlying urinary tract abnormality (e.g., infected calculus, necrotic papillae, foreign objects), which may shield the uropathogen from the effects of the antibiotic. It is important to identify these abnormalities, if present, given that many may be surgically treated.[26]

Reinfection also involves documentation of negative urine cultures after initial treatment, but in this case, subsequent infections are caused by organisms or strains that are different from the original pathogen isolated. Reinfection is usually acquired by periurethral colonization with perineal and rectal flora (i.e., retrograde ascent). Because *E. coli* is the most common infecting organism, distinguishing between reinfection and bacterial persistence can be challenging based on the many serotypes of *E. coli*. Serotyping the organism establishes reinfection if a different *E. coli* strain is isolated. However, serotyping is not commonly performed in routine clinical practice; therefore, a careful evaluation of antibiotic susceptibility patterns is helpful in distinguishing between reinfection versus bacterial persistence.[1,5,26]

CLINICAL PRESENTATION AND DIAGNOSIS

SIGNS AND SYMPTOMS

Children may not present with the classic UTI signs and symptoms reported by adults (e.g., urinary frequency, dysuria, hesitancy, flank pain, turbid urine). An atypical presentation is more common in younger age groups for whom nonspecific signs and symptoms are more prevalent. Neonates may present with jaundice, failure to thrive, fever, difficulty feeding, irritability, or gastrointestinal symptoms such as vomiting and diarrhea. Infants and children younger than 24 months may present with nonspecific signs and symptoms similar to those reported in neonates, with the exception of jaundice; but in this older age group, patient presentation may include cloudy or malodorous urine, hematuria, frequency, and dysuria. Children older than 2 years are more likely to present with fever, hematuria, frequency, dysuria, enuresis (in a previously toilet-trained child), costovertebral angle pain, and/or abdominal pain. Vomiting, diarrhea, and irritability are less common presentations for patients older than 2 years with UTI. The symptomatology of UTIs in adolescent patients is typically comparable to that of adults.[5-7,14,21]

DIAGNOSTIC CRITERIA

RAPID URINE TESTS

Early diagnosis and appropriate treatment are essential to produce a positive outcome in pediatric patients with UTIs, particularly in infants and younger children. Because it typically takes 24 hours or more for final urine culture results to be reported by the microbiology laboratory, clinicians often use rapid tests such as urine dipsticks or microscopy in the evaluation of children with symptomatology suggestive of UTI.[27] Urine dipstick tests are performed at the bedside, and results are available within minutes. For urine microscopy, the time it takes to receive the results varies because the sample is analyzed in the clinical laboratory; turnaround time generally ranges between 15 minutes and 2 hours.

Dipstick urinalysis measures urine-specific gravity and pH and detects the presence of glucose, protein, blood, nitrites, and leukocyte esterase (LE). For the presumptive diagnosis of UTI, only nitrites and LE are associated with relatively high sensitivity (low percentage of false negatives) and high specificity (low percentage of false positives), as confirmed by bacteriuria from quantitative urine cultures. Most gram-negative urinary bacteria reduce dietary nitrates to nitrites; the positive nitrite test detects the presence of this substance and suggests UTI. Gram-positive organisms (and some gram-negative organisms) do not reduce nitrates to nitrites. Therefore, a negative nitrite test does not rule out UTI. Mean sensitivity for the nitrate test is 53% with a specificity of 98%. Lysed white blood cells (WBCs) release esterases. The LE test detects these substances in the urine sample and is therefore a surrogate marker for the presence of WBCs in the urine. Average sensitivity and specificity for the LE test are reported to be 83% and 78%, respectively. The combination of LE and nitrite tests increases sensitivity but not specificity.[6,7,27]

Microscopic analysis directly identifies crystals, red blood cells (hematuria), WBCs (pyuria), casts, and bacteria. Quantification of WBCs and bacteria best correlates with a diagnosis of UTI. *Pyuria* is defined as 5 or more WBCs per high-power field of centrifuged urine or 10 or more WBCs per microliter of urine. The mean sensitivity and specificity for WBC microscopy are 73% and 81%, respectively.[6,7] Children with *Enterococcus* spp., *Klebsiella* spp. or *P. aeruginosa* UTIs have been reported to be less likely to exhibit pyuria than those infected with *E. coli*.[28] For bacterial microscopy, the reported mean sensitivity and specificity are 81% and 83%, respectively. Accuracy rates are higher when microscopy for bacteria is performed with a Gram stain.[6,7,14,29,30]

Rapid urine tests (whether dipstick urinalysis or microscopy) are not intended to replace urine culture as a diagnostic tool. Rapid tests do not identify the infecting pathogen or yield antibiotic susceptibility results to guide antibiotic selection.[29]

URINE CULTURES AND COLLECTION METHODS

A positive urine culture is required to make the UTI diagnosis; however, a positive culture alone (i.e., in the absence of pyuria or symptomatology) is insufficient to establish the diagnosis or initiate treatment, especially in the absence of urinary tract abnormalities. Asymptomatic bacteriuria represents uropathogen attenuation by the host or bladder colonization by nonvirulent bacteria.[1,25]

Urine cultures should be taken before initiating antimicrobial therapy. A urine culture may be obtained by a variety of techniques. Because the distal urethra is commonly colonized with the same pathogens that cause UTIs, the number of colony-forming units (CFUs) necessary to estimate infection probability depends on the method used to collect the urine sample.[2,5]

Suprapubic aspiration (SPA) is considered the gold standard for accurate UTI diagnosis. However, because SPA is an invasive technique, it is not routinely performed. The SPA technique involves the advancing of a 2- to 4-cm needle above the symphysis pubis through the bladder wall until urine flows into the syringe. Any number of gram-negative bacilli or greater than 10^3 gram-positive cocci is associated with a greater than 99% probability of infection.[1,5,14]

Even though transurethral catheterization is also an invasive technique, it is a commonly used method of obtaining a reliable urine sample (particularly in non-toilet trained children), provided that the initial aliquot of the sample is discarded to reduce the potential for culturing organisms introduced into the bladder on catheterization. For urine samples collected by transurethral catheterization, the probability of infection is 95% if 10^5 CFUs of bacteria or greater are recovered. A catheterized urine culture is considered suggestive of infection if 10^4–10^5 CFUs are quantified, and repeating a culture may be warranted to establish the diagnosis.[1,5,14]

The American Academy of Pediatrics (AAP) clinical practice guidelines for initial UTI in febrile children age 2–24 months recognize SPA and transurethral catheterization as the most reliable collection methods for diagnosing a UTI. To establish a UTI diagnosis, these guidelines recommend urinalysis results suggestive of UTI (i.e., pyuria and/or bacteriuria) plus the presence of 50,000 CFU/mL or more of uropathogen collected by SPA or catheterization for the target age group.[6,7]

Clean void urine samples are simple to perform and noninvasive. A clean void urine sample is obtained using the clean-catch midstream technique. It is the most commonly used collection method in toilet-trained children and adolescents. After appropriate topical disinfection of the genitalia, the patient urinates the first aliquot of the sample into the toilet, after which the collection cup is placed under the urine stream to collect the laboratory sample. Periurethral and preputial organisms contaminate clean-catch specimens in a significant percentage of samples, making interpretation of positive results challenging. In female patients, 10^5 CFUs or greater of bacteria confers a high probability of infection (i.e., 80% to 95%, depending on whether one, two, or three positive urine specimens were recovered). In male patients, greater than 10^4 CFUs of bacteria makes infection likely.[1,5,14]

A bagged specimen is an alternative method of urine collection and involves attaching a plastic bag to the perineum to collect the urine specimen; the bagged urine technique may be used to collect a sample from neonates, infants, and non-toilet trained children. Bagged urine samples are associated with an 85% rate of false-positive results and are therefore not reliable to establish a UTI diagnosis. However, a negative result from a bagged urine sample is helpful in ruling out a UTI.[6,7,14,20,25]

IMAGING STUDIES

In infants and young children, UTIs may serve as an indicator of urinary tract abnormalities; therefore, imaging studies have traditionally been recommended to identify potential urinary tract anomalies predisposing the young child to renal disease. Imaging studies performed in pediatric patients include renal and bladder ultrasonography (US), voiding cystourethrography (VCUG), radionuclide cystography, renal cortical scan, computed tomography, magnetic resonance imaging (MRI), and intravenous pyelography. Table 4 provides a summary of these imaging studies.[6,7,13,14]

Renal and bladder US offers a noninvasive method to evaluate anatomy (e.g., renal size and various aspects of the parenchyma); it may also reveal obstructive lesions. Ultrasonography identifies hydronephrosis, dilation of distal ureters, bladder wall hypertrophy, and presence of ureteroceles. Intravenous pyelography, which requires parenteral administration of iodinated contrast dye, was previously used to detect such anomalies; however, renal and bladder US is currently preferred to intravenous pyelography for anatomic evaluation of the urinary tract because it effectively reveals these abnormalities and is safer, less invasive, and more cost-effective. Ultrasonography does not reliably detect VUR.[6,7,13,14]

Table 4. Imaging Studies for Urinary Tract Infection in Pediatric Patients[6,7,12,14]

Study	Dye Administration	Catheterization	Diagnostic Use
Renal and bladder ultrasonography	No	No	Evaluate anatomy; may identify obstructions, hydronephrosis, distal ureter(s) dilation, bladder wall hypertrophy, ureteroceles
Voiding cystourethrography	Yes	Yes	Vesicoureteral reflux diagnosis and grading; obstructive lesions
Radionucleotide cystography	Yes	Yes	Vesicoureteral reflux diagnosis and grading; obstructive lesions
Renal cortical scans	Yes	No	Assess renal scarring, acute changes associated with pyelonephritis, mass lesions
Computed tomography	No	No	Renal abscesses
Magnetic resonance imaging	No	No	Renal abscesses; possible renal scarring
Intravenous pyelography	Yes	No	Evaluate anatomy

Both VCUG and radionuclide cystography are effective in diagnosing and grading VUR. Both of these imaging studies involve radiation exposure and catheterization. Radionuclide cystography, however, does not reveal male urethral or bladder abnormalities whereas VCUG does.[4,12]

Renal cortical scans, also known as *scintigraphy*, require injection of the radioisotope [99m]technetium dimercaptosuccinic acid (DMSA) or [99m]technetium glucoheptonate. It is a sensitive test for assessing renal scarring or identifying acute changes associated with pyelonephritis. Renal cortical scans are also useful in diagnosing mass lesions such as neoplasms and abscesses.[4,6,7,14]

Computed tomography and MRI studies best visualize renal abscesses. Computed tomography is more commonly used because it is readily available whereas MRI may yield better soft tissue resolution and diagnostic sensitivity.[14] Some evidence supports the use of MRI for the evaluation of renal scarring.[31,32]

The AAP clinical practice guidelines for febrile infants and children age 2–24 months recommend performing a renal and bladder US but not VCUG after the initial UTI; VCUG is recommended when US findings are suggestive of obstructive uropathy or high-grade VUR and in atypical or complex clinical circumstances, such as infection with non-*E. coli* organism, delayed response to appropriate antibiotics, presence of abnormal urine stream, or evidence of renal dysplasia or insufficiency.[4,6,7] A population-based comparative study concluded that the recommended imaging guidelines for patients age 2–24 months can be applied to infants younger than 2 months; the two groups were comparable with respect to clinical characteristics, predominant bacterium isolated, antibiotic resistance and bacteremia rates, grade III-V VUR diagnosis, imaging study findings, renal scarring incidence, and clinical outcomes after the first febrile UTI.[33]

Considerable discussion remains surrounding the use of imaging studies to evaluate pediatric UTIs in general. Questions about when to image, about the type of imaging to use, or whether to image at all are active topics under evaluation. More detailed reviews of the topic are found in other references.[15,34]

OTHER LABORATORY TESTS

Depending on clinical presentation and the patient's risk factors, a complete blood cell count, C-reactive protein, blood and/or cerebrospinal fluid cultures may provide valuable data when treating an acutely ill child or febrile infant younger than 2 months admitted for a sepsis workup. A basic metabolic panel may expose electrolyte abnormalities if the child is dehydrated or renally compromised.[2,5,25] Although not presently standard practice, serum procalcitonin has been evaluated as a surrogate marker for bloodstream infections and renal parenchymal inflammation in the setting of pediatric UTIs.[25,35-37]

TREATMENT

After reviewing the patient's allergy history and clinical presentation, a third-generation cephalosporin or a β-lactam/β-lactamase inhibitor combination is commonly selected for empiric UTI treatment based on local (or regional) susceptibility patterns of the selected antibiotic against the target organism(s). Patients with a history of anatomic or functional urinary tract abnormalities, recurrent UTIs, uncommon pathogens, catheter use, or immunodeficiency states may require more individualized antibiotic coverage. Antibiotic therapy is de-escalated accordingly once culture and susceptibility results are available.[2,6,7,38]

PARENTERAL ANTIBIOTICS

Children, particularly those younger than 2 years, may require administration of parenteral antibiotic therapy. Criteria for initiating parenteral antibiotic(s) include acutely ill or "toxic" children, hospitalized infants younger than 2 months, immunocompromised patients, children who are unable to retain oral intake or who are dehydrated, and patients for whom adherence to a treatment regimen or obtaining and/or administering oral antibiotics as an outpatient is uncertain.[1,4,6,7]

Table 5 lists commonly used parenteral antibiotics prescribed for the treatment of pediatric UTIs and pediatric dosing recommendations. The cephalosporins, aminoglycosides, and fluoroquinolone listed in Table 5 are generally active against uropathogens in the *Enterobacteriaceae* family (e.g., *E. coli, Klebsiella* spp., *Citrobacter* spp., *Enterobacter* spp., *M. morganii, P. mirabilis, P. stuartii,* and *Serratia* spp.). Third-generation cephalosporins are more β-lactamase stable than earlier generations and are thus more active against β-lactamase–producing pathogens and suitable for empiric therapy. Cefotaxime and ceftriaxone have comparable antimicrobial spectra of activity and may be used interchangeably in most instances; however, ceftriaxone is not routinely recommended for neonates. The drug is highly protein bound (more than 90% bound to albumin); in hyperbilirubinemic neonates, bilirubin displacement from its albumin binding sites increases the risk of kernicterus. In addition, ceftriaxone is contraindicated in neonates receiving or who may require calcium-containing intravenous solutions; crystalline material has been recovered at autopsy from the lungs and kidneys of a limited number of neonates administered this combination.[1,2,25]

If an anti-pseudomonal antibiotic is indicated, aminoglycosides, ciprofloxacin, ceftazidime, cefepime, and piperacillin/tazobactam are active against *P. aeruginosa,* an organism recovered in 13.1% of nosocomial UTIs.[5] Most gram-negative uropathogens produce β-lactamases; consequently, a significant percentage of these organisms are resistant to ampicillin. Ampicillin monotherapy is not a preferred empiric antibiotic selection for UTI. Ampicillin may be used empirically in combination with an aminoglycoside or a third-generation cephalosporin. Unlike cephalosporins, ampicillin is microbiologically active against enterococci, particularly *Enterococcus faecalis.*[1,6,7,39] Fluoroquinolones are a treatment option for pyelonephritis or complicated UTIs when conventional first-line antibiotics are not appropriate because of resistance, allergy, or adverse reaction history.[40]

Duration of parenteral therapy depends on the patient's clinical response to therapy. Parenteral antibiotics are continued until the patient is afebrile and clinically stable, after which the antibiotic is switched to an appropriate oral agent to complete the treatment course.[1]

ORAL ANTIBIOTICS

An oral antibiotic is typically prescribed to pediatric UTI patients for one of the two following reasons: to complete a treatment course for a patient initiated on parenteral antibiotics, or as initial treatment of the UTI in a child presenting to an emergency department or physician's office who does not meet criteria for the use of parenteral antibiotics. Advantages of oral antibiotic therapy include ease of administration and overall lower cost. Studies of children 1 month and older treated for pyelonephritis showed similar efficacy between oral and intravenous/oral sequential therapy. There was no statistical difference in renal scarring between oral and intravenous/oral treatment groups.[41-44] Historically, longer intravenous antibiotic courses (i.e., 7–14 days) were prescribed for neonates and younger infants. However, a cohort study of 12,333 neonates and infants younger than 6 months concluded that there was no difference in readmission rate at 30 days after discharge for patients administered antibiotics intravenously for 3 days or fewer versus 4 days or more, provided that the infants completed an antibiotic course that totaled 10 to 14 days.[45] Therefore, prolonged parenteral antibiotic therapy solely based on a patient's age is not warranted, and transition to oral therapy is a viable option in the younger age groups.

Table 6 identifies commonly used oral antibiotics for the treatment of pediatric UTIs in addition to dosing recommendations. Documented safety and efficacy are the primary considerations when selecting an oral antibiotic for the treatment of UTIs. The local susceptibility rate of the target organism(s) to the selected antibiotic for empiric use is an important consideration. The antibiotic selected should not have resistance rates of 20% or higher against the target organism.[2,46] Once the organism is identified in culture, de-escalating to the most appropriate, narrow-spectrum agent is recommended.[38] If a liquid formulation is indicated, its palatability must be considered because the formulation's taste influences patient adherence to the prescribed regimen. Studies evaluating the taste of pediatric antibiotic oral formulations report substantial variability in palatability for the products tested. In one study, which included some of the antibiotic suspensions listed in Table 6, the rankings in decreasing order of palatability are as follows: cefixime, ceftibuten, trimethoprim/sulfamethoxazole, amoxicillin-clavulanate, and cefpodoxime.[47] Cost and formulary status are additional considerations when selecting an oral antibiotic.[47]

Drug-specific properties are another important consideration. Use of trimethoprim/sulfamethoxazole should be avoided in children younger than 2 months because sulfonamides are highly protein bound, and, like ceftriaxone, may displace bilirubin and potentially cause kernicterus in hyperbilirubinemic patients. Nitrofurantoin should be avoided in patients with glucose-6-dehydrogenase deficiency because of the risk of precipitating hemolytic anemia. Per the manufacturer, nitrofurantoin is contraindicated if creatinine clearance is less than 60 mL/minute because therapeutic urine concentrations are not attained in renal insufficiency; however, data suggest safe and effective use in uncomplicated UTIs for creatinine clearances 30 mL/minute or greater.[39] Nitrofurantoin should also be avoided in the treatment of febrile infants with UTIs, pyelonephritis, or perinephric abscesses; parenchymal and serum concentrations attained may be insufficient to treat pyelonephritis or urosepsis. Nitrofurantoin use is not recommended in neonates (age younger than 30 days) because of increased risk of hemolysis.[6,7,39]

Table 5. Parenteral Antibiotics Commonly Used for Treatment of Urinary Tract Infection in Pediatric Patients[6,7,15,25,38,39]

Antibiotic	Pediatric Dosage[a,b]
Ampicillin[c]	100–200 mg/kg/day divided every 6 hr
Ampicillin/Sulbactam	200 mg/kg/day (ampicillin component) divided every 6 hr
Cefazolin[c]	50 mg/kg/day divided every 6–8 hr
Cefuroxime	150 mg/kg/day divided every 8 hr
Cefotaxime	100–150 mg/kg/day divided every 6–8 hr
Ceftriaxone	50–75 mg/kg/day divided every 12–24 hr
Ceftazidime	100–150 mg/kg/day divided every 8 hr
Cefepime	100 mg/kg/day divided every 12 hr
Ciprofloxacin	18–30 mg/kg/day divided every 8 hr
Gentamicin	5–7.5 mg/kg/day divided every 8–24 hr
Piperacillin/Tazobactam	300 mg/kg/day (piperacillin component) divided every 6-8 hr
Tobramycin	5–7.5 mg/kg/day divided every 8–24 hr

[a]Doses referenced assume normal renal function and are consistent with dosing recommendations for children older than the neonatal period. For neonatal dosing recommendations, consult an appropriate reference.
[b]Doses for higher-weight children and adolescents are typically limited to the adult dose when weight-based dosing results in a higher value than the standard adult dose for the indication.
[c]Not recommended for empiric therapy. Used for definitive therapy once susceptibility results are available.

DURATION OF TREATMENT

The AAP clinical practice guidelines recommend a 7- to 14-day treatment course for children between age 2 months and 2 years.[6,7] Antibiotic courses of 10–14 days are commonly prescribed for children and adolescents with a diagnosis of pyelonephritis. For uncomplicated lower UTIs (e.g., cystitis), shorter treatment courses (2–4 days) with oral antibiotics have been reported effective in children.[48,49]

PROPHYLAXIS

The antibiotics listed in Table 7 may be used for UTI prophylaxis in children. In patients with recurrent infections, careful evaluation of previous culture and susceptibility results serve as a valuable guide to antibiotic selection. Prophylactic antibiotics are generally continued until resolution of the underlying condition(s) predisposing the patient to UTIs. The rationale for antibiotic prophylaxis after active UTI treatment is maintaining sterilization of the urine. The goal is to prevent irreversible renal parenchymal damage (renal scarring) and its sequelae. The antibiotic selected for prophylaxis is administered at a reduced dose, achieving therapeutic urine concentrations while delivering low concentrations of antibiotic to the bowel to minimize its effect on normal intestinal flora.[1,13] Trimethoprim/sulfamethoxazole and nitrofurantoin are the preferred agents for prophylaxis.[15] Prophylactic cephalosporin use is associated with a greater likelihood of culturing extended-spectrum β-lactamase–producing organisms or non–E. coli multidrug-resistant uropathogens.[50,51]

The use of antibiotic prophylaxis is presently the subject of considerable debate. Traditionally, the following subgroups have been considered for antibiotic prophylaxis: neonates or infants being evaluated for anatomic or functional urinary tract abnormalities; children with a history of VUR grade III or higher, dysfunctional voiding, or partial urinary obstruction; immunosuppressed patients; and children with recurrent UTIs despite normal urinary anatomy and function.[1,13] Literature supporting the use of antibiotic prophylaxis to reduce renal scars or rate of recurrences has been published. In a Swedish study, prophylactic antibiotics were effective in reducing new renal scars in infant girls with grades III and IV reflux at DMSA scanning after a 2-year follow-up period.[52] Another trial reported a 50% reduced risk of recurrence in the trimethoprim/sulfamethoxazole prophylaxis group, but the rate of renal scarring did not differ between the prophylaxis and placebo groups.[53] A Cochrane Review of the pediatric literature concludes that prophylactic antibiotics reduce the risk of recurrent symptomatic UTIs; however, their benefit is limited, and the increased risk of bacterial resistance must be considered.[54]

Conversely, the AAP clinical practice guidelines do not recommend prophylactic antibiotics to prevent UTI recurrences. After the initial UTI, the clinician instructs the parents or guardians to seek prompt medical attention (i.e., within 48 hours) for any future febrile illness because early treatment is preferred to limit potential renal damage.[6,7] Moreover, a meta-analysis recommends against the routine use of antibiotic prophylaxis in children at risk of developing UTIs, citing lack of evidence supporting a positive benefit.[55] Another systematic review found no benefit of antibiotic prophylaxis in preventing renal scars in otherwise healthy children after an initial or a second febrile or symptomatic UTI.[56] An additional study reported an increased risk of resistant infections but no decrease in risk of recurrent UTIs associated with antibiotic prophylaxis.[57] Lastly, a more recent meta-analysis evaluated the 224 cases of UTIs among

Table 6. Oral Antibiotics Commonly Used for Treatment of Urinary Tract Infection in Pediatric Patients[15,25,38,39]

Antibiotic	Pediatric Dosage[a,b]
Amoxicillin[c]	40–50 mg/kg/day divided every 8–12 hr
Amoxicillin/clavulanate	40–50 mg/kg/day divided every 8–12 hr (Use 4:1 or 7:1 formulation)
Cefixime	8 mg/kg/day divided every 12-24 hr
Cefpodoxime proxetil	10 mg/kg/day divided every 12 hr
Cefprozil	30 mg/kg/day divided every 12 hr
Ceftibuten	9 mg/kg/dose once daily
Cefuroxime axetil	20–30 mg/kg/day divided every 12 hr
Cephalexin[c]	50 mg/kg/day divided every 6-8 hr
Ciprofloxacin	20–40 mg/kg/day divided every 12 hr
Nitrofurantoin[d]	5–7 mg/kg/day divided every 6 hr
Trimethoprim/sulfamethoxazole[c]	8–12 mg/kg/day trimethoprim divided every 12 hr

[a]Doses referenced assume normal renal function and are consistent with dosing recommendations for children older than the neonatal period. For neonatal dosing recommendations, consult an appropriate reference.

[b]Doses for higher-weight children and adolescents are typically limited to the adult dose when weight-based dosing results in a higher value than the standard adult dose for the indication.

[c]Not recommended for empiric therapy. Used for definitive therapy once susceptibility results are available.

[d]Nitrofurantoin should not be used for treatment of urinary tract infections in febrile infants and young children, in neonates (age younger than 30 days), or for pyelonephritis or perinephric abscesses.

1299 pediatric VUR patients who received continuous antibiotic prophylaxis for 3 months or more. A multidrug-resistant organism was recovered in 33% of first recurrent UTIs in the antibiotic prophylaxis group versus 6% in the placebo or no prophylaxis groups (p<0.001). Patients in the prophylaxis group were also more likely to be prescribed broad-spectrum antibiotics (68% vs. 49%, p<0.004) for the treatment of their recurrent UTI.[58]

In short, initiation of antibiotics for UTI prophylaxis requires careful consideration and accounts for the patient's underlying medical conditions and risk for serious adverse sequelae. Family involvement is imperative when deciding whether to initiate prophylactic antibiotics. Adherence to the prophylactic regimen varies between 17% and 69% and depends on patient and caregiver education.[25] Based on the Swedish study, infant girls with grade III or higher VUR may benefit from prophylaxis.[52] Patients with significant kidney and urinary tract abnormalities and recurrent UTIs may also benefit because of their increased risk for subsequent renal scarring or end stage renal disease.[52,59] Other indications for antibiotic prophylaxis may be identified in clinical practice and should be managed on an individual case basis, if benefits are expected to outweigh risks to the child.

Nonantibiotic approaches to reduce UTI recurrence have been described in the literature. Cranberry juice has been recommended for prevention of UTI recurrence, particularly for female adults. However, a meta-analysis concluded that cranberry products are not effective overall for preventing UTIs in children.[60] Probiotics have also been used in an attempt to reduce UTI recurrences, but two meta-analyses failed to demonstrate an advantage to probiotic use.[61,62] The effect of circumcision status on UTI incidence and prevalence is summarized in the Epidemiology section of this chapter. Male neonates with a diagnosis of urinary tract abnormalities benefit further from circumcision within the first 28 days of life. The number needed to treat (i.e., circumcised) to prevent one UTI is 83 in otherwise healthy boys but decreases to one in 6 to 13 in those with urinary tract abnormalities, depending on the specific diagnosis.[63] Managing bowel (e.g., constipation) and/or bladder dysfunction (e.g., dysfunctional or neurogenic bladder) is safe and effective in UTI prevention. Constipation may be treated with increased dietary fiber intake, optimal hydration, and laxatives such as polyethylene glycol 3350. Initial management of bladder dysfunction is nonpharmacologic and includes adequate hydration, timed voiding, biofeedback, and pelvic floor muscle retraining in older children and adolescents to improve relaxation and contraction of pelvic muscles.[64,65] For a more detailed discussion on bowel and bladder dysfunction, the reader is referred to a more comprehensive review of the subject.[65]

CONCLUSIONS

In infants and children, UTIs are a common diagnosis. This population is at increased risk for long-term morbidity, including irreversible renal damage and its sequelae. Signs and symptoms in the young child may be nonspecific, making diagnosis more challenging on presentation. Specific rapid urine tests are useful in the initial patient workup to support a presumptive diagnosis pending culture results. A positive urine culture is required to make the diagnosis of UTI. The predominant pathogen isolated is *E. coli*. Follow-up imaging studies may be necessary to identify anatomic or functional abnormalities, particularly in the young infant or child with recurrent UTIs. Prompt and effective antimicrobial treatment is indicated in acute infection to reduce the risk of subsequent complications.

Table 7. Oral Antibiotics Used for Urinary Tract Infection Prophylaxis in Pediatric Patients[14,25,39]

Antibiotic	Pediatric Dosage[a,b]
Trimethoprim/Sulfamethoxazole	2 mg/kg trimethoprim at bedtime OR 5 mg/kg trimethoprim twice weekly at bedtime
Nitrofurantoin	1-2 mg/kg once daily at bedtime
Amoxicillin	10–15 mg/kg once daily at bedtime
Cephalexin	12–15 mg/kg once daily at bedtime
Cefixime	2 mg/kg once daily at bedtime
Ceftibuten	2 mg/kg once daily at bedtime
Cefuroxime axetil	5 mg/kg once daily at bedtime

[a]Doses referenced assume normal renal function and are consistent with dosing recommendations for children older than the neonatal period. For neonatal dosing recommendations, consult an appropriate reference.
[b]Doses for higher-weight children and adolescents are typically limited to the adult dose when weight-based dosing results in a higher value than the standard adult dose for the indication.

An 8-month-old, 6-kg uncircumcised boy is brought to the pediatric emergency department with difficulty feeding, cloudy, malodorous urine, and a temperature of 102°F (38.9°C). The patient was born at full term, has no significant previous medical history, and has no known allergies. The physician orders a basic metabolic panel, complete blood count, C-reactive protein, urinalysis, and urine culture collected by transurethral catheterization. The following results are received 1 hour later.

Laboratory findings:

Glucose	85 mg/dL
Na	138 mEq/L
K	4.9 mEq/L
Cl	102 mEq/L
CO$_2$	27 mEq/L
BUN	7 mg/dL
SCr	0.3 mg/dL
WBC	19.6×10^3 cells/mm^3
Hgb	13.5 g/dL

Hct	41%
Plt	326×10^3 cells/mm^3
Neutrophils	70%
Bands	11%
CRP	5.7 mg/L

Urinalysis:

Color	Yellow
Appearance	Cloudy
Glucose	Negative

Ketones	Negative
Bilirubin	Negative
Specific gravity	1.015
Blood	2+
pH	5.5
Albumin	Negative
Nitrite	Positive
Leukocyte esterase	2+

Urine culture: Pending

1. Which of the laboratory and urinalysis findings support a diagnosis of urinary tract infection (UTI) in this infant?

An uncircumcised male infant who has difficulty feeding, cloudy, malodorous urine, and fever warrants a workup for UTI. The presence of increased white blood cell count, neutrophils and bands suggests infection, and an increased C-reactive protein indicates an ongoing acute inflammatory process. Positive nitrite and leukocyte esterase results in the urinalysis support a presumptive UTI diagnosis.

Case (continued). The physician decides to admit the infant to the hospitalists' service.

2. Which antibiotic(s) should be empirically started on pending urine culture and susceptibility results? Include dose, frequency, and duration of therapy.

This infection is the infant's first UTI. *Escherichia coli* is the predominant organism isolated, and antibiotic treatment must be microbiologically active against this organism. A parenteral, non-antipseudomonal third-generation cephalosporin, such as cefotaxime 100–150 mg/kg/day divided every 6–8 hours (in this patient, 200 mg intravenously every 8 hours) or ceftriaxone 50–75 mg/kg/day divided every 12–24 hours (in this patient, 300 mg intravenously every 24 hours), is an appropriate empiric selection. The patient has no known allergies. These third-generation cephalosporins are β-lactamase stable,

and the likelihood of isolating a resistant *E. coli* on the first UTI is low.

Case (continued). At 48 hours after admission, the infant has been afebrile for 24 hours, is feeding better, and is acting more playful. The urine culture is positive for *E. coli* susceptible to amoxicillin/clavulanate, cefazolin, cefuroxime, cefotaxime, ceftriaxone, gentamicin, and ciprofloxacin. The physician wants to transition to oral antibiotic therapy in preparation for discharge.

3. Which oral antibiotic would you recommend? Include dose, frequency, and duration of therapy.

Several options for oral antibiotics are available for the infant. Amoxicillin/clavulanate and first-, second-, and third-generation cephalosporins are active against the isolated organism and represent viable options. De-escalation to a first-generation cephalosporin (e.g., cephalexin 50 mg/kg/day divided every 6–8 hours to complete a 7- to 14-day course of treatment) is preferred in this case because it represents the narrowest spectrum antibiotic in the panel (for this patient, cephalexin 100 mg orally every 8 hours). Cephalexin is also associated with less gastrointestinal adverse drug events than amoxicillin/clavulanate. Aminoglycosides are not orally absorbed and are therefore not an option. Fluoroquinolones are not recommended as first-line treatment for pediatric UTIs and are reserved for the management of more resistant organisms.

REFERENCES

1. Chang SL, Shortliffe LD. Pediatric urinary tract infections. Pediatr Clin North Am 2006;53:379-400.

2. Lohr JA, Downs SM, Schlager TA. In: Long SS, Pickering LK, Prober CG, eds. Principles and Practice of Pediatric Infectious Diseases. Philadelphia: Churchill Livingstone, 2008:343-7.

3. Schroeder AR, Shen MW, Biondi EA, et al. Bacteraemic urinary tract infection: management and outcomes in young infants. Arch Dis Child 2016;101:125-30.

4. Montini G, Tullurs K, Hewitt I. Febrile urinary tract infections in children. N Engl J Med 2011;365:239-50.

5. Ma JF, Shortliffe LM. Urinary tract infection in children: etiology and epidemiology. Urol Clin North Am 2004;31:517-26.

6. American Academy of Pediatrics, Subcommittee on Urinary Tract Infection, Steering Committee on Quality Improvement and Management. Urinary tract infection: clinical practice guideline for the diagnosis and management of the initial UTI in febrile infants and children 2 to 24 months. Pediatrics 2011; 128:595-610.

7. AAP Subcommittee on Urinary Tract Infection. Reaffirmation of AAP clinical practice guideline: The diagnosis and management of the initial urinary tract infection in febrile infants and young children 2–24 months of age. Pediatrics 2016;138:e20163026.

8. Coulthard MG, Lambert HJ, Vernon SJ, et al. Does prompt treatment of urinary tract infection in preschool children prevent renal scarring: mixed retrospective and prospective audits. Arch Dis Child 2014;99;342-347.

9. Shaikh N, Mattoo TK, Keren R, et al. Early antibiotic treatment for pediatric urinary tract infection and renal scarring. JAMA Pediatr 2016;170:848-854.

10. Foxman B. Epidemiology of urinary tract infections: incidence, morbidity, and economic costs. Am J Med 2002;113:5S-13S.

11. Shaikh N, Morone NE, Bost JE, et al. Prevalence of urinary tract infection in childhood: a meta-analysis. Pediatr Infect Dis J 2008; 27:302-8.

12. White B. Diagnosis and treatment of urinary tract infection in children. Am Fam Physician 2011;83:409-15.

13. Krasinski KM. Urinary tract infections. In: Gershon AA, Hotez PJ, Katz SL, eds. Krugman's Infectious Diseases of Children. Philadelphia: Mosby, 2004:769-84.

14. Overturf GD. Urinary tract infection. In: Jenson HB, Baltimore RS, eds. Pediatric Infectious Diseases: Principles and Practice. Philadelphia: WB Saunders, 2002:983-91.

15. Wald ER. Cystitis and pyelonephritis. In: Cherry J, Demmler-Harrison GJ, Kaplan SL, et al., eds. Feigin and Cherry's Textbook of Pediatric Infectious Diseases, 7th ed. Philadelphia: Elsevier Saunders, 2014:535-53.

16. Friedman S, Reif S, Assia A, et al. Clinical and laboratory characterisics of non-E. coli urinary tract infections. Arch Dis Child 2006;91:845-6.

17. Shaikh N, Wald ER, Keren R, et al. Predictors of non-Escherichia coli urinary tract infection. Pediatr Infect Dis J 2016;35:1266-8.

18. Sobel JD. Pathogenesis of urinary tract infections: role of host defenses. Infect Dis Clin North Am 1997;11:531-49.

19. Flores-Mireles AL, Walker JN, Caparon M, et al. Urinary tract infections: epidemiology, mechanisms of infection and treatment options. Nature Rev Microbiol 2015;13:269-284.

20. Finnell SME, Carroll AE, Downs SM, et al. Technical report— diagnosis and management of an initial UTI in febrile infants and young children. Pediatrics 2011;128:e749-70.

21. Feld LG, Mattoo TK. Urinary tract infections and vesicoureteral reflux in infants and children. Pediatr Rev 2010;31:451-63.

22. Lebowitz RL, Olbing H, Parkkulainen KV, et al. International system of radiographic grading of vesicoureteral reflux: International reflux study in children. Pediatr Radiol 1985;15:105-9.

23. Stapleton AE. Urinary tract infection pathogenesis: Host factors. Infect Dis Clin N Am 2014;28:149-59.

24. Dielubanza EJ, Mazur DJ, Schaeffer AJ. Management of non-catheter-associated complicated urinary tract infection. Infect Dis Clin N Am 2014;28:121-34.

25. Stein R, Dogan HS, Hoebeke P, et al. Urinary tract infections in children: EAU/ESPU guidelines. Eur Urol 2015;67:546-58.

26. Chon CH, Lai FC, Shortliffe LM. Pediatric urinary tract infections. Pediatr Clin North Am 2001;48:1441-59.

27. Lohr JA. Use of routine urinalysis in making a presumptive diagnosis of urinary tract infection in children. Pediatr Infect Dis J 1991;10:646-50.

28. Shaikh N, Shope TR, Hoberman A, et al. Association between uropathogen and pyuria. Pediatrics 2016;138:e20160087.

29. Williams GJ, Macaskill P, Chan SF, et al. Absolute and relative accuracy of rapid urine tests for urinary tract infection in children: a meta-analysis. Lancet Infect Dis 2010;10:240-50.

30. Shah P, Cobb BT, Lower DR, et al. Enhanced versus automated urinalysis for screening of urinary tract infections in children in the emergency department. Pediatr Infect Dis J 2014;33:272-5.

31. Kavanagh EC, Ryan S, Awan A, et al. Can MRI replace DMSA in the detection of renal parenchymal defects in children with urinary tract infections? Pediatr Radiol 2005;35:275-81.

32. Rodriguez LV, Spielman D, Herfkens RJ, et al. Magnetic resonance imaging for the evaluation of hydronephrosis, reflux and renal scarring in children. J Urol 2001;166:1023-7.

33. Hsu CC, Tsai JD, Ku MS, et al. Antimicrobial resistance and diagnostic imaging in infants younger than 2 months old hospitalized with a first febrile urinary tract infection: A population-based comparative study. Pediatr Infect Dis J 2016;35:840-5.

34. Riccabona M. Imaging in childhood urinary tract infection. Radiol Med 2016;121:391-401.

35. Honkinen O, Jahnukainen T, Mertsola J, et al. Bacteremic urinary tract infection in children. Pediatr Infect Dis J 2000;19:630-4.

36. Averbuch D, Niz-Paz R, Tenenbaum A, et al. Factors associated with bacteremia in young infants with urinary tract infection. Pediatr Infect Dis J 2014;33:571-5.

37. Hernandez-Bou S, Trenchs V, Alarcon M, et al. Afebrile very young infants with urinary tract infection and the risk for bacteremia. Pediatr Infect Dis J 2014;33:244-7.

38. Robinson JL, Finlay JC, Lang ME, et al. Urinary tract infection in infants and children: Diagnosis and management. Paediatr Child Health 2014;19:315-9.

39. Taketomo CK, Hodding JH, Krauss DM. Pediatric & Neonatal Dosage Handbook, 23rd ed. Hudson, OH: Lexi-Comp, 2017.

40. Bradley JS, Jackson MA; Committee on Infectious Diseases. The use of systemic and topical fluoroquinolones. Pediatrics 2016;128:e1034-45.

41. Hoberman A, Wald ER, Hickey RW, et al. Oral versus initial intravenous therapy for urinary tract infections in young febrile children. Pediatrics 1999;104:79-86.

42. Montini G, Toffolo A, Zucchetta P, et al. Antibiotic treatment for pyelonephritis in children: multicentre randomised controlled non-inferiority trial. BMJ 2007;335:386-92.

43. Neuhaus TJ, Berger C, Buechner K, et al. Randomised trial of oral versus sequential intravenous/oral cephalosporins in children with pyelonephritis. Eur J Pediatr 2008;167:1037-47.

44. Bocquet N, Alaoui AS, Jais JP, et al. Randomized trial of oral versus sequential IV/oral antibiotic for acute pyelonephritis in children. Pediatrics 2012;129:e269-75.

45. Brady PW, Conway PH, Goudie A. Duration of inpatient intravenous antibiotic therapy and treatment failure in infants hospitalized with urinary tract infection. Pediatrics 2010;126:196-203.

46. Zorc JJ, Kiddoo DA, Shaw KN. Diagnosis and management of pediatric urinary tract infections. Clin Microbiol Rev 2005;18:417-22.

47. Steele RW, Estrada B, Begue RE, et al. A double-blind taste comparison of pediatric antibiotic suspensions. Clin Pediatr 1997; 36:193-9.

---

48. Fitzgerald A, Lee CW, Mori R. Antibiotics for treating uncomplicated urinary tract infection in children. Cochrane Database Syst Rev 2007;4:CD006857.

49. Michael M, Hodson EM, Craig JC, et al. Short versus standard duration oral antibiotic therapy for acute urinary tract infection in children. Cochrane Database Syst Rev 2003;1:CD003966.

50. Cheng CH, Tsai MH, Huang YC, et al. Antibiotic resistance patterns of community-acquired urinary tract infection in children with vesicoureteral reflux receiving prophylactic antibiotic therapy. Pediatrics 2008;122:1212-7.

51. Kizilca O, Siraneci R, Yilmaz A, et al. Risk factors for community-acquired urinary tract infection caused by ESBL-producing bacteria in children. Pediatr Int 2012;54:858-62.

52. Brandstrom P, Jodal U, Sillen U, et al. The Swedish reflux trial: Review of a randomized, controlled trial in children with dilating vesicoureteral reflux. J Pediatr Urol 2011;7:594-600.

53. RIVUR Trial Investigators; Hoberman A, Greenfield SP, Mattoo TK, et al. Antimicrobial prophylaxis for children with vesicoureteral reflux. N Engl J Med 2014;370:2367-76.

54. Williams G, Craig JC. Long-term antibiotics for preventing recurrent urinary tract infection in children. Cochrane Database Syst Rev 2011;3:CD001534.

55. Mori R, Fitzgerald A, Williams C, et al. Antibiotic prophylaxis for children at risk of developing urinary tract infection: a systematic review. Acta Pediatr 2009;98:1781-6.

56. Hewitt IK, Pennesi M, Morello W, et al. Antibiotic prophylaxis for urinary tract infection-related scarring: A systematic review. Pediatrics 2017:139:e20163145.

57. Conway PH, Cnaan A, Zaoutis T, et al. Recurrent urinary tract infections in children: risk factors and association with prophylactic antimicrobials. JAMA 2007;298:179-86.

58. Selekman RE, Shapiro DJ, Boscardin J, et al. Uropathogen resistance and antibiotic prophylaxis: A meta-analysis. Pediatrics 2018;142:e20180119.

59. Calderon-Margalit R, Golan E, Twig G, et al. History of childhood kidney disease and risk of adult end-stage renal disease. N Engl J Med 2018;378:428-38.

60. Jepson RG, Williams G, Craig JC. Cranberries for preventing urinary tract infections. Cochrane Database Syst Rev 2012:10: CD001321.

61. Schwenger EM, Tejani AM, Loewen PS. Probiotics for preventing urinary tract infections in adults and children. Cochrane Database Syst Rev 2015:12;CD008772.

62. Hosseini M, Yousefifard M, Ataei N, et al. The efficacy of probiotics in prevention of urinary tract infection in children: A systematic review and meta-analysis. J Pediatr Urol 2017:13:581-91.

63. Ellison JS, Dy GW, Fu BC, et al. Neonatal circumcision and urinary tract infections in infants with hydronephrosis. Pediatrics 2018;142:e20173703.

64. Balighian E, Burke M. Urinary tract infections in children. Pediatr Rev 2018;39:3-12.

65. Dos Santos J, Lopes RI, Koyle MA. Bladder and bowel dysfunction in children: An update on the diagnosis and treatment of a common, but underdiagnosed pediatric problem. Can Urol Assoc J 2017;11:S64-72.

CHAPTER 41

Skin and Soft Tissue Infections of Bacterial and Viral Etiology

M. Tuan Tran, Pharm.D., BCPS

LEARNING OBJECTIVES

1. Recognize common bacterial and viral skin and soft tissue infections (SSTIs) of childhood through an understanding of their definitions, epidemiology, and clinical presentation.

2. Select empiric and definitive antimicrobial therapy on the basis of the etiologic agent, antimicrobial resistance patterns, severity of illness, and clinical evidence.

3. Recommend supportive treatment to aid in the recovery from active illness and preventive strategies for avoiding disease transmission and outbreaks.

4. Recognize the increasing prevalence of community-acquired methicillin-resistant *Staphylococcus aureus* as a pathogen in pediatric SSTIs and its impact on antibiotic selection.

5. Monitor antimicrobial therapy to maximize effectiveness and safety.

ABBREVIATIONS IN THIS CHAPTER

BI	Bullous impetigo
CA-MRSA	Community-acquired methicillin-resistant *Staphylococcus aureus*
GAS	Group A β-hemolytic *Streptococcus*
HFMD	Hand, foot, and mouth disease
HHV	Human herpes virus
HSV	Herpes simplex virus
IC	Impetigo contagiosa
IVIG	Intravenous immunoglobulin
MRSA	Methicillin-resistant *Staphylococcus aureus*
MSSA	Methicillin-sensitive *Staphylococcus aureus*
NF	Necrotizing fasciitis
NSAID	Nonsteroidal anti-inflammatory drug
OC	Orbital cellulitis
PC	Periorbital cellulitis
SSSS	Staphylococcal scalded skin syndrome
SSTI	Skin and soft tissue infection
VZV	Varicella zoster virus

INTRODUCTION

Skin and soft tissue infections (SSTIs), a common reason for pediatric patients to receive medical attention, can range from a localized, superficial folliculitis, easily managed as an outpatient, to a life-threatening necrotizing fasciitis (NF), requiring immediate surgical intervention (Figure 1). Pharmacists should be familiar with the clinical presentation of common skin lesions and different pharmacologic treatment options so that they can refer patients to seek further treatment when necessary. A detailed history, time course, and physical examination are essential in making the proper diagnosis. Pharmacologic treatment is often empiric, requiring a general knowledge of common pathogens and local resistance patterns.

SUPERFICIAL BACTERIAL SKIN INFECTIONS

Historically, the most common pathogens responsible for SSTIs are *Staphylococcus aureus* and Streptococcus pyogenes, a group A β-hemolytic *Streptococcus* (GAS). Methicillin-resistant *S. aureus* (MRSA) develops by acquisition of *mec*A gene, a localized segment of DNA referred to as *staphylococcal chromosome cassette*, which encodes for penicillin-binding protein 2a and confers intrinsic resistant to β-lactams. In addition, an increasing prevalence in recent years of community-acquired methicillin-resistant *S. aureus* (CA-MRSA) has been observed in SSTIs.[1,2] Resistance is encoded for CA-MRSA by staphylococcal chromosome cassette *mec* type IV, a small, mobile genetic element that facilitates transfer of methicillin resistance more readily than the larger elements coding for strains often recovered from health care facilities—termed *health care-acquired MRSA*—making CA-MRSA isolates less prone to developing multidrug resistance. Another molecular feature specific to CA-MRSA is the expression of several virulence factors such as Panton-Valentine leukocidin, α-hemolysins, and phenol soluble modulins that can cause tissue necrosis and leukocyte destruction. Compared with methicillin-sensitive *S. aureus* (MSSA), CA-MRSA appears to cause deeper, more invasive necrotizing infections and has a higher rate of recurrence.

Table 1 summarizes pediatric antibiotic therapy for superficial bacterial skin infections.

FOLLICULITIS, FURUNCLES, CARBUNCLES, AND CUTANEOUS ABSCESSES

Folliculitis, furuncles, and carbuncles are a family of pyodermic infections that originate around a hair follicle. *Folliculitis* is the most superficial and least extensive of the three, resulting in the formation of a small follicular abscess in the epidermis. *Furuncles* (or *boils*) are characterized by a more widespread inflammatory response of adjacent follicles extending into the dermis and subcutaneous tissue. These suppurative lesions are painful, erythematous, fluctuant, and may cause cellulitis in the surrounding areas. *Carbuncles* represent a confluence of furuncles with still-wider infiltration that can spontaneously drain from many sites.[1,2] A *cutaneous abscess* is an encapsulated collection of pus within the dermis and deep skin tissues that is accompanied by swelling and an erythematous rim.

Children of all age groups can develop folliculitis. Furunculosis tends to occur in adolescents, whereas carbuncles are generally seen in adulthood. Risk factors include hyperhidrosis, obesity, diabetes, seborrhea, anemia, malnutrition, and immunodeficiency. Clusters of infections may occur in people who interact in close quarters, especially in settings where skin injury is common, or in those who share household items that can transfer infectious material.[3]

MICROBIOLOGIC ETIOLOGY

Staphylococcus aureus is the most common causative agent of purulent SSTIs, with rates of CA-MRSA surpassing MSSA and accounting for 61% of MRSA-associated SSTIs in children.[2] In addition, *S. aureus* accounts for 66% to 82% of all samples obtained through incision and drainage of cutaneous abscesses in three recent pediatric studies.[4-6] Colonization with *S. aureus* is likely a risk factor for recurrent infection because nasal carriage rates are twice as high in patients with recurrent infection as in the general population.[7,8] Because MRSA can also reside in other sites including the pharynx, axillae, rectum, and perineum, one pediatric study suggests a stronger correlation between rectal MRSA colonization and abscess development compared with nasal colonization.[4] Although most abscesses occurring above the trunk and extremities are caused by *S. aureus*, anaerobic organisms such as *Peptococcus* spp. and *Propionibacterium* spp. may also be involved. Gram-negative folliculitis typically infects buttock and axillary regions, as well as appearing on the faces of patients with a history of antibiotic therapy for acne.[3] *Pseudomonas aeruginosa* is less commonly isolated but can cause "hot tub" folliculitis affecting extremities, chest, back, and armpits from exposure to contaminated hot tub or whirlpool. Abscesses in the perineal region are often polymicrobial, containing anaerobic and aerobic bacteria that constitute the normal flora of regional skin and mucous membranes.[2,3]

CLINICAL PRESENTATION

Folliculitis occurs in hair-bearing areas and typically arises with no preexisting trauma to the skin. Inflammation along the hair shaft causes swelling and erythema that is accompanied by the formation of small dome-shaped pustules. Sites commonly affected include the scalp, extremities, buttocks, and areas of skin prone to moisture and friction (Figure 2). Furuncles and carbuncles can present as fluctuant masses that drain spontaneously. These infections are most often seen on the neck, breasts, face, buttocks, axillae, and groin.[3] Abscesses typically result from minor trauma to an area that becomes infected. The area may develop a nodule, which can become fluctuant or pustular and is surrounded by erythematous swelling. The abscess is usually painful and tender. Accompanying features can include local cellulitis, lymphangitis, regional lymphadenopathy, fever, and leukocytosis.[3]

DIAGNOSIS

The diagnosis of these conditions is largely based on clinical appearance. Assessment methods that are more objective, such as bedside ultrasonography, can help determine the presence of a drainable fluid collection.[9,10] Cultures are not routinely obtained, but assessment of drainage from a lesion or abscess may require a Gram stain and analysis to identify the causative organism.

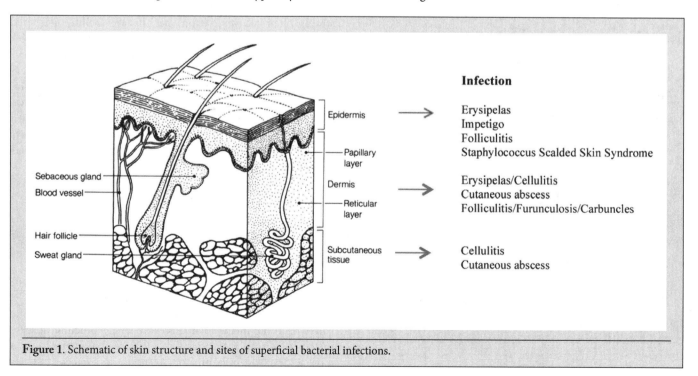

Figure 1. Schematic of skin structure and sites of superficial bacterial infections.

Table 1. Pediatric Antibiotic Therapy for Superficial Bacterial Skin Infections

| Infection and Pathogen | Daily Dose (Maximal Daily Dose) | | Comments |
	Oral	Parenteral	
Folliculitis, Furuncle, Carbuncle: *Staphylococcus aureus* (MRSA)	Cephalexin 25 mg/kg/day divided Q 6 hr (2 g) Dicloxacillin 12 mg/kg/day divided Q 6 hr (1 g) **MRSA coverage** Clindamycin 40 mg/kg/day divided Q 8 hr (1.35 g) TMP/SMX 12 mg/kg/day of TMP divided Q 12 hr (640 mg TMP)[a] Doxycycline 2–4 mg/kg/day divided Q 12 hr (200 mg)[b]	Cefazolin 75 mg/kg/day divided Q 8 hr (6 g) Oxacillin or nafcillin 150 mg/kg/day divided Q 4 hr (12 g) **MRSA coverage** Vancomycin 45–60 mg/kg/day divided Q 6–8h[c] Clindamycin 40 mg/kg/day divided Q 8 hr (1.8 g) Linezolid 20–30 mg/kg/day divided Q 8–12 hr (1.2 g)[d] Daptomycin 6–10 mg/kg/day once daily Ceftaroline 24–36 mg/kg/day divided Q 8 hr (1.2 g)	For frequent recurrences, reduce *Staphylococcus* colonization with nasal mupirocin 2% TID for 5–10 days For severe recurrent infections, rifampin 20 mg/kg/day divided Q 12 hr + doxycycline or TMP/SMX for 5–10 days
Erysipelas: GAS	Cephalexin 25 mg/kg/day divided Q 6 hr (2 g) Penicillin 50 mg/kg/day divided Q 6 hr (2 g) Erythromycin 40 mg/kg/day divided Q 6 hr (1 g) Clindamycin 30 mg/kg/day divided Q 8 hr (1.35 g)	Cefazolin 75 mg/kg/day divided Q 8 hr (6 g) Penicillin 250,000 units/kg/day divided Q 4–6 hr (24 MU) Azithromycin 10 mg/kg/day divided Q 24 hr (500 mg) Clindamycin 40 mg/kg/day divided Q 8 hr (1.8 g)	For MSSA coverage, use first-generation cephalosporin or add oxacillin in combination
Cellulitis: *S. aureus* (MRSA) GAS	Cephalexin 25 mg/kg/day divided Q 6 hr (2 g) Dicloxacillin 12 mg/kg/day divided Q 6 hr (2 g) Erythromycin 40 mg/kg/day divided Q 6 hr (1 g) **CA–MRSA coverage** Clindamycin 30 mg/kg/day divided Q 8 hr (1.35 g) TMP/SMX 12 mg/kg/day of TMP divided Q 12 hr (640 mg TMP)[a] Doxycycline 2–4 mg/kg/day divided Q 12 hr (200 mg)[b]	Cefazolin 75 mg/kg/day divided Q 8 hr (6 g) Oxacillin or nafcillin mg/kg/day divided Q 4 hr (12 g) Ampicillin/sulbactam 200 mg/kg/day of ampicillin divided Q 6 hr (12 g of ampicillin) **MRSA coverage** Vancomycin 45–60 mg/kg/day divided Q 6–8h[c] Clindamycin 40 mg/kg/day divided Q 8 hr (1.8 g) Linezolid 20–30 mg/kg/day divided Q 8–12 hr (1.2 g)[d] Daptomycin 6–10 mg/kg/day once daily Ceftaroline 24–36 mg/kg/day divided Q 8 hr (1.2 g)	Consider MRSA coverage if systemic illness or no improvement on initial therapy
Bullous Impetigo: *S. aureus* (MRSA)	Cephalexin 25 mg/kg/day divided Q 6 hr (2 g) Dicloxacillin 12 mg/kg/day divided Q 6 hr (1 g) Amoxicillin/clavulanate 30–45 mg/kg/day of amoxicillin divided Q 8–12 hr (1.75 g amoxicillin) Erythromycin 40 mg/kg/day divided Q 6 hr (1 g) **MRSA coverage** Clindamycin 30 mg/kg/day divided Q 8 hr (1.35 g) TMP/SMX 12 mg/kg/day of TMP divided Q 12 hr (640 mg TMP)[a]	—	Topical mupirocin 2% TID and retapamulin 1% BID for 7 days Recommended for localized disease

(continued)

Table 1. Pediatric Antibiotic Therapy for Superficial Bacterial Skin Infections *(continued)*

Infection and Pathogen	Daily Dose (Maximal Daily Dose)		Comments
	Oral	**Parenteral**	
Impetigo Contagiosa: *S. aureus* (MRSA) GAS	Same as for Bullous impetigo	—	—
Staphylococcus Scalded Skin Syndrome: *S. aureus*	Same as for Bullous impetigo	Clindamycin 40 mg/kg/day divided Q 8 hr (1.8 g) plus: Oxacillin or nafcillin 150 mg/kg ÷ Q 4 hr (12 g) —OR— Cefazolin 75 mg/kg/day divided Q 8 hr (6 g) Linezolid 20–30 mg/kg/day divided Q 8–12 hr (1.2 g)[d] Daptomycin 6–10 mg/kg/day once daily Ceftaroline 24–36 mg/kg/day divided Q 8 hr (1.2 g)	For secondary bacterial infection, add: Age-appropriate gentamicin —OR— Clindamycin + ceftriaxone IV 100 mg/kg/day divided Q 12 hr —OR— Cefotaxime IV 150 mg/kg/day divided Q 8 hr
Cutaneous Abscess MRSA	Clindamycin 30 mg/kg/day divided Q 8 hr (1.35 g) TMP/SMX 12 mg/kg/day of TMP divided Q 12 hr (640 mg TMP)[a] Doxycycline 2–4 mg/kg/day divided Q 12 hr (200 mg)[b] Linezolid 20–30 mg/kg/day divided Q 8–12 hr (1.2 g)[d]	Vancomycin 45–60 mg/kg/day divided Q 6–8h[c] Clindamycin 40 mg/kg/day divided Q 8 hr (1.8 g) Linezolid 20–30 mg/kg/day divided Q 8–12 hr (1.2 g)[d] Daptomycin 6–10 mg/kg/day once daily Ceftaroline 24–36 mg/kg/day divided Q 8 hr (1.2 g)	I&D is primary treatment Continue antibiotics only in high-risk patients Reserve linezolid for treatment failure because of high cost
Animal and Human Bites: *Pasteurella spp.* *Staphylococcus spp.* *Streptococcus spp.* *Eikenella corrodens,* anaerobes	Amoxicillin/clavulanate 45 mg/kg/day of amoxicillin divided Q 8–12 hr (1.75 g of amoxicillin) Clindamycin 30 mg/kg/day divided Q 8 hr (1.35 g) plus TMP/SMX 12 mg/kg/day of TMP divided Q 12 hr (640 mg TMP)[a] —OR— Cefuroxime 30 mg/kg/day divided Q 12 hr (1 g) Doxycycline 2–4 mg/kg/day divided Q 12 hr (200 mg)[b] Ciprofloxacin 30 mg/kg/day divided Q 12 hr (1 g)[e]	Ampicillin/sulbactam 200 mg/kg/day of ampicillin divided Q 6 hr (12 g of ampicillin) Clindamycin 40 mg/kg/day divided Q 8 hr (1.8 g) plus TMP/SMX 12 mg/kg/day of TMP divided Q 6 hr (640 mg TMP) Cefoxitin 100 mg/kg/day divided Q 4–6 hr (12 g) Meropenem 60 mg/kg/day divided Q 8 hr (3 g)	Reserve carbapenems for treatment failure or multidrug resistance

[a] Trimethoprim/sulfamethoxazole is contraindicated in children age < 2 months.

[b] Doxycycline can be administered for short durations (≤ 21 days) without regard to age[81]

[c] Target vancomycin to trough levels of 10–15 mcg/mL or AUC 400–600 mg × h/L

[d] Linezolid 10 mg/kg/dose Q 8 hr in children age < 5 years, 10 mg/kg/dose Q 12 in children age > 5 years.

[e] Fluoroquinolones should only be used when no safe and effective alternative exists or when oral treatment option represents a reasonable alternative to parenteral therapy.

BID = twice daily; GAS = group A β-hemolytic *Streptococcus;* I&D = incision and drainage; IV = intravenous; MRSA = community-acquired *Staphylococcus aureus;* MSSA = methicillin-sensitive *Staphylococcus aureus;* MU = million units; Q = every; TID = three times daily; TMP/SMX = trimethoprim/sulfamethoxazole.

TREATMENT

Most folliculitis cases will resolve spontaneously and will typically respond to warm compresses with or without topical antibiotics such as clindamycin, erythromycin, or mupirocin. Refractory, unresponsive to topical management, or deep lesions should be treated with a short course of oral antibiotics targeting *S. aureus*. Cephalexin and dicloxacillin are recommended for MSSA coverage, whereas clindamycin, trimethoprim/sulfamethoxazole, and minocycline are potential options for patients in areas with high MRSA prevalence.

Furuncles often rupture and drain spontaneously or with warm compresses. Large furuncles and carbuncles should be treated with incision and drainage. Parenteral antimicrobials are usually unnecessary, unless the patient presents with fever or other systemic symptoms. A parenteral penicillinase-resistant penicillin (e.g., oxacillin, nafcillin) or a first-generation cephalosporin should be used as initial treatment and then, once clinically improved, converted to oral therapy when appropriate for 5–10 days.[1] Empiric vancomycin should be considered in critically ill patients, especially those living in communities where CA-MRSA prevalence is high.

Incision and drainage is the cornerstone of therapy for the treatment of cutaneous abscesses.[1,11] The use of antimicrobial therapy with empiric coverage for *S. aureus* as an adjunct to incision and drainage should be based on the presence of systemic signs of infection. The 2014 Infectious Diseases Society of America guideline for the diagnosis and management of SSTIs recommends agents targeted against MRSA for patients with abscesses for whom initial treatment has failed, who are immunocompromised, or who are experiencing systemic inflammatory response syndrome and hypotension (Box 1).[1] Initial oral options may include dicloxacillin, cephalexin, amoxicillin-clavulanate, clindamycin, doxycycline, and trimethoprim/sulfamethoxazole. A recent study reported higher rates of treatment failure in patients who underwent a drainage procedure and received either trimethoprim/sulfamethoxazole (11.2%) or β-lactams (11.1%) compared with clindamycin (4.7%).[12] Furthermore, receipt of clindamycin

for treatment of CA-MRSA SSTI was associated with earlier clearance of colonization compared with other antibiotics, including trimethoprim/sulfamethoxazole and doxycycline.[13] In addition, for hospitalized children, vancomycin is the recommended first-line agent. Linezolid, given its wide spectrum of activity against other drug-resistant organisms and comparatively expensive cost, should be reserved as a last resort for outpatient management. Ceftaroline, a new broad-spectrum β-lactam with activity against many gram-positive (including MRSA) and gram-negative organisms, has approval for SSTIs in children older than 2 months.[1,11]

Treatments of chronic dermatologic conditions that predispose a patient to secondary bacterial infections and improvements in daily hygiene (e.g., antiseptic body washes, one-time use of washcloths, frequent dressing changes of draining lesions) are essential for preventing outbreaks. Topical anti-infective agents, such as chlorhexidine, are most effective when used in conjunction with other strategies; however, the risk of adverse neurologic effects should preclude the use of hexachlorophene in children younger than 2 months.[11] A 5-day decolonization with twice-daily intranasal mupirocin 2% or dilute (1/4–1/2 cup per full bath) bleach baths given daily for 15 minutes may be considered for prevention of recurrences.[1,11] Studies have demonstrated the effectiveness of decolonization with intranasal mupirocin and chlorhexidine wash in 50%–82% of carriers.[7,8] Yet, a recent survey showed only 3.7% of children undergoing incision and drainage in the emergency department had documentation of MRSA prevention and eradication, an important intervention for the pharmacist at discharge.[11] A short course (5–10 days) of an oral agent (trimethoprim/sulfamethoxazole or doxycycline) in combination with rifampin, if susceptible, may be considered for decolonization if infection recurs despite the measures just described.[11]

ERYSIPELAS AND CELLULITIS

Erysipelas and *cellulitis* are diffuse, spreading skin infections without a suppurative focus. Erysipelas disease is commonly seen among infants and among much older adults. Neonates and young children are particularly at risk in the pediatric age group. Immunosuppression is a risk factor for disease.

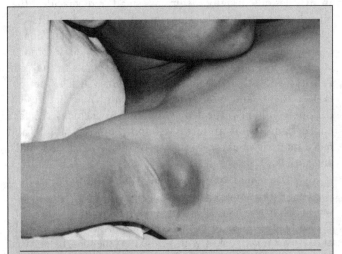

Figure 2. Erythematous, fluctuant abscess in the axilla.

Photo credit: Dr. James Korb, Children's Hospital of Orange County, Orange, CA.

Box 1. Patients Recommended for Antibiotic Therapy After Incision and Drainage of Simple Abscess[1,10]

Severe or extensive disease (e.g., involving many infection sites)

Rapid progression in the presence of associated cellulitis, signs and symptoms of systemic illness

Associated comorbidities or immunosuppression (diabetes mellitus, human immunodeficiency virus infection/AIDS, neoplasm)

Extremes of age

Abscess in area difficult to drain

Associated septic phlebitis

Lack of response to incision and drainage alone

MICROBIOLOGIC ETIOLOGY

The most common cause of erysipelas is GAS, or *S. pyogenes*, although groups B, C, and G have also been implicated. Historically, GAS and *S. aureus* have caused most cellulitis cases, with more than 70% of patients having serology consistent with GAS.[13] The contribution of MRSA relative to GAS and MSSA in nonpurulent cellulitis remains unknown; however, in cellulitis cases complicated by abscess formation, CA-MRSA should be strongly suspected, given its high prevalence as reported in epidemiologic studies of purulent SSTIs.[11]

CLINICAL PRESENTATION

Erysipelas and cellulitis typically present as painful, tender, and erythematous inflammation. Erysipelas is inflammation of the upper dermis, including superficial lymphatic vessels, and presents with a sharply demarcated border. Cellulitis involves the deeper dermis and subcutaneous fat with poorly defined borders. Vesicles or bullae formation may develop, and can rapidly progress to necrosis. In general, patients are not toxic appearing, and they lack systemic symptoms such as fever. Severe cases of cellulitis can be accompanied by fever, hemodynamic instability, and regional lymphadenopathy. The most common infection sites are the face (in a butterfly distribution) and lower extremities (legs and feet); in neonates, however, the periumbilical area is often the primary infection site.[14]

DIAGNOSIS

The diagnosis of erysipelas and cellulitis is largely based on the clinical appearance of the skin. Laboratory assessment may show an elevated leukocyte count with polymorphonuclear predominance. Blood cultures are not useful for diagnosis of uncomplicated cellulitis.[15] Invasive diagnostic procedures such as needle aspiration and skin biopsies are seldom performed because of their variable yield; however, they may be useful when it is necessary to identify the causative organism in patients with underlying comorbidities.[15,16]

TREATMENT

Initial treatment of erysipelas should include oral antibiotics with streptococcal coverage. Most GAS remains susceptible to β-lactams such as penicillin, cephalexin, and dicloxacillin. In patients with severe penicillin allergies, clindamycin and macrolides are reasonable alternatives, assuming that local resistance rates are low.[1] In hospitalized patients with suspected cellulitis requiring parenteral treatment, options include penicillinase-resistant penicillins (e.g., oxacillin, nafcillin), a first-generation cephalosporin (e.g., cefazolin), a combination β-lactam/β-lactamase inhibitor (e.g., ampicillin/sulbactam), clindamycin, or vancomycin.[1] The practice guidelines from the Infectious Diseases Society of America recommend broadening the scope of antibiotics to cover CA-MRSA in patients with complicated SSTIs, such as deep soft tissue infections, surgical/traumatic wound infection, major abscesses, infected ulcers, and burns; in patients who do not respond to initial therapy; and in patients who present with systemic toxicity. In addition to surgical debridement, antibiotic options specific to pediatrics include vancomycin (with a targeted trough of 10–15 mg/dL or an area-under-concentration curve, AUC 400-600 mg × h/L), clindamycin, linezolid, or ceftaroline.[1,11]

Treatment duration for erysipelas and uncomplicated cellulitis is typically 5–10 days. Longer therapy durations may be necessary for complicated cases and should be individualized on the basis of patient response. Elevation of the affected area to promote gravity drainage of edema and inflammatory substances is recommended.

IMPETIGO

Impetigo is an infection of the superficial dermis that results in purulent lesions. Nonbullous impetigo (also known as *impetigo contagiosa* [IC]) is characterized by a honey-colored crusted appearance. *Bullous impetigo* (BI), by contrast, is characterized by friable, fluid-filled vesicles or blisters.[17]

Impetigo is the third most common type of skin infection in children affecting mostly children age 2–5 years.[18] Of all impetigo cases 70% are nonbullous because of the high contagiousness of impetigo.[18] Transmission occurs through direct contact; thus, the conditions of crowding and poor hygiene, day care, and warm climates are risk factors for outbreaks. Colonization of the skin or nares typically precedes the development of impetigo. Bullous impetigo occurs more commonly in children younger than 5 years; however, most cases are diagnosed in neonates, possibly because of their lack of immunity against and impaired clearance of staphylococcal toxins.[17]

MICROBIOLOGIC ETIOLOGY

The most common causative organisms for IC are *S. aureus*, GAS, or a combination of the two. Bullous impetigo is almost exclusively caused by toxin-producing *S. aureus*.[1,19]

CLINICAL PRESENTATION

In IC, lesions usually begin as small red macules that quickly turn into vesicles surrounded by erythema. The vesicles become pustular and rupture to give a thick, honey-colored crust. Satellite lesions may appear when autoinoculation, or host reinfection, occurs at open breaks in the skin. Pruritus and other systemic complications, such as peripheral erythema and local lymphadenopathy, may be present. Lesions commonly affected in IC and BI includes the face and extremities, as are areas around the nose, mouth, and moist intertriginous zones, such as the diaper area, neck folds, and axillae.

Most impetigo cases are self-limiting and resolve without scarring within weeks. However, acute poststreptococcal glomerulonephritis may affect 1% to 5% of patients with IC.[20] Typically, BI evolves from rapidly enlarging vesicles to flaccid bullae over normal skin with limited erythema. The encased fluid turns turbid and often ruptures within 48 hours, resulting in thin brown to golden-yellow crusts. The formation of collarette scales in the periphery of a ruptured lesion is a pathognomonic finding of BI.[21]

DIAGNOSIS

Diagnosis is often made on clinical appearance alone. Microbiologic analysis and skin biopsies are rarely indicated, except to clarify cases of extensive involvement or in patients who do not respond to initial antibiotics. Bacteria may be cultured from the blister contents. Antistreptococcal antibody assays do not aid in diagnosing IC, but provide supporting evidence of recent systemic streptococcal infection in patients with suspected poststreptococcal glomerulonephritis.

TREATMENT

Topical antibiotics, such as mupirocin twice daily for 5 days, are recommended for uncomplicated impetigo cases.[1] Retapamulin is an additional topical agent in a new class of protein synthesis inhibitors (pleuromutilins) licensed for impetigo caused by MSSA or *S. pyogenes* in infants age 9 months or older.[22,23]

Oral antibiotics for 5–7 days should be reserved for cases of impetigo with more than a handful of lesions or in outbreaks setting affecting several people to help decrease transmission of infection. Because of the predominance of *S. aureus* in BI and

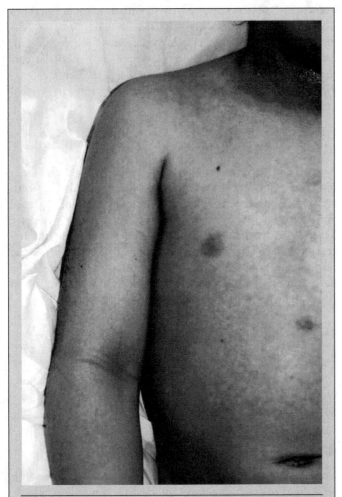

Figure 3. Erythematous patches on the torso, arm, and neck characteristic of staphylococcal scalded skin syndrome.

Photo credit: Dr. James Korb, Children's Hospital of Orange County, Orange, CA.

IC, penicillinase-resistant penicillins (dicloxacillin), β-lactam/β-lactamase combinations, or first-generation cephalosporins (cephalexin) are appropriate first-line oral antibiotic choices for the treatment of extensive impetigo. Macrolides may be substituted in patients with true penicillin allergies with confirmed macrolide susceptibility. When MRSA is suspected, doxycycline, clindamycin, or trimethoprim/sulfamethoxazole should be considered. Because no clinical trials have shown the superiority of one antibiotic over another, choice of an optimal regimen will depend on local susceptibility data and patient-specific factors, such as contraindications, allergies, and tolerance of adverse effects.[1,17]

STAPHYLOCOCCAL SCALDED SKIN SYNDROME

Staphylococcal scalded skin syndrome (SSSS) is a toxin-mediated epidermolytic disease that is associated with severe skin blistering and exfoliation caused by staphylococcal exfoliative toxins A and B, and is believed to be a generalized form of BI because of their shared virulence factor.[24] Typically SSSS presents in children younger than 5 years. Infants and young children are commonly affected because of waning immunity from maternal antibodies and impaired renal clearance of staphylococcal exfoliative toxins caused by immature renal function.[25] Disease transmission is likely through contact with asymptomatic carriers of *S. aureus*. Mortality in childhood SSSS is 5% but may exceed 60% in adults.[25-27]

MICROBIOLOGIC ETIOLOGY

In the spectrum of *S. aureus* exotoxin-mediated skin disease, SSSS is the most severe manifestation. A greater percentage of MRSA strains express toxin genes than do MSSA strains, although the clinical significance of this expression is unknown. Currently, very few cases of MRSA causing SSSS have been reported in the literature.[27,28]

CLINICAL PRESENTATION

Patients may present with a prodrome of sore throat and conjunctivitis, accompanied by constitutional symptoms of fever, malaise, and irritability. Within 48 hours, exquisitely tender erythematous patches, which rapidly erupt on the face, neck, axilla, and perineum, may develop into nontense bullae that rupture to reveal a friable, erythematous base that is susceptible to denuding by simple rubbing (e.g., positive Nikolsky sign) (Figure 3). Large areas of the skin may be involved, particularly in flexural and perioral regions. Mucous membranes are spared (Figure 4). Complications include secondary infections, electrolyte disturbances, and difficulties in temperature regulation.[25-27,29]

DIAGNOSIS

Diagnosis of SSSS is primarily based on clinical features supported by presence of *S. aureus* from culture report. Generalized SSSS is a manifestation of the hematogenous spread of staphylococcal exfoliative toxins produced by bacteria from a focus of colonization (nares, eye, umbilicus, groin, or wound site) or active infection (pneumonia, osteomyelitis, or endocarditis). The yield of bacterial cultures from blister aspirates and blood is generally poor because symptoms are mediated through toxins released by organisms residing in extracutaneous reservoirs.[25]

TREATMENT

A parenteral antibiotic with staphylococcal activity (i.e., penicillinase-resistant penicillin or a first- or second-generation cephalosporin) is recommended and should be initiated promptly. The addition of clindamycin as an adjunct to any regimen should be strongly considered because of its ability to attenuate toxin production.[25] Because patients with extensive exfoliation are at high risk of secondary gram-negative infections or septicemia, some experts recommend a third-generation cephalosporin plus clindamycin.[17,27] Lack of symptomatic improvement within 48 hours should also prompt expanded coverage to include MRSA.

Eroded areas are best covered with bland emollients, such as petrolatum, to prevent moisture loss and protect against bacterial infections. Topical antibiotic ointments may be prescribed for conjunctivitis and mupirocin for nasal decolonization. In outbreaks, carriers should be immediately identified and treated with antistaphylococcal antibiotics.

Exfoliation may continue for 24–48 hours after the initiation of appropriate antibiotic therapy until toxin production ceases. Thereafter, skin lesions should heal rapidly in 7–10 days with minimal scarring because only the superficial layers are affected.[27] Typical length of antibiotic treatment is at least 10 days.

ANIMAL AND HUMAN BITES

Animal and human bites are wounds that can result in infectious complications. The incidence of animal bites in the United States is estimated to be 2 million to 5 million per year, with most cases occurring in children. Around 85% to 90% of bite injuries are caused by dogs, followed by cats (5% to 10%), and then humans (2% to 3%).[30] About 1.3 in 1000 people with dog bites require medical treatment, with the highest incidence being among boys age 5–9 years (6 in 1000 people).[31]

MICROBIOLOGIC ETIOLOGY

Sources of bacteria recovered from a bite wound are those that colonize the victim's skin and those that derive from the oral cavity of the aggressor, as well as environmental organisms. In one study involving children who sustained injuries from animal bites (17 dogs, 4 cats), more than 66% of isolated organisms were a combination of aerobic and anaerobic bacteria.[32] In an adult study that analyzed the bacteriology of bite wounds from dogs and cats associated with clinical signs of infection, *Pasteurella* spp. was the most common isolate, followed by *Streptococcus* spp., *Staphylococcus* spp., *Moraxella* spp. Anaerobes included *Fusobacterium* spp., *Bacteroides* spp., and *Prevotella* spp.[33] Dogs and cats, as well as other feral animals, may be carriers of rabies. *Bartonella henselae*, a pathogen specific to cat bites, is associated with a febrile illness known as "cat scratch disease." Common aerobic microbes isolated from human bite injuries include *Streptococcus anginosis*, *S. aureus*, coagulase-negative *Staphylococcus*, *Enterococcus* spp., *Corynebacterium* spp., and *Eikenella corrodens*. *Prevotella* spp., *Porphyromonas* spp., *Bacteroides* spp., *Fusobacterium* spp., and *Peptostreptococcus* spp. are typical anaerobic pathogens.[34]

CLINICAL PRESENTATION

Anatomic differences in the tooth shapes of cats and dogs result in wound profiles specific to each animal. Cat teeth are long and slender, which are more likely to inflict small but deep puncture wounds. Most cat bites do not penetrate beyond the dermis. In contrast, dog bites are predominantly crush injuries, lacerations, or abrasions that result in partial skin penetration.[35] In children, the hands and arms are the most common wound sites for cat as well as human bites, compared with head and neck injuries with dog bites.[32,36]

Patients presenting 12 hours after the inciting event likely have established infection.[1] The wound site may appear edematous, erythematous, and bruised, and it may drain serosanguineous fluid. Pain is a common finding. Lymphadenopathy, streaking, and fever can signify more systemic complications such as cellulitis, subcutaneous abscesses, osteomyelitis, tendonitis, and, rarely, bacteremia.[1]

DIAGNOSIS

Diagnosis is based on a positive history of interaction with an animal or individual who inflicted the wound, as well as a clinical examination. Cultures should only be obtained for wounds more than 8–12 hours old or those that appear infected. Radiography is indicated if there is concern about injury to deep structures or if there is a need to assess foreign body inoculation.[37,38]

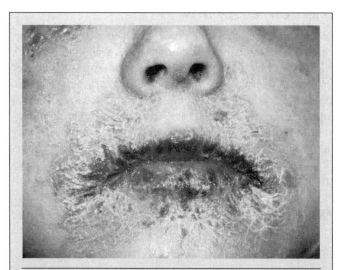

Figure 4. Perioral peeling from staphylococcal scalded skin syndrome.

Photo credit: Dr. James Korb, Children's Hospital of Orange County, Orange, CA.

TREATMENT

The goals of bite wound management are the treatment or prevention of infection and minimization of soft tissue damage. The wound should be cleansed with clean water and gentle soap to remove any visible dirt. Soaking the injury or using alcohol or peroxide is not recommended because of the potential for further tissue injury. Debridement is indicated for the removal of any foreign body or devitalized tissue. Edematous wounds should be passively elevated to encourage lymphatic drainage and accelerate healing. All wounds with established infection or at high risk of infection, including puncture wounds, crush injuries, wounds more than 12–24 hours old, hand or foot wounds, cat or human bites, or wounds in immunocompromised individuals, should not be sutured but kept well bandaged.[30] Tetanus prophylaxis in bite wounds should follow recommendations according to immunization status of the child. In addition, when the child has received fewer than three doses of tetanus toxoid-containing vaccine or when status is unknown, human tetanus immune globulin is indicated together with a dose of age-appropriate tetanus vaccine.[39] Exposure to rabies from rabid animal bites of bats, raccoons, or skunks can occur, and the decision to immunize the patient for potential exposure should be made in consultation with the local health department. There is no specific treatment for rabies; however, postexposure prophylaxis is recommended for an open wound or contaminated mucous membrane from rabid-animal bites from wild mammalian animals and should begin as soon as possible, ideally within 24 hours. A 1-mL intramuscular dose of vaccine (Imovax [Sanofi Pasteur SA, Lyon, France], RabAvert [GSK Vaccines, GmbH, Marburg, Germany]) should be given on day 0 and repeated on days 3, 7, and 14. A dose of rabies immune globulin should also be administered on day 0 at 20 international units/kg as an infiltrate around wound.[37,38]

Most uncomplicated bite injuries can be managed in the outpatient setting. Prophylactic antibiotics in low-risk wounds (early presenting, noninfected, nonpuncturing) have limited benefit and are not routinely recommended.[39] However, a 3- to 5-day oral course should be considered in selected cases (Box 2).[1,30,38] Close follow-up is indicated in the next 48 hours to monitor for signs of developing infection.

Patients presenting with signs of established infection after an animal bite should be empirically treated with antibiotics, which will cover the typical pathogens mentioned previously.

Box 2. Indications for Prophylactic Antibiotics After a Mammalian Bite[1,31,41]

Human bite wounds
Deep puncture wounds
Wounds with associated crush injury and edema
Wounds on hands/feet or in proximity to bone/joint
Moderate to severe injuries, especially to hand or face
Genital area bites
Wounds present in complicated hosts (extremes of age, immunocompromised or asplenic, advanced liver disease)

Empiric coverage for human bites should cover mixed flora, with special attention to *E. corrodens*, because it is not susceptible to first-generation cephalosporins. Outpatient management with oral amoxicillin/clavulanate is the first-line treatment for all mammalian bites, with trimethoprim/sulfamethoxazole or an extended-spectrum cephalosporin (e.g., cefuroxime) in combination with clindamycin as alternatives in patients with penicillin allergies.[37,38] Other oral alternatives include doxycycline and the fluoroquinolones, which—when dictated by cultures and sensitivities—may be used safely in children. Intravenous antimicrobials with activity against mixed flora such as β-lactam/β-lactamase inhibitor combinations, trimethoprim/sulfamethoxazole plus clindamycin, and second-generation cephalosporins with anaerobic activity (e.g., cefoxitin) are suitable empiric choices for severe infections. Broad-spectrum carbapenems should be reserved for treatment failure or drug-resistant isolates. Therapy duration will vary by the severity of injury, but it can range from 7–14 days for soft tissue infections to 3–6 weeks for involvement of the joints or bones.[1,37,38]

DEEP BACTERIAL TISSUE INFECTIONS

PERIORBITAL AND ORBITAL CELLULITIS

The orbital septum is a fibrous tissue that arises from the periosteum of the skull and continues into the eyelids. This anatomic landmark serves as a barrier to prevent superficial infections from penetrating deep into the orbit. Infections occurring in the soft tissue anterior to the septum are called *periorbital cellulitis* (PC), whereas those occurring posterior to the septum are considered *orbital cellulitis* (OC). Periorbital cellulitis is a disease that occurs in young children, particularly those younger than 5 years. In comparison, OC is only one-third as common as PC and tends to affect children age 5–7 years.[40-44] Because of its association with upper respiratory tract infections, OC tends to occur more often in the winter.[45] Predisposing factors for orbital infections include upper respiratory tract or sinus infections, extension of external ocular infections, dental abscesses, superficial breaks in the skin from underlying skin conditions, insect bites, penetrating injury to the orbit, periocular surgery, and hematogenous seeding.[45]

MICROBIOLOGIC ETIOLOGY

The organisms responsible for PC and OC have historically been the same bacteria implicated in respiratory tract and sinus infections; however, widespread administration of childhood *Haemophilus* and pneumococcal vaccines may shift the types of causative pathogens. Periorbital cellulitis seeded from minor trauma to the skin is often caused by staphylococcal and streptococcal species, which account for greater than 70% of positive cultures (e.g., orbital/sinus, conjunctiva, blood) obtained from infected children.[42,43,45] Often OC is a complication of acute sinusitis (specifically the ethmoid sinus); thus, respiratory organisms such as *Streptococcus pneumoniae*, GAS, other streptococcal species (*Streptococcus anginosus*), *S. aureus*, nontypeable *H. influenzae*, and

Moraxella catarrhalis are common pathogens. Mixed or polymicrobial infections, sometimes involving anaerobic organisms, tend to occur more commonly in older children because of the greater constriction between the sinus and their drainage passages, which impedes aeration and leads to an overgrowth of microbial flora.[40,41]

CLINICAL PRESENTATION

Both PC and OC can present with unilateral ocular erythema, edema, warmth, and tenderness (Figure 5). Fever and other systemic signs may also be seen. Other symptoms specific to OC, related to its invasiveness and potential to increase intraorbital pressure, include chemosis, blurred vision, impaired ocular movements, and proptosis (Figure 6). In general, markers for an inflammatory response are more robust in OC, manifested as higher fevers, greater elevation of C-reactive protein, and a more dramatic left shift.[45]

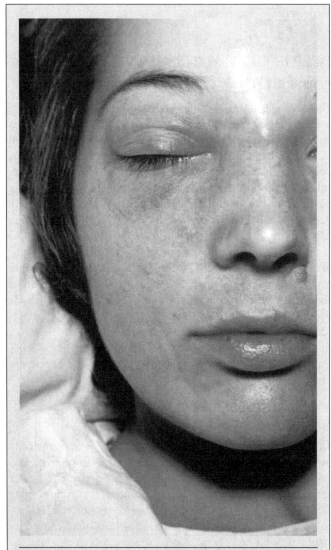

Figure 5. Periorbital and orbital cellulitis can present with fever, acute unilateral eyelid erythema, and limited extraocular motions.

Photo credit: Dr. Thomas F. Sellers, Centers for Disease Control and Prevention, Atlanta, GA.

DIAGNOSIS

Periorbital cellulitis and OC are diagnosed largely by physical examination. Positive computed tomography of sinusitis in the ethmoid and maxillary cavities, as well as subperiosteal or orbital abscesses and diffuse fat infiltration, is seen more often in cases of OC than PC. Microbiologic confirmation of orbital infections is best obtained by surgical sampling, whereby yields in excess of 80% are reported.[41,44]

TREATMENT

Simple PC without systemic involvement may be treated with empiric oral antibiotics that cover pathogens associated with the likely cause of infection. Local prevalence of MRSA should be considered when determining *S. aureus* coverage. A treatment course of 7–10 days is generally sufficient.[45]

Empiric parenteral antibiotics should cover *Streptococcus* spp., common respiratory pathogens, *S. aureus* (including MRSA when appropriate), and anaerobes. A β-lactam/β-lactamase inhibitor combination is a reasonable initial choice. If sinus involvement with respiratory pathogens is suspected, a second- or third-generation cephalosporin plus clindamycin or vancomycin can be tried. Parenteral antibiotics should be narrowed on the basis of susceptibility data and continued until systemic symptoms have resolved and significant improvement is seen in the eye, at which point an oral agent may be substituted to complete a 10- to 14-day course. Medical management alone may be adequate for treating OC, especially in children younger than 9 years or those presenting with no or only small subperiosteal abscesses.[43,46]

NECROTIZING FASCIITIS

Necrotizing fasciitis is a potentially life-threatening infection of the subcutaneous tissues comprising the superficial fascial plane, characterized by rapid and widespread inflammation and necrosis. The incidence of NF is 0.08 cases per 100,000 children, with a reported mortality rates of 5.4% in

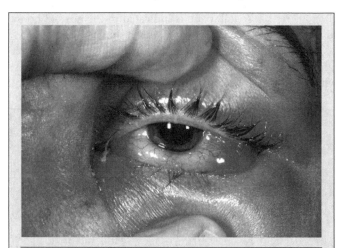

Figure 6. Orbital cellulitis with proptosis, ophthalmoplegia, and edema and erythema of the eyelids.

Image reprinted with permission from Medscape Drugs & Diseases. Orbital Cellulitis, 2018.

children.[47,48] Infections can be polymicrobial or monomicrobial, with most of the latter caused by GAS. In a prospective surveillance study of all Canadian children younger than 16 years, non-GAS–related NF and GAS-related NF accounted for 0.81 and 2.12 cases per 1 million children, respectively. Most children were younger than 5 years.[48]

General risk factors for NF include conditions that compromise skin integrity, such as recent trauma or skin lesions. Non-GAS–related NF is associated with chronic illnesses, malnutrition, obesity, immunosuppression, and intravenous drug use. In neonates, non-GAS-related NF can develop secondary to surgery, procedures, or necrotizing enterocolitis.[49]

In contrast, GAS-related NF generally affects healthy children. A strong correlation has been noted between GAS-related NF and varicella infection. In the Canadian study, 58% of the patients were recently given a diagnosis of varicella.[48] Although an association between nonsteroidal anti-inflammatory drugs (NSAIDs) and GAS-related NF has been reported in many case reports, a causal relationship has not been proved.[50]

MICROBIOLOGIC ETIOLOGY

Necrotizing fasciitis is generally classified into two types based on the causative organism with *polymicrobial NF* (*type 1*) more common, involving a combination of gram-positive cocci, gram-negative rods and anaerobic bacteria, such as *Bacteroides* and *Peptostreptococcus* spp., and bowel flora.[49] Critically ill neonates are especially vulnerable to polymicrobial NF involving *S. aureus* because of the variety of monitoring and surgical procedures they undergo.[51] The most common cause of *monomicrobial NF* (*type 2*) is GAS, although other bacteria have been implicated, such as *S. aureus*, *Vibrio vulnificus*, *Aeromonas hydrophila*, and *Peptostreptococcus* spp. Invasive GAS infections can occur from the translocation of colonized GAS in the pharynx through systemic spread to the site of minor trauma; however, more often than not, the infection occurs spontaneously with no preceding prodrome. The pathogenesis of GAS is facilitated by several important cell surface proteins that help it evade phagocytosis: proteases, which can precipitate intravascular occlusion; and pyrogenic exotoxins, which can act as superantigens.[52] Blood cultures have limited use because they may be negative in greater than 80% of cases.[53]

CLINICAL PRESENTATION

Patients with early stages of NF present with mild swelling and erythema over an affected site, but they may report pain seemingly out of proportion to the infection. High temperatures, tachycardia, altered mental status, and systemic toxicity are common. In children and neonates, the most common infection sites are the trunk, followed by the head and neck, limbs, lower extremities, and perineum.[48,51,54] Eventually, necrosis of the soft tissue, skin ischemia, and gangrene of the overlying skin ensue and can give rise to blister or bullae formation and skin ulceration. Damage to superficial nerves can lead to the loss of sensation. Rapidly advancing erythema without margins, lack of response to appropriate antibiotics,

and progression to systemic signs of sepsis should suggest NF. Symptoms generally progress for 2–4 days, but GAS-related NF tends to spread very quickly and can culminate in multisystem organ failure early in the disease process.[47,52,53]

DIAGNOSIS

Laboratory evaluation of patients with suspected NF is nonspecific but reflects evidence of systemic inflammation and organ dysfunction. Evidence of NF on ultrasonography may include the presence of fluid accumulation within thickened fascia or loculated abscesses. Gas in the soft tissue is a positive finding by plain radiography in 24% to 73% of patients, especially in patients with non-GAS–related NF.[52] Magnetic resonance imaging and computed tomography can be useful in distinguishing cellulitis from necrotizing infections.

TREATMENT

Surgical management is the first-line treatment in NF. Aggressive debridement of the wound up to the first margins of pink, viable tissues is required to control disease morbidity because NF can invade areas beyond the extent of visibly involved skin. Empiric coverage for polymicrobial infections should be broad with vancomycin or linezolid plus piperacillin/tazobactam or a carbapenem; or vancomycin or linezolid plus ceftriaxone and metronidazole. Empiric antibiotics should be continued until debridement is no longer needed, clinical improvement has been seen, and fever has subsided for at least 72 hours. If GAS is suspected, the combination of clindamycin and penicillin has shown superior clinical efficacy to penicillins alone.[1,55] Pharmacologically, clindamycin may suppress toxin production, modulate cytokine production, and sustain bacterial killing during slow phases of growth when penicillins are ineffective.

Given the suggested role of superantigens in the pathogenesis of GAS-related NF, intravenous immunoglobulin (IVIG) may help attenuate the untoward host inflammatory effect by neutralizing superantigens. Despite in vitro data and smaller case series that suggest benefit, this result has not been reproduced in larger-scale studies.[56-58] The routine use of IVIG remains controversial in the absence of substantial clinical benefits, high cost, and scarcity. In patients with polymicrobial NF, IVIG has not been studied and should not be recommended.

VIRAL SKIN INFECTIONS
HERPES SIMPLEX VIRUS

Herpes simplex viruses (HSV) belong to the family of human herpes viruses (HHV), all of which cause a primary infection and remain capable of reactivation later in life. Types 1 and 2 are the most pathogenic, and the dermatologic areas that they typically infect can distinguish the two types. The HSV-1 infections tend to occur "above the waist," involving the skin, oral cavity, lips, and face. Herpes labialis is the most common HSV-1 disease (also known as *orolabial HSV-1* or *gingivostomatitis*). The HSV-2 infections typically occur in the genital region ("below the waist") in teenagers and adults who are sexually active. Despite these generalizations, both viruses can cause disease in either area, as evidenced by the increasing incidence of orolabial HSV-2 and genital herpes caused by HSV-1.[59]

Among humans, HSV-1 is ubiquitous. Almost 60% to 90% of adults worldwide are infected with HSV-1 and are largely asymptomatic because of long latency periods in healthy individuals.[59] Unlike other childhood viral illnesses, which are acquired during day care or school outbreaks, primary HSV-1 infections occur early in life, between age 1 and 3 years by horizontal transmission, likely through close contact with family members who are contagious or on the verge of developing recurrent disease.[59] Among adolescents age 14–19 years, the HSV-1 seroprevalence has decreased by almost 23%, from 39% in 1999–2004 to 30.1% in 2005–2010, indicating declining orolabial infection in this age group. The HSV-2 seroprevalence in this age group was much lower, with less than 2% in both ranges of years.[60] The incidence of neonatal herpes infection is about 1 in every 3500–20,000 births.[59,61] Vertical perinatal transmission accounts for 85% of cases. Another 10% of cases are transmitted postnatally through horizontal transfer from caregiver, and less than 5% of infections are acquired from intrauterine transmission.[61] The disease carries high morbidity and mortality. Even with treatment, 15% of infants with encephalitis and 57% with disseminated disease die.[62]

MICROBIOLOGIC ETIOLOGY

Both HSV-1 and -2 are large DNA viruses with genomes that code for a variety of glycoproteins and polypeptides involved in viral replication. After multiplying in the epithelial cells, the virus invades local nerve endings and travels up to the neural cell bodies in the regional sensory ganglia, where it remains dormant until reactivation. The trigeminal ganglion

is the most common reservoir for oral-facial HSV-1 infection. Exposure to triggers such as trauma, ultraviolet light, fever, physical and emotional stress, radiotherapy, and organ transplants may result in disease reactivation.[63] Shedding of HSV from the oral cavity is observed in 2% to 9% of asymptomatic subjects. Horizontal transmission of HSV-2 infections can occur through skin contact or bodily fluids, including semen, cervical fluid, or vesicular fluid from active lesions. A person may be contagious even when clinically asymptomatic. The incubation period is typically from 2 days to 2 weeks after exposure.[59]

CLINICAL PRESENTATION

Primary HSV infection may result in the following: an asymptomatic course, resulting in antibody production; a localized or general eruption; or a serious systemic disease. Most healthy children who contract the herpes virus will present with a prodrome and develop lesions on the skin and mucous membranes in a variety of distributions, including the digits, knees, ear and face, mouth, and genital area (Figure 7 and Figure 8). Symptoms associated with primary infections will always be more severe than those associated with a recurrence. Immunocompromised patients most commonly present with

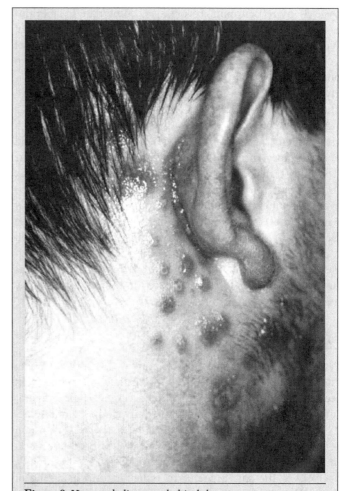

Figure 8. Herpes gladiatorum behind the ear.

Image reprinted with permission from Medscape Drugs & Diseases. Pediatric Herpes Simplex Virus Infection, 2019.

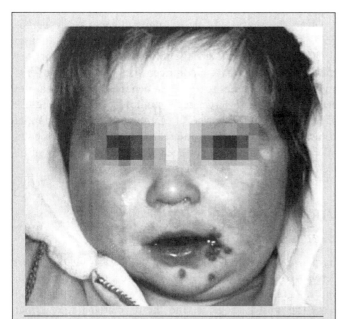

Figure 7. Primary herpes simplex virus gingivostomatitis in an infant.

Image reprinted with permission from Medscape Drugs & Diseases. Pediatric Herpes Simplex Virus Infection, 2019.

severe local lesions, although disseminated disease with generalized vesicular skin lesions and visceral involvement can also occur. Despite proper treatment, HSV infection acquired during the neonatal period is associated with significant morbidity and mortality because it can disseminate to the liver, lungs, and central nervous system. Skin lesions are present in 60% of cases with disseminated disease and in 85% of localized infection to the skin, eyes, and mouth.[59]

DIAGNOSIS

Most HSV-1 cases may be diagnosed by history and physical examination. Although a positive viral culture obtained from mucous membranes or lesions is considered confirmatory, this test is rarely performed. Immunologic assays are better at differentiating between different subtypes and confirming exposure.[59,61]

TREATMENT

The cornerstone of therapy is the purine nucleoside analog acyclovir, which limits viral replication but cannot eradicate cells that are already infected. Clinically, this limited replication translates into decreases in viral shedding, healing time, and disease severity. Oral acyclovir is effective for primary and recurrent genital herpes and orolabial herpes in immunocompetent hosts.[64,65] Parenteral acyclovir should be reserved for systemic disease requiring hospitalization, as well as for neonates or immunocompromised patients. Failure to respond to acyclovir may necessitate treatment with intravenous foscarnet, which carries significant renal toxicity.[59,66] Table 2 lists pediatric antiviral therapy for HSV-1 and -2.

Valacyclovir and famciclovir are oral prodrugs to acyclovir and penciclovir, respectively. Their enhanced bioavailability permits dosing less often with comparable efficacy to acyclovir for mucocutaneous herpetic disease, but not for systemic infections. In adolescents and adults, these drugs are indicated for primary and recurrent genital herpes and recurrent orolabial herpes.[66] Chronic suppressive therapy with these agents for up to 1 year is safe and effective in preventing recurrences and asymptomatic viral shedding in patients prone to frequent outbreaks.[64] Recent studies delineating their pharmacokinetic profiles and dosing recommendations in younger children may potentially allow their use in lieu of acyclovir in orolabial herpes.[64,67]

Topical formulations of acyclovir and penciclovir can be used in localized HSV disease to lessen disease severity, viral shedding, and associated discomfort, but are not as effective as oral regimens and should not be routinely recommended.[64] Docosanol is a biphenyl alcohol that is available as an over-the-counter topical cream. When applied early during the prodromal phase, docosanol can help reduce healing time and shorten the duration of painful symptoms in orolabial herpes.[68]

VARICELLA

Chicken pox is a ubiquitous childhood vesicular exanthema caused by the varicella zoster virus (VZV) (Figure 9 and Figure 10). Presentation and prevention with immunization are discussed in the Pediatric Vaccines chapter. Discussion of varicella in this chapter is limited to diagnostic and treatment strategies in children infected with chicken pox.

DIAGNOSIS

Diagnosis of varicella in healthy hosts is based on the appearance of the lesion, confirmed by a history of exposure. Laboratory analysis is not necessary but may reveal an initially depressed white blood cell count, decreased platelet

Table 2. Pediatric Antiviral Therapy for Superficial Skin Infections

Pathogen	Drug (Route)	Daily Oral Dose	Daily Parenteral Dose	Comments
HSV 1 and 2	Acyclovir (IV, PO)	80 mg/kg/day divided Q 6 hr Max 800 mg	15–30 mg/kg/day divided Q 8 hr	Obese patients are dosed using ideal body weight Nephrotoxicity risk increased with IV doses > 15 mg/kg/dose or 500 mg/m^2
	Valacyclovir (PO)	40 mg/kg/day divided Q 12 hr Max 1000 mg	—	—
	Famciclovir (PO)	250 mg TID	—	Indicated for genital herpes or herpes labialis Dose for children and adolescents ≥ 45 kg
Varicella zoster virus	Acyclovir (IV, PO)	80 mg/kg/day divided Q 6 hr Max 800 mg	30–45 mg/kg/day divided Q 8 hr	Obese patients are dosed using ideal body weight Nephrotoxicity risk increased with IV doses > 15 mg/kg/dose or 500 mg/m^2
	Valacyclovir (PO)	60 mg/kg/day divided Q 8 hr Max 1000 mg	—	—
	Famciclovir (PO)	500 mg TID	—	Dose for children and adolescents ≥ 45 kg

HSV = herpes simplex virus, IV = intravenous, max = maximum, PO = oral, Q = every, TID = three times daily.

count, and mildly elevated liver function tests. If central nervous system involvement is suspected, cerebrospinal fluid analysis may show mild lymphocytosis, slight elevation of protein, and near-normal glucose concentrations.[69] Polymerase chain reaction can also be used to identify VZV from fluid lesion or scabs and is more sensitive than viral culture or direct fluorescent antibody assay.

TREATMENT

In healthy children, supportive care is the primary treatment of varicella. Local therapy with drying agents such as calamine lotion or oatmeal soaks can be used on weeping lesions. Topical agents containing antihistamines should be avoided because of the increased risk of percutaneous absorption from loss of skin integrity. Daily baths with soap and water are recommended to destroy the virus's lipid envelope. Acetaminophen should be used for fever and analgesia because antipyretics, such as aspirin and NSAIDs, have been associated with an increased risk of Reye syndrome and invasive GAS disease, respectively.

Acyclovir is the antiviral drug of choice for treating primary VZV infection. When initiated within 24 hours of the onset of rash, oral acyclovir at 20 mg/kg/dose (maximum 800 mg/dose) four times/day for 5 days was safe and modestly effective in decreasing markers of VZV disease severity.[70] In particular, the clinical benefit seemed more pronounced in children older than 12 years and in patients who were secondary household cases tending to exhibit more serious dermatologic and constitutional symptoms.[69] Because of the self-limiting nature of VZV, the American Academy of Pediatrics does not recommend the routine use of antivirals for postexposure prophylaxis or treatment in otherwise young, healthy children; however, acyclovir may be useful for children with complicated disease (pneumonia, encephalitis, or hepatitis) or comorbid conditions (Table 3). Parenteral acyclovir should be initiated in any child who develops severe complications or in any high-risk patient with VZV. Acyclovir doses of 500 mg/m^2 (or a 10-mg/kg/dose in older children) administered intravenously every 8 hours for at least 7 days reduces the dissemination of varicella and hastens cutaneous healing in immunosuppressed patients.[69] Valacyclovir is the L-valine ester of acyclovir with improved bioavailability that is preferable compared with acyclovir, although at a higher cost. Famciclovir is an oral prodrug of penciclovir with similar activity to acyclovir against VZV; however, its efficacy and safety have not been established in children. Table 2 lists pediatric antiviral therapy for VZV.

OTHER VIRAL EXANTHEMS: HAND, FOOT, AND MOUTH DISEASE; FIFTH DISEASE; AND SIXTH DISEASE

Other common pediatric SSTIs include hand, foot, and mouth disease (HFMD), fifth disease, and sixth disease. These childhood exanthems are typified by a prodrome of fever and constitutional symptoms for several days, followed by the appearance of a characteristic rash in a specific distribution. Diagnosis is largely based on clinical presentation because serology may not always permit a distinction between previous and recent exposure. Polymerase chain reaction may be useful for confirming primary infection except in sixth disease, in which the herpes virus may remain dormant intracellularly. Treatment in otherwise healthy patients consists of supportive management and the occasional use of IVIG or other systemic antivirals in severe systemic disease.

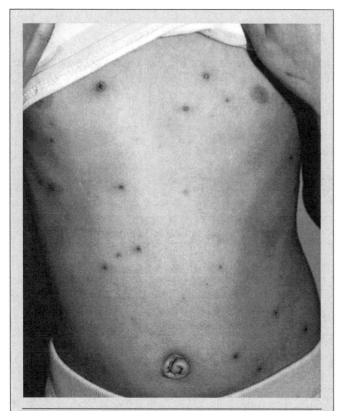

Figure 9. Vesicular rash from varicella zoster (chicken pox). Lesions usually begin on the trunk and spread to the face and limbs.

Photo credit: Dr. James Korb, Children's Hospital of Orange County, Orange, CA.

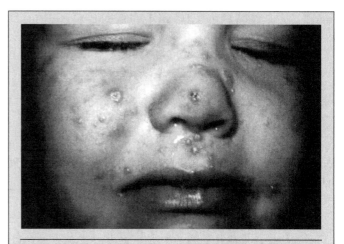

Figure 10. Varicella zoster lesions on the face.

Photo credit: Dr. John Noble Jr., Centers for Disease Control and Prevention, Atlanta, GA.

HAND, FOOT, AND MOUTH DISEASE

Hand, foot, and mouth disease is a highly contagious infection that presents with painful ulcerative lesions in the mouth, and rhomboid vesicles ("square blisters") on the palms, soles, and sides of fingers and toes. In the United States, outbreaks of HFMD are typically caused by coxsackievirus A16 or enterovirus 71.[71] Often HFMD occurs as an outbreak among collections of children in a school or childcare setting. Incidence is highest during the summer and fall months, with epidemics occurring in 3-year cycles in the United States.[71]

Enteroviruses spread primarily through contact with respiratory droplets or infectious fecal material, although vertical transmission from mother to child is also possible. Because of their resistance to environmental insults, enteroviruses can survive on fomites, adding to their contagiousness. Once infected, patients are contagious until the blisters have resolved.[72,73]

After the prodrome, patients develop large, painful oral lesions on the palate, tongue, and buccal mucosa in 1–2 days, followed by the presentation of peripheral skin lesions; however, not all patients will express both mucosal and dermatologic symptoms (Figure 11 and Figure 12).[73] Skin lesions are more commonly found on the dorsal surfaces and may present on the palms, fingers, toes, soles, buttocks, genitals, and limbs. The exanthem begins with red macules that evolve into gray vesicles surrounded by an erythematous halo, but they are not typically pruritic. Cutaneous lesions generally heal without scabbing in 1 week. Complications from coxsackievirus infection include myocarditis, pneumonia, and meningoencephalitis.

In a small case series, treatment with oral acyclovir provided symptomatic relief and improvement in lesions within 24 hours.[74] A trial of acyclovir may be considered in high-risk patients (e.g., immunocompromised hosts or neonates) or outbreaks. In patients hospitalized with systemic disease, IVIG has been used with some beneficial effects, but it should not be used routinely for HFMD.[73]

ERYTHEMA INFECTIOSUM (FIFTH DISEASE)

Fifth disease, or *erythema infectiosum*, is a ubiquitous, benign childhood viral exanthema caused by parvovirus B19, typically affecting children age 4–10 years. Antibody seroprevalence is 5%–10% in young children. Infection peaks during late winter to early spring, and secondary spread within a household occurs in up to 50% of individuals.[75] Spread of the virus is primarily through infected respiratory droplets, although transmission by blood products or vertical transmission can occur. The end of the incubation period, ranging from 4 to 14 days, is marked by the formation of immunoglobulin G and clearance of viremia, which precedes the characteristic rash. Thus, a patient who exhibits the diagnostic eruptions is not considered contagious.[71]

The rash associated with fifth disease typically develops on the cheeks and appears as if the patient was slapped (Figure 13). The exanthem may fade and recur when triggered by local irritation, high temperatures, or emotional stress, but this recurrence does not represent recrudescence of disease. Arthralgias involving the small joints of the hands, wrists, knees, or ankles can occur in 10% of patients.[75] Transient anemia is a complication that may develop in patients with limited red blood cell reserves, resulting in an aplastic crisis. Parvovirus B19 infection contracted during pregnancy can lead to nonimmune hydrops fetalis, a fetal complication resulting in profound anemia, heart failure, and occasionally the death of the fetus in utero.[76] For most patients, only supportive care is indicated. In chronically immunosuppressed patients with signs of anemia, IVIG may be considered, but it may precipitate the rash and joint symptoms of erythema infectiosum; also, no dosing has been established.[71]

ROSEOLA (SIXTH DISEASE/EXANTHEMA SUBITUM)

Roseola, also known as *sixth disease* or *exanthema subitum*, is a benign childhood exanthema caused by the sixth and seventh variants of HHV. Roseola is one of the most common

Table 3. Indications for Acyclovir Treatment in Varicella

Host Status	Treatment	Route
Healthy[a]	Optional	PO
Uncomplicated varicella, age 2–12 yr	Beneficial	PO
Secondary household contacts, age > 12 yr	Highly beneficial	PO
Complications Viral pneumonia Encephalitis Hepatitis	 Indicated Indicated Indicated	 IV IV IV
Immunocompromised Malignancy, transplant recipients, congenital immunodeficiency, HIV infection, neonates, steroid therapy	Indicated	IV
Chronic disease Cutaneous disorders, pulmonary disorders, diabetes mellitus, disease requiring chronic salicylate or intermittent steroid therapy	Recommended	PO or IV[b]

[a]Treatment must be initiated within 24 hours after rash for maximal benefit.
[b]Select patients considered at relatively low risk of varicella zoster virus dissemination can be treated by using acyclovir orally with careful monitoring for progression.
IV = intravenous, PO = oral.
Reprinted with permission of Elsevier. Arvin AM. Antiviral therapy for varicella and herpes zoster. Semin Pediatr Infect Dis 2002;13:12–21.

childhood exanthemas, affecting children between age 6–18 months.[71] Little is known about how the viruses are transmitted, and there seems to be no seasonal predilection for primary infections. Because herpes viruses may remain latent in bodily reservoirs years after the primary infection, the leading hypothesis is that young infants acquire disease through exposure to the saliva or oral secretions of an asymptomatic caretaker who is shedding virus. Vertical transmission of the virus from mother to baby is possible. In addition, HHV-6 can insert its genome into human chromosomes, enabling it to be passed on congenitally.[71,76,77]

The classic presentation permitting a clinical diagnosis of primary roseola is fever for 3–5 days that rapidly subsides, followed by the development of a rose-pink maculopapular rash on the neck and trunk that spreads to the extremities and face. Central nervous system complications, including febrile seizures, can occur in up to 15% of primary infections.[76] Examination of the oropharynx may reveal red papules on the soft palate and uvula (Nagayama spots), exudative tonsillar lesions, or herpangina. Other physical findings include mild upper respiratory congestion, otitis media, nausea, vomiting, cervical and post-occipital lymphadenopathy, and hepatosplenomegaly.[71,77] Reactivation from latent disease or reinfection may occur later in life, particularly in immunocompromised individuals such as transplant recipients. Serious manifestations of reactivated HHV-6 include bone marrow suppression, pneumonitis, encephalitis, hepatitis, and organ rejection. Reserved for only severe systemic infection, antivirals such as ganciclovir, foscarnet, and cidofovir show in vitro activity against HHV-6 and have resulted in viral clearance among immunocompromised patients with systemic disease.[78-80]

CONCLUSIONS

Bacterial and viral infections of the skin and soft tissue are common childhood illnesses that can develop into severe systemic complications without timely treatment, especially in an immunocompromised patient. The selection of antibiotics for treating bacterial infections must ensure adequate coverage of the most likely organisms based on a patient's risk factors, and these agents must show favorable absorption and penetration to the infected site. An understanding of local susceptibility patterns is crucial in light of the ever-increasing prevalence of resistant pathogens, such as CA-MRSA. Outpatient regimens with the greatest likelihood of patient acceptance are those that are palatable with simple administration schedules. Parents should be instructed to seek further medical attention if dermatologic and systemic symptoms do not improve within 48 hours. Although parenteral antibiotics should always be administered in a child exhibiting systemic complications from an SSTI, surgical drainage and intervention often plays an integral role in the overall treatment plan of a loculated soft tissue infection or NF. Empiric antibiotics should be narrowed once microbial

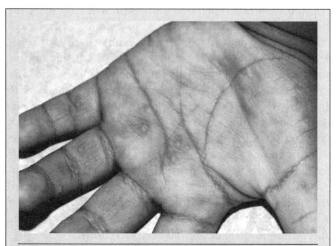

Figure 11. Small vesicles with an erythematous border on the palms and fingers characteristic of hand, foot, and mouth disease.

Photo credit: Dr. James Korb, Children's Hospital of Orange County, Orange, CA.

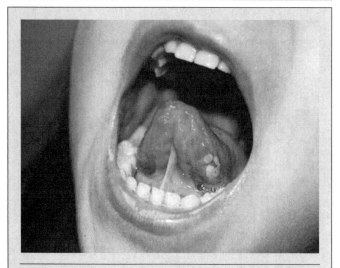

Figure 12. Painful oral lesions under the tongue from hand, foot, and mouth disease.

Photo credit: Dr. James Korb, Children's Hospital of Orange County, Orange, CA.

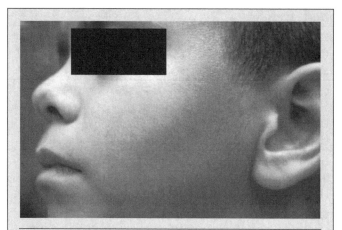

Figure 13. Erythematous rash resembling a slapped cheek associated with erythema infectiosum (fifth disease).

Photo credit: Centers for Disease Control and Prevention, Atlanta, GA.

susceptibilities are available to prevent the evolution of a drug-resistant organism.

Viral skin illnesses are ubiquitous and often acquired early in childhood without significant sequelae. Although the management of viral skin infections is largely supportive, aspirin and NSAIDs should be strictly avoided as antipyretics because of the risk of Reye syndrome and invasive GAS disease, respectively. Antivirals may be indicated in select cases of severe primary or recurrent infections in high-risk populations.

Patient Case ADOLESCENT WITH SKIN ABSCESS

A previously healthy 14-year-old boy weighing 52 kg, no known drug allergy, is brought to the emergency department with a 3-day history of increasing redness, swelling, and pain to his upper left thigh. His primary care pediatrician prescribed cephalexin 2 days prior, which he is still taking. He has no relevant medical or travel history. He feels well and has no fevers, chills, nausea, or vomiting. He is on the high school football team. A 2-by-3-cm fluctuant, tender, erythematous mass is palpable on physical examination. There is no drainage or associated open wound. A furuncle is diagnosed, and an antibiotic is initiated in the emergency department.

1. What is the most likely causative organism of the patient's skin infection?

Staphylococcus aureus is the most common cause of furunculosis. *Streptococcus pyogenes* is typically associated with nonpurulent and nonculturable skin infections, such as cellulitis and erysipelas. Although wound cultures can confirm the etiologic organism, cultures are only helpful for purulent infection; establishing the cause of nonpurulent skin infection is difficult. Infections with gram-negative organisms are seen in patients who are immunocompromised, with animal bites, or recent surgery. Polymicrobial skin infections involving aerobic and anaerobic organisms are typically seen in patients with diabetes mellitus, history of illicit drug use, or skin infections involving the gastrointestinal tract and perineal area, none of which are present for this patient.

2. The physician would like to prescribe an antibiotic for home and asks, what is your recommendation for this patient?

In this young boy presenting with a fluctuant furunculosis and not responding to cephalexin, methicillin-resistant *Staphylococcus aureus* (MRSA), especially community-acquired MRSA, which accounts for the majority of MRSA-associated skin and soft tissue infection in children, is the most likely cause of infection. An appropriate recommendation would be clindamycin 600 mg orally every 8 hours for 5 days because the patient appears to be clinically stable without systemic symptoms. Clindamycin is preferred for MRSA coverage as well as for toxin inhibition. Incision and drainage are also recommended.

3. What are some relevant counseling points for the patient at discharge?

The patient should be counseled to take clindamycin with or without meals, but with a full glass of water to avoid stomach irritation. He should also be instructed to seek medical attention with any of the following symptoms: fever or chills, increased pain, and redness or swelling of the infection site.

REFERENCES

1. Stevens DL, Bisno AL, Chambers HF, et al. Practice Guidelines for the diagnosis and management of skin and soft tissue infections. 2014 update by the Infectious Disease Society of America. Clin Infect Dis 2014;59:147-59.

2. Iwamoto M, Mu Y, Lynfield, R et al. Trends in invasive methicillin-resistant Staphylococcus aureus infections. Pediatrics 2013;132:e817-24.

3. Hedrick J. Acute bacterial skin infections in pediatric medicine. Pediatr Drugs 2003;5:35-46.

4. Faden H, Lesse A, Trask J, et al. Importance of colonization site in the current epidemic of staphylococcal skin abscesses. Pediatrics 2010;125:e618-24.

5. Olesevich M, Kennedy A. Emergence of community acquired methicillin-resistant *Staphylococcus aureus* soft tissue infections. J Pediatr Surg 2007;42:765-8.

6. Korczowski B, Antadze T, Giorgobiani M, et al. A multicenter, randomized, observer-blinded, active-controlled study to evaluate the safety and efficacy of ceftaroline versus comparator in pediatric patients with acute bacterial skin and skin structure infection. Pediatr Infect Dis J 2016;35:e239-47.

7. Fritz SA, Hogan PG, Hayek G, et al. Household versus individual approaches to eradication of community-associated Staphylococcus aureus in children: a randomized trial. Clin Infect Dis 2012;54:743-51.

8. Leung YH, Wong MM, Chuang SK. Effect of intranasal mupirocin and chlorhexidine body wash on decolonization of community-associated methicillin-resistant Staphylococcus aureus. Infect Control Hosp Epidemiol 2011;32:1048-50.

9. Adams CM, Neuman MI, Levy JA. Point-of-care ultrasonography for the diagnosis of pediatric soft tissue infection. J Pediatr 2016;169:122-7.

10. Marin JR, Dean AJ, Bilker WB, et al. Emergency ultrasound-assisted examination of skin and soft tissue infections in the pediatric emergency department. Acad Emerg Med 2013;20:545-53.

11. Liu C, Bayer A, Cosgrove S, et al. Clinical practice guidelines by the Infectious Diseases Society of America for the treatment of methicillin-resistant *Staphylococcus aureus* infections in adults and children. Clin Infect Dis 2011;52:1-38.

12. Williams DJ, Cooper WO, Kaltenbach LA, et al. Comparative effectiveness of antibiotic treatment strategies for pediatric skin and soft-tissue infections. Pediatrics 2011:128:e479-87.

13. Cluzet VC, Gerber JS, Nachamkin I, et al. Duration of colonization and determinants of earlier clearance of colonization with methicillin-resistant Staphylococcus aureus. Clin Infect Dis 2015;60:1489-96.

14. Martin JM, Green M. Group A Streptococcus. Semin Pediatr Infect Dis 2006;17:140-8.

15. Trenchs V, Hernandez-Bou S, Bianchi C, et al. Blood cultures are not useful in the evaluation of children with uncomplicated superficial skin and soft tissue infections. Pediatr Infect Dis J 2015;34:924.

16. Wilson ML, Winn W. Laboratory diagnosis of bone, joint, soft-tissue and skin infections. Clin Infect Dis 2008;46:453-7.

17. Sladden MJ, Johnston GA. Current options for the treatment of impetigo in children. Expert Opin Pharmacother 2005;6:2245-66.

18. Cole C, Gazewood J. Diagnosis and treatment of impetigo. Am Fam Physician 2007;75:859-64.

19. American Academy of Pediatrics. Group A Streptococcal Infections. In: Kimberlin DW, Brady MT, Jackson MA, et al., eds. Red Book: 2018 Report of the Committee on Infectious Diseases, 31st ed. American Academy of Pediatrics, 2018;750-7.

20. Brown J, Shriner DL, Schwartz RA, et al. Impetigo: an update. Int J Dermatol 2003;42:351-5.

21. Mancini AJ. Bacterial skin infections in children: the common and the not so common. Pediatr Ann 2000;29:26-35.

22. Pankuch GA, Lin G, Hoellman DB, et al. Activity of retapamulin against Streptococcus pyogenes and Staphylococcus aureus evaluated by agar dilution, microdilution, E-test, and disk diffusion methodologies. Antimicrob Agents Chemother 2006;50:1727-30.

23. Altabax [package insert]. Research Triangle Park, NC: Glaxo SmithKline, 2010.

24. Shi D, Higuchi W, Takano T, et al. Bullous impetigo in children infected with methicillin-resistant Staphylococcus aureus alone or in combination with methicillin-susceptible S. aureus: Analysis of genetic characteristics, including assessment of exfoliative toxin gene carriage. J Clin Micro 2011;49:1972.

25. Berk D, Bayliss S. MRSA, staphylococcal scalded skin syndrome, and other cutaneous bacterial emergencies. Pediatr Ann 2010;39:627-33.

26. Ladhani S. Recent developments in staphylococcal scalded skin syndrome. Clin Microbiol Infect 2001;7:301-7.

27. Patel GK, Finlay AY. Staphylococcal scalded skin syndrome. Am J Clin Dermatol 2003;4:165-75.

28. Yokota S, Imagawa T, Katakura S, et al. Staphylococcus scalded skin syndrome caused by exfoliative toxin B-producing methicillin-resistant Staphylococcus aureus [letter]. Eur J Paediatr 1996;155:722.

29. Antaya RJ, Robinson DM. Blisters and pustules in the newborn. Pediatr Ann 2010;39:635-45.

30. Kannikeswaran N, Kamat D. Mammalian bites. Clin Pediatr 2009;48:145-8.

31. Weiss HB, Friedman DI, Coben JH. Incidence of dog bite injuries treated in emergency departments. JAMA 1998;279:51-3.

32. Brook I. Microbiology of human and animal bite wounds in children. Pediatr Infect Dis J 1987;6:29-32.

33. Talan DA, Citron DM, Abrahamian FM, et al., Emergency Medicine Animal Bite Infection Study Group. Bacteriological analysis of infected dog and cat bites. N Engl J Med 1999;340:85-92.

34. Talan DA, Abrahamian FM, Moran GJ, et al. Clinical presentation and bacteriologic analysis of infected human bites in patients presenting to emergency departments. Clin Infect Dis 2003;37:1481-9.

35. Dire DJ, Hogan DE, Walker JS. Prophylactic oral antibiotics for low risk dog bite wounds. Pediatr Emerg Care 1992;8:194-9.

36. Daniel DM, Ritzi RB, O'Neil J, et al. Analysis of nonfatal dog bites in children. J Trauma 2009;66:S17-22.

37. American Academy of Pediatrics. Bite wounds. Kimberlin DW, Brady MT, Jackson MA, et al., eds. Red Book: 2018 Report of the Committee on Infectious Diseases. 31st ed. American Academy of Pediatrics; 2018:192-3.

38. Bula-Rudas FJ, Olcott JL, Human and animal bites. Pediatr Rev 2018;39:490-8.

39. Cummings P. Antibiotics to prevent infection in patients with dog bite wounds: a meta-analysis of randomized trials. Ann Emerg Med 1994;23:535-40.

40. Nageswaran S, Woods CR, Benjamin DK, et al. Orbital cellulitis in children. Pediatr Infect Dis J 2006;25:695-9.

41. McKinley SH, Yen MT, Miller AM, et al. Microbiology of pediatric orbital cellulitis. Am J Ophthalmol 2007;144:497-501.

42. Georgakopoulos CD, Eliopoulou MI, Stasinos S, et al. Periorbital and orbital cellulitis: a 10-year review of hospitalized children. Eur J Ophthalmol 2010;20:1066-72.

43. Yang M, Quah BL, Seah LL, et al. Orbital cellulitis in children - medical treatment versus surgical management. Orbit 2009;28:124-36.

44. Seltz LB, Smith J, Durairaj VD, et al. Microbiology and antibiotic management of orbital cellulitis. Pediatrics 2011;127:e-566-72.

45. Hauser A, Fogarasi S. Periorbital and orbital cellulitis. Pediatr Rev 2010;31:242-9.

46. Harris GJ. Subperiosteal abscess of the orbit: age as a factor in the bacteriology and response to treatment. Ophthalmology 1994;101:585-95.

47. Fustes-Morales A, Gutierrez-Castrellon P, Duran-McKinster C, et al. Necrotizing fasciitis: report of 39 pediatric cases. Arch Dermatol 2002;138:893-9.

48. Eneli I, Davies HD. Epidemiology and outcome of necrotizing fasciitis in children: an active surveillance study of the Canadian Paediatric Surveillance Program. J Pediatr 2007;151:79-84.

49. Hsieh WS, Yang PH, Chao HC, et al. Neonatal necrotizing fasciitis: a report of three cases and review of the literature. Pediatrics 1999;103:e53.

50. Holder EP, Moore PT, Browne B. Nonsteroidal anti-inflammatory drugs and necrotizing fasciitis. Drug Saf 1997;17:369-73.

51. Jamal E, Teach SJ. Necrotizing fasciitis. Pediatric Emer Care 2011;27:1195.

52. Fontes RA, Ogilvie CM, Miclau T. Necrotizing soft-tissue infections. J Am Acad Orthop Surg 2000;8:151-8.

53. Moss RL, Musemeche CA, Kosloske AM. Necrotizing fasciitis in children: prompt recognition and aggressive therapy improve survival. J Pediatric Surgery 1996;3:1142-6.

54. Leung AK, Eneli I, Davies HD. Necrotizing fasciitis in children. Pediatr Ann 2008;37:704-10.

55. Zimbelman J, Palmer A, Todd J. Improved outcome of clindamycin compared with beta-lactam antibiotic treatment for invasive Streptococcus pyogenes infection. Pediatr Infect Dis J 1999;18:1096-100.

56. Norrby-Teglund A, Muller MP, Mcgeer A, et al. Successful management of severe group A streptococcal soft tissue infections using an aggressive medical regimen including intravenous polyspecific immunoglobulin together with a conservative surgical approach. Scand J Infect Dis 2005;37:166-72.

57. Darenberg J, Ihendyane N, Sjolin J, et al. Intravenous immunoglobulin G therapy in streptococcal toxic shock syndrome: a European randomized, double-blind, placebo-controlled trial. Clin Infect Dis 2003;37:333-40.

58. Shah S, Hall M, Srivastava R, et al. Intravenous immune globulin in children with streptococcal toxic shock syndrome. Clin Infect Dis 2009;49:1369-76.

59. American Academy of Pediatrics. Herpes simplex. Kimberlin DW, Brady MT, Jackson MA, et al., eds. Red Book: 2018 Report of the Committee on Infectious Diseases, American Academy of Pediatrics, 2018:443.

60. Bradley H, Markowitz LE, Gibson T, et al. Seroprevalence of herpes simplex virus types 1 and 2—United States, 1999–2010. J Infect Dis 2014;209:325-33.

61. Wang A, Wohrley J, Rosebush J. Herpes Simplex in the neonates. Pediatr Ann 2017;46:e42-6.

62. Whitley R, Arvin A, Prober C, et al. Predictors of morbidity and mortality in neonates with herpes simplex virus infections. The National Institute of Allergy and Infectious Diseases Collaborative Antiviral Study Group. N Engl J Med 1991;324:450-4.

63. Kesson AM. Management of neonatal herpes simplex virus infection. Pediatr Drugs 2001;3:81-90.

64. Nasser M, Fedorowicz Z, Khoshnevisan MH, et al. Acyclovir for treating primary herpetic gingivostomatitis. Cochrane Database Syst Rev 2008;8:CD006700.

65. Kimberlin DW, Jacobs RF, Weller S, et al. Pharmacokinetics and safety of extemporaneously compounded valacyclovir oral suspension in pediatric patients from 1 month through 11 years of age. Clin Infect Dis 2010;50:221-8.

66. Cernik C, Gallina K, Brodell RT. The treatment of herpes simplex infections. An evidence-based review. Arch Intern Med 2008;168:1137-44.

67. Saez-Llorens X, Yogev R, Arguedas A, et al. Pharmacokinetics and safety of famciclovir in children with herpes simplex or varicella zoster virus infection. Antimicrob Agents Chemother 2009;53:1912-20.

68. Sacks SL, Thisted RA, Jones TM, et al. Clinical efficacy of topical docosanol 10% cream for herpes simplex labialis: A multicenter, randomized, placebo-controlled trial. J Am Acad Dermatol 2001; 45:222-30.

69. Arvin AM. Antiviral therapy for varicella and herpes zoster. Semin Pediatr Infect Dis 2002;13:12-21.

70. Dunkle LM, Arvin AM, Whitley RJ, et al. A controlled trial of acyclovir for chickenpox in normal children. N Engl J Med 1991;325:1539-44.

71. Dyer J. Childhood viral exanthems. Pediatr Ann 2007;36:21-9.

72. Biesbroeck L, Sidbury R. Viral exanthems: an update. Dermatol Ther 2013;26:433-8.

73. American Academy of Pediatrics. Enterovirus (nonpolio virus infections). In: Kimberlin DW, Brady MT, Jackson MA, et al., eds. Red Book: 2018 Report of the Committee on Infectious Diseases: American Academy of Pediatrics, 2018;332-5.

74. Shelley WB, Hashim M, Shelley ED. Acyclovir in the treatment of hand foot and mouth disease. Cutis 1996;57:232-4.

75. American Academy of Pediatrics. Parvovirus B19. In: Kimberlin DW, Brady MT, Jackson MA, et al., eds. Red Book: 2018 Report of the Committee on Infectious Diseases, American Academy of Pediatrics, 2018:602-5.

76. Koch WC. Fifth (human parvovirus) and sixth (herpesvirus 6) diseases. Curr Opin Infect Dis 2001;14:343-56.

77. American Academy of Pediatrics. Human herpes virus 6 (including roseola) and 7. In: Kimberlin DW, Brady MT, Jackson MA, et al., eds. Red Book: 2018 Report of the Committee on Infectious Diseases, American Academy of Pediatrics, 2018:454-7.

78. De Clercq E, Naesens L, De Bolle L, et al. Antiviral agents active against human herpes viruses HHV-6, HHV-7 and HHV-8. Rev Med Virol 2001;11:381-95.

79. Vinnard C, Barton T, Jerud E, et al. A report of human herpesvirus 6-associated encephalitis in a solid organ transplant recipient and a review of previously published cases. Liver Transpl 2009;15:1242-6.

80. Janoly-Duménil A, Galambrun C, Basset T, et al. Human herpes virus-6 encephalitis in a paediatric bone marrow recipient: successful treatment with pharmacokinetic monitoring and high doses of ganciclovir. Bone Marrow Transplant 2006;38:769-70.

81. American Academy of Pediatrics. Section 4. Antimicrobial Agents and Related Therapy. Tetracyclines. In: Kimberlin DW, Brady MT, Jackson MA, et al., eds. Red Book: 2018 Report of the Committee on Infectious Diseases, American Academy of Pediatrics, 2018:905-7.

CHAPTER 42

Bone and Joint Infections

Kalen Manasco, Pharm.D., FCCP, FPPA, BCPS

LEARNING OBJECTIVES

1. Describe the risk factors and mechanism of infection for bone and joint infections.

2. List the common etiologic organisms associated with osteomyelitis and infectious arthritis.

3. Distinguish between the clinical presentation and diagnosis of osteomyelitis and infectious arthritis.

4. Select appropriate antibiotic treatments for osteomyelitis and infectious arthritis.

5. Discuss monitoring guidelines in patients with osteomyelitis and infectious arthritis.

ABBREVIATIONS IN THIS CHAPTER

AUC/MIC	Area under the curve/minimum inhibitory concentration
CA-MRSA	Community-acquired methicillin-resistant *Staphylococcus aureus*
CRP	C-reactive protein
D-test	Double-disk diffusion
ESR	Erythrocyte sedimentation rate
MRI	Magnetic resonance imaging
MRSA	Methicillin-resistant *Staphylococcus aureus*
MSSA	Methicillin-susceptible *Staphylococcus aureus*
PVL	Panton-Valentine leukocidin
WBC	White blood cell

INTRODUCTION

Bone and joint infections are classified as *osteomyelitis* or *infectious arthritis (septic arthritis)*. These infections are usually associated with long treatment courses of antimicrobial agents and can lead to significant morbidity in some cases.[1] Bone and joint infections can affect patients of all ages, including children. The following sections will discuss osteomyelitis and infectious arthritis in detail.

OSTEOMYELITIS

DEFINITION

Osteomyelitis is defined as inflammation of the bone and/or bone marrow, usually accompanied by a microbial infection.[2,3] Although infection can occur with any bone throughout the body, the long bones are often affected in infants and children. Bacteria, fungi, and mycobacteria can cause infections. The infection in osteomyelitis is typically acute in origin, but all bone infections can progress to chronic osteomyelitis with a risk of necrosis of the bone.

EPIDEMIOLOGY AND CLASSIFICATION

The incidence of osteomyelitis has been reported as about 8 cases per 100,000 children per year.[4] It accounts for about 1% of all pediatric hospitalizations; 50% of the occurrences are in children younger than 5 years. Male children are more commonly affected than female children, with a ratio of about 2:1, respectively. Most infections involve one site, but up to 20% of children can present with multifocal osteomyelitis.[1,5] Neonatal osteomyelitis occurs in around 1 to 3 infants per 1000 neonatal intensive care admissions and is associated with a higher incidence of multifocal osteomyelitis compared with older children.[6]

The overall incidence of osteomyelitis has been decreasing during the past several decades.[7] However, the number of osteomyelitis cases is increasing because of resistant gram-positive organisms. In addition, more virulent strains of bacteria have emerged as causative organisms. In particular, Panton-Valentine leukocidin (PVL)-positive community-acquired methicillin-resistant *Staphylococcus aureus* (CA-MRSA) strains are of concern. Evidence has shown infections caused by these strains are associated with more severe disease and increased complications.[8]

Historically, osteomyelitis has been classified by symptom onset and duration. Patients were identified as having acute, subacute, or chronic osteomyelitis. Acute infections occur within 1–2 weeks of disease onset, subacute infections last for a few weeks but less than 1 month, and chronic infections last more than 1 month with the presence of bone necrosis.[9,10] Acute osteomyelitis accounts for 50% of infections and is more common in children.[1,9] Subacute and chronic osteomyelitis typically occur in adult patients.

WALDVOGEL CLASSIFICATION

In 1970, Waldvogel developed a classification system using both the pathogenesis and duration of the infection.[11-13] The Waldvogel system classifies osteomyelitis as hematogenous, contiguous, or chronic. *Hematogenous osteomyelitis* is spread through the bloodstream and is commonly seen in neonates, infants, and children. *Contiguous osteomyelitis* is spread through an adjacent soft tissue infection or by direct inoculation into the bone (e.g., trauma, puncture wounds, and surgery). Most contiguous infections in pediatric patients are associated with puncture wounds of the foot or patella.[9] Osteomyelitis of the foot after a puncture wound occurs in about 1.5% of cases.[14] *Chronic osteomyelitis* develops when the bone becomes necrotic because of the loss of blood supply. The disadvantage of the Waldvogel classification system is that it was not designed to guide surgical or antimicrobial therapy.

CIERNY-MADER STAGING SYSTEM

Cierny-Mader staging is another classification system for osteomyelitis that is based on anatomic location and physiologic status of the patient.[15] Initially established for adults, it can also be used to stage osteomyelitis in children. The staging, developed to allow guidance for treatment and/or surgical management, is particularly useful for infections involving long bones. There are four stages that describe the anatomic location and three host classifications (A, B, or C). *Stage 1* (*medullary*) is an infection entirely within the bone marrow from hematogenous spread. *Stage 2* (*superficial*) involves the surface of the bone, usually from a contiguous focus or direct inoculation. *Stage 3* (*localized*) involves both the surface of the bone and the bone marrow. *Stage 4* (*diffuse*) involves the entire thickness of the bone. The physiologic status is defined by the host's ability to mount an immune response (i.e., immunocompetent vs. immunocompromised). Patients are classified into the following categories: *healthy* (category A), *presence of local host compromise* (category BL), *presence of systemic host compromise* (category BS), *presence of both local and systemic compromise* (category BLS), and *presence of severe compromise that results in the treatment being worse than the disease* (category C). Systemic host factors include malnutrition, renal or hepatic failure, diabetes, and immunosuppression. The most common local host factors are venous stasis, major vessel compromise, arteritis, scarring, and neuropathy.

PATHOPHYSIOLOGY

Microorganisms can enter the bone through the bloodstream secondary to bacteremia, by direct inoculation (e.g., trauma, surgery), or from an adjacent soft tissue infection. Hematogenous spread to the bone occurs most commonly in pediatric patients because of the rich vascular supply and slow blood flow that is present in the metaphysis, particularly of long bones. The infecting organism initially affects the capillary loop near the epiphyseal growth plate to form a microabscess and localized inflammation. The organism then continues to travel through large venous sinusoids to areas of slow blood flow, where there is continued recruitment of inflammatory mediators, phagocytic cells, and toxins. Prostaglandins are produced in response to bone destruction and can decrease the amount of bacteria needed to cause infection.[2] Reactive bone formation occurs around the area of infection. The infection leads to edema and increased vascular permeability, which allows elevation of the periosteum. Eventually, the bacteria can enter the subperiosteal space and continue to form abscesses that become isolated from the blood supply within the bone. Once the blood supply is diminished, dead bone is formed, called *sequestra*. *Staphylococcus aureus* is of concern because it can express bacterial adhesion proteins, which promote attachment to the bone matrix (collagen, fibronectin, laminin) and cartilage.[16] In addition, *S. aureus* strains produce endotoxins capable of suppressing the local inflammatory response. If the infection spreads into the adjacent growth plate and epiphysis, joint damage and concomitant infectious arthritis can occur.

The most common cause of osteomyelitis in children is acute hematogenous osteomyelitis. Although the metaphysis of the long bones is most commonly affected, the bones of the hip, knee, and shoulder can also be involved, especially with a concomitant joint infection.[17] Osteomyelitis of the lower extremities has been reported in up to 72% of patients.[18] In neonatal osteomyelitis, there is a higher frequency of concomitant septic arthritis (up to 75% of cases), particularly in the hip, shoulder, and knee.[14] In children older than 1 month, adjacent infectious arthritis of the joint has been reported in up to 40% of patients.[19] Adjacent infectious arthritis of the joint is most common in patients younger than 18 months.

MICROORGANISMS

Typically only one infecting organism is involved in acute hematogenous osteomyelitis. The most common organism is *S. aureus*, which accounts for about 80% of cases. The percentage of infections caused by methicillin-resistant *S. aureus* (MRSA) strains varies greatly by region, but it may approach 50% in some areas.[1] Group A *Streptococcus* (*Streptococcus pyogenes*), *Streptococcus pneumoniae*, and *Kingella kingae* are also common causes in infants and children.[20-22] *Staphylococcus aureus*, *S. pyogenes*, and *S. pneumoniae* are gram-positive organisms found on the skin and in the oropharynx. *Kingella kingae* is a fastidious gram-negative coccobacillus that is part of the normal respiratory flora. *Haemophilus influenzae* type b is becoming rare because of universal childhood immunization against this pathogen. After age 4 years, the incidence of *H. influenzae* is dramatically decreased.[23] Table 1 and Table 2 list the most common organisms seen in osteomyelitis by patient age and clinical condition.[24-25]

Other organisms that less commonly cause osteomyelitis include *Mycobacterium* spp., *Bartonella henselae*, *Borrelia burgdorferi*, fungi (e.g., *Histoplasma*, *Cryptococcus*, *Blastomyces*, *Actinomyces*, *Coxiella*), *Pasteurella multocida*, and anaerobic

Table 1. Common Pathogens in Pediatric Osteomyelitis Based on Patient Age

Age	Organism
Neonate (< 1 mo)	*Staphylococcus aureus* Group B streptococci (*Streptococcus agalactiae*) Gram-negative enteric organisms (*Escherichia coli, Klebsiella oxytoca*) *Candida* spp.
1 mo to 5 yr	*Staphylococcus aureus* *Streptococcus pyogenes* *Streptococcus pneumoniae* *Kingella kingae*
> 5 yr	*Staphylococcus aureus* Streptococcus pyogenes

bacteria (e.g., *Bacteroides, Clostridium, Fusobacterium, Peptostreptococcus*).[26,27] In particular, *Mycobacterium, Bartonella*, and fungi are usually found in immunocompromised patients.

Contiguous osteomyelitis in children most often occurs after direct inoculation of bacteria from a traumatic wound. Anaerobic bacteria should be considered additional causative organisms in these cases. It is uncommon for children to develop osteomyelitis secondary to a contiguous infection. However, these cases usually involve a primary infection in the oromaxillary cavity (e.g., sinus, tooth, mastoid bone).[1]

The most common cause of chronic osteomyelitis in children is inadequate treatment of a hematogenous bone infection.[27] The presence of an orthopedic implant can also be associated with the development of chronic osteomyelitis.

RISK FACTORS

Risk factors for the development of hematogenous osteomyelitis include bacteremia, nonpenetrating trauma, and long-term, indwelling intravenous catheters. Pediatric patients are at increased risk of acute hematogenous osteomyelitis because the metaphyseal plate has a rich blood supply, and infectious spread from bacteremia is more likely. Additional risk factors specific for neonates include placement of an umbilical catheter and frequent heel stick blood draws. Risk factors for developing contiguous osteomyelitis include penetrating trauma, animal bites, puncture wounds, and adjacent soft tissue infections. Patients who are immunocompromised or have sickle cell disease are at higher risk of developing osteomyelitis caused by *Salmonella*.

CLINICAL PRESENTATION AND DIAGNOSIS

SIGNS AND SYMPTOMS

The clinical presentation usually involves local inflammation, pain and swelling, and systemic symptoms such as fever, irritability, and lethargy. Clinical presentation also depends on the origin of the infection and can vary with age. Pseudoparalysis is the cardinal sign in neonates and young children, although irritability is the most common symptom in this age group.[28] Pseudoparalysis occurs when the infant appears unable to move the affected arm or leg but has no true

Table 2. Common Pathogens in Pediatric Osteomyelitis Based on Comorbid Conditions[24,25]

Organism	Clinical Condition
Salmonella[24]	Sickle cell disease
Staphylococcus epidermidis	Foreign body
Pseudomonas aeruginosa[25]	Puncture wounds to feet Immunocompromised
Bartonella henselae	Human immunodeficiency virus Kitten exposure
Fungi	Immunocompromised
Anaerobic bacteria	Dental abscess
Pasteurella multocida	Human or animal bite

paralysis. In older children, the pain is usually more localized, and a common presentation is refusal to bear weight or presence of a limp. Fever is usually absent in most children with a diagnosis of osteomyelitis. Infections caused by *K. kingae* are usually preceded by an upper respiratory tract infection.

Clinically, patients with a PVL-positive strain of CA-MRSA present differently from those without the presence of PVL. Typical clinical manifestations associated with a PVL-positive strain include several infection sites, myositis, subperiosteal abscess, and severe life-threatening co-infections.[29] In addition, chronic osteomyelitis is more likely to be diagnosed on admission or to develop in patients with PVL-positive isolates compared with patients having PVL-negative strains.[30]

DIAGNOSTIC CRITERIA

Diagnosis of osteomyelitis is based on clinical presentation, presence of certain laboratory markers, and imaging studies to detect infection in the bone. Laboratory data indicative of osteomyelitis include an elevated white blood cell (WBC) count; increased procalcitonin; increased inflammatory markers, such as erythrocyte sedimentation rate (ESR) and C-reactive protein (CRP); presence of bacteria from a blood culture or biopsy of the bone of adjacent infected soft tissue; and abnormal physical examination, such as pain or tenderness. Blood cultures are only positive in about 50% of cases; thus, the presence of a negative blood culture cannot rule out osteomyelitis.[31] Polymerase chain reaction analyses have been useful in detecting *K. kingae* because it is difficult to culture using standard laboratory methods.[32]

The CRP, a nonspecific, acute inflammatory marker, is useful early in the disease process. It typically peaks a few days after an acute infection and normalizes once treatment has begun. A normal CRP value is less than 3.0 mg/L, but reference ranges can vary by laboratory. Values greater than 10.0 mg/L are considered indicative of infection or inflammation. The ESR is a marker of chronic inflammation and can be used to guide long-term treatment and disease management. Normal ESR values in pediatric patients are 3–20 mm/hour. Values greater than 60 mm/hour are associated with inflammation. The CRP better predicts recovery than WBC or ESR and is used more widely than ESR to trend during an acute bone or joint infection.[33] A normal WBC and CRP do not exclude a diagnosis of osteomyelitis. Patients with osteomyelitis caused by PVL-producing *S. aureus* have been found to have a higher mean ESR, CRP, and absolute neutrophil count compared with patients who do not have a PVL-producing strain.[34]

Procalcitonin is an acute phase reactant found be a useful biomarker for bacterial infections, particularly sepsis. In the past decade, studies have confirmed its usefulness as a diagnostic marker in osteomyelitis and septic arthritis.[35] A normal serum concentration is < 0.05 ng/mL. Concentrations are detectable within 4 hours and can peak within 6–24 hours, which is earlier than either CRP (rises within 12–24 hours and peaks in 2–3 days) or ESR (rises within 1–2 days and decreases slowly to normal values over time). The procalcitonin test is more expensive than a CRP and therefore used less often in the diagnosis of bone and joint infections.

If a biopsy of the infected bone is performed, histopathologic and microbiologic examinations of the bone are helpful diagnostic tools. The procedure is usually performed with guided computed tomography or ultrasonography. The presence of bacteria from a bone biopsy is diagnostic for osteomyelitis.

IMAGING PROCEDURES

Imaging studies are helpful in diagnosing osteomyelitis. Common studies include standard radiography, radionuclide imaging or scintigraphy, magnetic resonance imaging (MRI), computed tomography scan, and positron emission tomography. Standard radiographs can detect soft tissue swelling but are usually normal during the first 2–3 weeks of the infection (Figure 1). Standard radiographs are useful in detecting fractures or malignancies and thus in ruling out osteomyelitis. Radionuclide imaging (i.e., bone scan) is performed with an intravenous radiopharmaceutical (e.g., technetium-99m) administration. Radiography will show increased uptake of the technetium-99m in areas with inflammation. The

sensitivity of radionuclide imaging is between 80% and 100%, but the specificity is low because it cannot distinguish infection from trauma or malignancy.[1] This test is most useful when the exact infection site cannot be determined or when multifocal sites are suspected.

Magnetic resonance imaging has the best results for imaging, with 97% sensitivity and 92% specificity.[35,36] In fact, MRI is preferred to scintigraphy because of its ability to detect extraosseous complications such as subperiosteal abscesses, septic arthritis, and deep venous thrombosis (Figure 2).[37] Disadvantages of MRI compared with scintigraphy include high cost, inability to distinguish postsurgical inflammation from osteomyelitis, and the need for patient sedation. Computed tomography scans can also be performed to visualize bony structures, but they are less specific than MRI studies. Positron emission tomography is an imaging study that uses a nonspecific tracer that accumulates at infection or inflammation sites. In the management of osteomyelitis, positron emission tomography is useful in diagnosing chronic osteomyelitis and as a follow-up study to assess response to therapy.[38]

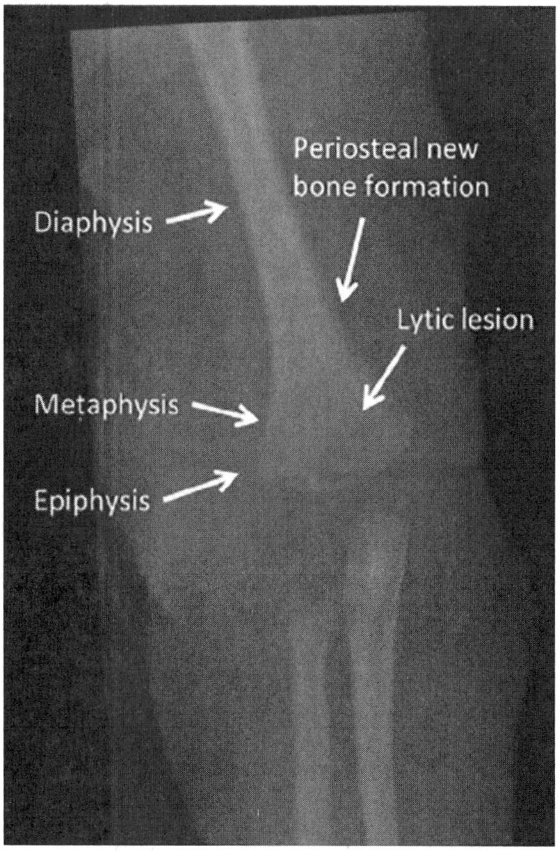

Figure 1. Radiographic image depicting long-bone regions (left labels) and bony changes (right labels) caused by *Staphylococcus aureus* osteomyelitis occurring in the distal right humerus of a 12-month-old infant.[17]

Reproduced with permission from Conrad DA. Acute hematogenous osteomyelitis. Pediatr Rev 2010;31:467. Copyright 2011 by the American Academy of Pediatrics.

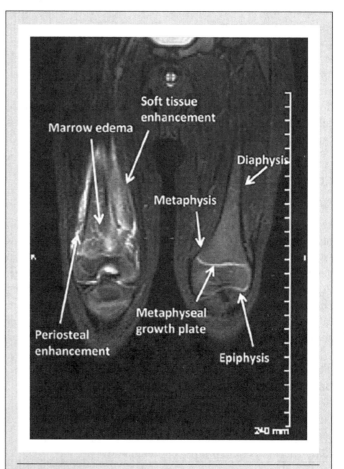

Figure 2. Magnetic resonance image depicting long-bone regions (left femur) and extensive marrow edema and significant enhancement of the periosteum and adjacent soft tissues (right femur) caused by *Staphylococcus aureus* osteomyelitis occurring in the distal right femur of a 26-month-old infant.[17]

Reproduced with permission from Conrad DA. Acute hematogenous osteomyelitis. Pediatr Rev 2010;31:467. Copyright 2011 by the American Academy of Pediatrics.

COURSE AND PROGNOSIS

Acute hematogenous osteomyelitis is associated with a favorable prognosis once bacteremia has cleared. Recurrence is reported in up to 5% of cases overall and in up to 50% of neonatal cases.[1] Relapse has been reported in 30% to 60% of children who did not have abscess drainage, if present, despite adequate antimicrobial therapy.[39] In one study, monitoring serial CRP values was helpful in identifying patients who might have a complicated course as well as in predicting outcomes.[40] If CRP values remained high on day 3 of treatment, the patient was more likely to have a complicated clinical course (determined at a follow-up visit 1–2 months after discharge). However, if CRP values fell to normal concentrations by day 5, patients were more likely to be asymptomatic at follow-up.

Complications of osteomyelitis include persistent bacteremia, subperiosteal abscesses, deep venous thromboembolism, and progression to chronic osteomyelitis.[36] Furthermore, permanent abnormalities of bone growth are possible. Chronic osteomyelitis, which may persist for several months, is usually managed with a combination of prolonged courses of antimicrobial therapy and surgical management. The prognosis of contiguous osteomyelitis depends on early diagnosis and aggressive therapy to avoid progression to chronic osteomyelitis.

TREATMENT

GOALS OF THERAPY

The goals of antimicrobial therapy are eradication of the organism, resolution of infection, and prevention of long-term sequelae. Because clinical practice guidelines for the management of osteomyelitis do not presently exist, the infection is best managed with a multidisciplinary team of clinicians. Recommendations for the diagnosis and treatment of pediatric osteomyelitis are based on expert opinion, case series, and small clinical trials. Early initiation of appropriate empiric antimicrobial therapy is crucial to prevent complications from osteomyelitis. Table 3 and Table 4 list treatment options and dosing information for specific organisms associated with

Table 3. Directed Antibiotic Therapy for Management of Bone and Joint Infections

Microorganism	Preferred Therapy	Alternative Therapies
MSSA	Nafcillin or oxacillin	Cefazolin Oral alternatives: dicloxacillin or cephalexin
MRSA	Vancomycin	Linezolid or daptomycin
CA-MRSA	Vancomycin or clindamycin	Linezolid or daptomycin
Streptococcus agalactiae	Penicillin G or ampicillin	Ceftriaxone
Staphylococcus epidermidis	Vancomycin	Daptomycin
Streptococcus pyogenes	Penicillin G	Clindamycin
Streptococcus pneumonia Penicillin-sensitive (MIC < 0.1 mg/L)	Penicillin G	Ceftriaxone
Streptococcus pneumonia Penicillin-intermediate (MIC 0.1–1 mg/L)	Ceftriaxone	Fluoroquinolone, clindamycin
Streptococcus pneumonia Penicillin-resistant MIC ≥ 2 mg/L)	Vancomycin	Linezolid
Kingella kingae	Cefuroxime or ceftriaxone	Penicillin, ampicillin, macrolide, fluoroquinolone
Salmonella spp.	Ampicillin (if susceptible) If ampicillin resistant: ceftriaxone	Ciprofloxacin
Pseudomonas aeruginosa or *Serratia marcescens*	Cefepime or piperacillin/tazobactam AND Gentamicin	Ceftazidime or meropenem AND Gentamicin
Escherichia coli	Ceftriaxone	Meropenem
Pasteurella multocida	Penicillin G or ampicillin	Doxycycline Ampicillin/sulbactam
Bacteroides fragilis	Clindamycin	Metronidazole Ampicillin/sulbactam Ticarcillin/clavulanate
Neisseria gonorrhoeae	Ceftriaxone	Amoxicillin or doxycycline
Bartonella henselae	Azithromycin	Doxycycline

CA-MRSA= community-acquired methicillin-resistant *Staphylococcus aureus;* MIC = minimum inhibitory concentration; MRSA = methicillin-resistant *Staphylococcus aureus;* MSSA = methicillin-susceptible *Staphylococcus aureus.*

osteomyelitis.[1,16,40,41] Important considerations when selecting an antibiotic for presumed osteomyelitis include infection type, etiologic organisms, availability of culture and sensitivity results, host factors, and antibiotic characteristics. The key antibiotic characteristics to consider include local resistance patterns, penetration into the bone, and potential for systemic toxicities.

PHARMACOLOGIC THERAPY

Specific considerations are necessary for both empiric and bacteria-specific treatment. Currently, there is no consensus on the appropriate duration of intravenous therapy or total duration of therapy for osteomyelitis. Clinicians must select treatment duration on the basis of clinical presentation, risk factors, infection site, and patient age. Therapy duration for acute osteomyelitis is typically 4–6 weeks. Chronic osteomyelitis requires treatment with both surgical and medical intervention. Patients may require antimicrobial therapy for up to 6–12 months.

Initial therapy typically includes intravenous antibiotics, which may be used for up to 2 weeks before switching to oral therapy. Recent evidence has shown that an earlier transition from intravenous to oral therapy results in clinical outcomes

Table 4. Antimicrobial Dosing for Specific Organisms in Osteomyelitis[1,16,40,41]

Agent	Neonates ≤ 7 days	Neonates > 7 days	Infants and Children	Comments
Ampicillin	75–150 mg/kg/day divided Q 8 hr	100–200 mg/kg/day divided Q 6 hr	150–200 mg/kg/day divided Q 6–8 hr	Max single dose 2000 mg
Cefazolin	40 mg/kg/day divided Q 12 hr	60 mg/kg/day divided Q 8 hr	100 mg/kg/day divided Q 6–8 hr	Max single dose 2000 mg
Cefepime	100 mg/kg/day divided Q 12 hr	100 mg/kg/day divided Q 12 hr	150 mg/kg/day divided Q 8 hr	Max single dose 2000 mg
Ceftazidime	100-150 mg/kg/day divided Q 8–12 hr	150 mg/kg/day divided Q 8 hr	150 mg/kg/day divided Q 8 hr	Max single dose 2000 mg Potential to induce β-lactamase production
Ceftriaxone	—	—	50 mg/kg/day Q 24 hr	Max single dose 2000 mg Avoid use in first 28 days of life
Cephalexin	—	—	100 mg/kg/day divided Q 6–8 hr	Max single dose 1000 mg
Ciprofloxacin	—	—	20–30 mg/kg/day divided Q 12 hr	—
Clindamycin	15 mg/kg/day divided Q 8 hr	20–30 mg/kg/day divided Q 6–8 hr	IV 40 mg/kg/day divided Q 6–8 hr Oral 30 mg/kg/day divided Q 8 hr	Only for cultures with negative D-test Max oral dose: 40 mg/kg/day or 600 mg Q 8 hr
Daptomycin	—	—	6–10 mg/kg/day	—
Dicloxacillin	—	—	100 mg/kg/day divided Q 6 hr	—
Doxycycline	—	—	2–4 mg/kg/day	Only for use in age > 8 yr
Gentamicin	5 mg/kg/day divided Q 12 hr	5–7.5 mg/kg/day divided Q 8 hr	7.5 mg/kg/day divided Q 8 hr	Monitor peak and trough concentrations
Linezolid	10 mg/kg/dose Q 12 hr	10 mg/kg/dose Q 8 hr	10 mg/kg/dose Q 8 hr	Max dose 600 mg twice daily
Meropenem	40 mg/kg/day divided Q 12 hr	60 mg/kg/day divided Q 8 hr	60 mg/kg/day divided Q 8 hr	Max single dose 2000 mg
Nafcillin	75 mg/kg/day divided Q 8 hr	100–150 mg/kg/day divided Q 6 hr	150–200 mg/kg/day divided Q 6 hr	Max daily dose 12 g
Oxacillin	150 mg/kg/day divided Q 8 hr	200 mg/kg/day divided Q 6 hr	200 mg/kg/day divided Q 6 hr	Max daily dose 12 g
Penicillin G	75,000 units/kg/day divided Q 8 hr	200,000 units/kg/day divided Q 6 hr	250,000–400,000 units/kg/day divided Q 4–6 hr	Max daily dose 24 million units
Vancomycin	15 mg/kg/dose Q 12 hr	45–60 mg/kg/day divided Q 6–8 hr	60 mg/kg/day divided Q 6 hr	Target trough concentration: 10–15 mg/L OR 15-20 mg/L in severe disease

D-test = double-disk diffusion; IV = intravenous; max = maximum; Q = every.

and treatment failures similar to those in prolonged intravenous therapy.[42-44] A recent systematic review of 15 studies (including almost 3600 patients) found that patients receiving shorts courses of intravenous therapy (2–3 weeks) followed by oral therapy had similar rates of treatment failure compared with patients receiving greater than 4 weeks of intravenous therapy (odds ratio 1.50; 95% confidence interval 0.97–2.34).[42] A study of 29 pediatric patients who were treated for acute osteomyelitis with a median of 4 days of intravenous therapy followed by 28 days of oral therapy showed no complications or treatment failures at the 6-month follow-up.[43] Another study of 131 pediatric patients with culture-positive acute hematogenous osteomyelitis showed a favorable outcome in patients who received 2–4 days of intravenous therapy followed by oral therapy for 20–30 days.[44] Furthermore, patients with prolonged home intravenous therapy are more likely to develop central venous catheter–associated complications (e.g., thrombosis, infection).[45]

Although there is no clear consensus on when to change from intravenous to oral therapy, most experts recommend a transition to oral therapy on the basis of clinical markers rather than number of days of intravenous therapy. When patients show normalizing temperature, improving physical examination, and decreasing inflammatory markers (ESR and CRP), they can be transitioned to oral therapy.

Empiric antimicrobial therapy. Because the most common cause of osteomyelitis is *S. aureus*, initial empiric therapy should be targeted against this organism. Monotherapy with an antistaphylococcal agent is appropriate for patients older than 5 years with no additional risk factors (e.g., immunocompromised, sickle cell disease). For patients at risk of other organisms (e.g., *Salmonella*, *Kingella*, or *Pseudomonas*) in addition to *S. aureus*, broad-spectrum antimicrobial therapy should be initiated with an antistaphylococcal agent plus a third-generation cephalosporin.

Intravenous penicillinase-resistant penicillins (e.g., nafcillin, oxacillin) or a first-generation cephalosporin (e.g., cefazolin) has historically been considered a first-line empiric agent because of its bactericidal activity against methicillin-susceptible *S. aureus* (MSSA). However, with an increasing prevalence of CA-MRSA, it is recommended to use vancomycin (60 mg/kg/day) or clindamycin (40 mg/kg/day), both intravenously, as first-line empiric therapy until culture and sensitivity results are available.[36] In addition, these two agents provide coverage against *S. pyogenes* and *S. pneumoniae*. According to the latest Infectious Diseases Society of America guidelines for the management of MRSA infections, clindamycin should only be used empirically if local resistance patterns are low (usually defined as less than 10%) and there is no evidence of bacteremia.[36] Otherwise, vancomycin is preferred. In patients with a severe clinical presentation, the addition of rifampin or gentamicin to vancomycin may also be considered.[46] Furthermore, vancomycin should be used as empiric therapy when other resistant gram-positive organisms (e.g., coagulase-negative staphylococci) are suspected.

Empiric therapy for neonates should cover both *S. aureus* and *Escherichia coli*. Therapy should be initiated with nafcillin or oxacillin plus gentamicin. A first-generation cephalosporin (e.g., cefazolin) or clindamycin can also be considered in place of nafcillin or oxacillin for neonates. Patients with sickle cell disease should receive a third-generation cephalosporin (e.g., ceftriaxone) for coverage against *Salmonella* spp. Empiric coverage against *K. kingae* is unnecessary in most patients unless there is a high clinical suspicion, such as in patients 5 years and younger who present after an upper respiratory tract infection. Figure 3 describes the empiric management of osteomyelitis in pediatric patients.

Definitive antimicrobial therapy. Once culture results and sensitivities are available, treatment should be directed

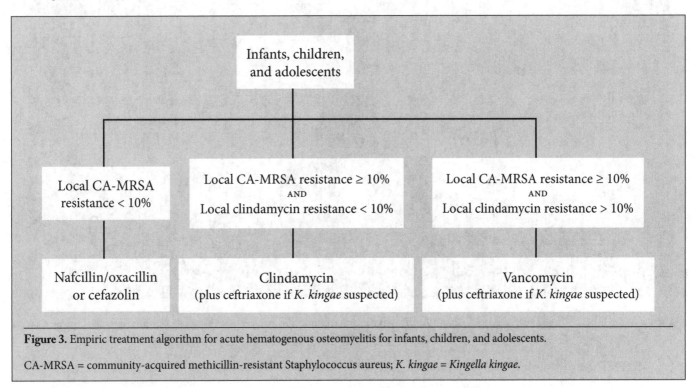

Figure 3. Empiric treatment algorithm for acute hematogenous osteomyelitis for infants, children, and adolescents.

CA-MRSA = community-acquired methicillin-resistant Staphylococcus aureus; *K. kingae* = Kingella kingae.

to provide coverage against the specific organism isolated. If no organisms are identified, then empiric coverage should be continued if the patient is improving. For patients who do not improve and have negative cultures, alternative or additional therapies and evaluation should be considered.

Gram-positive organisms. Vancomycin is the treatment of choice for MRSA osteomyelitis, especially for strains that are not susceptible to clindamycin and in critically ill patients. However, dosing vancomycin at 40 mg/kg/day is inadequate to achieve the pharmacokinetic and pharmacodynamic targets recently proposed for adults. An area under the curve/minimum inhibitory concentration (AUC/MIC) ratio of 400 or more in adults with MRSA bacteremia or pneumonia correlates to positive treatment outcomes.[36] Trough levels of 15–20 mg/L are recommended for invasive MRSA infections in adults, including osteomyelitis, because they correlate to an AUC/MIC ratio of 400 or more, increase tissue penetration, and minimize the selection of resistant strains of MRSA.[36] Doses of at least 60 mg/kg/day should be initiated in children to attain these trough targets, particularly in severe cases (e.g., with concurrent bacteremia), even though data are limited on the efficacy and safety of these serum concentrations in children.[39,47] It is important to achieve adequate vancomycin serum concentrations early in therapy to ensure a faster transition to oral therapy.[48] Recent evidence also suggests obtaining and monitoring AUC/MIC values for vancomycin.[49]

Clindamycin is an attractive option for CA-MRSA osteomyelitis because of its high bone concentrations; its efficacy, which is close to 100% (in the absence of inducible resistance); and its availability in both intravenous and oral preparations.[50-53] Clindamycin also has good activity against toxin-producing gram-positive organisms. The double-disk diffusion (D-test) is an important molecular test for the confirmation of inducible-resistant CA-MRSA strains (Figure 4).[54] This test identifies inducible clindamycin resistance among strains that initially show susceptibility to clindamycin, which is a lincosamide antibiotic similar to the macrolide class of antibiotics. The practitioner should be aware of the potential for inducible resistance when an MRSA isolate shows clindamycin susceptibility and erythromycin resistance. The D-test is performed by creating a bacterial lawn on an agar plate and placing a clindamycin and erythromycin disk 15 mm apart on the plate. If there is a uniform zone of inhibition around the clindamycin disk, then the test is negative (i.e., no inducible resistance). If there is blunting of the zone of inhibition on the side closest to the erythromycin disk that produced a D shape, then the test is positive (i.e., inducible resistance). For a positive D-test, the potential for treatment failure is increased, and clindamycin therapy should not be used. In an era of increasingly resistant gram-positive organisms, including vancomycin-intermediate and vancomycin-resistant

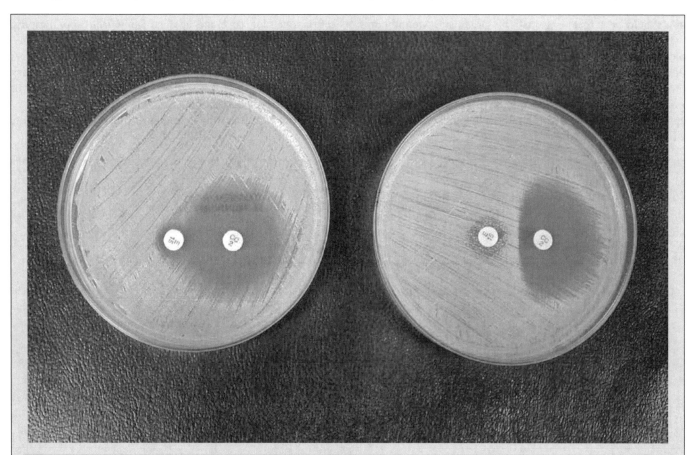

Figure 4. The D-test. A negative D-test is shown on the left, and a positive D-test is shown on the right. The erythromycin disk is located on the left of each agar plate, and the clindamycin disk is located on the right.

CC = clindamycin; D-test = double-disk diffusion; E = erythromycin. Photo courtesy of Julie Hixson-Wallace, Harding University, Arkansas.

staphylococci, clinical evidence is limited for the use of daptomycin and linezolid in pediatric osteomyelitis. These agents are not typically used for empiric therapy. Once culture results are known, they should be considered alternative therapy for MRSA osteomyelitis in patients who cannot receive vancomycin or clindamycin.[36]

Daptomycin is a lipopeptide antibiotic with bactericidal activity against sensitive and resistant gram-positive organisms. It is an option for osteomyelitis treatment as a parenteral alternative to vancomycin.[36] Evidence in children is limited; however, it has been found to be about 90% effective in adults for the treatment of osteomyelitis.[55,56] Daptomycin may have a role in the management of chronic osteomyelitis because of its ability to penetrate biofilm.[27] Daptomycin should not be used in the setting of osteomyelitis with concomitant pneumonia because it is inactivated by alveolar surfactants. Daptomycin is only available as an intravenous injection, but can be dosed once daily and may be a good choice for patients on prolonged courses of intravenous therapy as an alternative to vancomycin. It also has the advantage of no therapeutic drug monitoring and less incidence of acute kidney injury compared with vancomycin.

Linezolid is an oxazolidinone antibiotic with activity against MRSA and other resistant gram-positive organisms. Linezolid achieves high bone concentrations and inhibits toxins produced by gram-positive bacteria.[57,58] Linezolid is approved for use in pediatric patients, including neonates, and is available in intravenous and oral formulations with around 100% oral bioavailability. Therefore, transitioning patients to oral therapy can be considered early in the treatment course. Linezolid was reported to be effective (85% complete recovery) and safe for pediatric patients with osteomyelitis in a case series and one large clinical trial.[59,60] It is associated with a higher cost than some of the other oral alternatives.

If MSSA is identified, patients who were empirically initiated on vancomycin or clindamycin should change to a penicillinase-resistant penicillin or cefazolin. The bactericidal activity against MSSA is greater with the penicillinase-resistant penicillins than with vancomycin.[61] Cefazolin can be administered less often (every 8 hours) than either nafcillin or oxacillin (every 6 hours), which can be advantageous for outpatient use. In addition, there is a potential for thrombophlebitis with intravenous nafcillin administration. In patients with a serious hypersensitivity reaction to penicillin and a positive MSSA culture, clindamycin is the treatment of choice. Penicillin, clindamycin, or vancomycin may be used, depending on patient characteristics and microbial sensitivities to these agents, for the treatment of streptococcal species (e.g., *S. pyogenes* and *S. pneumoniae*).

Gram-negative organisms. *Kingella kingae*, if identified, can be treated with a β-lactam antibiotic such as a second- or third-generation cephalosporin. Alternative agents include penicillin, ampicillin, macrolides, or ciprofloxacin. Clindamycin should not be used if the organism is inherently resistant. If *E. coli* is identified as the cause of osteomyelitis, therapy should be guided by the susceptibility results, with the empiric agent continued if clinical improvement has been documented and the bacterial strain is susceptible. A complete list of bacteria-specific therapy is provided in Table 3.

First-line treatment of *Salmonella* is ampicillin if the organism is susceptible. For resistant strains, a third-generation cephalosporin (e.g., ceftriaxone) should be used. Fluoroquinolones (e.g., ciprofloxacin) are an alternative in patients with *Salmonella* osteomyelitis but are usually reserved for patients allergic to β-lactam antibiotics and as oral step-down therapy.

Pseudomonas aeruginosa is not a common organism in pediatric osteomyelitis, but if identified, therapy should include an antipseudomonal cephalosporin (e.g., ceftazidime, cefepime), antipseudomonal penicillin (e.g., piperacillin/tazobactam), or carbapenem (e.g., meropenem). Combination therapy with an antipseudomonal penicillin, carbapenem, or cephalosporin and an aminoglycoside may be considered in severe cases or with multidrug-resistant strains. The current American Academy of Pediatrics guidelines on the use of systemic fluoroquinolones in pediatric patients state that these agents can be used for definitive cases of acute or chronic osteomyelitis caused by *P. aeruginosa*.[62]

For an anaerobic infection, therapy can be continued with clindamycin if it was initiated as an empiric agent. Metronidazole, ampicillin/sulbactam, and ticarcillin/clavulanate are alternative agents with anaerobic activity.

Role of oral antimicrobial therapy. Oral antibiotics play a very important role in the medical management of pediatric patients with osteomyelitis. Oral therapy is usually initiated after adequate treatment of intravenous therapy, depending on the severity of the infection and the clinical response of the patient. Patients with osteomyelitis with no complications can be switched to oral therapy after they are afebrile for at least 48 hours; have decreased pain, swelling, and/or erythema; WBC normalization; and decrease in CRP. Although no specific duration of parenteral therapy is currently recommended, patients typically will be able to switch between 5–10 days after initiation.[63-64] Oral antibiotics can also be used as first-line agents in mild infections, but this choice is less common. Important considerations when initiating oral antibiotic therapy for the treatment of osteomyelitis in children include palatability, cost, availability of appropriate dosage forms, and ease of administration.[48] All of these characteristics are crucial in ensuring medication adherence for the treatment duration. Patient-specific factors to consider when initiating oral therapy are age 1 month or older, fully immunized for age, and ability to be adherent to the medication administration. Oral medications are typically initiated in the inpatient setting to demonstrate tolerability and adherence.

The most commonly used oral antibiotics in pediatric patients with osteomyelitis include clindamycin, linezolid, cephalexin, and dicloxacillin. Trimethoprim/sulfamethoxazole, doxycycline, or minocycline—alone or in combination with rifampin—and fluoroquinolones may also be considered, although data are limited. Trimethoprim/sulfamethoxazole has excellent activity against CA-MRSA and good oral palatability. Because of the risk of dental staining in younger children, tetracyclines can be used for CA-MRSA infections in patients after age 8 years. Table 3 lists oral alternatives for the most common intravenous therapies. Both clindamycin and linezolid have excellent oral bioavailability but poor palatability.[63] Oral β-lactam antibiotics must be given at high doses to achieve adequate bone penetration. Dosing is typically 2–3 times higher than recommended for other infections.

Outpatient parenteral antimicrobial therapy. Although sequential intravenous therapy to oral therapy is the preferred treatment of osteomyelitis, intravenous therapy must sometimes be continued for an extended period. Candidates for home parenteral therapy include the following: neonates; patients with infections caused by organisms for which no oral alternative exists; patients who cannot tolerate oral therapy; patients with chronic osteomyelitis; immunocompromised patients; patients with sickle cell anemia who have poor blood flow to the local area of infection; and patients in whom poor adherence to oral therapy is suspected.[64] In these cases, patients must have an indwelling central venous catheter inserted to continue intravenous therapy as an outpatient. Coordination for home parenteral therapy requires an interprofessional approach using the physician, pharmacist, nurse, and caregiver. Educating the caregiver is essential to preventing possible complications from home intravenous therapy, including catheter-related bacteremia and line malfunction.

Outpatient parenteral antimicrobial therapy for osteomyelitis can decrease health care costs associated with this infection by reducing the number of hospital days and possible exposure to additional hospital pathogens. However, this approach may affect patient and family quality of life because it may be associated with increased cost to the family and considerably affect the child's ability to attend school or perform daily activities. Both the benefits and possible risks and disadvantages need to be considered when selecting patients for outpatient parenteral therapy.

Localized antibiotic therapy. Localized antibiotic delivery directly to the infected bone provides the advantage of high local concentrations of the antibiotic with limited systemic toxicity. Cement beads made of polymethyl methacrylate are impregnated with antibiotics to allow drug release over several weeks to months.[65] These beads must be surgically placed at initiation and removed on therapy completion. Antibiotic-impregnated cement beads can be used in patients with difficult-to-treat infections and those with chronic osteomyelitis. They can be used in combination with systemic antibiotics or as an alternative. Antibiotics that have been used in this capacity include gentamicin, vancomycin, penicillins, and cephalosporins. In vitro evidence supports the use of daptomycin in polymethyl methacrylate beads and in calcium sulfate, which is another localized delivery matrix.[66]

NONPHARMACOLOGIC THERAPY

Nonpharmacologic therapy includes surgical debridement and the use of hyperbaric oxygen. Surgical debridement of the infected bone and drainage of adjacent soft tissue abscesses is a first-line treatment in addition to appropriate empiric antimicrobial therapy. Surgical drainage allows direct examination of the infected area, and, if debridement of bone occurs, direct histopathologic examination of the bone. This approach can help guide decisions about appropriate antimicrobial therapy. Some patients with CA-MRSA may require several incision and drainage procedures during the course of therapy.

Hyperbaric oxygen therapy. Hyperbaric oxygen therapy is used as an adjunctive treatment to surgery and antibiotics in patients with chronic osteomyelitis that is refractory to standard therapy. The procedure requires placement of the patient in an enclosed chamber where oxygen pressure is greater than sea level. The increased oxygen pressure enhances oxygen delivery to the infection site, leading to the formation of new capillaries, increased transport of antibiotics to the infected area, formation of a collagen matrix, suppression of anaerobic bacteria, and increased ability of phagocytes to target bacteria.[67] Disadvantages of this treatment approach include limited clinical experience in pediatric patients, increased cost, and adverse effects, such as barotraumas and reversible myopia.

MONITORING GUIDELINES

Because patients with osteomyelitis will require prolonged antibiotic therapy, it is very important that they be closely monitored throughout the treatment. Once the initial antimicrobial therapy is started, improvements in clinical signs and symptoms should occur within 48–72 hours. Patients should be monitored for clinical and laboratory response to therapy, especially when no organism is identified and for the presence of adverse drug reactions and adherence to outpatient therapy. Laboratory variables important for monitoring therapeutic response include culture and sensitivity results, improvement in markers of inflammation (e.g., CRP, ESR), and decrease in WBC. In patients with positive blood cultures, repeat cultures should be obtained to ensure eradication of the bacteremia. Patients receiving outpatient therapy should be monitored weekly for normalization of CRP and to ensure no toxicity is associated with the treatment. After 4–6 weeks of appropriate antimicrobial therapy, success can be defined by the resolution of clinical signs and symptoms and normalization of all laboratory tests.

Common adverse reactions in patients receiving β-lactam antibiotics include diarrhea and gastrointestinal upset. Patients receiving β-lactam antibiotics should be monitored closely for the development of a rash or other allergic reaction (e.g., urticaria). Clindamycin causes gastrointestinal upset, diarrhea (that may develop into pseudomembranous colitis), and nausea. Patients and their caregivers should be counseled on contacting their provider if diarrhea becomes severe or if bloody stools develop. Renal function should be monitored weekly in patients receiving vancomycin, and patients should be monitored for the development of red man syndrome on initiation of therapy. If red man syndrome occurs, then the infusion can be extended for a longer period (2 hours vs. 1 hour), and diphenhydramine can be administered before the infusion. Creatinine phosphokinase values should be monitored routinely in patients receiving daptomycin because rhabdomyolysis is associated with increased drug serum concentrations. Caution is advised with the use of linezolid for more than 2 weeks because of treatment duration–related adverse effects (e.g., thrombocytopenia, peripheral neuropathies, optic neuritis).[36,68] It is recommended to obtain weekly complete blood cell counts in patients receiving linezolid longer than 2 weeks and an ophthalmologic evaluation if therapy is continued for greater than 4 weeks. However, some data suggest that the hematologic effects of linezolid occur less often in children than in adults, especially in the first 2 weeks of therapy.[69]

INFECTIOUS ARTHRITIS

Infectious arthritis, commonly referred to as *pyogenic arthritis* or *septic arthritis*, is defined as an infection of the joint. It is much more common in pediatric patients than osteomyelitis. The infection usually begins in a monoarticular joint with inflammation of the joint space, synovium, synovial fluid, and surrounding cartilage. Prompt diagnosis and treatment is crucial in any patient with suspected infectious arthritis to prevent joint damage or spread of the infection to surrounding tissue or bone. In rare cases, if left untreated, the disease can be fatal. Many of the concepts previously introduced for osteomyelitis—the most common organisms and the treatments—also apply to infectious arthritis.

EPIDEMIOLOGY

The incidence of infectious arthritis is between 5 and 12 cases per 100,000 children; however, the incidence varies by age.[70] Children younger than 3 years and adolescents have the highest incidence.[1] Male children are affected twice as often as female children, perhaps because male children have more traumatic injuries during childhood. Infectious arthritis in children is almost exclusively from hematogenous spread and typically involves only one joint. The most common sites of infectious arthritis are the hip and knee, followed by the ankle.[70] The hip is most commonly affected in neonates and infants. Infections of the upper extremities are less common, with the elbow and shoulder being reported in less than 10% of cases.[71]

Although most cases of infectious arthritis are acute in nature, both chronic monoarticular arthritis and polyarticular arthritis can also occur. Mycobacteria, *B. burgdorferi*, and fungi typically present as chronic monoarticular arthritis. Polyarticular arthritis is most common after a viral infection.

PATHOPHYSIOLOGY

Infectious arthritis occurs secondarily to hematogenous seeding of an organism within the joint space. The synovial membrane is infected first. Edema and hypertrophy in the adjacent joint space lead to accumulation of exudative fluid in the synovium. Neutrophils, cytokines, and proteolytic enzymes are then recruited to the infection site. Pus accumulates in the joint space and leads to destruction of cartilage. Children younger than 18 months can develop infectious arthritis secondary to a bone infection because of the presence of transphyseal blood vessels that extend from the metaphysis to the epiphysis and growth plate.[1]

MICROORGANISMS

Bacteria are the most common cause of infectious arthritis, whereas fungi and mycobacteria are rarer. Bacterial infectious arthritis is commonly classified into nongonococcal or gonococcal etiologies. Gram-positive organisms are most commonly identified in nongonococcal cases. Pediatric patients can also develop reactive arthritis in a joint after infection at a distant site in the body.

Staphylococcus aureus is the most common bacterial cause of infectious arthritis in all age groups, followed by *S. pyogenes* and *K. kingae*. Similar to osteomyelitis, CA-MRSA strains have emerged as a common pathogen isolated from patients with infectious arthritis, but rates vary geographically. One small study of 45 patients in Texas found that one-third of isolates were positive for MRSA.[72] Strains of *S. aureus* associated with the PVL gene are associated with more severe disease (e.g., CRP of 10 mg/L or greater, longer duration of fever), the presence of concomitant abscess or cellulitis, and the possibility of a more difficult-to-treat infection.[73]

In neonates and infants younger than 2 months, common causes also include group B streptococci, *Neisseria gonorrhoeae*, gram-negative enteric bacteria (e.g., *E. coli*), and, rarely, *Candida*. *Staphylococcus aureus*, *S. pneumoniae*, *S. pyogenes*, and *K. kingae* are the most common organisms seen in children age 2 months to 5 years. Because of the increase in *H. influenzae* type b immunization rates during the past decade, this organism is now a rare cause of septic arthritis in an immunized child.

The most common cause of infectious arthritis in sexually active adolescents is *N. gonorrhoeae*. Other rare causes include *B. burgdorferi* (i.e., patients with tick exposure while in endemic areas), *Mycobacterium tuberculosis*, viruses (e.g., parvovirus B19, varicella, hepatitis B), and fungi.

Reactive arthritis is commonly seen in patients with gastrointestinal tract infections caused by *Salmonella*, *Shigella*, *Campylobacter*, or *Yersinia enterocolitis* or with genitourinary tract infections caused by *Chlamydia trachomatis* or *N. gonorrhoeae*. It may also occur after a group A streptococcal infection.

RISK FACTORS

Risk factors are associated with either systemic or host factors, such as age (younger than 3 years), preexisting joint disease, or immunosuppression. Local risk factors include recent joint trauma or surgery, presence of prosthetic joints, puncture wounds, recent administration of intra-articular corticosteroids, and rheumatoid arthritis. Although less common in the general pediatric population, intravenous drug abusers are also at increased risk of developing infectious arthritis.

CLINICAL PRESENTATION AND DIAGNOSIS

SIGNS AND SYMPTOMS

Patients with infectious arthritis typically present with an acute systemic infection. Fever, chills, and malaise are common symptoms. The joint is painful, hot, and edematous. It is important to distinguish patients with infectious causes of arthritis from those who have other causes. Transient synovitis is the most common cause of hip pain in children age 5–10 years. Although no exact cause is known, transient synovitis has been associated with trauma, preceding viral infections, and vaccine-mediated reactions.[1] The most common clinical presentation in these patients is unilateral pain and decreased range of motion. The patient may be afebrile or present with a low-grade fever. Other causes of joint pain (e.g., juvenile idiopathic arthritis, trauma, malignancy) should be considered if an infectious source cannot be identified.

DIAGNOSTIC CRITERIA

Clinical presentation is considered the gold standard diagnostic tool for infectious arthritis.[74] Laboratory findings that may suggest infectious arthritis include an increased WBC, procalcitonin, or increased inflammatory markers (e.g., ESR and CRP). Studies have shown the ESR and CRP to be elevated during septic arthritis in around 95% and 90% of patients, respectively.[75] In addition, procalcitonin is superior to CRP in distinguishing between septic and nonseptic arthritis.[76] Other diagnostic approaches include aspiration and culture of the synovial fluid. The synovial fluid should be collected for culture and sensitivity in any patient with a clinical presentation consistent with infectious arthritis. Typical findings suggestive of infectious arthritis on analysis of joint fluid include isolation of bacteria on the Gram stain, leukocytosis (50,000/mm³ or greater), decreased glucose (less than 50% of serum glucose), and increased lactate dehydrogenase, protein, or lactic acid. In addition, blood cultures should be performed to determine the presence of bacteremia. About 30% to 40% of patients will also have a positive blood culture.[70]

Radiography, ultrasonography, and MRI are used in diagnosis of infectious arthritis. Radiography is performed to rule out trauma or malignancy. A radiograph is useful in identifying any significant abnormalities on the adjacent bones to suggest the presence of a concomitant osteomyelitis. Ultrasonography is used to determine the presence of fluid within the joint space and can guide in joint aspiration. However, ultrasonography cannot discern whether fluid within the joint space is infected. An MRI should be considered for patients with suspected concomitant osteomyelitis.

COURSE AND PROGNOSIS

The overall prognosis is favorable for infectious arthritis with prompt initiation of antimicrobial therapy and adequate drainage. Infections of the hip are associated with the highest rates of long-term sequelae. Complications of infectious arthritis include abnormal bone growth, bony deformities at the femoral or humeral head, and local cartilage destruction. These occur more commonly in neonatal patients, patients with adjacent osteomyelitis, patients who do not seek immediate medical care after initiation of symptoms, and patients with S. aureus, including both MSSA and MRSA. If diagnosis is made promptly, the incidence of long-term sequelae after infectious arthritis is much lower.

TREATMENT

The goals of therapy for infectious arthritis include eradicating the infecting organism, resolving the infection and inflammation, and preventing long-term sequelae. Treatment of infectious arthritis is very similar to that of osteomyelitis because of the similarity of causative organisms. However, considerations should be made for patient-specific age, risk factors, and other disease-related issues. Once culture and sensitivity results are available, therapy can be tailored to the specific organism.

The minimum total duration of antibiotic therapy for septic arthritis is 2–3 weeks.[77] A sequential intravenous to oral therapy approach is similar to that for osteomyelitis. Studies have shown similar outcomes in patients treated with shorter courses of intravenous therapy (7 days or less) compared with prolonged courses (more than 10 days) for the treatment of infectious arthritis. Patients may be changed to oral therapy once they have been afebrile for at least 24 hours, the joint swelling has improved to allow better range of motion, and the CRP is decreasing.[78,79] A CRP value of 1.2 mg/L is considered the upper limit of normal. Once oral therapy is initiated, the highest recommended weight-based doses per day are required to achieve adequate joint tissue concentrations.[80]

PHARMACOLOGIC THERAPY

Empiric therapy should target S. aureus and usually includes vancomycin or intravenous clindamycin to provide coverage against MRSA. If K. kingae is strongly suggested (age younger than 5 years, preceding upper respiratory infection), then a β-lactam antibiotic (e.g., penicillin or cephalosporin) should be added to vancomycin or clindamycin.[81] Therapy for sexually active adolescents should include ceftriaxone to cover N. gonorrhoeae in addition to staphylococcal coverage. When culture and sensitivity results are available, treatment should be directed at the specific bacteria isolated from the joint fluid. Table 4 lists the most common organisms and corresponding antimicrobial therapy for infectious arthritis. Intraarticular antibiotics are not indicated for the management of infectious arthritis. Dexamethasone has been studied as an adjunctive agent in infectious arthritis. Studies have demonstrated potential benefits with the addition of dexamethasone; however, long-term outcomes were inconsistent, there were fewer patients in the studies with MRSA, and dexamethasone was not compared with other anti-inflammatory agents.[82-84]

NONPHARMACOLOGIC THERAPY

First-line therapy in the management of infectious arthritis is joint aspiration. This strategy is even more crucial than antimicrobial therapy to provide positive clinical outcomes. Closed-needle aspiration of the joint is indicated for all joints except the hip and shoulder, which require open drainage. Joint drainage can be repeated daily for 5–7 days. An alternative to needle aspiration is arthroscopy with placement of a drainage tube. Joint aspiration and drainage should always be performed in conjunction with antibiotic therapy. Aspiration not only aids in diagnosis but also helps in the therapeutic management of these patients. Antimicrobial therapy should be initiated, if possible, after joint aspiration. Variables to monitor after joint drainage include the volume of synovial fluid and the presence of WBCs, which should decrease with each subsequent drainage.

The key variables for monitoring in the management of infectious arthritis include laboratory and inflammatory markers and clinical signs and symptoms, particularly improvement in joint movement, and adherence to antimicrobial therapy. Routine monitoring of CRP is suggested to follow response to therapy. Patients may be safely transitioned to oral therapy once the CRP normalizes, even in the presence of continued fever. If CRP has not decreased after adequate microbial coverage for 72 hours, further studies are warranted to ensure appropriate drainage has occurred.

CONCLUSIONS

Bone and joint infections are common causes of invasive infections in the pediatric population. *Staphylococcus aureus* remains the most common causative organism in both osteomyelitis and infectious arthritis, with an increasing incidence of CA-MRSA seen in recent years. Prompt identification of bone or joint infection and prompt initiation of appropriate empiric antimicrobial therapy are keys in the management of these infections. Treatment courses are typically prolonged, 3–4 weeks for infectious arthritis and 4–6 weeks for osteomyelitis, with an early transition to oral antibiotic therapy becoming the standard of care. The management of these infections requires a multidisciplinary approach including infectious disease physicians, nurses, physical therapists, pharmacists, and surgeons. Pharmacists play a crucial role in assisting with determining cost-effective therapies, transitioning patients to appropriate oral therapy, ensuring adherence to outpatient therapy, monitoring for medication toxicities and adverse drug reactions, and assisting with discharge planning.

Patient Case — PAINFUL ANKLE

An 8-year-old girl is admitted to the hospital for right ankle pain, erythema, and swelling, in addition to confusion and dizziness. She is a previously healthy child who is up to date on all her immunizations.

The patient had impetigo 1 month ago. Two weeks ago, she developed a rash on her neck that subsided two days later. One week ago, she experienced bilateral ankle pain and had a subjective fever for which she was seen in her primary care physician's office. Radiography of the ankle was negative, and the physician advised over-the-counter pain medications. Two days after the primary care office visit, the patient developed right ankle pain and swelling with difficulty walking. By the day of admission, she had also developed a diffuse rash on her right ankle and became confused and dizzy. She was immediately taken to the emergency department and given a fluid bolus, then she was admitted to the pediatric intensive care unit. Blood cultures were drawn and fluid was aspirated from the joint and sent for culture.

Allergies: Naproxen (rash)

Vital signs: Tmax 102°F (39°C), HR 133 beats/minute, RR 15 breaths/minute, BP 94/46 mm Hg, Wt 50 kg

Laboratory findings:

Na	145 mEq/L
K	4 mEq/L
Cl	113 mEq/L
CO_2	19 mEq/L
BUN	14 mg/dL
SCr	0.7 mg/dL
Glucose	102 mg/dL

Ca, total serum	8.7 mg/dL
CRP	21.2 mg/L
Erythrocyte sedimentation rate	36 mm/hr
Hgb	10.1 g/dL
Hct	28.9%
Plt	78 × 10³ cells/mm³
WBC with differential	13.2 × 10³ cells/mm³: 36% neutrophils, 37% basophils, 23% lymphocytes, 2% eosinophils, 2% monocytes

Case (continued). Today in the emergency department, the patient's C-reactive protein (CRP) is 25.7 mg/L.

1. What is the most likely diagnosis based on the patient's clinical presentation?

The signs and symptoms and the clinical presentation indicate this patient has infectious arthritis. She has bilateral ankle pain and swelling, which indicates that a joint is involved. In addition, most cases of infectious arthritis are hematogenous, and this patient is also presenting with a fever, confusion, and likely sepsis.

2. What clinical and laboratory values need to be followed in this patient?

Clinical values to follow include pain and resolution of confusion. Laboratory values to follow include culture and sensitivity results, white blood cells, erythrocyte sedimentation rate, CRP, procalcitonin, signs of inflammation, and resolution of any abnormal imaging.

3. What empiric therapy should be chosen for this patient? Include the drug, patient-specific dosing, and monitoring guidelines.

This patient has several options for empiric therapy: vancomycin, a penicillinase-resistant penicillin (nafcillin or oxacillin), cefazolin, or clindamycin. Because the patient is confused, dizzy, and admitted to the pediatric intensive care unit, treatment with vancomycin 750 mg intravenously every 6 hours (15 mg/kg/dose) or clindamycin 500 mg intravenously every 6 hours (10 mg/kg/dose) is warranted to provide coverage against methicillin-resistant *Staphylococcus aureus*. Another option would be to initiate combination therapy with clindamycin or vancomycin plus nafcillin or oxacillin or cefazolin. Variables to monitor include renal function (which, if normal, can allow waiting for vancomycin trough level for up to 48 hours), clinical status, CRP, erythrocyte sedimentation rate, and culture results.

Case (continued). Two days after admission, the fluid from the joint aspiration is growing *S. aureus* with the following sensitivities:

Antibiotic	Minimum Inhibitory Concentration	Interpretation
Amoxicillin/clavulanate	≤ 4/2	Sensitive
Ampicillin	> 8	Resistant
Ampicillin/sulbactam	≤ 8/4	Sensitive
Cefazolin	≤ 4	Sensitive
Ceftriaxone	≤ 4	Sensitive
Chloramphenicol	≤ 8	Sensitive
Clindamycin	0.5	Sensitive
Erythromycin	> 4	Resistant
Gentamicin	≤ 1	Sensitive
Levofloxacin	≤ 0.5	Sensitive
Oxacillin	0.5	Sensitive
Penicillin	> 8	Resistant
Rifampin	≤ 1	Sensitive
Tetracycline	≤ 1	Sensitive
Trimethoprim/sulfamethoxazole	≤ 0.5/9.5	Sensitive

The initial blood culture drawn on the day of admission also is growing the same organism with the same sensitivities.

4. What changes to the empiric therapeutic regimen, if any, would you like to make at this time?

If vancomycin was started, changing to nafcillin or oxacillin (2 g intravenously every 6 hours) or cefazolin 1.5 g intravenously every 8 hours (around 100 mg/kg/day) is indicated because the patient is growing methicillin-susceptible *S. aureus* (MSSA). Because of its rapidly bactericidal activity, MSSA should always be treated with penicillinase-resistant penicillin or cefazolin versus vancomycin. If combination therapy was initially chosen, then the vancomycin component can be discontinued.

Case (continued). The patient is continued on inpatient intravenous therapy for the next 2 weeks. She had two subsequent blood cultures that were also positive for MSSA and one additional joint aspiration that also grew MSSA. All of her laboratory values have normalized, except her CRP is still elevated at 10.1 mg/L. The swelling and erythema have also subsided, but the patient is still having trouble bearing weight on her ankle. It is now time for her to be discharged.

5. What outpatient antibiotic therapy do you recommend for this patient and for how long?

The patient can safely be transitioned to a first-generation oral cephalosporin (cephalexin) at a higher dose four times daily (500 mg orally every 6 hours). The total treatment course for septic arthritis is 3–4 weeks; because this patient has already received 2 weeks of intravenous therapy, the oral therapy can be prescribed for 1 week. Antibiotic therapy can be discontinued even with an elevated CRP (as long as it is less than 20 mg/L).

REFERENCES

1. Paakkonen M, Peltola H. Bone and joint infections. Pediatr Clin North Am 2013;60:425-36.
2. Peltola H, Paakkonen M. Acute osteomyelitis in children. N Engl J Med 2014;370:352-60.
3. Waldvogel FA, Vasey H. Osteomyelitis: the past decade. N Engl J Med 1980;303:360-70.
4. Riise ØR, Kirkhus E, Handeland KS, et al. Childhood osteomyelitis-incidence and differentiation from other acute onset musculoskeletal features in a population-based study. BMC Pediatr 2008;8:45-54.
5. Castellazzi L, Mantero M, Esposito S. Update on the management of pediatric acute osteomyelitis and septic arthritis. Int J Mol Sci 2016;17:855.
6. Gutierrez KM. Osteomyelitis. In: Long SS, Pickering LK, Prober CG, eds. Principles and Practice of Pediatric Infectious Diseases. Philadelphia: Elsevier Churchill Livingstone, 1997:528-36.
7. Stanitski CL. Changes in pediatric acute hematogenous osteomyelitis management. J Pediatr Orthop 2004;24:444-5.
8. Bouras D, Doudoulakakis A, Tsolia M, et al. Staphylococcus aureus osteoarticular infections in children: an 8-year review of molecular microbiology, antibiotic resistance and clinical characteristics. J Med Microbiol 2018;67:1753-60.
9. Krogstad P. Osteomyelitis. In: Feigin RD, Cherry JD, Demmler-Harrison GD, et al, eds. Textbook of Pediatric Infectious Diseases, 6th ed. Philadelphia: Saunders Elsevier, 2009:725-42.
10. Carek PJ, Dickerson LM, Sack JL. Diagnosis and management of osteomyelitis. Am Fam Physician 2001;63:2413-20.
11. Waldvogel FA, Medoff G, Swartz MN. Osteomyelitis: a review of clinical features, therapeutic considerations and unusual aspects (first of three parts). N Engl J Med 1970;282:198-206.
12. Waldvogel FA, Medoff G, Swartz MN. Osteomyelitis: a review of clinical features, therapeutic considerations and unusual aspects (second of three parts). N Engl J Med 1970;282:260-6.
13. Waldvogel FA, Medoff G, Swartz MN. Osteomyelitis: a review of clinical features, therapeutic considerations and unusual aspects (third of three parts). N Engl J Med 1970;282:316-22.
14. Fitzgerald RJ, Cowan JD. Puncture wounds of the foot. Orthop Clin North Am 1975;6:965.
15. Cierny G, Mader JT, Pennick JJ. A clinical staging system for adult osteomyelitis. Contemp Orthop 1985;10:17-37.
16. Song KM, Sloboda JF. Acute hematogenous osteomyelitis in children. J Am Acad Orthop Surg 2001;9:166-75.
17. Conrad DA. Acute hematogenous osteomyelitis. Pediatr Rev 2010;31:464-71.
18. Peltola H, Unkila-Kallio L, Kallio MJ. Simplified treatment of acute staphylococcal osteomyelitis of childhood. The Finnish Study Group. Pediatrics 1997;99:846-50.
19. Perlman MH, Patzakis MJ, Kumar PJ, et al. The incidence of joint involvement with adjacent osteomyelitis in pediatric patients. J Pediatr Orthop 2000;20:40-3.
20. Ceroni D, Cherkaoui A, Ferey S, et al. Kingella kingae osteoarticular infections in young children: clinic features and contribution of a new specific real-time PCR assay to the diagnosis. J Pediatr Orthop 2010;30:301-4.
21. Ibia EO, Imoisili M, Pikas A. Group A β-hemolytic streptococcal osteomyelitis in children. Pediatrics 2003;112:e22-6.
22. Bradley JS, Kaplan SL, Tan TQ, et al. Pediatric pneumococcal bone and joint infections. Pediatrics 1998;102:1376-82.
23. Calhoun JH, Manring MM, Shirtliff M. Osteomyelitis of the long bones. Semin Plast Surg 2009;23:59-72.
24. Burnett MW, Bass JW, Cook BA. Etiology of osteomyelitis complicating sickle cell disease. Pediatrics 1998;101:296-7.
25. Jacobs RF, McCarthy RE, Elser JM. Pseudomonas osteochondritis complicating puncture wounds of the foot in children: a 10-year evaluation. J Infect Dis 1989;160:657-61.
26. Brook I. Joint and bone infections due to anaerobic bacteria in children. Pediatr Rehab 2002;5:11-9.
27. Harik NS, Smeltzer MS. Management of acute hematogenous osteomyelitis in children. Expert Rev Anti Infect Ther 2010;8:175-81.
28. Weichert S, Sharland M, Clarke NM, et al. Acute haematogenous osteomyelitis in children: is there any evidence for how long we should treat? Curr Opin Infect Dis 2008;21:258-62.
29. Bocchini CE, Hulten KG, Mason EO Jr, et al. Panton-Valentine leukocidin genes are associated with enhanced inflammatory response and local disease in acute hematogenous Staphylococcus aureus osteomyelitis in children. Pediatrics 2006;117:433-40.
30. Paakkonen M, Kallio PE, Kallio MJ, et al. Management of osteoarticular infections caused by Staphylococcus aureus is similar to that of other etiologies: analysis of 199 staphylococcal bone and joint infections. Pediatr Infect Dis J 2012;31:436-8.
31. Floyed RL, Steele RW. Culture negative osteomyelitis. Pediatr Infect Dis J 2003;22:731-6.
32. Moumile K, Merckx J, Glorion C, et al. Osteoarticular infections caused by Kingella kingae in children: contribution of polymerase chain reaction to the microbiologic diagnosis. Pediatr Infect Dis J 2003;23:255-7.
33. Unkila-Kallio L, Kallio MJ, Eskola J, et al. Serum C-reactive protein, erythrocyte sedimentation rate, and white blood cell count in acute hematogenous osteomyelitis of children. Pediatrics 1994;93:59-62.
34. McCaskill ML, Mason EO Jr, Kaplan SL, et al. Increase of the USA300 clone among community-acquired methicillin-susceptible Staphylococcus aureus causing invasive infections. Pediatr Infect Dis J 2007;26:1122-7.
35. Mazur JM, Ross G, Cummings J, et al. Usefulness of magnetic resonance imaging for the diagnosis of acute musculoskeletal infections in children. J Pediatr Orthop 1995;15:144-7.
36. Liu C, Bayer A, Cosgrove SE, et al. Clinical practice guidelines by the Infectious Diseases Society of America for the treatment of methicillin-resistant Staphylococcus aureus infections in adults and children. Clin Infect Dis 2011;52:e18-55.
37. Browne LP, Mason EO, Kaplan SL, et al. Optimal imaging strategy for community-acquired Staphylococcus aureus musculoskeletal infections in children. Pediatr Radiol 2008;38:841-7.
38. Jaramillo D, Dormans JP, Delgado J, et al. Hematogenous osteomyelitis in infants and children: imaging of a changing disease. Radiology 2017;283:629-43.
39. Dombrowski JC, Winston LG. Clinical failures of appropriately-treated methicillin-resistant Staphylococcus aureus infections. J Infect 2008;57:110-5.
40. Roine I, Faingezicht I, Arguedas A, et al. Serial serum C-reactive protein to monitor recovery from acute hematogenous osteomyelitis in children. Pediatr Infect Dis J 1995;14:40-4.
41. Taketomo CK, Hodding JH, Kraus DM. Pediatric & Neonatal Dosage Handbook, 25th ed. Hudson, OH: Lexi-Comp, 2018.
42. Huang C, Hsieh RW, Yen H, et al. Short- versus long-course antibiotics in osteomyelitis; a systematic review and meta-analysis. Int J Antimicrobial Agents 2019;246-50.
43. Bachur R, Pagon Z. Success of short-course parenteral antibiotic therapy for acute osteomyelitis of childhood. Clin Pediatr (Phila) 2007;46:30-5.
44. Peltola H, Paakkonen M, Kallio P, et al. Short- versus long-term antimicrobial treatment for acute hematogenous osteomyelitis of childhood: prospective, randomized trial on 131 culture-positive cases. Pediatr Infect Dis J 2010;29:1123-8.
45. Zaoutis T, Localio AR, Leckerman K, et al. Prolonged intravenous therapy versus early transition to oral antimicrobial therapy for acute osteomyelitis in children. Pediatrics 2009;123:636-42.
46. Kaplan SL. Osteomyelitis in children. Infect Dis Clin North Am 2005;19:787-97.

47. Frymoyer A, Hersh AL, Benet LZ, et al. Current recommended dosing of vancomycin for children with invasive methicillin-resistant *Staphylococcus aureus* infections is inadequate. Pediatr Infect Dis J 2009;28:398–402.

48. Geist A, Kuhn R. Pharmacological approaches for pediatric patients with osteomyelitis: current issues and answers. Orthopedics 2009;32:573–7.

49. Heil EL, Claeys KC, Mynatt RP, et al. Making the change to area under the curve-based vancomycin dosing. Am J Health Sys Pharm 2018;1986–95.

50. Martinez-Aguilar G, Hammerman WA, Mason EO Jr, et al. Clindamycin treatment of invasive infections caused by community-acquired, methicillin-resistant and methicillin-susceptible *Staphylococcus aureus* in children. Pediatr Infect Dis J 2003;22:593–8.

51. Frank AL, Marcinak JF, Mangat PD, et al. Clindamycin treatment of methicillin-resistant *Staphylococcus aureus* infections in children. Pediatr Infect Dis J 2002;21:530–4.

52. Thabit AK, Fatani DF, Bamakhrama MS, et al. Antibiotic penetration into bone and joints: an updated review. Int J Infect Dis 2019;81:128-136.

53. Joiner KA, Lowe BR, Dzink JL, et al. Antibiotic levels in infected and sterile subcutaneous abscesses in mice. J Infect Dis 1981;143:487–94.

54. Fiebelkorn KR, Crawford SA, McElmeel ML, et al. Practical disk diffusion method for detection of inducible clindamycin resistance in *Staphylococcus aureus* and coagulase-negative staphylococci. J Clin Microbiol 2003;41:4740–4.

55. Ardura MI, Mejias A, Katz KS, et al. Daptomycin therapy for invasive gram-positive bacterial infections in children. Pediatr Infect Dis J 2007;26:1128–32.

56. Crompton JA, North DS, McConnell SA, et al. Safety and efficacy of daptomycin in the treatment of osteomyelitis: results from the CORE registry. J Chemother 2009;21:414–20.

57. Rana B, Butcher I, Grigoris P, et al. Linezolid penetration into osteo-articular tissues. Antimicrob Agents Chemother 2002;50:747–50.

58. Dumitrescu O, Boisset S, Badiou C, et al. Effect of antibiotics on *Staphylococcus aureus* producing Panton-Valentine leukocidin. Antimicrob Agents Chemother 2007;51:1515–9.

59. Chen CJ, Chiu CH, Lin TY, et al. Experience with linezolid therapy in children with osteoarticular infections. Pediatr Infect Dis J 2007;26:985–8.

60. Chiappini E, Conti C, Galli L, et al. Clinical efficacy and tolerability of linezolid in pediatric patients: a systematic review. Clin Ther 2010;32:66–88.

61. Wood CA, Wisniewski RM. Beta-lactams versus glycopeptides in treatment of subcutaneous abscesses infected with *Staphylococcus aureus*. Antimicrob Agents Chemother 1994;38:1023–6.

62. Jackson MA, Schutze GE, Committee on Infectious Diseases. The use of systemic and topical fluoroquinolones. Pediatrics 2016;138:e20162706.

63. Steele RW, Russo TM, Thomas MP. Adherence issues related to the selection of antistaphylococcal or antifungal antibiotic suspensions for children. Clin Pediatr (Phila) 2006;45:245–50.

64. Steer AC, Carapetis JR. Acute hematogenous osteomyelitis in children: recognition and management. Pediatr Drugs 2004;6:333–46.

65. Henry SL, Galloway KP. Local antibacterial therapy for the management of orthopaedic infections. Clin Pharmacokinet 1995;29:36–45.

66. Weiss BD, Weiss EC, Haggard WO, et al. Optimized elution of daptomycin from polymethylmethacrylate beads. Antimicrob Agents Chemother 2008;53:264–6.

67. Lentrodt S, Lentrodt L, Kübler N, et al. Hyperbaric oxygen for adjuvant therapy for chronically recurrent mandibular osteomyelitis in childhood and adolescence. J Oral Maxillofac Surg 2007;65:186–91.

68. Frank G, Mahoney HM, Eppes SC. Musculoskeletal infections in children. Pediatr Clin North Am 2005;52:1083–106.

69. Messiner HC, Townsend T, Wenman W, et al. Hematologic effects of linezolid in young children. Pediatr Infect Dis J 2003;22:S186–92.

70. Wang CL, Wang SM, Yang YJ, et al. Septic arthritis in children: relationship of causative pathogens, complications, and outcome. J Microbiol Immunol Infect 2003;36:41–6.

71. Saisu T, Kawashima A, Kamegaya M, et al. Humeral shortening and inferior subluxation as sequelae of septic arthritis of the shoulder in neonates and infants. J Bone Joint Surg Am 2007;89:1784–93.

72. Carrillo-Marquez MA, Hulten KG, Hammerman W, et al. USA-300 is the predominant genotype causing *Staphylococcus aureus* septic arthritis in children. Pediatr Infect Dis J 2009;28:1076–80.

73. Caksen H, Oztürk MK, Uzüm K, et al. Septic arthritis in childhood. Pediatr Int 2000;42:534–40.

74. Mathews CJ, Kingsley G, Field M, et al. Management of septic arthritis: a systematic review. Ann Rheum Dis 2007;66:440–5.

75. Zhao J, Zhnag S, Zhang L, et al. Serum procalcitonin as a diagnostic marker for septic arthritis: a meta-analysis. Am J Emerg Med 2017;35:1166-71.

76. Khachatourians AG, Patzakis MJ, Roidis M, et al. Laboratory monitoring in pediatric acute osteomyelitis and septic arthritis. Clin Orthop Relat Res 2003;409:186–94.

77. Saavedra-Lozano, J, Falup-Pecurariu O, Faust SN, et al. Bone and Joint Infections. Pediatr Infect Dis J 2017;36:788-99.

78. Peltola H, Paakkonen M, Kallio P, et al. Prospective, randomized trial of 10 days versus 30 days of antimicrobial treatment, including a short-term course of parenteral therapy, for childhood septic arthritis. Clin Infect Dis 2009;48:1201–10.

79. Ballock RT, Newton PO, Evans SJ, et al. A comparison of early versus late conversation from intravenous to oral therapy in the treatment of septic arthritis. J Pediatr Orthop 2009;29:636–42.

80. Newton PO, Ballock R, Bradley JS. Oral antibiotic therapy of bacterial arthritis. Pediatr Infect Dis J 1999;18:1102–3.

81. Fogel I, Amir J, Bar-On E, et al. Dexamethasone therapy for septic arthritis in children. Pediatrics 2015;136:e776-82.

82. Harel L, Prais D, Bar-On E, et al. Dexamethasone therapy for septic arthritis in children: results of a randomized double-blind placebo-controlled study. Pediatr Orthop 2011;31:211-5.

83. Narayanan UG. Dexamethasone added to antibiotics improved clinical and laboratory outcomes in children with septic arthritis. J Bone Joint Surg Am 2011;93:2124.

84. Macchiaiolo M, Buonuomo PS, Mennini M, et al. Question 2: should steroids be used in the treatment of septic arthritis? Arch Dis Child 2014;99:785-7.

CHAPTER 43

LEARNING OBJECTIVES

1. Describe the epidemiology of and risk factors for infectious diarrhea in children.

2. Identify when oral rehydration solutions are appropriate for treating dehydration in children with infectious diarrhea.

3. Describe the clinical presentation of each gastrointestinal infection in children.

4. Recommend appropriate therapies and monitoring variables for children with infectious diarrhea.

5. Discuss preventive measures that can protect children from gastrointestinal infections.

ABBREVIATIONS IN THIS CHAPTER

CDI	*Clostridioides difficile* infection
EHEC	Enterohemorrhagic *Escherichia coli*
ETEC	Enterotoxigenic *Escherichia coli*
HUS	Hemolytic uremic syndrome
NTS	Nontyphoidal *Salmonella*
ORS	Oral rehydration solution
ORT	Oral rehydration therapy
PCR	Polymerase chain reaction

INTRODUCTION

Infectious diarrhea accompanied by dehydration is the second leading cause of global pediatric morbidity and mortality, resulting in more than 500,000 deaths annually in children younger than 5 years.[1] Almost 90% of pediatric deaths from infectious diarrhea occur in Africa and South Asia.[1] In the United States, acute gastrointestinal infections are less common than in the developing world, and older adults have the highest risk of death. However, infectious diarrhea and dehydration still account for almost 200,000 hospitalizations and 300 deaths annually among children in the United States.[2]

Diarrhea, defined as having unusually loose or watery stools at least three times per day or more than usual for an individual, is often a symptom of gastrointestinal infections. Viruses are the most common cause of pediatric infectious diarrhea worldwide, but bacteria and parasites also play a role. Significant diarrhea can lead to dehydration, which commonly occurs with cholera or after infection with rotavirus or enterotoxigenic *Escherichia coli* (ETEC). Management of infectious diarrhea focuses on preventing and treating dehydration and its complications in addition to limiting the spread of infection to others.

Several factors increase the risk of spreading gastrointestinal infections and developing diarrhea and its complications. Transmission occurs mainly by the oral–fecal route; therefore, the most significant risk factor for contracting infection is behavior that increases the likelihood of fecal contact. Examples include lack of handwashing after defecation or handling feces before handling food. In addition, day care attendance and living in crowded conditions increase the risk of contact with contaminated excrement. Ingestion of certain foods and exposure to reptiles or other pets increase the risk of exposure to specific infecting pathogens. In developing countries, polluted water sources, poor sanitation practices, contaminated food, and malnutrition contribute to the spread and severity of infectious diarrhea.[1] International travel to developing countries can result in traveler's diarrhea after the consumption of contaminated food or water.

Children and immunocompromised individuals have an increased risk of dehydration and severe disease from gastrointestinal infections. Compared with adults, children have a greater percentage of total body water and use more water to support metabolism and conserve less water through their kidneys. Thus, acute body water losses that occur with diarrhea have a greater effect of increasing the risk of dehydration in children. Immunocompromised conditions and the relatively immature immune system in young children contribute to more severe illness from gastrointestinal infections.

REHYDRATION THERAPY

Fluid replacement, electrolyte balance, and maintenance of normal feeding are vital components for managing dehydration from infectious diarrhea, regardless of the cause. The appropriate route of administration for replacement fluids depends on the severity of dehydration, as characterized by percent loss in body weight and clinical presentation. Table 1 displays the clinical signs and symptoms that are useful for categorizing dehydration in children and the recommended replacement fluids for each stage. Severe dehydration should be treated initially with intravenous fluids, whereas mild to moderate dehydration is best managed with oral rehydration therapy (ORT).[2-6]

SEVERE DEHYDRATION

Severe dehydration is a medical emergency that requires immediate and rapid rehydration to avoid vital organ damage from poor tissue perfusion. Intravenous resuscitation should occur with lactated Ringer solution or normal saline using an initial bolus dose of 20 mL/kg for most children. Children who are frail or malnourished should receive 10 mL/kg to avoid edema from reduced cardiac output.[2] Several bolus doses may be necessary and should be given until pulse, perfusion, and mental status are normalized. Once these variables have stabilized, intravenous rehydration is generally required to continue replenishing the fluid deficit and provide ongoing maintenance fluid needs. Specific calculations are recommended to determine fluid and electrolyte requirements; additional information can be found in the Fluids and Electrolytes chapter. Intravenous rehydration therapy can be switched to the oral route when clinically appropriate and able to be tolerated.

MILD TO MODERATE DEHYDRATION

Oral rehydration is highly effective for treating mild to moderate dehydration. This approach is the preferred route for rehydration because it is noninvasive, inexpensive, and administered at home.[2,3] Development of glucose-based oral rehydration solutions (ORS) was based on the principle of coupled glucose and sodium transport. These nutrients are co-absorbed across intestinal brush border luminal cell membranes into enterocytes, where they are then pumped into the bloodstream through different transmembrane transporter systems. Water reabsorption occurs because of the osmotic gradient generated by these transport systems, which remain intact even in severe diarrhea.[2] Mixtures of ORS, which contain water, electrolytes, and glucose, are recommended to have low osmolarity (e.g., 245 mmol/L) to reduce the stool output and vomiting associated with high-osmolarity solutions.[6] In a recent study in children age 6 to 60 months with gastroenteritis and mild dehydration, oral hydration with half-strength apple juice or other preferred fluids resulted in fewer treatment failures than electrolyte solutions.[7] Additional information on the management of dehydration from diarrhea can be found in the Diarrhea and Constipation chapter.

NONBACTERIAL CAUSES OF INFECTIOUS DIARRHEA

VIRAL GASTROENTERITIS

Viruses cause more than 50% of all pediatric diarrheal illnesses, which can occur in epidemics or as sporadic illnesses. Common viruses that cause gastroenteritis include rotavirus, noroviruses, enteric adenoviruses, astroviruses, and coronaviruses. Rotavirus is a predominant cause of infectious diarrhea worldwide, infecting almost all children by age 5 years; more information can be found in the Pediatric Vaccines chapter.[8] Immunity is usually incomplete after an initial rotavirus infection, but it may be protective against more severe illness from subsequent infection. Noroviruses are responsible for more than 50% of all gastroenteritis outbreaks and have been reported as the leading cause of acute infectious diarrhea in the United States in all age groups.[9] Noroviruses are highly contagious and are spread through contaminated food and water or through close personal contact. Outbreaks

Table 1. Clinical Signs and Symptoms and Fluid Replacement Therapies Associated with Degree of Dehydration in Children[2,3]

Sign or Symptom or Therapy	Severity of Dehydration (% Loss of Body Weight)		
	Minimal or None (< 3%)	Mild to Moderate (3%–9%)	Severe (> 9%)
Mental status	Normal; alert	Normal to fatigued or irritable	Lethargic, apathetic; unconscious
Fontanelle	Normal	Normal to sunken	Sunken
Eyes	Normal	Sunken orbits; decreased tears	Deeply sunken orbits; absent tears
Mucous membranes	Normal; moist	Slightly dry to dry	Parched
Thirst	Normal	Thirsty	Too lethargic to drink
Heart rate	Normal	Normal to increased	Increased; bradycardia in severe cases
Quality of pulse	Normal	Normal to decreased	Weak or not palpable
Blood pressure	Normal	Normal	Normal to reduced
Respirations	Normal	Normal to fast	Deep
Skin turgor	Normal recoil	Decreased recoil < 2 sec	Recoil > 2 sec
Extremities	Warm; normal capillary refill	Cool; delayed capillary refill	Cold, mottled, cyanotic; prolonged capillary refill
Urine output	Normal to decreased	Decreased	Minimal
Fluid replacement therapy	None	ORT 50–100 mL/kg over 2–4 hr	IV bolus of lactated Ringer solution or normal saline 20 mL/kg (over 15–30 min) until perfusion and mental status improve; then IV fluids (5% dextrose with normal saline [0.9%]) at twice maintenance fluid rate or ORT 100 mL/kg over 4 hr

IV = intravenous; ORT = oral rehydration therapy.

commonly occur in health care facilities, schools, child care centers, and cruise ships. Immunity to norovirus infection is complex and may depend more on innate host factors (such as cell receptor mutations that block viral entry into host cells) than on antibody development.

Ingestion of viruses through contaminated food or water or after contact with contaminated surfaces can lead to significant diarrhea and dehydration. Viruses directly damage the intestinal lining leading to impaired absorption and subsequent fluid and electrolyte loss. Brush border enzyme activity is reduced, which can result in transient lactose intolerance. After an incubation period of 12 hours to 3 days, clinical manifestations of viral gastroenteritis develop, which often begin with vomiting. Nonbloody diarrhea, abdominal cramping, and nausea are usually present. Viral gastrointestinal infection can also be asymptomatic or associated with extraintestinal symptoms such as fever, myalgia, headache, or malaise. Symptoms typically resolve in 1–3 days for norovirus infection or 3–7 days for rotavirus. Detecting stool viral antigens through enzyme immunoassay, latex agglutination assay, or polymerase chain reaction (PCR) confirms the diagnosis of viral gastroenteritis.

Treatment of viral diarrhea is mainly supportive. Rehydration with ORS or intravenous solutions replaces fluids and electrolytes lost through stool or vomitus. Children should continue their typical diet when possible, but foods and liquids high in simple sugars should be initially avoided because they can aggravate diarrhea. Probiotics containing *Lactobacillus rhamnosus* GG in doses of 10 billion colony-forming units have been shown to reduce the amount and duration of diarrhea by about 1 day when given to children early in the course of rotavirus infection.[10-12] Probiotics should not be used in certain patient populations, such as children with short bowel syndrome (short gut) or immunodeficiencies, because of the risk of developing bacteremia or sepsis from probiotic strains. Loperamide, an opioid antimotility agent, may reduce the duration of viral diarrhea, but it is not recommended for children who are younger than 3 years or in those who are malnourished, who are moderately to severely dehydrated, or who have bloody diarrhea.[13] These patient groups are at high risk of adverse events such as lethargy, ileus, and respiratory depression. Antimicrobials have no role in the management of viral gastroenteritis.

Zinc supplementation may reduce the duration of acute viral diarrhea in children who are at least age 6 months and at risk of zinc deficiency.[2,14] Zinc is poorly absorbed from grains, nuts, and legumes, whereas high concentrations of zinc are found in meat and fish. Zinc promotes a healthy gastrointestinal tract mucosa and restores brush border enzyme activity in addition to stimulating immunity against gastrointestinal pathogens.[6,14] Zinc doses of 10–20 mg/day given for 10–14 days should be considered for children with acute viral diarrhea, particularly those who are malnourished or at risk of zinc deficiency including those who live in developing countries.[6,14]

Prevention of viral gastroenteritis focuses on proper hygiene and vaccination. Handwashing with plain soap and running water for at least 20 seconds is essential for caregivers and individuals with diarrheal illness, particularly after defecation or potential contact with feces and before food preparation and ingestion. Hand sanitizers are an alternative to handwashing, but should not be considered a substitute.[9] Handwashing may be more effective at removing viral particles from the skin through its mechanical process than alcohol-based hand sanitizers. The only vaccine available to protect against diarrheal illness is the rotavirus vaccine recommended for infants, as detailed in the Pediatric Vaccines chapter.

PARASITIC GASTROINTESTINAL INFECTIONS

Parasitic diarrhea can arise in both the developing world and industrialized nations. In the United States, *Giardia lamblia* and *Cryptosporidium* are two protozoan parasites that commonly infect immunocompromised and immunocompetent children. Giardiasis is reviewed in the Parasitic Infections in Pediatric Patients chapter; thus, this chapter will focus on cryptosporidiosis.

Cryptosporidiosis is widespread across the United States with increasing rates over the past 10–20 years, particularly in the Midwest region.[15] Cases are most often reported in children between age 1 and 9 years, and the peak time for infection is during summer and early fall.[15] *Cryptosporidium* is often transmitted through recreational water such as swimming pools or through exposure to infected animals, particularly cattle. Risk factors for cryptosporidiosis include the use of public swimming pools or other freshwater sources, contact with livestock or incontinent children, international travel to areas of high endemicity, immunodeficiency, and consumption of a large amount of unboiled well water.

Cryptosporidiosis occurs after the ingestion of *Cryptosporidium* oocysts found in fecally contaminated food or water or through direct person-to-person contact. Infection is usually limited to the intestinal surface epithelia where the parasite attaches, causing a loss of microvilli, inflammation, and subsequent malabsorption and enhanced secretion. As few as 10–30 ingested oocysts can cause persistent infection in an individual because of repeated life cycles within the gastrointestinal tract.[16] Oocysts are shed in feces for up to 2 months after diarrhea subsides and are infectious immediately after excretion.[15] Although some infections may be asymptomatic, most individuals have profuse, watery diarrhea that contains mucus and lasts for about 2 weeks. Nausea, vomiting, abdominal cramping, and fever may also be present. Patients with HIV/AIDS can have a severe, cholera-like presentation that can persist for the patient's lifetime. Diagnosis of cryptosporidiosis is made when oocysts are identified on acid-fast staining of stool or when stool antigens are identified through immunoassay techniques.

Treatment of cryptosporidiosis does not routinely eradicate the infection, particularly in immunocompromised hosts. Immunocompetent individuals and those who are asymptomatic generally do not need antimicrobial therapy because the infection is self-limiting. Nitazoxanide (100 to 200 mg orally twice daily for 3 days) may be considered for treatment of malnourished immunocompetent children with prolonged diarrhea because it induces a positive parasitologic response and reduction in diarrhea.[17,18] Nitazoxanide has a unique mechanism of action involving interference with anaerobic energy metabolism through the disruption of electron transport, and it is not associated with any significant adverse effects. Optimal therapy in patients with HIV/AIDS is to restore immune function through the use of effective combination antiretroviral therapy; if this restoration is not possible or if it fails, antimicrobial and antidiarrheal therapies are recommended.[16,17] Paromomycin, azithromycin, and nitazoxanide have been used but are only modestly effective in this population because of a sustained immunodeficient state in HIV/AIDS.

Efforts to control cryptosporidiosis are best aimed at preventing oocyst transmission. Oocysts are resistant to many disinfectants and antiseptics, including chlorine, alcohol, and alkaline chemicals.[15] Severely immunocompromised patients should boil all water before consumption and avoid water from lakes or streams, contact with farm animals, and cleaning up after pets.[15] All individuals should practice proper hygiene to prevent the spread and ingestion of oocysts and avoid swallowing water from swimming pools, lakes, ponds, streams, or other untreated water sources.

BACTERIAL CAUSES OF INFECTIOUS DIARRHEA

Bacterial causes of infectious diarrhea are less common than viral causes, but their associated syndromes are well characterized. Two main categories of infection occur: *enterotoxigenic* (or watery diarrhea) and *dysentery* (or invasive diarrhea). Enterotoxigenic diarrhea is often self-limiting, whereas dysentery requires close monitoring of patients who have fever with stools containing blood and pus. Bacterial diarrhea is more common in summer months, whereas viral diarrhea is more common in winter and spring. Antibiotic therapy, outlined in Table 2, may be indicated for certain infections.

SHIGELLOSIS

Shigellosis, or bacillary dysentery, is a common cause of mortality from diarrhea. It affects around 165 million people worldwide, mostly children, and leads to more than 1 million deaths, 60% of which are in children younger than 5 years.[19,20] In the United States, almost 500,000 people are infected annually, with most cases caused by person-to-person transmission in day care centers, schools, and crowded living areas.[19] Transmission occurs easily, requiring as few as 10–100 organisms to cause infection after ingestion.[20] Shigellosis can also be spread through contaminated food and water, leading to large outbreaks.

Shigella spp. are nonmotile, gram-negative bacilli in the Enterobacteriaceae family. The four species most commonly associated with disease are *Shigella dysenteriae* type 1, *Shigella flexneri*, *Shigella boydii*, and *Shigella sonnei*. The most common species in the United States are *S. sonnei* and *S. flexneri*. After ingestion, bacterial replication and spread occur within intestinal epithelial cells and bowel mucosa and submucosa, leading to inflammation, ulceration, tissue sloughing, and bloody mucosal exudates. The entire colon is usually involved, but the infection seldom spreads to the bloodstream; bacteremia is more likely in malnourished and immunocompromised children. Certain *Shigella* strains (common in *S. dysenteriae*

type 1) produce Shiga toxin, a virulence factor that causes more severe disease. These strains are associated with complications such as toxic megacolon and hemolytic uremic syndrome (HUS). This syndrome is characterized by hemolytic anemia, thrombocytopenia, and renal failure. Although rare, HUS can be fatal.

Shigellosis usually follows a biphasic pattern, with initial signs and symptoms including abdominal pain and cramping, fever, and frequent watery diarrhea. Within 48 hours, severe abdominal pain and tenderness often develop, followed by mucoid or bloody diarrhea and tenesmus (a feeling of incomplete defecation with rectal pain). Vomiting may also be present. Fluid and electrolyte losses can be severe in infants and young children. If left untreated, shigellosis lasts about 1 week, but organisms can be excreted for up to 30 days after illness onset.[20] Postinfectious arthritis in conjunction with eye irritation and painful urination (Reiter syndrome) is a rare complication that occurs in genetically susceptible individuals and can lead to chronic arthritis. Other complications that are more common in children include rectal prolapse, seizures, and malnutrition. Diagnosis of shigellosis is made after the development of symptoms and is confirmed by stool culture or PCR.

Shigellosis is generally self-limiting and may require fluid replacement therapy if dehydration becomes significant. Antibiotic therapy is usually not indicated unless the infection is severe or occurs in a child who is immunocompromised or malnourished. Antibiotics shorten the duration of diarrhea and reduce infectivity by minimizing fecal shedding; however, antimicrobial resistance among *Shigella* is a growing concern and is well documented worldwide.[19-23] In 2014, more than 40% of strains in the United States were resistant to trimethoprim/sulfamethoxazole and more than 30% were resistant to ampicillin; however, there was minimal resistance to ceftriaxone and fluoroquinolones.[21] Reduced susceptibility to ciprofloxacin and azithromycin is reported more recently, so clinicians should request culture and susceptibility results when antibiotic therapy is indicated.[22,23] Empiric antibiotic regimens for shigellosis in children are shown in Table 2. Azithromycin is the empiric drug of choice, but the Clinical and Laboratory Standards Institute has not established susceptibility breakpoints. For azithromycin, epidemiologic cutoff values have been created to detect acquired resistance patterns for *S. sonnei* and *S. flexneri*, but these values should not be used to guide therapy because they do not incorporate clinical outcome data and pharmacologic drug properties.[21] If susceptible, ampicillin or trimethoprim/sulfamethoxazole can be used. Ciprofloxacin should be reserved for cases of multidrug resistance, and parenteral ceftriaxone should be reserved for children who are unable to tolerate oral antibiotics and for those with serious illness.[22] Clinicians should report treatment failures to the Centers for Disease Control and Prevention.[23] Antimotility agents are not recommended for shigellosis because they can worsen symptoms and increase the risk of complications such as toxic megacolon.

Preventing the spread of shigellosis is important to minimize outbreaks. Control measures should include strict hand hygiene; proper food cooking and storage; avoidance of recreational water while symptomatic, or day care attendance for at

Table 2. Antibiotic Therapy for Bacterial Infectious Diarrhea in Children

Infection and Indications	Antibiotic Regimens	Considerations
Shigellosis		
Severe infection, immunocompromised, malnourished	Azithromycin 10 mg/kg/day (max 500 mg) PO × 3 days	Empiric drug of choice; resistance rates unknown[a]
	Ciprofloxacin 10–15 mg/kg (max 750 mg) BID PO × 3–5 days	Reserve for cases of MDR
	Ceftriaxone 50 mg/kg (max 1 g) once daily IM or IV × 2–5 days	Must be given parenterally; reaches GI tract because of biliary excretion
Salmonellosis—Uncomplicated NTS Gastroenteritis		
Age < 3 mo, immunocompromised, hemoglobinopathies, malignancies, chronic GI diseases	Initial dose of ceftriaxone 75 mg/kg (max 2 g) IV; then one of the following PO options:	
	Azithromycin 10–20 mg/kg (max 1 g) PO once daily x 5–7 days	Preferred initial PO choice; resistance rates unknown[a]
	TMP/SMZ 4–5 mg/kg (TMP) (max 160 mg TMP/800 mg SMZ per dose) PO BID × 5 days	Avoid in children < 2 mo; increased risk of kernicterus
	Ampicillin 25 mg/kg (max 500 mg) PO QID × 5 days	Local resistance rates may be high
	Ciprofloxacin 10–15 mg/kg (max 750 mg) BID PO × 3–5 days	Reserve for cases of MDR
Salmonellosis—Enteric (Typhoid) Fever, Uncomplicated		
All patients, based on acquisition region and geographic susceptibility patterns	Ceftriaxone 75 mg/kg (max 2 g) IV once daily or azithromycin 10–20 mg/kg (max 1 g) PO once daily × 5–7 days	—
	Ciprofloxacin 10–15 mg/kg (max 750 mg) BID PO × 7–14 days	—
	Ampicillin 25 mg/kg (max 500 mg) PO QID × 7–14 days	Can be used if isolate is susceptible
Salmonellosis—Complicated Enteric Fever or Extraintestinal or Invasive NTS Infection		
All patients	Ceftriaxone 75–100 mg/kg (max 2 g) IV once daily × 10–14 days (4–6 wk if endovascular infection, osteomyelitis, or meningitis)	For bacteremia, ceftriaxone can be changed to PO azithromycin or ciprofloxacin once blood cultures are negative (total treatment duration 7–10 days)
Enterotoxigenic *Escherichia coli*		
Moderate to severe diarrhea	Azithromycin 10 mg/kg/day (max 500 mg) PO × 1–3 days	Drug of choice for children
	Rifaximin 200 mg TID PO × 3 days	Indicated only for children 12 yr and older; expensive alternative agent
Campylobacteriosis		
Severe bloody stools, elevated temperature, prolonged illness, pregnancy, immunocompromised	Azithromycin 10 mg/kg/day (max 500 mg) PO × 3 days (can use for 7–14 days if complicated or immunocompromised)	Drug of choice
Cholera		
Severe infection	Azithromycin 20 mg/kg (max 1 g) PO once	
	Doxycycline 4 mg/kg (max 300 mg) PO once	Often avoided in children < 8 yr because of potential effects on tooth formation and bone growth; resistance is common
***Clostridioides difficile* infection**		
Initial episode or first recurrence, nonsevere	Metronidazole 7.5 mg/kg (max 500 mg) PO TID to QID × 10 days	Drug of choice; can be given IV if PO administration is not an option
	Vancomycin 10 mg/kg (max 125 mg) PO QID × 10 days	Alternative first-line agent for children
Initial episode, severe/fulminant	Vancomycin 10 mg/kg (max 500 mg) PO or rectally QID × 10 days	Can be given with IV metronidazole 10 mg/kg (max 500 mg) TID × 10 days for fulminant infection

[a]Resistance rates unknown because of lack of reliable testing.
BID = twice daily; GI = gastrointestinal; IM = intramuscularly; IV = intravenously; MDR = multidrug resistance; NTS = non-typhoidal salmonella; PO = orally; QID = four times per day; SMZ = sulfamethoxazole; TID = three times daily; TMP = trimethoprim.

least 24 hours after diarrhea resolution; exclusion of infected individuals from handling food; and preventing child care workers from preparing food if they change diapers. No vaccines are currently available for preventing shigellosis.

SALMONELLOSIS

Salmonellosis is the most common foodborne illness in the United States in which nontyphoidal strains cause more than 1 million infections annually, leading to 20,000 hospitalizations and 400 deaths.[24] The rate of invasive salmonellosis is highest in infants, which may be related to their reduced gastric acidity, gut immaturity, or underdeveloped immune systems.[25] Outbreaks are associated with contaminated food or water, but fecal–oral transmission is also likely in children. Infection typically results from the ingestion of contaminated vegetables or fruits; undercooked pork, poultry, or beef; or unpasteurized dairy products. Accounting for up to 5% of cases, exotic pets, including snakes, turtles, and iguanas, are also an important source of infection because they are often carriers of *Salmonella* in their gastrointestinal tracts.

Salmonella enterica are motile, gram-negative bacilli in the Enterobacteriaceae family. The nontyphoidal strains, serotypes Enteritidis and Typhimurium, are the most common in the United States. These serotypes primarily cause gastroenteritis, but they can lead to bacteremia and localized extraintestinal infections. Serotypes Typhi and Paratyphi are more prevalent in certain parts of the world and cause enteric fever, or typhoid, from bacteremia. The infectious dose of *Salmonella* (around 1 million organisms) is higher than with *Shigella*, but it is lower in people with reduced gastric acidity. Once ingested, the organisms penetrate the epithelial lining of the distal ileum and colon, causing inflammation, tissue damage, and fluid secretion across the intestinal mucosa. In certain individuals or with certain serotypes, bacteremia may occur after translocation through the intestinal wall and can lead to localized extraintestinal infections in areas such as bone, heart, central nervous system, or spleen. Diagnosis of salmonellosis is made by isolating the organism through stool culture or PCR in patients with gastroenteritis, or from blood or bone marrow in those with enteric fever. Recovery of *Salmonella* from stool is most likely early in the course of illness, but bacteria may continue to be shed for up to 12 weeks in children.[26] About 1% of infected individuals become chronic carriers and shed organisms for more than 12 months because of biliary tract carriage.[26]

Clinical manifestations of salmonellosis depend on the infecting serotype and the host. After the ingestion of nontyphoidal *Salmonella* (NTS), symptoms typically occur within 36–72 hours. Most patients experience abdominal cramping, fever, and sudden diarrhea that is often nonbloody. Nausea, vomiting, and headache may also be present. Gastroenteritis is often self-limiting and resolves in 5–7 days, although it may take months for bowel movements to normalize completely. Invasive disease and extraintestinal infections are more common in infants younger than 3 months and in children with immunodeficiencies, malignancy, sickle-cell disease, or chronic gastrointestinal diseases. After typhoidal strains are ingested, fever and nonspecific systemic symptoms, including

profuse sweating, headache, chills, anorexia, myalgias, and malaise, develop within 7–14 days. Diarrhea may be present in enteric fever, and sequelae such as intestinal bleeding or perforation, delirium, or hepatosplenomegaly can develop within 3 weeks of illness onset. *Salmonella* infection can also be asymptomatic.

Treatment of *Salmonella* infection depends on the clinical severity and host. Uncomplicated gastroenteritis induced by NTS rarely requires intervention beyond hydration with ORS. Antibiotics may result in prolonged fecal shedding and a higher rate of short-term and chronic carriage, so they are recommended only for high-risk patients with NTS who may develop invasive or extraintestinal disease: children younger than 3 months or those with immunodeficiencies, hemoglobinopathies, malignancy, or chronic gastrointestinal tract disease.[26] For typhoid fever and invasive *Salmonella* infections, antibiotic therapy is warranted. Empiric regimens for salmonellosis are listed in Table 2. The choice of regimen should consider geographic resistance patterns. An initial dose of parenteral ceftriaxone should be given after blood cultures are obtained in high-risk patients with suspected NTS gastroenteritis. If disseminated infection is not present and the patient does not appear ill, then oral azithromycin can be used once blood culture results are available. Alternative agents for NTS gastroenteritis are based on susceptibility results. Patients who appear ill or have disseminated NTS infection should be hospitalized and treated with ceftriaxone with subsequent management as shown in Table 2. Typhoidal strains, which tend to be more drug resistant, should be treated empirically with broad-spectrum agents, but antibiotics should be streamlined when susceptibility results are available.[21] Chronic carriage (excretion longer than 1 year) is uncommon in children; however, when present, chronic carriage can be eradicated with 4 weeks of oral ciprofloxacin to prevent spread to others, such as in day care settings or immunosuppressed close contacts.[26]

Salmonella infection can be prevented with a variety of approaches. These methods include meticulous hand hygiene, sanitary food preparation and water supplies, and sanitary sewage and waste disposal, as well as excluding infected individuals from handling food or attending day care. Children younger than 5 years and immunocompromised patients should avoid contact with reptiles, amphibians, rodents, and live poultry. Eggs and meat should be cooked thoroughly, and ingestion of foods containing raw eggs or unpasteurized milk should be avoided. Breastfeeding is protective against infantile salmonellosis because it provides passive immunity and limits exposure to potentially contaminated formula or water. Typhoid fever can be prevented through vaccination using one of two typhoid vaccines: an oral live-attenuated vaccine or an injectable capsular polysaccharide vaccine. Vaccination is recommended for children who are traveling to an endemic area such as Africa, Asia, or Latin America, or who are household contacts of chronic typhoid carriers. The oral vaccine can be given to children 6 years and older (four doses given every other day), whereas the injectable vaccine can be administered to children as young as 2 years (a single dose). The oral vaccine should not be used in children who are immunocompromised or who have an active gastrointestinal tract illness.

ESCHERICHIA COLI

Infectious diarrhea caused by *E. coli* is categorized on the basis of pathogenic characteristics.[27] The most common form of *E. coli* diarrhea worldwide is ETEC, and it is the leading cause of traveler's diarrhea resulting from international travel. Enterotoxigenic *E. coli* causes watery diarrhea and is associated with food- and waterborne outbreaks in areas with inadequate sanitation. Person-to-person transmission is uncommon because infection requires a relatively large inoculum. In contrast, enterohemorrhagic *E. coli* (EHEC) causes bloody diarrhea, which can result in hemorrhagic colitis, HUS, and potentially death. Interpersonal spread occurs easily with EHEC because ingestion of only a few organisms can lead to infection. In the United States, EHEC is often caused by *E. coli* 0157:H7. Outbreaks of EHEC are associated with contaminated beef or vegetables, unpasteurized dairy products or apple cider, and exposure to animals in petting zoos. Enteroinvasive *E. coli* and enteropathogenic *E. coli* occur mainly in children in developing countries. Enteroaggregative *E. coli* is common in HIV infection and usually leads to persistent watery diarrhea.

Escherichia coli is a gram-negative bacillus found in the intestinal tract of humans, cattle and other farm animals, and deer. Gastrointestinal damage from *E. coli* infection varies depending on the infecting organism.[27] Enterotoxigenic *E. coli* have the ability to produce cholera-like enterotoxins that cause profuse secretory diarrhea. Enterohemorrhagic *E. coli* produces Shiga-like toxins that disrupt large intestinal mucosa, creating bloody diarrhea. These toxins can invade the bloodstream and damage the vascular supply to the gastrointestinal tract and kidneys, resulting in HUS. Enteroinvasive *E. coli* resemble *Shigella* and cause intestinal damage and symptoms similar to dysentery. Enteropathogenic *E. coli* adhere to intestinal epithelial cells, which disrupts their integrity, leading to watery diarrhea. Enteroaggregative *E. coli* adhere to mucosal cells in a biofilm layer that causes persistent colonization, epithelial damage, and watery diarrhea. Diagnosis of *E. coli* diarrhea is complicated by the inability to differentiate between normal *E. coli* stool flora and diarrhea-associated strains with use of stool cultures; therefore, PCR testing is often used. *Escherichia coli* 0157:H7 can be detected by its inability to ferment sorbitol, followed by subsequent serotyping. Shiga-like toxins from EHEC can be detected with immunologic assays.

Clinical presentation of *E. coli* diarrhea manifests in different ways. Enterotoxigenic *E. coli* and other nonhemorrhagic strains cause abrupt watery diarrhea, nausea, and abdominal cramping that usually resolve within 5 days. Enteropathogenic *E. coli* often cause low-grade fever and vomiting, whereas enteroaggregative *E. coli* diarrhea is persistent and watery with minimal or no vomiting. Enteroinvasive *E. coli* can present with dysentery symptoms of bloody diarrhea that contains mucus and pus, tenesmus, and fever. Enterohemorrhagic *E. coli* is associated with severe symptoms that begin as abdominal cramping and distension, watery diarrhea, and nausea or vomiting, but then progress to bloody diarrhea with increased abdominal pain within 48 hours. Fever is not a common feature of EHEC. Although most cases resolve after 1 week, HUS can develop in up to 6% of patients

with EHEC and is most common in children between age 1 and 5 years.[27] Typically, HUS develops 7 days after the onset of diarrhea, and up to 50% of children will require dialysis.[27]

All forms of *E. coli* diarrhea should be managed with fluid and electrolyte therapy to prevent dehydration. Enterohemorrhagic *E. coli* should not be treated with antibiotics because they may increase the release of toxins from bacterial lysis, increasing the risk of HUS.[28] Antimotility agents should also not be used in EHEC because they can reduce the clearance of the organisms and toxins. For other forms of *E. coli* diarrhea, particularly those associated with travel, antibiotics may be considered for moderate to severe diarrhea, but antimicrobial resistance can affect treatment success. Table 2 lists empiric agents that can be considered. Loperamide can reduce the severity of ETEC when taken in conjunction with antibiotics, but bismuth subsalicylate should be avoided in children younger than age 12 years because of the risk of Reye syndrome.

Preventing *E. coli* infection focuses on the avoidance of contaminated food and water sources. Methods to prevent infection include proper cooking of ground beef; ingestion of only pasteurized milk or apple juice or cider; and avoidance of tap water, uncooked or unpeeled foods, and inadequately stored foods during travel to developing countries. Use of proper hand hygiene and exclusion of symptomatic individuals from day care centers and recreational water sources are also helpful to prevent spread of infection. No vaccines are currently available to prevent *E. coli* infection.

CAMPYLOBACTERIOSIS

Campylobacter is a common bacterial cause of infectious diarrhea, accounting for almost 1 million cases annually in the United States.[24] The two peak age groups for infection are children younger than 1 year and individuals between age 15 and 44 years, with male children infected more commonly. Infection is transmitted through contaminated food or water and is often associated with poultry consumption. Risk factors for campylobacteriosis include exposure to chickens, other birds, or cats; consumption of undercooked poultry or other meats, unpasteurized milk, or contaminated water; and international travel.

Campylobacter spp. are motile, spiral-shaped, gram-negative bacilli that are sensitive to gastric acid. The two most common species to cause diarrhea are *Campylobacter jejuni* and *Campylobacter coli*. Infectious doses are around 500–800 organisms, but doses are lower in individuals with reduced gastric acidity. After ingestion, replication occurs in the small intestine, and organisms adhere to intestinal tissue in the jejunum, ileum, colon, and rectum, leading to local inflammation. Some strains of *C. jejuni* produce enterotoxins or cytotoxins that contribute to pathogenicity.[29] Host immunity plays a role in the development of campylobacteriosis, and frequent exposure provides short-term protection against infection but not colonization.[30] Diagnosis of campylobacteriosis is confirmed with stool culture, stool PCR, or enzyme immunoassay.

Common clinical manifestations of campylobacteriosis occur within 1–7 days of ingestion and include high fever, abdominal cramps, and diarrhea, which can be watery or bloody. Vomiting, headache, myalgia, malaise, and seizures can also be present. Some patients may experience only abdominal pain with minimal diarrhea. Gastrointestinal symptoms usually resolve within 1 week or less. Extraintestinal infections may occur and are more common in immunocompromised children and neonates and include the following: sepsis, septic arthritis, meningitis, pancreatitis, cholecystitis, and osteomyelitis. Campylobacteriosis leads to around 30% of Guillain-Barré syndrome cases, which occur within 3 weeks of infection, but the risk of developing this syndrome is less than 1 case per 1000 *C. jejuni* infections.[31]

The cornerstone of treatment of campylobacteriosis is ORT for hydration and electrolyte replacement. Antibiotics are usually unnecessary; they do not reduce illness duration or severity unless given within 3 days of symptom onset, but they can shorten the duration of bacterial shedding. Antibiotics should be considered in patients with severe bloody stools, elevated temperature, prolonged illness for longer than 1 week, pregnancy, and immunocompromised states (Table 2). Macrolides are the agents of choice because of increasing fluoroquinolone resistance from overuse in enteric infections and use of fluoroquinolones in poultry. Severely ill children with bacteremia can be treated with intravenous gentamicin or a carbapenem. Antimotility agents should be avoided because they prolong the duration of infection and enhance toxin retention.

Prevention of campylobacteriosis focuses on hand hygiene and avoiding contaminated food and water. Individuals should wash their hands, all utensils, and cutting boards after contact with uncooked poultry and avoid cross-contamination of vegetables and other foods with raw poultry juices. All poultry should be cooked thoroughly before eating. Hand hygiene is also important after defecation and contact with animal feces. Infected individuals should be excluded from food preparation and day care until asymptomatic. No vaccine is currently available to prevent *Campylobacter* infection.

CHOLERA

Cholera is uncommon in the United States but is endemic in areas of Asia and Africa. Some toxin-producing strains cause epidemics or pandemics, which have been reported in parts of Africa, Asia, the Middle East, and the Americas, including the Caribbean. This disease can be asymptomatic or mild, but classic cholera causes loss of large volumes of watery stool, severe dehydration, and shock. It is transmitted through water or contaminated foods, especially undercooked shellfish or fish. Cholera grows well in warm temperatures and appears in moist grains or vegetables stored at ambient temperatures. The infectious dose from environmental sources ranges from 10^6–10^{10} organisms but is lower in those with reduced gastric acidity. Risk factors for cholera include the ingestion of undercooked seafood or untreated water, low gastric acidity, and blood type O.[32]

Vibrio cholerae is a motile gram-negative bacillus similar to Enterobacteriaceae, with several serogroups known to cause pandemics. Infection occurs when organisms colonize the small intestine after ingestion and penetrate the mucosal layer. Enterotoxin production is an important pathogenic feature of cholera that leads to excessive isotonic fluid loss in the small intestine, exceeding colonic absorptive capacity. Electrolyte-rich watery diarrhea develops, which is highly infectious and allows for person-to-person spread. Diagnosis is made on request for isolation of vibrios from stool, which can be further serotyped at state laboratories.

Cholera occurs within a few hours to 5 days after ingestion. It is characterized by an abrupt onset of painless watery diarrhea and often vomiting. Stools are typically of large volume, reaching a loss of 1 L/hour, and have the consistency of rice water. Complications of cholera include hypoglycemia, seizures, renal failure, and mental status changes. Severe muscle cramps are common from electrolyte imbalances. Severe dehydration, metabolic acidosis, and shock occur rapidly and can progress to death within hours if untreated.

Rapid treatment of cholera with ORS is vital to replace fluids and electrolytes and thus prevent shock. Rice-based ORS is preferred by some experts because it may be more effective than glucose-based ORS in reducing stool output and because it reduces overall fluid requirements.[33] Intravenous rehydration with lactated Ringer solution may need to be given before ORS if shock is present. Antibiotics should be given to children with severe disease because they can shorten the duration of diarrhea and reduce fluid loss (Table 2). Oral antibiotics should be given after initial rehydration and cessation of vomiting. Antibiotic resistance is common among endemic strains and should be monitored during outbreaks to ensure that proper treatment is provided.

Prevention of cholera focuses on ensuring a safe water supply through proper sanitation, thorough cooking of seafood, and by appropriate hand hygiene after defecation and before food preparation. Antibiotic prophylaxis for household contacts is not recommended because of resistance concerns. Two oral vaccines are available in other countries but not in the United States. Vaccination is not recommended for most travelers to endemic areas because the risk of infection is low, and the immunity provided by the vaccines is incomplete.

CLOSTRIDIOIDES DIFFICILE INFECTION

Clostridioides difficile is the most common cause of nosocomial infectious diarrhea in the United States. Both the incidence of community-acquired disease and severe infection is increasing, and outbreaks from a single strain (North American pulsed-field type 1, or NAP-1) have emerged in recent years. *Clostridioides difficile* infection (CDI) is most common in adults, but the prevalence is increasing in children.[34] Pediatric risk factors for CDI include the following: age between 1 and 5 years; immunodeficiency; malignancy; inflammatory bowel disease; recent use of broad-spectrum antibiotics; abdominal surgery; presence of a gastrostomy or jejunostomy tube; and proton pump inhibitor or histamine-2 receptor blocker therapy.[34-36] In most community-acquired CDI, children do not have a previous history of antibiotic exposure.[34]

Clostridioides difficile is a gram-positive, spore-forming anaerobic bacillus that causes a toxin-mediated diarrhea. Infection occurs after the ingestion of organisms or spores that can survive harsh environmental conditions and are resistant to disinfectants, including alcohol. Ingested spores germinate in the small intestine and travel to the colon where they can produce toxins A and B, which are responsible for disease. Toxin A, an enterotoxin, causes fluid and mucus secretion, mucosal damage, and inflammation, whereas toxin B, a cytotoxin, is more potent and causes mucosal damage. Pseudomembranous plaques form in the colon and enlarge with disease progression to affect the entire colon and rectum.

Clostridioides difficile infection varies in severity from mild diarrhea to life-threatening pseudomembranous colitis and toxic megacolon. For antibiotic-associated infections, CDI can occur on the first day of antibiotic therapy or as late as several weeks after completing antibiotics. Diarrhea is usually watery and can be mild with only a few loose stools per day, accompanied by abdominal pain, low-grade fever, and mild leukocytosis. Colitis is characterized by frequent watery diarrhea (can also contain mucous or blood) with up to 15 bowel movements per day, abdominal pain and distension, nausea, anorexia, fever, and leukocytosis. Fulminant disease involves severe abdominal pain, profuse diarrhea, fever, dehydration, tachycardia, marked leukocytosis, and possibly hypotension. Toxic megacolon can develop with acute colonic dilation, signs of systemic disease (fever, tachycardia, hypotension), and cessation of bowel movements. Mortality is high if toxic megacolon develops. Some patients are asymptomatic carriers of *C. difficile*; up to 70% of neonates and young infants lack colonic toxin receptors and may be protected from CDI by antibodies found in breast milk.[34,37] Diagnosis of CDI is made by detecting toxin A or B in the stool of symptomatic individuals using either enzyme immunoassays or PCR. Endoscopy may be needed to diagnose CDI in individuals with an ileus. Because young children have a high rate of asymptomatic colonization with *C. difficile*, testing should only be performed if there is evidence of pseudomembranous colitis or toxic megacolon, or if there is significant diarrhea and other causes have been excluded.[37,38]

Initial treatment of CDI should include ORT and halting antibiotic therapy when possible. Although some patients may respond to discontinuing antibiotics alone, antimicrobial therapy directed at *C. difficile* is recommended for most cases (Table 2). Oral vancomycin or fidaxomicin are recommended as first-line agents for CDI in adults. In recent studies, oral vancomycin was superior to oral metronidazole for obtaining clinical cure in adults, regardless of disease severity.[38] Fidaxomicin achieves similar cure rates to vancomycin, but it is not currently approved for use in children. Oral metronidazole can be considered as a first-line alternative to vancomycin for children because data are lacking to support superiority of vancomycin in this population.[38] Newer antibiotics including rifaximin and nitazoxanide have been studied for CDI and may result in fewer recurrences; however, their role in therapy is yet to be defined. For fulminant CDI, oral high-dose vancomycin is recommended in conjunction with intravenous metronidazole with or without vancomycin enema, which is useful in cases of peristaltic ileus.[38]

Recurrent CDI occurs in up to 30% of children within 2–3 weeks of discontinuing antibiotic treatment.[34] Recurrence is associated with failure to eradicate spores or reinfection from an environmental source rather than from antibiotic

resistance. Treatment options for a first recurrence in children include a 10-day course of oral metronidazole or a 10-day course of oral vancomycin, particularly if metronidazole was used for the initial infection. Children with several recurrences are difficult to treat. Options to consider in these patients are extended courses of oral vancomycin, with pulse dosing and/or tapered dosing over 4–10 weeks; oral vancomycin followed by rifaximin; or fecal microbiota transplantation.[34,38] Adjunctive therapies for CDI, including cholestyramine and probiotics, have not consistently proven to be beneficial. Antiperistaltic agents are contraindicated because they increase the risk of toxic megacolon, which often requires surgical intervention.

Measures to prevent *C. difficile* transmission and infection must focus on proper infection control methods and antibiotic stewardship. Handwashing with soap and water is necessary to prevent spread because alcohol-based products are not effective at eliminating spores. Health care providers should use contact precautions and wear gowns and gloves while caring for *C. difficile*–infected patients. Isolating infected patients should also be practiced in institutional settings. Chlorine-containing cleaners at a concentration of at least 1000 parts per million are effective in minimizing environmental contamination. Infected individuals should be excluded from day care settings until diarrhea subsides. Rational use of antibiotics is vital for reducing CDI rates. In addition, mounting evidence suggests that probiotics, particularly *Saccharomyces boulardii*, may reduce the risk of CDI in children receiving antibiotics; however, their routine use is not recommended.[34]

TRAVELER'S DIARRHEA

Traveler's diarrhea occurs when people travel from industrialized nations to developing countries and consume contaminated water or food. Common pathogens include ETEC; *Campylobacter*, *Salmonella*, or *Shigella* spp.; and rotavirus or norovirus. Risk factors for developing traveler's diarrhea include ingesting tap water, uncooked foods, and foods that are stored inadequately, such as buffet-style meals. High-risk areas include South Asia, Africa, South and Central America, and Mexico. Most cases occur within 2 weeks of travel and resolve in a few days. Typical signs and symptoms are malaise, nausea, anorexia, abdominal cramps, and mild to moderate diarrhea that can interfere with planned activities. Traveler's diarrhea is rarely life threatening.

Treatment focuses on avoiding dehydration with the use of ORS or other fluids and returning to functional status as soon as possible. Antibiotics, which can reduce the duration of diarrhea, should be considered in children with severe diarrhea that is incapacitating and completely interfering with planned activities or in children who have fever plus blood, pus, or mucus present in stool.[39] Oral azithromycin 10 mg/kg/day (maximum 500 mg) for 3 days is recommended for treating children instead of fluoroquinolones, which have been historically used in adults.[39,40] Recent warnings about neurologic effects and tendinopathies from fluoroquinolone use in conjunction with increasing resistance rates have dampened enthusiasm for their use. In children 12 years and older, oral rifaximin (200 mg three times daily for 3 days) is an alternative agent for use in travelers to Mexico or Jamaica, where *E. coli* is predominant. Rifaximin is not recommended as an alternative agent in other areas because *Campylobacter* is generally resistant to this agent. Antimotility agents are not recommended unless they are administered with antibiotics, and they should be avoided if fever or bloody stools are present.

Prevention of traveler's diarrhea focuses on education and avoidance of high-risk foods and beverages. Antibiotic prophylaxis is not routinely recommended because of antimicrobial resistance concerns but can be considered in those with certain severe chronic medical conditions, such as inflammatory bowel disease. Bismuth subsalicylate taken four times per day for up to 3 weeks may inhibit enterotoxin activity, but it should not be used in children because of the risk of Reye syndrome. Probiotics may minimize infection from pathogenic organisms, but more studies are needed before they can be routinely recommended.[39]

CONCLUSIONS

Infectious diarrhea in children, which is caused by a variety of microorganisms, can result in significant dehydration, electrolyte disturbances, and additional complications. Although a large proportion of cases occur in developing countries, children in the United States are also susceptible because of contaminated food and water sources and international travel. Treatment should always involve rehydration, preferably with ORS, and antibiotics when appropriate. Knowledge regarding infectious sources and proper hygiene is vital to limiting the spread of infectious diarrhea.

Patient Case — INFECTIOUS DIARRHEA

A 13-month-old boy is brought to the emergency department (ED) with his mother for evaluation of fever and bloody diarrhea. Three days ago, the child began having watery, nonbloody diarrhea and a low-grade fever. He had three episodes of diarrhea on that day with no vomiting. Over the next 48 hours, he continued to have diarrhea and fever with a maximum recorded temperature of 101°F (38.3°C). He had several episodes of vomiting yesterday and has been eating and drinking a little less than usual. His mother took him to the ED last night where a diagnosis of viral gastroenteritis was made, and then the patient was discharged home. This morning, his mother noticed streaks of bright red blood in his stool, so she brought him back to the ED. She states that he has been sleeping more than usual and he "is not acting like himself." He has been refusing to drink all morning and has had very little urine output. She does not report any other concerns.

Medical history: Born at 41 weeks' gestation by normal spontaneous vaginal delivery, and no hospitalizations or complications since birth; one episode of acute otitis media at age 9 months

Family history: Father has hypertension; mother has allergic rhinitis and chronic sinusitis

Social history: Lives at home with parents, one dog, and one cat; attends day care 5 days a week; no passive smoke exposure; no recent travel; no known sick contacts, but lives in a community with recently reported cases of *Shigella* gastroenteritis

Allergies: None

Current medications: Acetaminophen 120 mg orally every 4-6 hours as needed for fever

Immunizations: Up to date

Vital signs: BP 90/56 mm Hg, HR 150 beats/minute, RR 25 breaths/minute, Tmax 101.9°F (38.8°C), Ht 30 inches, Wt 9.8 kg; his mother reports that

2 weeks ago he weighed 10.5 kg at his 12-month well-child office visit

Physical examination:

General: Tired and ill-appearing

Skin: No rashes; dry appearing skin; capillary refill 3-4 sec

HEENT: Pupils are equal, round, and reactive to light and accommodation; extraocular movements are intact; eyes sunken; dry, tacky mucous membranes; tympanic membranes normal; throat normal appearing

Neck and lymph nodes: Normal; nontender

Chest: Lungs clear to auscultation

CV: Normal heart sounds; tachycardia

Abdomen: Diffusely tender; no distension; hyperactive bowel sounds

Neuro: Grossly intact

Genitourinary/rectal: Perianal erythema; no fissures noted; rectal prolapse

Laboratory findings:

Glucose	65 mg/dL
Na	144 mEq/L
K	3.4 mEq/L
Cl	97 mEq/L
CO_2	12 mEq/L
Anion gap	21 mEq/L
BUN	25 mg/dL
SCr	0.6 mg/dL
WBC	18.6×10^3 cells/mm³; differential: 70% segmented neutrophils, 25% lymphocytes, 5% monocytes
Hgb	9.9 g/dL
Plt	350×10^3 cells/mm³
Stool	Heme-positive; multiplex PCR pending
Blood culture	Pending

Assessment: A 13-month-old boy with signs and symptoms consistent with infectious diarrhea, possibly *Shigella*, in addition to signs and symptoms consistent with moderate to severe dehydration

1. What information in this child's history and presentation is consistent with *Shigella* infection?

His initial presentation of fever with watery diarrhea is consistent with early *Shigella* infection, but it is also consistent with early infectious diarrhea caused by viruses, *Cryptosporidium*, *Salmonella*, *Escherichia coli*, *Campylobacter*, and *Clostridioides difficile*. Other features consistent with *Shigella* infection are the progression to bloody diarrhea, abdominal tenderness, persistent fever, vomiting, moderate to severe dehydration, and rectal prolapse. Although the child has no known sick contacts at home or at day care, there are recent reports of *Shigella* cases in his community. Shigellosis spreads easily from person to person and has a low infectious dose; it can also be spread by people who are asymptomatic or recovering from recent infection.

Case (continued). The decision is made to admit the child to the hospital.

2. What therapy should be initiated at this time?

Fluid replacement must be initiated to increase organ perfusion and prevent damage from hypovolemia. This child has signs and symptoms of moderate to severe dehydration: sleepiness, sunken eyes, dry and tacky mucous membranes, poor thirst despite dehydration, tachycardia, prolonged capillary refill, dry skin, and poor urine output. He has lost 0.7 kg since his well-child visit from 2 weeks ago, which equates to about 7% of his body weight and a fluid deficit of about 735 mL (7% dehydration × 10.5 kg × 1000 mL/kg). He also has some laboratory findings that suggest dehydration, including metabolic acidosis and elevated BUN and serum creatinine. He continues to have fever, poor oral intake, and increased stool output which all increase his risk of continued dehydration.

He should receive an intravenous bolus of either lactated Ringer solution or normal saline (200 mL, or 20 mL/kg) followed by intravenous maintenance fluids (typically given with 5% dextrose and normal saline, with addition of 20 mEq/L of potassium chloride once urinating) running between 1.5 and 2 times the maintenance fluid rate until he is able to tolerate oral fluid intake. Exact calculations for managing this child's isonatremic dehydration (as outlined in the Fluids and Electrolytes chapter) are:

Fluid deficit = 735 mL

Maintenance fluid requirements = [100 mL/kg/day × 10 kg] + [50 mL/kg/day × 0.5 kg] = 1025 mL

After the initial bolus to stabilize the child, intravenous fluids should continue to be given to replenish the fluid loss and provide for ongoing fluid needs. Over the first 8 hours, one-half of the deficit plus one-third of the daily maintenance should be given: 368 mL + 342 mL = 710 mL at a rate of 88 mL/hour. This amount is about equivalent to twice the maintenance rate calculated using the Holliday-Segar method ([4 mL/kg/hr × 10 kg] + [2 mL/kg/hr × 0.5 kg] = 41 mL/hr). Then, over the next 16 hours if intravenous fluids are still required, the remaining one-half of the deficit plus two-thirds of the daily maintenance should be

given: 368 mL + 683 mL = 1051 mL at a rate of around 65 mL/hour. This amount is around 1.5 times the maintenance rate calculated using the Holliday-Segar method.

Antibiotic therapy should be withheld until laboratory confirmation of *Shigella* or another infectious source for which antibiotics are recommended for use. Antibiotics are not recommended for most cases of nontyphoidal *Salmonella* gastroenteritis (unless the patient has a high-risk condition or has invasive infection) or campylobacteriosis (unless severe). Antibiotics should be avoided in enterohemorrhagic *E. coli* and *Shigella dysenteriae* type 1 infections because they can increase the risk of hemolytic uremic syndrome.

Case (continued). Laboratory results confirmed the presence of *Shigella* in the stool sample with negative blood cultures.

3. What antibiotic regimen should be recommended? How should this child be monitored? What adjunctive medications can be recommended?

Antibiotics are recommended for cases of severe shigellosis and in children who attend day care or are immunocompromised or malnourished. Antibiotics can reduce the duration of illness and limit infectivity; however, antibiotic resistance is a major concern. This child required hospitalization and attends day care; therefore, antibiotic therapy should be initiated. Antibiotic susceptibility testing is recommended to determine resistance patterns and to guide treatment if empiric therapy fails. Oral azithromycin (10 mg/kg/day for 3 days) is the empiric regimen of choice for children who can tolerate oral therapy. This child is not actively vomiting and does not have evidence of bacteremia; therefore, azithromycin 100 mg orally for 3 days can be initiated at this time. Improvements in stool output, bloody stools, appetite, and fever are expected within 1–2 days. If his fever persists or worsens, or his stool output and presence of blood does not change by day three of therapy, then treatment failure is probable, and antibiotic therapy should be changed according to susceptibility results and/or consultation with an infectious diseases specialist.

No good evidence exists to support the use of adjunctive therapies for most cases of gastroenteritis. Antimotility agents should be avoided for most bacterial causes because they can prolong the duration of symptoms and excretion of organisms in addition to increasing the risk of complications such as toxic megacolon.

4. What preventive measures should be discussed with this child's parents to limit the spread of infection to others?

It is essential to practice proper hand hygiene at all times, particularly after changing diapers and before food preparation and eating. Washing hands with soap and water for at least 20 seconds each time is preferred; hand sanitizers can be an alternative, but they should not be a substitute for soap and water washing. Soiled clothing should be washed with hot water, if possible. The child should be kept out of day care and recreational water sources (such as community pools) for at least 24 hours after diarrhea resolves.

REFERENCES

1. United Nations Children's Fund (UNICEF). One Is Too Many: Ending Child Deaths From Pneumonia and Diarrhoea. New York: UNICEF, 2016. Available at http://www.unicef.org/media/49816/file/UNICEF-Pneumonia-Diarrhoea-report-2016-ENG.pdf. Accessed January 23, 2020.
2. King CK, Glass R, Bresee JS, et al.; Centers for Disease Control and Prevention. Managing acute gastroenteritis among children: oral rehydration, maintenance, and nutritional therapy. MMWR Recomm Rep 2003;52:1-16.
3. Sentonga TA. The use of oral rehydration solutions in children and adults. Curr Gastroenterol Rep 2004;6:307-13.
4. Spandorfer PR, Alessandrini EA, Joffe MD, et al. Oral versus intravenous rehydration of moderately dehydrated children: a randomized, controlled trial. Pediatrics 2005;115:295-301.
5. Hartling L, Bellemare S, Wiebe N, et al. Oral versus intravenous rehydration for treating dehydration due to gastroenteritis in children. Cochrane Database Syst Rev 2006;9:CD004390.
6. World Health Organization. The Treatment of Diarrhoea: A Manual for Physicians and Other Senior Health Workers. Geneva: World Health Organization, 2005. Available at http://whqlibdoc.who.int/publications/2005/9241593180.pdf. Accessed September 17, 2019.
7. Freedman SB, Willan AR, Boutis K, et al. Effect of dilute apple juice and preferred fluids vs electrolyte maintenance solution on treatment failure among children with mild gastroenteritis: a randomized clinical trial. JAMA 2016;315:1966-74.
8. Bernstein DI. Rotavirus overview. Pediatr Infect Dis J 2009; 28:S50-3.
9. Division of Viral Diseases, National Center for Immunization and Respiratory Diseases, Centers for Disease Control and Prevention. Updated norovirus outbreak management and disease prevention guidelines. MMWR Recomm Rep 2011;60:1-15.
10. Thomas DW, Greer FR, American Academy of Pediatrics Committee on Nutrition, American Academy of Pediatrics Section on Gastroenterology, Hepatology, and Nutrition. Probiotics and prebiotics in pediatrics. Pediatrics 2010;126:1217-31.
11. Allen SJ, Martinez EG, Gregorio GV, et al. Probiotics for treating acute infectious diarrhoea. Cochrane Database Syst Rev 2010; 11:CD003048.
12. Van Niel CW, Feudtner C, Garrison MM, et al. *Lactobacillus* therapy for acute infectious diarrhea in children: a meta-analysis. Pediatrics 2002;109:678-84.
13. Li ST, Grossman DC, Cummings P. Loperamide therapy for acute diarrhea in children: systematic review and meta-analysis. PLoS Med 2007;4:e98.
14. Lazzerini M, Wanzira H. Oral zinc for treating diarrhoea in children. Cochrane Database Syst Rev 2016;12:CD005436.
15. Painter JE, Hlavsa MC, Collier SA, et al; Centers for Disease Control and Prevention. Cryptosporidiosis surveillance—United States, 2011-2012. MMWR Suppl 2015;64:1-14.
16. Shirley DA, Moonah SN, Kotloff KL. Burden of disease from cryptosporidiosis. Curr Opin Infect Dis 2012;25:555-63.
17. Siberry GK, Abzug MJ, Nachman S, et al. Guidelines for the prevention and treatment of opportunistic infections in HIV-exposed and HIV-infected children: recommendations from the National Institutes of Health, Centers for Disease Control and Prevention, the HIV Medicine Association of the Infectious Diseases Society of America, the Pediatric Infectious Diseases Society, and the American Academy of Pediatrics. Pediatr Infect Dis J 2013;32:i-KK4.
18. Gargala G. Drug treatment and novel drug target against *Cryptosporidium*. Parasite 2008;15:275-81.
19. Niyogi SK. Shigellosis. J Microbiol 2005;43:133-43.
20. Sur D, Ramamurthy T, Deen J, et al. Shigellosis: challenges and management issues. Indian J Med Res 2004;120:454-62.
21. Centers for Disease Control. National Antimicrobial Resistance Monitoring System for Enteric Bacteria (NARMS): Human Isolates Surveillance Report for 2015 (Final Report). Atlanta, GA: U.S. Department of Health and Human Services, CDC, 2018. Available at https://www.cdc.gov/narms/pdf/2015-NARMS-Annual-Report-cleared_508.pdf. Accessed September 17, 2019.
22. American Academy of Pediatrics. *Shigella* infections. In: Kimberlin DW, Brady MT, Jackson MA, et al., eds. Red Book: 2018 Report of the Committee on Infectious Diseases. 31st ed. Itasca, IL: American Academy of Pediatrics, 2018:723-7.
23. Centers for Disease Control and Prevention. Health Alert Network. Update—CDC Recommendations for Managing and Reporting *Shigella* Infections with Possible Reduced Susceptibility to Ciprofloxacin. Atlanta, GA: U.S. Department of Health and Human Services, CDC, 2018. Available at https://emergency.cdc.gov/han/han00411.asp. Accessed September 17, 2019.
24. Scallan E, Hoekstra RM, Angulo FJ, et al. Foodborne illness acquired in the United States—major pathogens. Emerg Infect Dis 2011;17:7-15.
25. Vugia DJ, Samuel M, Farley MM, et al. Invasive *Salmonella* infections in the United States, FoodNet, 1996-1999: incidence, serotype distribution, and outcome. Clin Infect Dis 2004;38:S149-56.
26. American Academy of Pediatrics. *Salmonella* infections. In: Kimberlin DW, Brady MT, Jackson MA, et al., eds. Red Book: 2018 Report of the Committee on Infectious Diseases. 31st ed. Itasca, IL: American Academy of Pediatrics; 2018:711-8.
27. American Academy of Pediatrics. *Escherichia coli* diarrhea. In: Kimberlin DW, Brady MT, Jackson MA, et al., eds. Red Book: 2018 Report of the Committee on Infectious Diseases. 31st ed. Itasca, IL: American Academy of Pediatrics; 2018:338-44.
28. Panos GZ, Betsi GI, Falagas ME. Systematic review: are antibiotics beneficial or detrimental for the treatment of patients with *Escherichia coli* 0157:H7 infection? Aliment Pharmacol Ther 2006;24:731-42.
29. Amieva MR. Important bacterial gastrointestinal pathogens in children: a pathogenesis perspective. Pediatr Clin North Am 2005;52:749-77.
30. Janssen R, Krogfelt KA, Cawthraw SA, et al. Host-pathogen interactions in *Campylobacter* infections: the host perspective. Clin Microbiol Rev 2008;21:505-18.
31. Poropatich KO, Walker CL, Black RE. Quantifying the association between *Campylobacter* infection and Guillain-Barré syndrome: a systematic review. J Health Popul Nutr 2010;28:545-52.
32. Sack DA, Sack RB, Nair GB, et al. Cholera. Lancet 2004;363:223-33.
33. Alam NH, Islam S, Sattar S, et al. Safety of rapid intravenous rehydration and comparative efficacy of 3 oral rehydration solutions in the treatment of severely malnourished children with dehydrating cholera. J Pediatr Gastroenterol Nutr 2009;48:318-27.
34. McFarland LV, Ozen M, Dinleyici EC, et al. Comparison of pediatric and adult antibiotic-associated diarrhea and *Clostridium difficile* infections. World J Gastroenterol 2016;22:3078-104.
35. Sandora TJ, Fung M, Flaherty K, et al. Epidemiology and risk factors for *Clostridium difficile* infection in children. Pediatr Infect Dis J 2011;30:580-4.
36. Turco R, Martinelli M, Miele E, et al. Proton pump inhibitors as a risk factor for paediatric *Clostridium difficile* infection. Aliment Pharmacol Ther 2010;31:754-9.
37. Wilson ME. *Clostridium difficile* and childhood diarrhea: cause, consequence, or confounder. Clin Infect Dis 2006;43:814-6.
38. McDonald LC, Gerding DN, Johnson S, et al. Clinical practice guidelines for Clostridium difficile infection in adults and children: 2017 update by the Infectious Diseases Society of America (IDSA) and Society for Healthcare Epidemiology of America (SHEA). Clin Infect Dis 2018;66:987-94.
39. Fox TG, Manaloor JJ, Christenson JC. Travel-related infections in children. Pediatr Clin North Am 2013;60:507-27.
40. Mackell S. Traveler's diarrhea in the pediatric population: etiology and impact. Clin Infect Dis 2005;41:S547-52.

CHAPTER 44

Parasitic Infections in Pediatric Patients
Tracy M. Hagemann, Pharm.D., FCCP, FPPA

INTRODUCTION

Parasitic infections are common worldwide and are associated with significant morbidity and mortality. Developing countries in Central and South America, Africa, and Asia are most affected by these infections.[1] In the United States, immigrants and travelers from endemic countries are likely to become infected, as are people with immunocompromised conditions such as AIDS.

Parasites are more common where sanitation is suboptimal, and they are spread through contact with food or water contaminated with fecal matter. However, other transmission routes include contact with infected dirt, contaminated freshwater, and an insect vector such as a mosquito bite. Although rare, parasites may also be transmitted through blood transfusion, by sharing of infected needles, and congenitally from mother to infant.

A parasite lives in or on another species (the host) to survive, using the host for food, water, or shelter. Parasites may infect their host by being ingested or through the external surface. Some parasites require several hosts of different species to complete their life cycles. Parasites typically cause some degree of injury to the host. The extent of injury depends on parasite load as well as on the nutritional status and immunologic competence of the host. Parasitic infections in children may lead to malnutrition and stunted growth and development, especially chronic infections in the gastrointestinal (GI) tract.[2,3]

Parasites are defined as eukaryotic unicellular or multicellular microorganisms. They are usually classified as single-celled protozoa or multicellular helminthes, including worms. Protozoa that multiply in their human hosts may increase to cause overwhelming infection. By contrast, helminthes have more complex life cycles that typically involve substantial time outside their human hosts. As they migrate through tissue, they may cause systemic reactions. This chapter will focus on the most common parasitic infections in children in the United States and will be divided into three main sections: protozoa, both GI and systemic; helminthes; and ectoparasites. Cryptosporidiosis is discussed in the Infectious Diarrhea chapter.

GASTROINTESTINAL PROTOZOA

GIARDIA

Giardiasis is caused by *Giardia duodenalis*, also known as *Giardia lamblia* and *Giardia intestinalis*. Humans, as well as domesticated animals and wildlife, can be infected with *Giardia*. The most common animal reservoirs include beaver, cattle, dogs, rodents, and bighorn sheep.[4] This flagellated protozoan is the most common intestinal parasitic cause of enteritis worldwide and the second most common cause in the United States; in 2012, 15,223 cases were reported to the Centers for Disease Control and Prevention (CDC).[5-7] Children age 1–9 years are considered a high-risk group, and they may transmit the infection to their caregivers.[6] With annual seasonal variation, cases in the United States spike between June and October.

Giardia is transmitted by the fecal–oral route; thus, the incidence is higher in populations with poor sanitation, and it may be contracted through close contact with infected individuals.[5] *Giardia* cysts are ingested through fecally contaminated sources, often water. *Giardia* is resistant to the chlorine levels in normal tap water. Because *Giardia* survives well in cold mountain springs for extended periods, giardiasis often occurs in those who camp, backpack, or hunt; it has been called "backpacker's diarrhea" or "beaver fever."[6] The relative infectious dose is small; as few as 10–25 cysts may cause infection in humans.[6] Once the cysts are ingested, they are activated in the acidic environment of the stomach, where they produce two trophozoites. These trophozoites migrate to the duodenum and proximal jejunum, attach to the mucosal wall, and replicate, resulting in malabsorption, dyspepsia, and diarrhea. Trophozoites can transform into cysts and pass back into the feces, where they are excreted. They can remain actively infectious for months in moist environments.[5,6]

Clinical presentation varies between individuals but typically includes symptoms of diarrhea, abdominal cramps, bloating, weight loss, and malabsorption that may have had a gradual onset and last for 2–4 weeks.[5,6,8] A 1- to 2-week incubation period typically precedes symptoms. Chronic giardiasis may develop after the acute infection, if not treated appropriately. Symptoms of chronic infection vary but may include loose stools, steatorrhea, malabsorption, weight loss of 10%–20%, fatigue, and malaise that may last for months.[6] Some patients have rash as part of a sensitivity reaction.

Because Giardia infection is noninvasive, the gold standard for diagnosing giardiasis is stool studies for ova and parasites. Cyst excretion can be found in both formed and loose stools, whereas trophozoites are mainly found in diarrhea. A single stool specimen has a sensitivity of 50%–70%, but the sensitivity increases to 85%–90% with three serial stool samples.[8] Fecal immunoassays, such as direct fluorescent antibody testing, immunochromatographic assays, and enzyme-linked immunosorbent assays (ELISA), have a faster turnaround time and greater sensitivity than stool microscopy.[7,9-11] Direct fluorescent antibody testing kits are available that have 100% sensitivity and specificity compared with microscopy.[9] Rates of ELISA kit sensitivity have been reported as 94%–100%, whereas specificity rates were all 100%.[9]

The treatment goal in Giardia infections is to eradicate the organism, which will resolve symptoms. The drug of choice is oral metronidazole, administered three times daily for 5–7 days (Table 1).[12,13] Typical cure rates with metronidazole are 80%–95%.[8,14] In pediatric patients too young or unable to swallow a tablet, a liquid preparation may be required; however, no preparation is commercially available. Metronidazole suspension can be extemporaneously compounded, but the taste of these preparations is often foul, and some children will not tolerate it. Using metronidazole benzoate, a salt of metronidazole with virtually no taste issues, for compounding a suspension can help with adherence, as can administering the dose with chocolate syrup. An alternative product, nitazoxanide, has a U.S. Food and Drug Administration (FDA) label for the treatment of Giardia infections in both pediatric and adult patients and is commercially available in both tablet and suspension formulations. Nitazoxanide should be administered every 12 hours for 3 days and may be taken with food to minimize GI upset. Other alternative products include albendazole and tinidazole. Albendazole is as effective as metronidazole in treating Giardia infections in pediatric patients.[15] This option is good in children with mixed helminth and Giardia infections. A single dose of tinidazole may be more effective than metronidazole or albendazole in children older than 3 years; however, like metronidazole, tinidazole is not commercially available as an oral liquid preparation and has to be extemporaneously compounded.

Patients treated for giardiasis should be monitored for symptom resolution, including reduction in diarrhea, resolution of bloating and abdominal cramps, and improved oral tolerance. It is especially important to monitor for signs and symptoms of dehydration and weight loss in children and to initiate oral rehydration as necessary. Diarrhea may begin to resolve in a few days but can take as long as 1–2 weeks for full resolution. Some patients may develop post-Giardia

Table 1. Drugs for Treatment of Giardia Infections[12,13,15,61]

Drug	Dosage (Oral)	Form	Common ADRs	Comments
Albendazole	10 mg/kg/day once daily for 5 days (max 400 mg/day)	Tablet: 200 mg	Abdominal pain, nausea, headache	Tablets may be crushed or chewed Take with food
Metronidazole	15–30 mg/kg/day in divided doses Q 8 hr for 5–7 days (max 250 mg/dose)	Capsule: 375 mg Tablet: 250 mg, 500 mg	Nausea, headache	May compound oral suspension 50 mg/mL[12]
Nitazoxanide	Children age 1–3 yr: 100 mg Q 12 hr for 3 days Children age 4–11 yr: 200 mg Q 12 hr for 3 days Adolescents age ≥ 12 yr: 500 mg Q 12 hr for 3 days	Suspension: 100 mg/ 5 mL Tablet: 500 mg	Abdominal pain, diarrhea, nausea, headache	Store reconstituted suspension at room temperature Discard unused portion after 7 days
Tinidazole	50 mg/kg once (max 2 g)	Tablet: 250 mg, 500 mg	Nausea, altered sense of taste	Only in children age > 3 yr Oral suspension 67 mg/mL can be compounded[13] Take with food

ADR = adverse drug reaction; max = maximum; Q = every.

lactose intolerance and will improve with the institution of a lactose-free diet. Patients who appear unresponsive to treatment should be evaluated for possible reinfection or antibiotic resistance. Patients with reinfection who initially received a course of metronidazole should receive a second course of 5–7 days, or they may be treated with one of the alternative drugs. Patients with a true antibiotic resistance to one drug should be treated with an alternative drug.[15,16] If two or more treatment courses with a given drug are unsuccessful, then another drug alone, or in combination with the first drug, is recommended.[16]

Strategies for preventing giardiasis include proper and frequent handwashing and use of proper sewage disposal and water treatment. In endemic areas, ingestion of bottled water is preferred to consumption of tap water or from freestanding bodies of water. In day care settings, proper disposal of diapers, as well as exceptional handwashing techniques when changing soiled diapers, should be used. When intake of potentially contaminated water is necessary, giardiasis may be prevented by boiling water for 1 minute (at altitudes higher than 6562 feet, boil for 3 minutes), heating water to 158°F (70°C) for 10 minutes, using portable camping filters, or using iodine purification tablets in potable water.[17]

AMEBIASIS

Entamoeba are nonflagellated protozoa that are ubiquitous worldwide, but they do not typically cause pathogenic diseases in human hosts. The exception is *Entamoeba histolytica*, which causes amebic colitis and liver abscess. *Entamoeba histolytica* is most prevalent in tropical and developing countries.[7] Worldwide, about 10% of the population is infected, 90% of whom are asymptomatic.[4] In the 10% who are symptomatic, around 100,000 deaths occur annually, making *E. histolytica* the world's second leading cause of protozoan-related death after malaria.[6] Most U.S. cases occur in travelers returning from endemic countries or in recent immigrants from Mexico, India, West and South Africa, and parts of Central and South America. In the United States, the prevalence of amebiasis is about 4% of the general population.[18] Infection is common in individuals with compromised immune systems.[6] Transmission is by the fecal–oral route and is increased by crowding and poor sanitation.

The infective cysts of *E. histolytica* are ingested and hatch into trophozoites in the small intestine, where they continue through the digestive tract to the colon. Some of these trophozoites become cysts that are passed into the feces; after they are excreted, they can survive for months in a moist environment, like *Giardia*. However, trophozoites can also invade the intestinal mucosa and produce flask-shaped ulcers in the submucosa; they may spread to the liver, lungs, and brain through the bloodstream.[6,8,18] The intestinal ulcerations may bleed and lead to colitis within 2–6 weeks of the initial infection.[17] Colitis is followed by weight loss, severe abdominal pain, bloody diarrhea, malaise, and fever. A chronic active infection of *E. histolytica* may mimic the symptoms of inflammatory bowel disease. In disseminated disease, trophozoites penetrate the mucosal wall, enter the liver, and release toxins that cause hepatocyte damage and lead to amebic liver

abscesses and periportal fibrosis, usually within 5 months of the initial infection.[6] Amebae are chemotactic, which may lead to a significant leukocytosis with left shift and high temperature. Other objective findings include elevated alkaline phosphatase, liver tenderness, dull pleuritic right upper quadrant pain that radiates to the right shoulder, and hepatomegaly.[6,18,19] Liver abscesses can spread to the lungs and pleura and may rupture into the pericardial, peritoneal, or pleural spaces.[6]

Effective diagnosis depends on a reliable patient history, including any recent international travel, as well as serial stool samples for ova and parasites and an *E. histolytica* stool antigen test.[6,9,18] Microscopy requires fresh stool samples and a high level of skill and typically has less than 60% sensitivity and 10%–50% specificity.[20] Tests with the greatest sensitivity and specificity include stool antigen detection with ELISA (greater than 95% sensitivity and specificity) and serum antibody detection with ELISA (greater than 90% sensitivity, greater than 85% specificity).[20] Because only 10%–35% of patients with liver abscesses have concomitant GI symptoms, magnetic resonance imaging, serology, and liver ultrasonography should be performed if amebic liver involvement is suspected.[18] Biopsy may be needed.

The goal of therapy for amebiasis is to eradicate the parasite by amebicides. However, supportive care may be necessary for 6 months to 1 year while the ulcerations and abscesses resolve and heal.[6] Amebiasis may manifest as invasive liver abscess, intraluminal colitis, and asymptomatic cyst carriage, and drug therapy may differ depending on the type and site of infection. Asymptomatic cyst carriers should receive oral paromomycin every 8 hours for 7 days (Table 2). This treatment has 84%–96% cure rates.[21] Paromomycin acts only in the lumen of the intestines and is only minimally absorbed by the GI tract. The mainstay for invasive amebiasis is oral metronidazole taken three times daily for 7–10 days. An alternative is once-daily tinidazole for 3–5 days. Tinidazole may be used in adults and children older than 3 years for both localized intestinal and invasive infections and may be better tolerated than metronidazole. Both erythromycin and tetracycline may be used in patients with contraindications to or intolerance of metronidazole or tinidazole. After completing treatment for invasive amebiasis, patients should receive a full course of a luminal amebicide (paromomycin) to ensure complete eradication (Table 2).

Drug effectiveness should be monitored by symptom resolution, and by repeat negative stool examinations after 5–7 days of treatment, at the end of the treatment course, and at 1 month after therapy ends. Intestinal symptoms abate within 3–5 days of treatment initiation. Patients with colitis may need a colonoscopy if serial stool samples are negative. Colonoscopy with tissue sample may identify amebiasis in patients with bloody diarrhea if other tests are inconclusive. In invasive disease, serology should be monitored for resolution at the end of treatment and 1 month after therapy ends. Patients with liver abscesses may require repeat imaging, although some radiographic evidence of liver abscesses may persist for up to 1 year after treatment ends.[21]

Prevention of amebiasis includes using proper sanitation to eradicate the carriage of cysts. Travelers to endemic areas should be cautioned to avoid consuming unpeeled fruit and vegetables, salads, ice cubes, and untreated water. If bottled water is unavailable, water should be boiled, which will eradicate *E. histolytica* cysts. Water may be disinfected with iodine or bleach solutions and may also be filtered.[6,18]

SYSTEMIC PROTOZOA

MALARIA

Malaria is a significant cause of morbidity and mortality in developing nations worldwide, with around 214 million clinical episodes in 2015 and 438,000 deaths, mainly in children younger than 5 years.[22] Although malaria is uncommon in the United States, 2078 cases of malaria in the United States were confirmed by the CDC in 2016, including 7 deaths.[23] Most of these cases occurred in people who had traveled to or came from endemic areas and did not adhere to chemoprophylaxis guidelines. In 2016, 17% of U.S. cases occurred in children younger than 18 years, accounting for 365 children total, mainly in those age 2–17 years.[23] Most of these infections were attributed to travel to Africa. Of the reported cases of malaria in U.S. residents, only 26.3% reported taking any chemoprophylaxis and adherence was very poor.[23]

Malaria in humans is caused by five different species of the *Plasmodium* parasite: *P. falciparum*, *P. vivax*, *P. ovale*, *P. malariae*, and *P. knowlesi*.[24,25] Presentation in humans is similar in all of these species, which can make it difficult to differentiate between species during diagnosis, but of these, *P. falciparum* is the most deadly. Although not often fatal, *P. vivax* and *P. ovale* are responsible for significant morbidity in endemic areas and may lie dormant in liver hepatocytes for months to years after exposure.[24] *Plasmodium vivax* is endemic to India, Pakistan, Bangladesh, Sri Lanka, and Central America, and it has the greatest burden of disease with a long incubation period but rarely causes severe complications. *Plasmodium falciparum* is endemic in Africa, Haiti, the Amazon region, the Dominican Republic, and New Guinea.[26] Infected individuals may progress to life-threatening illness within hours of infection.[26] *Plasmodium malariae* is distributed worldwide and often manifests with proteinuria. *Plasmodium ovale* infections mainly occur in Africa, and infections are usually less severe and relapse less often; spontaneous recovery is not uncommon.[27] *Plasmodium knowlesi* mainly occurs in certain countries in Southeast Asia, including Malaysia, Borneo, Philippines, Thailand, Singapore, and Cambodia, with high case-fatality rates, because of rapid replication and hyperparasitemia.[25]

Malaria is transmitted when an infected female *Anopheles* mosquito bites a human host. During the blood meal, the mosquito injects sporozoites of *Plasmodium* spp. into the individual's bloodstream.[27] These sporozoites travel to the liver, where asexual reproduction of the parasites enters a latent stage that lasts 8–30 days.[24] *Plasmodium vivax* and *P. ovale* form dormant hypnozoites that remain in the liver unless targeted therapy is administered. Without directed therapy to these dormant hypnozoites, a relapsing form of the disease can occur. After the latent stage, merozoites, or daughter cells, are released from the liver back into systemic circulation. The merozoites infect erythrocytes and begin another asexual reproductive cycle that results in lysing of the red blood cells within 2–6 days.[24]

Initial presentation of malaria may involve nonspecific symptoms such as fever, chills, malaise, diaphoresis, vomiting, and rigors.[24,27] Patients may have headache, myalgia, abdominal pain, arthralgia, cyclic shivering, and sweating. Anemia and splenomegaly may develop because of extensive hemolysis during the erythrocytic phase of infection. The most severe complications, including hypoglycemia, thrombocytopenia, acute renal failure, heart failure, seizures, and coma, occur in patients with *P. falciparum* infection because of its ability to invade erythrocytes of all ages, resulting in high levels of

Table 2. Drugs for Treatment of Amebiasis Infections[12,13,15,61]

Infection	Drug	Dosage (Oral)	Form	Common ADRs	Comments
Asymptomatic, Intraluminal	Paromomycin	25–35 mg/kg/day divided Q 8 hr for 5–10 days (max 4 g/day)	Capsule: 250 mg	Abdominal cramping, diarrhea, nausea	Usual duration is 7 days
Dysentery[a]	Metronidazole	35–50 mg/kg/day in divided doses Q 8 hr for 7–10 days (max 750 mg/dose)	Capsule: 375 mg Tablet: 250 mg, 500 mg	Nausea, headache	May need to compound oral suspension 50 mg/mL[12]
Extraluminal[a]	Metronidazole	35–50 mg/kg/day in divided doses Q 8 hr for 7–10 days (max 750 mg/dose)	Capsule: 375 mg Tablet: 250 mg, 500 mg	Nausea, headache	May need to compound oral suspension 50 mg/mL[12]
	Tinidazole	50 mg/kg/day for 3–5 days (max 2 g/day)	Tablet: 250 mg, 500 mg	Nausea, altered sense of taste	Only in children age > 3 yr Take with food Oral suspension 67 mg/mL can be compounded[13]

[a]After completing treatment for dysentery or extraluminal disease, patients should be treated with an intraluminal drug (paromomycin) to clear the intestinal organisms.
ADR = adverse drug reaction; max = maximum; Q = every.

parasitemia.[25] Patient groups at highest risk of these complications from *P. falciparum* are children younger than 5 years and pregnant women.[19] Most young children become restless or drowsy and have loss of appetite, persistent fever, flulike symptoms, seizures, vomiting, and/or diarrhea.[22,28] Typically, young children do not have the cyclic shivering and sweating, but older children may. Neonates with signs and symptoms of parasitemia within 1 week of birth have contracted malaria through transplacental transmission and have congenital malaria. They often present with fever and poor feeding in addition to objective findings of anemia, hepatosplenomegaly, and jaundice.[28,29] Treating pregnant women with malaria infection can decrease the risk of congenital malaria in the newborn.[29]

The gold standard for diagnosing malaria is the detection of parasites on blood smear by light microscopy.[23] Blood smears should be obtained every 12–24 hours on 3 consecutive days; a positive finding indicates infection.[24] Diagnosis of malaria can be difficult in children because only 50% of those infected have a positive blood smear, even with repeated examinations. Blood antigen capture tests have a high sensitivity and specificity and can produce rapid results. Both DNA and RNA probes, as well as polymerase chain reaction (PCR), also have good sensitivity and specificity and may be used to confirm a diagnosis.[24,27]

Pharmacotherapy for malaria can be grouped as follows: *chemoprophylaxis for travelers to endemic areas*, and *treatment of the active infection*. The goal of chemoprophylaxis is to lessen the likelihood of transmission because no preventive regimen is 100% effective. The goals of care are to quickly and effectively identify the infecting *Plasmodium* spp. and eradicate the infection to avoid complications.

PREVENTION

Prevention of malaria infection should consist of a combination of mosquito avoidance measures and chemoprophylaxis. Malarial transmission usually occurs between dusk and dawn in endemic areas, secondary to the feeding habits of the *Anopheles* mosquito. Contact with mosquitos may be reduced by wearing clothes that cover most areas of the body, remaining in well-screened areas, using mosquito bed nets, and using a pyrethroid-containing insect spray in both living and sleeping areas, especially during evening and nighttime hours.[30] Children older than 2 months should have a spray that contains up to 50% DEET (*N, N*-diethyl-meta-toluamide) applied to exposed parts of the skin when mosquito exposure is expected. The CDC also recommends a permethrin-containing product for applying to clothes and bed nets as additional protection.[30]

Before choosing a chemoprophylactic regimen, several patient-specific factors should be considered, including other medical conditions, concurrent drugs, and potential adverse effects of the antimalarial drug.[30] Chemoprophylactic regimens involve taking a drug before, during, and after leaving the endemic area.[30] The travel plan with respect to location and any known information on the area's transmission rates and antimalarial drug resistance patterns must be thoroughly assessed well in advance of departure. An excellent resource

on endemic area transmission rates and resistance is the *CDC Health Information for International Travel* (commonly called the *Yellow Book*), which is updated regularly and available online at https://wwwnc.cdc.gov/travel/page/yellowbook-home. Another helpful resource is the World Health Organization International Travel website at www.who.int/ith/en/.

Pediatric patients are at high risk of complications and transmission of malaria. Children traveling to endemic areas should take prophylactic antimalarial drugs (Table 3). Depending on the incidence of drug resistance at the destination, chloroquine and mefloquine are options. *Plasmodium falciparum* is chloroquine resistant in most endemic areas, except for Central America west of the Panama Canal, Haiti, the Dominican Republic, and most of the Middle East.[30] Where *P. falciparum* is resistant, mefloquine is an alternative option. However, mefloquine has severe neuropsychiatric adverse effects such as anxiety, paranoia, depression, hallucinations, confusion, and psychotic behavior. These effects can be difficult to identify in children, especially in those who are nonverbal, so another drug such as atovaquone/proguanil may be preferred. Children traveling to areas where *P. vivax* is predominant may use primaquine if they are not deficient in glucose-6-phosphate dehydrogenase.[30] Doxycycline is an option for children older than 8 years in chloroquine- or mefloquine-resistant malaria areas.[21,29]

Antimalarial drugs available in the United States come only in tablet form, and the taste can be quite bitter. If the child cannot swallow tablets, a compounding pharmacy may be able to produce an appropriate extemporaneous liquid formulation. Alternatively, the caregiver can crush and mix the tablet with a small amount of applesauce or syrup to ensure that the entire dose is delivered to the child.

TREATMENT

Treatment strategies depend on the species of malaria, drug resistance patterns in the area where the infection was acquired, age, pregnancy status, and disease severity.[29] Drugs used to treat malaria are active against the erythrocyte attack phase. Chloroquine, atovaquone/proguanil, artemether/lumefantrine, artesunate, mefloquine, quinine, doxycycline, and clindamycin are used for treatment. A new agent, tafenoquine, can be used in children age 16 years and older as a single dose to prevent relapse in those receiving appropriate antimalarial therapy for *P. vivax* infection.[31] Usually, when quinine is used, it is in combination with doxycycline and clindamycin. *Plasmodium vivax* and *P. ovale* have dormant stages in the liver, and their treatment regimens must include primaquine to eradicate these forms to prevent disease relapse (Table 4).[32,33] The CDC has a Malaria Hotline (toll-free at 855-856-4713) that helps clinicians with diagnosis or treatment of malaria.[30]

Children with fever who can still maintain adequate hydration and nutrition can be treated as outpatients. Oral acetaminophen can be used for fever. Although many children with malaria develop anemia, transfusions with packed red blood cells are rarely needed. Any child with vomiting, signs of dehydration, altered consciousness, convulsions, or difficulty breathing should be admitted to the hospital for treatment and supportive care.

Patients treated with antimalarial therapy should be monitored for symptom resolution. Prior malarial infection does not necessarily produce immunity in patients, and research has not yet provided an effective vaccine. Health care providers should stress the importance of prophylactic measures for travelers to malaria-endemic areas.

TRYPANOSOMIASIS (CHAGAS DISEASE)

Chagas disease is caused by infection with *Trypanosoma cruzi*, a protozoan parasite carried by reduviid bugs, also known as *kissing bugs* because of their propensity to feed at night, usually on an uncovered face.[34] Infection occurs when the bug defecates while feeding, and fecal material containing *T. cruzi* is introduced into the host through the bite or through mucous membranes.[35] Other methods of transmission are blood transfusion, congenital transfer from mother to fetus, and ingestion of food or water contaminated with bug feces.[34] Reduviid bugs live in the wall cracks of houses in rural areas of Central and South America, and 10 million people worldwide are estimated to be infected with *T. cruzi*.[15] Most individuals infected with *T. cruzi* in the United States are immigrants from endemic areas of Latin America, but eight vector-borne cases have been reported in the United States since 1995.[35]

The clinical course of Chagas disease consists of the acute and chronic phases. The acute phase in adults is mainly asymptomatic, but children are more likely to have a red nodule at the inoculation site within 1 week of infection.[15] If the inoculation site is the eye, unilateral orbital edema may result, also known as the *Romaña sign*. This manifestation is followed by fever, malaise, hepatosplenomegaly, and lymphadenopathy.[15,36] Complications from acute infection include myocarditis and meningoencephalitis.[37] The acute phase usually lasts 4–8 weeks, after which the parasitic load drops to undetectable levels, and is then followed by asymptomatic chronic infection.[38,39]

Most infected patients never develop symptoms but remain infected throughout their lives.[39] However, 20%–30% (mainly adults with long-term disease) develop manifestations of chronic Chagas disease, including cardiac aneurysms, megaesophagus, and megacolon. Infected mothers may pass the infection to their infants. In the United States, 65–315 congenital *T. cruzi* infections are estimated to occur annually.[35] Congenital infections cannot be prevented by treating pregnant women, given that the currently available drugs are not recommended in pregnancy because of the lack of safety data. However, a recent study of women with Chagas disease who had previously been treated with benznidazole did not show congenital transmission to their newborns, indicating that early treatment of women of childbearing age is important.[40]

Table 3. Prophylactic Antimalarial Drugs[15,22,30,61]

Drug	Dosage (Oral)	Form	Duration	Common ADRs
Chloroquine phosphate	5 mg/kg base once weekly (max 300 mg base) Chloroquine phosphate 16.6 mg = 10 mg chloroquine base	Tablet: 250 mg (150 mg base), 500 mg (300 mg base) Suspension (compounded): 15 mg/mL (9 mg base/mL)[30]	Start 2 wk before and continue for 4 wk after exposure	Nausea, abdominal pain, diarrhea, blurred vision
Chloroquine-Resistant Areas				
Atovaquone/ proguanil	5–8 kg: 31.25 mg/12.5 mg once daily 9–10 kg: 46.88 mg/18.75 mg once daily 11–20 kg: 62.5 mg/25 mg once daily 21–30 kg: 125 mg/50 mg once daily 31–40 kg: 187.5 mg/75 mg once daily > 40 kg: 250 mg/100 mg once daily	Pediatric tablet: atovaquone 62.5 mg/proguanil 25 mg Tablet: atovaquone 250 mg/proguanil 100 mg	Start 1-2 days before exposure and continue for 1 wk after exposure Tablet may be crushed or chewed	Photosensitivity, pruritus, abdominal pain, diarrhea, nausea, changes in liver function, headache, cough
Doxycycline[a]	2.2 mg/kg once daily (max 100 mg/day)	Tablet: 50 mg, 100 mg Capsule: 50 mg, 100 mg Suspension: 25 mg/5 mL Syrup: 50 mg/5 mL	Start 1–2 days before exposure and continue for 4 wk after exposure	Photosensitivity, diarrhea, nasopharyngitis
Mefloquine	≤ 9 kg: 5 mg/kg salt once weekly 10–19 kg: ¼ tablet once weekly (62.5 mg) 20–30 kg: ½ tablet once weekly (125 mg) 31–45 kg: ¾ tablet once weekly (187.5 mg) > 45 kg: 1 tablet once weekly (250 mg) (max 250 mg/wk)	Tablet: 250 mg 250 mg salt = 228 mg base	Start 2 wk before exposure and continue for 4 wk after exposure Take with food	Abdominal pain, diarrhea, nausea, vomiting, bradycardia Avoid in patients with seizures, cardiac conditions and those with psychiatric conditions
Primaquine[b]	0.5 mg/kg base once daily (max 30 mg base/day)	Tablet: 26.3 mg (15 mg base)	Start 1–2 days before and continue for 1 wk after exposure	Abdominal pain, nausea

[a]Only for use in children age ≥ 8 yr.
[b]Contraindicated in patients with deficiency of glucose-6-phosphate dehydrogenase.
ADR = adverse drug reaction; max = maximum.

Table 4. Drugs for Treatment of Malaria (*Plasmodium falciparum* or Unidentified Species)[22,30,32,33,61]

Drug	Dosage (Oral)	Form	Comments
Chloroquine Sensitive (Uncomplicated)			
Chloroquine phosphate	10 mg base/kg; then 5 mg base/kg at 6, 24, 48 hr Total 25 mg base/kg	Tablet: 250 mg (150 mg base); 500 mg (300 mg base)	Do not exceed 600 mg base for 1st dose and 300 mg base for subsequent doses Suspension (compounded): 15 mg/mL (9 mg base/mL)[32] Common ADRs: nausea, abdominal pain, diarrhea, blurred vision
Hydroxychloroquine	10 mg base/kg; then 5 mg base/kg at 6, 24, 48 hr Total 25 mg base/kg	Tablet: 200 mg (155 mg base)	Do not exceed 620 mg base for 1st dose and 310 mg base for subsequent doses Suspension (compounded): 25 mg/mL (19.4 mg base/mL)[33] Common ADRs: headache, abdominal pain, nausea, corneal disorders
Chloroquine Resistant[a] (Uncomplicated)			
Artemether/ lumefantrine	5 to < 15 kg: 1 tablet/dose 15 to < 25 kg: 2 tablets/dose 25 to < 35 kg: 3 tablets/dose ≥ 35 kg: 4 tablets/dose	Tablet: 20 mg of artemether/ 120 mg of lumefantrine	3-day treatment for a total of 6 oral doses: Initial dose; then 2nd dose in 8 hr; then 1 dose twice daily for next 2 days Common ADRs: diarrhea, vomiting, headache, cough, fever
Atovaquone/ proguanil	5–8 kg: 2 pediatric tablets once daily for 3 days 9–10 kg: 3 pediatric tablets once daily for 3 days 11–20 kg: 1 adult tablet once daily for 3 days 21–30 kg: 2 adult tablets once daily for 3 days 31–40 kg: 3 adult tablets once daily for 3 days > 40 kg: 4 adult tablets once daily for 3 days	Pediatric tablet: atovaquone 62.5 mg/proguanil 25 mg Adult tablet: atovaquone 250 mg/ proguanil 100 mg	May cause photosensitivity reactions Common ADRs: pruritus, abdominal pain, diarrhea, nausea, changes in liver function, headache, cough
Mefloquine	15 mg/kg salt for first dose, followed by 10 mg/kg salt given 6–12 hr after initial dose Total 25 mg/kg salt (max 750 mg first dose, 500 mg 2nd dose)	Tablet: 250 mg (228 mg base)	Take with food Common ADRs: abdominal pain, diarrhea, nausea, vomiting, bradycardia Not recommended unless other options unavailable
Quinine sulfate + one of the following: doxycycline, tetracycline, or clindamycin[b]	Quinine sulfate: 10 mg/kg Q 8 hr for 3 or 7 days[c] Doxycycline: 2.2 mg/kg Q 12 hr for 7 days Tetracycline: 25 mg/kg/day divided Q 6 hr for 7 days Clindamycin: 20 mg/kg/day divided Q 8 hr for 7 days	Quinine sulfate: capsule 324 mg Doxycycline: tablet: 50 mg, 100 mg Capsule: 50 mg, 100 mg Suspension: 25 mg/5 mL Syrup: 50 mg/5 mL Tetracycline: capsule: 250 mg, 500 mg Clindamycin: capsule: 75 mg, 150 mg, 300 mg Solution (oral): 75 mg/5 mL	Doxycycline and tetracycline should not be used in children age < 8 yr Common ADRs with quinine: syncope, photosensitivity, rash, diarrhea, nausea, vomiting, loss of appetite
Patients with Diagnosis of Severe Malaria[c,d] (Complicated)			
Artesunate	Intravenous therapy with IV artesunate ≥ 20 kg: 2.4 mg/kg per dose for 4 doses < 20 kg: 3 mg/kg per dose for 4 doses Follow artesunate treatment with one of the following: artemether-lumefantrine, atovaquone-proguanil, doxycycline, or clindamycin in doses as described above (or if unable to take oral medications, use IV formulation as below:	Solution for injection: 110 mg	Available under an expanded IND protocol through CDC Initial dose then repeat dose at 12, 24, and 48 hours for 4 total doses Interim treatment while waiting for artesunate to arrive, consider using artemether-lumefantrine, atovaquone-proguanil, or quinine PO or through a nasogastric tube. If no other options available may use mefloquine.

(continued)

Table 4. Drugs for Treatment of Malaria (*Plasmodium falciparum* or Unidentified Species)[22,30,32,33,61] *(continued)*

Drug	Dosage (Oral)	Form	Comments
Patients with Diagnosis of Severe Malaria[c,d] (Complicated)			
Artesunate *(continued)*	Doxycycline: 2.2 mg/kg IV Q 12 hr (< 45 kg), or 100 mg IV Q 12 hr (≥ 45 kg) for 7 days; then change to oral dosing as above, when possible Clindamycin: 10 mg/kg IV loading dose, followed by 5 mg/kg IV Q 8 hr for 7 days; then change to oral dosing as above, when possible	Doxycycline: IV: 100 mg of powder for reconstitution Clindamycin: IV: 150 mg/mL	Doxycycline should not be used in children age < 8 yr

[a]Treatment with atovaquone/proguanil, artemether/lumefantrine, or quinine + doxycycline, tetracycline, or clindamycin is equally recommended. Mefloquine should only be used when other preferred treatments have contraindications because of severe neuropsychiatric reactions with mefloquine at treatment doses.
[b]Quinine in combination with doxycycline or tetracycline is generally preferred to combination with clindamycin because of better efficacy data.
[c]Infections acquired in Southeast Asia should receive quinine/quinidine for 7 days; all others should continue for 3 days.
[d]Patients with a diagnosis of severe malaria should be aggressively treated with parenteral antimalarial therapy. Intravenous artesunate should be initiated as soon as diagnosis is confirmed. Consultation with the CDC or a physician experienced in treating malaria is recommended.
ADR = adverse drug reaction; IV = intravenous; max = maximum; PO = oral; Q = every.

Most infected newborns are asymptomatic, or they may have nonspecific symptoms such as low birth weight, low Apgar scores, prematurity, anemia, or thrombocytopenia.[38] Although serious complications, such as myocarditis, meningoencephalitis, and respiratory disease, are rare in newborns, they carry a high risk of mortality.[38] Before 2007, when widespread blood bank screening in the United States was initiated, *T. cruzi* could be contracted from infected donated blood products.[34] From 1993 to 2007, five transfusion-related cases were documented in the United States, all in immunocompromised individuals.[34] Reactivation of disease and symptoms may occur in chronically infected individuals who become immunocompromised.[39]

Diagnosis of acute trypanosomiasis is made through microscopically examining the blood for the presence of the parasite. Suspected cases of chronic trypanosomiasis infection should be evaluated through serologic testing for antibodies to *T. cruzi*. Because the available assays used alone may yield low sensitivity and/or specificity rates, World Health Organization experts in Chagas disease recommend that each specimen be tested with two types of assays, such as ELISA, indirect immunofluorescence, or indirect hemagglutination.[36,39] Use of two different assays has a sensitivity greater than 99.96% and a specificity greater than 99.93%.[41] Parasites are not detectable in peripheral blood during chronic-phase infections; therefore, PCR is not a useful diagnostic test during this phase.[39]

The goals of therapy for treating acute and congenital *T. cruzi* infections are to reduce disease duration and prevent chronic infection. Two drugs have proven efficacy against *T. cruzi*: nifurtimox and benznidazole. Only benznidazole has an FDA label for use in the United States, although nifurtimox may be obtained directly from the CDC under investigative protocols.[42] Drug treatment is always recommended for acute and reactivated *T. cruzi* infections in individuals of all ages, in early congenital infections, and in children younger than 18 years with chronic *T. cruzi* infection.[34,39] If treatment is initiated in the acute phase of infection, the parasitologic cure rate is about 85%, and in congenitally infected infants treated in the first year of life, the cure rate is about 90%.[38] In children younger than 18 years with chronic asymptomatic

disease, benznidazole has 60% efficacy in attaining cure and appears to slow the development and progression of Chagas cardiomyopathy in chronically infected older children and adults.[38] Benznidazole is given for 60 days and nifurtimox for 90 days. For children younger than 12 years, benznidazole should be dosed at 5–8 mg/kg orally in two divided doses; for those 12 years and older, it should be dosed at 5–7 mg/kg orally in two divided doses. For children who are unable to swallow tablets, a slurry can be made using the 12.5 mg or 100 mg tablets and water.[42] Common adverse effects include anorexia and weight loss, allergic dermatitis, peripheral neuropathy, and insomnia. Nifurtimox dosing for children 10 years and younger is 15–20 mg/kg orally in three or four divided doses/day; for those age 11–16 years, 12.5–15 mg/kg orally in three or four divided doses/day; and for those 17 years and older, 8–10 mg/kg orally in three or four divided doses/day. Common adverse effects of nifurtimox include anorexia, weight loss, nausea, vomiting, headache, dizziness, vertigo, and polyneuropathy. Both drugs are contraindicated in severe hepatic and renal disease and in breastfeeding.[39] Treatment efficacy can be assessed by monitoring for the disappearance of *T. cruzi*–specific antibodies, although this outcome may take up to several years in some patients. Treatment failures can be assessed by repeated hemoculture or PCR-based assay.[39]

Preventive measures of infection should include using insecticides in the sleeping areas of infested houses. Travelers to endemic areas are rarely at risk, but if they will be camping, sleeping outdoors, or sleeping in houses with poor construction, insecticide-impregnated bed nets are recommended.[39]

TOXOPLASMOSIS

Toxoplasma gondii exists worldwide in animals and birds, although felines are the most common source.[15] Oocytes of *T. gondii* can survive in moist soil for up to 18 months; however, their survival is decreased in dry, extremely cold, or hot climates and at higher altitudes. Human infection occurs through ingesting food or water that is contaminated with infected cat feces; ingesting undercooked infected animal meats from cattle, sheep, or pigs containing *T. gondii* sporozoites; or congenitally from an infected mother to fetus.[43,44] In the United States, it is estimated that 23% of the population older than 12 years has been infected with *Toxoplasma*.[44] Congenital toxoplasmosis occurs in 500–5000 newborns per year in the United States.[45] In most cases, infection is asymptomatic and resolves spontaneously without treatment; however, treatment is indicated for pregnant mothers, neonates, and immunocompromised individuals.[15]

Cats become infected with toxoplasmosis by eating infected birds, rodents, or other small animals. Sporozoites, which are eliminated in cat feces, must undergo sporulation to become infectious, which usually takes 2–3 days in temperate climates. Cats may shed 1–100 million sporozoites up to 3 weeks after their first infection. The risk of infection from cat litter boxes may be minimized if the litter is changed daily before this process occurs.[45] Human infection results from ingesting contaminated or inadequately cooked food infected with tissue cysts or sporozoites. Flies and cockroaches are thought to transport sporozoites to water and food. Once infected, only 10%–20% of acute infections produce symptoms, of which the most common is lymphadenopathy without fever.[43] Other physical findings may include fever, malaise, myalgia, hepatosplenomegaly, and lymphocytosis. Toxoplasmosis in immunocompetent individuals is self-limited, although lymphadenopathy may persist for several months.[43] In immunocompromised hosts, such as those undergoing chemotherapy for malignancy, those with HIV, or those who take immunosuppressive drugs post-transplantation, severe toxoplasmosis can follow acute infection or reactivation of prior infection.[43] Severe toxoplasmosis can lead to complications such as encephalitis, chorioretinitis, myocarditis, or pneumonia. Pregnant women who are infected are of special concern because they may pass the infection to their infant. Infection early in pregnancy may result in fetal demise, miscarriage, or severe congenital effects in the infant, whereas infection in the later stages of pregnancy is more likely associated with vertical transmission to the infant.[15] Although most neonates are asymptomatic at birth, symptoms may include the following: fever; microcephaly or hydrocephaly; hepatosplenomegaly; jaundice; chorioretinitis and/or blindness; seizures; intracranial calcifications; myocarditis; strabismus; thrombocytopenia; and an erythroblastosis-like syndrome.[46] The overall mortality rate of congenital toxoplasmosis is around 10%, and newborns with acute symptoms often die within the first month of life.[47]

Toxoplasmosis is diagnosed by identifying *Toxoplasma*-specific IgG, IgM, or IgA (immunoglobulin G, M, and A) antibodies, either through indirect fluorescent antibody test or ELISA. Direct observation of the parasite in biopsy tissue is also diagnostic.[44] In pregnant women, PCR can be performed on amniotic fluid at 18 weeks' gestation.[48]

The treatment goal is to eradicate the rapidly dividing parasitic organisms in acute infection. Treatment may not be needed in patients who are immunocompetent with acute infection because the infection is usually self-limited. Treatment of existing acute infection will not reverse central nervous system damage that is already present, but it may prevent further sequelae. Treatment of infected pregnant women may reduce vertical transmission to the fetus and the frequency of adverse outcomes.[43]

Children who are immunocompetent with toxoplasmic lymphadenopathy should not be treated unless the symptoms are severe because the disease is usually self-limited. Immunocompromised patients should receive a three-drug regimen of pyrimethamine with sulfadiazine plus leucovorin to prevent hematologic toxicity. Patients who are allergic to or cannot tolerate sulfadiazine can use clindamycin instead, in combination with pyrimethamine and leucovorin (Table 5). Alternative therapy with trimethoprim/sulfamethoxazole may be used, but it may not be as active in immunocompromised patients.[43]

Pregnant women in their first and early second trimester with acute toxoplasmosis should receive spiramycin 1 g orally every 8 hours without food until term or until fetal infection has been documented.[43] If fetal infection is documented after 18 weeks' gestation, the three-drug regimen of pyrimethamine with sulfadiazine plus leucovorin should be initiated and continued until term.[43,45] Because pyrimethamine has teratogenic effects, it cannot be used during the first trimester of pregnancy.[43,52]

Neonates and infants with congenital toxoplasmosis should be treated for 1 year with pyrimethamine and sulfadiazine plus leucovorin, although treatment practices may vary by neonatal center.[43,46] Treatment is generally discontinued when blood tests are negative for *Toxoplasma* antibodies.[46]

Prevention of toxoplasmosis includes proper handwashing techniques, especially for pregnant women and immunocompromised individuals. Hands should be thoroughly washed after handling raw meat and unwashed vegetables and fruits. Cutting boards, dishes, counters, and utensils should be washed in hot, soapy water after contact with raw meat. To limit environmental exposure, gloves should be worn when gardening or coming into contact with dirt or sand because hands may be contaminated with infected cat feces. Cat litter boxes should be changed daily but not by pregnant or immunocompromised individuals. To decrease transmission from cats, they should be kept indoors and fed only canned or dried commercial foods. All outdoor sandboxes should be covered when not in use.[52]

HELMINTHS

ASCARIASIS

Infection with the parasite *Ascaris lumbricoides*, the largest intestinal nematode found in humans, is distributed worldwide but is more common in Southeast Asia, Africa, and South and Central America, with more than 1.4 billion individuals infected worldwide.[53] Those living in tropical and subtropical areas with poor sanitation and poor personal hygiene and in places were human feces are used as fertilizer are commonly infected. Transmission is fecal–oral, through ingesting embryonic eggs in soil. In the United States, 4 million are thought to be infected, mainly immigrants from endemic countries. The southwestern states and those along the Gulf of Mexico were once endemic areas.[54] Although most cases are asymptomatic, morbidity is related to worm burden. Intestinal obstruction is the most common complication, followed by bile duct obstruction, GI perforation, peritonitis, and volvulus.[55] Children age

1–5 years are most likely to have intestinal obstruction, and all children are likely to have malnutrition, leading to growth retardation, cognitive impairment, and poor academic performance.[55,56] Some studies have linked *Ascaris* infection with an increased risk of allergic diseases and asthma, although this association is controversial.[56,57]

Ascaris lumbricoides is acquired through ingesting embryonated eggs, which hatch in the jejunum and release larvae that penetrate the intestinal wall and enter the portal venous circulation, migrating to the liver. From the liver, the larvae migrate to the lungs through the venous circulation, break into the alveolar spaces, ascend to the tracheobronchial tree, and pass the epiglottis, where they are swallowed. They return to the jejunum and mature into adult worms. The adult worms can live for 1–2 years and produce 240,000 eggs per day. The elapsed time from initial ingestion to development of mature adults is 18–24 days.[54,55,58] Eggs are excreted in feces, where they complete embryonization while in the soil.[55] Mature female worms are 20–40 cm long, whereas male worms may be 12–25 cm long.[55] Adult worms move through the GI tract and can move in and out of the biliary tract, pancreas, appendix, and diverticula, where they may create obstruction and cause inflammation, necrosis, infection, and abscess formation.[54]

Table 5. Drugs for Toxoplasmosis in Pediatric Patients and Pregnancy[15,43,52,61]

Infection	Drug	Dosage (Oral)	Form (Oral)	Common ADRs
Immunocompetent, nonsevere	No treatment needed			
Immunocompromised (not patients with HIV)	Pyrimethamine	2 mg/kg/day for 2 days (max dose 50 mg/day); then 1 mg/kg/day for 3–6 wk (max dose 25 mg/day) Adolescents: 200 mg on first day; then 50–75 mg once daily for 3–6 wk	Tablet: 25 mg Suspension (compounded): 2 mg/mL[49]	Rash
	Sulfadiazine	50 mg/kg Q 6 hr for 6 wk (max dose 6 g/day)	Tablet: 500 mg Suspension (compounded): 200 mg/mL[50]	Rash, abdominal pain, diarrhea, nausea
	Leucovorin	10–25 mg given with pyrimethamine	Tablet: 5 mg, 10 mg, 15 mg, 25 mg Suspension (compounded): 5 mg/mL[51]	Diarrhea, nausea, stomatitis, fatigue
Alternative	TMP/SMX	TMP 5 mg/kg, SMX 25 mg/kg BID for 4 wk	Tablet: 400 mg SMX/80 mg TMP, 800 mg SMX/160 mg TMP Suspension: 200 mg SMX/40 mg TMP per 5 mL	Rash, urticaria, nausea, loss of appetite
	Clindamycin	5–7.5 mg/kg QID (max dose 1.8 g/day)	Capsule: 75 mg, 150 mg, 300 mg Solution: 75 mg/5 mL	Rash, abdominal pain, diarrhea, nausea
Acute toxoplasmosis in pregnancy	Spiramycin	3 million units (1 g) Q 8 hr	Not commercially available in United States: may obtain through the FDA with an IND, after consultation[a]	Rash, abdominal pain, nausea, blurred vision
Fetal infection after 18 wk gestation	Pyrimethamine	50 mg BID for 2 days; then 50 mg once daily to term	Tablet: 25 mg Suspension (compounded): 2 mg/mL	Rash
	Sulfadiazine	75 mg/kg as initial dose; then 50 mg/kg BID to term (max dose 4 g/day)	Tablet: 500 mg Suspension (compounded): 200 mg/mL	Rash, abdominal pain, diarrhea, nausea
	Leucovorin	10–20 mg/day during treatment and for 1 wk after pyrimethamine	Tablet: 5 mg, 10 mg, 15 mg, 25 mg Suspension (compounded): 5 mg/mL	Diarrhea, nausea, stomatitis, fatigue
Congenital toxoplasmosis in neonates and infants[b]	Pyrimethamine	2 mg/kg/day for 2 days; then 1 mg/kg/day for 6 mo; then three times/wk for 1-yr total treatment (max dose 25 mg/day)	Tablet: 25 mg Suspension (compounded): 2 mg/mL	Rash
	Sulfadiazine	50 mg/kg BID for 1 yr (max dose 6 g/day)	Tablet: 500 mg Suspension (compounded): 200 mg/mL	Rash, abdominal pain, diarrhea, nausea
	Leucovorin	10 mg three times/wk during treatment and for 1 wk after pyrimethamine	Tablet: 5 mg, 10 mg, 15 mg, 25 mg Suspension (compounded): 5 mg/mL	Diarrhea, nausea, stomatitis, fatigue

[a]Palo Alto Medical Foundation Toxoplasma Serology Laboratory, telephone (650) 853-4828; or U.S. National Collaborative Trial Study, telephone (773) 834-4152, or the FDA (301) 796-1600.
[b]Practice varies among centers.
ADR = adverse drug reaction; BID = twice daily; FDA = U.S. Food and Drug Administration; IND = investigational new drug; max = maximum; Q = every; QID = four times daily; TMP/SMX = trimethoprim/sulfamethoxazole.

In most cases, individuals are asymptomatic but may have anorexia, abdominal discomfort, and diarrhea. In children, the most common complication is intestinal obstruction secondary to an entangled worm bolus. Symptoms include sharp, colicky abdominal pain; fever; diarrhea; and vomiting that may contain worms. Severely malnourished children may progress to sepsis and septic shock. Pulmonary ascariasis symptoms, which may develop 1–2 weeks after infection, are rarely life threatening, but they may include chest pain, dry cough, fever, dyspnea, and wheezing. However, most children with pulmonary ascariasis are asymptomatic.[54,55]

Diagnosis can be made by a microscopic examination of the feces for eggs. Adult worms may be coughed out or passed through the rectum. Eosinophilia may be evident, especially in the lung migration phase, and can be profound in pulmonary ascariasis cases. Abdominal ultrasonography helps identify worms in the biliary tree.[54]

The goal of therapy is to eradicate the worms from the intestinal tract; however, antihelminthic drugs are not recommended in patients with large worm burdens and abdominal pain because of the risk of precipitating intestinal obstruction as the worms die. The drugs of choice are albendazole, mebendazole, and pyrantel pamoate, with efficacy rates of 95%, 88%, and 88%, respectively (Table 6).[59] Albendazole is preferred as first-line treatment in pediatric patients because it is well tolerated; it has dosing for children younger than 2 years; and it has good efficacy when the patient is coinfected with hookworm or pinworm. An alternative option for children weighing at least 15 kg is ivermectin, which should only be used if other options are not available or tolerated. For both children and adults, the treatment course may be repeated if there is no cure within 3–4 weeks. In symptomatic pregnant women, the drug of choice is pyrantel pamoate, which should only be used when the patient's active symptoms have subsided.[60]

Children receiving these drugs should be monitored for adverse reactions, which are rare with short-term use. Pyrantel pamoate should be used with caution in patients with existing liver dysfunction. Patients with phenylketonuria should avoid the chewable tablet, which contains aspartame. Some suspensions of pyrantel pamoate contain sodium benzoate, a metabolite of benzyl alcohol, which has been associated with gasping syndrome in neonates if administered in large amounts. Although excessive amounts would unlikely be reached when treating ascariasis in neonates, caution is warranted. Other adverse effects in children taking pyrantel pamoate include GI upset, nausea, diarrhea, abdominal cramps, headache, and rash. Albendazole should be used with caution in patients with abnormal liver function tests and in those with a decreased leukocyte count. Other adverse effects include rash, urticaria, headache, abdominal pain, nausea, and vomiting. Adverse reactions with mebendazole include GI effects such as nausea, vomiting, diarrhea, and abdominal pain. Rash, pruritus, and headache also occur.[61]

Preventive measures include improved sanitation and the practice of good hygiene. In endemic areas, school screenings with subsequent treatment have helped identify asymptomatic carriers and improve the health and educational outcomes of school-age children.[54]

PINWORM

The most common helminth infection in U.S. school-age children is *Enterobius vermicularis*, or pinworm, with an estimated prevalence of 30% of children.[6] Pinworm, which is found worldwide, especially in temperate regions, occurs in children regardless of socioeconomic level, race, or culture. Humans are the only host of *E. vermicularis*, which does not spread through water or germinate in soil.[62] In addition to school-age children, other commonly infected groups

Table 6. Drugs for Pediatric Helminth Infections[15,61]

Parasite	Drug	Dosage	Form	Comments
Ascariasis (*Ascaris lumbricoides*)	Albendazole	400 mg once 200 mg once for age 1–2 yr	Tablet: 200 mg	Tablet may be crushed or chewed
	Mebendazole	100 mg twice daily for 3 days or 500 mg once as single dose	Chewable tablet: 100 mg	May repeat in 3 wk if not cured with initial treatment
	Pyrantel pamoate	11 mg/kg pyrantel base once (max 1 g)	Suspension: 144 mg/mL (50 mg/mL pyrantel base) Chewable tablet: 720.5 mg (250 mg pyrantel base)	Repeat dose in 2 wk
	Ivermectin	100–200 mcg/kg orally as a single dose	Tablet: 3 mg	For children ≥ 15 kg
Pinworm (*Enterobius vermicularis*)	Albendazole	400 mg once	Tablet: 200 mg	Repeat dose in 2 wk
	Mebendazole	100 mg once	Chewable tablet: 100 mg	Repeat dose in 2 wk
	Pyrantel pamoate	11 mg/kg pyrantel base once (max 1 g)	Suspension: 144 mg/mL (50 mg/mL pyrantel base) Chewable tablet: 720.5 mg (250 mg pyrantel base)	Repeat dose in 2 wk

include adult caretakers of infected children and institution-alized individuals.[63]

Pinworm is transmitted by several methods: finger to mouth, aerogenic, and retroinfection. Fingers become contaminated secondary to scratching in the anal area, and when infected fingers are placed in the mouth (through nail biting, poor hygiene, or inadequate handwashing), autoinfection occurs.[63] Infestation may also occur when eggs adhere to bed linens, soiled clothes, tabletops, and bathroom fixtures; once touched, they stick to fingers or are caught under fingernails. Some research also suggests that pinworm eggs are carried by cockroaches.[64] In aerogenic infestation, eggs are inhaled and ingested from airborne dust containing eggs that have been dislodged from bed linens and clothes.[62] Retroinfection occurs when a pinworm hatches at the opening to the anus and then reenters the rectum and bowel.[65]

Once the eggs are ingested, the larvae hatch in the duodenum and mature into adult worms within 1–2 months. Adult worms attach to the mucosa of the cecum, appendix, and bowel and live for up to 4–6 weeks.[62] Female pinworms, which are about 5–13 mm long, are threadlike and white. At night, the pregnant female migrates to the anus to deposit as many as 16,000 eggs in the perianal skin. In some cases, worms migrate into nearby orifices, usually in the female genitourinary tract, leading to symptoms of vulvovaginitis and urinary tract infection.[62] Within 6 hours of being deposited, the eggs become infective and can remain so for up to 14–20 days.[62]

Patients with pinworm infestation present with perianal and perineal pruritus, which is more intense at night as the worms migrate. Some individuals are asymptomatic, and in rare cases of heavy worm burden, bowel inflammation, perforation, and obstruction may occur. Children may have nausea or abdominal pain, as well as restless sleep, bedwetting, and irritability.[63] Severe itching may lead to anal excoriation and secondary bacterial infection. Infestation with pinworm may also lead to appendicitis.[66]

Diagnosis of pinworm is usually made by a careful clinical history and identification of pinworm eggs from the perianal area using the "tape test." A stool specimen is not very useful because E. vermicularis eggs are detectable in the stool in only 5%–15% of cases.[6] The tape test involves applying clear adhesive tape to the end of a cotton swab with the sticky side out. The tape should be touched to the areas around the anus in the morning before the child bathes or defecates. The tape should be preserved in a plastic bag and taken to a physician's office for microscopic examination.[62] To reduce false-negative results, this test should be done on 3 consecutive days, which yields a sensitivity of 90%.[63,67]

The treatment goal is to eradicate the infestation and reduce morbidity. Several antihelminthic drugs are available and are given as two doses, 2 weeks apart. Drugs of choice include pyrantel pamoate, albendazole, and mebendazole (Table 6). Because drugs are not completely effective against both eggs and larvae, re-treatment is recommended, which may decrease recurrence rates from 20% to 1%.[67] Although all three drugs have cure rates of up to 100% with two doses, pyrantel pamoate is the most common drug in the United States for treating pinworm because it is available without a prescription and is inexpensive. When treating the patient,

all infected household contacts should also be treated with the same agent. Personal hygiene, including changing under-clothes daily, using good handwashing, and changing bed linens and towels often, must be improved, and children should be discouraged from putting their fingers in their mouths.[63] Individuals at risk of infestation should bathe in the morning on awakening to reduce egg contamination.[63]

Patients should be reminded that recurrence is common if the dose is not repeated in 2 weeks. Therapy is much more effective if the patient's household contacts are treated at the same time. Patients should be reexamined after completing drug therapy to reevaluate for reinfection, especially if perianal itching or pain continues.[63]

ECTOPARASITES

PEDICULOSIS (HEAD LICE)

Head lice infestation (pediculosis) is caused by *Pediculus humanus capitis*. In the United States, head lice are most common in school-age children, especially those in preschool and elementary grades, age 3–12 years.[68] Household members of infested children, as well as other caretakers, may also contract lice. It is estimated that 6–12 million cases of head lice occur annually in the United States.[68] Treatment costs associated with head lice are estimated at $1 billion, and because of "no-nit" policies in U.S. schools, about 12–24 million days of school are lost each year.[69,70] Head lice are not known to spread disease. Pediculosis is much less common among African Americans.[71]

The adult head louse is about the size of a sesame seed (about 3–4 mm long), whereas the eggs (nits) are much smaller at only 1 mm. A female louse can live 3–4 weeks and lay up to 10 nits daily. Nits are attached to the base of the hair shaft near the scalp with a glue-like substance. Nits need the warmth of body heat to incubate, and in 7–12 days, they hatch, releasing a nymph that matures during the next 9–12 days to reach the adult stage. Lice feed on blood from the human host every few hours, injecting saliva into the scalp. Mature lice cannot survive for more than 1 day away from the scalp.[68]

Lice are transmitted only by direct close contact. Head-to-head contact is common in young and school-age children, through play activities, sports, slumber parties, and camp.[71] Less often, lice can be spread through the sharing of clothing such as hats, scarfs, and coats or through the sharing of other items that have been in recent contact with the infested person such as combs, brushes, towels, ribbons, and barrettes. Placing the head on a pillow, bed, carpet, or upholstered furniture that was recently used by an infested person may also promote transmission.[71]

Head lice are diagnosed by observing live lice on the scalp or hair, but this observation can be difficult. A lice comb or other fine-tooth comb can make this process easier.[72] Nits may be easier to find, especially close to the scalp, but finding nits does not always confirm that a child is infested. If the nits are attached to the hair more than ¼ inch from the scalp, they are usually dead or have already hatched. Nits can also be confused with dandruff particles or hair debris, but nits are usually difficult to remove from the hair. Although head lice may be found anywhere on the scalp, they are common in the postauricular and occipital areas.[68] Patients may or may not present with pruritus, and many children may be asymptomatic.[71] In some cases, pruritus may lead to excoriations on the scalp and secondary skin infections.

The treatment goal is to eradicate the infestation. Treatment is recommended for all individuals with an active infestation. Nonprescription topical drugs with pyrethroids, such as 1% permethrin or pyrethrins, can be first-line therapy unless there is proven resistance to these products in the community (Table 7). Pyrethroid resistance prevalence has marked geographic variability and, together with patient age, adverse effects, and treatment cost, should be considered when choosing a topical product.[73] Prescription products such as benzyl alcohol 5% can be used in children older than 6 months, and malathion 0.5% can be used in children older than 2 years. Spinosad 0.9% is a newer topical prescription product that may be used in children 6 months and older. It is ovicidal and does not require a nit comb after use.[74] Topical ivermectin lotion 0.5% may be used to treat head lice infestations in children 6 months and older. Like spinosad, it does not require nit combing after use.[75] These products may also be used when resistance to pyrethrins or permethrin is common or when a patient's nonprescription therapy has failed. If nonprescription treatment is used or if live lice are seen after malathion therapy, these products should be reapplied at the

Table 7. Drugs for Ectoparasite Infestations[61,68]

Drug	Instructions	Comments
Head lice		
Permethrin 1%[a]	Topical: Apply to clean, towel-dried hair; leave on for 10 min; rinse with water	Nonprescription Use in children age ≥ 2 mo May repeat in 1 wk, if needed
Pyrethrin	Topical: Completely wet hair with product, leave on for 10 min; wash; rinse well with warm water	Nonprescription Repeat in 7–10 days to kill newly hatched lice Use in children age ≥ 2 yr
Benzyl alcohol 5%	Topical: Apply to dry hair using enough product to completely saturate hair and scalp; leave on for 10 min and then rinse well with water; use fine-tooth comb to remove dead lice and eggs	Prescription only For children age ≥ 6 mo No ovicidal activity Repeat in 1 wk
Ivermectin 0.5%	Topical: Apply to dry hair using enough product to thoroughly coat the hair and scalp; leave on for 10 min and then rinse well with water	Prescription only Use in children age ≥ 6 mo Nit combing not required
Lindane	Topical: Apply 15–30 mL to head and lather for 4 min; rinse well; use fine-tooth comb to remove dead lice and eggs	Prescription only Not routinely recommended Last-line therapy Use extreme caution in patients weighing < 50 kg Prescription only
Malathion 0.5%	Topical: Sprinkle product on dry hair and rub in until scalp is moistened and then allow hair to dry naturally; wash hair after 8–12 hr with a non-medicated shampoo; rinse; use fine-tooth comb to remove dead lice and eggs	Prescription only May repeat application in 7–9 days, if needed Contraindicated in neonates and infants Use in children age ≥ 6 yr
Spinosad 0.9%	Topical: Apply sufficient amount to cover dry scalp and completely cover dry hair; leave on for 10 min; rinse thoroughly with warm water	Prescription only Use in children age ≥ 6 mo May repeat application in 7 days if live lice seen Nit combing not required Ovicidal
Scabies		
Permethrin 5%[a]	Topical: Apply head to toes; leave on for 8–14 hr; wash off with water	Prescription only May reapply in 1 wk if live mites present
Crotamiton 10%	Topical: Apply to entire body, neck to toes, once daily for 2 days; bathe 48 hr after last application	Prescription only May reapply after 7–10 days if mites reappear In infants and young children, may also apply to neck, head, and scalp; avoid face
Ivermectin	Oral: 200 mcg/kg as a single dose for children ≥ 15 kg	Prescription only May repeat dose in 10–14 days
Lindane	Topical: Apply thin layer to skin from neck to toes Infants: Wash off 6 hr after application Children: Wash off 6–8 hr after application	Prescription only Not routinely recommended Last-line therapy Use extreme caution in patients < 50 kg

[a]Drug of choice.

indicated intervals because they are not completely ovicidal.[68] Lindane, an organochlorine, is only available by prescription and was found to cause seizures in children.[68,71] The FDA recommends that it be used only for second-line treatment when treatment fails or in those who cannot tolerate other, safer agents. An FDA-issued public health advisory further emphasized that lindane should not be used in neonates and should be used with extreme caution in children and individuals who weigh less than 50 kg, who take drugs that may lower the seizure threshold, or who have HIV infection.[68] California has banned the use of lindane, and the American Academy of Pediatrics no longer recommends it as a pediculicide.[68] If treatment with a pediculicide is contraindicated or parents want a nontoxic alternative to pediculicides, "wet-combing" (using a fine-tooth comb on wet hair coated with conditioner) can be helpful, although it is time-consuming and difficult to perform on active young children. This process should take about 1 hour and should be repeated every 4 days until no more active lice are seen. Another nontoxic option is an occlusive product such as petroleum jelly or Cetaphil cream (Galderma Laboratories, Fort Worth, TX). Petroleum jelly is massaged into the hair and scalp and left on overnight with a shower cap. This treatment is thought to suffocate the adult louse and block air exchange in the eggs; it may need to be repeated within 2 weeks.[76] Cetaphil is applied to the hair and scalp, dried with a hair dryer, left on overnight, and then washed out in the morning. This process should be repeated once weekly for 3 weeks.[77]

Nit removal is not necessary, but it may be cosmetically desired. Because many U.S. schools have a "no-nit" policy requiring children to be free of nits before returning to school, parents may want to remove nits. Fine-tooth combs or special "nit combs" are used on wet hair, similar to the "wet-combing" process previously described. Some products claim to loosen the nits from the hair shaft, making the process easier, but no clinical benefit is proven.[68] Shaving the child's head is very effective in removing nits and lice, but it is generally not recommended because of the distress it may cause the child.[68]

Because head lice need a blood meal regularly and do not survive long after they fall off the scalp, aggressive cleaning is not necessary to prevent reinfestation. However, clothing or washable items that the infested person was in contact with during the 2 days before lice removal treatment should be machine washed in hot water and dried on high heat. Because adult lice do not survive long without a blood meal and their eggs typically hatch within 6–10 days, any clothing and items that cannot be washed may be dry-cleaned or tightly sealed in a plastic bag for 2 weeks. Brushes and combs should be washed in hot water for 5–10 minutes. Vacuuming the floor or furniture where an infested person has recently been may be helpful, but the risk of infestation in this circumstance is low.[71]

SCABIES

Scabies is caused by infestation with the human itch mite, *Sarcoptes scabiei* var. *hominis*, into the superficial layers of the skin. Scabies occurs worldwide and affects all age groups, races, and social classes. Risk factors include crowding, especially in poorer socioeconomic settings where proper hygiene is lacking. Scabies is transmitted through close body contact, and outbreaks often occur in nursing homes, extended care facilities, prisons, and child care facilities.[78]

Scabies mites are transmitted through prolonged direct human contact. The adult female mite is very small, 0.3–0.5 mm long, and can lay as many as 90 eggs after burrowing beneath the stratum corneum for a blood meal. When the female mite burrows, a trail of eggs, debris, and feces is left behind, which induces an immunologic response, manifested by intense pruritus. Larvae hatch under the skin within 3–4 days and mature over 2 weeks into adult mites. In a patient with classic scabies, the average mite population is 10–20 parasites.[78]

The main symptom of scabies is intense, distressing pruritus that worsens at night or with activities that elevate body temperature. Primary lesions include burrows, which look like faint white zigzags on the skin, papules, vesicles, and pustules.[78,79] Secondary lesions arise from scratching and may include crusted areas and nodules.[78] In infants, the palms, soles, axillae, and scalp are most commonly affected. In older children, lesions are usually below the neck, including the webbed spaces between the fingers; flexor surfaces of the arms, wrists, and axillae; and waistline. Other affected areas include the umbilicus, penis, nipples, and scrotum.[80] In new infestations, symptoms may take as long as 4–6 weeks to manifest.[79]

A definitive diagnosis of scabies is made by direct visualization of the mites, eggs, or feces in a skin scraping on low-power microscopy.[81] Because this visualization is not always feasible, the diagnosis is often based on clinical signs and symptoms, including the characteristic burrow pattern and history of pruritus that worsens at night.

The goal of therapy is to eradicate the infestation and minimize complications. Treatment of both the infested patient and all close contacts with scabicidal drugs is crucial. The drug of choice is permethrin, which has a 91% cure rate 28 days after a single whole-body application and a 96.8% cure rate with two doses at a 2-week interval.[82,83] Systemic ivermectin is preferred when an entire population has a high prevalence of scabies.[84] Scabicidal drugs are available only with a prescription, and the drug must be applied appropriately to ensure successful treatment (Table 7). The drug should be applied to clean skin and left on for the recommended time before it is washed off. In older children, the scabicide should be applied to all areas of the body from the neck to the toes, whereas in infants and young children, the head and neck should also be covered. After treatment, clean clothing should be worn. Because the pruritus is caused by a hypersensitivity reaction to the mites and their feces, patients may have itching for weeks after treatment, despite killing all mites and eggs. An oral antihistamine or a topical corticosteroid may help control the itching. A nonsedating antihistamine such as loratadine should be used during the daytime, whereas a sedating antihistamine such as hydroxyzine or diphenhydramine is used at night.[85] A medium- or high-potency topical corticosteroid should be used for mild to moderate itching, although in severe cases, an oral taper of prednisone over 1–2 weeks may be required.[86] Skin sores from itching may become infected and should be treated appropriately with antibiotics.[78,79] Patients should be examined 1 month after treatment for complete resolution of signs and symptoms.

Clothing, bedding, and towels used by the infested person should be washed in hot water and dried on the hot setting. Items that are non-washable should be dry-cleaned or placed in a sealed plastic bag and stored for a minimum of 72 hours because scabies mites can live for only 2–3 days without a host. Pesticide sprays or fogs are unnecessary.[79]

CONCLUSIONS

Parasitic infections in children can have a detrimental effect on a child's well-being, affecting nutritional status, growth, and development. It is vital that clinicians be aware of the signs and symptoms, complications, and available treatment options for the most prevalent parasites, even though they are not as common in the United States, except for head lice, as in other areas of the world. With increasing immigration and travel by children and their families to endemic areas of the world, the impact of parasites in children can be experienced in previously unaffected geographic locations in the United States. Public health awareness of transmission risks is important in both preventing and treating parasitic infections in pediatric patients.

Patient Case — PARASITES

A 4-year-old white girl is brought to the emergency department (ED) by her parents because of a high temperature, loss of appetite, and vomiting. She returned to the United States 10 days ago from an 8-day vacation to Africa with her family. They were in Madagascar and Mozambique exploring different cultures and the variety of animals. This trip was the family's first to a country outside the United States, and they did not know how to prepare or what to expect. The family stayed with local families during their vacation.

Medical history: None	patient attends preschool 5 days/week	**Laboratory findings:** Positive detection of Plasmodium falciparum in red blood cells on a blood smear detected by light microscopy
Family history: Insignificant	**Allergies:** No known drug allergies	
Social history: Father, mother, and 18-month-old sister are all healthy and have no past medical issues; the	**Vital signs:** Tmax 103.7°F (39.8°C), BP 98/68 mm Hg, HR 85 beats/minute, Ht 42 inches, Wt 19 kg	**Immunizations:** Up to date

1. Given the patient's recent history and other information presented, what disease has the patient most likely contracted and why?

Because *P. falciparum* was detected on a blood smear and given the patient's symptoms and other risk factors, she likely contracted malaria during her trip to Africa, which is an area with many parasitic infections, especially in the sub-Saharan region. The family was unprepared for the trip and was unaware of how to help prevent malaria transmission. Malaria normally presents as fever and flu-like symptoms such as chills, headaches, and tiredness. Nausea, vomiting, and diarrhea may also occur. Symptoms usually present around 10–28 days after infection. The patient presented to the ED 10 days after returning from Africa, meaning she was probably infected with malaria during the trip. The standard for diagnosing malaria is a positive detection of malarial parasites on a blood smear using a light microscope, which was confirmed for the patient.

2. What are the best ways to prevent a malarial infection? In this case, how can transmission to the younger sister and/or other children in the preschool best be prevented?

Preventing malaria transmission is not guaranteed, but two measures, which can be used in combination, can greatly reduce the risk. The first method is use of "mosquito avoidance measures" because malaria is transmitted by the *Anopheles* mosquito. These measures include wearing protective clothing to limit the amount of body surface area available for contact with mosquitos, using mosquito bed nets, staying in well-screened areas as much as possible, using a pyrethroid-containing insect spray in the living and sleeping area, and using spray containing up to 50% DEET (*N, N*-diethyl-meta-toluamide) on any exposed body area for children older than 2 months.

The second method is use of a prophylactic drug regimen. These regimens differ among patients, but all involve taking an appropriate drug about 1–2 weeks before, during, and up to 4 weeks after the expected exposure. In this patient case, her younger sister and the other children at the preschool are not at a significant risk of getting malaria from the patient because malaria is not transmitted person to person. However, the "mosquito avoidance measures" mentioned previously should be used until the patient's infection is fully treated.

Case (continued). After diagnosing uncomplicated malaria caused by *P. falciparum*, treatment was started. However, the infection was determined to be chloroquine resistant.

3. After identifying uncomplicated malaria caused by *P. falciparum* and determined to be chloroquine resistant, what are the available treatments and treatment regimens?

Given that she likely was infected in Africa, where the incidence of chloroquine-resistant *P. falciparum* is high, the initial treatment would be the same as if there was unknown resistance confirmed. Therefore, for this patient, the preferred treatment is atovaquone/proguanil because of the 3-day length of treatment and once-daily dosage regimen. There are two available strengths: an adult tablet of 250 mg/100 mg that is used for patients weighing more than 10 kg, and a pediatric tablet of 62.5 mg/25 mg that is used in patients weighing 10 kg or less. Given this patient's weight of 19 kg, she should take 1 adult tablet daily for 3 days. Because it is unlikely that a 4-year old is able to swallow a tablet whole, the tablet can be crushed and administered in a soft food.

Second-line treatment option for this patient is artemether/lumefantrine 20 mg/120 mg. The number of tablets needed for the treatment regimen is dependent on the patient's weight. Because this patient weighs between 15 and 25 kg, she should take 2 tablets now; then another 2 tablets 8 hours later on the first day; and then 2 tablets twice daily, in the morning and evenings, on days 2 and 3. This treatment course is a total of 12 tablets. Like other regimens, artemether/lumefantrine is available as oral tablets that may be crushed and mixed with soft foods if the child is not able to swallow whole tablets.

Mefloquine is considered a third-line option for this patient. Dosing is 13.7 mg base/kg (15 mg salt/kg) for the first dose and then 9.1 mg base/kg (10 salt/kg) 6–12 hours after the initial dose. This patient would require around 260 mg of mefloquine (285 mg) for the first dose and around 173 mg (190 mg) of mefloquine base for the second dose. Mefloquine tablets may be crushed if the child is unable to swallow whole tablets.

Regimens with quinine can be difficult in pediatric patients, because the only strength available of quinine, 324 mg capsules, cannot be crushed, opened, or chewed. The Centers for Disease Control and Prevention recommends that the other three available treatment options be used if dosing with quinine is problematic. Typically, quinine sulfate (10 mg/kg every 8 hours for 3–7 days) is combined with either doxycycline, tetracycline, or clindamycin. Because this patient weighs 19 kg and would need 190 mg of quinine, combination therapy with quinine sulfate is not recommended.

REFERENCES

1. Centers for Disease Control and Prevention (CDC). Parasites. Available at www.cdc.gov/parasites/. Accessed September 27, 2019.
2. Moore RS, Lima NL, Soares AM, et al. Prolonged episodes of acute diarrhea reduce growth and increase risk of persistent diarrhea in children. Gastroenterology 2010;139:1156-64.
3. Guerrant RL, Oria RB, Moore SR, et al. Malnutrition as an enteric infectious disease with long-term effects on child development. Nutr Rev 2008;66:487-505.
4. Glaser C, Lewis P, Wong S. Pet-, animal- and vector-borne infections. Pediatr Rev 2000;21:219-32.
5. Moffat T. Diarrhea, respiratory infections, protozoan gastrointestinal parasites, and child growth in Kathmandu, Nepal. Am J Phys Anthropol 2003;122:85-97.
6. Kucik CJ, Martin GL, Sortor BV. Common intestinal parasites. Am Fam Physician 2004;69:1161-8.
7. Centers for Disease Control and Prevention (CDC). Summary of notifiable diseases and conditions—United States, 2014. MMWR 2016;63:1-152.
8. Painter JE, Gargano JW, Collier SA, et al. Giardiasis surveillance—United States 2011–2012. MMWR Surveill Summ 2015; 64:15-25.
9. Katz DE, Taylor DN. Parasitic infections of the gastrointestinal tract. Gastroenterol Clin North Am 2001;30:795-815.
10. Centers for Disease Control and Prevention (CDC); DPDx—Laboratory Identification of Parasitic Diseases of Public Health Concern. Stool Specimens—Detection of Parasite Antigens Available at www.cdc.gov/dpdx/diagnosticprocedures/stool/antigendetection.html. Accessed September 27, 2019.
11. Johnston SP, Ballard MM, Beach MJ, et al. Evaluation of three commercial assays for detection of Giardia and Cryptosporidium organisms in fecal specimens. J Clin Microbiol 2003;4:623-6.
12. Allen LV, Erickson MA. Stability of ketoconazole, metolazone, metronidazole, procainamide hydrochloride and spironolactone in extemporaneously compounded oral liquids. Am J Health Syst Pharm 1996;53:2073-8.
13. Tinidazole [package insert]. Baltimore, MD: Lupin Pharmaceuticals, Inc. Available at www.lupinpharmaceuticals.com/pdf/17/02/tinidazole-tabs-pi-7-2013.pdf. Accessed September 27, 2019.
14. Gardner TB, Hill DR. Treatment of giardiasis. Clin Microbiol Rev 2001;14:114-28.
15. Moon TD, Oberhelman RA. Antiparasitic therapy in children. Pediatr Clin North Am 2005;52:917-48.
16. Leitsch D. Drug resistance in the microaerophilic parasite Giardia lamblia. Curr Trop Med Rep 2015;2:128-35.

17. Centers for Disease Control and Prevention (CDC). Parasites—Giardia. Available at www.cdc.gov/parasites/giardia/index.html. Accessed September 27, 2019.
18. Haque R, Huston CD, Hughes M, et al. Amebiasis. N Engl J Med 2003;348:1565-73.
19. Tanyuksel M, Petri WA. Laboratory diagnosis of amebiasis. Clin Microbiol Rev 2003;16:713-29.
20. Hughes MA, Petri WA Jr. Amebic liver abscess. Infect Dis Clin North Am 2000;14:565-81.
21. Petri WA, Haque R. Entamoeba species, including amebic colitis and liver abscess. In: Mandell GL, Dolin R, Blaser MJ, eds. Principles and Practice of Infectious Diseases, 8th ed. New York: Elsevier Saunders, 2015:3047-58.
22. Oramasionwu GE, Wootton SH, Edwards MS. Epidemiologic features impacting the presentation of malaria in children in Houston. Pediatr Infect Dis J 2010;29:28-32.
23. Mace KE, Arguin PM, Lucchi NW, et al. Malarial Surveillance – United States, 2016. MMWR Surveill Summ 2019;68(No. SS-5): 1-35.
24. World Health Organization (WHO). WHO Fact Sheet on Malaria. World Health Organization. Available at www.who.int/news-room/fact-sheets/detail/malaria. Accessed September 27, 2019.
25. Franco-Paredes C, Santos-Preciado JI. Problem pathogens: prevention of malaria in travelers. Lancet Infect Dis 2006;6:139-49.
26. Bledsoe GH. Malaria primer for clinicians in the United States. South Med J 2005;98:1197-204.
27. Fairhurst RM, Wellems RE. Malaria (Plasmodium species). In: Mandell GL, Dolin R, Blaser MJ, eds. Principles and Practice of Infectious Diseases, 8th ed. New York: Elsevier Saunders, 2015:3070-90.
28. Garcia LS. Malaria. Clin Lab Med 2010;30:93-129.
29. Hagmann S, Khanna K, Niazi M, et al. Congenital malaria, an important differential diagnosis to consider when evaluating febrile infants of immigrant mothers. Pediatr Emerg Care 2007; 23:326-9.
30. Tan KR, Arguin PM. Travel-Related Infectious Diseases: Malaria. Centers for Disease Control and Prevention. CDC Yellow Book 2020 Health Information for International Travel. Atlanta: U.S. Department of Health and Human Services, Public Health Service, 2019. Available at wwwnc.cdc.gov/travel/yellow-book/2020/travel-related-infectious-diseases/malaria. Accessed September 27, 2019.
31. Krintafel (tafenoquine) tablets [package insert]. Research Triangle Park, NC: GlaxoSmithKline, Inc., 2018.

32. Allen LV, Erickson MA. Stability of alprazolam, chloroquine phosphate, cisapride, enalapril maleate and hydralazine hydrochloride in extemporaneously compounded oral liquids. Am J Health Syst Pharm 1998;55:1915-20.

33. Pesko LJ. Compounding hydroxychloroquine. Am Druggist 1993;207:57.

34. Bern C, Montgomery SP, Katz L, et al. Chagas disease and the US blood supply. Curr Opin Infect Dis 2008;21:476-82.

35. Cantey PT, Stramer SL, Townsend RL, et al. The United States *Trypanosoma cruzi* Infection Study: evidence for vector-borne transmission of the parasite that causes Chagas disease among United States blood donors. Transfusion 2012;52:1922-30.

36. Barrett MP, Burchmore RJS, Stich A, et al. The trypanosomiases. Lancet 2003;362:1469-80.

37. Prata A. Clinical and epidemiological aspects of Chagas disease. Lancet Infect Dis 2001;1:92-100.

38. Bern C, Montgomery SP, Herwaldt BL, et al. Evaluation and treatment of Chagas disease in the United States: a systematic review. JAMA 2007;298:2171-81.

39. Centers for Disease Control and Prevention (CDC). Parasites—American Trypanosomiasis (also known as Chagas Disease). Available at www.cdc.gov/parasites/chagas/. Accessed September 27, 2019.

40. Moscatelli G, Moroni S, Garcia-Bournissen F, et al. Prevention of congenital Chagas through treatment of girls and women of childbearing age. Mem Inst Oswaldo Cruz 2015;110:507-9.

41. de Araujo Pereira G, Louzada-Neto F, de Fatima Barbosa V, et al. Performance of six diagnostic tests to screen for Chagas disease in blood banks and prevalence of *Trypanosoma cruzi* infection among donors with inconclusive serology screening based on the analysis of epidemiological variables. Rev Bras Hematol Hemoter 2012;34:292-7.

42. Benznidazole tablet [package insert]. Florham Park, NJ: Exeltis USA, Inc., 2019.

43. Montoya JG, Liesenfeld O. Toxoplasmosis. Lancet 2004;363:1965-76.

44. Jones JL, Dargelas V, Roberts J, et al. Risk factors for *Toxoplasma gondii* infection in the United States. Clin Infect Dis 2009; 49:878-84.

45. Hill DE, Chirukandoth S, Dubey JP. Biology and epidemiology of *Toxoplasma gondii* in man and animals. Anim Health Res Rev 2005;6:41-61.

46. Montoya JG, Rosso F. Diagnosis and management of toxoplasmosis. Clin Perinatol 2005;32:705-26.

47. Berrebi A, Assouline C, Bessieres MH, et al. Long-term outcome of children with congenital toxoplasmosis. Am J Obstet Gynecol 2010;203:e1-6.

48. Centers for Disease Control and Prevention (CDC). Parasites—Toxoplasmosis (*Toxoplasma* infection). Available at www.cdc.gov/parasites/toxoplasmosis. Accessed September 28, 2019.

49. Nahata MC, Morosco RS, Hipple TF. Stability of pyrimethamine in a liquid dosage formulation stored for three months. Am J Health Syst Pharm 1997;54:2714-6.

50. Allen Loyd V Jr. Sulfadiazine 100 mg/mL oral suspension. Intern J Pharm Compound 2011;15:426.

51. Lam MSH. Extemporaneous compounding of oral liquid dosage formulations and alternate drug delivery methods for anticancer drugs. Pharmacotherapy 2011;31:164-92.

52. Montoya JG, Remington JS. Management of *Toxoplasma gondii* infection during pregnancy. Clin Infect Dis 2008;47:554-66.

53. Valentine CC, Hoffner RJ, Henderson SO. Three common presentations of ascariasis infection in an urban emergency department. J Emerg Med 2001;20:135-9.

54. Centers for Disease Control and Prevention (CDC). Parasites—Ascariasis. Available at www.cdc.gov/parasites/ascariasis/index.html. Accessed September 28, 2019.

55. Crompton DW. *Ascaris* and ascariasis. Adv Parasitol 2001; 48:285-375.

56. Pinelli E, Willers SM, Hoek D, et al. Prevalence of antibodies against *Ascaris suum* and its association with allergic manifestations in 4-year-old children in the Netherlands: the PIAMA birth cohort study. Eur J Clin Microbiol Infect Dis 2009;28:1327-34.

57. Leonard-Bee J, Pritchard D, Britton J. Asthma and current intestinal parasite infection: systematic review and meta-analysis. Am J Respir Crit Care Med 2006;174:514-23.

58. Bethony J, Brooker S, Albonico M, et al. Soil-transmitted helminth infections: ascariasis, trichuriasis, and hookworm. Lancet 2006;367:1521-32.

59. Keiser J, Utzinger J. Efficacy of current drugs against soil-transmitted helminth infections: systematic review and meta-analysis. JAMA 2008;299:1937-48.

60. Jones JL, Schulkin J, Maguire JH. Therapy for common parasitic diseases in pregnancy in the United States: a review and a survey of obstetrician/gynecologists' level of knowledge about these diseases. Obstet Gynecol Surv 2005;60:386-93.

61. Taketomo CK, Hodding JH, Kraus DM, eds. Lexicomp Pediatric & Neonatal Dosage Handbook, 25th ed. Hudson, OH: Wolters Kluwer Clinical Drug Information, Inc., 2018.

62. Burkhart CN, Burkhart CG. Assessment of frequency, transmission, and genitourinary complications of enterobiasis (pinworms). Int J Dermatol 2005;44:837-40.

63. Centers for Disease Control and Prevention (CDC). Parasites—Enterobiasis (also known as Pinworm Infection). Available at www.cdc.gov/parasites/pinworm/index.html. Accessed September 27, 2019.

64. Chan TO, Lee EK, Hardman JM, et al. The cockroach as host for *Trichinella* and *Enterobius vermicularis*; implications for public health. Hawaii Med J 2004;63:74-7.

65. Tandan T, Pollard AJ, Money DM, et al. Pelvic inflammatory disease associated with *Enterobius vermicularis*. Arch Dis Child 2002;86:439-40.

66. Ajao OG, Jastaniah S, Malatani TS, et al. *Enterobius vermicularis* (pin worm) causing symptoms of appendicitis. Trop Doct 2007;27:182-3.

67. Capello M, Hotez PJ. Intestinal nematodes. In: Long SS, Pickering LK, Prober CG, eds. Principles and Practice of Pediatric Infectious Disease, 4th ed. New York: Elsevier Saunders, 2012:1326-34.

68. Frankowski BL, Bocchini JA. Clinical report—head lice. Pediatrics 2010;126:392-403.

69. Hansen RC, O'Harver J. Economic considerations associated with *Pediculus humanus capitis* infestation. Clin Pediatr 2004; 42:523-7.

70. Mumcuoglu KY, Meinking TA, Burkhart CN, et al. Head louse infestations: the "no nit" policy and its consequences. Int J Dermatol 2006;45:891-6.

71. Centers for Disease Control and Prevention (CDC). Parasites—Lice. Available at www.cdc.gov/parasites/lice/index.html. Accessed September 28, 2019.

72. Mumcuoglu KY, Friger M, Ioffe-Uspensky I, et al. Louse comb versus direct visual examination for the diagnosis of head louse infestations. Pediatr Dermatol 2001;18:9-12.

73. Lebwhol M, Clark L, Levitt J. Therapy for head lice based on life cycle, resistance, and safety concerns. Pediatrics 2007;119:965-74.

74. Cole SW, Lundquist LM. Spinosad for treatment of head lice infestation. Ann Pharmacother 2011;45:954-9.

75. SKLICE (ivermectin) lotion 0.5% [package insert]. Atlanta, GA: Arbor Pharmaceutical, LLC, 2017.

76. Schachner LA. Treatment resistant head lice: alternative therapeutic approaches. Pediatr Dermatol 1997;14:409-10.

77. Pearlman DL. A simple treatment for head lice: dry-on, suffocation-based pediculicide. Pediatrics 2004;114:e275-9.

78. Cestari TF, Martignago BF. Scabies, pediculosis, bedbugs and stinkbugs: uncommon presentations. Clin Dermatol 2005; 23:545-54.

79. Centers for Disease Control and Prevention (CDC). Parasites—Scabies. Available at www.cdc.gov/parasites/scabies/index.html. Accessed September 28, 2019.

80. Orion E, Marcos B, Davidovici B, et al. Itch and scratch: scabies and pediculosis. Clin Dermatol 2006;24:168-75.

81. Walton SF, Currie BJ. Problems in diagnosing scabies, a global disease in human and animal populations. Clin Microbiol Rev 2007;20:268-79.

82. Schultz MW, Gomez M, Hansen RC, et al. Comparative study of 5% permethrin cream and 1% lindane lotion for the treatment of scabies. Arch Dermatol 1990;126:167-70.

83. Ranjkesh MR, Naghili B, Goldust M, et al. The efficacy of permethrin 5% vs. oral ivermectin for the treatment of scabies. Ann Parasitol 2013;59:189-94.

84. Romani L, Whitfeld MJ, Koroivueta J, et al. Mass drug administration for scabies control in a population with endemic disease. N Engl J Med 2015;373:2305-13.

85. O'Donoghue M, Tharp MD. Antihistamines and their role as antipruritics. Dermatol Ther 2005;18:333-40.

86. Johnson G, Sladden M. Scabies: diagnosis and treatment. BMJ 2005;331:619-22.

CHAPTER 45

Human Immunodeficiency Virus

Rustin D. Crutchley, Pharm.D., AAHIVP; and
Amy C. Min, Pharm.D., BCACP, AAHIVP

LEARNING OBJECTIVES

1. Explain the routes of transmission for the human immunodeficiency virus (HIV).

2. Describe the life cycle of HIV.

3. Identify signs and symptoms of acute and chronic HIV infection, including the most common opportunistic infections.

4. Recommend appropriate prophylaxis for common opportunistic infections.

5. Identify goals of therapy for children living with HIV and recommend appropriate antiretroviral (ARV) therapy for treatment-naive children living with HIV.

6. Describe efficacy guidelines and adverse effects of ARV therapy.

7. Describe the importance of adherence to ARV therapy and strategies to improve adherence for children living with HIV.

8. Summarize important clinical pearls for children living with HIV using a patient case example.

ABBREVIATIONS IN THIS CHAPTER

AIDS	Acquired immunodeficiency syndrome
ART	Antiretroviral therapy
ARV	Antiretroviral
cART	Combination antiretroviral therapy
CCR5	C-C chemokine receptor type 5
CDC	Centers for Disease Control and Prevention
CMV	Cytomegalovirus
CYP	Cytochrome P450
CYP3A4	Cytochrome P450 3A4 isoenzyme
CXCR4	C-X-C motif chemokine receptor type 4
DHHS	U.S. Department of Health and Human Services
D/M	Dual/mixed
EIA	Enzyme immunoassay
FDA	U.S. Food and Drug Administration
FDC	Fixed-dose combination
HBV	Hepatitis B virus
HCV	Hepatitis C virus
HIV	Human immunodeficiency virus
INSTI	Integrase strand transfer inhibitor

MAC	*Mycobacterium avium* complex
MTCT	Mother-to-child-transmission
NNRTI	Nonnucleoside reverse transcriptase inhibitor
NRTI	Nucleoside reverse transcriptase inhibitor
OI	Opportunistic infection
PCP	*Pneumocystis jirovecii* pneumonia
PCR	Polymerase chain reaction
PI	Protease inhibitor
TAF	Tenofovir alafenamide
TDF	Tenofovir disoproxil fumarate
TDM	Therapeutic drug monitoring

INTRODUCTION

This chapter describes the current epidemiology of the human immunodeficiency virus (HIV), the genetic diversity of the virus, and the ways in which it affects the immune system, emphasizing prominent reservoirs of latent viral infection. The chapter also describes common routes of transmission and the signs and symptoms of acute and chronic HIV infection. Pertinent surrogate markers for HIV and the ways in which they pertain to HIV disease progression and the importance of resistance testing will be explained. With more than 25 antiretroviral (ARV) drugs available, the discussion focuses on the goals of treatment, including nonpharmacologic and pharmacologic approaches for treating HIV infection, with special attention to medication adherence. At the conclusion of this chapter, the reader will appreciate the complexity of the disease and have a clearer and more complete understanding of how to care for and optimize ARV treatment among children and adolescents living with HIV.

EPIDEMIOLOGY

About 37.9 million people worldwide in 2018 were living with HIV.[1] About two-thirds of the global burden of disease exists in sub-Saharan Africa. According to the World Health Organization, in 2018 an estimated 1.7 million children (younger than 15 years) were living with HIV globally, with 160,000 new HIV infections and 100,000 deaths occurring secondary to acquired immunodeficiency syndrome (AIDS).[1,2] In 2016, an estimated 2225 children younger than 13 years were living with HIV in the United States. Only one death, by any cause, in children living with HIV were recorded during this time in the United States.[3] In the 2017 Centers for Disease Control and Prevention (CDC) HIV Surveillance Report, the estimated number of new diagnoses of HIV infection among children younger than 13 years in the United States was 99; in contrast, 25 new cases appeared in children 13–14 years and 1711 new cases in adolescents age 15–19 years.[3]

Two different virus types exist for HIV: *HIV-1* and *HIV-2*; HIV type 1 is much more common worldwide than HIV-2. The first cases of HIV-1 infection were reported in the United States in 1981 among homosexual men in Los Angeles, California.[4] HIV type 1 is extremely diverse in its genetic composition and is classified into three groups: *M, N,* and *O*. The M group, which is the most common, consists of nine genetically distinct subtypes or clades designated by the letters *A–D, F–H,* and *J–K*. The geographic distribution of these different subtypes varies; for example, subtype B is common in the United States, and subtype C is common in Africa.[5]

In 1986, HIV-2 was isolated from patients with AIDS in West Africa, where it is still predominantly found. Most of the world's remaining burden of HIV-2 infection is reported among countries with historical socioeconomic ties to West Africa such as France, Spain, Portugal, and former Portuguese colonies Brazil, Angola, Mozambique, and parts of India near Goa. Although HIV-2 has modes of transmission similar to HIV-1, it is less virulent than HIV-1, and disease progresses more slowly. Compared with HIV-1, infection with HIV type 2 results in comparatively lower viral loads, less transmission, and fewer AIDS cases.[6]

ETIOLOGY

PATHOPHYSIOLOGY

The first HIV virus, HIV type 1, belongs to the lentivirus subfamily of retroviruses. It is a single-stranded RNA virus that uses reverse transcriptase to produce proviral DNA required for virus replication and persistent infection of CD4+ cells. In HIV type 1, nine separate genes are divided into three classes: *structural proteins* that encode for the viral core, the enzymes for viral replication and integration and for the structure of the viral envelope; *regulatory proteins* involved with viral transcription and protein synthesis; and *accessory proteins*.

During acute infection, HIV specifically infects CD4+ cells. The entry of HIV into the CD4+ cells is a multistep process. First, gp120, a trimer envelope glycoprotein on the HIV virion, binds to the CD4+ cell receptor. Once bound, a conformational change occurs in gp120, allowing additional binding to one of the co-receptors on the CD4+ cell: C-C chemokine receptor type 5 (CCR5) or C-X-C motif chemokine receptor type 4 (CXCR4). The CCR5 co-receptor is associated with early infection, and the CXCR4 co-receptor is more commonly found in treatment-experienced patients or in those with advanced stages of HIV disease. Antagonists of CCR5, such as maraviroc, bind to the CCR5 co-receptor, which thereby prevents HIV binding and subsequent fusion of the viral envelope and the cell membrane.

Once the HIV virion binds to one of the co-receptors, it enables the trimer gp41 to bind to the CD4+ cell membrane, facilitating the fusion of the virion with the CD4+ cell. The HIV entry inhibitor enfuvirtide is a fusion inhibitor that binds to gp41 and prevents fusion of the HIV virion with the CD4+ cell membrane. Uncoating of the capsid releases single-stranded HIV RNA into the cytoplasm of the CD4+ cell. This RNA strand is then transcribed into double-stranded HIV DNA by HIV reverse transcriptase. Because HIV reverse transcriptase is highly error prone with no proofreading mechanism, it permits the evolution of several mutations in HIV RNA as viral replication continues, thus contributing to its genetic variation. *Nucleoside reverse transcriptase inhibitors* (NRTIs) are nucleoside analogs that must be triphosphorylated (except for the ARV tenofovir, which is a nucleotide and requires only one additional phosphorylation) before incorporation by reverse transcriptase into the HIV DNA chain. These NRTIs then act as DNA chain terminators, inhibiting further synthesis of HIV DNA by competitive inhibition. *Nonnucleoside reverse transcriptase inhibitors* (NNRTIs) also inhibit reverse transcriptase by noncompetitive inhibition by binding directly to the enzyme, creating structural alterations that prevent the addition of nucleosides to the growing DNA chain.

Double-stranded HIV DNA is then transported to the nucleus and integrated into the genome of the CD4+ cell as proviral HIV DNA virus by HIV integrase. The mechanism of integrase strand transfer inhibitors (INSTIs) such as raltegravir prevent HIV integrase from inserting HIV proviral DNA into the host cell's DNA. The proviral DNA virus in HIV is representative of latent HIV viral reservoirs. Common sites of latent reservoir infection primarily include lymphoid tissue, as well as peripheral blood dendritic cells and monocytes, resting CD4+ lymphocytes, and microglial cells of the central nervous system, reproductive tract, and gastrointestinal tract. The establishment of these latent reservoirs of infection serves as one of the primary reasons for the difficulty in finding a cure for HIV.[7]

Once the proviral HIV DNA is activated in the CD4+ cell, it is transcribed and translated into a polyprotein, which is cleaved by HIV protease into several different smaller proteins or subunits that are responsible for assembling a new, mature HIV virion. Protease inhibitors (PIs) bind HIV protease, preventing the cleavage of the polyprotein into individual proteins, which makes the assembly of a mature and infectious HIV virion unlikely. This new HIV virion then buds off from the infected CD4+ cell and infects another CD4+ cell. The life cycle of HIV infection and replication just described is repeated 1–10 billion times/day.

GENETIC BASIS

The CCR5 co-receptor is a common host factor important for HIV transmission and pathogenesis. Not only do CD4+ cells have CCR5 co-receptors, but these co-receptors can also exist on macrophages. Therefore, HIV can also infect macrophages, which seem to act as one of the primary sources responsible for HIV transmission into the brain. About 3%–5% of patients with HIV infection can remain asymptomatic, maintaining normal CD4+ cell counts for several years without ARV therapy (ART); these patients are termed *long-term nonprogressors*. About 1% of patients living with HIV have undetectable viral loads with maintenance of high CD4+ cell counts; these patients are termed *elite controllers*.[8-10] Slow HIV disease progression in these patients may occur because of varying genotypes of the 32-bp deletion in the CCR5 co-receptor. Some patients who are homozygous for the CCR5 32-bp deletion do not express the co-receptor on CD4+ cells and are consequently resistant to HIV infection.[11] Those heterozygous for this CCR5 genetic mutation have slower disease progression than individuals without the mutation. Other genetic polymorphisms that may influence HIV infection and the rate of disease progression include *APOBEC3G*, *HLA-*B27*, and *HLA-*B57*.[12]

RISK FACTORS

One of the primary risk factors for HIV infection in infants and young children is the perinatal transmission of HIV from mother to child, also known as *mother-to-child-transmission* or MTCT. In 2017, the estimated number of new diagnoses of HIV from MTCT in the United States was 73.[3] The transmission risk of passing HIV from an untreated mother living with HIV to the fetus is about 20%. In these cases, elective caesarean section may be a suitable option to significantly reduce the rates of MTCT. For mothers who are taking ARVs and have excellent virologic control (defined as an undetectable viral load of less than 20–75 copies/mL), the risk of MTCT is reduced to less than 1%–2%. For older children and adolescents, risk factors may be similar to adults, especially for older adolescents who engage in sexual risk-taking behaviors. Table 1 is a comprehensive list of other risk factors (including more common and less common) for HIV transmission.[4,13-17]

CLINICAL PRESENTATION AND DIAGNOSIS

SIGNS AND SYMPTOMS

Infants and children infected with HIV often show signs of developmental delay (late to develop motor skills and cognitive ability). Weight gain or growth during the first year of life is usually absent, and children usually exhibit failure to thrive. Children with HIV may also develop opportunistic infections (OIs) or conditions that further affect growth and development. Encephalopathy in HIV can lead to microcephaly or brain atrophy. Motor impairments, such as gait abnormalities and ataxia, may also occur.[18] *Candida* infections (such as mucosal oropharyngeal thrush, vaginitis, and invasive esophageal candidiasis), cytomegalovirus (CMV), and *Pneumocystis jirovecii* pneumonia (previously termed *Pneumocystis carinii* pneumonia, or PCP) are common OIs and will be discussed in the following text. Children with HIV infection are also prone to recurrent bacterial infections and to lymphoid interstitial pneumonia, which is rare in the adult population.[19,20]

Adolescents who acquire HIV infection sexually or by intravenous drug use follow a clinical course similar to that of adults versus children who are perinatally infected with HIV and have a long and complicated treatment history. Acute HIV infection in adolescents who are infected through high-risk behaviors, such as sharing needles or unprotected sexual contact, may present with nonspecific symptoms, including fever, headache, sore throat, joint and/or muscle pain, lymphadenopathy, and generalized rash.[21-24] This acute retroviral syndrome typically occurs 2–4 weeks after infection. The persistence of these symptoms in the presence of ulcers on the mucosa of the mouth, anus, genitalia, or esophagus is suggestive of HIV infection. Gastrointestinal disturbances such as nausea, diarrhea, weight loss, and loss of appetite may also occur. Signs and symptoms of chronic HIV infection include continued weight loss, fatigue, recurrent yeast infections (vaginal or oral), and skin abnormalities (frequent rashes, psoriasis).[22]

Table 1. Risk Factors for HIV Transmission[13-17]

Risk Factor	Comment
More Common	
Breastfeeding	May be as high as 42% risk, depending on the duration
Injection drug use	Needle exchange programs and methadone maintenance programs reduce the risk of HIV transmission
Unprotected vaginal or anal sex	Men who have sex with men who engage in unprotected receptive anal sex have the highest risk of transmission
Multiple sex partners	Presence of other sexually transmitted infections (e.g., herpes simplex, syphilis) can increase the risk of HIV infection during sex
Substance abuse	Alcohol, crack cocaine, crystal methamphetamine, and opioids can lead to high-risk sexual behavior
Less Common	
Percutaneous exposure	Needle-stick or sharp object injury to a health care worker
Receipt of contaminated blood products	Through blood transfusion, organ/tissue transplantation
Unprotected oral sex	Extremely low risk compared to unprotected vaginal or anal sex
Receipt of pre-chewed food	Feeding infants food that is pre-chewed by person living with HIV
Being bitten by an person living with HIV or deep- or open-mouth kissing a person living with HIV whose mouth or gums are bleeding	HIV cannot reproduce outside the human body and is not spread by air or water; mosquitoes; saliva, tears, or sweat; shaking hands or sharing dishes; or closed-mouth or "social" kissing

DIAGNOSTIC CRITERIA

LABORATORY DATA

Infection with HIV is diagnosed by several methods, including detection of viral antibodies, p24 antigen, or HIV genetic material. Standard antibody testing is performed using enzyme immunoassay (EIA). Because of their high sensitivity and somewhat low specificity, positive EIA results must be confirmed by a Western blot, which uses antibodies to identify specific proteins after they are separated by gel electrophoresis. A negative EIA is typically considered a true negative; however, a false-negative result is possible if the test is performed in the "window period" of acute infection, describing the time it takes the body to produce antibodies to HIV. For indeterminate results, a repeat EIA is recommended as well as HIV RNA testing. Antibody testing may be performed by standard or rapid testing methods. Rapid tests offer the following advantages: the result can be read by a counselor/provider while the patient remains on site (results can be available in 40 minutes or less); patients can receive an immediate offer of or referral to medical care and/or counseling services; and these tests are performed using blood, plasma, serum, urine, or oral fluid samples.[25-27] The immediate results obtained from rapid testing have allowed more patients to be made aware of their infection status and expedited the care of patients with newly diagnosed HIV infection.[28-30] Many commercially available rapid tests can identify both HIV-1 and HIV-2. It is recommended to confirm a positive rapid test result with both the standard EIA and the Western blot tests. Criteria for interpreting a Western blot result have been offered by several national and international agencies, including the CDC and World Health Organization. The CDC criteria for a positive result include reactivity to either the gp41 or the p24 antigen, in addition to the gp120/160 antigens.

A polymerase chain reaction (PCR) test, a DNA test, or nucleic acid amplification can detect HIV antigens or isolate the virus. These methods are most useful to identify infection for those in the window period or for the diagnosis of HIV in infants. Virologic testing (for the presence of HIV RNA), rather than antibody testing, is recommended in infants because of the presence of maternal antibodies transferred by the placenta. Virologic testing for HIV should be performed in exposed infants within 14–21 days of birth, at age 1–2 months (2–4 weeks after the infant has completed ARV prophylaxis), and at age 4–6 months. Consideration may be given to performing the first round of testing at birth in infants who are at high risk of HIV infection, such as those born to mothers who did not receive antepartum ART for the prevention of MTCT or those whose mothers did not have a viral load less than 1000 copies/mL at delivery. An infant with an initial negative virologic test should be retested at age 1–2 months. Although infants should complete a 4- to 6-week course of zidovudine prophylaxis against HIV, this approach has not been shown to alter the time to detect HIV or alter the sensitivity of the testing method. A third virologic test is recommended at age 4–6 months in infants who have two previously negative tests to ultimately rule out the presence of HIV infection. Although not recommended at birth, two sets of negative antibody tests performed at a minimum by age 6 months may also rule out HIV infection in children in the absence of other clinical or virologic signs of infection. Antibody testing is also considered at age 12–18 months in patients with previous negative virologic testing to confirm that maternal antibodies are no longer present. Infection with HIV may be diagnosed by antibody testing and confirmatory Western blot in children 18 months and older.[31]

COURSE AND PROGNOSIS OF DISEASE

The highest risk of disease progression is in children younger than 5 years, regardless of immunologic status. For a child age 1 year compared with a child age 5 years at a similar CD4+ percentage, the risk of progression to AIDS is increased 4-fold and the risk of death is increased 6-fold. At CD4+ counts less than 350 cells/mm³, children who are at least age 5 years have a 12-month risk of death or progression to AIDS similar to that of young adults (around 20 years).[31,32] The difference in risk of disease progression and death between these age groups is likely multifactorial. High levels of HIV RNA can persist for a longer period in younger children, and although viral load levels may be low at birth, viral load can increase substantially by age 2 months to more than 100,000 copies/mL. The risk of HIV progressing to AIDS increases when viral loads are higher than this threshold. In addition, a young child's developing immune system may not be sufficiently robust to limit viral replication.

The *virologic set point* is the level of HIV RNA that is reached after a decline in viral load after acute infection; this point is typically set about 6–12 months after infection and shows a correlation with the risk of disease progression or death in adolescent patients. The application of this information to infants and young children is less clear because of the fluctuations in HIV viral load seen in this population. In infants, high viral loads (greater than 299,000 copies/mL) are associated with a greater risk of disease progression and death.[33,34] This increased risk is also present for perinatally and behaviorally infected adolescents with viral loads higher than 100,000 copies/mL.[35,36] The risk of progression to AIDS and death in children is greatest in the first year of life regardless of HIV RNA level, with the risk increasing at higher viral loads.[37] Given the potential for fluctuating HIV RNA levels in very young children as mentioned previously, it is important to consider both the immunologic and virologic status of a child when determining his or her risk of disease progression.[38]

OPPORTUNISTIC INFECTIONS

One of the most common OIs diagnosed in children living with HIV is PCP, with the highest rates of occurrence in infants up to age 12 months. The risk of PCP infection increases with a decrease in CD4+ count and CD4+ percentage. Distinguishing features of infection include fever, cough, dyspnea, and tachypnea. Pediatric patients older than 5 years typically also present with low oxygen saturation, a CD4+ count less than 200 cells/mm³, and/or a CD4+ percentage less than 15%. Chest radiographs may be normal or may show little infiltrate or bilateral parenchymal infiltrates. Although elevated lactate dehydrogenase and decreased serum albumin may also be present, they are not specific to PCP infection. To diagnose PCP, the organism must be identified in pulmonary tissue, preferably obtained by bronchoscopy with bronchoalveolar lavage. *Pneumocystis* organisms may be recognized through staining: methenamine-silver and toluidine blue stain the cyst wall, but immunofluorescent antibodies, which also stain the cyst wall, have higher specificity. Prophylaxis against PCP is highly recommended in children age 1–12 months regardless of CD4$^+$ count, in children 1–5 years with CD4$^+$ counts less than 500 cells/mm^3 or CD4$^+$ percentage less than 15%, and in children 6 years or older with CD4$^+$ counts less than 200 cells/mm^3 and/or CD4$^+$ percentage less than 15%. Primary prophylaxis should not be discontinued in patients younger than 1 year, but it may be discontinued in older children after they have received ARV treatment for at least 6 months and have met the following CD4$^+$ count thresholds: age 1–5 years—CD4$^+$ count of 500 cells/mm^3 or greater for more than 3 consecutive months; 6 years and older—CD4$^+$ count of 200 cells/mm^3 or greater for more than 3 consecutive months.[39]

Mycobacterium avium complex (MAC) is another common OI among children living with HIV. The risk of infection increases with varying levels of age-specific immunosuppression (Table 2). This infection colonizes the gastrointestinal and respiratory tracts; the presence of MAC in these locations can be predictive of disseminated MAC infection, which can involve the lungs, lymph nodes, liver, spleen, and bone marrow. Respiratory symptoms are rare, but cough may be present. Common signs and symptoms include fever, weight loss, muscle weakness, abdominal pain, diarrhea, chills, night sweats, fatigue, and hepatosplenomegaly. Laboratory

findings reveal anemia, neutropenia, and thrombocytopenia and may include elevated lactate dehydrogenase or alkaline phosphatase values. A blood culture or bone marrow biopsy is required for a diagnosis of MAC. Although a positive acid-fast bacillus test may be indicative of MAC in a symptomatic patient, it cannot be distinguished from *Mycobacterium tuberculosis* without a culture or confirmation with a PCR test. As with PCP, prophylaxis against MAC is highly recommended in patients meeting certain CD4$^+$ counts or CD4$^+$ percentage thresholds (Table 2). Prophylaxis is indicated in the following situations: in infants with CD4$^+$ counts less than 750 cells/mm^3; in children age 1–2 years with CD4$^+$ counts less than 500 cells/mm^3; in children 2–5 years with CD4$^+$ counts less than 75 cells/mm^3; and in children 6 years and older with CD4$^+$ counts less than 50 cells/mm^3. Primary prophylaxis should not be discontinued in patients younger than 2 years, but it may be discontinued in older children after they have received ARV treatment for at least 6 months and have met the following CD4$^+$ count thresholds: children age 2–5 years—CD4$^+$ count greater than 200 cells/mm^3 for more than 3 consecutive months; children 6 years and older—CD4$^+$ count greater than 100 cells/mm^3 for more than 3 consecutive months.[39]

Toxoplasma gondii infection in infants and children is usually the result of maternal infection present before or at birth. In older children and adolescents, acquisition is typically through ingesting parasite-containing raw or undercooked meat or water or soil contaminated with sporulated oocysts. Because cats are confirmed hosts for *T. gondii* and may excrete sporulated oocysts in their feces after early infection, contact with their feces can also be a risk factor for infection. In patients with AIDS, *T. gondii* usually presents with central

Table 2. Primary Prophylactic Drug Regimens for Common Opportunistic Infections in Children and Adolescents Living with HIV[39,78]

Pathogen	Indication by Age and CD4$^+$ (cells/mm^3) or CD4%	Children	Adolescents
Pneumocystis jirovecii pneumonia	1–12 mo 1–5 yr with CD4$^+$ < 500 or CD4% < 15% 6–12 yr with CD4$^+$ < 200 or CD4% < 15% Adolescents with CD4$^+$ < 200 or CD4% < 14%	TMP/SMX[a]: 150/750 mg/m^2 BSA/day, preferably as a daily dose OR every other day (e.g., Monday, Wednesday, Friday) OR single dose three times/wk on consecutive days MDD: 320/1600 mg	TMP/SMX: 160/800 mg once daily OR 80/400 mg once daily
Mycobacterium avium complex	< 1 yr with CD4$^+$ < 750 1–2 yr with CD4$^+$ < 500 2–5 yr with CD4$^+$ < 75 ≥ 6 yr with CD4$^+$ < 50	Azithromycin: 20 mg/kg once weekly Maximum weekly dose: 1200 mg Clarithromycin: 7.5 mg/kg BID MDD: 1000 mg	Azithromycin: 1200 mg once weekly OR 600 mg twice weekly Clarithromycin: 500 mg BID
Toxoplasma gondii	Positive for *Toxoplasma* antibody PLUS: < 6 yr with CD4% < 15% OR ≥ 6 yr with CD4$^+$ < 100	TMP/SMX: 150/750 mg/m^2 BSA/day, once daily MDD: 320/1600 mg	TMP/SMX: 160/800 mg once daily

[a]Patients who are allergic to sulfonamide antibiotics may take dapsone as an alternative to TMP/SMX for PCP prophylaxis; if so, they should be monitored for signs of cross-sensitivity. Additional alternatives to TMP/SMX include aerosolized pentamidine and atovaquone.
BID = twice daily; BSA = body surface area; HIV = human immunodeficiency virus; MDD = maximum daily dose; TMP/SMX = trimethoprim/sulfamethoxazole.

nervous system effects, including headache, confusion, neurologic deficiencies, and seizures. Fever may be present, and nausea or vomiting can occur with significant mental status changes. Diagnosis is confirmed by EIA testing for immunoglobulins specific to *Toxoplasma* (immunoglobulin A, E, or M up to age 6 months or G after age 1 year). Children 6 years and older with CD4$^+$ counts less than 100 cells/mm^3 and positive antibody tests should receive prophylaxis for *T. gondii*; children 5 years and younger with positive antibody testing should receive prophylaxis if the CD4$^+$ percentage is less than 15%. Primary prophylaxis should not be discontinued in patients younger than 1 year, but it may be discontinued in older children after they have received ARV treatment for at least 6 months if they meet the following CD4$^+$ count thresholds: children age 1–5 years—CD4$^+$ percentage of 15% or greater for more than 3 consecutive months; children 6 years and older—CD4$^+$ percentage of 15% or greater or CD4$^+$ count greater than 200 cells/mm^3 for more than 3 consecutive months.[39]

Transmission of CMV may occur perinatally or by ingesting CMV-containing bodily fluids (i.e., blood, breast milk, saliva, genital secretions) or through sexual contact. The risk of infection is highest during the first year of life. Symptoms of disease include microcephaly, hearing impairment, hepatosplenomegaly, and retinitis, which may be characterized by blurred vision or blind spots. Photopsia is highly associated with CMV retinitis in patients with AIDS.[41] Many children with CMV at birth subsequently acquire developmental delays, neurologic deficits, learning disabilities, ophthalmologic complications, or seizure disorders. Similar to HIV infection, CMV is difficult to diagnose in infants with antibody testing because maternal antibodies may be present throughout the first year of life. In children older than 12 months, a positive antibody test does not always indicate an active infection, but it is indicative of CMV exposure. Detection of CMV is by culture or a PCR test. Primary prophylaxis for CMV is not routinely recommended; however, yearly screenings are recommended for children who tested negative at birth and for children whose CD4$^+$ counts are less than 100 cells/mm^3 or who have a CD4$^+$ percentage less than 10%.[39]

Candida infections are common among children living with HIV and are most often caused by *Candida albicans*. These infections are found in the mucosa of the oral cavity, esophagus, and oropharynx (thrush, angular cheilitis) and as dermatitis in the diaper area; they may also be found in the vulvovaginal area of adolescent girls. Infants and toddlers with *Candida* infection may present with discomfort in the diaper area or difficulty or pain on swallowing. *Candida* infection can be diagnosed with a biopsy of infected tissue by staining or culture; by the presence of invasive disease, although not typically a significantly high-risk issue in patients living with HIV; or by blood culture. Although a low CD4$^+$ count, less than 100 cells/mm^3, increases the risk of developing a *Candida* infection, primary prophylaxis is rarely recommended because active infections respond well to existing treatment measures. Initiating antifungal prophylaxis also increases both the risk of developing antifungal drug resistance and the potential for drug–drug interactions with ARV medications.[39]

Table 2 provides a summary of recommended prophylaxis regimens for PCP, MAC, and toxoplasmosis. Resources are available that provide greater detailed information on alternative primary prophylaxis regimens, secondary prophylaxis, discontinuation of prophylaxis, and the treatment of active infection in children and adolescents living with HIV.[39,42]

TREATMENT

GOALS OF THERAPY

As a chronic infection, HIV requires lifelong therapy. Therefore, the goals of ARV treatment for children and adolescents living with HIV are the following: reduce HIV-related mortality and morbidity; preserve and restore immune function; achieve virologic suppression; prevent the emergence of drug resistance; minimize ARV adverse effects; maintain normal physical growth and neurocognitive development; improve quality of life; and prevent transmission to others.[31]

NONPHARMACOLOGIC THERAPY

Micronutrient (multivitamin and trace element) deficiencies are common in patients living with HIV, especially those with advanced disease progression and those living in developing countries. Therefore, vitamin supplementation has been explored as an avenue for reducing HIV disease burden. A Cochrane Review analysis showed that several micronutrient supplements reduced mortality and morbidity in pregnant women living with HIV and their children.[43] Multivitamin supplementation in African pregnant patients has also been associated with decreased adverse pregnancy outcomes such as fetal death, low birth weight, and severe preterm births. The children also had better growth, better micronutrient status, and higher CD4$^+$ counts in the first 6 months to 2 years of life.[43,44] Administration with oral cholecalciferol with calcium also adds additional benefit for skeletal and nonskeletal health, including innate immunity in children and adolescents living with HIV.[45] As a whole, multivitamin supplementation seems to be beneficial to patients living with HIV and may also serve as an indicator for assessing adherence to medications before considering the initiation of ARVs.

HERBAL THERAPY

Herbals may also play a role in the treatment of HIV infection. The catechins contained in green tea have been associated with several health benefits.[46] In vitro studies have shown that epigallocatechin gallate—the most plentiful catechin in green tea—inhibited gp120 of the HIV virion binding to the CD4$^+$ cell receptor.[47] However, studies of epigallocatechin gallate suggest that a significant quantity of green tea would need to be consumed to produce an in vivo effect.[48,49] Other potentially beneficial herbals include *Hypoxis hemerocallidea* (African potato) and *Sutherlandia frutescens*. The African potato is used as an immune-stimulant and has antioxidant properties. *Sutherlandia* possesses a constituent l-canavanine, which is thought to have antiviral activity.

One disadvantage of the *Hypoxis* and *Sutherlandia* spp. is the potential for drug interactions with ARVs because they may inhibit the cytochrome P450 (CYP) 3A4 isoenzyme (CYP3A4) and P-glycoprotein (an efflux transporter). Other herbals such as St. John's wort (*Hypericum perforatum*) or garlic supplements are inducers of CYP3A4 and may decrease the serum concentrations of the PIs, NNRTIs, INSTIs, and maraviroc.[50] Health care providers, especially pharmacists, are encouraged to ask patients about vitamin supplementation and herbal use to rule out any potential drug interactions with ARVs. Furthermore, another major limitation to using herbals for treating HIV infection is the lack of U.S. Food and Drug Administration (FDA) regulation and approval based on efficacy and safety. Thus, caution should be taken if children living with HIV are using herbals and ARVs concomitantly.

PREVENTION

Prevention of MTCT of HIV or prevention of vertical transmission include efforts to prevent transmission of HIV from a mother living with HIV to her infant during pregnancy, labor, delivery, and breastfeeding. A comprehensive approach to prevention of MTCT is advocated by the World Health Organization to include preventing new HIV infections among women of childbearing age and preventing unplanned pregnancies among women living with HIV.[51] The perinatal HIV guidelines discuss recommended ARV regimens for use during pregnancy in women living with HIV as well as intrapartum ART prophylaxis, mode of delivery, and management of infants born to women living with HIV including ARV prophylaxis.[52] Depending on the viral load of pregnant mothers living with HIV, intravenous zidovudine should be administered to the mother during labor if her HIV viral load is greater than 1000 copies/mL or unknown in late pregnancy or at delivery. For mothers for whom the clinician suspects challenges with adherence, the decision to use intrapartum intravenous zidovudine should be made based on clinical judgment. For pregnant mothers living with HIV who have an HIV viral load less than 1000 copies/mL, intravenous zidovudine is not required. Postpartum infant prophylaxis with oral zidovudine should be given to the neonate for 6 weeks unless a full-term infant's mother has been virally suppressed on ART during pregnancy with no concerns regarding maternal adherence, in which case a shortened course of 4 weeks of oral zidovudine can be given.

One of the best ways to prevent horizontal transmission of HIV is to use safe sex practices such as condoms. When latex condoms are used consistently and correctly, they are highly effective in preventing sexual transmission of HIV. One study found that consistent condom use resulted in an 80% reduction in HIV incidence in HIV serodiscordant heterosexual couples.[53] A review study also showed that among men who have sex with men, condom use reduced the per-contact risk of HIV infection by 78% compared with unprotected anal intercourse.[54] Furthermore, other methods to prevent HIV transmission have been explored, including male circumcision, vaccines, and microbicides. Male circumcision is associated with reduced transmission of sexually transmitted diseases, including HIV. Three large randomized controlled trials evaluated the impact of voluntary adult circumcision on HIV transmission rates in Kenya, South Africa, and Uganda. These trials showed a 50% to 60% reduction in the incidence of HIV infection for circumcised men compared with uncircumcised men.[55-57] Another clinical trial in Uganda evaluated male-to-female HIV transmission rates when the males were circumcised and had viral loads less than 50,000 copies/mL, showing a significantly lower rate of transmission in this group compared with the uncircumcised group.[58]

An effective HIV vaccine has yet to be found, despite decades of continuous research. Several types of vaccines are being studied, including protein vaccines, DNA vaccines, viral vector vaccines, and using antibodies for HIV prevention.[59] Several trials failed to show a protective benefit of vaccination.[58-62] However, a more recent study conducted in a community in a province in Thailand found a moderate short-lived protective effect for those who received a recombinant glycoprotein 120 subunit vaccine (AIDSVAX B/E) with or without a recombinant canarypox vector vaccine (ALVAC-HIV) regimen 6–8 years after initial vaccination compared with those on placebo.[63-66] Because of the success of this vaccine regimen, which produced broadly neutralizing antibodies, future research for HIV vaccine is focused on these antibodies. Obstacles that make it so difficult to find a successful HIV vaccine are the great genetic diversity of the virus, its ability to evade adaptive immune responses, its inability to induce a broadly reactive antibody response, and the establishment of latent reservoirs early in infection.

The benefits and the role of microbicides for preventing HIV transmission in adults was first studied in the CAPRISA (Centre for the AIDS Program of Research in South Africa) trial which found that a 1% tenofovir vaginal gel was associated with at least a 40% significantly reduced risk of transmission of HIV infection compared with placebo at 24 months.[67] Follow-up studies, including the VOICE trial and the FACTS 001 trial also studied 1% tenofovir vaginal gel but failed to show reduction in the rates of HIV-1 acquisition because of poor adherence to study drug (less than 30% adherence).[67-68] Additional studies are being conducted to evaluate the efficacy of rectal microbicides. The Microbicide Trials Network has conducted several phase I and phase II studies examining the safety and efficacy of various agents to be used as a rectal microbicide including tenofovir, maraviroc, and dapivirine gels; however, currently there are no rectal microbicides with an FDA label indication for the use of prevention of HIV infection.[69] Currently, no data support the use of microbicides to prevent HIV transmission in children.

In July 2012, the FDA approved emtricitabine/tenofovir disoproxil fumarate (TDF) to reduce the risk of HIV infection in uninfected individuals who are at high risk of HIV infection as HIV pre-exposure prophylaxis. The basis for the approval of emtricitabine/TDF as HIV pre-exposure prophylaxis is supported by results from various studies of emtricitabine/TDF in HIV uninfected individuals in different risk categories and older than 18 years.[70-74] In May 2018, the FDA approved an indication for emtricitabine/TDF in adults and adolescents weighing at least 35 kg. This expansion is based on the results of the Adolescent Medicine Trials Network

113 study, which enrolled 78 high-risk male adolescents age 15–17 years. Results suggest that at-risk youth may require closer and more frequent follow-up because their adherence decreased with quarterly visits.[75] The indications for pre-exposure prophylaxis, initial and follow-up prescribing recommendations, and recommendations for laboratory testing remain the same. The prescribing information of emtricitabine/TDF has been updated to reflect this new indication.[76] The CDC clinical practice guidelines on pre-exposure prophylaxis for the prevention of HIV infection will incorporate the change for use in adolescents weighing at least 35 kg into the next update.[77]

PHARMACOLOGIC THERAPY

Since the development of the first ARVs in the late 1980s, treatment of pediatric HIV infection has evolved tremendously, especially with the arrival of the first PI and now the INSTIs. Use of combination ART (cART) has improved survival; decreased the development and risk of OIs; improved growth and neurocognitive function; and enhanced the quality of life for children living with HIV. Treatment of pediatric HIV infection, however, is very complex and should

be tailored as well as possible to the patient's individual circumstances (Table 3).[31,78] Moreover, it is worth emphasizing that the monthly average wholesale price of individual ARVs is very expensive (ranging from $54 to $4303 depending on the choice of ARV).[78] Annual costs of cART using various coformulated combination products as single-tablet regimens may range in price from $36,000 to $40,000, whereas the monthly average wholesale price of NRTIs and NNRTIs tends to be considerably less than PIs and INSTIs. These average wholesale price costs, which are derived from September 2017 data, may not represent the pharmacy acquisition costs or price paid by consumers.[78] Affordability of cART may be considerably improved by insurance coverage as well as financial assistance programs such as AIDS drug assistance programs, funding through the Ryan White HIV/AIDS Program, and pharmaceutical company patient assistance programs. Furthermore, increasingly more ARVs—especially NRTIs and NNRTIs—are becoming available in their generic formulations. Although switching from branded coformulated products to using separate generic ART components may decrease costs, increased pill burden may lead to reduced medication adherence. Because very few randomized clinical trials have been conducted in children, most of the ARVs indicated for

Table 3. Factors in Choosing Antiretroviral Therapy for Children Living with HIV[31,78]

Factor	Comments
Age of child	Different levels of caregiver involvement
Severity of disease	Virologic, immunologic, and clinical status
Affordability of ARVs	Annual costs of ARVs are very expensive, but insurance coverage and AIDS drug assistance programs can help offset costs
Availability of appropriate dosage formulations	Liquid formulations including palatability Crushable/chewable/dissolvable tablets Powder/granule formulations
Availability of relevant PK data for different age groups	Limited PK data available for some more recently approved ARVs in pediatric and adolescent populations
Potency of ARV regimen	Use three fully active drugs if possible
Complexity of ARV regimen	Pill burden Dosing frequency Administration conditions, such as food considerations Medication storage conditions, such as refrigeration Expiration dates
Toxicity of ARV regimen	Minimization and management of adverse effects
Preservation of future ARV options	Maintain virologic control to avoid development of drug resistance/cross-resistance to other ARVs
ARV treatment history	Potential for cross-resistance to other ARVs and previous intolerance of specific ARVs
Presence of ARV drug-resistant virus	Knowledge of previous resistance tests including genotypes and phenotypes is useful to determine appropriate ARV regimen, although the complexity of regimen may be increased
Presence of comorbid conditions	Potential for drug–drug or drug–disease interactions, including overlapping toxicities of drugs
Potential drug–drug interactions	Dose adjustments may be necessary with some medications; however, some ARVs may need to be avoided if contraindicated
Adherence potential	Critical for determining choice of appropriate ARV therapy, with awareness that a good support system can greatly benefit a patient

ARV=antiretroviral; HIV = human immunodeficiency virus; PK = pharmacokinetic.

treatment of pediatric HIV infection derive their approval from efficacy data in adults, from pharmacokinetic and safety data from phase I/II trials of children, and from nonrandomized open-label studies. Furthermore, few phase III trials compare the effects of different ARV regimens in children living with HIV.

The decision about when to start treatment has been debated for adults living with HIV. However, recent clinical trials support initiation of cART for all individuals living with HIV, regardless of CD4+ cell count to reduce morbidity and mortality associated with HIV infection and to prevent HIV transmission.[79-82] There are both advantages and disadvantages to initiating ART earlier when the patient is asymptomatic versus delaying treatment until the patient becomes symptomatic. Advantages of initiating ART early include the following: having control of viral replication; allowing a lower viral load set point; reducing mutant viral strains; preserving immune function; preventing HIV disease progression; preventing sexual transmission of HIV; preventing non-AIDS malignancies and other complications; and improving overall quality of life. However, delaying ART may also have some advantages, such as reduced development of drug-resistant virus (because of no drug-selective pressure), improved adherence to ARV regimen because the patient is symptomatic, and reduced or delayed adverse effects of ART.

Although treatment is also recommended for all children living with HIV, the urgency for immediate initiation varies by age and pretreatment CD4+ cell count. This variation is because fewer data exist for the pediatric population versus adults regarding the risks and benefits of starting treatment immediately in asymptomatic children living with HIV. Of importance, CD4+ cell count and viral load show considerable variability by age in children. Although these surrogate markers are poorly predictive of mortality and disease progression in infants, it is recommended to start treatment for all infants with a diagnosis of HIV infection, regardless of symptoms and CD4+ cell count, because they are at greatest risk of rapid disease progression. In several studies infants who received early treatment had a significantly reduced risk of disease progression and achieved greater CD4+ cell recovery compared with those who received no ARV treatment.[83-85] In the HIV Pediatric Prognostic Markers Collaborative Study meta-analysis, both CD4+ percentage and HIV viral load were independent predictors of the risk of clinical progression or death in children older than 12 months.[32] Furthermore, an analysis of at least 21,000 pairs of CD4+ measurements from 3345 children (ranging in age from younger than 1 year up to 16 years) in the HIV Pediatric Prognostic Markers Collaborative Study concluded that CD4+ cell counts provide greater prognostic value over CD4+ percentage in terms of short-term disease progression for both children younger than 5 years and older children between 5 and 16 years.[86] Combined data from PENPACT-1 and PREDICT studies suggest that starting treatment at higher CD4+ cell count thresholds and at a younger age improves immunologic recovery.[87-88] Therefore, initiation of cART is recommended for all children living with HIV, regardless of clinical, immunologic, or virologic status. Figure 1 shows a summary of criteria and recommendations for when to initiate ART in children living with HIV.

When initiating ART in treatment-naive children living with HIV, the general approach is to use cART with at least three active ARV drugs from two different classes. Combination therapy is important because ARV resistance can develop more easily with monotherapy or dual therapy. The choice of initial cART for treatment-naive children living with HIV is critically important because the selection of the first regimen can affect the consideration of future treatment options. Before starting treatment, adherence barriers to ART should be fully assessed and discussed with both the patient and the parents or caregivers. If possible, identifying potential problems and resolving them before starting ART are ideal. Adherence to ARVs is the cornerstone for achieving the goals of therapy because poor adherence to ARVs can lead to subtherapeutic concentrations, which increases the risk of developing ARV resistance and virologic failure.

To date, more than 25 ARV drugs are approved for use in the treatment of HIV, most of which have an approved pediatric treatment indication. Currently, there are five ARV classes: NRTIs, NNRTIs, PIs, INSTIs, and entry inhibitors (including fusion inhibitors and attachment inhibitors such as CCR5 antagonists). The Pathophysiology section of this chapter provides for more information on the pharmacology of ARVs. Common ARV combinations for treatment-naive pediatric HIV infection include two NRTIs plus one NNRTI; two NRTIs plus one PI with ritonavir; or two NRTIs plus one INSTI. Although monotherapy for treatment of HIV infection is not recommended because of the potential for resistance development, one exception is zidovudine monotherapy for 6 weeks in infants of indeterminate HIV status to prevent perinatal HIV transmission. Should infants have a confirmation of HIV infection while receiving zidovudine monotherapy, zidovudine should be discontinued, and combination therapy with three active ARVs should be used for treatment (which may include zidovudine, if the genotype shows no resistance). Resistance testing for ARVs is always recommended before initiating therapy in treatment-naive children living with HIV because it is possible for infants to acquire drug resistance from their mothers living with HIV. For example, infants given single-dose peripartum nevirapine for prevention of transmission should not use nevirapine as combination therapy because if they are later given a diagnosis of HIV infection this maternal–infant prophylaxis could be associated with resistance to nevirapine and subsequent virologic failure.[89] Drug-resistant virus has been detected in 6% to 16% of ARV-naive adults and in 18% of adolescents with recent infection in both the United States and Europe.[90-93]

Recommendations for optimal ART among pediatric patients are continuously updated as new drug formulations are developed and more information regarding efficacy and safety becomes available. The U.S. Department of Health and Human Services (DHHS) guidelines are written by a panel of experts who assimilate data from all the clinical trials of adult and pediatric patients to date.[31,78] Their recommendations for specific ARV drugs or regimens are stratified into two different categories for treatment-naive pediatric patients living with HIV: preferred and alternative.[31] Updates to these guidelines can be found at https://aidsinfo.nih.gov. Table 3 shows some primary factors that may affect their recommendations for ARV use. Table 4 also provides a summary of various ARVs used to treat HIV infection, including dosing formulations, dosing, special instructions, and metabolism/mode of clearance for each ARV.

Most clinical data for pediatric and adult treatment-naive patients living with HIV include three basic regimens: *NNRTI-based*, with two NRTIs and an NNRTI; *PI-based*, with two NRTIs and a PI; or *INSTI-based*, with two NRTIs and an INSTI. All of these regimens are preferred as initial therapy. Advantages and disadvantages of NNRTI, PI, and INSTI ARV classes are shown in Table 5.[78] Both the regimens based on NNRTI (specifically, nevirapine) and INSTI (specifically, raltegravir) are preferred in infants younger than 14

days. The PI- and INSTI–based regimens are preferred over NNRTI-based regimens in children age 14 days or older and in children younger than 3 years because of superior virologic suppression.[89] For children 3 years and older, PI- and INSTI-based regimens are preferred as initial therapy. Available data on three clinical trials (P1060, PENPACT-1and PROMOTE) comparing PI- and NNRTI-based regimens in children living with HIV might also be useful in helping the clinician to choose between one of these two ARV class regimens.[94-96] The INSTI-based regimens have evolved to become an important and recommended component of initial therapy for children living with HIV. Although INSTIs have not yet been compared with other ARV regimens in clinical trials for treatment

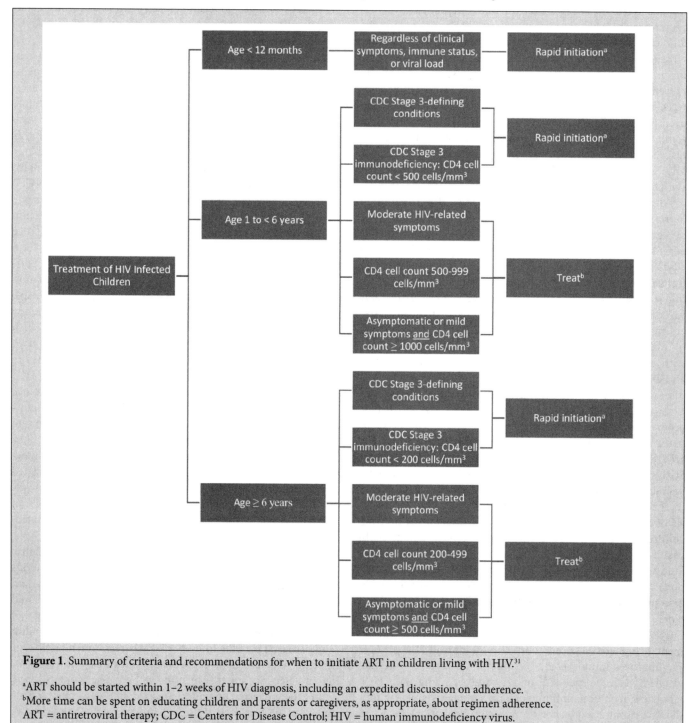

Figure 1. Summary of criteria and recommendations for when to initiate ART in children living with HIV.[31]

[a]ART should be started within 1–2 weeks of HIV diagnosis, including an expedited discussion on adherence.
[b]More time can be spent on educating children and parents or caregivers, as appropriate, about regimen adherence.
ART = antiretroviral therapy; CDC = Centers for Disease Control; HIV = human immunodeficiency virus.

of children living with HIV, they derive their preference for initial therapy based on noncomparative studies evaluating safety and pharmacokinetics of INSTIs. Furthermore, efficacy, tolerability, and fewer drug–drug interactions observed with INSTI-based regimens in comparative clinical trials demonstrated superiority over NNRTI- and PI-based regimens in adults. In addition, studies in adolescents supported the preferred use of INSTIs in children as young as birth.[97-100]

Regimens based on INSTIs include bictegravir, dolutegravir, elvitegravir, and raltegravir, which are all indicated for treatment-naive adults living with HIV. Raltegravir may be used in infants and children as young as birth; dolutegravir is used for children 3 years and older and weighing at least 25 kg; and elvitegravir—specifically, boosted with cobicistat in combination with tenofovir alafenamide (TAF) and emtricitabine—can be used in children living with HIV weighing at least 25 kg. Bictegravir coformulated with TAF and emtricitabine recently received FDA label approval for treatment of adults living with HIV only. Some advantages of this fixed-dose combination include one-tablet, once-daily dosing, a high genetic barrier to resistance, small pill size, and fewer drug–drug interactions, as well as coformulation with TAF, which provides reduced kidney and bone toxicities compared with TDF. Dolutegravir received FDA label approval for treatment of children living with HIV weighing at least 30 kg based on supportive studies including a total of 57 treatment-experienced children who had no previous treatment with INSTIs.[99,101,102] Dolutegravir has several advantages including the following: excellent efficacy; tolerability; few drug–drug interactions; a high genetic barrier, defined as the need to accumulate at least three mutations for it to not work effectively; dosage formulation as a relatively small, circular, pill-size, single tablet; and once-daily dosing for children and adolescents weighing at least 30 kg. As mentioned previously with respect to efficacy, dolutegravir was noninferior to raltegravir and superior to NNRTI-based (efavirenz) and PI-based (darunavir/ritonavir) cART regimens in clinical trials.[97,98,100,103] Elvitegravir is available only in fixed dose combination formulations (Genvoya and Stribild, both by Gilead Sciences, Inc., Foster City, CA). Genvoya (elvitegravir/cobicistat/emtricitabine/TAF) has FDA label approval for use in children and adolescents weighing at least 25 kg with any sexual maturity rating.[104] In comparison, Stribild has FDA label approval for use in adolescents weighing at least 35 kg and sexual maturity rating of 4 or 5. Based on efficacy and safety observed in clinical studies, the preferred recommendation for Genvoya is for children and adolescents age 12 years or older and weighing at least 25 kg who have creatinine clearance greater than 30 mL/minute/1.73 m².[105-107] Cobicistat does not have antiviral activity and acts similarly to ritonavir as a pharmacokinetic enhancer (CYP3A4 inhibitor) increasing the concentrations of elvitegravir. Genvoya tends to have better tolerability than Stribild because of the TAF component in its formulation, thus supporting its use earlier in children and adolescence. In clinical studies, patients taking Genvoya had significantly smaller increases in mean serum creatinine, less proteinuria, and smaller decreases in bone mineral density at both the hip and spine than those treated with Stribild.[106] The dosage formulation (tablet) of Genvoya is also smaller in size compared

with Stribild, which helps to improve overall adherence for some patients. However, one of the disadvantages of these fixed-dose combination formulations compared with other INSTIs such as dolutegravir and raltegravir is an increased potential for drug–drug interactions because of the cobicistat component. Raltegravir can be used for treatment of infants and children living with HIV weighing at least 2 kg and can be used as early as birth. According to the DHHS guidelines, raltegravir is recommended as a preferred INSTI in infants and children from birth up to older than 3 years and weighing less than 25 kg. Raltegravir has shown equivalent virologic efficacy as well as better tolerability than the comparative regimens for treatment of adults living with HIV in three large randomized clinical studies.[108-110] Raltegravir has also been evaluated in infants, children, and adolescents in an open-label trial (IMPAACT P1066), supporting its use in children as young as 4 weeks.[111-113] Numerous advantages regarding raltegravir use include the following: its availability in different dosage formulations—specifically a chewable tablet and oral suspension, which can facilitate adherence, especially in younger infants and children who have a problem swallowing pills; few drug–drug interactions; and favorable safety profile. Although twice-daily dosing with raltegravir is recommended in infants and children, the recent approval of the 600-mg high-dose tablet formulation permits once-daily dosing (two tablets) for children and adolescents weighing at least 40 kg.

The NNRTI-based regimens include one of these drugs: efavirenz, nevirapine, etravirine, or rilpivirine. All of these NNRTIs have FDA label approval for treatment of children living with HIV. Efavirenz is an alternative NNRTI recommended for initial treatment of children 3 years or older. Efavirenz has been evaluated in numerous clinical studies in both adults and children living with HIV and shows excellent virologic response rates.[114-127] It was also shown to be superior to nevirapine as first-line therapy in children and adolescents in Uganda.[128] One major limitation of efavirenz is increased discontinuation rates because of adverse effects on the central nervous system. Because of this limitation, efavirenz is no longer recommended as a preferred NNRTI for treatment of children and adults living with HIV in the United States. Efavirenz can be potentially used for treatment of children as young as age 3 months and who weigh at least 3.5 kg by opening efavirenz capsules and sprinkling the contents on food. However, many risks are associated with this administration in such a young population, including pharmacokinetic variability; therefore it is no longer recommended. If the use of efavirenz is unavoidable in such a young population, both CYP2B6 genotyping and follow-up therapeutic drug monitoring (TDM) are recommended to guide appropriate dosing to ensure therapeutic concentrations.

Nevirapine is another NNRTI that has been evaluated extensively in clinical studies demonstrating efficacy and safety in children living with HIV.[94-96,129-133] One of the advantages of nevirapine is its availability as a palatable liquid formulation, which may be an acceptable alternative to lopinavir/ritonavir in children older than 14 days to younger than 3 years if they cannot tolerate lopinavir/ritonavir. Furthermore, if treatment is planned before age 14 days, the DHHS panel recommends using nevirapine as a preferred agent.

Table 4. Summary of Antiretroviral Treatment for Pediatric Patients Living with HIV [a,31]

Generic (Brand, Abbreviation)	Dosage Formulation	Dosing by Age and Weight	Special Instructions	Mode of Clearance/ Metabolism	Adverse Effects	Management/ Monitoring
Nucleoside Reverse Transcriptase Inhibitors (NRTIs)						
Abacavir (Ziagen[b], ABC)	**Oral solution:** 20 mg/mL **Tablets:** 300 mg (scored)	**Note:** Initiation of 600 mg QD dosing is not recommended in infants and young children treated with liquid formulations; only after 6 mo of undetectable viral load and stable CD4+ count can BID dosing with oral liquid be changed to QD dosing with liquid or tablet **Infant/Child (≥ 3 mo):** Oral solution 8 mg/kg BID (max 300 mg BID) or 16 mg/kg QD (max 600 mg QD with undetectable viral load and stable CD4+ cell counts) Scored 300-mg tablet (Wt ≥ 14 kg) 	Wt (kg)	Dose
---	---
14–< 20	150 mg BID or 300 mg QD
≥ 20–< 25	150 mg QAM + 300 mg QPM or + 450 mg QD
≥ 25	300 mg BID or 600 mg QD	 **Adolescent (Wt ≥ 25 kg)/Adult:** 300 mg BID or 600 mg QD • Trizivir[b] (abacavir/lamivudine/zidovudine) 1 tablet BID (≥ 30 kg) • Epzicom[b] (abacavir/lamivudine) 1 tablet QD (≥ 25 kg) • Triumeq[b] (abacavir/lamivudine/dolutegravir) 1 tablet QD (≥ 40 kg)	• With or without food • Alcohol may increase ABC concentrations	Extensively metabolized by alcohol dehydrogenase and glucuronyl transferase—only a small % excreted unchanged	Hypersensitivity reaction (symptoms may include fever, rash, malaise or fatigue, and shortness of breath)	• Screen for *HLA-B*5701*; if positive, do not use ABC, but note ABC allergy in medical record • If hypersensitivity reaction is suspected, then discontinue immediately • Do not rechallenge if experienced previous hypersensitivity reaction • Adjust dose in hepatic failure

Didanosine (Videx[c], ddI)	**Oral solution:** 10 mg/mL **EC delayed-release capsules (beadlets):** • 125 mg 200 mg 250 mg 400 mg	**Note:** No longer recommended for use in children because of higher rates of adverse effects vs. other NRTIs **Neonate/Infant (2 wk–< 3 mo):** 50 mg/m² of BSA BID **Infant (≥ 3–8 mo):** 100 mg/m² of BSA BID **Infant/Child (> 8 mo):** Oral solution 120 mg/m² of BSA BID (range: 90–150 mg/m² of BSA BID; max 200 mg BID) **Child/Adolescent (6–18 yr and ≥ 20 kg):** Videx EC 	Wt (kg)	Dose
---	---
20–< 25 kg	200 mg QD
25–< 60	250 mg QD
≥ 60	400 mg QD | **Adolescent/Adult:** < 60 kg: 250 mg QD ≥ 60 kg: 400 mg QD	• Administer ddI on an empty stomach (30 min before or 2 hr after a meal) • Shake oral solution well; keep refrigerated; admixture is stable for 30 days • In treatment-naive pts 3–21 yr, 240 mg/m² BSA QD (oral solution or capsules) has resulted in viral suppression • Do not exceed max adult dose	• Peripheral neuropathy • Pancreatitis (dose related and less common in children than in adults) • Retinal changes (optic neuritis) • Noncirrhotic portal hypertension (rare) • Diarrhea, abdominal pain, nausea, and vomiting • Lactic acidosis and severe hepatomegaly with steatosis (increased risk when used with d4T) • Insulin resistance/ diabetes mellitus	• LFTs • Pancreatic enzymes lipase and amylase • Blood glucose • Adjust dose in renal failure Renal

(continued)

Table 4. Summary of Antiretroviral Treatment for Pediatric Patients Living with HIV [a,31] (*continued*)

Generic (Brand, Abbreviation)	Dosage Formulation	Dosing by Age and Weight	Special Instructions	Mode of Clearance/ Metabolism	Adverse Effects	Management/ Monitoring
Emtricitabine (Emtriva[d], FTC)	**Oral solution:** 10 mg/mL **Capsule:** 200 mg	**Neonate/Infant (0–< 3 mo):** Oral solution: 3 mg/kg QD **Infant/Child/Adolescent (≥ 3 mo–17 yr):** Oral solution: 6 mg/kg QD (max 240 mg QD) Capsules: 200 mg QD (> 33 kg) **Adolescent (≥ 18 yr)/Adult:** Oral solution: 240 mg (24 mL) QD Capsules: 200 mg QD • Truvada[d] (tenofovir disoproxil fumarate/ emtricitabine) QD dosing for Truvada low strength 	Wt (kg)	FTC (mg)	TDF (mg)
---	---	---
17–< 22	100	150
22–< 28	133	200
28–< 35	167	250
≥ 35 (Adult)	200	300 (Truvada) | • Descovy[d] (tenofovir alafenamide/emtricitabine) 1 tablet QD (≥ 25 kg) • Atripla[d] (tenofovir disoproxil fumarate/ emtricitabine/efavirenz) 1 tablet QD (≥ 40 kg) • Complera[d] (tenofovir disoproxil fumarate/ emtricitabine/rilpivirine) 1 tablet QD (≥ 35 kg) • Odefsey[d] (tenofovir alafenamide/emtricitabine/ rilpivirine) 1 tablet QD (≥ 35 kg) • Stribild[d] (elvitegravir/cobicistat/emtricitabine/ tenofovir disoproxil fumarate) 1 tablet QD (≥ 35 kg) • Genvoya[d] (elvitegravir/cobicistat/emtricitabine/ tenofovir alafenamide) 1 tablet QD (≥ 25 kg) • Biktarvy[d] (bictegravir/emtricitabine/tenofovir alafenamide) 1 tablet QD (≥ 18 yr) • Symtuza[e] (darunavir/cobicistat/emtricitabine/ tenofovir alafenamide) 1 tablet QD (≥ 18 yr)	• With or without food • Oral solution can be kept at RT if used within 3 mo; refrigerate if long-term storage is used	Renal	• Minimal toxicity • Nausea, diarrhea • Hyperpigmentation/ skin discoloration on palms and/or soles (mostly in nonwhite pts)	• Screen for HBV before use; severe acute exacerbation of hepatitis can occur when FTC is discontinued; monitor LFTs for several mo after FTC is discontinued • Adjust dose in renal failure

Lamivudine (Epivir[b], 3TC)	**Oral solution:** 10 mg/mL **Tablets:** 150 mg (scored) 300 mg	**Note:** Initiation of QD lamivudine is not recommended in infants and children treated with liquid formulations; pts ≥ 3 yr may be transitioned to QD treatment with oral solution once stable on BID dosing for 36 wk with undetectable viral load and stable CD4 count **Neonate/Infant:** Oral solution 	Age	Dose
≥ 32 wk gestation at birth	2 mg/kg BID
Birth–< 4 wk	2 mg/kg BID
≥ 4 wk–< 3 mo	4 mg/kg BID
≥ 3 mo–< 3 yr	5 mg/kg BID (max 150 mg)
≥ 3 yr	5 mg/kg BID (max 150 mg) or 10 mg/kg QD (max 300 mg)	 **Tablet:** Scored 150-mg tablet (Wt ≥ 14 kg) 	Wt (kg)	Dose
14–< 20	75 mg BID or 150 mg QD
≥ 20–< 25	75 mg QAM and 150 mg QPM or 225 mg QD
≥ 25	150 mg BID or 300 mg QD | **Child (≥ 25 kg)/Adolescent/Adult:** 150 mg BID or 300 mg QD • Cimduo[f] (lamivudine/tenofovir disoproxil fumarate) 1 tablet QD • Trizivir (abacavir/lamivudine/zidovudine) 1 tablet BID (≥ 30 kg) • Epzicom (abacavir/lamivudine) 1 tablet QD (≥ 25 kg) • Combivir[b] (lamivudine/zidovudine) 1 tablet BID (≥ 30 kg) • Triumeq (abacavir/lamivudine/dolutegravir) 1 tablet QD (≥ 40 kg) • Symfi[f] (efavirenz/lamivudine/tenofovir disoproxil fumarate) 1 tablet QD (≥ 40 kg) • Symfi Lo[f] (efavirenz/lamivudine/tenofovir disoproxil fumarate) 1 tablet QD (≥ 35 kg)	• With or without food • Store oral solution at RT		• Minimal toxicity • Headache • Nausea • Pancreatitis	• Pancreatic enzymes lipase and amylase • Screen for HBV before use; severe acute exacerbation of hepatitis can occur when 3TC is discontinued; monitor LFTs for several mo after 3TC is discontinued • Adjust dose in renal failure

(continued)

Table 4. Summary of Antiretroviral Treatment for Pediatric Patients Living with HIV [a,31] *(continued)*

Generic (Brand, Abbreviation)	Dosage Formulation	Dosing by Age and Weight	Special Instructions	Mode of Clearance/ Metabolism	Adverse Effects	Management/ Monitoring
Stavudine (Zerit[c], d4T)	**Oral solution:** 1 mg/mL **Capsules:** 15 mg 20 mg 30 mg 40 mg	**Note:** No longer recommended in children because of higher rates of adverse effects vs. other NRTIs **Infant (≥ 14 days and Wt < 30 kg):** 1 mg/kg BID **Adolescent (≥ 30 kg)/Adult:** 30–< 60 kg: 30 mg BID	• With or without food • Shake oral solution well; keep refrigerated; will remain stable for 30 days	Renal	• Peripheral neuropathy • Pancreatitis • Lipodystrophy • Lactic acidosis with hepatic steatosis (higher incidence than with other NRTIs) • Hyperlipidemia • Rapidly progressive ascending neuromuscular weakness (rare) • Insulin resistance/ diabetes mellitus	• LFTs • Pancreatic enzymes lipase and amylase • Lipids (especially triglycerides) • Blood glucose • Adjust dose in renal failure

| Tenofovir disoproxil fumarate (Viread[d], TDF) | Oral powder: 40 mg/g

Tablets:
150 mg
200 mg
250 mg
300 mg

Truvada low-dose strength tablet:
FTC 100 mg/TDF 150 mg
FTC 133 mg/TDF 200 mg
FTC 167 mg/TDF 250 mg | **Infant/Child (≥ 2 yr and < 12 yr): 8 mg/kg/dose QD**

Infant/Child (≥ 2 yr): Oral powder | • 1 level scoop = 40 mg of TDF in 1 g powder
• With or without food (for tablets only)
• Mix oral powder in a container with 2–4 oz of soft food (e.g., yogurt, applesauce, baby food) and ingest entire mixture immediately to avoid bitter taste
• Do not administer oral powder in liquid form
• Absorption is enhanced when administered with a high-fat meal | Renal | • Diarrhea, nausea, vomiting, flatulence
• Renal insufficiency, Fanconi syndrome
• Decreased bone mineral density, osteomalacia | • DEXA scan before initiating TDF and 6 mo later, especially in prepuberty and early puberty (Sexual Maturity Rating (SMR) 1 and 2)
• SCr/BUN
• Urinalysis (proteinuria/glycosuria)
• Decreased serum phosphate
• Screen for HBV before use; severe acute exacerbation of hepatitis can occur when TDF is discontinued; monitor LFTs for several mo after TDF is discontinued
• Adjust dose in renal failure |

Infant/Child (≥ 2 yr): Oral powder

Wt (kg)	Scoops	Dose (mg)
10–<12	2	80
12–<14	2.5	100
14–<17	3	120
17–<19	3.5	140
19–<22	4	160
22–<24	4.5	180
24–<27	5	200
27–<29	5.5	220
29–<32	6	240
32–<34	6.5	260
34–<35	7	280
≥35	7.5	300

Pediatric (≥ 2 yr and ≥ 17 kg): TDF tablets QD

Wt (kg)	Dose (mg)
17–<22	150
22–<28	200
28–<35	250
≥35	300

Truvada (FTC/TDF) tablets QD

Wt (kg)	FTC (mg)	TDF (mg)
17–<22	100	150
22–<28	133	200
28–<35	167	250
≥35	200	300

Adolescent (≥ 35 kg)/Adult: 300 mg QD
• Truvada (tenofovir/emtricitabine) 1 tablet QD
• Atripla (tenofovir/emtricitabine/efavirenz) 1 tablet QD (≥ 40 kg)
• Complera (tenofovir disoproxil fumarate/emtricitabine/rilpivirine) 1 tablet QD (≥ 35 kg)
• Stribild (elvitegravir/cobicistat/emtricitabine/tenofovir disoproxil fumarate) 1 tablet QD (> 35 kg)
• Symfi (efavirenz/lamivudine/tenofovir disoproxil fumarate) 1 tablet QD (≥ 40 kg)
• Symfi Lo (efavirenz/lamivudine/tenofovir disoproxil fumarate) 1 tablet QD (≥ 35 kg)

(continued)

Table 4. Summary of Antiretroviral Treatment for Pediatric Patients Living with HIV [a,31] *(continued)*

Generic (Brand, Abbreviation)	Dosage Formulation	Dosing by Age and Weight	Special Instructions	Mode of Clearance/ Metabolism	Adverse Effects	Management/ Monitoring
Tenofovir alafenamide (TAF)	**Fixed-dose combinations**	**Child and adolescent (Wt ≥ 25 kg):** Descovy (tenofovir alafenamide/emtricitabine) 1 tablet QD **Child (≥ 12 yr and Wt ≥ 35 kg):** Odefsey (tenofovir alafenamide/emtricitabine/rilpivirine) 1 tablet QD **Child (≥ 12 yr and Wt ≥ 25 kg):** Genvoya (elvitegravir/cobicistat/emtricitabine/tenofovir alafenamide) 1 tablet QD **Adolescent (≥ 18 yr)/Adult:** Biktarvy (bictegravir/emtricitabine/tenofovir alafenamide) 1 tablet QD **Adolescent (≥ 18 yr)/Adult:** Symtuza (darunavir/cobicistat/emtricitabine/tenofovir alafenamide) 1 tablet QD	• Available only in fixed-dose combinations • With or without food depending on the other ARVs in combination tablet	Renal	• Diarrhea, nausea, headache • Increased serum lipids	• SCr/BUN • Urinalysis (proteinuria/ glycosuria) • Screen for HBV before use; severe acute exacerbation of hepatitis can occur when TAF is discontinued; monitor LFTs for several mo after therapy with TAF is discontinued • Not recommended in renal failure

Zidovudine (Retrovir[g], AZT or ZDV)	**Oral Syrup:** 10 mg/mL **Concentrate for injection/IV infusion:** 10 mg/mL **Capsules:** 100 mg **Tablets:** 300 mg	**Gestational age ≥ 35 wk (oral syrup)** **Birth–4 wk:** 4 mg/kg or Wt-based dosing 	Wt or Age	Dose
2–< 3 kg	1 mL (10 mg) BID
3–< 4 kg	1.5 mL (15 mg) BID
4–< 5 kg	2 mL (20 mg) BID
> 4 wk	12 mg/kg BID	 **≥ 30–< 35 wk gestational age at birth:** 	Age	Dose
Birth–2 wk	2 mg/kg BID
2 to 6-8 wk	3 mg/kg BID
> 6-8 wk	12 mg/kg BID	 **< 30 wk gestational age at birth:** 	Age	Dose
Birth–4 wk	2 mg/kg BID
4 wk to 8-10 wk	3 mg/kg BID
> 8-10 wk	12 mg/kg BID	 **Infant (≥ 35 wk postconception–≥ 4 wk postdelivery, ≥ 4 kg)/Child:** 	Wt (kg)	Dose
4–< 9	12 mg/kg BID
9–< 30	9 mg/kg BID

≥ 30	300 mg BID |
	
	Alternative dosing based on BSA
	Oral syrup: 180–240 mg/m² BID
	
	Adolescent (≥ 18 yr)/Adult: 300 mg BID
	• Trizivir (abacavir/lamivudine/zidovudine) 1 tablet BID (≥ 30 kg)
	• Combivir (lamivudine/zidovudine) 1 tablet BID (≥ 30 kg)
		• With or without food
		• IV dose should be 75% of oral dose; use same dosing interval for infants who cannot tolerate oral agents
			Renal recovery of unchanged drug is < 20%; extensive liver metabolism, including glucuronide conjugates	• Macrocytic anemia
				• Granulocytopenia
				• Gastrointestinal intolerance
				• Headache
				• Fatigue
				• Myopathy
				• Lipodystrophy
				• Lactic acidosis with hepatic steatosis
				• Hyperlipidemia
					• Discontinue AZT if severe granulocytopenia or anemia; use of erythropoietin 50–200 international units/kg/dose TIW, filgrastim 5–10 mcg/kg QD, or transfusion may be necessary
					• If feasible, discontinue non ARV marrow-toxic drugs
					  • CBC
					  • LFTs
					  • Lipids
					  • Adjust dose in renal failure
					• May need to adjust dose in hepatic impairment

(continued)

Table 4. Summary of Antiretroviral Treatment for Pediatric Patients Living with HIV [a,31] (*continued*)

Generic (Brand, Abbreviation)	Dosage Formulation	Dosing by Age and Weight	Special Instructions	Mode of Clearance/ Metabolism	Adverse Effects	Management/ Monitoring
Non-Nucleoside Reverse Transcriptase Inhibitors (NNRTIs)						
Efavirenz (Sustiva[c], EFV)	**Capsules:** 50 mg 200 mg **Tablets:** 600 mg **Fixed-dose combination tablets:** Atripla (TDF 300 mg + emtricitabine 200 mg + efavirenz 600 mg) Symfi (TDF 300 mg + lamivudine 300 mg + efavirenz 600 mg) Symfi Lo (TDF 300 mg + lamivudine 300 mg + efavirenz 400 mg)	**Infant/Child (≥ 3 yr and ≥ 10 kg):** Wt (kg) | Dose 10–<15 | 200 mg QD 15–<20 | 250 mg QD 20–<25 | 300 mg QD 25–<32.5 | 350 mg QD 32.5–<40 | 400 mg QD ≥ 40 | 600 mg QD • Atripla (TDF/emtricitabine/efavirenz) 1 tablet QD (≥ 40 kg) • Symfi (efavirenz/lamivudine/tenofovir disoproxil fumarate) 1 tablet QD (≥ 40 kg) • Symfi Lo (TDF/lamivudine/efavirenz) 1 tablet QD (≥ 35 kg)	• Take on empty stomach at bedtime • Avoid administration with high-fat meal because it may increase EFV concentrations • Capsules can be opened and contents used as sprinkle preparation for pts unable to swallow capsules	Hepatic • CYP 3A4 and 2B6 inducer • CYP3A4 and 2B6 substrate	• CNS adverse effects (may include insomnia, abnormal dreams, dizziness, somnolence, depression, suicidal ideation) • Rash • Hepatotoxicity • Gynecomastia • Corrected QT prolongation	• May cause false-positive cannabinoid and benzodiazepine tests • LFTs • Lipids • Use with caution in hepatic impairment
Etravirine (Intelence[h], ETR)	**Tablets:** 25 mg 100 mg, 200 mg	*ARV-experienced* **Child/Adolescent (2–18 yr and Wt ≥ 10 kg):** Wt (kg) | Dose 10–<20 | 100 mg BID 20–<25 | 125 mg BID 25–<30 | 150 mg BID ≥ 30 | 200 mg BID *ARV-experienced* **Adult:** 200 mg BID	• Take after meals (AUC decreased by 50% on empty stomach) • Store at RT in original container with desiccant because of sensitivity to moisture • Tablets can be dispersed in small amount of water to make slurry: once dispersed, stir well and consume immediately • Rinse glass with water a few times, swallowing each rinse to make sure entire dose is taken	Hepatic • CYP3A4 inducer • CYP 2C9 and 2C19 inhibitor • CYP3A4, 2C9 and 2C19 substrate	• Nausea • Diarrhea • Rash • Hypersensitivity reaction (including rash and hepatic failure)	• LFTs • History of NNRTI-related rash with EFV or NVP does not increase risk of developing rash with ETR; however, avoid ETR if history of severe rash with EFV and NVP • No dosage adjustment in mild to moderate hepatic impairment

Drug	Formulations	Dose	Administration	Metabolism	Adverse Effects	Comments
Nevirapine (Viramune[i], NVP)	**Suspension:** 10 mg/mL **Tablets:** 200 mg IR 100 mg 400 mg XR	**Neonate < 1 mo gestational age:** IR and suspension (*investigational dosing*); no lead in dosing **Infant (34–37 wk):** 4 mg/kg/dose BID for 1st wk increasing to 6 mg/kg/dose BID thereafter **Infant (≥ 37 wk–< 1 mo):** 6 mg/kg/dose BID **Infant/Child (≥ 1 mo–< 8 yr):** 200 mg/m² BSA/dose BID after lead-in dosing (max dose 200 mg BID) **Child (≥ 8 yr):** 120–150 mg/m² BSA/dose BID after lead-in dosing (max dose 200 mg BID) XR formulation **Child (≥ 6 yr):** If already on immediate-release NVP BID can be switched to NVP XR without lead-in dosing BSA range dosing for XR formulation <table><tr><td>BSA</td><td>Dose</td></tr><tr><td>0.58 m²–0.83 m²</td><td>200 mg QD (2 × 100 mg)</td></tr><tr><td>0.84 m²–1.16 m²</td><td>300 mg QD (3 × 100 mg)</td></tr><tr><td>≥ 1.17 m²</td><td>400 mg QD (1 × 400 mg)</td></tr></table> **Lead-in dosing:** Initiate therapy with dose given QD for 1st 14 days; then increase to dose to BID if no rash or elevated LFTs **Adolescent/Adult:** 200 mg BID or 400 mg XR QD after lead-in	• With or without food • NVP is initiated at a lower dose and increased in a stepwise fashion because of autoinduction • Shake suspension well and store at RT	Hepatic • 80% excreted in urine as glucuronidated metabolites • CYP3A and 2B6 inducer	• Rash • Hepatotoxicity	• If rash occurs during 14-day lead-in period, do not increase dose until rash resolves • If discontinued for > 14 days, reinitiate as QD dosing for 2 wk, followed by full BID dosing • Avoid starting in female pts with CD4⁺ > 250 and in male pts with CD4⁺ > 400 cells/mm³ • LFTs at baseline, 2 wk, 4 wk, and then every 3 mo; if clinical hepatitis or hypersensitivity reactions occur, then permanently discontinue • Use with caution in elevated pretreatment LFTs • Do not use in moderate to severe hepatic impairment
Rilpivirine (Edurant[h], RPV)	**Tablets:** 25 mg	*ARV-naïve* **Adolescent (≥ 12 yr and Wt ≥ 35 kg)/Adult:** 25 mg QD **Wt ≥ 35 kg:** • Complera (TDF/emtricitabine/rilpivirine) 1 tablet QD • Odefsey (tenofovir alafenamide/emtricitabine/rilpivirine) 1 tablet QD • Juluca[b] (dolutegravir/rilpivirine) 1 tablet QD (≥ 18 yr)	Take with a meal of at least 500 calories	Hepatic • CYP3A substrate	• CNS adverse effects (depression, mood changes, insomnia) • Headache • Rash	• Use caution if taking with another drug that has known risk of torsades de pointes • Do not use rilpivirine in pts with viral load > 100,000 copies/mL because of increased risk of virologic failure • No dosage adjustment in mild to moderate hepatic impairment • Use caution in severe renal impairment or ESRD

(continued)

Table 4. Summary of Antiretroviral Treatment for Pediatric Patients Living with HIV [a,31] *(continued)*

Generic (Brand, Abbreviation)	Dosage Formulation	Dosing by Age and Weight	Special Instructions	Mode of Clearance/ Metabolism	Adverse Effects	Management/ Monitoring
Protease Inhibitors (PIs)						
Atazanavir (Reyataz[b], ATV)	**Capsules:** 150 mg 200 mg 300 mg **Oral powder (packet):** 50 mg/ packet **Fixed-dose combination tablets:** Evotaz[b] (atazanavir 300 mg + 150 mg COBI)	**Note:** Not approved for use in infants < 3 mo or Wt < 5 kg **Note:** Capsules and powder packets are not interchangeable **Note:** Atazanavir powder must be administered with RTV Powder formulation **Infant/Child (≥ 3 mo and Wt ≥ 5 kg):** 	Wt (kg)	ATV (mg)	+ RTV (mg)
---	---	---
5–<15	200 (4 packets)	80 (1 mL oral solution) QD
15–<25	250 (5 packets)	80 mg (1 mL oral solution) QD	 Capsules **Child/Adolescent (6–18 yr and Wt ≥ 15 kg):** 	Wt (kg)	Dose
---	---
<15	**Not recommended**
15–<35	ATV 200 mg + RTV 100 mg QD
≥ 35	ATV 300 mg + RTV 100 mg QD	 **Adolescent/Adult:** *Treatment naive:* ATV 300 mg + RTV 100 mg or ATV 400 mg QD with food or ATV 300 mg + COBI 150 mg QD 1 tablet QD *Treatment experienced* ATV 300 mg + RTV 100 mg QD with food or ATV 300 mg + COBI 150 mg (Evotaz) 1 tablet QD **Adult:** *Treatment naive* With EFV ATV 400 mg + RTV 100 mg + EFV 600 mg all QD at separate times With TDF • ATV 300 mg + RTV 100 mg + TDF 300 mg all QD with food because TDF can decrease ATV exposure • ATV 300 mg + COBI 150 mg + TDF 300 mg all QD	• Take with food to improve absorption of ATV • Do not open capsules • Mix oral powder in at least 1 tablespoon of soft food or at least 30 mL of beverage (milk or water) • Administer oral powder within 1 hr of preparation • Separate ATV dosing from acid-suppressive therapy (antacids should be separated by 1–2 hr; histamine-2 blockers should be separated by 12 hr) (if TDF is also used, use ATV 400 mg + RTV 100 mg QD); PPIs (≤ 20 mg equivalent dosing of omeprazole) should be separated by 12 hr from boosted ATV) • PPIs not recommended in treatment-experienced pts taking ATV	Hepatic • CYP1A2, CYP2C9, CYP3A4 and UGT1A1 inhibitor • CYP3A4 substrate • COBI: substrate of CYP3A, CYP2D6 (minor); CYP3A inhibitor	• Indirect hyperbilirubinemia (sclera icterus) • Nephrolithiasis (rare) • Rash • Increase in serum creatinine (with COBI) • Increased serum transaminases	• Hyperbilirubinemia may resolve with time (may discontinue if cosmetically unappealing) • Total bilirubin • Urinalysis • Adjust dose in hepatic failure; do not give in severe hepatic impairment • Do not use in treatment-experienced pts with ESRD on hemodialysis

| Darunavir (Prezista[h], DRV) | **Suspension:** 100 mg/mL

Tablets:
75 mg
150 mg
600 mg
800 mg

Fixed-dose combination tablets:
Prezcobix[h] (darunavir 800 mg + 150 mg COBI)

Symtuza (darunavir 800 mg + cobicistat + 200 mg emtricitabine + 10 mg TAF) | **Infant/Child (≥ 3–12 yr and Wt ≥ 10 kg):** DRV oral suspension/RTV oral solution

Treatment-naïve and treatment-experienced pts with or without ≥ 1 darunavir resistance mutations

Infant/Child (≥ 3–< 12 yr and Wt ≥ 10 kg): BID dosing with food

Treatment-naïve or treatment-experienced with no DRV resistance-associated mutations
Adolescent (≥ 12 yr and ≥ 40 kg)/Adult: DRV 800 mg + RTV 100 mg QD

Adult: Prezcobix (DRV 800 mg/COBI 150 mg): 1 tablet QD

Treatment-experienced with at ≥ 1 DRV resistance-associated mutation
Adolescent (≥ 12 yr and ≥ 30–< 40 kg): Darunavir 450 mg + RTV 100 mg BID with food

Adolescent (≥ 12 yr and ≥ 40 kg)/Adult: DRV 600 mg + RTV 100 mg BID with food

Note: Use of COBI is not recommended with DRV 600 mg BID

Symtuza (darunavir/cobicistat/emtricitabine/TAF): 1 tablet QD with food (adults only) | • Take with food; all oral suspension/solution doses are BID with food
• Because DRV has a sulfa moiety, use caution in pts with sulfonamide allergy
• Store tablets at RT
• Store oral suspension at RT in original container; shake well before dosing
• In pts with ≥ 1 DRV-associated mutation(s), DRV should only be used BID
• DRV resistance-associated mutations include any of the following: V11I, V32I, L33F, I47V, I50V, I54L, I54M, T74P, L76V, I84V, L89V | Hepatic
• CYP3A4 substrate and inhibitor
• CYP2C9 inducer
• COBI: substrate of CYP3A, CYP2D6 (minor); CYP3A inhibitor | • Rash
• Hepatotoxicity
• Headaches
• Diarrhea
• Nausea
• Vomiting
• Fatigue
• Abdominal pain
• Increase in serum creatinine (with COBI) | • LFTs
• Use caution in hepatic impairment; do not use in severe hepatic impairment)
• No pharmacokinetic data in severe renal impairment or ESRD |

Infant/Child (≥ 3–< 12 yr and Wt ≥ 10 kg): BID dosing with food

Wt (kg)	DRV	RTV
10–<11	200 mg (2 mL)	32 mg (0.4 mL)
11–<12	220 mg (2.2 mL)	2 mg (0.4 mL)
12–<13	240 mg (2.4 mL)	40 mg (0.5 mL)
13–<14	260 mg (2.6 mL)	40 mg (0.5 mL)
14–<15	280 mg (2.8 mL)	48 mg (0.6 mL)
15–<30	DRV 375 mg (combination of tablets or 3.8 mL)	48 mg (0.6 mL)
30–<40	450 mg (combination of tablets or 4.6 mL)	100 mg (tablet or 1.25 mL)
≥ 40	600 mg (tablet or 6 mL)	100 mg (tablet or 1.25 mL)

(continued)

Table 4. Summary of Antiretroviral Treatment for Pediatric Patients Living with HIV [a,31] (*continued*)

Generic (Brand, Abbreviation)	Dosage Formulation	Dosing by Age and Weight	Special Instructions	Mode of Clearance/ Metabolism	Adverse Effects	Management/ Monitoring
Fosamprenavir (Lexiva[g], FPV)	**Suspension:** 50 mg/mL **Tablets:** 700 mg	**Note:** QD dosing is not recommended for any pediatric pt Oral suspension: **Infant/Child (≥ 6 mo–18 yr):** Dose mg/kg/dose BID 	Wt (kg)	FPV	RTV
---	---	---
< 11	45	7
11–<15	30	3
15–<20	23	3
≥ 20	18	3
Max	700	100 | **Adolescents (> 18 yr)/Adult:** *Treatment naive* FPV 700 mg + RTV 100 mg BID or FPV 1400 mg + RTV 100–200 mg QD *PI experienced* FPV 700 mg + RTV 100 mg BID	• Take with food • Pts taking antacids or buffered formulations of ddI should take FPV at least 1 hr before or after antacid or ddI use • Because FPV has a sulfa moiety, use caution in pts with sulfonamide allergy • Shake oral suspension well before use (refrigeration not required)	Hepatic • FPV is a prodrug and is hydrolyzed to amprenavir • Amprenavir is a CYP3A4 inhibitor, inducer, and substrate	• Diarrhea • Nausea • Vomiting • Skin Rash (Stevens-Johnson syndrome) • Hyperlipidemia • Hyperglycemia • Fat maldistribution • Possible increased bleeding in pts with hemophilia • Transaminase elevation • Headache • Nephrolithiasis	• Urinalysis • Adjust dose in hepatic impairment
Indinavir (Crixivan[j], IDV)	**Capsules:** 100 mg 200 mg 400 mg	**Note:** Not approved for use in neonates/infants/children; a range of indinavir doses (234–500 mg/m² BSA) boosted with low-dose RTV has been studied in children **Note:** Should not be administered to neonates because of the risks associated with hyperbilirubinemia (kernicterus) **Note:** Not recommended in adolescents **Adolescent/Adult:** 800 mg IDV + 100 mg or 200 mg RTV BID	• IDV without RTV should be administered on an empty stomach • If coadministered with ddI, give IDV and ddI ≥ 1 hr apart on empty stomach • Adequate hydration is necessary to minimize nephrolithiasis (≥ 48 oz of daily fluid in adults) • Store at RT in original container with desiccant because capsules are sensitive to moisture	Hepatic • CYP3A4 substrate and inhibitor	• Nephrolithiasis • Gastrointestinal intolerance, nausea • Hyperlipidemia • Hyperglycemia • Fat maldistribution • Possible increased bleeding in pts with hemophilia • Hepatitis • Indirect hyperbilirubinemia (sclera icterus) • Headache • Metallic taste • Thrombocytopenia • Hemolytic anemia	• Hyperbilirubinemia may resolve with time (may discontinue if cosmetically unappealing) • Total bilirubin • Urinalysis • CBC • LFTs • Adjust dose in hepatic failure • Use decreased dosage in mild to moderate hepatic impairment; recommended dose for adults is 600 mg every 8 hr

(continued)

| Lopinavir/ ritonavir (Kaletra[k], LPV/RTV) | **Oral solution:** 80 mg/20 mg LPV/ RTV per mL **Film-coated tablets:** 100/25 mg 200/50 mg | **Neonate (< 14 days):** No data on appropriate dose or safety in this age group; do not administer to neonates < 42 wk postmenstrual and postnatal age ≥ 4 days because of toxicities Dosing for individuals not receiving concomitant nevirapine, efavirenz, FPV, or nelfinavir **Infant (14 days–12 mo): QD dosing is NOT recommended** Oral solution: LPV 300 mg/m²/RTV 75 mg/m² BSA BID or 16 mg/4 mg/kg BID **Child/Adolescent (> 12 mo–18 yr): QD dosing is NOT recommended** *Treatment-experienced* LPV 300 mg/RTV 75 mg per m² BSA BID Max LPV/RTV 400 mg/100 mg BID *Treatment-naive* LPV 230 mg/RTV 57.5 per m² BID Tablets: Recommended number of LPV/RTV 100 mg/25 mg tablets BID (Wt-based) with dosing target 300 mg/m²/dose BID | • Take tablets with or without food • Administration with or after meals may enhance GI tolerability • Tablets must be swallowed whole; do not crush or split • Solution should be refrigerated (expires after 60 days at RT) • Oral solution contains 42.4% alcohol by volume and 15.3% propylene glycol by Wt/volume • Oral solution should be administered with food because a high-fat meal enhances absorption | Hepatic • CYP3A4 substrate and inhibitor | • Nausea • Vomiting • Diarrhea • Headache • Rash • QT prolongation and torsades de pointes • Hyperlipidemia, especially hypertriglyceridemia • Postmarketing adverse effects of cardiac toxicity (complete AV block, bradycardia, and cardiomyopathy), lactic acidosis, acute renal failure, depression and respiratory problems in preterm neonates • Asthenia • Taste alteration | • ECG • Use in children ≥ 42 wk postmenstrual age and 14 days postnatal age • Use caution in hepatic impairment |

Wt (kg)	Tablets
15–20	2
> 20–25	3
> 25–30	3
> 30–35	4
> 35–45	4
> 45	4–5

Adult (> 45 kg) receiving concomitant nevirapine, efavirenz, FPV, or nelfinavir:
LPV 500 mg/RTV 125 mg as 2 LPV 200 mg/RTV 50 mg tablets and 1 LPV 100 mg/RTV 25 mg tablets or 3 tablets of LPV 200 mg/RTV 50 mg for ease of dosing

Adult (> 18 yr):
800 mg/200 mg LPV/RTV QD or 400 mg/100 mg LPV/RTV BID (especially if ≥ 3 LPV mutations)

Adults receiving concomitant nevirapine, efavirenz, FPV, or nelfinavir: LPV 500 mg/RTV 125 mg BID

Table 4. Summary of Antiretroviral Treatment for Pediatric Patients Living with HIV [a,31] (*continued*)

Generic (Brand, Abbreviation)	Dosage Formulation	Dosing by Age and Weight	Special Instructions	Mode of Clearance/ Metabolism	Adverse Effects	Management/ Monitoring
Nelfinavir (Viracept[l], NFV)	**Tablets:** 250 mg 625 mg	**Note:** No longer recommended for use in children because of inferior potency vs. other regimens **Child (≥ 2 yr):** 44–55 mg/kg BID **Adolescent/Adult:** 1250 mg BID	• Take with food • Tablets can be dissolved in a small amount of water to make slurry; must be consumed immediately • Tablets can also be crushed and administered with pudding or other nonacidic foods	Hepatic • CYP 2C19 and CYP3A4 substrate • Metabolized to active metabolite M8 • CYP3A4 inhibitor	• Diarrhea • Hyperlipidemia • Hyperglycemia • Abdominal pain • Serum transaminase elevations	Do not use in moderate to severe hepatic impairment
Ritonavir (Norvir[k], RTV)	**Oral solution:** 80 mg/mL (contains 43% ethanol by volume and approximately 27% (w/v) propylene glycol) **Oral powder (packet):** 100 mg per packet **Tablets:** 100 mg	• Used as a pharmacokinetic booster (increases concentrations of coadministered PIs) • Dosing varies with different PIs; individual PIs in this table can be used to determine dosing of RTV • Oral powder should only be used for dosing increments of 100 mg and cannot be used for doses < 100 mg	• May take with food to minimize GI intolerance and improve absorption • Tablets do not need to be refrigerated • Store oral solution at RT (must not be refrigerated); shake well before use • Use oral solution within 6 mo • To increase tolerability of oral solution in children: (1) Mix solution with soft foods or liquids (2) Administer or discard after 2 hr of mixing (3) Before administration, give the child a frozen substance to dull the taste buds or peanut butter to coat the mouth (4) After administration, give child strong-tasting foods such as maple syrup or cheese	Hepatic • CYP3A4 and CYP2D6 inhibitor • CYP2B6, 2C9, 2C19, 1A2, and UGT1A1 inducer	• Nausea • Vomiting • Diarrhea • Circumoral paresthesias • Hypertriglyceridemia • Taste perversion • Hepatitis • Abdominal pain • Anorexia • Headache	• Lipids • LFTs • Use caution in moderate to severe hepatic impairment

Drug	Formulations	Dosing	Administration/Notes	Metabolism	Adverse Effects	Monitoring/Comments
Saquinavir (Invirase[m], SQV)	**Capsules:** 200 mg **Tablets:** 500 mg	**Note:** Not approved for use in infants, children and adolescents < 16 yr SQV must be boosted with RTV **Adolescent (≥ 16 yr)/Adult:** SQV 1000 mg + RTV 100 mg BID	• Take within 2 hr after food to improve absorption • Always take with RTV (never unboosted because of poor bioavailability) • May cause photosensitivity reactions if exposed to sun; recommend protective clothing or sunscreen use	Hepatic • CYP3A4 substrate and inhibitor	• Headache • Abdominal discomfort • QT prolongation and torsades de pointes • Photosensitivity • Diarrhea • Nausea • Paresthesia • Skin rash • Lipid abnormalities	• ECG is recommended before initiation; pts with baseline QT intervals > 450 millisec should not receive SQV • Not recommended in pts taking other drugs that can cause QT prolongation • Use caution in mild to moderate hepatic impairment • Contraindicated in severe hepatic impairment
Tipranavir (Aptivus[i], TPV)	**Oral solution:** 100 mg/mL **Capsules:** 250 mg	**Note:** Not approved for children < 2 yr **Note:** Not recommended for treatment-naive pts **Child/Adolescent (2–18 yr):** BSA based TPV 375 mg/m² + RTV 150 mg/m² BID (max TPV 500 mg + RTV 200 mg BID) Wt-based TPV 14 mg/kg + RTV 6 mg/kg (max TPV 500 mg + RTV 200 mg BID) **Adult:** TPV 500 mg + RTV 200 mg BID	• Take with food • Oral solution contains vitamin E 116 international units/mL • Because TPV has a sulfa moiety, use caution in pts with sulfonamide allergy • Store oral solution at RT; do not refrigerate or freeze • Once oral solution is opened, it must be used within 60 days • Capsules can be kept at RT if used within 60 days; refrigerate capsules if longer storage is anticipated	Hepatic • CYP3A4 substrate and inducer • P-glycoprotein substrate	• Diarrhea • Rash • Hepatotoxicity • Intracranial hemorrhage (rare) • Hypertriglyceridemia • Fatigue • Headache • Nausea • Vomiting • Elevated transaminases, cholesterol and triglycerides	• LFTs • Use caution in pts at risk of increased bleeding from surgery, trauma, or other medical conditions or receiving drugs such as anti-platelets, anticoagulants, or excessive vitamin E supplemental doses • Lipids (especially triglycerides) • Contraindicated in moderate or severe hepatic impairment

(continued)

Table 4. Summary of Antiretroviral Treatment for Pediatric Patients Living with HIV[a,31] *(continued)*

Generic (Brand, Abbreviation)	Dosage Formulation	Dosing by Age and Weight	Special Instructions	Mode of Clearance/ Metabolism	Adverse Effects	Management/ Monitoring
Entry Inhibitors						
Enfuvirtide, (Fuzeon[n], ENF or T-20)	**Lyophilized powder for injection:** 108-mg vial reconstituted with 1.1 mL of sterile water will make 90 mg/mL **Convenience kit:** • 60 single-use vials of ENF (108-mg vial reconstituted as 90 mg/mL) • 60 vials of sterile water for injection • 60 reconstitution syringes (3 mL) • 60 administration syringes (1 mL) • Alcohol wipes	**Note:** Not approved for children < 6 yr **Child/Adolescent 6–16 yr:** 2 mg/kg SC BID (max 90 mg [1 mL]) **Adolescent (> 16 yr)/Adult:** 90 mg (1 mL) SC BID	• Inject SC in upper arm, anterior thigh, or abdomen • Allow up to 45 min for reconstituted powder to dissolve completely in solution; do not shake • Once reconstituted, inject immediately or keep refrigerated until use • Reconstituted vial must be used within 24 hr	Catabolism to constituent individual amino acids	• Injection site reactions • Bacterial pneumonia and local site cellulitis • Hypersensitivity reaction (rechallenge is not recommended)	• Rotate injection sites to minimize reactions • Local reactions may be minimized by applying heat or ice after injection, or gently massage injection site to better disperse dose • Discontinue if signs and symptoms of hypersensitivity reaction are suspected; seek medical attention immediately

| Maraviroc (Selzentry¹, MVC) | Oral solution: 20 mg/mL

Tablets:
25 mg
75 mg
150 mg
300 mg | Note: Not approved for neonates/infants

Child (≥ 2 yr and Wt ≥ 10 kg): Potent CYP3A inhibitors (with or without a CYP3A inducer) tablets (or oral solution)

Note: Not recommended for pts taking potent CYP3A inducers without a potent CYP3A inhibitor

Adolescent (> 18 yr)/Adult given with the following:

Potent CYP3A inhibitors (with or without CYP3A inducers) including PIs except TPV/RTV: 150 mg BID

NRTIs, enfuvirtide, TPV/RTV, NVP, RAL, and drugs that are not potent CYP3A inhibitors or inducers: ≥ 30 kg: 300 mg (15 mL) BID

Note: Not recommended in children, regardless of Wt

Adults, given with the following:

Potent CYP3A inducers including EFV and ETR (without a potent CYP3A inhibitor): 600 mg BID

Potent CYP3A inhibitors (with or without a potent CYP3A inducer) including PIs (except TPV/RTV): 150 mg BID

NRTIs, enfuvirtide, TPV/RTV, nevirapine, raltegravir, and other drugs that are not potent CYP3A inhibitors or inducers: 300 mg BID | • Use CCR5 tropism assay to determine whether child can use maraviroc (i.e., CCR5+ tropic-virus is present)
• Take with or without food | Hepatic
• CYP3A4 substrate | • Nausea/vomiting
• Abdominal pain
• Cough
• Dizziness
• Musculoskeletal symptoms
• Fever
• Rash
• Upper respiratory tract infections
• Hepatotoxicity
• Orthostatic hypotension | • LFTs
• Blood pressure if taking other antihypertensive drugs
• Caution in underlying cardiac disease
• Caution in hepatic impairment
• Do not use MVC in pts with CrCl < 30 mL/min/1.73 m² who are also taking other drugs that are potent CYP3A4 inhibitors or inducers |

Child (≥ 2 yr and Wt ≥ 10 kg) dosing:

Wt (kg)	Dose
10–< 20	50 mg (2.5 mL) BID
20–< 30	75 mg (4 mL) BID
30–< 40	100 mg (5 mL) BID
≥ 40	150 mg (7.5 mL) BID

(continued)

Table 4. Summary of Antiretroviral Treatment for Pediatric Patients Living with HIV [a,31] (*continued*)

Generic (Brand, Abbreviation)	Dosage Formulation	Dosing by Age and Weight	Special Instructions	Mode of Clearance/ Metabolism	Adverse Effects	Management/ Monitoring
Integrase Strand Transfer Inhibitors (INSTIs)						
Bictegravir (BIC)	**Note: bictegravir is only available in a fixed-dose combination tablet** Biktarvy: Bictegravir 50 mg + emtricitabine 200 mg + tenofovir alafenamide (TAF) 25 mg	**Note:** Not approved for use in pts < 18 yr **Child (< 12 yr):** No data available **Child/Adolescent (≥ 12–18 yr and Wt ≥ 35 kg):** 1 tablet QD (investigational dose) **Adult (≥ 18 yr):** 1 tablet QD	Take with or without food	UGT1A1 and CYP3A substrate	• Diarrhea • Nausea • Headache	• Screen for HBV infection before use of FTC or TAF • Not recommended for use with other ARV drugs • Not recommended in severe hepatic impairment • Not recommended with CrCl < 30 mL/min/1.73 m²
Dolutegravir (Tivicay[b], DTG)	**Tablets:** 10 mg 25 mg 50 mg Triumeq: dolutegravir 50 mg + abacavir 600 mg + lamivudine 300 mg Juluca: dolutegravir 50 mg + rilpivirine 25 mg	**Child (≥ 30–< 40 kg):** 35 mg QD **Child/Adolescent (≥ 40 kg)/Adult:** *Treatment-naive or treatment experienced/INSTI-naive* 50 mg QD *Treatment-naive or treatment experienced/INSTI-naive* when coadministered with following potent UGT1A/CYP3A inducers: EFV, FPV/r, TPV/r, or rifampin: 50 mg BID *INSTI-experienced with any INSTI-associated resistance* 50 mg BID Triumeq (abacavir/lamivudine/dolutegravir) 1 tablet QD (≥ 40 kg) Juluca (dolutegravir/rilpivirine): 1 tablet QD with a meal (adults only)	Take with or without food	UGT1A1 and CYP3A (minor) substrate	• Insomnia • Headache • Neuropsychiatric symptoms (depression; suicidal thoughts or actions) especially with history of psychiatric illness • Weight gain	• No dosage adjustment in renal impairment • Not recommended in severe hepatic impairment

| Elvitegravir (EVG) | **Fixed-dose combination tablets** | **Note:** Always used with a pharmacokinetic enhancer

Stribild (elvitegravir/cobicistat/emtricitabine/tenofovir disoproxil fumarate) 1 tablet QD
Pediatric (< 35 kg): No data available
Adolescent/Adult (≥ 35 kg): 1 tablet QD

Genvoya (elvitegravir/cobicistat/emtricitabine/tenofovir alafenamide)
Pediatric (< 25 kg): No data available

Child/Adolescent (≥ 25 kg)/Adult: 1 tablet QD

Stribild and Genvoya are only approved for ARV treatment-naive or to replace current ARV regimen in pts virologically suppressed on stable ARV regimen for at least 6 mo with no history of treatment failure and no known substitutions associated with resistance to individual drug components | CYP3A4 substrate and inducer of CYP2C9 | • Only available in fixed-dose combination tablets
• Take with food | • Diarrhea
• Nausea
• Headache
• Insomnia
• Fatigue | • Stribild should not be initiated with estimated CrCl < 70 mL/min/1.73 m² and should be discontinued with estimated CrCl < 50 mL/min/1.73 m² because dose adjustments required for FTC and TDF cannot be achieved with a fixed-dose combination tablet
• Genvoya should not be initiated with estimated CrCl < 30 mL/min/1.73 m²
• Do not use Stribild or Genvoya in severe hepatic impairment |
Raltegravir (Isentress, RAL)	**Tablets, chewable:** 25 mg 100 mg (scored) **Tablets, film-coated:** 400 mg 600 mg (HD tablets) **Granules for oral suspension:** single-use packet of 100 mg	**Full-Term Neonates (birth–4 wk [28 days]):** 	Age or Wt	Dose
Birth–1 wk	~1.5 mg/kg/dose QD
2–< 3 kg	0.4 mL (4 mg) QD
3–< 4 kg	0.5 mL (5 mg) QD
4–< 5 kg	0.7 mL (7 mg) QD
1–4 wk	~ 3mg/kg/dose BID
2–< 3 kg	0.8 mL (8 mg) BID
3–< 4 kg	1 mL (10 mg) BID
4–< 5 kg	1.5 mL (15 mg) BID | **Note:** If mother has taken RAL 2–24 hr prior to delivery, then delay neonate's first dose until 24–48 after birth **Note:** Children 11–20 kg can use oral suspension or chewable tablets	• UGT1A1 glucuronidation • UGT1A1 inhibitors such as ATV may increase RAL concentrations • UGT1A1 inducers such as TPV and rifampin may decrease RAL concentrations	• Take with or without food • Chewable tablets may be chewed or swallowed whole • Store at RT in original container with desiccant because of sensitivity to moisture • Chewable tablet, film-coated tablets, and oral suspension are not interchangeable • HD tablets must be swallowed whole • For oral suspension, suspend granules in 10 mL of water for final concentration of 10 mg/mL then gently swirl the mixing cup for 45 sec in a circular motion to mix powder into a uniform suspension (do not shake) • Dose should be administered within 30 min of mixing	• Insomnia • Headache • Nausea • Diarrhea • Muscle weakness and rhabdomyolysis	• Creatinine phosphokinase • No dosage adjustment in renal impairment or mild to moderate hepatic impairment; no data available for pts with severe hepatic impairment

(continued)

Table 4. Summary of Antiretroviral Treatment for Pediatric Patients Living with HIV [a,31] (*continued*)

Generic (Brand, Abbreviation)	Dosage Formulation	Dosing by Age and Weight	Special Instructions	Mode of Clearance/ Metabolism	Adverse Effects	Management/ Monitoring
Raltegravir (Isentress[j], RAL) (*continued*)		Oral suspension **Child (≥ 4 wk and ≥ 3 kg–< 20 kg):**				

Oral suspension dosing table:

Wt (kg)	Dose
3–< 4	2.5 mL (25 mg) BID
4–< 6	3 mL (30 mg) BID
6–< 8	4 mL (40 mg) BID
8–< 11	6 mL (60 mg) BID
11–< 14	8 mL (80 mg) BID
14–< 20	10 mL (100 mg) BID
Max	10 mL (100mg) BID)

Chewable tablets, film-coated tablets and HD tablets

Wt < 25 kg: chewable tablets BID (described in Table within this column)

Wt ≥ 25 kg: 400 mg film-coated tabled BID or chewable tablet BID

Child/Adolescent (≥ 40 kg): 1200 mg (2 600-mg tablets HD) QD

Treatment-naive or virologically suppressed on initial regimen of 400 mg BID

Chewable tablets:

Wt (kg)	Dose	Administration
11–< 14	75 mg BID	3 × 25 mg BID
14–< 20	100 mg BID	1 × 100 mg BID
20–< 28	150 mg BID	1.5 × 100 mg BID
28–< 40	200 mg BID	2 × 100 mg BID
≥ 40	300 mg BID	3 × 100 mg BID
Max	300 mg BID	

[a]Pediatric guidelines are updated at least annually and should be consulted for the most current recommendations and updates.
[b]ViiV Healthcare, Research Triangle Park, NC; [c]Bristol-Myers Squibb Company, Princeton, NJ; [d]Gilead Sciences, Inc., Foster City, CA; [e]Janssen Therapeutics, Titusville, NJ; [f]Mylan Specialty, Morgantown, WV; [g]GlaxoSmithKlein, Research Triangle Park, NC; [h]Janssen Therapeutics, Titusville, NJ; [i]Boehringer Ingelheim Pharmaceuticals Inc., Ridgefield, CT; [j]Merck, Whitehouse Station, NJ; [k]AbbVie Inc., North Chicago, IL; [l]Pfizer, New York, NY; [m]Roche Laboratories Inc., Nutley, NJ; [n]Genentech USA, Inc., South San Francisco, CA.

ARV = antiretroviral; AUC = area under the curve; AV = atrioventricular; BID = twice daily or every 12 hours; BSA = body surface area; CBC = complete blood cell count; CNS = central nervous system; CYP = cytochrome P450; DEXA = dual-energy x-ray absorptiometry; EC = enteric coated; ECG = electrocardiogram; ESRD = end-stage renal disease; GI = gastrointestinal; HBV = hepatitis B virus; HD = high-dose; HIV = human immuno-deficiency virus; IR = immediate release; IV = intravenous; LFT = liver function test; max = maximum; PPI = proton pump inhibitor; pts = patients; QAM = every morning; QD = once daily; QPM = every evening; RT = room temperature; SC = subcutaneously; TIW = three times/week; UGT1 = UDP glucuronosyltransferase 1 family; Wt = weight; XR = extended release.

Information from 2018 Panel on Antiretroviral Therapy and Medical Management of Children Living with HIV: Guidelines for the Use of Antiretroviral Agents in Pediatric HIV Infection.[31]

Etravirine is a second-generation NNRTI and can be used in treatment-experienced children and adolescents 2–18 years who weigh at least 10 kg. This drug may be effective in patients who may have acquired resistance to efavirenz or nevirapine because etravirine has a higher genetic barrier to developing resistance by retaining activity/potency until at least three mutations are acquired. Another advantage of etravirine is that children who are unable to swallow the tablets can disperse the contents into water, such that administration of this solution may facilitate higher adherence. One significant disadvantage of etravirine includes the potential for many drug–drug interactions because it is both an inducer of CYP3A4 and inhibitor of CYP2C9 and CYP2C19 enzymes.

Rilpivirine is a recently approved NNRTI and is indicated as an alternative for use in treatment-naive adolescents who are at least 12 years, weigh at least 35 kg, and have HIV viral load less than or equal to 100,000 copies/mL. Rilpivirine has been evaluated in several clinical studies in adolescents and adults living with HIV showing comparable efficacy and safety.[114,134-137] This NNRTI is also available as a one-tablet, once-daily, fixed-dose combination drug (Complera and Odefsey, both by Gilead Sciences; Juluca, ViiV Healthcare, Research Triangle Park, NC). However, Juluca is not approved for children or adolescents and is reserved for simplification of treatment in adults living with HIV who have been stable for at least 6 months on cART and have no resistance to the

Table 5. Advantages and Disadvantages of Non-Nucleoside Reverse Transcriptase Inhibitor, Protease Inhibitor, and Integrase Strand Transfer Inhibitor Antiretroviral Classes[31]

Advantages and Disadvantages	ARV Class		
	NNRTI	PI	INSTI
Advantages	• Reduced pill burden with use of 1 tablet, once-daily, FDC formulations[a] • Convenience of use • Fewer metabolic complications vs. PIs[b] • PI sparing • Long half-lives	• Reduced pill burden for adolescents ≥ 18 yr with one-tablet, once-daily, FDC formulations[c] • Reduced potential for multiple CYP–drug interactions for COBI-boosted atazanavir and darunavir vs. ritonavir-boosted PIs • Virologic and immunologic efficacy well established • Higher genetic barrier to resistance[d] • Different mechanism of action from NNRTIs[e] • NNRTI sparing	• Reduced pill burden with one-tablet, once daily, FDC formulations[f] • Reduced potential for multiple CYP–drug interactions[g] • Availability of formulations including oral suspension and chewable tablets (raltegravir) may improve adherence • Relatively good overall tolerability • Excellent efficacy[h] • High genetic barrier with dolutegravir and bictegravir use • Specific mechanism of action that may reduce latent viral reservoir size • NNRTI and PI sparing
Disadvantages	• Low genetic barrier to resistance[i] • Cannot use rilpivirine in children with viral load > 100,000 copies/mL • Rare but serious cases of rash and hepatotoxicity • Potential for several CYP–drug interactions[j]	• Higher pill burden (ritonavir-boosted PIs) • GI adverse effects • More metabolic complications vs. NNRTIs[k] • Potential for several CYP–drug interactions[l] • Poor palatability of liquid formulations, which may reduce adherence potential	• Insomnia and headache adverse effects • Reported worsening depression • Low genetic barrier to resistance[m] • Potential for several CYP–drug interactions with COBI-boosted elvitegravir • Potential for drug interactions between INSTIs and polyvalent cation[s]n

[a]NNRTIs with reduced pill burden are: Atripla (Gilead Sciences, Inc., Foster City, CA), Symfi (Mylan Specialty, Morgantown, WV), Symfi Lo (Mylan Specialty), Odefsey (Gilead Sciences), and Complera (Gilead Sciences).
[b]NNRTIs cause less dyslipidemia and fat maldistribution than PIs.
[c]PIs with reduced pill burden are: Evotaz (Bristol-Myers Squibb, Princeton, NJ), Prezcobix (Janssen Therapeutics, Titusville, NJ), and Symtuza (Janssen Therapeutics).
[d]PIs require the accumulation of several mutations for the ARV class not to work.
[e]PIs do not act on same enzyme reverse transcriptase as NNRTIs.
[f]INSTIs with reduced pill burden are: Stribild (Gilead Sciences), Genvoya (Gilead Sciences), Triumeq (ViiV Healthcare; Research Triangle Park, NC), and Biktarvy (Gilead Sciences).
[g]CYP–drug interaction potential is especially reduced for the UGT1A1-mediated and metabolized unboosted INSTIs raltegravir, dolutegravir and bictegravir.
[h]Efficacy for the INSTI dolutegravir is superior to PIs and NNRTIs in clinical trials, but non-inferior to raltegravir.
[i]A single mutation can confer resistance to class; the exception is etravirine, which has a higher genetic barrier.
[j]Rilpivirine is the exception to potential CYP–drug interactions with NNRTIs.
[k]PIs cause more dyslipidemia, fat maldistribution, and insulin resistance vs. NNRTIs.
[l]CYP–drug interactions are especially a concern for ritonavir-boosted PIs.
[m]A single mutation can confer resistance to raltegravir and elvitegravir; the exceptions are dolutegravir and bictegravir, which have a higher genetic barrier.
[n]INSTI–polyvalent-cation interactions are chelation with acid reducers and supplements (i.e. multivitamin), leading to reduced bioavailability of INSTIs.

ARV = antiretroviral; COBI = cobicistat; CYP = cytochrome P450; FDC = fixed-dose combination; GI = gastrointestinal; INSTI = integrase strand transfer inhibitor; NNRTI = non-nucleoside reverse transcriptase inhibitor; PI = protease inhibitor.

individual components of this combination drug. Although rilpivirine use is contraindicated with concomitant proton pump inhibitor use, one major advantage of rilpivirine compared with other NNRTIs is that it does not affect the metabolism of other medications, meaning that it does not induce or inhibit CYP enzymes and is therefore associated with fewer clinically relevant drug–drug interactions. Another advantage includes its small pill size as a single-agent formulation.

As previously noted, PI-based regimens are also effective for treatment-naive pediatric patients with HIV. Common PIs used for treatment of children living with HIV are atazanavir, darunavir, and lopinavir. The PIs are coadministered with ritonavir because of its advantageous pharmacokinetic properties. Ritonavir is referred to as a "booster" ARV drug because it is a strong CYP3A4 inhibitor that increases the concentrations of the other PIs by prolonging their half-life. Similarly, cobicistat is also used for its pharmacokinetic-enhancing properties to increase the concentrations of both atazanavir and darunavir. Because cobicistat has greater solubility than ritonavir, it can be coformulated with other ARVs such as atazanavir and darunavir as the simplified fixed-dose combinations in Evotaz (Bristol-Myers Squibb, Princeton, NJ) and Prezcobix/Symtuza (Janssen Therapeutics, Titusville, NJ), respectively.[138] However, these specific combinations only have FDA label approval for use in adult patients living with HIV (age 18 years and older). Atazanavir can be used for treatment of children living with HIV as young as 3 months and weighing more than 5 kg, but its recommendation as a preferred PI is for children 3 years and older and weighing less than 25 kg.

Atazanavir has been evaluated in many clinical studies demonstrating efficacy in infants, children, and adults living with HIV.[123, 139-145] However, a recent clinical study (ACTG 5257) showed more discontinuations secondary to toxicity (hyperbilirubinemia and gastrointestinal adverse events) in patients treated with atazanavir compared with those treated with either darunavir or raltegravir, leading to removal of atazanavir from the DHHS guidelines as a preferred treatment recommendation for initial therapy of adults living with HIV.[109] Atazanavir is available as both powder and capsule formulations for once-daily dosing, but because it cannot be coformulated with ritonavir, additional ritonavir liquid or tablets should be given simultaneously. One significant disadvantage for younger children who are unable to swallow tablets and are treated with atazanavir powder formulation is coadministration with ritonavir liquid, which can be challenging because of its very poor palatability.

Darunavir is recommended as a preferred PI regimen for children living with HIV older than 3 years and weighing less than 25 kg. Darunavir has been evaluated in many clinical studies in both children and adults living with HIV and shows efficacy and good tolerability.[103,109,146-150] Dosing frequency of darunavir varies depending on age and presence of darunavir resistance-associated mutations. Once-daily dosing of darunavir boosted with ritonavir is recommended for treatment-naive children and adolescents weighing at least 40 kg and who have no mutations associated with darunavir resistance. For children living with HIV age 3–6 years and weighing at least 10 kg, twice-daily dosing of darunavir boosted with ritonavir is preferred. Furthermore, twice-daily

dosing is also recommended for patients who have at least one of the following 11 mutations associated with darunavir resistance in the HIV protease gene: V11I, V32I, L33F, I47V, I50V, I54L, I54M, T74P, L76V, I84V, and L89V. Some disadvantages of darunavir include required twice-daily dosing in young children living with HIV, pill burden, and poor palatability of ritonavir liquid given with darunavir oral suspension for those who cannot swallow tablets. However, advantages of darunavir include its high genetic barrier to development of resistance, good tolerability, and its availability as a one-tablet, once-daily fixed-dose combination in Prezcobix and, most recently, in Symtuza for treatment of adults living with HIV.

Coformulated lopinavir/ritonavir has the most clinical pediatric data. Lopinavir/ritonavir is recommended as a preferred PI for treatment of infants with a postmenstrual age of at least 42 weeks and postnatal age greater than 14 days to 3 years. This PI has been evaluated extensively in children and adults living with HIV in many clinical studies showing comparable efficacy and tolerability to various different ART regimens.[120,142,143,149,151-162] Two major advantages of lopinavir/ritonavir are its different dosing formulations and its coformulation with ritonavir, including its availability for use at a very young age in infants. Some disadvantages of lopinavir/ritonavir include twice-daily dosing in children, pill burden, relatively poor palatability of oral suspension, increased risk for toxicities and drug–drug interactions compared with other PIs such as atazanavir and darunavir because of a higher required total daily dosing of ritonavir.

For those patients who are intolerant of ritonavir, both unboosted atazanavir and fosamprenavir are no longer recommended.[140,163] One of the major reasons for this lack of recommendation is the risk for lower therapeutic concentrations for children living with HIV who are not using ritonavir boosting, which could result in development of resistance mutations causing potential cross-resistance to other PIs (i.e., darunavir). Furthermore, when fosamprenavir is used without ritonavir boosting, the required volume of liquid medication is both high and associated with vomiting in young children. Extensive pediatric data exist for nelfinavir use, but because of its varying rates of virologic potency and the availability of more potent ART, including boosted PIs, INSTIs, and efavirenz, nelfinavir is also no longer recommended.[164] Saquinavir is not recommended in children because of the lack of a pediatric formulation and limited dosing information, although it provides virologic and immunologic outcomes similar to lopinavir/ritonavir in adult treatment-naive patients.[158] Indinavir is not recommended as initial therapy in children because there is no liquid formulation and it causes a high incidence of hematuria, sterile leukocyturia, and nephrolithiasis.[165-168] Although tipranavir is licensed for treatment-experienced children 2 years and older and has a high genetic barrier to development of resistance, it is not recommended for treatment because of increased dosing of ritonavir required for boosting and the rare, but severe, reported cases of intracranial hemorrhage.[31]

Two NRTIs form the backbone of ARV treatment in combination with either a boosted PI, NNRTI or INSTI. Eight NRTIs are approved for use in children younger than 13 years: didanosine, zidovudine, lamivudine, stavudine, abacavir, emtricitabine, TDF, and TAF. Preferred dual NRTI combinations include abacavir or zidovudine with either lamivudine or emtricitabine, or TAF together with emtricitabine. The most extensive clinical data in children are derived from the zidovudine and lamivudine combination, which is generally well tolerated.[169-172] This NRTI backbone is preferred in infants from birth and children to age 6 years or younger, but it is considered an alternative option for those older than 6 years and who are not sexually mature (sexual maturity rating 1-3) because of its requirement for twice-daily dosing. Emtricitabine and lamivudine are both cytosine NRTI analogs and can be substituted for one another. One advantage of emtricitabine compared with lamivudine includes its once-daily administration. Abacavir plus lamivudine or emtricitabine is another preferred NRTI combination for children older than 3 months.[171,173-179] Abacavir and lamivudine is a potent dual-combination NRTI for children, maintaining significantly better virologic suppression and growth rates (height and weight) than zidovudine and lamivudine or zidovudine and abacavir in 5 years of follow-up.[174] However, a primary limitation of abacavir is the requirement for *HLA-B*5701* genetic testing before its use because of its association with hypersensitivity reactions. Prevalence of this genetic polymorphism is more common in whites than in African Americans and Hispanics in the United States (8% vs. 2% to 2.5%, respectively). Genetic screening for *HLA-B*5701* before using abacavir has shown significant reductions in the hypersensitivity reaction from 7.8% to 3.4%.[180] This testing should be done before considering abacavir for treatment of children living with HIV, and abacavir should not be used in those who test positive for *HLA-B*5701*.

The oral prodrug of tenofovir, TAF, is associated with significantly fewer renal and bone toxicities compared with TDF.[106,181] This NRTI is available in several fixed-dose combination (FDC) tablets. One of these FDCs includes TAF/emtricitabine, which is a preferred NRTI combination recommended for use with either an INSTI or NNRTI in children and adolescents older than 6 years and weighing more than 25 kg, who have an estimated creatinine clearance greater than 30 mL/minute/1.73 m². For children and adolescents older than 12 years and weighing more than 35 kg, TAF/emtricitabine is recommended as a preferred combination as the FDC Genvoya or in combination with other INSTIs dolutegravir or raltegravir, NNRTI, or a boosted PI. One major advantage of the TAF/emtricitabine FDC includes its very small size compared with other NRTI FDCs, which may help to facilitate adequate adherence to ART. An alternative that is recommended as an NRTI backbone for children age 2-12 years is TDF plus lamivudine or emtricitabine.[175-177,182-191] Although TDF is associated with potential risks for decreased bone mineral density, one major benefit includes its ease of dosing because it is available in dosage formulations as an oral powder and numerous low-strength FDCs.[184,186-188,192,193] One other potential alternative NRTI combination includes zidovudine and abacavir for use in children older than 3 months. However, this combination had poorer efficacy and more toxicity resulting in ART modifications compared with one of the preferred recommended NRTI combinations of abacavir and lamivudine.[174,194]

Incorporating either stavudine or didanosine as part of any NRTI backbone is no longer recommended because of significant toxicities and availability of more tolerable NRTIs. Stavudine is associated with mitochondrial toxicity, which could lead to a higher risk of lipoatrophy and hyperlactatemia than with other NRTIs.[195-197] A stavudine and didanosine dual NRTI backbone is contraindicated because of the higher rates of toxicity observed in adults such as neurotoxicity, pancreatitis, hyperlactatemia and lactic acidosis, and lipodystrophy compared with those taking zidovudine and lamivudine.[198,199] Other dual NRTI combinations that are not recommended are abacavir and didanosine, abacavir and tenofovir, and didanosine and tenofovir because of insufficient data in children. Of note, these dual NRTI combinations are not recommended as initial treatment for newly infected adults living with HIV because of insufficient data and higher rates of resistance with some of the combinations. Furthermore, lamivudine and emtricitabine or stavudine and zidovudine combinations should not be coadministered because of competing pharmacologic activation pathways. Both maraviroc and enfuvirtide are reserved for treatment-experienced children living with HIV and will be briefly discussed in more detail in the following text.

If first-line therapy with ARVs fails, defined as having a suboptimal virologic response to the current cART regimen, the etiology of treatment failure must be assessed before considering changes in ART. Treatment failure in many cases could be multifactorial; some of the most common reasons for treatment failure are inadequate adherence to ARVs, drug intolerance, pharmacokinetic variability and drug–drug interactions, or the presence of drug-resistant virus. First, adherence to ARVs should be evaluated. *Adherence to therapy* refers not only to taking medications according to their prescribed schedules, but also to the timing of the doses, food considerations with certain ARVs, and the avoidance of drug–drug interactions, especially given the wide availability of some herbal and over-the-counter products that have important interactions with ARVs that could affect treatment response. Adherence plays a key role in the success of a treatment regimen because suboptimal adherence can lead to drug resistance and inadequate virologic control and has been associated with an increased risk of disease progression and mortality. If the patient has not been adherent to current ARVs, reasons for nonadherence should be addressed, and adherence to current ARVs should be reinforced, together with developing strategies to help patients overcome their adherence barriers. Drug intolerance may be one of the reasons for nonadherence to ARVs. If possible, adverse effects should be treated symptomatically, depending on severity. Pharmacokinetics, especially drug metabolism, may differ during puberty, necessitating a reevaluation of drug dosing, because some adolescents may require higher dosing by weight or by body surface area compared with adults. Concomitant drugs should be evaluated for each patient because drug–drug interactions could also be responsible for ARV treatment failure. If the patient has been adherent to ARVs and has not had a timely virologic response, then a genotype may be considered to determine whether the patient developed any resistance to current ARVs. However, if a patient is on a failing ARV regimen and no evidence of resistance is identified on a genotype, then poor adherence should be suspected.

Genotype resistance tests are recommended at baseline before starting ART. Genotypic assays can detect resistance to ARVs by PCR amplification and analysis of reverse transcriptase, protease, and integrase coding sequences from a patient's HIV viral load (if transmitted INSTI resistance is a concern). The HIV viral load should be greater than 1000 copies/mL for these tests to be performed. Some of these tests might also be considered if a patient's viral load is between 500 and 1000 copies/mL. A specialist in pediatric HIV infection should be consulted for appropriate interpretation of genotypic results. Furthermore, the International AIDS Society-USA and the Stanford University HIV Drug Resistance Database are two useful resources that compile significant resistance-associated mutations to current ARVs, and are available at https://www.iasusa.org/resources/hiv-drug-resistance-mutations/ and https://hivdb.stanford.edu. For the genotype to accurately reflect whether a patient may have resistance to the current ARV regimen, the patient must have been taking these ARVs within the past 4 weeks (i.e., drug-selective pressure). This point is very important because reversion from resistant virus to wild-type virus can occur in the first 4 weeks after ARVs are discontinued. The genotype test should help elucidate which ARVs are still active for the patient. It is also critical to review ARV history as well as all other resistance tests when selecting a new ARV regimen because previous resistance tests may reveal archived resistance that is not evident on current resistance tests.

Other resistance tests such as phenotypic assays are reserved for those who have developed resistance to previous ARV regimens, especially PIs. These assays are useful in deriving a direct assessment of the effect and interaction of mutations acquired by viral strains on viral replication. Phenotypic assays involve PCR amplification of HIV gene sequences from a patient's viral strain, which are then inserted into a laboratory HIV strain. Replications of this recombinant viral strain at varying ARV concentrations are compared with the replication of a reference or wild-type viral strain. Fold resistance change is reported as the ratio of IC_{50} (defined as the median inhibitory concentration of ARVs needed to inhibit 50% of viral replication) of a patient's viral strain to IC_{50} of a reference strain. The greater the fold change, the more likelihood of ARV resistance. Two advantages of a genotype over a phenotype are a quicker turnaround time (1–2 weeks vs. 2–3 weeks) and a lower price. Virtual phenotypes are another type of resistance test that predicts the likelihood of a drug-resistant phenotype from a genotype. This test takes the patient's genotype and predicts a phenotype from a large known database of matching genotypes and phenotypes. However, this test may be insufficient for reliably detecting predictable phenotypes, especially with newer ARV drugs, because there may be fewer matching genotypes and phenotypes available for these drugs.

In addition to resistance testing history, factors to consider in creating a new ARV regimen should include ARV treatment history and toxicities, CD4$^+$ and viral load trends, adherence potential, and available treatment options.

Furthermore, pill size, palatability, pill burden, and dosing frequency should be considered when developing a new ARV regimen. The goal of the new ARV regimen should be complete virologic suppression, ideally using three fully active drugs. If a child living with HIV were on an NNRTI-based regimen and developed resistance to the NNRTI, then a PI- or INSTI-based regimen would be recommended. If a child were on a PI-based regimen and developed resistance to the PI, then a NNRTI- or INSTI-based regimen or an alternative PI-based regimen would be recommended. With respect to using potential NRTIs, special attention should be given to ensure the correct combination is used. For example, some patients can easily develop resistance to either emtricitabine or lamivudine if they are nonadherent to these NRTIs. If the patient has very few other NRTI mutations (especially thymidine analog mutations), using lamivudine or emtricitabine in a future treatment regimen can be advantageous because selection of a common mutation by these drugs could increase susceptibility to concomitant NRTIs such as tenofovir or zidovudine.[200-202]

C-C chemokine receptor type 5 tropism assays should be considered in treatment-experienced children living with HIV who are as young as 2 years and weigh more than 10 kg to determine whether maraviroc is a feasible treatment option. Treatment-naive patients living with HIV usually have CCR5 (R5) tropic virus. However, a coreceptor switch from CCR5 to CXCR4 (X4) or CCR5 to CCR5 and CXCR4 dual/mixed (D/M) tropic viruses is possible with time, especially in treatment-experienced patients and those who have HIV disease progression. The Trofile (Monogram Biosciences, South San Francisco, CA) phenotypic assay is used in the United States to determine CCR5 tropism. This assay usually takes about 2 weeks to report results and requires that the patient's viral load be greater than 1000 copies/mL. Of note, these assays have good sensitivity in detecting X4 or D/M tropic virus, representing up to 0.3% of the patient's plasma virus. Genotypic assays (Trofile DNA) recently became available in the United States, which are useful for detecting mutations associated with X4 or D/M tropic viruses. These assays also have the advantage of being able to be performed in patients with an undetectable viral load. Because maraviroc is a CCR5 antagonist, it is only effective for patients who have R5 tropic virus. Limitations for using maraviroc include twice-daily dosing, potential for several drug–drug interactions, and requirement for tropism assays before use.

Enfuvirtide may also be considered in children with extensive treatment resistance. Enfuvirtide is approved for use in treatment-experienced children 6 years and older in combination with other ARVs, with evidence of continuing viral replication despite current ART. Some of the main limitations to using enfuvirtide are that it is the only ARV given subcutaneously (twice daily) and local injection site reactions are very common (98%). Other regimens such as dual PI combinations including lopinavir/ritonavir with saquinavir or atazanavir are no longer recommended in both adults and children.[158, 203-207] Some of the disadvantages of dual PI regimens are poor tolerability (particularly hyperlipidemia) and increased drug–drug interactions. If a patient has very limited treatment options, children should be considered for newer therapeutic

ARVs in clinical development. Information for clinical trials can be found at https://aidsinfo.nih.gov/clinical-trials. If a patient has extensive treatment resistance, a pediatric HIV specialist should also be consulted because of possible access to unpublished data regarding the efficacy and safety of newer agents approved for adults. Also worth noting is that off-label use of newer ARVs in children requires caution because the adverse effects of these agents are unknown and may have observable differences in children compared with adults. Furthermore, changing pharmacokinetics in a growing child makes the extrapolation of dosing from adults to children on the basis of body weight or body surface area unpredictable and often may underestimate appropriate pediatric dosing, potentially leading to ARV resistance.[208]

Considerations for ARV treatment may be different in certain special populations. The largest percentage of children living with HIV in the United States is composed of adolescents. Dosing of ARVs for adolescents can be complicated by factors such as sexual maturity rating of puberty and development of fat and muscles, which could influence drug pharmacokinetics. In children, dosing of ARVs may be higher than adult dosing to compensate for faster metabolism and/or higher drug clearance. Therefore, as a pediatric patient grows into adolescence, ARV dosing may be higher-than-usual adult dosing. Psychosocial and cognitive development may also present challenges for adolescents regarding adherence to ARVs. Some other challenges may be mood disorders and other mental illnesses that should be addressed adequately to ensure successful adherence to ARVs. Directly observed therapy may be useful in these situations. The transition from adolescent care to adult HIV care settings can also be complicated and difficult. General guidelines regarding transitional plans and those who may benefit from them are available.[209]

Female patients living with HIV may have greater risks of certain adverse effects than male patients. These effects may include nevirapine-associated hepatotoxicity; lactic acidosis caused by prolonged exposure to NRTIs such as stavudine, zidovudine, and didanosine; and metabolic complications such as central fat accumulation and propensity to osteopenia/osteoporosis postmenopause.[210-218] However, most of these differences do not require special treatment recommendations at this time. Sexually active girls or women living with HIV should be encouraged to use effective and consistent contraception methods. The FDA cautions that efavirenz should not be used in adolescent girls who are sexually active and not using reliable contraception, or who want to become pregnant, because of the potential for neural tube defects that could occur in the fetus if used in the first trimester. However, the perinatal guidelines do not restrict use of efavirenz in adolescent girls or adults who are pregnant or who may become pregnant based on updated data on potential teratogenicity.[52] In addition, PIs and NNRTIs may interact with oral contraceptives such as ethinyl estradiol, norethindrone, and norgestimate metabolites (norelgestromin and levonorgestrel).[78] Both NNRTIs and boosted PIs are more likely to cause decreases in these oral contraceptives versus unboosted PIs such as atazanavir and fosamprenavir, which may actually increase concentrations. Alternative or an additional contraceptive method should be used in women living with HIV who are using either NNRTIs or boosted PIs. Depot medroxyprogesterone acetate may also be an effective method of contraception because some studies have shown unaltered efficacy of this drug when coadministered with nelfinavir, efavirenz, or nevirapine regimens, as well as no additional adverse effects or significant changes in ARV drug concentrations.[219-222] Limited data exist for other forms of contraception such as vaginal rings and transdermal patches, but intrauterine devices have proven safe and effective in women living with HIV.[221,223,224]

Choice of ARVs for pregnant women living with HIV may be different from that for nonpregnant women.[52] Initiation of ARV treatment is necessary, regardless of immunologic and virologic values, to prevent vertical transmission to the fetus. The goal of therapy is virologic suppression by the time of delivery, when transmission is more likely. Baseline resistance testing is also recommended before starting therapy; however, testing should not delay therapy, and therapy should be initiated before the results of testing are available. If the pregnant mother living with HIV has no ARV resistance from genotypic assay, then abacavir/lamivudine or TDF with either emtricitabine or lamivudine should be selected as the preferred two-NRTI backbones with a third agent. Preferred third agent options include PIs such as boosted atazanavir or boosted darunavir, or integrase inhibitors such as raltegravir. Standard ARV dosing of some PIs such as boosted darunavir may need to be increased (to twice-daily dosing) during pregnancy to compensate for reduced bioavailability because of enhanced metabolism and increased clearance during pregnancy. Breastfeeding is also discouraged because it may continue to pose a transmission risk to the infant and also because of the availability of feeding alternatives. If ART must be stopped during pregnancy for reasons such as severe toxicity, abrupt discontinuation of ART for the mother living with HIV should be done cautiously. Certain ARVs such as NNRTIs have a long half-life, which must be taken into consideration. Some experts recommend discontinuing NNRTIs at least 1 week before discontinuing other ARVs, and others recommend substituting an NNRTI with a PI plus two other ARVs for at least 30 days to reduce the development of NNRTI resistance.[52]

If a child living with HIV is acutely infected with hepatitis B virus (HBV) infection, the risk of developing chronic HBV is markedly greater in infants than in older children and adolescents.[225-227] Very limited data exist for treatment of HIV/HBV-coinfected children. The American Association for the Study of Liver Disease HBV practice guidelines recommend standard interferon alfa-2b, entecavir, and TDF as preferred therapies in children older than 1 year, 2 years, and 12 years respectively.[228] If treatment of chronic HBV is indicated in an adult living with HIV, then HBV treatment should use fully suppressive cART with agents such as tenofovir and either emtricitabine or lamivudine, regardless of current CD4+ cell count, and should also be considered in older children. In this case cART is important to reduce the risk of developing resistance to ARVs. Caution must be used when discontinuing agents for treatment of chronic HBV because this change could potentially cause hepatic damage secondary to reactivation of HBV. Furthermore, caution should be used when discontinuing ARVs that have activity against HBV; if this is the case, then another active drug for HBV should be used to avoid a potential flare or reactivation of HBV. Alternative treatment strategies for chronic HBV may also include adefovir or tenofovir for older children who can receive adult dosing. Limited data on peginterferon alfa preclude its use in coinfected children at this time.

The prevalence of hepatitis C virus (HCV) in children living with HIV is as much as 3.1% in the United States.[229] Limited data exist for both HCV disease progression and treatment of HCV in coinfected children. Newer data suggest that children who are coinfected presented a lower rate of spontaneous clearance of HCV and were often viremic with elevated alanine aminotransferase concentrations compared with HCV-monoinfected children.[230] Coinfected adults with chronic HCV have a higher risk of progressing to cirrhosis and an overall higher mortality than do those with HCV infection alone. Because ART may slow the progression of liver disease, HIV ART should be initiated in all HCV/HIV coinfected patients regardless of CD4+ cell counts.[78] If CD4+ cell counts are less than 200 cells/mm[3], then ART should be initiated and HCV treatment may be deferred until CD4+ cell counts rebound. A recent pilot study identified differences in HIV viral evolution in the presence of HCV in pediatric patients, which suggests the possible relevance of virus–virus interactions.[230] Because few studies of coinfected children have been conducted, with only data from four case series available, recommendations are extrapolated from data in adults.[231] Treatment of HCV in coinfected adults has rapidly changed in the past few years with the advent of curative oral direct-acting antivirals. Despite the many newly approved direct-acting antivirals for adults older than 18 years who are infected with HCV, only two regimens (ledipasvir/sofosbuvir or glecaprevir/pibrentasvir) have been approved for use in pediatric patients. The American Association for the Study of Liver Disease HCV guidelines recommend deferring HCV treatment until interferon-free regimens are available for children younger than 11 years.[232] Didanosine and zidovudine should be avoided when using ribavirin because these NRTIs may lead to mitochondrial and hematologic toxicities.[39] Treating both HCV and HIV can result in drug-induced liver injury with substantially elevated liver enzymes; associated ARV agents include stavudine, didanosine, nevirapine, full-dose ritonavir, or tipranavir boosted with low-dose ritonavir.[233] Dose modification or avoidance of some hepatically metabolized ARV agents may be necessary, depending on the severity of liver disease (particularly Child-Pugh class B and C disease). In patients coinfected with HCV, ART may be beneficial because it may slow the progression to liver disease and reduce HIV-related inflammation associated with lower CD4+ cell counts. Although data exist on the treatment of HCV in adults living with HIV, few direct-acting antiviral options for treatment of HCV are available for pediatric patients living with HIV.

MONITORING OF THERAPY

THERAPEUTIC OUTCOMES

Before initiating ART, several variables related to laboratory testing and factors that may affect treatment adherence

should be assessed at baseline. Laboratory testing should include the following: CD4+ count and CD4+ percentage; HIV viral load; serum chemistries; lipid panel; hematologic panel; resistance testing (in some cases, it may be prudent to initiate therapy before resistance testing, understanding that therapy may require modification based on the results); and any other laboratory variable that may be affected by the choice of ARV regimen. For patients who are in acute or recent HIV infection and for pregnant women living with HIV, ARV initiation should not be delayed while awaiting the results of resistance testing. After ART is initiated or changed, children and adolescents living with HIV are monitored for the regimen's efficacy, safety (e.g., toxicity, adverse effects), tolerability (e.g., medication palatability, dosing frequency, pill burden), and adherence to the regimen. For pediatric patients on ART, the following laboratory tests are recommended for monitoring at baseline, at 2–4 weeks after ART initiation or modification, and then routinely every 3–4 months: CD4+ count, CD4+ percentage, HIV viral load, complete blood cell count with differential, and serum chemistries. Frequency of CD4 cell count monitoring can be extended to every 6–12 months in children who demonstrate adherence to ART with sustained viral suppression, have CD4 cell count values considerably higher than the threshold for developing OIs, and have a stable clinical status for greater than 2–3 years. However, viral load monitoring is generally recommended every 3-4 months to monitor adherence to ART and disease progression. A lipid panel, random plasma glucose, and urinalysis are usually required every 6–12 months. For adults on ART, the CD4+ count and percentage should be monitored at initiation; every 3–6 months during first 2 years of ART, or if viremia develops while the patient is on ART, or if CD4 count is less than 300 cells/mm[3]; and every 12 months after 2 years on ART with consistently suppressed viral load and CD4+ count 300–500 cells/mm[3] (monitoring is then optional if CD4+ count is greater than 500 cells/mm[3]). Furthermore, for adults living with HIV on ART, HIV viral load should be monitored at baseline, 2–8 weeks after initiation or modification of ART, and then every 3–6 months. Providers may extend this interval for monitoring viral load to every 6 months for adherent patients whose viral load has been suppressed for more than 2 years and whose clinical and immunologic status is stable. Monitoring of HIV surrogate markers may be required more often for patients who are experiencing virologic, immunologic, or clinical failure.

When monitoring the efficacy of ARV treatment, some patients may not have positive CD4+ and viral load trends. If this outcome occurs, then treatment failure may be considered and can be classified as *virologic, immunologic,* or *clinical*. The reader is encouraged to review the sections in the DHHS guidelines regarding recognizing and managing ARV treatment failure because the content and definition of these guidelines may be updated annually. *Virologic failure* occurs as an incomplete initial response to therapy or as a viral rebound after virologic suppression is achieved. Virologic failure may be defined for all children as a repeated plasma viral load more than 200 copies/mL after 6 months of therapy. An *incomplete virologic response* in children is defined as less than a 1-log decrease in viral load from baseline after

8–12 weeks of ART, a viral load greater than 400 copies/mL after 6 months of treatment, or a detectable viral load after 12 months of treatment (optimal viral suppression is less than 20–75 copies/mL, depending on the sensitivity of the assay used). *Viral rebound* is defined by repeated detectable viral loads after a period of viral suppression. Repeated viral loads greater than 200 copies/mL (especially more than 500 copies/mL) are indicative of virologic failure in children.[31]

Evaluation of immune response in children is complicated by the normal age-related changes in CD4+ count. Thus, the normal decline in CD4+ values with age must be considered when evaluating declines in CD4+ values. It is important to note that CD4+ percentage tends to vary less with age. At about age 5 years, absolute CD4+ cell count values in children approach those of adults; consequently, changes in absolute CD4+ count can be used in children older than 5 years.[31]

Immunologic failure may be classified as an incomplete response to ARV treatment. An incomplete response to treatment is characterized differently on the basis of age. Although there is no standardized definition, many experts consider suboptimal immunologic response to therapy as the failure to maintain or achieve CD4+ counts and percentage that is at least greater than the age-specific range for severe immunodeficiency.

Clinical failure may be identified through the presence of new OIs (excluding immune reconstitution inflammatory syndrome) or disease progression during ART. However, it is important to consider a patient's immunologic and virologic status in the presence of clinical symptoms because those symptoms may not necessarily represent treatment failure. Factors in disease progression that can represent treatment failure in children include failure to grow at a normal rate even when nutritional requirements are met, recurrent infections that may be indicative of progression to AIDS, and impairment in cognitive and motor skills development.[31]

When assessing treatment failure in children living with HIV, several factors should be considered before modifying ART. Some of these include pharmacokinetic variability, drug toxicity, and ARV resistance. However, one of the most significant factors affecting treatment outcome is adherence to ARVs. Low rates of adherence to ARVs have been linked to virologic failure, with that risk increasing as more ARV doses are missed. Low adherence rates can also increase the risk of developing ARV resistance, with the potential for cross-resistance if mutations continue to accumulate while a patient is on a suboptimal regimen. This consequence, in turn, could limit future treatment options. On the contrary, high adherence rates are associated with viral suppression, low rates of drug resistance, increased survival rates, and improved quality of life. Although a 95% adherence rate has historically been desired to achieve and maintain virologic suppression, it is possible to do so with lower rates, depending on the medications used for treatment, including some boosted PI-based regimens and those containing efavirenz plus two NRTIs.[41,234] It is difficult to predict high or low adherence rates in children because not only do they have their own adherence barriers to overcome, but they may also have to deal with any adherence barriers their own parents or caregivers introduce. Factors that influence adherence rates may include the following:

frequency of dosing, pill burden, ARV palatability, refusal of ARVs, forgetfulness, no established daily routine, ARV-related adverse effects, and psychosocial issues, which may include financial concerns, housing stability, transportation limitations, social/familial support, stigma, psychiatric disorders, and active substance abuse.[31] In hospitalization cases, it is important that the medical team be in contact with the patient's ambulatory HIV care provider to maintain appropriate HIV treatment (correct medications and doses), ensure continuity of care, recognize the potential for drug–drug interactions with ARVs (e.g., PIs, NNRTIs, and the INSTI elvitegravir are metabolized extensively through the CYP system), and discharge patients on appropriate therapy for HIV and any comorbid condition to maximize therapeutic benefit and minimize adverse events.

Children must depend on their parents or caregivers to administer their drugs appropriately; therefore, any adherence barriers that affect the individual who administers that drug may also directly affect the success or failure of the child's treatment regimen. Parents or caregivers may struggle with the decision to disclose a child's status to family or friends, which may lead to disguising or hiding prescription labels, not refilling medications in a timely manner, and skipping doses when away from the home. Furthermore, in vertical transmission, parents may have feelings of guilt or regret and seek to avoid reminders of their own HIV status.[31]

Adherence to ARVs in adolescents living with HIV may be influenced by various factors. These patients are very concerned with being perceived as different from their peers, and they may refuse to take their ARVs. They may skip doses to avoid disclosing their status to their peers. In vertical transmission, many adolescents have been taking ARVs for several years, and it is not unusual for them to experience pill fatigue. Instability in the home, mental health issues, neurocognitive delay, and active substance abuse may also negatively affect a patient's ability to remain adherent to a drug regimen. Educating patients, as well as parents and caregivers, on the need to maintain a consistently high rate of adherence to the ARV regimen for achieving therapeutic goals and to avoid the development of drug resistance in addition to providing them with strategic tools to help overcome adherence barriers are essential to achieving therapeutic goals, avoiding medication errors, and empowering patients to take control of their health care.

Because many of the adherence barriers previously described are perceived by patients and caregivers as of more immediate concern than taking their ARVs consistently, it is essential to work with them to overcome these barriers. Although studies of the adolescent population have used technology, peer support groups, and motivational interviewing techniques to improve adherence and virologic outcomes, their positive effects have been short lived.[235,236] Several strategies may still be used by the health care team to help patients and caregivers attain a higher rate of adherence to ARVs. Some of these strategies may include using a multidisciplinary approach to care, providing referrals for specialty services (medical and/or social), maintaining effective communication/follow-up, assessing adherence rates/barriers at each medical visit, and providing adherence tools (e.g., pillboxes, visual aids) to the patients. An interdisciplinary health care team including physicians, pharmacists, nurses, social workers/case managers, dietitians, and others working collectively and synergistically together is essential in optimizing care for children living with HIV. In addition, ARV regimens should be tailored to a patient's lifestyle with respect to dosing frequency, tolerability profile (e.g., potential adverse effects, drug interactions), and the patient's daily routine. Moreover, educating both patients and parents or caregivers on the importance of ARV adherence, interacting with them to establish a plan to manage potential adverse effects of ARVs, identifying adherence barriers and the reasons behind them, and encouraging a reliable support system are critical for optimizing adherence to ARVs.

THERAPEUTIC DRUG MONITORING

The use of TDM is to look at drug concentration measurements to determine appropriate drug dosing and to minimize adverse effects while also achieving or maintaining positive treatment outcomes. This monitoring is typically used as a therapeutic management strategy, with medications used to treat seizures, heart arrhythmias, and bacterial infections. Because of interpatient variability in plasma concentrations of certain NNRTIs, PIs, and INSTIs, low plasma concentrations of ARVs that can lead to decreased treatment response, and high concentrations that can lead to toxicities for certain ARVs, TDM may occasionally be used in the therapeutic management of pediatric patients with HIV. However, data are insufficient to correlate TDM with positive changes in virologic or clinical outcomes. Furthermore, definitive therapeutic ranges for maximizing clinical response and minimizing adverse effects are not well established for all ARVs, and few laboratory facilities within the United States are adequately equipped to perform TDM with ARVs. Although not recommended for routine use in HIV management, TDM may be useful in the following instances: as a tool to help explain a suboptimal treatment response; for a drug-resistant virus to compare drug concentration with virus susceptibility; for medication administration issues—crushing/chewing/dissolving a medication may change the pharmacokinetics of a drug, dietary habits may alter a medication's pharmacokinetic profile, and incorrect dosing may occur because of administration errors by caregivers; for problems related to adherence that lead to low plasma concentrations of ARVs such as missed doses or inconsistent dose timing; as a tool for identifying drug toxicity that may be caused by an agent exceeding the normal therapeutic range, such as the use of efavirenz in children younger than 3 years; and for identifying drug–drug interactions—many ARVs have significant interactions with other medications, herbals, and/or food that could lead to altered plasma concentrations.[31,78]

ADVERSE EFFECTS

Table 4 summarizes common adverse effects of ARVs and their management as well as relevant monitoring guidelines. Class-related adverse effects of NRTIs include lactic acidosis

and hepatic steatosis. These are commonly representative of prolonged stavudine, didanosine, or zidovudine use. Lactic acidosis is characterized by fatigue, weakness, myalgia, weight loss, and unexplained nausea or vomiting. Although it is rare, some patients present with acute organ failure such as fulminant hepatic, pancreatic, and respiratory failure. Blood lactate concentrations are considered in those with clinical signs and symptoms consistent with lactic acidosis. If lactic acidosis and hepatic steatosis occur with stavudine, zidovudine, or didanosine, switching to tenofovir or abacavir with either emtricitabine or lamivudine may be appropriate because these agents tend to have less mitochondrial toxicity. Some physicians will use an NRTI-sparing regimen, when possible, if the lactic acidosis is severe. Facial or peripheral lipoatrophy is also commonly associated with thymidine analog NRTIs such as stavudine and zidovudine, as well as didanosine. Lipoatrophy is manifested as a loss of subcutaneous fat in the face, buttocks, and extremities. If lipoatrophy is present, switching from zidovudine or stavudine to another NRTI that has less mitochondrial toxicity and is active against HIV may help reduce further progression of lipoatrophy. Diminished bone density (osteopenia and/or osteoporosis) is most often seen as a possible adverse effect with TDF. Compared with TDF, TAF has limited, if any effect on bone density because of its stability as the prodrug form in the plasma.[237] Monitoring should include serum 25-hydroxyvitamin D concentrations and dual-energy x-ray absorptiometry scans. Appropriate management may include sufficient calcium and vitamin D supplementation and avoidance of steroids and medroxyprogesterone, if possible. The role of bisphosphonates in children is not established, but considering ARVs other than TDF may reduce the incidence of osteopenia and osteoporosis.

Class-specific adverse effects of PIs include the following: dyslipidemia; hyperglycemia; prolonged PR interval as a manifestation of first-degree symptomatic atrioventricular block; fat maldistribution; increased bleeding episodes in patients with hemophilia; elevated liver enzymes; and gastrointestinal intolerance, such as diarrhea. Lipodystrophy and central lipohypertrophy are mostly associated with PIs. These may manifest as central fat accumulation in the abdomen, trunk (gynecomastia), or back of neck (buffalo hump). Lipodystrophy is more common in adolescents than in children. Lifestyle modification, including exercise and diet, or using other ARVs may help with the management of central lipohypertrophy. Of note, liposuction, metformin, and rosiglitazone are not useful for treatment in children. Tesamorelin was approved for treatment of lipodystrophy in adults living with HIV, but efficacy and safety have not been established in children. Effects of PIs on dyslipidemia are related to ritonavir dosing; higher ritonavir doses lead to worsening effects of dyslipidemia, especially hypertriglyceridemia. For PI use, the following should be monitored routinely: lipid panel, including total cholesterol, triglycerides, low-density lipoprotein cholesterol and high-density lipoprotein cholesterol; blood glucose; and liver enzymes. If triglycerides are greater than 500 mg/dL, the risk of pancreatitis is increased. Although fibrates are only approved for adults, one study showed that fibrates significantly decreased triglyceride concentrations among children in clinical practice.[238] Primary pharmacologic interventions used for the treatment of dyslipidemia in children living with HIV include fish oils and some statins. Fish oils containing n-3 polyunsaturated fatty acids may be considered, as well as pravastatin 20 mg once daily for children age 8–13 years and 40 mg once daily for adolescents age 14–18 years; atorvastatin 10–20 mg once daily for children older than 10 years; and rosuvastatin 5–20 mg once daily for those age 8–17 years.[31] Dyslipidemia should be appropriately treated with drugs when necessary, or ART may be switched if feasible to alternative ARVs that have less effect on dyslipidemia. Caution should also be used when taking ARVs with certain statins because drug–drug interactions are possible. Lovastatin and simvastatin are contraindicated with PI use. Also PIs should be used with caution in those with preexisting cardiac conduction problems or those taking other drugs such as calcium channel blockers, β-blockers, and digoxin because these are known to prolong the PR interval. Rash is also possible with some of the PIs, especially with fosamprenavir, tipranavir, and darunavir, which possess a sulfonamide moiety. Mild to moderate rash can be treated with antihistamines while continuing ARVs. For patients who develop a severe rash such as Stevens-Johnson syndrome, all ARVs should be discontinued. The FDA recently issued a new warning for labeling for lopinavir/ritonavir regarding a serious health problem reported in premature infants receiving lopinavir/ritonavir oral solution.[239] The oral solution contains alcohol and propylene glycol; premature infants have a decreased ability to eliminate propylene glycol, which has led to adverse events such as serious heart, kidney, or breathing problems.

Class-related adverse effects of NNRTIs include rash and elevated liver enzymes. Limitations for efavirenz use include central nervous system adverse effects such as fatigue, insomnia, vivid dreams, depression, suicidal ideation, poor concentration, and agitation. If any of these adverse effects occur, they are usually transient and should subside after 2–4 weeks. Some patients, particularly African Americans, may have a genetic polymorphism in the CYP2B6 enzyme, which could exacerbate the adverse effects of efavirenz.[240] In this case, patients who have these specific polymorphisms in CYP2B6 metabolism and require efavirenz for treatment may benefit from using a lower dose of efavirenz (400 mg once daily) to reduce the incidence of adverse effects.[241,242] If a patient has underlying depression or other preexisting psychiatric conditions, caution should be used when considering efavirenz or rilpivirine because both of these ARVs could exacerbate or worsen depression. Major limitations for nevirapine use in children are higher rates of toxicity, which may include rare cases of hypersensitivity reactions including Stevens-Johnson syndrome and life-threatening hepatitis. Hepatic toxicity tends to be less common in children than in adults who receive chronic nevirapine.[131,133] Rash and elevated liver enzymes occur more commonly in female patients than in male patients, and nevirapine should not be initiated in adult females whose CD4+ cell counts are greater than 250 cells/mm³ or in adult males whose CD4+ cell counts are greater than 400 cells/mm³ because of the increased risk of liver toxicity observed when nevirapine is initiated above these CD4+ cell thresholds.[243]

INSTIs are generally well tolerated with few class adverse effects, including insomnia and headache. Elvitegravir has a favorable metabolic profile with fewer adverse effects on serum lipids, with minimal effect on total cholesterol and low-density lipoprotein cholesterol compared with efavirenz-based therapies.[244] Elvitegravir and raltegravir may also be associated with mild diarrhea, but this adverse effect occurs minimally with dolutegravir. Raltegravir can also be associated with the development of rash.[112,113] Overall INSTIs have a better tolerability compared with other ART classes with minimal adverse effects.

The severity of adverse effects experienced with ARVs determines whether these medications are discontinued. Some mild or moderate adverse effects of ARVs such as diarrhea or mild rash can be treated symptomatically without discontinuation or substitution of ARVs. However, some adverse effects may be more severe and necessitate a change in ART. If the responsible ARV agent can be identified, caution should be taken to make sure that an active ARV is substituted. Careful attention should be given to history of treatment with ARVs and resistance testing when selecting an alternative ARV. If adverse effects are severe or life threatening, all ARVs should be discontinued at the same time. Once the patient is stabilized, implementation of a completely new ARV regimen that does not include the previous offending agent should be considered.

CONCLUSIONS

The availability of newer ARV agents in addition to the new research on the progression of disease and the efficacy and safety of treatment modalities will continue to affect the management of HIV infection in the pediatric and adolescent populations. It is important to consider a patient's individual characteristics—such as past ARV exposure, resistance profile, comorbid conditions, additional drug therapy, family/social situation—when determining an appropriate initial or modified treatment regimen to maximize the effect and minimize adverse events. Fortunately, a recent increased availability of once-daily fixed-dosed ART combinations approved for treatment of HIV infection in young adolescents has introduced greater opportunities for simplification, which will hopefully improve overall adherence to ART and lead to long-term positive treatment outcomes and a better quality of life. Finally, Box 1 presents the essential points to summarize as the clinical pearls for children living with HIV.

ADDITIONAL RESOURCES

U.S. Department of Health and Human Services AIDSinfo: www.aidsinfo.nih.gov

Centers for Disease Control and Prevention: www.cdc.gov

National Institutes of Health: www.nih.gov

HIV Medicine Association of the Infectious Diseases Society of America: www.hivma.org

Pediatric Infectious Diseases Society: www.pids.org

Box 1. Clinical Pearls for Children Living with HIV

Since the development of the first protease inhibitor in the mid-1990s, potent combination antiretroviral (ARV) therapy has transformed HIV infection from a death sentence to a chronic disease state

Children living with HIV are living longer and are able to experience a better quality of life because of an armamentarium of newer ARVs—many available as fixed-dose combinations—that are more potent, convenient, and tolerable

One of the best ways to prevent HIV transmission is to use safe sex practices such as condoms (which is especially important for adolescent population), including use of pre-exposure prophylaxis by the serodiscordant partner

Early initiation of ARV therapy leads to improved virologic, immunologic, and clinical outcomes

Many factors must be considered when initiating ARV therapy in children from both the medical and psychosocial standpoint, including the following:

> Appropriateness of certain medications for particular age groups
> Regimen complexity and palatability
> Adherence barriers
> Issues affecting parents and caregivers

Adherence to ARVs should be assessed and evaluated at every chance because this element is critical to ensure positive treatment outcomes

Treatment failure can be multifactorial, and the most common reasons are the following:

> Nonadherence to ARVs
> Drug intolerance
> Pharmacokinetic variability
> Drug–drug interactions
> Presence of drug-resistant virus

An interdisciplinary health care team approach including physicians, pharmacists, nurses, social workers, dietitians, and others is essential in optimizing care for children living with HIV

Patient Case

SWITCHING FROM A PROTEASE INHIBITOR-BASED TO AN INTEGRASE STRAND TRANSFER INHIBITOR-BASED REGIMEN FOR ANTIRETROVIRAL THERAPY

A perinatally infected 10-year-old boy living with HIV is brought to the clinic by his grandmother, who is his primary caretaker. They are here today for a 3-month follow-up visit to check routine laboratory tests and to review current adherence to antiretroviral therapy (ART). His grandmother tells you that now since the boy is older, he is fighting against taking his lopinavir/ritonavir solution because of the bitter taste. Because he is also now more involved with soccer after school, his schedule is busier, and administering a twice-daily liquid dose formulation is becoming more inconvenient. She is wondering when it would be possible for him to take just one pill for treatment of his HIV.

Medical history: HIV; attention deficit hyperactivity disorder; asthma; seasonal allergies

Family history:

Mother: Asthma, hypertension, HIV

Father: Hypertension, gastroesophageal reflux disease

Maternal grandmother: Diabetes mellitus, chronic obstructive pulmonary disease, hypertension

Maternal grandfather: Hypertension, congestive heart failure

Paternal grandmother: Glaucoma, chronic back pain

Paternal grandfather: Diabetes mellitus, hyperlipidemia, gout

Social history: In fifth grade now and will graduate next year to begin middle school; becoming more involved with after school soccer league

Current medications:

Lopinavir/ritonavir 80/20 mg/mL 4.2 mL by mouth twice daily (started 9 months ago)

Lamivudine/zidovudine 150/300 mg one tablet twice daily (started 9 months ago)

Fluticasone 88 mcg 2 actuations of 44 mcg inhaled twice daily

Methylphenidate 10 mg one immediate-release tablet twice daily

Loratadine 10 mg daily

Montelukast 5 mg every night before bed

Drug allergies: Penicillin (rash)

Immunizations: Up to date

Vital signs: Tmax 98.6°F (37°C), BP 110/74 mm Hg, HR 66 beats/minute, RR 17 breaths/minute, Ht 53 inches, Wt 31 kg

Laboratory markers:

Routine HIV Surrogate Marker	Jan. 15	Apr. 15	Jul. 15	Oct. 15
HIV viral load (copies/mL)	18,215	< 20	< 20	In process
CD4 (cells/mm³)	337	400	456	In process
CD4%	19	22	24	In process

Additional laboratory findings from 3 months ago (July 15):

Test	Results
Na	141 mEq/L
K	4.3 mEq/L
Cl	100 mEq/L
HCO$_3$	23 mEq/L
BUN	14 mg/dL
SCr	0.61 mg/dL
Glucose	90 mg/dL
Hgb	13.1 g/dL
Hct	35.5%
WBC	5.2 × 10³ cells/mm³
Plt	286 × 10³ cells/mm³
MCV	86 fL
AST	23 U/L
ALT	28 U/L
TC	120 mg/dL
HDL	50 mg/dL
LDL	85 mg/dL
TG	100 mg/dL

Resistance testing history: Genotype on January 15 non-nucleoside reverse transcriptase inhibitor (NNRTI) Y181C mutation (i.e., resistance to nevirapine) detected; no other resistance mutations noted to nucleoside reverse transcriptase inhibitor (NRTI), protease inhibitor (PI), and integrase strand transfer inhibitor (INSTI) classes

*HLA-B*5701:* Negative

ART history: Nevirapine liquid formulation + lamivudine + zidovudine

1. What interventions can be made to improve the child's adherence knowing that his grandmother says giving a liquid dose is inconvenient and that he has been fighting against taking his doses?

Some of the best interventions that may improve adherence for this child include changing current ART regimen completely to tablet formulations, and, if possible, also changing to a once-daily antiretroviral (ARV) regimen. Although the tolerability of the lopinavir/ritonavir solution could be potentially improved by mixing it with different foods (e.g., milk or pudding, or coating the mouth with peanut butter), a better alternative would be to switch to the lopinavir/ritonavir 100/25 mg pediatric tablet formulation (based on the patient's current weight, he would require four tablets twice daily). However, this change could introduce a considerably increased pill burden with 10 tablets daily, including the NRTI backbone of zidovudine/lamivudine. Darunavir boosted with ritonavir is another PI option but is also not ideal, since given the patient's weight and age, this regimen requires twice daily dosing and similar increased total daily pill burden associated with lopinavir/ritonavir.

An alternative once-daily PI-based regimen given his current weight might include a different two-NRTI backbone such as either Descovy (Gilead Sciences Inc., Foster City, CA) (emtricitabine 200 mg/ tenofovir alafenamide [TAF] 25 mg) one tablet once daily or Epzicom (ViiV Healthcare, Research Triangle Park, NC) (lamivudine 300 mg/abacavir 600 mg) one tablet once daily with atazanavir 200 mg as one capsule boosted with ritonavir 100 mg as one tablet, taken together once daily with food. Abacavir is a potential NRTI option given that the patient's *HLA-B* 5701* test is negative. These once-daily regimen changes would reduce overall pill burden to three pills/day, also maintaining the same ARV PI class.

Furthermore, a change to an INSTI-based regimen may also be considered to reduce overall pill burden and improve ease of use given that these agents are recommended as the first-line treatment in children, adolescents and adults living with HIV, and some are available as fixed-dose combination (FDCs) for the patient's current weight. Some suggested recommendations include Genvoya (Gilead Sciences) (elvitegravir 150 mg/cobicistat 150 mg/TAF 10 mg/emtricitabine 200 mg) one tablet once daily, or another INSTI dolutegravir 50 mg one tablet once daily together with either Descovy or Epzicom. To ensure adequate adherence, pill size can be very important. Descovy, dolutegravir, and Genvoya are relatively small in pill size compared with the lamivudine/zidovudine pill that the patient is currently taking. Therefore, a switch to Genvoya taken with food would be the best recommendation for this patient.

Lastly, another potential alternative is switching from lopinavir/ritonavir solution to chewable raltegravir as a 100-mg tablet (based on the patient's weight, he would require two chewable tablets twice daily), including continuation with the same lamivudine/zidovudine NRTI backbone. Although this raltegravir formulation has a better flavor, lower overall pill burden, and better adverse effect profile compared with lopinavir/ritonavir, the twice-daily dosing of raltegravir is still required and may not represent the best option.

2. How would you address the grandmother's question about when he can be simplified to a one-pill, once-daily ARV regimen?

Currently, very few available options are available with FDA label approval as a one-tablet FDC ARV regimen given the patient's weight of 31 kg; only Genvoya is approved and labeled for use in patients weighing at least 25 kg. Other future options might include INSTI-based Triumeq (ViiV Healthcare) and Biktarvy (Gilead Sciences) and PI-based Symtuza (Janssen Therapeutics, Titusville, NJ). When his weight increases to 40 kg and more, he could potentially take Triumeq (dolutegravir 50 mg/abacavir 600 mg/lamivudine 300 mg) one tablet once daily; however, Biktarvy and Symtuza are one-tablet once-daily ARV regimens only approved for use in adults 18 years and older. The NNRTI one-tablet once-daily regimens including Odefsey (Gilead Sciences) (if patient is at least 12 years and weighs 35 kg) and Atripla (Gilead Sciences) (if the patient weighs at least 40 kg) are NOT appropriate future options for this patient because he has previous NNRTI resistance which might reduce susceptibility to the NNRTIs rilpivirine and efavirenz in these one-tablet, once-daily FDCs.

3. What clinically relevant drug–drug interactions are currently present on the medication profile and how can they be best managed?

Clinically relevant drug–drug interactions present include fluticasone and lopinavir/ritonavir. Ritonavir is a cytochrome P450 (CYP) 3A4 isoenzyme (CYP3A4) inhibitor and may increase concentrations of fluticasone (CYP3A4 substrate). If the patient continues on lopinavir/ritonavir or changes to an alternative boosted PI atazanavir/ritonavir or to Genvoya, then the clinician should consider switching him to a different inhaled aerosol with fewer drug–drug interactions, such as beclomethasone 40 mcg twice daily. If the patient is switched from a PI-based ARV regimen to an INSTI-based regimen including either chewable raltegravir or dolutegravir, then he can continue his current aerosol inhaler fluticasone because the drug–drug interactions between fluticasone and these particular INSTIs are minimal—the predominant metabolism of raltegravir and dolutegravir is UGT1A1 mediated.

REFERENCES

1. World Health Organization. Global Health Observatory (GHO) data. Available at www.who.int/gho/hiv/en/. Accessed November 16, 2019.
2. UNAIDS. Fact sheet—Latest global and regional statistics on the status of the AIDS epidemic. Available at www.unaids.org/en/resources/documents/2019/UNAIDS_FactSheet. Accessed November 16, 2019.
3. Centers for Disease Control and Prevention. HIV Surveillance Report, vol. 29, 2017. Available at www.cdc.gov/hiv/library/reports/hiv-surveillance.html. Accessed November 16, 2019.
4. Centers for Disease Control and Prevention. Pneumocystis pneumonia–Los Angeles. MMWR. 1981;30:1-3.
5. Maartens G, Celum C, Lewin SR. HIV infection: epidemiology, pathogenesis, treatment, and prevention. Lancet 2014;384:258-71.

6. Campbell-Yesufu OT, Gandhi RT. Update on human immunodeficiency virus (HIV)-2 infection. Clin Infect Dis 2011;52:780-7.

7. Kulkosky J, Bray S. HAART-persistent HIV-1 latent reservoirs: their origin, mechanisms of stability and potential strategies for eradication. Curr HIV Res 2006;4:199-208.

8. Choudhary SK, Vrisekoop N, Jansen CA, et al. Low immune activation despite high levels of pathogenic human immunodeficiency virus type 1 results in long-term asymptomatic disease. J Virol 2007;81:8838-42.

9. Hunt PW, Brenchley J, Sinclair E, et al. Relationship between T cell activation and CD4+ T cell count in HIV-seropositive individuals with undetectable plasma HIV RNA levels in the absence of therapy. J Infect Dis 2008;197:126-33.

10. Sajadi M, Redfield RR. Long-term nonprogressive disease among individuals with untreated HIV infection. JAMA 2010; 3041784-86.

11. Paxton WA, Kang S, Koup RA. The HIV type 1 coreceptor CCR5 and its role in viral transmission and disease progression. AIDS Res Hum Retroviruses 1998;14:S89-92.

12. Carrington M, O'Brien SJ. The influence of HLA genotype on AIDS. Annu Rev Med 2003;54:535-51.

13. Coutsoudis A. Breastfeeding and HIV. Best Pract Res Clin Obstet Gynaecol 2005;19:185-96.

14. Gibson DR, Flynn NM, Perales D. Effectiveness of syringe exchange programs in reducing HIV risk behavior and HIV seroconversion among injecting drug users. AIDS 2001;15:1329-41.

15. Zaller ND, Bazazi AR, Velazquez L, et al. Attitudes toward methadone among out-of-treatment minority injection drug users: implications for health disparities. Int J Environ Res Public Health 2009;6:787-97.

16. Gaur AH, Dominguez KL, Kalish ML, et al. Practice of feeding premasticated food to infants: a potential risk factor for HIV transmission. Pediatrics 2009;124:658-66.

17. Patel P, Borkowf CB, Brooks JT, et al. Estimating per-act HIV transmission risk: a systematic review. AIDS 2014;28:1509-19.

18. Baillieu N, Potterton J. The extent of delay of language, motor, and cognitive development in HIV-positive infants. J Neurol Phys Ther 2008;32:118-21.

19. Scott GB, Hutto C, Makuch RW, et al. Survival in children with perinatally acquired human immunodeficiency virus type 1 infection. N Engl J Med 1989;321:1791-96.

20. Marolda J, Pace B, Bonforte RJ, et al. Pulmonary manifestations of HIV infection in children. Pediatr Pulmonol 1991;10:231-5.

21. Quinn TC. Acute primary HIV infection. JAMA 1997;278:58-62.

22. Niu MT, Stein DS, Schnittman SM. Primary human immunodeficiency virus type 1 infection: review of pathogenesis and early treatment intervention in humans and animal retrovirus infections. J Infect Dis 1993;168:1490-501.

23. Pedersen C, Lindhardt BO, Jensen BL, et al. Clinical course of primary HIV infection: consequences for subsequent course of infection. BMJ 1989;299:154-7.

24. Kelley CF, Barbour JD, Hecht FM. The relation between symptoms, viral load, and viral load set point in primary HIV infection. J Acquir Immune Defic Syndr 2007;45:445-8.

25. Reed JB, Hanson D, McNaghten AD, et al. HIV testing factors associated with delayed entry into HIV medical care among HIV-infected persons from eighteen states, United States, 2000-2004. AIDS Patient Care STDS. 2009;23:765-73.

26. Lubelchek R, Kroc K, Hota B, et al. The role of rapid vs conventional human immunodeficiency virus testing for inpatients: effects on quality of care. Arch Intern Med 2005;165:1956-60.

27. U.S. Food and Drug Administration. Complete List of Donor Screening Assays for Infectious Agents and HIV Diagnostic Assays. Available at https://www.fda.gov/vaccines-blood-biologics/complete-list-donor-screening-assays-infectious-agents-and-hiv-diagnostic-assays. Accessed August 1, 2018.

28. Kassler WJ, Dillon BA, Haley C, et al. On-site, rapid HIV testing with same-day results and counseling. AIDS 1997;11:1045-51.

29. Kendrick SR, Kroc KA, Withum D, et al. Outcomes of offering rapid point-of-care HIV testing in a sexually transmitted disease clinic. J Acquir Immune Defic Syndr 2005;38:142-6.

30. Myers JE, El-Sadr WM, Zerbe A, et al. Rapid HIV self-testing: long in coming but opportunities beckon. AIDS 2013;27:1687-95.

31. Panel on Antiretroviral Therapy and Medical Management of Children Living with HIV. Guidelines for the Use of Antiretroviral Agents in Pediatric HIV Infection. Available at https://aidsinfo.nih.gov/contentfiles/lvguidelines/pediatric-guidelines.pdf. Accessed August 1, 2018.

32. Dunn D, Woodburn P, Duong T, et al. Current CD4 cell count and the short-term risk of AIDS and death before the availability of effective antiretroviral therapy in HIV-infected children and adults. J Infect Dis 2008;197:398-404.

33. Abrams EJ, Weedon J, Steketee RW, et al. Association of human immunodeficiency virus (HIV) load early in life with disease progression among HIV-infected infants. New York City Perinatal HIV Transmission Collaborative Study Group. J Infect Dis 1998;178:101-8.

34. Shearer WT, Quinn TC, LaRussa P, et al. Viral load and disease progression in infants infected with human immunodeficiency virus type 1. Women and Infants Transmission Study Group. N Engl J Med 1997;336:1337-42.

35. Mofenson LM, Korelitz J, Meyer WA, et al. The relationship between serum human immunodeficiency virus type 1 (HIV-1) RNA level, CD4 lymphocyte percent, and long-term mortality risk in HIV-1-infected children. National Institute of Child Health and Human Development Intravenous Immunoglobulin Clinical Trial Study Group. J Infect Dis 1997;175:1029-38.

36. Palumbo PE, Raskino C, Fiscus S, et al. Predictive value of quantitative plasma HIV RNA and CD4+ lymphocyte count in HIV-infected infants and children. JAMA 1998;279:756-61.

37. Dunn D, Group HPPMCS. Short-term risk of disease progression in HIV-1-infected children receiving no antiretroviral therapy or zidovudine monotherapy: a meta-analysis. Lancet 2003;362:1605-11.

38. Hughes MD, Johnson VA, Hirsch MS, et al. Monitoring plasma HIV-1 RNA levels in addition to CD4+ lymphocyte count improves assessment of antiretroviral therapeutic response. ACTG 241 Protocol Virology Substudy Team. Ann Intern Med 1997;126:929-38.

39. Panel on Opportunistic Infections in HIV-Exposed and HIV-Infected Children. Guidelines for the Prevention and Treatment of Opportunistic Infections in HIV-Exposed and HIV-Infected Children. Department of Health and Human Services. Available at https://aidsinfo.nih.gov/contentfiles/lvguidelines/oi_guidelines_pediatrics.pdf. Section accessed August 1, 2018.

40. Chin DP, Hopewell PC, Yajko DM, et al. Mycobacterium avium complex in the respiratory or gastrointestinal tract and the risk of M. avium complex bacteremia in patients with human immunodeficiency virus infection. J Infect Dis 1994;169:289-95.

41. Hodge WG, Boivin JF, Shapiro SH, et al. Clinical risk factors for cytomegalovirus retinitis in patients with AIDS. Ophthalmology 2004;111:1326-33.

42. Panel on Opportunistic Infections in HIV-Infected Adults and Adolescents. Guidelines for the Prevention and Treatment of Opportunistic Infections in HIV-Infected Adults and Adolescents: Recommendations from the Centers for Disease Control and Prevention, the National Institutes of Health, and the HIV Medicine Association of the Infectious Diseases Society of America. Available at https://aidsinfo.nih.gov/contentfiles/lvguidelines/adult_oi.pdf. Accessed August 1, 2018.

43. Visser ME, Durao S, Sinclair D, et al. Micronutrient supplementation in adults with HIV infection. Cochrane Database Syst Rev 2017;12:CD003650.

44. McGrath N, Bellinger D, Robins J, et al. Effect of maternal multivitamin supplementation on the mental and psychomotor development of children who are born to HIV-1-infected mothers in Tanzania. Pediatrics 2006;117:e216-25.

45. Arpadi SM, McMahon D, Abrams EJ, et al. Effect of bimonthly supplementation with oral cholecalciferol on serum 25-hydroxyvitamin D concentrations in HIV-infected children and adolescents. Pediatrics 2009;123:e121-6.

46. Nance CL, Shearer WT. Is green tea good for HIV-1 infection? J Allergy Clin Immunol 2003;112:851-3.

47. Kawai K, Tsuno NH, Kitayama J, et al. Epigallocatechin gallate, the main component of tea polyphenol, binds to CD4 and interferes with gp120 binding. J Allergy Clin Immunol 2003;112:951-7.

48. Nance CL, Siwak EB, Shearer WT. Preclinical development of the green tea catechin, epigallocatechin gallate, as an HIV-1 therapy. J Allergy Clin Immunol 2009;123:459-65.

49. Williamson MP, McCormick TG, Nance CL, et al. Epigallocatechin gallate, the main polyphenol in green tea, binds to the T-cell receptor, CD4: Potential for HIV-1 therapy. J Allergy Clin Immunol 2006;118:1369-74.

50. Mills E, Montori V, Perri D, et al. Natural health product-HIV drug interactions: a systematic review. Int J STD AIDS 2005; 16:181-6.

51. World Health Organization (WHO). PMTCT Strategic Vision 2010–2015: Preventing Mother-to-Child Transmission of HIV to Reach the UNGASS and Millennium Development Goals. Available at www.who.int/hiv/pub/mtct/strategic_vision.pdf?ua=1. Accessed August 1, 2018.

52. Panel on Treatment of HIV-Infected Pregnant Women and Prevention of Perinatal Transmission. Recommendations for Use of Antiretroviral Drugs in Pregnant HIV-1-Infected Women for Maternal Health and Interventions to Reduce Perinatal HIV Transmission in the United States. Available at http://aidsinfo.nih.gov/contentfiles/lvguidelines/PerinatalGL.pdf. Accessed August 1, 2018.

53. Weller S, Davis K. Condom effectiveness in reducing heterosexual HIV transmission. Cochrane Database Syst Rev 2002; 1:CD003255.

54. Sullivan PS, Carballo-Diéguez A, Coates T, et al. Successes and challenges of HIV prevention in men who have sex with men. Lancet 2012;380:388-99.

55. Gray RH, Kigozi G, Serwadda D, et al. Male circumcision for HIV prevention in men in Rakai, Uganda: a randomised trial. Lancet 2007;369:657-66.

56. Auvert B, Taljaard D, Lagarde E, et al. Randomized, controlled intervention trial of male circumcision for reduction of HIV infection risk: the ANRS 1265 Trial. PLoS Med 2005;2:e298.

57. Bailey RC, Moses S, Parker CB, et al. Male circumcision for HIV prevention in young men in Kisumu, Kenya: a randomised controlled trial. Lancet 2007;369:643-56.

58. Gray RH, Kiwanuka N, Quinn TC, et al. Male circumcision and HIV acquisition and transmission: cohort studies in Rakai, Uganda. Rakai Project Team. AIDS 2000;14:2371-81.

59. HIV Vaccine Trials Network. Types of Vaccines. Available at www.hvtn.org/en/science/hiv-vaccine-basics/types-vaccines.html. Accessed August 1, 2018.

60. Buchbinder SP, Mehrotra DV, Duerr A, et al. Efficacy assessment of a cell-mediated immunity HIV-1 vaccine (the Step Study): a double-blind, randomised, placebo-controlled, test-of-concept trial. Lancet 2008;372:1881-93.

61. Flynn NM, Forthal DN, Harro CD, et al. Placebo-controlled phase 3 trial of a recombinant glycoprotein 120 vaccine to prevent HIV-1 infection. J Infect Dis 2005;191:654-65.

62. Hammer SM, Sobieszczyk ME, Janes H, et al. Efficacy trial of a DNA/rAd5 HIV-1 preventive vaccine. N Engl J Med 2013;369:2083-92.

63. Pitisuttithum P, Gilbert P, Gurwith M, et al; Bangkok Vaccine Evaluation Group. Randomized, double-blind, placebo-controlled efficacy trial of a bivalent recombinant glycoprotein 120 HIV-1 vaccine among injection drug users in Bangkok, Thailand. J Infect Dis 2006;194:1661-71.

64. Gray GE, Allen M, Moodie Z, et al; HVTN 503/Phambili study team. Safety and efficacy of the HVTN 503/Phambili study of a clade-B-based HIV-1 vaccine in South Africa: a double-blind, randomised, placebo-controlled test-of-concept phase 2b study. Lancet Infect Dis 2011;11:507–15.

65. Rerks-Ngarm S, Pitisuttithum P, Nitayaphan S, et al. Vaccination with ALVAC and AIDSVAX to prevent HIV-1 infection in Thailand. N Engl J Med 2009;361:2209-20.

66. Rerks-Ngarm S, Pitisuttithum P, Excler J, et al. Randomized, double-blind evaluation of late boost strategies for HIV-uninfected vaccine recipients in the RV144 HIV vaccine efficacy trial. J Infect Dis 2017;215:1255-63.

67. Abdool Karim Q, Abdool Karim SS, Frohlich JA, et al. Effectiveness and safety of tenofovir gel, an antiretroviral microbicide, for the prevention of HIV infection in women. Science 2010;329:1168-74.

68. Marrazzo JM, Ramjee G, Richardson BA, et al. Tenofovir-based preexposure prophylaxis for HIV infection among African women. N Engl J Med 2015;372:509-18.

69. Microbicide Trials Network (MTN). Rectal Microbicides Fact Sheet. Available at https://mtnstopshiv.org/news/rectal-microbicides-fact-sheet. Accessed August 1, 2018.

70. Grant RM, Lama JR, Anderson PL, et al. Preexposure chemoprophylaxis for HIV prevention in men who have sex with men. N Engl J Med 2010;363:2587-99.

71. Grohskopf LA, Chillag KL, Gvetadze R, et al. Randomized trial of clinical safety of daily oral tenofovir disoproxil fumarate among HIV-uninfected men who have sex with men in the United States. J Acquir Immune Defic Syndr 2013;64:79-86.

72. Baeten JM, Donnell D, Ndase P, et al. Antiretroviral prophylaxis for HIV prevention in heterosexual men and women. N Engl J Med 2012;367:399-410.

73. Thigpen MC, Kebaabetswe PM, Paxton LA, et al. Antiretroviral preexposure prophylaxis for heterosexual HIV transmission in Botswana. N Engl J Med 2012;367:423-34.

74. Choopanya K, Martin M, Suntharasamai P, et al. Antiretroviral prophylaxis for HIV infection in injecting drug users in Bangkok, Thailand (the Bangkok Tenofovir Study): a randomised, double-blind, placebo-controlled phase 3 trial. Lancet 2013;381:2083-90.

75. Hosek, SG, Landovitz RJ, Kapogiannis B, et al. Safety and feasibility of antiretroviral preexposure prophylaxis for adolescent men who have sex with men aged 15 to 17 years in the United States. JAMA Pediatr. 2017;171:1063-71.

76. Truvada [package insert] Foster City, CA: Gilead; 2018.

77. Centers for Disease Control and Prevention. US Public Health Service: Preexposure Prophylaxis for the Prevention of HIV Infection in the United States—2017 Update: A Clinical Practice Guideline. Available at https://www.cdc.gov/hiv/pdf/risk/prep/cdc-hiv-prep-guidelines-2017.pdf. Accessed August 1, 2018.

78. Panel on Antiretroviral Guidelines for Adults and Adolescents. Guidelines for the Use of Antiretroviral Agents in Adults and Adolescents Living with HIV. Department of Health and Human Services. Available at https://aidsinfo.nih.gov/contentfiles/lvguidelines/AdultandAdolescentGL.pdf. Accessed August 1, 2018.

79. Cohen MS, Chen YQ, McCauley M, et al. Prevention of HIV-1 infection with early antiretroviral therapy. N Engl J Med 2011;365:493-505.

80. Lundgren JD, Babiker AG, Gordin F, et al. Initiation of antiretroviral therapy in early asymptomatic HIV infection. N Engl J Med 2015;373:795-807.

81. Lifson AR, Grund B, Gardner EM, et al. Improved quality of life with immediate versus deferred initiation of antiretroviral therapy in early asymptomatic HIV infection. AIDS 2017;31:953-63.

82. Lodi S, Sharma S, Lundgren JD, et al. The per-protocol effect of immediate versus deferred antiretroviral therapy initiation. AIDS 2016;30:2659-63.

83. Abrams EJ, Wiener J, Carter R, et al. Maternal health factors and early pediatric antiretroviral therapy influence the rate of perinatal HIV-1 disease progression in children. AIDS 2003; 17:867-77.

84. Goetghebuer T, Haelterman E, Le Chenadec J, et al. Effect of early antiretroviral therapy on the risk of AIDS/death in HIV-infected infants. AIDS 2009;23:597-604.

85. Newell ML, Patel D, Goetghebuer T, et al. CD4 cell response to antiretroviral therapy in children with vertically acquired HIV infection: is it associated with age at initiation? J Infect Dis 2006;193:954-62.

86. Boyd K, Dunn DT, Castro H, et al. Discordance between CD4 cell count and CD4 cell percentage: implications for when to start antiretroviral therapy in HIV-1 infected children. AIDS 2010; 24:1213-1217.

87. Puthanakit T, Saphonn V, Ananworanich J, et al. Early versus deferred antiretroviral therapy for children older than 1 year infected with HIV (PREDICT): a multicentre, randomised, open-label trial. Lancet Infect Dis 2012;12:933-41.

88. Yin DE, Warshaw MG, Miller WC, et al. Using CD4 percentage and age to optimize pediatric antiretroviral therapy initiation. Pediatrics 2014;134:e1104-16.

89. Palumbo P, Violari A, Lindsey J, et al. Nevirapine (NVP) vs lopinavir-ritonavir (LPV/r)-based antiretroviral therapy (ART) in single dose nevirapine (sdNVP)-exposed HIV-infected infants: preliminary results from the IMPAACT P1060 trial. Presented at: 5th International AIDS Society (IAS) Conference on HIV Pathogenesis, Treatment and Prevention; July 19-22, 2009; Cape Town, South Africa.

90. Cane P, Chrystie I, Dunn D, et al. Time trends in primary resistance to HIV drugs in the United Kingdom: multicentre observational study. BMJ 2005;331:1368.

91. Novak RM, Chen L, MacArthur RD, et al. Prevalence of antiretroviral drug resistance mutations in chronically HIV-infected, treatment-naive patients: implications for routine resistance screening before initiation of antiretroviral therapy. Clin Infect Dis 2005;40:468-74.

92. Viani RM, Peralta L, Aldrovandi G, et al. Prevalence of primary HIV-1 drug resistance among recently infected adolescents: a multicenter adolescent medicine trials network for HIV/AIDS interventions study. J Infect Dis 2006;194:1505-09.

93. Weinstock HS, Zaidi I, Heneine W, et al. The epidemiology of antiretroviral drug resistance among drug-naive HIV-1-infected persons in 10 US cities. J Infect Dis 2004;189:2174-80.

94. Babiker A, Castro nee Green H, Compagnucci A, et al. First-line antiretroviral therapy with a protease inhibitor versus non-nucleoside reverse transcriptase inhibitor and switch at higher versus low viral load in HIV-infected children: an open-label, randomised phase 2/3 trial. Lancet Infect Dis 2011;11:273-83.

95. Ruel TD, Kakuru A, Ikilezi G, et al. Virologic and immunologic outcomes of HIV-infected Ugandan children randomized to lopinavir/ritonavir or nonnucleoside reverse transcriptase inhibitor therapy. J Acquir Immune Defic Syndr 2014;65:535-41.

96. Violari A, Lindsey JC, Hughes MD, et al. Nevirapine versus ritonavir-boosted lopinavir for HIV-infected children. N Engl J Med 2012;366:2380-9.

97. Molina JM, Clotet B, van Lunzen J, et al. Once-daily dolutegravir is superior to once-daily darunavir/ritonavir in treatment-naive HIV-1-positive individuals: 96 week results from FLAMINGO. J Int AIDS Soc 2014;17:19490.

98. Raffi F, Jaeger H, Quiros-Roldan E, et al. Once-daily dolutegravir versus twice-daily raltegravir in antiretroviral-naive adults with HIV-1 infection (SPRING-2 study): 96 week results from a randomised, double-blind, non-inferiority trial. Lancet Infect Dis 2013;13:927-35.

99. Viani RM, Alvero C, Fenton T, et al. Safety, Pharmacokinetics and efficacy of dolutegravir in treatment-experienced HIV-1 infected adolescents: forty-eight-week results from IMPAACT P1093. Pediatr Infect Dis J 2015;34:1207-13.

100. Walmsley S, Baumgarten A, Berenguer J, et al. Brief report: dolutegravir plus abacavir/lamivudine for the treatment of HIV-1 Infection in antiretroviral therapy-naive patients: week 96 and week 144 results from the SINGLE randomized clinical trial. J Acquir Immune Defic Syndr 2015;70:515-9.

101. Wiznia A, Alvero C, Fenton T, et al. IMPAACT 1093: Dolutegravir in 6- to 12-year-old HIV-infected children: 48-week results. Presented at: 23rd Conference on Retroviruses and Opportunistic Infections; February 22-25; Boston, MA.

102. Viani RM, Alvero A, Fenton T, et al. Safety, pharmacokinetics, and efficacy of dolutegravir in treatment-experienced HIV+ children. Presented at: 21st Conference on Retroviruses and Opportunistic Infections; March 3-6, 2014; Boston, MA.

103. Clotet B, Feinberg J, van Lunzen J, et al. Once-daily dolutegravir versus darunavir plus ritonavir in antiretroviral-naive adults with HIV-1 infection (FLAMINGO): 48 week results from the randomised open-label phase 3b study. Lancet 2014;383:2222-31.

104. Gaur AH, Kizito H, Prasitsueubsai W, et al. Safety, efficacy, and pharmacokinetics of a single-tablet regimen containing elvitegravir, cobicistat, emtricitabine, and tenofovir alafenamide in treatment-naive, HIV-infected adolescents: a single-arm, open-label trial. Lancet HIV 2016;3:e561-8.

105. Clumeck N, Molina JM, Henry K, et al. A randomized, double-blind comparison of single-tablet regimen elvitegravir/cobicistat/emtricitabine/tenofovir DF vs ritonavir-boosted atazanavir plus emtricitabine/tenofovir DF for initial treatment of HIV-1 infection: analysis of week 144 results. J Acquir Immune Defic Syndr 2014;65:e121-4.

106. Sax PE, Wohl D, Yin MT, et al. Tenofovir alafenamide versus tenofovir disoproxil fumarate, coformulated with elvitegravir, cobicistat, and emtricitabine, for initial treatment of HIV-1 infection: two randomised, double-blind, phase 3, non-inferiority trials. Lancet 2015; 385:2606-15.

107. Wohl DA, Cohen C, Gallant JE, et al. A randomized, double-blind comparison of single-tablet regimen elvitegravir/cobicistat/emtricitabine/tenofovir DF versus single-tablet regimen efavirenz/emtricitabine/tenofovir DF for initial treatment of HIV-1 infection: analysis of week 144 results. J Acquir Immune Defic Syndr 2014;65:e118-20.

108. Lennox JL, DeJesus E, Lazzarin A, et al. Safety and efficacy of raltegravir-based versus efavirenz-based combination therapy in treatment-naive patients with HIV-1 infection: a multicentre, double-blind randomised controlled trial. Lancet 2009;374:796-806.

109. Lennox JL, Landovitz RJ, Ribaudo HJ, et al. Efficacy and tolerability of 3 nonnucleoside reverse transcriptase inhibitor-sparing antiretroviral regimens for treatment-naive volunteers infected with HIV-1: a randomized, controlled equivalence trial. Ann Intern Med 2014;161:461-71.

110. Rockstroh JK, DeJesus E, Lennox JL, et al. Durable efficacy and safety of raltegravir versus efavirenz when combined with tenofovir/emtricitabine in treatment-naive HIV-1-infected patients: final 5-year results from STARTMRK. J Acquir Immune Defic Syndr 2013;63:77-85.

111. Briz V, Leon-Leal JA, Palladino C, et al. Potent and sustained antiviral response of raltegravir-based highly active antiretroviral therapy in HIV type 1-infected children and adolescents. Pediatr Infect Dis J 2012;31:273-7.

112. Nachman S, Alvero C, Acosta EP, et al. Pharmacokinetics and 48-week safety and efficacy of raltegravir for oral suspension in human immunodeficiency virus type-1-infected children 4 weeks to 2 years of age. J Pediatric Infect Dis Soc 2015;4:e76-83.

113. Nachman S, Zheng N, Acosta EP, et al. Pharmacokinetics, safety, and 48-week efficacy of oral raltegravir in HIV-1-infected children aged 2 through 18 years. Clin Infect Dis 2014;58:413-22.

114. Cohen CJ, Molina JM, Cahn P, et al. Efficacy and safety of rilpivirine (TMC278) versus efavirenz at 48 weeks in treatment-naive HIV-1-infected patients: pooled results from the phase 3 double-blind randomized ECHO and THRIVE Trials. J Acquir Immune Defic Syndr 2012;60:33-42.

115. Cooper DA, Heera J, Goodrich J, et al. Maraviroc versus efavirenz, both in combination with zidovudine-lamivudine, for the treatment of antiretroviral-naive subjects with CCR5-tropic HIV-1 infection. J Infect Dis 2010;201:803-13.

116. Fraaij PL, Neubert J, Bergshoeff AS, et al. Safety and efficacy of a NRTI-sparing HAART regimen of efavirenz and lopinavir/ritonavir in HIV-1-infected children. Antivir Ther 2004;9:297-9.

117. Funk MB, Notheis G, Schuster T, et al. Effect of first line therapy including efavirenz and two nucleoside reverse transcriptase inhibitors in HIV-infected children. Eur J Med Res 2005;10:503-8.

118. McKinney RE, Jr., Rodman J, Hu C, et al. Long-term safety and efficacy of a once-daily regimen of emtricitabine, didanosine, and efavirenz in HIV-infected, therapy-naive children and adolescents: Pediatric AIDS Clinical Trials Group Protocol P1021. Pediatrics 2007;120:e416-23.

119. Nunez M, Soriano V, Martin-Carbonero L, et al. SENC (Spanish efavirenz vs. nevirapine comparison) trial: a randomized, open-label study in HIV-infected naive individuals. HIV Clin Trials 2002;3:186-94.

120. Riddler SA, Haubrich R, DiRienzo AG, et al. Class-sparing regimens for initial treatment of HIV-1 infection. N Engl J Med 2008;358:2095-106.

121. Sax PE, DeJesus E, Mills A, et al. Co-formulated elvitegravir, cobicistat, emtricitabine, and tenofovir versus co-formulated efavirenz, emtricitabine, and tenofovir for initial treatment of HIV-1 infection: a randomised, double-blind, phase 3 trial, analysis of results after 48 weeks. Lancet 2012;379:2439-48.

122. Spector SA, Hsia K, Yong FH, et al. Patterns of plasma human immunodeficiency virus type 1 RNA response to highly active antiretroviral therapy in infected children. J Infect Dis 2000;182:1769-73.

123. Squires K, Lazzarin A, Gatell JM, et al. Comparison of once-daily atazanavir with efavirenz, each in combination with fixed-dose zidovudine and lamivudine, as initial therapy for patients infected with HIV. J Acquir Immune Defic Syndr 2004;36:1011-9.

124. Starr SE, Fletcher CV, Spector SA, et al. Efavirenz liquid formulation in human immunodeficiency virus-infected children. Pediatr Infect Dis J 2002;21:659-63.

125. Starr SE, Fletcher CV, Spector SA, et al. Combination therapy with efavirenz, nelfinavir, and nucleoside reverse-transcriptase inhibitors in children infected with human immunodeficiency virus type 1. Pediatric AIDS Clinical Trials Group 382 Team. N Engl J Med 1999; 341:1874-81.

126. Teglas JP, Quartier P, Treluyer JM, et al. Tolerance of efavirenz in children. AIDS 2001;15:241-3.

127. Torti C, Maggiolo F, Patroni A, et al. Exploratory analysis for the evaluation of lopinavir/ritonavir-versus efavirenz-based HAART regimens in antiretroviral-naive HIV-positive patients: results from the Italian MASTER Cohort. J Antimicrob Chemother 2005;56:190-5.

128. Kamya MR, Mayanja-Kizza H, Kambugu A, et al. Predictors of long-term viral failure among Ugandan children and adults treated with antiretroviral therapy. J Acquir Immune Defic Syndr 2007;46:187-93.

129. Bardsley-Elliot A, Perry CM. Nevirapine: a review of its use in the prevention and treatment of paediatric HIV infection. Paediatr Drugs 2000;2:373-407.

130. Luzuriaga K, Bryson Y, Krogstad P, et al. Combination treatment with zidovudine, didanosine, and nevirapine in infants with human immunodeficiency virus type 1 infection. N Engl J Med 1997;336:1343-9.

131. Luzuriaga K, McManus M, Mofenson L, et al. A trial of three antiretroviral regimens in HIV-1-infected children. N Engl J Med 2004;350:2471-80.

132. Palumbo P, Lindsey JC, Hughes MD, et al. Antiretroviral treatment for children with peripartum nevirapine exposure. N Engl J Med 2010;363:1510-20.

133. Verweel G, Sharland M, Lyall H, et al. Nevirapine use in HIV-1-infected children. AIDS 2003;17:1639-47.

134. Cohen CJ, Andrade-Villanueva J, Clotet B, et al. Rilpivirine versus efavirenz with two background nucleoside or nucleotide reverse transcriptase inhibitors in treatment-naive adults infected with HIV-1 (THRIVE): a phase 3, randomised, non-inferiority trial. Lancet 2011;378:229-37.

135. Cohen CJ, Molina JM, Cassetti I, et al. Week 96 efficacy and safety of rilpivirine in treatment-naive, HIV-1 patients in two phase III randomized trials. AIDS 2013;27:939-50.

136. Lombaard J, Bunupuradah T, Flynn PM, et al. Rilpivirine as a treatment for HIV-infected antiretroviral-naive adolescents: week 48 safety, efficacy, virology and pharmacokinetics. Pediatr Infect Dis J 2016;35:1215-21.

137. Molina JM, Cahn P, Grinsztejn B, et al. Rilpivirine versus efavirenz with tenofovir and emtricitabine in treatment-naive adults infected with HIV-1 (ECHO): a phase 3 randomised double-blind active-controlled trial. Lancet 2011;378:238-46.

138. Crutchley RD, Guduru RC, Cheng AM. Evaluating the role of atazanavir/cobicistat and darunavir/cobicistat fixed-dose combinations for the treatment of HIV-1 infection. HIV/AIDS (Auckl) 2016;8:47-65.

139. Kiser JJ, Fletcher CV, Flynn PM, et al. Pharmacokinetics of antiretroviral regimens containing tenofovir disoproxil fumarate and atazanavir-ritonavir in adolescents and young adults with human immunodeficiency virus infection. Antimicrob Agents Chemother 2008;52:631-7.

140. Kiser JJ, Rutstein RM, Samson P, et al. Atazanavir and atazanavir/ritonavir pharmacokinetics in HIV-infected infants, children, and adolescents. AIDS 2011;25:1489-96.

141. Malan DR, Krantz E, David N, et al. Efficacy and safety of atazanavir, with or without ritonavir, as part of once-daily highly active antiretroviral therapy regimens in antiretroviral-naive patients. J Acquir Immune Defic Syndr 2008;47:161-7.

142. Molina JM, Andrade-Villanueva J, Echevarria J, et al. Once-daily atazanavir/ritonavir versus twice-daily lopinavir/ritonavir, each in combination with tenofovir and emtricitabine, for management of antiretroviral-naive HIV-1-infected patients: 48 week efficacy and safety results of the CASTLE study. Lancet 2008;372:646-55.

143. Molina JM, Andrade-Villanueva J, Echevarria J, et al. Once-daily atazanavir/ritonavir compared with twice-daily lopinavir/ritonavir, each in combination with tenofovir and emtricitabine, for management of antiretroviral-naive HIV-1-infected patients: 96-week efficacy and safety results of the CASTLE study. J Acquir Immune Defic Syndr 2010;53:323-32.

144. Rutstein RM, Samson P, Fenton T, et al. Long-term safety and efficacy of atazanavir-based therapy in HIV-infected infants, children and adolescents: the Pediatric AIDS Clinical Trials Group Protocol 1020A. Pediatr Infect Dis J 2015;34:162-7.

145. Strehlau R, Donati AP, Arce PM, et al. PRINCE-1: safety and efficacy of atazanavir powder and ritonavir liquid in HIV-1-infected antiretroviral-naive and -experienced infants and children aged ≥3 months to <6 years. J Int AIDS Soc 2015;189467.

146. Blanche S, Bologna R, Cahn P, et al. Pharmacokinetics, safety and efficacy of darunavir/ritonavir in treatment-experienced children and adolescents. AIDS 2009;23:2005-13.

147. Flynn P, Komar S, Blanche S, et al. Efficacy and safety of darunavir/ritonavir at 48 weeks in treatment-naive, HIV-1-infected adolescents: results from a phase 2 open-label trial (DIONE). Pediatri Infect Dis J 2014;33:940-5.

148. Mills AM, Nelson M, Jayaweera D, et al. Once-daily daruna-vir/ritonavir vs. lopinavir/ritonavir in treatment-naive, HIV-1-infected patients: 96-week analysis. AIDS 2009;23:1679-88.

149. Ortiz R, Dejesus E, Khanlou H, et al. Efficacy and safety of once-daily darunavir/ritonavir versus lopinavir/ritonavir in treatment-naive HIV-1-infected patients at week 48. AIDS 2008;22:1389-97.

150. Violari A, Bologna R, Kumarasamy N, et al. Safety and efficacy of darunavir/ritonavir in treatment-experienced pediatric patients: week 48 results of the ARIEL trial. Pediatr Infect Dis J 2015;34:e132-7.

151. Chadwick EG, Capparelli EV, Yogev R, et al. Pharmacokinetics, safety and efficacy of lopinavir/ritonavir in infants less than 6 months of age: 24 week results. AIDS 2008;22:249-55.

152. Chadwick EG, Yogev R, Alvero CG, et al. Long-term outcomes for HIV-infected infants less than 6 months of age at initiation of lopinavir/ritonavir combination antiretroviral therapy. AIDS 2011;25:643-9.

153. De Luca M, Miccinesi G, Chiappini E, et al. Different kinetics of immunologic recovery using nelfinavir or lopinavir/ritonavir-based regimens in children with perinatal HIV-1 infection. Int J Immunopathol Pharmacol 2005;18:729-35.

154. Eron J, Jr., Yeni P, Gathe J, Jr., et al. The KLEAN study of fos-amprenavir-ritonavir versus lopinavir-ritonavir, each in combination with abacavir-lamivudine, for initial treatment of HIV infection over 48 weeks: a randomised non-inferiority trial. Lancet 2006;368:476-82.

155. Orkin C, DeJesus E, Khanlou H, et al. Final 192-week efficacy and safety of once-daily darunavir/ritonavir compared with lopinavir/ritonavir in HIV-1-infected treatment-naive patients in the ARTEMIS trial. HIV Med 2013;14:49-59.

156. Pulido F, Estrada V, Baril JG, et al. Long-term efficacy and safety of fosamprenavir plus ritonavir versus lopinavir/ritonavir in combination with abacavir/lamivudine over 144 weeks. HIV Clin Trials 2009;10:76-87.

157. Reitz C, Coovadia A, Ko S, et al. Initial response to protease-inhibitor-based antiretroviral therapy among children less than 2 years of age in South Africa: effect of cotreatment for tuberculosis. J Infect Dis 2010;201:1121-31.

158. Robbins BL, Capparelli EV, Chadwick EG, et al. Pharmacokinetics of high-dose lopinavir-ritonavir with and without saquinavir or nonnucleoside reverse transcriptase inhibitors in human immunodeficiency virus-infected pediatric and adolescent patients previously treated with protease inhibitors. Antimicrob Agents Chemother 2008;52:3276-83.

159. Saez-Llorens X, Violari A, Deetz CO, et al. Forty-eight-week evaluation of lopinavir/ritonavir, a new protease inhibitor, in human immunodeficiency virus-infected children. Pediatr Infect Dis J 2003;22:216-24.

160. Violari A, Cotton MF, Gibb DM, et al. Early antiretroviral therapy and mortality among HIV-infected infants. N Engl J Med 2008;359:2233-44.

161. Walmsley S, Avihingsanon A, Slim J, et al. Gemini: a noninferiority study of saquinavir/ritonavir versus lopinavir/ritonavir as initial HIV-1 therapy in adults. J Acquir Immune Defic Syndr 2009;50:367-74.

162. Walmsley S, Bernstein B, King M, et al. Lopinavir-ritonavir versus nelfinavir for the initial treatment of HIV infection. N Engl J Med 2002;346:2039-46.

163. Fortuny C, Duiculescu D, Cheng K, et al. Pharmacokinetics and 48-week safety and antiviral activity of fosamprenavir-containing regimens in HIV-infected 2- to 18-year-old children. Pediatr Infect Dis J 2014;33:50-6.

164. Scherpbier HJ, Bekker V, van Leth F, et al. Long-term experience with combination antiretroviral therapy that contains nelfinavir for up to 7 years in a pediatric cohort. Pediatrics 2006;117:e528-36.

165. Fraaij PL, Verweel G, van Rossum AM, et al. Indinavir/low-dose ritonavir containing HAART in HIV-1 infected children has potent antiretroviral activity, but is associated with side effects and frequent discontinuation of treatment. Infection 2007;35:186-9.

166. Jankelevich S, Mueller BU, Mackall CL, et al. Long-term virologic and immunologic responses in human immunodeficiency virus type 1-infected children treated with indinavir, zidovudine, and lamivudine. J Infect Dis 2001;183:1116-20.

167. van Rossum AM, Dieleman JP, Fraaij PL, et al. Persistent sterile leukocyturia is associated with impaired renal function in human immunodeficiency virus type 1-infected children treated with indinavir. Pediatrics 2002;110:e19.

168. van Rossum AM, Geelen SP, Hartwig NG, et al. Results of 2 years of treatment with protease-inhibitor–containing antiretroviral therapy in Dutch children infected with human immunodeficiency virus type 1. Clin Infect Dis 2002;34:1008-16.

169. Carr A, Workman C, Smith DE, et al. Abacavir substitution for nucleoside analogs in patients with HIV lipoatrophy: a randomized trial. JAMA 2002;288:207-15.

170. Moyle GJ, Sabin CA, Cartledge J, et al. A randomized comparative trial of tenofovir DF or abacavir as replacement for a thymidine analogue in persons with lipoatrophy. AIDS 2006;20:2043-50.

171. Mulenga V, Musiime V, Kekitiinwa A, et al. Abacavir, zidovudine, or stavudine as paediatric tablets for African HIV-infected children (CHAPAS-3): an open-label, parallel-group, randomised controlled trial. Lancet Infect Dis 2016;16:169-79.

172. Van Dyke RB, Wang L, Williams PL. Toxicities associated with dual nucleoside reverse-transcriptase inhibitor regimens in HIV-infected children. J Infect Dis 2008;198:1599-608.

173. DeJesus E, Rockstroh JK, Lennox JL, et al. Efficacy of raltegravir versus efavirenz when combined with tenofovir/emtricitabine in treatment-naive HIV-1-infected patients: week-192 overall and subgroup analyses from STARTMRK. HIV Clin Trials 2012;13:228-32.

174. Green H, Gibb DM, Walker AS, et al. Lamivudine/abacavir maintains virological superiority over zidovudine/lamivudine and zidovudine/abacavir beyond 5 years in children. AIDS 2007;21:947-55.

175. Post FA, Moyle GJ, Stellbrink HJ, et al. Randomized comparison of renal effects, efficacy, and safety with once-daily abacavir/lamivudine versus tenofovir/emtricitabine, administered with efavirenz, in antiretroviral-naive, HIV-1-infected adults: 48-week results from the ASSERT study. J Acquir Immune Defic Syndr 2010;55:49-57.

176. Sax PE, Tierney C, Collier AC, et al. Abacavir-lamivudine versus tenofovir-emtricitabine for initial HIV-1 therapy. N Engl J Med 2009;361:2230-40.

177. Smith KY, Patel P, Fine D, et al. Randomized, double-blind, placebo-matched, multicenter trial of abacavir/lamivudine or tenofovir/emtricitabine with lopinavir/ritonavir for initial HIV treatment. AIDS 2009;23:1547-56.

178. Technau KG, Lazarus E, Kuhn L, et al. Poor early virologic performance and durability of abacavir-based first-line regimens for HIV-infected children. Pediatr Infect Dis J 2013;32:851-5.

179. Technau KG, Schomaker M, Kuhn L, et al. Virologic response in children treated with abacavir-compared with stavudine-based antiretroviral treatment: a South African multi-cohort analysis. Pediatr Infect Dis J 2014;33:617-22.

180. Mallal S, Phillips E, Carosi G, et al. HLA-B*5701 screening for hypersensitivity to abacavir. N Engl J Med 2008;358:568-79.

181. Gaur A, Natukunda E, Kosalaraksa P, et al. Pharmacokinetics, safety & efficacy of E/C/F/TAF in HIV-infected children (6-12 yrs). Presented at: Conference on Retroviruses and Opportunistic Infections; February 13–16, 2017; Seattle, WA.

182. Andiman WA, Chernoff MC, Mitchell C, et al. Incidence of persistent renal dysfunction in human immunodeficiency virus-infected children: associations with the use of antiretrovirals, and other nephrotoxic medications and risk factors. Pediatr Infect Dis J 2009;28:619-25.

183. Arribas JR, Pozniak AL, Gallant JE, et al. Tenofovir disoproxil fumarate, emtricitabine, and efavirenz compared with zidovudine/lamivudine and efavirenz in treatment-naive patients: 144-week analysis. J Acquir Immune Defic Syndr 2008;47:74-8.

184. Gafni RI, Hazra R, Reynolds JC, et al. Tenofovir disoproxil fumarate and an optimized background regimen of antiretroviral agents as salvage therapy: impact on bone mineral density in HIV-infected children. Pediatrics 2006;118:e711-8.

185. Gallant JE, DeJesus E, Arribas JR, et al. Tenofovir DF, emtricitabine, and efavirenz vs. idovudine, lamivudine, and efavirenz for HIV. N Engl J Med 2006;354:251-60.

186. Giacomet V, Mora S, Martelli L, et al. A 12-month treatment with tenofovir does not impair bone mineral accrual in HIV-infected children. J Acquir Immune Defic Syndr 2005;40:448-50.

187. Hazra R, Balis FM, Tullio AN, et al. Single-dose and steady-state pharmacokinetics of tenofovir disoproxil fumarate in human immunodeficiency virus-infected children. Antimicrob Agents Chemother 2004;48:124-9.

188. Hazra R, Gafni RI, Maldarelli F, et al. Tenofovir disoproxil fumarate and an optimized background regimen of antiretroviral agents as salvage therapy for pediatric HIV infection. Pediatrics 2005;116:e846-54.

189. Papaleo A, Warszawski J, Salomon R, et al. Increased beta-2 microglobulinuria in human immunodeficiency virus-1-infected children and adolescents treated with tenofovir. Pediatr Infect Dis J 2007;26:949-51.

190. Pontrelli G, Cotugno N, Amodio D, et al. Renal function in HIV-infected children and adolescents treated with tenofovir disoproxil fumarate and protease inhibitors. BMC Infect Dis 2012; 12-8.

191. Riordan A, Judd A, Boyd K, et al. Tenofovir use in human immunodeficiency virus-1-infected children in the United Kingdom and Ireland. Pediatr Infect Dis J 2009;28:204-9.

192. Gallant JE, Staszewski S, Pozniak AL, et al. Efficacy and safety of tenofovir DF vs stavudine in combination therapy in antiretroviral-naive patients: a 3-year randomized trial. JAMA 2004;292:191-201.

193. Vigano A, Bedogni G, Manfredini V, et al. Long-term renal safety of tenofovir disoproxil fumarate in vertically HIV-infected children, adolescents and young adults: a 60-month follow-up study. Clin Drug Investig 2011;31:407-15.

194. Paediatric European Network for Treatment of AIDS (PENTA). Comparison of dual nucleoside-analogue reverse-transcriptase inhibitor regimens with and without nelfinavir in children with HIV-1 who have not previously been treated: the PENTA 5 randomised trial. Lancet 2002;359:733-40.

195. Dieterich DT. Long-term complications of nucleoside reverse transcriptase inhibitor therapy. AIDS Read 2003;13:176-184.

196. Falco V, Rodriguez D, Ribera E, et al. Severe nucleoside-associated lactic acidosis in human immunodeficiency virus-infected patients: report of 12 cases and review of the literature. Clin Infect Dis 2002 34:838-46.

197. Joly V, Flandre P, Meiffredy V, et al. Increased risk of lipoatrophy under stavudine in HIV-1-infected patients: results of a substudy from a comparative trial. AIDS 2002;16:2447-54.

198. Blanco F, Garcia-Benayas T, Jose de la Cruz J, et al. First-line therapy and mitochondrial damage: different nucleosides, different findings. HIV Clin Trials 2003;4:11-9.

199. Shafer RW, Smeaton LM, Robbins GK, et al. Comparison of four-drug regimens and pairs of sequential three-drug regimens as initial therapy for HIV-1 infection. N Engl J Med 2003;349:2304-15.

200. Campbell TB, Shulman NS, Johnson SC, et al. Antiviral activity of lamivudine in salvage therapy for multidrug-resistant HIV-1 infection. Clin Infect Dis 2005;41:236-42.

201. Nijhuis M, Schuurman R, de Jong D, et al. Lamivudine-resistant human immunodeficiency virus type 1 variants (184V) require multiple amino acid changes to become co-resistant to zidovudine in vivo. J Infect Dis 1997;176:398-405.

202. Ross L, Parkin N, Chappey C, et al. Phenotypic impact of HIV reverse transcriptase M184I/V mutations in combination with single thymidine analog mutations on nucleoside reverse transcriptase inhibitor resistance. AIDS 2004;18:1691-6.

203. Ananworanich J, Kosalaraksa P, Hill A, et al. Pharmacokinetics and 24-week efficacy/safety of dual boosted saquinavir/lopinavir/ritonavir in nucleoside-pretreated children. Pediatr Infect Dis J 2005;24:874-9.

204. Kosalaraksa P, Bunupuradah T, Engchanil C, et al. Double boosted protease inhibitors, saquinavir, and lopinavir/ritonavir, in nucleoside pretreated children at 48 weeks. Pediatr Infect Dis J 2008;27:623-8.

205. Ribera E, Azuaje C, Lopez RM, et al. Atazanavir and lopinavir/ritonavir: pharmacokinetics, safety and efficacy of a promising double-boosted protease inhibitor regimen. AIDS 2006;20:1131-9.

206. Stephan C, von Hentig N, Kourbeti I, et al. Saquinavir drug exposure is not impaired by the boosted double protease inhibitor combination of lopinavir/ritonavir. AIDS 2004;18:503-8.

207. van der Lugt J, Autar RS, Ubolyam S, et al. Pharmacokinetics and short-term efficacy of a double-boosted protease inhibitor regimen in treatment-naive HIV-1-infected adults. J Antimicrob Chemother 2008;61:1145-53.

208. Fletcher CV, Brundage RC, Fenton T, et al. Pharmacokinetics and pharmacodynamics of efavirenz and nelfinavir in HIV-infected children participating in an area-under-the-curve controlled trial. Clin Pharmacol Ther 2008;83:300-6.

209. Committee on Pediatric AIDS. Transitioning HIV-infected youth into adult health care. Pediatrics 2013;132:192-7.

210. Lactic Acidosis International Study Group. Risk factors for lactic acidosis and severe hyperlactataemia in HIV-1-infected adults exposed to antiretroviral therapy. AIDS 2007;21:2455-64.

211. Baylor MS, Johann-Liang R. Hepatotoxicity associated with nevirapine use. J Acquir Immune Defic Syndr 2004;35:538-9.

212. Brown TT, Qaqish RB. Response to Berg et al. Antiretroviral therapy and the prevalence of osteopenia and osteoporosis: a meta-analytic review. AIDS 2007;21:1830-1.

213. Dieterich DT, Robinson PA, Love J, et al. Drug-induced liver injury associated with the use of nonnucleoside reverse-transcriptase inhibitors. Clin Infect Dis 2004;38 Suppl 2:S80-9.

214. Galli M, Veglia F, Angarano G, et al. Gender differences in antiretroviral drug-related adipose tissue alterations. Women are at higher risk than men and develop particular lipodystrophy patterns. J Acquir Immune Defic Syndr 2003;34:58-61.

215. Leith J, Piliero P, Storfer S, et al. Appropriate use of nevirapine for long-term therapy. J Infect Dis 2005;192:545-6.

216. Thiébaut R, Dequae-Merchadou L, Ekouevi DK, et al. Incidence and risk factors of severe hypertriglyceridaemia in the era of highly active antiretroviral therapy: the Aquitaine Cohort, France, 1996-99. HIV Med 2001;2:84-8.

217. Wit FW, Kesselring AM, Gras L, et al. Discontinuation of nevirapine because of hypersensitivity reactions in patients with prior treatment experience, compared with treatment-naive patients: the ATHENA cohort study. Clin Infect Dis 2008;46:933-40.

218. Yin M, Dobkin J, Brudney K, et al. Bone mass and mineral metabolism in HIV+ postmenopausal women. Osteoporos Int 2005;16:1345-52.

219. Kourtis AP, Mirza A. Contraception for HIV-infected adolescents. Pediatrics 2016;138:e20161892.

220. Thurman AR, Anderson S, Doncel GF. Effects of hormonal contraception on antiretroviral drug metabolism, pharmacokinetics and pharmacodynamics. Am J Reprod Immunol 2014;71:523-30.

221. Curtis KM, Nanda K, Kapp N. Safety of hormonal and intrauterine methods of contraception for women with HIV/AIDS: a systematic review. AIDS 2009;23 Suppl 1:S55-67.

222. Watts DH, Park JG, Cohn SE, et al. Safety and tolerability of depot medroxyprogesterone acetate among HIV-infected women on antiretroviral therapy: ACTG A5093. Contraception 2008;77:84-90.

223. Robinson JA, Jamshidi R, Burke AE. Contraception for the HIV-positive woman: a review of interactions between hormonal contraception and antiretroviral therapy. Infect Dis Obstet Gynecol 2012;2012:890160.

224. Stringer EM, Kaseba C, Levy J, et al. A randomized trial of the intrauterine contraceptive device vs hormonal contraception in women who are infected with the human immunodeficiency virus. Am J Obstet Gynecol 2007;197:144 e141-8.

225. Chang MH, Sung JL, Lee CY, et al. Factors affecting clearance of hepatitis B e antigen in hepatitis B surface antigen carrier children. J Pediatr 1989;115:385-90.

226. Chu CM, Karayiannis P, Fowler MJ, et al. Natural history of chronic hepatitis B virus infection in Taiwan: studies of hepatitis B virus DNA in serum. Hepatology 1985;5:431-4.

227. Elisofon SA, Jonas MM. Hepatitis B and C in children: current treatment and future strategies. Clin Liver Dis 2006;10:133-48.

228. Terrault NA, Lock ASF, McMahon BJ, et al. Update on prevention, diagnosis, and treatment of chronic hepatitis B: AASLD 2018 hepatitis B guidance. Hepatology 2018;67:1560-99.

229. Toussi SS, Abadi J, Rosenberg M, et al. Prevalence of hepatitis B and C virus infections in children infected with HIV. Clin Infect Dis 2007;45:795-8.

230. Dominguez-Rodriguez S, Rojas P, McPhee CF, et al. Effect of HIV/HCV co-infection on the protease evolution of HIV-1B: A pilot study in a pediatric population. Nature 2018;8:2347.

231. Indolfi G, Bartolini E, Serranti D, et al. Hepatitis C in children co-infected with human immunodeficiency virus. J Pediatr Gastroenterol Nutr 2015;61:393-9.

232. American Association for the Study of Liver Diseases (AASLD)-Infectious Diseases Society of America (IDSA). HCV in Children. Available at www.hcvguidelines.org/unique-populations/children. Accessed August 1, 2018.

233. Nunez M. Hepatotoxicity of antiretrovirals: incidence, mechanisms and management. J Hepatol 2006; 44:S132-9.

234. Paterson DL, Swindells S, Mohr J, et al. Adherence to protease inhibitor therapy and outcomes in patients with HIV infection. Ann Intern Med 2000;133:21-30.

235. Naar-King S, Parsons JT, Murphy DA, et al. Improving health outcomes for youth living with the human immunodeficiency virus: a multisite randomized trial of a motivational intervention targeting multiple risk behaviors. Arch Pediatr Adolesc Med 2009;163:1092-8.

236. Simoni JM, Huh D, Frick PA, et al. Peer support and pager messaging to promote antiretroviral modifying therapy in Seattle: a randomized controlled trial. J Acquir Immune Defic Syndr 2009; 52:465-73.

237. Grant PM, Cotter AG. Tenofovir and bone health. Curr Opin HIV AIDS 2016;11:326-32.

238. Manlhiot C, Larsson P, Gurofsky RC, et al. Spectrum and management of hypertriglyceridemia among children in clinical practice. Pediatrics 2009;123:458-65.

239. US Food & Drug Administration. FDA Safety Communication: Serious Health Problems Seen in Premature Babies Given Kaletra (Lopinavir/Ritonavir) Oral Solution. Available at https://www.fda.gov/drugs/drug-safety-and-availability/fda-drug-safety-communication-serious-health-problems-seen-premature-babies-given-kaletra. Accessed August 1, 2018.

240. Saitoh A, Fletcher CV, Brundage R, et al. Efavirenz pharmacokinetics in HIV-1-infected children are associated with CYP2B6-G516T polymorphism. J Acquir Immune Defic Syndr 2007;45:280-5.

241. Carey D, Puls R, Amin J, et al. Efficacy and safety of efavirenz 400 mg daily versus 600 mg daily: 96-week data from the randomised, double-blind, placebo-controlled, non-inferiority ENCORE1 study. Lancet Infect Dis 2015;15:793-802.

242. Puls R, Amin J, Losso M, et al. Efficacy of 400 mg efavirenz versus standard 600 mg dose in HIV-infected, antiretroviral-naive adults (ENCORE1): a randomised, double-blind, placebo-controlled, non-inferiority trial. Lancet 2014;383:1474-82.

243. Yuan J, Guo S, Hall D, et al. Toxicogenomics of nevirapine-associated cutaneous and hepatic adverse events among populations of African, Asian, and European descent. AIDS 2011; 25:1271-80.

244. Dehority W, Abadi J, Wiznia A, et al. Use of integrase inhibitors in HIV-infected children and adolescents. Drugs 2015;75:1483-97.

CHAPTER 46

Pediatric Vaccines

Heather L. Girand, Pharm.D., BCPPS

LEARNING OBJECTIVES

1. Classify each of the routine childhood vaccines as a live or an inactivated vaccine.

2. Classify each inactivated vaccine as a polysaccharide, conjugate, toxoid, or subunit vaccine.

3. Given a clinical scenario, develop an immunization plan for a child or an adolescent.

4. Recognize clinical situations in which a vaccine is contraindicated or should be given with caution.

5. Describe appropriate methods to minimize vaccine-related adverse events.

6. Identify reliable electronic references for current vaccine information.

ABBREVIATIONS IN THIS CHAPTER

ACIP	Advisory Committee on Immunization Practices
CDC	Centers for Disease Control and Prevention
DTaP	Diphtheria, tetanus, and acellular pertussis
Hib	*Haemophilus influenzae* type b
HPV	Human papillomavirus
IIV	Inactivated influenza vaccine
IPV	Inactivated polio vaccine
LAIV	Live attenuated influenza vaccine
MMR	Measles, mumps, and rubella
MMRV	Measles, mumps, rubella, and varicella
PCV13	13-Valent pneumococcal conjugate vaccine
PPSV23	23-Valent pneumococcal polysaccharide vaccine
Td	Tetanus and diphtheria
Tdap	Tetanus, diphtheria, and acellular pertussis
VAERS	Vaccine Adverse Event Reporting System

INTRODUCTION

Vaccines are one of the most important advances in human medicine because of their dramatic impact on infectious disease morbidity and mortality. Since the famous work of Edward Jenner in the late 1700s, smallpox has been eradicated globally, and polio, diphtheria, tetanus, pertussis, measles, mumps, rubella, and *Haemophilus influenzae* type b (Hib) infections have significantly decreased. However, despite the widespread use of routine childhood vaccines in the Western Hemisphere, continued surveillance is necessary to detect disease outbreaks that occur from international travel and lack or underuse of vaccinations.

Vaccines are a form of active immunity in which an antigen is administered to induce antibody formation and protection against infection. The immune response occurs when antigens stimulate T cells that subsequently direct B cells to produce immunoglobulin G, which provides long-lasting protection in a future antigen exposure. Some antigens such as bacterial cell wall polysaccharides produce a T cell–independent immune response by directly stimulating B cells, but the antibody produced is less functional and consists mainly of immunoglobulin M, which provides temporary immunity.[1] Children younger than 2 years do not mount a sufficient response to these antigens because children at this age have immature immune systems. Conjugating a cell-wall polysaccharide to a protein molecule such as a nontoxic diphtheria toxin creates a T cell–dependent immune response that invokes a greater antibody response and provides a booster response when several vaccine doses are given over time.

Vaccines vary in their immunity potential depending on their classification. *Live vaccines* contain attenuated organisms that undergo limited replication, mimicking natural infection. Injectable live vaccines can confer lifelong immunity with one or two doses. However, immune protection from live vaccines can be reduced or completely hindered by the presence of circulating antibody to the vaccine antigens. Administering an antibody-containing blood product (e.g., immune globulin, packed red blood cells) within 2 weeks after a live injectable viral vaccine may interfere with viral replication; if this administration cannot be avoided, the vaccine dose should be repeated. Alternatively, if blood products are given first, then administering live vaccines may have to be postponed for up to 11 months. (Specific recommendations according to the type of blood product can be found on the Centers for Disease Control and Prevention [CDC] website at www.cdc.gov/vaccines/pubs/pinkbook/downloads/appendices/a/mmr_ig.pdf. Similarly, administering certain live viral vaccines can interfere with the patient's immunity to subsequently administered live vaccines. If two live vaccines are not administered simultaneously, then they must be separated by at least 4 weeks to ensure an adequate immune response to the second live vaccine.

In contrast, *inactivated vaccines* consist of killed whole organisms or specific antigens that require several doses to induce long-lasting immunity. In most cases, booster doses are also needed to maintain immunity. These vaccines are not inactivated by circulating antibodies and can be administered any time before or after other vaccines or blood products. Inactivated vaccines also differ in immunogenicity, depending on their composition. One type of inactivated vaccine, called *toxoids*, are inactive bacterial toxins that are usually combined with adjuvants, such as aluminum, to enhance antibody production against the toxin rather than the bacterial pathogen itself.

ROUTINE VACCINES

Childhood immunization schedules are published annually in January by the CDC Advisory Committee on Immunization Practices (ACIP). The currently recommended schedule for routine childhood and adolescent immunization is shown in Figure 1 and can be found on the CDC website at www.cdc. gov/vaccines. Schedule updates and new information are published throughout the year in the *Morbidity and Mortality Weekly Report*. Table 1 contains vaccine-specific information on administration schedules and requirements, adverse effects, precautions, and contraindications.

At each child health encounter, health care providers must consult the recommended dosing schedule and determine whether any vaccines should be given at that encounter. Recommended and minimum ages and intervals exist for all vaccines. Minimum ages are determined by the likelihood of inducing an immune response. Most inactivated vaccines do not induce a response before age 6 weeks, except for hepatitis B vaccine. Live vaccines such as the measles, mumps, and rubella (MMR) and varicella vaccines may not induce immunity if given before age 12 months because of the presence of maternal circulating antibodies. In general, increasing the interval between recommended doses does not reduce effectiveness, but decreasing the interval can reduce antibody response and interfere with immunity. Vaccine doses administered before the minimum recommended age or interval are not valid and must be repeated. Catch-up vaccine schedules, which incorporate the minimum ages and dosing intervals, can be used to update a child's immunization status that has lagged behind. These catch-up schedules are shown in Figure 2 and are also available on the CDC website at www.cdc.gov/ vaccines. Premature infants should be vaccinated at the same chronologic age as full-term infants and receive the full recommended doses.[2]

HEPATITIS B VACCINE

Hepatitis B virus is transmitted through parenteral, mucosal, perinatal, and sexual exposure, potentially leading to acute or chronic hepatitis, cirrhosis, and hepatocellular carcinoma. Children are most often infected during birth or from contact with infected household members and are at high risk of chronic infection and severe liver disease. Chronic infection is typically asymptomatic initially and can be spread to others by those who are unaware of their chronic viremia. In the United States, acute infection occurs mainly during adulthood but can become chronic in up to 5% of cases.[1,3] Because infants are at highest risk of acquiring asymptomatic chronic infection, vaccination efforts should focus on immunization

after birth and before hospital discharge. Catch-up vaccination should target all infants, children, and adolescents not previously vaccinated as well as high-risk unvaccinated adults.[3]

Hepatitis B vaccine is a recombinant vaccine in which hepatitis B surface antigen is harvested and purified after production in yeast. Hepatitis B vaccine is available as two single-antigen vaccines (Engerix-B [GlaxoSmithKline] and Recombivax HB [Merck & Co., Inc.]) and as a component of combination vaccines containing 10–40 mcg of hepatitis B surface antigen protein per milliliter. Table 2 and the Combination Vaccines section of this chapter provide more detail. More than 95% of infants, children, and adolescents develop protective antibody responses to the hepatitis B vaccine series, and its efficacy for protection against infection is 80%–100%.[1]

The recommended administration schedule varies according to patient age. Routine infant immunization with single-antigen vaccine should begin within 24 hours of birth to a hepatitis B surface antigen-negative mother (within 12 hours if mother is antigen-positive or status unknown) to prevent perinatal infection, followed by the second and third doses given at ages 1–2 months and 6–18 months. If a combination vaccine is used to complete the series after the birth dose, additional doses are given as shown in Table 2. Preterm infants weighing less than 2 kg do not mount a sufficient immune response to the birth dose; this dose can be delayed until age 1 month if the child is born to a hepatitis B surface antigen–negative mother. However, if a birth dose must be given, then it should not be counted as part of the recommended administration schedule, and the infant should receive three additional doses beginning at age 1 month.[3] Unvaccinated adolescents should receive a three-dose series of single-antigen vaccine (two doses separated by 4 weeks, with the third dose at least 8 weeks after the second dose and at least 16 weeks after the first dose); an alternative two-dose series with Recombivax HB (10-mcg/mL doses given 4–6 months apart) is approved for children age 11–15 years.

DIPHTHERIA AND TETANUS TOXOIDS AND PERTUSSIS VACCINE

Diphtheria is a toxin-mediated disease that destroys nasopharyngeal tissue; forms membranes covering the pharynx, uvula, tonsils, and soft palate; and can cause respiratory obstruction. *Corynebacterium diphtheriae* produces toxin only when infected by a bacteriophage carrying the *tox* gene. Systemic toxin absorption can lead to myocarditis, neuritis, and paralysis. Diphtheria is transmitted from person to person via the respiratory tract. Diphtheria disease is rare in the United States, with only five cases reported since 2000, but *C. diphtheriae* continues to circulate in previously endemic areas, particularly Native American communities.[1]

Diphtheria toxoid is an inactivated *C. diphtheriae* toxin adsorbed to aluminum to enhance immunogenicity. Diphtheria toxoid is only available in combination with either tetanus toxoid or both tetanus toxoid and pertussis vaccine. The pediatric diphtheria toxoid strength (designated by capital *D*) contains 3–4 times the amount of the adult diphtheria

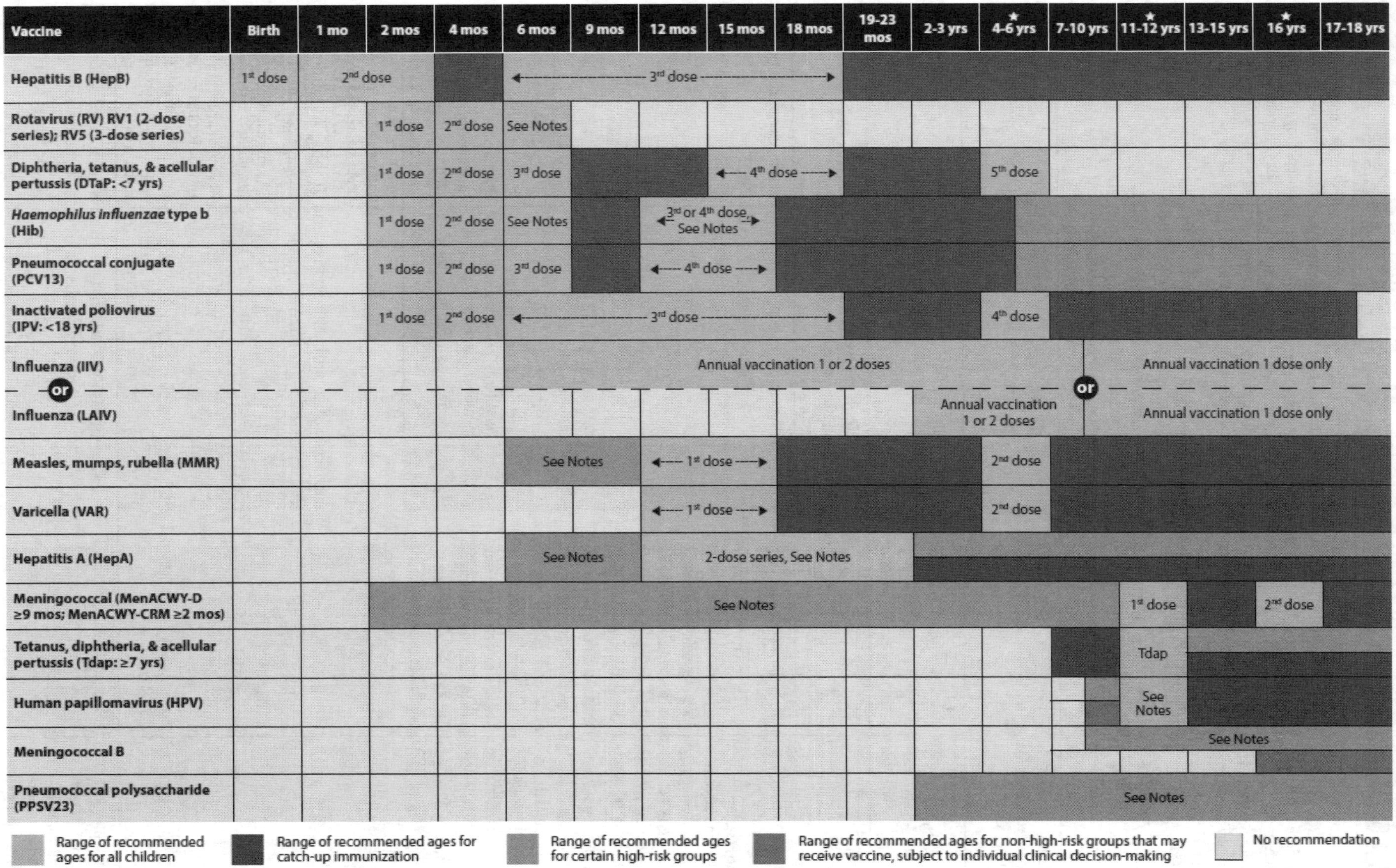

Figure 1. Recommended child and adolescent immunization schedule for children age 18 years or younger—United States, 2019

These recommendations must be read with the Notes that follow. For children who lag behind or start late, provide catch-up vaccination at the earliest opportunity as indicated by the dark gray bars in Figure 1. The catch-up schedule is shown in Figure 2 to determine minimum intervals between doses. School entry and adolescent vaccine age groups are marked with a star.

Table 1. Vaccine-Specific Administration Information, Adverse Effects, Precautions, and Contraindications

Vaccine	Administration	Route	Adverse Effects	Precautions	Contraindications
DTaP or Tdap Td or DT	DTaP: 2, 4, 6, 15–18 mo; 4–6 yr Tdap: Single dose at 11–18 yr (11–12 yr preferred) Td: Booster dose every 10 yr after adolescent Tdap dose DT: Not routinely recommended	IM	Exaggerated local (Arthus) reaction with limb swelling Pertussis-containing vaccines only: Moderate/severe systemic effects (temperature ≥ 105°F [40.6°C], febrile seizures, persistent crying ≥ 3 hr, hypotonic or hyporesponsive episode) Tdap only: Syncope in adolescents	GBS within 6 wk of prior tetanus-containing vaccine Arthus reaction after prior tetanus-containing vaccine; defer vaccine until > 10 yr elapsed since last tetanus-containing vaccine Pertussis-containing vaccines: Progressive or unstable neurologic disorder, uncontrolled seizures, or progressive encephalopathy; defer until condition stabilizes	Pertussis-containing vaccines only: encephalopathy within 7 days of prior vaccine dose with no other cause
Hib	2, 4, 6, 12–15 mo (no 6-mo dose needed if PedvaxHIB given at 2 and 4 mo)	IM	—	—	Age < 6 wk
Hepatitis A	2-dose series: 1st dose at 12–23 mo; 2nd dose 6–18 mo after 1st dose	IM	—	—	—
Hepatitis B	Birth, 1–2 mo, and 6–18 mo	IM	—	Newborns weighing < 2 kg if mother is hepatitis B surface antigen negative	—
HPV	1st dose at 11–12 yr (can give as early as 9 yr) 9–14 yr: 2-dose series (2nd dose 6–12 mo after 1st dose) 15–26 yr: 3-dose series (2nd dose 2 mo after 1st dose; 3rd dose 6 mo after 1st dose)	IM	Syncope in adolescents	Pregnancy	Severe allergic reaction to yeast
LAIV	Annually beginning at 2 yr Children 2–8 yr not vaccinated with at least 2 doses in previous years require 2 doses separated by at least 4 wk	NAS	Rhinorrhea or nasal congestion	GBS within 6 wk of prior influenza vaccine Asthma in children ≥ 5 yr Certain chronic medical conditions: pulmonary, renal, metabolic diseases Severe egg allergy other than hives—possible use if given by provider with severe allergy expertise	Age < 2 yr or > 50 yr Age 2–4 yr: asthma or history of wheezing in previous 12 mo Pregnancy Immunocompromised state Close contacts of severely immunocompromised children who require a protected environment; avoid contact with such people for 7 days after vaccination Chronic use of aspirin or salicylates Receipt of influenza antivirals 48 hr before vaccination; avoid these agents for 14 days after vaccination
IIV	Annually beginning at 6 mo Children 6 mo–8 yr not vaccinated with at least 2 doses in previous years require 2 doses separated by at least 4 wk	IM	GBS	GBS within 6 wk of prior influenza vaccine Severe egg allergy other than hives—possible use if given by provider with severe allergy expertise	—

(continued)

Table 1. Vaccine-Specific Administration Information, Adverse Effects, Precautions, and Contraindications *(continued)*

Vaccine	Administration	Route	Adverse Effects	Precautions	Contraindications
MMR MMRV	12–15 mo; 4–6 yr	SC	Transient rash 7–10 days after vaccination Arthralgias in women Thrombocytopenia Transient lymphadenopathy or parotitis MMRV: Febrile seizures MMRV: Varicella-like rash within 14 days of vaccine	Receipt of antibody-containing blood product (within up to 11 mo); defer for appropriate interval depending on product received[2] History of thrombocytopenia or thrombocytopenic purpura Need for tuberculin skin testing MMRV only: Personal or family history of febrile seizures or family history of epilepsy; administer MMR and varicella vaccines separately MMRV only: Chronic aspirin use; avoid salicylates for 6 wk after receipt of MMRV vaccine (per manufacturer)	Pregnancy Severe immunodeficiency or immunosuppression Severe allergic reaction to neomycin (both vaccines) or gelatin (MMRV only)
MCV; serogroups A, C, W, Y	11–12 yr; booster dose at 16 yr	IM	Syncope in adolescents GBS	History of GBS	—
MenB	16–23 yr Bexsero (2-dose series, 1 mo apart) Trumenba (2-dose series, 6 mo apart, or 3-dose series at 0, 1–2, 6 mo)	IM	Syncope in adolescents	—	—
PCV13	2, 4, 6, and 12–15 mo	IM	—	—	—
PPSV23	Not routinely recommended; use in high-risk groups only	IM	—	—	Children < 2 yr
IPV	2, 4, 6–18 mo; 4–6 yr	IM SC	—	—	Severe allergic reaction to neomycin, streptomycin, or polymyxin B
RV	2, 4, 6 mo (6-mo dose not needed if Rotarix given at 2 and 4 mo)	Oral	Intussusception (risk is unknown but is thought to be very low)	Immunocompromised state other than SCID Acute, moderate, or severe gastroenteritis Hospitalized infants Spina bifida (Rotarix only) Chronic gastrointestinal disease	Severe allergy to latex (Rotarix only) History of intussusception SCID Children < 6 wk
VAR	12–15 mo; 4–6 yr	SC	VAR-like rash within 14 days of vaccine	Receipt of antibody-containing blood product (within up to 11 mo); defer for appropriate interval based on product received[2] Receipt of antivirals (acyclovir, famciclovir, valacyclovir) 24 hr before vaccination; avoid these agents for 14 days after vaccination Chronic aspirin use; avoid salicylates for 6 wk after receipt of VAR vaccine (per manufacturer)	Pregnancy Severe immunodeficiency or immunosuppression Severe allergic reaction to neomycin or gelatin

DT = diphtheria and tetanus toxoids; DTaP = diphtheria, tetanus, and acellular pertussis; GBS = Guillain-Barré syndrome; Hib = Haemophilus influenzae type b; HPV = human papillomavirus; IIV = inactivated influenza vaccine; IM = intramuscular; IPV = inactivated polio vaccine; LAIV = live attenuated influenza vaccine; MCV = meningococcal conjugate vaccine; MenB = meningococcal serogroup B; MMR = measles, mumps, and rubella; MMRV = measles, mumps, rubella, and varicella; NAS = intranasal; PCV13 = pneumococcal conjugate vaccine 13-valent; PPSV23 = pneumococcal polysaccharide vaccine 23-valent; RV = rotavirus; SC = subcutaneous; SCID = severe combined immunodeficiency; Td = tetanus and diphtheria toxoids; Tdap = tetanus, diphtheria, and acellular pertussis; VAR = varicella.

Figure 2. Catch-up immunization schedule for children age 4 months through 6 years

Vaccine	Minimum Age for Dose 1	Dose 1 to Dose 2	Dose 2 to Dose 3	Dose 3 to Dose 4	Dose 4 to Dose 5
			Minimum Interval Between Doses		
Hepatitis B	Birth	**4 weeks**	**8 weeks and at least 16 weeks after first dose.** Minimum age for the final dose is 24 weeks.		
Rotavirus	6 weeks Maximum age for first dose is 14 weeks, 6 days	**4 weeks**	**4 weeks** Maximum age for final dose is 8 months, 0 days.		6 months
Diphtheria, tetanus, and acellular pertussis	6 weeks	**4 weeks**	**4 weeks**	**6 months**	6 months
Haemophilus influenzae type b	6 weeks	**No further doses needed** if first dose was administered at age 15 months or older. **4 weeks** if first dose was administered before the 1st birthday. **8 weeks (as final dose)** if first dose was administered at age 12 through 14 months.	**No further doses needed** if previous dose was administered at age 15 months or older. **4 weeks** if current age is younger than 12 months **and** first dose was administered at younger than age 7 months, **and** at least 1 previous dose was PRP-T (ActHIB, Pentacel, Hiberix) or unknown. **8 weeks and age 12 through 59 months (as final dose)** if current age is younger than 12 months **and** first dose was administered at age 7 through 11 months; **OR** if current age is 12 through 59 months **and** first dose was administered before the 1st birthday, **and** second dose administered at younger than 15 months; **OR** if both doses were PRP-OMP (PedvaxHIB; Comvax) **and** were administered before the 1st birthday.	**8 weeks (as final dose)** This dose only necessary for children age 12 through 59 months who received 3 doses before the 1st birthday.	
Pneumococcal conjugate	6 weeks	**No further doses needed** for healthy children if first dose was administered at age 24 months or older. **4 weeks** if first dose administered before the 1st birthday. **8 weeks (as final dose for healthy children)** if first dose was administered at the 1st birthday or after.	**No further doses needed** for healthy children if previous dose administered at age 24 months or older. **4 weeks** if current age is younger than 12 months and previous dose given at <7 months old. **8 weeks (as final dose for healthy children)** if previous dose given between 7–11 months (wait until at least 12 months old); **OR** if current age is 12 months or older and at least 1 dose was given before age 12 months.	**8 weeks (as final dose)** This **dose** only necessary for children age 12 through 59 months who received 3 doses before age 12 months or for children at high risk who received 3 doses at any age.	
Inactivated poliovirus	6 weeks	**4 weeks**	**4 weeks** if current age is < 4 years. **6 months** (as final dose) if current age is 4 years or older.	**6 months** (minimum age 4 years for final dose).	
Measles, mumps, rubella	12 months	**4 weeks**			
Varicella	12 months	**3 months**			
Hepatitis A	12 months	**6 months**			
Meningococcal	2 months MenACWY-CRM 9 months MenACWY-D	**8 weeks**	See Notes	See Notes	

Children and adolescents age 7 through 18 years

Vaccine	Minimum Age for Dose 1	Dose 1 to Dose 2	Dose 2 to Dose 3	Dose 3 to Dose 4	Dose 4 to Dose 5
Meningococcal	Not Applicable (N/A)	**8 weeks**			
Tetanus, diphtheria; tetanus, diphtheria, and acellular pertussis	7 years	**4 weeks** if first dose of DTaP/DT was administered before the 1st birthday. **6 months** (as final dose) if first dose of DTaP/DT or Tdap/Td was administered at or after the 1st birthday.	**4 weeks** if first dose of DTaP/DT was administered before the 1st birthday. **6 months** if first dose of DTaP/DT or Td was administered at or after the 1st birthday.	**6 months** if first dose of DTaP/DT was administered before the 1st birthday.	
Human papillomavirus	9 years	Routine dosing intervals are recommended.			
Hepatitis A	N/A	**6 months**			
Hepatitis B	N/A	**4 weeks**	**8 weeks and** at least 16 weeks after first dose.		
Inactivated poliovirus	N/A	**4 weeks**	**6 months** A fourth dose is not necessary if the third dose was administered at age 4 years or older and at least 6 months after the previous dose.	A fourth dose of IPV is indicated if all previous doses were administered at <4 years or if the third dose was administered <6 months after the second dose.	
Measles, mumps, rubella	N/A	**4 weeks**			
Varicella	N/A	**3 months** if younger than age 13 years. **4 weeks** if age 13 years or older.			

Figure 2. Catch-up immunization schedule for children age 4 months to 18 years who start late or who are more than 1 month behind—United States, 2019.

These data provide catch-up schedules and minimum intervals between doses for children whose vaccinations have been delayed. A vaccine series does not need to be restarted, regardless of the time that has elapsed between doses. Use the section appropriate for the child's age. Always use information in this figure in conjunction with the information in Figure 1 and the supplemental Notes in Figure 2.

For vaccine recommendations for persons 19 years of age and older, see the Recommended Adult Immunization Schedule.

Additional information

- Consult relevant ACIP statements for detailed recommendations at www.cdc.gov/vaccines/hcp/acip-recs/index.html.

- For information on contraindications and precautions for the use of a vaccine, consult the General Best Practice Guidelines for Immunization and relevant ACIP statements at www.cdc.gov/vaccines/hcp/acip-recs/index.html.

- For calculating intervals between doses, 4 weeks = 28 days. Intervals of ≥4 months are determined by calendar months.

- Within a number range (e.g., 12–18), a dash (–) should be read as "through."

- Vaccine doses administered ≤4 days before the minimum age or interval are considered valid. Doses of any vaccine administered ≥5 days earlier than the minimum age or minimum interval should not be counted as valid and should be repeated as age-appropriate. The repeat dose should be spaced after the invalid dose by the recommended minimum interval. For further details, see Table 3-1, Recommended and minimum ages and intervals between vaccine doses, in General Best Practice Guidelines for Immunization at www.cdc.gov/vaccines/hcp/acip-recs/general-recs/timing.html.

- Information on travel vaccine requirements and recommendations is available at wwwwnc.cdc.gov/travel/.

- For vaccination of persons with immunodeficiencies, see Table 8-1, Vaccination of persons with primary and secondary immunodeficiencies, in General Best Practice Guidelines for Immunization at www.cdc.gov/vaccines/hcp/acip-recs/general-recs/immunocompetence.html, and Immunization in Special Clinical Circumstances (In: Kimberlin DW, Brady MT, Jackson MA, Long SS, eds. *Red Book: 2018 Report of the Committee on Infectious Diseases*. 31st ed. Itasca, IL: American Academy of Pediatrics; 2018:67–111).

- For information regarding vaccination in the setting of a vaccine-preventable disease outbreak, contact your state or local health department.

- The National Vaccine Injury Compensation Program (VICP) is a no-fault alternative to the traditional legal system for resolving vaccine injury claims. All routine child and adolescent vaccines are covered by VICP except for pneumococcal polysaccharide vaccine (PPSV23). For more information, see www.hrsa.gov/vaccinecompensation/index.html.

Diphtheria, tetanus, and pertussis (DTaP) vaccination (minimum age: 6 weeks [4 years for Kinrix or Quadracel])

Routine vaccination

- 5-dose series at 2, 4, 6, 15–18 months, 4–6 years
  - Prospectively: Dose 4 may be given as early as age 12 months if at least 6 months have elapsed since dose 3.
  - Retrospectively: A 4th dose that was inadvertently given as early as 12 months may be counted if at least 4 months have elapsed since dose 3.

Catch-up vaccination

- Dose 5 is not necessary if dose 4 was administered at age 4 years or older.
- For other catch-up guidance, see Table 2.

Haemophilus influenzae type b vaccination (minimum age: 6 weeks)

Routine vaccination

- ActHIB, Hiberix, or Pentacel: 4-dose series at 2, 4, 6, 12–15 months
- PedvaxHIB: 3-dose series at 2, 4, 12–15 months

Catch-up vaccination

- Dose 1 at 7–11 months: Administer dose 2 at least 4 weeks later and dose 3 (final dose) at 12–15 months or 8 weeks after dose 2 (whichever is later).
- Dose 1 at 12–14 months: Administer dose 2 (final dose) at least 8 weeks after dose 1.
- Dose 1 before 12 months and dose 2 before 15 months: Administer dose 3 (final dose) 8 weeks after dose 2.
- 2 doses of PedvaxHIB before 12 months: Administer dose 3 (final dose) at 12–59 months and at least 8 weeks after dose 2.
- Unvaccinated at 15–59 months: 1 dose
- For other catch-up guidance, see Table 2.

Special situations

- Chemotherapy or radiation treatment:

  12–59 months
  - Unvaccinated or only 1 dose before age 12 months: 2 doses, 8 weeks apart
  - 2 or more doses before age 12 months: 1 dose at least 8 weeks after previous dose
  Doses administered within 14 days of starting therapy or during therapy should be repeated at least 3 months after therapy completion.

- Hematopoietic stem cell transplant (HSCT):
  - 3-dose series 4 weeks apart starting 6 to 12 months after successful transplant regardless of Hib vaccination history

- Anatomic or functional asplenia (including sickle cell disease):

  12–59 months
  - Unvaccinated or only 1 dose before 12 months: 2 doses, 8 weeks apart
  - 2 or more doses before 12 months:1 dose at least 8 weeks after previous dose
  Unvaccinated persons age 5 years or older
  - 1 dose

- Elective splenectomy:

  Unvaccinated persons age 15 months or older
  - 1 dose (preferably at least 14 days before procedure)

- HIV infection:

  12–59 months
  - Unvaccinated or only 1 dose before age 12 months: 2 doses, 8 weeks apart
  - 2 or more doses before age 12 months: 1 dose at least 8 weeks after previous dose
  Unvaccinated persons age 5–18 years
  - 1 dose

- Immunoglobulin deficiency, early component complement deficiency:

  12–59 months
  - Unvaccinated or only 1 dose before age 12 months: 2 doses, 8 weeks apart
  - 2 or more doses before age 12 months: 1 dose at least 8 weeks after previous dose

Unvaccinated = Less than routine series (through 14 months) OR no doses (14 months or older)

Figure 2. Catch-up immunization schedule for children age 4 months to 18 years who start late or who are more than 1 month behind—United States, 2019. *(continued)*

Notes — Recommended Child and Adolescent Immunization Schedule for ages 18 years or younger, United States, 2019

Hepatitis A vaccination
(minimum age: 12 months for routine vaccination)

Routine vaccination
- 2-dose series (Havrix 6–12 months apart or Vaqta 6–18 months apart, minimum interval 6 months); a series begun before the 2nd birthday should be completed even if the child turns 2 before the second dose is administered.

Catch-up vaccination
- Anyone 2 years of age or older may receive HepA vaccine if desired. Minimum interval between doses: 6 months
- Adolescents 18 years and older may receive the combined HepA and HepB vaccine, Twinrix, as a 3-dose series (0, 1, and 6 months) or 4-dose series (0, 7, and 21–30 days, followed by a dose at 12 months).

International travel
- Persons traveling to or working in countries with high or intermediate endemic hepatitis A (wwwnc.cdc.gov/travel/):
  - Infants age 6–11 months: 1 dose before departure; revaccinate with 2 doses, separated by 6–18 months, between 12 to 23 months of age.
  - Unvaccinated age 12 months and older: 1st dose as soon as travel considered

Special situations
At risk for hepatitis A infection: 2-dose series as above
- Chronic liver disease
- Clotting factor disorders
- Men who have sex with men
- Injection or non-injection drug use
- Homelessness
- Work with hepatitis A virus in research laboratory or nonhuman primates with hepatitis A infection
- Travel in countries with high or intermediate endemic hepatitis A
- Close, personal contact with international adoptee (e.g., household or regular babysitting) in first 60 days after arrival from country with high or intermediate endemic hepatitis A (administer dose 1 as soon as adoption is planned, at least 2 weeks before adoptee's arrival)

Hepatitis B vaccination
(minimum age: birth)

Birth dose (monovalent HepB vaccine only)
- Mother is HBsAg-negative: 1 dose within 24 hours of birth for all medically stable infants ≥2,000 grams. Infants <2,000 grams: administer 1 dose at chronological age 1 month or hospital discharge.

Human papillomavirus vaccination
(minimum age: 9 years)

Routine and catch-up vaccination
- HPV vaccination routinely recommended for all adolescents age 11–12 years (can start at age 9 years) and through age 18 years if not previously adequately vaccinated
- 2- or 3-dose series depending on age at initial vaccination:
  - Age 9 through 14 years at initial vaccination: 2-dose series at 0, 6–12 months (minimum interval: 5 months; repeat dose if administered too soon)
  - Age 15 years or older at initial vaccination: 3-dose series at 0, 1–2 months, 6 months (minimum intervals: dose 1 to dose 2: 4 weeks / dose 2 to dose 3: 12 weeks / dose 1 to dose 3: 5 months; repeat dose if administered too soon)
- If completed valid vaccination series with any HPV vaccine, no additional doses needed

Special situations
- Immunocompromising conditions, including HIV infection: 3-dose series as above
- History of sexual abuse or assault: Start at age 9 years
- Pregnancy: HPV vaccination not recommended until after pregnancy; no intervention needed if vaccinated while pregnant; pregnancy testing not needed before vaccination

Mother is HBsAg-positive:
- Administer HepB vaccine and 0.5 mL of hepatitis B immune globulin (HBIG) (at separate anatomic sites) within 12 hours of birth, regardless of birth weight. For infants <2,000 grams, administer 3 additional doses of vaccine (total of 4 doses) beginning at age 1 month.
- Test for HBsAg and anti-HBs at age 9–12 months. If HepB series is delayed, test 1–2 months after final dose.

Mother's HBsAg status is unknown:
- Administer HepB vaccine within 12 hours of birth, regardless of birth weight.
- For infants <2,000 grams, administer 0.5 mL of HBIG in addition to HepB vaccine within 12 hours of birth. Administer 3 additional doses of vaccine (total of 4 doses) beginning at age 1 month.
- Determine mother's HBsAg status as soon as possible. If mother is HBsAg-positive, administer 0.5 mL of HBIG to infants ≥2,000 grams as soon as possible, but no later than 7 days of age.

Routine series
- 3-dose series at 0, 1–2, 6–18 months (use monovalent HepB vaccine for doses administered before age 6 weeks)
- Infants who did not receive a birth dose should begin the series as soon as feasible (see Table 2).
- Administration of 4 doses is permitted when a combination vaccine containing HepB is used after the birth dose.
- Minimum age for the final (3rd or 4th) dose: 24 weeks
- Minimum intervals: dose 1 to dose 2: 4 weeks / dose 2 to dose 3: 8 weeks / dose 1 to dose 3: 16 weeks (when 4 doses are administered, substitute "dose 4" for "dose 3" in these calculations)

Catch-up vaccination
- Unvaccinated persons should complete a 3-dose series at 0, 1–2, 6 months.
- Adolescents age 11–15 years may use an alternative 2-dose schedule with at least 4 months between doses (adult formulation Recombivax HB only).
- Adolescents 18 years and older may receive a 2-dose series of HepB (Heplisav-B) at least 4 weeks apart.
- Adolescents 18 years and older may receive the combined HepA and HepB vaccine, Twinrix, as a 3-dose series (0, 1, and 6 months) or 4-dose series (0, 7, and 21–30 days, followed by a dose at 12 months).
- For other catch-up guidance, see Table 2.

Inactivated poliovirus vaccination
(minimum age: 6 weeks)

Routine vaccination
- 4-dose series at ages 2, 4, 6–18 months, 4–6 years; administer the final dose on or after the 4th birthday and at least 6 months after the previous dose.
- 4 or more doses of IPV can be administered before the 4th birthday when a combination vaccine containing IPV is used. However, a dose is still recommended after the 4th birthday and at least 6 months after the previous dose.

Catch-up vaccination
- In the first 6 months of life, use minimum ages and intervals only for travel to a polio-endemic region or during an outbreak.
- IPV is not routinely recommended for U.S. residents 18 years and older.

Series containing oral polio vaccine (OPV), either mixed OPV-IPV or OPV-only series:
- Total number of doses needed to complete the series is the same as that recommended for the U.S. IPV schedule. See www.cdc.gov/mmwr/volumes/66/wr/mm6601a6.htm?s_cid=mm6601a6_w.

Figure 2. Catch-up immunization schedule for children age 4 months to 18 years who start late or who are more than 1 month behind—United States, 2019. *(continued)*

Notes   Recommended Child and Adolescent Immunization Schedule for ages 18 years or younger, United States, 2019

- Only trivalent OPV (tOPV) counts toward the U.S. vaccination requirements. For guidance to assess doses documented as "OPV," see www.cdc.gov/mmwr/volumes/66/wr/mm6606a7.htm?s_cid=mm6606a7_w.
- For other catch-up guidance, see Table 2.

Influenza vaccination
(minimum age: 6 months [IIV], 2 years [LAIV], 18 years [RIIV])

Routine vaccination
- 1 dose any influenza vaccine appropriate for age and health status annually (2 doses separated by at least 4 weeks for children 6 months–8 years who did not receive at least 2 doses of influenza vaccine before July 1, 2018)

Special situations
- Egg allergy, hives only: Any influenza vaccine appropriate for age and health status annually
- Egg allergy more severe than hives (e.g., angioedema, respiratory distress): Any influenza vaccine appropriate for age and health status annually in medical setting under supervision of health care provider who can recognize and manage severe allergic conditions
- LAIV should not be used for those with a history of severe allergic reaction to any component of the vaccine (excluding egg) or to a previous dose of any influenza vaccine, children and adolescents receiving concomitant aspirin or salicylate-containing medications, children age 2 through 4 years with a history of asthma or wheezing, those who are immunocompromised due to any cause (including immunosuppression caused by medications and HIV infection), anatomic and functional asplenia, cochlear implants, cerebrospinal fluid-oropharyngeal communication, close contacts and caregivers of severely immunosuppressed persons who require a protected environment, pregnancy, and persons who have received influenza antiviral medications within the previous 48 hours.

Measles, mumps, and rubella vaccination
(minimum age: 12 months for routine vaccination)

Routine vaccination
- 2-dose series at 12–15 months, 4–6 years
- Dose 2 may be administered as early as 4 weeks after dose 1.

Catch-up vaccination
- Unvaccinated children and adolescents: 2 doses at least 4 weeks apart
- The maximum age for use of *MMRV* is 12 years.

Special situations
International travel
- Infants age 6–11 months: 1 dose before departure; revaccinate with 2 doses at 12–15 months (12 months for children in high-risk areas) and dose 2 as early as 4 weeks later.
- Unvaccinated children age 12 months and older: 2-dose series at least 4 weeks apart before departure

Meningococcal serogroup A,C,W,Y vaccination
(minimum age: 2 months [MenACWY-CRM, Menveo], 9 months [MenACWY-D, Menactra])

Routine vaccination
- 2-dose series: 11–12 years, 16 years

Catch-up vaccination
- Age 13–15 years: 1 dose now and booster at age 16–18 years (minimum interval: 8 weeks)
- Age 16–18 years: 1 dose

Special situations
Anatomic or functional asplenia (including sickle cell disease), HIV infection, persistent complement component deficiency, eculizumab use:
- Menveo
  - Dose 1 at age 8 weeks: 4-dose series at 2, 4, 6, 12 months
  - Dose 1 at age 7–23 months: 2-dose series (dose 2 at least 12 weeks after dose 1 and after the 1st birthday)
  - Dose 1 at age 24 months or older: 2-dose series at least 8 weeks apart
- Menactra
  - Persistent complement component deficiency:
    - Age 9–23 months: 2 doses at least 12 weeks apart
    - Age 24 months or older: 2 doses at least 8 weeks apart
  - Anatomic or functional asplenia, sickle cell disease, or HIV infection:
    - Age 9–23 months: Not recommended
    - 24 months or older: 2 doses at least 8 weeks apart
  - Menactra must be administered at least 4 weeks after completion of PCV13 series.

Travel in countries with hyperendemic or epidemic meningococcal disease, including countries in the African meningitis belt or during the Hajj (www.nc.cdc.gov/travel/):
- Children age less than 24 months:
  - Menveo (age 2–23 months):
    - Dose 1 at 8 weeks: 4-dose series at 2, 4, 6, 12 months
    - Dose 1 at 7–23 months: 2-dose series (dose 2 at least 12 weeks after dose 1 and after the 1st birthday)
  - Menactra (age 9–23 months):
    - 2-dose series (dose 2 at least 12 weeks after dose 1; dose 2 may be administered as early as 8 weeks after dose 1 in travelers)
- Children age 2 years or older: 1 dose Menveo or Menactra

First-year college students who live in residential housing (if not previously vaccinated at age 16 years or older) or military recruits:
- 1 dose Menveo or Menactra

Note: Menactra should be administered either before or at the same time as DTaP. For MenACWY booster dose recommendations for groups listed under "Special situations" above and additional meningococcal vaccination information, see meningococcal *MMWR* publications at www.cdc.gov/vaccines/hcp/acip-recs/vacc-specific/mening.html.

Meningococcal serogroup B vaccination
(minimum age: 10 years [MenB-4C, Bexsero; MenB-FHbp, Trumenba])

Clinical discretion
- MenB vaccine may be administered based on individual clinical decision to adolescents not at increased risk age 16–23 years (preferred age 16–18 years):
- Bexsero: 2-dose series at least 1 month apart
- Trumenba: 2-dose series at least 6 months apart; if dose 2 is administered earlier than 6 months, administer a 3rd dose at least 4 months after dose 2.

Special situations
Anatomic or functional asplenia (including sickle cell disease), persistent complement component deficiency, eculizumab use:
- Bexsero: 2-dose series at least 1 month apart
- Trumenba: 3-dose series at 0, 1–2, 6 months
Bexsero and Trumenba are not interchangeable; the same product should be used for all doses in a series.
For additional meningococcal vaccination information, see meningococcal *MMWR* publications at www.cdc.gov/vaccines/hcp/acip-recs/vacc-specific/mening.html.

Figure 2. Catch-up immunization schedule for children age 4 months to 18 years who start late or who are more than 1 month behind—United States, 2019. (*continued*)

Pneumococcal vaccination
(minimum age: 6 weeks [PCV13], 2 years [PPSV23])

Routine vaccination with PCV13
* 4-dose series at 2, 4, 6, 12–15 months

Catch-up vaccination with PCV13
* 1 dose for healthy children age 24–59 months with any incomplete* PCV13 series
* For other catch-up guidance, see Table 2.

Special situations
High-risk conditions below: When both PCV13 and PPSV23 are indicated, administer PCV13 first. PCV13 and PPSV23 should not be administered during same visit.

Chronic heart disease (particularly cyanotic congenital heart disease and cardiac failure); chronic lung disease (including asthma treated with high-dose, oral corticosteroids); diabetes mellitus:

Age 2–5 years
* Any incomplete* series with:
- 3 PCV13 doses: 1 dose PCV13 (at least 8 weeks after any prior PCV13 dose)
- Less than 3 PCV13 doses: 2 doses PCV13 (8 weeks after the most recent dose and administered 8 weeks apart)
* No history of PPSV23: 1 dose PPSV23 (at least 8 weeks after any prior PCV13 dose)

Age 6–18 years
* No history of PPSV23: 1 dose PPSV23 (at least 8 weeks after any prior PCV13 dose)

Cerebrospinal fluid leak, cochlear implant:

Age 2–5 years
* Any incomplete* series with:
- 3 PCV13 doses: 1 dose PCV13 (at least 8 weeks after any prior PCV13 dose)
- Less than 3 PCV13 doses: 2 doses PCV13, 8 weeks after the most recent dose and administered 8 weeks apart
* No history of PPSV23: 1 dose PPSV23 (at least 8 weeks after any prior PCV13 dose)

Age 6–18 years
* No history of either PCV13 or PPSV23: 1 dose PCV13, 1 dose PPSV23 at least 8 weeks later
* Any PCV13 but no PPSV23: 1 dose PPSV23 at least 8 weeks after the most recent dose of PCV13
* PPSV23 but no PCV13: 1 dose PCV13 at least 8 weeks after the most recent dose of PPSV23

Sickle cell disease and other hemoglobinopathies; anatomic or functional asplenia; congenital or acquired immunodeficiency; HIV infection; chronic renal failure; nephrotic syndrome; malignant neoplasms, leukemias, lymphomas, Hodgkin disease, and other diseases

associated with treatment with immunosuppressive drugs or radiation therapy; solid organ transplantation; multiple myeloma:

Age 2–5 years
* Any incomplete* series with:
- 3 PCV13 doses: 1 dose PCV13 (at least 8 weeks after any prior PCV13 dose)
- Less than 3 PCV13 doses: 2 doses PCV13 (8 weeks after the most recent dose and administered 8 weeks apart)
* No history of PPSV23: 1 dose PPSV23 (at least 8 weeks after any prior PCV13 dose) and a 2nd dose of PPSV23 5 years later

Age 6–18 years
* No history of either PCV13 or PPSV23: 1 dose PCV13, 2 doses PPSV23 (dose 1 of PPSV23 administered 8 weeks after PCV13 and dose 2 of PPSV23 administered at least 5 years after dose 1 of PPSV23)
* Any PCV13 but no PPSV23: 2 doses PPSV23 (dose 1 of PPSV23 administered 8 weeks after the most recent dose of PCV13 and dose 2 of PPSV23 administered at least 5 years after dose 1 of PPSV23)
* PPSV23 but no PCV13: 1 dose PCV13 at least 8 weeks after the most recent PPSV23 dose and a 2nd dose of PPSV23 administered 5 years after dose 1 of PPSV23 and at least 8 weeks after a dose of PCV13

Chronic liver disease, alcoholism:

Age 6–18 years
* No history of PPSV23: 1 dose PPSV23 (at least 8 weeks after any prior PCV13 dose)

*An incomplete series is defined as not having received all doses in either the recommended series or an age-appropriate catch-up series. See Tables 8, 9, and 11 in the ACIP pneumococcal vaccine recommendations (www.cdc.gov/mmwr/pdf/rr/rr5911.pdf) for complete schedule details.

Rotavirus vaccination
(minimum age: 6 weeks)

Routine vaccination
* **Rotarix:** 2-dose series at 2 and 4 months.
* **RotaTeq:** 3-dose series at 2, 4, and 6 months.
If any dose in the series is either **RotaTeq** or unknown, default to 3-dose series.

Catch-up vaccination
* Do not start the series on or after age 15 weeks, 0 days.
* The maximum age for the final dose is 8 months, 0 days.
* For other catch-up guidance, see Figure 2.

Tetanus, diphtheria, and pertussis (Tdap) vaccination
(minimum age: 11 years for routine vaccination, 7 years for catch-up vaccination)

Routine vaccination
* **Adolescents age 11–12 years:** 1 dose Tdap
* **Pregnancy:** 1 dose Tdap during each pregnancy, preferably in early part of gestational weeks 27–36
* Tdap may be administered regardless of the interval since the last tetanus- and diphtheria-toxoid-containing vaccine.

Catch-up vaccination
* **Adolescents age 13–18 years who have not received Tdap:** 1 dose Tdap, then Td booster every 10 years
* **Persons age 7–18 years not fully immunized with DTaP:** 1 dose Tdap as part of the catch-up series (preferably the first dose); if additional doses are needed, use Td.
* **Children age 7–10 years** who receive Tdap inadvertently or as part of the catch-up series should receive the routine Tdap dose at 11–12 years.
* **DTaP inadvertently given after the 7th birthday:**
- **Child age 7–10 years:** DTaP may count as part of catch-up series. Routine Tdap dose at 11–12 should be administered.
- **Adolescent age 11–18 years:** Count dose of DTaP as the adolescent Tdap booster.
* For other catch-up guidance, see Table 2.
* For information on use of Tdap or Td as tetanus prophylaxis in wound management, see www.cdc.gov/mmwr/volumes/67/rr/rr6702a1.htm.

Varicella vaccination
(minimum age: 12 months)

Routine vaccination
* 2-dose series: 12–15 months, 4–6 years
* Dose 2 may be administered as early as 3 months after dose 1 (a dose administered after a 4-week interval may be counted).

Catch-up vaccination
* Ensure persons age 7–18 years without evidence of immunity (see *MMWR* at www.cdc.gov/mmwr/pdf/rr/rr5604.pdf) have 2-dose series:
- **Ages 7–12 years:** routine interval: 3 months (minimum interval: 4 weeks)
- **Ages 13 years and older:** routine interval: 4–8 weeks (minimum interval: 4 weeks).
- The maximum age for use of *MMRV* is 12 years.

Figure 2. Catch-up immunization schedule for children age 4 months to 18 years who start late or who are more than 1 month behind—United States, 2019. *(continued)*

Table 2. Combination Vaccines and Indications

Brand Name	Components	Indications
Kinrix,[a] Quadracel[b]	DTaP, IPV	For 5th DTaP dose and 4th IPV dose at age 4–6 yr
		Quadracel can also be given for 4th or 5th IPV dose in children who received 4 doses of Pentacel and/or Daptacel (DTaP)
Pediarix[a]	DTaP, hepatitis B, IPV	For doses at age 2, 4, 6 mo; not for booster doses (4th and 5th doses)
Pentacel[b]	DTaP, IPV, Hib	For doses at age 2, 4, 6, 15–18 mo; 4th dose can be given as early as 12 mo if 6 mo elapsed since the 3rd dose
		Children need an additional IPV booster dose at 4–6 yr
ProQuad[c]	MMR, VAR	For age 1–12 yr; consider for only 2nd dose in series
Twinrix[a]	Hepatitis A, hepatitis B	Age ≥ 18 yr; 3-dose series
Vaxelis[c] (available in 2020)	DTaP, IPV, Hib, hepatitis B	For doses at age 2, 4, 6 mo

[a]GlaxoSmithKline, Research Triangle Park, NC
[b]Sanofi Pasteur Inc., Swiftwater, PA
[c]Merck & Co., Inc., Whitehouse Station, NJ
DTaP = diphtheria, tetanus, and acellular pertussis; Hib = Haemophilus influenzae type b; IPV = inactivated polio vaccine; MMR = measles, mumps, and rubella; VAR = varicella.

toxoid strength (designated by lowercase *d*). Routine vaccination begins as early as age 6 weeks and consists of a four-dose series given in combination with diphtheria, tetanus, and acellular pertussis vaccine (DTaP), as shown in Table 1. A booster dose should be given at age 4–6 years if the fourth dose in the primary series was given before age 4 years. Protective antibodies develop in more than 95% of infants after the four-dose series, with clinical efficacy estimated at 97%.[1] Additional booster doses of tetanus and diphtheria vaccine (Td) are given every 10 years after completion of the childhood DTaP series and the adolescent booster dose of tetanus, diphtheria, and acellular pertussis (Tdap) because of waning immunity during adulthood.

Tetanus, a toxin-mediated disease acquired from soil and animal feces, is the only vaccine-preventable disease that is not contagious. *Clostridium tetani* spores enter the body, usually through a wound, and germinate in anaerobic conditions, causing the production of neurotoxins that block neurotransmitter inhibitor impulses, causing severe muscle contractions and spasms. The most common form of tetanus is generalized; it begins with lockjaw and descends to the neck, esophagus, and abdomen. Additional manifestations include tachycardia, elevated blood pressure, fever, and sweating. Tetanus is rare in the United States, with fewer than 50 cases reported annually, but is common in developing countries and affects neonates whose mothers are not immune.[1,4]

Tetanus toxoid is a formalin-inactivated toxin that is available as an adsorbed toxoid (onto aluminum hydroxide) or a nonadsorbed toxoid. The adsorbed toxoid is preferred because it elicits a stronger and longer-lasting immune response.[1] The adsorbed toxoid is available as a single-antigen product, but it should be administered in combination with either diphtheria toxoid (either as DT or Td) or diphtheria toxoid and acellular pertussis vaccine (either as DTaP or Tdap) to protect against several infections with one vaccine dose. The primary childhood series should be given with DTaP (Table 1).

Protective antibody response and clinical efficacy are almost 100% after the primary series.[1] Booster doses should be given as Td every 10 years after the primary series and adolescent Tdap booster because of waning immunity. Patients who present with minor or uncontaminated wounds should receive a tetanus booster if it has been 10 years or more since their last tetanus-containing vaccine. Patients with moderate to severe or contaminated wounds should be vaccinated if they have not received a tetanus-containing vaccine in the preceding 5 years. Individuals who had an Arthus reaction (characterized by severe pain, swelling, and induration within 2–8 hours) after a tetanus vaccine should not receive a tetanus-containing vaccine any earlier than 10 years after the last tetanus dose, even for wound management.

Pertussis, or *whooping cough*, is a highly contagious respiratory infection caused by *Bordetella pertussis*. Pertussis is spread through airborne droplets that are inhaled or through direct contact with contaminated droplets. Pertussis toxins interfere with mucociliary clearance by paralyzing respiratory cilia and promoting inflammation. Classic pertussis occurs in three stages: *catarrhal*, *paroxysmal*, and *convalescence*. The catarrhal stage is characterized by rhinorrhea, sneezing, low-grade fever, and mild cough, lasting 1–2 weeks. The cough progressively worsens until coughing paroxysms become interrupted with the characteristic "whoop" sound on inspiration in the paroxysmal stage. In this stage, which can last up to 6 weeks, cyanosis, post-tussive vomiting, and exhaustion are common. Gradual improvement occurs in the convalescent stage, which can last a few months. Adolescents typically have a milder and shorter course of illness than infants and young children.

The incidence of pertussis in the United States has increased since the early 1980s, when around 3000 cases were reported annually.[1] More than 48,000 cases were reported in 2012, the largest number since 1959. Although infants younger than 6 months have the highest incidence, 60%

of cases are now reported in people age 11 years and older.[5] Increased disease recognition and waning immunity are possible causes for the many cases reported in this age group. Mortality, which remains highest in infants younger than 3 months, is usually caused by secondary bacterial pneumonia.[1]

Pertussis vaccines available in the United States are acellular, containing purified components of *B. pertussis* such as pertussis toxin, filamentous hemagglutinin, and pertactin. Acellular vaccines are less reactogenic than their predecessor whole-cell vaccines, which are no longer available in the United States. Whole-cell vaccines caused more local reactions, fevers, and systemic effects; however, they are still used in many countries. Two pediatric acellular vaccines are available (as DTaP) that contain different types and amounts of pertussis antigens: Daptacel (Sanofi Pasteur Inc., Swiftwater, PA) and Infanrix (GlaxoSmithKline). The primary series consists of five doses given between age 2 months and 4–6 years (Table 1). Protective antibody responses vary between vaccine products and by vaccine antigen components, but clinical efficacy of the available vaccines is estimated at 80%–85%.[1] The series should be completed with the same brand of DTaP, when possible, but they are considered interchangeable. The DTaP vaccines are also available in combination with other vaccines as detailed in the Combination Vaccines section of this chapter and in Table 2.

Two adolescent and adult acellular pertussis vaccines in combination with diphtheria and tetanus toxoids (Tdap, as Boostrix [GlaxoSmithKline] and Adacel [Sanofi Pasteur Inc.]) are available as booster doses to combat waning immunity after childhood and subsequent spread to unprotected infants. These vaccines contain reduced amounts of pertussis antigens (designated by lowercase *p*) compared with the pediatric formulations (designated by capital *P*), but they have the same amounts of diphtheria and tetanus toxoids as the Td vaccine. A single Tdap dose is recommended for all children age 11–18 years (preferably at 11–12 years) and for children age 7–18 years who are not fully vaccinated against pertussis.[6] A single Tdap dose should be given in place of Td for wound management in patients who have not previously received a Tdap dose. Others who should receive a single Tdap dose if they have not received one previously are health care personnel and those in close contact with infants age 12 months or younger, including child care providers and new parents and grandparents.[6] After Tdap is received, all subsequent booster doses should be with Td. An exception is for pregnant women, who should receive Tdap during each pregnancy, preferably in the early portion of gestational weeks 27–36, to provide passive immunity to the fetus.[6] No minimum interval is recommended between receipt of Tdap and the last tetanus- or diphtheria-containing vaccine.

HAEMOPHILUS INFLUENZAE TYPE B VACCINE

A common bacterial organism that causes otitis media, sinusitis, and invasive diseases such as meningitis, epiglottitis, pneumonia, and sepsis is *H. influenzae*, which is primarily transmitted through respiratory droplets. *Haemophilus influenzae* can be encapsulated with a polysaccharide capsule that contributes to its virulence, or it can be nonencapsulated. An encapsulated strain that causes invasive infections in children younger than 5 years, Hib, was historically the most common cause of bacterial meningitis. However, the incidence of invasive Hib disease in the United States has decreased by more than 99% since the Hib vaccine was introduced in the late 1980s. In 2003–2010, about 25 cases of invasive Hib disease were reported annually in children younger than 5 years.[1]

The Hib vaccines are conjugated vaccines in which polysaccharide capsular components are chemically linked to protein carriers that elicit a T cell–independent immune response, allowing for protection in young children. Three vaccines are available: two that use tetanus toxoid as the protein carrier (ActHIB [Sanofi Pasteur Inc.] and Hiberix [GlaxoSmithKline]) and one that uses *Neisseria meningitidis* group B outer membrane protein (PedvaxHIB [Merck & Co., Inc.]). In addition, there are combination vaccines that contain conjugated Hib vaccine, as shown in the Combination Vaccines section of this chapter and in Table 2. The primary childhood series is given at age 2, 4, and 6 months (with ActHIB or Hiberix) or at 2 and 4 months (with PedvaxHIB), followed by a booster dose at 12–15 months. Protective antibody response and clinical efficacy are 95%–100% after a primary series.[1] The Hib-containing vaccines should not be given to infants younger than 6 weeks because the immune response to subsequent doses is reduced.[1] The three Hib vaccines are considered interchangeable and can be given for any of the primary or booster doses; however, if PedvaxHIB is not given at age 2 and 4 months, then a 6-month dose of any Hib vaccine must be given.

Although Hib vaccines are only routinely recommended for children younger than 5 years, other patient populations may be at increased risk of infection. One dose of any Hib vaccine may be beneficial for patients who were not previously vaccinated in childhood and have sickle cell disease or asplenia, HIV infection, certain immunodeficiencies, or immunosuppression from cancer chemotherapy or in those who received a hematopoietic stem cell transplant.[1,2]

PNEUMOCOCCAL VACCINES

Streptococcus pneumoniae, a common cause of otitis media, sinusitis, pneumonia, bacteremia, and meningitis, is associated with significant morbidity and mortality in children younger than 2 years. Transmission is primarily through respiratory droplet spread. For *S. pneumoniae*, 90 capsular polysaccharide serotypes have been identified, and the 10 most common serotypes cause more than 60% of invasive disease.[1] Pneumococcal antibiotic resistance has escalated in recent years, and protection against invasive infection through vaccination is vital. Since the conjugated 7-valent vaccine (PCV7) was introduced in 2000, there has been a 99% reduction in invasive disease in young children caused by the vaccine serotypes and an additional serotype, 6A, for which the vaccine provided cross-protection.[1] Increased rates of invasive disease from non-vaccine serotypes (e.g., 19A) have emerged, leading to the introduction of an expanded multivalent vaccine in 2010.[7]

Two pneumococcal vaccines are currently available in the United States: a 13-valent pneumococcal conjugate vaccine (PCV13) and a 23-valent pneumococcal polysaccharide vaccine (PPSV23). These vaccines, which target different patient populations and age groups, are not interchangeable. Although children younger than 5 years are at increased risk of invasive disease, some factors increase the risk even further. Independent risk factors for invasive pneumococcal disease include the following: asplenia; HIV infection; patient race if Alaska Native, African American, or Native American; day care attendance; and cochlear implants.

The PCV13 elicits immunity in young children through a T cell–independent antibody response. The PCV13 contains a purified capsular polysaccharide of 13 serotypes (1, 3, 4, 5, 6A, 6B, 7F, 9V, 14, 18C, 19A, 19F, and 23F) conjugated to a nontoxic diphtheria toxin. Available since 2010 as a replacement for PCV7, administration of PCV13 is at age 2, 4, and 6 months, with a booster dose at 12–15 months. Protective antibody responses induced by PCV13 are similar to those induced by PCV7, which was more than 90% effective against invasive disease caused by vaccine serotypes.[8] Routine use of PCV13 is not recommended for healthy children 5 years and older, but incompletely vaccinated children with certain medical conditions should receive PCV13 at age 24–71 months, administered at least 8 weeks after the most recent pneumococcal vaccine dose. These conditions include the following: chronic heart or lung disease, diabetes, sickle cell disease or asplenia, cochlear implants, HIV infection, and other immunocompromised states. A single dose should also be given to children age 6–18 years with high-risk conditions (sickle cell disease or asplenia, immunocompromised states, cochlear implants, or cerebrospinal fluid leak) who have not previously received PCV13.[9]

The PPSV23 contains 23 capsular polysaccharides from the most prevalent pneumococcal serotypes. Children younger than 2 years do not mount a sufficient immune response to this vaccine. A single dose of PPSV23, administered at least 8 weeks after the most recent pneumococcal vaccine dose, is recommended for children 2 years and older with the following high-risk conditions: chronic cardiovascular, pulmonary, or liver disease; diabetes; asplenia or sickle cell disease; cochlear implants; cerebrospinal fluid leak; chronic renal failure; or immunocompromised conditions. This PPSV23 dose is administered in addition to the PCV13 vaccine series recommended previously. Protection against invasive infection from vaccine serotypes is 60%–70% overall, with conflicting results for clinical protection against nonbacteremic pneumococcal pneumonia.[1] Antibody response declines within 10 years of vaccination but can occur earlier in children. A second dose given 5 years after the first dose is recommended for children who remain at high risk of invasive disease caused by sickle cell disease or asplenia, immunocompromised conditions, or chronic renal failure.[9]

POLIO VACCINE

Polio is a highly contagious infection that, although usually asymptomatic, can rapidly deteriorate to potentially permanent flaccid paralysis. Polio is spread through the fecal–oral route and can be excreted in stool for several weeks, allowing easy spread to household contacts. After the first inactivated polio vaccine (IPV) was introduced in 1955 and the live oral polio vaccine was introduced in 1961, the incidence of paralytic polio in the United States dropped dramatically, from about 20,000 cases annually to less than 100 in 1965.[1] The last endemic case of paralytic polio in the United States was reported in 1979, but vaccine-acquired paralytic polio continued to occur because of oral polio vaccine use. In 2000, the oral polio vaccine was no longer recommended in the United States, but it is still necessary in areas of the world where polio continues to circulate.

The IPV contains three serotypes that are inactivated by formaldehyde. The IPV elicits a strong immune response but produces less gastrointestinal immunity than oral polio vaccine and has an unknown duration of protection. The childhood series should be given at age 2, 4, and 6–18 months with a booster dose at 4–6 years. Antibody response and clinical protection against infection are at least 99% after three doses.[1] This vaccine is commonly administered in combination with other antigens, as shown in the Combination Vaccines section of this chapter and in Table 2, but it is also available as a single vaccine.

ROTAVIRUS VACCINE

Rotavirus is a highly contagious virus spread through the fecal–oral route. Rotavirus is the most common cause of gastroenteritis in children worldwide, and most children are infected by age 5 years. Clinical manifestations range from asymptomatic to mild, watery diarrhea to severe dehydration from vomiting and diarrhea. Severe dehydration, which occurs mainly among children younger than 2 years, is associated with significant mortality in developing countries. Globally, more than 500,000 deaths occurred annually from rotavirus infection and dehydration, but in the United States, only 20–60 deaths occurred annually before routine rotavirus vaccination.[1,10] The first rotavirus vaccine, introduced in 1998, was associated with a markedly increased risk of intussusception and was withdrawn from the market in 1999. In 2006, a newer vaccine was reintroduced that led to a 90% reduction in rotavirus hospitalizations and almost a 50% reduction in emergency department visits for diarrhea over a 3-year period.[11]

Two live oral rotavirus vaccines are available in the United States: RotaTeq (Merck & Co., Inc.), which contains five live human-bovine reassortant rotavirus strains, and Rotarix (GlaxoSmithKline), which contains one live attenuated human rotavirus strain. These vaccines do not completely prevent infection, but studies report an 85%–98% reduction in severe gastroenteritis and a 96% reduction in hospitalization.[1] The vaccines have similar efficacy and safety data but different administration schedules. RotaTeq is given as a three-dose series and Rotarix as a two-dose series, both beginning at age 2 months, with subsequent doses given 1–2 months apart. The ACIP recommend that the maximum age for starting the vaccine series be 14 weeks and 6 days.[1] The maximum recommended age for any vaccine dose is 8 months and 0 days because intussusception is associated with increasing age at the time of vaccination. Although the vaccines are not considered interchangeable, the vaccine series can be continued or completed with either product. If any dose of RotaTeq is administered, then a three-dose series must be given. Rotavirus vaccine should not be administered to immunocompromised individuals without first consulting a specialist because rotavirus vaccine is a live viral vaccine that can cause rotavirus infection. The vaccine can be given to infants living with immunocompromised individuals as well as to infants regardless of antibody or blood product administration.

INFLUENZA VACCINE

Influenza is a highly contagious viral infection that causes significant morbidity and mortality among young children and older adults. Influenza is spread through airborne droplets or through direct contact with contaminated secretions that reach the mucus membranes. Infection usually occurs during the winter months in the Northern Hemisphere, and although all age groups are affected, children have the highest infection rate. Classic symptoms include rapid onset of fever, sore throat, myalgia, headache, nonproductive cough, malaise, and rhinorrhea, but children can also have nausea, vomiting, and otitis media (as described in the Lower Respiratory Tract Infections chapter). Pneumonia can result from primary influenza infection or secondary bacterial infection. Severe illness, hospitalization, and death are most likely in older adults, children younger than 2 years, and those with underlying conditions, including cardiopulmonary disease and pregnancy. An average of 42,000 deaths occur annually from influenza in the United States.[12] The best protection against influenza is vaccination.

Influenza A and B viruses that circulate concurrently cause human disease. Influenza A typically causes moderate to severe infection and affects all ages. Influenza A is further subtyped by its surface antigens hemagglutinin and neuraminidase. Human infections typically occur with subtypes categorized as hemagglutinin 1–3 and neuraminidase 1 or neuraminidase 2, but strains that usually infect animals (e.g., H5N1) can rarely infect humans. Influenza B usually causes milder infection and primarily infects children. Influenza B is not subtyped but is categorized as one of two lineages (Yamagata and Victoria) that have been circulating for many years. New variants are created by antigenic point mutations that evade host immunity and perpetuate the infectious cycle, known as *antigenic drift*. This variation occurs mainly with influenza A and is responsible for seasonal epidemics and the recommendation for annual vaccination. *Antigenic shift* occurs when influenza A virus acquires a new surface antigen as a result of genetic reassortment; these strains have pandemic potential because they are dissimilar to previously circulating influenza strains.

Two types of inactivated influenza vaccines (IIVs) are currently recommended to prevent seasonal influenza in children, both of which contain the same strains or subunit antigens of two influenza A subtypes and either one or two influenza B strains (trivalent or IIV3, or quadrivalent or IIV4, respectively). Currently, neither vaccine is preferred to the other. A cell culture–based inactivated quadrivalent vaccine (Flucelvax, Sequirus USA Inc., Summit, New Jersey) is a non–egg-based vaccine that is available for children 4 years and older. Other types of IIV, including an adjuvant trivalent vaccine, a high-dose trivalent vaccine, and a recombinant quadrivalent vaccine, are approved for use only in adults.

A live attenuated influenza vaccine (LAIV) is available that is cold adapted and administered intranasally, allowing local viral replication in the nasopharynx after administration but not in warm environments such as the lung. The current LAIV (FluMist Quadrivalent, MedImmune LLC, Gaithersburg, Maryland) is quadrivalent and is a vaccine option for those in whom it is appropriate (Table 1).[13]

Annual vaccination is recommended for all individuals 6 months and older because the duration of immunity is less than 1 year, given waning immunity and antigenic drift. Children age 6 months to 8 years who receive influenza vaccine for the first time or who have previously received only one vaccine dose should receive two doses, separated by at least 4 weeks.[13] The IIV can be administered to all patients, including those with high-risk conditions. Many manufacturers produce IIV annually, and each product has different age indications. Clinicians should see the CDC website at www.cdc.gov/flu on an annual basis for published tables listing influenza vaccine products and the age groups indicated for each vaccine because the products vary each year. Vaccine efficacy against laboratory-confirmed influenza infection also varies each year and has been 10%–60% since 2004–2005, depending on vaccine strain components and their match to circulating viruses each season.[14] Historically, influenza vaccine was contraindicated in individuals with egg allergies, but recent evidence suggests that any vaccine type can safely be given to patients who have only hives.[13] Referral to a health care provider who can manage severe allergic reactions is recommended when IIV or LAIV is administered to individuals who have had a serious reaction to eggs, including the following: angioedema, respiratory distress, lightheadedness, or recurrent emesis, or patients needing epinephrine or other emergency interventions.

HEPATITIS A VACCINE

Hepatitis A virus causes a self-limiting acute hepatitis characterized by fever, malaise, jaundice, and abdominal pain in adults and older children; however, hepatitis A is often asymptomatic in children younger than 6 years. Chronic infection does not occur, and death is extremely rare. Children may serve as a viral reservoir because of their lack of symptoms and prolonged viral shedding. Infection usually occurs by ingesting contaminated water or food or through the fecal-oral route. Hepatitis A is endemic in some areas of the world, but epidemics occurred about every 10 years in the United States in the prevaccine era, with the last increase reported in 1994–1995.[1] Children age 2–18 years and people living in Western states had the highest infection rates. Hepatitis A vaccine was initially recommended only for high-risk groups such as international travelers and for children who lived where infection rates were twice the U.S. average. In 2006, universal vaccination for all children was recommended, which has resulted in almost a 94% reduction in reported cases.[1,15]

Hepatitis A vaccine is an inactivated whole-virus vaccine that is available in two formulations as a single-virus vaccine (Havrix [GlaxoSmithKline] and Vaqta [Merck & Co., Inc.]). The two-dose series should begin at age 12–23 months, with the second dose given 6–18 months later. The single-virus vaccines are considered interchangeable. Protective antibodies develop in almost 100% of children after two doses, and clinical protection against infection occurs in 94%–100% of children.[1] Hepatitis A vaccine should also be strongly considered for anyone age 1 year or older with a high risk of infection including the following: homelessness; travel to a country with high or intermediate endemicity; close contact with an international adoptee from a country with high or intermediate endemicity; or a clotting factor disorder or chronic liver disease.[16-18] Hepatitis A vaccine is also available in combination with hepatitis B vaccine, but this vaccine is only approved for adults, as noted in the Combination Vaccines section of this chapter and in Table 2.

MEASLES, MUMPS, AND RUBELLA VACCINE

Measles, a highly contagious viral illness spread through respiratory droplets, leads to viremia and infection of the respiratory tract and other organs. Measles begins with a high temperature, cough, and rhinorrhea before progressing to its characteristic maculopapular rash, which begins at the hairline and spreads downward and outward. Koplik spots, which are pathognomonic for measles, are small blue-white spots that appear on the bright red buccal mucosa near the time the rash appears. Complications include diarrhea, pneumonia, encephalitis, and, rarely, death. In the prevaccine era, up to 4 million cases occurred annually in the United States, with more than 50% of cases reported in children age 5–9 years.[1] After the measles vaccine was introduced in 1963, the incidence decreased by more than 95% to a nadir of about 1500 cases in 1983. A resurgence occurred in 1989–1991, with a disproportionate number of cases reported in young children. Immunization efforts were subsequently enhanced in preschool-age children, and measles was declared eliminated in the United States in 2000. However, hundreds of cases per year are still reported because of importation from foreign countries, where unvaccinated travelers contract the infection and spread it to unvaccinated individuals when they return. There were 667 cases in 2014 and 372 cases in 2018, which were caused mainly by importation from the Philippines and Israel and subsequent spread to Amish and Orthodox Jewish communities with low vaccination rates.[19] In 2019, over 1200 cases were reported in 31 states, with 75% of cases linked to outbreaks in New York, which is the greatest number of cases in the United States since 1992.[19]

Measles vaccine is a live attenuated viral vaccine that is only available in combination with mumps and rubella vaccine (as MMR) or in combination with varicella vaccine (MMRV), as shown in the Combination Vaccines section of this chapter and in Table 2. After administration, measles vaccine produces a subclinical and noncommunicable infection that results in immunity in 95% of individuals. A second dose provides immunity to 99% of individuals and forms the basis for the two-dose series recommendation.[20]

Mumps is a viral illness spread through respiratory droplets that has a nonspecific prodrome of myalgia, headache, and low-grade fever, followed by its characteristic parotitis in 30%–65% of cases and aseptic meningitis in up to 10% of cases.[1] Orchitis occurs in up to 66% of postpubertal males, and rare complications include pancreatitis and deafness. After the mumps vaccine was introduced in 1967, the number of reported cases in the United States decreased by 99%, with annual reports of 200–2000.[1,21] Similar to the increase in measles, outbreaks of mumps continue to occur among those who are unvaccinated or who have received only one dose of mumps vaccine. Outbreaks are also increasingly being reported in fully immunized individuals, particularly on college campuses, because of crowded living conditions, frequent social gatherings that facilitate spread, and waning immunity. From January 2016 through June 2017, 9200 cases in 150 outbreaks were reported, with the largest outbreak occurring in an Arkansas community with almost 3000 cases.[21]

Mumps vaccine is a live attenuated vaccine containing the Jeryl Lynn strain, which is only available in combination with measles and rubella vaccine (as MMR) or in combination with varicella vaccine (MMRV), as shown in the Combination Vaccines section and in Table 2. After administration, mumps vaccine produces a subclinical and noncommunicable infection that is protective in 78% of individuals after one dose and in 88% of individuals after two doses.[20] Two doses of a mumps-containing vaccine are currently recommended, but a third dose is recommended for individuals who are identified by public health authorities as part of a group or population at increased risk of acquisition during an outbreak.[22]

Rubella is a viral infection that is often asymptomatic but can cause a maculopapular rash, lymphadenopathy, low-grade fever, and mild respiratory symptoms. Rubella is spread through airborne droplets or through direct contact with contaminated secretions. Rubella vaccination was developed to prevent congenital rubella syndrome, which occurred in up to 85% of infants whose mothers were infected during the first trimester of pregnancy.[1] Congenital rubella syndrome is characterized by congenital deafness, cataracts or glaucoma, heart disease, microcephaly and mental retardation, and other organ defects. Rubella acquired during pregnancy can also result in miscarriage or stillbirth. After rubella vaccination began in 1969, reported rubella cases were reduced by more than 98%.[1] Rubella is no longer considered endemic in the United States, although two or three congenital rubella cases are reported each year.

Rubella vaccine is a live attenuated vaccine that is only available in combination with measles and mumps vaccine (as MMR) or in combination with varicella vaccine (as MMRV), as detailed in the Combination Vaccines section of this chapter and in Table 2. More than 95% of people develop immunity after a single dose of rubella vaccine, and most are protected for at least 15 years.[1] At least one dose of rubella-containing vaccine is recommended to be given at age 12 months or older.

The MMR vaccine is given as a two-dose series to elicit an immune response in those who did not respond to the first dose. The first dose should be given no earlier than age 12 months, and the second dose should be given at age 4–6 years before the child enters elementary school. The second dose can be given as early as 28 days after the first dose. Children age 6–12 months who are traveling to endemic areas should be vaccinated before travel, but they must be revaccinated with two doses beginning at age 12 months or older. Because the MMR vaccine contains live viruses, it is contraindicated in pregnancy and immunosuppressed patients, except in asymptomatic patients or those with mild HIV infection. Measles can be severe in those infected with HIV; thus, the benefits outweigh the risks of vaccinating people with asymptomatic or mild HIV infection.

VARICELLA VACCINE

Varicella is a highly contagious airborne infection caused by varicella zoster virus. Primary infection causes chickenpox characterized by malaise, fever, and characteristic pruritic macules, which progress to vesicles that erupt and crust over during a period of several days (as detailed in the Skin and Soft Tissue Infections of Bacterial and Viral Etiology chapter). Secondary bacterial skin infections are a common complication. Adults and immunocompromised individuals have more severe illness, including pneumonia and encephalitis. After the primary infection resolves, the virus becomes dormant in the dorsal nerves and can reactivate as herpes zoster, or shingles, creating a pruritic, vesicular rash along a single nerve track. Zoster usually occurs in older adults and immunocompromised individuals. Up to 20% of individuals with zoster develop postherpetic neuralgia, a painful condition that persists for months after the zoster rash resolves. Before the varicella vaccine was introduced in 1995, varicella was endemic in the United States, infecting around 4 million individuals annually, leading to 11,000 hospitalizations and 100 deaths each year.[1] The highest incidence of infection was in children age 1–9 years, and near-universal infection occurred by adulthood. Routine vaccination has reduced infection rates by 97% and reduced hospitalizations and deaths by more than 70% and 88%, respectively.[1] The impact of varicella vaccination on zoster is not completely known, but the risk of zoster appears to be lower after vaccination than with natural infection and reported cases have been mild with no reported postherpetic neuralgia.[1]

Varicella vaccine is a live attenuated vaccine given as a two-dose series to enhance immunity and minimize the breakthrough disease that occurs with single doses.[23] Varicella vaccine is available as a single vaccine or in combination with MMR (as MMRV), presented in the Combination Vaccines section of this chapter and in Table 2. The first dose is given at age 12–15 months with a second dose at age 4–6 years, but the second dose can be given as early as 3 months after the first dose (for children younger than 13 years) or as early as 4 weeks (for children 13 years and older). Protective antibodies develop after one dose in 97% of children age 12 months to 12 years. Clinical efficacy against infection is estimated to be 70%–90%, and protection against severe disease is 90%–100%.[1] Varicella vaccine is contraindicated in pregnancy and in immunosuppressed patients, but it should be considered for children with HIV infection whose CD4 cell percentage is at least 15%.[23] Vaccine-strain varicella can be transmitted by individuals after vaccination, particularly by those who

develop a rash; these individuals should avoid contact with high-risk people who are not immune to varicella.

MENINGOCOCCAL VACCINE

Neisseria meningitidis is a common cause of meningitis and sepsis in children and adolescents in the United States. Most infections are caused by five encapsulated strains designated serogroups A, B, C, Y, and W-135. Infection is spread through respiratory droplets or contaminated secretions. Meningococcal sepsis is fatal in 40% of patients despite antibiotics and supportive therapy, and about 20% of survivors have permanent sequelae including deafness, neurologic damage, or loss of limbs.[1] Meningococcal disease rates have decreased, particularly for infections caused by serogroups C and Y among children age 11–14 years, since the routine adolescent meningococcal vaccine was introduced in 2005.[24] Individuals age 16–21 years still have high infection rates despite routine vaccination. Outbreaks of meningococcal disease continue, mainly caused by serogroups B and C, but outbreaks make up less than 2% of reported cases.

Two inactivated meningococcal vaccines containing serogroups A, C, Y, and W-135 are available that are conjugated to different protein carriers to enhance immunogenicity (Menactra [Sanofi Pasteur Inc.] and Menveo [GlaxoSmithKline]). These vaccines are licensed for individuals age 9 months to 55 years, but Menveo is also approved for children as young as 2 months. A protective immune response occurs in about 75% of adolescents, but antibody concentrations wane within 3–5 years of vaccination.[1] Routine vaccination with a single dose of either conjugate vaccine is recommended at age 11–12 years, with a booster dose at 16 years that is expected to provide immunity through the high-risk adolescent and early adult period.[24] Children with persistent complement component deficiency, asplenia, or HIV and children who receive eculizumab should also receive meningococcal conjugate vaccine beginning as early as age 2 months (with Menveo only), according to recommended schedules.[1,25,26] For these high-risk populations, booster doses should be given every 5 years; however, if the most recent dose was given before age 7 years, then the first booster dose should be given 3 years later. Individuals 9 months and older who travel to an endemic area should receive meningococcal conjugate vaccine before travel. These vaccines can also be used to control outbreaks caused by vaccine-specific strains.[1]

Two meningococcal serogroup B vaccines consisting of recombinant proteins are recommended for use in patients age 16–23 years, preferably at 16–18 years, to prevent invasive group B infection.[27] These meningococcal vaccines should also be given to children 10 years and older with risk factors for meningococcal disease, including asplenia and persistent complement component deficiency, or during a serogroup B outbreak. Bexsero (GlaxoSmithKline) is given as a two-dose series and Trumenba (Pfizer Inc., Philadelphia) as a two- or three-dose series; these vaccines are not considered interchangeable. Protective antibodies develop in 63%–88% of adolescents on completion of the series, but antibody concentrations wane over time.[27]

HUMAN PAPILLOMAVIRUS VACCINE

Human papillomavirus (HPV), the most common sexually transmitted disease in the United States, is associated with genital warts, cervical cancer, and other anogenital cancers. More than 120 different HPV types have been identified, but four are the most common causes of genital warts and cervical cancer: low-risk HPV types 6 and 11 cause 90% of genital warts, and high-risk HPV types 16 and 18 cause 70% of all cervical cancers.[1] Most infections are asymptomatic, which allows viral propagation to occur among unknowing partners. More than 14 million new infections are estimated to occur annually in the United States, most commonly among adolescents and young adults.[1]

An inactivated HPV vaccine is available that contains virus-like particles from nine HPV types: 6, 11, 16, 18, 31, 33, 45, 52, and 58 (HPV9 as Gardasil 9 [Merck & Co., Inc.]). This inactivated HPV vaccine is 97% effective in preventing precancerous lesions from vaccine types in females age 16–26 years.[28] The seroconversion rate to all vaccine types is almost 100% in males and females alike at age 9–26 years. Routine vaccination is recommended at age 11–12 years, but the series can be initiated at 9 years. Ideally, individuals should be vaccinated before exposure through sexual contact, but sexually active male and female adolescents and young adults age 13–26 years should still be vaccinated. A two-dose series is recommended for children age 9–14 years; a three-dose series is recommended for adolescents and young adults age 15–26 years and those who are immunocompromised. In 2018, Gardasil 9 was approved for use in male and female adults through age 45 years, but ACIP does not recommend routine catch-up vaccination for this age group and only recommends considering it in those not adequately vaccinated who are most likely to benefit (e.g., having new sex partners without prior sexual activity).[29]

COMBINATION VACCINES

Combination vaccines reduce the number of injections and increase the chances that the immunization schedule will be completed, particularly for infants who require several injections at each health encounter. Combination vaccines, which typically contain components that are given on a similar dosing schedule, result in immune responses similar to those of separately administered components. Several combination vaccines are available in the United States, with specific administration indications (Table 2). Despite their convenience, some of these vaccines cost $10–$25 more than single-component vaccines given separately, and they may result in up to 10% higher rates of fever and local skin reactions than single-component vaccines given separately. One combination vaccine, MMRV, is associated with a 2-fold higher rate of febrile seizures than the MMR and varicella vaccines given separately for the first dose in the series.[1,30] The ACIP recommends that the MMR and varicella vaccines be given separately for the first doses in the series, but MMRV is preferred for the second dose.

SPECIAL POPULATIONS

IMMUNOCOMPROMISED PATIENTS

A patient's response to a vaccine can be altered if the vaccine is given during an immunosuppressed state. All vaccines should be given before immunosuppression, when possible, and live vaccines should not be given to severely immunocompromised individuals. Live vaccines should not be given to patients within 3 months of chemotherapy or to patients receiving immunosuppressive doses of glucocorticoids (2 mg/kg/day of prednisone or an equivalent dose of another steroid for at least 2 weeks).[31] Live vaccines should not be given post-transplantation to patients with solid-organ transplants, but they can be considered 2 years after a hematopoietic stem cell transplant if the child is believed to be immunocompetent.[31] Inactivated vaccines may be less effective in these populations, but they can be given 6 months post-transplantation or 1 month after discontinuation of high-dose steroids.[1,31] Household contacts of immunosuppressed individuals should receive all routinely recommended vaccines.

PREGNANT WOMEN

Women who are pregnant or trying to become pregnant should receive all routinely recommended vaccines, when indicated, to ensure that sufficient antibodies are passed to the fetus to protect the infant after birth. Live vaccines should not be given during pregnancy to avoid the risk of transplacental infection of the fetus. Inactivated influenza vaccine should be given to women who are or will be pregnant during influenza season. For women during each pregnancy Tdap should be given, ideally in the early part of gestational weeks 27–36, to protect the infant after birth. Household contacts of pregnant women should be vaccinated according to usual schedules and recommendations.

VACCINE SAFETY

Vaccines are an important public health measure used to prevent disease, but they are not completely free of harm. Although most adverse reactions are acute, mild, and self-limiting, rarely occurring events can be serious and potentially fatal. Many people have not had a time when vaccine-preventable diseases were common in children, and the very low but potential risk of harm from vaccines may be perceived to outweigh their benefit. In the United States, vaccine information statements must be provided before vaccinations to give information on the risk–benefit of each vaccine. This information in turn gives health care providers an opportunity to discuss benefit–risk with patients and caregivers. Public education and vaccine safety surveillance are vital for public confidence in vaccines and the subsequent success of immunization programs.

Vaccine safety is monitored by the CDC and the U.S. Food and Drug Administration through the Vaccine Adverse Event Reporting System (VAERS), which captures adverse events that can be reported by health care providers, manufacturers, and the public. Reports to VAERS can occur by mail, by fax, or on the VAERS website at http://vaers.hhs.gov. Health care providers are mandated to report specific adverse events that are serious or life threatening. Some vaccine-specific adverse effects are included in Table 1.

MILD REACTIONS

The most common types of adverse reactions are local reactions and fever. Pain, swelling, and erythema at the injection site occur after up to 80% of vaccine doses.[1] These reactions are more common with repeated or booster doses because of the antibody presence and rapid immune response from previous doses. Local reactions are most common with inactivated adjuvant-containing vaccines, such as those containing diphtheria and tetanus toxoids. *Fever*, defined as a temperature higher than 100.4°F (38°C), occurs because of cytokine production during the immune response to a vaccine. Fever is most commonly reported after the administration of live vaccines. These vaccines can also produce symptoms similar to a mild form of the natural disease they protect against because the administered viruses must replicate to induce immunity. The MMR and varicella vaccines can cause rash (self-resolving) and fever within 7–21 days after vaccination.

Efforts to minimize pain and discomfort from vaccines can benefit both the vaccinee and the parent or caregiver. Effective methods for reducing distress and pain in infants and young children include the following: breastfeeding around the time of vaccination; having the child ingest 2 mL of 50% sucrose solution 1–2 minutes before vaccination with concomitant pacifier use; holding the child during vaccination; using topical anesthetics such as lidocaine/prilocaine; distracting the child with toys or videos led by a nurse; or combinations of these interventions.[2,32-34] In children 4 years and older, effective methods for reducing distress and pain include the following: deep-breathing exercises; child-directed distraction (e.g., music or stories played through headphones); nurse-led distraction; use of topical anesthetics; or combinations of these interventions.[32,34] Routine use of acetaminophen or ibuprofen before vaccination is discouraged; this practice does not prevent febrile reactions and may blunt the immune response to vaccines.[2,35] These medications can be considered for treating fever (e.g., temperature higher than 101.5°F [38.6°C]) or local discomfort that occurs after vaccination. Only acetaminophen should be used for children younger than 6 months.

THIMEROSAL AND AUTISM

Thimerosal was a commonly used mercury-based vaccine preservative until the late 1990s, when vaccine manufacturers began to produce thimerosal-free products in response to reports that children might receive unacceptably high amounts of mercury through routine vaccines. Methylmercury is neurotoxic at high doses and is found in the environment and in fish; moreover, it accumulates in the body. Ethylmercury is a metabolite of thimerosal for which the toxicities are not well studied, but it has no known limits of exposure and does not accumulate in the body. After concerns arose that thimerosal exposure could cause autism, several studies showed that children exposed to thimerosal-containing vaccines did not have a higher autism rate than children not exposed to thimerosal-containing vaccines, strongly suggesting that there is no association.[1,36,37] However, despite a lack of evidence linking thimerosal exposure to autism, all childhood vaccines now are either thimerosal free or contain only trace amounts of mercury (less than 0.3 mcg/0.5 mL), except for the multidose influenza vaccines, which contain no more than 25 mcg of mercury per 0.5 mL. Even with the removal of thimerosal from vaccines and the lack of evidence to support that vaccines cause autism, some people still believe there is a link between vaccination and autism, perhaps related to the number of antigens contained in vaccines or other ingredients such as aluminum. Yet large case-control and cohort studies have found no links between these proposed causes and development of autism spectrum disorder.[38-40]

SYNCOPE

Syncope after vaccination is a rare adverse event that can lead to considerable complications, including skull fracture and intracranial hemorrhage. Syncope is most likely in adolescents within 15 minutes after receiving HPV, Tdap, or meningococcal conjugate vaccines.[2] Adolescents should be vaccinated while seated and encouraged to remain seated for 15 minutes after vaccination to minimize injury, should fainting occur.

PRECAUTIONS AND CONTRAINDICATIONS

Precautions and contraindications are conditions in which vaccines should be avoided to prevent adverse events. *Precautions* are conditions in which the risk or severity of an adverse event may be increased or the ability for the vaccine to induce immunity may be compromised. Vaccination is often deferred in these conditions because such conditions are temporary; in some instances, the health care provider may opt to vaccinate the patient because the benefit outweighs the risk. Common precautions include minor acute illnesses with or without fever and mild to moderate local reactions or febrile response to a previous dose of the vaccine. *Contraindications* are conditions in which the risk of a serious adverse event is increased; vaccines are rarely administered when contraindications are present. A contraindication for every vaccine is a severe allergic reaction, such as anaphylaxis, to a previous dose of the vaccine or one of its components. Table 1 lists vaccine-specific precautions and contraindications for childhood and adolescent vaccines.

VACCINE INFORMATION SOURCES

Health care providers need to stay current with vaccination recommendations and updated schedules to best serve their patients. Many reliable Internet sources provide information on ACIP recommendations, schedules, vaccine safety, and links to other vaccination-related websites (Table 3). Many of these sites also provide information for parents or caregivers. However, hundreds of websites also exist that provide incorrect or misleading information on vaccines; thus, health care providers should direct the public to the proper websites for trustworthy vaccine information.

CONCLUSIONS

Vaccine-preventable diseases are at near-record low rates in the United States because of the successful implementation of routine childhood vaccinations. Health care providers involved in delivering immunization must be knowledgeable about vaccine schedules and recommendations and must evaluate patients for their vaccination status at every health care encounter. Efforts to educate the public about vaccine effectiveness and safety and successful vaccination programs are vital for maintaining widespread immunization coverage and preventing outbreaks of vaccine-preventable diseases.

Table 3. Reliable Vaccine Information Source Websites

Website	Source	Information
www.aimtoolkit.org	Alliance for Immunization in Michigan (AIM)	Free downloadable information for providers and parents; "quick-look" handouts useful for providers
www.cdc.gov/mmwr	*Morbidity and Mortality Weekly Report*, CDC	ACIP recommendations and updates; national immunization coverage rates and disease activity; free electronic subscription
www.cdc.gov/vaccines	Vaccines and Immunizations, CDC	Information for providers and parents on immunizations, schedules, safety; links to other websites
www.cdc.gov/vaccines/pubs/pinkbook/index.html	Epidemiology and Prevention of Vaccine-Preventable Diseases, CDC	Comprehensive information on vaccine-preventable diseases for providers
www.immunize.org	Immunization Action Coalition	Free downloadable information for providers and parents; subscription to free electronic newsletters
https://www.chop.edu/centers-programs/vaccine-education-center	Vaccine Education Center, Children's Hospital of Philadelphia	Vaccine information for parents and providers
www.vaccinesafety.edu	Institute for Vaccine Safety, Johns Hopkins Bloomberg School of Public Health	Objective and timely information on vaccine safety for providers and parents
http://vaers.hhs.gov/index	VAERS, CDC, and FDA	Reportable vaccine adverse events; forms to report adverse events to CDC and FDA; links to other vaccine safety websites

ACIP = CDC Advisory Committee on Immunization Practices; CDC = Centers for Disease Control and Prevention; FDA = U.S. Food and Drug Administration (FDA); VAERS = FDA Vaccine Adverse Event Reporting System.

A 6-month-old boy is brought to the pediatrician's office by his mother with concerns about a possible ear infection. She states that he did not sleep well last night because he woke up more than usual and appeared to be uncomfortable, and he has been fussy this morning and rubbing his right ear periodically. He did not eat as much as usual this morning, but he did take in his usual amount of formula. He felt warm to the touch, but his mother did not take his temperature because she could not find the thermometer. She reports no other concerns.

Medical history: Born at 38 weeks' gestation by normal spontaneous vaginal delivery; no hospitalizations or complications since birth; upper respiratory tract infection 2 months ago that resolved completely

Family history: Mother and 5-year-old sister have asthma; mother and father have allergic rhinitis

Social history: Lives at home with parents and sister; attends day care 3 days a week; no passive smoke exposure; no recent or planned travel

Allergies: None

Current medications: None

Immunizations:

Vaccine	Product	Age When Given
Hepatitis B	Engerix-B	Birth
	Pediarix	2 mo
Diphtheria, tetanus, and acellular pertussis (DTaP)	Pediarix	2 mo
Haemophilus influenzae type b (Hib)	ActHIB	2 mo
Polio	Pediarix	2 mo
Pneumococcal	Prevnar 13[a]	2 mo
Rotavirus	Rotarix	2 mo

[a]Pfizer Inc., Philadelphia

Vital signs: BP 85/55 mm Hg, HR 100 beats/minute, RR 25 breaths/minute, Tmax 99.5°F (37.5°C); Ht 26 inches; Wt 8.2 kg

Physical examination:

General: 6-Month-old boy who is fussy but in no acute distress

Skin: No abnormalities; normal skin turgor; capillary refill less than 3 seconds

HEENT: Pupils equal, round, and reactive to light and accommodation; extraocular movements intact; moist mucous membranes; slight erythema of right tympanic membrane without bulging or obvious effusion; left tympanic membrane not visible because of cerumen; slight rhinorrhea and minimal crusting of both nares; throat normal

Neck and Lymph Nodes: Normal; nontender

Pulmonary: Lungs clear to auscultation

Cardiovascular: Normal heart sounds; regular rate and rhythm

Abdomen: Nontender; no distension; positive bowel sounds

Neuro: Grossly intact

Genitourinary/Rectal: Deferred

Assessment: A 6-month-old boy with signs and symptoms consistent with an upper respiratory tract infection; immunizations are not up to date.

1. What vaccines should be considered for administration in this child, given the recommended schedule, and how can his immunizations be brought up to date?

The recommended vaccines that this patient did not receive at age 4 months are rotavirus, DTaP, Hib, 13-valent pneumococcal conjugate vaccine (PCV13), and inactivated polio vaccine (IPV); therefore, these vaccines should all be considered for administration at this visit. Because this boy is now age 6 months, he is also due for the third dose of hepatitis B vaccine and his first influenza vaccine. Today, he could receive all of these as single vaccines. Or, he could receive Pediarix, which contains hepatitis B, DTaP, and IPV, as an alternative to three separate injections; Hib, PCV13, rotavirus, and influenza vaccines. Pediarix is the preferred vaccine to minimize the number of intramuscular injections that this patient will receive at one time. To catch up with the recommended schedule, he should return in 4 weeks to receive DTaP (third dose), Hib (third dose), IPV (third dose), and PCV13 (third dose). These vaccines can be given using Pentacel (DTaP, IPV, and Hib) and PCV13 to minimize injections. He should also receive his second influenza vaccine in 4 weeks; this vaccination is recommended as a two-dose series for infants who are receiving influenza vaccine for the first time. He may also need a third dose of rotavirus vaccine in 4 weeks, but only if he does not receive Rotarix for his second dose. After that visit, his vaccinations will be up to date; he can resume the usual schedule beginning no earlier than age 13 months because he must wait at least 6 months after the third DTaP dose before he can receive the fourth DTaP dose. He could receive the measles, mumps, and rubella and varicella vaccines as early as age 12 months, but it would be more convenient to administer these vaccines when he returns for his fourth DTaP dose.

2. The child's mother states, "My mother told me that kids should not be immunized when they are sick. Won't giving all of these vaccines today be harmful?" How should you respond?

Vaccines can safely be given to children with mild illnesses with or without fever. Vaccines are contraindicated in only a few instances, none of which is present in this child. A temporary precaution to giving any vaccine is the presence of moderate or severe acute illness; however, there is no evidence that a concurrent illness reduces vaccine effectiveness or increases adverse events. Vaccines can cause fever, which may complicate the management of a severe illness. Mild illnesses such as upper respiratory tract infections, otitis media, mild gastroenteritis, or low-grade fevers are not valid indications for postponing vaccines; studies show that children with these conditions respond well to vaccines, with no increased risk of serious adverse events. There is no defined body temperature above which vaccines should be avoided, and the decision to vaccinate should not rely on body temperature alone. Giving these vaccines to the child today will not be harmful.

3. What adverse reactions could occur after administration of today's vaccines? What measures can be used to prevent or treat these reactions, if they occur?

The most common adverse reactions are local injection-site reactions (pain, swelling, and erythema) and fever. Ways to minimize distress and pain caused by injections include the following: feeding around the time of administration; giving 2 mL of 50% sucrose solution 1–2 minutes before vaccination with concomitant pacifier use; having a parent hold the child during vaccination; using topical anesthetics such as lidocaine/prilocaine; distracting the child with toys or videos led by a nurse; or combinations of these interventions. If pain (as evidenced by fussiness or crying) or fever (e.g., temperature higher than 101.5°F [38.6°C]) occurs over the 24–48 hours after vaccine administration, then acetaminophen or ibuprofen can be given to relieve these symptoms.

Although serious adverse reactions are uncommon, they should result in prompt medical attention. Examples of serious reactions include significant swelling of the extremity where the vaccines were administered, seizures, temperature greater than 105°F (40.6°C), lethargy, hives, swelling of the face or throat, and difficulty breathing. Rotavirus vaccine can also cause intussusception; warning signs include stomach pain with severe crying, significant vomiting, bloody stools, weakness, and extreme irritability.

4. What electronic resources can you refer the child's mother to for reliable information on vaccines and related information?

The child's mother can be referred to any of the following sites, which provide reliable vaccine information for patients and parents or caregivers: www.cdc.gov/vaccines, www.immunize.org, www.chop.edu/centers-programs/vaccine-education-center, and www.vaccinesafety.edu.

REFERENCES

1. Centers for Disease Control and Prevention (CDC). Hamborsky J, Kroger A, Wolfe S, eds. Epidemiology and Prevention of Vaccine-Preventable Diseases, 13th ed. Washington, DC: Public Health Foundation, 2015.
2. Kroger AT, Duchin J, Vázquez M. General Best Practice Guidelines for Immunization. Best Practices Guidance of the Advisory Committee on Immunization Practices (ACIP). Available at www.cdc.gov/vaccines/hcp/acip-recs/general-recs/index.html. Accessed September 27, 2019.
3. Centers for Disease Control and Prevention (CDC). A comprehensive immunization strategy to eliminate transmission of hepatitis B virus infection in the United States: recommendation of the Advisory Committee on Immunization Practices (ACIP). Part 1. Immunization of infants, children, and adolescents. MMWR Recomm Rep 2005;54:1-23.
4. Centers for Disease Control and Prevention (CDC). CDC Health Information for International Travel 2016. New York: Oxford University Press, 2016.
5. Broder KR, Cortese MM, Iskander JK, et al. Preventing tetanus, diphtheria, and pertussis among adolescents: use of tetanus toxoid, reduced diphtheria toxoid, and acellular pertussis vaccines. Recommendations of the Advisory Committee on Immunization Practices (ACIP). MMWR Recomm Rep 2006;55:1-34.

6. Liang JL, Tiwari T, Moro P, et al. Prevention of pertussis, tetanus, and diphtheria with vaccines in the United States: Recommendations of the Advisory Committee on Immunization Practices (ACIP). MMWR Recomm Rep2018;67:1-44.

7. Centers for Disease Control and Prevention (CDC). Invasive pneumococcal disease in young children before the licensure of 13-valent pneumococcal conjugate vaccine—United States, 2007. MMWR 2010;59:253-7.

8. Nuorti JP, Whitney GC, Centers for Disease Control and Prevention (CDC). Prevention of pneumococcal disease among infants and children—use of 13-valent pneumococcal conjugate vaccine and 23-valent pneumococcal polysaccharide vaccine. Recommendations of the Advisory Committee on Immunization Practices (ACIP). MMWR Recomm Rep 2010;59:1-18.

9. Centers for Disease Control and Prevention (CDC). Use of PCV-13 and PPSV-23 vaccines among children 6–18 years with immunocompromising conditions. MMWR 2013;62:521-4.

10. Cortese MM, Parashar UD, Centers for Disease Control and Prevention (CDC). Prevention of rotavirus gastroenteritis among infants and children. Recommendations of the Advisory Committee on Immunization Practices (ACIP). MMWR Recomm Rep 2009;58:1-25.

11. Cortes JE, Curns AT, Tate JE, et al. Rotavirus vaccine and health care utilization for diarrhea in U.S. children. N Engl J Med 2011;365:1108-17.

12. Centers for Disease Control and Prevention (CDC). Past seasons estimated influenza disease burden. Available at www.cdc.gov/flu/about/burden/past-seasons.html. Accessed September 27, 2019.

13. Grohskopf LA, Alyanak E, Broder KR, et al. Prevention and control of seasonal influenza with vaccines: recommendations of the Advisory Committee on Immunization Practices—United States, 2019–20 influenza season. MMWR Recomm Rep 2019;68:1-21.

14. Centers for Disease Control and Prevention (CDC). CDC seasonal influenza vaccine effectiveness. Available at https://www.cdc.gov/flu/vaccines-work/effectiveness-studies.htm. Accessed September 27, 2019.

15. Advisory Committee on Immunization Practices (ACIP), Fiore AE, Wasley A, et al. Prevention of hepatitis A through active or passive immunization. Recommendations of the Advisory Committee on Immunization Practices (ACIP). MMWR Recomm Rep 2006;55:1-23.

16. Doshani M, Weng M, Moore KL, et al. Recommendations of the Advisory Committee on Immunization Practices for use of hepatitis A vaccine for persons experiencing homelessness. MMWR 2019;68:153-6.

17. Nelson NP, Link-Gelles R, Hofmeister MG, et al. Update: recommendations of the Advisory Committee on Immunization Practices for use of hepatitis A vaccine for postexposure prophylaxis and for preexposure prophylaxis for international travel. MMWR 2018;67:1216-20.

18. Centers for Disease Control and Prevention (CDC). Updated recommendations from the Advisory Committee on Immunization Practices (ACIP) for use of hepatitis A vaccine in close contacts of newly arriving international adoptees. MMWR 2009;58:1006-7.

19. Centers for Disease Control and Prevention (CDC). Measles cases and outbreaks. Available at https://www.cdc.gov/measles/cases-outbreaks.html. Accessed September 27, 2019.

20. McLean HQ, Fiebelkorn AP, Temte JL, et al. Prevention of measles, rubella, congenital rubella syndrome, and mumps, 2013: summary recommendations of the Advisory Committee on Immunization Practices (ACIP). MMWR Recomm Rep 2013; 62:1-34.

21. Centers for Disease Control and Prevention (CDC). Mumps cases and outbreaks. Available at www.cdc.gov/mumps/outbreaks.html. Accessed September 27, 2019.

22. Marin M, Marlow M, Moore KL, et al. Recommendations of the Advisory Committee on Immunization Practices for use of a third dose of mumps virus-containing vaccine in persons at risk for mumps during an outbreak. MMWR 2018;67:33-8.

23. Marin M, Guris D, Chaves SS, et al. Prevention of varicella: recommendations of the Advisory Committee on Immunization Practices (ACIP). MMWR Recomm Rep 2007;56:1-40.

24. Cohn AC, MacNeil JR, Clark TA, et al. Prevention and control of meningococcal disease: recommendations of the Advisory Committee on Immunization Practices (ACIP). MMWR Recomm Rep 2013;62:1-28.

25. MacNeil JR, Rubin L, McNamara L, et al. Use of MenACWY-CRM vaccine in children aged 2 through 23 months at increased risk for meningococcal disease: recommendations of the Advisory Committee on Immunization Practices, 2013. MMWR 2014;63:527-30.

26. MacNeil JR, Rubin LG, Patton M, et al. Recommendations for use of meningococcal conjugate vaccines in HIV-infected persons—Advisory Committee on Immunization Practices, 2016. MMWR 2016;65:1189-94.

27. MacNeil JR, Rubin L, Folaranmi T, et al. Use of serogroup B meningococcal vaccines in adolescents and young adults: recommendations of the Advisory Committee on Immunization Practices, 2015. MMWR 2015;64:1171-6.

28. Petrosky E, Bocchini JA Jr., Hariri S, et al. Use of 9-valent human papillomavirus (HPV) vaccine: updated HPV vaccination recommendations of the Advisory Committee on Immunization Practices. MMWR 2015;64:300-4.

29. Meites E, Szilagyi PG, Chesson HW, et al. Human papillomavirus vaccination for adults: updated recommendations of the Advisory Committee on Immunization Practices. MMWR 2019; 68:698-702.

30. Marin M, Broder KR, Temte JL, et al. Use of combination measles, mumps, rubella, and varicella vaccine: recommendations of the Advisory Committee on Immunization Practices (ACIP). MMWR Recomm Rep 2010;59:1-12.

31. Casswall TH, Fischler B. Vaccination of the immunocompromised child. Expert Rev Vaccines 2005;4:725-38.

32. Shah V, Taddio A, Reider MJ; HELPinKIDS team. Effectiveness and tolerability of pharmacologic and combined interventions for reducing injection pain during childhood immunizations: systematic review and meta-analyses. Clin Ther 2009;31:s104-51.

33. Taddio A, Ilersich AL, Ipp M, et al.; HELPinKIDS team. Physical interventions and injection techniques for reducing injection pain during routine childhood immunizations: systematic review of randomized controlled trials and quasi-randomized controlled trials. Clin Ther 2009;31:s48-76.

34. Chambers CT, Taddio A, Uman LS, et al.; HELPinKIDS team. Psychological interventions for reducing pain and distress during routine childhood immunization: a systematic review. Clin Ther 2009;31:s77-103.

35. Prymula R, Siegrist CA, Chlibek R, et al. Effect of prophylactic paracetamol administration at time of vaccination on febrile reactions and antibody responses in children: two open-label, randomised controlled trials. Lancet 2009;374:1339-50.

36. Price CS, Thompson WW, Goodson B, et al. Prenatal and infant exposure to thimerosal from vaccines and immunoglobulins and risk of autism. Pediatrics 2010;126:656-64.

37. Parker SK, Schwartz B, Todd J, et al. Thimerosal-containing vaccines and autism spectrum disorder: a critical review of published original data. Pediatrics 2004;114:793-804.

38. DeStefano F, Price CS, Weintraub ES. Increasing exposure to antibody-stimulating proteins and polysaccharides in vaccines is not associated with autism. J Pediatr 2013;163:561-7.

39. Taylor LE, Swerdfeger AL, Eslick GD. Vaccines are not associated with autism: an evidence-based meta-analysis of case-control and cohort studies. Vaccine 2014;32:3623-9.

40. Hviid A, Hansen JV, Frisch M, et al. Measles, mumps, rubella vaccination and autism: a nationwide cohort study. Ann Intern Med 2019;170:513-20.

Section XII

Hematologic Disorders

CHAPTER 47

Pediatric Anemia

Teresa V. Lewis, Pharm.D., BCPS

INTRODUCTION

Anemia is characterized by a less-than-normal quantity of hemoglobin (Hgb) with an impaired capacity to transport oxygen.[1] The World Health Organization defines *anemia* as a Hgb concentration that is 2 standard deviations or more below the mean value for children of the same age and sex.[2]

The Centers for Disease Control and Prevention defines *anemia* as a Hgb value below the fifth percentile of the normal distribution in a healthy reference population.[3] Table 1 presents both sets of cutoff values used to diagnose anemia.

Infants and preschool children have increased risk of morbidity and mortality related to anemia. Anemia occurring during fetal development, particularly during the second trimester of gestation, can lead to low birth weight, which is a strong predictor of infant mortality.[4-6] In addition, anemia during peak growth periods can have adverse consequences on neurocognitive development.[7,8]

Anemia can be caused by nutritional deficiencies in iron, folate, vitamin B_{12}, and vitamin A. Other etiologies include blood loss, severe inflammation, infection, chronic kidney disease (CKD), and chronic illness.[1,8] Genetic mutations that are associated with impaired erythropoiesis can also cause anemia, including thalassemia, sickle cell trait, and Fanconi anemia.[8,9] This chapter will discuss anemia caused by deficiencies in folate, vitamin B_{12}, and iron, as well as anemia associated with CKD.

EPIDEMIOLOGY

Anemia affects around 800 million women and children worldwide, with the highest prevalence in children younger than 5 years.[8] The incidence of anemia in the United States attributable to all causes among infants and children is 3.6%. Iron-deficiency anemia (IDA), the most common type of anemia,[8,9] has a high prevalence among young children, adolescent girls, and pregnant women.[3,10] Risk factors include Hispanic ethnicity, younger age, and being overweight.[10] The prevalence of folate deficiency among American children age 4 years and older is less than 1%, whereas girls between age 12 and 19 years have the highest risk for deficiency.[11] The estimated incidence of neonatal B_{12} deficiency in the United States is around 0.88 per 100,000 newborns.[12]

PATHOPHYSIOLOGY AND DIAGNOSIS

The process by which new erythrocytes, or red blood cells (RBCs), are formed is termed *erythropoiesis*. Old erythrocytes are replaced by new erythrocytes daily, and the average life span of a normal RBC is 120 days.[13] In neonates, the life span of an RBC is 60–90 days.[5]

Erythropoietin plays a key role in the transformation of multipotent stem cells into erythroid progenitor cells and is produced primarily in the kidneys by specialized interstitial cells within the renal cortex.[13-15] The kidneys are extremely sensitive to changes in oxygen supply, and tissue hypoxia leads to an exponential increase in the amount of erythropoietin released.[14,15] This increase prolongs erythroid progenitor cell survival during the stem cell and progenitor cell stages. As erythrocyte production increases, delivery of oxygen to tissues is enhanced. When hypoxia is corrected, a negative feedback signal is created to decrease the release of erythropoietin to baseline concentrations.[14]

One or more factors that affect the sequence of events required for erythropoiesis may fail, leading to the development of anemia. Children are at increased risk of anemia from phlebotomy because of their small body size and decreased total blood volume.[16-18] Excessive blood loss from laboratory testing, without adequate replacement, is a significant contributor to the development of anemia in critically ill neonates and children.[16,17] Iron, folate, and vitamin B$_{12}$ deficiencies can lead to decreased Hgb and erythrocyte production, causing decreased oxygen delivery to tissues.[17] In the presence of kidney disease, erythropoietin production may be impaired. Abnormal hematopoietic tissue can lead to impaired responses to erythropoietin, contributing to impaired RBC formation.[15]

CLINICAL FEATURES AND COMPLICATIONS

Children who have anemia may be asymptomatic.[19,20] However, even with mild anemia, the oxygen transport capacity of the blood is reduced.[3] This reduction can lead to lethargy and decreased physical endurance. The clinical presentation of symptoms is related to the root cause of anemia. Common symptoms of anemia include irritability, lethargy, weakness, tachycardia, and pallor. Anemic infants may be irritable and have poor oral intake.[20] In addition, decreased attention span has also been reported in children with anemia.[3,7] Severe anemia can lead to impaired growth and development. Serious symptoms include arrhythmia, heart failure, and stroke.[19]

LABORATORY DATA

HEMOGLOBIN AND HEMATOCRIT

Assessments of Hgb and hematocrit are low-cost methods that provide rapid results for testing patients for anemia. Hematocrit measures the proportion of whole blood that is occupied by RBCs.[3] Its measurements are indirectly derived by automated analyzers, and values may differ among analytical instruments.[15] Thus, Hgb is considered the standard value for identifying anemia, but it is not the optimal test. Changes in Hgb typically do not occur until the late stages of iron deficiency.[3,15,19-21] The reference ranges of Hgb concentration for children vary according to the child's age and gender. The mean Hgb value for neonates born between 35- and 42-weeks' gestational age is about 18 g/dL,[22] and a cord blood Hgb value less than 12.5 g/dL indicates the presence of fetal anemia.[6]

MEAN CORPUSCULAR VOLUME

Erythrocyte size is often used to classify the type of anemia. Mean corpuscular volume (MCV) is the average size of erythrocytes. Erythrocyte size varies with age. In general, an MCV less than 78 fL suggests the presence of microcytic anemia[3,23]; specific MCV cutoff values for defining microcytic anemia among different age groups are listed in Table 2. An MCV greater than 100 fL suggests the presence of macrocytic anemia.[20] Macrocytic anemia can sometimes be megaloblastic or nonmegaloblastic. Megaloblastic anemia is characterized by the presence of unusually large and immature RBCs as well as hypersegmented neutrophils.[13,20] It is most commonly caused by folate deficiency and vitamin B$_{12}$ deficiency, whereas nonmegaloblastic anemia may be caused by hypothyroidism, liver disease, or bone marrow disorders (e.g. aplastic anemia, myelodysplasia, sideroblastic anemia).[20]

Changes in MCV are seen after long-standing nutrient deficiency.[15,24] One-third of patients with IDA have a normal MCV.[23] A peripheral blood smear will provide valuable information regarding the morphology of erythrocytes and assist with diagnosis.[19] Table 2 lists age-specific mean MCV cutoff values for defining IDA.[3]

TOTAL RETICULOCYTE COUNT

The total reticulocyte count is an indirect marker of erythropoietic activity that distinguishes anemia caused by hypoproduction from anemia caused by increased erythrocyte destruction. A low reticulocyte count may suggest an impaired production of erythrocytes, whereas a sustained high reticulocyte count may indicate active blood loss or increased erythrocyte destruction.[19]

Table 1. CDC and WHO Hemoglobin Cutoff Values to Diagnose Anemia[2,3]

Age and Sex	CDC Hemoglobin Cutoff (g/dL)	WHO Hemoglobin Cutoff (g/dL)
6 months to < 2 years	11	11
2 to < 5 years	11.1	11
5 to < 8 years	11.5	11.5
8 to < 12 years	11.9	11.5
Boys 12 to < 15 years	12.5	12
Girls 12 to < 15 years	11.8	12
Boys 15 to < 18 years	13.3	13
Girls 15 to < 18 years	12	12

CDC = Centers for Disease Control and Prevention; WHO = World Health Organization.

Table 2. MCV Cutoff Values for Microcytic Anemia[3]

Age (years)	MCV Cutoff (fL)
1–2	< 77
3–5	< 79
6–11	< 80
12–15	< 82
> 15	< 85

MCV = mean corpuscular volume.

SCREENING

The American Academy of Pediatrics recommends routine screening for anemia in infants ages 9 to 12 months.[18] The U.S. Preventive Services Task Force recommends expanding the routine screening age to include children up to 24 months.[25] Additional screening is recommended for children age 1 to 5 years who have risk factors for anemia (e.g., low socioeconomic status, Hispanic ethnicity, history of prematurity or low birth weight, lead exposure, exclusively breastfed, or inadequate dietary iron intake).[3,18]

Initial laboratory testing should include a complete blood count (CBC) that permits assessment of Hgb, hematocrit, and red cell indices (e.g., MCV, red cell distribution width). The need for further laboratory studies is dictated by the patient's history, physical examination, and results of initial testing.[3,18,19] As follow-up to abnormal CBC results, a reticulocyte count can help distinguish ineffective erythropoiesis from RBC destruction and a peripheral blood smear provides morphological details of anemic cells.[19] These additional analyses can help determine the underlying cause of anemia.

MACROCYTIC ANEMIA

PATHOPHYSIOLOGY AND DIAGNOSIS

Folate is critically important for nucleic acid synthesis. Deficiency during gestation can adversely affect cell replication and growth.[26] Folate is a water-soluble compound found in plant and animal tissues. Humans are entirely dependent on dietary sources for this nutrient. Primary sources are raw, green, leafy vegetables; beans; and fortified cereals. Animal sources include liver and kidney.[27] Cooking causes folate loss, with the extent of loss depending on the type of food and cooking method.[28] Milk is an important dietary source of folate during the first year of life. Most commercial infant formulas are fortified with folic acid and human breast milk contains sufficient concentrations of folate (50 mcg/L) for nursing infants.[27] The vitamin is excreted into breast milk in a continuous manner and is provided to the infant at the expense of maternal stores. Thus, breastfeeding women are at increased risk of folate deficiency and require folate supplementation.[29,30] Infants who are solely fed goat's milk are at risk of folate deficiency and anemia because of its very low folate content (6 mcg/L).[27,31]

Vitamin B_{12} is found in animal tissue. Pregnant women who adhere to a strictly vegetarian diet or who have had gastric bypass surgery are at risk of vitamin B_{12} deficiency, and the fetus is at risk of deficiency as well. Adults can withstand long-term vitamin B_{12} deficiency without significant physiologic impairment because reserves can last 3 to 5 years. Vitamin B_{12} composition of breast milk from mothers of term infants is highest in colostrum (0.49 mcg/L). Mature breast milk contains about 0.23 mcg/L of vitamin B_{12}.[32] Infants have limited hepatic reserves of vitamin B_{12} and are sensitive to deficiencies.[33]

Among individuals with normal dietary intake, impaired gastric acid secretion, loss of intrinsic factor as seen in pernicious anemia, or intestinal malabsorption can cause deficiency. Vitamin B_{12} in foods is protein bound. Stomach acids release the protein-bound vitamin. Once released, vitamin B_{12} is complexed to intrinsic factor that permits uptake of vitamin B_{12} in the distal ileum and subsequent transport to other cells by transcobalamin II.[13]

Folate and vitamin B_{12} are essential nutrients that are important in DNA production. A deficiency in one will alter the metabolism of the other.[33] Folate and/or vitamin B_{12} deficiency are common causes of megaloblastic anemia. The condition is characterized by impaired DNA synthesis resulting in abnormally large, immature, dysfunctional cells and subsequently increased rates of hematopoietic cell death through an unidentified mechanism.[13,14]

CLINICAL FEATURES AND COMPLICATIONS

FOLATE

Neural tube defects of the fetus (e.g., anencephaly, encephalocele, spina bifida cystica) are well-documented consequences of maternal folate deficiency.[26] Maternal folate deficiency may increase the risk of certain conditions such as abruptio placentae, preeclampsia, spontaneous abortion, preterm delivery, and low birth weight.[29] Individuals with an advanced stage of anemia may present with weakness, pallor, lethargy, and irritability.[24]

VITAMIN B_{12}

Breastfed infants of mothers who have vitamin B_{12} deficiency are at risk of severe developmental abnormalities, failure to thrive, and anemia.[30] The mothers may not have clinical symptoms of vitamin B_{12} deficiency. Infants may not have megaloblastic anemia, but will present with failure to thrive, have neurologic deficits, be irritable, and have abnormal reflexes and feeding difficulties.[29] If left untreated, almost all patients will eventually develop nervous system involvement before death occurs. Vitamin B_{12} deficiency lasting more than 3 months will lead to the development of irreversible central nervous system lesions.[34]

PREVENTION

FOLATE

Dietary folates (from natural sources) are found in a conjugated form in food. This characteristic contributes to decreased bioavailability of the nutrient.[35] In addition, dietary folates are prone to degradation from cooking, with spinach and broccoli retaining less than 50% of their folate content after boiling (49% and 44%, respectively). The extent of nutrient loss depends on the type of food and the cooking method.[28]

In 1998, the U.S. Food and Drug Administration (FDA) mandated the fortification of cereal products with 140 mcg of folic acid per 100 g of cereal/grain product. This mandate was targeted toward women of childbearing age to prevent neural tube defects. However, children who consume these products also benefit from folic acid fortification.[35]

The Institute of Medicine provides recommendations for adequate intake and recommended daily allowances (RDAs) of dietary folate. The term *dietary folate equivalent* (DFE) is used to describe the RDA of folate. One microgram of DFE (i.e., natural food folate) is equal to 0.6 mcg of folic acid from fortified foods.[24] The presence of food will affect the oral bioavailability of folic acid tablets.[35] If taken on an empty stomach, 1 mcg of DFE equals 0.5 mcg of folic acid, but when taken with food, 1 mcg DFE equals 0.6 mcg folic acid. The RDA for specified age groups is provided in Table 3.[24,36]

Pregnant and breastfeeding women may increase folic acid intake through supplements. For women with no previous history of neural tube defect affected pregnancy, folic acid 400 mcg daily taken at least 1 month before pregnancy and during pregnancy in addition to dietary folate intake minimizes the risk of fetal neural tube defects.[24,37] Lactating mothers require an additional 300 mcg of folic acid daily to maintain adequate serum folate concentrations.[29]

VITAMIN B₁₂

VITAMIN B$_{12}$

The best strategy to prevent vitamin B$_{12}$ deficiency is to encourage individuals to consume an adequate amount in their diet. Foods with the highest vitamin B$_{12}$ content include beef, liver, turkey, and chicken.[27] Fortified foods and oral supplements may provide alternative sources of vitamin B$_{12}$.[33] However, the ideal dose of vitamin B$_{12}$ for supplementation has not been established. Table 3 lists age-specific RDA values.[24,36]

DIAGNOSIS

MCV AND PERIPHERAL SMEAR

An MCV greater than 100 fL is a sensitive hematologic marker for folate and vitamin B$_{12}$ deficiency. A peripheral blood smear should be included in the workup. The presence of macroovalocytes and hypersegmented neutrophils indicates the presence of megaloblastic anemia.[20]

FOLATE AND VITAMIN B$_{12}$

Deficiencies may be determined by direct vitamin assays or indirectly by surrogate biochemical markers. Serum folate, RBC folate concentration, and serum vitamin B$_{12}$ are direct assays. Serum folate reflects short-term folate balance and is subject to diurnal and prandial variations. In contrast, RBC folate more accurately reflects average body folate concentrations when that particular population of erythrocytes was produced.[26,38]

Homocysteine and methylmalonic acid are surrogate biochemical markers that reflect the metabolic function of folate and vitamin B$_{12}$. Because the breakdown of homocysteine requires the presence of both folate and vitamin B$_{12}$, deficiencies of either vitamin lead to increased homocysteine concentrations.[26,38] However, only vitamin B$_{12}$ deficiency is associated with an elevation in methylmalonic acid concentration. Other disease states, such as renal failure or hypothyroidism, may also cause an increase in homocysteine and/or methylmalonic acid.[26,38] Direct measurement of vitamin B$_{12}$ and/or folate in conjunction with surrogate markers may provide a better diagnosis for deficiency. Reference ranges are listed in Table 4.[39]

SCHILLING TEST

The Schilling test is used to identify malabsorption of vitamin B$_{12}$. Individuals with malabsorption will have lower concentrations of radioactivity in their urine. This test is rarely used because of the high rate of indeterminate results.[38,40]

TREATMENT

FOLATE

Oxidative cleavage of dietary folate from cooking creates degradation products that are not active and cannot be converted by the body to active folate. Folate deficiency is treated with folic acid, which is more stable than dietary folate. Bioavailability of synthetic folic acid is twice the amount seen with dietary folate and gastrointestinal (GI) absorption is better at smaller doses. Folic acid is relatively well tolerated, and it may be given orally, intramuscularly, intravenously, or subcutaneously. The injectable form of folic acid is available as sodium folate. Dosage recommendations are 100 mcg/day for infants and 300 mcg/day for children younger than 4 years. Individuals older than 4 years are given a typical adult dose of 400 mcg/day. An extemporaneously prepared formulation can also be compounded.[41] Folate therapy should be continued for at least 3 to 4 weeks until a definite hematologic response is observed.[20]

Table 3. Recommended Daily Allowance[24,36]

Age and Sex	Folate (mcg)[a]	Vitamin B$_{12}$ (mcg)	Iron[b] (mg/day)	Ascorbic Acid (mg)
0–6 months	65[c] (9.4 mcg/kg)	0.4[c] (0.05 mcg/kg)	0.27[c]	40[c]
7–12 months	80[c] (8.8 mcg/kg)	0.5[c] (0.05 mcg/kg)	11	50[c]
1–3 years	150	0.9	7	15
4–8 years	200	1.2	10	25
Boys 9–13 years	300	1.8	8	45
Girls 9–13 years	300	1.8	8	45
Boys 14–18 years	400	2.4	11	75
Girls 14–18 years	400	2.4	15	65

[a]Amount listed as dietary folate equivalent.
[b]Elemental iron.
[c]Listed as recommendations for adequate intake.

VITAMIN B$_{12}$

Vitamin B$_{12}$ deficiency in children in the United States is uncommon. When supplementation is required, intramuscular or subcutaneous routes are preferred.[42,43] The dose used for children with vitamin B$_{12}$ deficiency is not well established, and a variety of dosing strategies have been used. Children who have pernicious anemia or deficiency caused by malabsorptive conditions may require life-long therapy.[42,43]

For the treatment of pernicious anemia, a starting dose of cyanocobalamin 0.2 mcg/kg administered as an intramuscular or a deep subcutaneous injection for 2 days followed by 1000 mcg/day for 2 to 7 days has been recommended. Dosing is then extended to the weekly administration of 100 mcg/week, with treatment spanning 1 month. Maintenance doses of 100 mcg/month have been recommended; however, some experts recommend doses as low as 50 mcg/month for infants and young children.[42]

To treat deficiency caused by malabsorption, cyanocobalamin intramuscular 250 to 1000 mcg daily or every other day may be administered for 1 week followed by weekly administration spanning 4 to 8 weeks. Dosing is then extended to monthly administration for maintenance therapy; however, some experts recommend doses as low as 50 mcg monthly for infants and young children.[42,43] Orally administered cyanocobalamin is not recommended for treating severe vitamin B$_{12}$ deficiency associated with lack of intrinsic factor because oral absorption is variable.[42] An intranasal formulation is also available; however, it does not have FDA label approval for use in children.[44]

MONITORING

All patients should have a baseline CBC. Vitamin B$_{12}$ and RBC folate concentrations can provide distinction between folate deficiency and vitamin B$_{12}$ deficiency.

Table 4. Reference Values for Folate and Vitamin B$_{12}$ Assays and Surrogate Markers[38]

Direct Vitamin Assays	Reference Range
Serum Vitamin B$_{12}$	
Newborn	160–1300 pg/mL
Child	200–835 pg/mL
Serum Folate	
Newborn	16–72 ng/mL
Child	4–20 ng/mL
Red Blood Cell Folate	
Newborn	150–200 ng/mL
Infant	74–995 ng/mL
2–16 years	> 160 ng/mL
> 16 years	140–628 ng/mL
Surrogate Markers	
Serum homocysteine	4.6–8.1 micromol/L
Methylmalonic acid	0.05–0.26 micromol/L

FOLATE

A decline in homocysteine concentrations may be observed within a few days after starting folic acid therapy and may be useful for assessing treatment response. A CBC drawn 8 weeks after initiation of folic acid therapy is also useful for determining response to therapy.[45] At a minimum, patients should be monitored 6 months after the start of therapy and annually thereafter.[33]

VITAMIN B$_{12}$

Vitamin B$_{12}$ concentrations and a CBC count should be performed 1 month after the start of cyanocobalamin and every 3 to 6 months thereafter to determine treatment efficacy.[43,44] Once therapy is initiated, it may take 1 to 4 months to achieve complete recovery of hematologic indices. When treating patients with severe vitamin B$_{12}$ deficiency, hypokalemia requiring replacement therapy and thrombocytosis may develop. Hypokalemia is caused by an intracellular shift of potassium after correction of anemia and can be severe and fatal.[43,44] Therefore, serum potassium and a CBC are particularly important during the initial treatment of vitamin B$_{12}$ deficiency. Laboratory values should be observed closely during the first 48 hours of treatment.

MICROCYTIC ANEMIA

PATHOPHYSIOLOGY AND DIAGNOSIS

Iron is an essential cofactor for many different cellular processes. Heme iron, or ferrous iron, is primarily from animal sources such as Hgb and myoglobin. It is well absorbed by the GI tract.[13,36,46] Non-heme iron, or ferric iron, is found in foods such as spinach, enriched cereals, and whole grains.[25,27] It is not efficiently absorbed because ferric iron must be reduced by brush border ferrireductase enzymes in the GI tract to ferrous iron for absorption to occur.[13,27,36,46,47] Reducing substances, such as ascorbic acid, facilitates the conversion of ferric iron to ferrous iron, enhancing GI absorption.[13,48] In addition, ascorbic acid has chelating properties that bind polyphenol (e.g., tannic acid) and phytates (e.g., bran, cereals), which inhibit iron absorption.[49]

Iron's ability to accept and donate electrons makes it a biologically useful element. However, this same characteristic gives iron the capacity for toxicity. The body tightly regulates iron by sequestering most of it within proteins.[47] Transferrin is the body's principle transport protein and tightly binds to iron for circulation throughout the body. Once inside erythroid cells, iron is cleaved from transferrin and transported to the mitochondria, where it can be made available for incorporation into protoporphyrin IX forming heme.[14,50] Heme may be incorporated into α-globin and β-globin chains to form Hgb.[14] Iron within Hgb functions as a carrier of oxygen.[3,50] Iron that is not readily used is complexed to ferritin and hemosiderin for storage within cells. In healthy individuals, most stored iron is bound to ferritin.[3,50]

When old RBCs are destroyed, the liberated iron is recycled for incorporation back into the Hgb. Iron deficiency slows Hgb synthesis and impairs erythropoiesis, causing fewer reticulocytes to be released by the bone marrow. Released reticulocytes are small with a decreased Hgb concentration and are described as *hypochromic* and *microcytic*.[50]

Iron status is a continuum. Individuals may have normal functional iron with varying concentrations of transport and stored iron. Iron depletion exists when the amount of stored iron is reduced while the amount of functional iron and transport iron are normal; however, the body may not have sufficient iron stores to mobilize if there is an increased need. Iron-deficient erythropoiesis may occur if the body continues to have a negative iron balance for a prolonged duration leading to low amounts of stored iron and low amounts of transport iron.[3] Iron-deficiency anemia is a more severe form of iron deficiency, in which functional, transport, and stored iron concentrations are all reduced. The lack of iron leads to impaired production of Hgb, myoglobin, and respiratory enzymes. Erythrocyte formation decreases, and organ systems can be adversely affected.[3]

Premature birth, low birth weight, and prolonged stay in the neonatal intensive care unit are risk factors for IDA. Preterm neonates possess lower total body iron than full-term neonates; however, the proportion of iron to body weight is similar between the two populations. The faster rate of postnatal growth experienced by preterm neonates places them at risk of rapidly depleting iron stores compared with their full-term counterparts. Preterm neonates can develop iron deficiency by age 2 to 3 months if adequate iron supplementation is not provided.[51]

Healthy term neonates are born with adequate iron stores for about 4 months of postnatal growth.[51] Infants who are exclusively breastfed and who do not receive iron supplementation are at increased risk of developing IDA.[3,18,23] Infants who are not fed iron-fortified formula during the first year of life and those who have an early introduction of cow's milk are also at increased risk.[3,18,23] Human breast milk and cow's milk have similarly low concentrations of elemental iron, about 0.5–1 mg/L.[3,52] However, human breast milk's bioavailability is around 50% compared with 10% with cow's milk.[3,52,53] High calcium and casein content of cow's milk can inhibit GI iron absorption, and early introduction of cow's milk during infancy can cause occult bleeding from the GI tract, both of which contribute to iron loss.[3,53,54]

Iron deficiency among children older than 3 years is usually caused by limited access to iron-rich foods, with African American or Hispanic ethnicity and those living in poverty having increased risk. Adolescent girls can become iron deficient because of regular blood loss during menstruation and limited dietary iron consumption.[3] Comorbidities such as cancer, CKD, bleeding disorders, inflammatory bowel disease, and other chronic inflammatory conditions may also increase risk for IDA.[3]

CLINICAL FEATURES AND COMPLICATIONS

Women who are iron deficient early during pregnancy have a higher risk of preterm delivery and of giving birth to babies with low birth weight.[55] Maternal IDA during the first half of pregnancy is associated with an increased risk of preterm delivery, despite correction of iron deficiency during the third trimester.[5] Pregnant women who present with IDA at their first prenatal visit are more likely to give birth to a baby with low birth weight. This risk is three times greater if the woman resides in a low-income household. The association between premature delivery and low birth weight has not been found with other types of maternal anemia.[56] Strong evidence supports the role of iron in neurologic development, and data suggest the causality of IDA with poor cognitive, neurologic, and motor development. Infants with IDA have lower motor function scores than infants who do not have IDA.[7] Some effects of IDA can be long lasting and irreversible.[7,57]

PREVENTION

The Department of Health and Human Services Healthy People 2020 includes objectives for reducing iron deficiency to less than 14.3% for children age 1–2 years, less than 4.3% for children 3–4 years, and less than 9.4% for females of childbearing age.[58] Moreover, the American Academy of Pediatrics has published guidance regarding the diagnosis and prevention of IDA, which recommends that all preterm infants receive elemental iron 2 mg/kg/day, the amount provided in iron-fortified formulas. This supplementation should be provided through 12 months of age. Preterm infants who are solely breastfed should be given oral iron supplementation by the age of 1 month with elemental iron at a dose of 2 mg/kg/day. This therapy should be continued until the infant is weaned to iron-fortified formula or is able to consume foods that supply elemental iron at 2 mg/kg/day. Healthy term infants who are exclusively breastfed should receive elemental iron at 1 mg/kg/day orally starting at age 4 months. Term, healthy infants who consume both breast milk and formula should be given elemental iron at 1 mg/kg/day orally starting at age 4 months if breast milk intake is greater than 50% of the infant's total daily intake. For infants who are solely formula fed, iron-fortified formulations are recommended until age 12 months and do not require additional iron supplementation.[18] Cow's milk should be avoided until after age 12 months.[3,18] Table 3 lists the RDA of iron for specified age groups.[36]

Ingesting foods that are rich in ascorbic acid increases the absorption of non-heme iron from the diet, and its effects are more pronounced when the meal contains inhibitors of iron absorption.[36,48] Synthetic ascorbic acid has a similar effect on improving dietary iron absorption.[36,48,49] For most people, taking ascorbic acid as a supplement to improve the absorption of dietary iron is unnecessary, and dietary sources of ascorbic acid are preferred. Health care professionals should advise patients and caregivers regarding RDA values of ascorbic acid if they are posed with questions about supplement use. The RDA for ascorbic acid is noted in Table 3.[36]

DIAGNOSIS

Hemoglobin alone may fail to identify children at risk of developing IDA because it does not detect iron deficiency in individuals who have normal-range Hgb values.[20] The American Academy of Pediatrics recommends obtaining serum ferritin and C-reactive protein or reticulocyte Hgb content concentration (CHr) for children who have a Hgb concentration less than 11 mg/dL and who have significant risk for IDA.[18]

IRON STATUS

An iron profile can confirm the presence of iron depletion, iron-deficient erythropoiesis, or IDA to guide therapy. Components of an iron profile include the following: serum iron concentration, total iron-binding capacity, transferrin saturation (TSAT), and serum soluble transferrin receptor. Serum iron concentration is the total amount of iron found in the serum. Total iron-binding capacity reflects the availability of iron-binding sites on transferrin. Transferrin saturation is serum iron divided by total iron-binding capacity. The value reflects the extent to which transferrin has "vacant" iron-binding sites. The National Kidney Foundation Kidney Disease Outcomes Quality Initiative (KDOQI) defines *absolute iron deficiency* as a TSAT less than 20%.[3] A serum-soluble transferrin receptor assay measures the expression of soluble transferrin receptors. This concentration is reciprocally related to the iron supply and increases markedly in the presence of iron deficiency.[59]

FERRITIN

Ferritin is an indicator of iron stores. Low serum ferritin is highly diagnostic for iron deficiency. In the absence of comorbidities, a ferritin value of 15 ng/mL or less indicates the absence of iron stores in children older than 6 months.[3,15] Individuals who have anemia from chronic disease may have normal or elevated serum ferritin, which is reflective of increased iron storage and retention in the reticuloendothelial system. Increased ferritin may also be caused by activation of the immune response.[59,60] The lower limit for serum ferritin is defined by the KDOQI workgroup as 200 ng/mL for individuals on hemodialysis and 100 ng/mL for those with CKD not on hemodialysis.[15]

LIMITATIONS TO SERUM IRON, TSAT, AND SERUM FERRITIN CONCENTRATION

Serum iron, TSAT, and serum ferritin concentrations may be affected by factors unrelated to iron. Diurnal variations have been observed with serum iron and TSAT. High estrogen or progesterone states (e.g., with pregnancy, oral contraceptive use) are associated with increased TSAT values. In addition, inflammatory states can cause elevations in serum ferritin.[50,59] Iron-deficient individuals on hemodialysis, chronically ill patients, or those with malnutrition, chronic infection, or inflammation can present with high serum ferritin concentrations.[3,15,50]

RETICULOCYTE HEMOGLOBIN CONTENT

Reticulocyte Hgb content (CHr) quantifies the amount of Hgb found in reticulocytes and is a direct measure of iron that is incorporated into newly formed RBCs. Because reticulocytes are typically 1–2 days old, this laboratory value reflects immediate availability of iron. Pediatric data are limited and reference ranges for children are not well defined. One pediatric study suggests a CHr value 26 pg/cell or less as the optimal cutoff value for detecting iron deficiency.[61]

ERYTHROCYTE PROTOPORPHYRIN

Erythrocyte protoporphyrin is the immediate precursor of Hgb and increases when insufficient iron is available for Hgb production. Erythrocyte protoporphyrin is more sensitive and is at least as specific for detecting IDA as Hgb and serum ferritin, making it a useful screening tool for detecting earlier stages of iron deficiency.[21] Early detection is important in children because of the developmental consequences associated with IDA. A whole-blood erythrocyte protoporphyrin value of 35 mcg/dL or greater suggests decreased Hgb production and iron deficiency.[62,63] Erythrocyte protoporphyrin is not widely used at this time because it is more expensive and complicated to perform compared with Hgb screening.

TREATMENT

If therapy is required, oral iron supplementation is preferred. Patients who have disease states associated with malabsorption of oral iron may benefit from intravenous therapy.[46] The ferrous salt form is often used because it is most readily absorbed, although only 10% to 35% of an oral dose of ferrous sulfate is absorbed by the GI tract, although the percentage of iron that is absorbed increases to 80% to 95% during iron deficiency.[64]

Most commercially available oral dosage formulations of iron are supplied as ferrous iron. The elemental iron content of each salt form varies. Table 5 and Table 6 list elemental iron content for single-ingredient oral iron preparations and multivitamins.[65-69]

Table 5. Iron Content of Select Single-Ingredient Pediatric Oral Supplements[65-68]

Drug	Elemental Iron (%)	Dosage Strength (elemental iron dose mg)
Ferrous gluconate	11.2	240-mg tablet (27 mg)
Ferrous fumarate	33	324-mg tablet (106 mg)
Ferrous sulfate, enteric-coated tablets	20	324-mg tablet (65 mg)
Ferrous sulfate, extended-release tablets	32.1	140-mg tablet (45 mg)
Ferrous sulfate, slow-release tablets (Slow FE)[a]	31.7	142-mg tablet (45 mg)
Ferrous sulfate, elixir	20	220 mg/5 mL (44 mg/5 mL)
Ferrous sulfate, liquid	20	300 mg/5 mL (60 mg/5 mL)
Ferrous sulfate, liquid drops (Fer-In-Sol)[b]	20	75 mg/mL (15 mg/mL)
Polysaccharide iron complex, capsules (various manufacturers)	100	150 mg per capsule

[a]GlaxoSmithKline, Philadelphia, PA; [b]Mead Johnson Nutrition, Evansville, IN.

For infants and children with mild IDA (Hgb 10–10.9 g/dL for children younger than 59 months; Hgb 11–11.9 g/dL for children age 5-14 years and non-pregnant females) to moderate IDA (Hgb 7–9.9 g/dL for children younger than 59 months; Hgb 8–10.9 g/dL for children age 5-14 years and non-pregnant females), elemental iron at a dose of 3 mg/kg given once daily or divided into two doses is recommended. Severe IDA (Hgb lower than 7 g/dL for children younger than 59 months; Hgb less than 8 g/dL for children age 5-14 years and non-pregnant females) is treated with elemental iron 4 to 6 mg/kg/day, usually given in three divided doses.[2,65] Liquid oral iron preparations are available for infants and young children who are unable to swallow tablets. This formulation may also be preferred for individuals who are unable to adequately absorb iron tablets because of poor dissolution of the film coating. Elemental iron concentrations vary among different liquid preparations and close attention should be given to interpreting iron content because some preparations provide details in the form of milligrams of the iron salt, whereas other preparations provide iron content as milligrams of elemental iron. Misinterpreting this information can lead to dosing errors. It is especially important to be aware of these issues when substituting one liquid preparation for another (Table 5).[65-68]

Oral iron supplements should be taken on an empty stomach, but this timing may not be possible because of the GI distress commonly associated with this therapy.[46,60] The most cited reasons for therapy nonadherence include the following: abdominal pain, epigastric pain, nausea, vomiting, and constipation. To alleviate constipation, adequate daily fluid intake should be encouraged and stool softeners may be considered. Diarrhea may occur, but to a lesser extent than constipation.[65-68] Administering the drug with meals may reduce GI symptoms at the expense of decreasing drug absorption. Instead, one may consider giving smaller doses more often.[60] Carbonyl iron, polysaccharide iron complex, or delayed-release formulations may have fewer GI effects.[70] Carbonyl iron is a pure form of iron that can be found in certain pediatric multivitamin formulations such as chewable tablets or as a gummy. This form of iron is more slowly absorbed and has a higher bioavailability than ferrous sulfate.[70,71] It also has a better safety profile than ferrous sulfate. The estimated median lethal dose (LD_{50}) of ferrous sulfate is ferrous iron at 250 mg/kg.[70] Fatal outcomes have arisen from children ingesting 30–40 ferrous sulfate 325 mg tablets, and very young children have died after consuming as few as five tablets.[71] Toxicity studies in animals estimate the lethal dose at which no deaths occurred (LD_0) for carbonyl iron to be a dose of

Table 6. Vitamin B, Folic Acid, and Elemental Iron Content of Select Multi-Ingredient Pediatric Oral Supplements[69]

Drug	Elemental Iron (%)	Elemental Iron Dosage Strength	Folic Acid Content (mcg per tablet or gummy)	Vitamin B_{12} (mcg per tablet, gummy, or mL)
Centrum Kids Complete[a] (Carbonyl iron)	100	18 mg/tablet	400 mcg/tablet	6 mcg/tablet
Flintstones Gummies Complete[b]	—	—	100 mcg/gummy	1.5 mcg/gummy
Flintstones Complete Chewables[b] (Ferrous fumarate)	100	18 mg/tablet	400 mcg/tablet	6 mcg/tablet
Flintstones with Iron Chewables[b] (Ferrous fumarate)	100	15 mg/tablet	300 mcg/tablet	4.5 mcg/tablet
L'il Critters Gummy Vites[c]	—	—	130 mcg/gummy	3 mcg/gummy
Nephro-Vite OTC[d]	—	—	800 mcg/tablet	6 mcg/tablet
Nephro-Vite Rx[d]	—	—	1000 mcg/tablet	6 mcg/tablet
One A Day Kids Scooby-Doo! Complete[b] (Ferrous fumarate)	100	18 mg/tablet	400 mcg/tablet	6 mcg/tablet
One A Day Teen Advantage for Her[b] (Ferrous fumarate)	100	18 mg/tablet	400 mcg/tablet	9 mcg/tablet
One A Day Teen Advantage for Him[b] (Ferrous fumarate)	100	9 mg/tablet	400 mcg/tablet	15 mcg/tablet
Poly-Vi-Sol[e]	—	—	—	2 mcg/mL
Poly-Vi-Sol with Iron[e] (Ferrous sulfate)	100	10 mg/mL	—	—
Tri-Vi-Sol with Iron[e] (Ferrous sulfate)	100	10 mg/mL	—	—

[a]Pfizer Inc., New York, NY; [b]Bayer Consumer Health, Morristown, NJ; [c]Church & Dwight Co., Inc., Ewing, NJ; [d]Allergan USA, Inc., Irvine, CA; [e]Mead Johnson Nutrition, Evansville, IN.

10,000–15,000 mg/kg.[70,71] Extrapolating these data to humans, a 10-kg child would consume around one-third of the LD$_{50}$ if the child ingests 63 carbonyl iron capsules, each containing 600 mg.[72] Caution should still be taken with carbonyl iron because an accidental overdose can occur. Polysaccharide iron complex is available as an elixir or tablet for use in children 6 years and older.[68] Enteric-coated iron preparations, which delay the dissolution of iron until it reaches the intestinal tract, may be considered for older children who are able to swallow tablets. Enteric-coated preparations may have lower bioavailability than film-coated preparations and oral solutions and should be considered when changing products.[72]

Iron supplementation can discolor urine and cause dark stools. Tooth discoloration observed with liquid iron preparations is superficial and not permanent. Diluting the oral liquid with water and giving the supplement through a straw can minimize contact of the solution with teeth. Proper oral hygiene can remove and prevent tooth discoloration.

MONITORING

Assessing Hgb changes, in combination with a reticulocyte count, may be useful in determining treatment response to IDA because changes in the reticulocyte count can be seen in the early stages of erythropoiesis. A Hgb increase of 1 g/dL should occur every 2–3 weeks after therapy initiation.[3,46] Some individuals may require up to 4 months of therapy for iron status to return to therapeutic range once Hgb has been corrected.[46] Hemoglobin values that increase by more than 1 g/dL or absolute reticulocyte count that increases by more than 100,000 cells/mm³ (100 × 10⁶/L) after 4 weeks of therapy indicate the patient is responding to therapy.[19]

ANEMIA OF CHRONIC KIDNEY DISEASE

PATHOPHYSIOLOGY AND DIAGNOSIS

Anemia in CKD is common. The cause of anemia may be erythropoietin deficiency, although there may be other causes as well, such as iron deficiency. Individuals on dialysis therapy have the highest risk of anemia secondary to regular blood loss to the dialysis circuit after each dialysis session. The use of anticoagulation associated with dialysis therapy increases the risk of GI bleeds, and frequent phlebotomy can contribute to blood loss and anemia.

CLINICAL FEATURES AND COMPLICATIONS

In general, complications in patients with CKD are similar to those in patients with IDA. Having CKD and anemia can decrease a patient's quality of life. These individuals have an increased risk of target organ damage. Impaired oxygen delivery increases the workload of the heart. Over time, this increased workload could lead to ventricular hypertrophy and decreased cardiac output.[73]

DIAGNOSIS

The *KDOQI* anemia workgroup recommends a CBC, TSAT, and serum ferritin for initial assessment of anemia in all children with a diagnosis of CKD.[15] Hemoglobin values should be measured at least annually. Children at a higher risk of anemia should be monitored more often, including children who have a greater disease burden, those who have an unstable clinical course, or those who have had a previous decrease in their Hgb concentration. A diagnosis of anemia should be made when the observed Hgb value is lower than the 5th percentile of normal when adjusted for age and sex.[3,15]

ERYTHROPOIETIN CONCENTRATION

Erythropoietin concentration testing is not routinely useful for differentiating erythropoietin deficiency from other types of anemia.[15] Erythropoietin concentrations are only useful when evaluating individuals with a Hgb value less than 10 g/dL because erythropoietin concentrations are typically within normal range in patients having Hgb values higher than 10 g/dL.[74]

RETICULOCYTE HEMOGLOBIN CONTENT

At this time CHr is not widely used to diagnosis anemia in children, and pediatric data are limited. The KDOQI recommends targeting CHr concentrations greater than 29 pg/cell as an alternative to TSAT for adult hemodialysis patients with anemia.[15]

TREATMENT

The goal of iron therapy is to avoid storage iron depletion, prevent iron-deficient erythropoiesis, and achieve and maintain erythropoiesis.[3] For patients on hemodialysis, sufficient iron should be given to maintain a serum ferritin greater than 200 ng/mL and TSAT greater than 20%. For patients who have CKD not requiring dialysis or those who require peritoneal dialysis, serum ferritin should be maintained greater than 100 ng/mL and TSAT greater than 20%.[3]

Although the absorption of oral iron may be slow, it remains an effective therapy and is preferred for children with anemia of CKD who are not on dialysis and children who are on peritoneal dialysis. The recommended dose of elemental iron is 2–3 mg/kg/day up to 6 mg/kg/day (maximum 150–300 mg/day) given in two or three divided doses. To optimize GI absorption, doses of oral iron preparations should be taken at least 1 hour before or 2 hours after ingesting any calcium-containing phosphate binders.[65-68] Patients may not respond to oral iron supplementation for several reasons, including therapy nonadherence, impaired GI absorption of iron, inflammation, and chronic bleeding. Furthermore, RBC transfusions are necessary if patients are symptomatic after experiencing acute bleeding, acute hemolysis, or blood loss from surgery.[3]

INTRAVENOUS IRON

Injectable iron therapy is generally reserved for oral therapy failure. However, it is the preferred route of administration for treating anemia in children on hemodialysis therapy. Current intravenous iron preparations consist of iron complexed to a carbohydrate moiety. In the body, the reticuloendothelial cells separate the iron from the iron–carbohydrate complex.[75] Free iron is then available for binding to transferrin and transport throughout the body. It may be incorporated into the body's total iron stores, or it may be used for Hgb synthesis.[75]

No adequately powered studies exist that directly compare efficacy between parenteral iron preparations. Hypersensitivity reactions can occur with all injectable iron preparations; however, they are most pronounced with iron dextran.[75] Iron toxicity can be detrimental in both acute and chronic settings. Care should be taken to monitor for iron overload in patients with predisposing conditions.

IRON DEXTRAN

Iron dextran is ferric hydroxide complexed with polymerized dextran.[76,77] Its use is associated with higher rates of adverse events and hypersensitivity reactions compared with newer parenteral iron preparations.[75] Avoid administering iron dextran to infants age 4 months or younger.[76,77] All patients should receive an intravenous test dose 1 hour before treatment doses to assess tolerability.[75-77] Weight-based test doses may be preferable, as follows: 10 mg (0.2 mL) for infants who weigh less than 10 kg; 15 mg (0.3 mL) for children who weigh 10–20 kg; 25 mg (0.5 mL) for children who weigh more than 20 kg.[77] Some patients may experience hypersensitivity reactions with treatment doses despite tolerating a test dose. Caution should be taken to maintain an administration rate less than 50 mg/minute when giving treatment doses.[75-77] The dosage calculation for intravenous infusion in an iron-deficient patient is described below.[76,77]

Calculation of iron dextran dose for children 5–15 kg is as follows:

Dose (mL) = 0.0442 [desired hemoglobin (g/dL) – observed hemoglobin (g/dL)] × W + (0.26 × W)

where W = weight in kg.

Weight in kg = weight (lb)/2.2

Desired hemoglobin = target hemoglobin (g/dL) (Normal hemoglobin for children 15 kg or less is 12 g/dL)

Calculation of iron dextran dose for children over 15 kg is as follows:

Dose (mL) = 0.0442 [desired hemoglobin (g/dL) – observed hemoglobin (g/dL)] × LBW + (0.26 × LBW)

where LBW = lean body weight in kg.

LBW (male sex) = 50 kg + 2.3 kg for each inch of the patient's height over 5 feet

LBW (female sex) = 45.5 kg + 2.3 kg for each inch of the patient's height over 5 feet

Weight in kg = weight (lb)/2.2

Desired hemoglobin = target hemoglobin (g/dL)

IRON SUCROSE (IRON SACCHARATE)

Iron sucrose is an aqueous complex of iron hydroxide in sucrose. It can be given undiluted by slow intravenous push or as an intravenous infusion. The dose for children age 2 years and older who are hemodialysis-dependent is 0.5 mg/kg/dose every 2 weeks for 12 weeks. The dose for children age 2 years and older with non-dialysis-dependent CKD or who are receiving peritoneal dialysis is 0.5 mg/kg/dose every 4 weeks for 12 weeks. The maximum single dose is 100 mg.[78] Iron sucrose has been successfully administered to adult patients with sensitivity to iron dextran and does not require a test dose before administration.[75]

FERRIC GLUCONATE

Ferric gluconate is a sodium ferric gluconate complex in sucrose. Ferric gluconate has FDA label approval for use in children 6 years and older undergoing hemodialysis and receiving epoetin therapy.[79] The recommended pediatric regimen is 1.5 mg/kg/dose of elemental iron at each dialysis session for eight doses total. The maximum single dose is 125 mg. A slow infusion rate is recommended over 60 minutes.[79,80] Hypersensitivity reactions are rare.[75,79]

FERUMOXYTOL

Ferumoxytol is a superparamagnetic iron oxide coated with a low-molecular-weight semisynthetic carbohydrate.[80] One study has evaluated the safety and efficacy of ferumoxytol for correcting IDA in 54 children between age 21 days and 19 years (mean age 11 years). Patients received ferumoxytol 10 mg/kg/dose (maximum dose 510 mg) diluted in 0.9% sodium chloride for a concentration of 5 mg/mL. Ferumoxytol was administered over 60 minutes for the first infusion and then over 15 minutes for subsequent infusions. Results were an increase in Hgb from 9.2–11.5 g/dL (p<0.001). More than 50% of patients in this study received epoetin concurrently. Most patients tolerated ferumoxytol; four children developed adverse effects that resulted in discontinuation of therapy.[81] Because of the potential for serious hypersensitivity reactions, the FDA recommend infusions lasting 15 minutes or longer and patients should be monitored for signs and symptoms of hypersensitivity reactions (e.g., pruritus, rash, urticarial, wheezing) for at least 30 minutes post infusion.[81]

RECOMBINANT HUMAN EPOETIN

Epoetin is used to stimulate erythropoiesis. Most literature for pediatric patients evaluate short-acting agents such as epoetin alfa. Pediatric observational trials suggest that short-acting epoetin given subcutaneously is more effective than intravenous administration.[15]

Patients receiving hemodialysis require higher starting doses of short-acting epoetin compared with individuals receiving peritoneal dialysis to achieve target Hgb values of 11–12 g/dL. The mean dose of short-acting epoetin for children on hemodialysis is 300 units/kg/week compared with 225 units/kg/week for peritoneal dialysis patients. Young children require higher doses per kilogram of body weight than older children, with infants typically requiring 350 units/kg/week and those between 2–5 years and 6–12 years requiring slightly lower doses, 275 units/kg/week and 250 units/kg/week, respectively. Children older than 12 years need about 200 units/kg/week.[15]

Data for the use of long-acting agents such as darbepoetin alfa for children are limited. One small study involving children on hemodialysis therapy proposed a dose conversion of 0.5 mcg of darbepoetin alfa for every 200 units of epoetin alfa.[15] For children with CKD who are not receiving dialysis, the mean dose of short-acting epoetin alfa required to maintain target Hgb values between 11.5 g/dL and 13.5 g/dL is 133 units/kg/week. The dose range is 75–300 units/kg/week, and darbepoetin alfa at a dose of 0.45 mcg/kg/week showed similar efficacy to short-acting epoetin alfa.[15]

Up to 10% of patients with CKD have a poor response to epoetin therapy. Hyporesponsiveness to epoetin therapy is defined as persistently low Hgb (less than 10 g/dL), despite treatment with clinically appropriate doses.[15] Initial steps in determining the cause include ensuring the patient has sufficient iron available for erythropoiesis and ruling out nonadherence. For sufficient iron, TSAT should be greater than 20% and serum ferritin should be higher than 100 ng/mL. Other potential causes of hyporesponsiveness include infection, inflammation, and inefficient dialysis. Furthermore, chronic inflammation can lead to impaired erythropoiesis.[14,15]

MONITORING

IRON THERAPY

An increase in the reticulocyte count is not observed for at least 4–7 days after starting therapy and decisions about the effectiveness of treatment should not be made until 3–4 weeks after treatment initiation.[15] Erythropoietic response to iron replacement is considered appropriate if the Hgb concentration increases by at least 2 g/dL or reaches normal values within 4 weeks of treatment. The Hgb target is 11–12 g/dL.[15] The 2 g/dL increase can be reached by intravenous iron therapy within 2–4 weeks.[15] Extending monitoring to every 1–3 months can be considered once the patient has achieved a stable iron dose. Monitoring is required more often for individuals who have experienced recent bleeding and for postsurgical or hospitalized patients.[15]

RECOMBINANT HUMAN EPOETIN

Monitoring intervals are the same for individuals who receive epoetin as with iron therapy. Similar to the monitoring recommendations for children receiving iron therapy, monitoring is required more often for those with a recent bleeding event, postsurgical or hospitalized patients, and for those who

are hyporesponsive to epoetin.[15] Guidelines defining appropriate responses to epoetin therapy vary among expert panels, with KDOQI recommending Hgb increases between 1 g/dL and 2 g/dL per month. The European Paediatric Peritoneal Dialysis Working Group suggests Hgb increases by at least 0.66 g/dL per month. However, an increase of 2.5 mg/dL or more per month is considered unacceptable. Epoetin doses should be adjusted for children who have a greater than 0.5 g/dL increase per week in Hgb to avoid exceeding the target value. Dose reductions are preferred over drug discontinuation when hemoglobin is above target range.[15] Hemoglobin concentrations greater than 13 g/dL are avoided because of increased risks for thrombosis. Assessment of blood pressures should occur regularly because hypertension in children receiving epoetin is an important concern.[15] In addition, iron status should be assessed monthly during initial treatment with epoetin to maintain serum ferritin greater than 100 ng/mL and TSAT greater than 20%. Monitoring intervals can be extended to every 3 months for children who are on a stable epoetin dose or for those who are on hemodialysis and are not receiving epoetin therapy.[15]

CONCLUSIONS

Anemia may be caused by nutritional deficiencies, severe inflammation, CKD, infections, and chronic illnesses. Iron deficiency is the most common form of nutritional deficiency. Children have increased risk for anemia because of rapid growth and decreased reserves of certain nutrients. Mild cases of anemia can still have effects on oxygen transport capacity of the blood and may produce symptoms such as irritability, lethargy, and decreased physical endurance. Iron deficiency is associated with poor cognitive and motor development, whereas vitamin B_{12} deficiency is associated with neurologic damage. Maternal folate deficiency can lead to neural tube defects in the fetus. Early detection of deficiency and prevention of anemia are essential. Hemoglobin is the standard laboratory assessment for detecting and monitoring anemia. Fortifying foods is one measure to prevent nutritional deficiencies.

Anemia of CKD may be caused by IDA in combination with erythropoietin deficiency. Oral iron supplementation is preferred, although children with malabsorptive disorders and those receiving dialysis may require intravenous iron. Epoetin, a recombinant erythropoiesis-stimulating glycoprotein, is commonly used and adequate iron status should be ensured before starting epoetin. Hemoglobin values while on epoetin therapy should not exceed 13 g/dL. Although untreated anemia of all types may result in considerable organ dysfunction, early detection and treatment can prevent complications.

A 3-month-old Hispanic girl is brought to the clinic for a well-child check-up. She was born preterm at 35 weeks gestation and is exclusively breastfed.

She has no current medications and no known drug allergies, and her immunizations are up to date. Her mother had very limited prenatal care, and her family medical history is otherwise noncontributory. She lives with her mother, father, and older brother.

Vital signs: Tmax 98°F (36.7°C), RR 30 breaths/minute, HR 165 beats/minute, BP 85/55 mm Hg, Ht 22 inches (10th percentile for age), Wt 5 kg (25th percentile for age).

Physical examination:

Appearance: Pale-appearing infant

HEENT: Normocephalic, pale conjunctiva, palate intact

Pulmonary: Lungs clear to auscultation bilaterally

Cardiovascular: Mild tachycardia, no murmur noted

Gastrointestinal: Nontender, nondistended, positive bowel sounds

---

1. What are the infant's risk factors for anemia?

Her risk factors for anemia include Hispanic ethnicity, premature birth, young age, and being exclusively breastfed.

2. What initial laboratory tests should be obtained to screen for anemia in this infant?

Initial laboratory testing should include a complete blood count that permits assessment of hemoglobin, hematocrit, and red cell indices. The need for additional laboratory studies is dictated by the patient's history, the physical examination, and the results of initial testing.

Case (continued). Laboratory analyses for this infant have returned and the findings confirm the presence of anemia. Her laboratory values are:

Hgb: 8.8 g/dL (range: 9–14 g/dL)

Hct: 25.8% (range: 32%–41%)

Mean corpuscular volume: 81.4 fL (range: 80–108 fL)

Red cell distribution width: 12.1% (range: 11%–15%)

3. The infant most likely has which type of anemia given her risk profile and clinical findings?

The infant most likely has iron deficiency anemia (IDA), which is the most common type of anemia among young children. Preterm neonates possess lower total body iron than full-term neonates. The faster rate of postnatal growth experienced by preterm neonates places them at risk of rapidly depleting iron stores compared with their full-term counterparts. Preterm neonates can develop iron deficiency by age 2 to 3 months if adequate

iron supplementation is not provided. Human breast milk has a low concentration of elemental iron, about 0.5–1 mg/L. Infants who are exclusively breastfed and who do not receive iron supplementation are at increased risk of developing anemia.

Case (continued). Additional laboratory analyses confirm the presence of iron deficiency anemia.

4. What pharmacologic intervention would be most appropriate for this infant based on the information provided within the case?

The infant has moderate anemia, defined as Hgb between 7 and 9.9 g/dL. The therapy of choice for managing IDA is oral iron supplementation. For infants and children with mild to moderate anemia, elemental iron at a dose of 3 mg/kg given once daily or divided into two doses is recommended. The total elemental iron dose for this infant is 15 mg per day given her weight of 5 kg. Any of the following oral iron supplements may be considered to treat the infant's IDA:

- Poly-Vi-Sol with iron (each 1 mL contains 10 mg of elemental iron): 1.5 mL orally once daily
- Tri-Vi-Sol with iron (each 1 mL contains 10 mg of elemental iron): 1.5 mL orally once daily
- Fer-in-sol drops (each 1 mL contains 15 mg of elemental iron): 1 mL orally once daily
- Ferrous sulfate liquid (each 1 mL contains 12 mg elemental iron): 1.25 mL orally once daily
- Ferrous sulfate elixir (each 1 mL contains 8.8 mg elemental iron): 1.7 mL orally once daily

REFERENCES

1. McLean E, Cogswell M, Egli I, et al. Worldwide prevalence of anaemia, WHO Vitamin and Mineral Nutrition Information System, 1993-2005. Public Health Nutr 2009;12:444-54.

2. World Health Organization (WHO). Haemoglobin Concentrations for the Diagnosis of Anaemia and Assessment of Severity. Vitamin and Mineral Nutrition Information System. Geneva, WHO, 2011. Available at https://www.who.int/vmnis/indicators/haemoglobin/en/. Accessed September 25, 2018.

3. Centers for Disease Control and Prevention. Recommendations to prevent and control iron deficiency in the United States. MMWR Recomm Rep 1998;47:1-36.

4. Menon KC, Ferguson EL, Thomson CD, et al. Effects of anemia at different stages of gestation on infant outcomes. Nutrition 2016;32:61-5.

5. Gairdner D, Marks J, Roscoe JD. Blood formation in infancy. Part II. Normal erythropoiesis. Arch Dis Child 1952;27:214-21.

6. Brabin BJ, Premji Z, Verhoeff F. An analysis of anemia and child mortality. J Nutr 2001;131:636S-45S; discussion 646S-8S.

7. Lozoff B, Beard J, Connor J, et al. Long-lasting neural and behavioral effects of iron deficiency in infancy. Nutr Rev 2006;64:S34-43.

8. Kassebaum NJ, Jasrasaria R, Naghavi M, et al. A systematic analysis of global anemia burden from 1990 to 2010. Blood 2014;123:615-24.

9. World Health Organization (WHO). The Global Prevalence of Anaemia in 2011. Geneva: WHO, 2015.

10. Brotanek JM, Gosz J, Weitzman M, et al. Secular trends in the prevalence of iron deficiency among US toddlers, 1976–2002. Arch Pediatr Adolesc Med 2008;162:374-81.

11. McDowell MA, Lacher DA, Pfeiffer CM, et al. Blood folate levels: the latest NHANES results. NCHS Data Brief 2008;6:1-8.

12. Hinton CF, Ojodu JA, Fernhoff PM, et al. Maternal and neonatal vitamin B12 deficiency detected through expanded newborn screening—United States, 2003-2007. J Pediatr 2010;157:162-3.

13. Koury MJ, Ponka P. New insights into erythropoiesis: the roles of folate, vitamin B12, and iron. Annu Rev Nutr 2004;24:105-31.

14. Koury MJ. Abnormal erythropoiesis and the pathophysiology of chronic anemia. Blood Rev 2014;28:49-66.

15. KDOQI clinical practice guidelines and clinical practice recommendations for anemia in chronic kidney disease. Am J Kidney Dis 2006;47:S11-145.

16. Bateman ST, Lacroix J, Boven K, et al. Anemia, blood loss, and blood transfusions in North American children in the intensive care unit. Am J Respir Crit Care Med 2008;178:26-33.

17. Lin JC, Strauss RG, Kulhavy JC, et al. Phlebotomy overdraw in the neonatal intensive care nursery. Pediatrics 2000;106:E19.

18. Baker RD, Greer FR. Diagnosis and prevention of iron deficiency and iron-deficiency anemia in infants and young children (0-3 years of age). Pediatrics 2010;126:1040-50.

19. Irwin JJ, Kirchner JT. Anemia in children. Am Fam Physician 2001;64:1379-86.

20. Janus J, Moerschel SK. Evaluation of anemia in children. Am Fam Physician 2010;81:1462-71.

21. Mei Z, Parvanta I, Cogswell ME, et al. Erythrocyte protoporphyrin or hemoglobin: which is a better screening test for iron deficiency in children and women? Am J Clin Nutr 2003;77:1229-33.

22. Jopling J, Henry E, Wiedmeier SE, et al. Reference ranges for hematocrit and blood hemoglobin concentration during the neonatal period: data from a multihospital health care system. Pediatrics 2009;123:e333-7.

23. Segel GB, Hirsh MG, Feig SA. Managing anemia in pediatric office practice. Part 1. Pediatr Rev 2002;23:75-84.

24. Institute of Medicine (U.S.). Dietary Reference Intakes for Thiamin, Riboflavin, Niacin, Vitamin B, Folate, Vitamin B12, Pantothenic Acid, Biotin, and Choline. Washington, DC: National Academy Press, 1998.

25. Siu AL and USPS Task Force. Screening for Iron Deficiency Anemia in Young Children: USPSTF Recommendation Statement. Pediatrics 2015;136:746-52.

26. Scholl TO, Johnson WG. Folic acid: influence on the outcome of pregnancy. Am J Clin Nutr 2000;71:1295S-1303S.

27. U.S. Department of Agriculture. USDA National Nutrient Database for Standard Reference [online database] 2018. Washington, DC. Available at www.ars.usda.gov/Services/docs.htm?docid=8964. Accessed September 27, 2018.

28. McKillop DJ, Pentieva K, Daly D, et al. The effect of different cooking methods on folate retention in various foods that are amongst the major contributors to folate intake in the UK diet. Br J Nutr 2002;88:681-8.

29. Molloy AM, Kirke PN, Brody LC, et al. Effects of folate and vitamin B12 deficiencies during pregnancy on fetal, infant, and child development. Food Nutr Bull 2008;29:S101-11.

30. Stabler SP, Allen RH. Vitamin B12 deficiency as a worldwide problem. Annu Rev Nutr 2004;24:299-326.

31. Basnet S, Schneider M, Gazit A, et al. Fresh goat's milk for infants: myths and realities—a review. Pediatrics 2010;125:e973-7.

32. Ford JE, Zechalko A, Murphy J, et al. Comparison of the B vitamin composition of milk from mothers of preterm and term babies. Arch Dis Child 1983;58:367-72.

33. Folate and vitamin B12 deficiencies. Proceedings of a WHO technical consultation held 18-21 October 2005, in Geneva, Switzerland. Food Nutr Bull 2008;29:S1-246.

34. Reynolds E. Vitamin B12, folic acid, and the nervous system. Lancet Neurol 2006;5:949-60.

35. Brouwer IA, van Dusseldorp M, West CE, et al. Bioavailability and bioefficacy of folate and folic acid in man. Nutr Res Rev 2001;14:267-94.

36. Institute of Medicine (U.S.). Dietary Reference Intakes for Vitamin A, Vitamin K, Arsenic, Boron, Chromium, Copper, Iodine, Iron, Manganese, Molybdenum, Nickel, Silicon, Vanadium, and Zinc. Washington, DC: National Academy Press, 2001.

37. US Preventive Services Task Force. Folic Acid Supplementation for the Prevention of Neural Tube Defects: US Preventive Services Task Force Recommendation Statement. JAMA 2017;317:183-9.

38. Green R. Indicators for assessing folate and vitamin B12 status and for monitoring the efficacy of intervention strategies. Food Nutr Bull 2008;29:S52-63; discussion S64-6.

39. Tschudy MM, Arcara KM, eds. Johns Hopkins: The Harriet Lane Handbook, 19th ed. Philadelphia: Elsevier, 2012.

40. Snow CF. Laboratory diagnosis of vitamin B12 and folate deficiency: a guide for the primary care physician. Arch Intern Med 1999;159:1289-98.

41. Lexi-Comp Online, Lexi-Drugs Online [Internet database]. Folic Acid. Hudson, OH: Lexi-Comp, Wolters Kluwer Clinical Drug Information, Inc. Updated periodically.

42. Lexi-Comp Online, Pediatric and Neonatal Lexi-Drugs Online [Internet database]. Cyanocobalamin. Hudson, OH: Lexi-Comp, Wolters Kluwer Clinical Drug Information, Inc. Updated periodically.

43. Cyanocobalamin injection [package insert]. Shirley, NY: American Regent, 2015.

44. Cyanocobalamin nasal spray [package insert]. Spring Valley, NY: Par Pharmaceuticals, 2015.

45. Koury M, Wheeler AP, Sika M. Folate deficiency. BMJ Best Practice. June 2018. Available at https://bestpractice.bmj.com/topics/en-us/823. Accessed September 27, 2018.

46. Killip S, Bennett JM, Chambers MD. Iron deficiency anemia. Am Fam Physician 2007;75:671-8.

47. Andrews NC. Iron metabolism: iron deficiency and iron overload. Annu Rev Genomics Hum Genet 2000;1:75-98.

48. Teucher B, Olivares M, Cori H. Enhancers of iron absorption: ascorbic acid and other organic acids. Int J Vitam Nutr Res 2004;74:403-19.

49. Siegenberg D, Baynes RD, Bothwell TH, et al. Ascorbic acid prevents the dose-dependent inhibitory effects of polyphenols and phytates on nonheme-iron absorption. Am J Clin Nutr 1991;53:537-41.

50. Adamson JW. Normal iron physiology. Semin Dial 1999; 12:219-23.

51. Oski FA. Iron deficiency in infancy and childhood. N Engl J Med 1993;329:190-3.

52. McMillan JA, Oski FA, Lourie G, et al. Iron absorption from human milk, simulated human milk, and proprietary formulas. Pediatrics 1977;60:896-900.

53. Hallberg L, Rossander-Hulten L, Brune M, et al. Bioavailability in man of iron in human milk and cow's milk in relation to their calcium contents. Pediatr Res 1992;31:524-7.

54. Ziegler EE. Adverse effects of cow's milk in infants. Nestle Nutr Workshop Ser Pediatr Program 2007;60:185-96.

55. Rasmussen K. Is there a causal relationship between iron deficiency or iron-deficiency anemia and weight at birth, length of gestation and perinatal mortality? J Nutr 2001;131:590S-601S.

56. Allen LH. Folate and vitamin B12 status in the Americas. Nutr Rev 2004;62:S29-33.

57. Andrews NC, Schmidt PJ. Iron homeostasis. Annu Rev Physiol 2007;69:69-85.

58. U.S. Department of Health and Human Services. Healthy People 2020. Topics and Objectives: Nutrition and Weight Status. Available at https://www.healthypeople.gov/2020/topics-objectives/topic/nutrition-and-weight-status/objectives. Accessed September 27, 2018.

59. Wish JB. Assessing iron status: beyond serum ferritin and transferrin saturation. Clin J Am Soc Nephrol 2006;1:S4-8.

60. Umbreit J. Iron deficiency: a concise review. Am J Hematol 2005;78:225-31.

61. Brugnara C, Zurakowski D, DiCanzio J, et al. Reticulocyte hemoglobin content to diagnose iron deficiency in children. JAMA 1999;281:2225-30.

62. Kazal LA Jr. Prevention of iron deficiency in infants and toddlers. Am Fam Physician 2002;66:1217-24.

63. Deinard AS, Schwartz S, Yip R. Developmental changes in serum ferritin and erythrocyte protoporphyrin in normal (nonanemic) children. Am J Clin Nutr 1983;38:71-6.

64. Harju E. Clinical pharmacokinetics of iron preparations. Clin Pharmacokinet 1989;17:69-89.

65. Lexi-Comp Online, Pediatric and Neonatal Lexi-Drugs Online [Internet database]. Ferrous Sulfate. Hudson, OH: Lexi-Comp, Wolters Kluwer Clinical Drug Information, Inc. Updated periodically.

66. Lexi-Comp Online, Pediatric and Neonatal Lexi-Drugs Online [Internet database]. Ferrous Fumarate. Hudson, OH: Lexi-Comp, Wolters Kluwer Clinical Drug Information, Inc. Updated periodically.

67. Lexi-Comp Online, Pediatric and Neonatal Lexi-Drugs Online [Internet database]. Ferrous Gluconate. Hudson, OH: Lexi-Comp, Wolters Kluwer Clinical Drug Information, Inc. Updated periodically.

68. Lexi-Comp Online, Lexi-Drugs Online [Internet database]. Polysaccharide-Iron Complex. Hudson, OH: Lexi-Comp, Wolters Kluwer Clinical Drug Information, Inc. Updated periodically.

69. Lexi-Comp Online, Pediatric and Neonatal Lexi-Drugs Online [Internet database]. Multivitamin Product Table. Hudson, OH: Lexi-Comp, Wolters Kluwer Clinical Drug Information, Inc. Updated periodically.

70. Gordeuk VR, Brittenham GM, Hughes M, et al. High-dose carbonyl iron for iron deficiency anemia: a randomized double-blind trial. Am J Clin Nutr 1987;46:1029-34.

71. Fine JS. Iron poisoning. Curr Probl Pediatr 2000;30:71-90.

72. Walker SE, Paton TW, Cowan DH, et al. Bioavailability of iron in oral ferrous sulfate preparations in healthy volunteers. CMAJ 1989;141:543-7.

73. Pendse S, Singh AK. Complications of chronic kidney disease: anemia, mineral metabolism, and cardiovascular disease. Med Clin North Am 2005;89:549-61.

74. Krafte-Jacobs B, Williams J, Soldin SJ. Plasma erythropoietin reference ranges in children. J Pediatr 1995;126:601-3.

75. Silverstein SB, Rodgers GM. Parenteral iron therapy options. Am J Hematol 2004;76:74-8.

76. INFeD [package insert]. Parsippany, NJ: Actavis Pharma, Inc., 2018.

77. Lexi-Comp Online, Pediatric Lexi-Drugs Online. Iron dextran. Hudson, OH: Lexi-Comp Online, Wolters Kluwer, Inc. Updated periodically.

78. Lexi-Comp Online, Pediatric Lexi-Drugs Online. Iron sucrose. Hudson, OH: Lexi-Comp Online, Wolters Kluwer, Inc. Updated periodically.

79. Ferrlecit [package insert]. Bridgewater, NJ: Sanofi-Aventis, 2015.

80. Feraheme [package insert]. Waltham, MA: AMAG Pharmaceuticals, 2018.

81. Hassan N, Boville B, Reischmann D, et al. Intravenous ferumoxytol in pediatric patients with iron deficiency anemia. Ann Pharmacother 2017;51:548-54.

CHAPTER 48

Anticoagulation

Brady S. Moffett, Pharm.D., MPH, MBA

LEARNING OBJECTIVES

1. Understand the epidemiology, pathophysiology, and common risk factors for pediatric thrombosis.

2. Understand the pharmacology and therapeutics of antithrombotic agents including unfractionated heparin, warfarin, low molecular weight heparin, and direct thrombin inhibitors.

3. Establish monitoring for pediatric patients receiving anticoagulant medications for the treatment and prevention of thrombosis.

ABBREVIATIONS IN THIS CHAPTER

ACT	Activated clotting time
Anti-Xa	Antifactor Xa
aPTT	Activated partial thromboplastin time
CYP	Cytochrome P450
DVT	Deep venous thrombosis
HIT	Heparin-induced thrombocytopenia
INR	International normalized ratio
PE	Pulmonary embolism
UFH	Unfractionated heparin

INTRODUCTION

This chapter will focus on the pharmacologic treatment and prophylaxis of thrombosis in pediatric patients, with a brief review of the etiology and pathophysiology of thrombosis that is common to the pediatric population. This chapter will focus on the following: deep venous thrombosis (DVT), arterial thrombosis, pulmonary embolism (PE), ischemic stroke, and intravascular catheter patency in the pediatric population. Patients undergoing anticoagulation for hemodialysis, anticoagulation in the cardiac catheterization laboratory, and anticoagulation in the operating room are smaller subsets of patients that will not be covered in this review. The intention is that the information provided in this chapter will cover most clinical situations that a pediatric pharmacist will encounter.

DEEP VENOUS THROMBOSIS

Pediatric DVT has distinct characteristics compared with adult DVT. Unlike in adults, the etiology of pediatric DVT is rarely idiopathic. Pediatric patients have a lower thrombotic potential compared with adults because of their decreased concentrations of plasma procoagulant factors, decreased thrombotic potential of the vascular endothelium, and increased inhibition of thrombin by α-2 macroglobulin.[1,2] Most adult DVTs occur in the lower extremities, whereas pediatric DVTs can occur in both the upper and lower extremities.

The incidence of pediatric DVT has been increasing over time, with an incidence of 5.3 per 10,000 pediatric hospital admissions in the year 2000, to a recent incidence as high 58 per 10,000 pediatric hospital admissions.[1-4] In general, infants and adolescents have the highest incidence of DVT compared with toddlers and young children.[4] Central venous catheters account for most DVTs in the upper parts of the vasculature, particularly in younger and critically ill children. Adolescent girls also have a higher risk of developing a DVT, likely because of oral contraceptive use.[1-5] Sepsis, nephrotic syndrome, malignancy, surgery, congenital heart disease (with or without prosthetic materials), antiphospholipid antibody syndrome, L-asparaginase therapy, and congenital or acquired prothrombotic conditions also contribute to DVT formation.

Patients with a DVT note symptoms of pain, discoloration, and swelling in the area distal to the DVT; however, many patients are asymptomatic.[2,6] Intravascular catheter dysfunction is often the initial symptom for catheter-related DVTs.[1,2,6] Imaging can be useful for detection of thrombus including the use of Doppler ultrasonography, echocardiography (for intracardiac thrombi), or computed tomography scan for abdominal thrombi.[1,2,6] D-dimer tests can be used for DVT detection, and platelet counts can be useful for detection of DVT in neonates with thrombocytopenia secondary to thrombus consumption of platelets.

Mortality rates for venous thromboembolism have been reported at 1%–8%.[2,3,6] Recurrence rates for DVT range from 9%–21%, and are higher in patients with chronic conditions.[5] Postthrombotic syndrome, consisting of pain, swelling, altered skin pigmentation, and skin ulceration near the site of the DVT, can occur in pediatric patients after resolution of a DVT.[2,7]

Enoxaparin or warfarin is typically indicated for 3–6 months for treatment of an uncomplicated DVT in the outpatient setting.[8] Laboratory monitoring of antifactor-Xa (anti-Xa) or international normalized ratio (INR) should occur regularly throughout therapy to ensure attainment of therapeutic end points, especially in younger patients.[9] Unfractionated heparin (UFH) titrated to therapeutic activated partial thromboplastin time (aPTT) or anti-Xa concentration is often used for inpatients before transition to enoxaparin or warfarin.

PULMONARY EMBOLISM

Pulmonary embolism in pediatric patients is reported at less than 1 per 100,000 children per year; however, most patients are asymptomatic, and symptomatology occurs in patients with very large thrombi (obstructing more than 50% of the pulmonary circulation).[10-12] The percentage of patients who were asymptomatic but had a PE was as high as 50% in pediatric populations with risk factors, which are similar to the risk factors associated with DVTs.[13]

Primary symptoms of PE include dyspnea, cough, hemoptysis, and chest pain.[12] Arrhythmias and even sudden death have occurred in pediatric patients with a PE. Ventilated patients may have a sudden increase in oxygen requirements. Elevated right ventricular pressures or tricuspid regurgitation may occur because of increased pulmonary vascular resistance. Ventilation and perfusion mismatch may occur resulting in decreased arterial oxygen saturation. Diagnosis can be made by the use of noninvasive imaging, such as magnetic resonance imaging, computed tomography scan, ventilation perfusion lung scanning, or pulmonary angiography.[12]

The goal of treatment is to eradicate the PE and prevent recurrence or propagation of the embolus. Nonpharmacologic therapies for PE include surgical embolectomy and interventional procedures, but these interventions require significant expertise and can have high morbidity.[14,15]

Unfractionated heparin is often the first-line agent for acute treatment of PE in children. Alteplase for thrombolysis is an option, but definitive recommendations for the use of alteplase in pediatric patients are unavailable because of a paucity of data, and therefore this treatment should be evaluated on a case-by-case basis because of the high risk of hemorrhage.[16-20] Patients will often be treated for at least 6 months after receiving a diagnosis of a PE with enoxaparin or warfarin; however, the optimal treatment duration in pediatric patients is currently unknown.[8]

ARTERIAL THROMBOSIS

Arterial thrombosis occurs because of indwelling arterial catheters or after cardiac catheterization at the arterial access point of catheter insertion.[21,22] The primary pathophysiology for arterial thrombosis is damage to the endothelium of the artery, resulting in inflammation and clotting cascade activation.[8] The length of time of catheter placement and younger age are both risk factors for arterial thrombus.[23] Indwelling catheters in septic patients and patients with underlying coagulopathies are also at increased risk of arterial thrombosis.[8,21,24,25]

Acute loss of circulation to a limb or region of the body is the hallmark of arterial thrombus. An affected limb may become cool, pale, have a sluggish capillary refill, or lack of distal pulses. Doppler ultrasonography can be useful to assess the clinical severity of the thrombus. Contrast angiography is the gold standard for assessing arterial thrombosis but is not commonly used.[26]

If possible, the first step for treatment of arterial thrombosis is to remove the offending catheter. Nonpharmacologic treatment of arterial thrombosis is typically reserved for life- or limb-threatening conditions. Thrombectomy, either surgically or interventionally, can be performed for large thrombi. Devices to mechanically destroy a thrombus have also been used. However, these devices have the disadvantage of potentially causing trauma to the vessel wall and are sometimes unable to extract free-floating thrombus.[27]

Pharmacologic therapy is started on the basis of the severity of arterial blockage. Enoxaparin or UFH is typically a first-line agent for arterial thrombus that is not immediately life or limb threatening.[26,28] Alteplase has been used in emergency cases for the dissolution of an arterial thrombus.[29] The use of alteplase has a high bleeding risk, and caution should be exercised in patients with the potential for hemorrhage, such as premature infants, patients who have undergone recent major surgery, or patients with baseline bleeding disorders.[8]

ISCHEMIC STROKE

Acute ischemic stroke has a very low annual incidence in the United States, ranging from 2 to 8 per 100,000 children. However, the morbidity with stroke is high with reports of 70% of patients having a persistent neurologic deficit. Cardiovascular disease (congenital or acquired), sickle cell disease, and other coagulopathies are risk factors for stroke, with 30% of children presenting with an ischemic stroke having no identifiable risk factors.[30-33]

The symptoms associated with ischemic stroke in adults are similar to those in the pediatric population, and will vary depending on the age of the child and other comorbidities: monoparesis or hemiparesis, vision changes, numbness, ataxia, headache, seizures, and/or altered mental status.[30-34]

Aside from basic interventions to support life, hematologic studies in the pediatric stroke patient are warranted to evaluate for baseline coagulopathies. Brain computed tomography or magnetic resonance imaging can be useful to characterize the etiology of the stoke (hemorrhagic or ischemic).[35] Patients with hypotension or hyperglycemia have been identified to have worse outcomes, and these symptoms should be managed.[36,37] Fever can often be present and should be treated with acetaminophen, avoiding nonsteroidal anti-inflammatory medications for their risk of bleeding.[36,37] Fosphenytoin and levetiracetam have been used to treat seizures in this population.[37]

No current standard for treatment of pediatric ischemic stroke has been published. Enoxaparin or UFH has traditionally been a first-line treatment option, as well as antiplatelet medications, such as aspirin.[36,38] Warfarin or enoxaparin can be used as long-term therapy for stroke after the acute period. Limited data are available for the use of either clopidogrel and dipyridamole.[39,40] Etiology of the stroke and patient comorbidities will influence the duration and intensity of anticoagulant or antiplatelet therapy.

MAINTENANCE OF ARTERIAL OR VENOUS CATHETER PATENCY

As previously mentioned, the main cause of thromboembolism in pediatric patients is the presence of an indwelling venous or arterial catheter. Several different strategies have been used to prevent catheter-related thrombosis; however, definitive recommendations for prophylaxis are currently unavailable. Adverse events can occur even with the routine use of UFH for flushing of catheters, and care should be taken when implementing recommendations or practices for line maintenance.[41-44] Data for the use of UFH boluses or continuous infusions show conflicting results in the pediatric population.[45-47] Other methods of preventing catheter-related thrombosis have also had unclear results, such as routine low-dose anticoagulation of critically ill pediatric patients (not directed through the catheter).[44] Reports of using heparin-bonded catheters have shown promise in preventing thromboembolism in pediatric patients; however, this reduction may be the result of prevention of infection, and not a direct anticoagulant effect.[48-53] In the outpatient setting, prevention of catheter-related thrombosis has been evaluated in patients receiving warfarin and long-term total parenteral nutrition.[54] A Cochrane Review suggests that using a low concentration of UFH as a continuous infusion through a central venous catheter in neonates prevents thrombosis.[55] Overall, the use of anticoagulation directed through a central venous catheter appears to have benefit in the neonatal population, although other methods of anticoagulation for prevention of catheter thrombus do not share the same degree of support. Alteplase has shown safety and efficacy in clearing catheter occlusions, whether by instilling in the catheter or using interventional catheter-directed methods.[56-65]

PHARMACOLOGY

ASPIRIN

Aspirin mediates antiplatelet effects by irreversibly acetylating cyclooxygenase-1 and decreasing the amount of thromboxane A2 generated, subsequently decreasing platelet aggregation.[66] Absorption is primarily in the stomach and small intestines, with greater absorption in the small intestines for enteric-coated formulations.[67] Peak serum concentrations for nonenteric-coated or nondelayed-release aspirin formulations occur about 1–2 hours after oral ingestion. Aspirin is primarily hepatically metabolized and renally eliminated as unchanged drug or as metabolites and is dialyzable.[67] Aspirin dosing in pediatric patients, which is not well defined, is often rounded to the nearest one-quarter tablet because of unavailability of a commercially produced suspension (Table 1).

Adverse events with aspirin include bleeding, and enteric-coated formulations have been developed to avoid gastrointestinal bleeding.[67] Reye syndrome, a form of noninflammatory hepatic encephalopathy, has been linked to aspirin therapy in patients with viral illness. However, data supporting the link between aspirin use, viral illness, and Reye syndrome are weak, and the true etiology of Reye syndrome likely has a strong genetic component and is multifactorial.[68]

DIPYRIDAMOLE

Dipyridamole inhibits platelet aggregation by decreasing phosphodiesterase and releasing prostacyclin, resulting in decreased platelet aggregation and mild vasodilation.[67] Few data are available regarding the pharmacokinetics of dipyridamole in pediatric patients, and most dosing has been extrapolated from adult data (Table 1).[69-72] Dipyridamole is primarily hepatically metabolized, and, when administered enterally, has slow and variable enteric absorption. Adverse events with dipyridamole include bleeding, and events related to vasodilation, such as syncope, dizziness, and hypotension.[67] These data are extrapolated from the adult population because pediatric data are limited.

CLOPIDOGREL

Clopidogrel is extensively hepatically metabolized into an active thiol compound, which irreversibly binds to the P2Y12 platelet receptors and prevents activation of the glycoprotein IIb/IIIa platelet-binding complex (Table 1).[73-75] The metabolism of clopidogrel involves cytochrome P450 (CYP) enzymes, particularly CYP2C19 and CYP3A4. Platelet inhibition can be variable, and it is based on enzyme expression to transform clopidogrel into the active form.[76] Practitioners should be aware of the potential for significant drug interactions with clopidogrel, such as concomitant use of proton pump inhibitors.[77,78]

WARFARIN

Warfarin has been widely used in both adult and pediatric patients for many years and extensive guidelines for dosing have been published.[8] Anticoagulation occurs through inhibition of vitamin K epoxide reductase, which converts vitamin K–dependent clotting factors (II, VII, IX, X) to active forms. Warfarin also inhibits the anticoagulant proteins C and S.

Warfarin dosing in pediatric patients is on a milligram per kilogram basis, with reductions in dose for drug interactions or disease states (Table 1).[9] The full effect of warfarin will typically not be seen until after 5–7 days of therapy because of the differing half-lives of the vitamin K–dependent clotting factors. Dosing algorithms or guidelines that incorporate pharmacogenomic testing can assist with identifying appropriate warfarin doses.[79,80] Pharmacogenomic testing has recently come to the forefront as a method for improving warfarin dosing and identifying patients at risk of warfarin-related morbidity.[79,81-85] Specifically, Asian patients require lower doses of warfarin because of the underexpression of VKORC1.[86] Polymorphisms in CYP2C9 have been shown to affect a patient's response to warfarin therapy.[81] These data are now available to assist in dosing of warfarin in the pediatric patient.[87-89]

In addition, factors other than pharmacogenomics may better explain the variation in warfarin dose in the pediatric patient population.[82] Drug interactions play a role in the morbidity of pediatric patients receiving warfarin.[90,91] Younger patients often require higher warfarin doses per kilogram of body weight to achieve therapeutic INR values (Table 1).[9,92-94] The effect of vitamin K supplementation in diets as well as enteral feeding formulas or breastfeeding should be considered when evaluating warfarin therapy in pediatric patients.[9]

The INR is used to monitor warfarin therapy, but most pediatric goal INR ranges have been extrapolated from adult data. Variation in INR values is high in pediatric patients, and close monitoring is warranted.[9,95,96] Significant morbidity associated with warfarin therapy has driven the development of methods to improve warfarin dosing and monitoring.

Table 1. Dosing and Monitoring of Commonly Used Anticoagulant and Antiplatelet Agents in Pediatric Patients[67]

Medication	Dosing and Administration	Suggested Monitoring Variables
Abciximab	Infants, children, adolescents **Treatment:** Bolus IV 0.25 mg/kg/dose; continuous IV infusion 0.125 mcg/kg/min	aPTT; PT; fibrinogen; platelet count; bleeding
Alteplase[a]	Infants, children, adolescents **Treatment of systemic thrombus:** Continuous IV infusion 0.1–0.6 mg/kg/hr for 6 hr **Treatment of catheter thrombus (low dose):** Continuous IV infusion 0.01–0.05 mg/kg/hr **Catheter clearance:** 0.5–2 mg in 1–3 mL of normal saline instilled into catheter and aspirated after a 1- to 2-hr dwell time; NOT infused into patient	aPTT; anti-Xa; plasminogen; fibrinogen; bleeding
Argatroban[b]	Infants, children, adolescents **Treatment:** Continuous IV infusion 1.75 mcg/kg/hr	aPTT; platelet count; bleeding; serum creatinine; liver function
Aspirin	Infants, children, adolescents **Prophylaxis:** Oral 1–5 mg/kg/day once daily; max 81 mg/day **Kawasaki disease:** Oral 80–100 mg/kg/day divided QID for 14 days, or until defervescence; then 3–5 mg/kg/day once daily	Platelet count; bleeding
Bivalirudin	Infants, children, adolescents **Treatment:** Bolus IV 0.75 mg/kg/dose; continuous IV infusion 1.75 mg/kg/hr	aPTT; ACT; platelet count; serum creatinine; bleeding
Clopidogrel	**Treatment and prophylaxis** Infants < 24 mo: Oral 0.2 mg/kg/dose once daily Children > 2 yr: Oral 1 mg/kg/dose once daily; max 75 mg once daily	Platelet count; bleeding
Dipyridamole	Infants, children, adolescents **Treatment and prophylaxis:** Oral 3–6 mg/kg/day divided TID; max 400 mg/day	Platelet count; bleeding
Enoxaparin[c,d]	**Treatment** Preterm neonates: SC 2 mg/kg/dose BID Term neonates: SC 1.7 mg/kg/dose BID Infants 1 to < 2 mo: SC 1.5 mg/kg/dose BID Children > 2 mo: SC 1 mg/kg/dose BID Adolescents, adults: SC 1 mg/kg/dose BID	Anti-Xa; platelet count; serum creatinine; bleeding Goal anti-Xa concentrations for treatment of thrombus are typically 0.5–1 unit/mL, drawn 4–6 hr after a dose
	Prophylaxis Neonates, infants, children: SC 0.75 mg/kg/dose BID Adolescents, adults: SC 0.5 mg/kg/dose BID	
Unfractionated heparin	**Treatment of venous or arterial thrombus**—starting dose Infants < 1 yr: Bolus IV 75 units/kg/dose; continuous infusion IV 28 units/kg/hr Children > 1 yr: Bolus IV 75 units/kg/dose; continuous IV infusion 20 units/kg/hr Adolescents and adults: Bolus IV 80 units/kg/dose (max 5000 units); continuous IV infusion 18 units/kg/hr	aPTT; anti-Xa; platelet count; bleeding; thrombosis; serum creatinine Infusions should be titrated to a therapeutic aPTT or anti-Xa values, which may be institution-specific aPTT values are typically calibrated to achieve an anti-Xa concentration of 0.35–0.7 unit/mL
	Maintenance of catheter patency **Arterial catheter:** Neonates: 5 units/mL infused at 1 mL/hr Infants and children: 1 unit/mL infused at 1 mL/hr **Venous catheter:** Neonates: 10 units/mL as a bolus flush Infants and children: 10–100 units/mL as a bolus flush	UFH use to maintain catheter patency will vary based on patient- and institution-related factors Caution is warranted to ensure young patients do not receive therapeutic doses of UFH from several flushes or infusions

(continued)

Table 1. Dosing and Monitoring of Commonly Used Anticoagulant and Antiplatelet Agents in Pediatric Patients[67] *(continued)*

Medication	Dosing and Administration	Suggested Monitoring Variables
Warfarin	**Treatment and prophylaxis**—starting dose[e] Infants, children, adolescents: Oral 0.2 mg/kg/dose; max 5 mg/day Patients with drug interactions, Fontan-associated liver disease, or hepatic disease: Oral 0.1 mg/kg/dose	PT; INR; bleeding; thrombosis; dietary intake of vitamin K; drug-drug interactions
	Usual therapeutic doses Infants < 1 yr: 0.34 mg/kg/day Children 1–12 yr: 0.15–0.19 mg/kg/day Adolescents: 0.14 mg/kg/day	Dose should be titrated to goal INR value for the patient

[a] UFH infusion is typically continued during alteplase infusion to prevent rethrombosis.
[b] Argatroban dose may need to be reduced in patients with hepatic dysfunction.
[c] Prophylaxis for adolescents and adults may be a standard dose (40 mg SC) and can depend on indication for prophylaxis.
[d] Injection sites should be rotated (abdomen, thigh, upper arm) to prevent injection site bruising and lipomas.
[e] Loading doses of > 5 mg are generally not recommended.
ACT = activated clotting time; anti-Xa = antifactor Xa; aPTT = activated partial prothrombin time; BID = twice daily; INR = international normalized ratio; IV = intravenous; PT = prothrombin time; QID = four times daily; SC = subcutaneous; TID = three times daily; UFH = unfractionated heparin.

The use of standardized guidelines, health care provider and family education programs, computerized algorithms, and home INR monitoring are examples of interventions used to improve warfarin dosing and monitoring.[80,96-98]

Adverse events with warfarin primarily consist of bleeding complications, with other complications (thrombosis, "purple toe syndrome") occurring rarely.[9] Studies evaluating the outpatient management of warfarin in pediatric patients have reported the incidence of bleeding caused by warfarin at around 0.5% per patient-year, although this rate can vary because of differing management strategies.[9,69,93,99] Guidelines for the reversal of warfarin therapy have been published, and reversal can be accomplished with the administration of enteral or intravenous vitamin K (Table 2).[8] Severe bleeding events may require the administration of blood products or recombinant clotting factors.[8,100] Routine administration of vitamin K for the management of elevated INR values without bleeding symptoms is discouraged. Holding warfarin therapy for a period is often as effective as administering reversal agents and prevents resistance to warfarin when therapy is reinitiated.[101]

UNFRACTIONATED HEPARIN

Unfractionated heparin is a glycosaminoglycan that potentiates the action of antithrombin III on thrombin (factor II) to inhibit the conversion of fibrinogen to fibrin, which leads to decreased formation of thrombi. In addition, UFH releases tissue factor pathway inhibitor, which has antithrombotic effects, and inhibits the activated factors IX, X, XI, and XII and plasmin.[102] Metabolism of UFH is thought to occur by the reticuloendothelial system with minimal elimination by renal routes.[102]

The dosing for UFH is often dependent on laboratory monitoring variables, patient factors, and pathophysiology (Table 1). Primarily, UFH is given as an intravenous continuous infusion for the treatment of thrombi, with loading doses given as a bolus. The subcutaneous route has been used for DVT prophylaxis in adults, but it is not typically recommended in children. Continuous infusions of UFH are dosed as units per kilogram per hour, with neonates requiring larger per kilogram doses compared with older children and adults, likely because of differences in the characteristics of heparin-protein binding (Table 1).[102,103] Obese patients have been noted to require lower doses of UFH.[104] Institutional guidelines and policies should be developed regarding the use of UFH for treatment and prophylaxis to enhance safety and efficacy of therapies.

Laboratory monitoring of UFH can vary markedly depending on patient care setting and availability of tests; the ideal approach for laboratory monitoring of UFH in pediatric patients is unclear (Table 1). Most often, the aPTT has been the standard for laboratory measurement of therapeutic effect of UFH. The aPTT is titrated to an anti-Xa concentration of 0.3–0.7 unit/mL (chromogenic assay). Monitoring anti-Xa concentrations in pediatric patients is used in some institutions, but it is not routinely available because of cost and labor.[105-107] The activated clotting time (ACT) is used when heparin concentrations are high, as in patients in the cardiac catheterization laboratory or patients on cardiopulmonary bypass or extracorporeal membrane oxygenation. The use of the aPTT or the ACT for children has not been shown to correlate well with anti-Xa concentrations.[108] Finally, no data are available to correlate beneficial outcomes with the achievement of goal aPTT values in pediatric patients.[109]

Primary adverse events with UFH are bleeding and heparin-induced thrombocytopenia (HIT). Bleeding rates in pediatric patients receiving UFH are high (ranging from 1% to 56% of patients), but they are difficult to interpret because of the variety of definitions used and the relative paucity of data.[109] Clinically significant hemorrhage can be treated with protamine sulfate and by discontinuing the UFH infusion (Table 2). Osteoporosis has been noted as a potential adverse event in patients who are receiving prolonged therapy with UFH.[109,110]

Because HIT can occur with UFH, patients should have platelet counts monitored while receiving therapy. Heparin-induced thrombocytopenia type II is an immune-mediated reaction to platelets, whereas HIT type I is a much milder form of thrombocytopenia that is not immune mediated. The data for HIT type II in pediatric patients are scarce, but it is thought to occur at a much lower incidence than in adult patients.[111] Heparin-induced thrombocytopenia type II is characterized by a greater than 50% decrease in platelets and/or a new thrombotic event after the initiation of UFH, typically 5–14 days after starting.[112] Clinical confirmation of HIT type II can occur with laboratory testing, including serotonin tests, platelet factor 4, and ELISA (enzyme-linked immunoassay); however, the sensitivity and specificity of these tests are often low, and the results can be inconclusive. When a patient is given a diagnosis of HIT type II, removal of UFH from all sources, including flushes, must occur. Low molecular weight heparins should not be used because of a high incidence of cross-reactivity.[112] A direct thrombin inhibitor can be used, if anticoagulant therapy is necessary.

LOW MOLECULAR WEIGHT HEPARIN

The primary low molecular weight heparin used in pediatric patients is enoxaparin. Other low molecular weight heparins, such as dalteparin and tinzaparin, have limited data for use in pediatric patients.[113,114] Enoxaparin primarily inhibits factor X and, to a lesser degree, factor II, by potentiating the action of antithrombin III on those factors. Factor X is inhibited to a 4-times-greater extent than factor II. Enoxaparin is renally eliminated, with as much as 40% of the drug eliminated unchanged in the urine.[115-117] Enoxaparin has high bioavailability (about 100%) when administered subcutaneously.[67]

Dosing of enoxaparin for treatment of thrombosis is on a milligram per kilogram basis for children (Table 1).[67,115] An upper limit of dosing has not been determined, but morbidly obese patients may require empiric decreases in dose.[118,119] Dosage requirements to attain therapeutic concentrations decrease with age, with neonates requiring higher doses per kilogram than older children and adults.[117-126] However, the dose requirements for neonates and infants can vary widely.[117-126] To decrease the pain associated with several injections, subcutaneous catheters have been used.[120-122] Dilutions of enoxaparin made from commercially available concentrations and the use of insulin syringes have been proposed to ensure adequate delivery of small volumes for subcutaneous injection.[127,128]

Concentrations of anti-Xa should be measured in pediatric patients, patients with renal dysfunction, patients who

Table 2. Reversal of Supratherapeutic Anticoagulant Effect[67]

Anticoagulant	Laboratory Values	Clinical Evidence of Bleeding	Reversal Agent and Dosing
Low molecular weight heparin (enoxaparin)	Elevated aPTT or anti-Xa	Dependent on patient—clinical evidence of bleeding not necessary to administer reversal agents	Protamine sulfate Dose for correction of enoxaparin overdose is 1 mg protamine per 1 mg enoxaparin Additional doses of 0.5 mg protamine per 1 mg enoxaparin can be administered at 2- to 4-hr intervals if necessary
Unfractionated heparin	Elevated aPTT or anti-Xa	Dependent on patient—clinical evidence of bleeding not necessary to administer reversal agents	Protamine sulfate Dose for immediate correction of UFH overdose is 1–1.5 mg protamine per 100 units UFH, with max 50 mg UFH is rapidly eliminated, and protamine dose should be decreased based on time after UFH administration
Warfarin	INR < 5	No evidence of bleeding	Hold doses; no reversal agent necessary
	INR ≥ 5 and < 9	No factors for increased bleeding risk and no evidence of bleeding	Hold doses; no reversal agent necessary
	INR ≥ 9	Factors that increase risk of bleeding but no evidence of bleeding	Hold doses; administer enteral vitamin K at 1–2.5 mg/dose daily until INR is within normal limits
	Any INR value	Serious or life-threatening bleeding	Hold doses; administer IV vitamin K, fresh frozen plasma, cryoprecipitate Recombinant factor VIIa (10-100 mcg/kg/ dose) may also be used; lower doses are initially preferred

aPTT = activated partial thromboplastin time; anti-Xa = antifactor Xa; INR = international normalized ratio; max = maximum; UFH = unfractionated heparin.

are pregnant, and obese patients.[67] Therapeutic concentrations often become more difficult to achieve in neonates and infants.[123,124] An anti-Xa concentration of 0.5–1 unit/mL drawn 4–6 hours after a dose at steady state is generally considered a therapeutic concentration, although pediatric data for confirming the efficacy of this range are limited (Table 1).[129]

Bleeding has been associated with enoxaparin use, but at a much lower rate than with UFH. Hematoma development at the site of subcutaneous injection has been noted to occur, and appropriate administration techniques can minimize this adverse event.[130] Protamine sulfate can be used to reverse the effects of enoxaparin (Table 2).[67] Finally, HIT has been noted with enoxaparin, at a lower incidence than with UFH, but should not be used in patients with HIT secondary to UFH.[67]

ALTEPLASE

Alteplase is a recombinant form of serine protease that activates the conversion of plasminogen to plasmin within a fibrin clot. The plasmin degrades the fibrin and other procoagulant materials into soluble materials reducing the fibrin thrombus. Adult data suggest that alteplase has a very short half-life (from a few minutes to an hour) with primary hepatic metabolism. Few pharmacokinetic data are available in the pediatric population.[67]

Alteplase dosing for the treatment of a thrombus in pediatric patients is controversial. High- and low-dose regimens have been reported (Table 1).[67,131-140] The clinical condition of the patient, size and location of the thrombus, and available expertise will influence use of alteplase in the pediatric patient.

Alteplase is often given as an adjunct to continuous-infusion UFH therapy to prevent the re-formation of thrombus after lysis. Patient platelet counts, plasminogen concentrations, fibrinogen concentrations, aPTT, and anti-Xa concentrations should be monitored during the course of alteplase therapy. Evaluation of bleeding risk should occur before the administration of alteplase, and patients should be monitored for signs and symptoms of bleeding.

When alteplase is used to clear an occluded arterial or venous catheter, standard doses and concentrations are often instilled into the occluded catheter, with lower doses/concentrations administered to younger patients. The alteplase is instilled into the catheter, left to dwell for about 2 hours, and then aspirated from the catheter and not given to the patient.[67] Laboratory monitoring is not indicated when alteplase is used in this situation.

BIVALIRUDIN

Bivalirudin is an intravenous direct thrombin inhibitor, with an immediate onset of action and a half-life of about 25 minutes in adults.[67] The primary reported adverse events have been bleeding and hypotension in adults. The dose should be reduced for patients with kidney dysfunction to prevent accumulation of the drug (Table 1). Therapy should be monitored using the ACT, particularly in areas where that test is the standard of care (i.e., cardiac catheterization laboratory).

Bivalirudin has shown promise in pediatric patients as an alternative to UFH in patients with HIT or other coagulopathies.[67,141-143] Dosing of bivalirudin in pediatric patients appears to be similar to that of adult patients, with good evidence of efficacy in treating thrombi (Table 1).[144-148]

ARGATROBAN

Argatroban is an intravenous direct thrombin inhibitor with a rapid onset of action and a short half-life.[67] About 20% of the drug is eliminated through the urine unchanged, with no empiric adjustment needed for kidney dysfunction, but dose adjustment for severe hepatic dysfunction is recommended.[67] It has been noted that critically ill pediatric patients have a lower clearance (up to 50% lower) than a relatively healthy adult patient; these patients may therefore require dose adjustments accordingly.[149-151]

The literature for pediatric patients has primarily been in the form of case reports or series of patients with HIT requiring mechanical circulatory support (Table 1).[152-156] Other reports have shown its use in pediatric patients in the cardiac catheterization laboratory.[157] Higher-goal INR values must be used when changing a patient from argatroban to warfarin because argatroban will elevate INR values.[67] Argatroban therapy should be monitored with aPTT, in general, or with ACT if used in the cardiac catheterization laboratory, in patients on extracorporeal membrane oxygenation, or during cardiopulmonary bypass.[67]

FUTURE DIRECTIONS

RIVAROXABAN

Rivaroxaban is an oral direct inhibitor of factor Xa that inhibits platelet activation and fibrin clot formation.[158-160] It is rapidly absorbed, highly protein bound, and metabolized via CYP3A4/5 and CYP2J2. Rivaroxaban is renally eliminated, and patients with kidney dysfunction should have doses decreased. Assays for anti-Xa and other traditionally used anticoagulant laboratory tests are not useful for monitoring therapy.[159] Pharmacokinetic data for use in pediatric patients have been published for future use in clinical trials.[160,161]

CONCLUSIONS

Safe and efficacious application of anticoagulant pharmacotherapy requires that pediatric pharmacists understand the pharmacology, potential for adverse events, and appropriate monitoring of anticoagulant and antiplatelet agents in infants and children.

Patient Case

ARTERIAL THROMBOSIS

A 4-day-old, term infant is admitted to the cardiovascular intensive care unit after a surgical procedure for transposition of the great arteries. An arterial catheter was placed intraoperatively for invasive blood pressure monitoring in the right radial artery. The immediate postoperative course is uneventful. On postoperative day 2, the patient appears warm and well perfused, with the exception of his right hand, which is pale and cool with sluggish capillary refill. He is intubated and sedated, and is in no acute distress. He has two thoracostomy tubes with moderate drainage. An ultrasound of the catheter site is performed and shows a blockage of the radial artery with minimal flow distal to the blockage. The hematology service is consulted and a diagnosis of right radial artery thrombosis is made. The recommendation is to remove the catheter and initiate anticoagulation therapy.

Medications:

Milrinone 0.5 mcg/kg/min IV

Epinephrine 0.02 mcg/kg/min IV

Fentanyl 1 mcg/kg/hr IV

Midazolam 0.05 mg/kg/ hr IV

Ranitidine 1 mg/kg/dose IV every 6 hr

Cefazolin 50 mg/kg/day IV divided every 8 hr at maintenance values

Furosemide 1 mg/kg/dose every 8 hr IV

Fluids: 5% Dextrose with 0.45% sodium chloride at 50%

Laboratory findings:

Na	144 mEq/L
K	3.2 mEq/L
HCO$_3$	29 mEq/L
Cl	97 mEq/L
SCr	0.3 mg/dL
Serum lactate	1.4 mg/dL (stable)

Vital signs: BP (arterial line) 110/62 mm Hg, HR 120 beats per minute

Physical examination: Capillary refill is brisk (2–3 seconds), except for right upper extremity distal to the arterial catheter; urine output 0.9 ml/kg/hr

---

1. What would be the appropriate initial anticoagulation therapy for this patient?

The use of medications in this scenario should be based on the urgency with which the thrombus should be treated. An arterial thrombus can be life- or limb-threatening; therefore, a medication that can be easily and quickly titrated to therapeutic values should be initiated. Unfractionated heparin (UFH) initiated at 28 units/kg/hour would be the best initial choice in this scenario because it can be titrated every 4–6 hours to goal factor Xa or aPTT values. The use of tissue plasminogen activator should be considered, particularly if the thrombus were in the extremities (i.e., appendage loss is likely) or if the use of UFH does not achieve perfusion to the extremity. However, the risk of bleeding with tissue plasminogen activator is very high, particularly in a newly postoperative cardiac surgical patient, and this risk should be balanced with the patient's current condition. Enoxaparin would be an acceptable choice for therapy after perfusion to the limb has been established, but would not be a good initial choice. Anticoagulant therapy would need to be rapidly titrated to effect/goal laboratory values in this patient, and enoxaparin typically requires laboratory evaluation (anti-Xa) 4 hours after two or more doses, which would be an unacceptably long

time for this patient. In addition, enoxaparin is difficult to initially dose in neonates and infants with very wide dose ranges, and identifying an appropriate dose would take time. Warfarin would not be a good choice because data in infants is sparse; the ability to titrate in the smallest patients is limited because there is no formulation for a suspension; and management of INR values in this patient population is difficult.

Case (continued). After 24 hours of therapy with continuous infusion UFH, perfusion to the limb has been restored. The hematology service recommends continuation of therapy for 6 months after discharge.

2. What anticoagulation therapy would you recommend?

Enoxaparin would be the most appropriate choice for long-term therapy in this patient. Titration of enoxaparin can occur as an inpatient to achieve a therapeutic dose, and parental instruction can be given so the drug can be administered at home. As mentioned previously, warfarin is difficult to titrate and manage in the infant population, and the use of continuous infusion UFH on an outpatient basis is impractical. Aspirin, although used as prophylaxis for thrombus development in many patients with congenital heart disease, would not be as effective for an arterial thrombus.

REFERENCES

1. McCrory MC, Brady KM, Takemoto C, et al. Thrombotic disease in critically ill children. Pediatr Crit Care Med 2011;12:80-9.

2. Parasuraman S, Goldhaber SZ. Venous thromboembolism in children. Circulation 2006;113:e12-6.

3. Raffini L, Huang YS, Witmer C, et al. Dramatic increase in venous thromboembolism in children's hospitals in the United States from 2001 to 2007. Pediatrics 2009;124:1001-8.

4. Stein PD, Kayali F, Olson RE. Incidence of venous thromboembolism in infants and children: data from the National Hospital Discharge Survey. J Pediatr 2004;145:563-5.

5. Nowak-Gottl U, Junker R, Kreuz W, et al. Risk of recurrent venous thrombosis in children with combined prothrombotic risk factors. Blood 2001;97:858-62.

6. Monagle P, Adams M, Mahoney M, et al. Outcome of pediatric thromboembolic disease: a report from the Canadian Childhood Thrombophilia Registry. Pediatr Res 2000;47:763-6.

7. Goldenberg NA, Donadini MP, Kahn SR, et al. Post-thrombotic syndrome in children: a systematic review of frequency of occurrence, validity of outcome measures, and prognostic factors. Haematologica 2010;95:1952-9.

8. Holbrook A, Schulman S, Witt DM, et al. Evidence-based management of anticoagulant therapy: antithrombotic therapy and prevention of thrombosis, 9th ed: American College of Chest Physicians evidence-based clinical practice guidelines. Chest 2012;141:e152S-84.

9. Streif W, Andrew M, Marzinotto V, et al. Analysis of warfarin therapy in pediatric patients: A prospective cohort study of 319 patients. Blood 1999;94:3007-14.

10. Andrew M, David M, Adams M, et al. Venous thromboembolic complications (VTE) in children: first analyses of the Canadian Registry of VTE. Blood 1994;83:1251-7.

11. van Ommen CH, Heijboer H, Buller HR, et al. Venous thromboembolism in childhood: a prospective two-year registry in The Netherlands. J Pediatr 2001;139:676-81.

12. van Ommen CH, Peters M. Acute pulmonary embolism in childhood. Thromb Res 2006;118:13-25.

13. Buck JR, Connors RH, Coon WW, et al. Pulmonary embolism in children. J Pediatr Surg 1981;16:385-91.

14. Putnam JB, Jr., Lemmer JH, Jr., Rocchini AP, et al. Embolectomy for acute pulmonary artery occlusion following Fontan procedure. Ann Thorac Surg 1988;45:335-6.

15. Uflacker R. Interventional therapy for pulmonary embolism. J Vasc Interv Radiol 2001;12:147-64.

16. Beitzke A, Zobel G, Zenz W, et al. Catheter-directed thrombolysis with recombinant tissue plasminogen activator for acute pulmonary embolism after fontan operation. Pediatr Cardiol 1996;17:410-2.

17. Cannizzaro V, Berger F, Kretschmar O, et al. Thrombolysis of venous and arterial thrombosis by catheter-directed low-dose infusion of tissue plasminogen activator in children. J Pediatr Hematol Oncol 2005;27:688-91.

18. Nowak-Gottl U, Auberger K, Halimeh S, et al. Thrombolysis in newborns and infants. Thromb Haemost 1999;82:112-6.

19. Pugh KJ, Jureidini SB, Ream R, et al. Successful thrombolytic therapy of pulmonary embolism associated with urosepsis in an infant. Pediatr Cardiol 2002;23:77-9.

20. Pyles LA, Pierpont ME, Steiner ME, et al. Fibrinolysis by tissue plasminogen activator in a child with pulmonary embolism. J Pediatr 1990;116:801-4.

21. Monagle P, Newall F, Barnes C, et al. Arterial thromboembolic disease: a single-centre case series study. J Paediatr Child Health 2008;44:28-32.

22. King MA, Garrison MM, Vavilala MS, et al. Complications associated with arterial catheterization in children. Pediatr Crit Care Med 2008;9:367-71.

23. Sellden H, Nilsson K, Larsson LE, et al. Radial arterial catheters in children and neonates: a prospective study. Crit Care Med 1987;15:1106-9.

24. Butt W, Shann F, McDonnell G, et al. Effect of heparin concentration and infusion rate on the patency of arterial catheters. Crit Care Med 1987;15:230-2.

25. de NM, Heijboer H, van Woensel JB, et al. The efficacy of heparinization in prolonging patency of arterial and central venous catheters in children: a randomized double-blind trial. Pediatr Hematol Oncol 2002;19:553-60.

26. Revel-Vilk S, Sharathkumar A, Massicotte P, et al. Natural history of arterial and venous thrombosis in children treated with low molecular weight heparin: a longitudinal study by ultrasound. J Thromb Haemost 2004;2:42-6.

27. Coombs CJ, Richardson PW, Dowling GJ, et al. Brachial artery thrombosis in infants: an algorithm for limb salvage. Plast Reconstr Surg 2006;117:1481-8.

28. Bontadelli J, Moeller A, Schmugge M, et al. Enoxaparin therapy for arterial thrombosis in infants with congenital heart disease. Intensive Care Med 2007;33:1978-84.

29. Manco-Johnson MJ, Grabowski EF, Hellgreen M, et al. Recommendations for tPA thrombolysis in children. On behalf of the Scientific Subcommittee on Perinatal and Pediatric Thrombosis of the Scientific and Standardization Committee of the International Society of Thrombosis and Haemostasis. Thromb Haemost 2002;88:157-8.

30. Chong WK, Saunders DE, Ganesan V. Stroke is an important paediatric illness. Pediatr Radiol 2004;34:2-4.

31. Deveber GA, MacGregor D, Curtis R, et al. Neurologic outcome in survivors of childhood arterial ischemic stroke and sinovenous thrombosis. J Child Neurol 2000;15:316-24.

32. Fullerton HJ, Chetkovich DM, Wu YW, et al. Deaths from stroke in US children, 1979 to 1998. Neurology 2002;59:34-9.

33. Ganesan V, Chong WK, Cox TC, et al. Posterior circulation stroke in childhood: risk factors and recurrence. Neurology 2002;59:1552-6.

34. Lynch JK, Hirtz DG, deVeber G, et al. Report of the National Institute of Neurological Disorders and Stroke workshop on perinatal and childhood stroke. Pediatrics 2002;109:116-23.

35. Jones BP, Ganesan V, Saunders DE, et al. Imaging in childhood arterial ischaemic stroke. Neuroradiology 2010;52:577-89.

36. Goldenberg NA, Bernard TJ, Fullerton HJ, et al. Antithrombotic treatments, outcomes, and prognostic factors in acute childhood-onset arterial ischaemic stroke: a multicentre, observational, cohort study. Lancet Neurol 2009;8:1120-7.

37. Nowak-Gottl U, Gunther G, Kurnik K, et al. Arterial ischemic stroke in neonates, infants, and children: an overview of underlying conditions, imaging methods, and treatment modalities. Semin Thromb Hemost 2003;29:405-14.

38. Burak CR, Bowen MD, Barron TF. The use of enoxaparin in children with acute, nonhemorrhagic ischemic stroke. Pediatr Neurol 2003;29:295-8.

39. Finkelstein Y, Nurmohamed L, Avner M, et al. Clopidogrel use in children. J Pediatr 2005;147:657-61.

40. Soman T, Rafay MF, Hune S, et al. The risks and safety of clopidogrel in pediatric arterial ischemic stroke. Stroke 2006;37:1120-2.

41. Anon. Heparin overdose scare in 14 babies at Texas hospital. Healthcare Benchmarks Qual Improv 2008;15:89-90.

42. Alsoufi B, Boshkov LK, Kirby A, et al. Heparin-induced thrombocytopenia (HIT) in pediatric cardiac surgery: an emerging cause of morbidity and mortality. Semin Thorac Cardiovasc Surg Pediatr Card Surg Annu 2004;7:155-71.

43. Novak M, Cvitkovic M, Galic S, et al. The life-threatening hemodialysis catheter heparin lock caused bleeding in a child after peritoneal catheter removal. J Pediatr Surg 2008;43:E41-4.

44. Schroeder AR, Axelrod DM, Silverman NH, et al. A continuous heparin infusion does not prevent catheter-related thrombosis in infants after cardiac surgery. Pediatr Crit Care Med 2010;11:489-95.

45. Jonker MA, Osterby KR, Vermeulen LC, et al. Does low-dose heparin maintain central venous access device patency?: a comparison of heparin versus saline during a period of heparin shortage. JPEN J Parenter Enteral Nutr 2010;34:444-9.

46. Klenner AF, Fusch C, Rakow A, et al. Benefit and risk of heparin for maintaining peripheral venous catheters in neonates: a placebo-controlled trial. J Pediatr 2003;143:741-5.

47. Kotter RW. Heparin vs saline for intermittent intravenous device maintenance in neonates. Neonatal Netw 1996;15:43-7.

48. Anton N, Cox PN, Massicotte MP, et al. Heparin-bonded central venous catheters do not reduce thrombosis in infants with congenital heart disease: a blinded randomized, controlled trial. Pediatrics 2009;123:e453-8.

49. Birch P, Ogden S, Hewson M. A randomised, controlled trial of heparin in total parenteral nutrition to prevent sepsis associated with neonatal long lines: the Heparin in Long Line Total Parenteral Nutrition (HILLTOP) trial. Arch Dis Child Fetal Neonatal Ed 2010;95:F252-7.

50. Krafte-Jacobs B, Sivit CJ, Mejia R, et al. Catheter-related thrombosis in critically ill children: comparison of catheters with and without heparin bonding. J Pediatr 1995;126:50-4.

51. Long DA, Coulthard MG. Effect of heparin-bonded central venous catheters on the incidence of catheter-related thrombosis and infection in children and adults. Anaesth Intensive Care 2006;34:481-4.

52. Pierce CM, Wade A, Mok Q. Heparin-bonded central venous lines reduce thrombotic and infective complications in critically ill children. Intensive Care Med 2000;26:967-72.

53. Shah PS, Shah N. Heparin-bonded catheters for prolonging the patency of central venous catheters in children. Cochrane Database Syst Rev 2007;4:CD005983.

54. Newall F, Barnes C, Savoia H, et al. Warfarin therapy in children who require long-term total parenteral nutrition. Pediatrics 2003;112:e386.

55. Shah PS, Shah VS. Continuous heparin infusion to prevent thrombosis and catheter occlusion in neonates with peripherally placed percutaneous central venous catheters. Cochrane Database Syst Rev 2008;2:CD002772.

56. Blaney M, Shen V, Kerner JA, et al. Alteplase for the treatment of central venous catheter occlusion in children: results of a prospective, open-label, single-arm study (The Cathflo Activase Pediatric Study). J Vasc Interv Radiol 2006;17:1745-51.

57. Choi M, Massicotte MP, Marzinotto V, et al. The use of alteplase to restore patency of central venous lines in pediatric patients: a cohort study. J Pediatr 2001;139:152-6.

58. Davis SN, Vermeulen L, Banton J, et al. Activity and dosage of alteplase dilution for clearing occlusions of venous-access devices. Am J Health Syst Pharm 2000;57:1039-45.

59. Fisher AA, Deffenbaugh C, Poole RL, et al. The use of alteplase for restoring patency to occluded central venous access devices in infants and children. J Infus Nurs 2004;27:171-4.

60. Kerner JA, Jr., Garcia-Careaga MG, Fisher AA, et al. Treatment of catheter occlusion in pediatric patients. JPEN J Parenter Enteral Nutr 2006;30:S73-81.

61. Khan JU, Takemoto CM, Casella JF, et al. Catheter-directed thrombolysis of inferior vena cava thrombosis in a 13-day-old neonate and review of literature. Cardiovasc Intervent Radiol 2008;31:S153-60.

62. Lee EK. Alteplase use for prevention of central line occlusion in a preterm infant. Ann Pharmacother 2002;36:272-4.

63. Ruud E, Holmstrom H, Aagenaes I, et al. Successful thrombolysis by prolonged low-dose alteplase in catheter-directed infusion. Acta Paediatr 2003;92:973-6.

64. Semba CP, Deitcher SR, Li X, et al. Treatment of occluded central venous catheters with alteplase: results in 1,064 patients. J Vasc Interv Radiol 2002;13:1199-205.

65. Timoney JP, Malkin MG, Leone DM, et al. Safe and cost effective use of alteplase for the clearance of occluded central venous access devices. J Clin Oncol 2002;20:1918-22.

66. Israels SJ, Michelson AD. Antiplatelet therapy in children. Thromb Res 2006;118:75-83.

67. Taketomo C, Hodding J, Kraus D. Pediatric Dosage Handbook. Hudson, OH: Lexi-Comp, 2018.

68. Schror K. Aspirin and Reye syndrome: a review of the evidence. Paediatr Drugs 2007;9:195-204.

69. Bradley LM, Midgley FM, Watson DC, et al. Anticoagulation therapy in children with mechanical prosthetic cardiac valves. Am J Cardiol 1985;56:533-5.

70. Bradley SM, Sade RM, Crawford FA, Jr., et al. Anticoagulation in children with mechanical valve prostheses. Ann Thorac Surg 1997;64:30-4.

71. Rao PS, Solymar L, Mardini MK, et al. Anticoagulant therapy in children with prosthetic valves. Ann Thorac Surg 1989;47:589-92.

72. Ziegler JW, Ivy DD, Wiggins JW, et al. Effects of dipyridamole and inhaled nitric oxide in pediatric patients with pulmonary hypertension. Am J Respir Crit Care Med 1998;158:1388-95.

73. Gentilomo C, Huang YS, Raffini L. Significant increase in clopidogrel use across U.S. children's hospitals. Pediatr Cardiol 2011;32:167-75.

74. Maltz LA, Gauvreau K, Connor JA, et al. Clopidogrel in a pediatric population: prescribing practice and outcomes from a single center. Pediatr Cardiol 2009;30:99-105.

75. Skillman KL, Caruthers RL, Johnson CE. Stability of an extemporaneously prepared clopidogrel oral suspension. Am J Health Syst Pharm 2010;67:559-61.

76. Angiolillo DJ, Fernandez-Ortiz A, Bernardo E, et al. Contribution of gene sequence variations of the hepatic cytochrome P450 3A4 enzyme to variability in individual responsiveness to clopidogrel. Arterioscler Thromb Vasc Biol 2006;26:1895-900.

77. Liu TJ, Jackevicius CA. Drug interaction between clopidogrel and proton pump inhibitors. Pharmacotherapy 2010;30:275-89.

78. Pasquali SK, Yow E, Jennings LK, et al. Platelet activity associated with concomitant use of clopidogrel and proton pump inhibitors in children with cardiovascular disease. Congenit Heart Dis 2010;5:552-5.

79. Klein TE, Altman RB, Eriksson N, et al. Estimation of the warfarin dose with clinical and pharmacogenetic data. N Engl J Med 2009;360:753-64.

80. Moffett BS, Parham AL, Caudilla CD, et al. Oral anticoagulation in a pediatric hospital: impact of a quality improvement initiative on warfarin management strategies. Qual Saf Health Care 2006;15:240-3.

81. Lenzini P, Wadelius M, Kimmel S, et al. Integration of genetic, clinical, and INR data to refine warfarin dosing. Clin Pharmacol Ther 2010;87:572-8.

82. Nowak-Gottl U, Dietrich K, Schaffranek D, et al. In pediatric patients, age has more impact on dosing of vitamin K antagonists than VKORC1 or CYP2C9 genotypes. Blood 2010;116:6101-5.

83. Samardzija M, Topic E, Stefanovic M, et al. Association of CYP2C9 gene polymorphism with bleeding as a complication of warfarin therapy. Coll Antropol 2008;32:557-64.

84. Takahashi H, Ishikawa S, Nomoto S, et al. Developmental changes in pharmacokinetics and pharmacodynamics of warfarin enantiomers in Japanese children. Clin Pharmacol Ther 2000;68:541-55.

85. Visscher H, Amstutz U, Sistonen J, et al. Pharmacogenomics of cardiovascular drugs and adverse effects in paediatrics. J Cardiovasc Pharmacol 2011;58:228-39.

86. Ross KA, Bigham AW, Edwards M, et al. Worldwide allele frequency distribution of four polymorphisms associated with warfarin dose requirements. J Hum Genet 2010;55:582-9.

87. Biss TT, Avery PJ, Brandao LR, et al. VKORC1 and CYP2C9 genotype and patient characteristics explain a large proportion of the variability in warfarin dose requirement among children. Blood 2012;119:868-73.

88. Hawcutt DB, Ghani AA, Sutton L, et al. Pharmacogenetics of warfarin in a paediatric population: time in therapeutic range, initial and stable dosing and adverse effects. Pharmacogenomics J 2014;14:542-8.

89. Vear SI, Ayers GD, Van Driest SL, et al. The impact of age and CYP2C9 and VKORC1 variants on stable warfarin dose in the paediatric population. Br J Haematol 2014;165:832-5.

90. Johnson MC, Wood M, Vaughn V, et al. Interaction of antibiotics and warfarin in pediatric cardiology patients. Pediatr Cardiol 2005;26:589-92.

91. Ruud E, Holmstrom H, Bergan S, et al. Oral anticoagulation with warfarin is significantly influenced by steroids and CYP2C9 polymorphisms in children with cancer. Pediatr Blood Cancer 2008;50:710-3.

92. Doyle JJ, Koren G, Cheng MY, et al. Anticoagulation with sodium warfarin in children: effect of a loading regimen. J Pediatr 1988;113:1095-7.

93. Tait RC, Ladusans EJ, El-Metaal M, et al. Oral anticoagulation in paediatric patients: dose requirements and complications. Arch Dis Child 1996;74:228-31.

94. Thornburg CD, Jones E, Bomgaars L, et al. Pediatric warfarin practice and pharmacogenetic testing. Thromb Res 2010; 126:e144-6.

95. Andrew M, Marzinotto V, Brooker LA, et al. Oral anticoagulation therapy in pediatric patients: a prospective study. Thromb Haemost 1994;71:265-9.

96. Bauman ME, Black KL, Massicotte MP, et al. Accuracy of the CoaguChek XS for point-of-care international normalized ratio (INR) measurement in children requiring warfarin. Thromb Haemost 2008;99:1097-103.

97. Bauman ME, Black K, Bauman ML, et al. EMPoWarMENT: Edmonton pediatric warfarin self-management pilot study in children with primarily cardiac disease. Thromb Res 2010; 126:e110-5.

98. Bauman ME, Black K, Kuhle S, et al. KIDCLOT: the importance of validated educational intervention for optimal long term warfarin management in children. Thromb Res 2009;123:707-9.

99. Stewart S, Cianciotta D, Alexson C, et al. The long-term risk of warfarin sodium therapy and the incidence of thromboembolism in children after prosthetic cardiac valve replacement. J Thorac Cardiovasc Surg 1987;93:551-4.

100. Young G, Wicklund B, Neff P, et al. Off-label use of rFVIIa in children with excessive bleeding: a consecutive study of 153 off-label uses in 139 children. Pediatr Blood Cancer 2009;53:179-83.

101. Bauman ME, Black K, Bauman ML, et al. Warfarin induced coagulopathy in children: assessment of a conservative approach. Arch Dis Child 2011;96:164-7.

102. Newall F, Ignjatovic V, Johnston L, et al. Age is a determinant factor for measures of concentration and effect in children requiring unfractionated heparin. Thromb Haemost 2010;103:1085-90.

103. Ignjatovic V, Furmedge J, Newall F, et al. Age-related differences in heparin response. Thromb Res 2006;118:741-5.

104. Riney JN, Hollands JM, Smith JR, et al. Identifying optimal initial infusion rates for unfractionated heparin in morbidly obese patients. Ann Pharmacother 2010;44:1141-51.

105. Ignjatovic V, Summerhayes R, Gan A, et al. Monitoring unfractionated heparin (UFH) therapy: which anti-factor xa assay is appropriate? Thromb Res 2007;120:347-51.

106. Khaja WA, Bilen O, Lukner RB, et al. Evaluation of heparin assay for coagulation management in newborns undergoing ECMO. Am J Clin Pathol 2010;134:950-4.

107. Newall F, Ignjatovic V, Summerhayes R, et al. In vivo age dependency of unfractionated heparin in infants and children. Thromb Res 2009;123:710-4.

108. Kuhle S, Eulmesekian P, Kavanagh B, et al. Lack of correlation between heparin dose and standard clinical monitoring tests in treatment with unfractionated heparin in critically ill children. Haematologica 2007;92:554-7.

109. Newall F, Johnston L, Ignjatovic V, et al. Unfractionated heparin therapy in infants and children. Pediatrics 2009;123:e510-e8.

110. Murphy MS, John PR, Mayer AD, et al. Heparin therapy and bone fractures. Lancet 1992;340:1098.

111. Newall F, Barnes C, Ignjatovic V, et al. Heparin-induced thrombocytopenia in children. J Paediatr Child Health 2003;39:289-92.

112. Warkentin TE, Greinacher A, Koster A, et al. Treatment and prevention of heparin-induced thrombocytopenia: American College of Chest Physicians evidence-based clinical practice guidelines (8th edition). Chest 2008;133:340S-80.

113. Kuhle S, Massicotte P, Dinyari M, et al. Dose-finding and pharmacokinetics of therapeutic doses of tinzaparin in pediatric patients with thromboembolic events. Thromb Haemost 2005; 94:1164-71.

114. Nohe N, Flemmer A, Rumler R, et al. The low molecular weight heparin dalteparin for prophylaxis and therapy of thrombosis in childhood: a report on 48 cases. Eur J Pediatr 1999;158:S134-9.

115. Ho SH, Wu JK, Hamilton DP, et al. An assessment of published pediatric dosage guidelines for enoxaparin: a retrospective review. J Pediatr Hematol Oncol 2004;26:561-6.

116. O'Brien SH, Lee H, Ritchey AK. Once-daily enoxaparin in pediatric thromboembolism: a dose finding and pharmacodynamics/pharmacokinetics study. J Thromb Haemost 2007;5:1985-7.

117. Trame MN, Mitchell L, Krumpel A, et al. Population pharmacokinetics of enoxaparin in infants, children and adolescents during secondary thromboembolic prophylaxis: a cohort study. J Thromb Haemost 2010;8:1950-8.

118. Deal EN, Hollands JM, Riney JN, et al. Evaluation of therapeutic anticoagulation with enoxaparin and associated anti-Xa monitoring in patients with morbid obesity: a case series. J Thromb Thrombolysis 2011;32:188-94.

119. Lewis TV, Johnson PN, Nebbia AM, et al. Increased enoxaparin dosing is required for obese children. Pediatrics 2011;127:e787-e90.

120. Crary SE, Van OH, Journeycake JM. Experience with intravenous enoxaparin in critically ill infants and children. Pediatr Crit Care Med 2008;9:647-9.

121. Dix D, Andrew M, Marzinotto V, et al. The use of low molecular weight heparin in pediatric patients: a prospective cohort study. J Pediatr 2000;136:439-45.

122. Dunaway KK, Gal P, Ransom JL. Use of enoxaparin in a preterm infant. Ann Pharmacother 2000;34:1410-3.

123. Malowany JI, Knoppert DC, Chan AK, et al. Enoxaparin use in the neonatal intensive care unit: experience over 8 years. Pharmacotherapy 2007;27:1263-71.

124. Malowany JI, Monagle P, Knoppert DC, et al. Enoxaparin for neonatal thrombosis: a call for a higher dose for neonates. Thromb Res 2008;122:826-30.

125. Massicotte P, Adams M, Marzinotto V, et al. Low-molecular-weight heparin in pediatric patients with thrombotic disease: a dose finding study. J Pediatr 1996;128:313-8.

126. Sanchez de TJ, Gunawardena S, Munoz R, et al. Do neonates, infants and young children need a higher dose of enoxaparin in the cardiac intensive care unit? Cardiol Young 2010;20:138-43.

127. Bauman ME, Black KL, Bauman ML, et al. Novel uses of insulin syringes to reduce dosing errors: a retrospective chart review of enoxaparin whole milligram dosing. Thromb Res 2009;123:845-7.

128. Dager WE, Gosselin RC, King JH, et al. Anti-Xa stability of diluted enoxaparin for use in pediatrics. Ann Pharmacother 2004;38:569-73.

129. Ignjatovic V, Summerhayes R, Newall F, et al. The in vitro response to low-molecular-weight heparin is not age-dependent in children. Thromb Haemost 2010;103:855-6.

130. Obaid L, Byrne PJ, Cheung PY. Compartment syndrome in an ELBW infant receiving low-molecular-weight heparins. J Pediatr 2004;144:549.

131. Amlie-Lefond C, deVeber G, Chan AK, et al. Use of alteplase in childhood arterial ischaemic stroke: a multicentre, observational, cohort study. Lancet Neurol 2009;8:530-6.

132. Guerin V, Boisseau MR, Fayon M. Efficiency of alteplase in the treatment of venous and arterial thrombosis in neonates. Am J Hematol 1993;42:236-7.

133. Gupta AA, Leaker M, Andrew M, et al. Safety and outcomes of thrombolysis with tissue plasminogen activator for treatment of intravascular thrombosis in children. J Pediatr 2001;139:682-8.

134. Hartmann J, Hussein A, Trowitzsch E, et al. Treatment of neonatal thrombus formation with recombinant tissue plasminogen activator: six years experience and review of the literature. Arch Dis Child Fetal Neonatal Ed 2001;85:F18-22.

135. Levy M, Benson LN, Burrows PE, et al. Tissue plasminogen activator for the treatment of thromboembolism in infants and children. J Pediatr 1991;118:467-72.

136. Olarte JL, Glover ML, Totapally BR. The use of alteplase for the resolution of an intravesical clot in a neonate receiving extracorporeal membrane oxygenation. ASAIO J 2001;47:565-8.

137. Tzifa A, Joashi U, Slavik Z. Recombinant t-PA in myocardial ischemia after switch operation. Pediatr Cardiol 2004;25:417-20.

138. Weiner GM, Castle VP, DiPietro MA, et al. Successful treatment of neonatal arterial thromboses with recombinant tissue plasminogen activator. J Pediatr 1998;133:133-6.

139. Zenz W, Muntean W, Beitzke A, et al. Tissue plasminogen activator (alteplase) treatment for femoral artery thrombosis after cardiac catheterisation in infants and children. Br Heart J 1993;70:382-5.

140. Zenz W, Zoehrer B, Levin M, et al. Use of recombinant tissue plasminogen activator in children with meningococcal purpura fulminans: a retrospective study. Crit Care Med 2004;32:1777-80.

141. Almond CS, Harrington J, Thiagarajan R, et al. Successful use of bivalirudin for cardiac transplantation in a child with heparin-induced thrombocytopenia. J Heart Lung Transplant 2006;25:1376-9.

142. Breinholt JP, Moffett BS, Texter KM, et al. Successful use of bivalirudin for superior vena cava recanalization and stent placement in a child with heparin-induced thrombocytopenia. Pediatr Cardiol 2008;29:804-7.

143. Gates R, Yost P, Parker B. The use of bivalirudin for cardiopulmonary bypass anticoagulation in pediatric heparin-induced thrombocytopenia patients. Artif Organs 2010;34:667-9.

144. Rayapudi S, Torres A, Jr., Deshpande GG, et al. Bivalirudin for anticoagulation in children. Pediatr Blood Cancer 2008;51:798-801.

145. Young G, Tarantino MD, Wohrley J, et al. Pilot dose-finding and safety study of bivalirudin in infants <6 months of age with thrombosis. J Thromb Haemost 2007;5:1654-9.

146. Bingham KR, Riley JB, Schears GJ. Anticoagulation management during first five days of infant-pediatric extracorporeal life support. J Extra Corpor Technol 2018;50:30-7.

147. Sanfilippo F, Asmussen S, Maybauer DM, et al. Bivalirudin for alternative anticoagulation in extracorporeal membrane oxygenation: a systematic review. J Intensive Care Med. 2017;32:312-9.

148. Zaleski KL, DiNardo JA, Nasr VG. Bivalirudin for pediatric procedural anticoagulation: a narrative review. Anesth Analg 2019; 128:43-55.

149. John TE, Hallisey RK, Jr. Argatroban and lepirudin requirements in a 6-year-old patient with heparin-induced thrombocytopenia. Pharmacotherapy 2005;25:1383-8.

150. Madabushi R, Cox DS, Hossain M, et al. Pharmacokinetic and pharmacodynamic basis for effective argatroban dosing in pediatrics. J Clin Pharmacol 2011;51:19-28.

151. Young G, Boshkov LK, Sullivan JE, et al. Argatroban therapy in pediatric patients requiring nonheparin anticoagulation: an open-label, safety, efficacy, and pharmacokinetic study. Pediatr Blood Cancer 2011;56:1103-9.

152. Ciccolo ML, Bernstein J, Collazos JC, et al. Argatroban anticoagulation for cardiac surgery with cardiopulmonary bypass in an infant with double outlet right ventricle and a history of heparin-induced thrombocytopenia. Congenit Heart Dis 2008; 3:299-302.

153. Dyke PC, Russo P, Mureebe L, et al. Argatroban for anticoagulation during cardiopulmonary bypass in an infant. Paediatr Anaesth 2005;15:328-33.

154. Malherbe S, Tsui BC, Stobart K, et al. Argatroban as anticoagulant in cardiopulmonary bypass in an infant and attempted reversal with recombinant activated factor VII. Anesthesiology 2004;100:443-5.

155. Mejak B, Giacomuzzi C, Heller E, et al. Argatroban usage for anticoagulation for ECMO on a post-cardiac patient with heparin-induced thrombocytopenia. J Extra Corpor Technol 2004;36:178-81.

156. Potter KE, Raj A, Sullivan JE. Argatroban for anticoagulation in pediatric patients with heparin-induced thrombocytopenia requiring extracorporeal life support. J Pediatr Hematol Oncol 2007;29:265-8.

157. Cetta F, Graham LC, Wrona LL, et al. Argatroban use during pediatric interventional cardiac catheterization. Catheter Cardiovasc Interv 2004;61:147-9.

158. Chan A, Lensing AWA, Kubitza D, et al. Clinical presentation and therapeutic management of venous thrombosis in young children: a retrospective analysis. Thromb J 2018;16:29.

159. Kubitza D, Willmann S, Becka M, et al. Exploratory evaluation of pharmacodynamics, pharmacokinetics and safety of rivaroxaban in children and adolescents: an EINSTEIN-Jr phase I study. Thromb J 2018;16:31.

160. Willmann S, Thelen K, Kubitza D, et al. Pharmacokinetics of rivaroxaban in children using physiologically based and population pharmacokinetic modelling: an EINSTEIN-Jr phase I study. Thromb J 2018;16:32.

161. Lensing AWA, Male C, Young G, et al. Rivaroxaban versus standard anticoagulation for acute venous thromboembolism in childhood. Design of the EINSTEIN-Jr phase III study. Thromb J 2018;16:34.

CHAPTER 49

Hemophilia A and B

Heidi Trinkman, Pharm.D.

INTRODUCTION

Hemophilia A and B are genetic bleeding disorders that result from decreased or absent circulating concentrations of functional factor VIII (FVIII) or factor IX (FIX), respectively. These deficiencies can ultimately lead to prolonged and excessive bleeding and result in poor-quality clot formation. Hemophilia A (also known as *classic hemophilia*) is more common and accounts for 80%–85% of cases or 1 in 5000–10,000 males. Hemophilia B (also known as *Christmas disease*, named for the first patient identified) constitutes the remaining 15%–20% of cases or 1 in 30,000–50,000 males.[1-3] Hemophilia A and B occur in all ethnic groups.

ETIOLOGY

Both hemophilia A and B are genetically inherited X-linked recessive disorders primarily expressed in males. Females have two X chromosomes; therefore, if one chromosome is affected, the other chromosome carries the information for normal factor production, and the female does not exhibit signs or symptoms of the disease. Any female children from a mother who is a carrier have a 50% chance of also being a carrier for the disease. Any male children have a 50% chance of receiving the affected X chromosome resulting in hemophilia. Every female child from a father with hemophilia will be a carrier for the disease. Despite the genetic inheritance of hemophilia, about one-third of patients with newly diagnosed hemophilia have no family history of the disease, indicating a spontaneous genetic mutation.[1]

The FVIII and FIX genes are located on the long arm of the X chromosome. These genes are very long and complex, representing around 0.1% of the X chromosome. Many mutations have been identified, including gene deletions, stop codon abnormalities, frameshift mutations, and inversion mutations. The inversion of intron 22 is the most common mutation found in hemophilia A (about 50% of cases) and can be identified using Southern blot analysis.[1] Independent mutations account for greater than 95% of all families with severe or moderate hemophilia B. Missense mutations are the most common mutations in patients with hemophilia B, accounting for 60% of FIX defects.[4] Knowledge of the gene mutations may be used for determining carrier status and prenatal assessment. Major alterations to either gene will lead to a more severe disease versus minor defects in the gene. Mutations in the 5' promoter region can result in the hemophilia B Leiden phenotype. This phenotype is characterized by very low concentrations of FIX activity at birth and through childhood and increases in adolescence to greater than 60% after puberty in response to androgens.[1]

Acquired hemophilia is an autoimmune disease targeting FVIII and is very uncommon in children. The production of autoantibodies leads to FVIII proteolysis, thus increasing plasma clearance.[5] Bleeding complications, which present similarly to classic hemophilia, are unpredictable. Of these cases, 50% occur spontaneously, whereas 10% occur postpartum within 3 months of delivery.[5] Autoantibodies can be transferred to the neonate across the placenta, which can result in clinically significant bleeding. The incidence of acquired hemophilia is equally distributed between men and women. Outcomes are generally better in children because of the quicker resolution of autoantibodies in cases secondary to infections or antibiotic use.[5]

PATHOPHYSIOLOGY

Both FVIII and FIX are crucial for normal thrombin formation. The classic representation of hemostasis is through activation of factor X by factor VII and tissue-activating factor. However, recent studies suggest that FIX plays a role in this activation sequence. Through the intrinsic pathway, activated FIX complexes with activated FVIII, calcium, and phosphatidylserine on the membrane surface to generate activated factor X. The activation of factor X initiates the common pathway of the coagulation cascade, leading to normal thrombin and fibrin generation.[4] A deficiency of FVIII or FIX results in delayed formation of a clot caused by a lack of normal thrombin and fibrin production (Figure 1). The resulting clots are friable, and re-bleeding is common. About 50% of patients with hemophilia B produce a nonfunctional FIX protein, whereas the other 50% of patients lack production of the protein entirely.

DIAGNOSIS

Mothers with known familial hemophilia may have sons tested with a cord blood FVIII or FIX activity assay obtained at the time of delivery because neither FVIII nor FIX crosses the placenta. Prenatal testing may be performed using chorionic villus sampling or amniocentesis.[1] These invasive techniques are not without risk to the mother and the fetus and should be discussed with the parents before the procedure.

About one-third of patients with a new diagnosis have no known family members with the disease. Children with signs of bleeding that are suggestive of hemophilia are evaluated further to make the diagnosis. These signs may include prolonged bleeding in newborns with circumcision or heel sticks; intracranial hemorrhage (ICH) or large cephalohematomas after difficult vaginal deliveries (e.g., use of forceps or vacuum extraction); or large, raised bruising and/or many bruises. Common laboratory assessments include a complete blood cell count, coagulation studies, and FVIII and FIX assays. Most patients with hemophilia have significantly prolonged partial thromboplastin time.[5] In general, the partial thromboplastin time is thought to be the most sensitive measure of defects in the intrinsic pathway of the coagulation cascade.

The severity of hemophilia is based on the patient's baseline circulating functional FVIII or FIX activity (Table 1). One unit is defined as the amount of factor found in 1 mL of normal plasma. Factor concentrations are often expressed as *a percentage of activity*. A concentration of 100% (1 IU/mL) is equal to the activity in 1 mL of normal plasma.[4] For hemophilia A, around 70% of patients have the severe form of the disease.

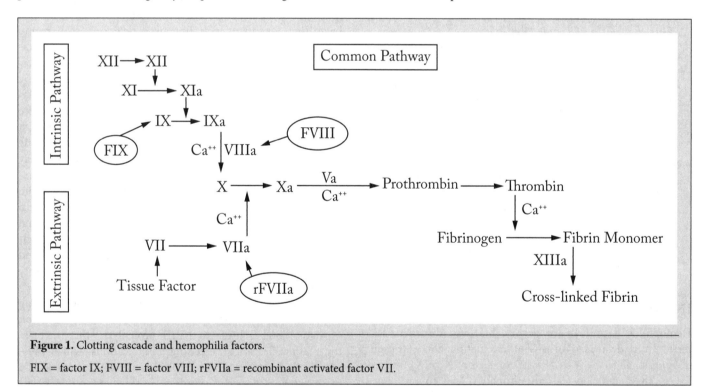

Figure 1. Clotting cascade and hemophilia factors.

FIX = factor IX; FVIII = factor VIII; rFVIIa = recombinant activated factor VII.

Table 1. Categorization of the Severity of Hemophilia[20]

Severity	Clotting Factor Concentration % Activity (IU/mL)	Bleeding Risk
Mild	5%–40% (0.05–0.40)	Prolonged bleeding only with severe trauma or surgery
Moderate	1%–5% (0.01–0.05)	Spontaneous bleeding is rare; prolonged bleeding with trauma or surgery
Severe	< 1% (< 0.01)	Spontaneous bleeding

For hemophilia B, the prevalence of the severe form is around 50%.[6] The diagnosis of mild hemophilia in a newborn may be delayed because vitamin K–dependent factors are reduced in this patient population, and therefore they would naturally have a slightly prolonged partial thromboplastin time.[5]

CLINICAL MANIFESTATIONS

The clinical manifestations of hemophilia A and B are all associated with bleeding. Patients with the severe form of the disease often have bleeding episodes from minor or unknown trauma. These children will often have spontaneous bleeding into muscle or joints from one to six times per month. If bleeding occurs in a closed space, such as a joint, cessation is aided by tamponade. In contrast, an open wound in which tamponade cannot occur may result in substantial blood loss.[4] Patients with the moderate classification of the disease will not spontaneously bleed but can have significant bleeding with mild to moderate trauma. Those with only mild hemophilia may be undiagnosed for many years and have significant bleeding only with severe trauma or surgery.[4] The significance of the bleeding will be determined by the location and severity of disease.

CENTRAL NERVOUS SYSTEM BLEEDS

Bleeding into the central nervous system can be a life-threatening situation for a patient with hemophilia. Because FVIII and FIX do not cross the placenta, male infants with the severe form of the disease will have either no or very little FVIII or FIX at birth. Newborns who are delivered after a long, difficult labor, or after a vaginal delivery aided by the use of forceps or vacuum extraction, are at risk of developing large cephalohematomas or ICHs. The signs of ICH can include pallor, lethargy, neurologic deficits, unequal pupils, tense fontanelle, or vomiting. If the type of hemophilia is not known and FVIII or FIX assays are not immediately available, fresh frozen plasma should be administered at a dose of 10 mL/kg of body weight.[1] In some reports, around 1% to 2% of neonates with hemophilia experience an ICH.

MUCOCUTANEOUS/SOFT TISSUE BLEEDS

In children without a family history of hemophilia, the disease is often diagnosed when the child begins to crawl or walk. Tongue and mouth ulcerations may occur around this time caused by the child's propensity for putting objects in his or her mouth. Soft tissue bruising is also more common during this first year of life, but it is often more alarming in appearance than clinically serious. If a diagnosis of hemophilia has not yet been made, these patients may be mistaken for child abuse victims. Around 30% of patients with hemophilia have bleeding with circumcision.[5]

HEMARTHROSIS

As an infant starts to maintain an upright position and transitions to walking, more pressure is placed on the ankles, making this joint one of the more common bleeding sites.

After the ankles, the knees are the most common sites of joint bleeding. As the child ages, more bleeding will occur in the knees and elbows. When bleeding into a joint occurs, patients have described a sensation of tingling or warmth followed by increasing pain and decreased range of motion. In older children and adolescents, the risk of bleeding comes from sports-related activities and risk-taking behaviors. It usually takes 3–4 weeks for the blood to be reabsorbed from the joint and the fluid to be removed by the synovium.[6]

When repeated bleeding occurs at a rate that does not allow resolution to baseline, the joint becomes a "target" for rebleeding, which is then identified as a *target joint*. These joints show a chronic inflammation of the synovium, which increases the volume of the joint. A new network of capillaries forms underneath the inflamed synovium to increase the blood flow for the removal of the breakdown products of the blood. The surface of the synovium becomes friable and irregular, increasing the likelihood of being caught in the sliding surfaces of the joint and causing more bleeding. This self-perpetuating process can lead to irreversible damage to the joint, resulting in loss of mobility, chronic pain, and ultimately destruction of the joint.[6] Splinting and application of ice packs to the affected joint may provide some pain relief, but these are no substitutes for factor replacement therapy.[5] Nonsteroidal anti-inflammatory medications, such as aspirin and ibuprofen, inhibit platelet function and can further hinder hemostasis in patients with hemophilia; therefore, these medications should be avoided. Early and aggressive management of these bleeds is the best approach for preventing the bleed–synovitis–bleed cycle that characterizes a target joint. In patients with target joint bleeds that cannot be controlled with appropriate prophylactic factor administration, it may be necessary to remove the affected synovium, allowing a new, normal synovial layer to form within a few weeks. This intervention can be accomplished through surgical removal of the affected synovium or through injection of a chemical, such as rifampin, or a radioactive agent, such as yttrium.[6]

INTRAMUSCULAR HEMORRHAGE

Muscle hematomas may be difficult to diagnose because the bleeds are generally deep within the tissue and not easily palpable. Some children with severe hemophilia may have excessive bleeding after intramuscular vaccinations. The bleeding occurs in the body of the muscle, causing the affected area to swell. Patients report a vague feeling of pain with motion. Bleeding into muscles is as serious as bleeding into joints. Repeated muscle bleeds can result in severe muscle contractures caused by fibrosis and atrophy. Muscle weakness is also a risk factor for joint bleeds, thus continuing the cycle of complications. Appropriate factor replacement is necessary to stop the bleed and reduce the size of the hematoma, whereas physical therapy can restore range of motion and prevent fibrosis of the muscle.[5]

One muscle that is particularly worrisome for bleeding is the iliopsoas muscle. Symptoms may be vague, including lower abdominal or upper thigh pain, pain with passive extension of the thigh, and paresthesias below the inguinal ligament from femoral nerve compression. The clinical diagnosis should be confirmed with either ultrasonography or computed tomography. Iliopsoas muscle hemorrhages can be life-threatening because of the large amount of blood volume that can be lost into the retroperitoneal space.

Bleeding into other flexor muscles such as the calf or forearm can lead to a process called *compartment syndrome*, named because of the limited space in the compartment where these muscles are located. When hemorrhage and swelling occur in this space, pressure compresses nerves and blood vessels that travel through the same compartment. This compression is manifested as paresthesias or numbness. Immediate factor replacement is indicated, and fasciotomy may be necessary if vascular supply and nerve function become compromised.[7]

TREATMENT

The fundamental treatment of both hemophilia A and B is replacement of the deficient factor. The first recorded successful treatment of hemophilia using a blood transfusion was in 1840.[1] Since then, the treatment has evolved from the infusion of pork or bovine plasma, which caused allergic responses that limited its usefulness, to human pooled plasma products, which may expose the patient to transmission of bloodborne infectious risks such as hepatitis and HIV, to the current practice of infusing safer, more pure factor concentrates produced through recombinant DNA technologies.

The improvements in replacement factors have made a dramatic impact on life expectancy for patients with hemophilia. The life expectancy before 1960 was a dismal 11 years for patients with severe hemophilia. From the 1960s to the early 1980s, life expectancy increased dramatically—to about 60 years—because of the development of replacement factors. During the 1980s, viral contamination of plasma-derived factor products became a problem. Many patients treated with these products became infected with HIV or hepatitis A, B, or C. The most serious of these infections was HIV, with 75% seroconversion in patients with severe hemophilia. In the United States, the mortality rates for patients with hemophilia tripled from 0.4 deaths per 1 million people (1979–1981) to 1.2 deaths per 1 million people (1987–1989). Of all hemophilia deaths, AIDS accounted for 55%. With improved screening of donors, new purification methods, and recombinant factor production, much of this risk has been removed.[8-10]

Despite these advances, apprehension remains because prions, such as Creutzfeldt–Jakob disease, are emerging as a threat to patients with hemophilia who use blood- and plasma-derived products. Immunoaffinity and other chromatography techniques for preventing the transmission of prions are not well defined, and the use of pasteurization and solvent/detergent techniques is probably ineffective at preventing the transmission of these types of pathogens. In addition, other pathogens such as parvovirus B19 are resistant to many purification measures. A concern is that as-yet unidentified pathogens may exist and can still be transmitted, even through highly purified products.[11]

EARLY THERAPIES

Fresh frozen plasma was the only product available to treat hemophilia B until the introduction of prothrombin complex concentrates (PCCs) and activated PCCs (aPCCs) in 1972.[2] The PCCs contain only the factors themselves, whereas the aPCCs contain the factors as well as other activating components that allow hemostasis to occur through the common coagulation pathway. These hemostatic agents are intermediate-purity pooled plasma products containing FIX and a variety of other vitamin K–dependent clotting factors (II, VII, and X). Although these agents are highly effective for both hemophilia A and B, the PCCs, and especially the aPCCs, have been associated with thrombotic complications, such as disseminated intravascular coagulation and myocardial infarction.[2] Factor eight inhibitor bypass activity (FEIBA) is one of the most commonly used aPCCs currently on the market. It has been activated during the fractionation process to achieve increased amounts of activated FVII, FX, and thrombin.[4] The simultaneous use of antifibrinolytic therapy should be avoided in patients receiving this product because of an increased risk of thrombosis.

FACTOR REPLACEMENT PRODUCTS

The cloning of the FVIII and FIX genes in the 1980s, combined with the explosion of recombinant technologies, led to the development of much safer, more consistent factor replacement products.[12] Recently, newer techniques have been developed that allow recombinant FVIII (rFVIII) and recombinant factor IX (rFIX) to be produced through a virtually plasma-free process. First-generation recombinant factor products used viral removal or inactivation techniques, such as immunoaffinity or ion exchange chromatography.[11] Second-generation recombinant factor products combined solvent/detergents and the use of ultrafiltration or nanofiltration in their manufacturing process for the removal of enveloped viruses, such as HIV and hepatitis B and C.[12] Third-generation recombinant factor products are manufactured through a process that is free of both human albumin and plasma (Table 2). Since 1999, rFIX has become the mainstay of therapy for hemophilia B.

A significant amount of research has been dedicated to the improvement of the pharmacokinetic profiles for these factor products. This research has led to several new recombinant factor products becoming commercially available with enhanced pharmacokinetic characteristics (Table 3). Most of these products have an extended half-life (EHL) compared with plasma-derived or standard recombinant factor products. One approach to improving factor products is through modification of the factor molecule to include polyethylene glycol (PEGylation). Polyethylene glycol can enhance the pharmacokinetics and pharmacodynamics of the factor product. These molecules are less susceptible to proteolytic cleavage and degradation and undergo slower clearance from the circulation, resulting in a longer half-life. The PEGylation of rFVIII has resulted in the first PEGylated product (Adynovate, Takeda, Deerfield, IL) to be commercially available. The half-life could be extended to between 14 and

Table 2. Comparison of Recombinant Factor VIII Products[11,18]

Product	Generation	Producing Cell Line	Stabilizing Agent	Purification Method
Recombinate[a]	First	Chinese hamster ovary	Human albumin	Immunoaffinity, ion exchange
Kogenate FS[b]	Second	Baby hamster kidney	Sucrose	Immunoaffinity, ion exchange, solvent/detergent, ultrafiltration
ReFacto[c]	Second	Chinese hamster ovary	Sucrose	Immunoaffinity, ion exchange, solvent/detergent, nanofiltration
Advate[d]	Third	Chinese hamster ovary	Trehalose	Immunoaffinity, ion exchange, solvent/detergent, plasma/albumin-free culture medium
Xyntha[c]	Third	Chinese hamster ovary	Sucrose	Immunoaffinity, ion exchange, solvent/detergent, nanofiltration

[a]Baxalta, Lexington, MA; [b]Bayer, Whippany, NJ; [c]Pfizer, Andover, MA; [d]Takeda, Deerfield, IL.

19 hours (1.4 times longer than rFVIII). Phase II and III studies are under way researching PEGylated products of rFVIII, rFIX, and recombinant activated factor (rFVIIa).[13]

Another new approach to improving the pharmacokinetic profile of factor products is binding them to large proteins commonly found in the blood such as albumin or immunoglobulins. These proteins have a much longer half-life in the circulation and can protect the factor molecule from proteolytic degradation and reduce its clearance, thus prolonging the half-life of the factor, hopefully without increasing immunogenicity.[14] Several of these products have already been approved and are commercially available, such as Eloctate, and Alprolix (Sanofi Genzyme, Cambridge, MA) and more products are in clinical phase III trials.

An alternative approach to extending the half-life of rFVIII has to do with increasing the stability of the molecule as well as enhancing its binding to von Willebrand factor (VWF), which has a much longer half-life (around 19 hours). This approach uses a covalent bond to join the heavy and light chains of a B-domain truncated rFVIII resulting in a single chain that has greater stability as well as a higher binding affinity for VWF. Because of the stability of the covalent bond, this molecule is less likely to disassociate than other rFVIII products. The increased binding affinity for VWF is protective to the molecule against proteolysis, resulting in a slightly EHL to about 12 hours in children and 14 hours in adults.[15-17] An example of a product that uses this approach is Afstyla (CSL Behring, King of Prussia, PA).

Table 3. Commercially Available Extended Half-Life Products[13,15]

Factor VIII	Mechanism of Prolongation	Age: Half-Life (hr)	Recovery (IU/dL)
Adynovate[a] (rFVIII-P)	PEGylation	12–18 yr: 13.43 ± 4.05 Adults: 14.69 ± 3.79	12–18 yr: 2.12 ± 0.6 Adults: 2.66 ± 0.68
Afstyla[b] (rFVIII-SC)	Single chain	0–6 yr: 12.4 6–12 yr: 12.3 12–18 yr: 14.2 Adults: 14.3	0–6 yr: 1.60 6–12 yr: 1.66 12–18 yr: 1.69 Adults: 2.00
Eloctate[c] (BDD-rFVIII-Fc)	Fc Fusion (IgG)	1–5 yr: 12.7 6–11 yr: 14.9 12–17 yr: 16.4 Adults: 19.7	1–5 yr: 1.92 6–11 yr: 2.44 12–17 yr: 1.85 Adults: 2.26
Factor IX			
Alprolix[c] (rFIX-Fc)	Fc Fusion (IgG)	2–5 yr: 66.4 6–11 yr: 72.23 12–17 yr: ~83.5 Adults: ~87	2–5 yr: 0.598 6–11 yr: 0.7422 12–17 yr: 0.8929 Adults: 1.0154
Idelvion[d] (rFIX-FP)	Fusion protein (Albumin)	< 18 yr: 87 to 93 Adults: 104 to 118	< 18 yr: not reported Adults: 1.27

[a]Takeda, Deerfield, IL; [b]CSL Behring, King of Prussia, PA; [c]Sanofi Genzyme, Cambridge, MA; [d]CSL Behring, King of Prussia, PA.

BDD = B-domain deleted; Fc = crystallizable fragment; FP = Fusion Protein; IgG = immunoglobulin G; P = Plasma Derived; PEGylation = modification of the factor molecule to include polyethylene glycol; rFIX = recombinant FIX; rFVIII = recombinant factor VIII; SC = Single Chain.

ADJUVANT THERAPIES

A nonpharmacologic adjuvant therapy for bleeds is easily remembered by the acronym *RICE*: *rest, ice, compression, and elevation*. Resting the joint or muscle associated with the bleed can be accomplished through splinting or the assistance of crutches or a wheelchair. Ice is helpful in reducing inflammation and causing vasoconstriction and should be applied to the area with a towel or wrap. It is recommended to apply ice or an ice pack for 20 minutes every 4–6 hours until pain and swelling begin to decrease.[18]

The role of desmopressin in the treatment of hemophilia A pertains to patients with the mild to moderate form of the disease. Desmopressin causes bound FVIII to be released into the systemic circulation, elevating the concentration available for coagulation. This agent can be a useful home treatment for mild bleeds. However, many patients may experience tachyphylaxis (diminishing response) with often-repeated dosing. This diminished response can occur after just a few doses; therefore, if the bleeding does not resolve after one or two doses, replacement of FVIII is indicated. Because of the potential for hyponatremia and water intoxication, fluids should be restricted for at least 12 hours after a desmopressin dose. Because of the difficulty in restricting fluids in very young children, this drug is not recommended for use in children younger than 2 years. Desmopressin can be administered intravenously, orally, or intranasally. The last form is most often used for home therapy for hemophilia A. The concentrated nasal spray desmopressin (Stimate, CSL Behring) delivers 150 mcg per activation. One spray of this product (one nostril) is recommended for patients weighing less than 50 kg and two sprays (one in each nostril) for those weighing 50 kg or more.[19-21]

Antifibrinolytic agents may be used in combination with factor replacement to help maintain a clot that has formed. This effect is most often seen with bleeds that occur in the oral cavity because these tissues are rich in fibrinolytic materials. The two products currently used are aminocaproic acid and tranexamic acid. They should be started the evening before any planned invasive dentistry and should be continued for 7–10 days. A mouthwash can also be made by mixing tranexamic acid with sterile water to make a 10% solution. This approach may be helpful after permanent tooth extractions.[19]

THERAPEUTIC APPROACHES

ON-DEMAND

One approach to hemophilia treatment is the "on-demand" administration of replacement factors. Bleeding episodes are treated with factor replacement at a dose that is based on the bleeding site and the patient's weight. The desired percent correction of factor activity varies by location of bleeding or procedure. The most severe bleeding associated with ICH or surgical procedures would require a 100% correction. The amount of FVIII product required to achieve this goal is calculated on the basis that 1 international unit/kg will raise the serum FVIII activity by 2%. Using this formula, the desired dose of FVIII replacement can be determined as follows[20]:

Units of FVIII required = weight (kg) × desired concentration (%) × 0.5

Because FIX binds to sites in the endothelium, more of the product is required to achieve the same rise in activity. Therefore, the amount of FIX product required to raise the activity to a desired concentration is twice that of the FVIII product as follows:

Weight (kg) × desired concentration (%) × 1

The rFIX products require an additional step in calculating the dose needed to raise the activity by a value of 1%. The result of the weight–desired concentration equation should be multiplied by the *reciprocal of the recovery rate* (the percentage of factor recovered 5 minutes after the administration of the dose), which is reported as units/dL per units/kg infused. For example, if using the recombinant product BeneFIX

(Pfizer, Andover, MA), the recovery is reported as 0.8 in adults and 0.7 for those younger than 15 years. Therefore, the dose calculated would need to be multiplied by 1.2 for adults or 1.4 for patients younger than 15 years.[15,22]

The dosing schedule at standard half-life (SHL) FVIII and FIX is influenced by their respective half-lives. Infused FVIII has a half-life of between 3 and 6 hours during the initial equilibration with the extravascular spaces. The half-life then becomes closer to 12 hours. Dosing initially can be as often as every 8 hours until good hemostasis is achieved. The schedule can then be extended to every 12 hours, followed by every 24 hours as the patient recovers. The SHL-FIX products have a half-life of about 18–24 hours, allowing once-daily dosing except before surgery, when a twice-daily dose is required for the first day of the procedure.[20] Table 4 shows the common dosing goals. All factor products can be administered as rapid intravenous infusions over several minutes. Maximum infusion rates are specific to each product. Continuous infusion of FVIII is an approach that has been used in the treatment of moderate and severe bleeds. Using a continuous infusion of factor after initial homeostasis is achieved can result in less overall factor consumption by avoiding the peaks and troughs associated with bolus dosing.[23] An infusion rate of 2–3 international units/kg/hour can maintain an activity value of a concentration around 50% to 60%.[4] The concentrations of FVIII should be monitored periodically to ensure goal concentrations are reached.

PROPHYLAXIS

Another approach to therapy for hemophilia A and B is the prophylactic administration of factor concentrates. The European Paediatric Network for Haemophilia Management has suggested several definitions based on the initiation of therapy. They describe *primary prophylaxis* as continuous therapy starting before age 2 years (solely on the basis of age) or after the first episode of hemarthrosis and before age 2 years. *Secondary prophylaxis* can be a long-term continuous treatment started after 2 years and two or more joint bleeds, or it can be an intermittent periodic treatment approach.[24] The ultimate goal of primary prophylaxis is to prevent the formation of target joints and subsequent chronic arthropathy. Secondary prophylaxis is intended to prevent the progression of joint disease.[25] It is important to remember that even one severe hemarthrosis is enough to start the cycle of bleeding and synovial hypertrophy that leads to the formation of a target joint.[20] However, magnetic resonance imaging examinations have shown that sometimes abnormalities have already occurred, even if no hemarthrosis event has been clinically recognized. The efficacy of this approach largely depends on the patient's adherence.[26]

Prophylaxis is now recommended by the World Health Organization and the World Federation of Hemophilia.[18,20] Historically, the dosing strategy of prophylactic therapy has been to maintain the patient's factor activity at a concentration greater than 1% (0.01 IU/mL), with the goal to convert disease severity from severe to moderate, thereby eliminating spontaneous bleeding. Unfortunately, there are no specific guidelines endorsed by either agency to guide product selection or dosing approach. For hemophilia A patients, this strategy could be to use a regimen of SHL-FVIII dosed 20–40 international units/kg every other day or three times/week.[26-28] A prophylactic dose for hemophilia B would be SHL-FIX 25–40 international units/kg twice weekly because of the longer half-life.[5,20] In long-term follow-up studies, this treatment strategy was highly successful when the annual bleeding rate (ABR) is compared with that of patients treated with the on-demand approach.[28] However, despite some patients having adequate concentrations of 1% or greater, breakthrough bleeding still can occur. Joint bleeds may still occur, although less commonly, when factor concentrations are between 1% and 4% until the baseline concentration is greater than 10% to 15%.[28] This potential for bleeding has sparked the discussion that factor concentrations required to prevent bleeding into joints varies between patients, and perhaps the goals set for prophylaxis should be tailored to individual patients, their pharmacokinetics, and their degree of physical activity, as well as the cost and feasibility of the dose required to achieve it.[14,28] This variance is where the benefit of the EHL factors may begin to play a significant role.

With the introduction of EHL factors into the market is the hope that these agents would increase the feasibility of prophylaxis by decreasing the frequency of dosing needed to achieve the same concentrations, leading to fewer instances for intravenous access, less factor consumed, and better patient compliance and satisfaction. The current EHL factors on the market have been studied in prophylactic regimens using different dosing regimens and intervals based on the half-life of each product. In general, common findings are that children had shorter half-lives than adults, no inhibitors were seen, and the dosing intervals for prophylaxis were able to be extended.[29] *Inhibitors* are antibodies that can develop against the exogenously administered factor products, significantly

decreasing their efficacy. The impact of EHL on the dosing interval was more pronounced for patients with hemophilia B because of the greater than 2.5-fold increase in half-life of these products compared with their SHL counterparts.[30] The EHL-FVIII product achieved a modest extension of 1.5-fold in adults and slightly less in children, which allowed the extension of dosing to twice weekly versus three to four times weekly dosing with SHL-FVIII. Dosing was able to be extended to once every 2 weeks from once weekly in many adults using an EHL-FIX product, whereas children were able to be dosed once weekly to every 10 days.[14] The pharmacokinetic variability between patients is even more pronounced with the EHL products, especially in children, making it even more critical to monitor these patients and their concentrations of these agents when switching products. All of these trials were in previously treated patients, so the lack of inhibitor formation finding is promising, but not surprising. These trials have extension arms and arms evaluating use in previously untreated patients. The results will provide a better understanding of the risk with these newer agents of causing inhibitor formation.

The studies have assessed ABRs compared with the same product used in on-demand therapy.[14] It is difficult from these data to determine the impact on ABRs by switching from an effective SHL factor prophylaxis regimen to one using an EHL product. Only the B-LONG study had a post hoc arm that estimated the impact of 39 adult patients who switched from an SHL-FIX prophylactic regimen to the EHL-FIX product.[30] Findings showed that weekly consumption of factor could be decreased by 30% to 50% and that ABRs would be less than pre-study estimated mean ABRs using pharmacokinetic models.[14] The benefit of decreased factor consumption could potentially be muted by an increased cost of these EHL factor products. Longer, more-inclusive studies are needed to

Table 4. Treatment of Specific Hemorrhages in Hemophilia[4,19]

Event	Hemophilia A FVIII Dosing international units/kg (% Correction)		Hemophilia B FIX Dosing international units/kg (% Correction)		Comments
	First Dose	Subsequent Dosing Every 12–24 hr	First Dose	Subsequent Dosing Every 12–24 hr	
Hemarthrosis	40–50 (80%–100%)	20–35 (40%–70%)	20–50 (20%–50%)	30–50 (30%–50%)	Ice for 20 min; immobilize for 48 hr
Muscle or soft tissue hematoma	25–50 (50%–100%)	20–25 (40%–50%)	20–30 (20%–30%)	20–30 (20%–30%)	Ice for 20 min
Hematuria	20–35 (40%–70%)	25–30 (50%–60%)	25–50 (25%–50%)	30 (30%)	Bed rest; prednisone 1–2 mg/kg/day
Gastrointestinal	35–50 (70%–100%)	25–35 (50%–70%)	50–100 (50%–100%)	50–100 (50%–100%)	Monitor complete blood cell count
Mucosal/dental	35–50 (70%–100%)	25–35 (50%–70%)	25–50 (25%–50%)	25–50 (25%–50%)	Local ice; aminocaproic acid 100 mg/kg every 6 hr
Head trauma, major surgery	50–75 (100%–150%)	25–35 (50%–70%)	50–100 (50%–100%)	50–100 (50%–100%)	Monitor factor activity concentrations

FIX = factor IX; FVIII = factor VIII.

determine the true overall benefit that these products may have regarding prophylaxis and the impact that they make on inhibitor formation, overall outcomes, patient compliance, and cost.

Previously, primary prophylaxis was reserved for patients without inhibitors. A study compared on-demand therapy with prophylaxis using an aPCC (FEIBA) for patients with inhibitors and found an overall reduction in bleeding of 84%, reduction in joint bleeds of 61%, with target joint bleeds reduced by 71% during the prophylactic period.[31] These findings give clinical support to the use of bypassing agents for prophylaxis in children who develop inhibitors.

Despite the many studies establishing prophylaxis as a superior approach to treatment and recommended as standard of care versus on-demand therapy, prophylaxis is still a challenge in developing countries. The main deterrents continue to be cost and complications. The costs of prophylaxis versus those of on-demand therapy are difficult to quantify. The SHL factor consumed during on-demand therapy tends to be one-third of that consumed with the prophylactic approach using SHL products.[31,32] The cost impact of using EHL factor products has yet to be quantified. However, when assessing the pharmacoeconomics of prophylaxis, the approach must be a view from a long-term outcome perspective, including variables such as quality of life; potential benefits of avoiding hospitalizations and days lost from school or work; and prevention of long-term complications, such as worsening joint disease and disability.

Another obstacle to prophylactic therapy is the need for venous access for factor administration. Peripheral venous access is preferred for the infusion of factor products; however, for patients receiving continuous prophylactic or immune tolerance induction (ITI) therapy, a central venous access device may be required. These devices are especially useful in infants and children whose small veins are difficult to access and who tend to be intolerant of frequent needle sticks.[33] Central venous access devices are used in about 30% of children receiving prophylactic therapy with SHL products and in 90% of those receiving daily ITI. The biggest drawback to these devices is the risk of infection. A meta-analysis performed on 48 studies found a 44% incidence of infection in patients with hemophilia with central venous access devices.[33-35] These devices also require comprehensive education of the family/caregivers on proper aseptic technique as well as maintenance and monitoring of the central line.

THERAPEUTIC MONITORING

Most therapeutic monitoring of effective treatment for acute bleeding episodes is based on overall clinical response.[35] The clinical monitoring of a patient with an acute bleed includes surrogate markers such as pain levels, range of motion if the acute bleed is in a joint, swelling, and laboratory values such as hemoglobin. Although serum factor concentrations can be measured, the results can vary widely, and the clinical correlation is inconsistent. This variance and inconsistency are thought to result from the variable effect of FVIII on endogenous thrombin generation.[36] The monitoring of FVIII concentrations is warranted in the setting of surgical procedures. In some cases, homeostasis is achieved using a continuous

infusion of factor product. Daily monitoring of factor concentrations during the continuous infusion is beneficial to ensure a consistent degree of factor activity.[37] Research continues into identifying the most appropriate surrogate marker for monitoring therapy. Assessments such as thrombin generation tests and endogenous thrombin potential are being studied to determine their degree of clinical correlation to outcomes.[38,39] If the patient is not clinically responding to adequate doses of factor replacement, serum should be sent for testing to determine whether an inhibitor is present.

COMPLICATIONS OF THERAPY

A serious complication of hemophilia therapy is the formation of antibodies against FVIII and FIX. These antibodies, called *inhibitors*, neutralize the procoagulant activity of FVIII and FIX, leading to the failure of routine factor replacement therapy. About 14% to 35% of patients with severe hemophilia A and up to 3% of patients with severe hemophilia B will develop inhibitors.[2,4,40] Most inhibitor development occurs in patients with severe hemophilia around age 1–2 years with about nine to 12 treatments with factor product. The highest risk of developing inhibitors occurs within the first 50 exposures to FVIII, with the risk rapidly reducing after 200 treatment days.[41] Risk factors for developing inhibitors include genetic factors such as the type of mutation on the FVIII or FIX gene, polymorphisms in genes that regulate the immune system, family history of inhibitors, and African heritage.[42-45] Environmental risk factors for inhibitor development include intensive factor exposure caused by serious injury, surgery, or immunologic challenge such as infection or immunizations.[46] Another risk factor to consider is the type of factor product administered during those first early exposures. Recently the results from the Survey of Inhibitors in Plasma Products in Exposed Toddlers (SIPPET) trial were released. This trial was a large randomized, multicenter, prospective study in children evaluating the incidence of inhibitor formation between those who received recombinant factor replacement and those receiving plasma-derived products. Patients receiving recombinant products had almost twice the risk of developing inhibitors than those receiving plasma-derived factor products.[47] Despite these findings, several limitations preclude its generalizability to patients in the United States.[48] In addition to the loss of therapeutic response to factor replacement, patients with hemophilia B with inhibitor development may experience anaphylaxis associated with FIX administration.[49]

Inhibitors can be categorized into two groups: low responding and high responding. Inhibitors are measured by the Bethesda assay. One *Bethesda unit* (*BU*) is defined as the amount of inhibitor needed to inactivate 50% of FVIII or FIX in pooled normal plasma. *Low-responding inhibitors* are defined by a peak historical titer of less than 5 BU/mL, resulting in a very low or attenuated response to FVIII or FIX.[20] Patients with low-responding inhibitors may still respond to factor replacement therapy at higher doses and/or more frequent dosing intervals. *High-responding inhibitors* are those with a titer greater than 5 BU/mL or a brisk anamnestic response to FVIII challenge. Patients can convert from low-responding inhibitors to high-responding inhibitors over time. All patients should be monitored for inhibitor formation every 6 months or in the setting of a decreased clinical or laboratory response to therapy.[20]

Patients with high-responding inhibitors usually will not respond to FVIII or FIX replacement therapy, even at high doses, and alternative approaches to treatment of acute bleeds must be used, such as rFVIIa (90 mcg/kg every 2–3 hours) or aPCCs (FEIBA 50–100 international units/kg every 6–12 hours).[50,51] The effect of rFVIIa is to achieve homeostasis without requiring FVIII or FIX by using the extrinsic coagulation pathway and binding to tissue factor at the site of injury, which then triggers coagulation through the common pathway. In addition, rFVIIa can also cause activation of FIX and factor X on the surface of activated platelets.[20]

Once an inhibitor has formed, ITI may be initiated in an attempt to decrease or eliminate the antibodies. The use of ITI involves frequent, continuing exposure to the deficient clotting factor to achieve tolerance by antigen overload, resulting in restoration of normal factor replacement pharmacokinetics.[2] This approach was first attempted in the 1970s and was achieved by the administration of high doses of FVIII (100–150 international units/kg) twice daily with the combination of aPCCs for control of acute bleeds. After a period of months to years, the FVIII antibodies were markedly reduced, and the dose could be decreased to a smaller daily dose or even administered every other day.[5] A variety of different ITI regimens have been developed, with some using varied doses of FVIII given less often and others combining the use of intravenous gamma globulin and immunosuppressants (cyclophosphamide, rituximab).[50] The success rates for ITI are generally higher in patients with lower inhibitor titers (preferably less than 10 BU) at the initiation of therapy.[51,52] A meta-analysis of the North American Immune Tolerance Registry (NAITR) and the International Immune Tolerance Registry (IITR) determined that for patients with inhibitor titers less than 200 BU and pre-ITI titers less than 10 BU, FVIII dose did not affect ITI outcome. The IITR study protocol is presently comparing high-dose ITI (200 units/kg/day) with low-dose ITI (50 units/kg three times/week). The data are undergoing final analysis.[51] In patients with hemophilia A, ITI is unsuccessful in 30% to 50% of individuals. In patients with hemophilia B, ITI is much less effective, with a high incidence of allergic reaction. It is important to be aware that ITI is demanding and expensive, exceeding $1.2 million for an average 5-year-old patient.[53] The need for central venous access is another factor to consider when deciding whether to initiate ITI. However, the cost of successful ITI can decrease the overall lifetime cost of hemophilia therapy.[20,53,54]

Some studies report better success rates for ITI in patients receiving plasma-derived factor products containing VWF, which is thought to be because of the role of VWF in FVIII function, stabilization, and immunogenicity.[55] By the binding of VWF to the C2 domain of FVIII, a common site for inhibitor formation, epitope masking and decreased inhibitor activity may result. The use of VWF-containing products may also extend the plasma half-life of FVIII during ITI, thus increasing antigen presentation and possibly contributing to its overall success.[55] If no response is seen after 2 years of ITI, then the treatment approach is usually discontinued.[20]

FUTURE CONSIDERATIONS

Gene therapy for hemophilia A and B is considered to be the only approach with curative potential. Great strides have been made over the past 10 years, resulting in several phase III trials currently under way for patients with hemophilia B. The results of the longest-running trial of gene therapy for hemophilia B have been very promising. A total of 10 patients have been treated in this trial conducted jointly by St. Jude Children's Research Hospital (Memphis, TN) and the University College London (London, UK). The six patients treated with the highest doses of viral vector are still maintaining concentrations of FIX at around 5% after almost 4 years. There have been no signs of decreasing expression in these patients, and no serious adverse effects have been reported. Four of these six patients did experience an asymptomatic rise in their liver transaminases between 7 and 11 weeks after vector infusion. This transaminase increase corresponded to a decrease in factor expression when left untreated. Prompt treatment with corticosteroids seemed to treat the inflammatory response and prevent a decline in the FIX production.[53]

Gene therapy for hemophilia A has been more challenging for researchers because of the size of FVIII. Efficient packaging into the viral vector requires the transgene to be the same size or smaller than the viral vector genome, in this case 4.7 kb. For FIX, this size is not an issue because its transgene is only 1.4 kb; however, for FVIII, which is around 9 kb, this size was a limitation. By modifying the molecule and deleting the B-domain together with its promoter region, researchers could yield a B-domain deleted FVIII that was only 4.4 kb which would fit into the viral vector. Other strategies are also being studied, such as splitting the FVIII and packaging into two different vectors.[56,57] Another approach being studied includes an attempt to correct the gene in situ using gene editing techniques.[58] Stem cell-directed gene therapy is also being explored as a potential option for patients with hemophilia.[59] These alternative approaches are still early in development. It will take time to determine which, if any, of these approaches will advance into clinical trials.

In an effort to think beyond the factor replacement approach to therapy for these patients, some researchers are pursuing alternative targets in the clotting cascade where they could possibly make a therapeutic impact. One such approach is to inhibit the inhibitors of coagulation, which would enhance the involved hemostatic pathways. An example of this approach is the tissue factor pathway inhibitor, which inhibits the extrinsic pathway for hemostasis. By inhibiting this inhibitor in animal models, the hemostatic cascade involving the extrinsic pathway can be enhanced. This effect causes an increase in tenase and thrombin formation.[60,61] There is currently a monoclonal antibody (concizumab) in clinical trials that targets this inhibitor. The same approach is being studied for the inhibition of antithrombin.[61] Products are being studied to mimic the function of cofactors in the coagulation cascade as well as bioengineered factor Va and factor Xa variants in the preclinical phase which may increase thrombin generation.[61]

CONCLUSIONS

From the transfusion of blood products to the development of recombinant factors to the creation of genetic therapies, the treatment of hemophilia continues to evolve. It has changed from a childhood disease with early mortality to a chronically managed disease with a significantly improved life span. As the options for therapy continue to grow, the life span and quality of life continue to improve for patients affected by the disease.

It is essential that pharmacists take an active role in understanding the treatment regimens as well as the products available for managing hemophilia A and B. A complete understanding of the pathophysiology of the disease is also necessary to assist patients with supportive care both inside and outside the hospital setting. Important advances in hemophilia A and B therapies have occurred during the past 25 years, resulting in safer treatment options, better quality of life for patients, and, with improvements in gene therapy on the horizon, a hope for a cure in the future.

Patient Case — HEMOPHILIA

A 5-year-old boy (22 kg) with a history of severe hemophilia A is brought to the emergency department after his youth soccer game. He reports pain and tingling in his calf. On examination his calf is swollen, warm, and tender to the touch.

1. What is your recommended therapeutic approach, and why?

Replacement of factor VIII is the correct approach for this patient because he has signs and symptoms of a muscle bleed with the potential for compartment syndrome resulting in nerve and vascular compromise. Because of the severity of this complication, it is important to gain hemostasis quickly. A goal of 100% correction (50 international unit/kg) is appropriate. The calculated dose is 1100 international units. The patient's pain should also be addressed but nonsteroidal anti-inflammatory drugs should be avoided because of the risk of inhibition of platelet aggregation, which could worsen bleeding.

Case (continued). After 24 hours on appropriate aggressive therapy, the patient has clinical signs of a worsening bleed evident by more pain and swelling. An inhibitor concentration was checked and found to be 15 BU.

2. What is an appropriate adjustment to the therapy for this patient, and why?

The patient should be switched to recombinant activated factor VII or an activated prothrombin complex concentrate such as factor eight inhibitor bypass activity because they both use alternate means of activating the common pathway to encourage clot formation. Either of these factors are approved approaches for treating acute bleeds in hemophilia A patients with inhibitors.

REFERENCES

1. Lusher JM. Hemophilia A and B. In: Lilleymann J, Hann I, Blanchette V, eds. Pediatric Hematology. Edinburgh, UK: Churchill Livingstone, 1999:585-600.

2. Valentino LA, Ismael Y, Grygotis M. Novel drugs to treat hemophilia. Expert Opin 2010;15:597-613.

3. Van den Berg HM, Fischer K. Phenotypic-genotypic relationship. In: Lee C, Berntorp E, Hoots K, eds. Textbook of Hemophilia. West Sussex, UK: Wiley-Blackwell, 2010:33-7.

4. Montgomery RR, Gill JC, Di Paola J. Hemophilia and von Willebrand disease. In: Orkin SH, Nathan DG, Ginsburg D, et al., eds. Hematology of infancy and childhood. Philadelphia: Saunders Elsevier, 2009:1487-513.

5. Franchini M, Zaffanello M, Lippi G. Acquired hemophilia in pediatrics: a systematic review. Pediatr Blood Cancer 2010;55:606-11.

6. Mulder K, Llinas A. The target joint. Haemophilia 2004;10:152-6.

7. Journeycake J, Miller K, Anderson A, et al. Arthroscopic synovectomy in children and adolescents with hemophilia. J Pediatr Hematol Oncol 2003;25:726-32.

8. Chorba T, Holman R, Strine T, et al. Changes in longevity and causes of death among persons with hemophilia A. Am J Hematol 1994;45:112-21.

9. Jones P, Ratnoff O. The changing prognosis of classic hemophilia (factor VIII "deficiency"). Ann Intern Med 1991;114:641-8.

10. Darby S, Kan S, Spooner R, et al. Mortality rates, life expectancy, and causes of death in people with hemophilia A or B in the United Kingdom who were not infected with HIV. Blood 2007;110:815-25.

11. Josephson CD, Abshire T. The new albumin-free recombinant factor VIII concentrates for treatment of hemophilia: do they represent an actual incremental improvement? Clin Adv Hematol Oncol 2004;2:441-6.

12. Franchini M, Lippi G. Recombinant factor VIII concentrates. Semin Thromb Hemost 2010;36:493-7.

13. Young G, Mahlangu JN. Extended half-life clotting factor concentrates: results from published clinical trials. Haemophilia 2016;22:25-30.

14. Berntorp E, Andersson NG. Prophylaxis for hemophilia in the era of extended half-life factor VIII/factor IX products. Semin Thromb Hemost 2016;42:518-25.

15. Lexi-Comp Online [Internet database]. Pediatric & Neonatal Lexi-Drugs, version 3.0.1. Hudson, OH: Lexi-Comp. Updated periodically.

16. Pabinger-Fasching I. The story of a unique molecule in hemophilia A: recombinant single-chain factor VIII. Thromb Res 2016;141:S2-4.

17. Klamroth R, Simpson M, Von Depka-Prondzinski M, et al. Comparative pharmacokinetics of rVIII-single-chain and octocog alfa (Advate) in patients with severe hemophilia A. Haemophilia 2016;1-9.

18. World Federation of Hemophilia. Guidelines for the Management of Hemophilia. Montreal, Quebec, Canada: World Federation of Hemophilia, 2005.

19. Micromedex Healthcare Series. [Internet database]. Greenwood Village, CO: Thomson Reuters (Healthcare). Updated periodically.

20. Smith J, Smith OP. Hemophilia A and B. In: Arceci RJ, Hann IM, Smith OP, eds. Pediatric Hematology. Malden, MA: Blackwell, 2006:585-97.

21. Castaman G. Desmopressin for the treatment of haemophilia. Haemophilia 2008;14:15-20.

22. Negrier C. Entering new areas in known fields: recombinant fusion protein linking recombinant factor VIIa with recombinant albumin (rVIIa-FP)—advancing the journey. Thromb Res 2016;141:S9-12.

23. Stachnik JM, Gabay MP. Continuous infusion of coagulation factor products. Ann Pharmacother 2002;36:882–91.

24. Donadel S. Current co-ordinated activities of the PEDNET (European Paediatric Network for Haemophilia Management). Haemophilia 2006;12:124-7.

25. Fischer K, Van Den Berg HM, Thomas R, et al. Dose and outcome of care in haemophilia—how do we define cost-effectiveness? Haemophilia 2004;10:216-20.

26. Blanchette VS. Prophylaxis in the haemophilia population. Haemophilia 2010;16:181-8.

27. Manco-Johnson MJ, Abshire TC, Shapiro AD, et al. Prophylaxis versus episodic treatment to prevent joint disease in boys with severe hemophilia. N Engl J Med 2007;357:535-44.

28. Collins PW. Personalized prophylaxis. Haemophilia 2012;18:131-5.

29. Mahlangu J, Powell JS, Ragni MV, et al; A-LONG Investigators. Phase 3 study of recombinant factor VIII Fc fusion protein in severe hemophilia A. Blood 2014;123:317-25.

30. Powell JS, Pasi KJ, Ragni MV, et al; B-LONG Investigators. Phase 3 study of recombinant factor IX Fc fusion protein in hemophilia B. N Engl J Med 2013;369:2313-23.

31. Leissinger C, Gringeri A, Antmen B, et al. Anti-inhibitor coagulant complex prophylaxis in hemophilia with inhibitors. N Engl J Med 2011;365:1684-92.

32. Ljung R. Prophylactic therapy in haemophilia. Blood Rev 2009;23:267-74.

33. Valentino L, Kawji M, Grygotis M. Venous access in the management of hemophilia. Blood Rev 2011;25:11-5.

34. Valentino L, Ewenstein B, Navickis R, et al. Central venous access devices in haemophilia. Haemophilia 2004;10:134-46.

35. Ahnstrom J, Berntorp E, Lindvall K, et al. A 6-year follow-up of dosing, coagulation factor levels and bleedings in relation to joint status in the prophylactic treatment of haemophilia. Haemophilia 2004;10:689-97.

36. Lewis SJ, Stephens E, Florou G, et al. Measurement of global haemostasis in severe haemophilia A following factor VIII infusion. Br J Haematol 2007;138:775-82.

37. Dingli D, Gastineau DA, Gilchrist GS, et al. Continuous factor VIII infusion therapy in patients with haemophilia A undergoing surgical procedures with plasma-derived or recombinant factor VIII concentrates. Haemophilia 2002;8:629-34.

38. Dargaud Y, Lienhart A, Negrier C. Prospective assessment of thrombin generation test for dose monitoring of bypassing therapy in hemophilia patients with inhibitors undergoing elective surgery. Blood 2010;116:5734-7.

39. Shima M, Matsumoto T, Ogiwara K. New assays for monitoring haemophilia treatment. Haemophilia 2008;14:83-92.

40. Saint-Remy JMR, Lacroix-Desmazes S, Oldenburg J. Inhibitors in haemophilia: pathophysiology. Haemophilia 2004;10:146-51.

41. Chambost H. Assessing risk factors: prevention of inhibitors in haemophilia. Haemophilia 2010;16:10-5.

42. Oldenburg J, Pavlova A. Genetic risk factors for inhibitors to factors VIII and IX. Haemophilia 2006;12:15-22.

43. Astermark J, Oldenburg J, Pavlova A, et al. Polymorphisms in the IL 10 but not the IL1beta and IL4 genes are associated with inhibitor development in patients with hemophilia A. Blood 2006;107:3167-72.

44. Astermark J, Oldenburg J, Carlson J, et al. Polymorphisms in the TNFA gene and the risk of inhibitor development in patients with hemophilia. Blood 2006;108:3739-45.

45. Astermark J, Wang X, Oldenburg J, et al. Polymorphisms in the CTLA-4 gene and inhibitor development in patients with severe hemophilia A. J Thromb Haemost 2007;5:263-5.

46. Gouw S, van der Born J, Marijke van den Berg H. Treatment-related risk factors of inhibitor development in previously untreated patients with hemophilia A: the CANAL cohort study. Blood 2007;109:4648-54.

47. Peyvandi F, Mannucci PM, Garagiola I, et al. A randomized trial of factor VIII and neutralizing antibodies in hemophilia A. N Engl J Med 2016;374:2054-64.

48. National Hemophilia Foundation [homepage on the Internet]. MASAC recommendation on SIPPET (survey of inhibitors in plasma-product-exposed toddlers): results and recommendations for treatment products for previously untreated patients with hemophilia A. Available at www.hemophilia.org/Researchers-Healthcare-Providers/Medical-and-Scientific-Advisory-Council-MASAC/MASAC-Recommendations/MASAC-Recommendation-on-SIPPET-Survey-of-Inhibitors-in-Plasma-Product-Exposed-Toddlers-Results-and-Recommendations-for-Treatment-Products-for-Previously. Accessed January 17, 2020.

49. Chitlur M, Warrier I, Rajpurkar M, et al. Inhibitors in factor IX deficiency a report of the ISTH-SSC international FIX inhibitor registry (1997–2006). Haemophilia 2009;15:1027-31.

50. Aggarwal A, Grewal R, Green RJ, et al. Rituximab for autoimmune haemophilia: a proposed treatment algorithm. Haemophilia 2005;11:13-9.

51. Di Michele D, Hoots W, Pipe S, et al. International workshop on immune tolerance induction: consensus recommendations. Haemophilia 2007;13:1-22.

52. Di Michele D. Immune tolerance induction in haemophilia: evidence and the way forward. J Thromb Haemost 2011;9:216-25.

53. Colowick A, Bohn R, Avorn J, et al. Immune tolerance induction in hemophilia patients with inhibitors: costly can be cheaper. Blood 2000;96:1698-702.

54. Astermark J, Santagostino E, Hoots KW. Clinical issues in inhibitors. Haemophilia 2010;16:54-60.

55. Coppola A, Di Minno MN, Santagostino E. Optimizing management of immune tolerance induction in patients with severe haemophilia A and inhibitors: towards evidence-based approaches. Br J Hematol 2010;150:515-28.

56. Giangrande P. The future of hemophilia treatment: longer-acting factor concentrates versus gene therapy. Semin Thromb Hemost 2016;42:513-17.

57. Ward P, Walsh CE. Current and future prospects for hemophilia gene therapy. Exp Rev of Hemat 2016;9:649-59.

58. Park CY, Lee DR, Sung JJ, et al. Genome-editing technologies for gene correction of hemophilia. Hum Gennet 2016;135:977-81.

59. Spencer HT, Riley BE, Doering CB. State of the art: gene therapy of haemophilia. Haemophilia 2016;22:66-71.

60. Peterson JA, Maroney SA, Mast AE. Targeting TFPI for hemophilia treatment. Thromb Res 2016;141:S28-30.

61. Mannucci PM, Manusco ME, Santagostino E, et al. Innovative pharmacological therapies for the hemophilias not based on deficient factor replacement. Semin Thromb Hemost 2016;42:526-32.

CHAPTER 50

Sickle Cell Disease

Tracy M. Hagemann, Pharm.D., FCCP, FPPA

LEARNING OBJECTIVES

1. Discuss the role of newborn screening in sickle cell disease (SCD).

2. List the signs and symptoms of SCD for infants, children, and adolescents.

3. Recognize the clinical characteristics associated with an acute SCD crisis.

4. Identify patients who require penicillin prophylaxis.

5. Review vaccination recommendations for patients with SCD.

6. Explain the rationale for using hydroxyurea in pediatric patients with SCD.

7. Identify appropriate hydroxyurea regimens and monitoring values.

8. Discuss the risks and benefits of chronic transfusion therapy in patients with SCD.

9. Select appropriate empiric antimicrobial coverage for children with SCD who present with fever.

10. Develop a treatment plan for chelation therapy in pediatric patients receiving chronic transfusion therapy.

11. Create a treatment plan for children and adolescents with SCD who present with acute chest syndrome, priapism, and SCD crisis.

12. Devise a pain management plan for pediatric patients presenting with vaso-occlusive pain crisis.

ABBREVIATIONS IN THIS CHAPTER

ACS	Acute chest syndrome
CBC	Complete blood count
FDA	U.S. Food and Drug Administration
HbA	Normal adult hemoglobin
HbC	Hemoglobin C
HbF	Fetal hemoglobin
HbS	Sickle hemoglobin
HbS βthal	Sickle cellβ-thalassemia
HbSC	Compound heterozygous hemoglobin (sickle hemoglobin and hemoglobin C)
HbSS	Homozygous form of sickle cell disease
Hib	*Haemophilus influenzae* type B
HLA	Human leukocyte antigen
PCA	Patient-controlled analgesia
PPSV23	23-Valent pneumococcal polysaccharide vaccine
RBC	Red blood cell
SCD	Sickle cell disease
SCT	Sickle cell trait

INTRODUCTION

Sickle cell disease (SCD) is one of the most commonly inherited diseases in the United States, primarily affecting African Americans. About 2000 confirmed cases are reported through neonatal screening in the United States each year. Sickle cell disease is estimated in 1 of 346 African American infants and in 1 of 1114 Hispanic infants in the eastern United States.[1] Although childhood morbidity and mortality have dramatically decreased because of standardized newborn screening, advances in preventive therapy, and acute complication management, children with SCD are often hospitalized, usually for severe pain, fever, or acute complications. Sickle cell disease is a chronic illness that can have a detrimental effect on a child's quality of life and, because of its unpredictability, can interrupt a child's physical, family, and academic functioning as well as emotional and social well-being.[2] Most children with SCD require several hospitalizations because of severe pain crises, and almost 1 in 10 have a sickle-related stroke.[3]

EPIDEMIOLOGY AND NOMENCLATURE

Normal adult hemoglobin (HbA) is composed of two α-globin chains and two β-globin chains. Sickle hemoglobin (HbS) occurs when the branched-chain amino acid valine is substituted for glutamic acid at position 6 of the β-polypeptide chain. Hemoglobin C (HbC) is another genetic variant that occurs when amino acid lysine is substituted for glutamic acid as the sixth amino acid in the β-globin chain. Changes in the β-globin chain are primarily responsible for the sickling of the red blood cells (RBCs); however, the α-globin chain structure is identical in all forms (HbA, HbS, and HbC).

Sickle cell syndromes can be divided into sickle cell trait (SCT) and SCD. Sickle cell trait is the heterozygous form of SCD in which the individual inherits one HbA gene and one HbS gene. Patients with SCT are usually asymptomatic or mildly symptomatic and are carriers of the sickle cell gene. Because *Plasmodium falciparum* cannot invade sickled RBCs easily, SCT offers protection against clinical infections of malaria. Therefore, the HbS gene is more prevalent in tropical areas with a higher incidence of malaria. In the homozygous form of SCD (HbSS), also called *sickle cell anemia*, the patient inherits both abnormal genes, one from each parent. Compound heterozygous inheritance of HbS with another mutation results in sickle cell hemoglobin C (HbSC) or one of two types of sickle cellβ-thalassemia (HbS β+thal and HbS β0thal). Patients with HbSS and HbS β0thal typically have a more severe disease course than patients with other types because patients with HbSS and HbS β0thal do not have normal β-globin production.[4]

Two million people in the United States carry the sickle cell gene. Most are of African ancestry, although those of Mediterranean and Middle Eastern descent may also have sickle cell mutations. More than 50,000 Americans have SCD, and for every infant with SCD, 50 infants are identified as carriers. About 9% of African Americans carry the HbS gene. The most common variant of SCD in the United States is HbSS at 45%, followed by HbSC (25%), HbS β+thal (8%), and HbS β0thal (2%).[5]

PATHOPHYSIOLOGY

In the fetus, fetal hemoglobin (HbF) is the predominant oxygen transport protein, which constitutes 60%–90% of RBC hemoglobin at birth. Fetal hemoglobin contains two γ chains instead of β chains; therefore, RBCs with HbF do not sickle. Before birth, HbF undergoes a conversion from γ chains to β chains; after birth, only a few RBC clones remain to produce HbF. Infants with SCD typically have few symptoms of the disease until their HbF concentrations fall, usually by age 6 months. In an adult, RBCs contain less than 1% HbF.[6]

Because of high hemoglobin concentrations, RBCs are extremely flexible. The HbA and HbS have the same solubility when they are oxygenated, and HbS carries the oxygen normally. As oxygen is unloaded from the cell, HbS solubility decreases, leading to valine binding to sites on adjacent globin chains. The deoxygenated HbS begins to form a gel-like substance that distorts RBCs into the classic *crescent* or *sickle* shape. When HbS is reoxygenated, the RBC resumes its normal shape; however, as this sickle/unsickle process is repeated, membrane damage occurs, and the cell loses its flexibility as well as its potassium and water. This change leads to dehydrated, dense sickled cells that cannot resume their original shape and that remain sickled, even when oxygenated. Vaso-occlusion occurs as the blood becomes more viscous and as sickled RBCs adhere to the vascular endothelium, blocking small blood vessels and resulting in local tissue hypoxia. A normal RBC lives 100–120 days. An irreversibly sickled RBC lives only 10–20 days, leading to anemia, which is common in patients with SCD.[7]

In addition to the local tissue damage caused by vaso-occlusive crises, sickled cells may obstruct the spleen, leading to functional asplenia and splenomegaly. Patients with SCD are at an increased risk of infections from encapsulated bacteria (e.g., *Streptococcus pneumoniae*) because of this effect on the spleen. They may also have coagulation abnormalities because of decreased concentrations of protein C, protein S, and antithrombin III, as well as increased thrombin generation and platelet aggregation.[8,9]

CLINICAL PRESENTATION AND DIAGNOSIS

NEWBORN SCREENING

Most infants with SCD appear healthy at birth and begin to have symptoms only as their HbF concentrations decrease during the first 6 months of life. Newer therapies and interventions have dramatically decreased morbidity in infants and children with SCD, so identifying these children before age 2 months is important. Neonatal screening for SCD is required in all 50 of the United States so that caregiver education can begin and care plans can be developed for these children. Newborns are screened using high-performance liquid chromatography or thin-layer isoelectric focusing, both of which have high sensitivity and specificity for SCT and SCD. Positive tests should be confirmed with a second test within 2 months. Because HbF is the primary hemoglobin in fetuses and other hemoglobins (HbA, HbC, or HbS) are not produced until the last trimester of pregnancy, very premature neonates (those born at less than 28 weeks' gestation) may have false negative test results.[10,11]

SIGNS AND SYMPTOMS

Children with SCT are typically asymptomatic, although female children with SCT may have more urinary tract infections.[12] Because of RBC sickling in the renal medulla, patients with SCT may be unable to maximally concentrate their urine, leading to an increased risk of dehydration. Although microscopic hematuria is rare, patients with SCT may have gross hematuria after very high-intensity exercise.[13]

The most common signs and symptoms of SCD are pain and anemia, which usually manifest early in childhood. In children with HbS, anemia occurs within 6 months of birth. Anemia is chronic and hemolytic with hemoglobin concentrations of 7–10 g/dL. These children typically tolerate the anemia well. Anemia may be complicated by megaloblastic changes caused by folate deficiency. As HbS concentrations increase, so do the episodes of pain, usually together with fever. Splenomegaly is common during the first year of life, as well as functional asplenia. The spleen becomes fibrotic and eventually shrinks, leading to an increased risk of infection with encapsulated bacteria. A painful splenic sequestration crisis may occur, in which the spleen is suddenly enlarged because of the pooling of many sickled RBCs. Infants may also present with dactylitis, also known as hand-foot syndrome, a painful swelling of the hands and feet.[4,10,12,14] Clinical presentation of SCD in children may differ depending on the age at symptom onset. Infants and younger children may have dactylitis, pneumococcal sepsis, meningitis, severe anemia, acute chest syndrome (ACS), pallor, jaundice, or splenomegaly. Older children may have anemia, aplastic crisis, ACS, splenomegaly or splenic sequestration, cholelithiasis, and severe or recurrent abdominal or musculoskeletal pain.[12] Children with HbSC usually have a less severe presentation, with fewer pain episodes and a mild anemia in which the hemoglobin is greater than 9 g/dL. These children may also have splenomegaly that persists into adulthood.[4,12,14]

LABORATORY DIAGNOSIS

Low hemoglobin counts (usually less than 10 g/dL) are common in patients with SCD. Typically, RBC transfusions are not used unless the patient is being treated for an acute complication such as ACS, a pain crisis, or an infection.[12] Increased reticulocyte counts, platelet counts, and white blood cell counts are common findings in a complete blood count (CBC). Peripheral blood smears reveal sickle cell forms.[12]

DISEASE COURSE AND PROGNOSIS

GROWTH AND DEVELOPMENT

Decreases in growth velocity and growth delays during puberty are common in children with SCD. Children and adolescents with SCD may also be below average for both height and weight, although this finding is independently associated with decreased hemoglobin concentrations, increased total energy expenditures, and nutritional intake.[15] In adolescents, the onset of puberty is slow, and delayed sexual maturation is common.

MORBIDITY AND MORTALITY

Morbidity and mortality in SCD are caused by complications of the disease. In the past, 50% of patients with SCD did not survive to adulthood. However, recent reports suggest that 85% of children with SCD will survive to age 18 years because of improved comprehensive care and early screening and intervention.[12] Median survival is about 42 years for men and 48 years for women.[12] Children younger than 3 years are more likely to die of infectious causes. Children who have dactylitis before age 1 year, severe anemia in the second year of life (hemoglobin concentrations less than 7 g/dL), and signs of leukocytosis without infection have higher morbidity and mortality. Morbidity and mortality in later years are secondary to chronic complications such as repeated pain crises, anemia, ACS, kidney dysfunction, and cerebrovascular complications, including stroke and lung disease.[12,16,17]

COMPLICATIONS

Acute complications of SCD are unpredictable, and rate and occurrence vary between patients. Because of functional asplenia, the risk of overwhelming sepsis from encapsulated microorganisms is high, especially from *S. pneumoniae*, *Haemophilus influenzae*, and *Salmonella* spp., which highlights the need for patient adherence to the vaccination schedule. Viral infections can also result in significant morbidity, especially from influenza and parvovirus B19.[12,14,18] By age 20 years, about 11% of patients with SCD will have had a stroke, with the highest incidence of stroke in children age 2–5 years.[19] Symptoms of stroke in children with SCD may include aphasia or dysphasia, hemiparesis, severe headache, cranial nerve palsy, seizures, stupor, and coma. Nonfocal signs, such as developmental delay and poor academic performance, may indicate ischemic central nervous system injury. The leading cause of death in patients with SCD is ACS. Patients with a new infiltrate on chest radiography, together with symptoms of a lower respiratory tract infection and hypoxia, should be treated immediately. Acute chest syndrome may occur while patients are undergoing general anesthesia, during an acute illness, or 2–3 days after a severe vaso-occlusive pain crisis. Routine incentive spirometry is vital during hospital admissions to help prevent ACS. Early signs of ACS (e.g., cough, dyspnea, chest pain) should be assessed immediately and treated to prevent deterioration to respiratory failure. Priapism, a prolonged painful penile erection, is a common complication in males with SCD, occurring in 90% of male patients by age 18 years. Vaso-occlusive pain crises are the most common SCD crisis and are characterized by acute pain (often deep and throbbing) with tenderness, erythema, and swelling in the affected area. Recurrent acute pain crises can lead to bone, joint, and organ damage, as well as chronic pain. These acute crises may be precipitated by infection, dehydration, extreme weather changes, and stress.[12,14] Aplastic crisis, usually caused by parvovirus B19 infection, occurs when hemoglobin decreases, with an acute, rapid decrease in the patient's reticulocyte count, usually to less than 1%.[12] Patients in acute aplastic crisis may present with severe pain, ACS, and splenic sequestration. Splenic sequestration in young children may lead to an acutely enlarged spleen, together with a rapid decrease in the patient's hemoglobin concentration, leading to hypovolemia, shock, and death.

Chronic complications are usually a result of organ damage, affecting the heart, lung, brain, bones and joints, eyes, kidneys, and gallbladder. Although these chronic complications are much more common in adult patients with SCD, children and adolescents with poorly managed disease or severe repeated acute complications may also have them (Table 1).[4,10,12,14,20]

TREATMENT

THERAPY GOALS

Therapy goals for children and adolescents with SCD are to decrease complications and morbidity to improve quality of life. This strategy requires a comprehensive multidisciplinary approach, including medication, regular examinations, education of both patients and caregivers, and psychosocial support.[12] Preteens and adolescents should actively be involved in managing their disease. Medications are aimed at maintaining health through prophylactic measures and treating acute complications and crises as they arise.

PREVENTIVE THERAPY

IMMUNIZATIONS

Children with SCD should receive all routine immunizations recommended by the Advisory Committee on Immunization Practices of the Centers for Disease Control and Prevention and the American Academy of Pediatrics (Pediatric Vaccines chapter). The impaired splenic function that develops in these children during childhood increases the risk of infection with encapsulated bacteria (e.g., *S. pneumoniae*, *H. influenzae*, *Salmonella* spp.). Children with SCD are up to 600 times more likely to have invasive pneumococcal disease, especially if they are younger than 2 years.[21] Vaccination with the 13-valent pneumococcal vaccine and *H. influenzae* type B vaccine (Hib) is crucial in this population and has significantly decreased morbidity and mortality in children younger than 2 years with SCD. However, despite appropriate vaccination, some children with SCD still have high rates of invasive pneumococcal disease. The 23-valent pneumococcal polysaccharide vaccine (PPSV23) contains the most common pneumococcal isolates in older children and adults. Children older than 2 years should also receive the PPSV23, with the first dose separated from the last dose of the 13-valent pneumococcal vaccine by at least 2 months. A second dose of the PPSV23 is recommended 5 years after the initial dose. In addition to pneumococcal vaccine, children with SCD older than 2 years who are scheduled for surgical splenectomy or who have functional asplenia should receive a dose of the meningococcal conjugate vaccine (Menactra, Sanofi Pasteur, Inc., Swiftwater, PA, and Menveo, GSK Vaccines, Srl, Research Triangle Park, NC) at least 2 weeks before the surgical procedure. When the first dose of meningococcal conjugate vaccine is administered at age 2–6 years, a second dose of meningococcal conjugate vaccine is recommended 3 years after the initial dose.[22] Meningococcal serogroup B vaccine (Trumenba, Pfizer Inc., Philadelphia, PA, and Bexsero, GSK Vaccines, Srl, Research Triangle Park, NC) is also recommended in patients 10 years and older with SCD.

PENICILLIN PROPHYLAXIS

Despite appropriate vaccination against pneumococcal disease, the available vaccines do not cover all *S. pneumoniae* serotypes. Use of prophylactic penicillin has dramatically decreased mortality from invasive pneumococcal infections in young children.[12] Prophylactic penicillin used in children with SCD reduces the incidence of pneumococcal bacteremia by about 85%.[23] Children with SCD should be initiated on prophylactic penicillin by age 2 months and continued until they are at least age 5 years.[12] Penicillin V potassium 125 mg orally twice daily is given until age 3 years; then, the dose

is increased to 250 mg orally twice daily until the child is at least age 5 years. Amoxicillin 20 mg/kg/day divided every 12 hours (maximum 250 mg/dose) can also be used. Benzathine penicillin 600,000 units intramuscularly every 4 weeks beginning at age 6 months and continued to age 6 years is an option when adherence to the oral regimen is a concern. Penicillin-allergic children can receive erythromycin orally at 10 mg/kg twice daily.[12,14] Some children develop invasive pneumococcal infections despite use of prophylactic penicillin. Penicillin prophylaxis should be continued indefinitely in children with a history of severe invasive pneumococcal infections and in those with asplenia. In these patients, the dose remains 250 mg orally twice daily.[12,14]

FOLIC ACID SUPPLEMENTATION

Folic acid supplementation is generally recommended in children with SCD who have chronic hemolysis. Infants should receive 0.1 mg orally once daily, and children 1–4 years of age should receive 0.3 mg orally once daily. Children older than 4 years and adolescents should receive 0.4–1 mg orally once daily.[24]

HYDROXYUREA

Hydroxyurea is a ribonucleotide reductase inhibitor that prevents DNA synthesis, increases HbF production, and decreases neutrophils in patients with SCD. Hydroxyurea also decreases RBC adhesion to the intravascular endothelium and increases nitric oxide concentrations, which is a regulator involved in physiological disturbances. In landmark studies of adults with SCD who received hydroxyurea, the pain crises, hospitalization rates, RBC transfusions, ACS incidence, and mortality were reduced. The HbF concentrations increased, and hemolysis decreased.[25,26] Results of studies of children and adolescents with SCD are similar to those of adults in adult hydroxyurea trials, with no adverse effects on growth and development.[12,27,28] In a long-term follow-up study of 93 children with severe SCD, 84% and 74% were free

Table 1. Body Systems Affected by Sickle Cell Disease and Complications[4,10,12,14,20]

System	Complication
Cardiovascular	Myocardial infarction, anemia
Gastrointestinal	Acute hepatic ischemia, cholestasis, acute or chronic cholelithiasis, acute or chronic liver disease (caused by drug toxicity or hepatitis C contracted from transfusions)
Genitourinary	Priapism, infertility
Musculoskeletal	Acute pain crises, vaso-occlusive pain crises, chronic pain, bone infarcts, osteonecrosis, dactylitis, osteomyelitis, septic arthritis, growth delays
Neurological	Transient ischemic attacks, silent ischemic lesions, stroke, neurocognitive compromise
Ocular	Eye vessel occlusion, proliferative sickle retinopathy
Pulmonary	Acute chest syndrome, hypoxemia
Renal	Hematuria, proteinuria, renal infarct, focal segmental glomerulosclerosis, renal medullary carcinoma, enuresis
Skin	Leg ulcers
Other	Delayed puberty, splenomegaly, infectious complications secondary to *Haemophilus influenzae*, *Streptococcus pneumoniae*, *Salmonella* spp., leukocytosis

of vaso-occlusive crises during the first and fifth year of treatment, respectively. The median number of hospitalizations decreased from two per year before the study to zero during the 6-year follow-up.[29] In very young children with SCD, hydroxyurea significantly decreased pain, dactylitis, ACS, hospitalization rates, and need for transfusion while increasing hemoglobin and HbF.[30]

Hydroxyurea treatment should be considered in infants 9 months and older and children and adolescents with SCD, regardless of clinical severity, to reduce SCD-related complications.[12] Hydroxyurea can be used in children as young as 6 months. Therapy goals with hydroxyurea are to reduce the number and severity of acute SCD complications, including pain crises, and to improve the patient's quality of life. Hydroxyurea dosing should be individualized according to the patient's HbF concentration and hematologic response (Box 1). [31-33]

Box 1. Hydroxyurea Dosing and Monitoring[12,31-33]

Dosing (Infants Age ≥ 6 Mo, Children, Adolescents)

20 mg/kg orally once daily

Increase by 5 mg/kg every 8 wk until mild myelosuppression, defined as absolute neutrophil count (ANC) 2000–4000 cells/mm^3

Maximum dose 35 mg/kg/day

Monitoring

CBC with differential and reticulocytes every 2 wk while titrating dose; then every 4–6 wk once dosing is stabilized

If inadequate response, evaluate for adherence to therapy

If hemoglobin (Hgb) < 5 g/dL, ANC < 2000 cells/mm^3, platelet count < 80 × 10^3 cells/mm^3, or reticulocyte < 80 × 10^3 cells/mm^3 when Hgb < 9 g/dL, discontinue hydroxyurea until recovery of at least 1 of the cell counts

Monitor counts weekly until dose can be reinitiated

After recovery, reinitiate at 2.5–5 mg/kg less than last total daily dose when toxicity occurred

Titrate dose by 2.5–5 mg/kg every 8 wk until stable for 24 wk of therapy

Adverse Effects

Mild to moderate neutropenia

Mild thrombocytopenia

Severe anemia

Rash

Nail changes

Headache

Notes

Adjust doses for renal dysfunction

Clinical response may take up to 6 mo

Children and adolescents receiving hydroxyurea should be closely monitored for both safety and efficacy (Box 1). Mean corpuscular volume will increase as HbF concentration increases. If mean corpuscular volume does not increase with hydroxyurea use, the bone marrow may be unable to respond, the dose may be inadequate, or patients may not be adherent to their therapy. Monitoring the HbF concentrations, which should increase by 15%–20%, can also assess response to therapy.

Hydroxyurea is commercially available in a solid oral dosage form as 200-, 300-, 400-, and 500-mg capsules, and as a 100- and 1000-mg tablet. The 1000-mg tablet is triple scored for ease in providing smaller doses: each tablet can be divided into four equal parts of 250 mg each.[34] The tablet dosage forms can be dissolved with a small amount of water and administered. An extemporaneous suspension can also be compounded for younger children who cannot swallow a capsule and cannot tolerate the dissolved tablets. Doses for patients taking solid dosage forms should be rounded to the nearest available capsule or capsule combination. The most common adverse effect of hydroxyurea is mild to moderate neutropenia; other reported effects include mild thrombocytopenia, severe anemia, rash, nail changes, and headaches. Adverse effects are reversible on product discontinuation. Hydroxyurea is teratogenic in high doses in animal studies, so female patients should be counseled to use effective contraception. Studies are evaluating hydroxyurea use in children with SCD who have had a stroke to reduce the need for chronic RBC transfusions and prevent end-organ damage in young children with SCD.

TRANSFUSION THERAPY

Transfusions are indicated in children and adolescents with SCD for acute exacerbations of anemia that require supplemental oxygen; with aplastic crisis, stroke, symptomatic severe ACS, acute splenic sequestration plus severe anemia, symptomatic anemia, or acute multiorgan failure; and in those who are preparing for surgery involving general anesthesia or radiologic procedures requiring ionic contrast. Hyperviscosity may occur if the hemoglobin concentration is increased to greater than 10–11 g/dL. Volume overload is a concern if the anemia is corrected too rapidly, which may lead to congestive heart failure.[12]

Studies show that in children, chronic RBC transfusions decrease stroke recurrence from 50% to 10% over a period of 3 years.[35] In addition, chronic transfusions are used in children and adolescents to reduce certain SCD complications such as vaso-occlusive pain crises and ACS. Without chronic transfusion therapy, up to 93% of children with SCD who have had a stroke will have a recurrence. Several transfusion methods have been used, including simple transfusion, exchange transfusion, and erythrocytapheresis. The goal of chronic transfusion therapy is to reduce erythropoiesis and maintain the HbS concentration at less than 30% of the total hemoglobin concentration.[12] Depending on the HbS concentrations, transfusions are administered every 3–4 weeks. For secondary stroke prevention, lifelong transfusions are required; stroke risk increases once the transfusions are discontinued.[12] Although chronic transfusion therapy is not standard, observational and retrospective evidence shows that in children and adolescents with SCD for whom hydroxyurea therapy has failed, chronic transfusion therapy may help with severe or recurrent ACS, recurrent priapism, debilitating chronic pain, chronic organ failure, transient ischemic attacks, and intractable leg ulcers, as well as with severe chronic anemia accompanied by heart failure.[36-39]

Risks associated with transfusions include alloimmunization, hyperviscosity, viral transmission, volume overload, transfusion reactions, and iron overload. Alloimmunization can be minimized with leukocyte-reduced RBCs or human leukocyte antigen (HLA)-matched units. Although the risk of viral transmission through transfusion is low, patients with SCD should be immunized against hepatitis B and monitored for hepatitis C and other bloodborne pathogens. Parvovirus is associated with aplastic crisis and may be present in 1 of every 40,000 units of RBCs. Sickle cell hemolytic transfusion reaction syndrome is a distinct condition that occurs because of alloimmunization and may lead to acute or delayed transfusion reactions. Symptoms of hemolytic transfusion reaction syndrome mimic pain crises. Delayed reactions occur 5–20 days post-transfusion. Severe anemia may occur after the transfusion because of a rapid decrease in hemoglobin and hematocrit with the suppression of erythropoiesis. Additional transfusions may worsen the clinical picture because of the presence of autoimmune antibodies. Recovery occurs only after all transfusions are discontinued and is evidenced by a gradual increase in hemoglobin and reticulocytes.[12,22,40]

Iron chelation. Iron overload is a concern in patients maintained on chronic transfusions for more than 1 year because humans lack an effective means to excrete excess iron.[41,42] There is no consensus on the best way to estimate iron overload in children with SCD maintained on chronic transfusion therapy. Most comprehensive SCD centers in the United States use a combination of serum ferritin concentrations, cumulative RBC transfusion volumes, and liver biopsy to determine the patient's iron status. Each milliliter of packed RBCs contains about 1 mg of elemental iron. Chelation therapy should be considered when the child or adolescent has received a cumulative total of 120 mL/kg of RBCs (around 20 units) and/or when the serum ferritin concentration is greater than 1500–2000 ng/mL.[42] If a liver biopsy is completed, chelation should start when the liver tissue iron content is greater than 7 mg/g of dry tissue weight.[43]

The three medications available in the United States for iron chelation are deferoxamine, deferasirox, and deferiprone (Table 2). Deferoxamine is a parenteral iron chelator that complexes with trivalent ferric ions to form ferrioxamine, which is then removed by the kidneys. Deferoxamine is superior to the other approved agents in removing cardiac iron. However, its poor oral bioavailability and short half-life necessitate an 8- to 12-hour subcutaneous infusion. Patients receiving deferoxamine should also receive supplemental ascorbic acid starting 1 month after deferoxamine initiation. Ascorbic acid increases the availability of iron for chelation. Children with preexisting cardiac conditions should not receive supplemental ascorbic acid. Contraindications include those with renal impairment. Complications of deferoxamine

therapy may include ototoxicity, allergic reactions, growth failure, ocular disturbances, pulmonary hypersensitivity, and arthralgias. Adherence to deferoxamine can be an issue because of its route of administration. Children and adolescents receiving chelation with deferoxamine should have regular eye and auditory examinations.

Deferasirox is an oral iron chelator that selectively binds iron, forming complexes that are excreted through the feces. Deferasirox (Exjade, Novartis, East Hanover, NJ) is available in a tablet for oral suspension that should be dissolved in water, orange juice, or apple juice and should be consumed 30 minutes before eating. Deferasirox (Jadenu, Novartis) is also available as a tablet that can be swallowed whole. Of note, a 30% lower dose should be used if converting a patient from Exjade to Jadenu. Deferasirox has a U.S. Food and Drug Administration (FDA) label for use in children 2 years and older. Serum ferritin concentrations should be monitored closely in patients receiving deferasirox. If serum ferritin decreases to less than 500 ng/mL, deferasirox should be discontinued and then reinitiated once the serum ferritin concentration increases to 500 ng/mL or higher.[32] Adverse effects include headache, rash, abdominal pain, nausea, diarrhea, arthralgia, increased serum hepatic transaminases and creatinine, and visual and auditory disturbances. As with deferoxamine, regular annual eye and auditory examinations are recommended. Deferasirox doses should be decreased if the patient's serum creatinine increases above the age-appropriate upper limit of normal on two consecutive measurements. If the patient's serum creatinine increases to more than two times the upper limit of normal for age or the creatinine clearance is less than 40 mL/minute/1.73 m², then deferasirox should be discontinued until measurements return to baseline.[42,44,45]

Deferiprone has label approval by the FDA for the treatment of transfusional iron overload in adults with thalassemia syndromes who experienced an inadequate response to other chelation therapies. Deferiprone binds to ferric ions and forms a complex, which is excreted in the urine. Deferiprone is an oral agent administered three times daily. Agranulocytosis has occurred in patients receiving deferiprone; therefore, careful monitoring is necessary. Studies of deferiprone use in children are limited, but trials are ongoing.[46,47]

Recent studies have evaluated the combination of chelation agents in patients with excess iron overload. Deferoxamine and deferiprone have synergistic effects.[48] Studies of pediatric patients with transfusion-related iron overload that has been unsuccessfully treated with monotherapy have shown safety and efficacy with chelation combinations; however, these studies were small, and more research is warranted.[49,50]

L-Glutamine. L-glutamine is an essential amino acid that, although synthesized endogenously, may not be efficiently used during times of stress. Evidence suggests that L-glutamine can reduce the incidence of SCD-related vaso-occlusive crises. Red blood cells from patients with SCD who received glutamine showed reduced sickling and the cells were less adherent to the vascular walls.[51] In children younger than 5 years with SCD, severe complications were reduced with the administration of L-glutamine including fewer hospital visits for pain crises, fewer hospitalized days, fewer episodes of ACS, and fewer sickle cell pain crises overall.[52] The product is provided as an oral powder and is dosed based on body weight, 0.3 g per kg, twice daily for a total daily dose of 10, 20, or 30 g/day.[53] The dose should be mixed in 8 ounces of cold or room-temperature beverage or food such as applesauce or yogurt, and then should be ingested immediately. Adverse effects include constipation, nausea, headache, abdominal pain and cough, and are considered mild. There is no adjustment for renal or hepatic dysfunction.

ACUTE COMPLICATION MANAGEMENT

INFECTION AND FEVER

Children with SCD who have a temperature of 101.3°F (38.5°C) or higher should seek immediate medical attention because their condition may deteriorate rapidly. Because of splenic dysfunction, children with SCD are at high risk of complications from encapsulated bacteria such as *S. pneumoniae*. Hospital admission is necessary, especially in children younger than 1 year, patients with elevated white blood cell counts, patients with a history of sepsis or bacteremia, or patients who appear acutely ill. Physical examination, blood cultures, CBCs including reticulocyte count, and chest radiographs if cough is present or if the child has difficulty breathing should be completed. Patients should immediately be initiated on empiric broad-spectrum intravenous antibiotics such as cefotaxime, ceftriaxone, or cefuroxime. Patients who have a true allergy to cephalosporins may be treated with clindamycin. Vancomycin should be initiated if the patient has a history of a staphylococcal infection or is severely ill. If *Mycoplasma pneumoniae* pneumonia is suspected, a macrolide such as azithromycin may be initiated. Pain and swelling in an extremity may indicate bone infarct, and osteomyelitis

Table 2. Iron Chelators Used in Children with Sickle Cell Disease and Iron Overload

Drug	Route	Dosage Regimen	Toxicities	Notes
Deferoxamine	SC	20–50 mg/kg/day for 4–7 days/wk Max 2 g/day Infuse over 8–12 hr	Ototoxicity Visual impairment Arthralgia Headache ARDS Hypersensitivity	Supplement with PO ascorbic acid 50–150 mg/day[a] Do not use in severe kidney dysfunction
Deferasirox	PO (Exjade)[b]	20 mg/kg once daily Titrate every 3–6 mo by 5–10 mg/kg/day Max 40 mg/kg/day Round to available whole-tablet dose: 125, 250, 500 mg	Headache Rash Abdominal pain Nausea Arthralgia Visual impairment Increased hepatic transaminases Increased SCr	Disperse tablet in water or orange or apple juice before administration Adjust dose in kidney or hepatic dysfunction
	PO (Jadenu)[b]	14 mg/kg once daily Titrate every 3–6 mo by 3.5 or 7 mg/kg/day Max < 28 mg/kg/day Round to available whole-tablet dose: 90, 180, 360 mg	Headache Rash Abdominal pain Nausea Arthralgia Visual impairment Increased hepatic transaminases Increased SCr	Give on empty stomach or with light meal Administer with water or other liquids Adjust dose in kidney or hepatic dysfunction
Deferiprone	PO	25 mg/kg TID Titrate based on patient response and therapeutic goals Max 99 mg/kg/day Round to the nearest 250 mg (tablet) or 2.5 mL (PO solution)	Agranulocytosis Neutropenia Nausea Vomiting Abdominal pain Increased hepatic transaminases Arthralgia	May be taken with food to decrease nausea

[a]Do not use supplemental ascorbic acid in patients with preexisting cardiac conditions.
[b]Novartis, East Hanover, NJ
ARDS = acute respiratory distress syndrome; max = maximum; PO = oral; SC = subcutaneous; TID = three times daily.
Adapted with permission from: Hagemann T. Sickle cell disease. In: Richardson M, Chant C, Chessman KH, et al., eds. Pharmacotherapy Self-Assessment Program, 7th ed. Pediatrics. Lenexa, KS: American College of Clinical Pharmacy, 2010:35.

should be considered. The most common cause of osteomyelitis in this population is *Salmonella* spp., followed by *Staphylococcus aureus*.[12] Prophylactic penicillin regimens should be held while the patient receives broad-spectrum antibiotics. Intravenous fluids to prevent dehydration may also be indicated, as well as treatment of fever with appropriate doses of ibuprofen or acetaminophen.[4,10,14]

ACUTE CHEST SYNDROME

Patients with ACS require hospitalization because their condition may rapidly deteriorate into respiratory failure and death. Acute chest syndrome may present during an acute illness or 2–3 days after a severe vaso-occlusive pain crisis. A patient receives a diagnosis of ACS when a new infiltrate is revealed on chest radiograph, together with symptoms of a lower respiratory infection and possibly hypoxemia.[12] Acute chest syndrome may be caused by a viral or bacterial infection, a pulmonary infarct, and pulmonary fat emboli. Gram-negative, gram-positive, and atypical bacteria should be suspected, and early use of appropriate empiric parenteral antibiotics such as a cephalosporin and a macrolide is important. Oxygen therapy may be indicated if the patient is hypoxic or in respiratory distress. Oxygen saturations measured with pulse oximetry should be maintained at 95% or greater. Intravenous fluid use should be monitored closely to avoid fluid overload, which may cause pulmonary edema and increase respiratory distress. Patients may require an RBC transfusion, depending on their hemoglobin concentration, to improve oxygenation. Incentive spirometry is encouraged every 2–4 hours to help prevent atelectasis and to help with lung expansion. Appropriate pain management is crucial, but care should be taken to prevent opioid-induced hypoventilation. Corticosteroid use is controversial because it is associated with higher complication rates and readmission.[12,44,45,54,55]

CEREBROVASCULAR ACCIDENTS

Initial assessment of stroke in a child with SCD should include a physical examination, a CBC including a reticulocyte count, and noncontrast computed tomography or magnetic resonance imaging. Close monitoring every 2 hours with both physical and neurologic examinations is recommended. Treatment may include transfusion to maintain a hemoglobin concentration at 10 g/dL and an HbS concentration at less than 30%. Patients who seize may require anticonvulsants, and interventions may be needed to decrease intracranial pressure. Children with a history of stroke should be initiated on chronic transfusion therapy.[12] Use of clopidogrel and other antiplatelet agents has not been studied in children with SCD and is not recommended.

Early screening for ischemic events with transcranial Doppler ultrasonography is recommended for children with SCD beginning at age 2 years, and children should be screened annually. In the Stroke Prevention Trial in Sickle Cell Anemia (STOP) study, screening followed by chronic transfusion therapy significantly reduced the incidence of primary stroke.[56] Children with positive findings may be candidates for chronic transfusion therapy for primary stroke prevention.[57,58]

PRIAPISM

Children and adolescents with SCD have two types of priapism. Stuttering episodes, which last from a few minutes to less than 2 hours, recur and resolve spontaneously. Severe episodes may last longer than 2–4 hours and require medical attention to prevent complications that lead to impotence. Therapy goals for priapism are to provide pain relief, provide detumescence, and preserve fertility. Patients can self-treat initially by increasing oral fluid intake, urinating, taking warm baths, and using analgesics. If the episode continues for more than 2 hours, patients should be instructed to seek medical attention.

Initial treatment of severe prolonged episodes should include intravenous fluids and analgesics. Patients may require RBC transfusion if their current hemoglobin concentration is less than their baseline concentration. Both vasodilators and vasoconstrictors have been used to treat severe episodes. Aspiration of penile blood, followed by intracavernous irrigation with epinephrine (1:1,000,000), has been used effectively with minimal complications.[59,60]

Several medications have been used to prevent or decrease episodes of priapism. First-line therapy is pseudoephedrine 30–60 mg orally at bedtime. Terbutaline 5 mg orally at bedtime has been used, but the evidence is inconsistent. In severe cases, initiating hydroxyurea or chronic transfusion therapy may be beneficial.[12,59]

CRISIS MANAGEMENT

APLASTIC CRISIS

Treatment of aplastic crisis is generally supportive because most patients spontaneously recover. Patients may require pain management and transfusion if the anemia is severe or if they are symptomatic. The most common cause of aplastic crisis is human parvovirus B19 infection. These patients should be isolated from other individuals with SCD, immunocompromised individuals, and pregnant women because parvovirus is highly contagious.[4,10,12]

SEQUESTRATION CRISIS

In young children, splenic sequestration of RBCs can lead to a rapid decrease in hemoglobin concentration, usually more than 2 mg/dL below the baseline, and an acutely enlarged spleen. This shift can result in hypovolemia, shock, and death. Treatment should include RBC transfusions to correct the hypovolemia in addition to broad-spectrum antibiotics because infections can precipitate the sequestration crisis.[4,12] Management of recurrent episodes involves chronic RBC transfusions and splenectomy. Splenectomy is usually delayed in children until after age 2 years because of the risk of post-splenectomy septicemia.[12,14]

VASO-OCCLUSIVE PAIN CRISIS

Most cases of mild to moderate pain in children and adolescents with SCD can be managed at home. Patients should be instructed to increase their oral fluid intake, rest, apply warm compresses to the painful areas, and take oral analgesics such as acetaminophen or ibuprofen with or without an opioid (hydrocodone). In moderate to severe cases, patients should be hospitalized for treatment. Intravenous or oral fluids at 1.5 times maintenance should be initiated, with careful monitoring to prevent fluid overload.[12] Transfusion may be required in patients who are anemic to bring their hemoglobin concentration back to their baseline concentration if they are symptomatic. Patients presenting with fever should be initiated on broad-spectrum antibiotics empirically because infection may lead to a pain crisis. Aggressive pain management is required and should be individualized and titrated to achieve the best patient response (Table 3). Patients admitted to the hospital with a vaso-occlusive crisis require continuous 24-hour pain medication with as-needed analgesics for breakthrough pain. This control can be achieved through a continuous patient-controlled analgesia pump or through scheduled intravenous pain medications. Pain control should be assessed regularly with a self-reported pain scale. Patients receiving intravenous opioids should be encouraged to use incentive spirometry to prevent atelectasis. Nausea and vomiting are common adverse effects of the opioid analgesics and can be managed with antiemetics such as promethazine or ondansetron. However, promethazine is contraindicated in children younger than 2 years and should be used with caution in young children because of the increased risk of

respiratory depression. Patients receiving opioids should be assessed for stool frequency and initiated on prophylactic stool softeners and stimulant laxatives. Pruritus can be severe in patients taking higher doses of opioids, and an antihistamine such as diphenhydramine on a scheduled routine may be necessary. A low-dose continuous infusion of naloxone may help when other agents inadequately relieve pruritus.[61]

Many patients with SCD have some degree of chronic pain, especially as they age or their condition advances. The lowest dose of an oral analgesic, usually a combination of hydrocodone and acetaminophen, is typically available for these patients on an as-needed basis. Some patients may require the addition of ketamine or use of a lidocaine patch for appropriate pain control when in vaso-occlusive crisis. Neuropathic pain from repeated vaso-occlusive crises may necessitate the regular use of medications such as gabapentin, amitriptyline, or pregabalin (Pain Management chapter).

HEMATOPOIETIC STEM CELL TRANSPLANTATION

The only cure for SCD is hematopoietic stem cell transplantation using marrow from a donor who does not have SCD, ideally an HLA-matched sibling. In a recent review of children with SCD who received a transplant from an HLA-matched

Table 3. Drug Regimens for Vaso-Occlusive Pain Crises in Children with Sickle Cell Disease

Treatment Goal	Drug Regimen
Mild to moderate pain	Acetaminophen: 10–15 mg/kg PO every 6 hr (max dose ≤ 75 mg/kg/day in ≤ 5 divided doses)
	Hydrocodone with acetaminophen: 0.2 mg/kg (based on hydrocodone) PO every 6 hr
	Ibuprofen: 10 mg/kg PO every 6–8 hr[a]
	Naproxen: 5 mg/kg PO every 12 hr[a]
Severe pain	Morphine: Intermittent doses: 0.05–0.15 mg/kg IV every 3–4 hr CI: 0.02–0.05 mg/kg/hr; titrate to effect PCA: 0.02–0.03 mg/kg/hr basal + 0.02–0.06 mg/kg IV every 10 min
	Hydromorphone: Intermittent doses: 0.005–0.015 mg/kg IV every 3–4 hr CI: 0.003–0.005 mg/kg/hr IV; titrate to effect PCA: 0.003–0.005 mg/kg/hr basal + 0.003–0.005 mg/kg IV every 10 min
	Fentanyl: Intermittent doses: 1–2 mcg/kg/dose IV every 30–60 min PCA: 0–1 mcg/kg/hr basal + 0.5–1 mcg/kg IV every 6–8 min
	Ketorolac: 0.5 mg/kg up to 30 mg per dose IV every 6 hr[a,b,c]
Adjunctive treatment	Docusate: 5 mg/kg/day PO divided in 1-4 doses
	Diphenhydramine: 1 mg/kg/dose IV/PO every 6 hr
	Naloxone (for itching): 0.25–1 mcg/kg/hr IV infusion
	Promethazine: 0.25 mg/kg IV/PO every 6 hr (max dose 25 mg)[d]
	Ondansetron: 0.15 mg/kg/dose IV/PO every 8 hr

[a]Use with caution in patients with kidney failure, dehydration, thrombocytopenia, or bleeding.
[b]Use in children age ≥ 1 yr; use with caution in children age 6–12 mo.
[c]Limit use to 5 days max.
[d]Contraindicated in children < 2 yr because of potential for severe and potentially fatal respiratory depression.
CI = continuous infusion; IV = intravenous; max = maximum; PCA = patient-controlled analgesia; PO = oral.
Adapted with permission from: Hagemann T. Sickle cell disease. In: Richardson M, Chant C, Chessman KH, eds. Pharmacotherapy Self-Assessment Program, 7th ed. Pediatrics. Lenexa, KS: American College of Clinical Pharmacy, 2010:37.

sibling, overall survival was 95%, and event-free survival was 92%.[62] Ideal SCD transplant recipients are younger than 16 years, with an HLA-identical donor and at least one of the following:

- Stroke
- ACS
- Recurrent severe pain episodes
- Impaired neurological function with an abnormal magnetic resonance imaging
- Mild to moderate chronic sickle lung disease
- Sickle nephropathy
- Bilateral proliferative retinopathy
- Osteonecrosis of several joints
- RBC alloimmunization secondary to long-term transfusion treatment[12,47]

An international expert panel recently recommended that young patients with symptomatic SCD who have an HLA-identical sibling donor should undergo transplantation as early as possible, preferably at preschool age; however, additional research is needed.[63] Although outcomes have been positive, potential risks are associated with transplantation, including failure of engraftment and chronic graft-versus-host disease. Moreover, many of the preparatory regimens used pretransplantation lead to loss of fertility; thus, cryopreservation of ovarian tissue pretransplantation is being evaluated.[64] Less than 1% of children with SCD have an HLA-identical sibling who does not have SCD, which is the main barrier to transplantation in SCD.

EMERGING TREATMENTS

Because SCD has a complex pathophysiology, emerging treatments are largely focused on preventing or treating acute complications. Investigations of these treatments include ongoing phase I, II, or III studies targeting RBC adhesion or inflammation leading to a vaso-occlusive crisis using rivipansel (GMI 1070), a selectin inhibitor; poloxamer 188 (MST 188); regadenoson, an adenosine A2A agonist; ω-3 docosahexaenoic acid; propranolol; leukotriene inhibitors, such as montelukast; simvastatin; and arginine. Other ongoing studies are investigating HbF induction (decitabine, tetrahydrouridine); anti-sickling agents SCD-101, and Sanguinate (Prolong Pharmaceuticals, South Plainfield, NJ); anticoagulation with unfractionated heparin in ACS, rivaroxaban, apixaban, or acetylcysteine; and ticagrelor, an antiplatelet agent.[65] The registered clinical trial number identifiers for these agents are shown in Box 2.

Gene therapy for SCD continues to be investigated. Sickle cell disease is monogenetic, and the causative point mutation has been well characterized. Thus, several trials are actively recruiting patients with SCD, including studies using a vector that expresses a non-sickling β-globin mutation, T87Q; a γ-globin–expressing vector; and a triple β-globin mutant, which has an increased affinity for α-globin subunits.[66-68]

CONCLUSIONS

Caring for children with SCD requires a comprehensive, multidisciplinary approach to prevent long-term complications and to improve or maintain the patient's quality of life. Children with SCD should have regularly scheduled assessments and treatment plans available if fever, pain, or symptoms of infection occur. Education of both the patient and the caregivers should routinely be updated.

Box 2. Clinical Trial Numbers for Emerging Sickle Cell Disease Treatments

---

NCT 010800526: Acetylcysteine

NCT 01685515: Fetal hemoglobin induction (decitabine, tetrahydrouridine)

NCT 01702246: Simvastatin

NCT 01737814: Poloxamer 188 (MST 188)

NCT 01788631: Regadenoson, an adenosine A2A agonist

NCT 01960413: Leukotriene inhibitors, such as montelukast

NCT 02012777: Propranolol

NCT 02072668: Rivaroxaban

NCT 02098993: Anticoagulation with unfractionated heparin in acute chest syndrome

NCT 02179177: Apixaban

NCT 02187003: Rivipansel (GMI 1070), a selectin inhibitor

NCT 02214121 and NCT 02482298: Ticagrelor, an antiplatelet agent

NCT 02380079: Anti-sickling agents SCD-101

NCT 02411708: Sanguinate[a]

NCT 02536170: Arginine

NCT 02604368: ω-3 Docosahexaenoic acid

[a]Prolong Pharmaceuticals, South Plainfield, NJ

An 11-year-old African American boy with sickle cell disease (SCD) is brought to the emergency department with a fever. His mother reports persistent and nonproductive cough for the past 48 hours and temperature reaching 101.5°F (38.6°C) using an oral thermometer. The patient reports deep and pulsating pain in his left knee (7/10 verbal pain scale). His pain and fever were unaffected by hydrocodone/acetaminophen 5/325 mg given 4 hours before and ibuprofen 300 mg given 6 hours before his emergency department visit. His left knee appears to be irritated, swollen, and tender to the touch. He has a history of vaso-occlusive pain crises and has had a splenectomy. The primary concerns are his cough, fever, and pain in extremities for 2 days.

Medical history: SCD diagnosed at birth as a homozygous form of SCD (HbSS), splenectomy (at age 5 years), hospitalized for pain crisis 3 months ago and 9 months ago (average of three per year)

Family history: Both his mother and father have sickle cell trait

Allergies: No known drug allergies

Vital signs: BP 125/80 mm Hg, HR 90 beats/minute, Tmax 102°F (38.9°C), Wt 29.5 kg, Ht 55 inches

Laboratory findings:

CBC	Value	Range
WBC	19.1	4.5–11.0 × 10³ cells/mm³
RBC	2.1	4.2–5.1 × 10⁶ cells/mm³
Hgb	7	12.0–14.0 g/dL
Hct	21	35.8%–42.4%
MCV	103	76.5–90.6 fL
Plt	160	150-450 × 10³ cells/mm³

Medications: Penicillin 250 mg orally twice daily, folic acid 1 mg orally daily, ibuprofen 300 mg orally every 6–8 hours as needed for pain (maximum four doses/day), hydrocodone/acetaminophen 5/325 mg 1 tablet orally every 4–6 hours as needed for pain (maximum six doses/day)

Immunizations: Pneumococcal 13-valent conjugate vaccine (age 2, 4, 6, and 13 months of age); *Haemophilus influenzae* type B (Hib) (age 5 years); 23-valent pneumococcal polysaccharide vaccine (ages 2 and 7 years); meningococcal (ages 5 and 8 years); influenza (yearly); diphtheria, tetanus, and pertussis; inactivated polio; hepatitis B; Hib; measles, mumps, and rubella; varicella; and hepatitis A (in childhood)

1. What are the clinical characteristics of an acute SCD crisis in this patient?

The patient presents with fever, cough, and pain, which indicate an infection that could lead to an acute pain crisis. After the physical examination, the patient's symptoms of swelling, tenderness, and erythema in his left knee suggest a vaso-occlusive crisis.

2. What would you recommend to manage the patient's acute crisis?

The patient should be hospitalized for treatment. Intravenous fluids should be initiated at 1.5 times the maintenance dose. The strategy is to start with a solution of dextrose 5% in water with half-normal saline, 3000 mL/day, to run at 125 mL/hour. After the first 24 hours, this rate can be decreased to 83 mL/hour with careful monitoring to prevent fluid overload (urinary output, weight, oral and intravenous intake). Once the patient can maintain adequate oral intake, the intravenous fluids can be discontinued.

A physical examination should be completed, as well as laboratory tests including blood cultures and a complete blood count (CBC) that includes a reticulocyte count. Blood cultures should be monitored for the presence of bacteria, and antibiotics should be adjusted based on the culture results. Daily CBCs with reticulocyte counts should be followed until the patient's values are within the normal range. Also, an initial chest radiograph should be performed, which may or may not reveal an infiltrate indicative of pneumonia. Chest radiography should be repeated if there is an acute change in the patient's condition. Infection and fever must be treated immediately to prevent deterioration to respiratory failure. Temperature should be monitored and treated if the patient's temperature is higher than 100.9°F (38.3°C). Acetaminophen 400 mg orally every 4-6 hours as needed should be used to treat fever. It is important to monitor the total number of doses of acetaminophen used in 24 hours, which should not exceed 5 doses per day. Empiric broad-spectrum intravenous antibiotics (cefotaxime, ceftriaxone, cefuroxime) should be used, such as ceftriaxone 1 g intravenously every 12 hours for 7–10 days. Adding azithromycin should be considered to cover for atypical organisms. The dose for this patient is azithromycin suspension, 300 mg orally on admission, followed by 150 mg orally once daily for 5 days total. Prophylactic penicillin should be held while patient is receiving intravenous antibiotics.

For the patient's vaso-occlusive pain crisis, patient-controlled analgesia (PCA) should be initiated with morphine at 0.8 mg/hour plus 1.6 mg every 10 minutes with a 1-hour lockout limit of 8.8 mg. The patient's pain control can be monitored through the use of a self-reported pain scale. The basal rate is adjusted based on the average 1-hour totals over the first 12 hours; it may also be necessary to adjust the dose according to the use of breakthrough doses as well as the trends in the patient's self-ratings of pain. The PCA can be continued until the patient's self-reported pain ratings are back to the patient's usual baseline; then the approach is to stop the basal rate and reinitiate the patient's home analgesia regimen, with the PCA demand dose, for 12-24 hours. After 12-24 hours, the PCA is discontinued and the patient's home regimen is continued. Ketorolac 15 mg intravenously every 6 hours should be added to the regimen and continued until the pain crisis resolves, or for 5 days, whichever is first. It is also important to monitor pain ratings and urinary output.

If nausea or vomiting occurs, ondansetron can be administered 4 mg intravenously or orally every 8 hours as needed. The patient should be assessed for stool frequency because opioids may cause constipation. When opioids are initiated, prophylactic stool softeners and stimulant laxatives should be given on a scheduled basis. For this patient, a good choice is docusate 50-100 mg orally three times daily. These agents should be continued until intravenous opioids are discontinued or until the patient is discharged. Finally, because the patient is anemic and symptomatic, packed red blood cells should be administered.

3. What preventive therapy would most benefit the patient, and what should be monitored post-discharge?

Because of the patient's history of frequent vaso-occlusive crises, hydroxyurea should be initiated to reduce pain crises and prevent hospitalization. Hydroxyurea should be initiated at 20 mg/kg orally once daily, then increased in increments of 5 mg/kg every 12 weeks to a maximal dose of 35 mg/kg/day. Because hydroxyurea is available in 200-, 300-, 400- and 500-mg capsules, this patient's starting dose should be 500 mg orally daily. A CBC should be obtained every 2 weeks during dose titration, and then every 4-6 weeks once the dose is stabilized. The patient should be closely monitored for both safety and efficacy. Mean corpuscular volume will increase as the fetal hemoglobin (HbF) concentration increases; if HbF does not increase, then the patient's bone marrow may be unable to respond, the dose may be inadequate, or the patient may not be adherent to therapy. A HbF concentration should be used to assess response to therapy. Over the course of treatment, HbF should increase by 15%–20%. If hemoglobin is less than 9 g/dL and reticulocyte count is less than 80×10^3 cells/mm^3 or if absolute neutrophil is less than 2000/mm^3, platelet count is less than 80×10^3 cells/mm^3, or reticulocyte count is less than 80×10^3 cells/mm^3, then hydroxyurea should be discontinued until recovery. Patients who are sexually active should be counseled on the teratogenic properties of hydroxyurea and to use protection against pregnancy during and at least 1 year after treatment with hydroxyurea.

Immunization is also necessary: The patient will need a dose of meningococcal serogroup B vaccine. After discharge, penicillin prophylaxis should be continued to prevent invasive pneumococcal infections. Counseling the patient on home treatment for pain should specify to increase oral fluid intake, rest, apply warm compress to painful areas, and take oral analgesics as prescribed. Finally, folic acid supplementation should be continued for chronic hemolysis.

REFERENCES

1. National Newborn Screening & Global Resource Center (NNSGRC). Newborn Screening Information. Available at http://genes-r-us.uthscsa.edu/. Accessed January 20, 2020.

2. Panepinto JA. Health-related quality of life in sickle cell disease. Pediatr Blood Cancer 2008;51:5-9.

3. Quinn CT, Rogers ZR, Buchanan GR. Survival of children with sickle cell disease. Blood 2004;103:4023-7.

4. Stuart MJ, Nagel RL. Sickle-cell disease. Lancet 2004;364:1343-60.

5. Ashley-Koch A, Yang Q, Olney RS. Sickle hemoglobin (HbS) allele and sickle cell disease: a huge review. Am J Epidemiol 2000;151:839-44.

6. Trompeter S, Roberts I. Haemoglobin F modulation in childhood sickle cell disease. Br J Haematol 2008;144:308-16.

7. Bunn HF. Pathogenesis and treatment of sickle cell disease. N Engl J Med 1997;337:762-9.

8. Inwald DP, Kirkham FJ, Peters MJ, et al. Platelet and leucocyte activation in childhood sickle cell disease; association with nocturnal hypoxaemia. Br J Haematol 2000;111:474-81.

9. Westerman MP, Green D, Gilman-Sachs A, et al. Antiphospholipid antibodies, proteins C and S, and coagulation changes in sickle cell disease. J Lab Clin Med 1999;134:352-62.

10. Ad Hoc Writing Committee, American Academy of Pediatrics. Health supervision for children with sickle cell disease. Pediatrics 2002;109:526-35.

11. Anonymous. Newborn screening for sickle cell disease and other hemoglobinopathies. Natl Inst Health Consensus Dev Conf Consens Statement 1987;6:1-8.

12. National Heart, Lung, and Blood Institute (NHLBI). Evidence-Based Management of Sickle Cell Disease: Expert Panel Report, 2014. Bethesda, MD: National Institutes of Health, 2014. Available at www.nhlbi.nih.gov/health-topics/evidence-based-management-sickle-cell-disease. Accessed January 20, 2020.

13. Key NS, Derebail VK. Sickle-cell trait: novel clinical significance. Hematology 2010;2010:418-22.

14. Fixler J, Styles L. Sickle cell disease. Pediatr Clin North Am 2002;49:1193-210.

15. Bennett EL. Understanding growth failure in children with homozygous sickle cell disease. J Pediatr Oncol Nurs 2001;28:67-74.

16. Quinn CT, Rogers ZR, Buchanan GR. Survival of children with sickle cell disease. Blood 2004;103:4023-7.

17. Dabari DS, Kple-Faget P, Kwagyan J, et al. Circumstances of death in adult sickle cell patients. Am J Hematol 2006;81:858-63.

18. Smith-Whitley K, Zhao H, Hodinka RL, et al. Epidemiology and human parvovirus B19 in children with sickle cell disease. Blood 2004;103:422-7.

19. Ohene-Frempong K, Weiner SJ, Sleeper LA, et al. Cerebrovascular accidents in sickle cell disease: rates and risk factors. Blood 1998;91:288-94.

20. Vichinsky EP. Overview of the clinical manifestations of sickle cell disease. In: Basow DS, ed. UpToDate. Waltham, MA: UpToDate, 2011.

21. Battersby AJ, Knox-Macaulay HHM, Carrol ED. Susceptibility to invasive bacterial infections in children with sickle cell disease. Pediatr Blood Cancer 2010;55:401-6.

22. Centers for Disease Control and Prevention (CDC). Vaccines and Preventable Diseases: Meningococcal Vaccination. Available at www.cdc.gov/vaccines/vpd-vac/mening/default.htm. Accessed January 20, 2020.

23. Gaston MH, Verter JI, Woods G, et al. Prophylaxis with oral penicillin in children with sickle cell anemia. A randomized trial. N Engl J Med 1986;314:1593-9.

24. Kennedy TS, Fung EB, Kawchak DA, et al. Red blood cell folate and serum vitamin B12 status in children with sickle cell disease. J Pediatr Hematol Oncol 2001;23:165-9.

25. Charache S, Terrin ML, Moore RD, et al. Effect of hydroxyurea on the frequency of painful crises in sickle cell anemia. N Engl J Med 1995;332:1317-22.

26. Steinberg MH, Bartin F, Castro O, et al. Effect of hydroxyurea on mortality and morbidity in adult sickle cell anemia: risks and benefits up to 9 years of treatment. JAMA 2003;289:1645-51.

27. Kinney TR, Helms RW, O'Branski EE, et al. Safety of hydroxyurea in children with sickle cell anemia: results of the HUG-KIDS study, a phase I/II trial. Blood 1999;94:1550-4.

28. Zimmerman SA, Schultz WH, Davis JS, et al. Sustained long-term hematologic efficacy of hydroxyurea at maximum tolerated dose in children with sickle cell disease. Blood 2004;103:2039-45.

29. Ferster A, Tahriri P, Vermylen C, et al. Five years of experience with hydroxyurea in children and young adults with sickle cell disease. Blood 2001;97:3628-32.

30. Wang WC, Ware RE, Miller ST, et al. Hydroxycarbamide in very young children with sickle-cell anaemia: a multicenter, randomized, controlled trial (BABY HUG). Lancet 2011;377:1663-72.

31. Yawn BP, Buchanan GR, Afenyi-Annan AN, et al. Management of sickle cell disease: summary of the 2014 evidence-based report by expert panel members. JAMA 2014;312:1033-48.

32. Lexi-Comp Online [Internet database]. Pediatric and Neonatal Lexi-Drugs Online. Hudson, OH: Wolters Kluwer Clinical Drug Information, Inc., 2020.

33. Strouse JJ, Lanzkron S, Beach MC, et al. Hydroxyurea for sickle cell disease: a systematic review for efficacy and toxicity in children. Pediatrics 2008;122:1332-42.

34. Siklos (hydroxyurea) tablets [package insert]. Bryn Mawr, PA: Medunik USA, 2017.

35. Wang WC. The pathophysiology, prevention, and treatment of stroke in sickle cell disease. Curr Opin Hematol 2007;14:191-7.

36. Hankins J, Jeng M, Harris S, et al. Chronic transfusion therapy for children with sickle cell disease and recurrent chest syndrome. J Pediatr Hematol Oncol 2005;27:158-61.

37. Miller ST, Wright E, Abboud M, et al. Impact of chronic transfusion on incidence of pain and acute chest syndrome during the Stroke Prevention Trial (STOP) in sickle cell anemia. J Pediatr 2001;139:785-9.

38. DeBaun MC, Gordon M, McKinstry RC, et al. Controlled trial of transfusions for silent cerebral infarcts in sickle cell anemia. N Engl J Med 2014;371:699-710.

39. Howard J, Robinson SE. Transfusion therapy for sickle cell disease. ISBT 2016;11:263-70.

40. Ballas SK, Mohandas N. Sickle red cell microrheology and sickle blood rheology. Microcirculation 2004;11:209-25.

41. Wanko SO, Telen MJ. Transfusion management in sickle cell disease. Hematol Oncol Clin North Am 2005;19:803-26.

42. Brittenham GM. Iron-chelating therapy for transfusional iron overload. N Engl J Med 2011;364:146-56.

43. Adamkiewicz TV, Abboud MR, Paley C, et al. Serum ferritin level changes in children with sickle cell disease on chronic blood transfusion are nonlinear and are associated with iron load and liver injury. Blood 2009;114:4632-8.

44. Vichinsky E, Onyekwere O, Porter J, et al. A randomized comparison of deferasirox versus deferoxamine for the treatment of transfusional iron overload in sickle cell disease. Br J Haematol 2007;136:510-8.

45. Stumpf JL. Deferasirox. Am J Health Syst Pharm 2007;64:6006-16.

46. Elalfy MS, Sari TT, Lee CL, et al. Safety, tolerability, and efficacy of a liquid formulation of deferiprone in young children with transfusional iron overload. J Pediatr Hematol Oncol 2010;32:601-5.

47. Adhikari D, Roy TB, Biswas A, et al. Efficacy and safety of oral iron chelating agent deferiprone in beta-thalassemia and hemoglobin E-beta thalassemia. Indian Pediatr 1995;32:855-61.

48. Tanner MA, Galanello R, Dessi C, et al. A randomized, placebo-controlled, double-blind trial of the effect of combined therapy with deferoxamine and deferiprone on myocardial iron in thalassemia major using cardiovascular magnetic resonance. Circulation 2007;115:1876-84.

49. Totadri S, Bansal D, Bhatia P, et al. The deferiprone and deferasirox combination is efficacious in iron overloaded patients with beta-thalassemia major: a prospective, single center, open label study. Pediatr Blood Cancer 2015;62:1592-6.

50. Elalfy MS, Adly AM, Wali Y, et al. Efficacy and safety of a novel combination of two oral chelators deferasirox/deferiprone over deferoxamine/deferiprone in severely iron overloaded young beta thalassemia major patients. Eur J Haematol 2015;95:411-20.

51. Niihara Y, Matsui NM, Shen YM, et al. L-glutamine therapy reduces endothelial adhesion of sickle red blood cells to human umbilical vein endothelial cells. BMC Blood Disord 2005;5:4.

52. Niihara Y, Miller ST, Kanter J, et al. A phase 3 trial of L-Glutamine in sickle cell disease. N Engl J Med 2018;379:226-35.

53. Endari (L-Glutamine) powder [package insert]. Torrance, CA: Emmaus Medical, 2017.

54. Caboot JB, Allen JL. Pulmonary complications of sickle cell disease in children. Curr Opin Pediatr 2008;20:279-87.

55. Johnson CS. The acute chest syndrome. Hematol Oncol Clin North Am 2005;198:857-79.

56. Adams RJ, Brambilla DJ, Granger S, et al. Stroke and conversion to high risk in children screened with transcranial Doppler ultrasound during the STOP study. Blood 2004;103:3689-94.

57. Lee MT, Piomelli S, Granger S, et al. Stroke Prevention Trial in Sickle Cell Anemia (STOP): extended follow-up and final results. Blood 2006;108:847-52.

58. Kwiatkowski JL, Granger S, Brambilla DJ, et al. Elevated blood flow velocity in the anterior cerebral artery and stroke risk in sickle cell disease; extended analysis from the STOP trial. Br J Haematol 2006;134:333-9.

59. Maples BL, Hagemann TM. Treatment of priapism in pediatric patients with sickle cell disease. Am J Health Syst Pharm 2004;61:355-63.

60. Fuh BR, Perkin RM. Sickle cell disease emergencies in children. Pediatr Emerg Med Rep 2009;14:145-55.

61. Maxwell LG, Kaufmann SC, Bitzer S, et al. The effects of a small-dose naloxone infusion on opioid-induced side effects and analgesia in children and adolescents treated with intravenous patient-controlled analgesia: a double-blind, prospective, randomized, controlled study. Anesth Analg 2005;100:953-8.

62. Walters MC, De Castro LM, Sullivan KM, et al. Indications and results of HLA-identical sibling hematopoietic cell transplantation for sickle cell disease. Biol Blood Marrow Transplant 2016;22:207-11.

63. Angelucci E, Matthes-Martin S, Baronciani D, et al. Hematopoietic stem cell transplantation in thalassemia major and sickle cell disease: indications and management recommendations from an international expert panel. Haematologica 2014;99:811-20.

64. Dovey S, Krishnamurti L, Sanfilippo J, et al. Oocyte cryopreservation in a patient with sickle cell disease prior to hematopoietic stem cell transplantation: first report. J Assist Reprod Genet 2012;29:265-9.

65. Clinical Trials.gov. A Service of the U.S. National Institutes of Health. Available at www.clinicaltrials.gov. Accessed January 20, 2020.

66. Negre O, Eggimann AV, Beuzard Y, et al. Gene therapy of the beta-hemoglobinopathies by lentiviral transfer of the (ß(A(T87Q))-globin gene. Hum Gen Ther 2016;27:148-65.

67. Orkin SH. Recent advances in globin research using genome-wide association studies and gene editing. Ann N Y Acad Sci 2016;1368:5-10.

68. Hoban MD, Orkin SH, Bauer DE. Genetic treatment of a molecular disorder: gene therapy approaches to sickle cell disease. Blood 2016;127:839-48.

Section XIII

Oncologic Disorders

CHAPTER 51

Childhood Acute Lymphoblastic Leukemia

Alix A. Dabb, Pharm.D.; and
Nicole M. Arwood, Pharm.D., BCPPS

INTRODUCTION

Acute lymphoblastic leukemia (ALL) is the most common malignancy during childhood and is responsible for around 75% of all childhood leukemias, resulting in an annual incidence of 30–40 new cases per 1 million children in the United States.[1] Survival has drastically improved because of a better understanding of the biology of the disease as well as the therapeutic advances made through clinical trials, as shown by improved 5-year survival rates from 55% in the 1970s to 85%–90% in the most recently reported period (Figure 1).[1-5] Although ALL can occur anytime during childhood development, presentation is usually at age 1–4 years.[1] In the United States, childhood ALL occurs with the highest incidence in Hispanic children, followed by white and African American children.[6,7] The incidence of ALL is higher in boys than in girls, and boys tend to present with more high-risk features than girls.[6,8]

Although the exact factors leading to the development of ALL remain unknown, much research has investigated risk factors that may contribute. However, the contribution of these risk factors remains controversial because many of the trials have produced conflicting results. From the environmental perspective, exposure to ionizing radiation has been linked with the development of ALL.[9] Other environmental factors studied include exposure to electromagnetic fields, cigarette smoke, hydrocarbons, and pesticides.[6,9-11] Certain genetic factors can increase a child's likelihood of developing ALL. The leukemia concordance rate in identical twins is high and rates of leukemia are increased in siblings of patients with childhood ALL; however, these factors does not translate to a high likelihood of ALL developing among siblings, given the overall low incidence of ALL.[6,9] In addition,

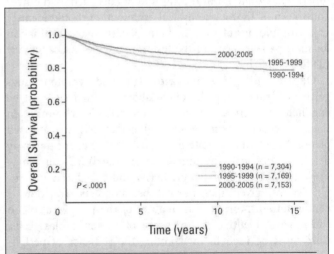

Figure 1. Overall survival probability by treatment era for patients enrolled in Children's Oncology Group trials in 1990–1994, 1995–1999, and 2000–2005.

children with other types of inherited diseases such as Fanconi anemia, ataxia telangiectasia, Down syndrome, and neurofibromatosis are at an increased risk of developing ALL.[6,9]

To better understand the pathogenesis of ALL, the normal hematopoietic process must be understood. In brief, hematopoiesis begins with a pluripotent stem cell that can differentiate into myeloid and lymphoid stem cells. The lymphoid progenitor cell then further differentiates into T cells and B cells. In the development of ALL, the lymphoid progenitor cell is defective such that it does not undergo terminal differentiation, leading to uncontrolled proliferation of immature lymphoblasts in the bone marrow.[12,13] This uncontrolled proliferation results in expanded populations of leukemia blast cells (termed *lymphoblasts*), which in turn can cause a decrease in normal hematopoiesis, leading to signs of bone marrow suppression. Lymphoblasts can be either T cells or B cells, determined by analyzing the antigen expression on the surface of the lymphoblasts. Identifying the lineage involved is important for appropriate therapy decisions, risk stratification, and prognostic implications.[14]

CLINICAL PRESENTATION AND DIAGNOSTIC EVALUATION

The clinical presentation of a child with ALL varies depending on the duration of symptoms and the degree of involvement of the bone marrow, central nervous system (CNS), and extramedullary sites. Common symptoms that may be reported on presentation include bone pain, pallor, bruising, fatigue, weight loss, fever, and potentially an enlargement of the liver, lymph nodes, and spleen.[15] Symptoms can arise from increased lymphoblasts reducing normal hematopoietic function, as well as infiltrating into organs such as the liver and spleen. A thorough physical examination should identify objective findings of ALL, including a testicular examination for male patients because the testes may serve as a sanctuary site for lymphoblasts.

Once a patient presents with signs and symptoms suggestive of leukemia, a thorough laboratory analysis must be conducted in a timely fashion. A complete blood count often shows decreased hemoglobin and hematocrit, a decreased platelet count, and a white blood cell (WBC) count that may be elevated or low. The differential on the WBC count may show the presence of lymphoblasts and a reduced neutrophil count, given that normal hematopoietic function is compromised. Morphologic analysis of the peripheral blood smear can identify the presence of leukemic blast cells. Care must be used in interpreting the presence of peripheral blasts because other causes may exist for the presence of these immature cells, such as a viral infection.[16] In addition, a comprehensive metabolic panel and uric acid concentration should be obtained to monitor the patient's renal function and evaluate electrolyte abnormalities that may suggest tumor lysis syndrome (TLS). Because the signs, symptoms, and clinical presentation of childhood leukemia are often nonspecific, other disease states should be included in the differential diagnosis. Nonmalignant diseases that might have similar presenting features include but are not limited to the

following: juvenile rheumatoid arthritis, infectious mononucleosis, osteomyelitis, aplastic anemia, and idiopathic thrombocytopenic purpura.[16]

Next in the diagnostic evaluation, a bone marrow aspirate, a biopsy, or both should be obtained to confirm the suggestion of ALL. A diagnostic lumbar puncture is also done to evaluate CNS involvement.[15] Intrathecal chemotherapy may be given during the diagnostic lumbar puncture if the diagnosis of ALL has already been confirmed on the basis of peripheral blood analysis. The specimens obtained during these procedures are analyzed by various techniques including flow cytometry, immunophenotyping, and cytogenetic studies. These techniques are used to identify leukemic blasts, determine the extent of involvement, and learn more specific details about the leukemia such as antigen expression and cytogenetic abnormalities.[15] These test results are important to determine the prognosis and to stratify the patient's therapy on the basis of risk of relapse.

CLASSIFICATION

Childhood ALL can be classified on the basis of morphology, immunophenotype, and cytogenetic abnormalities. The French–American–British system was used in the past to categorize ALL into three categories, L1, L2, and L3, according to cytologic features of the lymphoblasts in the bone marrow biopsy specimen.[6] This system is no longer used to classify leukemia because it does not correlate well with risk stratification, and there are now more advanced and more accurate methods for classification.[6,17] Immunophenotyping is one such method that uses antigens and other markers expressed on the cell surface to categorize the ALL subtype. Bone marrow samples are analyzed for cytogenetic abnormalities to better assess risk factors and prognosis.[6]

PROGNOSTIC FACTORS

Throughout decades of clinical trials, much knowledge has been gained about risk stratification for children with ALL. Prognostic factors affect treatment decisions such that more intensive therapy is provided to patients with poor prognostic features such as those stratified to high risk or very high risk to maximize outcomes, whereas therapy is often minimized for patients with favorable features such as low- or standard-risk groups to eliminate excessive toxicity in the patient subset likely to have good long-term survival.[18] Table 1 provides an overview of some of the main prognostic factors, both favorable and unfavorable.

Age and WBC count at diagnosis are two strong prognostic factors that help determine the patient's initial therapy during induction. Infants (younger than 1 year at diagnosis) and children 10 years and older are at a higher risk of relapse and need more intensive therapy to overcome this high-risk factor.[15,18,19] A presenting WBC count of 50×10^3 cells/mm^3 or more has been associated with a poor outcome, so these patients will also be considered high risk and receive more intensive therapy.[15,18,19]

Chromosomal abnormalities in the leukemic blast cell have prognostic importance. The two main types of chromosomal abnormalities are structural changes (i.e., translocations, insertions, inversions, and deletions) and changes in the number of chromosomes (i.e., gains and losses).[20] A translocation occurs when genetic material is rearranged between chromosomes. An example of a translocation is t(9;22)(q34;q11), which identifies the presence of the Philadelphia chromosome (Ph). In this case, "t" identifies that it is a translocation, (9;22) identifies that chromosomes 9 and 22 are involved, and (q34;q11) identifies the specific sections of each chromosome that are involved. The "q" refers to the long arm of the chromosome, whereas the "p" would identify the short arm of the chromosome. Thus, in this example of the Ph, genetic material on the long arm of chromosome 9 at segment 3, band 4 has changed places with the genetic material on the long arm of chromosome 22, segment 1, band 1.[20] Additions occur when genetic material is gained. The most common example of this is trisomy 21, indicative of Down syndrome, in which there are three copies of chromosome 21 rather than the normal two copies. Finally, a deletion occurs when there is a loss of genetic material. Deletions can affect a section of a chromosome or an entire chromosome. For example, monosomy 7 describes the presence of only one copy of chromosome 7. Table 1 reviews some of the main chromosomal abnormalities with prognostic importance.

The *DNA index* refers to the number of chromosomes in the leukemic blast cell compared with normal cells.[20] A DNA index of 1.0 identifies that there is the same number of chromosomes in blast cells as in normal cells. A DNA index of more than 1, termed *hyperdiploidy*, means that the blast cells have more chromosomes than normal cells.[21] Hyperdiploidy has been associated with a favorable prognosis, partly because of the increased sensitivity to chemotherapy agents, and generally occurs in patients with other favorable prognostic factors such as age and WBC count.[21-23] *Pseudodiploidy* (DNA index 1.0) describes blast cells with a normal number of chromosomes but with abnormalities such as translocations. Finally, a DNA index of less than 1, termed *hypodiploidy*, shows that the blast cell contains fewer chromosomes than

Table 1. Selected Prognostic Factors in Infant and Childhood ALL

	Favorable	Unfavorable	Application/Comments
Age at diagnosis	1 to < 10 years of age	≥ 10 years of age	Informs traditional risk group assignment (NCI risk grouping)
		≤ 1 year of age	Treated on separate, more intensive regimens
		For infants, < 6 months of age	Informs risk group assignment in infant ALL
Presenting WBC count	< 50 × 10³ cells/mm³	≥ 50 × 10³ cells/mm³	Informs traditional risk group assignment (NCI risk grouping)
		Within infant group, ≥ 300 × 10³ cells/mm³	Informs risk group assignment in infant ALL
Immunophenotype	B ALL	T ALL	Informs treatment selection. With current regimens, outcome of B ALL and T ALL appears to be similar
		ETP	Associated with inferior prognosis in initial assessments. May be associated with poorer early response and higher rates of induction failure but overall similar long-term outcomes within contemporary treatment regimens
Cytogenetic and genomic features	Hyperdiploidy (favorable trisomies), ETV6-RUNX1		"Low-risk" feature on some treatment protocols, treated in low-intensity regimens
		BCR-ABL1	Designates use of higher intensity treatment regimens with use of TKI
		MLL gene rearrangements; hyperdiploidy	Inform very high-risk status and intensification of therapy within some treatment protocols
		iAMP21	Associated with inferior outcome in some reports; informs the use of non-standard risk therapy within some treatment protocols
		IKZF1 deletions	Application under active investigation
		Philadelphia chromosome-like ALL	Application under active investigation
End-induction MRD response	Undetectable or low[a]	High[a] end-induction MRD	Incorporated into risk group assignment in modern treatment protocols

[a]Thresholds defined differently based on MRD assessment methodology, on different protocols, and at different time points.

ALL = acute lymphoblastic leukemia; ETP = early T cell precursor; MLL = mixed lineage leukemia; MRD = minimal residual disease; NCI = National Cancer Institute; TKI = tyrosine kinase inhibitor; WBC = white blood cell.
Reprinted with permission from Springer: Vrooman LM, Silverman LB. Treatment of childhood acute lymphoblastic leukemia: prognostic factors and clinical advances. Curr Hematol Malig Rep 2016;11:385-94.

normal cells, which has been associated with a poorer prognosis and very high risk stratification.[24]

Childhood ALL is more common in boys, and male sex has been associated with a poorer prognosis than female sex.[8,18] Through clinical trials and risk-adapted therapy, the impact of male sex has largely disappeared as a prognostic factor. Male patients are, however, at risk of testicular relapse as an additional site of disease. Historically, race has been identified as a factor affecting outcomes, with African American children having a poorer outcome from therapy than white children.[18] Results from a retrospective study showed that, although these patients were more likely to have unfavorable prognostic factors, their outcomes were similar to those of white children when treated with appropriate therapy.[25]

Response to therapy is the most significant prognostic factor in childhood ALL.[26] This factor has traditionally been measured by examining the bone marrow for the morphologic presence of leukemic blasts (greater than 5% blasts has been associated with a poorer response to therapy) at various times during induction and throughout therapy.[27-30] In addition, the clearance of blasts from the peripheral blood helps predict a favorable outcome.[31] Most recently, measuring minimal residual disease (MRD) has become standard practice to better assess response to therapy.[32] Detected by flow cytometry or polymerase chain reaction, MRD enables the identification of leukemic disease in the bone marrow or peripheral blood that would not have been detected morphologically. Thus, patients can now be identified as having a poor or suboptimal response when they would otherwise have been considered to have a complete response morphologically.[26] The presence of MRD (defined as MRD of 0.01% or greater) is predictive of an increased risk of relapse or poor response to therapy. The higher the MRD, the worse the prognosis because patients with high levels of MRD of 1% or greater at the end of induction have an estimated 5-year event-free survival (EFS) of 30%.[26,32-34] The same has been true for use of pretransplant MRD to predict the risk of relapse after transplantation.[35] Use of MRD to risk-stratify patients during or at the end of induction according to MRD has been effective in clinical trials.[36-38] For example, patients with high-risk ALL who are MRD positive at the end of induction are reclassified as very high risk and receive therapy thereafter designed for that group.

TREATMENT

Therapy for childhood ALL lasts 2–3 years, with increasingly complex treatment protocols as clinical trial results are incorporated into front-line therapy. Table 2 presents information on the chemotherapeutic agents used in therapy.[39] Traditionally, therapy has been divided into three phases—*induction*, *consolidation/intensification*, and *maintenance/ continuation*—with CNS-directed therapy provided throughout each phase. Certain clinical trials and therapeutic regimens may have additional phases or different treatment approaches, but most center on the backbone of the three general phases described. Therapy is stratified according to a patient's risk of relapse, with patients at a high risk of

relapse receiving more intense therapy than patients at a low or standard risk of relapse. For this discussion on treatment approaches, we will focus on therapy for patients with precursor B cell leukemia.

DOSING CHEMOTHERAPEUTIC AGENTS

Chemotherapy doses are usually calculated using a patient's body surface area, except in the infant population, for which doses are usually calculated using a patient's weight. Many formulas are available to calculate body surface area, all of which use height and weight in the calculation. Intrathecal chemotherapy is dosed not according to weight or body surface area but according to patient age. Some oral chemotherapy agents are administered as a flat dose for the adolescent and young adult population. The dosing for a given regimen should be carefully reviewed to ensure safety and efficacy.

INDUCTION

The goal of induction is to induce a complete remission, broadly defined as the absence of leukemia cells in the bone marrow, which occurs successfully in around 98% of patients.[39] A three-drug induction with a glucocorticoid, asparaginase, and vincristine is used for patients with low- and standard-risk ALL (WBC count less than 50×10^3 cells/ mm^3; age 1–9 years at presentation), whereas an anthracycline is added as the fourth drug in induction for high-risk and very high-risk patients.[39] In addition to the systemic agents, patients receive intrathecal chemotherapy as prophylaxis against CNS relapse or treatment of CNS involvement, if present.[39-43] The typical 4-week induction regimen can be extended an additional 2 weeks for patients who do not achieve a complete remission at the end of induction. Response to therapy at various times during, at the end of, and after induction is the most important prognostic factor.

Glucocorticoids are used throughout most phases of ALL therapy.[44] The choice of glucocorticoid varies between prednisone, prednisolone, methylprednisolone, and dexamethasone, depending on the protocol. Clinical trials have shown that dexamethasone has an advantage over prednisone by improving EFS and decreasing the rate of CNS relapses.[45-47] In vitro, dexamethasone has a higher antileukemic potency than prednisone.[44,45,48,49] In addition, dexamethasone has a longer half-life and can better cross the blood-brain barrier.[45-47] However, dexamethasone is also associated with an increased risk of infectious complications and avascular necrosis compared with prednisone.[44,45,50,51] The risk of developing avascular necrosis increases with age, with patients age 10–20 years at highest risk.[52] Moreover, development of avascular necrosis may be related to specific genetic polymorphisms, including *SERPINE1* and *ACP1*.[51,53,54] Although the optimal glucocorticoid is not known, several approaches are being investigated in clinical trials to maximize outcome and minimize toxicity.

Asparaginase is an essential component of ALL therapy that improves outcomes.[55,56] Asparaginase is very effective because leukemia blast cells rely on exogenous asparagine for protein synthesis, so when asparaginase is administered, the asparagine available for use by these cells is reduced.[57] Asparaginase can be derived from either *Escherichia coli* or *Erwinia chrysanthemi*.[57,58] *Escherichia coli* asparaginase, also called "native" asparaginase, has a half-life of about 1.4 days. Its use in therapy is limited by the inconvenience of three-times-weekly intramuscular dosing and the incidence of hypersensitivity reactions, which have been reported in as many as 60% of patients in clinical trials.[57,59-62] PEGylated asparaginase, termed *pegaspargase*, also derived from *E. coli* but with a half-life of about 6 days, was introduced as an option for patients with a hypersensitivity reaction to native asparaginase.[57,58,63] Initial data showed that the incidence of hypersensitivity reactions with pegaspargase was lower than with *E. coli* native asparaginase; however, clinical experience has seemed to favor a more pronounced incidence of these reactions with pegaspargase than reported. Development of a hypersensitivity reaction may be delayed and the duration prolonged, given the half-life of the pegylated preparation.[57,63]

Table 2. Chemotherapy Commonly Used in the Treatment of ALL[a]

Drug Name	Class	Major Adverse Effects	Other Notes
Cyclophosphamide	Alkylating agent	Nausea, vomiting, myelosuppression, hemorrhagic cystitis, SIADH, sterility, secondary malignancy	May be used during consolidation or for relapsed disease
Cytarabine	Antimetabolite (pyrimidine analog)	Nausea, vomiting, myelosuppression, rash, neurotoxicity, hemorrhagic conjunctivitis	May be used during consolidation or for relapsed disease May be given intrathecally
Daunorubicin/ doxorubicin	Anthracycline	Red discoloration of urine, myelosuppression, mucositis, cardiomyopathy, secondary malignancy	Added to induction mainly for high-risk patients
Etoposide	Topoisomerase II inhibitor	Myelosuppression, transient hypotension, anaphylaxis, secondary malignancy	May be used during consolidation or for relapsed disease
Imatinib/dasatinib	BCR-ABL TKI	Fluid retention, peripheral edema, myelosuppression, peripheral neuropathies, hepatotoxicity, cardiotoxicity, growth retardation (imatinib), pulmonary arterial hypertension (dasatinib)	Ph-positive ALL only, added to existing treatment plan
Mercaptopurine	Antimetabolite (purine analog)	Myelosuppression, immunosuppression, secondary malignancy, hepatotoxicity	Oral drug for maintenance therapy Minimal or no TPMT activity increases the risk of severe toxicity
Methotrexate	Antimetabolite	Hepatotoxicity, nausea, vomiting, mucositis, photosensitivity, osteonecrosis, nephrotoxicity, infertility, secondary malignancy	For high-dose IV methotrexate, ensure hyperhydration, urinary alkalinization, and leucovorin administration; monitor methotrexate pharmacokinetics May be given intrathecally
Nelarabine	Antimetabolite (purine analog)	Myelosuppression, neurotoxicity	T cell ALL only
Pegaspargase/ Erwinia asparaginase	Miscellaneous	Hypersensitivity, pancreatitis, rash, coagulation abnormalities, thrombotic events, hyperglycemia, liver function test abnormalities, hypertriglyceridemia	Staple of induction therapy Pegaspargase is produced by *Escherichia coli* and administered every 14 days Erwinia asparaginase is administered three times weekly as an alternative product for patients with hypersensitivity to pegaspargase (not *E. coli* based)
Prednisone or dexamethasone	Glucocorticoid	Hyperglycemia, hypertension, Cushing syndrome, immune suppression, gastritis, infections, osteopenia, avascular necrosis	Integral part of induction and maintenance therapy
Vincristine	Vinca alkaloid	Peripheral neuropathy, constipation, jaw pain, SIADH, foot drop, hepatotoxicity	Fatal if administered intrathecally Integral part of induction and maintenance therapy

[a]This information is intended to summarize adverse effects that occur commonly or are of major significance and is not meant to be inclusive of all adverse effects or other pertinent information.

ALL = acute lymphoblastic leukemia; IV = intravenous; Ph = Philadelphia chromosome; SIADH = syndrome of inappropriate secretion of antidiuretic hormone; TKI = tyrosine kinase inhibitor; TPMT = thiopurine S-methlytransferase.
Information from: Micromedex Solutions. Ann Arbor, MI: Truven Health Analytics. Available at www.micromedexsolutions.com. Accessed March 1, 2020.

Pegaspargase has replaced native asparaginase in clinical trials because pegaspargase is more convenient to administer, data support administering pegaspargase intravenously rather than intramuscularly, and native asparaginase is no longer available on the U.S. market.[64,65] If a patient cannot tolerate pegaspargase, then Erwinia asparaginase can be considered. Erwinia asparaginase is better tolerated after hypersensitivity reactions to native asparaginase or pegaspargase because it is not *E. coli* based, with overall hypersensitivity reaction rates as low as 5%–33%.[57] Erwinia asparaginase has a short half-life of about 0.6 day, requiring three-times-weekly administration, thus six intramuscular or intravenous doses replace one pegaspargase dose.[58,66] Some data show inferior outcomes from therapy when *Erwinia* is used in place of an *E. coli* asparaginase product, but other trials have not confirmed this finding.[59,60] The pharmacokinetics, pharmacodynamics, and dosing schemas differ between these products, so care must be taken when a different product is used to ensure the appropriate dose, route, and administration schedule.[57,58,62,63] In addition, toxicities that may occur with asparaginase products should be monitored for, including pancreatitis, thromboembolism, hypertriglyceridemia, hyperglycemia, and liver dysfunction.[57,67] The role of therapeutic drug monitoring of asparaginase products is emerging because efficacy has been linked to achieving a minimum serum asparaginase activity concentration of at least 0.1 IU/mL at 14 days after a pegaspargase dose or before the next dose of Erwinia asparaginase when given three times weekly.[66,68-71] Monitoring of serum asparaginase activity also assists in differentiating between an antibody-mediated hypersensitivity reaction versus a nonallergic infusion reaction to the asparaginase product.[72] In the setting of a clinical reaction with asparaginase administration, an antibody-mediated hypersensitivity reaction would result in a low serum asparaginase activity concentration, whereas a nonallergic infusion reaction would result in a normal serum asparaginase activity concentration, greater than 0.1 IU/mL. With the use of serum asparaginase activity concentrations, one study found more than half of the reactions to pegaspargase did not necessitate the change to the more expensive and more frequent Erwinia asparaginase product.[72] Therapeutic drug monitoring of asparaginase allows providers to premedicate patients with H1 and H2 antagonists, as one might for other biologic products, decreasing the clinical significance of asparaginase infusion reactions and ensuring that the asparaginase product administered is effective.[72]

CNS THERAPY

The CNS is a sanctuary site for leukemia cells.[73] The blood-brain barrier acts as an effective obstacle over which many systemically administered chemotherapy agents do not adequately cross; therefore, leukemia can reside in the CNS virtually free from exposure to therapy.[74] Relapse of disease in the CNS is a primary cause of treatment failure when adequate therapy is not provided to this site.[40,74] All patients are screened at diagnosis for CNS involvement by a lumbar puncture, in which the cerebrospinal fluid (CSF) is analyzed for the presence of WBCs and leukemic blasts. Because the results of the diagnostic lumbar puncture will affect the patient's

CNS-directed therapy, the procedure should be completed by an experienced practitioner with good technique to avoid potential contamination with leukemia cells from the peripheral blood.[75,76] Patients are further classified as having CNS-1, CNS-2, or CNS-3 disease. Patients with CNS-1 have no leukemic blasts in the CSF; patients with CNS-2 have blasts in the CSF with a WBC count less than 5 cells/mm^3; and patients with CNS-3 have leukemic blasts in the CSF with a WBC count of 5 cells/mm^3 or more.[6] This CNS classification helps determine the risk of CNS relapse as well as the amount and intensity of CNS-directed therapy a patient will require.

Patients with childhood ALL are at risk of CNS involvement and CNS relapse, but certain features increase that risk, including patients with T cell ALL, a WBC count greater than 50×10^3 cells/mm^3, certain cytogenetic abnormalities such as t(9;22) or t(4;11), and CNS involvement at diagnosis.[40] *Intrathecal chemotherapy*, which is chemotherapy that is delivered directly into the CSF by a lumbar puncture or by a reservoir that is placed under the scalp (Ommaya reservoir), is given to all patients concurrently with systemic chemotherapy administration as a prophylactic approach to preventing CNS relapse or to treat active CNS involvement. In a patient who presents with CNS disease, therapy is intensified using a triple intrathecal consisting of methotrexate, hydrocortisone, and cytarabine, with intrathecal therapy administered more commonly than in children without CNS disease at presentation. The choice of systemic glucocorticoid used in therapy can play a role in preventing CNS relapses because dexamethasone has been associated with fewer CNS relapses than prednisone. The dosing for intrathecal therapy is based on age, not on body surface area as for most other chemotherapy agents. Age-based dosing of intrathecal therapy allows more accurate dosing as the CSF volume changes with age, making age a much better predictor for exposure than weight, height, or body surface area (Figure 2).[77]

In the past, cranial irradiation was effectively used as prophylaxis and treatment of ALL in the CNS. However, cranial

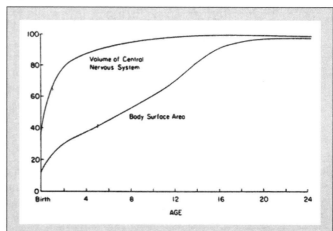

Figure 2. Relationship between body surface area and central nervous system volume as a function of age.

Reprinted with permission from: Bleyer AW. Clinical pharmacology of intrathecal methotrexate. II. An improved dosage regimen derived from age-related pharmacokinetics. Cancer Treat Rep 1977;61:1419-25.

irradiation, especially in children, is associated with many short- and long-term toxicities, including secondary malignancies, neurocognitive dysfunction, learning disabilities, effects on growth and development, and neurotoxicity.[40] Data now support that intrathecal therapy, together with intensive systemic therapy, can either replace cranial irradiation in most patients or allow the dose of cranial irradiation to be markedly reduced.[4,40-43,78,79] Cranial irradiation should be reserved for patients at an extremely high risk of CNS relapse or in the setting of CNS relapse.[40]

POST-REMISSION THERAPY

Post-remission therapy, generally consisting of two main phases, consolidation and maintenance/continuation, begins after the successful completion of induction therapy with a complete remission. As more knowledge has been gained about prognostic factors and risk stratification, additional treatment phases have been added throughout to further intensify therapy and improve outcomes.

Consolidation begins after the successful completion of induction therapy and usually lasts 2–6 months. Consolidation therapy is meant to introduce medications with mechanisms of action different from those used during induction to treat any remaining undetectable disease. If post-remission therapy is not administered and completed, the patient will experience a relapse of leukemia, despite achieving a complete remission after induction. Typical agents used during the consolidation phase include cytarabine, methotrexate, anthracyclines, etoposide, cyclophosphamide, and intrathecal chemotherapy. The drug dosing and administration schedules vary depending on the protocol or treatment plan.[2,3,80,81]

Methotrexate has antileukemic activity and is available orally, intramuscularly, intravenously, and intrathecally. High-dose intravenous methotrexate (at least 1 g/m²) during consolidation improves outcomes and requires pharmacokinetic drug level monitoring.[81-83] A methotrexate serum concentration within a specific range after an infusion of high-dose methotrexate is also associated with positive outcomes.[84] In addition, another study showed that the duration of the methotrexate infusion can affect efficacy.[85] In this study, patients were randomized to receive 1 g/m² of methotrexate intravenously over either 4 hours or 24 hours. The intracellular concentration of active drug, methotrexate polyglutamates, was higher in the patients receiving the 24-hour infusion, which correlated with a lower risk of relapse. In addition, another study showed that a high-dose infusion of methotrexate (5 g/m² per dose) had superior survival outcomes in a population of high-risk patients with ALL compared with low-dose, escalating methotrexate (Capizzi style) plus asparaginase.[86] In addition, EFS was improved, and the incidence of other toxicities did not increase in the patients receiving high-dose methotrexate. These are two recent examples of using information gleaned from clinical trials to support seemingly minor modifications to drug therapy to maximize outcomes with currently available agents.

Some childhood ALL treatment protocols also include intensification of consolidation therapy, often called *delayed intensification*, which improves EFS.[87-92] More intensive

therapy is delivered in one or two short phases consisting of 5–8 weeks of treatment. Delayed intensification is administered during the first 6 months of post-remission therapy, using agents consistent with those used during induction and other phases of consolidation. Because of the success of these intensification regimens during consolidation and continuation, most protocols and standard treatment regimens now routinely include these additional phases of therapy.

Maintenance therapy, also called *continuation therapy*, begins after the completion of consolidation and continues to complete a 2- to 3-year overall treatment from the time of initial diagnosis. This longest phase of therapy is intended to maintain a complete remission and prevent relapse. Maintenance therapy is less intense and delivered mainly in the outpatient and home settings. Maintenance therapy relies primarily on antimetabolite administration consisting of daily oral mercaptopurine and weekly low-dose oral/parenteral methotrexate together with periodic vincristine, glucocorticoids, and continued intrathecal chemotherapy.[39] Maintenance therapy can be very myelosuppressive, increasing the risk of infectious complications such as febrile neutropenia, so antimetabolite doses may need to be modified or held because of cytopenias.[39] Adding short pulses of more intense therapy during maintenance with vincristine and a glucocorticoid improves the continuous complete remission rate and disease-free survival and is therefore included in most treatment regimens.[93-95] Adherence to these oral medications is extremely important because patients with a lower adherence rate are at an increased risk of relapse.[96]

TREATMENT OF SELECT PATIENT SUBGROUPS

T CELL ALL

T cell ALL represents about 10%–15% of childhood ALL cases and has historically been associated with worse outcomes than precursor B cell ALL.[97] Reports from the late 1970s showed 3-year survival rates of around 56%, which increased to almost 80% in the early 1990s because of the intensification of therapy.[97,98] These patients are at an increased risk of induction failure, death during induction, early relapse, and isolated CNS relapses.[98] Patients with a diagnosis of T cell ALL are more likely to present with high-risk features including the following: older age, an elevated WBC count greater than 50 × 10³ cells/mm³, hepatosplenomegaly, the presence of a mediastinal mass, and CNS involvement.[97,99] Because of the high rates of CNS involvement at diagnosis and the increased risk of CNS relapse, prophylactic and therapeutic cranial irradiation has routinely been administered to these patients.[97] However, recent trials have shown that the dose of radiation delivered to the CNS can be minimized or even omitted without affecting overall EFS when intrathecal chemotherapy is incorporated into the treatment plan.[97,100-102]

Current therapy regimens for patients with T cell ALL include intensive, multiagent, systemic chemotherapy similar to that for patients with precursor B cell ALL, in addition to CNS-directed therapy in the form of intrathecal chemotherapy, cranial irradiation, or both.[100,102] Areas that differ include the use of low-dose, escalating methotrexate (Capizzi style) rather than high-dose infusion of methotrexate (5 g/m² per dose) and the addition of nelarabine to upfront therapy, both of which showed superior survival outcomes patients in with T cell ALL.[103-107] However, the most troublesome adverse effect of nelarabine is neurotoxicity, manifested mainly as somnolence and peripheral neuropathies.[108]

INFANT ALL

Infant ALL, defined as ALL arising in children younger than 1 year at diagnosis, accounts for about 5% of childhood ALL and is associated with a worse prognosis than ALL in older children and stratified as very high risk.[109-118] Clinical trials in this population have shown a 5-year EFS reaching only about 50%. Although this survival rate has improved, it continues to be substantially lower than the survival rate in children older than 1 year at diagnosis. A potential explanation for this difference in outcome is that infant ALL is biologically different from the ALL in other pediatric age groups.[119] First, the rate of chromosomal translocations with the mixed-lineage gene is very high, which has been implicated as a poor prognostic indicator.[120] Second, blast cells in infant ALL are often resistant to glucocorticoid and asparaginase therapy, two of the mainstays of therapy for childhood ALL, but they appear to be more sensitive to cytarabine.[120]

Mutations that lead to the development of infant ALL may occur completely or partly in utero. Leukemic clones have been identified in blood obtained from neonatal heel sticks (Guthrie cards) in patients who later developed ALL, showing that some or all of these genetic events occur in utero.[121] Epidemiologic studies have implicated many factors that may be associated with the development of infant ALL; however, the literature remains conflicting on most of these factors.

The clinical presentation of infant ALL is similar to that in other children. However, these patients are more likely to present with an elevated WBC count, hepatosplenomegaly, and CNS involvement.[119,120] One-half of the patients receiving a diagnosis in the first month of life will present with a condition known as *leukemia cutis*, which is the presence of leukemic infiltrates in the skin, resulting in a bluish purple cutaneous lesion.[120]

Given the rarity of ALL in infants, it is highly recommended that patients with infant ALL be enrolled and treated in a clinical trial available through a cooperative group. Therapy for infant ALL has been modeled after therapy for older children with the addition of high-dose cytarabine, but outcomes from early treatment failure are still poorer, namely bone marrow relapse.[119,120] Attempts have been made to use more aggressive chemotherapy dosing, a hematopoietic stem-cell transplantation (HSCT), or both for infant ALL. However, a report investigating the role of HSCT in infants with the mixed-lineage gene rearrangements found no survival advantage with HSCT compared with intensified chemotherapy.[122] Targeted therapy for infant ALL is under investigation.[123] The FMS-like tyrosine kinase-3 (FLT3), a receptor tyrosine kinase, is of particular interest in infant ALL because this mutation has been associated with poor outcomes.[124] However, lestaurtinib, an oral FLT3 inhibitor, did not improve outcomes when combined with chemotherapy in infant ALL.[125] Hypermethylation of DNA which silences tumor suppressor genes has also been shown to play a critical role in chemoresistance and relapse in infant ALL. Thus, azacitidine, a hypomethylating agent, in combination with chemotherapy is currently under investigation in infant ALL.[126]

DOWN SYNDROME

Patients with Down syndrome, a genetic disorder characterized by a trisomy of chromosome 21, are at a markedly increased risk of developing childhood ALL.[127-130] The reason behind this increased risk has not yet been identified.[128] Although the clinical presentation of patients with Down syndrome is similar to that of patients without Down syndrome, there are some important differences. Patients younger than 1 year with Down syndrome rarely develop ALL,[128] making the age distribution of ALL different in patients with Down syndrome. In addition, patients with Down syndrome and ALL have a lower incidence of high-risk features such as T cell ALL, CNS involvement, hyperdiploidy, and other cytogenetic abnormalities.[128] Historically, EFS rates in patients with Down syndrome were inferior to those in patients without Down syndrome.[128,129] With risk-adapted therapy, patients with ALL and Down syndrome can now be expected to have outcomes from therapy similar to those of patients with precursor B cell ALL without Down syndrome.[130,131]

Patients with Down syndrome and ALL are also at an increased risk of developing toxicity from therapy, especially mucositis and infections.[128,132] Although ALL therapy for patients with Down syndrome is similar to that for patients without Down syndrome, the Down syndrome cohort is exquisitely sensitive to the effects of methotrexate.[128,129] The exact reason for this excess toxicity is unknown; however, potential reasons include delayed methotrexate clearance and other alterations in drug handling secondary to involvement of chromosome 21.[128,129,133] In some instances, this sensitivity to methotrexate may require dose reductions, more intensive rescue therapy with leucovorin, or both. Other supportive care approaches to optimize care in the Down syndrome population include enteral or parenteral nutrition and opioids for pain management during periods of mucositis. Because these patients are at an increased risk of infections, infection-related complications, and infection-related mortality, prophylaxis with antibiotics, supplementation with immune globulins, close monitoring, and early initiation of empiric broad-spectrum antibiotics should be considered.[127,128,130]

PHILADELPHIA CHROMOSOME

Classified by the translocation between chromosomes 9 and 22, the Philadelphia chromosome is present in 3%–5% of children with a diagnosis of ALL.[134] The presence of t(9;22) has been deemed a high-risk feature because it correlates with poor outcomes in patients with traditional chemotherapy compared with patients with ALL lacking the Philadelphia chromosome.[135-140]

Early studies that treated Ph-positive patients with intensive chemotherapy regimens had an EFS rate of only up to 38%.[135,137-140] Attempts to identify high-risk features within the subset of Ph-positive patients have revealed that increased age, WBC count greater than 50×10^3 cells/mm^3 at diagnosis, and poor response to induction therapy are associated with a poorer outcome.[137-140] Imatinib, a tyrosine kinase inhibitor that competes for binding at the *BCR-ABL* site, has improved the dismal outcome of patients with Ph-positive ALL. A recent clinical trial showed the benefit of imatinib together with standard chemotherapy, as evidenced by the 3-year EFS rate of the patients receiving imatinib, which increased to 80%.[141] This trial also questioned the role of HSCT in this patient population in first complete remission. Outcomes of patients who received imatinib plus chemotherapy were similar to those of patients who received stem-cell transplants, with sustained results at 5 years.[141,142] Patients with Ph-positive ALL should have a BCR-ABL tyrosine kinase inhibitor added to their standard treatment regimen.

Although adding imatinib to therapy for Ph-positive patients has dramatically improved outcomes, resistance to imatinib has developed, rendering patients refractory to this therapy.[143] To address this resistance issue, second- and third-generation tyrosine kinase inhibitors such as dasatinib, nilotinib, and ponatinib have been developed and are being investigated in pediatric Ph-positive ALL.[134,143,144] Dasatinib is more potent than imatinib and has expanded activity against other tyrosine kinases.[134,143,145] Nilotinib is under investigation and may have benefit in pediatric patients with Ph-positive ALL.[134,143,145] Ponatinib, the third-generation tyrosine kinase inhibitor, has efficacy in overcoming the T315I mutation that confers resistance to imatinib, dasatinib, and nilotinib.[134] It is not yet known which of the second- or third-generation tyrosine kinase inhibitors provide the most benefit to childhood patients with ALL while causing the least toxicity. The most commonly reported toxicities of the tyrosine kinase inhibitors include the following: fluid retention, peripheral edema, myelosuppression, peripheral neuropathies, and potential cardiotoxicity.[108]

ADOLESCENTS AND YOUNG ADULTS

Adolescent and young adult patients with ALL, generally defined as those age 15–39 years at diagnosis, have been identified as a population with lower survival outcomes.[146] These patients have a higher incidence of T cell ALL; have a higher presenting WBC count; are more likely to have chromosomal abnormalities associated with a poor outcome, such as t(9;22); are less likely to have favorable prognostic features such as hyperdiploidy; and have a lower induction remission rate.[147,148] Other potential reasons for the differences in outcome may include decreased adherence to medications, presence of comorbidities, and increased toxicity from therapy.[147,149,150]

Given their age, young adults may be treated by either a pediatric oncologist or an adult oncologist, which means these patients may receive therapy designed either for pediatric ALL or adult ALL. Pediatric regimens rely on long-term continuous therapy, which is heavily based on asparaginase, vincristine, and glucocorticoids, whereas adult therapy uses higher doses of myelosuppressive agents such as cyclophosphamide and cytarabine, which are given intermittently for a shorter period.[149,151] Several studies conducted in the United States and Europe have shown superior outcomes in the young adult population when treated with pediatric ALL regimens rather than adult-based regimens.[152-155] Most recently, a comparison of young adult patients treated with intensive, response-based therapy had an improved outcome with chemotherapy alone and did not require stem-cell transplantation.[150] Thus, adolescent and young adult patients are currently advised to be treated at a pediatric center on a pediatric clinical trial or receive pediatric-based therapy.

The adolescent and young adult population also has increased toxicity from therapy compared with younger children.[50,150,156,157] Deaths during induction, avascular necrosis, and hyperglycemia are more common in this patient subset, potentially because of the decreased clearance rate of glucocorticoid.[50,150,156-158] These toxicities often necessitate that therapy be modified or delayed.

RELAPSE

Even with major improvements in outcome over time for childhood ALL, disease relapse remains a serious problem, with survival rates in the relapsed setting reaching only 50%.[159,160] The most recent data show rates of relapse disease in patients with B cell and T cell ALL as low as 12% and 11%, respectively; however, relapse disease in infant ALL remains higher at 35%.[160] The main sites of relapse include the bone marrow, presenting with persistent cytopenias; the CNS, which may manifest as headaches or intractable nausea/vomiting; and, to a much lesser extent, the testes, with a painless unilateral testicular enlargement.[159,161] The sites involved in the relapse and the time at which the relapse occurs must be considered because the prognosis and therapeutic approach will change, depending on these factors.[159,161] The longer the time from diagnosis to relapse, the better the survival rate.[160,162] *Early relapses*, defined as those that occur less than 36 months from initial diagnosis, have been associated with poor outcomes and often require intensive chemotherapy, likely with agents not used before to induce a second remission and then continue to allogeneic HSCT.[160,161,163-167] *Late relapses*, defined as those that occur 36 months or more from the initial diagnosis, usually respond well to conventional multiagent chemotherapy, making a stem-cell transplant potentially unnecessary.[160,161,166,168] Emerging treatment regimens for relapsed ALL include novel biologic agents such as blinatumomab, CD-19 directed chimeric antigen receptor (CAR) T cells, and inotuzumab.[169-173]

Blinatumomab, a novel antineoplastic agent for relapsed or refractory Ph-negative B cell precursor ALL, is associated with favorable overall response rates.[174-176] Blinatumomab is a bispecific T cell engager that links CD19 (antigen present on B cells) and CD3 (a T cell receptor), resulting in the lysis of CD19 cells. Administration of blinatumomab is complex and requires a continuous infusion for 28 days because of the drug's very short half-life. This infusion can be administered through home care but requires intense coordination; depending on preparation, the blinatumomab infusion must be changed every 1-7 days. The role of blinatumomab together with standard chemotherapy as first-line therapy for B cell ALL is under investigation in clinical trials.

CD-19 directed CAR T cell therapy has shown promising response rates in the relapse setting.[177-179] Similar to blinatumomab, CD-19 CAR T cells redirect T cells to lyse CD19 B cells. However, the CAR T cells themselves are engineered to incorporate this linking receptor into their cell membrane and are a living persisting drug.[180] Since a patient's own T cells are modified to create CAR T cells, each patient's drug product is unique and the manufacturing process takes up to 3 weeks. Tisagenlecleucel is the first FDA CD19 CAR T cell therapy approved for patients with pediatric ALL and has a Risk Evaluation and Mitigation Strategy (REMS) because of the potential severe adverse effects, the most acute adverse effect being cytokine release syndrome (CRS), which occurs as CAR T cells become activated and release inflammatory cytokines. This immune response has a similar presentation to sepsis with fever, hypotension, tachycardia, and capillary leak, which can progress to respiratory failure, shock, and ultimately multiorgan system dysfunction if left untreated.[181,182] With tisagenlecleucel, up to 80% of patients develop CRS and 50% require admission to the intensive care unit for management.[177] Severe CRS should be treated with tocilizumab, an IL-6 antagonist, as IL-6 is one of the main cytokines involved in CRS. Per the FDA REMS program, hospitals are required to have at least two doses of tocilizumab on site for each patient receiving tisagenlecleucel.[183] CRS is a medical emergency, and prompt administration of toclizumab is essential. Patients remain at risk of infections at this time and, in addition to management for CRS, a standard fever workup should be completed with antibiotic administration in a timely manner. Additionally, CAR T cells also present a risk of CAR T cell–related encephalopathy syndrome (CRES), which typically presents as either delirium or seizures and in rare cases cerebral edema. The mechanism of CRES is not known and tocilizumab is ineffective because it is unable to cross the blood-brain barrier. Antiseizure prophylaxis is recommended and patients should be screened for delirium at least daily until 4 weeks after the CAR T cell infusion.[181] Most patients with CRES can be treated with supportive care; however, in severe cases, corticosteroids should be considered to suppress this immune reaction.[181] An oncologist should always be involved when administering corticosteroids to a patient who has recently received CAR T cells because corticosteroids are potent immunosuppressants and the efficacy of CAR T cells are dependent on an immune response.[184] In the long term, CAR T cells cause B cell aplasia and patients will require intravenous immunoglobulins for hypogammaglobulinaemia.[181]

Isolated extramedullary relapses are those outside the bone marrow. An isolated extramedullary relapse is generally associated with better outcomes than an isolated marrow relapse or a relapse involving the marrow combined with other sites.[161,166] Around 5%–10% of patients with a diagnosis of childhood ALL will have an isolated CNS relapse. Patients at an increased risk of CNS relapse include those with T cell ALL, CNS involvement at diagnosis, and certain cytogenetic abnormalities, as well as those considered high risk by age and WBC count at diagnosis.[166] Historically, patients with an isolated CNS relapse have been treated with intensive intrathecal and systemic chemotherapy together with CNS radiation.[185-187]

New literature supports delaying the implementation of cranial irradiation so that adequate systemic and intrathecal therapy can be delivered up front.[185-187] About 2% of patients with childhood ALL have isolated testicular relapses, which tend to occur late.[166] Testicular relapses are managed with testicular radiation and systemic chemotherapy.[166]

SUPPORTIVE CARE

The pediatric patient with ALL will be treated, on average, with 2–3 years of therapy. During this time, each patient must receive appropriate supportive care so that outcomes can be maximized. The pharmacist should screen for drug–drug interactions, especially with patients receiving high-dose methotrexate; counsel the patient and family on the prescribed medication regimen; and provide supportive care recommendations to the medical team through suggesting appropriate antiemetics, identifying when prophylactic anti-infectives are necessary, and developing plans to mitigate drug-induced toxicities such as mucositis.[188]

At initial diagnosis, patients with a high tumor burden are at risk of developing TLS. In ALL, a high tumor burden is usually characterized by an increased WBC count. Tumor lysis syndrome occurs as leukemic cells lyse, releasing their intracellular contents into the vasculature, which may cause serious electrolyte abnormalities such as hyperuricemia, hyperkalemia, hyperphosphatemia, and hypocalcemia. This syndrome can occur spontaneously because of rapid cell turnover or on starting therapy with chemotherapy, radiation, or even targeted therapy. The consequences of inadequate prophylaxis, identification, and treatment of TLS include acute renal failure from uric acid precipitating in the renal tubules, arrhythmias, and possibly even death. Published guidelines provide a thorough discussion on determining a patient's risk of TLS and the literature supporting the current prevention and treatment strategies.[189-191] Prophylactic therapies for a patient at risk of TLS include aggressive intravenous hydration and agents to reduce the production of uric acid accumulating in the renal tubules such as allopurinol or rasburicase.

Patients with ALL may experience myelosuppression from therapy, resulting in the need for platelet and red blood cell transfusions. Because neutropenia occurs during ALL therapy, the prophylactic use of granulocyte colony-stimulating factor (G-CSF) has been investigated in several clinical trials for pediatric ALL. Prolonged neutropenia can place the patient at risk of infections and compromise the ability to deliver dose-intensive therapy. Prophylactic use of G-CSF shortens the duration of neutropenia from chemotherapy, but this shortened duration has generally not been associated with clinically meaningful results.[192,193] Most clinical trials have shown that adding prophylactic G-CSF does not decrease the incidence of neutropenic fever episodes, incidence of documented culture-proven infections, or cost associated with therapy.[192-196] Therefore, routine prophylactic use of G-CSF is not indicated. Use of G-CSF may be considered in patients with a documented, severe infection in which the timely recovery of neutrophils is critical for outcomes.

Patients with ALL are at an increased risk of infections because of the myelosuppressive effects of drug therapy as well as the suppression of normal hematopoiesis from increased leukemic clones within the bone marrow. *Febrile neutropenia*, defined as an oral temperature of 38°C or higher lasting at least an hour or a single temperature of 38.3°C or higher in the presence of an absolute neutrophil count less than 500 cells/mm[3] or an absolute neutrophil count that is expected to be less than 500 cells/mm[3] within 48 hours, should be managed as a medical emergency.[197] Appropriate, broad-spectrum antibiotic therapy must be initiated rapidly. Patients and their caregivers need to be appropriately educated about monitoring for fevers and transporting the patient to a hospital as soon as possible. *Pneumocystis jiroveci* (formerly *Pneumocystis carinii*), is one of the specific infections these patients are at increased risk of developing. Patients should receive prophylaxis against *P. jiroveci* beginning by the end of induction and continuing for 6 months after therapy ends. Successful prophylaxis is achieved with sulfamethoxazole/trimethoprim (gold standard), atovaquone, dapsone, and pentamidine.[198-202]

Nutritional status plays an important role in the body's ability to fight infections and tolerate intensive chemotherapy.[203] Nutritional status should be monitored at baseline and throughout therapy, implementing nutritional supplements, appetite stimulants, and enteral or parenteral nutrition as appropriate when a problem has been identified. To this extent, a dietitian must be a member of the multidisciplinary health care team. On the other end of the spectrum is the emerging problem of treating overweight patients or patients with obesity.[204] The obesity pandemic has led to new challenges regarding appropriate dosing of chemotherapy. It is currently unknown whether chemotherapy in the pediatric population should be dosed on body surface area calculated from actual body weight, ideal body weight, adjusted ideal body weight, or some other metric, although adult literature recommends dosing based on actual body weight in patients who are obese.[205] Pharmacokinetic and pharmacodynamic studies are lacking in this area, especially for the pediatric population.

SURVIVORSHIP

Late effects from childhood cancer therapy are defined as toxicities that become apparent over time after therapy ends, as a result of the body's inability to compensate for the increased demands that occur as a person ages.[206] Development of late effects is a serious problem in childhood ALL because more than 80% of patients can be expected to become long-term survivors.[207] Late adverse effects associated with ALL treatment can include the development of the following: neurocognitive deficits/learning disabilities, hypothyroidism, precocious puberty, hypogonadism, growth deficiency, obesity, infertility, cardiotoxicity, secondary malignancies, and cataracts.[208] However, because use of cranial irradiation has been minimized in ALL, the incidence of many neurocognitive deficits has significantly decreased.[208] Patients who receive anthracyclines as part of their therapy are at an increased risk of developing cardiac dysfunction in the form

of increased left ventricular afterload and decreased contractility.[209,210] Most patients who receive anthracyclines for ALL do not exceed lifetime cumulative doses greater than 300 mg/m[2], doses above which have been associated with a markedly increased incidence of cardiotoxicity.[207] Development of secondary malignancies in childhood ALL survivors, namely acute myeloid leukemia, myelodysplastic syndrome, or solid tumors, occurs at a low incidence of 1.4%–4.2%.[207,211] Patients at highest risk of developing a secondary malignancy include those with the following characteristics: female, relapsed disease, or treatment with radiation, anthracyclines, cyclophosphamide, and etoposide.[207,211-213] Infertility is not a major problem in survivors of childhood ALL.[207] Patients at high risk of developing infertility include those who received testicular irradiation or who received total body irradiation or high-dose alkylating agents in the HSCT setting.[207,214] Survivors of childhood ALL require lifelong monitoring and medical care to screen for, prevent, identify early, and treat these late complications.[215]

FUTURE CONSIDERATIONS

The future of ALL therapy will continue to involve the development of new targeted agents used in upfront therapy to maximize outcomes and minimize toxicity, particularly in certain patient subsets with suboptimal outcomes.[123,143] Agents currently under investigation include carfilzomib, blinatumomab, inotuzumab, daratumumab, CAR T cells, mTOR (mammalian target of rapamycin) inhibitors (sirolimus and temsirolimus), Janus kinase (JAK) inhibitors (ruxolitinib), hypomethylating agents in infant ALL (azacitidine), and newer tyrosine kinase inhibitors in Ph-positive ALL.[123,143,216] In addition, the use of pharmacogenomics to tailor therapy will likely become more common as research in this field advances. *Pharmacogenomics* or *pharmacogenetics* refers to the knowledge and use of genetic polymorphisms in drug-metabolizing enzymes to better understand and characterize the differences between individual responses to specific drugs and therapy.[6,217] The most well-established example of pharmacogenomics in childhood ALL is the knowledge of thiopurine S-methlytransferase (TPMT) polymorphisms to predict response to mercaptopurine therapy.[217-220] Mercaptopurine undergoes a complex metabolic pathway to be converted from a prodrug to its active moieties, thioguanine nucleotides, and inactive nontoxic compounds.[219] The metabolism of mercaptopurine occurs through activity of the enzyme TPMT. Ninety percent of the population have high TPMT activity (homozygous wild type), 10% have intermediate TPMT activity (heterozygous), and 0.3% have low or no measurable enzyme activity (homozygous TPMT-deficient).[219] An increased TPMT activity level was associated with lower levels of thioguanine nucleotide accumulation.[219] Conversely, lower TPMT activity was associated with very high concentrations of thioguanine nucleotides, which led to increased bone marrow suppression and a lower rate of MRD positivity.[221,222] Therefore, the *TPMT* genotype can be used to identify patients at increased risk of toxicity from mercaptopurine therapy. Rather than using the surrogate markers of absolute neutrophil count and platelet count to determine the mercaptopurine dose adjustments mentioned previously, one institution took the prospective approach of using the *TPMT* genotype to initially dose mercaptopurine.[223] The practice in most institutions is to analyze for *TPMT* polymorphisms either initially at diagnosis or when a patient has severe myelosuppression to empiric dosing of mercaptopurine. Guidelines are available, which include dosing recommendations according to genotype.[224]

CONCLUSIONS

The pharmacist's role on a multidisciplinary pediatric oncology team includes but is not limited to the following: verifying the accuracy of drug dosing while considering organ function and developmental concerns; confirming the point in therapy; ensuring that appropriate supportive care measures are addressed and maximized; providing education to the medical team; providing patient and caregiver education about drug therapy; and monitoring for expected responses and toxicities. Pharmacists can contribute to the medical team, given their specific education and training. In addition, pharmacists can play a vital role in contributing to clinical trial design as it pertains to drug therapy and in aiding in the conduct of these clinical trials at an institution.

Pharmacists who practice in the pediatric oncology setting should become familiar with the trials being conducted and the chemotherapeutic agents being used so that they can aid in the safe and effective delivery of therapy to these patients.

The outcomes for childhood ALL have improved drastically because of a better understanding of the biology of the disease, the significance of prognostic factors, and the development of risk-adapted therapy to maximize outcomes while minimizing toxicity. Although the overall survival rates for childhood ALL are close to 90%, certain patient subgroups still have a less favorable prognosis and outcome. Clinical trials continue to be conducted, especially in these subgroups, to advance the knowledge and to design increasingly effective therapeutic regimens that will allow more patients to be long-term survivors. As the long-term survivor population continues to grow, it is important that these patients receive adequate long-term follow-up by experienced medical teams. The survivors need to have a thorough and complete medical history and therapeutic summary so that they can be appropriately monitored and screened for the late effects that may arise over time after therapy ends. With all the advances in therapy and the potential role for targeted therapy, pharmacogenomics, and response-based therapy stratification, the outlook for childhood ALL remains promising.

Patient Case — ACUTE LYMPHOBLASTIC LEUKEMIA

A 4-year-old previously healthy Hispanic girl is evaluated for a 2-week history of leg pain, low-grade fevers, and fatigue. Her mother reports that she has refused to walk because of the pain, which she experiences even when at rest. Her pediatrician orders a complete blood count, and the results show pancytopenia. She is referred to the emergency department for further workup and evaluation.

Medical history: Full-term birth by spontaneous vaginal delivery without complications

Family history: Father has hypertension

Social history: Lives with mother, father, and sister; none are smokers; has one dog; attends day care full time

Allergies: No known drug allergies

Home medications: Daily multivitamin

Immunizations: Up to date for age

Vital signs: Tmax 38.5°C, HR 120 beats/minute, RR 28 breaths/minute, BP 88/45 mm Hg, Wt 18 kg, Ht 36 inches

Review of systems: Ill-appearing, pale 4-year-old girl with obvious bruising on trunk and extremities

Physical examination: Palpable hepatosplenomegaly; all other systems within normal limits

Laboratory findings:

WBC	62 × 10³ cells/mm³
Hgb	5.4 g/dL
Hct	16.2%
Plt	4 × 10³ cells/mm³
Absolute neutrophil count	800 cells/mm³
Peripheral blood blasts	78%
Bone marrow aspiration	Consistent with acute lymphoblastic leukemia precursor B cell

1. What therapy should this patient receive for leukemia?

The patient should receive a four-drug induction regimen consisting of vincristine 1.5 mg/m²/dose (maximum dose 2 mg) intravenously weekly, daunorubicin 25 mg/m²/dose intravenously weekly, pegaspargase 2,500 units/m²/dose intravenously once on day 4, and dexamethasone 5 mg/m²/dose orally twice daily for the first 14 days of induction. Anthracycline is added as the fourth drug because the patient is considered at high risk, given her presenting white blood cell count of 62×10^3 cells/mm³. Dexamethasone was selected as the glucocorticoid in this regimen, given that the patient is at high risk but is younger than 10 years because this population benefits from the effects of dexamethasone but is not at as high a risk of developing avascular necrosis. Enrollment on an open, accruing clinical trial should be considered. In addition, she should receive central nervous system (CNS)-directed therapy in the form of intrathecal chemotherapy dosed according to her age rather than her weight or body surface area. At this point, we do not know the results of her initial lumbar puncture to identify CNS involvement, but once these results are known, her plan for CNS-directed therapy can be defined. The cytogenetic features of her leukemia should be assessed, as should her response to therapy measured by minimal residual disease at specific time points: early, during, and at the end of induction. These factors may change her prognosis and necessitate intensification of her therapeutic plan. The patient should receive consolidation and maintenance therapy for about 2 years; at this point she is unlikely to need a hematopoietic stem-cell transplantation.

Case (continued). The patient receives vincristine, methotrexate, and pegaspargase today as part of interim maintenance therapy. While in the clinic, she develops severe urticaria and difficulty breathing.

2. Provide recommendations to manage the patient's hypersensitivity reaction, assuming that her treatment plan consists of these agents in future cycles.

The patient is most likely experiencing a hypersensitivity reaction to pegaspargase that is presenting as anaphylaxis, given her difficulty breathing. If she received pegaspargase as an intravenous infusion, the infusion should be stopped immediately on development of these symptoms and not resumed. The patient should receive continuous monitoring of her vital signs and be observed in a location equipped to handle a medical emergency. Her symptoms should be treated with diphenhydramine and hydrocortisone, plus or minus epinephrine. Other supportive measures for anaphylaxis should be considered, including oxygen, albuterol, and fluid resuscitation. Monitoring serum asparaginase activity is not necessary after anaphylaxis because the severity of this reaction necessitates changing to Erwinia asparaginase for any future doses. However, monitoring serum asparaginase activity during and after Erwinia asparaginase is recommended to ensure adequate activity levels, especially given the different pharmacokinetic profiles of intramuscular and intravenous Erwinia asparaginase.

REFERENCES

1. Howlader N, Noone A, Krapcho M, et al. SEER Cancer Statistics Review, 1975-2016. Bethesda, MD: National Cancer Institute. Based on November 2018 SEER data submission, posted to the SEER website, April 2019. Available at http://seer.cancer.gov/csr/1975_2016/. Accessed March 5, 2020.
2. Gaynon PS, Angiolillo AL, Carroll WL, et al. Long-term results of the children's cancer group studies for childhood acute lymphoblastic leukemia 1983-2002: a Children's Oncology Group Report. Leukemia 2010;24:285-97.
3. Silverman LB, Stevenson KE, O'Brien JE, et al. Long-term results of Dana-Farber Cancer Institute ALL Consortium protocols for children with newly diagnosed acute lymphoblastic leukemia (1985-2000). Leukemia 2010;24:320-34.
4. Pui CH, Campana D, Pei D, et al. Treating childhood acute lymphoblastic leukemia without cranial irradiation. N Engl J Med 2009;360:2730-41.
5. Hunger SP, Lu X, Devidas M, et al. Improved survival for children and adolescents with acute lymphoblastic leukemia between 1990 and 2005: a report from the children's oncology group. J Clin Oncol 2012;30:1663-9.
6. Margolin J, Rabin K, Steuber C, Poplack D. Acute Lymphoblastic Leukemia. In: Pizzo P, Poplack D, editors. Principles and Practice of Pediatric Oncology. 6th ed. Philadelphia: Lippincott Williams & Wilkins; 2011.
7. Pollock BH, DeBaun MR, Camitta BM, et al. Racial differences in the survival of childhood B-precursor acute lymphoblastic leukemia: a Pediatric Oncology Group Study. J Clin Oncol 2000;18:813-23.
8. Pui CH, Boyett JM, Relling MV, et al. Sex differences in prognosis for children with acute lymphoblastic leukemia. J Clin Oncol 1999;17:818-24.
9. Belson M, Kingsley B, Holmes A. Risk factors for acute leukemia in children: a review. Environ Health Perspect 2007;115:138-45.
10. Kleinerman RA, Kaune WT, Hatch EE, et al. Are children living near high-voltage power lines at increased risk of acute lymphoblastic leukemia? Am J Epidemiol 2000;151:512-5.
11. Brondum J, Shu XO, Steinbuch M, et al. Parental cigarette smoking and the risk of acute leukemia in children. Cancer 1999; 85:1380-8.
12. Pui CH. Recent research advances in childhood acute lymphoblastic leukemia. J Formos Med Assoc 2010;109:777-87.
13. Cline MJ. The molecular basis of leukemia. N Engl J Med 1994;330:328-36.
14. Pui CH, Evans WE. Acute lymphoblastic leukemia. N Engl J Med 1998;339:605-15.
15. Stanulla M, Schrappe M. Treatment of childhood acute lymphoblastic leukemia. Semin Hematol 2009;46:52-63.
16. Hutter JJ. Childhood leukemia. Pediatr Rev 2010;31:234-41.
17. Hayhoe FG. Classification of acute leukaemias. Blood Rev 1988; 2:186-93.
18. Pui CH, Evans WE. Treatment of acute lymphoblastic leukemia. N Engl J Med 2006;354:166-78.
19. Smith M, Arthur D, Camitta B, et al. Uniform approach to risk classification and treatment assignment for children with acute lymphoblastic leukemia. J Clin Oncol 1996;14:18-24.
20. Robinson DL. Childhood leukemia: Understanding the significance of chromosomal abnormalities. J Pediatr Oncol Nurs 2001; 18:111-23.
21. Trueworthy R, Shuster J, Look T, et al. Ploidy of lymphoblasts is the strongest predictor of treatment outcome in B-progenitor cell acute lymphoblastic leukemia of childhood: a Pediatric Oncology Group study. J Clin Oncol 1992;10:606-13.

22. Look AT, Roberson PK, Williams DL, et al. Prognostic importance of blast cell DNA content in childhood acute lymphoblastic leukemia. Blood 1985;65:1079-86.

23. Pui CH. Acute lymphoblastic leukemia. Pediatr Clin North Am 1997;44:831-46.

24. Heerema NA, Nachman JB, Sather HN, et al. Hypodiploidy with less than 45 chromosomes confers adverse risk in childhood acute lymphoblastic leukemia: a report from the children's cancer group. Blood 1999;94:4036-45.

25. Pui CH, Sandlund JT, Pei D, et al. Results of therapy for acute lymphoblastic leukemia in black and white children. JAMA 2003;290:2001-7.

26. Campana D. Role of minimal residual disease monitoring in adult and pediatric acute lymphoblastic leukemia. Hematol Oncol Clin North Am 2009;23:1083,98, vii.

27. Miller DR, Coccia PF, Bleyer WA, et al. Early response to induction therapy as a predictor of disease-free survival and late recurrence of childhood acute lymphoblastic leukemia: a report from the Childrens Cancer Study Group. J Clin Oncol 1989;7:1807-15.

28. Gaynon PS, Bleyer WA, Steinherz PG, et al. Day 7 marrow response and outcome for children with acute lymphoblastic leukemia and unfavorable presenting features. Med Pediatr Oncol 1990;18:273-9.

29. Gaynon PS, Desai AA, Bostrom BC, et al. Early response to therapy and outcome in childhood acute lymphoblastic leukemia: a review. Cancer 1997;80:1717-26.

30. Sandlund JT, Harrison PL, Rivera G, et al. Persistence of lymphoblasts in bone marrow on day 15 and days 22 to 25 of remission induction predicts a dismal treatment outcome in children with acute lymphoblastic leukemia. Blood 2002;100:43-7.

31. Gajjar A, Ribeiro R, Hancock ML, et al. Persistence of circulating blasts after 1 week of multiagent chemotherapy confers a poor prognosis in childhood lymphoblastic leukemia. Blood 1995;86:1292-5.

32. Conter V, Bartram CR, Valsecchi MG, et al. Molecular response to treatment redefines all prognostic factors in children and adolescents with B-cell precursor acute lymphoblastic leukemia: results in 3184 patients of the AIEOP-BFM ALL 2000 study. Blood 2010;115:3206-14.

33. Campana D. Progress of minimal residual disease studies in childhood acute leukemia. Curr Hematol Malig Rep 2010;5:169-76.

34. Borowitz MJ, Devidas M, Hunger SP, et al. Clinical significance of minimal residual disease in childhood acute lymphoblastic leukemia and its relationship to other prognostic factors: a Children's Oncology Group study. Blood 2008;111:5477-85.

35. Uckun FM, Kersey JH, Haake R, et al. Pretransplantation burden of leukemic progenitor cells as a predictor of relapse after bone marrow transplantation for acute lymphoblastic leukemia. N Engl J Med 1993;329:1296-301.

36. Vora A, Goulden N, Mitchell C, et al. Augmented post-remission therapy for a minimal residual disease-defined high-risk subgroup of children and young people with clinical standard-risk and intermediate-risk acute lymphoblastic leukaemia (UKALL 2003): a randomised controlled trial. Lancet Oncol 2014;15:809-18.

37. Pui CH, Pei D, Coustan-Smith E, et al. Clinical utility of sequential minimal residual disease measurements in the context of risk-based therapy in childhood acute lymphoblastic leukaemia: a prospective study. Lancet Oncol 2015;16:465-74.

38. Bartram J, Wade R, Vora A, et al. Excellent outcome of minimal residual disease-defined low-risk patients is sustained with more than 10 years follow-up: results of UK paediatric acute lymphoblastic leukaemia trials 1997-2003. Arch Dis Child 2016; 101:449-54.

39. Jeha S, Pui CH. Risk-adapted treatment of pediatric acute lymphoblastic leukemia. Hematol Oncol Clin North Am 2009;23:973-90.

40. Pui CH. Central nervous system disease in acute lymphoblastic leukemia: prophylaxis and treatment. Hematology Am Soc Hematol Educ Program 2006:142-6.

41. Nachman J, Sather HN, Cherlow JM, et al. Response of children with high-risk acute lymphoblastic leukemia treated with and without cranial irradiation: a report from the Children's Cancer Group. J Clin Oncol 1998;16:920-30.

42. Tubergen DG, Gilchrist GS, O'Brien RT, et al. Prevention of CNS disease in intermediate-risk acute lymphoblastic leukemia: comparison of cranial radiation and intrathecal methotrexate and the importance of systemic therapy: a Childrens Cancer Group report. J Clin Oncol 1993;11:520-6.

43. Sullivan MP, Chen T, Dyment PG, et al. Equivalence of intrathecal chemotherapy and radiotherapy as central nervous system prophylaxis in children with acute lymphatic leukemia: a pediatric oncology group study. Blood 1982;60:948-58.

44. McNeer JL, Nachman JB. The optimal use of steroids in paediatric acute lymphoblastic leukaemia: no easy answers. Br J Haematol 2010;149:638-52.

45. Inaba H, Pui CH. Glucocorticoid use in acute lymphoblastic leukaemia. Lancet Oncol 2010;11:1096-106.

46. Bostrom BC, Sensel MR, Sather HN, et al. Dexamethasone versus prednisone and daily oral versus weekly intravenous mercaptopurine for patients with standard-risk acute lymphoblastic leukemia: a report from the Children's Cancer Group. Blood 2003;101:3809-17.

47. Mitchell CD, Richards SM, Kinsey SE, et al. Benefit of dexamethasone compared with prednisolone for childhood acute lymphoblastic leukaemia: results of the UK Medical Research Council ALL97 randomized trial. Br J Haematol 2005;129:734-45.

48. Ito C, Evans WE, McNinch L, et al. Comparative cytotoxicity of dexamethasone and prednisolone in childhood acute lymphoblastic leukemia. J Clin Oncol 1996;14:2370-6.

49. Kaspers GJ, Veerman AJ, Popp-Snijders C, et al. Comparison of the antileukemic activity in vitro of dexamethasone and prednisolone in childhood acute lymphoblastic leukemia. Med Pediatr Oncol 1996;27:114-21.

50. Mattano LA,Jr, Sather HN, Trigg ME, et al. Osteonecrosis as a complication of treating acute lymphoblastic leukemia in children: a report from the Children's Cancer Group. J Clin Oncol 2000;18:3262-72.

51. Kawedia JD, Kaste SC, Pei D, et al. Pharmacokinetic, pharmacodynamic, and pharmacogenetic determinants of osteonecrosis in children with acute lymphoblastic leukemia. Blood 2011;117:2340-7; quiz 2556.

52. Kunstreich M, Kummer S, Laws HJ, et al. Osteonecrosis in children with acute lymphoblastic leukemia. Haematologica 2016;101:1295-305.

53. French D, Hamilton LH, Mattano LA, Jr, et al. A PAI-1 (SERPINE1) polymorphism predicts osteonecrosis in children with acute lymphoblastic leukemia: a report from the Children's Oncology Group. Blood 2008;111:4496-9.

54. Patel B, Richards SM, Rowe JM, et al. High incidence of avascular necrosis in adolescents with acute lymphoblastic leukaemia: a UKALL XII analysis. Leukemia 2008;22:308-12.

55. Sallan SE, Hitchcock-Bryan S, Gelber R, et al. Influence of intensive asparaginase in the treatment of childhood non-T-cell acute lymphoblastic leukemia. Cancer Res 1983;43:5601-7.

56. Silverman LB, Gelber RD, Dalton VK, et al. Improved outcome for children with acute lymphoblastic leukemia: results of Dana-Farber Consortium Protocol 91-01. Blood 2001;97:1211-8.

57. Raetz EA, Salzer WL. Tolerability and efficacy of L-asparaginase therapy in pediatric patients with acute lymphoblastic leukemia. J Pediatr Hematol Oncol 2010;32:554-63.

58. Asselin BL, Whitin JC, Coppola DJ, et al. Comparative pharmacokinetic studies of three asparaginase preparations. J Clin Oncol 1993;11:1780-6.

59. Vrooman LM, Supko JG, Neuberg DS, et al. Erwinia asparaginase after allergy to E. coli asparaginase in children with acute lymphoblastic leukemia. Pediatr Blood Cancer 2010; 54:199-205.

60. Duval M, Suciu S, Ferster A, et al. Comparison of Escherichia coli-asparaginase with Erwinia-asparaginase in the treatment of childhood lymphoid malignancies: results of a randomized European Organisation for Research and Treatment of Cancer-Children's Leukemia Group phase 3 trial. Blood 2002;99:2734-9.

61. Avramis VI, Sencer S, Periclou AP, et al. A randomized comparison of native Escherichia coli asparaginase and polyethylene glycol conjugated asparaginase for treatment of children with newly diagnosed standard-risk acute lymphoblastic leukemia: a Children's Cancer Group study. Blood 2002;99:1986-94.

62. Hak LJ, Relling MV, Cheng C, et al. Asparaginase pharmacodynamics differ by formulation among children with newly diagnosed acute lymphoblastic leukemia. Leukemia 2004;18:1072-7.

63. Panetta JC, Gajjar A, Hijiya N, et al. Comparison of native E. coli and PEG asparaginase pharmacokinetics and pharmacodynamics in pediatric acute lymphoblastic leukemia. Clin Pharmacol Ther 2009;86:651-8.

64. Silverman LB, Supko JG, Stevenson KE, et al. Intravenous PEG-asparaginase during remission induction in children and adolescents with newly diagnosed acute lymphoblastic leukemia. Blood 2010;115:1351-3.

65. Place AE, Stevenson KE, Vrooman LM, et al. Intravenous pegylated asparaginase versus intramuscular native Escherichia coli L-asparaginase in newly diagnosed childhood acute lymphoblastic leukaemia (DFCI 05-001): a randomised, open-label phase 3 trial. Lancet Oncol 2015;16:1677-90.

66. Vrooman LM, Kirov II, Dreyer ZE, et al. Activity and Toxicity of Intravenous Erwinia Asparaginase Following Allergy to E. coli-Derived Asparaginase in Children and Adolescents With Acute Lymphoblastic Leukemia. Pediatr Blood Cancer 2016;63:228-33.

67. Stock W, Douer D, DeAngelo DJ, et al. Prevention and management of asparaginase/pegasparaginase-associated toxicities in adults and older adolescents: recommendations of an expert panel. Leuk Lymphoma 2011;52:2237-53.

68. van der Sluis IM, Vrooman LM, Pieters R, et al. Consensus expert recommendations for identification and management of asparaginase hypersensitivity and silent inactivation. Haematologica 2016;101:279-85.

69. Tong WH, Pieters R, Kaspers GJ, et al. A prospective study on drug monitoring of PEGasparaginase and Erwinia asparaginase and asparaginase antibodies in pediatric acute lymphoblastic leukemia. Blood 2014;123:2026-33.

70. Bleyer A, Asselin BL, Koontz SE, et al. Clinical application of asparaginase activity levels following treatment with pegaspargase. Pediatr Blood Cancer 2015;62:1102-5.

71. Asselin B, Rizzari C. Asparaginase pharmacokinetics and implications of therapeutic drug monitoring. Leuk Lymphoma 2015;56:2273-80.

72. Cooper SL, Young DJ, Bowen CJ, et al. Universal premedication and therapeutic drug monitoring for asparaginase-based therapy prevents infusion-associated acute adverse events and drug substitutions. Pediatr Blood Cancer 2019;66:e27797.

73. Bleyer WA. Biology and pathogenesis of CNS leukemia. Am J Pediatr Hematol Oncol 1989;11:57-63.

74. Ruggiero A, Conter V, Milani M, et al. Intrathecal chemotherapy with antineoplastic agents in children. Paediatr Drugs 2001; 3:237-46.

75. Howard SC, Gajjar AJ, Cheng C, et al. Risk factors for traumatic and bloody lumbar puncture in children with acute lymphoblastic leukemia. JAMA 2002;288:2001-7.

76. Rech A, de Carvalho GP, Meneses CF, et al. The influence of traumatic lumbar puncture and timing of intrathecal therapy on outcome of pediatric acute lymphoblastic leukemia. Pediatr Hematol Oncol 2005;22:483-8.

77. Bleyer AW. Clinical pharmacology of intrathecal methotrexate. II. An improved dosage regimen derived from age-related pharmacokinetics. Cancer Treat Rep 1977;61:1419-25.

78. Pui CH. Toward optimal central nervous system-directed treatment in childhood acute lymphoblastic leukemia. J Clin Oncol 2003;21:179-81.

79. Schrappe M, Reiter A, Ludwig WD, et al. Improved outcome in childhood acute lymphoblastic leukemia despite reduced use of anthracyclines and cranial radiotherapy: results of trial ALL-BFM 90. German-Austrian-Swiss ALL-BFM Study Group. Blood 2000;95:3310-22.

80. Moricke A, Zimmermann M, Reiter A, et al. Long-term results of five consecutive trials in childhood acute lymphoblastic leukemia performed by the ALL-BFM study group from 1981 to 2000. Leukemia 2010;24:265-84.

81. Salzer WL, Devidas M, Carroll WL, et al. Long-term results of the pediatric oncology group studies for childhood acute lymphoblastic leukemia 1984-2001: a report from the children's oncology group. Leukemia 2010;24:355-70.

82. Mahoney DH,Jr, Shuster J, Nitschke R, et al. Intermediate-dose intravenous methotrexate with intravenous mercaptopurine is superior to repetitive low-dose oral methotrexate with intravenous mercaptopurine for children with lower-risk B-lineage acute lymphoblastic leukemia: a Pediatric Oncology Group phase III trial. J Clin Oncol 1998;16:246-54.

83. Arico M, Baruchel A, Bertrand Y, et al. The seventh international childhood acute lymphoblastic leukemia workshop report: Palermo, Italy, January 29-30, 2005. Leukemia 2005;19:1145-52.

84. Evans WE, Crom WR, Abromowitch M, et al. Clinical pharmacodynamics of high-dose methotrexate in acute lymphocytic leukemia. Identification of a relation between concentration and effect. N Engl J Med 1986;314:471-7.

85. Mikkelsen TS, Sparreboom A, Cheng C, et al. Shortening infusion time for high-dose methotrexate alters antileukemic effects: a randomized prospective clinical trial. J Clin Oncol 2011; 29:1771-8.

86. Larsen EC, Devidas M, Chen S, et al. Dexamethasone and High-Dose Methotrexate Improve Outcome for Children and Young Adults With High-Risk B-Acute Lymphoblastic Leukemia: A Report From Children's Oncology Group Study AALL0232. J Clin Oncol 2016;34:2380-8.

87. Seibel NL, Steinherz PG, Sather HN, et al. Early postinduction intensification therapy improves survival for children and adolescents with high-risk acute lymphoblastic leukemia: a report from the Children's Oncology Group. Blood 2008; 111:2548-55.

88. Lange BJ, Bostrom BC, Cherlow JM, et al. Double-delayed intensification improves event-free survival for children with intermediate-risk acute lymphoblastic leukemia: a report from the Children's Cancer Group. Blood 2002;99:825-33.

89. Hutchinson RJ, Gaynon PS, Sather H, et al. Intensification of therapy for children with lower-risk acute lymphoblastic leukemia: long-term follow-up of patients treated on Children's Cancer Group Trial 1881. J Clin Oncol 2003;21:1790-7.

90. Tubergen DG, Gilchrist GS, O'Brien RT, et al. Improved outcome with delayed intensification for children with acute lymphoblastic leukemia and intermediate presenting features: a Childrens Cancer Group phase III trial. J Clin Oncol 1993; 11:527-37.

91. Arico M, Valsecchi MG, Conter V, et al. Improved outcome in high-risk childhood acute lymphoblastic leukemia defined by prednisone-poor response treated with double Berlin-Frankfurt-Muenster protocol II. Blood 2002;100:420-6.

92. Nachman JB, Sather HN, Sensel MG, et al. Augmented post-induction therapy for children with high-risk acute lymphoblastic leukemia and a slow response to initial therapy. N Engl J Med 1998;338:1663-71.

93. Conter V, Valsecchi MG, Silvestri D, et al. Pulses of vincristine and dexamethasone in addition to intensive chemotherapy for children with intermediate-risk acute lymphoblastic leukaemia: a multicentre randomised trial. Lancet 2007;369:123-31.

94. De Moerloose B, Suciu S, Bertrand Y, et al. Improved outcome with pulses of vincristine and corticosteroids in continuation therapy of children with average risk acute lymphoblastic leukemia (ALL) and lymphoblastic non-Hodgkin lymphoma (NHL): report of the EORTC randomized phase 3 trial 58951. Blood 2010;116:36-44.

95. Bleyer WA, Sather HN, Nickerson HJ, et al. Monthly pulses of vincristine and prednisone prevent bone marrow and testicular relapse in low-risk childhood acute lymphoblastic leukemia: a report of the CCG-161 study by the Childrens Cancer Study Group. J Clin Oncol 1991;9:1012-21.

96. Bhatia S, Landier W, Hageman L, et al. 6MP adherence in a multiracial cohort of children with acute lymphoblastic leukemia: a Children's Oncology Group study. Blood 2014;124:2345-53.

97. Uckun FM, Sensel MG, Sun L, et al. Biology and treatment of childhood T-lineage acute lymphoblastic leukemia. Blood 1998; 91:735-46.

98. Goldberg JM, Silverman LB, Levy DE, et al. Childhood T-cell acute lymphoblastic leukemia: the Dana-Farber Cancer Institute acute lymphoblastic leukemia consortium experience. J Clin Oncol 2003;21:3616-22.

99. Shuster JJ, Falletta JM, Pullen DJ, et al. Prognostic factors in childhood T-cell acute lymphoblastic leukemia: a Pediatric Oncology Group study. Blood 1990;75:166-73.

100. Schorin MA, Blattner S, Gelber RD, et al. Treatment of childhood acute lymphoblastic leukemia: results of Dana-Farber Cancer Institute/Children's Hospital Acute Lymphoblastic Leukemia Consortium Protocol 85-01. J Clin Oncol 1994;12:740-7.

101. Uyttebroeck A, Suciu S, Laureys G, et al. Treatment of childhood T-cell lymphoblastic lymphoma according to the strategy for acute lymphoblastic leukaemia, without radiotherapy: long term results of the EORTC CLG 58881 trial. Eur J Cancer 2008;44:840-6.

102. Reiter A, Schrappe M, Ludwig WD, et al. Intensive ALL-type therapy without local radiotherapy provides a 90% event-free survival for children with T-cell lymphoblastic lymphoma: a BFM group report. Blood 2000;95:416-21.

103. Winter SS, Dunsmore KP, Devidas M, et al. Improved survival for children and young adults with T-lineage acute lymphoblastic leukemia: results from the Children's Oncology Group AALL0434 methotrexate randomization. J Clin Oncol 2018;36:2926-34.

104. Dunsmore KP, Winter S, Devidas M, et al. COG AALL0434: A randomized trial testing nelarabine in newly diagnosed t-cell malignancy. J Clin Oncol 2018;36(suppl 15):10500.

105. Reilly KM, Kisor DF. Profile of nelarabine: use in the treatment of T-cell acute lymphoblastic leukemia. Onco Targets Ther 2009;2:219-28.

106. DeAngelo DJ. Nelarabine for the treatment of patients with relapsed or refractory T-cell acute lymphoblastic leukemia or lymphoblastic lymphoma. Hematol Oncol Clin North Am 2009;23:1121,35,vii-viii.

107. Winter SS, Dunsmore KP, Devidas M, et al. Safe integration of nelarabine into intensive chemotherapy in newly diagnosed T-cell acute lymphoblastic leukemia: Children's Oncology Group Study AALL0434. Pediatr Blood Cancer 2015;62:1176-83.

108. Micromedex Solutions. Truven Health Analytics, Inc. Ann Arbor, MI. Available at www.micromedexsolutions.com. Accessed March 1, 2020.

109. Pieters R, Schrappe M, De Lorenzo P, et al. A treatment protocol for infants younger than 1 year with acute lymphoblastic leukaemia (Interfant-99): an observational study and a multicentre randomised trial. Lancet 2007;370:240-50.

110. Reaman G, Zeltzer P, Bleyer WA, et al. Acute lymphoblastic leukemia in infants less than one year of age: a cumulative experience of the Children's Cancer Study Group. J Clin Oncol 1985;3:1513-21.

111. Silverman LB, McLean TW, Gelber RD, et al. Intensified therapy for infants with acute lymphoblastic leukemia: results from the Dana-Farber Cancer Institute Consortium. Cancer 1997; 80:2285-95.

112. Ferster A, Bertrand Y, Benoit Y, et al. Improved survival for acute lymphoblastic leukaemia in infancy: the experience of EORTC-Childhood Leukaemia Cooperative Group. Br J Haematol 1994; 86:284-90.

113. Chessells JM, Harrison CJ, Watson SL, et al. Treatment of infants with lymphoblastic leukaemia: results of the UK Infant Protocols 1987-1999. Br J Haematol 2002;117:306-14.

114. Chessells JM, Eden OB, Bailey CC, et al. Acute lymphoblastic leukaemia in infancy: experience in MRC UKALL trials. Report from the Medical Research Council Working Party on Childhood Leukaemia. Leukemia 1994;8:1275-9.

115. Frankel LS, Ochs J, Shuster JJ, et al. Therapeutic trial for infant acute lymphoblastic leukemia: the Pediatric Oncology Group experience (POG 8493). J Pediatr Hematol Oncol 1997;19:35-42.

116. Lauer SJ, Camitta BM, Leventhal BG, et al. Intensive alternating drug pairs after remission induction for treatment of infants with acute lymphoblastic leukemia: A Pediatric Oncology Group Pilot Study. J Pediatr Hematol Oncol 1998;20:229-33.

117. Reaman GH, Sposto R, Sensel MG, et al. Treatment outcome and prognostic factors for infants with acute lymphoblastic leukemia treated on two consecutive trials of the Children's Cancer Group. J Clin Oncol 1999;17:445-55.

118. Hilden JM, Dinndorf PA, Meerbaum SO, et al. Analysis of prognostic factors of acute lymphoblastic leukemia in infants: report on CCG 1953 from the Children's Oncology Group. Blood 2006;108:441-51.

119. Pieters R. Infant acute lymphoblastic leukemia: Lessons learned and future directions. Curr Hematol Malig Rep 2009;4:167-74.

120. Zweidler-McKay PA, Hilden JM. The ABCs of infant leukemia. Curr Probl Pediatr Adolesc Health Care 2008;38:78-94.

121. Taub JW, Konrad MA, Ge Y, et al. High frequency of leukemic clones in newborn screening blood samples of children with B-precursor acute lymphoblastic leukemia. Blood 2002;99:2992-6.

122. Dreyer ZE, Dinndorf PA, Camitta B, et al. Analysis of the role of hematopoietic stem-cell transplantation in infants with acute lymphoblastic leukemia in first remission and MLL gene rearrangements: a report from the Children's Oncology Group. J Clin Oncol 2011;29:214-22.

123. Smith MA. Update on developmental therapeutics for acute lymphoblastic leukemia. Curr Hematol Malig Rep 2009;4:175-82.

124. Brown P, Levis M, Shurtleff S, et al. FLT3 inhibition selectively kills childhood acute lymphoblastic leukemia cells with high levels of FLT3 expression. Blood 2005;105:812-20.

125. Brown P, Kairalla J, Wang C, et al. Addition of FLT3 Inhibitor Lestaurtinib to Post-Induction Chemotherapy does not Improve Outcomes in Mll-Rearranged Infant Acute Lymphoblastic Leukemia (ALL): AALL0631, A Children's Oncology Group Study. Pediatr Blood Cancer 2016;63(S3).

126. Kostadinov R, Scharpf, Brown P. Identifying subclonal epigenetic changes driving chemoresistance in infant MLL-r acute lymphoblastic leukemias. Blood 2015;126:809.

127. Shah N, Al-Ahmari A, Al-Yamani A, et al. Outcome and toxicity of chemotherapy for acute lymphoblastic leukemia in children with Down syndrome. Pediatr Blood Cancer 2009;52:14-9.

128. Whitlock JA. Down syndrome and acute lymphoblastic leukaemia. Br J Haematol 2006;135:595-602.

129. Zwaan CM, Reinhardt D, Hitzler J, et al. Acute leukemias in children with Down syndrome. Hematol Oncol Clin North Am 2010;24:19-34.

130. Dordelmann M, Schrappe M, Reiter A, et al. Down's syndrome in childhood acute lymphoblastic leukemia: clinical characteristics and treatment outcome in four consecutive BFM trials. Berlin-Frankfurt-Munster Group. Leukemia 1998;12:645-51.

131. Bassal M, La MK, Whitlock JA, et al. Lymphoblast biology and outcome among children with Down syndrome and ALL treated on CCG-1952. Pediatr Blood Cancer 2005;44:21-8.

132. Christensen MS, Heyman M, Mottonen M, et al. Treatment-related death in childhood acute lymphoblastic leukaemia in the Nordic countries: 1992-2001. Br J Haematol 2005;131:50-8.

133. Garre ML, Relling MV, Kalwinsky D, et al. Pharmacokinetics and toxicity of methotrexate in children with Down syndrome and acute lymphocytic leukemia. J Pediatr 1987;111:606-12.

134. Bleckmann K, Schrappe M. Advances in therapy for Philadelphia-positive acute lymphoblastic leukaemia of childhood and adolescence. Br J Haematol 2016;172:855-69.

135. Fletcher JA, Lynch EA, Kimball VM, et al. Translocation (9;22) is associated with extremely poor prognosis in intensively treated children with acute lymphoblastic leukemia. Blood 1991;77:435-9.

136. Crist W, Carroll A, Shuster J, et al. Philadelphia chromosome positive childhood acute lymphoblastic leukemia: clinical and cytogenetic characteristics and treatment outcome. A Pediatric Oncology Group study. Blood 1990;76:489-94.

137. Schrappe M, Arico M, Harbott J, et al. Philadelphia chromosome-positive (Ph+) childhood acute lymphoblastic leukemia: good initial steroid response allows early prediction of a favorable treatment outcome. Blood 1998;92:2730-41.

138. Ribeiro RC, Broniscer A, Rivera GK, et al. Philadelphia chromosome-positive acute lymphoblastic leukemia in children: durable responses to chemotherapy associated with low initial white blood cell counts. Leukemia 1997;11:1493-6.

139. Arico M, Schrappe M, Hunger SP, et al. Clinical outcome of children with newly diagnosed Philadelphia chromosome-positive acute lymphoblastic leukemia treated between 1995 and 2005. J Clin Oncol 2010;28:4755-61.

140. Arico M, Valsecchi MG, Camitta B, et al. Outcome of treatment in children with Philadelphia chromosome-positive acute lymphoblastic leukemia. N Engl J Med 2000;342:998-1006.

141. Schultz KR, Bowman WP, Aledo A, et al. Improved early event-free survival with imatinib in Philadelphia chromosome-positive acute lymphoblastic leukemia: a children's oncology group study. J Clin Oncol 2009;27:5175-81.

142. Schultz KR, Carroll A, Heerema NA, et al. Long-term follow-up of imatinib in pediatric Philadelphia chromosome-positive acute lymphoblastic leukemia: Children's Oncology Group study AALL0031. Leukemia 2014;28:1467-71.

143. Lee-Sherick AB, Linger RM, Gore L, et al. Targeting paediatric acute lymphoblastic leukaemia: novel therapies currently in development. Br J Haematol 2010;151:295-311.

144. Aplenc R, Blaney SM, Strauss LC, et al. Pediatric phase I trial and pharmacokinetic study of dasatinib: a report from the children's oncology group phase I consortium. J Clin Oncol 2011;29:839-44.

145. Schultz KR, Prestidge T, Camitta B. Philadelphia chromosome-positive acute lymphoblastic leukemia in children: new and emerging treatment options. Expert Rev Hematol 2010; 3:731-42.

146. Burkart M, Sanford S, Dinner S, et al. Future health of AYA survivors. Pediatr Blood Cancer 2019;66:e27516.

147. Crist W, Pullen J, Boyett J, et al. Acute lymphoid leukemia in adolescents: clinical and biologic features predict a poor prognosis—a Pediatric Oncology Group Study. J Clin Oncol 1988;6:34-43.

148. Advani AS, Hunger SP, Burnett AK. Acute leukemia in adolescents and young adults. Semin Oncol 2009;36:213-26.

149. Nachman J. Clinical characteristics, biologic features and outcome for young adult patients with acute lymphoblastic leukaemia. Br J Haematol 2005;130:166-73.

150. Nachman JB, La MK, Hunger SP, et al. Young adults with acute lymphoblastic leukaemia have an excellent outcome with chemotherapy alone and benefit from intensive postinduction treatment: a report from the children's oncology group. J Clin Oncol 2009;27:5189-94.

151. Mattison R, Stock W. Approaches to treatment for acute lymphoblastic leukemia in adolescents and young adults. Curr Hematol Malig Rep 2008;3:144-51.

152. Stock W, La M, Sanford B, et al. What determines the outcomes for adolescents and young adults with acute lymphoblastic leukemia treated on cooperative group protocols? A comparison of Children's Cancer Group and Cancer and Leukemia Group B studies. Blood 2008;112:1646-54.

153. de Bont JM, Holt B, Dekker AW, et al. Significant difference in outcome for adolescents with acute lymphoblastic leukemia treated on pediatric vs adult protocols in the Netherlands. Leukemia 2004;18:2032-5.

154. Boissel N, Auclerc MF, Lheritier V, et al. Should adolescents with acute lymphoblastic leukemia be treated as old children or young adults? Comparison of the French FRALLE-93 and LALA-94 trials. J Clin Oncol 2003;21:774-80.

155. Ramanujachar R, Richards S, Hann I, et al. Adolescents with acute lymphoblastic leukaemia: outcome on UK national paediatric (ALL97) and adult (UKALLXII/E2993) trials. Pediatr Blood Cancer 2007;48:254-61.

156. Rubnitz JE, Lensing S, Zhou Y, et al. Death during induction therapy and first remission of acute leukemia in childhood: the St. Jude experience. Cancer 2004;101:1677-84.

157. Barry E, DeAngelo DJ, Neuberg D, et al. Favorable outcome for adolescents with acute lymphoblastic leukemia treated on Dana-Farber Cancer Institute Acute Lymphoblastic Leukemia Consortium Protocols. J Clin Oncol 2007;25:813-9.

158. Yang L, Panetta JC, Cai X, et al. Asparaginase may influence dexamethasone pharmacokinetics in acute lymphoblastic leukemia. J Clin Oncol 2008;26:1932-9.

159. Ko RH, Ji L, Barnette P, et al. Outcome of patients treated for relapsed or refractory acute lymphoblastic leukemia: a Therapeutic Advances in Childhood Leukemia Consortium study. J Clin Oncol 2010;28:648-54.

160. Rheingold SR, Ji L, Xu X, et al. Prognostic factors for survival after relapsed acute lymphoblastic leukemia (ALL): A Children's Oncology Group (COG) study. J Clin Oncol 2019; 37(suppl 15): 10008.

161. Gaynon PS, Qu RP, Chappell RJ, et al. Survival after relapse in childhood acute lymphoblastic leukemia: impact of site and time to first relapse—the Children's Cancer Group Experience. Cancer 1998;82:1387-95.

162. Tallen G, Ratei R, Mann G, et al. Long-term outcome in children with relapsed acute lymphoblastic leukemia after time-point and site-of-relapse stratification and intensified short-course multidrug chemotherapy: results of trial ALL-REZ BFM 90. J Clin Oncol 2010;28:2339-47.

163. Gaynon PS, Harris RE, Altman AJ, et al. Bone marrow transplantation versus prolonged intensive chemotherapy for children with acute lymphoblastic leukemia and an initial bone marrow relapse within 12 months of the completion of primary therapy: Children's Oncology Group study CCG-1941. J Clin Oncol 2006;24:3150-6.

164. Barrett AJ, Horowitz MM, Pollock BH, et al. Bone marrow transplants from HLA-identical siblings as compared with chemotherapy for children with acute lymphoblastic leukemia in a second remission. N Engl J Med 1994;331:1253-8.

165. Uderzo C, Valsecchi MG, Bacigalupo A, et al. Treatment of childhood acute lymphoblastic leukemia in second remission with allogeneic bone marrow transplantation and chemotherapy: ten-year experience of the Italian Bone Marrow Transplantation Group and the Italian Pediatric Hematology Oncology Association. J Clin Oncol 1995;13:352-8.

166. Jacobs JE, Hastings C. Isolated extramedullary relapse in childhood acute lymphocytic leukemia. Curr Hematol Malig Rep 2010;5:185-91.

167. Balduzzi A, Valsecchi MG, Uderzo C, et al. Chemotherapy versus allogeneic transplantation for very-high-risk childhood acute lymphoblastic leukaemia in first complete remission: comparison

by genetic randomisation in an international prospective study. Lancet 2005;366:635-42.

168. Sadowitz PD, Smith SD, Shuster J, et al. Treatment of late bone marrow relapse in children with acute lymphoblastic leukemia: a Pediatric Oncology Group study. Blood 1993;81:602-9.

169. Raetz EA, Borowitz MJ, Devidas M, et al. Reinduction platform for children with first marrow relapse of acute lymphoblastic Leukemia: A Children's Oncology Group Study[corrected]. J Clin Oncol 2008;26:3971-8.

170. Buie LW, Pecoraro JJ, Horvat TZ, et al. Blinatumomab: a first-in-class bispecific T-cell engager for precursor B-cell acute lymphoblastic leukemia. Ann Pharmacother 2015;49:1057-67.

171. Maude SL, Teachey DT, Porter DL, et al. CD19-targeted chimeric antigen receptor T-cell therapy for acute lymphoblastic leukemia. Blood 2015;125:4017-23.

172. Maude SL, Frey N, Shaw PA, et al. Chimeric antigen receptor T cells for sustained remissions in leukemia. N Engl J Med 2014;371:1507-17.

173. O'Brien MM, Ji L, Shah NN, et al. A phase 2 trial of inotuzumab ozogamicin (InO) in children and young adults with relapsed or refractory (R/R) CD22+ B-acute lymphoblastic leukemia (B-ALL): results from Children's Oncology Group Protocol AALL1621. Blood 2019;134(Supplement_1):741.

174. von Stackelberg A, Locatelli F, Zugmaier G, et al. Phase I/phase II study of blinatumomab in pediatric patients with relapsed/refractory acute lymphoblastic leukemia. J Clin Oncol 2016;34:4381-9.

175. Handgretinger R, Zugmaier G, Henze G, et al. Complete remission after blinatumomab-induced donor T-cell activation in three pediatric patients with post-transplant relapsed acute lymphoblastic leukemia. Leukemia 2011;25:181-4.

176. Brown P, Ji L, Xu X, et al. A randomized phase 3 trial of blinatumomab vs chemotherapy as post-reinduction therapy in high and intermediate risk (HR/IR) first relapse of B-acute lymphoblastic leukemia (B-ALL) in children and adolescents/young adults (AYAs) demonstrates superior efficacy and tolerability of blinatumomab: a report from Children's Oncology Group Study AALL1331. Blood 2019;134(suppl 2):LBA-1.

177. Maude SL, Laetsch TW, Buechner J, et al. Tisagenlecleucel in children and young adults with B-cell lymphoblastic leukemia. N Engl J Med 2018;378:439-48.

178. Gardner RA, Finney O, Annesley C, et al. Intent-to-treat leukemia remission by CD19 CAR T cells of defined formulation and dose in children and young adults. Blood 2017;129:3322-31.

179. Park JH, Riviere I, Gonen M, et al. Long-term follow-up of CD19 CAR therapy in acute lymphoblastic leukemia. N Engl J Med 2018;378:449-59.

180. Maude SL, Teachey DT, Porter DL, et al. CD19-targeted chimeric antigen receptor T-cell therapy for acute lymphoblastic leukemia. Blood 2015;125:4017-23.

181. Mahadeo KM, Khazal SJ, Abdel-Azim H, et al. Management guidelines for paediatric patients receiving chimeric antigen receptor T cell therapy. Nat Rev Clin Oncol 2019;16:45-63.

182. Fitzgerald JC, Weiss SL, Maude SL, et al. Cytokine release syndrome after chimeric antigen receptor T cell therapy for acute lymphoblastic leukemia. Crit Care Med 2017;45:e124-31.

183. Approved Risk Evaluation and Mitigation Strategies (REMS) for Kymriah (tisagenlecleucel) [homepage on the Internet]. 2019. Silver Spring, MD: U.S. Food and Drug Administration. Available at www.accessdata.fda.gov/Scripts/Cder/Rems/index.cfm?event=IndvRemsDetails.page&REMS=368. Accessed March 6, 2020.

184. Davila ML, Riviere I, Wang X, et al. Efficacy and toxicity management of 19-28z CAR T cell therapy in B cell acute lymphoblastic leukemia. Sci Transl Med 2014;6:224ra25.

185. Barredo JC, Devidas M, Lauer SJ, et al. Isolated CNS relapse of acute lymphoblastic leukemia treated with intensive systemic chemotherapy and delayed CNS radiation: a pediatric oncology group study. J Clin Oncol 2006;24:3142-9.

186. Ribeiro RC, Rivera GK, Hudson M, et al. An intensive re-treatment protocol for children with an isolated CNS relapse of acute lymphoblastic leukemia. J Clin Oncol 1995;13:333-8.

187. Ritchey AK, Pollock BH, Lauer SJ, et al. Improved survival of children with isolated CNS relapse of acute lymphoblastic leukemia: a pediatric oncology group study. J Clin Oncol 1999;17:3745-52.

188. Haidar C, Jeha S. Drug interactions in childhood cancer. Lancet Oncol 2011;12:92-9.

189. Coiffier B, Altman A, Pui CH, et al. Guidelines for the management of pediatric and adult tumor lysis syndrome: an evidence-based review. J Clin Oncol 2008;26:2767-78.

190. Cairo MS, Coiffier B, Reiter A, et al. Recommendations for the evaluation of risk and prophylaxis of tumour lysis syndrome (TLS) in adults and children with malignant diseases: an expert TLS panel consensus. Br J Haematol 2010;149:578-86.

191. Howard SC, Jones DP, Pui CH. The tumor lysis syndrome. N Engl J Med 2011;364:1844-54.

192. Welte K, Reiter A, Mempel K, et al. A randomized phase-III study of the efficacy of granulocyte colony-stimulating factor in children with high-risk acute lymphoblastic leukemia. Berlin-Frankfurt-Munster Study Group. Blood 1996;87:3143-50.

193. Bessmertny O, Cairo MS. Prophylactic use of myelopoietic growth factors in children after myelosuppressive chemotherapy: does it pay? J Pediatr Hematol Oncol 2003;25:435-40.

194. Ozkaynak MF, Krailo M, Chen Z, et al. Randomized comparison of antibiotics with and without granulocyte colony-stimulating factor in children with chemotherapy-induced febrile neutropenia: a report from the Children's Oncology Group. Pediatr Blood Cancer 2005;45:274-80.

195. Heath JA, Steinherz PG, Altman A, et al. Human granulocyte colony-stimulating factor in children with high-risk acute lymphoblastic leukemia: a Children's Cancer Group Study. J Clin Oncol 2003;21:1612-7.

196. Pui CH, Boyett JM, Hughes WT, et al. Human granulocyte colony-stimulating factor after induction chemotherapy in children with acute lymphoblastic leukemia. N Engl J Med 1997;336:1781-7.

197. Freifeld AG, Bow EJ, Sepkowitz KA, et al. Clinical practice guideline for the use of antimicrobial agents in neutropenic patients with cancer: 2010 Update by the Infectious Diseases Society of America. Clin Infect Dis 2011;52:427-31.

198. Hughes WT, Kuhn S, Chaudhary S, et al. Successful chemoprophylaxis for Pneumocystis carinii pneumonitis. N Engl J Med 1977;297:1419-26.

199. Madden RM, Pui CH, Hughes WT, et al. Prophylaxis of Pneumocystis carinii pneumonia with atovaquone in children with leukemia. Cancer 2007;109:1654-8.

200. Blum RN, Miller LA, Gaggini LC, et al. Comparative trial of dapsone versus trimethoprim/sulfamethoxazole for primary prophylaxis of Pneumocystis carinii pneumonia. J Acquir Immune Defic Syndr 1992;5:341-7.

201. Weinthal J, Frost JD, Briones G, et al. Successful Pneumocystis carinii pneumonia prophylaxis using aerosolized pentamidine in children with acute leukemia. J Clin Oncol 1994;12:136-40.

202. Kim SY, Dabb AA, Glenn DJ, et al. Intravenous pentamidine is effective as second line Pneumocystis pneumonia prophylaxis in pediatric oncology patients. Pediatr Blood Cancer 2008;50:779-83.

203. Sala A, Pencharz P, Barr RD. Children, cancer, and nutrition—a dynamic triangle in review. Cancer 2004;100:677-87.

204. Rogers PC, Meacham LR, Oeffinger KC, et al. Obesity in pediatric oncology. Pediatr Blood Cancer 2005;45:881-91.

205. Griggs JJ, Mangu PB, Temin S, et al. Appropriate chemotherapy dosing for obese adult patients with cancer: American Society of Clinical Oncology clinical practice guideline. J Oncol Pract 2012;8:e59-61.

206. Schwartz CL. Long-term survivors of childhood cancer: the late effects of therapy. Oncologist 1999;4:45-54.

207. Nathan PC, Wasilewski-Masker K, Janzen LA. Long-term outcomes in survivors of childhood acute lymphoblastic leukemia. Hematol Oncol Clin North Am 2009;23:1065,82, vi-vii.

208. Bhatia S. Late effects among survivors of leukemia during childhood and adolescence. Blood Cells Mol Dis 2003;31:84-92.

209. Lipshultz SE, Colan SD, Gelber RD, et al. Late cardiac effects of doxorubicin therapy for acute lymphoblastic leukemia in childhood. N Engl J Med 1991;324:808-15.

210. Sorensen K, Levitt G, Bull C, et al. Anthracycline dose in childhood acute lymphoblastic leukemia: issues of early survival versus late cardiotoxicity. J Clin Oncol 1997;15:61-8.

211. Bhatia S, Sather HN, Pabustan OB, et al. Low incidence of second neoplasms among children diagnosed with acute lymphoblastic leukemia after 1983. Blood 2002;99:4257-64.

212. Neglia JP, Meadows AT, Robison LL, et al. Second neoplasms after acute lymphoblastic leukemia in childhood. N Engl J Med 1991;325:1330-6.

213. Kimball Dalton VM, Gelber RD, Li F, et al. Second malignancies in patients treated for childhood acute lymphoblastic leukemia. J Clin Oncol 1998;16:2848-53.

214. Relander T, Cavallin-Stahl E, Garwicz S, et al. Gonadal and sexual function in men treated for childhood cancer. Med Pediatr Oncol 2000;35:52-63.

215. Long-Term Follow-Up Guidelines for Survivors of Childhood, Adolescent, and Young Adult Cancer [homepage on the Internet]. Version 5.0 - October 2018. Available at www.survivorshipguidelines.org. Accessed March 6, 2020.

216. Annesley CE, Brown P. Novel agents for the treatment of childhood acute leukemia. Ther Adv Hematol 2015;6:61-79.

217. Evans WE, Relling MV. Pharmacogenomics: translating functional genomics into rational therapeutics. Science 1999;286: 487-91.

218. Mehta PA, Davies SM. Pharmacogenetics of acute lymphoblastic leukemia. Curr Opin Hematol 2004;11:434-8.

219. McLeod HL, Krynetski EY, Relling MV, et al. Genetic polymorphism of thiopurine methyltransferase and its clinical relevance for childhood acute lymphoblastic leukemia. Leukemia 2000;14:567-72.

220. Relling MV, Hancock ML, Rivera GK, et al. Mercaptopurine therapy intolerance and heterozygosity at the thiopurine S-methyltransferase gene locus. J Natl Cancer Inst 1999;91:2001-8.

221. Stanulla M, Schaeffeler E, Flohr T, et al. Thiopurine methyltransferase (TPMT) genotype and early treatment response to mercaptopurine in childhood acute lymphoblastic leukemia. JAMA 2005;293:1485-9.

222. Relling MV, Hancock ML, Boyett JM, et al. Prognostic importance of 6-mercaptopurine dose intensity in acute lymphoblastic leukemia. Blood 1999;93:2817-23.

223. Meeker ND, Yang JJ, Schiffman JD. Pharmacogenomics of pediatric acute lymphoblastic leukemia. Expert Opin Pharmacother 2010;11:1621-32.

224. Relling MV, Gardner EE, Sandborn WJ, et al. Clinical Pharmacogenetics Implementation Consortium guidelines for thiopurine methyltransferase genotype and thiopurine dosing. Clin Pharmacol Ther 2011;89:387-91.

CHAPTER 52

Acute Myelogenous Leukemia

*M. Brooke Bernhardt, Pharm.D., MS, BCOP, BCPPS;
and Tara E. Wright, Pharm.D., BCOP, BCPPS*

LEARNING OBJECTIVES

1. Understand the epidemiology and etiology of childhood acute myelogenous leukemia (AML).

2. Describe the standard approach to treating children with AML.

3. Discuss the potential role of targeted therapy in the treatment of pediatric AML.

4. Identify critical supportive care issues when treating children with AML.

ABBREVIATIONS IN THIS CHAPTER

ALL	Acute lymphoblastic leukemia
AML	Acute myelogenous leukemia
APL	Acute promyelocytic leukemia
CBF	Core-binding factor
CEBPA	CCAAT/enhancer binding protein alpha
CINV	Chemotherapy-induced nausea and vomiting
CNS	Central nervous system
CYP	Cytochrome P450
FLT3-/ITD	FMS-like tyrosine kinase 3 internal tandem duplication
GATA1	GATA-binding protein 1 (globin transcription factor 1 or GATA1 gene)
MLL	Mixed lineage leukemia
TMD	Transient myeloproliferative disorder
WBC	White blood cell

INTRODUCTION

Acute myelogenous leukemia (AML) is a term used to describe a diverse group of disorders that arise from the proliferation of abnormal myeloid, erythroid, monocytic, and megakaryocytic cell precursors.[1] Although the disease-free survival of patients with AML has improved during the past three decades, only about 60% of patients with AML will achieve long-term survival.[2-15] The focus of this chapter is to review the epidemiology, etiology, prognosis, diagnosis, and treatment of childhood AML.

EPIDEMIOLOGY

About 11,000 children in the United States younger than 15 years receive a diagnosis of cancer each year.[16] Over one-fourth of these children have a diagnosis of leukemia, making it the most common type of cancer overall in children.[16] Most patients with leukemia have a diagnosis of acute lymphoblastic leukemia (ALL), and about 20% have a diagnosis of AML, reflecting an incidence of about 7 patients per 1 million individuals younger than 19 years.[17]

No known differences in incidence have been found between male and female patients. The incidence of AML appears to be highest in children of Hispanic ethnicity compared with African American or white children. Children of Hispanic descent also appear to have the highest incidence of the subtype known as *acute promyelocytic leukemia* (APL).[18-21]

ETIOLOGY

Several inherited conditions and environmental exposures have been associated with the development of de novo and secondary AML. In many cases of childhood AML, a potential cause is unknown; however, at least one known genomic alteration can be found in more than 90% of cases.[22] Inherited conditions associated with the development of de novo childhood AML are identified in Box 1.[19,23-38]

Environmental exposures generally associated with the development of AML include benzene, organic solvents, herbicides, pesticides, petroleum products, maternal use of marijuana during pregnancy, and previous use or exposure to chemotherapy or ionizing radiation. Except for ionizing radiation, however, a definitive association of these factors with childhood AML is difficult to establish.[19,39-41] Maternal consumption of fresh fruits and vegetables that contribute to DNA topoisomerase II inhibition (e.g., apples, berries, canned or dried legumes, onions, soy products) may increase the risk of infant AML with rearrangements of the mixed lineage leukemia (*MLL*) gene.[42] Chemotherapeutic agents most notably

---

Box 1. Inherited Conditions Associated with Childhood Acute Myelogenous Leukemia[19,23-38]

Bloom syndrome
Diamond-Blackfan anemia
Down syndrome
Dyskeratosis congenital
Familial platelet disorder with a predisposition to acute myelogenous leukemia
Fanconi anemia
Kostmann syndrome
Li-Fraumeni syndrome
Neurofibromatosis type 1
Noonan syndrome
Shwachman-Diamond syndrome

associated with the development of secondary AML include etoposide, topoisomerase II inhibitors (e.g., doxorubicin), and alkylating agents (e.g., mechlorethamine, cyclophosphamide). The median time between diagnosis of primary malignancy and secondary AML varies based on initial chemotherapy exposure—2–3 years for secondary AML related to topoisomerase II inhibitors and etoposide versus 5–7 years for alkylating agents.[43-47] Finally, AML may also develop after an acquired predisposing condition, such as aplastic anemia or myelodysplastic syndrome.[48-50]

BIOLOGY AND PATHOPHYSIOLOGY

Genetic mutations or chromosomal rearrangements may result in abnormal hematopoietic precursors. Clonal transformation, replication, and proliferation of abnormal myeloid, erythroid, monocytic, or megakaryocytic precursors can result in the development of AML. Differentiation and apoptosis of these precursors is impaired, resulting in dysregulation of normal hematopoiesis. Acute myeloid leukemia develops when at least one class I mutation and one class II mutation in a host's hematopoietic precursor cells occur. Class I mutations do not affect cellular differentiation, but they do confer a proliferative or survival advantage to hematopoietic precursor cells. Examples of clinically relevant class I alterations include FMS-like tyrosine kinase 3 internal tandem duplications (*FLT3-*/ITD) and oncogenic *ras* mutations. Class II mutations impair the normal precursor cell differentiation and apoptosis; treatment-related examples include the *PML/RARA* fusion gene, which is the translocation of chromosomes 15 and 17, or t(15;17), and *MLL* gene rearrangements, for example, t(4;22), t(11;19), t(9;11).[1,22] The prognostic significance of these alterations will be discussed later in this chapter.

CLASSIFICATION OF AML

The French–American–British or FAB classification system has been used historically to describe seven subtypes of AML (M1–M7) based on morphologic, histochemical, immunophenotypic, and cytogenetic features of the abnormal clone.[51] The M0 subtype has been used to describe undifferentiated AML. The goal of this classification system was to create uniformity in diagnosing and categorizing AML in patients. The specific criteria for each subtype will not be discussed in this chapter, which will instead focus on the subtypes of clinical importance (M0, M4, and M7) with respect to differences in therapy.

The concept of classification based on cytogenetic subtypes is still relatively new. In 2008, the World Health Organization, the European Association for Haematopathology, and the Society for Hematopathology released a revised fourth edition of their classification system of hematopoietic and lymphoid tissues. In general, AML is defined as the presence of at least 20% myeloblasts in the peripheral blood or among all nucleated bone marrow cells. This presence can occur de novo or through evolution from a previously diagnosed myelodysplastic syndrome or neoplasm. However, the presence of certain translocations, such as t(8;21)(q22;q22), t(16;16)(p13.1;q22), or t(15;17)(q22;q12), or the inversion of chromosome 16, which is the inv(16)(p13.1;q22) translocation, is definitive for a diagnosis of AML, regardless of the blast count or percent.[52] The traditional World Health Organization classification was not as applicable to children; therefore a revised classification was published.[53] The groupings now included in the classification are AML with recurrent genetic abnormalities, AML with myelodysplasia-related features, therapy-related myeloid neoplasms, AML new onset/de novo, myeloid sarcoma, and myeloid proliferations related to Down syndrome.

PROGNOSIS

For the past several decades, intensified chemotherapy has led to complete remission rates of 68%–93%.[3-15] However, relapse is relatively common, occurring in 30%–40% of patients. The 5-year event-free and overall survival rates vary on the basis of the treatment protocol used, with these rates ranging from 31%–54% and from 36%–66%, respectively, as represented in Table 1 for patients without Down syndrome across several international cooperative groups.[3-15]

The prognosis for patients with AML is affected by a variety of clinical features as well as genetic factors. In children and adolescents, age older than 10 years at diagnosis has been associated with a poorer outcome, even when controlling for potential confounding features.[54] Ethnicity may also play a role in predicting prognosis. African American children have worse outcomes than white children undergoing treatment for AML. This disparity is thought to be a product of potential pharmacogenetic differences among ethnic groups—and not access to care, based on the nature and delivery of cooperative group care to children with cancer.[55,56] Body mass index may also play a role in predicting prognosis; children who are underweight or overweight have a significantly lower chance of survival than patients who are of normal weight. This difference in survival is largely because of the increased risk of treatment-related mortality in underweight and overweight patients.[57]

A retrospective evaluation of children with AML by the Children's Oncology Group revealed an 11% incidence of central nervous system (CNS) disease at presentation; children with Down syndrome–associated AML, APL, myelodysplastic syndrome, secondary AML, and isolated extramedullary AML were excluded from the analysis. Factors associated with CNS disease at presentation included younger age, hepatosplenomegaly, elevated white blood cell (WBC) count, M4 morphology, abnormalities in chromosome 16, and hyperdiploidy.[58] Disease of the CNS at diagnosis increases the risk of relapse (including either isolated CNS relapse or marrow plus CNS relapse) and shortens disease-free survival.[58]

Pathologic disease-related features may also play a role in predicting survival. Children with AML of the M0 or M7 subtype (without Down syndrome) may have worse outcomes than those with other subtypes of AML.[59,60] Historically, children with Down syndrome typically experienced a greater event-free survival rate and a lower relapse rate than children without Down syndrome, especially with respect to the M7 subtype of AML. This enhanced response seen in children with Down syndrome AML may be a result of the greater sensitivity to chemotherapy, specifically cytarabine.[61,62]

Children with APL who receive treatment with standard chemotherapy and tretinoin (all–*trans*-retinoic acid) may have complete remission rates greater than 95%, 5-year event-free survival greater than 70%, and overall survival of about 90%.[63-65] Within this subgroup, an elevated WBC at diagnosis (specifically, WBC greater than 10×10^3 cells/mm^3) is considered a major, adverse prognostic factor with a reduced event-free survival of about 60%.[22,64] A small percentage of patients die during induction; about 50% of deaths occur because of coagulopathy and hemorrhagic complications. Other factors associated with a poor prognosis in childhood APL include the presence of *FLT3-/ITD* , a *bcr3 PML* breakpoint, or the microgranular variant (M3v) of the disease.[22,63]

Cytogenetic abnormalities have been evaluated as both prognostic indicators and as a means to guide therapy. At present, molecular abnormalities are associated with both favorable and unfavorable prognoses. Box 2 details some of the more common mutations; this list is not comprehensive. In some patients, one or more of these cytogenetic abnormalities or a variety of other abnormalities may be present, making prognostic prediction and treatment decisions difficult.

Some of the more notable karyotypes of blast cells that typically confer a more positive outcome include t(8;21) and inv(16). These two alterations are typically referred to as the *core-binding factor (CBF) leukemias*, which are characterized by *RUNX1-RUNX1T1* and *CBFB-MYH11* fusion genes that disrupt the activity of core-binding factor. About 20% of children with AML have CBF AML. For this group, reported 5-year overall survival rates range from 75%–90%. Patients with t(8;21) may have a lower overall survival compared with those with inv(16) because of a lower salvage rate after relapse. In patients with t(8;21), race may also play an important prognostic role.[1,66-68] Mutations in the *CEBPA* gene, which provides instructions for making a protein called CCAAT enhancer-binding protein alpha, occur in about 5%–8% of children with AML. Most children have biallelic mutations in *CEBPA,* which is associated with a significantly improved survival rate; similar survival rates may not carry over to children with single-allele mutations.[69-71]

Up to 20% of patients have *KMT2A* (*MLL*) gene rearrangements at chromosome band 11q23; these patients are traditionally classified as having intermediate-risk disease.[63,72-74] However, more recent work has demonstrated that the prognosis of *KMT2A* rearrangements may be dependent on accompanying fusion partners. For example, children with t(6;11)(q27;q23) and t(4;11)(q21;q23) are expected to have a poor outcome, with 5-year EFS of 11% and 29%, respectively. In contrast, children with t(1;11)(q21;q23) have much higher expected 5-year EFS at 92%.[75]

Karyotypes associated with a less favorable outcome include monosomy 5, del(5q), monosomy 7, and 3q abnormalities.[63] Also in children *FLT3-ITD* is associated with unfavorable outcomes and is a strong predictor of relapse. Event-free survival rates for children with *FLT3-/ITD* overall may be as low as 7%–29%.[76,77] However, like other mutations, the prognostic significance of *FLT3-/ITD* is modified by other concomitant genomic alterations. Co-existing *FLT3-/ITD* and NPM1 mutations may extend a more favorable prognosis,

Table 1. International Cooperative Group Outcome Data for Pediatric AML[1,3-15]

Study	n	CR (%)	5-yr EFS (%)	5-yr OS (%)
AIEOP92	160	89	54	60
AML-BFM93	427	83	51	58
CCG2891	750	78	34	47
DCOG-ALL 92/94	78	82	42	42
EORTC-CLG 58,921	166	84	48	62
GATLA-AML90	179	70	31	41
LAME91	247	91	48	62
NOPHO-AML93	223	92	50	66
PINDA-92	151	68	36	36
POG8821	511	77	31	42
PPLSG98	104	80	47	50
St. Jude-AML91	62	79	44	57
UK MRC AML10	303	93	49	58
UK MRC AML12	455	92	56	66

AIEOP = Associazione Italiana Ematologia Oncologia Pediatrica; AML = acute myelogenous leukemia; ALL = acute lymphoblastic leukemia; BFM = Berlin–Frankfurt–Munster; CCG = Children's Cancer Group; CR = complete remission; DCOG = Dutch Childhood Oncology Group; EFS = event-free survival; EORTC–CLG = European Organization for the Research and Treatment of Cancer–Children Leukemia Group; GATLA = Argentine Group for the Treatment of Acute Leukemia; LAME = Leucémie Aiguë Myéloblastique Enfant; NOPHO = Nordic Society of Pediatric Haematology and Oncology; OS = overall survival; PINDA = National Program for Antineoplastic Drugs for Children; POG = Pediatric Oncology Group; PPLLSG = Polish Pediatric Leukemia/Lymphoma Study Group; UK MRC = United Kingdom Medical Research Council.

Reprinted with permission from WB Saunders Co., from Rubnitz JE, Gibson B, Smith FO. Acute myeloid leukemia [review]. Hematol Oncol Clin North Am 2010;24:35-63.

whereas patients with *FLT3-/ITD* and *NUP98-NSD1* have a poorer prognosis.[78,79]

Many other pathogenic mutations have been discovered in pediatric AML; however, their prognostic importance has yet to be defined clearly. For example, the prognostic significance of *KIT, RAS,* and *WT1* mutations in childhood AML are still unclear, and may be dependent on other presenting aberrations.[80-83]

Finally, the response to initial therapy is of great prognostic significance. Complete remission after induction is traditionally defined as normalizing peripheral blood counts (ANC greater than 1000/mcL, platelet count greater than 100×10^3 cells/mm³), mildly hypocellular or normal cellularity marrow with less than 5% blasts, and no evidence of extramedullary disease. The presence of minimum residual disease (defined as the presence of 0.1% or more leukemic cells) is also a critical marker. Children with detectable disease after the first course of induction therapy are 4.8 times more likely to relapse and 3.1 times more likely to die than those who achieve remission at the end of induction.[84]

CLINICAL PRESENTATION AND DIAGNOSIS

SIGNS AND SYMPTOMS

Leukemic infiltration of the bone marrow and extramedullary sites is responsible for most of the commonly seen signs and symptoms of AML. Children may present with fever, fatigue, pallor, bleeding, bone pain, or infection as some of the initial symptoms. Anemia, neutropenia, and thrombocytopenia occur as the normal hematopoietic cells within the bone marrow are replaced by the abnormal clone. In some cases, patients may present with hyperleukocytosis at diagnosis instead of neutropenia or leukopenia. Lymphadenopathy, hepatosplenomegaly, chloromas, leukemia cutis, gum swelling and/or bleeding, and orbital swelling can result from extramedullary involvement of the leukemic clone.[1]

Patients with Down syndrome may initially present with transient myeloproliferative disorder (TMD) weeks to months before AML develops. Also referred to as *transient abnormal myelopoiesis* or *transient leukemia*, TMD may present on a spectrum from an incidental finding of blasts in the blood in a well-appearing child to a variety of severe complications including effusions, hydrops fetalis, and multi-organ system failure.[28]

Patients with APL may present with signs and symptoms similar to those of children with AML. In addition, they often present with a specific coagulopathy that is a combination of fibrinolysis and disseminated intravascular coagulation.[85] Emergency management of the presenting coagulopathy and underlying disease state is critical.

DIAGNOSTIC CRITERIA

A diagnosis of AML is based on a combination of tests that are typically performed on a sample obtained during a bone marrow aspirate and biopsy. Diagnostic tests include morphologic evaluation, cytogenetic and cytochemical analysis, fluorescence in situ hybridization, immunophenotyping by flow cytometry, and molecular testing.[1] Lumbar puncture should be performed to determine the presence and extent of any abnormal myeloblasts in the CNS.

TREATMENT

CHEMOTHERAPY OVERVIEW

Chemotherapy for the treatment of AML is typically divided into two phases: *induction therapy* and *post-remission therapy*, also called *consolidation therapy*. In addition, *maintenance therapy*, although typically used in ALL, is not used routinely but will be discussed briefly. A general schematic of the treatment of AML is provided in Table 2. Selected common and unique toxicities of chemotherapy used in the treatment of AML are provided in Table 3.

Improvement in the survival of children with AML is partly a result of refinement in the use of conventional chemotherapeutic agents. Each of the international cooperative groups in Table 1 stratified therapy on the basis of various risk classifications and features. Therapy for each group involved intensive induction chemotherapy, followed by aggressive post-remission chemotherapy. Similar agents were used throughout each phase of therapy, including cytarabine, etoposide, and an anthracycline (i.e., daunorubicin, idarubicin, or mitoxantrone).

Doses of each of the agents varied widely across groups. Among the 14 cooperative groups, cumulative doses (for all phases of therapy combined) of cytarabine ranged from

---

Box 2. Prognosis-Related Molecular Abnormalities in Acute Myelogenous Leukemia (AML)

Favorable Prognosis

AML with t(8;21)(q22;q22.1); *RUNX1-RUNX1T1*

AML with inv(16)(p13.1;q22) or t(16;16)(p13.1;q22); *CBFB-MYH11*

AML with t(16;21)(q24;q22); *RUNX1-CBFA2T3*

Acute promyelocytic leukemia with *PML-RARA*

AML with mutated *NPM1*

AML with biallelic mutations of *CEBPA*

Myeloid leukemia associated with Down syndrome (*GATA1* mutations)

Unfavorable Prognosis

Chromosomes 5 and 7: monosomy 5, monosomy 7, and del(5q)

AML with inv(3)(q21.3;q26.2) or t(3;3)(q21.3;q26.2); *GATA2, MECOM*

FMS-like tyrosine kinase 3 (*FLT3)* mutations

AML with t(16;21)(p11;q22); *FUS-ERG*

CBF = core-binding factor; *CEBPA* = CCAAT/enhancer binding protein alpha; GATA = GATA-binding protein.

3.8 to 55.7 grams/m², with about one-third of the groups giving cumulative cytarabine doses exceeding 30 grams/m². Cumulative doses of etoposide over the entire treatment plan varied as well, from 400 to 2250 mg/m². Lastly, cumulative doses of anthracyclines varied from 180 to 610 mg/m² (expressed in daunorubicin dosing equivalents); almost all groups used doses exceeding 300 mg/m², with some using cumulative doses as high as 610 mg/m². In some patients, myeloablative hematopoietic stem cell transplantation was used as a component of post-remission therapy.[1-15]

INDUCTION THERAPY

The goal of the induction phase of therapy is to eliminate the disease to the point of remission, as previously defined. Standard induction therapy consists of an anthracycline (daunorubicin, idarubicin, or mitoxantrone) and cytarabine. A third drug such as etoposide or thioguanine may be added to the induction backbone.[86-88] Although the cumulative dose of cytarabine given for the duration of therapy appears to be important, the specific dose and frequency of cytarabine during induction do not appear to significantly affect outcomes. Various doses of cytarabine have resulted in similar complete response rates.[1-15,89]

Most North American protocols use a dose of 100 mg/m²/dose given every 12 hours for 8 to 10 days with each of the two courses of induction. The dose of the anthracycline used during induction appears to be of critical importance.[1-15,90] In previously untreated adults with AML, a higher dose of daunorubicin (90 mg/m²) given as three daily doses during the induction phase of therapy provided a statistically higher complete remission rate and overall survival compared with a lower dose of 45 mg/m².[91] The optimal dose of anthracycline for children with AML is unclear; it is possible that doses of 375–550 mg/m² are necessary because protocols using anthracycline doses (in daunorubicin equivalents) of less than 375 mg/m² report lower event-free survival.[1] Most North American studies incorporate daunorubicin at 50 mg/m²/dose on days 1, 3, and 5 of each induction course. However, the optimal anthracycline and its corresponding dose recommended for use in pediatric AML are not known. The use of idarubicin has shown faster cellular uptake, increased retention, and reduced susceptibility to resistance in preclinical and in vitro studies.[92,93] In a clinical trial using cytarabine and etoposide, the addition of idarubicin showed statistically greater blast clearance at induction day 15 compared with daunorubicin, yet it did not result in a greater event-free or overall survival at 5 years. In this study, patients who received idarubicin experienced more bone marrow toxicity and exhibited a longer time to bone marrow recovery than patients who received daunorubicin.[90] A later trial indicated that daunorubicin and idarubicin were similarly effective when a daunorubicin dose of 50 mg/m² was compared with an idarubicin dose of 10 or 12 mg/m². This trial also showed that at these comparable doses, the use of idarubicin resulted in more renal, gastrointestinal, and pulmonary toxicities.[86] Daunorubicin and mitoxantrone have shown similar efficacy, yet slightly different toxicity profiles, with mitoxantrone being more myelosuppressive.[15] Pediatric patients may be at a greater risk of developing cardiotoxicity from anthracyclines; therefore, some

Table 2. Overview of the Treatment of Acute Myelogenous Leukemia[1-15,60, 62-64,85,91]

Subgroup	Phase	Agents[a]
Non–Down syndrome	Induction (two cycles)	Standard- or high-dose cytarabine + etoposide + anthracycline
	Post-remission/Consolidation (two or three cycles[b])	High-dose cytarabine + one of the following (per cycle): • Etoposide • Mitoxantrone OR idarubicin • L-Asparaginase
Down syndrome	Induction (two to four cycles)	Standard-dose cytarabine + daunorubicin (or mitoxantrone) + thioguanine High-dose cytarabine + L-asparaginase[c]
	Consolidation/Intensification (two or three cycles[a])	Standard-dose cytarabine + one of the following (per cycle): • Etoposide • Mitoxantrone • L-Asparaginase
Acute promyelocytic leukemia	Induction	ATRA + idarubicin
	Consolidation	ATRA + one of the following (per cycle): • High-dose cytarabine + mitoxantrone • Mitoxantrone + etoposide • High-dose cytarabine + idarubicin ± thioguanine • Arsenic trioxide (investigational)
	Maintenance (if used)	ATRA + mercaptopurine + methotrexate

[a]Agents used vary based on institutional practice and clinical protocol or trial. These agents are representative of some of the types of combinations used in the respective disease state.
[b]Patients at a high risk of relapse with a matched donor may undergo hematopoietic stem cell transplantation based on institutional practice or protocol-directed therapy.
[c]May be used in some centers for one cycle.
ATRA = all-*trans*-retinoic acid.

investigators have sought to determine whether the cumulative dose of anthracycline used can be reduced.[1] To date, this dose has yet to be defined. Dexrazoxane is another option for reducing cardiotoxicity associated with anthracyclines. Dexrazoxane is a topoisomerase II inhibitor that interferes with iron-dependent free radical generation. In the past, the use of this agent in pediatrics was limited because of risk of secondary malignancies, specifically AML.[87,94-100] However, a number of more recent studies have found this agent to be safe in pediatrics with no increased risk for secondary malignant neoplasms, and many clinicians incorporate this agent as part of front-line therapy.[97-100]

In some populations, other adjunct agents may be used. Specifically, a recently completed study evaluated the effect of sorafenib as an added agent for pediatric patients with *FLT3-ITD*; data collection is still ongoing. In addition, post-hoc data analysis of the Children's Oncology Group AML0531 study demonstrated the potential role of gemtuzumab/ozogamicin in a subset of patients. In this study, multivariate analysis revealed that patients with a single nucleotide polymorphism resulting in the CC genotype for CD33 had a significantly improved 5-year disease-free survival and reduced 5-year relapse risk.[101]

POST-REMISSION/CONSOLIDATION THERAPY

Post-remission therapy, or consolidation therapy, is given to all patients with the goal of eliminating any residual disease. For many patients, chemotherapy given in the post-remission phase will include two or three additional courses of high-dose cytarabine with other active agents, such as etoposide, mitoxantrone, idarubicin, or L-asparaginase. Asparaginases are bacterial enzymes that primarily act by depleting plasma asparagine, which is essential to the survival of leukemia cells.[102] L-Asparaginase preparations are derived from either *Escherichia coli* or *Erwinia chrysanthemi*. In the post-remission/consolidation setting, the use of high-dose cytarabine appears to be of greater benefit than standard or low-dose cytarabine in some patients with AML. Specifically, adult patients with t(8;21) who were given three or more courses of chemotherapy with high-dose cytarabine in the post-remission period had improved failure-free and overall survival compared with those who received only one course of post-remission chemotherapy that included high-dose cytarabine.[103] Similarly, adult patients with inv(16) and t(16;16) had a significantly lower cumulative incidence of relapse and a trend toward a reduction in relapse-free survival with three or four

Table 3. Common and Unique Toxicities of Chemotherapy for Acute Myelogenous Leukemia[86]

Agent	Toxicities[a]
Arsenic trioxide	Tachycardia, prolongation of the QT interval, edema, hypotension, insomnia, anxiety, dizziness, depression, dermatitis, bruising, hypokalemia, hyperglycemia, hypomagnesemia, nausea, vomiting, sore throat, constipation, anorexia, leukocytosis, acute promyelocytic leukemia syndrome, anemia, transaminitis, pain, rigors, paresthesias, cough, dyspnea, hypoxia, pleural effusion, epistaxis, sinusitis, diarrhea, fatigue, fever, headache, pruritus
L-Asparaginase	Anaphylaxis, fever, chills, nausea, vomiting, abdominal cramping, seizures, coma, azotemia, coagulopathy, hypofibrinogenemia, decreased clotting factors, decreased antithrombin III, hepatotoxicity, pancreatitis, hyperglycemia
All–*trans*-retinoic acid	Arrhythmias, chest discomfort, dyspnea, respiratory insufficiency, pleural effusion, edema, weight gain, shivering, dizziness, pain, pruritus, nausea, vomiting, diarrhea, earache/ear fullness, fever, malaise, flushing, rash, headache, hypercholesterolemia, hypertriglyceridemia, leukocytosis, mucositis, hemorrhage, disseminated intravascular coagulation, retinoic acid syndrome, skin/mucous membrane dryness, increased liver function tests, infection
Cytarabine	Conjunctivitis (with high-dose use steroid eye drops), rash, alopecia, anorexia, diarrhea, fever, malaise, nausea, vomiting, mucositis, myelosuppression, neurotoxicity (cerebellar toxicity, confusion, seizures, tremor), hepatotoxicity, thrombophlebitis
Daunorubicin and idarubicin	Cardiomyopathy (may be delayed), transient electrocardiogram changes, mucositis, myelosuppression, radiosensitizer, vesicant if extravasated, nausea, vomiting, red discoloration of urine
Etoposide	Anaphylaxis, hypotension, irritant if extravasated, mucositis (with higher doses), myelosuppression, alopecia, nausea, vomiting
Mercaptopurine and thioguanine	Hepatotoxicity, myelosuppression, pancreatitis (mercaptopurine), sinusoidal obstruction syndrome (thioguanine), drug fever, alopecia, hyperpigmentation, rash, diarrhea, hyperuricemia, anorexia
Methotrexate	Nausea, vomiting, diarrhea, anorexia, mucositis, myelosuppression, neurotoxicity, rash or reddening of skin, renal failure, nephropathy, transient transaminitis
Mitoxantrone	Cardiomyopathy (may be delayed), arrhythmia, edema, fever, pain, fatigue, alopecia, nausea, vomiting, diarrhea, anorexia, mucositis, amenorrhea, myelosuppression, hyperglycemia, transaminitis, increased BUN, bluish discoloration of sclera, fingernails, and urine
Sorafenib	QT prolongation, hypertension, hand–foot skin reaction, hepatotoxicity, fatigue, headache, diarrhea

[a]This list is not inclusive but notes the more common or distinguishing toxicities of each agent.

courses of high-dose cytarabine-containing chemotherapy compared with one course in the post-induction period.[104] A clinical trial involving both children and adults with previously untreated AML found no difference in relapse rate, relapse-free survival, death in complete remission, or overall survival when patients were administered four versus five courses of chemotherapy (i.e., two vs. three courses of chemotherapy in the post-remission or consolidation phase).[105]

Considerable controversy still exists regarding the appropriate type and use of stem cell transplantation in children with AML in first remission (as a consolidating regimen). Complicating matters, international cooperative groups use various risk criteria and stratification to determine which patients should receive a transplant in first remission as part of post-remission or consolidation therapy. It is generally accepted that children with APL, Down syndrome, inv(16), or t(8;21) have considerably better outcomes than other patients with AML and that stem cell transplants in first remission could result in excess toxicity without a survival advantage.[1] Retrospective data suggest that allogeneic stem cell transplantation from a matched sibling donor provides a survival benefit over additional chemotherapy for patients with intermediate-risk AML. On the basis of these data, it is assumed that the same would be true for patients with high-risk disease (e.g., patients with deletions of 5q, monosomy 5 or 7, or more than 15% blasts remaining after the first course of chemotherapy).[106-108] It is possible that patients who receive a matched sibling transplant have a reduced risk of relapse without a corresponding improvement in overall survival.[15] The risk of secondary malignancy and the potentially severe toxicities incurred because of stem cell transplantation should be balanced with a significant survival advantage; to date, this transplant advantage is unclear in any subgroups of children with AML.[106-108]

MAINTENANCE THERAPY

Historically maintenance therapy has not played a role in the treatment of most types of pediatric AML.[109] However, there has been a long-standing interest in the use of maintenance therapies to prolong remission and improve survival.[110] Sorafenib, a multi-tyrosine kinase inhibitor, has shown promising results in adult *FLT3-ITD*-positive AML patients in the period after stem cell transplantation or who relapsed after hematopoietic stem cell transplantation, suggesting sorafenib may synergize with allogeneic immune anti-leukemic effects to induce remission.[111,112] Currently a phase III clinical trial by the Children's Oncology Group is evaluating the efficacy of sorafenib in addition to conventional chemotherapy for children with newly diagnosed, previously untreated AML. Patients with high risk *FLT3/ITD+* AML stratified to arm C will receive sorafenib maintenance therapy for 1 year.[113] Although early data showed maintenance therapy was important for maintaining remission with APL, recent data suggest that maintenance therapy in APL does not affect overall survival, particularly when arsenic trioxide is added in consolidation.[63,114-117] An ongoing phase III study is evaluating the combination of arsenic trioxide and all-*trans*-retinoic acid in newly diagnosed patients with APL as a means to reduce the exposure to anthracyclines and, as a result, to reduce the risk of late effects of anthracyclines in patients with a low risk of relapse and high risk of survival.[117]

CNS THERAPY

Unlike its role in the treatment of pediatric ALL, the role of CNS-directed therapy in pediatric AML is unclear. Most contemporary studies will include between two to six doses of intrathecal cytarabine for patients with CNS disease. The use of systemic high-dose cytarabine and idarubicin is thought to contribute to the treatment or prophylaxis of CNS disease in pediatric AML.[118] Up-front cranial irradiation is not widely used by various international cooperative groups and is not used for the treatment of pediatric AML in the United States.[1,119] It is used in some patients who do not clear leukemic blasts from the CNS after systemic and intrathecal chemotherapy.[5,12,14] In the setting of relapsed or refractory disease, triple-agent (cytarabine, hydrocortisone, and methotrexate) intrathecal chemotherapy may be used for CNS prophylaxis.[1]

SPECIAL EXCEPTIONS

CHILDREN WITH DOWN SYNDROME

Down syndrome is the most common inherited condition associated with AML in children younger than 19 years in the United States. These children have a 10- to 20-fold increased risk of developing some type of leukemia compared with children without Down syndrome.[28] About 10% of newborn children with Down syndrome or mosaicism may develop TMD. This incidence may be underestimated because the screening of blood counts at birth is not routine. In most patients, abnormal blasts will spontaneously disappear, and the remaining components of the blood count will normalize.[38] However, almost 20% of children with TMD will develop leukemia by a median age of 20 months; of those children, most will develop the M7 subtype of AML, or acute megakaryocytic leukemia.[28] One study documented that 16% of patients with TMD developed AML or myelodysplastic syndrome at a median time of 441 days (range, 118–1085 days).[38] As a result, children with Down syndrome have a 500-fold higher risk of developing acute megakaryocytic leukemia than do children without Down syndrome within the first few years of life.[28] Although not fully understood, it is thought that mutation in the GATA-binding protein 1 (globin transcription factor 1, or *GATA1* gene) on the X chromosome may be an initiating factor in the development of leukemia in patients with Down syndrome. This gene is responsible in part for normal erythroid and megakaryocytic differentiation. Mutations in this gene have been identified exclusively in Down syndrome–associated TMD and acute megakaryocytic leukemia.[26-28]

Children with Down syndrome are uniquely sensitive to chemotherapeutic agents active in the treatment of AML. Myeloblasts in children with Down syndrome and AML exhibit enhanced activation and reduced metabolism of cytarabine. These effects are likely the result of the mutant *GATA1* gene seen in these patients, which results in the increased expression of deoxycytidine kinase and cystathionine β-synthase together with decreased expression of cytidine deaminase.[60,120,121] This enhanced sensitivity is likely related to the greater treatment-related toxicity and mortality seen in children with Down syndrome. A reduction in the dosing of conventional chemotherapy—specifically, the omission of high-dose cytarabine (3000 mg/m²/dose in four doses) in favor of intermediate, fractionated dosing (100 mg/m²/dose every 12 hours for 8 to 10 doses)—may result in improved survival because of a reduction in treatment-related mortality.[122]

ACUTE PROMYELOCYTIC LEUKEMIA

Historically, APL has been treated with standard chemotherapy (cytarabine plus anthracyclines) in induction and consolidation/post-remission therapy, similar to other types of AML. Some studies have used daunorubicin as the anthracycline of choice, whereas other studies have used idarubicin or mitoxantrone. Tretinoin has been added to standard chemotherapy with success.[62,64] Tretinoin is recognized as the first molecularly targeted pharmacologic agent in the treatment of acute leukemias because of its ability to destabilize the *PML-RARA* complex, permitting the expression of genes that allow differentiation of the abnormal clone.[22]

Patients with APL treated with tretinoin may experience a specific set of adverse events in the first few days to weeks after beginning therapy. This condition, *retinoic acid syndrome*, may occur in 6% to 27% of patients and be more pronounced in children than in adults. Retinoic acid syndrome has been associated with increasing WBCs, fever, weight gain, dyspnea, pleural effusion, pulmonary infiltrates, and pseudotumor cerebri.[85] Characterized by increased intracranial pressure, visual abnormalities, and papilledema, pseudotumor cerebri may occur without other complications of retinoic acid syndrome and may be more common in children.[62,63,123] In some patients, renal failure, hypotension, and pericardial effusion may also occur. The mechanism of this syndrome is not well understood, but it is speculated to involve the release of cytokines from the APL cells undergoing differentiation.[84] The management of pseudotumor cerebri may require the dose reduction or discontinuation of tretinoin and the administration of corticosteroids, analgesics, and mannitol.[123] Dose modification of tretinoin should follow the specific protocol or clinical trial recommendations. However, it is common practice to hold tretinoin until symptoms resolve and then reinitiate at a 25% dose reduction. If tretinoin is tolerated for 1 week, then the dose can be re-escalated. If tretinoin is not tolerated, then it may be held again and reduced by another 25%. The use of acetazolamide and therapeutic CSF removal may also be considered. Medical management of the patient in the critical care unit is often required.

Improved outcomes through the years have been associated with intensive treatment with anthracyclines, including cumulative doses as high as 400–750 mg/m².[124] These higher doses of anthracyclines increase the risk of late cardiotoxicity in children and have led investigators to examine ways to reduce total anthracycline exposure.[22] Of particular interest is the utility of arsenic trioxide in the management of relapsed/refractory and children with newly diagnosed APL.[125-130] A recent cooperative

group clinical trial evaluated the effect of arsenic in the consolidation phase in lieu of an anthracycline-containing course with the aim of reducing anthracycline exposure while maintaining a high survival rate.[131] Preliminary data from this study of children with APL suggest that the substitution of arsenic in the consolidation phase has similar efficacy with respect to event-free and overall survival; in adult patients, the addition of arsenic significantly improved event-free and overall survival.[132] This trial also used high-dose cytarabine on the basis of data showing a higher event-free and overall survival together with a reduced relapse rate in patients receiving cytarabine plus daunorubicin.[131] Tretinoin is used in the maintenance phase together with chemotherapy.[22,63]

THERAPY FOR RELAPSED DISEASE

Survival after relapse is low. Only 21% to 33% of patients who receive chemotherapy for the treatment of relapse survive.[133-138] Agents that have been used in the treatment of relapsed disease include fludarabine, clofarabine, and cladribine as well as the agents used during the initial treatment of the disease (e.g., cytarabine, etoposide, daunorubicin, idarubicin, and mitoxantrone). Various combinations have been studied, including fludarabine plus cytarabine, fludarabine plus cytarabine and idarubicin, clofarabine monotherapy, clofarabine plus cytarabine, and clofarabine plus cytarabine and etoposide.[139-144]

The length of first remission is an important predictor of long-term survival.[134-136] An evaluation of prognostic factors for survival in children with relapsed AML found that the only independent variable associated with outcome was the time to relapse. Specifically, children who relapsed after a disease-free period of at least 18 months (1.5 years) had a statistically higher long-term survival, regardless of whether they received chemotherapy alone or chemotherapy plus stem cell transplantation.[134] Children with a late relapse had a 5-year survival estimate of 40% (standard error 10%), whereas those relapsing earlier (i.e., within 1.5 years from the end of previous therapy) had a 5-year survival estimate of 10% (standard error 5%).[134] Patients who receive a stem cell transplant after an early relapse can be expected to have a 56% chance of survival at 5 years compared with 65% at 5 years for late relapse.[138]

FUTURE APPROACHES

Future approaches to improving outcomes in childhood AML may include novel or targeted agents, enhanced supportive care techniques to support intensive chemotherapy, and further refinement of the role and timing of stem cell transplantation. Additional approaches should focus on a greater understanding of the biologic and genetic features of the disease that may be used for treatment and prognostic purposes. Agents under consideration include tyrosine kinase inhibitors (e.g., sorafenib) and liposomal doxorubicin/cytarabine.[113]

SUPPORTIVE CARE

Supportive care is critical to minimize toxicities and treatment delays. As for patients with other hematologic malignancies, patients with newly diagnosed AML must receive close monitoring and treatment for tumor lysis syndrome, infection, and various hematologic complications. *Clinical tumor lysis syndrome* is defined as laboratory findings of tumor lysis syndrome plus at least one of the following clinical complications: cardiac arrhythmias/sudden death, renal insufficiency, or seizures. Electrolyte abnormalities associated with TLS includes hyperkalemia, hyperphosphatemia, hypocalcemia, and hyperuricemia.[145,146] Clinical TLS has been reported to occur in 3.4% to 5% of children with AML; this percentage is slightly less than the incidence of tumor lysis syndrome in children with ALL (5.2%) and non-Hodgkin lymphoma (6.1%).[144] Children with newly diagnosed AML and a total WBC greater than 100×10^3 cells/mm^3 have been characterized as being at high risk of developing tumor lysis syndrome.[146] Tumor lysis syndrome can be prevented or managed through the aggressive use of hydration, electrolyte monitoring and prompt correction. Either rasburicase or allopurinol is used in the treatment of tumor lysis syndrome on the basis of risk of developing tumor lysis syndrome. Current evidenced-based guidelines recommend rasburicase for patients at high risk of developing tumor lysis syndrome.[146,147] Hematologic variables may require correction through packed red blood cell or platelet transfusions and, in some cases, exchange transfusions or leukapheresis. The Tumor Lysis Syndrome and Febrile Neutropenia in Children chapter provides further detail.

Patients with AML are at an increased risk of a variety of infectious complications because of prolonged periods of neutropenia. Patients with AML who develop febrile neutropenia should receive treatment with broad-spectrum antibiotics in a closely monitored inpatient setting.[148,149] Empiric antibiotics administered to the febrile, neutropenic patient with AML should at minimum include appropriate coverage for gram-negative enteric bacteria and viridans streptococci. Of note, patients who have recently received high-dose cytarabine are at increased risk of developing sepsis from viridans streptococci.[150] A retrospective analysis of the use of prophylactic antibiotics revealed that the use of cefepime and vancomycin can significantly reduce the risk of general bacterial sepsis as well as streptococcal sepsis.[151]

Pediatric cooperative group trial data show invasive fungal infection rates of 10%–27% per AML chemotherapy phase.[152] Because of the high risk of invasive fungal infection in patients with AML, many treatment protocols now recommend or require the use of an antifungal agent as prophylaxis. Recent data indicate pediatric patients with AML receiving antifungal prophylaxis during induction are at significantly reduced risk of infection-related mortality. This cohort was also found to have less exposure to gram-positive antibiotics and β-lactam antipseudomonal antibiotics.[151] The preferred antifungal agent for prophylaxis is generally accepted to be fluconazole (6–12 mg/kg/day; maximum 400 mg/day), when no known contraindication or drug interaction exists.[153] For patients age 13 years and older, posaconazole suspension 200 mg by mouth three times daily may also be considered—and is guideline-recommended—in settings with a high risk of mold disease; drug interactions and absorption issues must also be considered.[153] For patients who develop febrile neutropenia, broad-spectrum antifungal agents (e.g., caspofungin or liposomal amphotericin B) should be considered as empiric therapy.[149] For severe cases of sepsis or prolonged neutropenia, the addition of granulocyte colony-stimulating factors should be considered.[1] In some cases, granulocyte transfusions have been used.[154]

One of the greatest concerns for patients with cancer is the development of chemotherapy-induced nausea and vomiting (CINV). The introduction of serotonin-3 receptor blockers (e.g., granisetron, ondansetron, palonosetron) has improved the prevention and treatment of CINV.[155] These agents are now routinely used as front-line agents to manage this complication in children with cancer. Although dexamethasone is an effective antiemetic, many centers may avoid its use in patients with AML because of the potential to increase the already high risk of invasive fungal disease. In adult patients with CINV, the neurokinin 1 receptor antagonist, aprepitant, has significantly improved CINV management.[156] Aprepitant capsules have label approval by the U.S. Food and Drug administration for patients 12 years and older.[157-159] Aprepitant oral suspension has been approved for use in children 6 months of age and older.[160,161] However, the concern for potential drug-drug interactions cannot be ignored because of the effect of aprepitant as an inhibitor of the cytochrome P450 3A4 isoenzyme.[162]

LATE EFFECTS

All children who receive chemotherapy for the treatment of a malignancy should receive long-term monitoring. Long-term follow-up should include plans to monitor for treatment-related toxicities as well as disease recurrence. Children with AML who are in remission after treatment with chemotherapy are at an increased risk of developing several late effects, depending on the agents included in the treatment regimen. For any child who receives an anthracycline, long-term follow-up must include monitoring for cardiac toxicities, specifically left ventricular hypertrophy. Most children will require a vaccination "catch-up" schedule based on the time of diagnosis and the number of vaccines missed during the treatment period. Children who receive a stem cell transplant will require additional interventions, such as revaccination with any vaccines received before transplantation. Clinicians are encouraged to refer to the publicly available Children's Oncology Group *Long-Term Follow-Up Guidelines for Survivors of Childhood, Adolescent, and Young Adult Cancers* for additional information on the appropriate timing and selection of evaluation criteria and markers for survivors of childhood cancer.[163]

CONCLUSIONS

Childhood AML continues to be a difficult malignancy to treat. Merely half of patients with newly diagnosed AML can be expected to have a long-term survival. Significant progress in recent years has occurred in the treatment of APL, a subtype of AML. Survival in these patients exceeds that of other subtypes because of the development of targeted therapy for the specific genetic alteration seen in the disease. Although genetic associations have been seen in other patients with

AML, a successful targeted therapy has yet to be discovered. Further refinement and understanding of the genetic alterations responsible for disease development and progression are necessary for targeted drug development. Future clinical trials will focus on the treatment of childhood AML with various targeted therapies and other investigational agents, techniques to minimize the late effects of chemotherapy, and the role and timing of hematopoietic stem cell transplantation.

Patient Case | IDENTIFYING LEUKEMIA IN A PEDIATRIC PATIENT

A previously healthy 2-year-old girl presented to the clinic with a complaint of a persistent ear infection. She had been prescribed 2 courses of antibiotics (amoxicillin/clavulanate and cefixime) with no resolution of symptoms following completion of therapy. Her mother noted that the girl had been bruising more than usual over the past two weeks. Her mother also reported that she had become persistently fussy and irritable and refused to bear weight on her left leg. Results of a complete blood count suggested leukemia with anemia, thrombocytopenia, and leukocytosis with an absolute myeloblast count of 32,000 cells/mm³. The pediatrician referred the child to an oncologist for further evaluation and management.

Medical history: Gastroesophageal reflux; recurrent otitis media

Social history: Lives with both parents; has no siblings; has two indoor cats

Family history: Lung cancer (grandfather); no family history of childhood cancers or bleeding disorders

Medications: Ibuprofen 70 mg orally every 6 hours as needed for mild pain; famotidine 5 mg orally every 12 hours

Allergies: No known drug allergies

Vital signs: Tmax 100.8°F (38.2°C), HR 119 beats/minute, BP 108/61 mm Hg, RR 28 breaths/minute, peripheral capillary oxygen saturation 100%, Wt 14.2 kg

Immunizations: Up to date

Physical examination:

General: Fatigue, fever, activity change, and unexpected weight change

HEENT: No congestion, facial swelling, mouth sores, rhinorrhea, or sore throat

Pulmonary: No cough or wheezing

Cardiovascular: Regular rate and rhythm

Abdomen: Nontender and nondistended; positive for bowel sounds

Neuro: Alert and awake; cranial nerves intact

Musculoskeletal: Capillary refill < 2 seconds

Skin: Pallor; petechiae on left proximal arm

Hematologic: Adenopathy; bruises and bleeds easily

Laboratory findings:

Test	Result
Na	142 mEq/L
K	4.2 mEq/L
Cl	107 mEq/L
CO_2	20 mEq/L
BUN	12 mg/dL
SCr	0.38 mg/dL
Glucose	102 mg/dL
Ca (total serum)	9.7 mg/dL
PO_4	5.3 mg/dL
Mg	2.0 mg/dL
LDH	2819 U/L
Uric acid	2.3 mg/dL
WBC	61.72×10^3 cells/mm³
Hgb	3.8 g/dL
Hct	10.9%
Plt	25×10^3 cells/mm³
Albumin	3.8 g/dL
AST	46 U/L
ALT	28 U/L
γ-Glutamyltransferase	13 U/L

Cytogenetic studies: inv(16)(p13.1q22); del(6)(q14q21); del(7)t(7;7); positive for FMS-like tyrosine kinase 3 internal tandem duplications (*FLT3*-ITD)

Flow cytometry: Myeloblasts (52%) show the presence of a myeloid disease with granulocytic differentiation, consistent with acute myeloid leukemia (AML)

1. What risk factors have been associated with developing AML? What do the results of this patient's cytogenetic studies indicate regarding risk stratification?

Environmental exposures have been associated with the development of AML including benzene, organic solvents, herbicides, pesticides, petroleum products, maternal use of marijuana during pregnancy, and previous use or exposure to chemotherapy or ionizing radiation. Maternal consumption of fresh fruits and vegetables such as apples, berries, canned or dried legumes, onions, and soy products may increase the risk of infant AML. Certain chemotherapeutic agents have also been associated with the development of secondary AML include etoposide, topoisomerase II inhibitors (e.g., doxorubicin), and alkylating agents (e.g., mechlorethamine, cyclophosphamide). Finally, AML may also develop after an acquired predisposing condition, such as aplastic anemia or myelodysplastic syndrome.

In addition, risk stratification in AML can be determined by cytogenetics, indicating three general categories: low risk, high risk, and a third group with no low-risk or no high-risk features. Low-risk cytogenetics include t(8:21), inv(16) or t(16;16), *CEBPA* mutations, and NPM1 mutations. High-risk cytogenetics include t(6:9), t(8:16), t(16-21), chromosomes 5 and 7: monosomy 5, monosomy 7, and del(5q), and FLT3/ITD mutations (Box 2 shows more molecular abnormalities). This patient has inv(16) (p13.1q22), which is considered diagnostic for AML. It is also a molecular abnormality with a favorable prognosis.

2. Describe the induction treatment regimen for this patient, including relevant adverse effects of each chemotherapy agent.

Induction I therapy is commonly referred to as *ADE 10+3+5*. The patient may receive cytarabine intravenously 100 mg/m² every 12 hours on days 1–10, daunorubicin 50 mg/m² favorable on days 1, 3, 5, and etoposide 100 mg/m² on days 1–5. Common adverse effects of cytarabine include fever, diarrhea, palmar–plantar erythema, nausea and vomiting at higher doses, chemical conjunctivitis at higher doses, and rash. Adverse effects of daunorubicin include mucositis, myelosuppression, and most significantly acute and chronic cardiotoxicity. Dexrazoxane may be added to this chemotherapy regimen as a cardioprotectant, and is dosed as 500 mg/m² intravenously on days 1, 3, and 5, given immediately before the daunorubicin. The most common adverse effect of etoposide is hypotension during administration. Slowing the infusion can mitigate this effect. Long-term effects of etoposide include secondary malignancies, particularly AML. The median time between the primary malignancy diagnosis and secondary diagnosis is 2–3 years. Cytogenetic results are not often available at the time of treatment initiation. This patient's cytogenetics showed *FLT3*-ITD; based on this finding, it would be appropriate to add a tyrosine kinase inhibitor, such as sorafenib. In general, all patients will receive the same induction I therapy, and then will be stratified to higher risk treatment if determined to be high risk based on cytogenetics and response to induction I chemotherapy.

3. What supportive care, particularly infectious disease prophylaxis, should be provided for this patient?

There is a high risk of fungal infections in patients with AML with rates of 10%–27% reported in pediatric cooperative group trials. Because of this high risk, AML patients should be initiated on antifungal prophylaxis. The current guidelines recommend fluconazole. An appropriate regimen for this patient would be fluconazole 6 mg/kg orally daily. It is important to consider cytochrome P450 (CYP) 3A4 drug interactions when initiating azole therapy. Fluconazole is a CYP3A4 inhibitor, which interacts with sorafenib (a CYP3A4 substrate). Another appropriate option for antifungal prophylaxis is an echinocandin, such as micafungin. An appropriate regimen for this patient would be micafungin 1 mg/kg intravenously daily. In addition, prophylaxis for *Pneumocystis jirovecii* pneumonitis should be initiated for this patient. Appropriate options would include sulfamethoxazole/trimethoprim, pentamadine, dapsone, or atovaquone. Although bacterial prophylaxis is not currently recommended, it is important to consider the appropriate antibiotic choice if this patient experiences fever and neutropenia. Broad-spectrum antibiotics should be initiated for fever and neutropenia. Also adequate viridans streptococci coverage is needed because this patient is receiving cytarabine. Appropriate options include cefepime or ceftazidime plus clindamycin, among other options.

REFERENCES

1. Rubnitz JE, Gibson B, Smith FO. Acute myeloid leukemia. Hematol Oncol Clin North Am 2010;24:35-63.

2. Kaspers GJ, Creutzig U. Pediatric acute myeloid leukemia: international progress and future directions. Leukemia 2005;19:2025-9.

3. Pession A, Rondelli R, Basso G, et al. Treatment and long-term results in children with acute myeloid leukaemia treated according to the AIEOP AML protocols. Leukemia 2005;19:2043-53.

4. Creutzig U, Zimmermann M, Ritter J, et al. Treatment strategies and long-term results in paediatric patients treated in four consecutive AML-BFM trials. Leukemia 2005;19:2030-42.

5. Smith FO, Alonzo TA, Gerbing RB, et al. Long-term results of children with acute myeloid leukemia: a report of three consecutive phase III trials by the Children's Cancer Group: CCG 251, CCG 213 and CCG 2891. Leukemia 2005;19:2054-62.

6. Kardos G, Zwaan CM, Kaspers GJ, et al. Treatment strategy and results in children treated on three Dutch Childhood Oncology Group acute myeloid leukemia trials. Leukemia 2005;19:2063-71.

7. Entz-Werle N, Suciu S, van der Werff ten Bosch J, et al. Results of 58872 and 58921 trials in acute myeloblastic leukemia and relative value of chemotherapy vs allogeneic bone marrow transplantation in first complete remission: the EORTC Children Leukemia Group report. Leukemia 2005;19:2072-81.

8. Armendariz H, Barbieri MA, Freigeiro D, et al. Treatment strategy and long-term results in pediatric patients treated in two consecutive AML-GATLA trials. Leukemia 2005;19:2139-42.

9. Perel Y, Auvrignon A, Leblanc T, et al. Treatment of childhood acute myeloblastic leukemia: dose intensification improves outcome and maintenance therapy is of no benefit—multicenter studies of the French LAME (Leucémie Aiguë Myéloblastique Enfant) Cooperative Group. Leukemia 2005;19:2082-9.

10. Lie SO, Abrahamsson J, Clausen N, et al. Long-term results in children with AML: NOPHO-AML Study Group—report of three consecutive trials. Leukemia 2005;19:2090-100.

11. Quintana J, Advis P, Becker A, et al. Acute myelogenous leukemia in Chile PINDA protocols 87 and 92 results. Leukemia 2005;19:2143-6.

12. Ravindranath Y, Chang M, Steuber CP, et al. Pediatric Oncology Group (POG) studies of acute myeloid leukemia (AML): a review of four consecutive childhood AML trials conducted between 1981 and 2000. Leukemia 2005;19:2101-16.

13. Dluzniewska A, Balwierz W, Armata J, et al. Twenty years of Polish experience with three consecutive protocols for treatment of childhood acute myelogenous leukemia. Leukemia 2005;19:2117-24.

14. Ribeiro RC, Razzouk BI, Pounds S, et al. Successive clinical trials for childhood acute myeloid leukemia at St. Jude Children's Research Hospital, from 1980 to 2000. Leukemia 2005;19:2125-9.

15. Gibson BE, Wheatley K, Hann IM, et al. Treatment strategy and long-term results in paediatric patients treated in consecutive UK AML trials. Leukemia 2005;19:2130-8.

16. American Cancer Society. Cancer facts and figures 2019. Atlanta: American Cancer Society, 2019. Available at www.cancer.org/research/cancer-facts-statistics/all-cancer-facts-figures/cancer-facts-figures-2019.html. Accessed October 18, 2019.

17. Xie Y, Davies SM, Xiang Y, et al. Trends in leukemia incidence and survival in the United States (1973-1998). Cancer 2003;97:2229-35.

18. Gurney JG, Severson RK, Davis S, et al. Incidence of cancer in children in the United States. Sex-, race-, and 1-year age-specific rates by histologic type. Cancer 1995;75:2186-95.

19. Bhatia S, Neglia JP. Epidemiology of childhood acute myelogenous leukemia [Lange B. comment: progress in acute myelogenous leukemia: the one hundred years' war]. J Pediatr Hematol Oncol 1995;17:94-100.

20. Ross JA, Davies SM, Potter JD, et al. Epidemiology of childhood leukemia, with a focus on infants. Epidemiol Rev 1994;16:243-72.

21. Sandler DP, Ross JA. Epidemiology of acute leukemia in children and adults. Semin Oncol 1997;24:3-16.

22. Pui CH, Carroll WL, Meshinchi L, et al. Biology, risk stratification, and therapy of pediatric acute leukemias: an update. J Clin Oncol 2011; 29:551-65.

23. German J. Bloom's syndrome. XX. The first 100 cancers. Cancer Genet Cytogenet 1997;93:100-6.

24. Halperin DS, Freedman MH. Diamond-Blackfan anemia: etiology, pathophysiology, and treatment. Am J Pediatr Hematol Oncol 1989; 11:380.

25. Alter BP, Giri N, Savage SA, et al. Malignancies and survival patterns in the National Cancer Institute inherited bone marrow failure syndromes cohort study. Br J Haematol 2010;150:179-88.

26. Robison LL, Nesbit ME Jr, Sather HN, et al. Down syndrome and acute leukemia in children: a 10-year retrospective survey from Children's Cancer Study Group. J Pediatr 1984;105:235-42.

27. Zipursky A, Poon A, Doyle J. Leukemia in Down syndrome: a review. Pediatr Hematol Oncol 1992;9:139-49.

28. Massey GV, Zipursky A, Chang MN, et al. A prospective study of the natural history of transient leukemia (TL) in neonates with Down syndrome (DS): Children's Oncology Group (COG) study and POG-9481. Blood 2006;107:4606-13.

29. Alter BP, Giri N, Savage SA, et al. Cancer in dyskeratosis congenita. Blood 2009;113:6549-57.

30. Liew E, Owen CJ. Familial myelodysplastic syndromes—a review of the literature. Haematologica 2011;96:1536-42.

31. Rosenberg PS, Greene MH, Alter BP. Cancer incidence in persons with Fanconi anemia. Blood 2003;101:822-6.

32. Butturini A, Gale RP, Verlander PC, et al. Hematologic abnormalities in Fanconi anemia: an International Fanconi Anemia Registry study. Blood 1994;84:1650.

33. Dong F, Brynes RK, Tidow N, et al. Mutations in the gene for the granulocyte colony-stimulating-factor receptor in patients with acute myeloid leukemia preceded by severe congenital neutropenia. N Engl J Med 1995;333:487-93.

34. Phillips CL, Gerbing R, Alonzo T, et al. MDM2 polymorphism increases susceptibility to childhood acute myeloid leukemia: a report from the Children's Oncology Group. Pediatr Blood Cancer 2010;55:248-53.

35. Bader JL, Miller RW. Neurofibromatosis and childhood leukemia. J Pediatr 1978;92:925-9.

36. Shannon KM, O'Connell P, Martin GA, et al. Loss of the normal NF1 allele from the bone marrow of children with type 1 neurofibromatosis and malignant myeloid disorders. N Engl J Med 1994;330:597-601.

37. Bader-Meunier B, Tchernia G, Mielot F, et al. Occurrence of myeloproliferative disorder in patients with Noonan syndrome. J Pediatr 1997; 130:885-9.

38. Gamis AS, Alonzo TA, Gerbing RB. Natural history of transient myeloproliferative disorder clinically diagnosed in Down syndrome neonates: a report from the Children's Oncology Group Study A2971. Blood 2011;118:6752-9; quiz 6996.

39. Eden T. Aetiology of childhood leukemia. Cancer Treat Rev 2010; 36:286-97.

40. Korte JE, Hertz-Picciotto I, Schulz MR, et al. The contribution of benzene to smoking-induced leukemia. Environ Health Perspect 2000;108:333-9.

41. McBride ML. Childhood cancer and environmental contaminants. Can J Public Health 1998;89:S53-62, S58-68.

42. Spector LG, Xie Y, Robison LL, et al. Maternal diet and infant leukemia: the DNA topoisomerase II inhibitor hypothesis: a report from the Children's Oncology Group. Cancer Epidemiol Biomarkers Prev 2005;14:651-5.

43. Pui CH, Ribeiro RC, Hancock ML, et al. Acute myeloid leukemia in children treated with epipodophyllotoxins for acute lymphoblastic leukemia. N Engl J Med 1991;325:1682-7.

44. Le Deley MC, Leblanc T, Shamsaldin A, et al. Risk of secondary leukemia after a solid tumor in childhood according to the dose of epipodophyllotoxins and anthracyclines: a case-control study by the Société Française d'Oncologie Pédiatrique. J Clin Oncol 2003;21:1074-81.

45. Le Deley MC, Vassal G, Taïbi A, et al. High cumulative rate of secondary leukemia after continuous etoposide treatment for solid tumors in children and young adults. Pediatr Blood Cancer 2005;45:25-31.

46. Sandoval C, Pui CH, Bowman LC, et al. Secondary acute myeloid leukemia in children previously treated with alkylating agents, intercalating topoisomerase II inhibitors, and irradiation. J Clin Oncol 1993;11:1039-45.

47. Hijiya N, Ness KK, Ribeiro RC, et al. Acute leukemia as a secondary malignancy in children and adolescents: current findings and issues. Cancer 2009;115:23-35.

48. Socié G, Henry-Amar M, Bacigalupo A, et al., European Bone Marrow Transplantation–Severe Aplastic Anaemia Working Party. Malignant tumors occurring after treatment of aplastic anemia. N Engl J Med 1993;329:1152-7.

49. Ohara A, Kojima S, Hamajima N, et al. Myelodysplastic syndrome and acute myelogenous leukemia as a late clonal complication in children with acquired aplastic anemia. Blood 1997;90:1009-13.

50. Niemeyer CM, Baumann I. Myelodysplastic syndrome in children and adolescents. Semin Hematol 2008;45:60-70.

51. Bennett JM, Catovsky D, Daniel MT, et al. Proposed revised criteria for the classification of acute myeloid leukemia. Ann Intern Med 1985;103:626-9.

52. Vardiman JW, Thiele J, Arber DA, et al. The 2008 revision of the World Health Organization classification of myeloid neoplasms and acute leukemia: rationale and important changes. Blood 2009;114:937-51.

53. Arber DA, Orazi A, Hasserjian R, et al. The 2016 revision to the World Health Organization classification of myeloid neoplasms and acute leukemia. Blood 2016;127: 2391-405.

54. Razzouk BI, Estey E, Pounds S, et al. Impact of age on outcome of pediatric acute myeloid leukemia: a report from 2 institutions. Cancer 2006;106:2495-502.

55. Rubnitz JE, Lensing S, Razzouk BI, et al. Effect of race on outcome of white and black children with acute myeloid leukemia: the St. Jude experience. Pediatr Blood Cancer 2007;48:10-5.

56. Aplenc R, Alonzo TA, Gerbing RB, et al. Effect of race on outcome of white and black children with acute myeloid leukemia: a report from the Children's Oncology Group. Blood 2006;108:74-80.

57. Lange BJ, Gerbing RB, Feusner J, et al. Mortality in overweight and underweight children with acute myeloid leukemia. JAMA 2005;293:203-11.

58. Johnston DL, Alonzo TA, Gerbing RB, et al. The presence of central nervous system disease at diagnosis in pediatric acute myeloid leukemia does not affect survival: a Children's Oncology Group study. Pediatr Blood Cancer 2010;55:414-20.

59. Athale UH, Razzouk BI, Raimondi SC, et al. Biology and outcome of childhood acute megakaryoblastic leukemia: a single institution's experience. Blood 2001;97:3727-32.

60. Barbaric D, Alonzo TA, Gerbing R, et al. Minimally differentiated acute myeloid leukemia (FAB AML-0) is associated with an adverse outcome in children: a report from the Children's Oncology Group, studies CCG-2891 and CCG-2961. Blood 2007;109:2314-21.

61. Rao A, Hills RK, Stiller C, et al. Treatment for myeloid leukemia of Down syndrome: population-based experience in the UK and results from the Medical Research Council AML 10 and AML 12 trials. Br J Haematol 2005;132:576-83.

62. Al-Ahmari A, Shah N, Sung L, et al. Long-term results of an ultra low-dose cytarabine-based regimen for the treatment of acute megakaryoblastic leukemia in children with Down syndrome. Br J Haematol 2006;133:646-8.

63. de Botton S, Coiteux V, Rayon C, et al. Outcome of childhood acute promyelocytic leukemia with all-trans-retinoic acid and chemotherapy. J Clin Oncol 2004;22:1404-12.

64. Testi AM, Biondi A, Lo Coco F, et al. GIMEMA-AIEOP AIDA protocol for the treatment of newly diagnosed acute promyelocytic leukemia (APL) in children. Blood 2005;106:447-53.

65. Ortega JJ, Madero L, Martin G, et al. Treatment with all-trans-retinoic acid and anthracyclines monochemotherapy for children with promyelocytic leukemia: a multicenter study by the PETHEMA Group. J Clin Oncol 2005;23:7632-40.

66. Grimwade D, Walker H, Oliver F, et al. The importance of diagnostic cytogenetics on outcome in AML: analysis of 1,612 patients entered into the MRC AML 10 trial. The Medical Research Council Adult and Children's Leukemia Working Parties. Blood 1998;92:2322-33.

67. Raimondi SC, Chang MN, Ravindranath Y, et al. Chromosomal abnormalities in 478 children with acute myeloid leukemia: clinical characteristics and treatment outcome in a cooperative Pediatric Oncology Group study-POG 8821. Blood 1999;94:3707-16.

68. Marcucci G, Mrozek K, Ruppert AS, et al. Prognostic factors and outcome of core binding factor acute myeloid leukemia patients with t(8;21) differ from those of patients with inv(16): a Cancer and Leukemia Group B Study. J Clin Oncol 2005;24:5705-17.

69. Harrison CJ, Hills RK, Moorman AV, et al. Cytogenetics of childhood acute myeloid leukemia: United Kingdom Medical Research Council Treatment trials AML 10 and 12. J Clin Oncol 2010;28:2674-81.

70. von Neuhoff C, Reinhardt D, Sander A, et al. Prognostic impact of specific chromosomal aberrations in a large group of pediatric patients with acute myeloid leukemia treated uniformly according to trial AML-BFM 98. J Clin Oncol 2010;28:2682-9.

71. Klein K, Kaspers G, Harrison CJ, et al. Clinical impact of additional cytogenetic aberrations, cKIT and RAS mutations, and treatment elements in pediatric t(8;21)-AML: results from an international retrospective study by the International Berlin–Frankfurt–Münster Study Group. J Clin Oncol 2015; 33:4247-58.

72. Dimartino JF, Cleary ML. MLL rearrangements in haematological malignancies: lessons from clinical and biological studies. Br J Haematol 1999;106:614-26.

73. Rubnitz JE, Raimondi SC, Tong X, et al. Favorable impact of the t(9;11) in childhood acute myeloid leukemia. J Clin Oncol 2002;20:2302-9.

74. Schoch C, Schnittger S, Klaus M, et al. AML with 11q23/MLL abnormalities as defined by the WHO classification: incidence, partner chromosomes, FAB subtype, age distribution, and prognostic impact in an unselected series of 1897 cytogenetically analyzed AML cases. Blood 2003;102:2395-402.

75. Balgobind BV, Raimondi SC, Harbott J, et al. Novel prognostic subgroups in childhood 11q23/MLL-rearranged acute myeloid leukemia: results of an international retrospective study. Blood 2009;114:2489-96.

76. Zwaan CM, Meshinchi S, Radich JP, et al. FLT3 internal tandem duplication in 234 children with acute myeloid leukemia: prognostic significance and relation to cellular drug resistance. Blood 2003;102:2387-94.

77. Meshinchi S, Woods WG, Stirewalt DL, et al. Prevalence and prognostic significance of FLT3 internal tandem duplication in pediatric acute myeloid leukemia. Blood 2001;97:89-94.

78. Ostronoff F, Othus M, Gerbing RB, et al. NUP98/NSD1 and FLT3/ITD coexpression is more prevalent in younger AML patients and leads to induction failure: a COG and SWOG report. Blood 2014;124: 2400-7.

79. Bolouri H, Farrar JE, Triche T Jr, et al. The molecular landscape of pediatric acute myeloid leukemia reveals recurrent structural alterations and age-specific mutational interactions. Nat Med 2018;24:103-12.

80. Ho PA, Zeng R, Alonzo TA, et al. Prevalence and prognostic implications of WT1 mutations in pediatric acute myeloid leukemia (AML): a report from the Children's Oncology Group. Blood 2010;116:702-10.

81. Pollard JA, Alonzo TA, Gerbing RB, et al. Prevalence and prognostic significance of KIT mutations in pediatric patients with core binding factor AML enrolled on serial pediatric cooperative trials for de novo AML. Blood 2010;115:2372-9.

82. Goemans BF, Zwaan CM, Miller M, et al. Mutations in KIT and RAS are frequent events in pediatric core-binding factor acute myeloid leukemia. Leukemia 2005;19:1536-42.

83. Shimada A, Taki T, Tabuchi K, et al. KIT mutations, and not FLT3 internal tandem duplication, are strongly associated with a poor prognosis in pediatric acute myeloid leukemia with t(8;21): a study of the Japanese Childhood AML Cooperative Study Group. Blood 2006;107:1806-9.

84. Sievers EL, Lange BJ, Alonzo TA, et al. Immunophenotypic evidence of leukemia after induction therapy predicts relapse: results from a prospective Children's Cancer Group study of 252 patients with acute myeloid leukemia. Blood 2003;101:3398-406.

85. De Botton S, Dombret H, Sanz M, et al. Incidence, clinical features, and outcome of all-trans-retinoic acid syndrome in 413 cases of newly diagnosed acute promyelocytic leukemia. Blood 1998;92:2712-8.

86. O'Brien TA, Russell SJ, Vowels MR, et al. Results of consecutive trials for children newly diagnosed with acute myeloid leukemia from the Australian and New Zealand Children's Cancer Study Group. Blood 2006;107:1315-24.

87. Creutzig U, van den Heuvel-Eibring M, Gibson B, et al. Diagnosis and management of acute myeloid leukemia in children and adolescents: recommendations from an international expert panel. Blood 2012;120:3187-205.

88. Kaspers GJ. Pediatric acute myeloid leukemia. Expert Rev Anticancer Ther 2012;12:405-13.

89. Rubnitz JE, Inaba H, Dahl G, et al. Minimal residual disease-directed therapy for childhood acute myeloid leukaemia: results of the AML02 multicentre trial. Lancet Oncol 2010;11:543-52.

90. Creutzig U, Ritter J, Zimmerman M, et al. Idarubicin improves blast cell clearance during induction therapy in children with AML: results of study AML-BFM 93. AML-BFM Study Group. Leukemia 2001;15:348-54.

91. Fernandez HR, Sun Z, Yao X, et al. Anthracycline dose intensification in acute myeloid leukemia. N Engl J Med 2009;361:1249-59.

92. Carella AM, Berman E, Maraone MP, et al. Idarubicin in the treatment of acute leukemias: an overview of preclinical and clinical studies. Haematologica 1990;75:159-69.

93. Berman E, McBride M. Comparative cellular pharmacology or daunorubicin and idarubicin in human multidrug leukemia cells. Blood 1992;79:3267-73.

94. U.S. Food and Drug Administration. FDA statement on dexrazoxane. Available at http://web.archive.org/web/20131216191210/http://www.fda.gov/Drugs/DrugSafety/ucm263729.htm. Accessed October 18, 2019.

95. Shaikh F, Dupuis L, Alexander S, et al. Cardioprotection and second malignant neoplasms associated with dexrazoxane in children receiving anthracycline chemotherapy: a systematic review and meta-analysis. JNCI J Natl Cancer Inst 2016;108:1-11.

96. Tebbi C, London W, Friedman D, et al. Dexrazoxane-associated risk for acute myeloid leukemia/myelodysplastic syndrome and other secondary malignancies in pediatric Hodgkin's disease. J Clin Oncol 2007;25:493-500.

97. Barry E, Vrooman L, Dahlberg S, et al. Absence of secondary malignant neoplasms in children with high-risk acute lymphoblastic leukemia treated with dexrazoxane. J Clin Oncol 2008;26:1106-11.

98. Vrooman L, Neuberg D, Stevenson K, et al. The low incidence of secondary acute myelogenous leukemia in children and adolescents treated with dexrazoxane for acute lymphoblastic leukemia: a report from the Dana-Farber Cancer Institute ALL Consortium. Eur J Cancer 2011;47:1373-9.

99. Seif A, Walker D, Li Y, et al. Dexrazoxane exposure and risk of secondary acute myeloid leukemia in pediatric oncology patients. Pediatr Blood Cancer 2015;62:704-09.

100. Sánchez-Medina J, Gonzalez-Ramella O, Gallegos-Castorena S. The effect of dexrazoxane for clinical and subclinical cardiotoxicity in children with acute myeloid leukemia. J Pediatr Hematol Oncol 2010; 32:294-97.

101. Lamba JK, Chauhan L, Shin M, et al. CD33 Splicing polymorphism determines gemtuzumab ozogamicin response in de novo acute myeloid leukemia: report from randomized phase III Children's Oncology Group Trial AAML0531. J Clin Oncol 2017;35:2674-82.

102. Shinnick SE, Browning ML, Koontz SE. Managing hypersensitivity to asparaginase in pediatrics, adolescents, and young adults. J Ped Onc Nurs 2013;30:63-77.

103. Byrd JC, Dodge RK, Carroll A, et al. Patients with t(8;21)(q22,q22) and acute myeloid leukemia have superior failure-free and overall survival when repetitive cycles of high-dose cytarabine are administered. J Clin Oncol 1999;17:3767-75.

104. Byrd JC, Ruppert AS, Mrózek K, et al. Repetitive cycles of high-dose cytarabine benefit patients with acute myeloid leukemia and inv(16)(p13q22) or t(16;16)(p13;q22): results from CALGB 8461. J Clin Oncol 2004;22:1087-94.

105. Burnett AK, Hills RK, Milligan DW, et al. Attempts to optimize induction and consolidation treatment in acute myeloid leukemia: results of the MRC AML12 trial. J Clin Oncol 2010;28:586-95.

106. Alonzo TA, Wells RJ, Woods WG, et al. Postremission therapy for children with acute myeloid leukemia: the children's cancer group experience in the transplant era. Leukemia 2005; 19:965-70.

107. Horan JT, Alonzo TA, Lyman GH, et al. Impact of disease risk on efficacy of matched related bone marrow transplantation for pediatric acute myeloid leukemia: the Children's Oncology Group. J Clin Oncol 2008;26:5797-801.

108. Niewerth D, Creutzig U, Bierings MB, et al. A review on allogeneic stem cell transplantation for newly diagnosed pediatric acute myeloid leukemia. Blood 2010;116:2205-14.

109. Perel Y, Auvrignon A, Leblanc T, et al. Impact of addition of maintenance therapy to intensive induction and consolidation chemotherapy for childhood acute myeloblastic leukemia: results of a prospective randomized trial, LAME 89/91. J Clin Oncol 2002;20:2774-82.

110. Rashidi A, Walter R, Tallman M, et al. Maintenance therapy in acute myeloid leukemia: an evidence-based review of randomized trials. Blood 2016;128:763-73.

111. Metzelder S, Wang Y, Wollmer E, et al. Compassionate use of sorafenib in FLT3-ITD-positive acute myeloid leukemia: sustained regression before and after allogeneic stem cell transplantation. Blood 2009;113:6567-71.

112. Metzelder SK, Schroeder T, Finck A, et al. High activity of sorafenib in FLT3-ITD-positive acute myeloid leukemia synergizes with allo-immune effects to induce sustained responses. Leukemia 2012;26:2353-59.

113. Bortezomib and sorafenib tosylate in patients with newly diagnosed acute myeloid leukemia with or without mutations. Clinicaltrials.gov identifier: NCT01371981. Available at https://clinicaltrials.gov/ct2/show/NCT01371981. Accessed October 18, 2019.

114. Avvisati G, Lo-Coco F, Paoloni FP, et al. AIDA 0493 protocol for newly diagnosed acute promyelocytic leukemia: very long-term results and role of maintenance. Blood 2011; 117:4716-25.

115. Powell BL, Moser BK, Stock W, et al. Adding mercaptopurine and methotrexate to alternate week ATRA maintenance therapy does not improve the outcome for adults with acute promyelocytic leukemia (APL) in first remission: results from North American Leukemia Intergroup Trial C9710. Blood 2011;118:258.

116. Muchtar E, Vidal L, Ram R, et al. The role of maintenance therapy in acute promyelocytic leukemia in the first complete remission. Cochrane Database of Systematic Reviews 2013;3: CD009594.

117. Tretinoin and arsenic trioxide in treating patients with untreated acute promyelocytic leukemia. Clinicaltrials.gov identifier: NCT02339740. Available at https://clinicaltrials.gov/ct2/show/NCT02339740. Accessed October 18, 2019.

118. Reid JM, Pendergrass TW, Krailo MD, et al. Plasma pharmacokinetics and cerebrospinal fluid concentrations of idarubicin and idarubicinol in pediatric leukemia patients: a Children's Cancer Study Group report. Cancer Res 1990;50:6525-8.

119. Creutzig U, Zimmermann M, Bourquin JP, et al. CNS irradiation in pediatric acute myeloid leukemia: equal results by 12 or 18 Gy in studies AML-BFM98 and 2004. Pediatr Blood Cancer 2011;57:986-92.

120. Ge Y, Jensen TL, Stout ML, et al. The role of cytidine deaminase and GATA1 mutations in the increased cytosine arabinoside sensitivity of Down syndrome myeloblasts and leukemia cell lines. Cancer Res 2004;64:728-35.

121. Ge Y, Stout ML, Tatman DA, et al. GATA1, cytidine deaminase, and the high cure rate of Down syndrome children with acute megakaryocytic leukemia. J Natl Cancer Inst 2005;97:226-31.

122. Sorrell AD, Alonzo TA, Hilden JM, et al. Favorable survival maintained in children who have myeloid leukemia associated with Down syndrome used with reduced-dose chemotherapy on Children's Oncology Group trial A2971: a report from the Children's Oncology Group. Cancer 2012;118:4806-14.

123. Sanz MA, Tallman MS, Lo Coco F. Tricks of the trade for the appropriate management of newly diagnosed acute promyelocytic leukemia. Blood 2005;105:3019-25.

124. Sanz MA, Grimwade D, Tallman MS, et al. Management of acute promyelocytic leukemia: recommendations from an expert panel on behalf of the European Leukemia Net. Blood 2009;113:1875-91.

125. Niu C, Yan H, Yu T, et al. Studies on treatment of acute promyelocytic leukemia with arsenic trioxide: remission induction, follow-up, and molecular monitoring in 11 newly diagnosed and 47 relapsed acute promyelocytic leukemia patients. Blood 1999;94:3315-24.

126. Shen ZX, Chen GQ, Ni JH, et al. Use of arsenic trioxide (As2O3) in the treatment of acute promyelocytic leukemia (APL) II: clinical efficacy and pharmacokinetics in relapsed patients. Blood 1997;89:3354-60.

127. Soignet SL, Frankel SR, Douer D, et al. United States multicenter study of arsenic trioxide in relapsed acute promyelocytic leukemia. J Clin Oncol 2001;19:3852-60.

128. Zhang L, Zhu X, Zou Y, et al. Effect of arsenic trioxide on the treatment of children with newly diagnosed acute promyelocytic leukemia in China. Int J Hematol 2011;93:199-205.

129. Zhou J, Zhang Y, Li J, et al. Single-agent arsenic trioxide in the treatment of children with newly diagnosed acute promyelocytic leukemia. Blood 2010;115:1697-702.

130. Gore SD, Gojo I, Sekeres MA, et al. Single cycle of arsenic trioxide-based consolidation chemotherapy spares anthracycline exposure in the primary management of acute promyelocytic leukemia. J Clin Oncol 2010;28:1047-53.

131. Adès L, Chevret S, Raffoux E, et al. Is cytarabine useful in the treatment of acute promyelocytic leukemia? Results of a randomized trial from the European Acute Promyelocytic Leukemia Group. J Clin Oncol 2006;24:5703-10.

132. Powell BL, Moser B, Stock W, et al. Effect of consolidation with arsenic trioxide (As2O3) on event-free survival (EFS) and overall survival (OS) among patients with newly diagnosed acute promyelocytic leukemia (APL): North American Intergroup Protocol C9710. J Clin Oncol [2007 ASCO Annual Meeting Proceedings, part I] 2007;25:2.

133. Webb DK, Wheatley K, Harrison G, et al. Outcome for children with relapsed acute myeloid leukaemia following initial therapy in the Medical Research Council (MRC) AML 10 trial. MRC Childhood Leukaemia Working Party. Leukemia 1999;13:25-31.

134. Stahnke K, Boos J, Bender-Gotze C, et al. Duration of first remission predicts remission rates and long-term survival in children with relapsed acute myelogenous leukemia. Leukemia 1998;12:1534-8.

135. Aladjidi N, Auvrignon A, Leblanc T, et al. Outcome in children with relapsed acute myeloid leukemia after initial treatment with the French Leucémie Aiguë Myéloïde Enfant (LAME) 89/91 protocol of the French Society of Pediatric Hematology and Immunology. J Clin Oncol 2003; 21:4377-85.

136. Wells RJ, Adams MT, Alonzo TA, et al. Mitoxantrone and cytarabine induction, high-dose cytarabine, and etoposide intensification for pediatric patients with relapsed or refractory acute myeloid leukemia: Children's Cancer Group Study 2951. J Clin Oncol 2003;21:2940-7.

137. Rubnitz JE, Razzouk BI, Lensing S, et al. Prognostic factors and outcome of recurrence in childhood acute myeloid leukemia. Cancer 2007;109:157-63.

138. Abrahamsson J, Clausen N, Gustafsson G, et al. Improved outcome after relapse in children with acute myeloid leukaemia. Br J Haematol 2007;136:222-36.

139. Leahey A, Kelly K, Rorke L, et al. A phase I/II study of idarubicin with continuous infusion fludarabine (F-ara-A) and cytarabine (ara-C) for refractory or recurrent pediatric acute myeloid leukemia (AML). J Pediatr Hematol Oncol 1997;19:304-8.

140. Montillo M, Mirto S, Petti C, et al. Fludarabine, cytarabine, and G-CSF (FLAG) for the treatment of poor risk acute myeloid leukemia. Am J Hematol 1998;58:105-9.

141. Jeha S, Razzouk B, Rytting M, et al. Phase II study of clofarabine in pediatric patients with refractory or relapsed acute myeloid leukemia. J Clin Oncol 2009;27:4392-7.

142. Hijiya N, Gaynon P, Barry E, et al. A multi-center phase I study of clofarabine, etoposide and cyclophosphamide in combination in pediatric patients with refractory or relapsed acute leukemia. Leukemia 2009;23:2259-64.

143. Sander A, Zimmerman M, Dworzak M, et al. Consequent and intensified relapse therapy improved survival in pediatric AML: results of relapse treatment in 379 patients of three consecutive AML-BFM trials. Leukemia 2010;24:1422-8.

144. Ravandi F, Cortes JE, Jones D, et al. Phase I/II study of combination therapy with sorafenib, idarubicin, and cytarabine in younger patients with acute myeloid leukemia. J Clin Oncol 2010;28:1856-62.

145. Coiffier B, Altman A, Pui CH, et al. Guidelines for the management of pediatric and adult tumor lysis syndrome: an evidence-based review. J Clin Oncol 2008;26:2767-78.

146. Cairo M, Coiffier B, Reiter A , et al. Recommendations for the evaluation of risk and prophylaxis of tumour lysis syndrome (TLS) in adults and children with malignant diseases: an expert TLS panel consensus. Br J Haematol 2010;149:578-86.

147. Jones G, Will A, Jackson G, et al. Guidelines for the management of tumour lysis syndrome in adults and children with haematological malignancies on behalf of the British Committee for Standards in Haematology. Br J Haematol 2015;169:661-71.

148. Freifeld AG, Bow EJ, Sepkowitz KA, et al. Clinical practice guideline for the use of antimicrobial agents in neutropenic patients with cancer: 2010 update by the Infectious Diseases Society of America. Clin Infect Dis 2011;52:e56-93.

149. Lehrnbecher T, Phillips R, Alexander S, et al. Guideline for the management of fever and neutropenia in children with cancer and/or undergoing hematopoietic stem-cell transplantation. J Clin Oncol 2012;30:4427-38.

150. Gamis AS, Howells WB, DeSwarte-Wallace J, et al. Alpha hemolytic streptococcal infection during intensive treatment for acute myeloid leukemia: a report from the Children's Cancer Group Study CCG-2891. J Clin Oncol 2000;18:1845-55.

151. Kurt B, Flynn P, Shenep JL, et al. Prophylactic antibiotics reduce morbidity due to septicemia during intensive treatment for pediatric acute myeloid leukemia. Cancer 2008;113:376-82.

152. Fisher BT, Kavcic M, Li Y, et al. Antifungal prophylaxis associated with decreased induction mortality rates and resources utilized in children with new-onset acute myeloid leukemia. Clin Infect Dis 2014;58:502-8.

153. Science M, Robinson PD, MacDonald T, et al. Guideline for primary antifungal prophylaxis for pediatric patients with cancer or hematopoietic stem cell transplant recipients. Pediatr Blood Cancer 2014;61:393-400.

154. Díaz R, Soundar E, Hartman SK, et al. Granulocyte transfusions for children with infection and neutropenia or granulocyte dysfunction. Pediatr Hematol Oncol 2014;31:425-34.

155. de Boer-Dennert M, de Wit R, Schmitz PI, et al. Patient perceptions of the side-effects of chemotherapy: the influence of 5HT3 antagonists. Br J Cancer 1997;76:1055-61.

156. Hesketh PJ, Grunberg SM, Gralla RJ, et al. The oral neurokinin-1 antagonist aprepitant for the prevention of chemotherapy-induced nausea and vomiting: a multinational, randomized, double-blind, placebo-controlled trial in patients receiving high-dose cisplatin—the Aprepitant Protocol 052 Study Group. J Clin Oncol 2003;21:4112-9.

157. Smith AR, Repka TL, Weigel BJ. Aprepitant for the control of chemotherapy induced nausea and vomiting in adolescents. Pediatr Blood Cancer 2005;45:857-60.

158. Gore L, Chawla S, Petrilli A, et al. Aprepitant in adolescent patients for prevention of chemotherapy-induced nausea and vomiting: a randomized, double-blind, placebo-controlled study of efficacy and tolerability. Pediatr Blood Cancer 2009;52:242-7.

159. Choi MR, Jiles C, Seibel NL. Aprepitant use in children, adolescents, and young adults for the control of chemotherapy-induced nausea and vomiting (CINV). J Pediatr Hematol Oncol 2010;32:e268-71.

160. Emend [package insert]. Whitehouse Station, NJ: Merck Sharp & Dohme Corp; 2016.

161. Jin Kang H, Loftus S, DiCristina C, et al. Randomized, placebo-controlled, phase III study of aprepitant in preventing chemotherapy-induced nausea and vomiting in children: analysis by age group. J Clin Oncol 2016;34:abstr 10579.

162. Jarkowski A. Possible contribution of aprepitant to ifosfamide-included neurotoxicity. Am J Health Syst Pharm 2008;65:2229-31.

163. Survivorshipguidelines.org [homepage on the Internet]. Children's Oncology Group. Available at www.survivorshipguidelines.org/. Accessed October 18, 2019.

CHAPTER 53

Tumor Lysis Syndrome and Febrile Neutropenia in Children

Joanie Spiro Stevens, Pharm.D., BCPS, BCPPS

LEARNING OBJECTIVES

1. Recognize the presentation of tumor lysis syndrome and febrile neutropenia in the pediatric population.

2. Describe risk factors for developing tumor lysis syndrome and febrile neutropenia.

3. Recommend the appropriate drug therapy to manage and prevent tumor lysis syndrome and febrile neutropenia.

ABBREVIATIONS IN THIS CHAPTER

ALL	Acute lymphoblastic leukemia
AML	Acute myeloid leukemia
ANC	Absolute neutrophil count
CYP	Cytochrome P450
ECG	Electrocardiogram; electrocardiographic
G-CSF	Granulocyte colony-stimulating factor
G6PD	Glucose-6-phosphate dehydrogenase
HSCT	Hematopoietic stem-cell transplantation
LDH	Lactate dehydrogenase
TLS	Tumor lysis syndrome
WBC	White blood cell

INTRODUCTION

An oncologic emergency is an acute condition caused by cancer or its treatment that requires an intervention to avoid death or permanent damage.[1] Tumor lysis syndrome (TLS) and febrile neutropenia represent two common oncologic emergencies that occur in pediatric oncology patients. *Tumor lysis syndrome* is defined as a group of metabolic derangements caused by rapid tumor cell death resulting in the release of intracellular contents into the bloodstream.[2] This syndrome occurs most often in patients with hematologic malignancies, which are the most common types of malignancy in pediatric patients.[3] *Febrile neutropenia* is defined as the presence of fever in a neutropenic cancer patient. The recognition of fever in these patients is essential because other signs and symptoms of infection are typically not present in the setting of chemotherapy-induced neutropenia.[4] Prompt recognition and treatment of TLS and febrile neutropenia are required to prevent significant morbidity and mortality. This chapter will review the presentation, management, and prevention of TLS and febrile neutropenia in the pediatric population.

TUMOR LYSIS SYNDROME

CLASSIFICATION

In 1993, Hande and Garrow developed a TLS classification system to distinguish patients with life-threatening clinical abnormalities from those with laboratory changes that do not require therapeutic intervention. They classified TLS into two categories: laboratory TLS or clinical TLS.[5] In 2004, Cairo and Bishop modified this system and further defined laboratory and clinical TLS as shown in Table 1. *Laboratory TLS* is defined as a change in two or more of the following: serum uric acid, potassium, phosphorus, or calcium; whereas *clinical TLS* is the presence of at least one clinical complication in addition to laboratory TLS.[6] Clinical complications include renal insufficiency, cardiac arrhythmia/sudden death, and seizure. Even after this modification a classification system is still not universally accepted.[2]

EPIDEMIOLOGY

The incidence of TLS varies depending on the patient's underlying malignancy and the definition used to classify TLS.[7,8] In absence of an accepted classification system, determining the true incidence of TLS is challenging.[9] The syndrome most often occurs in patients with hematologic malignancies such as non-Hodgkin lymphoma, Burkitt lymphoma, acute lymphoblastic leukemia (ALL), and acute myeloid leukemia (AML).[2] One study evaluated 1791 pediatric patients with non-Hodgkin lymphoma and reported the incidence of TLS to be 4.4% (78 patients). Subgroup analysis found the incidence highest among patients with either Burkitt lymphoma (8.4%) or B cell ALL (26.4%).[10] Although less common, TLS may also occur in patients with solid tumors.[2,3,9]

PATHOPHYSIOLOGY

Tumor lysis syndrome consists of several metabolic disturbances resulting from the rapid lysis of malignant cells. Cell lysis causes the release of intracellular contents, including nucleic acids, proteins, phosphorus, and potassium, into the bloodstream.[11] The rate of release can overwhelm the body's homeostatic mechanisms leading to the development of hyperuricemia and electrolyte disturbances including hyperphosphatemia, hyperkalemia, and hypocalcemia. Without recognition and management, TLS can progress to renal failure, cardiac arrhythmias, seizures, and death caused by multi-organ failure.[9]

Hyperuricemia results from the release and subsequent breakdown of nucleic acids into hypoxanthine and xanthine in the bloodstream. Xanthine is further broken down by xanthine oxidase into uric acid, as displayed in Figure 1.[2,12,13] Uric acid is cleared through the kidneys but is poorly soluble in water. Increasing amounts of uric acid will exceed the kidney's ability to excrete and may result in uric acid crystal formation within the renal tubules. Uric acid crystals can cause uremia, tubular injury, and renal insufficiency and failure. Uremia and kidney damage may also result from calcium phosphate precipitation, xanthine crystallization, infiltration of the kidney by the tumor, tumor-associated obstructive uropathy, drug-associated nephrotoxicity, and/or acute sepsis.[2]

Hyperphosphatemia is caused by the release of phosphorus from lysed malignant cells, which contain about four times the concentration of phosphorus found in healthy cells.[14] In an effort to maintain homeostasis, the kidney's tubular transport mechanisms will increase urinary excretion of phosphorus and decrease tubular resorption. When these mechanisms become overwhelmed, as in the case of acute renal dysfunction, hyperphosphatemia results.[15] Symptoms of severe

hyperphosphatemia include nausea, vomiting, diarrhea, lethargy, and seizures. In addition, increased serum concentrations of phosphorus increase the risk of calcium phosphate precipitation. These precipitates increase toxicity by depositing in the renal tubules, which worsen renal failure and further perpetuate the cycle.[2,16]

Hyperkalemia results from the rapid release of potassium from lysed cells and is worsened in the setting of renal failure or the administration of exogenous potassium.[17] Symptoms of hyperkalemia include muscle cramps, paresthesia, cardiac arrhythmias, ventricular tachycardia, fibrillation, and sudden death.[2,9,18]

Hypocalcemia occurs secondary to hyperphosphatemia and results from the formation of calcium phosphate precipitates. Symptoms of hypocalcemia include cardiac arrhythmias, hypotension, tetany, and muscle cramps.[2,18]

Table 1. Cairo-Bishop Definitions of Laboratory and Clinical Tumor Lysis Syndrome[2,6,7]

Laboratory TLS Defined by Serum Values[a]	Clinical TLS Defined by Clinical Conditions[b]
Uric acid ≥ 476 mcmol/L or 8 mg/dL Potassium ≥ 6 mmol/L or 6 mEq/L Phosphorus ≥ 2.1 mmol/L or 6.5 mg/dL Calcium ≤ 1.75 mmol/L or 7 mg/dL	Renal insufficiency (defined as creatinine ≥ 1.5 × upper limit of normal for patient age and sex) Cardiac arrhythmia/sudden death Seizure

[a]Laboratory TLS defined as the presence of ≥ 2 of the listed serum values outside the normal range or ≥ 25% change from baseline within 3 days before or up to 7 days after treatment initiation.
[b]Clinical TLS defined as the presence of laboratory TLS and ≥ 1 of the listed clinical conditions.
TLS = tumor lysis syndrome.

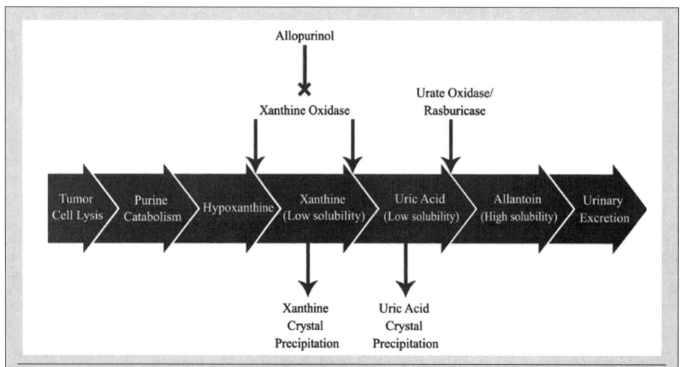

Figure 1. Purine catabolism.[2,3,23,24]

The lysis of tumor cells causes the release of cellular contents into the blood stream. Purines are released from the cells and catabolized to hypoxanthine, xanthine, and uric acid by the enzyme xanthine oxidase. Both xanthine and uric acid are poorly soluble in water. If the amount of uric acid exceeds the kidney's ability to excrete it, then uric acid crystals may develop, leading to kidney damage and potentially kidney failure. Allopurinol inhibits xanthine oxidase, which inhibits the conversion of xanthine to uric acid. Allopurinol leads to an increase in hypoxanthine and xanthine levels, which may lead to the precipitation of xanthine crystals and subsequent kidney injury. The enzyme urate oxidase is present in most mammals other than humans. The recombinant form of urate oxidase, rasburicase, can be administered to humans to convert uric acid to allantoin. Allantoin is much more soluble in water and is readily excreted through the urine.

CLINICAL PRESENTATION

Tumor lysis syndrome commonly occurs during the initial presentation of cancer or relapse. Patients may present with spontaneous TLS occurring before treatment initiation because of high tumor burden and rapid cell proliferation.[2,9] Others may develop TLS after initial exposure to chemotherapy, radiation, or steroids.[2,7] Patients may present with an array of symptoms, many of which are a result of hyperuricemia and electrolyte disturbances. These symptoms may include the following: nausea, vomiting, diarrhea, anorexia, lethargy, edema, fluid overload, hematuria, congestive heart failure, cardiac dysrhythmias, seizures, muscle cramps, tetany, and syncope.[2,18] Symptoms may be present before chemotherapy initiation but usually occur within 12 to 72 hours after the start of treatment.[2,3,19]

RISK STRATIFICATION

Factors contributing to increased risk of developing TLS include high rates of tumor-cell proliferation, large tumor burden, increased tumor sensitivity to chemotherapy, and increased concentrations of lactate dehydrogenase (LDH) on initial presentation of malignancy or relapse.[2,9,19] Concurrent complications such as renal insufficiency, dehydration, oliguria, hypotension, and acidic urine are associated with an increased risk for TLS.[2] In addition, certain cytogenetic mutations linked to more aggressive disease, such as the presence of *MYCN* amplification in neuroblastoma, translocation t(8;14)(q24;32) in ALL, or an inversion of chromosome 16 [inv(16)(p13;q22)] in AML, may increase a patient's risk for TLS.[8] Patients can be stratified into three risk groups for the development of TLS based on the type of malignancy, tumor burden (stage and LDH concentration), white blood cell (WBC) count, and renal function, as shown in Table 2.[2,19]

PREVENTION AND MANAGEMENT

Prompt recognition and management are critical to preventing potentially life-threatening consequences of TLS. Management consists of aggressive hydration, maintenance of adequate urine output, and interventions to correct or prevent hyperuricemia and electrolyte imbalances. Patients at low risk should be monitored but rarely require intervention. Allopurinol and hydration are recommended for these patients only if they develop metabolic derangements. Intermediate-risk patients should receive hydration and allopurinol as prophylaxis or treatment for TLS. Those at high risk should receive hydration and are recommended to receive allopurinol or one dose of rasburicase as prophylaxis.[2,19] Some institutions reserve the use of rasburicase for patients requiring treatment of hyperuricemia. Monitoring frequency of electrolytes, uric acid, creatinine, LDH, and urine output depends on the risk or severity of TLS. In patients being treated for hyperuricemia, monitoring is recommended as often as every 4 to 6 hours, depending on the patient's clinical condition and risk of TLS.[2] Monitoring should be continued until approximately 24 hours after the administration of the final agent of the first chemotherapy cycle.[2]

HYDRATION

Aggressive hydration is the mainstay of TLS prophylaxis and treatment. Increased hydration and urine output promote the elimination of uric acid and phosphate.[2] Hydration

Table 2. Risk Stratification for Tumor Lysis Syndrome[2,8,19]

Risk Stratification	Chance of Developing TLS	Type of Malignancy
Low[a]	< 1%	Indolent NHL Most solid tumors Slowly proliferating malignancies Diffuse large-cell lymphoma stage I/II Anaplastic large-cell lymphoma stage I/II AML + WBC < 25 × 10³ cells/mm³ + LDH < 2 × ULN
Intermediate[a]	1–5%	Burkitt lymphoma/leukemia + early stage + LDH < 2 × ULN Diffuse large-cell lymphoma stage III/IV + LDH < 2 × ULN Anaplastic large-cell lymphoma stage III/IV Rapidly proliferating malignancies ALL + WBC < 100 × 10³ cells/mm³ + LDH < 2 × ULN AML + WBC < 25 × 10³ cells/mm³ + LDH ≥ 2 × ULN OR WBC ≥ 25–100 × 10³ cells/mm³

High[a]	> 5%	Burkitt lymphoma/leukemia + early stage + LDH ≥ 2 × ULN OR
		    advanced stage
		Diffuse large-cell lymphoma stage III/IV + LDH ≥ 2 × ULN
		ALL + WBC < 100 × 10³ cells/mm³ + LDH ≥ 2 × ULN OR
		    WBC ≥ 100 × 10³ cells/mm³
		AML + WBC ≥ 100 × 10³ cells/mm³

[a]Presence of renal dysfunction and/or renal involvement increases the patient's risk to the next level (from low to intermediate risk or intermediate to high risk). ALL = acute lymphoblastic leukemia; AML= acute myeloid leukemia; LDH = lactate dehydrogenase; NHL = non-Hodgkin lymphoma; TLS = tumor lysis syndrome; ULN = upper limit of normal; WBC = white blood cell.

recommendations for pediatric patients are to administer 2 to 3 L/m^2/day (or 200 mL/kg/day for those weighing 10 kg or less) of dextrose 5% and one-quarter normal saline, unless the patient's clinical condition requires volume restriction (such as in acute kidney injury or cardiac dysfunction). Additional electrolytes should not be added because of the increased risk of hyperkalemia, hyperphosphatemia, and calcium phosphate precipitation.[2] If the patient develops hyperglycemia, adjustments to the fluid composition should be made accordingly.

It is imperative to maintain urine output between 80 to 100 mL/m^2/hour (or 4 to 6 mL/kg/hour for those weighing 10 kg or less) in pediatric patients at risk of developing or those receiving treatment for TLS.[6] If appropriate output is not achieved with hydration alone, then loop diuretics may be given unless the patient has an obstruction or is hypovolemic.[19] Loop diuretics are preferred because of their ability to induce diuresis and reduce potassium reabsorption. In addition to urine output, urine specific gravity should be monitored. Hydration should be adjusted to maintain the urine specific gravity at 1.010 or less.[6] The optimal duration of hydration has yet to be determined. The patient's ability to tolerate oral fluids and produce adequate urine output should be taken into consideration before discontinuing intravenous hydration.

Although historically used to promote uric acid excretion, urinary alkalinization is no longer recommended as part of TLS management. The rationale for urinary alkalinization was based on the fact that uric acid is more than 10 times more soluble at pH 7.0 than pH 5.0. Therefore, sodium bicarbonate was added to intravenous fluids to alkalinize the urine. The data evaluating this practice lack evidence of efficacy and show administration of saline alone equally effective as urinary alkalinization at reducing uric acid precipitation. The study also found increased urine flow rate to be the most effective strategy to prevent urate-induced obstructive uropathy.[2,20] Urinary alkalinization has also fallen out of favor because of the potential risk of increased calcium phosphate precipitation. Lastly, when sodium bicarbonate is administered to a patient receiving allopurinol, xanthine crystals can precipitate in the renal tubules because of the low solubility of xanthine at either pH.[2] Based on guideline recommendations, alkalinization should be reserved for patients requiring management of metabolic acidosis and is not recommended to prevent or treat TLS.[2,8]

DIALYSIS

A nephrologist should be consulted to assist with the management of a patient experiencing TLS in the event of oliguria, renal failure, or persistent hyperphosphatemia or hypocalcemia.[2] The number of patients requiring dialysis has decreased since the introduction of rasburicase; however, about 1.5% of pediatric patients still require dialysis.[21] Studies estimate that the average length of stay triples and medical costs increase 5-fold in patients who develop acute kidney injury requiring dialysis compared with those who do not.[22] The impact of acute kidney injury and the need for dialysis reinforce the importance of recognition and prevention of TLS.

CORRECTION OF HYPERURICEMIA

Whereas management of TLS starts with hydration, allopurinol and rasburicase are the two medications used to prevent and correct hyperuricemia in pediatric patients. The indications for their use vary based on their mechanisms of action and the patient's risk of developing or severity of TLS.

Allopurinol. The enzyme xanthine oxidase converts hypoxanthine to xanthine and xanthine to uric acid. Allopurinol, a xanthine analog, inhibits xanthine oxidase, thereby blocking the conversion of hypoxanthine to xanthine and, ultimately, xanthine to uric acid as shown in Figure 1.[23,24]

Efficacy. Since 1965, allopurinol has played an important role in TLS prevention and management by decreasing the incidence of obstructive uropathy.[23] In one study, the efficacy of allopurinol to treat TLS in pediatric patients was demonstrated with serum uric acid improvement and stabilization in 88% and 7% of patients, respectively. The mean time to treatment response was 1 day. When used prophylactically, 92% of pediatric patients did not experience an increase in serum uric acid concentrations.[25]

Dosing and duration of therapy. Allopurinol can be administered orally or intravenously. Oral administration is preferred unless the patient is unable to tolerate this route. Guidelines recommend reduction of the dose of allopurinol for renal impairment.[2] However, because the use of allopurinol to prevent or treat TLS is only for a few days and the most common and severe adverse effects of allopurinol are not dose related, the need for dose reductions have been questioned.[7] Table 3 provides the dosing recommendations and renal dose adjustments.

Allopurinol is recommended as prophylaxis in patients at intermediate risk of developing TLS. This agent may also be considered for prophylaxis in patients at high risk of TLS especially if rasburicase is unavailable. Allopurinol can also be used for the treatment of laboratory or clinical TLS in patients with a uric acid concentration less than 8 mg/dL. Allopurinol should be initiated 12 to 24 hours before the start of induction chemotherapy. Administration may be discontinued once uric acid concentrations and other laboratory values have normalized and the tumor burden and WBC count have decreased. This state usually occurs within 3 to 7 days after the start of chemotherapy.[2]

Limitations. Allopurinol works well to reduce the formation of uric acid but requires around 24 to 72 hours to do so.[2,26] In addition, allopurinol is unable to reduce concentrations of existing uric acid. It is important to consider the limitations of allopurinol, the time to effect, and the patient's clinical condition when determining which therapy is best. Also, by blocking xanthine oxidase, the administration of allopurinol causes an increase in hypoxanthine and xanthine. The low solubility of xanthine and increased concentrations can lead to xanthine crystal precipitation in the renal tubules and, ultimately, obstructive nephropathy.[13,27,28]

Adverse effects. The most common adverse effect of allopurinol is the development of a hypersensitivity reaction that may manifest as a rash or fever. Allopurinol is contraindicated in those with a known allergy to allopurinol or who develop a severe hypersensitivity reaction while receiving allopurinol. Bone marrow suppression has been reported in patients concomitantly receiving cytotoxic medications but is uncommon when allopurinol is used for the short-term management of TLS.[2,29]

Drug interactions. Although the short duration of allopurinol administration will limit the risk for drug interactions, it is important to be aware of the medications that may interact with allopurinol and to take necessary precautions. Mercaptopurine degradation may be reduced when administered concurrently with allopurinol, resulting in higher serum concentrations of mercaptopurine and the active metabolites of azathioprine. If the combination cannot be avoided, mercaptopurine and azathioprine dose reductions by 66% to 75% are necessary when either is administered with allopurinol.[30,31] Loop and thiazide diuretics may increase the allergic or hypersensitivity reactions patients have to allopurinol. They may also increase the active metabolite of allopurinol, oxypurinol, resulting in an increased therapeutic effect.[31] Other medications that may interact with allopurinol include but are not limited to the following: amoxicillin,

ampicillin, cyclosporine, cyclophosphamide, and high-dose methotrexate.[2]

Rasburicase. The enzyme urate oxidase converts uric acid into allantoin, which is 5 to 10 times more soluble in urine. Although urate oxidase is present in most mammals, it is not present in humans. Rasburicase is a recombinant urate oxidase enzyme produced by a genetically modified yeast strain, *Saccharomyces cerevisiae.*[32] Before the development of rasburicase, a nonrecombinant form of urate oxidase was available in Europe, but it was associated with hypersensitivity reactions and has since been replaced by rasburicase.[33] Unlike allopurinol, which helps prevent future production of uric acid, rasburicase reduces the amount of existing uric acid, as shown in Figure 1.[34]

Efficacy. The United States Food and Drug Administration approved rasburicase in 2002 for use in pediatric patients as part of initial management of elevated uric acid concentrations. In one study, pediatric patients treated with rasburicase experienced an 86% decrease in their uric acid concentrations

Table 3. Antihyperuricemic Agents Used in Pediatric Patients[2,19,25,29,31,32]

Variable	Allopurinol	Rasburicase
Mechanism of action	Inhibits xanthine oxidase, thereby decreasing uric acid formation by blocking the conversion of hypoxanthine to xanthine, and ultimately xanthine to uric acid	Recombinant urate oxidase enzyme that converts uric acid into more soluble allantoin
Dose	50–100 mg/m^2/dose PO every 8 hr or 10 mg/kg/day PO divided every 8 hr (max daily dose 800 mg) 200–400 mg/m^2/day IV over ≥ 30 min divided in 1–3 doses (max dose 300 mg; max daily dose 600 mg)	0.1–0.2 mg/kg IV over 30 min every 24 hr for 1–5 days Single fixed doses of 1.5–7.5 mg have been used in adults
Renal dose adjustment	GFR 10–50 mL/min/m^2 = 50% dose GFR < 10 mL/min/m^2 = 30% dose Dialysis CRRT = 50% dose HD or PD = 30% dose	Not required
Place in therapy	Prophylaxis: LR (if needed), IR, HR Treatment: Uric acid < 8 mg/dL	Prophylaxis: IR (if patient intolerant to allopurinol), HR Treatment: Uric acid ≥ 8 mg/dL
Monitoring	No special monitoring required	Serum uric acid samples must be collected in pre-chilled tubes containing heparin, kept on ice, and tested within 4 hr of collection
Common adverse effects	Hypersensitivity reactions (fever, rash)	Vomiting, nausea, fever, peripheral edema, anxiety, headache, abdominal pain, and increased alanine aminotransferase
Drug interactions	Mercaptopurine, azathioprine, loop diuretics, thiazide diuretics, amoxicillin, ampicillin, cyclosporine cyclophosphamide, high-dose methotrexate	No clinically relevant interactions
Notes	Contraindicated in patients with known allergy to or who develop severe hypersensitivity to allopurinol	Time to effect is within 4 hr from initial administration Contraindicated in patients with G6PD deficiency

CRRT = continuous renal replacement therapy; G6PD = glucose-6-phosphate dehydrogenase; GFR = glomerular filtration rate; HD = hemodialysis; HR = high risk; IR = intermediate risk; IV = intravenous; LR = low risk; max = maximum; PD = peritoneal dialysis; PO = oral.

within 4 hours of the first dose, compared with a 12% decrease in patients treated with allopurinol.[35] Another study reported dramatic reductions in uric acid concentrations after rasburicase administration in patients up to age 20 years presenting with either hyperuricemia or uric acid concentrations within normal limits who were at risk of developing hyperuricemia. Median reductions reported were 9.7 mg/dL to 1 mg/dL and 4.3 mg/dL to 0.5 mg/dL, respectively. These reductions persisted throughout the treatment period.[36] In addition to reductions in uric acid concentrations, these studies also reported reductions in serum creatinine and/or phosphorus concentrations after the administration of rasburicase.[2,35,36]

Dosing and duration of therapy. Rasburicase is recommended for patients requiring treatment for hyperuricemia associated with TLS, those at high risk of TLS, or those at intermediate risk who develop hyperuricemia while receiving prophylactic allopurinol administration.[2] The recommended dose of rasburicase varies depending on the reference used. The package insert recommends a dose of 0.2 mg/kg as a 30-minute intravenous infusion daily for up to 5 days; several studies have demonstrated efficacy using lower doses and shorter durations of therapy, generating significant cost savings.[2,32] Weight-based doses as low as 0.1 mg/kg have been used in pediatric studies.[19,37] A small study of eight patients age 18 months to 72 years evaluated the effect of a single dose of 0.15 mg/kg using actual body weight or adjusted body weight for obese patients, and rounded to the nearest vial size. The uric acid concentrations remained less than 4 mg/dL for up to 96 hours while the patients received chemotherapy, and a second dose of rasburicase was not needed.[38] Table 3 lists the dosing and administration recommendations.

An alternative dosing method that has been studied is the administration of a single fixed dose. A case report of three pediatric patients age 4 to 13 years demonstrated the effect of a single fixed dose of 4.5 mg of rasburicase to manage hyperuricemia in patients at risk of TLS.[39] Several studies evaluating the effect of a single fixed dose ranging from 1.5 to 7.5 mg have been reported in adult patients with varied success.[40-42] Some questions that still remain after the results of these studies include the optimal dose, dose adjustment in obese patients, the optimal time and dose if a second dose is needed, and the need for allopurinol after rasburicase administration.[2,40] Regardless of the method used, the lowest effective dose should be administered for the shortest duration of time. Additional doses may be administered once daily, as needed, for persistently elevated uric acid concentrations. Rasburicase should be discontinued when concentrations are within the normal range or undetectable.[2] Dose adjustments for renal impairment are not necessary with rasburicase.

The need for allopurinol after management with rasburicase is unclear.[26] Although the current guidelines for management of TLS in pediatric patients suggest that it is not necessary, no data are available to determine whether the addition of allopurinol after rasburicase leads to a better clinical outcome.[2]

Limitations. The use of rasburicase in patients with a known glucose-6-phosphate dehydrogenase (G6PD) deficiency is contraindicated. Administration of rasburicase to patients with G6PD deficiency can lead to hemolytic anemia, which is caused by the inability to break down the hydrogen

peroxide byproduct released when uric acid is converted to allantoin.[43] Because TLS can rapidly progress, it is not always possible to rule out G6PD deficiency before initiating rasburicase. It is important to obtain a thorough history of the patient, taking note of the patient's ethnic background and any previous occurrences of drug-induced hemolytic anemia, as well as family history of the deficiency.[2] Deficiency in G6PD has been found to be more common in male patients and those of African American or Mediterranean descent.[43] Close monitoring of a peripheral blood smear and complete blood count should be performed to identify hemolysis.[43] If identified, rasburicase should be permanently discontinued.[32]

Adverse effects. The most common adverse effects of rasburicase include vomiting, nausea, fever, peripheral edema, anxiety, headache, abdominal pain, and increased alanine aminotransferase.[32] Serious adverse effects have rarely been reported after the administration of rasburicase. Potential serious reactions include the following: anaphylaxis, rash, hemolysis, methemoglobinemia, fever, neutropenia, respiratory distress, sepsis, and mucositis.

Drug interactions. No clinically relevant drug interactions have been identified with the use of rasburicase.[31,32]

Monitoring considerations. Rasburicase has the ability to cause further degradation of uric acid at room temperature. Special handling of uric acid blood samples is necessary to prevent misleading laboratory results. A pre-chilled collection tube containing heparin should be used to collect serum uric acid samples. The samples must be kept on ice and tested within 4 hours of collection. The duration of time needed to continue this special handling procedure after a dose of rasburicase is unclear, but one source recommends continuing for 4 days after the last dose of rasburicase.[34]

Future agent. Febuxostat has not yet been approved for use in pediatric patients but has been studied in adults as an alternative to allopurinol for TLS prophylaxis in patients deemed to be at intermediate or high risk.[44] Like allopurinol, febuxostat is a xanthine oxidase inhibitor, but it is metabolized by the liver and does not require dose adjustments for patients with renal impairment.[7] Another benefit over allopurinol is the lack of hypersensitivity reactions with febuxostat use.[7] The FLORENCE study compared the efficacy of daily fixed dose febuxostat to three different doses of allopurinol in lowering of serum uric acid and creatinine concentrations. The study reported a sustained, significant difference in the reduction of serum uric acid in the febuxostat arm within 24 hours of treatment initiation. No significant difference was found in the degree of creatinine reduction between the two arms.[44] Febuxostat may represent an alternative to allopurinol for patients with renal dysfunction, hypersensitivity to allopurinol, or those requiring a rapid decrease in uric acid concentrations, but its cost compared with that of allopurinol will likely limit its use.[7] Further studies must be done to establish an effective dosing regimen in pediatric patients.

ELECTROLYTE CORRECTION

Patients can experience asymptomatic or symptomatic hyperphosphatemia. Management of asymptomatic hyperphosphatemia includes maintaining recommended hydration and eliminating additional sources of phosphorus through the administration of phosphate binders. Aluminum hydroxide is a commonly used phosphate binder, but use must be limited to 1 to 2 days to avoid cumulative aluminum toxicity. Alternative options include sevelamer hydroxide and calcium carbonate; the latter must be avoided in the presence of elevated calcium concentrations.[2] Severe, symptomatic hyperphosphatemia necessitates the use of dialysis because phosphate binders do not bind serum phosphorus. Hemodialysis has demonstrated better phosphate clearance than continuous venovenous hemofiltration or peritoneal dialysis.[2,45-47]

To prevent hyperkalemia, exogenous sources of potassium should be eliminated through the period of possible TLS development. Immediate intervention is needed if the potassium concentration exceeds 7 mEq/L or if a widening of the QRS complex is recognized on an electrocardiogram (ECG). Sodium polystyrene sulfonate is the recommended treatment for asymptomatic hyperkalemia. Symptomatic patients require more intense intervention, which may include rapid-acting insulin and glucose infusion. Sodium bicarbonate may be given as an alternative to insulin to drive potassium intracellularly. In the event of life-threatening arrhythmias, calcium gluconate may be administered by slow infusion with ECG monitoring.[2]

Hypocalcemia should only be treated in symptomatic patients. Treatment includes the administration of calcium gluconate slowly with continuous ECG monitoring. When clinically indicated, the smallest effective calcium replacement dose should be used to decrease the risk of calcium phosphate precipitation and subsequent development of obstructive uropathy.[2,6]

CONCLUSIONS

Tumor lysis syndrome is one of the most common oncologic emergencies and requires prompt recognition and management to prevent severe morbidity and mortality. Risk of TLS is highest before and within the first few days of treatment initiation. Familiarity with the risk factors and options for prevention and treatment are necessary for pharmacists involved in the management of pediatric oncology patients.

FEBRILE NEUTROPENIA

DEFINITION

The definition of febrile neutropenia is consistent among adult and pediatric patients. Guidelines define *fever* as a single oral temperature of at least 101°F (38.3°C) or a sustained temperature of 100.4°F (38°C) or greater for 1 hour.[4,48] To define febrile neutropenia, it is necessary to understand how to calculate the absolute neutrophil count (ANC). The ANC quantifies the number of WBCs that are neutrophils. To calculate ANC, the number of WBCs is multiplied by the percentage of granulocytes, which are made up of segmented neutrophils and bands. *Neutropenia* is defined as an ANC less than 500 cells/mm³ or expected to decrease to less than 500 cells/mm³ during the next 48 hours.[4] *Severe neutropenia* is defined

as an ANC less than 100 cells/mm³. The *nadir* refers to the lowest value to which blood counts fall after the administration of chemotherapy. Depending on the type of chemotherapy administered, the nadir is reached around 10 to 14 days after chemotherapy.[49] During the period of neutropenia, as the ANC falls to its nadir and slowly recovers, the patient is at increased risk for developing an infection.

EPIDEMIOLOGY

The incidence of febrile neutropenia is higher in hematologic malignancies than in solid tumors. About 80% of patients with hematologic malignancies and 10% to 50% of patients with solid tumors will develop febrile neutropenia during at least one cycle of chemotherapy.[4,50]

CLINICAL PRESENTATION

Fever is often the only sign of infection in neutropenic patients because of the body's inability to mount a robust immune response given the lack of neutrophils. Other symptoms are rare but may include the following: erythema, dysuria, cough, dyspnea, or localized pain or tenderness. Patients may present with signs of clinical instability such as hypotension, tachycardia, mental status changes, or organ dysfunction.[4,48]

DIAGNOSIS

Diagnostic workup for patients presenting with febrile neutropenia should include the following: physical examination, blood cultures, chest radiography (if the patient presents with respiratory signs or symptoms), complete blood count, basic metabolic panel, liver function tests, urinalysis, and urine culture.[4,48] Many pediatric cancer patients have a central venous catheter, which presents a potential source of infection. It is recommended to draw blood cultures from all lumens of a central venous catheter, if present. In an effort to balance the ability to detect infection against an increase in pain and potential contamination, the pediatric febrile neutropenia guidelines leave the decision to draw a peripheral blood culture, in addition to cultures from the central catheter, to the treating physician's discretion.[48]

ETIOLOGY

Neutropenia results from the administration of myelosuppressive chemotherapy. Fever may be caused by a bacterial, viral, or fungal infection or a noninfectious cause.[48] The most common source of infection is the patient's own flora, particularly in patients with indwelling central venous access.[4] Common sites of infection include the alimentary tract, lungs, sinus, and skin.[51] Catheters and central lines present increased risk for infection. Viral infections are common and should be considered when evaluating the patient.[48] Fungal infections are generally associated with prolonged neutropenia and should be considered after persistent fever beyond 96 hours of antibiotic treatment.[4,48]

About 50% of patients who develop febrile neutropenia will have an undetermined cause of infection.[52] One study evaluated the etiology of febrile neutropenia in 337 pediatric patients. A *proven infection*, defined as a pathogen identified by a laboratory test, was found in only 25% of episodes of febrile neutropenia. *Probable infections*, defined as clinical or radiologic findings of infections showing a rapid response to antimicrobials, were identified in 22% of patients. Most proven infections (63%) were bacterial infections, with bacteremia identified in 76%. Viruses were found to cause about one-third of febrile neutropenia cases, and fungi caused 2.4%.[52]

Per guidelines, the most common gram-negative pathogens identified include *Escherichia coli*, *Klebsiella* spp., *Enterobacter* spp., and *Pseudomonas aeruginosa*. Typical gram-positive organisms identified include: coagulase-negative staphylococci, *Staphylococcus aureus* (including methicillin-resistant strains), viridans group streptococci, and *Enterococcus* spp. (including vancomycin resistant strains).[4,51] Potential viral pathogens include herpes simplex virus, respiratory syncytial virus, parainfluenza, and influenza A and B.[51] Bloodstream infections caused by *Candida* spp. may result from the development of thrush in the setting of chemotherapy-induced mucositis.[4,51] Molds, such as *Aspergillus* spp., and other filamentous fungi, have severe and potentially life-threatening consequences for patients with severe and prolonged neutropenia.[51] Molds are typically found in the sinuses or lungs after 2 weeks of neutropenia.[4] Antibiotic resistant bacteria, fungi, and viruses are usually identified as the cause of subsequent episodes of febrile neutropenia.[51]

RISK ASSESSMENT

Treatment decisions are best determined by an assessment of the patient's risk of developing severe complications from infection. Adult patients are evaluated using the Multinational Association for Supportive Care in Cancer risk index.[50] Unfortunately, criteria in this validated tool do not apply to pediatric patients and therefore prevent its use in this population.

Although there is a lack of consensus regarding a standardized approach to risk assessment for pediatric patients, several studies have suggested validated risk stratification methods to identify pediatric patients at low risk of developing significant complications from infection.[48,53-59] Among the many stratification methods, the following factors are commonly considered when determining a patient's risk: *patient-specific factors*, such as age, malignancy type, and disease status; *treatment-specific factors*, such as type and timing of chemotherapy; and *episode-specific factors*, including maximum temperature, hypotension, mucositis, blood counts, and C-reactive protein. Patients receiving highly myelosuppressive treatment, such as treatment for AML, and patients undergoing hematopoietic stem-cell transplantation (HSCT) are excluded from the low-risk category. Pediatric guidelines recommend each institution adopt a validated risk-stratification scheme that applies to their patient population and can feasibly be implemented at the institution.[48]

One such stratification scheme that may be applicable to institutions in the United States is the method developed by Alexander et al.[48,55] Low-risk patients in this study were defined as those with anticipated neutropenia less than 7 days and no significant comorbidities at presentation. Anticipated neutropenia less than 7 days included patients who did not have AML, Burkitt lymphoma, ALL in induction therapy, or progressive or relapsed disease with bone marrow involvement. Significant comorbid conditions included hypotension, tachypnea or hypoxia (oxygen saturation less than 94% on room air), new infiltrates on chest radiography, altered mental status, mucositis requiring intravenous narcotics, vomiting, abdominal pain, evidence of a significant focal infection (tunnel infection, perirectal abscess, or cellulitis), or other clinical reasons beyond febrile neutropenia requiring inpatient treatment. Using these criteria, a significantly lower rate of adverse events was observed in the low-risk group at 4% versus 41% in the high-risk group (p<0.001) and no deaths in the low-risk group.[55] The results from this study and other studies demonstrate the ability to separate patients based on risk status and have led to the differentiation of treatment methods based on risk.[53-59]

TREATMENT

INITIAL

It is imperative to start empiric broad-spectrum antibiotics urgently (within 2 hours) in all patients presenting with febrile neutropenia immediately after blood cultures are drawn.[4] The goal of empiric therapy is to prevent morbidity and mortality caused by the most likely and most virulent pathogens while also reducing exposure to unnecessary antibiotics.[48] The choice of antibiotic therapy depends on the patient's risk status for complications of severe infections, clinical condition, history of resistant organisms, and the prevalence of bacterial resistance at the institution.[4] Treatment should be selected that covers for gram-negative organisms in all patients, as well as viridans group streptococci and *Pseudomonas aeruginosa* in high-risk patients, as shown in Figure 2.[48] Table 4 presents a list of antibiotics commonly used to treat febrile neutropenia.[31,60,61]

High-risk patients require hospitalization and empiric intravenous antibiotic therapy.[4] These patients should be initiated on monotherapy with an antipseudomonal β-lactam or carbapenem.[48] Several prospective trials have evaluated the efficacy of various empiric antibiotic regimens; however, no one regimen has demonstrated superiority.[48,62-64] The selected monotherapy regimen should be based on the patient's characteristics and clinical presentation, drug availability and cost, and the institution's resistance patterns. Monotherapy regimens that have been evaluated and recommended in pediatric patients include antipseudomonal penicillins (piperacillin/tazobactam), antipseudomonal cephalosporins (cefepime), and carbapenems (meropenem or imipenem/cilastatin). Because of increasing gram-positive and gram-negative resistance, ceftazidime monotherapy is no longer recommended.[48,65] Consideration should be given before selecting therapy with a carbapenem because study findings suggest use of carbapenems may be associated with a higher incidence of pseudomembranous colitis.[48,66] In addition, unless required, carbapenem use should be limited in an effort to decrease antimicrobial resistance.

Studies have failed to show a benefit with the routine use of combination therapy and have revealed an increased risk of toxicity.[48,62-64,67] The addition of vancomycin or a second gram-negative agent should be reserved for clinically unstable patients, those with an increased risk of resistant organisms, or patients in centers with high rates of resistant pathogens.[48] Antibiotics with activity against aerobic gram-positive cocci, such as vancomycin, should be considered for patients with suspected catheter-related infections, skin and soft tissue infections, pneumonia, or hemodynamic instability.[4]

Close attention must be paid to identify resistant organisms. If a patient becomes clinically unstable or has a blood culture positive for resistant bacteria, modifications must be made to the patient's treatment regimen; Table 5 shows the treatment recommendations. Previous infection or colonization with a resistant organism or treatment in an institution with high rates of resistance are risk factors for resistant organisms and should be considered when selecting treatment for a patient. Use of the institution's antibiogram is necessary to help guide therapy selection, especially when resistant organisms are of concern.

Low-risk patients may be managed in the inpatient or outpatient setting depending on the infrastructure in place to ensure careful monitoring and follow-up.[48] One study compared the inpatient and outpatient administration of cefepime and found equal length of fever duration and no serious adverse events between groups.[68] Study results show an increase in quality of life, a large reduction in costs, and similar rates of treatment failure and mortality with outpatient management compared with those treated as inpatients.[68-74] To successfully manage patients on an outpatient basis, patients and their families must understand the need to immediately seek medical attention if the patient's clinical condition worsens.

Treatment with oral antibiotics may also be considered for patients at low risk. Consideration must be given to the following factors before making the selection of oral therapy: availability of the medication as a liquid if the patient cannot swallow tablets or capsules, palatability of the formulation, ability of the patient to adhere to the dosing regimen, presence of mucositis, and presence of impaired gastrointestinal absorption.[48] Several trials have found no significant difference in the rates of treatment failure, overall mortality, or antibiotic adverse effects when oral antibiotic therapies were

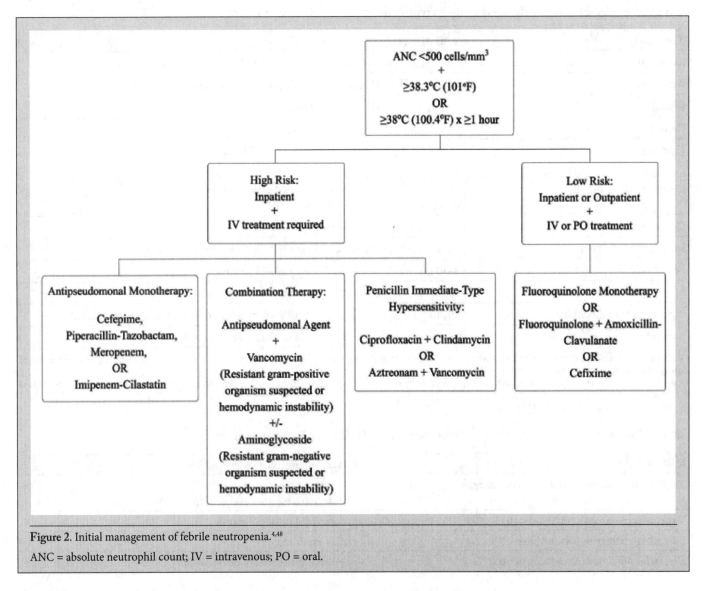

Figure 2. Initial management of febrile neutropenia.[4,48]

ANC = absolute neutrophil count; IV = intravenous; PO = oral.

compared with parenteral options.[69,72,75] Fluoroquinolone monotherapy, combination therapy with a fluoroquinolone and amoxicillin-clavulanate, and cefixime have all been evaluated for use as oral options and demonstrated no significant differences in treatment failure or infection-related deaths.[69]

Most patients with an allergy to penicillin will tolerate cephalosporins, unless the allergic reaction consists of immediate-type hypersensitivity, such as anaphylaxis or hives. In this case, both β-lactams and carbapenems should be avoided because they have a similar incidence of cross-reactivity. A combination regimen of ciprofloxacin and clindamycin or aztreonam and vancomycin may be used.[4]

BEYOND 24 TO 72 HOURS

Initial empiric therapy selection should be reevaluated within the first 24 to 72 hours after treatment initiation. If added, vancomycin or double coverage for gram-negative organisms should be discontinued after 24 to 72 hours of therapy if the patient is responding to treatment and there is no indication for the added therapy based on culture results.[48] Therapy should be modified if the causative organism or source of infection is identified, if the infection site worsens, or if the patient develops hypotension or other signs of clinical instability.[48] In the setting of clinical instability, the regimen should be broadened to ensure coverage for resistant gram-negative, gram-positive, and anaerobic bacteria.[4,48,62] Consideration of nonbacterial causes such as viruses and fungi is also necessary.[48] Based on culture and susceptibility results and the patient's clinical response, antibiotics should be de-escalated to decrease potential adverse effects and minimize the development of resistance. Figure 3 and Figure 4 outline the management for high- and low-risk patients, respectively, after the initiation of empiric therapy.

PERSISTENT FEVER

Therapy adjustment for persistent fever in the absence of other symptoms or microbiologic culture results represents an area of controversy. Evidence of improved clinical outcomes after the escalation of antibiotic therapy caused by fever alone is lacking.[76] The guidelines recommend adjusting therapy for patients with persistent fevers who either become unstable or have new culture results.[4,48] Regardless of the therapy selected,

Table 4. Antibiotics Frequently Used for the Treatment of Febrile Neutropenia[31,60,61]

Antibiotic	Pediatric Dosage[a,b]
Amoxicillin-clavulanate	40–50 mg/kg/day PO divided every 8–12 hr (max 875 mg/dose)
Aztreonam	30 mg/kg/dose IV every 6–8 hr (max 8000 mg/day)
Cefepime	50 mg/kg/dose IV every 8 hr (max 2000 mg/dose)
Cefixime	8 mg/kg/day PO divided every 12–24 hr
Ciprofloxacin	10–15 mg/kg/dose IV every 8 hr (max 400 mg/dose)[a] 15–20 mg/kg/dose PO every 12 hr (max 750 mg/dose)
Clindamycin	20–40 mg/kg/day IV or PO divided every 6–8 hr (max 4800 mg/day IV, 1800 mg/day PO)
Gentamicin	5–10.5 mg/kg/day divided every 8–24 hr
Imipenem/Cilastatin	60–100 mg/kg/day divided every 6–8 hr (max 4000 mg/day)
Levofloxacin	8–10 mg/kg/dose IV or PO every 12–24 hr (max 750 mg/day)
Meropenem	20 mg/kg/dose IV every 8 hr (max 1000 mg/dose)
Piperacillin/Tazobactam	80–100 mg/kg/dose piperacillin IV every 6 hr (max 4000 mg piperacillin/dose)
Vancomycin	15–20 mg/kg/dose IV every 6–8 hr (max 4000 mg/day)

[a]Doses referenced assume normal renal function and are consistent with dosing recommendations for children outside of the neonatal period. For neonatal dosing recommendations, consult appropriate reference.
[b]Doses for larger children and adolescents are typically capped at the adult dose when weight-based dosing results in a higher value than the standard adult dose for the indication.
IV = intravenous; max = maximum; PO = oral.

Table 5. Resistant Pathogens in Febrile Neutropenia and Treatment Recommendations[4]

Resistant Pathogens	Treatment Recommendations
Methicillin-resistant *Staphylococcus aureus*	Vancomycin Alternatives: linezolid or daptomycin
Vancomycin-resistant enterococcus	Linezolid or daptomycin
Extended-spectrum β-lactamase	Carbapenem
Klebsiella pneumoniae carbapenemase	Polymyxin-colistin or tigecycline

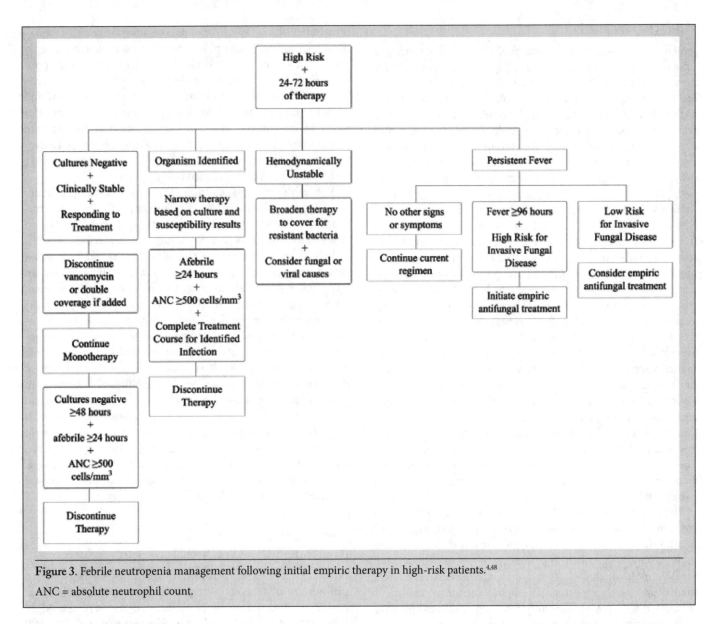

Figure 3. Febrile neutropenia management following initial empiric therapy in high-risk patients.[4,48]

ANC = absolute neutrophil count.

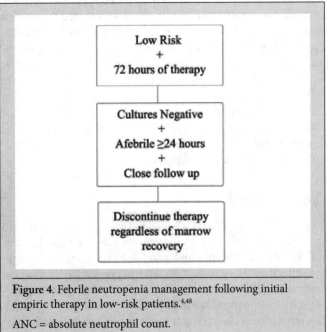

Figure 4. Febrile neutropenia management following initial empiric therapy in low-risk patients.[4,48]

ANC = absolute neutrophil count.

patients with persistent fever after treatment initiation should have additional blood cultures drawn each day that the patient has a fever for the first 72 hours of treatment. Beyond 72 hours, it is recommended to only obtain blood cultures if the patient becomes hemodynamically unstable or has a new physical finding.[4]

A study evaluated the incidence of positive blood culture findings in persistently febrile pediatric oncology patients on subsequent days after an initial negative result drawn before the initiation of empiric antibiotics. The reported incidence was low, with only 4.21% of patients (four of 95 patients) having a positive blood culture. Furthermore, only two of the four patients had positive cultures identified after the third day of treatment. The decision to continue to repeat blood cultures after the first 72 hours of treatment for febrile neutropenia is challenging. The risk of potential contamination, added blood loss, and pain that may result from additional blood cultures must be weighed against the missed opportunity to detect a resistant or uncovered pathogen, which could result in the development of sepsis and death if left untreated.[77]

FUNGAL COVERAGE

Patients can be stratified as either high or low risk for invasive fungal disease based on their underlying malignancy, treatment, or laboratory factors. Patients with any of the following are considered high risk for invasive fungal disease: AML, high-risk ALL, relapsed acute leukemia, allogeneic HSCT recipient, prolonged neutropenia, or high-dose corticosteroid exposure.[78] All other patients are considered to be at low risk.

Consideration should be given to the addition of antifungal agents in patients at high risk for invasive fungal disease, with persistent fever at or beyond 96 hours of broad-spectrum antibacterial therapy and neutropenia expected to continue beyond 7 to 10 days.[4,48] Fungal infections may be considered in patients at low risk in the setting of persistent febrile neutropenia, but evidence to support the need for empiric treatment is weak.[78,79] A computed tomography of the lungs and imaging of other suspected areas, such as the abdomen or sinuses, may be used to identify fungal disease.[78] Previously, guidelines recommended for hospitalized children at high risk for invasive fungal disease to be monitored for invasive aspergillosis through the use of twice-weekly serum galactomannan screening.[48] Poor positive predictive values of galactomannan testing led to a change in this recommendation against testing because of the risk of false-positive results and limited value of a negative result. Similarly, the updated guidelines recommend against fungal polymerase chain reaction testing because of the high risk of false-positive results. Therefore, current recommendations suggest prolonged fever alone indicates the need for empiric antifungal therapy in patients at high risk.[78]

The agent's spectrum of activity, potential toxicities, and cost must be considered when selecting an empiric antifungal agent. Whereas Candida and Aspergillus spp. are the most common pathogens identified in patients with febrile neutropenia, invasive molds including Zygomycetes and Fusarium spp. are increasingly being reported.[4] If empiric antifungal treatment is initiated for a patient currently receiving antifungal prophylaxis, it is important to select an agent in a different class.

Three different classes of antifungals have demonstrated efficacy as empiric antifungal treatment and include amphotericin B, azoles, and echinocandins. Liposomal amphotericin B is preferred over conventional amphotericin B deoxycholate because of its reduced adverse effect profile and similar efficacy.[80] Liposomal amphotericin B is active against Candida and most molds, including Aspergillus, but resistance is of growing concern. It is given intravenously at a dose of 3–5 mg/kg/day and is not available in an oral formulation.[81,82]

The azole antifungals represent a less toxic alternative to amphotericin B. Attention must be paid to avoid possible drug interactions because they are metabolized hepatically through the cytochrome P450 (CYP) system. Fluconazole, although useful for Candida prophylaxis, lacks anti-mold activity and should not be used for empiric treatment. Compared with amphotericin B, voriconazole demonstrated efficacy in adult patients, good central nervous system penetration, low renal toxicity, and a broad spectrum of activity. It is also available in an oral formulation.[81,82] Voriconazole is given as a loading dose on day 1 of 6–9 mg/kg/dose every 12 hours for two doses, followed by 4–8 mg/kg/dose every 12 hours for the remainder of therapy. Voriconazole may be given intravenously or orally. Voriconazole is extensively metabolized by CYP2C19. Genetic polymorphisms in CYP2C19 are responsible for interindividual variability in voriconazole serum concentrations. Because of the variation of metabolism and potential for drug interactions, it is recommended to monitor voriconazole trough values and adjust the dose to maintain a target trough of 1–6 mcg/mL.[83] Posaconazole use is recommended in pediatric patients age 13 years and older as salvage treatment for infections caused by Zygomycetes.[80,84]

The echinocandins caspofungin and micafungin represent another alternative to amphotericin B or azole antifungals. Although they have activity against Candida and Aspergillus, they lack activity against other molds, specifically Zygomycetes, Cryptococcus neoformans, and Fusarium spp. Caspofungin and micafungin are only available in intravenous formulations but are generally well tolerated. Caspofungin 70 mg/m^2 on day 1 followed by 50 mg/m^2 daily (maximum 70 mg per day) demonstrated comparable tolerability, safety, and efficacy compared with liposomal amphotericin B as empiric antifungal therapy for febrile neutropenic pediatric patients.[85] Small studies have reported efficacy of micafungin when used as empiric antifungal treatment in pediatric patients. Doses ranged from 1 to 6 mg/kg daily to a higher max than traditionally recommended of 300 mg.[86] Regardless of the agent selected, empiric antifungal treatment should be continued until the resolution of neutropenia (ANC greater than 100 to 500 cells/mm^3) or until the treatment course is complete for those with suspected or proven fungal infections, whichever is longer.[48]

CONSIDERATIONS FOR TREATMENT DISCONTINUATION

Before discontinuing therapy, cultures must be negative for a minimum of 48 hours, the patient should be afebrile for at least 24 hours, and evidence of marrow recovery should be demonstrated by the resolution of neutropenia (ANC 500 cells/mm^3 or more).[48] Therapy can be discontinued in low-risk patients after 72 hours of therapy if blood cultures are negative and the patient has been afebrile for at least 24 hours, regardless of marrow recovery.[48,87] Close follow-up is essential for patients at low risk when therapy is discontinued before marrow recovery because rare instances of recurrent fever and bacteremia have been reported.[48,87] For patients with a documented infection, length of therapy is dependent on the causative organism and source of infection but must also continue until neutropenia resolves.

PROPHYLAXIS

It is important to recognize when patients being treated with chemotherapy are most vulnerable to developing infections and to educate patients and caregivers on methods to prevent infection. The primary method to prevent infections is to practice good hand hygiene. The role of routine antibiotic prophylaxis is controversial in the pediatric oncology population. The strongest evidence supporting the use of antibiotic prophylaxis comes from adult data and uses a fluoroquinolone, either ciprofloxacin or levofloxacin. Although adult data have demonstrated a significant reduction in all cause and infection-related mortality with the use of fluoroquinolone prophylaxis compared with placebo, concerns of musculoskeletal adverse effects and growing bacterial resistance have limited fluoroquinolone use in pediatric populations.[80,88] Guidelines recommend considering the use of fluoroquinolone prophylaxis in patients at very high risk of febrile neutropenia. These patients are expected to experience prolonged, profound neutropenia with an ANC less than 100 cells/mm^3 for more than 7 days, such as allogeneic HSCT recipients and patients receiving induction therapy for acute leukemia.[4]

Prophylaxis with combination regimens to increase activity against gram-positive organisms is not recommended by the current published guidelines.[4] A study conducted at St. Jude Children's Research Hospital evaluated the use of a variety of agents as prophylactic therapy in pediatric AML patients and found the use of oral cephalosporins to be ineffective at reducing the incidence of bacteremia when used alone. In a comparison of the use of intravenous cefepime to combination therapy with intravenous vancomycin plus an oral cephalosporin (cefpodoxime or cefuroxime), oral ciprofloxacin (250 mg/m^2 every 12 hours), or intravenous cefepime, the study found no difference in the incidence of clinically or microbiologically documented infection. Compared with oral cephalosporins or no prophylaxis, patients receiving intravenous cefepime or combination vancomycin regimens had significantly fewer documented infections.[89] Regardless of the therapy selected, close monitoring of resistance patterns is necessary when deciding to use antibiotic prophylaxis and selecting a regimen.[4,89]

Guidelines recommend antifungal prophylaxis for pediatric patients receiving treatment for AML or myelodysplastic syndrome and for those undergoing HSCT (Table 6).[90]

Fluconazole is recommended as the primary agent used for prophylaxis in these patients. Posaconazole is preferred for patients age 13 years and older undergoing allogeneic HSCT who have acute grade II to IV graft-versus-host disease or chronic graft-versus-host disease. Posaconazole is also preferred for patients receiving treatment at centers with high local incidence of mold infections. An echinocandin is recommended for patients who have a contraindication to fluconazole.[90] Prophylaxis with micafungin was compared with fluconazole in two randomized controlled trials in both adult and pediatric allogeneic HSCT recipients. The trials found micafungin to be well tolerated and not inferior to fluconazole.[91,92] Limited data supporting the use of micafungin for prophylaxis in pediatrics make it difficult to determine the optimal dose. Although the guidelines recommend doses of 1 mg/kg/day to a maximum of 50 mg/day, it is suggested that higher weight-based doses may be required for children with lower weights.[90] Caspofungin may represent an alternative to fluconazole when used as prophylaxis in patients with AML undergoing chemotherapy. A trial compared the use of caspofungin 70 mg/m^2 (maximum 70 mg) on day 1 followed by 50 mg/m^2 (maximum 50 mg) intravenously over 1 hour daily to fluconazole 12 mg/kg (maximum 400 mg) for ages 3 months to less than 18 years and 6 mg/kg (maximum 400 mg) for ages 18 years and above given intravenously or orally daily. The trial reported significantly lower incidence of invasive fungal disease in the caspofungin arm; however, the interpretation of the findings is limited because of early termination of the study.[93] Other antifungals have been reviewed by current guidelines and are not recommended for prophylaxis because of the lack of a significant difference in efficacy compared with fluconazole, in addition to their cost, potential drug interactions, limited evidence, or adverse effects.[90]

Table 6. Antifungal Prophylaxis Recommendations[90]

Diagnosis	Age	Recommended Regimen	Recommendation
Allogeneic HSCT	1 mo–18 yr	Fluconazole 6–12 mg/kg/day IV or PO (max 400 mg/day)	Administer from start of conditioning until engraftment
		Echinocandin	If fluconazole is contraindicated
Allogeneic HSCT + acute grade II–IV GVHD or chronic extensive GVHD	1 mo–12 yr	Fluconazole 6–12 mg/kg/day IV or PO (max 400 mg/day)	Administer from GVHD diagnosis until resolution
	≥ 13 yr	Posaconazole 200 mg PO TID	Administer from GVHD diagnosis until resolution
		Fluconazole 6–12 mg/kg/day IV or PO (max 400 mg/day)	If posaconazole is contraindicated
Autologous HSCT + anticipated neutropenia > 7 days	1 mo–18 yr	Fluconazole 6–12 mg/kg/day IV or PO (max 400 mg/day)	Administer from start of conditioning until engraftment
AML or myelodysplastic syndrome	1 mo–18 yr	Fluconazole 6–12 mg/kg/day IV or PO (max 400 mg/day)	Administer during chemotherapy-associated neutropenia
	≥ 13 yr	Posaconazole 200 mg PO TID	Alternative to fluconazole in centers with a high local incidence of mold infections or if fluconazole is not available

AML = acute myeloid leukemia; GVHD = graft-versus-host disease; HSCT = hematopoietic stem-cell transplantation; IV = intravenous; max = maximum; PO = oral; TID = three times daily.

ROLE OF GRANULOCYTE-COLONY STIMULATING FACTOR

The impact of granulocyte colony-stimulating factors (G-CSFs) in preventing and treating febrile neutropenia in patients with a variety of malignancies has been evaluated. By stimulating the proliferation and maturation of progenitor cells, G-CSFs increase the number of circulating neutrophils.[94] The use of G-CSF in the setting of leukemia remains controversial because studies have conflicting results regarding the potential to induce leukemic blast proliferation.[94] The G-CSF product, filgrastim, has been used in pediatric patients at doses of 5 and 10 mcg/kg/day without significant differences found between the two doses in time to recovery after intensive chemotherapy administration.[95,96]

Prophylaxis with G-CSF has shown a decrease in the duration of neutropenia in both pediatric and adult patients but with variable clinical benefit. The impact of G-CSF administration on the duration of hospitalization or frequency of severe infection varies widely among study results. Furthermore, studies have found G-CSF to have little, if any, positive effect on overall survival, disease survival, or likelihood of complete remission.[94,96] The evidence supporting the use of G-CSF in the treatment of febrile neutropenia is conflicting. Because of limited evidence of clinical benefit and the increased cost, recommendations for the use of G-CSF in established febrile neutropenia are limited to the setting of serious infections or not recommended at all.[4,51]

CONCLUSIONS

Febrile neutropenia is an oncologic emergency that requires immediate initiation of antibiotics to avoid increased morbidity and mortality in pediatric cancer patients. Treatment selection and duration of therapy are dependent on the patient's risk of developing severe complications from infection and the causative suspected or identified organism.

Patient Case 1 — TUMOR LYSIS SYNDROME

A 15-year-old boy (Wt 60 kg, Ht 68 inches, body surface area 1.7 m²) is brought to the emergency department with a 2-week history of fatigue, decreased appetite, and malaise. He is noted to be pale and has a temperature of 101.3°F (38.5°C) and a white blood cell count (WBC) of 78×10^3 cells/mm³. Work-up for acute lymphoblastic leukemia (ALL) is started.

Laboratory findings:

Na	140 mEq/L	CO₂	27 mEq/L	PO₄	6 mg/dL
K	6.1 mEq/L	BUN	26 mg/dL	LDH	956 U/L
Cl	108 mEq/L	SCr	1.4 mg/dL	Uric acid	15 mg/dL
		Calcium (total serum)	8.2 mg/dL		

1. What is this patient's risk of developing TLS?

Patients with ALL and either a WBC of less than 100×10^3 cells/mm³ plus a lactate dehydrogenase of twice or more the upper limit of normal or a WBC 100×10^3 cells/mm³ or more are at high risk of developing tumor lysis syndrome (TLS).

2. Based on clinical and laboratory data, is this patient currently experiencing TLS? If so, what type?

Yes, this patient is experiencing laboratory TLS. He has two serum values, potassium and uric acid, outside the normal range, which meets criteria for laboratory TLS. He does not meet criteria for clinical TLS at this time.

3. What medical intervention(s) should be recommended for this patient at this time?

The intervention for this patient is to initiate hydration and administer a single dose of intravenous rasburicase 6 mg (0.1–0.2 mg/kg or as a fixed dose, depending on institutional guidelines). Intravenous hydration consisting of dextrose 5% in 0.225% sodium chloride should be started on this patient at 213 mL/hr (3 L/m²/day) because this approach is the mainstay of prevention and treatment for TLS. Rasburicase is the TLS treatment of choice for patients presenting with a uric acid greater than 8 mg/dL. Allopurinol would not be recommended as initial treatment in this patient because of his elevated uric acid concentration. Febuxostat is not recommended in pediatric patients and is not preferred over rasburicase for the treatment of TLS.

An 8-year-old, 30-kg boy is evaluated after recently receiving a diagnosis of acute myeloid leukemia (AML). He completed induction I with cytarabine and daunorubicin 9 days ago and has an absolute neutrophil count (ANC) of 20 cells/mm³. He currently has a central venous catheter. His maximum temperature has been 101.3°F (38.5°C); he has no other signs or symptoms of infection, and he has no other significant medical history.

1. What is the most appropriate initial empiric regimen for this patient and why?

The appropriate initial regimen for this patient is to start cefepime 1500 mg (50 mg/kg) intravenously and administer every 8 hours as soon as blood cultures are drawn. Treatment with antipseudomonal monotherapy is recommended for hemodynamically stable patients at high risk of febrile neutropenia. Cefepime is an appropriate antipseudomonal agent. Fever is defined as a sustained fever of 100.4°F (38°C) or greater for 1 hour or a single fever of 101°F (38.3°C) or greater. Treatment should be initiated after the single fever this patient had of 101.3°F (38.5°C). This patient is not a candidate to be managed on oral therapy or as an outpatient because of the fact that he is at high risk for febrile neutropenia. Antifungal treatments are not recommended as initial empiric therapy.

2. What criteria must this patient meet before therapy should be discontinued?

High-risk patients, such as this patient, must be afebrile for at least 24 hours, have negative blood cultures for at least 48 hours, and have evidence of marrow recovery before treatment discontinuation.

REFERENCES

1. Cervantes A, Chirivella I. Oncological emergencies. Ann Oncol 2004;15 Suppl 4:iv299-306.
2. Coiffier B, Altman A, Pui CH, et al. Guidelines for the management of pediatric and adult tumor lysis syndrome: an evidence-based review. J Clin Oncol 2008;26:2767-78.
3. Burns RA, Topoz I, Reynolds SL. Tumor lysis syndrome risk factors, diagnosis, and management. Pediatr Emer Care 2014;30:571–9.
4. Freifeld AG, Bow EJ, Sepkowitz KA, et al. Clinical practice guideline for the use of antimicrobial agents in neutropenic patients with cancer: 2010 update by the Infectious Diseases Society of America. Clin Infect Dis 2011;52:e56–93.
5. Hande KR, Garrow GC. Acute tumor lysis syndrome in patients with high-grade non-Hodgkin's lymphoma. Am J Med 1993;94:133-9.
6. Cairo MS, Bishop M. Tumour lysis syndrome: new therapeutic strategies and classification. Br J Haematol 2004;127:3–11.
7. Wilson FP, Berns JS. Tumor lysis syndrome: new challenges and recent advances. Adv Chronic Kidney Dis 2014;21:18–26.
8. Edeani A, Shirali A. Tumor Lysis Syndrome. In: Online Curricula: Onco-Nephrology Introduction to the American Society of Nephrology Onco-Nephrology Curriculum. 2016;1-8. Available at https://www.asn-online.org/education/distancelearning/curricula/onco/Chapter4.pdf. Accessed July 11, 2018.
9. Howard SC, Jones DP, Pui CH. The tumor lysis syndrome. N Engl J Med 2011;364:1844–54.
10. Wossmann W, Schrappe M, Meyer U, et al. Incidence of tumor lysis syndrome in children with advanced stage Burkitt's lymphoma/leukemia before and after introduction of prophylactic use of urate oxidase. Ann Hematol 2003;82:160–5.
11. Seegmiller JE, Laster L, Howell RR. Biochemistry of uric acid and its relation to gout. N Engl J Med 1963;268:712-6.
12. Van den Berghe G. Purine and pyrimidine metabolism between millennia: what has been accomplished, what has to be done? Adv Exp Med Biol 2000;486:1-4.
13. Hande KR, Hixson CV, Chabner BA. Postchemotherapy purine excretion in lymphoma patients receiving allopurinol. Cancer Res 1981;41:2273-9.
14. Arseneau JC, Canellos GP, Banks PM, et al. American Burkitt's lymphoma: a clinicopathologic study of 30 cases—I. Clinical factors relating to prolonged survival. Am J Med 1975;58:314-21.
15. McCroskey RD, Mosher DF, Spencer CD, et al. Acute tumor lysis syndrome and treatment response in patients treated for refractory chronic lymphocytic leukemia with short-course, high-dose cytosine arabinoside, cisplatin, and etoposide. Cancer 1990;66:246-50.
16. Gomez GA, Han T. Acute tumor lysis syndrome in prolymphocytic leukemia. Arch Intern Med 1987;147:375-6.
17. Kunkel L, Wong A, Maneatis T, et al. Optimizing the use of rituximab for treatment of B-cell non-Hodgkin's lymphoma: a benefit-risk update. Semin Oncol 2000;27:53-61.
18. Cheson BD, Frame JN, Vena D, et al. Tumor lysis syndrome: an uncommon complication of fludarabine therapy of chronic lymphocytic leukemia. J Clin Oncol 1998;16:2313-20.
19. Cairo MS, Coiffier B, Reiter A, et al., TLS Expert Panel. Recommendations for the evaluation of risk and prophylaxis of tumour lysis syndrome (TLS) in adults and children with malignant diseases: an expert TLS panel consensus. Br J Haematol 2010;149:578–86.
20. Conger JD, Falk SA. Intrarenal dynamics in the pathogenesis and prevention of acute urate nephropathy. J Clin Invest 1977;59:786-93.
21. Jeha S, Kantarjian H, Irwin D, et al. Efficacy and safety of rasburicase, a recombinant urate oxidase (Elitek), in the management of malignancy-associated hyperuricemia in pediatric and adult patients: final results of a multicenter compassionate use trial. Leukemia 2005;19:34-8.
22. Candrilli S, Bell T, Irish W, et al. A comparison of inpatient length of stay and costs among patients with hematological malignancies (excluding Hodgkin's disease) associated with and without acute renal failure. Clin Lymph Myeloma 2008;8:44-51.
23. Krakoff IH, Meyer RL. Prevention of hyperuricemia in leukemia and lymphoma: use of allopurinol, a xanthine oxidase inhibitor. JAMA 1965;193:1-6.
24. Spector T. Inhibition of urate production by allopurinol. Biochem Pharmacol 1977;26:355-8.

25. Smalley RV, Guaspari A, Haase-Statz S, et al. Allopurinol: intravenous use for prevention and treatment of hyperuricemia. J Clin Oncol 2000;18:1758-63.

26. Cortes J, Moore JO, Maziarz RT et al. Control of plasma uric acid in adults at risk for tumour lysis syndrome: efficacy and safety of rasburicase alone and rasburicase followed by allopurinol compared with allopurinol alone—results of a multicenter phase III study. J Clin Oncol 2010;28:4207–13.

27. Landgrebe AR, Nyhan WL, Coleman M. Urinary-tract stones resulting from the excretion of oxypurinol. N Engl J Med 1975;292:626-7.

28. Band PR, Silverberg DS, Henderson JF, et al. Xanthine nephropathy in a patient with lymphosarcoma treated with allopurinol. N Engl J Med 1970;283:354-7.

29. Allopurinol tablets [package insert]. Huntsville, AL: Qualitest Pharmaceuticals, 2017.

30. Conger JD. Acute uric acid nephropathy. Med Clin North Am 1990;74:859-71.

31. Taketomo CK, Hodding JH, Krauss DM. Pediatric & Neonatal Dosage Handbook, 24th ed. Hudson, OH: Lexi-Comp, 2017.

32. Elitek [package insert]. Bridgewater, NJ: Sanofi-Aventis, 2017.

33. Cheuk DK, Chiang AK, Chan GC, et al. Urate oxidase for the prevention and treatment of tumor lysis syndrome in children with cancer. Cochrane Database Syst Rev 2014;8:CD006945.

34. Ueng S. Rasburicase (Elitek): a novel agent for tumor lysis syndrome. Proc (Bayl Univ Med Cent) 2005;18:275-9.

35. Goldman SC, Holcenberg JS, Finklestein JZ, et al. A randomized comparison between rasburicase and allopurinol in children with lymphoma or leukemia at high risk for tumor lysis. Blood 2001;97:2998-3003.

36. Pui CH, Mahmoud HH, Wiley JM, et al. Recombinant urate oxidase for the prophylaxis or treatment of hyperuricemia in patients with leukemia or lymphoma. J Clin Oncol 2001;19:697-704.

37. Henry M, Sung L. Supportive care in pediatric oncology: oncologic emergencies and management of fever and neutropenia. Pediatr Clin North Am 2015;62:27-46.

38. Liu CY, Sims-McCallum RP, Schiffer CA. A single dose of rasburicase is sufficient for the treatment of hyperuricemia in patients receiving chemotherapy. Leuk Res 2005;29:463-5.

39. Lee AC, Li CH, So KT, et al. Treatment of impending tumor lysis with single-dose rasburicase. Ann Pharmacother 2003;37:1614-7.

40. Patel KS, Lau JE, Zembillas AS, et al. Single 4.5 mg fixed-dose of rasburicase for hyperuricemia associated with tumor lysis syndrome. J Oncol Pharm Pract 2017;23:333-7.

41. Coutsouvelis J, Wiseman M, Hui L, et al. Effectiveness of a single fixed dose of rasburicase 3 mg in the management of tumour lysis syndrome. Br J Clin Pharmacol 2013;75:550–3.

42. Knoebel RW, Lo M, Crank CW. Evaluation of a low, weight-based dose of rasburicase in adult patients for the treatment or prophylaxis of tumor lysis syndrome. J Oncol Pharm Pract 2011;17:147–54.

43. Nguyen AP, Ness GL. Hemolytic anemia following rasburicase administration: a review of published reports. J Pediatr Pharmacol Ther 2014;19:310–6.

44. Spina M, Nagy Z, Ribera JM, et al. FLORENCE: a randomized, double-blind, phase III pivotal study of febuxostat versus allopurinol for the prevention of tumor lysis syndrome (TLS) in patients with hematologic malignancies at intermediate to high TLS risk. Ann Oncol 2015;26:2155-61.

45. DeConti RC, Calabresi P. Use of allopurinol for prevention and control of hyperuricemia in patients with neoplastic disease. N Engl J Med 1966;274:481-6.

46. Sakarcan A, Quigley R. Hyperphosphatemia in tumor lysis syndrome: the role of hemodialysis and continuous veno-venous hemofiltration. Pediatr Nephrol 1994;8:351-3.

47. Heney D, Essex-Cater A, Brocklebank JT, et al. Continuous arteriovenous haemofiltration in the treatment of tumour lysis syndrome. Pediatr Nephrol 1990;4:245-7.

48. Lehrnbecher T, Phillips R, Alexander S, et al. Guideline for the management of fever and neutropenia in children with cancer and/or undergoing hematopoietic stem-cell transplantation. J Clin Oncol 2012;30:4427–38.

49. Shord SS, Cordes LM. Cancer Treatment and Chemotherapy. In: DiPiro JT, Talbert RL, Yee GC, et al., eds. Pharmacotherapy: A Pathophysiologic Approach, 10th ed. New York: McGraw-Hill.

50. Klastersky J, Paesmans M, Rubenstein EB, et al. The multinational association for supportive care in cancer risk index: a multinational scoring system for identifying low-risk febrile neutropenic cancer patients. J Clin Oncol 2000;18:3038–51.

51. National Comprehensive Cancer Network. Prevention and treatment of cancer-related infections (Version 1.2019). Available at www.nccn.org/professionals/physician_gls/pdf/infections.pdf. Accessed November 18, 2019.

52. Hakim H, Flynn PM, Knapp KM, et al. Etiology and clinical course of febrile neutropenia. J Pediatr Hematol Oncol 2009;31:623–9.

53. Phillips B, Wade R, Stewart LA, et al. Systematic review and meta-analysis of the discriminatory performance of risk prediction rules in febrile neutropaenic episodes in children and young people. Eur J Cancer 2010;46:2950-64.

54. Rackoff WR, Gonin R, Robinson C, et al. Predicting the risk of bacteremia in children with fever and neutropenia. J Clin Oncol 1996;14:919-24.

55. Alexander SW, Wade KC, Hibberd PL, et al. Evaluation of risk prediction criteria for episodes of febrile neutropenia in children with cancer. J Pediatr Hematol Oncol 2002;24:38-42.

56. Rondinelli PI, Ribeiro Kde C, de Camargo B. A proposed score for predicting severe infection complications in children with chemotherapy-induced febrile neutropenia. J Pediatr Hematol Oncol 2006;28:665-70.

57. Santolaya ME, Alvarez AM, Becker A, et al. Prospective, multi-center evaluation of risk factors associated with invasive bacterial infection in children with cancer, neutropenia, and fever. J Clin Oncol 2001;19:3415-21.

58. Ammann RA, Hirt A, Lüthy AR, et al. Identification of children presenting with fever in chemotherapy-induced neutropenia at low risk for severe bacterial infection. Med Pediatr Oncol 2003;41:436-43.

59. Ammann RA, Bodmer N, Hirt A, et al. Predicting adverse events in children with fever and chemotherapy-induced neutropenia: the prospective multicenter SPOG 2003 FN study. J Clin Oncol 2010;28:2008-14.

60. Infectious Diseases Society of America. Fever and Neutropenia GUIDELINES Pocket Card. Available at http://eguideline.guidelinecentral.com/i/53994-fever-and-neutropenia. Accessed November 23, 2019.

61. Inparajah M, Wong C, Sibbald C, et al. Once daily gentamicin dosing in children with febrile neutropenia resulting from antineoplastic therapy. Pharmacotherapy 2010;30:43-51.

62. Downes KJ, Zaoutis TE, Shah SS. Guidelines for management of children with fever and neutropenia. J Pediatric Infect Dis Soc 2013;2:281-5.

63. Manji A, Lehrnbecher T, Dupuis LL, et al. A systematic review and meta-analysis of antipseudomonal penicillins and carbapenems in pediatric febrile neutropenia. Support Care Cancer 2012;20:2295-305.

64. Manji A, Lehrnbecher T, Dupuis LL, et al. A meta-analysis of antipseudomonal penicillins and cephalosporins in pediatric patients with fever and neutropenia. Pediatr Infect Dis J 2012;31:353-8.

65. Marron A, Carratalà J, Alcaide F, et al. High rates of resistance to cephalosporins among viridans-group streptococci causing bacteraemia in neutropenic cancer patients. J Antimicrob Chemother 2001;47:87-91.

66. Paul M, Yahav D, Bivas A, et al. Antipseudomonal beta-lactams for the initial, empirical, treatment of febrile neutropenia:

comparison of beta-lactams. Cochrane Database Syst Rev 2010; 11:CD005197.

67. Vardakas KZ, Samonis G, Chrysanthopoulou SA, et al. Role of glycopeptides as part of initial empirical treatment of febrile neutropenic patients: a meta-analysis of randomised controlled trials. Lancet Infect Dis 2005;5:431-9.

68. Orme LM, Babl FE, Barnes C, et al. Outpatient versus inpatient IV antibiotic management for pediatric oncology patients with low risk febrile neutropenia: a randomised trial. Pediatr Blood Cancer 2014;61:1427-33.

69. Manji A, Beyene J, Dupuis LL, et al. Outpatient and oral antibiotic management of low-risk febrile neutropenia are effective in children—a systematic review of prospective trials. Support Care Cancer 2012;20:1135-45.

70. Teuffel O, Amir E, Alibhai SM, et al. Cost-effectiveness of outpatient management for febrile neutropenia in children with cancer. Pediatrics 2011;127:e279-86.

71. Speyer E, Herbinet A, Vuillemin A, et al. Agreement between children with cancer and their parents in reporting the child's health-related quality of life during a stay at the hospital and at home. Child Care Health Dev 2009;35:489-95.

72. Teuffel O, Ethier MC, Alibhai SM, et al. Outpatient management of cancer patients with febrile neutropenia: a systematic review and meta-analysis. Ann Oncol 2011;22:2358-65.

73. Ahmed N, El-Mahallawy HA, Ahmed IA, et al. Early hospital discharge versus continued hospitalization in febrile pediatric cancer patients with prolonged neutropenia: a randomized, prospective study. Pediatr Blood Cancer 2007;49:786-92.

74. Santolaya ME, Alvarez AM, Avilés CL, et al. Early hospital discharge followed by outpatient management versus continued hospitalization of children with cancer, fever, and neutropenia at low risk for invasive bacterial infection. J Clin Oncol 2004;22:3784-9.

75. Vidal L, Ben Dor I, Paul M, et al. Oral versus intravenous antibiotic treatment for febrile neutropenia in cancer patients. Cochrane Database Syst Rev 2013;10:CD003992.

76. Cometta A, Kern WV, De Bock R, et al. Vancomycin versus placebo for treating persistent fever in patients with neutropenic cancer receiving piperacillin-tazobactam monotherapy. Clin Infect Dis 2003;37:382-9.

77. Neemann K, Yonts AB, Qui F, et al. Blood cultures for persistent fever in neutropenic pediatric patients are of low diagnostic yield. J Pediatric Infect Dis Soc 2016;5:218-21.

78. Lehrnbecher T, Robinson P, Fisher B, et al. Guideline for the management of fever and neutropenia in children with cancer and hematopoietic stem-cell transplantation recipients: 2017 update. J Clin Oncol 2017;35:2082-94.

79. Caselli D, Cesaro S, Ziino O, et al. A prospective, randomized study of empirical antifungal therapy for the treatment of chemotherapy-induced febrile neutropenia in children. Br J Haematol 2012;158:249-55.

80. Koh AY. Prolonged febrile neutropenia in the pediatric patient with cancer. Am Soc Clin Oncol Educ Book 2012:565-9.

81. Cesaro S, Strugo L, Alaggio R, et al. Voriconazole for invasive aspergillosis in oncohematological patients: a single-center pediatric experience. Support Care Cancer 2003;11:722-7.

82. Walsh TJ, Pappas P, Winston DJ, et al. Voriconazole compared with liposomal amphotericin B for empirical antifungal therapy in patients with neutropenia and persistent fever. N Engl J Med 2002;346:225-34.

83. Choi SH, Lee SY, Hwang JY, et al. Importance of voriconazole therapeutic drug monitoring in pediatric cancer patients with invasive aspergillosis. Pediatr Blood Cancer 2013;60:82-7.

84. Lüer S, Berger S, Diepold M, et al. Treatment of intestinal and hepatic mucormycosis in an immunocompromised child. Pediatr Blood Cancer 2009;52:872-4.

85. Maertens JA, Madero L, Reilly AF, et al. A randomized, double-blind, multicenter study of caspofungin versus liposomal amphotericin B for empiric antifungal therapy in pediatric patients with persistent fever and neutropenia. Pediatr Infect Dis J 2010;29:415-20.

86. Kobayashi R, Suzuki N, Yoshida M, et al. Efficacy and safety of micafungin for febrile neutropenia in pediatric patients with hematological malignancies: a multicenter prospective study. J Pediatr Hematol Oncol 2013;35:e276-9.

87. Santolaya ME, Villarroel M, Avendano LF, et al. Discontinuation of antimicrobial therapy for febrile, neutropenic children with cancer: a prospective study. Clin Infect Dis 1997;25:92-7.

88. Sung L, Manji A, Beyene J, et al. Fluoroquinolones in children with fever and neutropenia: a systematic review of prospective trials. Pediatr Infect Dis J 2012;31:431-5.

89. Inaba H, Gaur AH, Cao X, et al. Feasibility, efficacy, and adverse effects of outpatient antibacterial prophylaxis in children with acute myeloid leukemia. Cancer 2014;120:1985-92.

90. Science M, Robinson PD, MacDonald T, et al. Guideline for primary antifungal prophylaxis for pediatric patients with cancer or hematopoietic stem cell transplant recipients. Pediatr Blood Cancer 2014;61:393-400.

91. van Burik JA, Ratanatharathorn V, Stepan DE, et al. Micafungin versus fluconazole for prophylaxis against invasive fungal infections during neutropenia in patients undergoing hematopoietic stem cell transplantation. Clin Infect Dis 2004;39:1407-16.

92. Hiramatsu Y, Maeda Y, Fujii N, et al. Use of micafungin versus fluconazole for antifungal prophylaxis in neutropenic patients receiving hematopoietic stem cell transplantation. Int J Hematol 2008;88:588-95.

93. Fisher BT, Zaoutis T, Dvorak CC, et al. Effect of caspofungin vs fluconazole prophylaxis on invasive fungal disease among children and young adults with acute myeloid leukemia: a randomized clinical trial. JAMA 2019;322:1673-81.

94. Lehrnbecher T, Zimmermann M, Reinhardt D, et al. Prophylactic human granulocyte colony-stimulating factor after induction therapy in pediatric acute myeloid leukemia. Blood 2007;109:936-43.

95. Levine JE, Boxer LA. Clinical applications of hematopoietic growth factors in pediatric oncology. Curr Opin Hematol 2002;9:222-7.

96. Inaba H, Cao X, Pounds S, et al. Randomized trial of two dosages of prophylactic granulocyte colony-stimulating factor after induction chemotherapy in pediatric acute myeloid leukemia. Cancer 2011;117:1313-20.

Section XIV

Immunologic Disorders

CHAPTER 54

Allergies and Anaphylaxis

Stephanie D. Natale, Pharm.D.

INTRODUCTION

An *allergic reaction* is defined as an undesired immunologic response to an allergen. Allergic reactions require a previous sensitization to the offending allergen, which on future exposure gives rise to an immunologic-mediated hypersensitivity reaction. Reactions may manifest as a broad spectrum of symptoms from runny nose to gastrointestinal upset to full airway obstruction and death. Allergic diseases in the United States are increasing, especially in children. With such a widespread scope, it is important to recognize and treat the different types of allergic diseases most prevalent in children to minimize their psychological and medical impact. The objective of this chapter is to discuss allergic rhinitis (AR), drug and food allergies, and anaphylaxis with a primary focus on the pharmacotherapy for these conditions.

EPIDEMIOLOGY AND ETIOLOGY

Allergic rhinitis is the most common allergic disease in children, affecting up to 40% of children in the United States.[1-3]

Allergic rhinitis is an immunoglobulin E (IgE)-mediated inflammatory immune response, usually to inhaled allergens, in the nasal and sinus passageways. Symptoms may appear seasonally or persist year-round, depending on the triggering allergen. The prevalence of AR is almost nonexistent in children younger than 2 years, but it steadily increases, with bimodal peaks during the early school and adolescent periods. Prevalence decreases with age after adolescence.[4] Box 1 shows other associated risk factors for developing AR.[5-7]

Allergic rhinitis profoundly affects a child's everyday activities, sleep habits, and quality of life. Children with AR are more likely to experience a variety of cognitive and psychiatric issues including poor concentration, attention-deficit/hyperactivity disorder, poor academic and athletic performance during peak pollen season, and low self-esteem.[8-13] In older children and adults, anxiety and depression rates are higher among those with AR than among those without.[14] Children with AR also more commonly experience other allergic diseases such as asthma and atopic dermatitis. Although AR is not directly associated with fatal reactions, patients with poorly controlled AR are at higher risk of experiencing severe and possibly fatal exacerbations of other allergic conditions such as food allergies and asthma.[13,15]

Food allergies also profoundly affect children's lives and well-being. They are the most common cause of anaphylaxis in children.[16] Fear of severe reactions, combined with ubiquitous exposure to possible food allergens, cause a high level of anxiety and create a social stigma around children with food allergies. Food allergies involve an immune response to an ingested food and affect anywhere from 4%–10% of children in the United States.[17-22] The most common food allergens, accounting for more than 85% of children with food allergies, are peanuts (1%–2% of all children), milk (1.7%), shellfish (1.4%), tree nuts (1%), and eggs (0.8%).[22] The most common causes of fatal reaction are peanuts (50%–62%) and tree nuts (15%–30%).[23]

Box 1. Risk Factors Associated with Allergic Rhinitis[5-7]

Family history of allergic diseases
Male sex
Birth during the pollen season
Firstborn
Early introduction of formula and food (age < 6 mo)
Early use of antibiotics
Maternal smoking exposure in the first year of life
Exposure to indoor allergens (e.g., dust mites, mold)
Serum immunoglobulin E (IgE) > 100 IU/mL before age 6 yr
Presence of allergen-specific IgE

The risk of developing food allergies appears to be greatest in children of Asian or African American descent.[22] The presence of another preexisting allergic disease (e.g., AR, asthma, atopic dermatitis) or a biologic parent or sibling with a history of allergic disease is also associated with an increased risk of developing food allergies.[24]

Allergic reactions from drugs are a subset of adverse drug reactions that are immunologically mediated responses. It is important to distinguish the term *allergic drug reaction* from the more general term *adverse drug reaction*, which may or may not be immune-mediated. The incidence of drug allergies in children is likely to be overestimated because both children and their parents are often unaware of the differences.[25] This lack of knowledge can lead to the unnecessary exclusion of a drug class that would otherwise be preferred.

The incidence of allergic drug reactions in the pediatric population is unknown. A 10-year retrospective cohort study found that only 51% of all pharmacist-reviewed adverse drug events among hospitalized children were determined to be of allergic origin or idiosyncratic.[26] The most common causes of the adverse drug reactions in this study were antibiotics (33%), narcotic analgesics (12%), anticonvulsants (11%), and anxiolytic agents (10%). Nonsteroidal anti-inflammatory drugs have also been implicated in an elevated risk of developing Stevens-Johnson syndrome.[27]

In the most severe allergic reactions, anaphylaxis may develop. A commonly accepted definition of *anaphylaxis* is lacking, but it generally includes an acute onset of systemic symptoms involving the skin, respiratory compromise, decreased blood pressure, gastrointestinal symptoms, and/ or other symptoms of end-organ dysfunction.[28] With the increasing prevalence of all pediatric allergies, it is not surprising that anaphylactic allergic reactions are also rising. The mortality from anaphylactic reactions is low, ranging from 100 to 150 cases in the United States per year. However, anaphylaxis causes more than 30,000 emergency department visits each year.[29] Risks of developing anaphylaxis are highest in males, in adolescents, and in children with several allergic diseases.[22] In a series of epidemiologic evaluations of fatalities from anaphylactic reactions, almost all had a positive history for asthma.[30-33]

PATHOPHYSIOLOGY

Allergic reactions occur through a variety of immunologically mediated mechanisms. Most allergic reactions may be classified as one of four types of hypersensitivity reactions (Table 1). Although type I hypersensitivity is the only type associated with an IgE response to a drug, food, or other allergen, and is equated with allergic reaction, types II–IV are significant causes of adverse drug events (often interpreted as an allergy by parents) and other common "allergies" such as those to metals, gluten, and topical contact with plants.

Type I hypersensitivity reactions are the immediate reactions usually associated with anaphylaxis. Type I hypersensitivity has a 15- to 30-minute onset and is associated with IgE production in response to a particular allergen. The IgE antibody antigen-mediated degranulation of cells releases histamine, which produces cutaneous, gastrointestinal, respiratory, and cardiovascular symptoms such as flushing, nausea, bronchospasm, and hypotension. First exposure to an allergen does not usually produce enough IgE to create a clinical response; therefore, most patients presenting with a type I reaction are sensitized from a previous exposure.[34]

Type II hypersensitivity or antibody-dependent cytolytic reactions occur when IgM and IgG are produced in response to an allergen binding to a host cell (usually a blood cell). In these cases, the allergen binds as a hapten to a cell and elicits an IgM or IgG response to the allergen-cell complex. For example, penicillin attaches to Coombs-positive red blood cell surface proteins. An IgG then binds to the penicillin and red blood cell protein complex, allowing complement to cross-link and destroy the red blood cell, resulting in hemolytic anemia.[35,36] This type of reaction usually targets blood cells and is a common cause of drug-induced agranulocytosis, thrombocytopenia, and hemolytic anemia. The onset of type II hypersensitivity reactions is usually 5–12 hours after drug exposure.

Type III or immune complex hypersensitivities are similar to type II hypersensitivities. In type III, antibody-antigen complexes form and deposit along blood vessels and in various organs and tissues. The complexes may activate complement, cause platelet aggregation, and activate macrophages, all of which result in local tissue damage. Many types of medication-induced kidney and joint damage result from

Table 1. Types of Allergic Reactions

Type	Mechanism	Examples
I	Allergen binds to specific IgE, which causes degranulation of basophils and mast cells, resulting in release of inflammatory mediators	IgE-mediated anaphylaxis from an antibiotic; localized allergic rhinitis
II	Allergen binds to a cell and elicits an IgG or IgM response to the antigen-cell complex, resulting in cell destruction	Hemolysis secondary to penicillin exposure
III	Antigen-antibody complexes form and deposit on blood vessel walls and in various organs, resulting in complement activation and platelet aggregation	Serum sickness from IVIG
IV	Antigen recognition activates a memory T cell, initiating an inflammatory response	Poison ivy–induced contact dermatitis; gluten sensitivity

IgE = immunoglobulin E; IgG = immunoglobulin G; IgM = immunoglobulin M; IVIG = intravenous immunoglobulin.

these immune complexes. Examples of these medications include quinine, salicylates, and sulfonamides. Onset is usually 3–8 hours after first exposure but may present as late as 7–10 days.

Type IV, also known as delayed type hypersensitivity, is a reaction caused by memory T-cell recognition of an antigen. On antigen recognition, T cells initiate an inflammatory response, resulting in neutrophil and macrophage influx. Onset is 24–48 hours after antigen exposure. Most allergic cutaneous reactions are type IV hypersensitivity reactions. This phenomenon occurs commonly in patients given a β-lactam antibiotic during a concurrent mononucleosis infection.[22,36]

CLINICAL PRESENTATION AND DIAGNOSIS

ALLERGIC RHINITIS

Clinical manifestations of AR include conjunctivitis, nasal congestion, rhinorrhea, sneezing, cough, wheezing, or headache. Clinical findings may include dark circles under the eyes from sinus congestion (commonly known as "allergic shiners") and nasal creases from frequent rubbing of the nose. Diagnosis is largely based on patient history and physical examination. It can be difficult to differentiate symptoms of allergies from congestion and rhinitis secondary to viral illness. Triggers can often be identified when symptoms present concurrently with pollen seasons or exposure to cockroaches, dust, and pets. Symptoms of rhinitis in children younger than 2 years are rarely allergy based because sensitization to environmental allergens takes at least one or two seasons. Other potential etiologies, such as infection, should be ruled out before considering AR in very young children.

Allergy skin testing may help determine whether a patient's rhinitis is an allergic response and can identify the allergen or allergens. Skin testing involves introducing an allergen percutaneously by a prick or intracutaneously by intradermal injection. This testing creates an in vivo IgE response on mast cells that releases histamine. This histamine release creates a wheal and flare that can be measured. However, patients who take commonly prescribed second-generation antihistamines (SGAs) must discontinue them for at least 10 days before testing, and certain skin conditions (e.g., dermatographia) may affect skin test results. The Allergic Rhinitis and its Impact on

Asthma (ARIA) guidelines suggest that AR be subdivided as intermittent or persistent disease and as mild or as moderate to severe disease based on the frequency and severity of symptoms as a basis for selecting treatment (Table 2).[37]

FOOD ALLERGIES

Food allergies can manifest as a wide range of symptoms including dermatitis, emesis, diarrhea, abdominal pain, and anaphylaxis. The diagnosis of food allergies is based mainly on symptomatic reports from parents or a clinical history obtained on acute presentation. A confirmed diagnosis requires a food challenge, but this testing is not routinely recommended because of the risk of anaphylaxis. Skin testing is a widely used option, as discussed previously. Assays for testing serum for the presence of allergen-specific IgE is another option for diagnosing food allergies, but these assays are best used as screening tools because the positive presence of IgE may not indicate a true allergy. A positive result simply implies the patient has been sensitized to the food. Patients may use their serum test results as a guide for avoiding or eliminating certain foods from the diet.

DRUG ALLERGIES

Allergic drug reactions can be difficult to diagnose because of their broad and fairly common range of symptoms. However, several criteria may help support an immunologically mediated reaction as follows: (1) the reaction does not resemble the drug's pharmacologic or adverse effects; (2) there is a delay, usually ranging from hours to days between the drug exposure and the reaction (unless previous sensitization has occurred, in which case the reaction occurs in minutes to hours); (3) reactions occur with even a small amount of the drug; (4) the symptoms are characteristic of an allergic reaction (e.g., anaphylaxis, pruritus); (5) the reaction resolves after the drug is discontinued; and (6) the reaction can be reproduced on subsequent exposure.[38]

Drug allergies manifest as a wide variety of symptoms that are associated with specific drugs (Table 3). The most common manifestation of an allergic drug reaction is cutaneous. Although most skin reactions are mild, severe and life-threatening cutaneous reactions can rarely occur, usually in the form of Stevens-Johnson syndrome or toxic epidermal

Table 2. Allergic Rhinitis and Its Impact on Asthma Classification of Allergic Rhinitis[37]

Intermittent		Persistent

Symptoms occur (one of the following):
    < 4 days/wk
    < 4 wk/yr
	OR	Symptoms occur (*both* of the following):
		    ≥ 4 days/wk
		    ≥ 4 wk/yr

AND		
Mild		**Moderate to Severe**

All of the following apply:
    Normal sleep
    No impairment in daily activities, sports, or leisure
    No impairment with work or school
    No troublesome symptoms
	OR	One or more of the following apply:
		    Impaired sleep
		    Impaired daily activities, sports, or leisure
		    Impaired performance at work or school
		    Troublesome symptoms

necrolysis. Stevens-Johnson syndrome is a widespread rash with characteristic blistering of the mucosal membranes. Fever may be present. Toxic epidermal necrolysis is similar to Stevens-Johnson syndrome, but it involves the breakdown of skin layers and subsequent blistering and the sloughing of large areas of skin.

Skin testing can be a useful diagnostic tool; however, penicillin is one of the few agents used in the skin test with a well-validated predictive value. Skin testing is most appropriate for patients with a history of severe type I penicillin reactions or a vague history of penicillin reactions. The methods for diagnosing drug allergies are similar to those for food allergies because the diagnosis is based heavily on symptoms at acute presentation and clinical history. Skin testing may assist in diagnosis, but only penicillin and a few other protein-based agents (e.g., insulin) have well-validated predictive values. A positive response to a skin test indicates that the patient has specific IgE antibodies, but its correlation to a clinical allergic reaction is unclear. Assays for the presence of serum IgE are available, but as with food allergies, their clinical application is limited.[39]

ANAPHYLAXIS

Anaphylaxis is a systemic allergic reaction that occurs within minutes to hours after allergen exposure. The more severe the reaction, the more quickly it will occur. The first signs are often warm skin with flushing, itching, and a tingling sensation. Skin examination reveals the classic wheal and flare associated with urticaria. In mild reactions, the skin is often the only organ involved. The upper airway is the second most commonly involved organ, especially if the patient also has AR or asthma. Angioedema of the tongue, pharynx, larynx, and uvula can lead to shortness of breath, voice hoarseness, and rarely apnea.

Symptoms of wheezing and airway edema occur as the reaction progresses to the lower airways. Patients with underlying asthma have more severe bronchoconstriction and lower airway symptoms. A similar process of intestinal edema can result in nausea, vomiting, and abdominal pain. Tachycardia or cardiac arrhythmias may manifest with dizziness and chest pain. Even after initial symptoms resolve, in severe cases a biphasic response can occur 6–8 hours after allergen exposure. Therefore, after any anaphylactic event, the patient should be closely observed for at least 6 hours. Rapid decline in blood pressure is the most worrisome complication of anaphylaxis. Patients can experience rapid vasodilation and collapse of the circulatory system. Most fatal anaphylactic reactions occur within minutes of exposure and involve laryngeal or pulmonary edema.

Diagnosis is primarily based on history and physical examination; however, some laboratory tests can aid in diagnosis. Serum tryptase, a mediator released from mast cells, is elevated in anaphylaxis. Blood should be drawn within 6 hours of symptom onset because tryptase has a 2- to 6-hour half-life. Histamine and N-methylhistamine can be measured in urine samples several hours after symptom onset. Plasma histamine is not practical to measure because its half-life is about 2 minutes. Identifying the causative allergen is very important to patient education on avoiding triggers. In rare cases of idiopathic anaphylaxis, the causative agent is never identified, yet these patients often have a history of atopy.

TREATMENT

ALLERGIC RHINITIS

The goal of AR treatment is to minimize or prevent symptoms so that quality of life and cognitive function are improved. Initial treatment of AR should always be removing or avoiding the offending allergen. This strategy can be managed by performing more frequent and thorough household cleanings, remaining indoors as much as reasonably possible during peak pollen seasons, and avoiding pets, cigarette smoke, perfumes,

Table 3. Common Manifestations of Drug Allergies

Manifestation	Clinical Symptoms	Common Causative Agents
Anaphylaxis (type I reactions)	Rapid onset of cutaneous symptoms associated with respiratory compromise, low blood pressure, and/or persistent gastrointestinal symptoms	Penicillins, cephalosporins
Drug-induced autoimmune disorders (hemolytic anemia, nephritis, hepatitis) (type II reactions)	Arthralgias, myalgias, polyarthritis, and specific organ involvement (e.g., proteinuria, elevated transaminases, jaundice)	Phenytoin, penicillins, sulfonamides
Serum sickness (type III reactions)	Fever, malaise, and lymphadenopathy occurring 1–2 wk after drug exposure. Cutaneous symptoms such as urticaria and rash may/may not be present	Penicillins, sulfonamides, cephalosporins, radiocontrast dyes
Respiratory	Rhinitis, asthma	NSAIDs, aspirin
Cutaneous	Mild to severe rash, blistering of the mucosal membranes	Penicillins, cephalosporins, NSAIDs, phenytoin, carbamazepine

NSAIDs = nonsteroidal anti-inflammatory drugs.

and poor air-quality conditions.[40] Box 2 lists avoidance techniques for common specific allergens.[41] Although these are likely the safest and most cost-effective options for managing allergies, they require significant lifestyle changes for both patients and their families.

The histamine-1 (H_1)-antihistamines (e.g., diphenhydramine) function as direct competitive inhibitors between histamine and the H_1-receptors. The H_1-antihistamines are effective, inexpensive, and convenient therapy for alleviating the sneezing, itching, rhinorrhea, and conjunctival symptoms of AR. For children with only mild, intermittent symptoms of AR, H_1-antihistamines are preferred on an as-needed basis. Nonsedating SGAs, such as loratadine, cetirizine, and fexofenadine, are strongly preferred over first-generation antihistamines (FGAs).[42,43] The sedating effects of the FGAs can further diminish cognitive function in children affected with AR.[42] If symptoms are present for more than 4 days/week or for more than 4 weeks/year, or if they begin to affect daily activities, then therapy should be advanced according to the ARIA guidelines for AR treatment (Table 4).[37,43] Dosing recommendations for the various antihistamines are found in Table 5.[46-55]

First-generation antihistamines have a significant adverse effect profile because they are lipophilic and readily cross the blood-brain barrier, resulting in sedation and cognitive impairment. They are also powerful anticholinergic agents that help alleviate symptoms such as runny, watery nose and eyes, but can cause other undesired effects such as sedation, difficulty urinating, constipation, and dry mouth. A paradoxical hyperstimulation, in addition to seizures, arrhythmias, apnea, and dosing errors, has led the U.S. Food and Drug Administration (FDA) to recommend that over-the-counter cough and cold medications, including antihistamines, not be used in children younger than 2 years and to discourage their use in children younger than 4 years.[44] Manufacturers of some over-the-counter cough and cold medications have followed this recommendation, also in accordance with the American Academy of Pediatrics' position, and labeled these products as not for use in children younger than 4 years. First-generation antihistamines should not be used to sedate or promote sleep in children younger than 12 years. For the adolescent population, it is important to educate patients and parents about associated residual daytime sedation caused by a slow elimination of active metabolites.

Second-generation antihistamines are generally preferred over FGAs because they do not have the same central nervous system effects. They are lipophobic, thereby limiting penetration across the blood-brain barrier. Second-generation antihistamines are also preferred over the FGAs because they can be dosed less often.

Because neither FGAs nor SGAs affect nasal congestion, both are less effective as monotherapy than intranasal corticosteroids (INCSs). Second-generation antihistamines may be used as a primary therapy for mild, intermittent AR but should be reserved as an adjunctive treatment for moderate to severe intermittent or mild-severe persistent symptoms. The evidence is unclear whether an H_1-antihistamine in addition to an INCS offers more effective symptom management than an INCS alone, and the decision to add one of these agents should be based on a patient's symptoms and tolerance.

Box 2. Avoidance Techniques for Common Allergens That Cause Allergic Rhinitis[41]

Pollen
Stay inside and keep windows and doors closed during the pollen season
Shower and wash clothes after outdoor activities
Dry clothes and bedding indoors

Mold
Clean indoor moldy surfaces with 5% bleach; then dry thoroughly
Keep damp areas of the house well ventilated and clean regularly
Fix and seal all leaky faucets and pipes
Avoid carpet on concrete or damp floors

Dust Mites
Use "allergen-proof" covers on all pillows, mattresses, and box springs
Wash bedding in hot water (at least 130°F [54.4°C]) weekly
Maintain an indoor humidity < 50%
Remove or minimize carpets and/or upholstered furniture in bedrooms
Wash and dry throw rugs on a regular basis
Remove or minimize any stuffed animals or toys
Use a vacuum with a HEPA (high-efficiency particulate air) filter or a double-layer bag

Animals
Remove the pet from the home, if possible
Do not allow pets into bedrooms
If possible, do not allow pet on/near carpet or upholstered furniture
Have a nonallergic relative clean the animal's house, litter box, and/or cage

Cockroaches
Seal off any area where a cockroach could potentially enter the home
Fix and seal all leaky faucets and pipes
Keep food and garbage in tightly sealed containers and put pet food away as soon as pets are finished eating
Take out garbage and recyclables regularly
Wash dishes immediately after use
Clean under stoves, refrigerators, and toasters regularly
Wipe off all kitchen surfaces on a regular basis

Smoke
Avoid smoking during pregnancy
Do not allow smoking inside the house or car
Do not allow smoking around the allergic child
Avoid wood-burning stoves, fireplaces, or fires

Insect Stings
Stay away from nests
Have any nests around the home destroyed
Remain calm and move away slowly if stinging insects are close by
Avoid brightly colored clothing and perfume
Keep food and drinks covered outdoors
Avoid loose-fitting clothes, open toe shoes, or going barefoot

---

Table 4. ARIA Guidelines for Allergic Rhinitis Treatment[37,43]

Intermittent Allergic Rhinitis		Persistent Allergic Rhinitis	
Mild	Moderate to Severe	Mild	Moderate to Severe

Allergen avoidance
 	
Select ≥ 1 of the following based on symptoms and tolerability:
 	
   Antihistamine (second-generation oral or nasal) or leukotriene inhibitor
   Mast cell stabilizer
 	
If conjunctivitis, consider an intraocular agent based on symptoms
	Allergen avoidance
	
	Intranasal corticosteroid ± antihistamine (second-generation or nasal) or leukotriene inhibitor
	
	If nasal congestion, consider a short-term nasal decongestant
	
	If rhinorrhea, consider ipratropium
	
	If conjunctivitis, consider an intraocular agent based on symptoms
	
	Consider immunotherapy if (any of the following):
	   Prolonged season or symptoms induced by succeeding pollen seasons
	   Lower airway symptoms
	   Insufficiently controlled symptoms on maximal therapy
	   Patient does not want to be on constant or long-term pharmacotherapy
	   Pharmacotherapy induces undesirable adverse effects
	
	Consider omalizumab if ≥ 6 yr, nonresponsive to previous therapies, and severe asthma is also present		

ARIA = Allergic Rhinitis and its Impact on Asthma.

An intranasal antihistamine spray (azelastine or olopatadine) offers an alternative route of administration if a child does not tolerate oral antihistamines. Adverse effects are minimal as long as the drug is not swallowed, but may include bitter taste, headache, dysesthesia, rhinitis, epistaxis, sinusitis, and somnolence.[45] Intranasal antihistamines are inferior to INCSs as a monotherapy for persistent and/or moderate to severe AR, but they may be considered for mild, intermittent AR (Table 4).

Intranasal corticosteroids inhibit the recruitment of inflammatory cells and the release of proinflammatory mediators. Therapy is best initiated before allergen exposure, but if symptoms are already troublesome, then the maximal dose for age should be used initially until symptoms are adequately controlled. Once the child's symptoms are controlled, a step-down therapy should be used to the lowest effective dose. Efficacy does not vary markedly between the various INCSs (Table 5).

Adverse effects of INCSs include mainly local irritation (dryness, burning, and irritation); however, a major concern, especially for the long-term treatment of children, is hypothalamic–pituitary–adrenal axis suppression and growth retardation. Although substantial evidence exists to suggest that these agents have a minimal effect on growth rates, some literature suggests the preferred use of the newer INCSs with low-to-undetectable bioavailability in children to minimize any potential long-term effects.[13,56-58] Table 6 lists the bioavailability of available INCSs.[13,59-62] Oral corticosteroids carry a significant adverse effect profile and are not preferred for the routine treatment of AR.

The ARIA guidelines support the use of an INCS as the first-line therapy after allergen avoidance for persistent AR and moderate to severe intermittent AR.[37] The superior efficacy of INCSs over H_1-antihistamines, both oral and intranasal formulations, on the nasal symptoms of AR is supported by extensive literature.[13,63-65]

Decongestants (e.g., pseudoephedrine) are highly effective for relieving nasal congestion. They act by vasoconstriction through α-receptor stimulation. Oral decongestants are widely available over the counter both as single agents and combined with antihistamines (Table 5). Because of significant adverse effects (e.g., insomnia, agitation, urinary retention), they are recommended only for the temporary relief of nasal obstruction.[37,43] Topical decongestants generally have fewer adverse effects than oral agents, but topical agents should not be used for more than 3 days. Therapy extending beyond 3 days can result in rebound congestion and overall worsening of symptoms.

Mast cell stabilizers are available over the counter (as cromolyn nasal spray) and by prescription (as several ophthalmic solutions). They are most effective if initiated before the start of allergen exposure and may take up to 2–4 weeks for full effectiveness if begun after symptoms develop. Their efficacy is less than that of INCSs or antihistamines; they may therefore be an option for children who cannot tolerate these other therapies. In addition, they have an excellent safety profile, causing mainly local irritation; however, their frequent dosing limits their practicality in children (Table 5).

Montelukast is the only leukotriene inhibitor approved for treating AR (Table 5). Leukotriene inhibitors are competitive antagonists that prevent the binding of cysteinyl leukotrienes (pro-inflammatory mediators released by eosinophils and mast cells) to the CysLT_1 receptor, thus inhibiting inflammatory reactions in the upper respiratory passageways. Some evidence suggests that leukotriene inhibitors are as efficacious as H_1-antihistamines for relieving nasal symptoms, although less so than INCSs.[43,66] Leukotriene inhibitors may carry an additional benefit in patients with asthma because they also inhibit airway smooth muscle contraction. Montelukast is generally well tolerated with minimal adverse effects, with the most common adverse effects being mild headache, ear infection, and nausea.[56] In 2009, the FDA recommended

Table 5. Pharmacologic Agents for Management of Allergic Rhinitis[46-55]

Medication	Dosing by Patient Age	
	Pediatric	Adolescent and Adult
First-Generation Antihistamines		
Brompheniramine	2–5 yr: 1 mg PO every 4–6 hr 6–11 yr: 2 mg PO every 4–6 hr	≥ 12 yr: 4 mg PO every 4–6 hr
Chlorpheniramine maleate	2–5 yr: 1 mg PO every 4–6 hr 6–11 yr: 2 mg PO every 4–6 hr (max 12 mg/day) or ER: 8 mg PO every 12 hr Alternative dosing: 0.35 mg/kg/day PO divided every 4–6 hr	≥ 12 yr: 4 mg PO every 4–6 hr or ER: 8–12 mg PO every 12 hr; max 24 mg/day
Clemastine fumarate	< 6 yr: 0.11–0.34 mg PO every 8–12 hr, max 1.34 mg/day 6–11 yr: 0.34–0.67 mg PO every 12 hr, max 4.02 mg/day	≥ 12 yr: 0.67–1.34 mg PO every 8–12 hr, max 8.04 mg/day
Diphenhydramine (Benadryl[a])	2–5 yr: 6.25 mg PO/IM/IV every 4–6 hr, max 37.5 mg/day 6–11 yr: 12.5–25 mg PO/IM/IV every 4–6 hr, max 150 mg/day Alternative dosing: 1 mg/kg PO/IM/IV every 4–6 hr, up to 50 mg/dose	≥ 12 yr: 25–50 mg PO/IM/IV every 4–6 hr, max 300 mg/day
Second-Generation Antihistamines		
Cetirizine (Zyrtec[a])	6–12 mo: 2.5 mg PO once daily 12 mo–5 yr: 2.5 mg PO every 12–24 hr	≥ 6 yr: 5 mg PO every 12–24 hr or 10 mg PO once daily
Desloratadine	6–11 mo: 1 mg PO once daily 1–5 yr: 1.25 mg PO once daily 6–11 yr: 2.5 mg PO once daily	≥ 12 yr: 5 mg PO once daily
Fexofenadine (Allegra[b])	6–23 mo: 15 mg PO every 12 hr 2–11 yr: 30 mg PO every 12 hr	≥ 12 yr: 60 mg PO every 12 hr or 180 mg PO once daily
Levocetirizine (Xyzal[c])	6 mo–5 yr: 1.25 mg PO once daily 6–11 yr: 2.5 mg PO once daily	≥ 12 yr: 5 mg PO once daily
Loratadine (Claritin[d])	2–5 yr: 5 mg PO daily	≥ 6 yr: 10 mg PO once daily
Oral Decongestants		
Pseudoephedrine (Sudafed[a])	Not recommended for children < 2 yr 2–5 yr: 15 mg PO every 6 hr, max 60 mg/day 6–12 yr: 30 mg PO every 6 hr, max 120 mg/day	≥ 12 yr: 60 mg PO every 6 hr as needed or ER: 120 mg PO every 12 hr or 240 mg PO once daily
Phenylephrine (Sudafed PE[a])	4–6 yr: 2.5 mg PO every 4 hr, max 15 mg/day 7–12 yr: 5 mg PO every 4 hr, max 30 mg/day	≥ 12 yr: 10 mg PO every 4 hr, max 60 mg/day
Topical Decongestants		
Naphazoline 0.05%	6–12 yr: 1 drop or spray in each nostril every 6 hr as needed Therapy should not exceed 3–5 days	≥ 12 yr: 1–2 drops or sprays in each nostril every 3–6 hr as needed Therapy should not exceed 3–5 days
Phenylephrine	≥ 6–11 mo: 0.16% solution: 1–2 drops in each nostril every 3 hr as needed 1–5 yr: 0.125% solution: 2–3 drops in each nostril every 4 hr as needed 6–11 yr: 0.25% solution: 2–3 drops in each nostril every 4 hr as needed Therapy should not exceed 3 days	0.25%–0.5% solution: ≥ 12 yr: 2–3 drops or 1–2 sprays in each nostril every 4 hr as needed Therapy should not exceed 3–5 days
Oxymetazoline 0.05% (Afrin[e])	≥ 6 yr: 2–3 drops or sprays in each nostril every 12 hr Therapy should not exceed 3 days	
Xylometazoline 0.1%	≥ 12 yr: 2–3 drops into each nostril every 8–10 hr as needed Therapy should not exceed 3 days	
Nasal Corticosteroids		
Beclomethasone (Beconase AQ[f]) 42 mcg/spray	≥ 6 yr: 1–2 sprays in each nostril every 12 hr After symptoms are controlled, titrate to lowest effective dose	
Budesonide (Rhinocort Aqua[g]) 32 mcg/spray	6–11 yr: 1–2 sprays in each nostril once daily After symptoms are controlled, titrate to lowest effective dose	≥ 12 yr: 1–4 sprays in each nostril once daily After symptoms are controlled, titrate to lowest effective dose
Ciclesonide (Omnaris[h]) 50 mcg/spray	> 6 yr: 2 sprays in each nostril once daily After symptoms are controlled, titrate to lowest effective dose	
Fluticasone propionate (Flonase[i]) 50 mcg/spray	≥ 4 yr: 1–2 sprays in each nostril once daily After symptoms are controlled, titrate to lowest effective dose	Adult: 2 sprays in each nostril once daily Alternative dosing: 1 spray in each nostril every 12 hr After symptoms are controlled, titrate to lowest effective dose
Fluticasone furoate (Flonase Sensimist[j]) 27.5 mcg/spray	≥ 2 yr: 1–2 sprays in each nostril once daily After symptoms are controlled, titrate to lowest effective dose	

(continued)

Table 5. Pharmacologic Agents for Management of Allergic Rhinitis[46-55] *(continued)*

Medication	Dosing by Patient Age	
	Pediatric	**Adolescent and Adult**
Nasal Corticosteroids *(continued)*		
Flunisolide 29 mcg/spray	6–14 yr: 1 spray in each nostril every 8–24 hr Alternative dosing: 2 sprays in each nostril every 12 hr, max 4 sprays/nostril/day After symptoms are controlled, titrate to lowest effective dose	≥ 15 yr: 2 sprays in each nostril every 8–12 hr, max 8 sprays/nostril/day After symptoms are controlled, titrate to lowest effective dose
Mometasone (Nasonex[j]) 50 mcg/spray	2–11 yr: 1 spray in each nostril once daily After symptoms are controlled, titrate to lowest effective dose	≥ 12 yr: 2 sprays in each nostril once daily After symptoms are controlled, titrate to lowest effective dose
Triamcinolone (Nasacort[b]) 55 mcg/spray	2–5 yr: 1 spray in each nostril once daily 6–11 yr: 1–2 sprays in each nostril once daily After symptoms are controlled, titrate to lowest effective dose	≥ 12 yr: 1–2 sprays in each nostril once daily After symptoms are controlled, titrate to lowest effective dose
Nasal Antihistamine		
Azelastine 0.1% intranasal solution	5–11 yr: 1 spray in each nostril every 12 hr	≥ 12 yr: 1–2 sprays in each nostril every 12 hr
Olopatadine (Patanase[k]) 0.6% intranasal solution	6–11 yr: 1 spray in each nostril every 12 hr	≥ 12 yr: 2 sprays in each nostril every 12 hr
Nasal Mast Cell Stabilizer		
Cromolyn	≥ 2 yr: 1 spray in each nostril every 6–8 hr	
Nasal Anticholinergic		
Ipratropium (Atrovent[l]) 0.03%, 0.06%	≥ 6 yr: 0.03%: 2 sprays in each nostril every 8–12 hr ≥ 5 yr: 0.06%: 2 sprays in each nostril every 6–8 hr	
Ophthalmic Antihistamines		
Azelastine (Optivar[m]) 0.05% solution	≥ 3 yr: 1 drop into each affected eye every 12 hr	
Emedastine 0.05% solution	≥ 3 yr: 1 drop into each affected eye up to four times/day	
Ophthalmic Antihistamines/Decongestant Combinations		
Antazoline 0.05% + naphazoline 0.05% solution	≥ 6 yr: 1–2 drops into affected eye(s) as needed, max four times/day	
Pheniramine 0.3% + naphazoline 0.025% (Naphcon-A[k]) solution	≥ 6 yr: 1–2 drops into affected eye(s) as needed, max four times/day	
Ophthalmic Antihistamine/Mast Cell Stabilizers		
Ketotifen (Zaditor[k]) 0.025% solution	≥ 3 yr: 1 drop into lower conjunctival sac of affected eye(s) twice daily at an interval of 8–12 hr	
Olopatadine (Patanol[k]) 0.1% solution	≥ 3 yr: 1 drop into each affected eye twice daily at an interval of 6–8 hr	
Olopatadine (Pataday[k]) 0.2% solution	≥ 2 yr: 1 drop into each affected eye once daily	
Olopatadine (Pazeo[k]) 0.7% solution	≥ 2 yr: 1 drop into each affected eye once daily	
Ophthalmic Mast Cell Stabilizers		
Cromolyn 4% solution	≥ 4 yr: 1–2 drops in affected eye(s) every 4–6 hr	
Lodoxamide 0.1% solution	≥ 2 yr: 1–2 drops in affected eye(s) every 6 hr for up to 3 mo	
Nedocromil 2% solution	≥ 3 yr: 1–2 drops in affected eye(s) every 12 hr	
Ophthalmic Nonsteroidal Anti-inflammatory Drugs (NSAIDs)		
Ketorolac (Acular[n]) 0.5% solution	≥ 3 yr: 1 drop in affected eye(s) every 6 hr	
Leukotriene Inhibitors		
Montelukast (Singulair[j])	6 mo–5 yr: 4 mg PO once daily 6–14 yr: 5 mg PO once daily	≥ 15 yr: 10 mg PO once daily
Monoclonal Antibodies		
Omalizumab (Xolair[o])	≥ 6 yr: 75 – 375mg by subcutaneous injection every 2-4 weeks Dose (mg) and dosing frequency are determined by IgE levels measured before start of treatment and body weight	

[a]McNeil Consumer Healthcare, Fort Washington, PA; [b]Chattem, Inc., Chattanooga, TN; [c]UCB, Inc., Smyrna, GA; [d]Bayer Healthcare, LLC, Whippany, NJ; [e]Lil' Drug Store Products, Inc., Cedar Rapids, IA; [f]GlaxoSmithKline, Research Triangle Park, NC; [g]AstraZeneca, Wilmington, DE; [h]Sunovion Pharmaceuticals Inc., Marlborough, MA; [i]GSK Consumer Healthcare, Warren, NJ; [j]Merck Sharp & Dohme Corp., Whitehouse Station, NJ; [k]Alcon Laboratories, Inc., Fort Worth, TX; [l]Boehringer Ingelheim Pharmaceuticals, Inc., Ridgefield, CT; [m]Meda Pharmaceuticals, Inc., Somerset, NJ; [n]Allergan, Inc., Irvine, CA; [o]Genentech, Inc., South San Francisco, CA
ER = extended release; IM = intramuscularly; IV = intravenously; max = maximum; PO = orally.

precautionary warning labeling for all leukotriene inhibitors to include the following neuropsychiatric events: agitation, aggression, anxiousness, depression, dream abnormalities, hallucinations, insomnia, restlessness, suicidal ideation, and tremor. The warning was not exclusive to the pediatric population; however, case reports of neuropsychiatric events in children do exist.[67,68]

Although generics are now available, leukotriene inhibitors still carry a higher drug cost, and they are not recommended over an H_1-antihistamine. If a patient has elevated leukotriene levels, leukotriene inhibitors may be beneficial either as a primary therapy or in addition to an H_1-antihistamine or INCS, but there is not currently a way to predict this benefit. If a patient has not responded sufficiently to either an H_1-antihistamine or INCS, it may be worth either adding or replacing with a leukotriene receptor. Some benefit may occur in patients with concomitant asthma, but the role of leukotriene inhibitors in AR has yet to be clearly defined.[43]

Ophthalmic therapies are excellent options for patients with conjunctivitis symptoms (Table 5). They act locally, often with minimal adverse effects aside from local irritation. These therapies are excellent options for children with symptoms limited to the eye area.

Ipratropium is an anticholinergic agent that relieves rhinorrhea (Table 5). When applied topically, it has an antisecretory effect but does not offer relief for other symptoms. Because ipratropium is a topical agent, it has a minimal adverse effect profile, with the most common adverse effects being epistaxis and nasal dryness.

Immunotherapy should be reserved for patients with severe symptoms not well controlled under standard therapy. It is typically a two-phase process. The first phase of immunotherapy consists of subcutaneous injections or sublingual tablets of diluted allergen extracts given at frequent intervals and increasing in concentration until a predetermined target dose is reached, typically over 3–4 months. Once the target dose is reached, maintenance injections are given as the second phase every 2–3 months for 3–5 years. The first injection or tablet is typically given in the medical office setting followed by observation of the patient for an hour or more. If no reaction occurs, then the dose may be raised and repeated that same day or the patient may be asked to return at a later time, typically 1 week, for more doses. Subcutaneous therapy is typically given weekly with in-office dose escalations occurring as tolerated. Sublingual therapy is typically taken daily by the patient at home with weekly dose escalation done in the office setting, again, as tolerated. Over time, the patient's immune system becomes tolerant of the allergens and stops producing hypersensitivity reactions. There is evidence that subcutaneous therapy is more effective in reducing symptoms; however, sublingual therapy involves less pain on the patient's part (typically preferred in pediatrics) and has a lower risk of anaphylaxis.[69] More study is needed to recommend one form over another.

Although well established in adults, the efficacy and safety of immunotherapy is controversial in the pediatric population.[13] Immunotherapy can result in life-threatening anaphylactic reactions, requiring that most treatments be administered in an office setting with an adequate observation period. The ARIA guidelines set the same indications for immunotherapy in both children 5 years or older and adults as follows: patients with symptoms induced predominantly by allergen exposure; patients with a prolonged pollen season or with symptoms induced by succeeding pollen seasons; patients with rhinitis and symptoms from the lower airways during peak allergen exposure; patients in whom antihistamines and moderate-dose topical glucocorticoids insufficiently control symptoms; patients who do not want to be on constant or long-term pharmacotherapy; and patients in whom pharmacotherapy induces undesirable adverse effects.[37] It is important to weigh the benefits and risks of immunotherapy before therapy is initiated. Immunotherapy is a long-term, costly investment; a typical course involves one or two treatments per week for 8–12 weeks and then every 4 weeks for 3–5 years.

An alternative agent in the treatment of AR is omalizumab (Xolair, Genentech, Inc., South San Francisco, CA), a monoclonal antibody that binds to circulating IgE. The IgE-omalizumab complex cannot interact with mast cells or basophils, thus inhibiting IgE-mediated allergic reactions. The label approval by the FDA is for patients 6 years or older with moderate to severe persistent asthma who have a positive skin test or in vitro reactivity to a perennial aeroallergen and whose symptoms are inadequately controlled with inhaled corticosteroids.[55] Omalizumab carries a black box warning for potentially life-threatening allergic reactions after any dose, even if there is no history of a reaction. Because of its significant cost and potentially life-threatening allergic reactions, omalizumab should be reserved for patients 6 years or older who have not adequately responded to other AR treatments.

Table 6. Bioavailability of Intranasal Corticosteroids[13,59–62]

Medication	Bioavailability (%)
Beclomethasone	44
Fluticasone propionate	< 2
Flunisolide	50
Triamcinolone	< 1
Mometasone	< 0.1
Ciclesonide	< 1
Budesonide	34
Fluticasone furoate	< 1

FOOD ALLERGIES

The goals for managing food allergies are primarily to minimize the effect on quality of life and reduce anxiety. The best treatment is prevention, and children and their parents should receive instruction on the importance of avoiding allergens. Referral to an allergist can assist in specifically identifying the offending food or foods, which can help prevent an overly restrictive diet. Consulting with a nutritionist may also help ensure adequate nutrition in conjunction with the dietary limitations.

In 2015, the landmark LEAP (Learning Early about Peanut Allergy) trial suggested that early introduction to peanuts was safe in infants at high risk of developing a peanut allergy and reduced the risk of developing a subsequent peanut allergy by 81%. The LEAP trial—and also later, the National Institute of Allergy and Infectious Diseases and the American Academy of Pediatrics—recommends introducing age-appropriate peanut foods as early as 4–6 months in infants with severe eczema, egg allergy, or both to reduce the risk of peanut allergy. Serum peanut IgE should be tested before introduction in these most high-risk infants. Results will determine if the infant should be referred to a specialist or is able to continue with the introduction. In children with no to moderate eczema, peanut foods should be introduced around age 6 months in the home setting in accordance with family preferences and cultural practices. Other solid foods should be introduced before peanut foods to demonstrate developmental readiness.[70,71]

The focus of pharmacologic treatment is purely symptomatic management (e.g., diphenhydramine for hives) because no recommended pharmacologic treatment currently exists for preventing food allergies. Food-induced anaphylactic reactions should be treated as a life-threatening emergency in which treatment is initiated as quickly as possible. The treatment of anaphylaxis is discussed later in this chapter.

DRUG ALLERGIES

The goal of treating allergic drug reactions is symptomatic management. Oral antihistamines can be used for treating cutaneous pruritus and rashes. Topical corticosteroids are an option if the reaction is localized to a small area. Topical steroids should not be used over extensive areas, particularly in children, because of the risk of significant systemic absorption.

Anaphylaxis triggered by any drug should be treated as outlined in the following Treatment of Anaphylaxis section. The offending drug should be discontinued immediately. For nonlife-threatening reactions, the benefits and risks should be considered before discontinuing the medication.

Ultimately, when a clinician is deciding whether to use an agent to which a patient has a documented or suspected allergy, it is best to consider the severity of the previous reaction, the specific symptoms present during the previous reaction, and the timing of the reaction relative to the trigger exposure. Delayed cutaneous reactions, especially to antibiotics, have a low probability of recurring on rechallenge.[72,73]

ANAPHYLAXIS

Promptly initiating treatment is vital to minimizing anaphylactic-related morbidity and preventing death.[30,31,74] If possible, the allergic trigger should be avoided or discontinued as quickly as possible. The primary goal should always be to restore and maintain airway, breathing, and circulation, although the emphasis in this chapter will be on treatments specific to anaphylaxis.

It is also important to consider the possibility of a biphasic anaphylactic reaction. This type of reaction occurs in up to 20% of anaphylactic cases and can be as severe as the initial reaction.[18] The patient will appear to have recovered from the initial episode and suddenly develop a second acute episode of bronchospasm that does not respond as well to initial therapies. Thus, it is important to observe patients before discharge for at least 4–6 hours with moderate reactions and for up to 8–24 hours with severe refractory reactions.[75-77]

Epinephrine is well supported as the primary pharmacologic intervention for treating anaphylaxis and should be administered as soon as anaphylaxis is suspected (Table 7).[28,75,76] Despite strong evidence in favor of using epinephrine, other evidence suggests that this treatment is vastly underused in both the community and emergency settings, with less than 50% of all anaphylactic cases receiving an epinephrine intramuscular injection.[78] An optimal window for epinephrine administration has not been studied; however, delaying epinephrine treatment may be severely detrimental because the lack of prompt treatment with epinephrine is a major risk factor for anaphylactic-related death.[30,31,74] It is worth noting that delayed epinephrine administration is likely to offer some benefit over no administration, so epinephrine should be given as soon as it becomes available.

The action of epinephrine during anaphylaxis is 3-fold: it is an α_1-agonist causing increased blood pressure and decreased vascular permeability by vasoconstriction of vascular smooth muscle, a β_1-agonist causing increased inotropic and chronotropic effects (increased heart rate and cardiac contractility), and a β_2-agonist resulting in bronchodilation.[79,80] Administering intramuscular epinephrine to the anterior lateral thigh is preferred because of its more rapid absorption and attainment of higher peaks compared with subcutaneous injections.[65,81] Subcutaneous injection has slow absorption because of local vasoconstriction.[75] Intravenous administration carries a high risk of dosing errors, particularly in children; it is not practical in most community settings; and it is generally not recommended except when intramuscular epinephrine is ineffective or in an acute care setting with continuous cardiac monitoring.[75,82] Epinephrine 1:1000 is dosed at 0.01 mg/kg intravenously/intramuscularly, up to 0.3 mg in children and 0.5 mg in older children and adults. Autoinjectors for intramuscular administration are commercially available in 0.15-mg and 0.3-mg doses. Children who weigh 10–25 kg should receive 0.15 mg, and 0.3 mg is indicated for children weighing 25 kg or more.[34] Several doses may be necessary in severe reactions and can be given every 5–15 minutes, as necessary.[24,75] Patient education on using an autoinjector is discussed later in the Patient Education section.

Although β-blocker use is uncommon in the pediatric population, the response to epinephrine could theoretically be reduced if the patient is concomitantly taking β-blockers.[75,83] Although largely unsupported in the literature, the use of glucagon in children could be useful if epinephrine is having a reduced effect in a patient known to be using a β-blocker. At high doses, glucagon is thought to produce a positive cardiac inotropic effect independent of β-receptors. The recommended dose in children is a 20- to 30-mcg/kg bolus dose up to a maximum of 1 mg administered intravenously over 5 minutes, followed by a continuous infusion of 5–15 mcg/minute titrated to clinical effect.[75] Vomiting is a common adverse effect, so the airway should be secured before administration.

Aggressive fluid resuscitation (10–20 mL/kg) with a crystalloid intravenous solution such as 0.9% saline or (lactated) Ringer solution may be required to support cardiovascular function if initial doses of epinephrine are ineffective. Other vasopressors, such as dopamine or norepinephrine, may be required if fluid resuscitation and epinephrine are inadequate. Patients should be placed in a supine position with legs raised to maximize blood flow to vital organs.[28,75] Supplemental oxygen may also be of use to patients experiencing respiratory symptoms and wheezing. Endotracheal intubation should be used if the patient is unable to maintain a patent airway.

The H_1-antihistamines are the most commonly used pharmacologic intervention for anaphylaxis, but they are not effective as a primary therapy.[78] These agents have a much

Table 7. Management of Anaphylaxis[24]

First-Line Therapies	
Epinephrine IM (autoinjector or 1:1000 solution)	10–25 kg: 0.15 mg IM autoinjector > 25 kg: 0.3 mg IM autoinjector Alternative: 0.01 mg/kg/dose, max 0.5 mg/dose May repeat every 5–15 min as needed
Adjunctive Therapies	
Fluid resuscitation	10–20 mL/kg
Supine position with lower extremities elevated	
Supplemental oxygen	
Glucagon	IV bolus: 20–30 mcg/kg over 5 min, max 1 mg over 5 min ≥ 12 yr: 1–5 mg May follow with continuous IV infusion of 5–15 mcg/min
H_1-Antihistamines	
Diphenhydramine	1–2 mg/kg/dose PO/IM/IV every 4–6 hr, up to 50-mg/dose
Chlorpheniramine	2–5 yr: 1 mg PO every 4–6 hr 6–11 yr: 2 mg PO every 4–6 hr ≥ 12 yr: 4 mg PO every 4–6 hr
Cetirizine	6–12 mo: 2.5 mg PO once daily 12 mo–5 yr: 2.5 mg PO every 12–24 hr > 6 yr: 5 mg PO every 12–24 hr or 10 mg PO once daily
Levocetirizine	6 mo–5 yr: 1.25 mg PO once daily 6–11 yr: 2.5 mg PO once daily ≥ 12 yr: 5 mg PO once daily
Loratadine	2–5 yr: 5 mg PO daily ≥ 6 yr: 10 mg PO once daily
Desloratadine	6–11 mo: 1 mg PO once daily 1–5 yr: 1.25 mg PO once daily 6–11 yr: 2.5 mg PO once daily ≥ 12 yr: 5 mg PO once daily
Fexofenadine	6–23 mo: 15 mg PO every 12 hr 2–11 yr: 30 mg PO every 12 hr ≥ 12 yr: 60 mg PO every 12 hr or 180 mg PO once daily
H_2-Antihistamines	
Ranitidine	1–2 mg/kg/dose PO/IV, maximum 150 mg
Short-Acting β-Agonist	
Albuterol nebulized solution	≤ 11 yr: 0.15 mg/kg every 20 min × 3 doses; then 0.15–0.3 mg/kg every 1–4 hr, max 10 mg/dose ≥ 12 yr: 2.5–5 mg every 20 min × 3 doses; then 2.5–10 mg every 1–4 hr Alternative: 0.5 mg/kg/hr continuous nebulization (Adults: 10–15 mg/hr)
Albuterol MDI	4–8 puffs every 20 min × 3 doses; then every 1–4 hr as needed (same dosing for adults)
Glucocorticoids	
Prednisone Methylprednisolone	1 mg/kg PO, max 80 mg 1 mg/kg IV, max 80 mg

H_1 = histamine-1; H_2 = histamine-2; IM = intramuscular; IV = intravenous; max = maximum dose; MDI = metered dose inhaler; PO = oral.

slower onset of action than epinephrine and do not affect the life-threatening cardiovascular or pulmonary symptoms of anaphylaxis. The H_1-antihistamines should be used only as an adjuvant therapy for the relief of anaphylactic-related cutaneous and nasal symptoms (e.g., urticarial, flushing, rhinorrhea). Some evidence exists that H_1- and H_2-antihistamines given together are more effective at treating the cutaneous symptoms of anaphylaxis versus H_1-antihistamines alone.[24,75,83] Dosing information on various antihistamines is presented in Table 7.

Inhaled short-acting β-agonists such as albuterol may be used as an adjunct to epinephrine for bronchospasm. However, their efficacy for anaphylaxis is not well supported, and delivery may be impaired in severe reactions.

Glucocorticoids have not been evaluated for use in anaphylactic reactions. Because of their usefulness in other allergic reactions (drug-mediated and AR), however, they are commonly used in treating acute anaphylaxis. Prednisone 1 mg/kg orally (maximum 80 mg) or methylprednisolone 1 mg/kg intravenously (maximum 80 mg) may be used as single one-time doses during acute anaphylaxis and repeated every 6 hours if symptoms require. Some evidence suggests they help prevent a biphasic reaction, although the evidence is minimal.[30,84]

Table 8. Sample Desensitization Protocol for 1 Gram of Intravenous Penicillin[85]

Step	Drug (mg/mL)	Amount (mL)	Total Amount of Penicillin (mg)
1	0.1	0.1	0.01
2	0.1	0.2	0.02
3	0.1	0.4	0.04
4	0.1	0.8	0.08
5	1	0.16	0.16
6	1	0.32	0.32
7	1	0.64	0.64
8	10	0.12	1.2
9	10	0.24	2.4
10	10	0.48	4.8
11	100	0.1	10
12	100	0.2	20
13	100	0.4	40
14	100	0.8	80
15	1000	0.16	160
16	1000	0.32	320
17	1000	0.64	640
18	1000	1	1000

Instructions:

Protocol must be performed in an intensive care unit setting with intravenous line and continuous monitoring in place

15 Minutes should elapse between doses

Between Steps 17 and 18, 30 minutes should elapse

If a dose is missed, protocol must be restarted from the beginning

DESENSITIZATION

Patients may require treatment with a medication known to induce anaphylaxis. Desensitization can be performed by gradually exposing the patient to small doses of the medication according to a strict protocol. The protocol must be started from the beginning if a dose is missed. The full dose of the medication must be given on completing the protocol; otherwise, it must be repeated. Ultimately, this desensitization allows the temporary administration of necessary medication with few adverse effects. Table 8 provides an example desensitization protocol for penicillin.[85] For initial desensitization, patients must be monitored in an inpatient setting with intravenous access and cardiopulmonary monitoring. Often, after the initial desensitization, patients can be desensitized in an outpatient setting. These protocols are commonly used for patients with cystic fibrosis who are colonized with several drug-resistant organisms for whom maximizing antibiotic choices through desensitization is often the only choice.

PATIENT/CAREGIVER EDUCATION

For patients who have experienced severe allergic reactions, prevention education for future episodes must be discussed with each parent with an emphasis on parents in turn educating each caregiver, including day care staff, grandparents, teachers, coaches, and babysitters. This approach includes a prescription for self-injectable epinephrine and instructions on its use and storage. All patients should have action plans in place at school and extracurricular events. Precautions must be taken to avoid known allergens, and caretakers of children should be aware of this importance.

For patients being treated for milder allergic reactions, education regarding prevention is also vital. For severe reactions, both the child and caregivers should take precautions to avoid known triggers. Even children with a history of only mild allergic reactions should be given a prescription for an epinephrine autoinjector because most severe reactions occur in children with no history of allergy.

Proper education is critical for appropriate and accurate use of an epinephrine autoinjector. Children and their parents should be counseled not to delay injection if anaphylaxis is suspected because delayed injections are associated with worse outcomes. The commercially available autoinjectors are designed to work through clothing, so clothing removal is unnecessary before administration. Doses should only be injected into the outer thigh, never into the buttock. In addition, most of the liquid stays in the autoinjector after administration; thus, even if a decreased amount is not visible, patients should be assured they received the correct dose. It is also important to counsel patients never to put thumbs, fingers, or hands over the tip of the autoinjector because accidental injection might occur. If the patient does accidentally inject the liquid into the hands or feet, immediate medical attention should be sought because this injection may result in local vasoconstriction and loss of blood flow to the affected extremity. Box 3 provides instructions for using an epinephrine autoinjector.[86]

The importance of seeking immediate medical attention should also be stressed, as should the fact that the epinephrine injection is not a replacement for medical evaluation and treatment. Medical attention or an emergency 911 notification should be sought immediately after epinephrine is administered. The patient should bring the used autoinjector to the emergency department and alert the medical providers that a dose of epinephrine was administered.

Patients receiving a prescription or over-the-counter recommendation for a nasal spray should be counseled on appropriate technique. Proper technique can help maximize efficacy and minimize local irritation and adverse effects. Sprays should always be primed before first use or if stored unused for more than 1 week. Patients should blow their nose, if possible, before use. If considerable crusting or mucous is present, patients should be encouraged to use a saline nasal spray or irrigation before using the medication. This approach will allow a maximum application of spray to the nasal membranes. Sprays should always be directed away from the nasal septum to avoid the risk of perforation and irritation. The patient should breathe gently inward through the nostril after each spray and out through the mouth. Nasal applicators

should be wiped clean after use and recapped. Adults should assist young children who may have difficulty with these steps.

CONCLUSIONS

Diagnosing AR, drug allergies, and food allergies involves a combination of history and laboratory testing. Drug and food allergies can be managed through recognizing and avoiding triggers. Although AR may be managed through avoiding allergens, it often requires pharmacologic intervention. Pharmacologic treatment of AR should be selected on the basis of a child's specific symptoms and optimized for quality of life. For the treatment of mild, intermittent AR, SGAs are the first-line agent. For patients with moderate to severe or persistent rhinitis, INCSs should be given with FGAs or SGAs added if needed. Other pharmacologic agents may be added to treat specific symptoms as need arises (e.g., ophthalmic agents, nasal decongestants). Finding the most effective combination while minimizing the adverse effects of therapies can be challenging because so many effective pharmacologic options are available for physicians and patients to consider.

The pharmacologic treatment of anaphylaxis is difficult to study in a standardized manner. It is unethical to conduct a placebo-controlled trial of epinephrine administration and dosing; therefore, clinicians continue to use the guidelines established from years of clinical experience. It is important to remember that anaphylaxis is a potentially fatal reaction that may occur within minutes of drug or allergen exposure. Medical treatment should be sought immediately if anaphylaxis is suspected. Intramuscular epinephrine should be administered as soon as possible because prompt delivery results in a dramatic improvement in symptoms and reduced morbidity. In the acute care setting, additional measures such as fluid resuscitation and vasopressor use may be required. Antihistamines (first or second generation) should never be considered a first-line agent for anaphylaxis treatment because they have no effect on the life-threatening cardiovascular or pulmonary symptoms. Finally, providing education about avoiding triggers is very important in all allergic diseases, as is ensuring that patients have medications such as epinephrine available and instructions on their proper use.

Box 3. Instructions for Use of an Epinephrine Autoinjector[86]

Flip open the cap of the epinephrine autoinjector of the carrier tube

Remove the autoinjector from the carrier tube

Form a fist around the unit with the orange end pointed downward

Pull off the blue safety release—do NOT remove the blue safety release until ready to use

Hold the orange tip near the outer thigh

Swing and FIRMLY PUSH the orange tip against the outer thigh until a click is heard; the unit should be at a 90-degree angle to the outer thigh

Hold FIRMLY against the thigh for about 10 seconds

Remove unit from thigh; the orange tip will extend to cover the needle

Massage injection area for 10 seconds

A 10-year-old boy is evaluated for increasing problems with stuffy nose, coughing, and "allergies." His mother reports that symptoms have always seemed to worsen in the late summer/early fall with the start of each school year, but since they moved and he started at a new school this year, his symptoms did not improve as the school year continued. She has become increasingly concerned because his symptoms have persisted for several months now and have worsened to the point of affecting his school performance and sleep. The patient reports that he has had a runny nose, sneezing, and coughing in previous school years, but "never as bad as this year." He also reports that he is awoken at night by coughing and that the nasal congestion makes it hard to him to breathe. He reports feeling tired during the day despite an adequate amount of sleep. His mother states that she had given him some over-the-counter diphenhydramine 25 mg, but it made him sleepy and unable to concentrate during the daytime.

The patient's mother says that he received a diagnosis of asthma as a young child, but he has mainly experienced symptoms when exercising or during a viral illness. His symptoms have always been well controlled with an albuterol metered dose inhaler, using two inhalations no sooner than every 4 hours as needed. His mother denies that he has any known drug or food allergies. His immunizations are up to date. He takes no medications other than the occasional albuterol.

His family history is positive for a grandfather with asthma and a maternal aunt with severe seasonal allergies. He lives with both parents and has no pets. He has carpet in his bedroom, a 7-year-old mattress, and a 1-year-old pillow. There are no smokers at home.

1. What signs and symptoms of allergic rhinitis (AR) are present in this patient?

This patient has the classic symptoms of AR, including a runny, stuffy nose and sneezing and coughing that worsen predictably during allergen season. Starting a new school in a new area could likely have triggered sensitivities to existing allergens that are more common in his new school environment. Also, the carpet in his bedroom could be exacerbating his symptoms if he is sensitive to dust mites or mold. His history of asthma and his family history of allergic disease (asthma and seasonal allergies) further strengthen the case for AR versus a viral illness.

This patient meets the Allergic Rhinitis and its Impact on Asthma classification for moderate to severe, persistent AR. His symptoms have been present for more than 4 weeks/year. He is also experiencing impaired sleep, decreased performance at school, and other negative symptoms.

2. What nonpharmacologic measures would you recommend to prevent symptoms?

First-line therapy for treating AR should always include avoiding or removing the offending allergen. Regular and thorough cleanings of the patient's house should be performed and his mother should consider removing the carpet from his bedroom, if possible. Clothes and bedding should be washed in hot water weekly and "allergen-proof" covers should be used on all of the patient's pillows and mattresses. Special care should be taken to perform the most frequent and more thorough cleanings during the late summer and early fall when his symptoms seem to peak. It is also advisable to refer him for skin testing because this information may help him identify and avoid his particular triggering allergens.

3. What pharmacologic therapy would you recommend and why?

Pharmacotherapy should be initiated with an intranasal corticosteroid. One with a low bioavailability such as mometasone or fluticasone is preferred to minimize any potential effect on the patient's growth. Because he is already experiencing severe symptoms, the maximum dose should be initiated until his symptoms are well controlled. Once symptoms are under control, a step-down dose should be used down to the lowest effective dose for symptom management. The addition of a second-generation antihistamine (SGA) should be considered at least until his symptoms are under control. A first-generation antihistamine should be avoided because of their sedating effects and lack of efficacy over SGAs. All the SGAs listed in Table 5 are considered equally effective. If the intranasal corticosteroid and SGA do not yield satisfactory symptom control, the addition of the leukotriene inhibitor, montelukast, may be considered. Montelukast carries a significant increased cost compared with the SGA.

Case (continued). The patient has returned for evaluation after 6 months of continuous therapy on mometasone 0.05% nasal spray 1 spray in each nostril once daily, loratadine 10 mg once daily, and montelukast 5 mg once daily. He has experienced moderate relief, but his mother is still concerned that symptoms are interfering with his schoolwork and sleep throughout the year. She reports that the patient has had skin testing, which demonstrated ragweed and pollen allergies. She recently heard about "allergy shots" and asks if they would be a good option for her son.

4. Is immunotherapy appropriate for this patient? What are the advantages and disadvantages of this therapy?

Because this patient's symptoms are not satisfactorily controlled on his current therapy and he is experiencing the symptoms year-round, immunotherapy is an appropriate next step. His mother should be counseled that immunotherapy is effective in the long-term reduction of symptoms, but requires a minimum 3- to 5-year commitment of once- to twice-weekly office visits. Adverse reactions can include local skin reactions (redness, swelling, itching) if subcutaneous therapy is chosen. Sublingual therapy may be preferred given the patient's age. In both subcutaneous and sublingual therapy, there is risk of anaphylaxis (although the risk is low). Cost of medications and office visits should be considered before choosing to initiate therapy.

REFERENCES

1. U.S. Department of Health and Human Services, Agency for Healthcare Research and Quality (AHRQ). Management of Allergic and Non-Allergic Rhinitis. AHQR Publication No. 02: E023. Summary, Evidence Report/Technology Assessment: No. 54. Boston: AHRQ, 2002. Available at https://archive.ahrq.gov/clinic/tp/rhintp.htm. Accessed October 5, 2019.

2. Settipane RA. Demographics and epidemiology of allergic and nonallergic rhinitis. Allergy Asthma Proc 2001;22:185-9.

3. Singh K, Axelrod S, Bielory L. The epidemiology of ocular and nasal allergy in the United States, 1988-1994. J Allergy Clin Immunol 2010;126:778-83.

4. Simola M, Holopainene E, Malmberg H. Changes in skin and nasal sensitivity to allergens and the course of rhinitis; a long-term follow-up study. Ann Allergy Asthma Immunol 1999;82:152-6.

5. Matheson MC, Dharmage SC, Abramson MJ, et al. Direct expenditures for the treatment of allergic rhinoconjunctivitis in 1996, including the contributions of related airway illnesses. J Allergy Clin Immunol 1999;103:401-7.

6. Frew AJ. Advances in environmental and occupational disease 2003. J Allergy Clin Immunol 2004;113:1161-6.

7. Watson WT, Becker AB, Simons FE. Treatment of allergic rhinitis with intranasal corticosteroids in patients with mild asthma: effect on lower airway responsiveness. J Allergy Clin Immunol 1993;91:97-101.

8. Brawley A, Silverman B, Kearney S, et al. Allergic rhinitis in children with attention-deficit/hyperactivity disorder. Ann Allergy Asthma Immunol 2004;92:663-7.

9. Vuurman EF, Van Veggel LM, Uiterwijk MM, et al. Seasonal allergic rhinitis and antihistamine effects on children's learning. Ann Allergy 1993;71:121-6.

10. Marshall PS, O'Hara C, Steinberg P. Effects of seasonal allergic rhinitis on selected cognitive abilities. Ann Allergy Asthma Immunol 2000;84:403-10.

11. Walker S, Khan-Wasti S, Fletcher M, et al. Seasonal allergic rhinitis is associated with a detrimental effect on examination performance in United Kingdom teenagers: case-control study. J Allergy Clin Immunol 2007;120:381-7.

12. Meltzer EO, Blaiss MS, Derebery MJ, et al. Burden of allergic rhinitis: results from the Pediatric Allergies in America survey. J Allergy Clin Immunol 2009;124:S43-70.

13. Georgalas C, Terreehorst I, Fokkens W. Current management of allergic rhinitis in children. Pediatr Allergy Immunol 2010; 21:e119-26.

14. Cuffel B, Wamboldt M, Borish L, et al. Economic consequences of comorbid depression, anxiety, and allergic rhinitis. Psychosomatics 1999;40:491-6.

15. Baena-Cagnani CE. Allergic rhinitis and asthma in children: disease management and outcomes. Curr Allergy Asthma Rep 2001; 1:515-22.

16. Rudders SA, Banerji A, Vassallo MF, et al. Trends in pediatric emergency department visits for food-induced anaphylaxis. J Allergy Clin Immunol 2010;126:385-8.

17. Branum AM, Lukacs SL. Food allergy among children in the United States. Pediatrics 2009;124:1549-55.

18. Sicherer SH. Epidemiology of food allergy. J Allergy Clin Immunol 2011;127:594-602.

19. Liu AH, Jaramillo R, Sicherer SH, et al. National prevalence and risk factors for food allergy and relationship to asthma: results from the National Health and Nutrition Examination Survey 2005–2006. J Allergy Clin Immunol 2010;126:798-806.

20. Boyce JA, Assa'ad A, Burks AW, et al. Guidelines for the diagnosis and management of food allergy in the United States: summary of the NIAID-sponsored expert panel report. J Allergy Clin Immunol 2010;126:1105-18.

21. Chafen JJ, Newberry SJ, Riedl MA, et al. Diagnosing and managing common food allergies: a systematic review. JAMA 2010; 303:1848-56.

22. Gupta RS, Springston EE, Warrier MR, et al. The prevalence, severity, and distribution of childhood food allergy in the United States. Pediatrics 2011;128:e9-17.

23. Keet CA, Wood RA. Food allergy and anaphylaxis. Immunol Allergy Clin North Am 2007;27:193-212.

24. Burks AW, Jones SM, Boyce JA, et al. NIAID-sponsored 2010 guidelines for managing food allergy: applications in the pediatric population. Pediatrics 2011;128:955-65.

25. Thong BY, Tan TC. Epidemiology and risk factors for drug allergy. Br J Clin Pharmacol 2011;71:684-700.

26. Le J, Nguyen T, Law AV, Hodding J. Adverse drug reactions among children over a 10-year period. Pediatrics 2006;118:555-62.

27. Sethuraman G, Sharma VK, Pahwa P, et al. Causative drugs and clinical outcome in Stevens-Johnson syndrome (SJS), toxic epidermal necrolysis (TEN), and SJS-TEN overlap in children. Indian J Dermatol 2012;57:199-200.

28. Lieberman P, Nicklas RA, Oppenheimer J, et al. The diagnosis and management of anaphylaxis practice parameter: 2010 update. J Allergy Clin Immunol 2010;126:477-80.

29. Munoz-Furlong A, Weiss CC. Characteristics of food-allergic patients placing them at risk for a fatal anaphylactic episode. Curr Allergy Asthma Rep 2009;9:57-63.

30. Sampson HA, Mendelson L, Rosen JP. Fatal and near-fatal anaphylactic reactions to food in children and adolescents. N Engl J Med 1992;327:380-4.

31. Pumphrey RS. Lessons for management of anaphylaxis from a study of fatal reactions. Clin Exp Allergy 2000;30:1144-50.

32. Bock SA, Munoz-Furlong A, Sampson HA. Fatalities due to anaphylactic reactions to foods. J Allergy Clin Immunol 2001; 107:191-3.

33. Bock SA, Munoz-Furlong A, Sampson HA. Further fatalities caused by anaphylactic reactions to food, 2001-2006. J Allergy Clin Immunol 2007;119:1016-8.

34. Castells M. Desensitization for drug allergy. Curr Opin Allergy Clin Immunol 2006;6:476-81.

35. Martelli A, Ghiglioni D, Sarratud T, et al. Anaphylaxis in the emergency department: a paediatric perspective. Curr Opin Allergy Clin Immunol 2008;8:321-9.

36. Lieberman P, Camargo C, Bohlke K, et al. Epidemiology of anaphylaxis: findings of the American College of Allergy, Asthma and Immunology Epidemiology of Anaphylaxis Working Group. Ann Allergy Asthma Immunol 2006;97:596-602.

37. Bousquet J, Khaltaev N, Cruz AA, et al. Allergic Rhinitis and its Impact on Asthma (ARIA) 2008 update (in collaboration with the World Health Organization, GA(2)LEN and AllerGen). Allergy 2008;63:8-160.

38. Demoly P, Hillaire-Buys D. Classification and epidemiology of hypersensitivity drug reactions. Immunol Allergy Clin North Am 2004;24:345-56.

39. Aberer W, Bircher A, Romano A, et al. Drug provocation testing in the diagnosis of drug hypersensitivity reactions: general considerations. Allergy 2003;58:854-63.

40. Scadding GK. Corticosteroids in the treatment of pediatric allergic rhinitis. J Allergy Clin Immunol 2001;108:S59-64.

41. American Academy of Allergy, Asthma, and Immunology [homepage on the Internet]. Available at www.aaaai.org. Accessed October 5, 2019.

42. Das RR. Treatment of allergic rhinitis in children: what's new? J Paediatr Child Health 2012;48:366.

43. Brozek JL, Bousquet J, Baena-Cagnani CE, et al. Allergic Rhinitis and its Impact on Asthma (ARIA) guidelines: 2010 revision. J Allergy Clin Immunol 2010;126:466-76.

44. U.S. Food and Drug Administration (FDA). Use Caution When Giving Cough and Cold Products to Kids [monograph on the Internet]. Available at https://www.fda.gov/drugs/special-features/use-caution-when-giving-cough-and-cold-products-kids. Accessed October 5, 2019.

45. Astelin [package insert]. Somerset, NJ: Meda Pharmaceuticals Inc., 2011.

46. Taketomo CK, Hodding JH, Kraus DM. Pediatric Dosage Handbook, 26th ed. Hudson, OH: Lexi-Comp, 2019.

47. Omnaris [package insert]. Marlborough, MA: Sunovion Pharmaceuticals, 2013.

48. Patanase [package insert]. Fort Worth, TX: Alcon Laboratories, 2012.

49. Emadine (emedastine difumarate) solution [package insert]. Fort Worth, TX: Alcon Laboratories, 2009.

50. Patanol [package insert]. Fort Worth, TX: Alcon Laboratories, 2018.

51. Pataday [package insert]. Fort Worth, TX: Alcon Laboratories, 2010.

52. Pazeo [package insert]. Fort Worth, TX: Alcon Laboratories, 2016.

53. Alomide [package insert]. Fort Worth, TX: Alcon Laboratories, 2015.

54. Alocril [package insert]. Irvine, CA: Allergan, 2012.

55. Xolair [package insert]. East Hanover, NJ: Novartis Pharmaceuticals Corporation, 2016.

56. Meltzer EO, Caballero F, Fromer LM, et al. Treatment of congestion in upper respiratory diseases. Int J Gen Med 2010;3:69-91.

57. Murphy K, Uryniak T, Simpson B, et al. Growth velocity in children with perennial allergic rhinitis treated with budesonide aqueous nasal spray. Ann Allergy Asthma Immunol 2006;96:723-30.

58. Schenkel EJ, Skoner DP, Bronsky EA, et al. Absence of growth retardation in children with perennial allergic rhinitis after one year of treatment with mometasone furoate aqueous nasal spray. Pediatrics 2000;105:E22.

59. LaForce C. Use of nasal steroids in managing allergic rhinitis. J Allergy Clin Immunol 1999;103:S388-94.

60. Onrust SV, Lamb HM. Mometasone furoate. A review of its intranasal use in allergic rhinitis. Drugs 1998;56:725-45.

61. Juniper EF, Ståhl E, Doty RL, et al. Clinical outcomes and adverse effect monitoring in allergic rhinitis. J Allergy Clin Immunol 2005;115:S390-413.

62. Zitt M, Kosoglou T, Hubbell J. Mometasone furoate nasal spray: a review of safety and systemic effects. Drug Saf 2007;30:317-26.

63. Bender BG, Milgrom H. Comparison of the effects of fluticasone propionate aqueous nasal spray and loratadine on daytime alertness and performance in children with seasonal allergic rhinitis. Ann Allergy Asthma Immunol 2004;92:344-9.

64. Weiner JM, Abramson MJ, Puy RM. Intranasal corticosteroids versus oral H1 receptor antagonists in allergic rhinitis: systematic review of randomized controlled trials. BMJ 1998;317:1624-9.

65. Ratner PH, van Bavel JH, Martin BG, et al. A comparison of the efficacy of fluticasone propionate aqueous nasal spray and loratadine, alone and in combination, for the treatment of seasonal allergic rhinitis. J Fam Pract 1998;47:118-25.

66. Wilson AM, O'Byrne PM, Parameswaran K. Leukotriene receptor antagonists for allergic rhinitis: a systematic review and meta-analysis. Am J Med 2004;116:338-44.

67. U.S. Food and Drug Administration (FDA). Updated Information on Leukotriene Inhibitors: Montelukast (Marketed as Singulair), Zafirlukast (Marketed as Accolate), and Zileuton (Marketed as Zyflo and Zyflo CR). Available at https://wayback.archive-it.org/7993/20170404172438/https://www.fda.gov/Drugs/DrugSafety/PostmarketDrugSafetyInformationforPatientsandProviders/DrugSafetyInformationforHeathcareProfessionals/ucm165489.htm. Accessed October 5, 2019.

68. Callero-Viera A, Infante S, Fuentes-Aparicio V, et al. Neuropsychiatric reactions to montelukast. J Investig Allergol Clin Immunol 2012;22:452-3.

69. Wang C, Zhang L. Specific immunotherapy for allergic rhinitis in children. Curr Opin Orolaryngol Head Neck Surg 2014;22:487-94.

70. Togias A, Cooper SF, Acebal ML, et al. Addendum guidelines for the prevention of peanut allergy in the United States. Ped Derm 2017;34:5-12.

71. Du Toit G, Roberts G, Sayre PH, et al. Randomized trial of peanut consumption in infants at risk for peanut allergy. N Engl J Med 2015;372:803-13.

72. Romano A, Gaeta F, Valluzzi RL, et al. Diagnosing hypersensitivity reactions to cephalosporins in children. Pediatrics 2008;122:521-7.

73. Lammintausta K, Kortekangas-Savolainen O. The usefulness of skin tests to prove drug hypersensitivity. Br J Dermatol 2005;152:968-74.

74. Yunginger JW, Sweeney KG, Sturner WQ, et al. Fatal food-induced anaphylaxis. JAMA 1988;260:1450-2.

75. Sampson HA, Munoz-Furlong A, Campbell RL, et al. Second symposium on the definition and management of anaphylaxis: summary report—Second National Institute of Allergy and Infectious Disease/Food Allergy and Anaphylaxis Network symposium. J Allergy Clin Immunol 2006;117:391-7.

76. Joint Task Force on Practice Parameters; American Academy of Allergy, Asthma and Immunology; American College of Allergy, Asthma and Immunology; Joint Council of Allergy, Asthma and Immunology. The diagnosis and management of anaphylaxis: an updated practice parameter. J Allergy Clin Immunol 2005;115:S483-523.

77. Muraro A, Roberts G, Clark A, et al. The management of anaphylaxis in childhood: position paper of the European Academy of Allergology and Clinical Immunology. Allergy 2007;62:857-71.

78. Rudders SA, Banerji A, Corel B, et al. Multicenter study of repeat epinephrine treatments for food-related anaphylaxis. Pediatrics 2010;125:e711-8.

79. Brunton L, Lazo J, Parker K. Goodman & Gilman's the pharmacological basis of therapeutics, 11th ed. New York: McGraw-Hill, 2005.

80. Sicherer SH, Simons FE. Self-injectable epinephrine for first-aid management of anaphylaxis. Pediatrics 2007;119:638-46.

81. Simons FE, Roberts JR, Gu X, et al. Epinephrine absorption in children with a history of anaphylaxis. J Allergy Clin Immunol 1998;101:33-7.

82. Simons FE, Gu X, Simons KJ. Epinephrine absorption in adults: intramuscular versus subcutaneous injection. J Allergy Clin Immunol 2001;108:871-3.

83. Keet C. Recognition and management of food-induced anaphylaxis. Pediatr Clin North Am 2011;58:377-88.

84. Lieberman P. Biphasic anaphylactic reactions. Ann Allergy Asthma Immunol 2005;95:217-26.

85. Gilbert DN, Elipoulos GM, Chamber HF, et al. The Sanford guide to antimicrobial therapy 2019. Sperryville, VA: Antimicrobial Therapy, Inc., 2019.

86. EpiPen [patient information]. Napa, CA: Dey Pharma, 2018.

Kawasaki Disease

Jennifer Le, Pharm.D., MAS, BCPS AQ-ID

INTRODUCTION

Kawasaki disease (KD) is a multisystem vasculitis of infancy and early childhood, classified as a mucocutaneous lymph node syndrome. Kawasaki disease is characterized by fever, pleomorphic rash, and several other symptoms and laboratory abnormalities suggestive of inflammation. The walls of the blood vessels throughout the body become inflamed in patients with KD. Of particular concern, KD may affect the coronary arteries and thereby progress to serious complications, including coronary artery aneurysms or ectasia, which may result in myocardial infarction or sudden death.[1] In fact, KD is the leading cause of acquired heart disease in children in the United States.[2] Furthermore, KD mortality and recurrence rates are less than 1% and 2%, respectively.[3,4]

ETIOLOGY

Although the cause of KD remains unknown, infectious as well as immunologic and genetic factors are thought to result in the disease's immune-mediated vascular inflammation and damage.[5,6] Selective expansion of specific T-cell receptors on monocytes in patients with KD suggests that KD is caused by superantigen-producing microorganisms.[7] In addition, the clinical manifestation of fever and rash, seasonal increase in

incidence during winter and spring months, age distribution (e.g., rare in infants younger than 6 months, possibly because of passive immunity from residual maternal antibodies), spatial and temporal clustering, and laboratory features suggest an infectious cause.[1,8,9]

Because no infectious source has been identified definitively, KD appears to result from an immunologic response that is caused by several infecting organisms.[5] Pathologically, neutrophils predominate in the early course of KD.[10,11] This is followed by the formation of large mononuclear cells jointly with CD8+ T lymphocytes and immunoglobulin A (IgA) plasma cells to stimulate fibroblastic proliferation.[1] In addition to these cells, macrophages – a unique feature evident in KD unlike in other types of vasculitis – contribute to coronary arteritis.[1,12]

The striking increase in KD in Asian and Asian American populations and their family members suggests that the disease has a genetic predisposition.[13-15] In fact, several genes have been associated with KD, including a single nucleotide polymorphism of the inositol 1,4,5-trisphosphate 3-kinase C gene on chromosome 19q13.2, an array of *HLA* genes, and the angiotensin-1-converting enzyme gene.[16-19] Furthermore, patients with the allelic change on the inositol 1,4,5-trisphosphate 3-kinase C gene have an increased risk of coronary artery lesions, possibly because of their heightened T-cell response.

Ethnicity, age, and male sex are the most common risk factors for KD. The epidemiologic variation of this syndrome indicates that ethnicity is one risk factor for KD. The incidence of KD is highest among children of Asian or Pacific Islander descent, followed by non-Hispanic African Americans, Hispanics, and whites.[9,20] Up to 90% of KD cases are in patients older than 6 months and younger than 5 years.[21,22] According to the CDC, the estimated annual incidence of KD is 17–27 per 100,000 U.S. children younger than 5 years.[20,23] Cases of KD are rarely reported in late childhood (older than 12 years) and adulthood. From the Pediatric Health Information System (PHIS), the median age at first hospital admission for KD is 3.4 years, with 60% of patients age 1–4 years.[3] Furthermore, in the PHIS study, 60% of the patients were male, another risk factor consistently reported.[3,21,22]

CLINICAL PRESENTATION

Three clinical phases – acute, subacute, and convalescent – describe the course of KD.[24] The acute phase is marked by fever that usually persists for 1–2 weeks, together with bilateral, nonexudative conjunctivitis; lip and tongue changes ("strawberry" tongue); swelling and erythema of the hands and feet; polymorphous rash; and cervical lymphadenopathy.[1] Resolution of fever completes this acute phase and denotes the beginning of the subacute phase, which occurs in weeks 2 and 3 after initial fever onset.[24] During this phase, patients may have periungual peeling of fingers and toes, arthritis, arthralgia, diarrhea, vomiting, and thrombocytosis.[1,24] Finally, recovery from the clinical symptoms signifies the convalescent phase, which continues until the erythrocyte sedimentation rate (ESR) normalizes (usually during weeks 6–8 of illness).[24]

DIAGNOSIS

The signs and symptoms associated with KD are nonspecific; thus, diagnosing KD requires excluding other potential diseases that cause similar clinical presentations. The clinical and laboratory criteria for diagnosing KD, created by Tomisaku Kawasaki in 1967 and updated in 2004, are presented in Table 1. Symptoms may not occur simultaneously, necessitating close monitoring while waiting for clinical presentation. Prolonged, unexplained fever for 5 days or more (the most consistent feature) and at least four other primary clinical signs of mucocutaneous inflammation are required for a diagnosis of typical or classic KD.[1,25] However, in the presence of coronary artery disease, only four or less primary clinical features, together with fever for 5 days or more, are needed for KD diagnosis. In addition, KD can be diagnosed on day 4 of fever or earlier by an expert clinician when four or more primary clinical symptoms are present. Finally, in a young child with an unexplained fever for 5 days or more and any of the principal clinical features, KD should be considered.

Although laboratory findings are not required for a diagnosis of typical KD, some are highly suggestive of KD and can be useful for ambiguous cases. Markers for systemic inflammation indicative of KD include elevation in acute-phase reactants (e.g., elevated ESR, CRP) and leukocytosis with a left shift in the WBC. Normocytic, normochromic anemia, sterile pyuria, hypoalbuminemia, and thrombocytosis are other laboratory abnormalities in patients with KD (Table 1).

Incomplete (also called atypical) KD occurs when the five clinical diagnostic criteria are not fulfilled, common in infants younger than 12 months.[26] Infants 6 months and younger with an unexplained fever for 7 days or more and no other clinical signs should therefore be assessed for incomplete KD. In addition, children older than 5 years are more likely to have incomplete KD than are children age 1–4 years.[27] Laboratory findings and echocardiography prove invaluable in the differential diagnostic workup for incomplete KD (Table 1). In fact, the American Heart Association and the American Academy of Pediatrics recommend the following laboratory tests: acute-phase reactants (e.g., CRP, ESR), CBC, urinalysis by clean catch, ALT concentration, and serum albumin.[1] Nonetheless, improvements in diagnosing incomplete KD are essential to ensure timely treatment because cardiac complications can develop.

Although a self-limiting disease, KD can progress to cardiac complications that result in significant morbidity and mortality. Cardiac sequelae consist of coronary artery aneurysms, congestive heart failure, myocarditis, pericarditis, and arrhythmias. Extensive or large coronary artery aneurysms (i.e., greater than 8 mm) considerably increase the risk of occlusion and myocardial infarction.[28] Prompt initiation of appropriate therapy, particularly within 10 days of fever onset, may prevent cardiac morbidity progression and mortality.[1] Coronary artery aneurysms, the major cardiac complication, occur in 25% of untreated children with KD compared with 4% of children receiving therapy, emphasizing the importance of adequate treatment.[1] Despite treatment, infants younger than 1 year have the highest risk of cardiac complications.[29] Additional risk factors for coronary artery lesions include male sex, fever for 14 days or more, hyponatremia (serum sodium less than 135 mEq/L), anemia (Hct less than 35%), leukocytosis (WBC more than 12×10^3 cells/mm^3), and certain ancestries (American Indians, whites, and non-Hispanics).[3,30,31] Other complications of KD are peripheral arterial occlusion, painful arthritis or arthralgias usually in the lower extremities, and shock.

Kawasaki disease recurs when the second episode follows the first incident by at least 3 months. The recurrence rate is 1%–3%, usually within the first 2 years after initial diagnosis.[22,30,32]

Table 1. Clinical and Laboratory Signs of KD[1,25]

Primary Clinical Signs[a,b]	Laboratory Abnormalities
Fever ≥ 5 days	Leukocytosis with neutrophilia
Bilateral, nonexudative conjunctivitis	Normocytic, normochromic anemia (appropriate for age)
Changes in lips and oral cavity (cracked, red lips; strawberry tongue; discrete oral vesicles or ulcers)	Thrombocytosis (Plt ≥ 450 x 10^3 cells/mm^3) after weeks 1–2 of illness onset
Polymorphous rash	Elevated ESR (≥ 40 mm/hr) and/or CRP (≥ 3.0 mg/L)
Extremity changes (edema of hands and feet; palmar erythema)	Sterile pyuria (≥ 10 WBC per high-power field)
Cervical lymphadenopathy (≥ 1.5 cm, usually unilateral)	Hypoalbuminemia (≤ 3.0 g/dL)
	Elevated serum aminotransaminases (> 50 U/L)

[a]Persistent fever for ≥ 5 days, with ≥ 4 primary clinical features, is diagnostic criteria for classic KD. In the presence of coronary artery abnormalities, fever for ≥ 5 days and only ≤ 4 primary clinical signs are required for diagnosis of KD. In addition, KD can be diagnosed on day 4 of fever or earlier by an expert clinician when ≥ 4 primary clinical symptoms are present.

[b]Other clinical signs include cardiovascular (coronary artery aneurysms, congestive heart failure, myocarditis, pericarditis, and arrhythmias); diarrhea, vomiting, or abdominal pain; arthritis; CNS (irritability and aseptic meningitis); and mild uveitis.

ESR = erythrocyte sedimentation rate; KD = Kawasaki disease.

TREATMENT

The severity and range of clinical presentations and potential for serious cardiac complications from KD necessitate hospitalization for a diagnostic workup and subsequent treatment. Early diagnosis of KD to allow prompt initiation of appropriate therapy can prevent or ameliorate progression toward cardiac complications, an important goal of therapy. Nonetheless, late diagnosis, defined as more than 10 days after illness onset, occurs in 16% of patients, especially young infants and incomplete KD cases.[33] Pharmacologic treatment is required for all cases of classic KD as well as for incomplete KD in the presence of an abnormal echocardiograph. Treatment should also be considered in incomplete KD cases without cardiac abnormalities because it may prevent progression to coronary artery aneurysms.[25] Even with adequate treatment, coronary artery aneurysms can still occur in 4% of KD cases.[34]

PHARMACOLOGIC THERAPY

The goal of pharmacologic treatment during the acute phase is to alleviate inflammation in the coronary artery wall and prevent coronary thrombosis. In children with coronary aneurysms who require long-term treatment, prevention of myocardial ischemia or infarction is another therapeutic goal.[1] Aspirin and intravenous immunoglobulin (IVIG) are the mainstays of KD treatment. From guidelines by the American Heart Association and the American Academy of Pediatrics, standard KD therapy includes a single dose of IVIG and high-dose aspirin initiated as soon as KD is diagnosed or within the first 10 days of illness. Such therapy optimally decreases the risk of subsequent coronary artery aneurysms (Table 2).[1,26,34,35] Additional IVIG doses may be needed in patients who do not respond (e.g., do not defervesce) to initial therapy.[1] Long-term use of antiplatelet and/or anticoagulation therapies may be warranted when the risk of thrombotic events is high, particularly in patients with rapidly enlarging coronary aneurysms.

The anti-inflammatory properties of IVIG – possibly derived from cytokine production modulation, enhanced T-cell suppressor activity, and neutralization of bacterial superantigens – help resolve fever and other acute inflammatory processes in response to disease.[1] In addition, IVIG prevents coronary artery aneurysms, improves left ventricular contractility, and normalizes serum lipoproteins.[36,37] A single, high-dose infusion of IVIG at 2 g/kg, compared with low doses over 4–5 days, produces a greater decrease in the duration of fever and length of hospital stay as well as faster resolution of laboratory findings for acute inflammation.[35,38] Ideally, IVIG should be initiated within the first 10 days after the initial symptoms, though data analyses to suggest benefit with earlier treatment within 4–6 days are conflicting.[39,40] However, patients who receive a diagnosis of KD on day 3 or 4 of illness are most likely to have very severe disease that warrants immediate treatment to prevent coronary aneurysms. In fact, they may require retreatment with IVIG. In some patients with KD, treatment beyond day 10 of illness may be appropriate, particularly in the presence of an elevated ESR or CRP (greater than 3 mg/L) with persistent fever or any coronary artery aneurysm.

Different IVIG formulations vary in biologic effects because they are from donor plasma that undergoes different sterilization processes (Table 3). Risk of coronary artery aneurysms, resolution of fever, and duration of hospital stay differ with brands of IVIG.[35,41,42] Although different IVIG brands appear to affect the clinical outcome, no single brand has been proven superior. Insufficient efficacy data, concerns for fluid overload, product availability, and cost are reasons not to exceed the recommended dose of 2 g/kg, even though IVIG shows a dose-response effect.[38]

Although aspirin does not appear to decrease the development of coronary abnormalities, its anti-inflammatory and antiplatelet activities underscore its role in KD treatment. Initially, high-dose aspirin (80–100 mg/kg/day, not to exceed 4 g/day) continued until 48–72 hours after fever resolves is recommended to achieve additive anti-inflammatory effects with IVIG (Table 2). Alternatively, high-dose aspirin can be continued until 14 days after illness onset, with at least 48–72 hours after fever cessation. The prevalence of coronary artery aneurysm is similar between moderate-dose aspirin (i.e., 30–50 mg/kg/day, which is used in Japan and Western Europe), and high-dose aspirin, though there have been no randomized controlled studies to date.[1]

With the unavailability of liquid aspirin, the baby aspirin tablet formulation should be used because it is chewable and/or crushable for delivery to infants and young children. This is followed by low-dose aspirin for its antiplatelet effect and is continued until resolution of laboratory markers of acute inflammation, or until 6–8 weeks after illness onset to rule out cardiac abnormalities (Table 2). However, in patients who develop coronary abnormalities, aspirin may be continued indefinitely. Although children with a diagnosis of KD have decreased aspirin exposure because of reduced absorption and increased clearance, drug monitoring is not necessary. Aneurysm formation and resolution of fever seem to be unaffected by aspirin use alone. In fact, most patients who received a single, high dose of IVIG without aspirin had resolution of fever within 24 hours after completing therapy.[43] Other antiplatelet drugs, including clopidogrel, dipyridamole, and ticlopidine, have been used in KD.[35]

Adding prednisolone to standard therapy should be considered in KD cases at high risk of cardiac involvement (Table 2).[44] Factors contributing to a significant risk of cardiac abnormalities include a CRP of 7 mg/L or greater, a total bilirubin of 0.9 mg/dL or greater, and an AST of 200 U/L or greater.[45] In Japanese children at risk of IVIG resistance but without initial coronary artery damage, adding a corticosteroid to IVIG improves clinical outcomes.[46]

RESISTANT CASES

About 10%–20% of patients treated with standard therapy have persistent or recrudescent fever for at least 36 hours and within 7 days after completing the first IVIG administration, placing these patients at a 9-fold increased risk of cardiac abnormalities.[29] Models to predict initial treatment response are not available in the United States. Nonetheless, fever of any grade indicates unresolved vasculitis, and its duration indicates coronary artery damage. Risk factors associated

Table 2. Treatment of KD[1]

Disease Type	Standard Therapy	Alternative Therapy	Comment
Newly diagnosed, including incomplete type with cardiac abnormality	IVIG 2 g/kg/day infused over 8–12 hr as a single dose[a,b] PLUS	Prednisolone 2 mg/kg/day divided every 8 hr intravenously for 5 days or until afebrile, plus standard therapy[c]	IVIG – Toxicities: infusion-related adverse effects, possible transmission of bloodborne pathogens; different brands affect clinical efficacy, but no single product has been proven superior
	High-dose aspirin 80–100 mg/kg/day orally in four divided doses[a,b] until afebrile for 48–72 hr (or until 14th day of illness), followed by 3–5 mg/kg/day[d] until no evidence of coronary changes (total duration ~6–8 wk)[e]	Ibuprofen 5–10 mg/kg every 6–8 hr, or naproxen 10–15 mg/kg/day in two or three divided doses for several weeks can be used for prolonged arthritis or arthralgia Clopidogrel 0.2 mg/kg/dose for ≤ 2 yr or 1 mg/kg/day for > 2 yr (maximum 75 mg) once daily if allergic to, or intolerant of, aspirin	Aspirin – Toxicities: aminotransaminase elevation, transient hearing loss, and Reye syndrome (not associated with low-dose); annual influenza vaccination recommended; avoid aspirin during acute viral illness (varicella and flu)
Resistant[f]	IVIG 1–2 g/kg/day infused over 8–12 hr as a second dose[a,g]	Prednisolone 2 mg/kg/day divided every 8 hr intravenously for 5 days or until afebrile, plus second dose of IVIG[h] Infliximab 5 mg/kg intravenously over 2 hr as a single dose Cyclosporine 3 mg/kg/day divided every 12 hr intravenously, or 4–8 mg/kg/day divided every 12 hr orally; adjust dose to achieve trough 50–150 ng/mL[i] Anakinra 2–6 mg/kg/day subcutaneously[i] Cyclophosphamide 2 mg/kg/day intravenously[i]	Prednisolone – Toxicities: cardiac arrhythmias, infarction and arrest at high doses and rapid infusion, decreased lymphocyte and monocyte counts, most other adverse effects (including growth suppression, glucose intolerance) are associated with long-term use Infliximab – Toxicities: rash, flushing, pruritus, and other dermatologic reactions (including Stevens-Johnson syndrome and toxic epidermal necrolysis), hepatotoxicity with particular increase in ALT, transient hepatomegaly, anemia Cyclosporine – Toxicities: cardiovascular (hypertension), hirsutism, nephrotoxicity, neurotoxicity (tremor), and leukopenia and other hematologic effects Anakinra – Toxicities: injection site reaction, anaphylaxis and hypersensitivity, GI disturbance, thrombocytopenia and neutropenia, infections (including opportunistic) Cyclophosphamide – Toxicities: dermatologic (including Stevens-Johnson syndrome, alopecia), GI disturbance, hematologic effects (including leukopenia and neutropenia), nephrotoxicity, pulmonary fibrosis

[a]Anti-inflammatory action.
[b]Initiate immediately upon diagnosis in the acute phase to prevent coronary artery aneurysms.
[c]Consider for cases at highest risk of coronary artery aneurysms.
[d]Antiplatelet action.
[e]Duration of aspirin can be indefinite in cases with cardiac abnormalities.
[f]Other alternative treatments for resistant cases include cyclosporine 3 mg/kg/day divided every 12 hr intravenously or 4–8 mg/kg/day·divided every 12 hr orally; anakinra 2–6 mg/kg/day subcutaneously; and cyclophosphamide 2 mg/kg/day intravenously.
[g]Cumulative doses > 4 g/kg have not been studied.
[h]For continued resistant cases after completing two courses of IVIG.
[i]Reserved for highly resistant cases failing other alternative therapies because of significant adverse effects.
IVIG = intravenous immunoglobulin.

Table 3. IVIG Product Comparison (available in the United States)[a]

Trade Name	Bivigam	Carimune NF	Flebogamma DIF	Gammagard Liquid	Gammagard S/D (less IgA)	Gammaked	Gammaplex	Gamunex-C	Octagam	Privigen[b]
Formulation	Liquid	Lyophilized	Liquid	Liquid	Lyophilized	Liquid	Liquid	Liquid	Liquid	Liquid
Concentration (%, g IgG per 100 mL)	10	3, 6, 12	5, 10	10	5, 10	10	5, 10	10	5, 10	10
IgA content	≤ 200 mcg/mL	1000–2000 mcg/ mL	5%: < 50 mcg/mL 10%: < 100 mcg/mL	37 mcg/mL	5%: < 1 mcg/mL	46 mcg/mL (average)	5%: < 10 mcg/mL 10%: < 20 mcg/mL	46 mcg/mL	5%: ≤ 200 mcg/mL 10%: 106 mcg/mL (average)	≤ 25 mcg/mL
Sugar content	None	1.67 g of sucrose per gram of protein	50 mg/mL sorbitol	None	5%: 20 mg/mL of glucose	None	5%: 50 mg/mL D-sorbitol 10%: None	None	5%: 100 mg/mL maltose 10%: 90 mg/mL	None
Sodium content	Sodium chloride 0.1–0.14 mol/L	Sodium chloride < 20 mg per gram of IgG	Trace	Not detectable	5%: 8.5 mg/mL	Trace < 7 mEq/L	5%: Sodium acetate 2 mg/mL Sodium chloride 3 mg/mL 10%: < 0.3 mmol/mL	Trace < 7 mEq/L	≤ 30 mmol/L	Trace ≤ 1 mmol/L
Other content	Glycine 0.20– 0.29 mol/L Polysorbate 80 1.5–2.5 mg/mL	None	5%: PEG ≤ 3 mg/mL 10%: PEG ≤ 6 mg/mL	Glycine 0.25 mol/L	5%: Glycine 22.5 mg/mL PEG 2 mg/mL Polysorbate 80–100 mcg/mL Albumin 3 mg/mL	Glycine 0.16– 0.24 mol/L	5%: Glycine 6 mg/mL Polysorbate 80 at ~0.05 mg/mL 10%: Glycine 0.2–0.3 mmol/mL Polysorbate 80 ~0.01–0.06 mg/mL	Glycine 0.15 g/kg	Not reported	L-Proline 250 mmol/L
Osmolality (mOsm/L)	< 510 mOsm/kg	192–1074 mOsm/kg	240–370 mOsm/kg	240–300 mOsm/kg	5%: 636 mOsm/L	258 mOsm/kg	5%: 420–500 mOsm/kg 10%: ~280 mOsm/kg	258 mOsm/kg	310–380 mOsm/kg	220–440 mOsm/kg

[a]Although products available in the United States are not identical or approved for similar indications, they are generally considered interchangeable. However, some clinically relevant differences may affect product selection (i.e., osmolarity differences, sucrose content, fluid volume, product pH, and IgA content).
[b]Contraindicated in patients with hyperprolinemia.
IgG = immunoglobulin G; PEG = polyethylene glycol.

with resistance to standard therapy that therefore necessitates retreatment are as follows: age younger than 1 year, early diagnosis with initial treatment after 5 days or less of symptoms, bands of 20% or greater, CRP of 8 mg/L or greater, elevation in liver enzymes (ALT of 80 U/L or greater or γ-glutamyl transferase of 60 U/L or greater), thrombocytopenia (Plt 30×10^3 cells/mm³ or less), and hyponatremia (serum sodium of 133 mEq/L or less).[46-49]

To minimize cardiac complications, further therapy should be considered in the presence of any of these risk factors. For patients with persistent or recrudescent fever after receiving standard therapy, additional therapy is necessary and should be initiated at least 36 hours after IVIG completion to allow the exclusion of drug-related fever.

Repeated courses of IVIG or other anti-inflammatory agents for vasculitis (including corticosteroids, inhibitors of tumor necrosis factor alpha [TNFα], and plasmapheresis) have been used in refractory cases, usually marked by persistent or recurrent fever that indicates continued vasculitis and increased risk of coronary artery aneurysms.[3] In limited studies, retreatment with a second dose of IVIG 2 g/kg resolved fever in some patients.[29,50,51] The rationale for retreatment with IVIG, particularly with the high dose, is its dose-response effect.[38] When therapeutic response is not achieved even after two IVIG courses, corticosteroids can be used until fever resolves (Table 2).[51,52] According to a meta-analysis of the treatment of primary and refractory KD, steroid use was associated with improved coronary artery abnormalities, decreased hospital stay, and decreased duration of clinical symptoms. For resistant KD unresponsive to the first or second course of IVIG and corticosteroids, infliximab (a TNFα inhibitor) may be considered because TNF concentrations appear to be elevated in KD.[53-56] Infliximab is the first anti-TNF approved for pediatric use that appears to be safe and well tolerated in children as young as 1 year.[57] According to case reports and clinical trials, adding infliximab to the first course of IVIG appears safe but does not relieve persistent fever. As such, infliximab should be reserved for patients with refractory disease. Etanercept 0.8 mg/kg/dose has been evaluated in one study and should also be reserved for refractory IVIG-resistant cases.[57,58]

Other therapies that are neither well studied nor supported for routine use include plasmapheresis and cytotoxic agents (cyclophosphamide and cyclosporine) (Table 2).[1,56,59] Plasmapheresis is reserved for patients in whom all pharmacotherapy has failed. Significant adverse drug effects limit the use of cytotoxic agents to the most severe and highly resistant cases. Further studies are necessary to understand the benefits of cytotoxic agents in KD, particularly because some of these drugs are associated with significant toxicities. Early-phase clinical trials are under way to evaluate atorvastatin for ending the progression of arterial wall damage and anakinra (a recombinant human interleukin-1 receptor antagonist) for patients with KD having existing coronary artery abnormalities.[60,61]

Surgical intervention may be necessary in some cases, depending on the severity of cardiac abnormalities. Because surgical procedures are beyond the scope of this chapter, more information can be obtained elsewhere.[1]

PREVENTION OF CORONARY THROMBOSIS

In children with coronary involvement, additional medications may be necessary for thrombosis. In fact, another goal of KD treatment in patients with coronary abnormalities is to prevent thrombosis. Because platelet activation occurs during all disease phases, antiplatelet therapy is crucial at every stage. Use of antiplatelet, anticoagulation, or combination therapies depends on the degree of coronary involvement. For mild, asymptomatic cases, low-dose aspirin is recommended. Adding other antiplatelet drugs (e.g., clopidogrel and dipyridamole) to low-dose aspirin to further enhance activity through the adenosine-5-diphosphate antagonism may be more effective in moderate cases with evidence of moderate coronary artery aneurysm.[1] This dual antiplatelet therapy may be considered as an alternative to anticoagulation therapy for small aneurysms.

Anticoagulation therapy, particularly in combination with low-dose aspirin, is indicated when the risk of thrombosis is high, as in rapidly enlarging coronary aneurysms with abnormal flow conditions and stenoses at the proximal or distal end of the aneurysms. Warfarin with low-dose aspirin is the most common combination therapy used. The targeted range for warfarin's activity is an INR of 2–2.5.[1] Because warfarin's full therapeutic effect may take several days, unfractionated heparin can be initiated first to bridge the gap in therapy. Alternatively, low-molecular-weight heparin can be substituted for warfarin, though it requires subcutaneous injections compared with oral warfarin administration. Triple therapy that incorporates both anticoagulation and dual antiplatelet therapy can be considered for large aneurysms.

MONITORING OF THERAPY

Therapeutic outcomes for KD are to achieve defervescence, reverse presenting symptoms, normalize any irregular laboratory tests, prevent cardiac abnormalities, prevent coronary thrombosis, and prevent mortality from myocardial infarction or arrhythmias. Hospitalization is required for diagnostic workup and treatment, especially for IVIG administration. Clinical evaluations for the first 2 months after the KD diagnosis are needed for information on changes from baseline presentation and treatment response.

To ascertain the degree of cardiac involvement, an echocardiogram should be done within 2 weeks after fever onset and repeated 6–8 weeks later to confirm therapeutic response.[1] As such, referral to pediatric cardiology is required for all patients with KD, particularly after hospital discharge, for close monitoring. Classification of coronary artery abnormalities involves assessing luminal dimensions and using Z-scores (preferably adjusted for body surface area to improve evaluation of severity; Table 4). Additional echocardiographic evaluations are imperative for children at high risk of cardiac effects, including those with persistent fevers or coronary abnormalities. Follow-up echocardiograms every 1–2 years after the diagnosis may be warranted to determine the status (e.g., improving or worsening) of coronary aneurysms and to evaluate for other cardiac conditions, including ventricular dysfunction and pericardial effusions. Long-term

KD management depends on the severity of coronary artery involvement and consists of antiplatelet therapy, anticoagulation, restriction in physical activity, precautions for pregnancy, cardiac evaluation, and echocardiogram (Table 4).[1,62]

Overall, IVIG is generally well tolerated and less likely to cause adverse effects if infused at the recommended minimum concentration and infusion rate. Infusion-related reactions consisting of flushing, hypotension, nausea, vomiting, fever, chills, pruritus, malaise, myalgia, and chest tightness have been reported with IVIG administration. These reactions usually occur 30 minutes to 1 hour after initiation of the infusion and usually resolve when the infusion is slowed or temporarily discontinued. Pretreatment with acetaminophen and diphenhydramine may help decrease these infusion-related reactions.

Serious adverse effects have been reported with IVIG administration. Anaphylactoid reactions, though rare, are likely in patients who have selective IgA deficiency with serum antibodies to IgA and have not received IVIG within the preceding 8 weeks. Products with the lowest IgA content may be used with caution in these patients (Table 3). In addition, nephrotoxicity, including acute renal failure as evidenced by increases in SCr and BUN, can occur as soon as 1–2 days after IVIG administration. Reports of renal dysfunction have mainly been associated with IVIG products containing sucrose. Finally, aseptic meningitis syndrome, marked by headache, nuchal rigidity, drowsiness, fever, photophobia, and GI intolerance, has been reported from several hours to 2 days after IVIG administration.[63,64] Infusions should be discontinued in patients with aseptic meningitis syndrome or acute hypersensitivity reactions. Epinephrine and diphenhydramine should also be initiated in children with severe hypersensitivity reactions.

Another major concern with IVIG is transmission of bloodborne pathogens, including parvovirus. Once problematic, hepatitis C virus cannot be transmitted under current sterilization methods. In addition, antibodies contained in IVIG may interfere with the immune response to certain live

Table 4. Classification of Coronary Artery Abnormality and Long-term Management of KD[1,62]

Type of Coronary Artery Abnormality[a]	Z-Score[b]	Management
No coronary artery abnormality or transient ectasia/dilation	< 2, no involvement 2–2.5, dilation only	• Low-dose aspirin for 2–3 mo[c] • Follow-up monitoring in 1 yr to assess for cardiovascular risk • Normal physical activities and regular age-appropriate reproductive counseling
Small coronary aneurysm (< 4 mm)	2.5 to < 5	• Low-dose aspirin until regression is documented with echocardiogram[c] • Assess for cardiovascular risk once yearly and myocardial ischemia every 2–5 yr • Normal physical activities (unless receiving dual antiplatelet therapy where overexertion should be avoided) and precautions for pregnancy
Medium coronary aneurysm (4–8 mm)	5 to < 10	• Low-dose aspirin until regression is documented with echocardiogram[c] • Consider dual antiplatelet therapy using low-dose aspirin with clopidogrel • Assess for cardiovascular risk once yearly and myocardial ischemia every 2–4 yr • Limited physical activities without overexertion and precautions for pregnancy
Large or giant coronary aneurysm (≥ 8 mm)	≥ 10	• Triple therapy using anticoagulation (warfarin therapy with INR at 2.0–2.5; alternative is subcutaneous low-molecular-weight heparin) and low-dose aspirin[c] with clopidogrel • Immediate referral to pediatric cardiologist[d] • Assess for cardiovascular risk every 6 mo to once yearly and myocardial ischemia every 6 mo to 3 yr • Limited physical activities without overexertion and precautions for pregnancy
Coronary artery obstruction or ischemia	—	• Evaluate for angioplasty, bypass grafting, stent placement, or cardiac transplantation

[a]Size of aneurysm for children < 5 yr.
[b]Z-score should be adjusted to body surface area.
[c]Low-dose aspirin 3–5 mg/kg/day.
[d]Referral to pediatric cardiology is necessary for all patients with KD, particularly after hospital discharge, for close monitoring. However, immediate referral upon diagnosis of KD is necessary for patients who initially present with a significant coronary aneurysm.

virus vaccines (e.g., measles, mumps, and rubella). As such, these vaccinations should be deferred for at least 11 months in patients receiving IVIG treatment. Repeat immunization is necessary if the live virus vaccine was administered within 14 days or at the same time of IVIG administration.[26]

Patients with KD may be at an increased risk of adverse effects from aspirin use, consisting of GI intolerance, elevation in transaminases, transient hearing loss, and Reye syndrome. Altered protein binding to augment free drug concentrations as a result of hypoalbuminemia in children with KD is the potential mechanism for increased toxicity.[44] Children undergoing long-term aspirin therapy and their household contacts should receive the annual influenza vaccine.[65] In addition, aspirin, including the low-dose therapy, should be discontinued in patients with influenza or varicella infection to avoid Reye syndrome. Furthermore, aspirin should be avoided in the 6 weeks after varicella vaccination. Clopidogrel 0.2–1 mg/kg/day (maximum 75 mg) can temporarily be substituted for aspirin in these situations, as well as in patients who are allergic to or intolerant of aspirin. Ibuprofen and other NSAIDs should be avoided in combination with aspirin because they can interfere with the action of aspirin.

Adverse effects of other KD therapies are provided in Table 3. Further studies are needed to evaluate corticosteroids as a first-line treatment together with IVIG and aspirin in certain high-risk KD cases. Other agents, including antioxidants and neutrophil elastase inhibitors, are being evaluated for the treatment of refractory KD, but their efficacy remains unclear.

CONCLUSION

Kawasaki disease is a vasculitis that appears primarily in infancy and early childhood. Current diagnostic criteria for KD consist of clinical symptoms; therefore, diagnosing KD can be challenging because of the unusual clinical presentations in certain pediatric patients. Aspirin and IVIG are the mainstays of therapy for their anti-inflammatory and antiplatelet effects. Refractory KD cases require additional therapies, including an additional dose of IVIG, corticosteroids, and/or infliximab. Although KD is self-limiting, cardiac complications can result in significant morbidity and mortality. Prompt diagnosis and treatment of KD with appropriate follow-up monitoring are critical to improve patient outcomes.

Patient Case — NEWLY DIAGNOSED KAWASAKI DISEASE

A 2-year-old Asian boy was admitted to the hospital with a 5-day history of daily fevers (temperature 102.5°F [39.2°C]). Four days before admission, the primary pediatrician diagnosed mild acute otitis media (noted as inflamed tympanic membrane) and prescribed a course of high-dose amoxicillin. Within 1 day of receiving the high-dose amoxicillin, the patient developed a maculopapular rash that was attributed to a penicillin allergy. The same primary pediatrician discontinued amoxicillin and replaced it with cefdinir. During this clinic visit, a urinalysis showed 20 WBCs with no bacteria. The patient continued to have fevers daily and developed red eyes and lips with remarkable irritability. On admission, the patient had additional symptoms of palmar and plantar swelling, with palmar erythema.

Family history: Noncontributory. No sudden infant death syndrome or congenital heart disease

Social history: Lives with both parents. No pets. No exposure to smoking

Allergies: No known food allergies. Rash to amoxicillin

Home medications:

Medication	Sig	Taking	Authorizing Provider
Amoxicillin	480 mg orally every 12 hr for 7 days (12 mL of 200 mg/5 mL suspension)	No, discontinued by physician because of rash	Dr. Chen
Acetaminophen	160 mg (5 mL) orally every 4–6 hr as needed for fever (the mother brought bottle of 160 mg/5 mL suspension)	Yes	Dr. Chen

Immunizations: Up to date. Received seasonal influenza vaccine

Vital signs: BP 95/42 mm Hg, HR 145 beats/minute, RR 40 breaths/minute, Tmax 102.2°F (39.0°C), Wt 12 kg, Ht 35.4 inches, 98% Sao_2 on room air

Review of systems: Positive for fever, conjunctivitis, and swollen hands and feet (bilateral). No emesis or recent sick contacts. Remaining 12-systems review was negative

Physical examination:

General: Nontoxic, no acute distress. Crying on examination. Extremely fussy and irritable

HEENT: Head: Normocephalic, atraumatic. Eyes: Positive red reflex. Bilateral nonexudative redness. Nose: Nares are patent without gross rhinorrhea. Ears: Tympanic membranes intact, slightly red. Mouth: Moist mucous membrane. Erythema on lips. No exudates

Neck: Supple. No marked masses

Respiratory: Clear to auscultation bilaterally. Good equal air movement

Cardiovascular: RRR. No murmurs, rubs, or gallops. Normal S1 and S2

Abdomen: Soft, nontender, nondistended. Positive bowel sounds. No masses appreciated

Skin: Diffuse blanching macular rash over abdomen. No vesicles, no lesions and with some associated dry skin

MS: Warm and well-perfused. Edema of hands/feet and palmar erythema noted

Neuro: Positive Moro, suck, and grasp reflex. Patient moving all four extremities equally and spontaneously

Laboratory findings:

Component	Results	Normal Range
Basic Metabolic Panel		
Glucose	89	60–110 mg/dL
BUN	10	7–17 mg/dL
Na	141	137–145 mEq/L
K	4.7	3.6–5.0 mEq/L
Cl	101	98–107 mEq/L
HCO_3	25	22–30 mEq/L
Anion gap	8	6–16 mEq/L
SCr	0.67	0.60–1.00 mg/dL
Calcium	9.9	8.4–10.2 mg/dL
Calculated Osmolality		
Calculated osmolality	269	263–273 mOsm/kg
CBC with Differential		
WBC	16,700	$4.5–11 \times 10^3$ cells/mm³
RBC	3.9	$4.30–5.10 \times 10^6$ cells/mm³
Hgb	10.3	11.4–15.4 g/dL
Hct	30.4	36.0%–49.0%
MCV	95	78.0–98.0 fL
MCH	31	26.0–34.0 pg
MCHC	32	32.0–35.0 g/dL
RBC distribution width	13.5	11.5%–14.5%
Plt	480	$150-450 \times 10^3$ cells/mm³
Mean platelet volume	11.3	9.4–12.4 fL
Neutrophils	75	34.0%–71.1%
Immature granulocytes	1	0.0%–0.5%
Neutrophils, absolute	7.50	$1.56–6.13 \times 10^3$ cells/mm³
Lymphocytes	39	19.3%–51.7%

Laboratory findings: *(continued)*

Component	Results	Normal Range
Lymphs, absolute	2.9	$1.18–3.74 \times 10^3$ cells/mm³
Monocytes	10.0	3.0%–13.0%
Monocytes, absolute	0.59	$0.24–0.86 \times 10^3$ cells/mm³
Eosinophils	3.5	0.7%–5.8%
Eosinophils, absolute	0.29	$0.04–0.36 \times 10^3$ cells/mm³
Basophils	1.0	0.1%–1.2%
Basophils, absolute	0.07	$0.01–0.08 \times 10^3$ cells/mm³
Blood, Other		
CRP	15.2	0–1.0 mg/L
ESR	49	3–13 mm/hr
Albumin	2.6	3.5–5.5 g/dL
Bilirubin, total	0.9	0–1.5 mg/dL
ALT	32	8–35 U/L
AST	45	15–46 U/L
Urinalysis		
Color	Cloudy	
RBC	3	0–3/high-power field
WBC	26	0–2/high-power field
Glucose	Negative	Negative
Nitrite	Negative	Negative
Protein	Trace	0–20 mg/dL
Gram stain	Negative	Negative
Microbiology		
Culture - Blood	Pending	
Culture - Urine	Pending	

1. Explain the benefits of a pharmacologic treatment that incorporates IVIG and aspirin during hospitalization and at home. Provide the patient's therapeutic goals and monitoring plans.

Standard KD therapy is a single dose of IVIG and high-dose aspirin, initiated within the first 10 days of illness. The benefits of IVIG are its anti-inflammatory properties to resolve fever and prevent coronary artery aneurysm. Although it does not decrease coronary abnormalities, aspirin is used for its additive anti-inflammatory and antiplatelet activities. Alleviation of inflammation in the coronary artery wall and prevention of coronary thrombosis are the primary therapeutic goals. Other targeted therapeutic outcomes are to achieve defervescence, reverse presenting symptoms, normalize any irregular laboratory tests, and prevent mortality from myocardial infarction or arrhythmias.

A single, high-dose infusion of IVIG at 2 g/kg (24 g infused over 8–12 hours for this patient) compared with low doses over 4–5 days would produce a greater decrease in the duration of fever and length of hospital stay as well as a faster resolution of laboratory findings for acute inflammation. In addition, high-dose aspirin 80–100 mg/kg/day administered orally (240–300 mg in this patient, which equates to three 81-mg chewable tablets every 6 hours, not to exceed 4 g/day) is recommended for 48–72 hours until after fever resolves. Alternatively, high-dose aspirin can be continued until 14 days after illness onset, with at least 48–72 hours after fever cessation. This is followed by low-dose aspirin 3–5 mg/kg/day (i.e., around 40 mg [½ of an 81-mg chewable tablet] orally once daily), continued until resolution of ESR or 6–8 weeks after illness onset.

Case (continued). A 2-D echocardiogram 2 weeks after onset of fever revealed, at the precordial short axis, the formation of a small 2-mm uniform aneurysm at the proximal right coronary artery. The Z-score was 3.

2. Provide the rationale for using antithrombotic agents in this patient.

Medications to prevent thrombosis formation may be necessary, on the basis of the echocardiogram (which was correctly done in this patient) and clinical progress. Use of antiplatelet, anticoagulation, or combination therapies (dual or triple) depends on the degree of coronary involvement. For a small coronary artery aneurysm less than 4 mm with a Z-score less than 5, low-dose aspirin is adequate. Adding other antiplatelet drugs (e.g., clopidogrel) to low-dose aspirin for dual therapy may be effective for cases with a moderate (or medium) coronary artery aneurysm with a Z-score of 5 to less than 10. Anticoagulation using warfarin (with initial unfractionated heparin as bridge therapy), in combination with low-dose aspirin and clopidogrel, is indicated when the risk of thrombosis is high, particularly for large coronary aneurysms with a Z-score of 10 or greater. In this patient, the echocardiogram reveals a small aneurysm of the right coronary artery. As such, low-dose aspirin until regression is documented with echocardiogram.

To ensure regression of aneurysm, an echocardiogram should be repeated in 6–8 weeks. Referral to pediatric cardiology is required for all patients with KD, particularly after hospital discharge for close monitoring. Follow-up echocardiograms every 1–2 years after diagnosis may be warranted to determine the status (e.g., improving or worsening) of the coronary aneurysm and to evaluate for other cardiac conditions, including myocardial ischemia.

3. What educational points should you provide to the parents regarding the safe use of intravenous immunoglobulin and aspirin and future vaccinations?

IVIG is generally well tolerated, but infusion-related reactions (consisting of flushing, hypotension, nausea, vomiting, fever, chills, pruritus, malaise, myalgia, and chest tightness) may occur within 30 minutes to 1 hour after initiation of the infusion. These reactions usually resolve when the infusion is slowed or discontinued, or when the patient is pretreated with acetaminophen and diphenhydramine. In addition, antibodies in IVIG may interfere with the immune response to certain live virus vaccines (e.g., varicella). As such, live vaccines should be deferred for at least 11 months. Repeat immunization is necessary if the live virus vaccine was administered within 14 days before, or at the same time as, IVIG. Other routine childhood vaccinations (e.g., pneumococcal conjugate vaccine) should be administered with no change.

The parent should be instructed to use baby aspirin (because it is chewable and/or crushable) and to administer it with food to minimize stomach upset. The patient may be at risk of adverse effects from aspirin use, consisting of elevated transaminases, transient hearing loss, and Reye syndrome. To avoid Reye syndrome, parents should be instructed to report any episode of influenza or varicella infection to health care providers. Furthermore, aspirin should be avoided in the 6 weeks after varicella vaccination. The patient should receive specifically the inactivated influenza vaccine, whereas household contacts can use any formulation. Ibuprofen and other NSAIDs should be avoided because they interfere with the antiplatelet cardioprotective action of aspirin.

REFERENCES

1. McCrindle BW, Rowley AH, Newburger JW, et al. Diagnosis, treatment, and long-term management of Kawasaki disease: a scientific statement for health professionals from the American Heart Association. Circulation 2017;135:e927-e99.
2. Taubert KA, Rowley AH, Shulman ST. Nationwide survey of Kawasaki disease and acute rheumatic fever. J Pediatr 1991;119: 279-82.
3. Son MB, Gauvreau K, Ma L, et al. Treatment of Kawasaki disease: analysis of 27 US pediatric hospitals from 2001 to 2006. Pediatrics 2009;124:1-8.
4. Hirata S, Nakamura Y, Yanagawa H. Incidence rate of recurrent Kawasaki disease and related risk factors: from the results of nationwide surveys of Kawasaki disease in Japan. Acta Paediatr 2001;90:40-4.
5. Burgner D, Harnden A. Kawasaki disease: what is the epidemiology telling us about the etiology? Int J Infect Dis 2005;9:185-94.
6. Burns JC, Glode MP. Kawasaki syndrome. Lancet 2004;364:533-44.
7. Abe J, Kotzin BL, Jujo K, et al. Selective expansion of T cells expressing T-cell receptor variable regions V beta 2 and V beta 8 in Kawasaki disease. Proc Natl Acad Sci U S A 1992;89:4066-70.
8. Burns JC, Cayan DR, Tong G, et al. Seasonality and temporal clustering of Kawasaki syndrome. Epidemiology 2005;16:220-5.
9. Kao AS, Getis A, Brodine S, et al. Spatial and temporal clustering of Kawasaki syndrome cases. Pediatr Infect Dis J 2008;27:981-5.
10. Naoe S, Takahashi K, Masuda H, et al. Kawasaki disease. With particular emphasis on arterial lesions. Acta Pathol Jpn 1991;41: 785-97.
11. Popper SJ, Shimizu C, Shike H, et al. Gene-expression patterns reveal underlying biological processes in Kawasaki disease. Genome Biol 2007;8:R261.
12. Jennette JC. Implications for pathogenesis of patterns of injury in small- and medium-sized-vessel vasculitis. Cleve Clin J Med 2002;69(suppl 2):SII33-8.
13. Fujita Y, Nakamura Y, Sakata K, et al. Kawasaki disease in families. Pediatrics 1989;84:666-9.
14. Uehara R, Yashiro M, Nakamura Y, et al. Clinical features of patients with Kawasaki disease whose parents had the same disease. Arch Pediatr Adolesc Med 2004;158:1166-9.
15. Yeung RS. Kawasaki disease: update on pathogenesis. Curr Opin Rheumatol 2010;22:551-60.
16. Onouchi Y, Gunji T, Burns JC, et al. ITPKC functional polymorphism associated with Kawasaki disease susceptibility and formation of coronary artery aneurysms. Nat Genet 2008;40:35-42.
17. Huang Y, Lee YJ, Chen MR, et al. Polymorphism of transmembrane region of MICA gene and Kawasaki disease. Exp Clin Immunogenet 2000;17:130-7.
18. Lin YJ, Wan L, Wu JY, et al. HLA-E gene polymorphism associated with susceptibility to Kawasaki disease and formation of coronary artery aneurysms. Arthritis Rheum 2009;60:604-10.
19. Wu SF, Chang JS, Peng CT, et al. Polymorphism of angiotensin-1 converting enzyme gene and Kawasaki disease. Pediatr Cardiol 2004;25:529-33.
20. Holman RC, Curns AT, Belay ED, et al. Kawasaki syndrome hospitalizations in the United States, 1997 and 2000. Pediatrics 2003;112(3 pt 1):495-501.
21. Huang WC, Huang LM, Chang IS, et al. Epidemiologic features of Kawasaki disease in Taiwan, 2003-2006. Pediatrics 2009;123: e401-5.
22. Yanagawa H, Yashiro M, Nakamura Y, et al. Epidemiologic pictures of Kawasaki disease in Japan: from the nationwide incidence survey in 1991 and 1992. Pediatrics 1995;95:475-9.
23. Okubo Y, Nochioka K, Sakakibara H, et al. National survey of pediatric hospitalizations due to Kawasaki disease and coronary artery aneurysms in the USA. Clin Rheumatol 2017;36:413-9.
24. Taubert KA, Shulman ST. Kawasaki disease. Am Fam Physician 1999;59:3093-102, 107-8.
25. Yellen ES, Gauvreau K, Takahashi M, et al. Performance of 2004 American Heart Association recommendations for treatment of Kawasaki disease. Pediatrics 2010;125:e234-41.
26. American Academy of Pediatrics (AAP). Kawasaki syndrome. In: Pickering LK, ed. Red Book: 2009 Report of the Committee on Infectious Diseases, 28th ed. Elk Grove Village, IL: AAP, 2009:413.
27. Manlhiot C, Yeung RS, Clarizia NA, et al. Kawasaki disease at the extremes of the age spectrum. Pediatrics 2009;124:e410-5.
28. Kato H, Ichinose E, Kawasaki T. Myocardial infarction in Kawasaki disease: clinical analyses in 195 cases. J Pediatr 1986; 108:923-7.
29. Burns JC, Capparelli EV, Brown JA, et al. Intravenous gammaglobulin treatment and retreatment in Kawasaki disease. US/Canadian Kawasaki Syndrome Study Group. Pediatr Infect Dis J 1998;17:1144-8.
30. Belay ED, Maddox RA, Holman RC, et al. Kawasaki syndrome and risk factors for coronary artery abnormalities: United States, 1994-2003. Pediatr Infect Dis J 2006;25:245-9.
31. Suzuki A, Kamiya T, Kuwahara N, et al. Coronary arterial lesions of Kawasaki disease: cardiac catheterization findings of 1100 cases. Pediatr Cardiol 1986;7:3-9.
32. Nakamura Y, Hirose K, Yanagawa H, et al. Incidence rate of recurrent Kawasaki disease in Japan. Acta Paediatr 1994;83:1061-4.
33. Minich LL, Sleeper LA, Atz AM, et al. Delayed diagnosis of Kawasaki disease: what are the risk factors? Pediatrics 2007; 120:e1434-40.
34. Terai M, Shulman ST. Prevalence of coronary artery abnormalities in Kawasaki disease is highly dependent on gamma globulin dose but independent of salicylate dose. J Pediatr 1997;131:888-93.
35. Oates-Whitehead RM, Baumer JH, Haines L, et al. Intravenous immunoglobulin for the treatment of Kawasaki disease in children. Cochrane Database Syst Rev 2003;4:CD004000.

36. Newburger JW, Sanders SP, Burns JC, et al. Left ventricular contractility and function in Kawasaki syndrome. Effect of intravenous gamma-globulin. Circulation 1989;79:1237-46.

37. Newburger JW, Burns JC, Beiser AS, et al. Altered lipid profile after Kawasaki syndrome. Circulation 1991;84:625-31.

38. Newburger JW, Takahashi M, Beiser AS, et al. A single intravenous infusion of gamma globulin as compared with four infusions in the treatment of acute Kawasaki syndrome. N Engl J Med 1991;324:1633-9.

39. Muta H, Ishii M, Egami K, et al. Early intravenous gamma-globulin treatment for Kawasaki disease: the nationwide surveys in Japan. J Pediatr 2004;144:496-9.

40. Tse SM, Silverman ED, McCrindle BW, et al. Early treatment with intravenous immunoglobulin in patients with Kawasaki disease. J Pediatr 2002;140:450-5.

41. Tsai MH, Huang YC, Yen MH, et al. Clinical responses of patients with Kawasaki disease to different brands of intravenous immunoglobulin. J Pediatr 2006;148:38-43.

42. Manlhiot C, Yeung RS, Chahal N, et al. Intravenous immunoglobulin preparation type: association with outcomes for patients with acute Kawasaki disease. Pediatr Allergy Immunol 2010;21:515-21.

43. Hsieh KS, Weng KP, Lin CC, et al. Treatment of acute Kawasaki disease: aspirin's role in the febrile stage revisited. Pediatrics 2004;114:e689-93.

44. Newburger JW, Sleeper LA, McCrindle BW, et al. Randomized trial of pulsed corticosteroid therapy for primary treatment of Kawasaki disease. N Engl J Med 2007;356:663-75.

45. Okada K, Hara J, Maki I, et al. Pulse methylprednisolone with gammaglobulin as an initial treatment for acute Kawasaki disease. Eur J Pediatr 2009;168:181-5.

46. Kobayashi T, Inoue Y, Takeuchi K, et al. Prediction of intravenous immunoglobulin unresponsiveness in patients with Kawasaki disease. Circulation 2006;113:2606-12.

47. Egami K, Muta H, Ishii M, et al. Prediction of resistance to intravenous immunoglobulin treatment in patients with Kawasaki disease. J Pediatr 2006;149:237-40.

48. Tremoulet AH, Best BM, Song S, et al. Resistance to intravenous immunoglobulin in children with Kawasaki disease. J Pediatr 2008;153:117-21.

49. Uehara R, Belay ED, Maddox RA, et al. Analysis of potential risk factors associated with nonresponse to initial intravenous immunoglobulin treatment among Kawasaki disease patients in Japan. Pediatr Infect Dis J 2008;27:155-60.

50. Sundel RP, Burns JC, Baker A, et al. Gamma globulin re-treatment in Kawasaki disease. J Pediatr 1993;123:657-9.

51. Hashino K, Ishii M, Iemura M, et al. Re-treatment for immune globulin-resistant Kawasaki disease: a comparative study of additional immune globulin and steroid pulse therapy. Pediatr Int 2001;43:211-7.

52. Furukawa T, Kishiro M, Akimoto K, et al. Effects of steroid pulse therapy on immunoglobulin-resistant Kawasaki disease. Arch Dis Child 2008;93:142-6.

53. Sonoda K, Mori M, Hokosaki T, et al. Infliximab plus plasma exchange rescue therapy in Kawasaki disease. J Pediatr 2014;164:1128-32 e1.

54. Burns JC, Best BM, Mejias A, et al. Infliximab treatment of intravenous immunoglobulin-resistant Kawasaki disease. J Pediatr 2008;153:833-8.

55. de Magalhaes CM, Alves NR, de Melo AV, et al. Catastrophic Kawasaki disease unresponsive to IVIG in a 3-month-old infant: a diagnostic and therapeutic challenge. Pediatr Rheumatol Online J 2012;10:28.

56. Furukawa S, Matsubara T, Umezawa Y, et al. Pentoxifylline and intravenous gamma globulin combination therapy for acute Kawasaki disease. Eur J Pediatr 1994;153:663-7.

57. Tremoulet AH, Jain S, Jaggi P, et al. Infliximab for intensification of primary therapy for Kawasaki disease: a phase 3 randomised, double-blind, placebo-controlled trial. Lancet 2014;383:1731-8.

58. Choueiter NF, Olson AK, Shen DD, et al. Prospective open-label trial of etanercept as adjunctive therapy for kawasaki disease. J Pediatr 2010;157:960-6 e1.

59. Imagawa T, Mori M, Miyamae T, et al. Plasma exchange for refractory Kawasaki disease. Eur J Pediatr 2004;163:263-4.

60. Tremoulet AH, Jain S, Kim S, et al. Rationale and study design for a phase I/IIa trial of anakinra in children with Kawasaki disease and early coronary artery abnormalities (the ANAKID trial). Contemp Clin Trials 2016;48:70-5.

61. Tremoulet AH, Jain S, Burns JC. Evaluating a novel treatment for coronary artery inflammation in acute Kawasaki disease: a phase I/IIa trial of atorvastatin. Expert Opin Orphan Drugs 2015;3:967-70.

62. Shulman, ST, Rowley AH. Kawasaki disease. In: Cherry JD, Demmler-Harrison GJ, Kaplan SL, et al., eds. Textbook of Pediatric Infectious Diseases, 8th ed. Philadelphia: Saunders, 2018:759.

63. Carbone J. Adverse reactions and pathogen safety of intravenous immunoglobulin. Curr Drug Saf 2007;2:9-18.

64. Sekul EA, Cupler EJ, Dalakas MC. Aseptic meningitis associated with high-dose intravenous immunoglobulin therapy: frequency and risk factors. Ann Intern Med 1994;121:259-

65. Koren G, Silverman E, Sundel R, et al. Decreased protein binding of salicylates in Kawasaki disease. J Pediatr 1991;118:456-9.

Section XV

Dermatologic Disorders

CHAPTER 56

Pediatric Dermatology

Jamie L. Miller, Pharm.D., FPPA, BCPS, BCPPS; and
Michelle Condren, Pharm.D., FPPA, BCPPS, CDE, AE-C

LEARNING OBJECTIVES

1. Identify topical products that should typically be avoided in infants and children.

2. Create pharmacologic and nonpharmacologic treatment plans for diaper dermatitis.

3. Recommend treatment for seborrheic dermatitis.

4. Recommend pharmacologic and nonpharmacologic treatment for atopic dermatitis in children.

5. Recommend treatment for acne in adolescence.

6. Recommend pharmacologic and nonpharmacologic treatment for dermatophytic fungal infections in children.

7. Describe the role of propranolol in the treatment of infantile hemangioma.

ABBREVIATIONS IN THIS CHAPTER

IH	Infantile hemangioma

INTRODUCTION TO SKIN CARE FOR INFANTS AND CHILDREN

Skin disorders in childhood are a common reason for health care use and self-care worldwide. Although some dermatologic conditions are unique to pediatric patients, many continue into adulthood. However, the approach to therapy for skin disorders in children differs from that in adults because skin structure and function differ.

Skin is composed of the epidermis, dermis, and hypodermis. The outer layer of the epidermis, the stratum corneum, prevents water loss and serves as the primary barrier to the penetration of medications and irritants. Children younger than 2 years are especially susceptible to skin damage, irritation, and systemic absorption of medications because they have a thinner and weaker stratum corneum and total skin layer.[1] In addition, infants and children have a larger skin surface area/body weight ratio than adults. Preterm and term neonates are at increased risk because of an underdeveloped stratum corneum. The increased surface area, increased skin hydration, and underdeveloped stratum corneum help improve the absorption of topical agents. In addition, differences in the lipid component of the stratum corneum occur until puberty, placing children at higher risk of bacterial and fungal skin infections.[1]

General skin care for infants involves maintaining adequate hydration and avoiding products that can cause skin irritation.

Gentle, fragrance-free soaps and emollients are recommended, with emollients applied after bathing. Products should be avoided that can cause irritant dermatitis or harmful systemic absorption. Table 1 includes a list of ingredients that should not be applied topically to children younger than 2 years or those with skin disorders, when possible.[1,2]

Common dermatologic conditions in childhood include diaper dermatitis, atopic dermatitis, acne, warts, birthmarks, seborrheic dermatitis, and fungal or bacterial skin infections. This chapter will focus on the common disorders requiring pharmacologic interventions. Treatment of bacterial skin infections is discussed in detail in the Skin and Soft Tissue Infections of Bacterial and Viral Etiology chapter. For images of the conditions described, see www.visualdx.com for helpful examples.

DIAPER DERMATITIS

Diaper dermatitis, commonly called diaper rash, is a nonspecific term used to describe inflammatory skin eruptions in the diaper region. Diaper dermatitis is one of the most common skin disorders affecting infants and toddlers, with an overall reported prevalence of 50%–65%,[3,4] but diaper dermatitis is likely underreported.

Diaper dermatitis is usually the result of irritant contact dermatitis secondary to a combination of the following factors: occlusiveness of the diaper, friction of the diaper, maceration of the skin, presence of feces/urine, and alkaline pH of the skin.[5-7] The occlusiveness of the diaper results in a moist environment, causing maceration of the skin and, in turn,

Table 1. Topical Products to Avoid in Neonates and Infants

Products That Can Cause Local Irritation	Products That Can Cause Systemic Effects
Cod liver oil	Betamethasone
Hexachlorophene	DEET (> 10%)
Iodine	Hexachlorophene, resorcinol
Isopropyl alcohol (> 4%)	High-potency topical
Lanolin	corticosteroids
Neomycin	Isopropyl alcohol
Nickel	Mercury
Phenol	Methylene blue
Propylene glycol	Neomycin
Resorcinol	Povidine-iodine
Thimerosal	Salicylic acid
Topical antihistamines	Silver sulfadiazine
	Tacrolimus, pimecrolimus
	Topical anesthetics
	(e.g., benzocaine, prilocaine)
	Urea

DEET = *N,N*-diethyl-*m*-toluamide.

decreasing the integrity of the skin barrier function. The decreased barrier function allows an increased permeability of irritants and microbial flora. Friction from movement, together with moisture in the diaper environment, further serves to physically break down the skin. The presence of feces (i.e., fecal enzymes), bile acid salts, and urine also promotes the development of diaper dermatitis by acting as a direct irritant to the skin. In the presence of fecal urease, the urine is broken down to ammonia, contributing to the basic pH of the diapered skin. The increase in pH subsequently causes an increased activity of the fecal enzymes (i.e., proteases and lipases) and further disruption of the barrier function of the skin. Secondary infection by either bacteria (e.g., Staphylococcus aureus) or yeast is thought to occur because of the decreased barrier function of the stratum corneum. Candida albicans can be present on the skin of infants with and without diaper dermatitis; however, extensive colonization can increase the severity of diaper dermatitis. Candida albicans can be isolated in up to 80% of cases in which diaper dermatitis persists for 3 days or more.[7]

Several risk factors for developing diaper dermatitis have been identified and include the type of diaper used, the infant's diet, and antibiotic exposure. Infants in cloth diapers are at greater risk of developing moderate or severe diaper dermatitis because cloth diapers do not have the absorption capacity of disposable diapers and do not wick away the moisture as efficiently. By absorbing the urine, disposable diapers prevent its interaction with fecal enzymes, thereby decreasing the ammonia produced. Another risk factor is exposure to infant formula versus breast milk, because formula-fed infants are more likely to develop moderate to severe diaper dermatitis.[5] Antibiotic-associated diarrhea increases the incidence of diaper dermatitis because of repeated exposure of the skin to feces.[4]

Simple diaper dermatitis presents as erythema and scaling on the skin that is in direct apposition with the diaper, sparing the skinfolds. The severity of diaper dermatitis can be categorized as mild (some erythema with minimal scaling), moderate (more pronounced erythema with papules, scaling, and/or edema), or severe (very intense erythema with severe desquamation, edema, erosion, and ulceration). Mild and moderate cases of diaper dermatitis are often self-limiting, with a mean of 2–3 days per episode.[5] Severe dermatitis (i.e., Jacquet diaper dermatitis) may take longer for resolution and healing. Secondary infection with C. albicans presents as an intense erythematous rash, often accompanied by papules and pustules called satellite lesions that are often described as beefy-red. Unlike contact dermatitis, the infection is present in the skinfolds and perianal skin. In most cases, a clinical diagnosis can be made on the basis of presentation; however, a diagnosis can be confirmed by culture or by doing a potassium hydroxide preparation of a scraping from the lesion.

Secondary bacterial infections are usually S. aureus or group A Streptococcus. Staphylococcus aureus may present as small papules and pustules or as bullous impetigo. When the bullae erupt, they form superficial erosions with a honey-colored crust. Group A Streptococcus presents as perianal patchy erythema. If a bacterial cause is suspected, cultures can be obtained to provide targeted antimicrobial therapy.

If the diaper rash remains after 1 month of vigilant treatment for irritant, bacterial, and yeast dermatitis, a further workup should be done to rule out immunodeficiency, nutritional deficiency, metabolic disorders, and abuse/neglect.[7] Other diagnoses that should be considered in the differential diagnosis include allergic contact dermatitis, seborrheic dermatitis, intertrigo, psoriasis, and infection (e.g., candidiasis, bullous impetigo, scabies, folliculitis).

Prevention of diaper dermatitis begins with educating the caregiver/parent on proper diaper hygiene. Removing the diaper immediately after defecation is optimal to prevent interaction of the urine and feces and a subsequent increase in skin pH. The diaper area should be gently cleansed with water and a cotton cloth or commercial baby wipes to remove the irritants. If commercial products are used, products containing preservatives, fragrances, alcohol, or aloe should be avoided because they can cause further irritation. After cleansing, the diaper area should be patted dry. If feasible, daily diaper-free time should be implemented to allow exposure of the diaper area to the air. Use of superabsorbent disposable diapers decreases the frequency and severity of diaper dermatitis. Not all infants need empiric application of a barrier protectant as a preventive measure. If the infant is prone to develop diaper rash or at increased risk, barrier protectants such as zinc oxide or petrolatum can be used prophylactically. Barrier preparations protect the skin from irritants by coating it with a water-repellent barrier and serve to reduce friction by providing lubrication. Ointments and pastes provide better protection because they are not as easily removed. The product selected should have minimal ingredients and no other additives, which can lead to sensitization of the skin. Use of talcum powder, baby powder, or cornstarch should be discouraged because of the risk of aspirating airborne particles and developing pneumonitis.

Treatment of diaper dermatitis involves both nonpharmacologic and pharmacologic therapy. Barrier protectants should be initiated at the first sign of erythema to prevent further irritation to the area. The barrier protectant should be applied with each diaper change. The nonpharmacologic measures recommended for preventing diaper dermatitis are also recommended for treating diaper dermatitis.

Patients whose diaper rash does not respond to barrier protectants after 3 days should be referred to their primary care provider. In these cases, if the diaper rash involves the skinfolds, a topical antifungal agent such as nystatin, miconazole, or clotrimazole should be initiated. The antifungal agent should be applied twice daily, as described in Table 2, until 1 week after the eruption has cleared.[5,8] Some experts recommend applying four times daily or with every diaper change.[3] Miconazole 2% and clotrimazole 1% are both available over the counter. Although not specifically labeled for candidal diaper dermatitis, nystatin ointment is available as a prescription product. An additional prescription product with specific labeling for candidal diaper dermatitis in children older than 4 weeks is a combination of miconazole 0.25%, zinc oxide 15%, and white petrolatum. Oral antifungal medications are not routinely recommended. However, if an infant has concomitant oral thrush, oral nystatin suspension should also be initiated.

For cases that do not respond to barrier protectants after 3 days and do not involve the skinfolds, the primary care provider can recommend topical corticosteroids to reduce the inflammation and pain. Only low-potency corticosteroids such as hydrocortisone 1%, hydrocortisone 2.5%, or desonide 0.05% should be used, with application once or twice daily. Table 3 includes potency ratings for topical corticosteroids.[8-10] The topical corticosteroid should be discontinued on resolution of the erythema and should not be continued for longer than 14 days. Mid- and high-potency steroids should not be applied underneath a diaper because the occlusive environment increases the systemic absorption of corticosteroids and the risk of systemic adverse effects. In addition, the occlusive environment results in increased skin atrophy. If combination therapy with both a topical corticosteroid and a barrier protectant is used, the topical corticosteroid should be applied first. In severe cases, both corticosteroids and antifungal agents can be used. If the provider recommends this, combination antifungal-corticosteroid products should be avoided because they contain high-potency corticosteroids and are contraindicated for use in the diaper area. If both antifungal and anti-inflammatory activity is desired, separate administration of the agents is required.

If a secondary bacterial infection is suspected or no improvement in the rash is noted, the addition of topical mupirocin 2% should be considered. Mupirocin provides gram-positive antibacterial activity, as well as some antifungal activity. For diaper dermatitis, mupirocin should be applied three times daily for 7 days. For more severe cases, an oral antibiotic with activity against group A *Streptococcus* and *S. aureus* is recommended.

For severe irritant dermatitis and excoriation secondary to diarrhea, liquid antacids, sucralfate, or a compounded cholestyramine paste can be prescribed.[11,12] Liquid antacids, though not evaluated in clinical studies, have been used anecdotally to neutralize the pH of the acidic stools. However, there is no evidence regarding efficacy or frequency and duration of use with liquid antacids. Use of topical sucralfate has been reported in adults, with a compounded 4% topical sucralfate preparation applied four times daily.[11] The severe erosive diaper dermatitis resolved after 2 months. Topical sucralfate is thought to act as a physical barrier to protect the damaged skin. One case report described the use of a compounded preparation of cholestyramine 5% in Aquaphor ointment (Beiersdorf, Inc., Wilton, CT) after each bowel movement, with significant improvement within 2 days.[12] Although data are limited, anecdotally, cholestyramine is prepared at 5%–20% compounded preparations. Cholestyramine is thought to be beneficial because of its mechanism of action of binding bile acid salts.

SEBORRHEIC DERMATITIS

Seborrheic dermatitis is an inflammatory skin condition that can affect areas of the skin with increased sebaceous gland activity (e.g., nasolabial folds, eyebrows, scalp, ears). Seborrheic dermatitis can occur at any age but often has a bimodal presentation in children. In infants, specifically within the first 3 months of life, seborrheic dermatitis typically presents as "cradle cap," whereas in adolescents, it presents as scalp scaling (i.e., dandruff) or erythema and scaling on the scalp, face, and trunk. The overall prevalence of

Table 2. Topical Antifungal Agents[8]

Antifungal	Dosing Frequency	Indications	Therapy Duration
Butenafine 1% cream	Once daily	Tinea pedis Tinea cruris Tinea corporis	7–14 days or 1 wk after resolution of symptoms 14 days or 1 wk after resolution of symptoms 14 days or 1 wk after resolution of lesion
Clotrimazole 1% cream	Twice daily	Diaper dermatitis Tinea pedis Tinea corporis	14 days or 1 wk after resolution of lesion 28 days or 1 wk after resolution of symptoms 14 days or 1 wk after resolution of lesion
Econazole 1% cream	Once daily	Tinea pedis Tinea cruris Tinea corporis	28 days or 1 wk after resolution of symptoms 14 days or 1 wk after resolution of lesion 14 days or 1 wk after resolution of lesion
Ketoconazole 2% foam, cream, gel	Once or twice daily	Adolescent seborrheic dermatitis	28 days or 1 wk after resolution of symptoms
Miconazole 2% cream, powder	Twice daily	Diaper dermatitis Tinea pedis Tinea corporis	14 days or 1 wk after resolution of lesion 14–28 days or 1 wk after resolution of symptoms 14 days or 1 wk after resolution of lesion
Nystatin cream or ointment	Twice daily	Diaper dermatitis	14 days or 1 wk after resolution of lesion
Terbinafine 1% cream, spray	Once or twice daily	Tinea pedis Tinea cruris Tinea corporis	7–14 days or 1 wk after resolution of symptoms 7 days 14 days or 1 wk after resolution of lesion
Tolnaftate 1% cream	Twice daily	Tinea pedis Tinea cruris Tinea corporis	28 days or 1 wk after resolution of symptoms 14 days or 1 wk after resolution of symptoms 14 days or 1 wk after resolution of lesion

seborrheic dermatitis is 42% in infants, 10% in male children, and 9.5% in female children.[13]

The exact cause of seborrheic dermatitis is unknown; however, it has been associated with fungal infections (i.e., *Malassezia furfur,* previously *Pityrosporum ovale*), increased hormone concentrations, nutritional deficiencies, and neurogenic factors.[14] Support for the potential link with hormone activity is that it presents in early infancy when transplacental hormones are elevated, resolves spontaneously, and then returns around puberty when another hormonal flux occurs. No firm linkage has been established with the other proposed causes (i.e., nutritional deficiencies, altered essential fatty acid patterns, or neurogenic factors).

Infantile seborrheic dermatitis (i.e., cradle cap) presents as thick, greasy scales that are white, off-white, or yellow on the vertex of the scalp. This condition is not pruritic and does not cause the infant discomfort, though it can be bothersome to the caregiver. In addition, some infants may present with mild scaling of the face, ears, and forehead and on the flexural folds (e.g., antecubital region, popliteal region). The prognosis of infantile seborrheic dermatitis is usually benign and resolves within the first year of life, though there is some association with development of seborrheic dermatitis as an adult.[15]

Adolescent seborrheic dermatitis presents as mild, greasy scaling of the scalp (i.e., dandruff). In addition, an oily complexion with scaling and erythema can be present in the nasolabial folds, eyebrows, postauricular skin, glabella (i.e., T-zone), and trunk. Unlike infantile seborrheic dermatitis, adolescent seborrheic dermatitis can be pruritic.

Table 3. Potency Ratings of Selected Topical Corticosteroids[8-10]

Potency (group)	Selected Representative Corticosteroids	Brand (dosage form)
Super (I)	Augmented betamethasone dipropionate Clobetasol propionate Fluocinonide, optimized vehicle Halobetasol propionate	Diprolene 0.05% (ointment)[a] Clobex 0.05% (lotion, shampoo, spray)[b] Olux 0.05% (foam)[c] Temovate E 0.05% (cream)[d] Cormax 0.05% (ointment, solution)[e] Temovate 0.05% (gel, ointment, solution)[f] Vanos 0.1% (cream)[g] Ultravate 0.05% (cream, ointment)[h]
High (II)	Augmented betamethasone dipropionate Betamethasone dipropionate Betamethasone valerate Fluocinonide Mometasone furoate	Diprolene AF 0.05% (cream), Diprolene 0.05% (lotion)[a] [0.05%, ointment] [0.1%, ointment] [0.05%, ointment, gel, cream] Elocon 0.1% (ointment)[a]
Upper mid (III)	Betamethasone dipropionate Triamcinolone acetonide Fluticasone propionate	[0.05%, cream] Kenalog 5% (ointment)[i] Cutivate 0.005% (ointment)[j]
Mid (IV)	Betamethasone valerate Hydrocortisone valerate Mometasone furoate Triamcinolone acetonide	Luxiq 0.12% (foam)[c] [0.2% ointment] Elocon 0.1% (cream, lotion)[a] Kenalog 0.025%, 0.1% (ointment)[i]
Low mid (V)	Betamethasone valerate Fluticasone propionate Hydrocortisone valerate Triamcinolone acetonide	[0.1%, cream, lotion] Cutivate 0.05% (cream)[j] [0.2%, cream] Triderm 0.1% (cream) [cream 0.025%][k]
Mild (VI)	Desonide Fluocinolone acetonide Hydrocortisone butyrate	Verdeso 0.05% (foam)[c] DesOwen 0.05% (cream, ointment, lotion)[l] Desonate 0.05% (gel)[m] Derma-Smoothe FS 0.01% (oil, shampoo)[n] [cream 0.01%, 0.025%] Locoid 0.1% (cream, solution)[h]
Low (VII)	Hydrocortisone	[0.5%, cream] Cortisone-10 Maximum Strength 1% (cream, lotion, ointment) [2.5% cream, ointment, lotion][o]

[a]Merck & Co., Inc., Whitehouse Station, NJ; [b]DPT Laboratories, Ltd., San Antonio, TX; [c]Connetics Corporation, Palo Alto, CA; [d]Fougera Pharmaceuticals, Inc., Melville, NY; [e]ECR Pharmaceuticals, Richmond, VA; [f]Glaxo Wellcome, Inc., Research Triangle Park, NC; [g]Patheon, Inc., Mississauga, Ontario, Canada; [h]Ferndale Laboratories, Inc., Ferndale, MI; [i]Bristol-Myers Squibb Company, Princeton, NJ; [j]Nycomed US Inc., Melville, NY; [k]Crown Laboratories, Johnson City, TN; [l]Stiefel Laboratories, Inc., Research Triangle Park, NC; [m]Bayer HealthCare Pharmaceuticals, Inc., Whippany, NJ; [n]Hill Dermaceuticals, Inc., Sanford, FL; [o]Sanofi-Aventis, Paris, France.

Cradle cap typically resolves spontaneously; however, if treatment is needed, nonpharmacologic therapy that includes nonmedicated, mild shampoo and loosening of scales with a soft brush should be initiated first. If this is ineffective, emollients such as petrolatum or mineral oil can be applied to the scalp. The emollient should be applied for at least 20 minutes before washing the hair with a mild shampoo. After removing the emollient, the scales can gently be removed by scratching the scales with a soft brush or fingertips. For more severe cases that do not resolve with nonpharmacologic treatment, antidandruff shampoos containing selenium sulfide or pyrithione zinc can be recommended by a provider. Selenium sulfide shampoo can safely be applied twice weekly for 2 weeks and then once weekly until resolution. However, parents/caregivers should be informed that selenium sulfide can stain the scalp reddish brown, which resolves shortly after discontinuation.[16] In addition, ketoconazole shampoo has been shown safe and effective in infants for the treatment of infantile seborrheic dermatitis when used twice weekly for 1 month.[17] If erythema is present, a prescriber may recommend topical hydrocortisone. However, because of the potential for increased systemic absorption and skin atrophy when topical hydrocortisone is applied to the thin skin of the head and face, application should be limited to a small area and discontinued after the erythema resolves.

Management of adolescent dermatitis differs from that of infantile dermatitis because of differences in presentation. As a preventive measure, adolescents with seborrheic dermatitis should be instructed to cleanse the affected areas regularly to remove excess oil from the skin. In addition, emollients can be applied for relief of dry skin. Treatment options differ, depending on the location of the affected area. Antifungal creams (e.g., clotrimazole, miconazole, ketoconazole) are first-line pharmacologic therapy for application to the face and can be applied once or twice daily. For scalp involvement, antidandruff shampoos (i.e., selenium sulfide, pyrithione zinc) are first-line nonprescription pharmacologic therapy for dandruff in adolescents. These agents should be applied to wet hair and massaged into the scalp and rinsed at least twice weekly for best results. An alternative first-line nonprescription option is the antifungal ketoconazole 1% shampoo. This agent should be applied twice weekly, with at least 3 days between shampoos, for 8 weeks.[8] The shampoo should be applied to wet hair and massaged over the entire scalp for 1 minute, after which it should be rinsed out and reapplied for another 3 minutes before rinsing again. If the seborrheic dermatitis affects areas other than the scalp, nonprescription ketoconazole 2% shampoo can be applied body-wide to the damp skin of the affected area and left in place for 5 minutes before rinsing.[8] A 2% ketoconazole gel has also received FDA labeling for the treatment of seborrheic dermatitis in children 12 years and older; this is a prescription product that is applied once daily for 2 weeks.[8]

Other agents can be considered for seborrheic dermatitis in adolescents whose conditions do not respond to the therapies listed earlier. A short course of a topical corticosteroid can be used to relieve erythema and pruritus. In patients with scalp involvement, fluocinolone 0.01% solution or shampoo can be prescribed. For body and face involvement, low- to mid-potency topical corticosteroid creams or ointments can be used. In addition, topical calcineurin inhibitors (i.e., tacrolimus and pimecrolimus) have been evaluated in adults as a steroid-sparing therapy for resistant seborrheic dermatitis; however, further studies to evaluate efficacy are needed in adolescents.[18] Of note, up to 1 week of daily use of topical calcineurin inhibitors is required before efficacy is noticeable.

ATOPIC DERMATITIS

Atopic dermatitis, also known as atopic eczema, is the most common dermatologic condition in children, with an overall prevalence of 8.7%–18.1% across the United States.[19] In affected children, onset is typically at 3–6 months of age, with 60% developing symptoms within the first year of life.[20,21]

The cause of atopic dermatitis is multifactorial, with skin barrier dysfunction, genetics, environment, and immunologic factors playing a role. In recent years, greater emphasis has been placed on skin barrier dysfunction in the pathogenesis of atopic dermatitis. Patients with atopic dermatitis have inherent abnormalities in the barrier function of their skin, which allows greater penetration of allergens and increased irritation. In addition, they have decreased ability to retain moisture in the stratum corneum secondary to decreased intracellular lipids and ceramides. Overall, patients with atopic dermatitis have a decreased threshold to pruritus that is typically worse in the nighttime hours. The mechanism of pruritus is not completely understood, but histamine is not thought to play a major role.

Risk factors for developing atopic dermatitis include a family history of atopy, exposure to allergens (e.g., pollen, mites, cow's milk), irritants (e.g., soap, wool), microbial colonization, and hard water. Children are at a 2- to 3-fold and a 3- to 5-fold higher risk if one or both parents are atopic, respectively.[21] Studies linking environmental factors (e.g., pet exposure, dust mite exposure, tobacco smoke exposure) to development of atopic dermatitis are less conclusive and may have conflicting data. Likewise, withholding of allergenic foods has not been shown to alter the risk of atopic dermatitis.[21]

The prognosis for atopic dermatitis depends on the disease severity and age at onset. This disease often involves chronic relapses. Children with atopic dermatitis are at risk of the atopy triad of atopic dermatitis, allergic rhinitis, and asthma. One-half of children with atopic dermatitis in the first 2 years of life have asthma in the following years.[22] Atopic dermatitis can significantly affect both the child's and the caregiver's quality of life. Itching at nighttime can affect sleep, which in turn can cause daytime sleepiness and irritability. In addition, because of the visibility of the condition, children may feel the stigma of being different.

The clinical presentation of atopic dermatitis may differ depending on the patient's age and the disease stage.[23] In the first 2 years of life, atopic dermatitis is characterized by pruritic, eczematous lesions that typically occur on the face, scalp, and flexor regions (i.e., antecubital space, popliteal region). The lesions become more lichenified in the childhood phase, from age 2 years to puberty, and may involve the hands, feet, wrists, ankles, and flexor regions. The adult phase begins at puberty and affects similar regions, but the lesions are characterized by dry, scaling erythematous papules and plaques, and the lichenified areas are larger.

Atopic dermatitis has no cure; treatment is aimed at relieving symptoms. The key to treatment is preventing an exacerbation. Emollients are the mainstay of prevention, which increase hydration of the skin and provide a barrier. Emollients are most effective when applied continuously, regardless of whether inflammatory lesions are present. The maximal duration of benefit for emollients is about 6 hours; therefore, they should be applied often throughout the day.[24] Ointments and creams should be recommended because they have greater occlusive properties than lotions. Products that contain lanolin and fragrances should be discouraged because of the risk of contact sensitization, which can exacerbate the dermatitis. Other preventive strategies include avoiding or minimizing exposure to irritating factors. Bath time should be limited (i.e., 5 minutes or less), and tepid water and mild fragrance-free soaps should be used. After bathing, the skin should be gently patted dry and an emollient applied immediately to trap in the remaining moisture. Furthermore, because scratching perpetuates dry, broken skin and can introduce bacteria, fingernails should be cut short to prevent damage from scratching. In addition, cotton gloves can be worn to bed to prevent unintentional scratching while sleeping.

Acute flare-ups can be managed with mild- to moderate-potency topical corticosteroids as first line.[25,26] Topical corticosteroids are often underused.[27] Underuse of topical corticosteroids may be because of concern for the adverse effects associated with these agents (e.g., skin atrophy, striae, systemic effects). The American Academy of Dermatology guidelines suggest that, if used appropriately, these agents have a low risk of significant adverse effects.[25] During the acute phase of the exacerbation, topical corticosteroids should be applied no more than twice daily because there is no further benefit with more frequent application, only an increased risk of adverse effects. Once the exacerbation is controlled (i.e., resolution of pruritus), therapy can be stepped down to a less potent preparation or tapered to once- or twice-weekly application to known problem areas to reduce the rate of relapse.[25] Once- or twice-weekly applications to prevent relapse for up to 40 weeks have not been associated with adverse effects.[28] If chronic corticosteroid therapy is required, the least potent corticosteroid that is effective is recommended. Topical corticosteroids, summarized in Table 3, are grouped according to potency, with group I being the most potent and group VII being the least potent. The vehicle in which the drug is contained can increase the potency. Ointments compared with creams of the same corticosteroid have increased potency because of their occlusiveness and hydration of the skin. Increasing the corticosteroid's solubility by adding propylene glycol can also increase the potency by increasing the drug that is absorbed. These agents are often called augmented. In children younger than 12 years, only low-mid to low-potency (i.e., groups V–VII) topical corticosteroids should be used. When selecting the appropriate potency, an agent with the lowest potency that is effective for the condition should be considered.

Wet-wrap therapy can be used in patients with acute, oozing, and erosive lesions who cannot tolerate standard topical therapy. Wet-wrap therapy consists of applying a layer of ointment or cream. The ointment or cream can be an emollient only, or it can contain a topical corticosteroid that is diluted. Applying a diluted topical steroid has greater efficacy than applying emollient alone.[29] The area is then covered with a double layer of cotton bandages, with the first layer being moist. Recommended time for application is 3–24 hours.

Topical calcineurin inhibitors (i.e., tacrolimus, pimecrolimus) are considered second line for short-term, intermittent treatment of moderate to severe atopic dermatitis; however, some experts now consider calcineurin inhibitors an alternative first-line agent.[30] Calcineurin inhibitors target the inflammatory pathogenesis of atopic dermatitis by preventing the release of inflammatory cytokines and mediators. However, unlike corticosteroids, topical calcineurin inhibitors are not associated with skin atrophy, which allows their use on the face, eyelids, and intertriginous areas. As a result, these agents may be an appropriate alternative in children with facial atopic dermatitis or those with significant adverse effects from topical corticosteroids. Topical calcineurin inhibitors should be applied twice daily to the affected area. Of note, only tacrolimus 0.03% ointment and pimecrolimus 1% cream are labeled for children 2 years and older, and tacrolimus 0.1% ointment should not be used in these patients. However, recent data analyses have shown that pimecrolimus is safe in children 3 months and older for use up to 5 years.[31] The most common adverse effect of these agents is a burning sensation at the application site in the first week of use. Use of these agents has been associated with an increased risk of infection and photocarcinogenicity. In addition, malignancy and lymphoma are listed in a black box warning included in the agents' FDA-approved labeling.[8] This warning is primarily the result of a lack of sufficient long-term safety data; no direct evidence of a causal link with cancer exists.[32] Because of the concern for developing cutaneous malignancy, patients should be encouraged to apply sunscreen regularly (sun protection factor [SPF] of 15 or greater) if exposed to UV radiation.

Crisaborole ointment 2%, a phosphodiesterase type 4 inhibitor, received FDA approval in 2016 and is labeled for the treatment of atopic dermatitis in children 2 years and older.[8] This agent is applied twice daily to affected areas. Crisaborole's role in therapy has not currently been fully established because it has not been extensively compared with topical steroids or calcineurin inhibitors.[33] The most common adverse effect with crisaborole is application site pain and infection.[34] Crisaborole is safe with long-term use in children 2 years and older for use up to 48 weeks.[34]

Systemic agents play a limited role in the treatment of atopic dermatitis. Systemic antimicrobials should not routinely be used for infection prophylaxis. Rather, these agents should be reserved for diagnosed secondary infections (e.g., S. aureus). Likewise, use of systemic corticosteroids as long-term maintenance therapy should be avoided because the risks of therapy exceed the benefits. Oral antihistamines play a limited role in the treatment of atopic dermatitis because the pruritus is not necessarily histamine related. A sedating antihistamine (e.g., hydroxyzine, diphenhydramine) can be recommended for use at bedtime to aid sleep. Second-generation, nonsedating antihistamines (e.g., loratadine, cetirizine) have no firm evidence of efficacy in managing atopic dermatitis.[35,36]

Immunomodulating agents such as cyclosporine, azathioprine, and methotrexate have been efficacious in severe cases of atopic dermatitis that are refractory to conventional therapy and are recommended in the American Academy of Dermatology guidelines.[36] Efficacy data for mycophenolate mofetil are more inconsistent, and this agent is considered an alternative, according to the guidelines. Therapies that have not been proven efficacious for atopic dermatitis include delayed introduction of solid foods in infants, dietary restrictions, homeopathy, prolonged breastfeeding, and Chinese herbal therapy.[37]

PEDIATRIC ACNE

Acne vulgaris is a common dermatologic condition that affects up to 87% of teenagers.[38] Although typically thought of as an adolescent condition, acne can affect children of any age.[39] Pediatric acne is classified according to age and presentation and includes neonatal, infantile, mid-childhood, preadolescent, and adolescent acne. Neonatal acne (i.e., acne neonatorum) presents within the first 4 weeks of life and affects up to 20% of neonates.[38] Neonates usually present with open or closed comedones on the forehead, nose, and cheeks. The exact cause of acne lesions in neonates is controversial, but acne neonatorum with comedones is believed to be caused by increased androgens.[1] Infantile acne presents at 3–16 months of age and is much less common than neonatal acne.[38] Compared with neonatal acne, infantile acne has lesions that are more inflamed and that appear predominantly on the cheeks. In addition to comedones, papules, and pustules, infantile acne is associated with the development of cystic lesions, which can cause scarring. Mid-childhood acne presents at 1–7 years of age and involves comedones and inflammatory lesions on the face.[38] If acne occurs in this age group, an endocrine abnormality should be suspected, and further workup is needed. Preadolescent acne presents with comedones on the forehead and central face in children 7–12 years of age. Adolescent acne involves patients 12–18 years of age and presents with comedones, papules, and pustules that can vary in severity.

Acne is thought to be caused by four primary factors: sebum production, *Propionibacterium acnes* colonization, alteration in the keratinization process, and release of inflammatory mediators.[40] These four factors are interrelated and interact in a complex manner to promote the characteristic and inflammatory lesions of acne (i.e., comedone, papules, pustules, or nodules). Family history of acne, onset of puberty, and overweight/obese status have been identified as risk factors for developing acne.[41]

Assessment of acne involves rating disease severity, which in turn drives the treatment pathway. Proposed strategies rate acne severity on the basis of lesion count or on a grading system of the total clinical presentation by accounting for lesion type, location of lesion, and involvement. To date, there are more than 25 acne-grading systems[42]; however, there is no consensus on a single classification or grading system for acne.

The American Academy of Pediatrics endorsed treatment recommendations for pediatric acne by the American Acne and Rosacea Society in 2013.[38] In addition, the American Academy of Dermatology established treatment guidelines and recommendations for adolescent and adult acne in 2015.[43] Acne in neonates is typically self-limiting and does not require pharmacologic treatment. Parents can be instructed to cleanse the face with a gentle soap and water. In more severe cases, neonates can be treated with 2.5% benzoyl peroxide lotion. If colonization with *Malassezia* is suspected, 2% ketoconazole cream twice daily for 1 week can be prescribed.[38] Infantile acne is also typically self-limiting; however, more severe cases can be managed first line with a topical retinoid with or without benzoyl peroxide plus or minus a topical antibiotic. A small open-label study has shown that adapalene gel is both safe and efficacious for mild to moderate acne in children younger than 24 months.[44] If an oral antibiotic is necessary, macrolides are the medication of choice in these children because of the relative contraindication of tetracyclines. For severe, recalcitrant cases of infantile acne associated with scarring, use of oral isotretinoin has been reported in infants as young as 5 months, with doses of 0.2–2 mg/kg/day in two divided doses.[39] Administering oral isotretinoin in infants may present some technical difficulties because this medication is commercially available only in tablet and capsule forms.

Treatment of mid-childhood and preadolescent acne is similar to that of adolescent and adult acne.[38] Figure 1 summarizes a general treatment approach that is based on acne severity, and Table 4 summarizes the medications used for acne. Topical retinoids (e.g., tretinoin, adapalene, tazarotene) are considered first line for acute management of mild to moderate cases of acne because they reduce the formation of microcomedones and comedones, have anti-inflammatory activity, and promote normal desquamation of the skin. The safety and efficacy of topical retinoids have been well established in studies including children.[38] For individuals with papular/pustular eruptions of mild to moderate severity, a topical antimicrobial agent (e.g., erythromycin, clindamycin) added to a topical retinoid is recommended for acute treatment. The combination of a topical retinoid with an antibacterial agent will address three of the four major pathogenic factors of acne. These antimicrobial agents have activity against *P. acnes* and decrease the colonization of the skin. However, development of antimicrobial resistance is a concern with antibiotic therapy, and antibiotic monotherapy is strongly discouraged. Adding topical benzoyl peroxide decreases the likelihood that *P. acnes*–resistant strains will emerge. In addition, benzoyl peroxide provides antibacterial activity. Benzoyl peroxide is available in strengths of 2.5%–10% and is available as a nonprescription product. Benzoyl peroxide is the most commonly studied nonprescription product and been shown both safe and effective.[38] Because benzoyl peroxide can be irritating and drying to the skin, therapy should be initiated with a lower concentration. Stronger concentrations tend to be more irritating and may not necessarily be more efficacious. Topical dapsone 5% gel can also be used in mild, moderate, or severe acne. Topical dapsone 5% gel is most effective against inflammatory lesions. Patients should be informed that co-application with benzoyl peroxide can result in temporary orange-brown skin discoloration.

For individuals with moderate to moderately severe acne, an oral antibiotic (e.g., doxycycline, minocycline, erythromycin) is recommended in addition to a topical retinoid. Minocycline and doxycycline are considered the most efficacious oral antibiotics for decreasing *P. acnes* colonization.[43] However, the tetracycline antibiotics should not be used in children younger than 8 years because of the potential for binding to calcium and being incorporated in the tooth and bone matrix, resulting in tooth discoloration, enamel hypoplasia, and decreased bone development. For children younger than 8 years, erythromycin is the oral antibiotic of choice. If oral antibiotics are used, duration should be limited to 3 months, and the need for continuation should be assessed every 6–12 weeks.[40] Many experts recommend against the concomitant use of oral and topical antibiotic therapy because of the increased risk of resistance and the minimal increase in therapeutic benefit.[40]

Fixed-dose topical products are commercially available that contain a combination of therapeutic agents (e.g., clindamycin 1%/benzoyl peroxide 5%, adapalene 0.1%/benzoyl peroxide 2.5%, clindamycin 1.2%/tretinoin 0.025%). These products are proposed to be more convenient for patient use by decreasing the time involved in product application and thus promoting greater adherence to therapy. A common adverse effect with combination therapy is increased skin irritation, including burning and peeling. Some data analyses suggest that, among the retinoids, combination therapy with adapalene is best tolerated.[40] Other topical therapies with limited benefit in managing acne include salicylic acid, azelaic acid, sulfur, resorcinol, aluminum chloride, and topical zinc.

Severe recalcitrant nodular acne requires treatment with isotretinoin. Isotretinoin decreases comedone formation by decreasing sebum production and has some anti-inflammatory activity. The FDA-labeled dose of isotretinoin for children 12 years and older is 0.5–2 mg/kg/day in two divided doses for a maximum of 20 weeks, though this agent has been studied in younger children.[30] This duration can be exceeded if lower doses are used, with a maximal total cumulative dose of 150 mg/kg.[43] The recommendation from the American Acne and Rosacea Society is to start at 0.5 mg/kg/day for 4 weeks and then increase to 1 mg/kg/day in preadolescents and adolescents.[38] Isotretinoin has several adverse

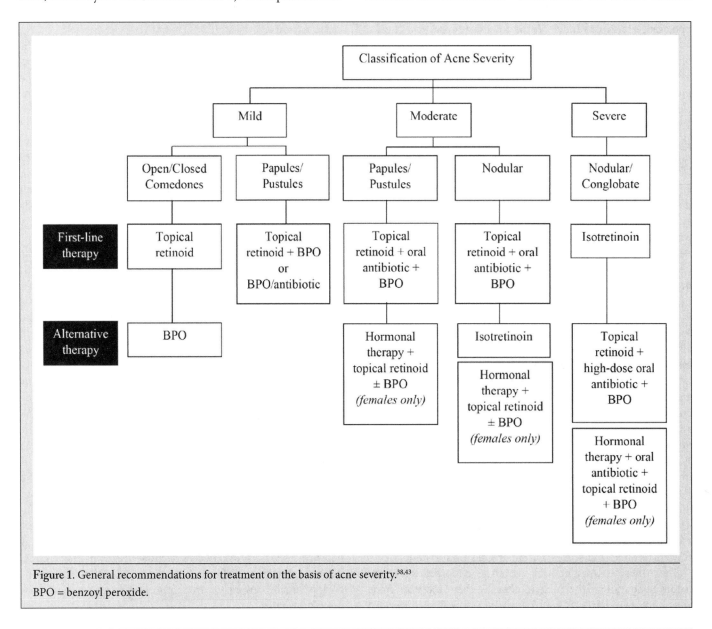

Figure 1. General recommendations for treatment on the basis of acne severity.[38,43]
BPO = benzoyl peroxide.

Table 4. Acne Products[8]

Class/Selected Agents	Brand Name(s)	Dosing	Comments
Topical Agents			
Retinoids			
Adapalene 0.1%, 0.3%	Differin[a]	Apply once daily in the evening	Increased risk of photosensitivity reactions. Recommend sunscreen (SPF ≥ 15)
Tazarotene 0.05%, 0.1%	Tazorac[b]	Apply 2 mg/cm² once daily in the evening	
Tretinoin 0.025%, 0.05%, 0.1%, 0.01%	Retin-A, Avita[c]	Apply once daily in the evening; start with 0.025% cream or 0.01% gel and increase concentration as tolerated	
Antibiotics			
Clindamycin 1%	Cleocin T[d]	Apply a thin film twice daily	Should not be used as monotherapy
Dapsone 5%, 7.5%	Aczone[e]	Apply pea-sized amount once (7.5%) or twice (5%) daily	Temporary orange staining will occur if applied with benzoyl peroxide
Erythromycin 2%	—	Apply twice daily	Should not be used as monotherapy
Benzoyl peroxide 2.5%, 4%, 5%, 8%, 10%	Multiple nonprescription products	Apply once daily; can gradually increase to two or three times daily, if needed	If excessive dryness or peeling occurs, reduce dose frequency or concentration. Recommend sunscreen (SPF ≥ 15)
Keratolytic Agent			
Salicylic acid 0.5%–2.0%	Multiple nonprescription products	Apply once or twice daily	Available in a variety of dosage forms. Recommended in patients who cannot tolerate benzoyl peroxide. Do not use in children < 2 yr
Combination Products			
Erythromycin/ benzoyl peroxide	Benzamycin[f]	Apply twice daily	
Clindamycin/ benzoyl peroxide	Acanya,[f] BenzaClin[f]	Apply pea-sized amount once daily (Acanya) Apply twice daily (BenzaClin)	
Clindamycin/tretinoin	Veltin,[e] Ziana[f]	Apply once daily	Increased risk of photosensitivity reactions. Recommend sunscreen (SPF ≥ 15)
Adapalene/ benzoyl peroxide	Epiduo[a]	Apply once daily	Increased risk of photosensitivity reactions. Recommend sunscreen (SPF ≥ 15)
Systemic Agents			
Antibiotics			
Tetracycline	—	Children ≥ 8 yr: 500 mg twice daily	Should not be used in children < 8 yr because of effects on teeth and bone; increased risk of photosensitivity reactions. Recommend sunscreen (SPF ≥ 15). Avoid taking with calcium- or iron-containing products
Doxycycline	Vibramycin	Children ≥ 8 yr: 50–100 mg/dose once or twice daily	
Minocycline	Minocin,[f] Solodyn,[f] Ximino (extended release)[g]	Children ≥ 8 yr: 50–100 mg/dose once or twice daily Extended-release product (Solodyn): Children > 12 yr: About 1 mg/kg daily: 45–49 kg: 45 mg once daily 50–59 kg: 55 mg once daily 60–71 kg: 65 mg once daily 72–84 kg: 80 mg once daily 85–96 kg: 90 mg once daily 97–110 kg: 105 mg once daily 111–125 kg: 115 mg once daily 126–136 kg: 135 mg once daily	
Erythromycin	EryPed[h]	Children: 250–500 mg once or twice daily (maximum daily dose: 50 mg/kg/day)	Several drug interactions, CYP3A4 inhibitor

(continued)

Table 4. Acne Products[8] *(continued)*

Class/Selected Agents	Brand Name(s)	Dosing	Comments
Hormonal Therapy			
Oral contraceptives	Multiple prescription products	Females ≥ 14 yr (drospirenone/ethinyl estradiol) or ≥ 15 yr (norethindrone/ethinyl estradiol or norgestimate/ethinyl estradiol): Take 1 tablet daily	May take up to 4 mo for efficacy
Spironolactone	Aldactone[d]	Females ≥ 15 yr: 50–100 mg twice daily	Potassium-sparing, can cause hyperkalemia
Retinoic Acid Derivative			
Isotretinoin	Claravis,[i] Amnesteem,[c] Absorica[j]	Children ≥ 12 yr: 0.25–0.5 mg/kg/dose twice daily; maximal dose of 1 mg/kg twice daily	Do not use in pregnancy, iPLEDGE registration. Recommend sunscreen (SPF ≥ 15)

[a]Galderma Laboratories, LP, Ft. Worth, TX; [b]Allergan, Irvine, CA; [c]Mylan Pharmaceuticals Inc., Morgantown, WV; [d]Pfizer, Inc., New York, NY; [e]Almirall, LLC., Exton, PA; [f]Bausch Health Companies, Inc., Laval, Quebec, Canada; [g]Journey Medical Corporation, Scottsdale, AZ; [h]Arbor Pharmaceuticals, LLC, Atlanta, GA; [i]Teva Pharmaceuticals USA, Inc, Salt Lake City, UT; [j]Sun Pharmaceutical Industries, Inc., Princeton, NJ.

effects, including hypertriglyceridemia, hypercholesterolemia, and elevation of hepatic enzymes, which require monitoring throughout therapy. Recommendations for monitoring frequency vary; however, recent studies have shown that baseline laboratory values and repeat laboratory values after 2 months of therapy are sufficient if no abnormalities are noted.[45] Although rare, neutropenia can occur, which should be monitored at baseline and after 2 months of therapy, with continued monitoring in those with abnormal values.[45] A causal link exists between isotretinoin and ulcerative colitis.[38,43] The risk increases with higher doses and longer use. Overall, the absolute risk for patients who are exposed to isotretinoin is very low; however, patients should be made aware of this association. In addition, isotretinoin has been associated with depression, aggressive behavior, and suicidal ideation. Although no direct relationship has been established in clinical studies, patients and caregivers should monitor for changes in behavior and mood. Isotretinoin is rated pregnancy category X and has a warning against use in pregnancy. Because of this teratogenic risk, all patients (male and female), prescribers, manufacturers, wholesalers, and dispensing pharmacies must be registered in the iPLEDGE risk management program. Females of childbearing age should have two negative pregnancy tests, at least 19 days apart, before therapy initiation. According to the iPLEDGE program, two forms of contraception should be used 1 month before, during, and 1 month after isotretinoin therapy. Prescriptions can only be written for a 30-day supply, and a pregnancy test should be completed monthly.

Hormone therapy with estrogen-containing contraceptive agents can be considered second line in pubertal female patients with mild to moderate acne because of these agents' antiandrogenic effects. Oral contraceptives with FDA labeling for managing acne in females 15 years and older include ethinyl estradiol/norgestimate and ethinyl estradiol/norethindrone, and in females 14 years and older for ethinyl estradiol/drospirenone, though it is expert opinion that any estrogen-containing contraceptive would be as effective.[43] Patients should be educated that improvement in acne lesions may take up to 4 months with these agents.[46] Another agent that has been evaluated for acne because of its antiandrogen activity is spironolactone at doses of 50–200 mg/day. Patients

receiving this therapy should be monitored for hyperkalemia, specifically when higher doses are used.

After initial treatment of active lesions, maintenance therapy should be initiated to prevent a rebound exacerbation of acne. For all acne types, a topical retinoid should be recommended for maintenance therapy, with the addition of benzoyl peroxide if more antibacterial activity is needed. Adapalene 0.3% and adapalene 0.1%/benzoyl peroxide 2.5% have been studied most extensively for long-term use up to 1 year.[40] Experts recommend applying the maintenance product to the entire area, not just the area of concern. This is because microcomedones are not detectable by the naked eye, and topical retinoid therapy will decrease the formation of microcomedones. Use of antibiotics for maintenance therapy should be discouraged. Nonpharmacologic recommendations should include washing the skin with a gentle cleanser twice daily and applying a noncomedogenic moisturizer. Individuals should avoid too frequent or too harsh washing because this can worsen the acne. Consumption of certain foods has anecdotally been associated with worsening acne; however, no studies support this belief. Therefore, according to the guidelines, dietary restriction is of no benefit in managing acne.[43]

DERMATOPHYTE FUNGAL INFECTIONS

Ringworm fungi are dermatophytes that include species of *Microsporum*, *Trichophyton*, and *Epidermophyton*. These fungi can typically survive only in the stratum corneum, hair, and nails. The infections described in the following sections are considered *tinea*, or fungal infections that are further classified by the body region infected.

TINEA CORPORIS

Tinea corporis, or ringworm that presents on the body, is typically caused by *Trichophyton* spp. Tinea corporis presents as a round, but irregular, scaly spot that develops a raised border and central clearing. The border may be red with raised papules. Lesions may be small or may appear to spread.

Topical antifungals, summarized in Table 2, are sufficient to treat most cases of tinea corporis. The antifungal should be applied to the lesion and the 2 cm surrounding it. Therapy continues for 14 days, or for 1 week after clinical resolution, to ensure fungal eradication. Newer therapies, terbinafine and butenafine, are fungicidal and considered more effective than miconazole and clotrimazole.[47] Combination products containing corticosteroids and antifungals are not recommended or necessary. More extensive cases can be treated with systemic fluconazole, itraconazole, or terbinafine.

TINEA PEDIS

Tinea pedis, or athlete's foot, is caused by *Trichophyton* or *Epidermophyton* spp. Tinea pedis is less common in prepubertal children. Tinea pedis presents as a white area between the toes, or dry scaling accompanied by itching. Exposure to a moist environment predisposes the feet to fungal infections. Terbinafine and butenafine have higher cure rates and more rapid resolution than miconazole or clotrimazole.[48] Treatment with terbinafine and butenafine typically requires 1–2 weeks. Miconazole and clotrimazole require 2–4 weeks of treatment. As with tinea corporis, treatment should continue for 1 week beyond clinical resolution. Antifungal powders can be applied to the feet to decrease moisture. Nonpharmacologic therapy includes exposing the feet to air as often as possible.

TINEA CRURIS

Tinea cruris, also known as jock itch, is an infection of the groin caused by *Trichophyton* or *Epidermophyton* spp. Although tinea cruris is most common in postpubertal males, it also occurs in females. The rash is typically reddish brown and symmetric with defined borders, typically sparing the scrotum. The rash is usually pruritic and may burn.

Treatment should consist of either terbinafine cream or spray for 1 week or butenafine cream for 2 weeks.[47] Agents such as miconazole, clotrimazole, econazole, and ciclopirox are generally not recommended for tinea cruris because their fungistatic nature requires a longer treatment, which may present a problem with adherence to the regimen.

TINEA CAPITIS

The most common fungal infection in children is tinea capitis, or tinea of the scalp, occurring in an estimated 4% of the U.S. population, with a higher incidence in those of African American descent and in developing countries.[49] In the United States, most tinea capitis cases are caused by *Trichophyton tonsurans*, with some cases caused by *Microsporum* spp. Other countries typically have a predominance of *Microsporum* spp.

Children with tinea capitis present with itching, scaling of the scalp, or circular patches of hair loss. When more inflammation is present, there are pustules as well. Those with more persistent infection and inflammation may present with kerion lesions, which are boggy, tender, and pustular.[49] A diagnosis can typically be made from clinical presentation, but a fungal culture can confirm the diagnosis and identify the infecting fungus.

Tinea capitis requires prolonged systemic therapy to penetrate the infected hair shaft. Griseofulvin is considered the drug of choice in children, but fluconazole, terbinafine, and itraconazole are effective alternatives. Each agent has similar efficacy when treating *Trichophyton* spp., but terbinafine is inferior to griseofulvin, fluconazole, and itraconazole for *Microsporum* spp.[50] Treatment of *Microsporum* infections requires longer than does treatment of *Trichophyton*. Treatment regimens for tinea capitis are summarized in Table 5.[49-51]

Griseofulvin is available in microsize suspension and tablets and in ultramicrosize tablets. Because of poor water solubility, griseofulvin should be given with a fatty meal to increase absorption. Common adverse effects include GI upset (often leading to treatment discontinuation), headache, and rash. Dividing the daily dose can decrease the incidence of GI complaints. More rarely, elevated liver function tests and granulocytopenia are reported. Monitoring a CBC and liver function is recommended for treatment lasting longer than 8 weeks.

Terbinafine is available as a 250-mg tablet. Historically, 125- and 187.5-mg packets of granules for sprinkling were available, but production recently stopped, creating a challenge

Table 5. Treatment Regimens for Tinea Capitis[49-51]

Antifungal	Dose	Treatment Duration (wk)	Treatment Considerations
Griseofulvin microsize	20–25 mg/kg/day in one or two divided doses up to 1000 mg/day	6–12	Monitor liver function if duration > 8 wk
Griseofulvin ultramicrosize	10–15 mg/kg/day in one or two divided doses up to 750 mg/day	6–12	Monitor liver function if duration > 8 wk
Terbinafine	< 25 kg: 125 mg/day 25–35 kg: 187.5 mg/day > 35 kg: 250 mg/day	2–6	Monitor liver function before treatment and if duration > 6 wk
Fluconazole	6 mg/kg/day OR 8 mg/kg once weekly	3–6 6–12	Limited data available
Itraconazole	Capsules: 5 mg/kg/day Oral solution: 3 mg/kg/day	2–6	Monitor liver function before treatment and if duration > 4 wk A pulse regimen of daily dosing 1 wk each month for 2–4 mo has been studied in adults

for using terbinafine in children who cannot swallow tablets. An advantage of terbinafine is the shorter therapy duration required for *Trichophyton* spp., which can improve adherence. Common adverse effects include vomiting, nausea, loss of appetite, and itching. More rarely, elevated liver function tests and hepatic failure in those with preexisting liver disease have been reported. Liver function tests are recommended before initiating therapy and if terbinafine is continued for longer than 6 weeks.

Fluconazole has a favorable safety profile in children and is available in liquid and tablet formulations, making it a reasonable alternative to griseofulvin. Common adverse effects include GI issues, headache, and rash. Elevated hepatic enzymes are a rare complication of fluconazole therapy.

Itraconazole is available as capsules and liquid. The capsules should be given with food, and the liquid should be given on an empty stomach. Although an intermittent regimen involving daily dosing for 1 week each month for a total of two or four cycles has been studied in adults, no pediatric data are available to confirm this regimen's efficacy. Common adverse effects include headache, rash, and GI complaints. Elevated liver function tests were a rare complication of itraconazole therapy in tinea capitis studies. Because of its adverse effect and drug interaction profile, itraconazole should be reserved for cases not responding to other treatment options.

Treatment should generally be continued until hair regrowth is evident or about 2 weeks after clinical resolution. Long therapy often results in nonadherence and treatment failure. Topical treatment with selenium sulfide or ketoconazole shampoo may decrease the carriage of spores, thus reducing transmission to others and reinfection. Shampoos should be used twice weekly for 2–4 weeks as an adjunct to systemic therapy.

TINEA UNGUIUM

Tinea unguium is a type of onychomycosis affecting the fingernails or toenails, usually caused by *Trichophyton rubrum* in children.[52] Although tinea unguium is generally considered a cosmetic problem, it can cause a loss of self-esteem and cause complications in those with underlying diseases such as diabetes. Tinea unguium is less common in prepubertal children and has a higher incidence in children with Down syndrome.[52]

The clinical presentation includes discoloration and possibly flaking or dystrophy of the nail. Children typically have a distal presentation called distal lateral subungual onychomycosis.[52] Other types of onychomycosis include proximal subungual and superficial white onychomycosis. Superficial white onychomycosis affects only the nail plate, not the nail bed.

In children with superficial onychomycosis and distal involvement not exceeding one-third of the nail bed, topical therapy with ciclopirox 8% nail lacquer can be tried. The lacquer is applied daily, with removal once a week, for 48 weeks.[53] The cure rate is low, and relapse is common. In infants and young children, the nail bed is thinner, and topical therapies may be more effective.[52] Topical therapy is also recommended for anyone who is not an appropriate candidate for systemic therapy. Two topical agents, tavaborole and efinaconazole, have recently entered the market for adults and are effective when less than 50% of the nail is affected.

Systemic therapy is recommended for most cases of onychomycosis. Treatment of the toenails requires longer than treatment of the fingernails. The most effective therapy is terbinafine. Additional treatment options include itraconazole and fluconazole, with fluconazole as the least effective option. The fingernail usually looks normal before the fungus is eradicated, making it very important to emphasize that treatment should continue for the complete duration to avoid relapse. Table 6 summarizes treatment regimens for tinea unguium in children.[52,53]

MOLLUSCUM CONTAGIOSUM

Molluscum contagiosum is a localized skin infection caused by a virus in the poxvirus family. Molluscum contagiosum usually occurs in children but can present in adults more commonly as a sexually transmitted variant. Infection occurs after contact with an infected individual or an object harboring the virus. Swimming pools and baths are another source of transmission. Molluscum contagiosum is most common in children 2–5 years old and has a reported prevalence of 5%–7% in elementary schools, resulting in almost 300,000 office visits each year.[54]

Molluscum typically presents as one or many shiny, white or flesh-colored papules with a dimple in the center. With time, there may be crusting or fluid production as the lesion begins to destruct. Most cases resolve spontaneously, but this may take up to 9 months because of the spread of the virus. In some cases, the lesions may persist for up to 4 years. Lesions are usually not harmful, except that they can be spread to others. In addition, in individuals with atopic dermatitis, local irritation and inflammation often occur.

In those with normal immune function, therapy is not typically indicated. However, treatment may help in the following situations: lesions associated with discomfort or itching, cosmetic reasons or social stigma, limiting spread to others, and secondary infections. Therapy may consist of physically destroying the lesions, applying topical

Table 6. Systemic Treatment Regimens for Tinea Unguium in Children[52,53]

Antifungal	Dose	Duration
Terbinafine	< 20 kg: 62.5 mg/day 20–40 kg: 125 mg/day > 40 kg: 250 mg/day	Toenail: 12 wk Fingernail: 6 wk
Itraconazole capsules	Pulse with 5 mg/kg/day, 1 wk/mo Up to 400 mg/day	Toenail: 3 pulses Fingernail: 2 pulses
Itraconazole solution	Pulse therapy 3–5 mg/kg/day, 1 wk/mo	Toenail: 3 pulses Fingernail: 2 pulses
Fluconazole	3–6 mg/kg, one dose per week	Toenail: 26 wk Fingernail: 12 wk

treatments, or using systemic treatment. Physical removal with a sharp curette or liquid nitrogen is most effective, but this can be painful and can lead to scarring. Topical treatments can include cantharidin or imiquimod. Cantharidin is applied in the medical provider's office; it is then washed off after 4–6 hours and repeated every 2–4 weeks until resolved.[48] Imiquimod is applied nightly, 5–7 days/week, for at least 12 weeks. Imiquimod is slower acting, but provides the advantage of being painless compared with physical removal. Other topical agents that have been used, but that are generally not recommended, are podofilox, retinoids, salicylic acid, and potassium hydroxide. Systemic cimetidine has been studied using 35 mg/kg/day for 4 months; however, no significant difference from placebo was observed. Currently, evidence is insufficient to choose one therapy over another,[54] but a recent survey showed that dermatologists usually use no intervention, cantharidin, imiquimod, curettage, or cryotherapy.[55] Given that many clinic-based treatments are painful, imiquimod is the least invasive of all the options but takes weeks to be efficacious.

INFANTILE HEMANGIOMAS

Infantile hemangiomas (IHs) are the most common benign childhood tumor, but they can cause tissue damage, infection, bleeding, pain, and functional impairment, depending on their size and location. Around 5% of children have IHs, with a higher prevalence in white infants and females.[56] Infantile hemangiomas are typically visible early in life and reach about 80% of their final size by 3–5 months of age.[56] Infantile hemangiomas can be described as superficial, deep, or mixed lesions and are often bright red and dome shaped. The involution rate is estimated at 10% per year, resulting in lesions that persist into early childhood.[57] Because of their

rapid growth rate and potential involvement of underlying structures, rapid recognition, specialist evaluation, and possibly treatment are essential. The treatment approach to IHs depends on the lesion's size and location, with goals of preventing life-threatening complications, preventing permanent scarring, decreasing psychosocial stress, and minimizing pain and infection. Lesions that obstruct the airway or affect visual function require surgical intervention. Other lesions may be treated with systemic and/or topical therapies to control the spread of the lesion or promote faster involution.

A meta-analysis estimated the clearance rate of IHs without intervention at 6%.[56] Oral propranolol had the highest expected clearance rate at 95%, followed by topical timolol at 62%, intralesional triamcinolone at 58%, and oral steroids at 43%.[56] Despite significant variability in study design and patient characteristics, oral propranolol is considered superior to other treatment modalities in efficacy and safety. Although atenolol and nadolol are shown to provide benefit, data are limited. If propranolol is used for IHs, it is initiated at 1 mg/kg/day and titrated to 3.4 mg/kg/day in two or three divided doses.[58] Improvement is expected within 3–4 months, with treatment continuing until 8–12 months of age, followed by a taper over 3 weeks to prevent rebound tachycardia. Adverse effects include hypotension, bradycardia, hypoglycemia, and bronchospasm.

CONCLUSIONS

Given the high prevalence of dermatologic conditions in childhood, pharmacists have an opportunity to help determine age-appropriate therapy and provide patient and caregiver education. Knowledge of the unique aspects of topical medication delivery and common irritants to avoid in infants and children will help ensure the best care for these patients.

A 6-month-old infant is brought to the community pharmacy by her mother. The mother states that her child has redness in the diaper area.

Family history: Noncontributory

Social history: Lives at home with mother and father, no siblings. The mother reports use of cloth diapers.

Home medications: None

Immunizations: Up to date for age

Vital signs: The mother states that the infant is afebrile; no other vital signs are known at this time.

Review of symptoms: Redness in the diaper area has been present for 3 days, and the infant cries and screams when her diaper is changed. The mother

states that the redness is present on the surfaces that contact the diaper and not in the skinfolds. The mother has applied baby powder for the past 48 hours with no relief for the child.

Medical history: Late preterm (born at 36 weeks' gestation)

1. What is the most appropriate recommendation for treating this infant's diaper dermatitis?

A barrier cream (e.g., zinc oxide) should be recommended with each diaper change. Because the erythema is not present in the skinfolds, this is more likely a simple diaper dermatitis and not secondary to *C. albicans*. Baby powder is not appropriate for diaper dermatitis for two reasons. First, it does not serve as a protective barrier like creams or ointments. Second, there is a risk of aspirating the airborne particles and developing pneumonitis. The first recommendation should be to use a barrier cream (e.g., zinc oxide) with every diaper change. If the erythema does not resolve after 3 days of a barrier cream, a low-potency corticosteroid can be recommended (e.g., hydrocortisone 1%), applied

two or three times daily. If used, the corticosteroid should be discontinued immediately after resolution of erythema, not to exceed 14 days.

2. What are nonpharmacologic recommendations for managing this child's diaper dermatitis?

Nonpharmacologic recommendations include removing the diaper immediately after defecation and allowing for diaper-free time. During diaper changes, the area should be cleansed with water and a cotton cloth or commercially available wipes that contain no preservatives or fragrances. For this child who wears cloth diapers, temporarily changing to superabsorbent disposable diapers may also be beneficial until the erythema resolves.

REFERENCES

1. Paller AS, Mancini AJ. Cutaneous disorders of the newborn. In: Paller AS, Mancini AJ, eds. Hurwitz Clinical Pediatric Dermatology, 4th ed. Edinburgh: Elsevier, 2011.
2. Metry D, Hebert A. Topical therapies and medications in the pediatric patient. Pediatr Clin North Am 2000;47:867-75.
3. Adalat S, Wall D, Goodyear H. Diaper dermatitis-frequency and contributory factors in hospital attending children. Pediatr Dermatol 2007;24:483-8.
4. Blume-Peytavi U, Hauser M, Lunnemann L, et al. Prevention of diaper dermatitis in infants – a literature review. Pediatr Dermatol 2014;31:413-29.
5. Shin H. Diaper dermatitis that does not quit. Dermatol Ther 2005;18:124-35.
6. Stamatas GN, Tierney NK. Diaper dermatitis: etiology, manifestations, prevention, and management. Pediatr Dermatol 2014; 31:1-7.
7. Nield L, Kamat D. Prevention, diagnosis, and management of diaper dermatitis. Clin Pediatr 2007;46:480-6.
8. Taketomo C, Hodding J, Kraus D. Pediatric Dosage Handbook, 24th ed. Hudson, OH: Lexi-Comp, 2017.
9. Ference J, Last A. Choosing topical corticosteroids. Am Fam Physician 2009;29:135-40.
10. Valencia I, Kerder F. Topical corticosteroids. In: Wolff K, Goldsmith L, Katz S, et al., eds. Fitzpatrick's Dermatology in General Medicine, 7th ed. New York: McGraw-Hill, 2008:2102-6.
11. Markham T, Kennedy F, Collins P. Topical sucralfate for erosive irritant diaper dermatitis. Arch Dermatol 2000;136:1199-200.
12. White C, Gailey R, Lippe S. Cholestyramine ointment to treat buttocks rash and anal excoriation in an infant. Ann Pharmacother 1996;30:954-6.
13. Foley P, Zuo Y, Plunkett A, et al. The frequency of common skin conditions in preschool-aged children of Australia: seborrheic dermatitis and pityriasis capitis (cradle cap). Arch Dermatol 2003;139:318-22.
14. Schwartz R, Janusz C, Janniger C. Seborrheic dermatitis: an overview. Am Fam Physician 2006;74:125-30.
15. Mimouni K, Mukamel M, Zeharia A, et al. Prognosis of infantile seborrheic dermatitis. J Pediatr 1995;127:77406.
16. Gilbertson K, Jarrett R, Bayliss SJ, et al. Scalp discoloration from selenium sulfide shampoo: a case series and review of the literature. Pediatr Dermatol 2012;29:84-8.
17. Clark GW, Pope SM, Jaboori KA. Diagnosis and treatment of seborrheic dermatitis. Am Fam Physician 2015;91:185-90.
18. Shaw TE, Currie GP, Koudeika CW, et al. Eczema prevalence in the United States: data from the 2003 National Survey of Children's Health. J Invest Dermatol 2011;131:670-3.
19. Fleischer A. Diagnosis and management of common dermatoses in children: atopic, seborrheic, and contact dermatitis. Clin Pediatr 2008;47:332-46.
20. Eichenfield LF, Tom WL, Chamlin SL, et al. Guidelines of care for the management of atopic dermatitis: section 1. Diagnosis and assessment of atopic dermatitis. J Am Acad Dermatol 2014;70:338-51.
21. Greer FR, Sicherer SH, Burks AW; American Academy of Pediatrics Section on Allergy and Immunology. Effects of early nutritional interventions on the development of atopic disease in infants and children: the role of maternal dietary restriction, breastfeeding, timing of introduction of complementary foods, and hydrolyzed formulas. Pediatrics 2008;121:183-91.

22. Warner J, Group ES. A double-blinded, randomized, placebo-controlled trial of cetirizine in preventing the onset of asthma in children with atopic dermatitis: 18 months' treatments and 18 months' post-treatment follow-up. J Allergy Clin Immunol 2001;108:929-37.

23. Siegfried EC, Jaworski JC, Kaiser JD, et al. Systematic review of published trials: long-term safety of topical corticosteroids and topical calcineurin inhibitors in pediatric patients with atopic dermatitis. BMC Pediatrics 2016;16:75.

24. Eichenfield L, Hanifin J, Luger T, et al. Consensus conference on pediatric atopic dermatitis. J Am Acad Dermatol 2003;49:1088-99.

25. Eichenfield LF, Tom WL, Berger TG, et al. Guidelines of care for the management of atopic dermatitis: section 2. Management and treatment of atopic dermatitis with topical therapies. J Am Acad Dermatol 2014;71:116-32.

26. Eichenfield LF, Ahluwalia J, Waldman A, et al. Current guidelines for the evaluation and management of atopic dermatitis: a comparison of the Joint Task Force Practice Parameter and American Academy of Dermatology guidelines. J Allergy Clin Immunol 2017;139:S49-57.

27. Horii K, Simon S, Liu D, et al. Atopic dermatitis in children in the United States, 1997-2004: visit trends, patient and provider characteristics, and prescribing patterns. Pediatrics 2007;120:e527-34.

28. Devillers A, Oranje A. Efficacy and safety of "wet-wrap" dressings as an intervention treatment in children with severe and/or refractory atopic dermatitis: a critical review of the literature. Br J Dermatol 2006;154:579-85.

29. Luger T, Boguniewicz M, Carr W, et al. Pimecrolimus in atopic dermatitis: consensus on safety and the need to allow use in infants. Pediatr Allergy Immunol 2015;26:306-15.

30. Sigurgeirsson B, Boznanski A, Todd G, et al. Safety and efficacy of pimecrolimus in atopic dermatitis: a 5-year randomized trial. Pediatrics 2015;135:597-606.

31. Siegfried EC, Jaworski JC, Kaiser JD, et al. Systematic review of published trials: long-term safety of topical corticosteroids and topical calcineurin inhibitors in pediatric patients with atopic dermatitis. BMC Pediatr 2016;16:75.

32. Simpson E, Udkoff J, Borok J, et al. Atopic dermatitis: emerging therapies. Semin Cutan Med Surg 2017;36:124-30.

33. Eichenfield LF, Call RS, Forsha DW, et al. Long-term safety of crisaborole ointment 2% in children and adults with mild to moderate atopic dermatitis. J Am Acad Dermatol 2017;77:641-9.

34. Diepgen T. Early treatment of the Atopic Child Study Group. Long-term treatment with cetirizine of infants with atopic dermatitis: a multi-country, double-blind, randomized, placebo-controlled trial (the ETAC trial) over 18 months. Pediatr Allergy Immunol 2002;13:278-86.

35. Sidbury R, Davis DM, Cohen DE, et al. Guidelines for care for the management of atopic dermatitis. Section 3. Management and treatment with phototherapy and systemic agents. J Am Acad Dermatol 2014;71:327-49.

36. Buys L. Treatment options for atopic dermatitis. Am Fam Physician 2007;75:523-8.

37. Eichenfield LF, Krakowski AC, Piggott C, et al. Evidence-based recommendations for the diagnosis and treatment of pediatric acne. Pediatrics 2013;131:S163-86.

38. Antoniou C, Dessinioti C, Stratigos A, et al. Clinical and therapeutic approach to childhood acne: an update. Pediatr Dermatol 2009;26:373-80.

39. Thiboutot D, Gollnick H, Bettoli V, et al. New insights into the management of acne: an update from the Global Alliance to Improve Outcomes in Acne Group. J Am Acad Dermatol 2009;60:S1-S50.

40. Karciauskiene J, Valiukeviciene S, Gollnick H, et al. The prevalence and risk factors of adolescent acne among schoolchildren in Lithuania: a cross-sectional study. J Eur Acad Dermatol Venereol 2014;28:733-40.

41. Tan J. Current measures for the evaluation of acne severity. Expert Rev Dermatol 2008;3:595-603.

42. Zaenglein AL, Pathy AL, Schlosser BJ, et al. Guidelines of care for the management of acne vulgaris. J Am Acad Dermatol 2016;74:945-73.e33.

43. Kose O, Koc E, Arca E. Adapalene gel 0.1% in the treatment of infantile acne: an open clinical study. Pediatr Dermatol 2008;25:383-6.

44. Hansen TH, Lucking S, Miller JJ, et al. Standardized laboratory monitoring with use of isotretinoin in acne. J Am Acad Dermatol 2016;75:323-8.

45. Krakowski A, Stendardo S, Eichenfield L. Practical considerations in acne treatment in the clinical impact of topical combination therapy. Pediatr Dermatol 2008;25:1-14.

46. Andrews M, Burns M. Common tinea infections in children. Am Fam Physician 2008;77:1415-20.

47. Habif T. Superficial fungal infections. In: Habif T, ed. Clinical Dermatology, 5th ed. Oxford: Elsevier, 2009.

48. Ali S, Graham T, Forgie S. The assessment and management of tinea capitis in children. Pediatr Emerg Care 2007;23:662-5.

49. Kakourou T, Uksal U. Guidelines for the management of tinea capitis in children. Pediatr Dermatol 2010;27:226-8.

50. Chen X, Jiang X, Yang M, et al. Systemic antifungal therapy for tinea capitis in children. Cochrane Database Syst Rev 2016;12:1-121.

51. Gupta A, Skinner A. Onychomycosis in children: a brief overview with treatment strategies. Pediatr Dermatol 2004;21:74-9.

52. deBerker D. Fungal nail disease. N Engl J Med 2009;360:2108-16.

53. van der Wouden JC, van der Sande R, Suijlekom-Smit LV, et al. Interventions for cutaneous molluscum contagiosum. Cochrane Database Syst Rev 2009;4:1-48.

54. Coloe J, Morrell D. Cantharidin use among pediatric dermatologists in the treatment of molluscum contagiosum. Pediatr Dermatol 2009;26:405-8.

55. Chinnadurai S, Fonnesbeck C, Snyder K, et al. Pharmacologic interventions for infantile hemangioma: a meta-analysis. Pediatrics 2016;137:e1-10.

56. Paller AS, Mancini AJ. Vascular disorders in infancy and childhood. In: Paller AS, Mancini AJ, eds. Hurwitz Clinical Pediatric Dermatology, 4th ed. Edinburgh: Elsevier, 2011.

57. Darrow D, Green AK, Mancini AJ, et al. Diagnosis and management of hemangioma. Pediatrics 2015;136:e1060-1104.

Note: Page numbers followed by *b, f,* or *t* indicate material in boxes, figures, or tables, respectively.

oncology. *See* cancer
ondansetron, 467, 595, 610, 871, 907
ontogeny
    absorption and, 21, 34–37
    distribution and, 21–22
    dosing and, 44–45
    elimination and, 22, 42–43
    metabolism and, 21, 22, 40, 41
    organ function and, 21–22
onychomycosis, 976
ophthalmic antihistamines, 942t, 943
ophthalmic infections, 25
opioid abstinence syndrome, 505
opioids
    abuse of, 604t, 606, 608t, 609–610
    acetaminophen with, 503–504
    acute kidney injury and, 361
    adverse effects of, 504–505, 504t
    child-specific dosing for, 494
    continuous infusions of, 501
    dependence on, 505
    for diarrhea, 257
    dosage forms, 501, 504
    education on use of, 505, 506
    equianalgesic doses for, 501, 502t
    mechanism of action, 257, 501
    medication errors involving, 71
    for migraines, 467
    nurse-controlled, 505–506
    for pain management, 498, 501–506,
        502t, 508
    patient-controlled, 498, 501, 505–506,
        505t, 508
    taper schedules for, 505
    tolerance to, 504t, 505
    toxicity of, 82, 83–84t
    for vaso-occlusive pain crises, 871,
        871t
    withdrawal from, 84t, 504t, 505, 606,
        606b, 609–610
opportunistic infections (OIs), 751–754,
    753t
Ora-Blend, 54
Ora-Blend SF, 54
oral administration, 34–37. *See also*
    extemporaneous formulations
oral antihyperglycemic agents, 403–406,
    405t
oral contraceptives. *See* contraceptives
oral poliovirus vaccine, 813
oral rehydration therapy (ORT)
    acute kidney injury and, 362
    commercially available products, 307
    for diarrhea, 256–257, 256t, 720
    for hyponatremia, 310
    intravenous therapy vs., 307
    severity of dehydration and, 720t
oral temperature, 8
Ora-Plus, 53–55
Ora-Sweet, 53, 54
Ora-Sweet SF, 53, 54
orbital cellulitis (OC), 691–692, 692f
orexigenic neurons, 335, 337t
organic anion transporters (OATs), 43,
    43t, 44f
organic cation transporters (OCTs), 43,
    43t, 44f
organ ontogeny and function, 21–22
organophosphate toxicity, 82t

orlistat, 344–345, 347, 595
Orphan Drug Act of 1983, 10
ORT. *See* oral rehydration therapy
orthodromic tachycardia, 126–127, 126f
orthopedic injuries, NSAID precautions
    in, 500
orthopedic surgery, 429
orthotics, for cerebral palsy, 477
oseltamivir, 41, 657–659, 658t
osmolality, 302–304, 304t
osmoreceptors, 302
osmotic diarrhea, 252
osmotic laxatives, 263, 265–266, 291, 293t
osteogenesis imperfecta (OI), 427–433
    classification of, 427–428
    clinical presentation of, 427–428
    diagnosis of, 428
    epidemiology of, 427
    nonpharmacologic therapy for, 429
    pathophysiology of, 427
    patient case study, 432–433
    pharmacotherapy for, 429–432, 430t
    prognosis for patients, 428
    therapeutic goals for, 428
osteomyelitis, 703–713
    acute, 703
    chronic, 703–705, 708
    classification of, 703–704
    complications of, 707
    contiguous, 703, 705
    course and prognosis for, 707
    defined, 703
    diagnosis of, 705–706
    empiric treatment algorithm for, 709,
        709f
    epidemiology of, 703
    hematogenous, 703, 704, 707, 709f
    imaging studies in, 706, 706f
    monitoring of therapy for, 712–713
    nonpharmacologic therapy for, 712
    pathophysiology of, 704–705,
        704–705t
    patient case study, 46
    pharmacotherapy for, 707–708t,
        708–712
    risk factors for, 705
    sickle cell disease and, 869–870
    signs and symptoms of, 705
    subacute, 703
    therapeutic goals for, 707–708
osteonecrosis of the jaw, 431
osteopenia
    antiretroviral drugs and, 788
    cystic fibrosis and, 221, 223
    diuretic use and, 174
    eating disorders and, 588
    parenteral nutrition and, 329
osteoporosis
    anticonvulsants and, 456
    antiretroviral drugs and, 788
    cerebral palsy and, 486–487, 486f
    cystic fibrosis and, 221
    parathyroid hormone therapy for, 432
    unfractionated heparin and, 843
ostomy, 266
otitis media. *See* acute otitis media
overweight, 335, 341–342, 341t. *See also*
    obesity
oxacillin

adverse effects of, 628t
    for carbuncles, 687
    for cellulitis, 688
    for furuncles, 687
    for meningitis, 626t
    for osteomyelitis, 708t, 709
    pediatric dosing of, 664t
oxazolidinone antibiotics, 39
oxcarbazepine
    for autism spectrum disorder, 542t,
        544
    for bipolar disorder, 573, 573t, 579
    interactions with, 419
    for seizure disorders, 447t, 452, 455,
        456
oxycodone, 502t, 503–504, 604t, 608t
oxygen therapy
    for anaphylaxis, 945, 945t
    for apnea of prematurity, 183
    for bronchiolitis, 653
    for bronchopulmonary dysplasia, 169,
        173
    for cardiac output manipulation, 105
    for osteomyelitis, 712
    for respiratory distress syndrome,
        170–171
    for sickle cell disease, 870
    for tetralogy of Fallot, 109
oxymetazoline, 941t
oxytocin, 545
ozogamicin/gemtuzumab, 904

P

PA. *See Pseudomonas aeruginosa*
pacifiers, for pain management, 497
pain. *See also* pain management
    abdominal, 287, 288, 290–292, 290b,
        293t
    acute, 493, 498–505, 511
    assessment of, 8, 463, 494–496, 495t
    burn-related, 508–509
    cancer-related, 508
    chronic, 493, 506–509, 507t, 512
    clinical presentation of, 494–496
    defined, 493
    as fifth vital sign, 494
    indicators of, 8
    mild, moderate, and severe
        categorization, 498
    neuropathic, 506–508, 507t, 871
    perceptions of, 493–494
    physiology of pain transmission,
        493–494
    procedural, 509–510
    vaso-occlusive pain crises, 865, 868,
        870–874, 871t
pain management, 493–512. *See also*
    analgesics
    acute, 498–505, 511
    in acute otitis media, 639
    adjuvant agents for, 498, 506–508,
        507t
    for cancer, 498, 504, 506, 508
    in children vs. adults, 494
    child-specific dosing in, 494
    chronic, 506–509, 507t, 512
    inadequacy of, 493

medication errors in, 493

nonpharmacologic therapy for, 497, 508

nurse-controlled, 505–506

patient case studies, 511–512

patient-controlled, 498, 501, 505–506, 505*t*, 508

pharmacokinetic considerations in, 497–498

pharmacotherapy for, 493, 497–510

procedural, 509–510

in vaso-occlusive pain crises, 870–871, 871*t*

pain receptors, 494

palatability of medications, 10, 12, 34, 54, 677

paliperidone, 544

palivizumab, 652, 652*t*

palonosetron, 907

pamidronate, 429–431, 430*t*, 487

pancolitis, 273

pancreatic enzyme replacement therapy (PERT), 221–222, 222*t*, 225

pancreatic insufficiency, 221–222, 225, 251

pancreatic peptide, 336

Pancreaze, 222*t*

Panton-Valentine leukocidin (PVL), 683, 703, 705, 713

pantoprazole, 242, 243, 245*t*

para-aminohippurate, 42

parainfluenza viruses, 640, 642, 651, 656, 659, 922

parasites, defined, 731

parasitic infections, 731–746

diarrhea and, 719, 721–722

ectoparasites, 742–745, 743*t*

gastrointestinal protozoa, 731–734

helminths, 731, 739–742, 741*t*

patient case study, 745–746

routes of transmission, 731

systemic protozoa, 734–739

parathyroid hormone therapy, 432

paregoric, 257, 258*t*

parenteral drugs, 52, 55, 676–677, 677*t*

parenteral nutrition (PN), 323–332

additives in, 328

calculations for, 326, 327*f*

carbohydrates in, 324–326

complications of, 328–330

components of, 323–328

defined, 320

drug–nutrient considerations in, 328, 329*t*

electrolytes in, 323, 325–328

fluid and caloric requirements in, 320–321, 320*t*

formula considerations in, 323

indications for, 320

intravenous lipid emulsion in, 323, 326, 329

minerals in, 323, 326–327

patient case study, 331–332

pharmacist's role in, 319, 330

protein in, 323–324

for refractory celiac disease, 295

safety considerations in, 330

trace elements in, 323, 328

vitamins in, 323, 328

parenteral nutrition–associated liver disease (PNALD), 326, 329

parents. *See* caregivers

A Parent's Guide to Poison Prevention (Texas Poison Center Network), 92

Paris Classification of IBD, 273, 274

paromomycin, 722, 733, 734*t*

paroxetine

for autism spectrum disorder, 544

interactions with, 560

for major depressive disorder, 558–560, 561*t*

for migraine prophylaxis, 469

paroxysmal stage of pertussis, 654, 811

partial seizures. *See* focal seizures

parvovirus, 697, 854, 865, 870, 957

Pasteurella, in animal and human bites, 690

Pasturella multocida, osteomyelitis and, 704

patch repair technique, 111

patent ductus arteriosus (PDA)

anatomic description of, 106, 106*f*

diagnosis of, 28–29

pharmacotherapy for, 29

preoperative pharmacotherapy for, 106–107, 500

prostaglandin E_2 in, 29, 106, 107

sequelae of, 100*t*

signs and symptoms of, 106

surgical repair of, 29, 100*t*, 106

patent foramen ovale (PFO), 106

pathologic jaundice, 27

patient-centered care, 73

patient-controlled analgesia (PCA), 498, 501, 505–506, 505*t*, 508

patient education. *See* education

Patient Health Questionnaire-9 Item (PHQ-9), 555–556

PC (periorbital cellulitis), 691–692, 692*f*

PCCs (prothrombin complex concentrates), 854

PCDAI. *See* pediatric Crohn disease activity index

PCP (phencyclidine), 605*t*, 607

PCR. *See* polymerase chain reaction

PD (peritoneal dialysis), 364–365, 365–367*t*

PDA. *See* patent ductus arteriosus

PDDs (pervasive development disorders), 535

peak flow meters, 198

peanut allergies, 935, 943–944

Pedialyte, 256*t*, 307

Pediarix vaccine, 811*t*

Pediatric Advanced Life Support guidelines, 82, 129

Pediatric & Neonatal Dosage Handbook, 8, 52, 441

pediatric Crohn disease activity index (PCDAI), 274, 274*t*, 275, 280, 281

Pediatric Drug Formulations, 52

Pediatric Endocrine Society, 421

Pediatric Health Information System (PHIS), 951

Pediatric Migraine Disability Assessment Score (PedMIDAS), 461

pediatric patients. *See also* adolescents; children; infants; neonates; *specific conditions*

classification of, 3–4, 4*t*, 69

communication with, 59–64

data differences in, 5, 8–9

distinctness of, 4

education for, 13–14

epidemiology of, 4–5

fundamentals of care for, 12–14

growth and development in, 5, 6–7*f*

medication use among, 51

pediatric pharmacists, 3, 14

Pediatric Pharmacy Association (PPA), 3, 14, 14*b*, 71

Pediatric Practice Research Network, 3

Pediatric Pulmonary Centers, 227

Pediatric Quality of Life inventory (PedsQL), 461–462

Pediatric Research Equity Act of 2003 (PREA), 10, 51

pediatric resources, 14, 14*b*

Pediatric Rule (1994), 10

pediatric ulcerative colitis activity index (PUCAI), 273–275, 274*t*, 280, 281

pediculosis (head lice), 742–744, 743*t*

PedMIDAS (Pediatric Migraine Disability Assessment Score), 461

PedsQL (Pediatric Quality of Life inventory), 461–462

PedvaxHIB vaccine, 812

pegaspargase, 883–884, 883*t*

peginterferon alfa, 786

penciclovir, 695, 696

penicillins

absorption of, 34, 34*f*

acute kidney injury and, 360, 360*t*

adverse effects of, 628*t*

allergies to, 638–639, 936, 938

for carbuncles, 687

for cellulitis, 688

for cystic fibrosis, 219

desensitization protocol for, 946, 946*t*

for erysipelas, 688

for febrile neutropenia, 922

for furuncles, 687

for impetigo, 689

for meningitis, 625–627, 626*t*

for necrotizing fasciitis, 693

for osteomyelitis, 708*t*, 709, 711, 712

for peritoneal dialysis, 367*t*

for pharyngitis, 643, 644

for pneumonia, 661–662

resistance to, 634, 642, 661, 662

in sickle cell disease prophylaxis, 866, 870

for staphylococcal scalded skin syndrome, 690

Pentacel vaccine, 811*t*

pentamidine, 889

pentobarbital, 454

peppermint oil capsules, 292

peptide YY, 336, 337*t*

Peptococcus, cutaneous abscesses and, 684

Peptostreptococcus

in animal and human bites, 690

in necrotizing fasciitis, 693

osteomyelitis and, 705